Nathan and Oski's
Hematology
of Infancy
and Childhood

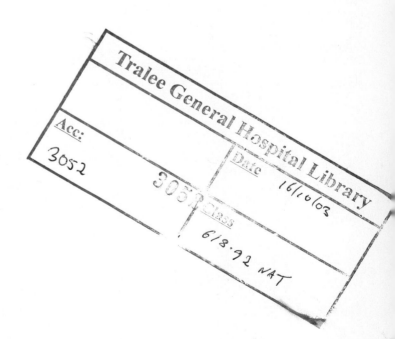

Nathan and Oski's
Hematology of Infancy and Childhood

5th EDITION

VOLUME

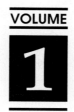

David G. Nathan, M.D.
Richard and Susan Smith Professor
   of Medicine and Professor of
   Pediatrics
Harvard Medical School
President, Dana-Farber Cancer
   Institute
Boston, Massachusetts

Section XI edited
with the assistance of
David Ginsburg, M.D.

Stuart H. Orkin, M.D.
Leland Fikes Professor of Pediatric
   Medicine
Harvard Medical School
Investigator, Howard Hughes
   Medical Institute
Division of Hematology/Oncology
Children's Hospital
Boston, Massachusetts

Managing Editor
Cathryn J. Lantigua

W.B. SAUNDERS COMPANY
A Division of Harcourt Brace & Company
Philadelphia   London   Toronto   Montreal   Sydney   Tokyo

W.B. SAUNDERS COMPANY
A Division of Harcourt Brace & Company

The Curtis Center
Independence Square West
Philadelphia, Pennsylvania 19106

Library of Congress Cataloging-in-Publication Data

Nathan and Oski's hematology of infancy and childhood / [edited by] David G. Nathan, Stuart H. Orkin; managing editor, Cathryn J. Lantigua.—5th ed.

p.   cm.

Rev. ed. of: Hematology of infancy and childhood / [edited by] David G. Nathan, Frank A. Oski. 4th ed. c1993. Includes bibliographical references and index.

ISBN 0-7216-5951-9

1. Pediatric hematology.   I. Nathan, David G.   II. Orkin, Stuart H.
III. Oski, Frank A.   [DNLM: 1. Hematologic Diseases—
in infancy & childhood.   WS 300 N273 1998]

RJ411.H46 1998   618.92′15—dc20

DNLM/DLC   96-41120

Set ISBN 0–7216–5951–9
Volume One ISBN 0–7216–5952–7
Volume Two ISBN 0–7216–5953–5

NATHAN AND OSKI'S HEMATOLOGY OF INFANCY AND CHILDHOOD

Printed in the United States of America.

Last digit is the print number: 9   8   7   6   5   4   3   2   1

Contributors

Abul K. Abbas, M.D.
Professor of Pathology, Harvard Medical School; Head, Immunology Research Division, Department of Pathology, Brigham and Women's Hospital, Boston, Massachusetts
Humoral Immunity and the Development and Regulation of Immune Responses

Estella M. Alonso, M.D.
Assistant Professor of Pediatrics, Pritzker School of Medicine, University of Chicago, and Section of Pediatric Gastroenterology, Hepatology, and Nutrition, The University of Chicago Hospitals, University of Chicago Children's Hospital, Chicago, Illinois
Disorders of Bilirubin Metabolism

Blanche P. Alter, M.D.
Professor of Pediatrics and Chief, Division of Pediatric Hematology/Oncology, The University of Texas Medical Branch, Galveston, Texas
The Bone Marrow Failure Syndromes

Arnold J. Altman, M.D.
Hartford Whalers Professor of Childhood Cancer, University of Connecticut School of Medicine Farmington; Head, Division of Hematology/Oncology, Connecticut Children's Medical Center, Hartford, Connecticut
Management of Malignant Solid Tumors

Maureen Andrew, M.D.
Professor of Pediatrics, McMaster University, Hamilton Civic Hospitals Research Centre, Hamilton and Hospital for Sick Children, Toronto, Ontario, Canada
Developmental Hemostasis: Relevance to Newborns and Infants; Acquired Disorders of Hemostasis

Nancy C. Andrews, M.D., Ph.D.
Assistant Professor of Pediatrics, Harvard Medical School; Assistant Investigator, Howard Hughes Medical Institute; Assistant in Medicine, Children's Hospital, Boston, Massachusetts
Disorders of Iron Metabolism and Sideroblastic Anemia

Frank M. Balis, M.D.
Senior Investigator and Head, Pharmacology and Experimental Therapeutics Section, Pediatric Branch, National Cancer Institute, Bethesda, Maryland
Cancer Chemotherapy

Kenneth A. Bauer, M.D.
Associate Professor of Medicine, Harvard Medical School, Boston; Chief, Hematology-Oncology Section, Brockton-West Roxbury VA Medical Center, West Roxbury, Massachusetts
Rare Hereditary Coagulation Factor Abnormalities

Diana Schultz Beardsley, M.D., Ph.D.
Associate Clinical Professor of Pediatrics and Internal Medicine, Yale University School of Medicine; Attending Physician and Director, Yale Hemophilia Center, Yale-New Haven Hospital, New Haven, Connecticut
Platelet Abnormalities in Infancy and Childhood

Stacey L. Berg, M.D.
Assistant Professor of Pediatrics, Texas Children's Cancer Center, Texas Children's Hospital, Baylor College of Medicine, Houston, Texas
Cancer Chemotherapy

Barbara E. Bierer, M.D.
Associate Professor of Medicine, Harvard Medical School; Director, Pediatric Bone Marrow and Stem Cell Transplantation, Dana-Farber Cancer Institute, Boston, Massachusetts
Principles of Bone Marrow and Stem Cell Transplantation; Cell-Mediated Immunity and the Regulation of Immune Responses

Francisco A. Bonilla, M.D., Ph.D.
Instructor in Pediatrics, Harvard Medical School; Assistant in Medicine, Children's Hospital, Boston, Massachusetts
Primary Immunodeficiency Diseases

John M. Bowman, M.D.
Professor, Department of Pediatrics and Child Health, and Department of Obstetrics, Gynecology and Reproductive Sciences, University of Manitoba Faculty of Medicine; Medical Director, Rh Laboratory, Department of Pediatrics and Child Health and Division of Laboratory Medicine and Pathology, Health Sciences Centre, Winnipeg, Manitoba, Canada
Immune Hemolytic Disease

Kenneth R. Bridges, M.D.
Associate Professor of Medicine, Harvard Medical School; Associate Physician, Brigham and Women's Hospital, Boston, Massachusetts
Disorders of Iron Metabolism and Sideroblastic Anemia

Carlo Brugnara, M.D.
Associate Professor of Pathology, Harvard Medical School; Director of the Hematology Laboratory, Department of Laboratory Medicine, Children's Hospital, Boston, Massachusetts
The Neonatal Erythrocyte and Its Disorders; A Diagnostic Approach to the Anemic Patient; Appendix: Reference Values in Infancy and Childhood

H. Franklin Bunn, M.D.
Professor of Medicine, Harvard Medical School; Research Director, Hematology-Oncology Division, Brigham and Women's Hospital, Boston, Massachusetts
Human Hemoglobins: Normal and Abnormal

Curt I. Civin, M.D.
Professor, Oncology and Pediatrics, Johns Hopkins University School of Medicine; Director, Pediatric Oncology Division, The Johns Hopkins Hospital, Baltimore, Maryland
Myeloid Leukemias, Myelodysplasia, and Myeloproliferative Diseases in Children

Steven C. Clark, Ph.D.
Senior Vice President, Research, Genetics Institute, Inc., Cambridge, Massachusetts
The Anatomy and Physiology of Hematopoiesis

Bernard A. Cooper, M.D.
Clinical Professor of Medicine (Hematology), Stanford University, Palo Alto, California; Professor of Medicine, McGill University, Montreal, Quebec, Canada
Megaloblastic Anemia

Lisa Diller, M.D.
Assistant Professor of Pediatrics, Harvard Medical School; Pediatric Oncologist, Dana-Farber Cancer Institute, Children's Hospital, Boston, Massachusetts
Epidemiology of Cancer in Childhood

Mary C. Dinauer, M.D., Ph.D.
Associate Professor of Pediatrics, and Medical and Molecular Genetics, Indiana University School of Medicine; Attending Physician, Section of Pediatric Hematology/Oncology, James Whitcomb Riley Hospital for Children, Indianapolis, Indiana
The Phagocyte System and Disorders of Granulopoiesis and Granulocyte Function

Sarah S. Donaldson, M.D.
Professor of Radiation Oncology, Stanford University School of Medicine; Professor of Radiation Oncology, Stanford Health Services, Stanford, California
The Lymphomas and Lymphadenopathy

George J. Dover, M.D.
Professor of Pediatrics, Medicine, and Oncology, and Director, Department of Pediatrics, Johns Hopkins University School of Medicine; Pediatrician-in-Chief, The Johns Hopkins Hospital, Baltimore, Maryland
Sickle Cell Disease

Charles T. Esmon, Ph.D.
Adjunct Professor of Pathology and Biochemistry, University of Oklahoma; Member and Head, Cardiovascular Biology, Oklahoma Medical Research Foundation; Investigator, Howard Hughes Medical Institute, Oklahoma City, Oklahoma
Blood Coagulation

R. Alan B. Ezekowitz, M.B.Ch.B., D.Phil.
Charles Wilder Professor of Pediatrics, Harvard Medical School; Chief, Pediatric Service, Massachusetts General Hospital, Boston, Massachusetts
Hematologic Manifestations of Systemic Diseases

Bernard G. Forget, M.D.
Professor of Medicine and Genetics and Chief, Hematology Section, Yale University School of Medicine; Attending Physician, Yale-New Haven Hospital, New Haven, Connecticut
Disorders of the Erythrocyte Membrane

Patrick G. Gallagher, M.D.
Assistant Professor, Department of Pediatrics, Yale University School of Medicine; Attending Physician, Yale-New Haven Hospital, New Haven, Connecticut
Disorders of the Erythrocyte Membrane

Raif S. Geha, M.D.
Prince Turki bin Abdul Aziz Al-Saud Professor of Pediatrics, Harvard Medical School; Chief, Division of Immunology, Children's Hospital, Boston, Massachusetts
Primary Immunodeficiency Diseases

Joan Cox Gill, M.D.
Professor of Pediatrics, Medical College of Wisconsin; Medical Director, Comprehensive Center for Bleeding Disorders, The Blood Center of Southeastern Wisconsin, Milwaukee, Wisconsin
Hemophilia and von Willebrand Disease

D. Gary Gilliland, M.D., Ph.D.
Associate Professor of Medicine, Harvard Medical
School; Assistant Investigator, Howard Hughes
Medical Institute; Physician, Brigham and Women's
Hospital, Boston, Massachusetts
The Molecular Biology of Cancer

David Ginsburg, M.D.
Professor, Department of Internal Medicine and
Human Genetics, University of Michigan; Investigator,
Howard Hughes Medical Institute, Ann Arbor,
Michigan
Section XI: Hemostasis

Todd R. Golub, M.D.
Assistant Professor, Department of Pediatrics,
Harvard Medical School; Assistant Professor,
Department of Pediatric Oncology, Dana-Farber
Cancer Institute, Boston, Massachusetts
The Molecular Biology of Cancer

Jed B. Gorlin, M.D.
Assistant Professor, University of Minnesota Medical
School; Associate Medical Director, Memorial Blood
Centers of Minnesota, Minneapolis, Minnesota
*Red Cell Transfusion; Therapeutic Plasma Exchange and
Cytapheresis*

Holcombe E. Grier, M.D.
Associate Professor of Pediatrics, Harvard Medical
School; Clinical Director, Pediatric Oncology, Dana-
Farber Cancer Institute, Boston, Massachusetts
*Myeloid Leukemias, Myelodysplasia, and
Myeloproliferative Diseases in Children*

Stephan A. Grupp, M.D., Ph.D.
Assistant Professor, Department of Pediatrics,
University of Pennsylvania School of Medicine;
Division of Oncology, Children's Hospital of
Philadelphia, Philadelphia, Pennsylvania
*Humoral Immunity and the Development and
Regulation of Immune Responses*

Eva C. Guinan, M.D.
Associate Professor of Pediatrics, Harvard Medical
School; Clinical Director, Bone Marrow and Stem Cell
Transplantation, Dana-Farber Cancer Institute/
Children's Hospital, Boston, Massachusetts
*Principles of Bone Marrow and Stem Cell
Transplantation*

Katherine A. Hajjar, M.D.
Stavros S. Niarchos Professor of Pediatrics in
Medicine, Cornell University Medical College;
Attending Pediatrician, New York Hospital, New
York, New York
The Molecular Basis of Fibrinolysis

Robert I. Handin, M.D.
Professor of Medicine, Harvard Medical School; Chief,
Hematology-Oncology Division, Brigham and
Women's Hospital, Boston, Massachusetts
Blood Platelets and the Vessel Wall

Catherine P. M. Hayward, M.D., Ph.D.
Assistant Professor of Medicine and Pathology,
Faculty of Health Sciences; Director, Residency
Training Program in Hematology, McMaster
University; Hematologist and Director of Coagulation
Laboratory, Chedoke-McMaster Hospitals, Hamilton,
Ontario, Canada
*Destruction of Red Cells by the Vasculature and
Reticuloendothelial System*

Attallah Kappas, M.D.
Sherman Fairchild Professor and Physician-in-Chief
Emeritus, The Rockefeller University, New York, New
York
The Porphyrias

John G. Kelton, M.D., F.R.C.P.C.
Professor of Medicine and Pathology, Faculty of
Health Sciences, Chief of Medicine, Chedoke-
McMaster Hospitals, and Discipline Chair,
Hematology, McMaster University Medical Center,
Hamilton, Ontario, Canada
*Destruction of Red Cells by the Vasculature and
Reticuloendothelial System*

Sherwin V. Kevy, M.D.
Associate Professor, Pediatrics, Harvard Medical
School; Director Emeritus, Transfusion Service and
Therapeutic Apheresis, Children's Hospital, Boston,
Massachusetts
Red Cell Transfusion

Edwin H. Kolodny, M.D.
Bernard A. and Charlotte Marden Professor and
Chairman, Department of Neurology, New York
University School of Medicine; Vice-Chairman,
Executive Committee of the Medical Board, and
Attending Physician, Tisch Hospital, New York, New
York
Storage Diseases of the Reticuloendothelial System

Dominic Kwiatkowski, M.D., F.R.C.P.
MRC Senior Clinical Fellow, Institute of Molecular
Medicine, Oxford University; Honorary Consultant,
Department of Paediatrics, John Radcliffe Hospital,
Oxford, England
*Hematologic Manifestations of Systemic Diseases in
Children of the Developing World*

Diana Lebron, M.D.
Clinical Instructor, New York University School of
Medicine, New York; Junior Attending, The Brooklyn
Hospital Center, and Woodhull Hospital, Brooklyn,
New York
Storage Diseases of the Reticuloendothelial System

Frederick P. Li, M.D.
Professor of Clinical Cancer Epidemiology, Harvard
School of Public Health; Chief, Division of Cancer
Epidemiology and Control, Dana-Farber Cancer
Institute, Boston, Massachusetts
Epidemiology of Cancer in Childhood

Michael P. Link, M.D.
Professor of Pediatrics, Stanford University School of
Medicine, Stanford; Staff Physician, Lucile Salter
Packard Children's Hospital at Stanford, Palo Alto,
California
The Lymphomas and Lymphadenopathy

Jeanne M. Lusher, M.D.
Marion I. Barnhart Hemostasis Research Professor
and Professor of Pediatrics, Wayne State University
School of Medicine; Co-Director, Division of
Hematology-Oncology, and Director, Coagulation
Laboratories, Children's Hospital of Michigan, Detroit,
Michigan
Approach to the Bleeding Patient

Samuel E. Lux, M.D.
Robert A. Stranahan Professor of Pediatrics, Harvard
Medical School; Chief, Division of Hematology/
Oncology, Children's Hospital, Boston, Massachusetts
Disorders of the Erythrocyte Membrane

Lucio Luzzatto, M.D.
Professor of Genetics and Medicine, Cornell
University Medical College; Courtney Steel Professor
of Genetics and Chairman, Department of Human
Genetics, Memorial Sloan-Kettering Cancer Center,
New York, New York
*Glucose-6-Phosphate Dehydrogenase Deficiency and
Hemolytic Anemia*

Karen Chayt Marcus, M.D.
Assistant Professor, Joint Center for Radiation
Therapy, Harvard Medical School; Chief, Division of
Radiation Oncology, Dana-Farber Cancer Institute,
Boston, Massachusetts
Principles of Pediatric Radiation Therapy

William C. Mentzer, M.D.
Professor and Director, Division of Hematology/
Oncology, Department of Pediatrics, University of
California, San Francisco; Attending Pediatrician,
University of California Hospitals and San Francisco
General Hospital, San Francisco, California
Pyruvate Kinase Deficiency and Disorders of Glycolysis

Robert R. Montgomery, M.D.
Professor of Pediatrics, Medical College of Wisconsin;
Director of Research and Executive Vice President,
Blood Research Institute of The Blood Center of
Southeastern Wisconsin, Milwaukee, Wisconsin
*Hemophilia and von Willebrand Disease; Acquired
Disorders of Hemostasis*

Brigitta U. Mueller, M.D.
Assistant Professor of Pediatrics, Harvard Medical
School; Assistant in Medicine, Children's Hospital,
Boston, Massachusetts
*Infectious Complications in Children with Hematologic
Disorders*

David G. Nathan, M.D.
Richard and Susan Smith Professor of Medicine and
Professor of Pediatrics, Harvard Medical School;
President, Dana-Farber Cancer Institute, Boston,
Massachusetts
*The Anatomy and Physiology of Hematopoiesis; A
Diagnostic Approach to the Anemic Patient; The
Thalassemias; Platelet Abnormalities in Infancy and
Childhood*

Charlotte M. Niemeyer, M.D.
Privatdozentin and Attending Physician, University
Children's Hospital, Freiburg, Germany
Acute Lymphoblastic Leukemia

Diane J. Nugent, M.D.
Clinical Professor, Department of Pediatrics,
University of California, Irvine; Director, Hematology-
Oncology, Children's Hospital of Orange County,
Orange, California
Platelet Transfusion

Stuart H. Orkin, M.D.
Leland Fikes Professor of Pediatric Medicine, Harvard
Medical School; Investigator, Howard Hughes
Medical Institute; and Senior Associate in Medicine,
Children's Hospital, Boston, Massachusetts
The Thalassemias

Frank A. Oski, M.D.†
Distinguished Service Professor, Johns Hopkins
University School of Medicine, Baltimore, Maryland
A Diagnostic Approach to the Anemic Patient

†Deceased.

Lisa G. Payne, M.D.
Research Fellow, Howard Hughes Medical Institute,
University of Michigan, Ann Arbor, Michigan
*Destruction of Red Cells by the Vasculature and
Reticuloendothelial System*

Howard A. Pearson, M.D.
Professor of Pediatrics, Yale University School of
Medicine; Attending Physician, Yale-New Haven
Hospital, New Haven, Connecticut
The Spleen and Disturbances of Splenic Function

Sergio Piomelli, M.D.
James A. Wolff Professor of Pediatrics, Columbia
University; Director, Pediatric Hematology, Babies and
Children's Hospital of New York, New York, New
York
Lead Poisoning

Philip A. Pizzo, M.D.
Thomas Morgan Rotch Professor of Pediatrics,
Harvard Medical School; Physician-in-Chief and
Chair, Department of Medicine, Children's Hospital,
Boston, Massachusetts
*Infectious Complications in Children with Hematologic
Disorders*

Orah S. Platt, M.D.
Associate Professor of Pediatrics, Harvard Medical
School; Director, Department of Laboratory Medicine,
Children's Hospital, Boston, Massachusetts
*The Neonatal Erythrocyte and Its Disorders; Sickle Cell
Disease*

David G. Poplack, M.D.
Elise C. Young Professor of Pediatric Oncology and
Head, Hematology/Oncology Section, Department of
Pediatrics, Baylor College of Medicine; Director, Texas
Children's Cancer Center and Hematology Service,
Texas Children's Hospital, Houston, Texas
Cancer Chemotherapy

John J. Quinn, M.D.
Professor of Pediatrics, University of Connecticut
School of Medicine, Farmington; Senior Attending
Pediatrician, Connecticut Children's Medical Center,
Hartford, Connecticut
Management of Malignant Solid Tumors

Marion E. Reid, Ph.D.
Director, Immunohematology Laboratory, New York
Blood Center, New York, New York
Erythrocyte Blood Groups in Transfusion

Fred S. Rosen, M.D.
James L. Gamble Professor of Pediatrics, Harvard
Medical School; Senior Associate in Medicine,
Children's Hospital; and President, Center for Blood
Research, Boston, Massachusetts
Primary Immunodeficiency Diseases

**David S. Rosenblatt, M.D.C.M.,
F.R.C.P.(C), F.C.C.M.G.**
Professor of Human Genetics, Medicine, and
Pediatrics, McGill University; Director, Division of
Medical Genetics, and Director, The Hess B. and
Diane Finestone Laboratory in Memory of Jacob and
Jenny Finestone, Royal Victoria Hospital and Montreal
General Hospital, Montreal, Quebec, Canada
Megaloblastic Anemia

Wendell F. Rosse, M.D.
Florence McAlister Professor of Medicine, and
Professor of Immunology, Duke University Medical
Center, Durham, North Carolina
Autoimmune Hemolytic Anemia

Janet D. Rowley, M.D., Ds.C.
Blum-Riese Distinguished Service Professor,
Departments of Medicine and of Molecular Genetics
and Cell Biology, University of Chicago, Chicago,
Illinois
*Chromosomal Abnormalities in Childhood Hematologic
Malignant Diseases*

Stephen E. Sallan, M.D.
Professor of Pediatrics, Harvard Medical School; Chief
of Staff, Dana-Farber Cancer Institute, Boston,
Massachusetts
Acute Lymphoblastic Leukemia

Shigeru Sassa, M.D., Ph.D.
Associate Professor, Physician, and Head of
Laboratory for Biochemical Hematology, The
Rockefeller University, New York, New York
The Porphyrias

Yuko Sato, M.D., Ph.D.
Division of Intractable Diseases, Department of
Intractable Diseases, Research Institute, International
Medical Center of Japan, Tokyo, Japan
*Chromosomal Abnormalities in Childhood Hematologic
Malignant Diseases*

J. Paul Scott, M.D.
Professor of Pediatrics, Medical College of Wisconsin;
Investigator, Blood Research Institute of The Blood
Center of Southeastern Wisconsin, Milwaukee,
Wisconsin
Hemophilia and von Willebrand Disease

Colin A. Sieff, MB.BCh., F.R.C.Path.

Associate Professor of Pediatrics, Harvard Medical School; Associate Professor, Department of Pediatric Oncology, Dana-Farber Cancer Institute; Senior Associate in Medicine, Children's Hospital, Boston, Massachusetts

The Anatomy and Physiology of Hematopoiesis; Principles of Stem Cell Therapy

Jeffrey Sklar, M.D., Ph.D.

Professor of Pathology, Harvard Medical School; Director, Divisions of Molecular Oncology and Diagnostic Molecular Biology, Brigham and Women's Hospital, Boston, Massachusetts

Antigen Receptor Genes and Lymphocytic Neoplasia

Barbara M. Sourkes, Ph.D.

Assistant Professor of Pediatrics, McGill University; Psychologist, Intensive Ambulatory Care Service and Palliative Care Service, Montreal Children's Hospital, Montreal, Quebec, Canada

Psychologic Aspects of Leukemia and Other Hematologic Disorders

James A. Stockman III, M.D.

Clinical Professor of Pediatrics, University of North Carolina School of Medicine, Chapel Hill; Consultant Professor of Pediatrics, Duke University School of Medicine, Durham; President, American Board of Pediatrics, Chapel Hill, North Carolina

Hematologic Manifestations of Systemic Diseases

John L. Sullivan, M.D.

Professor of Pediatrics and Division Director, Department of Pediatric Immunology/Rheumatology, University of Massachusetts Medical Center, Worcester, Massachusetts

Lymphohistiocytic Disorders

Nancy J. Tarbell, M.D.

Associate Professor, Harvard Medical School; Chief, Division of Radiation Oncology, Children's Hospital, Boston, Massachusetts

Principles of Pediatric Radiation Therapy

Pearl T. C. Y. Toy, M.D.

Professor, Department of Laboratory Medicine, University of California, San Francisco; Chief, Blood Bank and Donor Center, University of California Medical Center, San Francisco, California

Erythrocyte Blood Groups in Transfusion

Russell E. Ware, M.D., Ph.D.

Associate Professor of Pediatrics, Duke University Medical Center, Durham, North Carolina

Autoimmune Hemolytic Anemia

David Weatherall, M.D., F.R.C.P., F.R.S.

Regius Professor of Medicine, and Honorary Director, Institute of Molecular Medicine, University of Oxford, Oxford, England

Hematologic Manifestations of Systemic Diseases in Children of the Developing World

Daniel C. West, M.D.

Assistant Professor of Pediatrics, Department of Pediatrics, Hematology/Oncology, University of California, Davis, Sacramento, California

Antigen Receptor Genes and Lymphocytic Neoplasia

V. Michael Whitehead, M.A.(Cantab), M.D.C.M., F.R.C.P.C.

Professor of Pediatrics, Medicine and Oncology, Faculty of Medicine, McGill University; Director of Hematology, Coordinator of Oncology, Montreal Children's Hospital, Montreal, Quebec, Canada

Megaloblastic Anemia

Peter F. Whitington, M.D.

Professor of Pediatrics and Medicine, Pritzker School of Medicine, The University of Chicago; Section Chief, Section of Pediatric Gastroenterology, Hepatology, and Nutrition, The University of Chicago Hospitals, University of Chicago Children's Hospital, Chicago, Illinois

Disorders of Bilirubin Metabolism

Bruce A. Woda, M.D.

Professor of Pathology, Vice-Chairman, Department of Pathology, and Director, Anatomic Pathology and Laboratory of Hematopathology, University of Massachusetts Medical Center, Worcester, Massachusetts

Lymphohistiocytic Disorders

Neal S. Young, M.D.

Chief, Hematology Branch, National Heart, Lung, and Blood Institute, Bethesda, Maryland

The Bone Marrow Failure Syndromes

Wolf W. Zuelzer, M.D.†

Emeritus Professor of Pediatric Research, Wayne State University School of Medicine; Emeritus Director of Laboratories and Hematologist-in-Chief, Children's Hospital of Michigan, Detroit, Michigan; Emeritus Director, Division of Blood Diseases and Resources, National Heart, Lung and Blood Institute, National Institutes of Health, Bethesda, Maryland

Pediatric Hematology in Historical Perspective

---

†Deceased.

Preface

This is the fifth edition of our attempt to collate the rapidly growing scientific information that supports clinical judgment in pediatric hematology and oncology, and to translate that judgment into modern diagnosis and therapy. We are proud of this edition, but it marks a particularly sad and simultaneously a joyous transfer of responsibility for the book.

Twenty-five years ago, Frank A. Oski and I decided to create this textbook together. We had met a decade earlier when Frank was a first-year hematology fellow at Children's Hospital. I believe that he was the brightest and most visionary of the remarkable legion of young hematologists trained by Louis K. Diamond. I was then a young faculty member in hematology in the Department of Medicine at the then Peter Bent Brigham Hospital. Pediatrics was far from my mind. But time spent with Frank in Boston and my continued collaboration with him when he returned to Children's Hospital of Philadelphia persuaded me that pediatric hematology is the locus of action in the modern world of genetics and medicine. Frank's enthusiastic capacity to define new biological concepts in patients with obscure hemolytic anemias easily tore me away from myeloma, vitamin B_{12} deficiency, and the anemia of renal failure. Before long I was ensnared, and later found myself at Children's Hospital trying to continue Diamond's great tradition.

Thus we began this book, separated only geographically, with Blanche P. Alter, new in her fellowship, helping us to organize the text in a comprehensible fashion. The first edition was published in 1974, and in 1975 we won a Book Award of the American Medical Writers Association. Other reviews were also superlative, and we were launched into a partnership that carried through three more editions. While the first edition was in progress, Frank's career began to change. He had always been devoted to General Pediatrics. He loved teaching, and he particularly enjoyed working with young house officers. When an opportunity arose for him to become Chair of Pediatrics at Syracuse, he took it and transformed that Department into a vibrant and excellent program. But that decision decreased his ability to work on the book. This is not to say that he was not working on other books. Frank was a prodigious writer. His own book on the hematology of the newborn is a medical classic. But he had to define his priorities, and, after the second edition, I found myself increasingly on my own.

In 1985, Frank was called to the Chair at Johns Hopkins. I was delighted for him, but the decision forced him to avoid any significant editing responsibilities for the book. He had become completely committed to General Pediatrics, and his stupendous text on the principles and practice of Pediatrics is a testimony to that commitment. Sadly, Frank become mortally ill while at the pinnacle of his career. Afflicted with cancer of the prostate, he died in early December of 1996. Pediatrics has lost a great clinician, teacher, and clinical investigator, and I have lost a stimulating colleague and a wonderful friend. Barbara Oski and the Oski children have lost a marvelous husband and father, but they can be proud in the knowledge that they lived with one of the truly great figures in American Pediatrics. We shall all miss him. This fifth edition is dedicated to him.

When Frank told me that he could not participate at all in this edition, I made two decisions. The first was to retain and enhance his chapter on the differential diagnosis of anemia so that he would remain part of the book. The second was to ask Stuart H. Orkin to become my co-editor. That is the joyful part of this preface. I have known Stuart since he was an intern at Children's Hospital in Boston. A graduate of Massachusetts Institute of Technology, Stuart was a brilliant Harvard Medical School student and a fine house officer at Children's. When I recruited him into pediatric hematology, Charles A. Janeway wrote a letter on his behalf. In typical Janeway fashion the letter begins, "Dr. Orkin is a somewhat small man with a very large mind. . ."

When Stuart began his laboratory work at Children's Hospital, little was known of the molecular basis of thalassemia. Today, we know more about that disease than any of the genetic disorders described in this volume, and much of that knowledge has been acquired by Stuart. Not content with that feat, Stuart uncovered the genetic mystery that surrounded chronic granulomatous disease and went on to define the transcription factors that control the regulation of hematopoiesis. I can speak of his contributions with some knowledge because I have devoted much of my own career to all three of those areas. But Stuart dislodged me from them one after another, not by force, but by the simple fact that I could not catch him! I am trying gene replacement therapy now, but I fear that Stuart will be along soon, and my bags are packed!

On the simple theory that "if you can't beat 'em, join 'em," I have persuaded Stuart to join me as my co-editor for this fifth edition and to remain as an editor thereafter. He has begun with supervision of the hemostasis section of the book. Stuart and David Ginsburg, who helped him enormously, can be blamed for that, but for nothing else. The rest of the editing has been my responsibility. In the next edition, Stuart will take over much more of the leadership. For now, we are fortunate to welcome him to the book.

Pediatric hematology and oncology has grown prodigiously during the past five years of the continued revolution in molecular medicine. Accordingly, this fifth edition is massively revised and bears little resemblance to its predecessor. Most of the chapters are totally rewritten, and new authors have taken responsibility for more than a third of them. This is appropriate because the scientific underpinnings of this vibrant field are constantly changing. For example, the genetic basis of cancer is unfolding as we go to press. New and exciting therapies for bone marrow failure, cancer, and inherited diseases are virtually upon us. The rapidly emerging biotechnical industry that has such an important symbiotic relationship with academic medicine is beginning to produce remarkable new products. Recombinant factor VIII, erythropoietin, and the interferons are but a few exciting examples.

So Stuart Orkin and I begin this next new adventure together, with confidence in the future of pediatric hematology and oncology. We have labored to produce this book for the benefit of our students and research faculty members throughout the world who will continue the great progress that is recorded here. We offer the book as well to young and more experienced practitioners of the art and science of pediatric hematology and oncology who give their best for the patients who depend on their skills. Finally, we provide this book for the many basic scientists whose efforts have helped so much to unfold the mysteries that seemed completely elusive when Frank Oski and I began to collaborate 35 years ago.

Stuart and I could not have produced this large book without a great deal of help—our authors are of course paramount in our minds. They have put up with our tiresome critiques and exhortations with uncommon patience. We thank them and the staff at our publisher W.B. Saunders Company, who have made a volume out of mere chapter outlines. But the fundamental accomplishments that made this edition a viable enterprise were those of Cathryn Lantigua, our managing editor. We have worked with Cathy for more than a decade. Her skills, her persistence, and her warm smile have made our efforts productive and brightened our days. Supporting Cathy has been Janet Cameron, my administrative assistant, in charge of hounding truant authors and connecting my pen to Cathy's computer. Without her, I would have failed at this and many other tasks.

Finally, I want to thank the staffs and trustees of Dana-Farber Cancer Institute, Children's Hospital, Howard Hughes Medical Institute, and Harvard Medical School for providing environments in which scholarly work is valued and supported. I appreciate as well the inspiring memory of the late Samuel A. Levine, William B. Castle, and Charles A. Janeway. I only want to continue their tradition.

DAVID G. NATHAN, M.D.

Contents

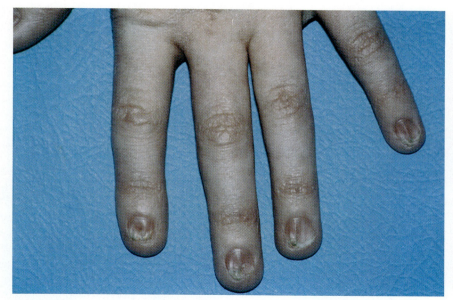

Figure 7-16. Dystrophic nails in dyskeratosis congenita. (From Drachtman RA, Alter BP: Dyskeratosis congenita. Dermatol Clin 1995; 13:33.)

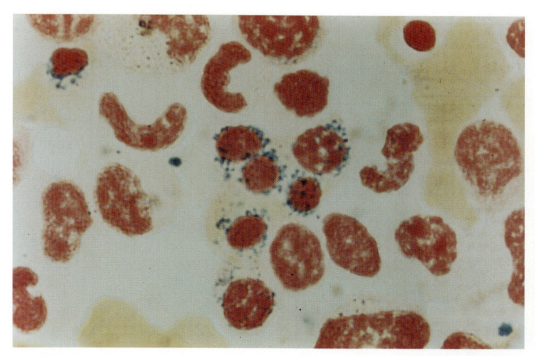

Figure 11-6. Prussian blue stain of a bone marrow aspirate from a patient with sideroblastic anemia. The greenish blue flecks that circle the nucleus of the normoblasts are iron-laden mitochondria.

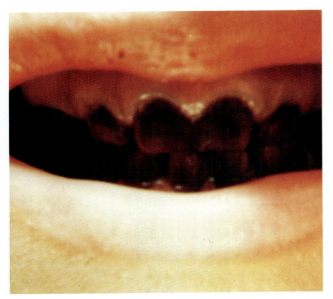

Figure 12–4. Erythrodontia of a patient with CEP. Dark reddish brown discoloration of teeth is noted. When the teeth are exposed to ultraviolet light, they emit the intense red fluorescence of porphyrins. Discoloration is usually more pronounced in decidual teeth than in permanent teeth. (Courtesy of H.M. Nitowsky, MD.)

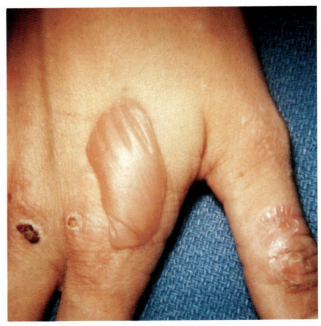

Figure 12–5. A large fluid-like bulla, crusted erosions, and unsightly scarring are typical findings in patients with PCT. These changes may also be seen in other forms of cutaneous porphyrias, but adult onset of lesions suggests either PCT, HEP, HCP, or VP. (From Poh-Fitzpatrick MB: Porphyrin-sensitized cutaneous photosensitivity: pathogenesis and treatment. Clin Dermatol 1985; 3:41.)

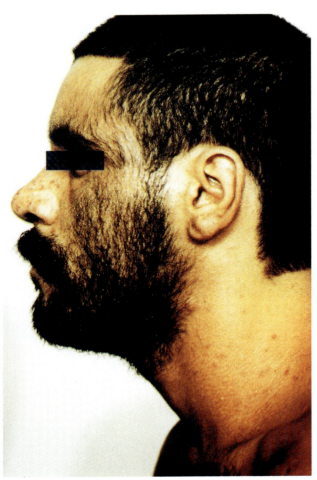

Figure 12-6. Hypertrichosis of the face of a patient with PCT. Note the erosions and pigmentations over the nose and cheeks. (From Poh-Fitzpatrick MB: Porphyrin-sensitized cutaneous photosensitivity: pathogenesis and treatment. Clin Dermatol 1985; 3:41.)

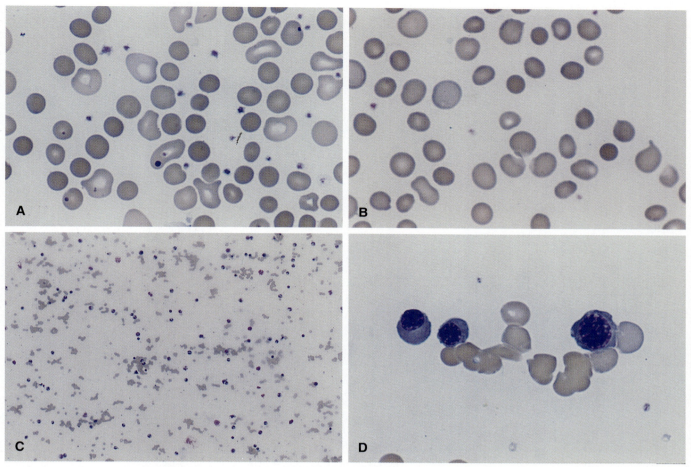

Figure 14-1. Examination of the peripheral blood in autoimmune hemolytic anemia (AIHA). *A,* Blood from a patient with IgG (warm-reactive) AIHA illustrates many small microspherocytes and larger reticulocytes (× 1000). *B,* Blood from a patient with hereditary spherocytosis illustrates the morphologic similarities between spherocytosis and AIHA. *C,* Agglutinated erythrocytes from a patient with IgM (cold-reactive) AIHA are clearly visible at low power (× 100). *D,* At higher power in this patient (× 1000), the nucleated cells in the peripheral blood are identified as erythroid progenitor cells prematurely released from the bone marrow.

I

History

1

Pediatric Hematology in Historical Perspective

Wolf W. Zuelzer

Wolf W. Zuelzer, who died on March 19, 1987 at the age of 77, wrote the history of pediatric hematology for the first edition of this book. We reprint it here in his memory.

As a subspecialty of pediatrics and a *sine qua non* of the modern teaching institution, pediatric hematology is a latecomer, naturally enough, for diseases of the blood were a minor problem—one is tempted to say a mere hobby of a few inquisitive and farseeing minds—compared with the great challenges of infectious and nutritional disorders that faced the pioneers of pediatrics. As a serious concern of investigators, however, pediatric hematology is as old as scientific pediatrics as a whole, though its early history is too closely interwoven with that of general hematology to be traced separately. Its tools as well as its basic concepts came largely from internal medicine and from the experimental sciences, and one needs only to mention such names as Ehrlich, Metchnikoff, Landsteiner, Chauffard, Downey, Minot, Castle, Whipple, and Wintrobe to appreciate the magnitude of this debt.

The discoveries of these and many other men were applied to the special problems of infancy and childhood by investigators who, with few exceptions, were pediatricians with diverse interests rather than hematologists with a specialized background. This is true even of those whose names are familiar through eponymic usage, such as von Jaksch, Lederer, Cooley, Blackfan, and Fanconi. Those who labored patiently in the vineyards without stumbling on a buried syndrome are mostly forgotten, though it is among them that one finds the first true pediatric hematologists. A case in point is that of Heinrich Lehndorff, who grew up in the Vienna of von Pirquet and Escherich and devoted his life to the study of both normal and abnormal hematologic conditions in childhood, publishing his first paper at the age of 29 in 1906 and his last at the age of 86 in 1963. His interest was in the blood of the newborn, in the anemias of infancy, and in leukemia. Like that of most of his contemporaries, his work was almost entirely descriptive, but he was a good morphologist and clinical observer. Lehndorff was forced to leave Vienna in 1939 at the age of 63, found temporary shelter in Birmingham with Leonard Parsons (then the leading figure in pediatric hematology in England), came to the United States during World War II, and

ended his career as an octogenarian with an honorary appointment at the New York Medical College. *Sic transit gloria mundi.*

From the very beginning, the unique blood picture of the newborn received special attention. In one of the oldest hematologic texts, *Du Sang et de ses Altérations Anatomiques,* published in Paris in 1889, Hayem—known to this day as the inventor of Hayem's solution but deserving to be remembered for more important contributions—discussed the blood at birth in great detail, giving the number of red and white corpuscles and platelets on the basis of his own counts; describing macrocytosis, anisocytosis, and a tendency toward spherocytosis; and attributing the high hemoglobin level of the newborn to hyperactivity of the bone marrow. The title of a paper by E. Schiff in the *Jahrbuch für Kinderheilkunde* in 1892, "Newer contributions to the hematology of the neonate, with special reference to the time of ligation of the umbilical cord," implies the existence of earlier studies and anticipates those of Windle and his associates some 50 years later.

The hematology of the neonate remained a cardinal concern of investigators for many decades. Progress was slow, perhaps in part because of the tediousness of the methods used and in part because of variables in obstetric and pediatric practice and differences in the timing of observations. Schiff himself, working successively in Prague and Budapest, found hemoglobin levels on the first day after birth to average 104 per cent in one city and 144 per cent in the other. Much controversy arose over normal values because the early workers did not come to grips with the problems of individual variation and frequency distribution. A German author, H. Flesch,[1] wrote despairingly in 1909, "The differences in the hemoglobin values of different observers according to the ages of the children are so considerable that one is really in no position to give definite normal figures." It was difficult, moreover, to draw a line between normal and abnormal conditions. ABO hemolytic disease, for example, was unknown until 1944, when Halbrecht[2] in Hadera recognized the relationship between "icterus praecox" and incompatibility of the major blood groups of mother and child. Prior to the studies of Lippman[3] in 1924, on the other hand, the transient normoblastemia of normal full-term infants was considered pathologic, although Neumann[4] had observed it in 1871 and König[5] had written about it in 1910. Supravital staining, introduced by Ehrlich in 1880, was not used until 1925, when Friedländer and Wiedemer,[6] writing in the *American Journal of Diseases of Children*—then the only major pediatric journal in the United States—reported reticulocytosis as a regular feature of neonatal blood. Although it was known by then that reticulocytes were young cell forms, the belief still prevailed that the high hemoglobin level at birth was due solely to hemoconcentration rather than to active erythropoiesis, as postulated by Hayem.

Conversely, the postnatal drop in hemoglobin concentration was taken as evidence of accelerated hemolysis, which in turn was held by some to be the cause of physiologic jaundice. That puzzling phenomenon was long thought to signify the entry of bile into the blood as a result of temporary mechanical obstruction by a mucous plug in the common bile duct or a "desquamative catarrh" of the small radicles, or liver damage from bacterial toxins from the recently colonized intestine of the newborn. The noted Finnish neonatologist Ylppö,[7] however, had demonstrated increased bilirubin levels in the cord blood as early as 1913 and had concluded that icterus neonatorum was due to a "functional inferiority" of the liver. All theories involving the regurgitation of bile became untenable in 1922, when Erwin Schiff and E. Färber,[8] pupils of the renowned Adalbert Czerny, showed that "during the period of bilirubinemia only the indirect van den Bergh reaction is positive." The alternative that the jaundice was due to increased blood destruction, however, could not be proved. Summarizing the argument in 1928, the Viennese pediatric hematologist Eugen Stransky[9] wrote, "Although the morphologic stigmata of a hemolytic icterus (i.e., spherocytosis) are lacking and the red blood counts do not permit a firm explanation, a hematogenous origin of icterus neonatorum nevertheless seems likely. Why destruction of red corpuscles takes place is still an unsolved question."

One must sympathize with these early investigators who formulated the alternatives clearly enough but could not solve the riddle of neonatal jaundice with the means at their disposal. To them icterus meant either regurgitation of bile or increased destruction of blood. Hemolysis seemed indeed a plausible explanation for the combination of bilirubinemia of the indirect variety with a falling hemoglobin level and a regenerative blood picture, all the more because mild forms of hemolytic disease were undoubtedly included in studies of infants presumed to be normal. The life span of fetal—or, for that matter, adult—red cells remained an unknown quantity, even after Winifred Ashby in 1919 had measured it in adults, using the differential agglutination technique, as the range of 30 to 100 days reported by her was too great to be of practical value. This was also true of the blood volume of the newborn, which William Palmer Lucas and B. F. Dearing[10] of San Francisco had actually attempted to measure in the same year, using the brilliant vital red dilution method. They obtained a range of values from 107 to 195 mL per kg of body weight, almost twice that found in 1950 by Mollison and his associates[11] with a method

combining isotope and dye dilution. The mere fact that they concerned themselves with such questions in 1919 puts them ahead of their pediatric contemporaries. Neither of the first two books devoted specifically to pediatric hematology, that of Ferruccio Zibordi of Modena, *Ematologia Infantile Normale e Patologica*,[12] which appeared in 1925, and that of Baar and Stransky of Vienna, *Die Klinische Hämatologie des Kindesalters*,[1] published in 1928, mentioned blood volume or red cell survival. The name of Lucas deserves recognition in any survey of pediatric hematology, for, apart from looking after patients with blood diseases in the Children's Department of the University of California before such specialization had become accepted elsewhere, he was an enterprising and thoughtful investigator. His chapters on blood in Abt's *Pediatrics* of 1924, written with E. C. Fleischner,[13] are outstanding in their emphasis on physiologic processes, clarity of thought, and absence of semantic claptrap, and in these respects are superior to the two works just cited.

As for the solution to the puzzle of neonatal jaundice, the functional inferiority of the liver postulated so long ago by Ylppö could not be defined, of course, until Hijmans van den Bergh's two pigments had been identified as free and glucuronide-conjugated bilirubin by the independent studies of Billing and Lathe,[14] Schmid,[15] and Talafant[16] in 1956. The results of the preceding demonstration of the role of uridine diphosphate glucuronic acid (UDPGA) as a glucuronide donor by Dutton[17] and others could be applied to bilirubin, and the enzymatic reactions involved in the conjugation process could be investigated as a function of hepatic maturation by Brown and co-workers.[18]

Traditionally, the history of pediatric hematology begins in 1889 with von Jaksch's report[19] on the condition that bears his name, which he designated *anemia pseudoleucaemica infantum*. By an irony of fate, not only the term but the very syndrome has long since vanished from the horizon, although in its day it had an enormous vogue and was considered by some to be the anemia of infancy *par excellence*. In 1891, the condition was described independently by Hayem[20] and his compatriot Luzet,[21] so that their names were also attached to it. The clinical picture was overshadowed by severe nutritional disturbances, wasting, diarrhea, rickets, and, as a rule, chronic infections of the respiratory tract, otitis media, pyoderma, and the like. The findings suggestive of leukemia were marked splenomegaly, anemia, and that which later hematologists would call a leukemoid reaction, characterized by leukocytosis and immature granulocytes. It was Luzet who noted the normoblastemia that led to the use of the term "erythroblastic anemia," until that term was temporarily pre-empted by Cooley for the anemia that *he* described. At that time, the combination of splenomegaly and leukocytosis meant leukemia, and von Jaksch's paper was therefore a distinct step forward, though its essence was the simple observation that some of the patients survived, a remarkable fact in itself given their general condition and the paucity of therapeutic means then available.

Von Jaksch was not a hematologist, and except for a

follow-up report in 1890, he made no further contributions to the understanding of the disease that made him famous. He practiced pediatrics in Prague, then the capital of the Austrian province of Bohemia, and held an appointment at the Charles University, where, as a legendary octogenarian, he was pointed out to this writer in 1934, a tall aristocratic figure with a massive white head who bore his fame with a casual elegance reminiscent of the old Hapsburg Empire. The riddle of von Jaksch's anemia was never properly solved. It was at one time common in central Europe and in France, less so in England, and still less so in the United States. Its disappearance paralleled the gradual improvement in child health and care. As Lehndorff[22] wrote many years afterward in an almost nostalgic epitaph on the extinct entity, it had been "a poor people's disease." In truth, it was not an entity at all but a convenient diagnostic wastebasket, though an interesting one. The contemporaries finally agreed that it was a nonspecific response of the infantile organism to the horrendous combinations of infectious and nutritional insults that were so common at the time and so difficult to sort out.

More lasting and far more important, of course, was the contribution made to pediatric hematology—and indeed to medical science as a whole—by Thomas B. Cooley of Detroit in 1925,[23] when he salvaged from this wastebasket the distinct entity now known as thalassemia. He soon abandoned his original designation of "erythroblastic anemia," for he realized that the conspicuous normoblastemia that had first attracted his attention was neither a specific nor a central feature of the disorder, and in his later publications he emphasized the fragmentation and shape anomalies of the red cells and the paucity and uneven distribution of the hemoglobin. He did not know, of course, that the ultimate disturbance was one of hemoglobin, let alone β chain synthesis, but he came to conceive of the disease as a fundamental disorder of hematopoiesis and was fully aware of its genetic nature from the beginning. He himself had originally proposed a recessive mode of inheritance, anticipating the classic study of Valentine and Neel of 1944.[24] Strangely enough, he failed to investigate the seemingly normal parents and siblings of the propositi. Later, unverified reports of hereditary transmission of the disorder by a single affected parent seemed to militate against a recessive mode and left him uncertain.

Cooley was, in any case, profoundly interested in the genetic aspects of the anemias and was in this respect far ahead of most contemporary hematologists. He corresponded with geneticists, used such terms as "heterozygote" for humans at a time when their use was still largely restricted to plants and *Drosophila*, and for years pondered the then wholly puzzling relationship between "sicklemia" and sickle cell anemia. He reported the first instance of sickle cell disease (which this writer later had occasion to identify as a case of sickle-thalassemia) in a Greek family.[25] He also proposed an X-linked mode of inheritance, backed by pedigree studies over five generations, for a familial hypochromic anemia in a kindred first described by him[26] and later restudied by Rundles and Falls[27] at Ann Arbor, Michigan. In accepting the term "Mediterranean anemia," which Whipple had suggested at a time when the known cases were restricted to Italian and Greek families, Cooley[28] made an interesting and prophetic reservation: "We are not inclined," he wrote in 1932, "to lay great stress on the limitation of this or any similar disease to a particular race. We have found that sickle cell anemia, formerly supposed to be peculiar to Negroes, occurs in Greeks, and it seems likely to us that any disease in which there is a hereditary element, as presumably there is in this disease, is limited more by locality and association than by race."

The style is as characteristic of the man as the thought. Cooley was articulate, well educated—he spoke or at least read four languages and maintained a global correspondence—and highly intelligent. He came from a family of distinguished jurists, the only one to eschew the law and enter the medical profession. Born in Ann Arbor, the son of a future justice of the Michigan Supreme Court, he obtained his degree in medicine at the University of Michigan, worked for 3 years in "clinical chemistry," interned at Boston City Hospital, spent a year visiting clinics in Germany, returned to Boston for prolonged training in contagious diseases, and then was appointed Assistant Professor of Hygiene at his *alma mater*. Except for a stint with the Children's Bureau of the American Red Cross during World War I, he remained in Michigan for the rest of his life, first as a practicing pediatrician and, after the death of Raymond Hoobler in 1936, as a professor of pediatrics in Detroit. Throughout these years he was closely associated with The Children's Hospital of Michigan, whose pediatrician-in-chief he ultimately became.

As mentioned, Cooley had no formal training in hematology and very little technical help. He and his faithful associate of many years, Pearl Lee, examined blood smears, roentgenograms, and, of course, the patients themselves, making sketchy notes on index cards and keeping the bulk of their observations in their heads. His equipment consisted of a monocular microscope of ancient vintage, a staining rack, a rather small card file, and—in an otherwise vacant room upstairs intended for the affairs of the Child Research Council of the American Academy of Pediatrics—a couch on which he took siestas and did much of his thinking. His daughter Emily, a gifted and artistic young woman, made the beautiful camera lucida and freehand drawings with which he illustrated his papers. She also chauffeured him about town, went to the library for him, and accompanied him to meetings. His home in Detroit's "Indian Village" and his garden, professionally landscaped by Emily, were oases of good taste. He owned a cottage on the coast of Maine where he spent his summers. He loved music, knew his wines, enjoyed good food, and was an excellent conversationalist. He knew how to live.

At times, his penchant for conversation got him into trouble. Old-time Detroiters recall the story of his house call to a well-to-do family whose child had contracted an undiagnosed illness. As a social acquaintance Dr. Cooley was led into the living room, offered refreshments, and asked his opinion on some topic of current interest. A lively discussion ensued, at the end of which the doctor, having forgotten the original purpose of his visit, grabbed his hat and coat and was out of the house before the astonished parents could remind him of the patient upstairs.

Cooley's influence extended well beyond the field of hematology. His was the conception behind a series of studies on the chemical composition of the red cell stroma carried out in the 1930s by Erickson and associates in the laboratories of Icie Macy Hoobler of the Children's Fund of Michigan, which earned high praise from Eric Ponder. He was one of the founders of the Academy of Pediatrics and, long before the time was ripe, saw the role of pediatrics in terms of preventive medicine. Politically he was a liberal, scientifically a radical, personally a patrician. Combined with a rather haughty expression, an irrepressible wit, and an utter lack of reverence for established authority, these traits were bound to earn him enmities on the part of town and gown alike, but his enemies respected and his friends admired him. He was well ahead of his time, a lucid thinker and a giant in the history of pediatric hematology.

An entirely different personality was George Guest, for many years one of the mainstays of the Children's Hospital Research Foundation in Cincinnati, whose contributions were equally important, if less spectacular. Guest was as much a physiologist as a hematologist, interested in the basic aspects of blood during growth, a stickler for precise measurements, a patient investigator who set himself longterm goals and took a systematic approach to reaching them. The meticulous studies he conducted between 1932 and 1942 on the hemoglobin levels, red blood counts, and packed cell volumes of a large group of infants and young children of widely different social and economic backgrounds are a model of intelligent and purposeful data-gathering, the purpose being both physiologic and clinical. In the face of the rather arbitrary definitions and therapeutic practices then prevailing, Guest set out to ascertain the range of normal variation and to delineate optimal values against hypoferric states. Such data were badly needed then and have remained valid to this day. In serial studies[29] involving, among other things, intrafamily and twin comparisons, he showed convincingly that a fall of the mean corpuscular volume (MCV) and mean corpuscular hemoglobin (MCH) in the presence of seemingly adequate hemoglobin levels could be reversed or altogether prevented by the administration of iron and is therefore a sensitive indicator of an incipient deficiency state rather than a physiologic phenomenon. He concluded that iron deficiency anemia was far more common among infants than had been previously thought, and advocated the general use of prophylactic measures. His earlier observations on glycolysis and the rise of inorganic phosphorus levels in stored blood[30] and his joint observations with Sam Rapoport[31] on the role of the pH in the breakdown of diphosphoglycerate were milestones in the understanding of red cell metabolism. He also made significant contributions to the knowledge of the osmometric properties of erythrocytes,[32] both normal and abnormal, devising a method that was, typically, both practical and precise and permitted simultaneous determinations of hemolysis and red cell volume at each stage of the procedure.

Apart from these accomplishments, George Guest was a delightful friend and, with the help of his wife, a perfect host, so that the house on Dana Avenue in Cincinnati became a kind of unofficial headquarters for the entertainment of the many visitors to the Children's Hospital. Here they were offered the *vin d'honneur* from a well-stocked wine cellar decorated with frescoes by an artist friend—the owners' pride and the first and last stop for the visitor—and here they would find good conversation, interesting people, and exquisite cuisine. The Guests were passionate Francophiles, and the cooking was French, unless a keg of oysters had just arrived from the East to be prepared in endless variations, or unless Jesse, the houseman, more friend than butler, just happened to have shot—illegally, of course—a fat squirrel from one of the magnificent old trees in the garden. George, a short, stocky, quiet-spoken man, understood the art of good fellowship, but the soul of the house and its social genius was his wife "M.L.," a handsome woman with red hair who had a passion for poetry and a gift for conversation. They had met in Europe after World War I as young and idealistic members of the Hoover Relief team, were drawn together by their love for all things French, and remained deeply devoted to one another. A large part of every summer was spent in France visiting friends, traveling through the countryside, and sampling wines. George Guest was the only American member of the French Pediatric Society, a fact in which he took greater pride than in all his other achievements, and though his French accent left much to be desired, he liked to attend meetings and even present papers in such delightful places as Bordeaux, Lyon, and Paris. When M.L. died about 1964, the house was sold and an era passed.

It would be instructive to trace in detail the thinking of earlier observers concerning the iron deficiency anemia of infancy, to whose definition Guest made such a solid contribution, but which remained an object of controversy, confusion, and neglect for generations of pediatricians. Although Bunge had proposed an essentially correct explanation as early as 1889, the nature of the most common anemia of infancy eluded investigators for many years. The reasons for this paradox are enlightening. One was the belief that not only mild anemia but also hypochromasia was a physiologic phenomenon. "That the hemoglobin content suffers more than the red blood count," Heinrich Baar wrote in 1928,[33] "is surely a purposeful mechanism, for the same quantity of hemoglobin can serve its function better when it is distributed over a larger number of red corpuscles." More important, no doubt, is the fact that among the clinic patients on whom most studies were conducted, pure iron deficiency anemia was rare. In the face of the multiple ailments to which such patients were prone, failure to respond to iron alone was common, and it was easy to draw erroneous conclusions from therapeutic trials. Conversely, of course, a rise of the hemoglobin level following the administration of iron was just as uncritically taken as proof of its efficacy on the principle of *post hoc propter hoc,* though it was believed that iron was a bone marrow "stimulant" rather than a specific substance effective only when correcting or preventing a deficiency.

Much of the problem was semantic in nature. Whereas French pediatricians described iron-responsive hypochromic anemia in infants as *"chlorose due jeune âge"* or *"chlorose alimentaire,"* most German and Austrian authors rejected this concept, if only because "chlorosis occurs only during puberty and only in females." The highly influential Czerny, in particular, set the clock back by stating categorically that an entire group of alimentary anemias existed that could be influenced by diet but in which iron was utterly ineffective. Baar wrote: "If it appears, *a priori,* unjustified to group together, and attribute to direct or indirect lack of iron, anemias of the most diverse origin solely because they are all hypochromic, fail to show nucleated red cells in the peripheral blood and lack splenomegaly, the notion of chlorosis of alimentary origin was definitely refuted by Czerny's findings." If this was to pour the baby out with the bathwater, Baar retreated from his a prioristic position to the extent of recognizing a "pseudochlorosis infantum," or infantile iron deficiency anemia, as an "etiologically uniform type to be separated from the rest of the alimentary anemias of infancy." This was rare, however, he asserted, in comparison with "the overwhelming majority [which] remains uninfluenced by iron administration, though nevertheless improved or cured by appropriate changes in diet." In reading such statements, one must remember that even fresh air and sunshine were still considered essential adjuncts to the treatment of anemia. Moreover, no less an authority than Haldane[34] had asserted earlier that "recovery affords no ground for assuming that iron is built up into hemoglobin," and that "in typical cases [of chlorosis] the curative factor of iron salts must be exercised otherwise than simply in building up the hemoglobin." Haldane went on to say that "The essential process in the cure of chlorosis is the reduction in the volume of the plasma [*sic*]." In addition, the notion of toxic hemolysis due to the fatty acids in cow's milk and especially in goat's milk had a prolonged vogue on the Continent, where "cow's milk anemia" and "goat's milk anemia" were accepted entities.

Related to the semantic difficulties was the problem of classification. Ever since Hayem had introduced the color index in 1877, hypochromasia had been used to characterize certain anemias. It was soon apparent that most anemias of older infants were of this type, but the difficulty of relating morphologic criteria to pathogenetic mechanisms and of recognizing in turn that different etiologic factors could operate through identical pathways proved too much. Not until the work of Minot and Castle established the characteristic response of hemoglobin and reticulocytes to specific hematinics, and Wintrobe put the morphologic classification on the firm basis of red cell measurements, did

pediatric hematologists gradually abandon terms such as "alimentary-infectious" anemia. In 1936, Hugh Josephs[35] still used this term as a common denominator that, to him, included deficient hemoglobin formation, deficient erythropoiesis and deficient stimulation of erythropoiesis, deficient maturation (the "erythroblastoses"), and blood destruction. Such usage, apart from the vagueness of the etiologic concept, was bound to delay both the understanding of the pathogenesis and the development of a workable classification of the anemias. It was an internist who said that "the infant bleeds into its own increasing blood volume," and the importance of the hemoglobin mass at birth was not appreciated until later. When Blackfan and Diamond's *Atlas of the Blood in Children* finally appeared in 1944,[36] it used Wintrobe's classification and described the principal anemia of infancy under the title "iron deficiency anemia."

One cannot leave the subject of iron deficiency without reference to Hugh Josephs, a strange figure, and in his day an authority in the field of American pediatric hematology. It is remarkable that this should have been the case, for he published little and confined his work primarily to the relationship between iron metabolism and anemia in infancy. His chapters on diseases of the blood in Holt and McIntosh's textbook were excellent, but his mind had a somewhat pedantic cast and a tendency to look for profound meanings underneath simple facts. His forte was a thorough knowledge of the literature, which he analyzed in erudite but unconscionably lengthy reviews, complete with foreword, statement of scope and purpose, introduction, presentation of fundamental concepts, summary, table of contents, and a bibliography that in one instance exceeded 750 titles. He was Associate Professor of Pediatrics in Dr. Park's department at Johns Hopkins University and published mostly in the Johns Hopkins Bulletin. His manner and appearance were those of a college professor or a don—mild, pleasant, serious, single-minded, a slight, gray-haired man who smoked a pipe, wore soft collars and a velvet jacket with elbow patches, and received his visitors in a drab office in the old Harriet Lane Home cluttered with books, magazines, and reprints.

By means of a curious logic, Josephs came to the unshakable conclusion that the hypochromic iron deficiency anemia of infants was not due to depletion of iron but to its diversion to unknown sites by unknown mechanisms.[37] He based this hypothesis on theoretical calculations that proved that an anemic baby of 18 months *should* have an excess of 200 mg of unused iron—other than the necessary tissue iron—somewhere in his body; *ergo* the baby suffered from "iron deficiency without depletion." This hypothetical baby, Josephs said, "is starving in the midst of plenty. Give this baby a small amount of iron by mouth and he will utilize it avidly for hemoglobin formation, and may as a result use even more than he was given." In the absence of infection, the unavailability of iron might be due, he thought, to hormonal, histotrophic, or even emotional factors. But in 1956, 3 years after these speculations, Philip Sturgeon[38] calculated on the basis of the same data that had been available to Josephs that a seemingly normal newborn could easily have a hemoglobin mass low enough to account for severe anemia in later infancy, reflecting the expansion of the blood volume with growth. Earlier, Bruce Chown[39] of Winnipeg had documented the occurrence of massive transplacental hemorrhage. Soon afterward, Kleihauer and Betke[40] devised their ingenious method for demonstrating fetal cells in maternal blood by the acid elution technique. Subsequent studies by Cohen, Zuelzer, and associates[41] and others showed that moderate and repeated fetal bleeds were not at all rare. A mechanism for depriving the fetus of hemoglobin iron without necessarily causing overt anemia at birth but capable of explaining the later development of iron deficiency in the absence of further blood loss seemed to offer a simpler solution than the tortuous hypothesis of "iron deficiency without depletion." The modern age had arrived.

Their semantic difficulties did not keep the earlier pediatricians from devising eminently practical methods of treatment, as exemplified by the story of pediatric transfusion therapy. The technical problems of transfusing infants were overcome in various ways. In 1915, Helmholz of the Mayo Clinic advocated the use of the superior sagittal sinus, and in 1925 Hart of the Sick Children's Hospital of Toronto used this route for the first exchange transfusion ever given for "icterus gravis."[42] Though his patient recovered, exchange transfusion was not again used for this indication until Wallerstein revived it in 1946 on the grounds that "the removal of most of the Rh-positive cells and of the circulating antibody shortly after birth prevents the incidence of the more severe pathological and physiological changes." Wallerstein,[43] then Director of the Erythroblastosis Fetalis Clinic of the Jewish Memorial Hospital in New York, had used the sagittal sinus for most of his cases, but stated that "the umbilical vessels should be an excellent route for both the withdrawal and replacement procedures," with the strange proviso that they could be used "only if the decision to perform the substitution is made before birth. . . ." J. B. Sidbury,[44] a pediatrician at the Babies' Hospital in Wrightsville, North Carolina, in a little-noticed report had described a simple transfusion via the umbilical vein in the case of a bleeding newborn in 1923. It was Diamond[45] who later established the umbilical route as the safest and simplest for exchange transfusion in hemolytic disease and who, with Allen and Vaughan,[46] was the first to recognize that the prevention of kernicterus was the main rationale of the procedure. It is interesting to recall that exsanguination transfusion through the fontanelle or the femoral vein was used on a large scale at the Sick Children's Hospital in Toronto for the treatment of burns, erysipelas, and other conditions since 1921. This procedure was introduced by Bruce Robertson, who in 1916 during the campaign in France had observed two soldiers recover from severe carbon monoxide poisoning after venesections followed by transfusions. By March of 1924, when Robertson was already dead, 501 exsanguination trans-

fusions had been performed at the Sick Children's Hospital.[47]

In the late 1950s there was a small flurry of papers reporting successful transfusions by the intraperitoneal route. This subject had been thoroughly explored in two studies, one experimental,[48] the other clinical,[49] in 1923 by a young pediatric resident in Minneapolis, David Siperstein, whose concise and accurate summary read as follows: "1. The intraperitoneal transfusion of citrated blood is a therapeutic procedure of possible merit. 2. It can apparently be utilized in cases in which transfusion is indicated, when other routes are unavailable." The author documented the effective reabsorption of the transfused cells not only with serial red counts and hemoglobin determinations but also with photomicrographs showing the dual population of hypochromic recipient and normochromic donor cells. In his review of the literature, he found that intraperitoneal transfusion was first used by Ponfick of Berlin in 1875, and that Hayem in 1884 had performed ingenious experiments involving cross transfusions of dog and rabbit blood in order to prove absorption from the peritoneal cavity. Although technical progress has since made the procedure obsolete, Siperstein's work deserves to be rescued from oblivion, if only to show that there is nothing new under the sun. He recognized a potential need, defined the problem, and solved it with an enviable economy of means (and words).

Passing mention should also be made of the use of bone marrow transfusions as a means of side-stepping technical difficulties in transfusing infants, especially for the general pediatrician with little practice in "needlework." The method had its day in England and particularly in Denmark, where Heinild[50] in 1947 described the experience of 4 years, during which 686 blood transfusions were given via the bone marrow without a single mishap. He stated that the risk of osteomyelitis was limited to patients receiving continuous infusions. One hesitates to argue with success and realizes that, in places and under conditions in which the required skills or supplies are lacking, it is better to apply unorthodox methods than to let a baby die for lack of blood.

A less desirable development that took place in the late 1920s and continued until the early 1940s was the practice of giving newborn infants intramuscular injections of adult blood as a prophylactic measure against hemorrhagic disease of the newborn. During those years, according to recollections provided by James L. Wilson, who for many years was Dr. Blackfan's right arm at The Children's Hospital in Boston, hemorrhagic disease was becoming so great a problem that this practice seemed justified. The blood was given without typing or crossmatching, and the procedure undoubtedly was responsible for a significant number of sensitizations against the Rh factor that did not come to light until these infants had grown up (and the Rh factor had meanwhile been discovered). The subsequent decline in hemorrhagic disease of the newborn coincided with both the introduction of vitamin K and a significant improvement in obstetric practices. Since the condition has now become rare and its definition was always vague and without clear distinction between traumatic hemorrhages and those primarily attributable to a coagulation difficulty, the mystery of its upsurge and the reasons for its virtual disappearance have never become quite clear.

If pediatricians proved resourceful in the matter of blood transfusions, it must be said that they showed little innovative spirit in certain other respects. It is a curious fact that the study of the bone marrow in children was neglected, especially in the United States, long after its usefulness had been amply demonstrated in adults. Thus Cooley, for example, never looked at anything but the peripheral blood, and Blackfan and Diamond's otherwise exhaustive *Atlas* of 1944 appeared without a single illustration of bone marrow. This writer remembers visiting a major pediatric center on the East Coast about 1946 and being shown half a dozen patients on the wards suspected of having leukemia and awaiting *surgical* biopsies—to be performed when and if they stopped bleeding. His own interest in the cytology of the bone marrow, which led to the recognition of megaloblastic anemia of infancy and its reversal by folic acid,[51] had been stimulated by many "curb-stone" discussions with Lawrence Berman, a student of Downey and himself an outstanding morphologist. It should be noted that Amato of Naples, Italy,[52] gave an excellent description of infantile megaloblastic anemia independently in the same year as Zuelzer and Ogden,[51] though he did not have folic acid at his disposal and concluded from the response to potent liver extract that he was dealing with true pernicious anemia or at least with a temporary deficiency of intrinsic factor. An even earlier report by Veeneklaas of Holland[53] had the misfortune of being prevented from reaching readers abroad because of World War II.

This is the place to pay tribute to the memory of Katsuji Kato, pupil and associate of Downey, a superb morphologist and illustrator, who was the first student of the infantile bone marrow in the United States. In 1937, Kato[54] published a definitive study based on bone marrow aspirations in 51 normal infants and children. He commented on the lymphocytosis in the younger subjects and gave the myeloid-erythroid ratios for the various ages. He also illustrated the diagnostic value of the procedure by citing a case of leukemia and one of Niemann-Pick disease. Kato was on the staff of Bobs Roberts Memorial Hospital in Chicago and often made the long trek to the North Side to participate in Dr. Brennemann's grand rounds at the Children's Memorial Hospital. One remembers him, a jolly, round-faced, smiling figure reminiscent of the *Hotei-Sama* statuettes of his native Japan, a rapid speaker with an atrocious accent but interesting ideas, showing off his delicate colored drawings with as much aesthetic pleasure as scientific pride and at the same time implying by his self-deprecating manner that it was all quite simple and hardly worth the honorable listener's attention. World War II put an end to his career. He returned to Japan and was lost from sight.

Perhaps it was Kato's unfortunate choice of the sternum as the site for diagnostic punctures, making the procedure unnecessarily difficult and unpleasant in pe-

diatric practice, that kept others from emulating him. American authors virtually ignored Kato's work, except for the enterprising Peter Vogel at Mount Sinai Hospital in New York, whose study with Frank Bassen[55] in 1939 covered 113 examples of diverse conditions, including leukemia, Gaucher's disease, and metastatic neuroblastoma, illustrated with excellent photomicrographs. In Europe, and especially in Switzerland under the influence of Rohr and Moeschlin, pediatric hematologists were more curious. Zürich, where Naegeli had created a strong tradition, had already become a mecca of Continental hematology. Writing in 1937, Guido Fanconi[56] declared: "The painstaking exploration of every case [of unexplained anemia] with old and new methods, which include bone marrow puncture, handled at the Zürich [Children's] Clinic with consummate skill by my *Oberarzt*, *Dozent* Willi, promises to uncover new, sharply defined entities." In the short span between 1935 and 1938, H. Willi[57] published four excellent studies on the bone marrow in thrombocytopenic purpura, leukemia, and various anemias of childhood. Fanconi had the satisfaction of seeing his prophecy fulfilled, in part by his next *Oberarzt*, Conrad Gasser. In addition to megaloblastic anemia of infancy, a whole series of conditions came to light or were clarified by bone marrow studies, among them the acute erythroblastopenia described in 1949 by Gasser[58]; chronic benign neutropenia, also studied by Gasser[59] and later by Zuelzer and Bajoghli[60]; Kostmann's infantile genetic agranulocytosis[61]; "myelokathexis"[62] or "ineffective granulopoiesis"[63]; and the aplastic and hypoplastic anemias.

Hematology occupied a special place among Fanconi's far-flung interests, and in giving encouragement and support to his associates—in this respect not unlike Blackfan—he contributed as much to progress in this field as he had done earlier with the recognition of the anemia that bears his name.[64] A tall, handsome man, every inch the professor yet gracious and outgoing, capable of charming an audience in six languages, a lively and eclectic spirit, Fanconi was a superb clinician and an excellent organizer to whom pediatric hematology owes much. With Fanconi one must rank his colleague in Bern, Glanzmann,[65] whose report in 1918 on "hereditary hemorrhagic thrombasthenia" as a condition characterized by prolonged bleeding time and poor clot retraction in the presence of a normal platelet count opened the era of platelet function studies. Glanzmann postulated the existence of a platelet factor specifically involved in clot retraction. He contributed greatly to the knowledge of the various purpuras. The term "anaphylactoid purpura" stems from his studies[66] and was based partly on clinical observations and similarities with human serum sickness and partly on his interpretation of Hayem's findings in dogs injected intravenously with bovine serum.

Conrad Gasser, one of the ablest and most productive pediatric hematologists in Europe, deserves more than passing mention in this narrative. Apart from his discovery of acute erythroblastopenia—known until then only from the report of Owren[67] as a complication of congenital spherocytosis—and his study of chronic neutropenia, he added greatly to our knowledge of hemolytic anemias in childhood. His monograph *Die Hämolytischen Syndrome des Kindesalters,*[68] which appeared in 1951, ranks in quality if not in scope with Dacie's well-known book. In 1948, in a paper with Grumbach,[69] Gasser described spherocytosis as a feature of ABO hemolytic disease. In the same year he gave a detailed report of anemia with spontaneous Heinz body formation in a premature infant,[70] a condition then unknown except for a brief note by Willi. In his book, and in subsequent publications, he added a large compilation of case material, described the detailed morphologic picture of the abnormal red cells—which were identical with the "pyknocytes" later observed in full-term infants by Tuffy, Brown, and Zuelzer,[71] but which he called more graphically "ruptured eggshells"—and determined their incidence in the blood of normal premature infants. He coined the term "hemolytic-uremic syndrome," being among the first to recognize that condition.

One reports with regret that so fruitful a career was disrupted by the exigencies of an academic system that, at the time at least, provided insufficient "room at the top" and effectively eliminated key people upon the retirement of their chief (unless they happened to be chosen to succeed him). Such a system was, and to a large extent still is, in force in Switzerland and elsewhere on the Continent. Fanconi's retirement from the *Kinderspital* in Zürich almost automatically entailed that of his *Oberarzt* Gasser. The latter, a modest man with a quiet sense of humor and a *gemütlich* Alemannic temperament, maintained his interest in hematology, which came to include the treatment of childhood leukemia, but he did so as a practicing pediatrician in a private office. Similar reasons prematurely ended the academic career of Sansone in Genoa, author of a book on favism and one of the most promising pediatric hematologists in Italy.

It is manifestly impossible in the allotted space to do justice to, or even name, all those who contributed to the evolution of pediatric hematology. Among European workers one would like to dwell on the achievements of Sir Leonard Parsons of Birmingham, England, the Grand Old Man of British pediatric hematology, founder of a veritable school that attracted students from many countries, including the United States. Parsons was an original thinker who refused to accept the confused semantics of childhood anemias and created his own system along pathophysiologic lines. He was the first to recognize, in 1933, the hemolytic nature of erythroblastosis fetalis and to defend that concept[72] even against the authority of Castle and Minot. These men, along with Diamond, Blackfan and Baty, Josephs, and others, regarded erythroblastosis fetalis as a defect of hematopoiesis in a class with Cooley's anemia and other "erythroblastoses." One would like to describe the achievements of Parson's associates, Hawksley and Lightwood; of Cathie, Gairdner, Walker, Hardisty, and so many other British colleagues of Lichtenstein in Sweden—an early student of the anemia of prematurity, which he was the first to call physiologic and to separate from the later phase of iron deficiency; of

his compatriots Wallgren and Vahlquist; of Plum in Copenhagen, the discoverer of vitamin K and originator of the thesis of a temporary deficiency of this substance as the cause of hemorrhagic disease of the newborn; of van Crefeld of Amsterdam, a pioneer in the study of coagulation factors in the newborn; of Betke, then in Tübingen, who with Kleihauer developed the acid elution technique for the demonstration of fetal hemoglobin in individual cells and who later, in Munich, made his department into a strong base of pediatric hematology; of Jonxis in Leyden, an imaginative investigator, who among other things organized a comparative study of the incidence of sickling in Curaçao and Dutch Guiana (now Surinam) to test Allison's hypothesis of the selective effect of malaria on two genetically similar populations exposed for centuries to different risks of the infection.

To return closer to home, credit must be given to James M. Baty as a member, with Blackfan and Diamond, of the triumvirate at Children's Hospital, Boston, that set the pattern for the development of pediatric hematology in the United States. Their collaborative effort resulted in, among other things, the recognition that hydrops fetalis, icterus gravis, and hemolytic anemia of the newborn, in spite of the differences in their clinical manifestations, were etiologically related conditions.[73] This was truly a breakthrough in the understanding of hemolytic disease. After Baty moved to the Floating Hospital and Blackfan died an untimely death, Diamond emerged as the American pediatric hematologist *par excellence*. His role cannot be described solely in terms of his publications, which are too numerous to be listed here. He became the mentor of a whole generation of pediatric hematologists who later held, and in most instances still hold, key positions in teaching institutions throughout the United States. Directly or indirectly we all owe him a debt of gratitude, even those of us who from time to time disagreed with some of his ideas. This writer vividly remembers his first meeting with Dr. Diamond, when as a lowly intern in 1935 he consulted him in connection with a case of Cooley's anemia, then an unheard-of rarity in the small New England hospital where he served. This writer made the pilgrimage to Children's Hospital—which under Blackfan was forbidden territory to those who were not graduates of Harvard, Yale, Columbia, or Johns Hopkins—with some trepidation. His fears were not allayed when he laid eyes on Dr. Diamond, rather fierce-looking in a dark, Assyrian sort of way. But Diamond proved to be a gracious consultant, willing to discuss the case at hand without condescension or conceit with an insignificant beginner, to listen to the history and examine the blood films, and above all to confirm the beginner's diagnosis. Over the years, hundreds of colleagues and young would-be hematologists came to appreciate "L.K.'s" kindness and unfailing courtesy. Of his numerous contributions one need mention here only the "Diamond-Blackfan" syndrome of hypoplastic anemia,[74] the studies on the nature, diagnostics, and treatment of hemolytic disease, and the *Atlas,* an outstanding achievement for its day, which was his work rather than Blackfan's. But perhaps even more important was the guidance and encouragement he provided for pediatric hematologists of the next generation, of whom—at the risk of being selective—we can name here only a few: Fred ("Hal") Allen, Park Gerald, Frank Oski, N.T. Shahidi, Victor Vaughan, and William Zinkham.

Less influential, though no less respected, was the late Carl Smith of New York. His book, *Blood Diseases of Infancy and Childhood*,[75] was the first of its kind in the United States and for many years served as the major reference work in the field. Smith's most important contribution was the description of infectious lymphocytosis, an essentially asymptomatic condition associated with a blood picture reminiscent of that of whooping cough (or chronic lymphocytic leukemia), endemic and probably of viral origin. He took a great interest in thalassemia and established a model outpatient transfusion service at The New York Hospital. Carl Smith was a modest and generous man, always willing to praise and give credit, even when credit was not due. Through his untiring efforts, Cornell became one of the important centers of pediatric hematology on the East Coast.

The prime mover in the field on the West Coast was Philip Sturgeon, who created the hematology service at the Children's Hospital of Los Angeles. He emerged about 1950 as an independent investigator interested in the study of the infantile bone marrow. His research provided quantitative measurements, then badly needed,[76] and stimulated the diagnostic use of bone marrow aspiration. A great traveller and sportsman in private life, Sturgeon combined in his work the elements of common sense and scientific curiosity, establishing the outstanding hematology clinic that was later carried on by his successor, Dennis Hammond. In the midst of a productive career, Sturgeon surprised his friends and colleagues by retiring to Zermatt in Switzerland, but skiing and hiking even in the most glorious of landscapes was not enough to fill his existence, and after a few years he returned to his work, and California.

The fact that a major pediatric teaching institution in the United States (or in many European countries, for that matter) today is almost unthinkable without a pediatric hematologist reflects the influence of a few model institutions in the post–World War II era. We have noted the importance of a Diamond "school" of pediatric hematology. During this same critical era, the only other center of comparable importance was the Hematology Service at the Children's Hospital of Michigan in Detroit, which this writer was privileged to direct, and which over a quarter of a century turned out well over 100 fellows, many of them today directing services of their own in the United States and abroad, among them Audrey Brown, Flossie Cohen, Eugene Kaplan, Sanford Leikin, Jeanne Lusher, and William A. Newton. The work of this group includes contributions to the knowledge of ABO hemolytic disease, fetal-maternal hemorrhage, immune hemolytic anemia, the hemoglobinopathies, purpura and other bleeding disorders, and the therapy of childhood leukemia. The creation some time ago of a subspecialty board in pediatric hematology, whether or not it serves a practical purpose, is a sure indication that among Boston, Detroit, Los Angeles and San Francisco, New York, and more recently New Haven, Cincinnati and Syracuse, Minneapolis and Memphis, and Seattle and Houston, a sufficiency of man- (and woman-) power exists to provide service, teaching, and research at a high level of excellence today and in the future.

Throughout its history, pediatric hematology has benefited from the advances of adult hematology, and in fact some of its major achievements rest on contributions made by scientists in other fields (e.g., immunology, chemistry, genetics, and physiology). A striking example is the history of hemolytic disease of the newborn. In 1938, Ruth Darrow, a pathologist who had a deep personal interest in the subject, having experienced a series of stillbirths, reflected on the pathogenesis of what was then called erythroblastosis fetalis.[77] Assembling all of the then known facts, notably the sparing of the first child, the involvement of all or most children born after the first afflicted baby, and the range of clinical and hematologic manifestations, she discarded all the current theories and concluded that the disease could be explained only as the result of maternal sensitization to an as yet unknown fetal antigen—a splendid example of the value of intelligent speculation.

Within 3 years Darrow's hypothesis was confirmed, and the Rh factor, described in a brief communication by Landsteiner and Wiener[78] in 1940, was identified as the offending antigen. Wiener,[79] and independently Levine,[80] observed transfusion reactions after administration of ABO-compatible blood that could be attributed to Rh antibodies. It was Levine, observing such a reaction in a woman who had received no prior transfusions[81] but had received blood from her husband after delivering a stillborn fetus, who recognized the relationship between the Rh factor and hemolytic disease of the newborn.[82] He showed that mothers of affected infants possessed antibodies that reacted with most random blood samples and with blood samples of their husbands and children but not with each other's. Gentle, unassertive, and scholarly, Levine characteristically sought the opinions of those experienced in neonatal pathology before publishing his revolutionary conclusion. This writer remembers Levine's visit to his laboratory in Detroit in this connection, which took place sometime in 1941. Bubbling with excitement yet reluctant to overturn established dogma and aware that he was venturing into uncharted seas, Levine was visibly reassured when his attention was called to Ruth Darrow's paper in the *Archives of Pathology*. But the serologic evidence was conclusive in itself, and the paper Levine and his associates published the same year bore the title "The role of isoimmunization in the pathogenesis of erythroblastosis." Levine had been an associate of Landsteiner at the Rockefeller Institute, but by this time he had withdrawn from that prestigious institution and was working at a hospital in Elizabeth, New Jersey, a modest, unpretentious man, content to pursue his research in any setting. When this writer first knew him, he was a devoted *paterfamilias*, amateur pianist, and bridge player. After the death of his wife he moved to New York City and continued his work at the Sloan-Kettering Institute, where he remains active to this day. The scope and the fruitfulness of his investigations, which extend from fetal-maternal isoimmunization to the relationship between blood group and cancer antibodies, have made him one of the most creative scientists of our time.

The names of Levine and Alexander Wiener were antithetically linked for the generation that witnessed their ascent, largely because both had been associates of Landsteiner and both contributed enormously to the knowledge of immunohematology and of human genetics, but above all because their views often clashed. This was confusing for the bystanders but in no way detracts from the achievements of each man. Wiener's role in the technical and conceptual understanding of hemolytic disease, both Rh and ABO, cannot be underestimated, but his obsession with nomenclature, his tendency to pile hypothesis upon hypothesis, usually without bothering to inform the reader that he was discarding pieces from the bottom without toppling the edifice, and most of all his imperviousness to the needs of clinicians unfamiliar with the mysteries of blood group immunology isolated him from the mainstream of clinical investigation. Of Wiener's enormous output—by 1954, when the theory of Rh isoimmunization was essentially complete, he had published more than 333 papers, and a typical Wiener bibliography might contain 60 references by A. S. Wiener (with or without et al.)—the contributions relevant to pediatric and obstetric practice were above all those dealing with the "blocking" Rh antibodies,[83] which he discovered and named "univalent," recognizing that they alone could pass the placental barrier and cause disease in the fetus.[84] He was one of the pioneers of exchange transfusion[85] and personally performed the procedure countless times at the Brooklyn Jewish Hospital, but his technique involving transection of the radial artery and the use of heparinized blood did not gain general acceptance. Less reticent to invade the domain of the clinician and the clinical pathologist than his rival Levine, he proposed ingenious but purely speculative theories of the pathophysiology of hemolytic disease that did not stand the test of time and tended to detract from his brilliant achievements in his proper field of blood group immunology. Personally a likable, friendly, unassuming man, he was always in the thick of a battle in which he was his own worst enemy.

Rh hemolytic disease has become a rarity. Within the life span of one generation the condition was defined, its etiology and pathogenesis identified, effective treatment devised, and a program of prophylaxis instituted that prevents maternal sensitization and has virtually eliminated the disease. This crowning achievement rests on the work of two teams of investigators working independently in Britain and the United States: Clarke and Finn in Liverpool,[86] and Freda, Gorman, Pollack, and their associates in New York.[87] Starting from different theoretical premises, both groups, by 1967, had demonstrated the effectiveness of passive isoimmunization of previously unsensitized mothers by means of a potent anti-Rh gamma globulin. The story of the conquest of hemolytic disease of the newborn is matched by few other chapters in the history of medicine.

The modern era of leukemia therapy begins in the 1940s with the work of Sidney Farber,[88] then pathologist at Children's Hospital of Boston and the leading pediatric pathologist in the United States and indeed the world, who in 1948 developed the concept of cancer chemotherapy. Farber had the good fortune of finding, in Subarov of Lederle Laboratories, a chemist able to give him the "antifol" compounds he needed, but the idea of disrupting the growth of malignant cells with antimetabolites was his, and he pursued and promoted it with single-minded energy. It led him to the creation of the Children's Cancer Research Foundation and to the organization of a vast program of clinical and fundamental research that in turn gave rise to the nationwide collaborative studies sponsored by the National Cancer Institute and to the efforts of countless institutions and individuals the world over. Although married to a charming woman of great artistic talent, and the father of gifted and lively children, Farber was a man of almost monastic dedication to his work, a magnificent hermit who spent day and night in his rather resplendent cell in the Jimmy Fund building planning new approaches, an indefatigable optimist who was convinced from the beginning that a cure for leukemia would come forth and who did much to bring it nearer.

It is a little known irony of fate that Farber's concept of antimetabolite therapy evolved as the result of a faulty—or at least doubtful—observation, namely the impression that the administration of folic acid accelerated the growth of leukemic cells in the bone marrow. This writer became privy to this information because it was he who, during a visit to Boston in 1946, showed his former chief slides of aspirated bone marrow from leukemic children. Farber, hitherto strictly a "tissue pathologist," became very interested in the cytologic method and switched from surgical biopsies to needle aspirations. At that time folic acid had just become available, and in view of its striking effects on the bone marrow in megaloblastic anemia, Farber decided to investigate its effects on leukemia. From sequential examinations he gained the—probably erroneous—impression that the administration of folic acid per os led to more rapid growth of the leukemic cell population. It seems unlikely that the difference, if any, between treated and untreated patients was real, given the pitfalls of quantitating the cellular elements of aspirated bone marrow, but correct or not, the observation gave rise to the idea of using folic acid antagonists, of which aminopterin was the first, and the era of cancer chemotherapy had begun.

Shortly afterward, in 1949, new ground was broken in another field. In that year, by coincidence, two papers bearing on the same subject from different angles appeared within a few months of each other; they were destined to revolutionize the study of what became known as the "hemoglobinopathies." One was the report of Linus Pauling, Harvey Itano, and their co-workers[89] identifying sickle hemoglobin as a discrete protein separable by electrophoresis from normal hemoglobin, and characterizing sickle cell anemia as a "molecular disease." The other was James V. Neel's study of the genetics of sickle cell anemia and the sickle trait, establishing the former as the homozygous and the latter as the heterozygous state for the sickling gene.[90] The findings of the two reports meshed and became the fountainhead of a veritable flood of investigations leading to the discovery of other hemoglobinopathies and enormously widening the scope of human genetics. The next major achievement was Vernon Ingram's demonstration, by means of the "fingerprinting" of hemoglobin fragments obtained by tryptic digestion, that sickle hemoglobin differs from normal adult hemoglobin (HbA) only in the replacement of a single amino acid among the more than 300 components of the half-molecule, and his subsequent identification of the abnormality as the substitution of a valine for a glutamic acid residue.[91, 92] Since then, abnormalities in the amino acid sequence of the hemoglobin molecule (for the most part involving β chain mutations) have been found in hundreds of variants, and amino acid sequencing has become a basic tool of molecular genetics.

Following the identification of point mutations affecting the amino acid skeleton of globin molecules as the basis of sickling and other hemoglobinopathies, it seemed logical to search for similar structural anomalies of hemoglobin in thalassemia and, when none were found, to postulate "silent" mutations (i.e., amino acid substitutions that did not alter the electrophoretic behavior of the hemoglobin, but inhibited the rate of its synthesis).[93] While this hypothesis proved to be incorrect, it implied the valid assumption that, in analogy to the known structural mutants, the abnormality would be specific for either the α or β chain synthesis. This assumption was made explicit in 1959 by Ingram and Stretton,[94] when they postulated two classes of thalassemia, α- and β-thalassemias, corresponding to the α and β chain variants, respectively, of the hemoglobinopathies proper. This concept proved to be extraordinarily fruitful. It soon became apparent that the thalassemias constitute a highly heterogeneous group of disorders, and that these disorders generally can be classified as either α- or β-thalassemias. Following the development of a method for separating α and β (as well as γ and δ) chains by Weatherall and co-workers,[95] it became possible—by means of incorporating radioactive amino acids into the hemoglobin of reticulocytes *in vitro*—to determine the rate of synthesis of these chains directly and to identify α- and β-thalassemias as disorders of globin chain production of one or the other type. A new explosion of knowledge began with the demonstrations by Nienhuis and Anderson,[96] and Benz and Forget[97] of reduced β chain synthesis by β messenger RNA from β-thalassemic patients, measured in a cell-free heterologous system. The emphasis now shifted to the investigation of quantitative and qualitative defects of mRNA. As additional new techniques became available—e.g., the use of DNA polymerase

(reverse transcriptase) to make complementary DNA from mRNA templates, the mapping of DNA sequences by means of restriction endonucleases, and the cloning of DNA fragments—it was possible to identify coding, transcription, translation, and many other defects in the genetic machinery of both α- and β-thalassemic cells. This writer cannot trace the ramifications of this work, which is still ongoing and is discussed elsewhere in this book, nor would I presume to select the names of the investigators from among the many—in the United States, Great Britain, Greece, Thailand, and many other countries—who deserve special recognition. Suffice it to say that the elucidation of the defects in the various forms of thalassemia constitutes one of the great triumphs of biomedical and genetic research. The hoped-for conquest of these disorders surely will come from the application of this knowledge.

In yet another field, that of the enzymopathies, the red cell proved to be an almost inexhaustible source of information of equal interest to the hematologist and the geneticist. The point of departure was the 1956 report of Carson and associates[98] of a deficiency of glucose-6-phosphate dehydrogenase (G-6-PD) in primaquine-sensitive erythrocytes. Not only did this prove to be the explanation for the acute severe hemolytic anemia seen in certain adults who had received the antimalarial drug but, as shown within 2 years by Zinkham and Childs,[99] it also accounted for the then common hemolytic anemia associated with naphthalene poisoning in infants and young children (described in 1949 by this writer and Leonard Apt[100]), as well as for the previously mysterious hemolysis associated with favism, elucidated by Sansone in Genoa.[101] Through the investigations of Kirkman and co-workers[102] and those of Marks and associates,[103] it was soon apparent that G-6-PD deficiency is genetically as heterogeneous (and geographically as widespread) as are the thalassemias. Of special interest to the pediatric hematologist and to the neonatologist are the numerous reports of an association of G-6-PD deficiency and neonatal hyperbilirubinemia in certain Mediterranean and African countries, as well as in China. In addition to the many mutants of G-6-PD, all under the control of genes located on the X chromosome, other defects of the pentose pathway inherited as autosomal recessives were found, but these proved to be rare and chiefly of theoretical interest. Of greater importance for the understanding of the hereditary nonspherocytic hemolytic anemias was the discovery of a whole series of defects in the glycolytic pathway, beginning with pyruvate kinase deficiency, by Tanaka and Valentine and their co-workers.[104] Here too, an association with severe neonatal hyperbilirubinemia was observed. Here too, a high degree of genetic polymorphism soon became apparent. Today, when the well-equipped pediatric hematology laboratory must be able to perform a whole range of red cell enzyme studies as a matter of course, it seems strange that less than a generation ago the entire field of the enzymopathies was *terra incognita.*

The same can be said for several other areas of

hematology that are today considered essential, but that were hardly dreamed of a few decades ago. One example is cellular immunity. During much of this writer's early career the thymus was a wholly mysterious organ, "status thymico-lymphaticus" was a widely accepted entity (and an indication for the ill-founded practice of "prophylactic" irradiation), and the different classes and functions of lymphocytes, T and B cells, and helper, suppressor, and killer cells were unknown. Similarly, immunologic tolerance, self-recognition and graft-versus-host disease, the HLA system, and the importance of these observations for bone marrow transplantation (and transplantation in general) are now such well-established concepts that it is easy to forget how recently they were elaborated. Still another example involves the origin of the various lines of blood cells. The existence of a common ancestral cell in the bone marrow, which earlier generations of hematologists so heatedly debated for so many years, was not established until the 1960s, when morphologic arguments suddenly became irrelevant in the face of Till and McCulloch's[105] demonstration of pluripotential colony-forming cells, and the subsequent studies of these and many other workers elucidating the conditions of amplification and differentiation of these precursors. A comparable quantum jump occurred in the field of blood coagulation. Only those who had to deal with the horrendous problems of hemophiliacs in the days before cryoprecipitates and factor VIII (and IX) concentrates made replacement therapy and home care possible can truly appreciate the magnitude of this progress.

It cannot be our purpose here to give a complete overview of our subject. To do so would require a book of its own and duplicate much of the information contained in the following chapters. From what has been said it is clear that pediatric hematology has come into its own. After a prolonged infancy beset by semantic and morphologic woes, it has moved out of the descriptive and empirical phase into an era of functional and physiologic concepts well beyond the fondest dreams of the pioneers. In the process, it has again become part of the mainstream of hematology, yet preserved its identity and its impetus. It seems fitting that this text, which represents the sum of current knowledge, should begin with an account of this evolution and a tribute to those who brought it about, the men and women who did the best they could with the tools available to them and on whose work the new generation is building.

ADDENDUM

Wolf W. Zuelzer was a remarkable clinical scholar. He ends his history by reminding us that it is important to remember the investigators of an earlier period who built the foundations upon which we now do our work. Frank Oski and I were fortunate to enter pediatric hematology during a very fascinating period. When we began our work in the late 1950s and early 1960s, Cooley, Zuelzer, Blackfan, Diamond, and Smith had described nearly all the diseases with which this book is concerned. They were superb pediatricians with elephantine memories who could collect and accurately codify information about patients. We knew Dr. Diamond best and were stunned by his ability to remember almost every detail of a patient that he might have seen a decade or more before. Because he and his colleagues could reliably and reproducibly categorize their patients by clinical characteristics, we could begin to apply the rapidly developing fields of cell biology, protein chemistry, and enzymology to sort them out at a more fundamental level. We were helped immeasurably by our environment. For example, it was extraordinarily valuable to work in a hospital a block or so away from the Harvard Medical School laboratory in which Arthur K. Solomon and his students were defining the mechanisms by which water and salt are transported across the red cell membrane. At that time, unusual cases of hemolytic anemia came to our attention that could not be fitted into the categories that had been carefully established by Diamond and his aforementioned colleagues. To determine that these patients had most unusual defects in red cell water and electrolyte metabolism, we established collaborations with members of Solomon's laboratory and discovered the conditions that are today referred to as "erythrocyte hydrocytosis" and "xerocytosis." In another example of the collaboration of basic science with clinical pediatric hematology, I was introduced by my colleague Fred S. Rosen to patients with X-linked susceptibility to staphylococcal and certain gram-negative infections. These cases had already been described by Charles A. Janeway and Robert Good, but their metabolic basis was unknown. Naively wondering whether G-6-PD deficiency of the leukocyte might have something to do with the defect, Robert Baehner and I added nitroblue tetrazolium to normal and chronic granulomatous disease (CGD) leukocytes. The CGD leukocytes failed to reduce the dye. We immediately began to collaborate with Manfred L. Karnovsky, Professor of Biological Chemistry at the Harvard Medical School, who specializes in the study of the leukocyte oxidases, and discovered that CGD leukocytes are oxidase deficient. Many years later, Stuart Orkin cloned the gene for the heavy chain of the particular antimicrobial oxidase that is deficient in X-linked CGD.

Three years before I began to work at Children's Hospital, Park S. Gerald had set about to sort out the various cases of Cooley's anemia that Dr. Diamond had collected. He collaborated with Vernon Ingram at the Massachusetts Institute of Technology (MIT), who had recently discovered the molecular defect in sickle hemoglobin. Gerald's application of starch block electrophoresis to hemolysates of thalassemic blood led to the measurement of hemoglobin A_2 levels in the diagnosis of the various forms of the disorder. A burst of work in many laboratories followed. John Clegg and David Weatherall showed that one could measure the relative rates of the synthesis of hemoglobin chains in hemolysates, and this led Yuet Wai Kan, Blanche Alter, and me to the first successful application of this technique in the prenatal diagnosis of the hemoglobinopathies. However, it is the explosion in molecular biology that has been the most exciting of all. With the discoveries of restriction enzymes by Daniel Nathans and reverse transcriptase by Howard Temin and David Baltimore and the many important contributions of others, it became possible to analyze the thalassemias on a molecular level. Members of our own laboratory, including Bernard Forget, Edward Benz, and I, established most important collaborations with David Baltimore, Harvey Lodish, David Housman, and others at MIT. As a result of those collaborations and brilliant studies by Stuart Orkin, Yuet Wai Kan, Haig Kazazian, Arthur Nienhuis, and members of David Weatherall's laboratory in Oxford, huge strides were made. We now understand the various forms of thalassemia at the molecular level and have excellent molecular techniques for prenatal diagnosis. As a result of the transfer of technology, a marked decline in the incidence of new cases is already being observed in Sardinia and Greece.

Though Dr. Diamond's greatest contributions were made in erythroblastosis, he remained vitally concerned with and vexed by the problem of bone marrow failure. From the latter concern has arisen a commitment to research in experimental hematopoiesis and its clinical application in bone marrow transplantation. Today, the growth factors and receptors that govern the behavior of stem cells and committed progenitors are being identified and used to treat patients, with great effect.

So, the recent history of pediatric hematology is one of collaboration of clinical investigators with basic scientists. Our field arches into all of biology. No single individual can possibly encompass all of it. Teams are needed to solve the fundamental problems of today; but Wolf Zuelzer was right: we would have no basis to move, no logical framework with which to extend these fundamental studies, were it not for the superb clinical definitions that Zuelzer, Diamond, and the others provided. They gave us a framework without which all of our work would have been without meaning. This book is due to the great clinicians who preceded us, and its future editions will depend upon the productivity of the next generation of their students.

DAVID G. NATHAN

References

1. Flesch H, quoted by Baar H, and Stransky E: Die Klinische Hämatologie des Kindesalters. Leipzig, Franz Deuticke, 1928.
2. Halbrecht I: Role of hemo-agglutinins anti-A and anti-B in pathogenesis of the newborn (icterus neonatorum praecox). Am J Dis Child 1964; 45:1.
3. Lippman HS: A morphologic and quantitative study of the blood corpuscles in the new-born period. Am J Dis Child 1924; 27:473.
4. Neumann NA, quoted by Baar H, and Stransky E: Die Klinische Hämatologie des Kindesalters. Leipzig, Franz Deuticke, 1928.
5. König H: Die Blutbefunde bei Neugeborenen. Folia Haematol (Leipz) 1910; 9:278.
6. Friedländer A, and Wiedemer C, quoted by Baar H, and Stransky E: Die Klinische Hämatologie des Kindesalters. Leipzig, Franz Deuticke, 1928.
7. Ylppö A: Icterus neonatorum. Z Kinderheilk 1913; 9:208.
8. Schiff E, Färber E: Beitrag zur Lehre des Icterus Neonatorum. Jb Kinderheilk 1922; 97:245.
9. Stransky E: In Baar H, Stransky E (eds): Die Klinische Hämatologie des Kindesalters. Leipzig, Franz Deuticke, 1928.
10. Lucas WP, Dearing BF: Blood volume in infants estimated by the vital dye method. Am J Dis Child 1921; 21:96.
11. Mollison PO, Veall W, et al: Red cell volume and plasma volume in newborn infants. Arch Dis Child 1950; 24:242.
12. Zibordi F: Ematologia Infantile Normale e Patologica. Milano, Instituto Editoriale Scientifico, 1925.
13. Lucas WP, Fleischner EC: In Abt IA (ed): Pediatrics. Philadelphia, W. B. Saunders Co., 1924, p 406.
14. Billing BH, Lathe GH: The excretion of bilirubin as an ester glucuronide, giving the direct van den Bergh reaction. Biochem J 1956; 63:68.
15. Schmid R: Direct-reacting bilirubin, bilirubin glucuronide in serum, bile and urine. Science 1956; 124:76.
16. Talafant E: On the nature of direct and indirect bilirubin. V. The presence of glucuronic acid in the direct bile pigment. Chem Listy 1956; 50:1329.
17. Dutton GJ: Uridine-diphosphate-glucuronic acid and ester glucuronide synthesis. Biochem 1955; 60:XIX.
18. Brown AK, Zuelzer WW, et al: Studies on the neonatal development of the glucuronide conjugating system. J Clin Invest 1958; 37:332.
19. von Jaksch R, quoted by Baar H, and Stransky E: Die Klinische Hämatologie des Kindesalters. Leipzig, Franz Deuticke, 1928.
20. Hayem G, quoted by Baar H, and Stransky E: Die Klinische Hämatologie des Kindesalters. Leipzig, Franz Deuticke, 1928.
21. Luzet C: Etude sur L'Anémie de la Première Enfance et sur l'Anémie Enfantile Pseudoleucémique. Thèse de Paris, 1891.
22. Lehndorff H: Jaksch-Hayem anaemia pseudoleucaemica infantum. Helv Paediatr Acta 1963; 18:1.
23. Cooley TB, Lee P: Series of cases of splenomegaly in children with anemia and peculiar bone changes. Trans Am Pediatr Soc 1925; 37:29.
24. Valentine WN, Neel JV: Hematologic and genetic study of the transmission of thalassemia (Cooley's anemia: Mediterranean anemia). Arch Intern Med 1944; 74:185.
25. Cooley TB, Lee P: Sickle cell anemia in a Greek family. Am J Dis Child 1929; 38:103.
26. Cooley TB: A severe type of hereditary anemia with elliptocytosis. Am J Med Sci 1945; 209:561.
27. Rundles LW, Falls HF: Hereditary (sex-linked) anemia. Am J Med Sci 1946; 211:641.
28. Cooley TB, Lee P: Erythroblastic anemia, additional comments. Am J Dis Child 1932; 43:705.
29. Guest GM: Hypoferric Anemia in Infancy. Symposium on Nutrition, Robert Gould Research Foundation, Inc., Cincinnati, Ohio, 1947.
30. Guest GM: Studies of blood glycolysis: sugar and phosphorus relationships during glycolysis in normal blood. J Clin Invest 1932; 11:555.
31. Guest GM, Rapoport S: Organic acid-soluble phosphorus compounds of the blood. Physiol Rev 1941; 21:410.
32. Guest GM: Osmometric behavior of normal and abnormal human erythrocytes. Blood 1948; 3:541.
33. Baar H: Die Anämien. In Baar H, Stransky E (eds): Die Klinische Hämatologie des Kindesalters. Leipzig, Franz Deuticke, 1928.
34. Haldane and Smith, quoted by Lucas WP, and Fleischner EC: In Abt IA (ed): Pediatrics. Philadelphia, W. B. Saunders Co., 1924, pp 406–623.
35. Josephs HW: Anaemia of infancy and early childhood. Medicine 1936; 15:307.
36. Blackfan KD, Diamond LK: Atlas of the Blood in Children. New York, The Commonwealth Fund, 1944.
37. Josephs HW: Iron metabolism and the hypochromic anemia of infancy. Medicine 1953; 22:125.
38. Sturgeon P: Iron metabolism: a review. Pediatrics 1956; 18:267.
39. Chown B: Anaemia in a newborn due to the fetus bleeding into the mother's circulation: proof of the bleeding. Lancet 1954; 1:1213.
40. Kleihauer E, Betke K: Praktische Anwendung des Nachweises von Hb F-haltigen Zellen in fixierten Blutausstrichen. Internist 1960; 6:292.
41. Cohen F, Zuelzer WW, et al: Mechanisms of isoimmunization. I. The transplacental passage of fetal erythrocytes in homospecific pregnancies. Blood 1964; 23:621.
42. Hart AP: Familial icterus gravis of the newborn and its treatment. Can Med Assoc 1925; 15:1008.
43. Wallerstein H: Erythroblastosis foetalis and its treatment. Lancet 1946; 2:922.
44. Sidbury JB: Transfusion through the umbilical vein in hemorrhage of the newborn. Am J Dis Child 1923; 25:290.
45. Diamond LK, Allen FH Jr, et al: Erythroblastosis fetalis. VII. Treatment with exchange transfusion. N Engl J Med 1951; 244:39.
46. Allen FH Jr, Diamond LK, et al: Erythroblastosis fetalis. VI. Prevention of kernicterus. Am J Dis Child 1950; 80:779.
47. Robertson B: Exsanguination—transfusion: a new therapeutic measure in the treatment of severe toxemias. Arch Surg 1924; 9:1.
48. Siperstein DM, Sansby TM: Intraperitoneal transfusion with citrated blood: an experimental study. Am J Dis Child 1923; 25:107.
49. Siperstein DM: Intraperitoneal transfusion with citrated blood: a clinical study. Am J Dis Child 1923; 25:203.
50. Heinild S, Søndergaard T, et al: Bone marrow infusion in childhood. J Pediatr 1947; 30:400.
51. Zuelzer WW, Ogden F: Megaloblastic anemia in infancy. Am J Dis Child 1946; 71:211.

52. Amato M: Rilievi anamnesto-clinici . . . su 25 casi di anemie ipercromiche megaloblastiche osservate in bambini della prima infanzia. Pediatria 1946; 54:71.

53. Veeneklaas GMH: Über Megalozytäre Mangelanämien bei Kleinkindern. Folia Haematol (Leipz) 1940; 65:203.

54. Kato K: Sternal marrow puncture in infants. Am J Dis Child 1937; 54:209.

55. Vogel P, Bassen FA: Sternal marrow of children in normal and in pathologic states. Am J Dis Child 1939; 57:246.

56. Fanconi G: Die primären Anämien und Erythroblastosen im Kindesalter. Monatsschr Kinderheilkd 1937; 68:129.

57. Willi H, quoted by Rohr K: Das Menschliche Knochenmark. Stuttgart, Georg Thieme Verlag, 1949.

58. Gasser C: Akute Erythroblastopenie. Helv Paediatr Acta 1949; 4:107.

59. Gasser C: Die Pathogenese der essentiellen chronischen Granulocytopenie. Helv Paediatr Acta 1952; 7:426.

60. Zuelzer WW, Bajoghli M: Chronic granulocytopenia in childhood. Blood 1964; 23:359.

61. Kostmann R: Infantile genetic agranulocytosis (agranulocytosis infantilis hereditaria). A new recessive lethal disease in man. Acta Paediatr 1956; 45(Suppl 105):1.

62. Zuelzer WW: "Myelokathexis"—A new form of chronic granulocytopenia. Report of a case. N Engl J Med 1964; 270:699.

63. Krill CE Jr, Smith HD, et al: Chronic idiopathic granulocytopenia. N Engl J Med 1964; 270:973.

64. Fanconi F: Familiäre infantile perniciosa-artige Anämie (Perniziöses Blutbild und Konstitution). Jb Kinderheilk 1927; 117:257.

65. Glanzmann E: Hereditäre hämorrhagische Thrombasthenie. Jb Kinderheilk 1918; 88:113.

66. Glanzmann E: Die Konzeption der Anaphylaktoiden Purpura. Jb Kinderheilk 1920; 91:371.

67. Owren PA: Congenital hemolytic jaundice. The pathogenesis of the "hemolytic crisis." Blood 1948; 3:231.

68. Gasser C: Die Hämolytischen Syndrome des Kindesalters. Stuttgart, Georg Thieme Verlag, 1951.

69. Grumbach A, Gasser C: ABO-Inkompatibilitäten und Morbus Hemolyticus Neonatorum. Helv Paediatr Acta 1948; 3:447.

70. Gasser C, Karrer J: Deletäre Hämolytische Anämie mit "Spontan-Innen-Körper" Bildung bei Frühgeburten. Helv Paediatr Acta 1948; 3:387.

71. Tuffy P, Brown AK, et al: Infantile pyknocytosis, a common erythrocyte abnormality of the first trimester. Am J Dis Child 1959; 98:227.

72. Parsons LG: The haemolytic anaemias of childhood. Lancet 1938; 2:1395.

73. Diamond LK, Blackfan FD, et al: Erythroblastosis foetalis and its association with universal edema of the fetus, icterus gravis neonatorum and anemia of the newborn. J Pediatr 1932; 1:269.

74. Diamond LK, Blackfan KD: Hypoplastic anemia. Am J Dis Child 1938; 54:464.

75. Smith CH: Blood Diseases of Infancy and Childhood. 2nd ed. St. Louis, C. V. Mosby Co., 1966.

76. Sturgeon P: Volumetric and microscopic pattern of bone marrow in normal infants and children. II. Cytologic pattern. Pediatrics 1951; 7:642.

77. Darrow RR: Icterus gravis neonatorum. An examination of etiologic considerations. Arch Pathol 1938; 25:378.

78. Landsteiner K, Wiener AS: An agglutinable factor in human blood recognized by human sera for rhesus blood. Proc Soc Exp Biol Med 1940; 43:223.

79. Wiener AS, Peters HR: Hemolytic reactions following transfusions of blood of the homologous group with 3 cases in which the same agglutinogen was responsible. Ann Intern Med 1946; 13:2306.

80. Levine P, Katzin EM, et al: Atypical warm isoagglutinins. Proc Soc Exp Biol Med 1940; 45:346.

81. Levine P, Katzin EM, et al: Isoimmunization in pregnancy, its possible bearing on the etiology of erythroblastosis fetalis. JAMA 1941; 116:825.

82. Levine P, Burnham L, et al: The role of isoimmunization in the pathogenesis of erythroblastosis fetalis. Am J Obstet Gynecol 1941; 42:825.

83. Wiener AS: A new test (blocking test) for Rh sensitization. Proc Soc Exp Biol Med 1944; 56:173.

84. Wiener AS: Pathogenesis of congenital hemolytic disease (erythroblastosis fetalis) I. Theoretic considerations. Am J Dis Child 1946; 71:14.

85. Wiener AS, Wexler IB: The use of heparin in performing exchange transfusions in newborn infants. J Lab Clin Med 1946; 31:1016.

86. Clarke CA: Prevention of Rh hemolytic disease. Br Med J 1967; 4:7.

87. Freda VJ, Gorman JG, et al: Prevention of Rh isoimmunization. JAMA 1967; 199:390.

88. Farber S, Diamond LK, et al: Temporary remissions in acute leukemia in children produced by folic acid antagonist, 4-aminopteroylglutamic acid (aminopterin). N Engl J Med 1948; 238:787.

89. Pauling L, Itano AH, et al: Sickle cell anemia, a molecular disease. Science 1949; 110:543.

90. Neel JV: The inheritance of sickle cell anemia. Science 1949; 110:64.

91. Ingram VM: A specific chemical difference between the globins of normal human and sickle cell anaemia haemoglobin. Nature 1956; 178:792.

92. Ingram VM: The chemical difference between normal human and sickle cell anaemia haemoglobins. Conference on Hemoglobin. Publication No. 557, National Academy of Sciences—National Research Council, 1958, pp 233–238.

93. Itano HA: The human hemoglobins: their properties and genetic control. Adv Protein Chem 1957; 12:216.

94. Ingram VM, Stretton AOW: Genetic basis of the thalassaemia diseases. Nature 1959; 184:1903.

95. Weatherall DJ, Clegg JB, et al: Globin synthesis in thalassaemia. Nature 1965; 208:1061.

96. Nienhuis AW, Anderson WF: Isolation and translation of hemoglobin messenger RNA from thalassemia, sickle cell anemia, and normal human reticulocytes. J Clin Invest 1971; 50:2458.

97. Benz EJ, Forget BC: Defect in messenger RNA for human hemoglobin synthesis in beta thalassemia. J Clin Invest 1971; 50:2755.

98. Carson PE, Flanagan CL, et al: Enzymatic deficiency in primaquine-sensitive erythrocytes. Science 1956; 124:484.

99. Zinkham WH, Childs B: A defect of glutathione metabolism in erythrocytes from patients with a naphthalene-induced hemolytic anemia. Pediatrics 1958; 22:461.

100. Zuelzer WW, Apt L: Acute hemolytic anemia due to naphthalene poisoning, a clinical and experimental study. JAMA 1949; 141:185.

101. Sansone G, Piga AM, et al: Favismo. Torino, Minerva Medica, 1958.

102. Kirkman HW, Riley FD Jr, et al: Different enzymic expressions of mutants of human glucose-phosphate dehydrogenase. Proc Natl Acad Sci USA 1960; 46:938.

103. Marks PA, Szeinberg A, et al: Erythrocyte glucose phosphate dehydrogenase of normal and mutant subjects. Properties of the purified enzymes. J Biol Chem 1961; 236:10.

104. Tanaka KR, Valentine WN, et al: Pyruvate kinase (PK) deficiency hereditary nonspherocytic hemolytic anaemia. Blood 1962; 19:267.

105. Till JE, McCulloch EA: Direct measurement of the radiation sensitivity of normal mouse bone marrow cells. Radiation Res 1961; 14:213.

II

Neonatal Hematology

The Neonatal Erythrocyte and Its Disorders

Immune Hemolytic Disease

Disorders of Bilirubin Metabolism

Developmental Hemostasis: Relevance to
Newborns and Infants

The Neonatal Erythrocyte and Its Disorders

Carlo Brugnara • Orah S. Platt

THE NEONATAL ERYTHROCYTE

At no other time in the life of the patient is the physician confronted with as many diagnostic considerations in the interpretation of apparent disturbances in the erythrocyte as during the neonatal period.

The erythrocytes produced by the human fetus are fundamentally different from the red cells produced by older infants and children. These cells possess different membrane properties, different hemoglobins, a unique metabolic profile, and a much shorter red cell life span. In a variety of pathologic conditions, erythrocytes bearing some of the properties of fetal erythrocytes again appear in the circulation. A better understanding of the factors that regulate fetal erythropoiesis and a precise definition of the fetal erythrocyte may eventually result in the development of a unifying hypothesis that explains these acquired disorders of erythropoiesis. The interpretation of hematologic abnormalities in the neonate is confounded by the interactions of genetics, acquired disease in the neonate, and maternal factors with the gestationally related peculiarities of the fetal erythrocyte.

Development of Erythropoiesis
(See also Chapter 6)

Hematopoiesis in the embryo and fetus can be conceptually divided into three periods: mesoblastic, hepatic, and myeloid.[1] All blood cells are derived from the embryonic connective tissue—the mesenchyme—and blood formation can first be detected by the fourteenth day of gestation. Isolated foci of erythropoiesis can be observed throughout the extraembryonic mesoblastic

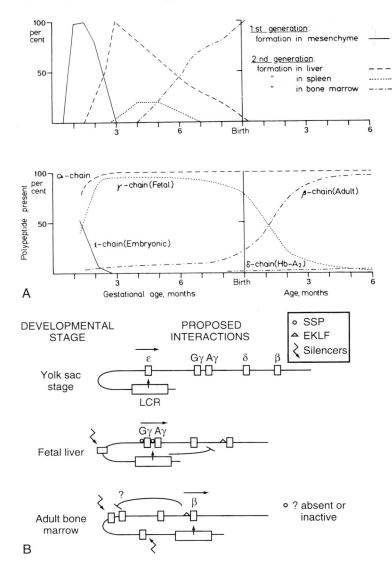

Figure 2-1. *A,* Hematopoietic sites and development of different globin chains during fetal life and early infancy. (*A,* After Knoll W, Pingel E: Der Gang der Erythropoese beim menschlichen Embryo. Acta Haematol 1949; 2:369, with permission of Karger, Basel; and Huehns ER, Dance, N, et al: Human embroyonic hemoglobins. Symp Quant Biol 1964; 29:327.) *B,* Globin gene switching in the human β-globin gene cluster. Some of the postulated interactions at each developmental stage of the human are indicated. *Arcs* ending in *oblique lines* are meant to depict competitive interactions. In the fetal liver stage, interaction of the γ-globin genes with the locus control region (LCR) prevents β-globin expression, despite the presence of EKLF, a β-globin gene–specific activator. In adult bone marrow erythroid cells, interaction of the β-globin gene with the LCR may facilitate shutoff of the γ-globin gene (as indicated by ?). Although it is not established, EKLF is shown bound to the β-globin promoter at the fetal stage to emphasize that transcription of the γ-genes prevails even in its presence. The status of the stage-selector protein (SSP) complex, and the postulated embryonic/fetal-specific subunit, in adult cells is unknown (as shown at the bottom). It is likely that SSP is present at the yolk sac stage. If this is the case, interactions between the ε-globin gene and the LCR presumably are dominant to γ-globin expression. (*B,* From Orkin SH: Regulation of globin gene expression in erythroid cells. Eur J Biochem 1995; 231:271.)

tissue in the area vasculosa of the yolk sac at 3 to 4 weeks after conception. Blood islands in the yolk sac differentiate in two directions. Peripheral cells in the islands form the walls of the first blood vessels, whereas the centrally located cells become the primitive blood cells, or hematocytoblasts.[2, 3]

The first blood cells produced by the embryo belong to the red cell series. Two distinct generations of erythrocytes can be observed in the developing embryo. Red cells arise as a result of either primitive megaloblastic erythropoiesis or definitive normoblastic erythropoiesis. Both megaloblasts and normoblasts apparently derive from similar-appearing hematocytoblasts and develop through roughly similar but morphologically distinct series of erythroblasts. In the very early embryo, the red cells arise from the primitive erythroblasts. These cells were termed "megaloblasts" by Ehrlich[4] because of their resemblance to the erythroid precursors found in patients with pernicious anemia. Megaloblasts are large cells with abundant polychromatophilic cytoplasm, and they possess a nucleus in which fine chromatin is widely dispersed. Megaloblasts give rise to large, irregularly shaped, somewhat hypochromic erythrocytes that can be seen in circulating blood 4 to 5 weeks after conception. The primitive erythroblasts arise primarily from intravascular sites; as development continues, these cells gradually are replaced by smaller cells of the definitive or normoblastic series.

Normoblastic erythropoiesis begins at about the sixth gestational week, and enucleated macrocytes enter the circulation by the eighth week; by the tenth week of development, normoblastic erythropoiesis accounts for more than 90% of the circulating erythrocytic cells. Maturation of normoblastic erythroid cells resembles that seen in postnatal life, giving rise to enucleated erythrocytes and being primarily extravascular.

By about the fifth to sixth week of gestation, blood formation begins in the liver. In the period between the fifth and tenth weeks, the liver undergoes a substantial increase in size, with an associated increase in the total nucleated cell count from 2.3×10^6 to 1.7×10^8 cells.[5] The fetal liver appears to be a site of pure erythropoiesis, and during the third to fifth months of gestation, erythroid precursors represent approximately 50% of the total nucleated cells of this organ.[6] Migration via the blood stream of pluripotent cells and early progenitors is probably responsible for the yolk sak to liver transition.[5] The liver is the chief organ of hematopoiesis from the third to the sixth fetal month and continues to produce formed elements into the first postnatal week (Fig. 2–1). During the third fetal month, hematopoiesis also can be detected in the spleen and the thymus, and shortly afterward in the lymph nodes. Blood cell formation can still be observed in the spleen during the first week of postnatal life.

Fukuda[7] employed electron microscopy to examine the characteristics of hepatic hematopoiesis in 26 human embryos and fetuses from 26 days after conception to 30 weeks of gestation. The development of hepatic hematopoiesis appeared to correlate closely with the histologic development of the liver. In the earliest stages of hepatic hematopoiesis, undifferentiated mononuclear cells, presumably stem cells, were present in the intercellular spaces of the hepatocytes. With maturation of the fetus, the number of erythroid cells in the hepatic parenchyma increased, and stem cells diminished in number and eventually disappeared. These stem cells were exclusively observed in the extravascular spaces and were considered to be derived from the septum transversum.

The ultrastructure of the hepatic erythroid cells was found to be quite distinct from the yolk sac–derived erythroblasts and the erythroblasts observed in the bone marrow of normal adults. The microtubules characteristic of normal bone marrow–derived erythroblasts were rarely observed in the hepatic erythroblasts.

Erythropoietic progenitors from livers of fetuses studied between 13 and 23 weeks of gestation appear more sensitive to humoral stimuli—colony-forming units–erythrocyte (CFU-E) for erythropoietin, and burst-forming units-erythrocyte (BFU-E) for burst-promoting activity—than do the progenitors from adult bone marrow.[8] Large numbers of committed erythroid and granulocytic-monocytic progenitor cells have been found in blood obtained by fetoscopy at 12 to 19 weeks of gestation. These fetal progenitor cells are more sensitive to appropriate stimuli than are adult progenitor

cells grown under the same conditions, presumably as a consequence of intrinsic differences in the progenitor cells of fetal origin.[9, 10] Functional and genetic differences between fetal and adult stem cells indicate that the hematopoietic stem cell is not an invariable cell type.[11]

The myeloid period of hematopoiesis commences during the fourth to fifth fetal month and becomes quantitatively important by the sixth fetal month. During the last 3 months of gestation, the bone marrow is the chief site of blood cell formation. Marrow cellularity becomes maximal at about the 30th gestational week, although the volume of marrow occupied by hematopoietic tissue continues to increase until term.[12] A summary of the time of first appearance of the different blood cells in the various fetal hematopoietic organs, based on the observations of Kelemen and associates from an analysis of 190 fetuses and embryos,[13] is provided in Table 2–1.

Cord blood is rich in bone marrow progenitor cells and contains multipotential CFU granulocyte-erythroid-monocyte-macrophage (CFU-GEMM), erythroid BFU-E, and CFU granulocyte-macrophage (CFU-GM) cell lines.[14] The frequency of circulating CFU-GMs from the 23rd week of gestation to full term is consistently high and provides evidence that CFU-GMs are produced in the yolk sac as well as at other hematopoietic sites.[15] The frequency of BFU-E[8] is highest at midgestation, with values being threefold greater than those for cord blood and 10-fold greater than those for adult bone marrow.[16] The in vitro behavior of progenitor cells obtained from umbilical cord blood is substantially different from that of progenitor cells in the bone marrow of adults. In contrast to adult progenitors, which require the presence of multiple growth factors, fetal progenitors can mature in vitro with no growth factors present or with the addition of only one. Recombinant human erythropoietin (r-HuEPO), [17, 18] interleukin-6,[19] interleukin-9,[20] and interleukin-11[21] are active as single agents in fetal but not adult progenitors. It has been shown that in vitro cultures of CD34+ fetal hematopoietic progenitors produce hematopoietic factors such as granulocyte-macrophage colony-stimulating factor (GM-CSF) and interleukin-3, which can sustain their

Table 2–1. THE FIRST APPEARANCE OF DIFFERENT BLOOD CELL TYPES IN HEMATOPOIETIC ORGANS AND IN CIRCULATING BLOOD, GIVEN BY FERTILIZATION AGE IN WEEKS

	Extraembryonic*	Liver	Thymus	Spleen	Lymph Nodes	Bone Marrow	Blood
Primitive erythroblasts	3–4	5	—	8	—	—	3–4
Definitive erythroblasts	6–7†	5	10	8	11	8–9	6–7
Granulocytes	3–4‡	5	10	8	12	8–9	7–8
Monocytes (classic)	—	?	—	11	12–13	11	7–8
Histiocytes, macrophages	3–4	5	10	8	11	8–9	3–4
Megakaryocytes, platelets	5†	5	—	11	—	8–9	6–7
Lymphocytes	6	6	8	8	9–12	10–12	7–9
Mast cells§	—	—	—	—	—	—	—

*Yolk sac, chorion, allantois, and body stalk.
†From the circulating blood?
‡Maternal origin is possible.
§The bone marrow was the only site where substantial amounts of mast cells were distinguished.
From Kelemen E, Calvo W, Filedner TM: Atlas of Human Hemopoietic Development. Berlin, Springer-Verlag, 1979.

growth factor–independent proliferation.[22] The exit from the G0/G1 phase of the cell cycle in response to stem cell factor also is accelerated in umbilical cord blood CD34$^+$ cells.[23]

The number of hematopoietic progenitors in cord blood is in the range of the requirements for successful engraftment by bone marrow cells.[14] Although the average cord blood collection contains only 14% of the nucleated cells present in an autologous bone marrow collection, it contains 91.6% of the CFU-GM colonies, 24% of the CFU-GEMM colonies, and 29% of the BFU-E colonies.[14] Studies of long-term cultures initiating cells have indicated that the number of putative stem cells in cord blood is comparable to that of allogeneic bone marrow or peripheral stem cell collections.[24]

Human umbilical cord blood has been successfully employed for hematopoietic reconstitution in patients with Fanconi's anemia,[25] aplastic anemia, X-linked lymphoproliferative disease, leukemia, immune deficiency, genetic and metabolic diseases (e.g., Hunter's syndrome),[26, 27] and severe hemoglobin E-β-thalassemia disease.[28]

Following birth, the amount of marrow tissue continues to grow, with no apparent increase in cellular concentration. The only way for an infant to increase cell production is to effect a more rapid turnover of cells or to increase the volume of hematopoietic tissue. This increase in tissue produces the marrow expansion that is most readily observed in the calvaria.

An increasing role for erythropoietin is observed during the hepatic and myeloid phases of erythropoiesis. Erythropoietin is detectable in the cord blood of nonanemic premature infants in quantities that are comparable to or greater than those in the blood of normal adults.[29] Fetal erythropoiesis is only partially influenced by maternal factors and is primarily under the control of the fetus. In the mouse, suppression of maternal erythropoiesis by hypertransfusion does not suppress fetal erythropoiesis,[30] nor does stimulation of maternal erythropoietin production result in stimulation of fetal red cell production; these findings indicate that erythropoietin is incapable of crossing the placenta.[31] The exact site of erythropoietin production in the fetus is unknown, but the liver is a likely candidate. In other animal species, nephrectomy of the fetus does not influence erythropoietin production or the erythropoietic responses to stresses such as bleeding.[32]

The development of hematopoiesis is controlled by the effect of growth factors on cell proliferation and the activation of lineage-specific genes by transcription factors (nuclear regulators).[33] For each cell lineage, cell specific transcription depends on critical deoxyribonucleic acid–binding motifs in promoters or enhancers. Differentiation in the erythroid series depends on the presence of GATA-binding and AP-1/NFE2 binding proteins, and on the presence of TAL1/SCL, EKLF, and RBTN2 factors.[33] The crucial role of these factors has been established with gene targeting and generation of knockout animals.[34, 35]

Erythroid progenitors found in the liver, bone marrow, or peripheral blood of the fetus appear to produce identical quantities of fetal hemoglobin.[36] Fetal erythropoiesis results in the orderly evolution of a series of different hemoglobins. Developmentally, there are embryonic, fetal, and adult hemoglobins (Table 2–2). Globin genes are arranged in order of expression in the α- and β-globin clusters and are selectively activated and silenced at the various stages of erythroid development. Distal, cis-regulatory elements in the β-globin–like cluster are contained in the locus control region, which comprises four hypersensitivity sites.[37] Figure 2–1 presents some of the postulated interactions involved in gene switching for the human β-globin gene cluster.

The first globin chains to be produced are the ε chains, which appear to be similar to β chains in certain aspects of their structural sequences.[38] Before the onset of other chain formation, these unpaired globin chains may form tetramers (ϵ_4), resulting in the presence of hemoglobin (Hb) Gower-1. Almost immediately thereafter, α and ζ chain production begins, and Hb Gower 2 ($\alpha_2\epsilon_2$) and Hb Portland ($\zeta_2\gamma_2$) are formed. Early γ chain formation also results in the presence of fetal hemoglobin ($\alpha_2\gamma_2$). By the time the fetus has a crown-rump length of about 16 mm (about 37 days of gestation), Hbs Gower-1 and Gower-2 constitute 42% and 24% of the total hemoglobin, respectively, with fetal hemoglobin making up the remainder.[39] At a crown-rump length of about 30 mm, Hb F represents 50% of the total hemoglobin, and at a length of 50 mm it forms more than 90% of the hemoglobin. Very small quantities of Hb A are found beginning at 6 to 8 weeks of gestation.

Although Hb Portland may constitute as much as 20% of the hemoglobin at 10 weeks of gestation, only trace amounts are normally present at birth. The ζ chain is quite similar to the α chain in its amino acid sequences.[40] Studies of steady-state liver messenger ribonucleic acid globin levels in human embryos (gestational age, 10 to 25 weeks) indicate that levels of globin proteins are regulated by the relative amounts of each globin messenger ribonucleic acid.[41]

The absolute rate of synthesis of hemoglobin or formation of red cells during fetal life is difficult to estimate, because neither the absolute increase in circulating hemoglobin or red cells nor the absolute destruction rate is known. The absolute rate of production of red cells at birth, however, can be estimated fairly well. A value of 2.5% to 3.0% per day of the circulating red cell mass, or about 4.5 mL per day in a 3.5-kg infant, can be calculated on the basis of determinations of the relative number of circulating reticulocytes and determinations of the in vitro mean life span

Table 2-2. GLOBIN CHAIN DEVELOPMENT

Stage	Hemoglobin	Composition
Embryo	Gower 1	ϵ_4 or $\zeta_2\epsilon_2$
Embryo	Gower 2	$\alpha_2\epsilon_2$
Embryo	Portland	$\zeta_2\gamma_2$
Embryo	Fetal	$\alpha_2\gamma_2$
Fetus	Fetal	$\alpha_2\gamma_2$
Fetus	A	$\alpha_2\beta_2$
Adult	A	$\alpha_2\beta_2$
Adult	A$_2$	$\alpha_2\delta_2$
Adult	F	$\alpha_2\gamma_2$

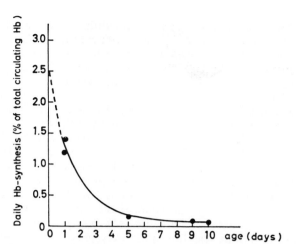

Figure 2–2. The relative rate of hemoglobin synthesis at birth and during the first 10 days of life. (From Garby L, Sjölin S, et al: Studies on erythrokinetics in infancy. III. Plasma disappearance and red cell uptake of intravenously injected radioiron. Acta Paediatr 1963; 52:537.)

of reticulocytes obtained from cord blood.[42] A very similar figure was obtained on the basis of an analysis of the distribution kinetics of radioiron in the plasma and in the red cells[43] (Fig. 2–2).

Measurements of the circulating red cell volume in newborn infants at various gestational ages shown in Figure 2–3 demonstrated an increase in the red cell volume of about 1.5% per day. Assuming a mean life span of these cells of 45 to 70 days (discussed later in this chapter), these data show a production rate of 3.6% to 4.2% per day of the red cell volume 2 months before term and a rate of 2.5% to 3.5% per day of the red cell volume at term. The combined data, therefore, indicate very strongly that the rate of red cell production during the latter part of fetal life is quite high—about three-

to fivefold that of a normal adult subject. This finding is in agreement with the well-established facts that, at the same period of development, all of the bones are filled with red marrow, the concentration of red cell precursors per unit volume of marrow is markedly increased,[44–46] and the number of erythroid and granulocyte-monocyte progenitors in cord blood is greater than that of normal adult blood.[47]

Erythropoiesis After Birth

The rate of hemoglobin synthesis and red cell production decreases dramatically during the first few days after delivery. The production of red cells (or hemoglobin) decreases by a factor of 2 to 3 during the first few days after birth, and by a factor of about 10 during the first week of life. This sudden and marked decrease in red cell production is undoubtedly initiated by the equally sudden increase in the tissue oxygen level that takes place at birth. This is reflected by the virtual disappearance of erythropoietin in the plasma.[48] At the time of birth, between 55% and 65% of the total hemoglobin synthesis consists of Hb F.[49] Thereafter, the synthesis of Hb F decreases much more rapidly than that of Hb A; the time course is shown in Figure 2–4. The switching from Hb F to Hb A is delayed in infants of diabetic mothers,[50] in metabolic diseases characterized by the inability to metabolize propionic acid,[51] and in chronic bronchopulmonary dysplasia.[52] Hb F synthesis can also be "reactivated" in severe cases of anemia of prematurity.[53] The rate of production of red cells (and of hemoglobin), which reaches a minimum during the second week of life, increases during the following months and reaches a maximum, at about 3 months of age, of approximately 2 mL of packed red cells per day, or about 2% of the circulating red cell mass per day.

Figure 2–3. The circulating red blood cell mass in newborn infants in relation to the gestational age. ● = by ^{51}Cr-dilution method; △, □, = from plasma volume measurements. (From Bratteby L-E: Studies on erythrokinetics in infancy. X. Red cell volume of newborn infants in relation to gestational age. Acta Pediatr Scand 1968; 57:132.)

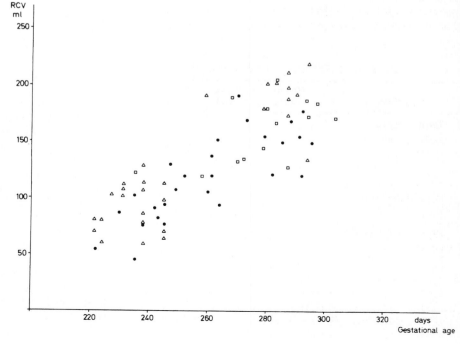

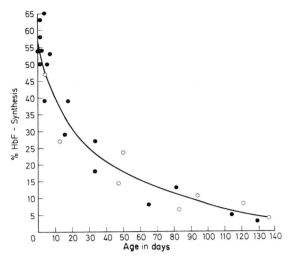

Figure 2–4. The time course of the relative synthesis of hemoglobin F (HbF) in normal infants during the first 140 days of life. ● = Radioiron method; ○ = reticulocyte method. (From Garby L, Sjölin S, et al: Studies on erythrokinetics in infancy. II. The relative rate of synthesis of haemoglobin F and haemoglobin A during the first months of life. Acta Paediatr 1962; 51:245.)

Life Span of the Erythrocyte

The life span of erythrocytes obtained from term infants is somewhat shorter than that of red cells from the adult, whereas the life span of red cells obtained from premature infants is considerably shorter. The more immature the infant, the greater the degree of reduction.

Because of their relative simplicity, studies employing ^{51}Cr have been used most extensively. Results of numerous investigators are summarized in Table 2–3. These data indicate that the mean ^{51}Cr half-life of erythrocytes from term infants is 23.3 days (range, 13 to 35 days), whereas the mean value for red cells from premature infants is 16.6 days (range, 9 to 26 days). These values contrast with a half-life of 26 to 35 days

Table 2–3. REPORTED ^{51}Cr SURVIVAL DATA

Author(s)	No. of Cases	Range (d)	Average (d)
Term Infants			
Hollingsworth	6	13–23	18.2
Giblett	10	—	20.0
Foconi and Sjölin	10	17–25	22.8
Vest	8	20–27	23.5
Gilardi and Miescher	3	21–26	23.5
Kaplan and Hsu	14	21–35	26.8
Total	51	13–35	23.3
Premature Infants			
Foconi and Sjölin	6	10–18	15.8
Kaplan and Hsu	11	9–26	17.8
Vest	7	15–19	16.0
Gilardi and Miescher	7	15–19	16.1
Total	31	9–26	16.6

From Pearson HA: Life span of the fetal red blood cell. J Pediatr 1967; 70:166.

obtained in studies on normal adults. Conversion of these fetal red cell life spans for term infants from ^{51}Cr half-life to true red cell survival indicates an actual life span of approximately 60 to 70 days. Similar calculations for the red cells of premature infants yield values of 35 to 50 days.

Wranne,[49] using the carbon monoxide technique, found that 1.5% of the term infant's red cell mass was broken down daily during the first week of life. Wranne concluded that the life span of most erythrocytes formed during the late fetal and early neonatal period is only 90 days. Equations derived from accumulated data led Bratteby and Garby[54] to the conclusion that the mean life span of cells produced during the last 60 days of fetal life was between 45 and 70 days and that the life span frequency was skewed, with a majority of the cells dying before the mean life span was achieved.

No unifying hypothesis has been presented to explain why the red cells produced in fetal life have a shortened life span. Landaw and Guancial[55] demonstrated a similar shortening of life span of erythrocytes obtained from the fetal rat. In their studies, the decrease in life span correlated with red cell rigidity, as reflected by red cell filtration studies.[56] These observations suggest that alterations in membrane function may ultimately be responsible for the decreased life span of the fetal erythrocytes obtained from humans.

Unique Characteristics of the Neonatal Erythrocyte

The Red Cell Membrane

Simple clinical laboratory studies as well as sophisticated biochemical procedures have provided evidence that the red cell membrane of fetal erythrocytes differs from that of its adult counterpart.

The red cells from normal newborns are slightly more resistant to osmotic lysis than are those of adults.[57] A minor population of cells with increased osmotic fragility also is present; however, these cells appear to be selectively destroyed within the first several days after birth.[58] The mechanical fragility of cord blood red cells also is increased.[59, 60] Neonatal reticulocytes are mostly composed of motile R1 reticulocytes,[61] which have been shown to be capable of performing receptor-mediated endocytosis.[62] Neonatal red cells have increased total and membrane-associated myosin content compared with adult red cells[63]; possibly, this increased content is a remnant of these cells' motile machinery.

Figure 2–5 presents flow cytometric measurements of cell volume and hemoglobin concentration in neonatal red cells compared with adult red cells. Measurements of reticulocyte indices in neonatal and adult blood also are presented. Neonatal red cells have larger volumes and lower cell hemoglobin concentrations than do adult cells. Neonatal reticulocytes also have larger volumes and lower hemoglobin concentrations than do adult reticulocytes.

The red cells of normal newborns also appear differ-

RED CELLS

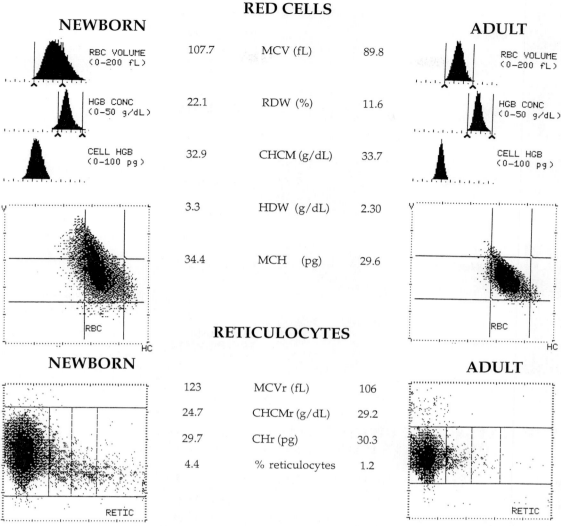

NEWBORN				ADULT
107.7	MCV (fL)	89.8		
22.1	RDW (%)	11.6		
32.9	CHCM (g/dL)	33.7		
3.3	HDW (g/dL)	2.30		
34.4	MCH (pg)	29.6		

RETICULOCYTES

NEWBORN   ADULT

123	MCVr (fL)	106
24.7	CHCMr (g/dL)	29.2
29.7	CHr (pg)	30.3
4.4	% reticulocytes	1.2

Figure 2-5. Red blood cell and reticulocyte indices in neonatal and adult blood. *Top,* Histograms for red blood cell (RBC) volume, RBC hemoglobin (Hb) concentration, and RBC Hb content obtained in a newborn *(left)* and an adult *(right)*. *Bottom,* Reticulocyte analysis for newborn and adult RBCs. The staining intensity of reticulocytes (x-axis) is plotted against the cell Hb concentration (y-axis).

ent by conventional light microscopy, interference phase microscopy, and electron microscopy. Zipursky and co-workers,[64] employing careful analysis of wet preparations suspended in 0.2% glutaraldehyde, observed that 78% of erythrocytes from adults appeared as biconcave discs and 18% as "bowl" forms; in contrast, only 43% of cells from term infants appeared as discs and 40% appeared as bowl forms. In addition, only up to 3% of cells from normal adults appeared as assorted spherocytes and poikilocytes of various types, whereas up to 14% of cells from term infants showed these morphologic distortions.

In premature infants, the departure from normal adult cells was even more marked. In these infants, 40% of the cells were discs, 30% were bowls, and 27% displayed a variety of morphologic disturbances (Fig. 2–6). The high frequency of dysmorphology in hematologically normal neonates creates great difficulty in diagnosing specific disorders of the red cell at birth.

When the dysmorphology is severe, the condition is sometimes called "infantile pyknocytosis." In this usually transient disorder, the red cell life span is even shorter than normal,[65] and the disorder may represent a neonatal form of hereditary ovalocytosis (see Chapter 16). Using interference phase microscopy, Holroyde and associates[66] observed that the red cells from both premature and term infants displayed the "pocked" appearance that was first observed by Nathan and Gunn in splenectomized patients with thalassemia.[67] These surface alterations are believed to reflect the presence of vacuoles and internal structures just below the red cell membrane. They were observed in greatest numbers among the most immature infants. Similar surface abnormalities are seen in patients without spleens and in patients with sickle cell hemoglobinopathies with reduced splenic function.[66, 68] The presence of these red cell "pocks" is presumed to reflect impaired splenic function in the immature infant but also may

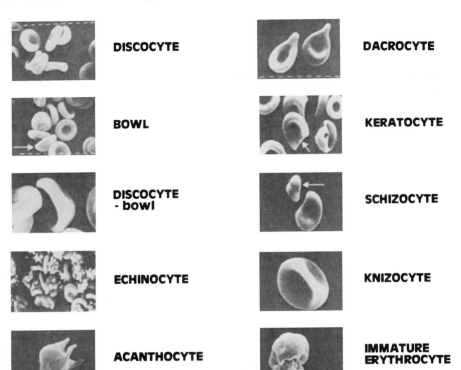

Figure 2-6. The variety of morphologic abnormalities of the erythrocyte observed in premature infants, term infants, and normal adults. (Photomicrographs courtesy of Zipursky, Brown, and Brown.) (Adapted from Zipursky A, Brown E, et al: The erythrocyte differential count in newborn infants. Am J Pediatr Hematol Oncol 1983; 5:45.)

THE ERYTHROCYTE DIFFERENTIAL COUNT
(Median and 5% to 95% range)

Cell Type	Premature Infant	Term Infant	Normal Adult
Discocyte	39.5 (18-57)	43 (18-62)	78 (42-94)
Bowl	29.0 (13-53)	40 (14-58)	18 (4-50)
Discocyte-Bowl	3.0 (0-10)	2 (0-5)	2 (0-4)
Spherocyte	0.0 (0-3)	0 (0-1)	0 (0-0)
Echinocyte	5.5 (1-23)	1 (0-4)	0 (0-3)
Acanthocyte	0.0 (0-2)	1 (0-2)	0 (0-1)
Dacrocyte	1.0 (0-5)	1 (0-3)	0 (0-1)
Keratocyte	3.0 (0-7)	2 (0-5)	0 (0-1)
Schizocyte	2.0 (0-5)	0 (0-2)	0 (0-1)
Knizocyte	3.0 (0-11)	3 (0-8)	1 (0-5)
Immature erythrocyte	1.0 (0-6)	0 (0-2)	0 (0-0)

be a reflection of the tendency of fetal erythrocytes for increased vesicle formation, which overwhelms the clearance capacity of the spleen.[69, 70]

Examination of fetal red cells with electron microscopy also reveals the presence of vacuoles and internal structures just below the cell membrane.[71, 72] Freeze-etching and transmission electron microscopy of fetal erythrocyte membranes indicate that the protoplasmic fracture faces have 24% more intramembrane particles than do those of adult cells and that the number of particles on exoplasmic fracture faces exceeds that of the adult by 45%.[73]

The membrane of the fetal erythrocytes also appears to be more fluid than that of adult cells. Both ferritin-labeled anti-A antibodies[72] and concanavalin A[74] are taken up by endocytosis in the mature erythrocytes of newborn infants but not by cells from normal adults. This unique phenomenon does not appear to be the result of differences in the lipid viscosity of the membrane.[75]

Compared with adult cells, the membrane of the erythrocytes of the newborn has more binding sites for insulin,[76] more insulin-like growth factor,[77] and more prolactin[78]; however, it has fewer digoxin receptor sites[79] and reduced membrane acetylcholinesterase.[80] The membrane proteins from both premature and term infants are indistinguishable from those from the normal adult when solubilized in sodium dodecyl sulfate and analyzed with polyacrylamide gel electrophoresis.[74, 75]

The red cells of the cord blood of full-term infants contain increased quantities of total lipid, lipid phosphorus, and cholesterol per cell, although the percentages of total lipid composed of lipid phosphorus and cholesterol are similar to those found in the adult.[81] These erythrocytes have a greater percentage of their phospholipid as sphingomyelin and a lesser portion as lecithin. Phospholipid fatty acid patterns in cord blood erythrocytes have a greater percentage of palmitic, stearic, arachidonic, and combined 22- and 24-carbon fatty acids and a lesser proportion of oleic and linoleic acid. The cells are much more prone to lipid peroxidation on oxidant challenge.[82] It is likely that the relative hyposplenism of the neonate contributes to these membrane alterations.

From an immunologic perspective, the erythrocyte membrane of the newborn also is different from that of the adult. At birth, the Lewis system of absorbed serum antigens is incompletely expressed, partly because the receptor sites of the membrane are weak or absent. In the ABO system, the A antigen, particularly the A_1 antigen, and the B antigen sites are weakly expressed, and in the Ii system, the I antigen is either weak or absent. Other weakly expressed antigens are Sd^a, P1, Lu^a, Lu^b, Yt^a, Xg, and Vel.[83]

The cells are less permeable to the nonelectrolytes glycerol and thiourea[84]; they display a reduced potassium influx via the Na^+,K^+-ATPase and the Na^+, K^+,Cl^- cotransport systems[85] and altered kinetics of glucose transfer[86]; and they are prone to acid lysis.[87] The number of Na^+-K^+ pumps, estimated from ouabain binding, is increased in premature infants compared with term infants.[87a] Chloride and bicarbonate transport systems of fetal and adult red cells are similar.[88]

The filtration rate of red blood cells from preterm and term infants is lower than that of adults.[89–91] This decreased filterability may be a manifestation of the larger size of the erythrocytes from the newborn rather than of their different lipid composition.

Metabolism of the Erythrocytes of the Newborn Infant

(Table 2–4)

Enzymes of the Embden-Meyerhof Pathway. Numerous investigators[92–96] are in agreement that the activities of the enzymes phosphoglycerate kinase and enolase in the red cells of the newborn infant are much more intense than would be anticipated from their young cell age. The activity of the enzymes glyceraldehyde-3-phosphate dehydrogenase and glucose phosphate isomerase also is probably significantly greater than would be anticipated from the cell age.[94]

The activity of phosphofructokinase (PFK), a rate-controlling enzyme in glycolysis, has repeatedly been found to be lower than normal in the red cells of newborn infants.

The decreased PFK activity so characteristic of fetal red cells may reflect the accelerated decay of an unstable enzyme. Travis and Garvin[97] fractionated cord blood red cells into cohorts of varying cell age and compared them with adult red cells that were fractionated in a similar fashion. The rate of decline of pyruvate kinase activity was essentially the same in neonates and adults, whereas PFK activity in cord erythrocytes decreased at a significantly greater rate when compared with that of adults.

The studies of Vora and Piomelli[98] have provided a clear understanding of the nature of PFK in the fetal erythrocyte. They found that human muscle and liver PFKs are homotetramers, each of which is composed of identical subunits, which they termed "M_4" and "L_4."

Study of adult erythrocytes revealed the presence of three heterotetramers—M_3L, M_2L_2, and ML_3. Analysis of cord blood erythrocytes revealed the presence of the three heterotetramers in the adult erythrocytes; the L_4 isoenzyme was also identified. The presence of the liver homotetramer in the fetal erythrocytes may be responsible for the decreased PFK stability observed by Travis and Garvin.[97]

Differences in the distribution of other red cell isoenzymes have also been described. Hemolysates normally contain two isoenzymes of hexokinase, types I and III. Holmes and co-workers[99] found that in the cells of the newborn infant, type II hexokinase was the predominant isoenzyme. Schroter and Tillman,[100] in contrast, observed that type I predominated, although the predominance of type I was not characteristic of young cells in general but was a unique feature of the red cells of the newborn infant. Chen and associates[101] also observed differences in the distribution of hexokinase isoenzymes obtained from first trimester and midtrimester fetuses.

Enolase also exists as multiple isoenzymes in erythrocytes, and the distribution of enolase isoenzymes appears to be a unique characteristic of fetal erythrocytes.[102]

Chen and associates[101] studied a total of 26 enzyme patterns in hemolysates prepared from 11 fetuses that ranged in gestational age from 65 to 138 days. Six enzymes—enolase, guanylate kinase, lactate dehydrogenase, nucleoside phosphorylase, PFK, and the previously mentioned hexokinase—showed differences in the staining intensity of certain isoenzyme zones as compared with adult controls. The fetal red cell zymograms contained the mitochondrial forms of isocitric dehydrogenase and aspartate transaminase as well as more definite zones of phosphoglucomutase type 3.

Glucose Consumption. Glucose consumption by the erythrocytes of both the term and the premature infant has generally been found to be greater than that observed in the cells of the normal adult.[103, 104] This would be anticipated in view of the fact that young red cells consume more glucose. However, when the cells from infants are compared with adult cell populations of similar young age, their rate of glucose consumption appears to be less than would be expected.[103]

Table 2-4. METABOLIC CHARACTERISTICS OF THE ERYTHROCYTES OF THE NEWBORN

Carbohydrate Metabolism

Glucose consumption increased
Galactose more completely utilized as substrate both under normal circumstances and for methemoglobin reduction*
Decreased activity of sorbitol pathway*
Decreased triokinase activity*

Glycolytic Enzymes

Increased activity of hexokinase, phosphoglucose isomerase,* aldolase, glyceraldehyde 3-phosphate,* phosphoglycerate
   kinase,* phosphoglycerate mutase, enolase,* pyruvate kinase, lactate dehydrogenase, glucose-6-phosphate
   dehydrogenase 6-phosphogluconic dehydrogenase, galactokinase, and galactose 1-phosphate uridyltransferase
Decrease activity of phosphofructokinase*
Different distribution of hexokinase isoenzymes*

Nonglycolytic Enzymes

Increased activity of aspartate transaminase and glutathione reductase
Decreased activity of NADP-dependent methemoglobin reductase,* catalase,* gluthathione peroxidase, superoxide
   dismutase, carbonic anhydrase,* adenylate kinase,* and glutathione synthetase*
Presence of α-glycerol-3-phosphate dehydrogenase*

ATP and Phosphate Metabolism

Decreased phosphate uptake,* slower incorporation into ATP and 2,3-diphosphoglycerate*
Accelerated decline of 2,3-diphosphoglycerate upon red blood cell incubation*
Increased ATP and 2,3-diphosphoglycerate levels
Accelerated decline of APT during brief incubation

Storage Characteristics

Increased potassium efflux and greater degrees of hemolysis during short periods of storage
More rapid assumption of altered morphologic forms upon storage or incubation*

Membrane

Decreased ouabain-sensitive Na^+, K^+-ATPase*; decreased ouabain-resistant potassium influx*
Decreased permeability to glycerol and thiourea*
Decreased membrane deformability*
Increased sphingomyelin, decreased lecithin content of stromal phospholipids
Decreased content of linoleic acid*
Increased lipid phosphorus and cholesterol per cell
Greater affinity for glucose*
Increased number of insulin, insulin-like growth factor, and prolactin binding sites
Increased membrane-associated myosin
Reduced membrane acetylcholinestrase activity

Other

Increased methemoglobin content*
Increased affinity of hemoglobin for oxygen*
Glutathione instability*
Increased tendency for Heinz body formation in presence of oxidant compounds*

NADP = nicotinamide-adenine dinucleotide phosphate; ATP = adenosine triphosphate; ATPase = adenosine triphosphatase.
*Appears to be a unique characteristic of the newborn's erythrocytes and not merely a function of the presence of young red blood cells.

Circumstantial evidence exists to suggest that the relative deficiency of PFK may be responsible for this relative impairment of glycolysis. All strategies designed to maximize PFK activity produce a far greater augmentation of glucose consumption in the cells of the neonate. Incubation of cells at high phosphate concentration[105] causes cells of both premature and term infants to consume glucose at rates commensurate with their age. Increasing the pH of the incubation media produces a much greater increase in red cell glucose consumption[106] in cells from the newborn infant. Analysis of glycolytic intermediates reveals that as the pH increases, there is a decrease in the levels of glucose-6-phosphate and fructose-6-phosphate and an increase in the concentration of fructose 1,6-diphosphate, glyceraldehyde 3-phosphate, dihydroxyacetone phosphate, and 2,3-diphosphoglycerate (2,3,-DPG). All of these changes are consistent with an activation of PFK. It would appear that this pH-induced augmentation of

PFK obscures the relative deficiency that manifests itself as a lower-than-expected glucose consumption at pH 7.4.

Further evidence that the relative deficiency of PFK may play the major role in depressing glucose consumption in the newborn comes from incubation of neonatal red cells with methylene blue, 10^{-6} mol. At this concentration of methylene blue, 90% of glucose consumption proceeds via the pentose-phosphate pathway, which bypasses the PFK step. The incubation of red cells from newborn infants in the presence of methylene blue produces a far greater acceleration of glycolysis than is observed either in the red cells of normal adults or in those of subjects with reticulocytosis.[107]

Finally, when one examines the oldest cells from the cord blood of the newborn infant, the profound PFK deficiency that was previously described is found to be associated with a marked decrease in glucose consumption and a pattern of glycolytic intermediates that suggests that a relative block in glycolysis is present at this step.

2,3-Diphosphoglycerate Metabolism. When the red cells of infants and adults are incubated under identical conditions, the concentration of 2,3 DPG declines far more rapidly in the erythrocytes of the newborn than in those of the adult.[108, 109] Three postulates have been advanced to explain this 2,3-DPG instability. Zipursky and co-workers[108] presented evidence to suggest that a relative block in glycolysis, proximal to the formation of glyceraldehyde-3-phosphate, was responsible for the failure to maintain 2,3-DPG levels. Schröter and Winter[109] proposed that in the red cells of the newborn, the synthesis of 3-phosphoglycerate was favored over the synthesis of 2,3-DPG because of the increased glycolytic rate, the increased activity of phosphoglycerate kinase, and the slight elevation in the red cell adenosine diphosphate concentration. Trueworthy and Lowman[110] proposed that the instability of 2,3-DPG was a result of an accelerated rate of hydrolysis as a consequence of increased 2,3-DPG phosphatase activity. The 2,3-DPG content of normal fetal red cells is greater than that of adult cells and is further increased in anemic fetuses, possibly as a consequence of the relative preponderance of PFK activity over pyruvate kinase activity.[111]

The Pentose-Phosphate Pathway and Response to Oxidant-Induced Injury. Oxidative stress induced by the formation of O_2, H_2O_2, or related species is handled within the red cell by the combined activities of hexose monophosphate shunt (NADPH [nicotinamide-adenine dinucleotide phosphate, reduced] generation), glutathione peroxidase, catalase, and superoxide dismutase. There is general agreement that the red cells from newborn infants are more susceptible to oxidant induced injury than adult cells.[112–114]

Fetal hemoglobin is more prone than adult hemoglobin to denaturation; however, there is no relationship between the fetal hemoglobin content of the cell and the tendency to form Heinz bodies. The pentose-phosphate pathway in the cells of both the term and the premature infant is intact and responds appropriately to oxidant-induced stimulation.[107, 115] The cell content of glutathione is normal in neonatal erythrocytes.[116] The activity of glutathione peroxidase is decreased in comparison with that of adult cells[117, 118]; however, metabolic studies have failed to demonstrate a convincing direct relationship between this relative deficiency and the oxidant vulnerability.[115, 119] A slight decrease in superoxide dismutase activity has been observed in fetal red cells.[120] It would appear that the relative deficiencies of glutathione peroxidase and catalase[121] may act in concert with plasma factors[122] to produce this metabolic handicap. Vitamin E plays a crucial role in limiting membrane lipid auto-oxidation. Vitamin E deficiency has been observed in the plasma of full-term and premature newborns.[123]

Suggestions that other factors are implicated come from the observations that the red cells of the newborn infant, when compared with those of adults, have a decreased number of membrane SH groups,[124] that the membranes isolated from them contain more residual hemoglobin and form Heinz bodies faster,[125] and that, following the transfusion of adult cells into newborn infants, these cells also appear to be more prone to develop Heinz bodies.[126, 127]

The red cells from newborn infants, like other young red cells, consume more oxygen and produce more hydrogen peroxide[128, 129] than do the red cells of adults.

Cord blood erythrocytes have been demonstrated to possess L-α-glycerol-3-phosphate dehydrogenase activity, whereas this enzyme is lacking in the red cells of normal adults.[130] Although the reticulocytes of normal adults appear to lack this enzyme, it seems to be present in the erythrocytes of patients with both β-thalassemias minor and major.[131]

HEMATOLOGIC VALUES AT BIRTH

Several variables influence the interpretation of what might be considered normal values for hemoglobin, hematocrit, red cell indices, and reticulocyte count at the time of birth and during the early weeks of life. These variables include the gestational age of the infant, the conduct of labor and the treatment of the umbilical vessels, the site of sampling, and the time of sampling. The Appendix of this text contains a series of tables describing representative norms that have appeared in the literature. A few of these norms are highlighted in the following discussion to illustrate pertinent points.

Site of Sampling

Capillary samples obtained by skin prick, generally from the heel or toe, have a higher hemoglobin concentration than do simultaneously collected venous samples. During the first hours of life, this difference averages approximately 3.5 g/dL,[131] as is illustrated in Figure 2–7. In some instances, the capillary hemoglobin–venous hemoglobin difference may exceed 10 g/dL.[132]

The clinical importance of the site of sampling was illustrated by Moe[132] in a study of 54 infants with erythroblastosis fetalis. Simultaneously obtained cord blood and capillary samples were compared. In this study, 41 infants eventually required exchange transfusion for hyperbilirubinemia. Of these 41 infants, 25 were found to be anemic, based on determinations performed on cord blood samples, whereas only 14 could be considered anemic on the basis of the results of capillary sample analysis.

In virtually all infants, the capillary-to-venous hematocrit ratio is greater than 1.00. The greatest ratios, often in excess of 1.20, are observed in infants born before 30 weeks of gestation, infants with arterial blood pH values below 7.20, infants with hypotension, and infants with a red cell mass of less than 35 mL/kg.[133] In other words, the capillary hemoglobin values are falsely elevated in the sickest infants. These are the same infants in whom an accurate determination of hemoglobin concentration is most important in clinical

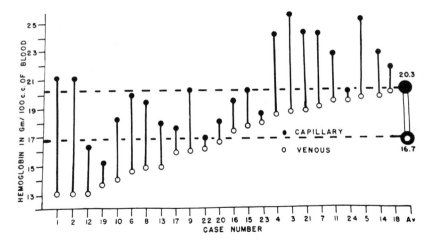

Figure 2-7. Simultaneous capillary and venous Hb determinations in 24 newborn infants. (From Oettinger L, Mills W B: Simultaneous capillary and venous hemoglobin determinations in newborn infants. J Pediatr 1949; 35:362.)

management. The capillary-to-venous hematocrit ratio gradually decreases with increasing gestational age.[133] Infants born between 26 and 30 weeks of gestation have a mean ratio of 1.21; infants born at 31 to 32 weeks, 1.12; infants born at 33 to 35 weeks, 1.16; and infants born between 36 and 41 weeks, 1.12. By the fifth day of life, the capillary-to-venous difference has decreased in healthy infants, and capillary samples may have a hematocrit that is only 2.5% higher when blood is obtained by deep stick from a well-warmed heel.

Treatment of the Umbilical Vessels

At birth, the blood volume of the infant may be increased by as much as 61% if complete emptying of the placental vessels is allowed before the cord is clamped.[134, 135] It has been estimated that the placental vessels contain 75 to 125 mL of blood at birth—or one quarter to one third of the fetal blood volume. Under normal circumstances, about one quarter of the placental transfusion takes place within 15 seconds of birth and one half by the end of the first minute. The ratio of blood in the neonatal and the placental circulations

has been found to average 67:33 at birth, 80:20 at 1 minute, and 87:13 at the end of the placental transfusion.[135]

The umbilical arteries generally constrict shortly after birth, so that no blood flows from the infant to the mother; however, the umbilical vein remains dilated, permitting blood to flow in the direction of gravity. Infants held below the level of the placenta continue to gain blood; infants held above the placenta may bleed into it.[136] Yao and co-workers[135] demonstrated that hydrostatic pressure, produced by placing the infant 40 cm below the mother's introitus, hastened placental transfusion to virtual completion in 30 seconds. In infants delivered at term with cesarean section, maximal placental transfusion is achieved within 40 seconds after birth; however, net blood flow reverses, with blood traveling from the infant back to the placenta, if the clamping is delayed for longer than 40 seconds.[137]

The effects of placental transfusion on the total blood volume of the infant show wide variability. This is partially because of the techniques employed and partially because of the time at which the samples were taken. During the first hours after birth, plasma apparently leaves the circulation. It seems that the greater

Table 2-5. EFFECT OF CORD CLAMPING ON HEMATOCRIT AND HEMOGLOBIN CONCENTRATION AT VARIOUS TIMES AFTER DELIVERY

| | Early Clamping | | Delayed Clamping | | |
Reference	Hb (g/dL)	Hct (%)	Hb (g/dL)	Hct (%)	Time of Study
Phillips (1941)	15.6	—	19.3	—	20–30 h
Marsh et al. (1948)	17.4	—	20.8	—	3rd day
Colozzi (1954)	14.7	—	17.3	—	72 h
Lanzkowsky (1960)	18.1	—	19.7	—	72–96 h
	11.1	—	11.1	—	3 mo
Linderkamp et al. (1992)[138]		48 ± 4		50 ± 4	At birth
		47 ± 5		63 ± 5	2 h
		43 ± 6		59 ± 5	24 h
		44 ± 5		59 ± 6	120 h
Kinmond et al. (1993)[141]		50.9 ± 4.5		56.4 ± 4.8	Not standardized
Nelle et al. (1993)[139]		48 ± 6		58 ± 6	2 h
		44 ± 5		56 ± 7	24 h
		44 ± 5		54 ± 8	5 d

Hb = hemoglobin; Hct = hematocrit.

Table 2-6. HEMATOLOGIC VALUES FOR NORMAL CORD BLOOD*

Parameter	Mean ± SD
Hb (g/dL)	15.3 ± 1.3
Hct (%)	49 ± 5
RBC count (× 10⁶/mm³)	4.3 ± 0.4
MCV (fL)	112 ± 6
MCH (pg)	36.2 ± 2.2
MCHC (g/dL)	30.9 ± 1.3
CHCM (g/dL)	30.4 ± 1.2
% Hypo (MCHC < 28 g/dL)	17.3 ± 11.9
% Hyper (MCHC > 41 g/dL)	0.6 ± 0.3
% Micro (MCV < 61 fL)	0.8 ± 0.3
% Macro (MCV > 120 fL)	31.8 ± 9.7
Reticulocytes	
%	3.63 ± 1.11
MCVr (fL)	125.8 ± 7.3
CHCMr (g/dL)	25.6 ± 1.2
CHr (pg)	31.3 ± 1.4

RBC = red blood cell; MCV = mean corpuscular volume; MCVr = mean corpuscular volume, reticulocytes; MCH = mean corpuscular hemoglobin; MCHC = mean corpuscular hemoglobin volume; CHCM = cell hemoglobin concentration, mean; CHCMr = CHCM of reticulocytes; CHr = cell hemoglobin content of reticulocytes.
*Values obtained with Technicon H•2 and H•3 hematology analyzers (Bayer Diagnostics) in neonates delivered at term with weight ≥2500 g. These data were kindly provided by Dr. Gil Tchernia, Laboratoire d'Hématologie, Centre Hospitalier de Bicêtre, Bicêtre, France.

the placental transfusion, the greater the plasma loss. Thus, by the third day of life, there are only small differences in total blood volume, regardless of the method of cord clamping. Usher found that infants with delayed cord clamping had an average blood volume of 93 mL/kg at an age of 72 hours; infants with immediate cord clamping had a blood volume of 82 mL/kg.[134] Although the total blood volume may be only slightly altered by the timing of the cord clamping, more significant differences can be observed in the red cell mass or hemoglobin concentration. In the study of Usher and associates,[134] infants with delayed cord clamping had an average red cell mass of 49 mL/kg at 72 hours of age, as compared with a red cell mass of only 31 mL/kg in infants with immediate cord clamping. The results of other investigators are listed in references[138, 139] and in Table 2–5.

These data indicate that infants with delayed cord clamping tend to have higher hemoglobin values during the first week of life than those whose clamping was not delayed. A reduced volume of red blood cells is associated with an increase in mortality among premature infants affected by respiratory distress syndrome.[140] Thus, delayed cord clamping could be particularly indicated for premature births. Studies have shown that delayed cord clamping in premature infants is associated with a significant reduction in transfusion requirements and improved outcome,[141] but not with reduced incidence of periventricular/intraventricular hemorrhages.[142]

There have been reports of circulatory overload and congestive cardiac failure in the settings of delayed cord clamping. "Symptomatic neonatal plethora" was observed in eight premature and three full-term infants.[143] Radiologic findings of volume overload[144] and reduced left ventricular performance[145] have been reported in infants with delayed cord clamping. For cesarean sections, a delay of 3 minutes in cord clamping has been associated with signs of respiratory and metabolic acidosis (reduced oxygen tension, pH, and elevated plasma lactate levels), indicating that earlier clamping may be preferable in this setting.[146]

Blood Volume

Both blood volume and red cell mass are influenced by the treatment of the cord vessels and by the clinical condition of the infant. Shortly after birth, the blood volume of term infants may range from 50 to 100 mL/kg, with the mean value being 85 mL/kg.[134, 147, 148] As previously discussed, the blood volume in infants with early cord clamping averages 78 mL/kg at 30 minutes of age, in contrast to a value of 98.6 mL/kg in infants with cords that were clamped late. By 72 hours of age, these differences are not as great; infants with early clamping have an average blood volume of 82 mL/kg, whereas infants with late clamping have an average of 93 mL/kg.

The blood volume of the premature infant ranges from 89 to 105 mL/kg during the first few days of life.[149, 150] This increased blood volume is primarily the result of an increase in plasma volume, with the total red cell volume per kilogram of body weight being quite similar to that of the term infant. The plasma volume decreases with increasing gestational age, except in infants with intrauterine growth retardation.[151]

For infants born at term, blood volumes are approximately 73 to 77 mL/kg by 1 month of life.[152, 153]

A reduced blood volume and a reduced red cell mass are frequently observed in infants with hyaline membrane disease[154] and in newborns delivered with a tight nuchal cord.[155] Approximately 16% of infants born with a nuchal cord are anemic in the neonatal period.[156] Infants born following late intrauterine asphyxia tend to have a greater blood volume and red cell mass.[155]

Hemoglobin, Hematocrit, Red Cell Count, and Red Cell and Reticulocyte Indices

Representative values for these hematologic measurements are presented in Tables 2–6 to 2–9. The hemoglo-

Table 2-7. NORMAL HEMATOLOGIC VALUES DURING FIRST 2 WEEKS OF LIFE IN TERM INFANT

	Cord Blood	Day 1	Day 3	Day 7	Day 14
Hb (g/dL)	16.8	18.4	17.8	17.0	16.8
Hct (%)	53.0	58.0	55.0	54.0	52.0
RBC count (mm³ × 10⁶)	5.25	5.8	5.6	5.2	5.1
MCV (fL)	107.0	108.0	99.0	98.0	96.0
MCH (pg)	34.0	35.0	33.0	32.5	31.5
MCHC (g/dL)	31.7	32.5	33.0	33.0	33.0
Reticulocytes (%)	3–7	3–7	1–3	0–1	0–1
Nucleated RBC/(mm³)	500.0	200.0	0–5	0	0
Platelets (1000/mm³)	290.0	192.0	213.0	248.0	252.0

Table 2–8. RED BLOOD CELL VALUES ON FIRST POSTNATAL DAY

	Gestational Age (wk)							
	24–25 (7)*	26–27 (11)	28–29 (7)	30–31 (25)	32–33 (23)	34–35 (23)	36–37 (20)	Term (19)
RBC count ($\times 10^6$/mm³)	4.65† ± 0.43†	4.73 ± 0.45	4.62 ± 0.75	4.79 ± 0.74	5.0 ± 0.76	5.09 ± 0.5	5.27 ± 0.68	5.14 ± 0.7
Hb (g/dL)	19.4 ± 1.5	19.0 ± 2.5	19.3 ± 1.8	19.1 ± 2.2	18.5 ± 2.0	19.6 ± 2.1	19.2 ± 1.7	19.3 ± 2.2
Hct (%)	63 ± 4	62 ± 8	60 ± 7	60 ± 8	60 ± 8	61 ± 7	64 ± 7	61 ± 7.4
MCV (fL)	135 ± 0.2	132 ± 14.4	131 ± 13.5	127 ± 12.7	123 ± 15.7	122 ± 10.0	121 ± 12.5	119 ± 9.4
Reticulocytes (%)	6.0 ± 0.5	9.6 ± 3.2	7.5 ± 2.5	5.8 ± 2.0	5.0 ± 1.9	3.9 ± 1.6	4.2 ± 1.8	3.2 ± 1.4
Weight (g)	725 ± 185	993 ± 194	1174 ± 128	1450 ± 232	1816 ± 192	1957 ± 291	2245 ± 213	—

*Number of infants.
†Mean values ± SD.
From Zaizov R, Matoth Y: Red cell values on the first postnatal day during the last 16 weeks of gestation. Am J Hematol 1976; 1:276. Copyright © 1976 Wiley-Liss. Reprinted by permission of Wiley-Liss, A Division of John Wiley and Sons, Inc.

Table 2–9. NORMAL HEMATOLOGIC VALUES DURING FIRST 12 WEEKS OF LIFE IN TERM INFANT

Age	No. of Cases	Hb (g/dL) ± 1 SD	RBC ($\times 10^6$/mm³) ± 1 SD	Hct (%) ± 1 SD	MCV (fL) ± 1 SD	MCHC (g/dL) ± 1 SD	Reticulocytes (%) ± 1 SD
Days							
1	19	19.0 ± 2.2	5.14 ± 0.7	61 ± 7.4	119 ± 9.4	31.6 ± 1.9	3.2 ± 1.4
2	19	19.0 ± 1.9	5.15 ± 0.8	60 ± 6.4	115 ± 7.0	31.6 ± 1.4	3.2 ± 1.3
3	19	18.7 ± 3.4	5.11 ± 0.7	62 ± 9.3	116 ± 5.3	31.1 ± 2.8	2.8 ± 1.7
4	10	18.6 ± 2.1	5.00 ± 0.6	57 ± 8.1	114 ± 7.5	32.6 ± 1.5	1.8 ± 1.1
5	12	17.6 ± 1.1	4.97 ± 0.4	57 ± 7.3	114 ± 8.9	30.9 ± 2.2	1.2 ± 0.2
6	15	17.4 ± 2.2	5.00 ± 0.7	54 ± 7.2	113 ± 10.0	32.2 ± 1.6	0.6 ± 0.2
7	12	17.9 ± 2.5	4.86 ± 0.6	56 ± 9.4	118 ± 11.2	32.0 ± 1.6	0.5 ± 0.4
Weeks							
1–2	32	17.3 ± 2.3	4.80 ± 0.8	54 ± 8.3	112 ± 19.0	32.1 ± 2.9	0.5 ± 0.3
2–3	11	15.6 ± 2.6	4.20 ± 0.6	46 ± 7.3	111 ± 8.2	33.9 ± 1.9	0.8 ± 0.6
3–4	17	14.2 ± 2.1	4.00 ± 0.6	43 ± 5.7	105 ± 7.5	33.5 ± 1.6	0.6 ± 0.3
4–5	15	12.7 ± 1.6	3.60 ± 0.4	36 ± 4.8	101 ± 8.1	34.9 ± 1.6	0.9 ± 0.8
5–6	10	11.9 ± 1.5	3.55 ± 0.2	36 ± 6.2	102 ± 10.2	34.1 ± 2.9	1.0 ± 0.7
6–7	10	12.0 ± 1.5	3.40 ± 0.4	36 ± 4.8	105 ± 12.0	33.8 ± 2.3	1.2 ± 0.7
7–8	17	11.1 ± 1.1	3.40 ± 0.4	33 ± 3.7	100 ± 13.0	33.7 ± 2.6	1.5 ± 0.7
8–9	13	10.7 ± 0.9	3.40 ± 0.5	31 ± 2.5	93 ± 12.0	34.1 ± 2.2	1.8 ± 1.0
9–10	12	11.2 ± 0.9	3.60 ± 0.3	32 ± 2.7	91 ± 9.3	34.3 ± 2.9	1.2 ± 0.6
10–11	11	11.4 ± 0.9	3.70 ± 0.4	34 ± 2.1	91 ± 7.7	33.2 ± 2.4	1.2 ± 0.7
11–12	13	11.3 ± 0.9	3.70 ± 0.3	33 ± 3.3	88 ± 7.9	34.8 ± 2.2	0.7 ± 0.3

From Matoth Y, Zalzov R, et al: Postnatal changes in some red cell parameters. Acta Paediatr Scand 1971; 60:317.

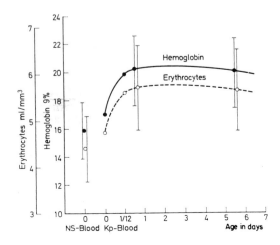

Figure 2–8. Hb concentration and RBC count in cord blood and in venous blood in normal infants during the first week of life. NS-Blood = cord blood; Kp-Blood = capillary blood; ml = million. (After Künzer, W: In Kepp R, Oehlert G (eds). Blutbildung und Blutumsatz beim Feter und Neugeborenen. Stuttgart, Ferdinand Enke, 1962, p 4.)

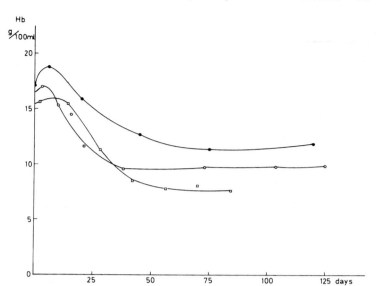

Figure 2–9. Hb concentration in infants of different degree of maturation at birth. ● = full-term infants; ○ = premature infants with birth weights of 1200 to 2350 g; □ = premature infants with birth weights less than 1200 g.

bin values increase gradually until approximately 32 to 33 weeks of gestation and remain relatively constant until term. The mean red cell volume (MCV) and mean reticulocyte count decline continuously during the course of gestation. Hematologic values from normal fetuses with gestational ages between 18 to 30 weeks reflect this trend.[157]

In healthy term infants, no measurable decrease in hemoglobin values occurs during the first week of life (Fig. 2–8); in contrast, in infants born weighing less than 1500 g but of appropriate weight for gestational age, the hemoglobin concentration may decrease by as much as 1.0 to 1.5 g/dL during this interval (Fig. 2–9).

Considerable differences are present in the peripheral blood cell counts and indices of infants born in developing countries. A study carried out by Tchernia's group in 199 newborns in Bomako (Mali) indicated that 32% were anemic (hemoglobin level < 13 g/dL).[158] When compared with a control group of French newborns, the Bamako groups had lower hemoglobin levels (13.9 ± 2.0 g/dL versus 15.1 ± 1.4 g/dL), lower mean corpuscular hemoglobin levels (32.9 ± 3.0 pg versus 35 ± 1.9 pg), lower serum ferritin levels (97.5 μg/L versus 135 mg/L, geometric means), and lower erythrocyte ferritin levels (244.7 ag per cell versus 348 ag per cell, geometric means). These differences cannot be explained by hemoglobinopathies, malaria, or folate deficiency, and they are probably due to iron deficiency.

FETAL ANEMIA

Improved diagnostic and therapeutic techniques have made possible the early identification and treatment of anemia in the fetus. The experience gained in the treatment *in utero* of hemolytic diseases of the fetus has been applied to a wide spectrum of pathologic conditions. Normal fetal hematologic values also are available[159] as a consequence of the development of percutaneous umbilical blood sampling and prenatal diagnosis (Table 2–10). A substantial portion of the cases of nonimmune fetal hydrops are due to chromosomal abnormalities[160] and thus presently are not treatable. Fetuses with hydrops fetalis and anemia have characteristic sonographic abnormalities (thickened placenta, less pleural effusion, less marked edema); these abnormalities aid in the distinction of infants with hydrops fetalis without anemia from those with anemia.[161] The major causes of treatable fetal anemias are listed in Table 2–11. Most of them are related to hemolytic disease of the fetus, hemoglobinopathies or severe red cell enzyme defects. A case of severe fetal anemia due to maternal acquired chronic pure red cell aplasia has also been described.[162] However, other pathologic conditions have been associated with anemia during the fetal period, such as hydrops fetalis in combination with either cystic hygroma[163] or placental chorioangioma,[164] parvovirus B19 infection,[165] and ma-

Table 2-10. EVOLUTION OF HEMATOLOGIC VALUES OF 163 FETUSES DURING PREGNANCY*

Week of Gestation	Hb (g/dL)	Hct (%)	RBC (10^9/L)	MCV (fL)	RDW (%)	MCH (pg)
18–20 (n = 25)	11.47 ± 0.78	35.86 ± 3.29	2.66 ± 0.29	133.92 ± 8.83	20.64 ± 2.28	43.14 ± 2.71
21–22 (n = 55)	12.28 ± 0.89	38.53 ± 3.21	2.96 ± 0.26	130.06 ± 6.17	20.15 ± 1.92	41.39 ± 3.32
23–25 (n = 61)	12.40 ± 0.77	38.59 ± 2.41	3.06 ± 0.26	126.19 ± 6.23	19.29 ± 1.62	40.48 ± 2.88
26–30 (n = 22)	13.35 ± 1.17	41.54 ± 3.31	3.52 ± 0.32	118.17 ± 5.75	18.35 ± 1.67	37.94 ± 3.67

RDW = red cell distribution width.
*Data ± SD. Studies performed with a Coulter Hematology Analyzer, model S-PLUS II.
Modified from Forestier F, Daffos F, et al: Hematological values of 163 normal fetuses between 18 and 30 weeks of gestation. Pediatr Res 1986; 20:342.

Table 2–11. FETAL ANEMIAS TREATABLE WITH
INTRAUTERINE TRANSFUSION

Immune
Hemolytic disease of the fetus
Nonimmune
Hemolytic: hemoglobinopathies (e.g., α-thalassemia
  (four-gene deletion)), G6PD deficiency
Nonhemolytic: acquired chronic pure red cell aplasia
Other
Severe antepartum fetomaternal hemorrhage
Twin-to-twin transfusion syndrome
Cystic hygroma with hydrops fetalis
Placenta chorioangioma
Intrauterine parvovirus B19 infection
Malaria

G6PD = glucose-6-phosphate dehydrogenase.

laria.[166] The literature on nonimmune hydrops fetalis also has been reviewed.[167]

ANEMIA IN THE NEONATE

Anemia present at birth or appearing during the first week of life can be broadly classified into three major categories: anemia as a result of blood loss, anemia as a result of a hemolytic process, or anemia secondary to less-than-normal red cell production. Many of the disorders producing a hemolytic process are discussed in greater detail in other sections of this text (see Chapter 3, Immune Hemolytic Disease; Chapter 16, Disorders of the Red Cell Membrane; Chapter 17, Pyruvate Kinase Deficiency and Disorders of Glycolysis; Chapter 18, Glucose-6-Phosphate Dehydrogenase Deficiency and Hemolytic Anemia; and Section VI, Disorders of Hemoglobin).

Anemias that are unique to the newborn and are not the result of isoimmunization are the focus of the following discussion. The reader is encouraged to consult other monographs in which the primary focus is anemia in the newborn period.[168–177]

BLOOD LOSS AS A CAUSE OF ANEMIA

Blood loss resulting in anemia may occur prenatally, at the time of delivery, or in the first few days of life. Blood loss may be the result of occult hemorrhage prior to birth, obstetric accidents, internal hemorrhages, or excessive blood sampling by physicians.

The multiple causes of blood loss in the newborn period are listed in Table 2–12. Faxelius and associates[178] estimated the red cell volume in 259 infants admitted to a high-risk unit in an attempt to determine which clinical events were frequently associated with a reduction in red cell mass. A low red cell volume was frequently associated with a maternal history of vaginal bleeding, with placenta previa or abruptio placentae, with nonelective cesarean section, and with deliveries associated with cord compression. Asphyxiated infants (Apgar score at 1 minute of 6 or less) often had low red cell volume. An early central venous hematocrit level below 45% correlated with a low red cell volume, but a normal or even high early hematocrit concentration did not exclude the possibility that the infant was hypovolemic. Infants with mean arterial pressures of less than 30 mm Hg and infants in whom the hematocrit value fell by more than 10 percentage points during the first 6 hours of life were also frequently found to have a reduced red cell mass. These findings serve to underscore the fact that much anemia in early life is the result of obstetric factors that produce blood loss in the infant.

Occult Hemorrhage Prior to Birth

Occult hemorrhage prior to birth may be caused by bleeding of the fetus into the maternal circulation or by bleeding of one fetus into another when multiple fetuses are present.

Fetal-to-Maternal Hemorrhage

In approximately 50% of all pregnancies, some fetal cells can be demonstrated in the maternal circulation.[179] Nucleated fetal erythrocytes can be detected in the maternal circulation as early as the fifth gestational

Table 2–12. TYPES OF HEMORRHAGE IN THE NEWBORN

Occult Hemorrhage Prior to Birth
Fetomaternal
Abdominal or multiple trauma
Amniocentesis in third trimester
Following external cephalic version
Placental tumors
Spontaneous
Twin-to-Twin
Velamentous cord insertion
''Stuck twin'' phenomenon
Obstetric Accidents, Malformation of the Placenta and Cord
Rupture of a normal umbilical cord (precipitous
  delivery, entanglement)
Hematoma of the cord or placenta
Rupture of an abnormal umbilical cord (varices,
  aneurysm)
Rupture of anomalous vessels (aberrant vessels,
  velamentous insertion; communicating vessels in
  multilobed placenta)
Intrauterine manipulation*
Manual removal of placenta*
Cesarean section*
Incision of placenta during cesarean section
Placenta previa*
Abruptio placentae*
Internal Hemorrhage
Intracranial
Giant cephalohematoma, caput succedaneum
Retroperitoneal
Ruptured liver
Ruptured spleen

*Defined by the American College of Obstetrics and Gynecology (ACOG) as conditions associated with high risk for the development of fetomaternal hemorrhages of 30 mL or more. Additional high risk conditions are antepartum fetal death and antepartum bleeding.

Table 2–13. CHARACTERISTICS OF ACUTE AND CHRONIC BLOOD LOSS IN THE NEWBORN

Characteristics	Acute Blood Loss	Chronic Blood Loss
Clinical	Acute distress; pallor; shallow, rapid, and often irregular respiration; tachycardia; weak or absent peripheral pulses; low or absent blood pressure; no hepatosplenomegaly	Marked pallor disproportionate to evidence of distress; on occasion, signs of congestive heart failure may be present, including hepatomegaly
Venous pressure	Low	Normal or elevated
Laboratory Values		
Hb concentration	May be normal initially; then drops quickly during first 24 h of life	Low at birth
RBC morphology	Normochromic and macrocytic	Hypochromic and microcytic; anisocytosis and poikilocytosis
Serum iron level	Normal at birth	Low at birth
Course	Prompt treatment of anemia and shock necessary to prevent death	Generally uneventful
Treatment	Intravenous fluids and whole blood; iron therapy later	Iron therapy; packed RBCs may be necessary on occasion

week,[180] and efforts to isolate these cells for prenatal diagnosis of genetic disease are in progress.[181] The estimated volume of fetal blood present in the maternal circulation is less than 2 mL in 98% of the pregnancies.[182] Fetal-to-maternal hemorrhages of 30 mL or more are observed in 3 of 1000 women, and they are most common following traumatic diagnostic amniocentesis or external cephalic version prior to delivery. A study of 30,944 Rh-negative mothers showed that 1 out of 1146 had fetal bleedings of at least 80 mL, whereas 1 out of 2813 had bleedings of 150 mL or more.[183] The risk factors for fetal to maternal bleeding are summarized in Table 2–12. Traumatic injuries to the mother during pregnancy (e.g., injury secondary to motor vehicle accidents, falls, abdominal trauma),[184] third-trimester amniocentesis, placental abnormalities (abruptio placentae and placental tumors[185]), and manual removal of the placenta have also been associated with fetal-to-maternal hemorrhages.[182]

The clinical manifestations of fetal-to-maternal hemorrhages depend on the volume of the hemorrhage and the rapidity with which it has occurred. If the hemorrhage has been prolonged or repeated during the course of the pregnancy, anemia develops slowly, giving the fetus an opportunity to develop hemodynamic compensation. Such an infant may manifest only pallor at birth. Following acute hemorrhage, just prior to delivery, the infant may be pale and sluggish, have gasping respirations, and manifest signs of circulatory shock. The typical physical findings and laboratory data that are useful in distinguishing the acute and chronic forms of fetal-to-maternal blood loss are described in Table 2–13.

The degree of anemia is quite variable. Usually, the hemoglobin value is less than 12 g/dL before signs and symptoms of anemia are recognized by the physician. Hemoglobin values as low as 3 to 4 g/dL have been recorded in infants who were born alive and survived. If the hemorrhage has been acute, and particularly when hypovolemic shock is present, the hemoglobin value may not reflect the magnitude of the blood loss. In such instances, several hours may elapse before hemodilution occurs and the magnitude of the hemor-

rhage is appreciated. In general, an acute loss of 20% of the blood volume is sufficient to produce signs of shock and is reflected in a decrease in hemoglobin levels within 3 hours of the event.

Examination of a peripheral blood smear provides useful diagnostic information. In acute hemorrhage, the red cells appear normochromic and normocytic, whereas in chronic hemorrhage the cells are generally hypochromic and microcytic.

In anemia that is a direct result of a fetal-to-maternal hemorrhage, Coombs' test yields a negative result, and the infants are not jaundiced. Infants with anemia secondary to blood loss generally have much lower bilirubin values throughout the neonatal period as a consequence of their reduced red cell mass.

The diagnosis of a fetomaternal hemorrhage of sufficient magnitude to result in anemia at birth can be made with certainty only through demonstration of the presence of fetal cells in the maternal circulation. Techniques for demonstrating these cells include differential agglutination, mixed agglutination, fluorescent antibody techniques, and the acid elution method of staining for cells containing fetal hemoglobin.

The Kleihauer and Betke technique[186] of acid elution is the simplest of these methods and the one most commonly employed for the detection of fetal cells. The test is based on the resistance of fetal hemoglobin to elution from the intact cell in an acid medium. The acid elution technique can be relied on with certainty for diagnosis only when other conditions capable of producing elevations in maternal fetal hemoglobin levels are absent. These include maternal thalassemia minor, sickle cell anemia, hereditary persistence of fetal hemoglobin, and, in some normal women, a pregnancy-induced increase in fetal hemoglobin production. In the presence of these conditions, other techniques based on differential agglutination should be employed.[187] Flow cytometry has been shown to be an acceptable alternative to the acid elution test in the detection of fetomaternal hemorrhages.[188] However, most of the flow cytometric tests are designed to quantify D-positive fetal cells in D-negative mothers[189, 190] and are not applicable to D-positive mothers.

Diagnosis of a fetomaternal hemorrhage may be missed in situations in which the mother and infant are incompatible for the ABO blood group system. In such instances, the infant's A or B cells are rapidly cleared from the maternal circulation by the maternal anti-A or anti-B antibodies and are not available for staining. A presumptive diagnosis may be made through demonstration of either marked erythrophagocytosis in smears of the maternal buffy coat or an increase in maternal immune anti-A or anti-B titers in the weeks following delivery.

Fetal-to-Fetal Hemorrhage

This form of hemorrhage is observed only in monozygotic multiple births with monochorial placentas. In approximately 70% of monozygotic twin pregnancies, a monochorial placenta exists.[191] It has been estimated that from 13% to 33% of all twin pregnancies in which a monochorial placenta is present are associated with a twin-to-twin transfusion.[192, 193] Velamentous cord insertions are associated with an increased risk of twin-to-twin transfusion syndrome, possibly as a result of compression forces, which reduce blood flow to one twin.[194] This blood exchange can produce anemia in the donor and polycythemia in the recipient. When a significant hemorrhage has occurred, the difference in hemoglobin concentration between the twins exceeds 5.0 g/dL. This is in contrast to a maximal discrepancy of 3.3 g/dL in cord blood hemoglobin in dizygotic twins. The survival rate for twin-to-twin transfusion syndromes diagnosed before the 28th week of gestation is 21%.[193, 195] Clinical characteristics of and diagnostic modalities for this syndrome and the possible therapeutic role of amniocentesis and cordocentesis with fetal transfusion in reducing the high perinatal mortality of this syndrome have been reviewed.[196–198]

The anemic infant may develop congestive heart failure, whereas the plethoric twin may manifest symptoms and signs of the hyperviscosity syndrome, disseminated intravascular coagulation, and hyperbilirubinemia.[199]

The hemorrhage may be acute or chronic. Tan and associates[200] reviewed 482 twin pairs, among which 35 pairs were found to have this syndrome. They pointed out how the difference in weight of the twins could be used for establishing the timing of the hemorrhage. When the weight difference exceeded 20% of the weight of the larger twin, the transfusion was chronic and the smaller infant was invariably the donor. The anemic smaller twin displayed reticulocytosis. When the difference in the weight of the twins did not exceed 20% of the weight of the larger twin, the larger twin was the donor in almost 50% of all instances. In these presumably acute transfusions, significant reticulocytosis was not observed in the anemic donor. Although hemoglobin values of the recipient were increased equally with both acute and chronic transfusions, the donor twin in the chronic transfusion group was found to be more anemic than the donor in the acute transfusion group. These findings support and extend the original proposal of Klebe and Ingomar,[201] who suggested these two types of transfusions on the basis of a review of previously documented cases.

Obstetric Accidents and Malformations of the Placenta and Cord

The normal umbilical cord may rupture during precipitous deliveries. The cord also may rupture during a normal delivery when it is unusually short or is entangled around the fetus, or when traction is applied to the infant with forceps.[202]

Other abnormalities of the umbilical cord that predispose to hemorrhage and the development of anemia in the infant include vascular abnormalities such as umbilical venous tortuosity and arterial aneurysm. Inflammation of the cord can weaken vessels and predispose them to rupture.

Velamentous insertion of the umbilical cord is observed in approximately 1% of all pregnancies. It appears to be most common in twin pregnancies and in pregnancies accompanied by low-lying placentas. It is estimated that 1% to 2% of pregnancies associated with velamentous insertion of the cord result in fetal blood loss.[202] The perinatal death rate in such circumstances ranges from 58% to 80%, with many of the infants being stillborn. Approximately 12% of those infants who are born alive will be anemic.

The placenta may be inadvertently incised during a cesarean section, with the incision producing a fetal hemorrhage.[203] As previously mentioned, placenta previa or abruptio placentae often results in fetal hemorrhage.[204] In women with late third-trimester bleeding, the physician may anticipate the birth of an anemic infant by examining the vaginal blood for the presence of fetal erythrocytes, employing the acid elution technique of Kleihauer and Betke.[205]

Internal Hemorrhage

When internal hemorrhage takes place in the newborn, it may not be recognized until shock has occurred.

Anemia that appears in the first 24 to 72 hours after birth and that is not associated with jaundice is commonly due to internal hemorrhages. It is well recognized that traumatic deliveries may result in subdural or subarachnoid hemorrhages of sufficient magnitude to result in anemia. Cephalohematomas may be of giant size and result in anemia.[206]

Blood loss into the subaponeurotic area of the scalp tends to be greater than that observed with cephalohematomas. The bleeding is not confined by periosteal attachments and thus is not limited to an area overlying a single skull bone. A subaponeurotic hemorrhage usually extends through the soft tissue of the scalp and covers the entire calvaria. Blood loss in this area can result in exsanguination.[207] Packman[208] observed a hemoglobin value of 2.2 g/dL in an infant 48 hours of age in whom a massive hemorrhage into the scalp had occurred. This form of hemorrhage most commonly occurs after difficult deliveries or vacuum extractions.[209] It also appears with vitamin K deficiency and may be more frequent in infants of black parentage than in those of other ethnicity. Examination of the infant reveals a boggy edema of the head extending into the frontal region and to the nape of the neck. The edema, which may have bluish coloration, obscures the fontanelles and swells the eyelids. The infant may be in shock. Robinson and Rossiter[207] have developed a formula for predicting the volume of blood loss in this condition. For each centimeter of increase in head circumference above that expected, a 38-mL loss of blood has occurred. When the products of red cell breakdown are absorbed from these entrapped hemorrhages, hyperbilirubinemia may develop.[210]

Breech deliveries may be associated with hemorrhage into the adrenal glands, kidneys, spleen, or retroperitoneal area. Blood loss of this type should be suspected in infants found to be anemic during the first few days of life following a traumatic delivery. Hemorrhage into the adrenal glands may also be observed after any difficult delivery or following the birth of a large infant. In adrenal hemorrhage, the clinical picture may include sudden collapse, cyanosis, limpness, jaundice, irregular respirations, elevated or subnormal temperatures, and the presence of a flank mass accompanied by bluish discoloration of the overlying skin.

Rupture of the liver, with resultant anemia, appears to occur more frequently than is clinically appreciated. In stillbirths and neonatal deaths, the incidence of hepatic hemorrhages found at autopsy ranges from 1.2% to 5.6%.[211] In approximately half of the cases reviewed by Henderson,[212] the hemorrhage was subcapsular only; in the remainder, the capsule had ruptured, and free blood was present in the peritoneal cavity.

An infant with a ruptured liver generally appears to be well for 24 to 48 hours and then suddenly goes into shock. The moment of onset of shock appears to coincide with the time when the gradually increasing hematoma finally ruptures the hepatic capsule, causing hemoperitoneum. At this time, the upper abdomen may appear distended, and often a mass contiguous with the liver is palpable. Shifting dullness can be demonstrated on abdominal percussion. Flat films of the abdomen taken with the patient in both the erect and supine positions frequently confirm the presence of free fluid in the abdomen. Paracentesis, performed with the infant in the lateral position, reveals free blood in the abdomen. The prognosis is poor, but infants have been saved following multiple blood transfusions and prompt surgical repair of the laceration.

Splenic rupture may also occur after a difficult delivery[213] or as a result of the extreme distention of the spleen that often accompanies severe erythroblastosis fetalis.[214] The physician should always suspect a rupture of the spleen with associated hemorrhage when, at the time of exchange transfusion, the anemic and hydropic infant with erythroblastosis fetalis is found to have a decreased, rather than an increased, venous pressure. Rupture of the spleen may also occur during the exchange transfusion.

Splenic rupture occurs, although uncommonly, in healthy infants born after seemingly normal deliveries.[215] Many of these infants are of large size. Pallor, abdominal distention, scrotal swelling, and radiographic evidence of peritoneal effusion without free air should alert the physician to the presence of splenic rupture.

Other less common causes of neonatal bleeding include maternal treatment with antiepileptic drugs during pregnancy associated with vitamin K deficiency,[216] neonatal adenovirus infection,[217] fetal cytomegalovirus infection,[218] hemangiomas of the gastrointestinal tract, and hemangioendotheliomas of the skin.[219, 220]

Bleeding into the ventricles and subarachnoid space also can produce significant anemia. Intraventricular hemorrhage may occur in half of all infants with birthweights of less than 1500 g and with even greater frequency when the mother has ingested aspirin in the week prior to the birth of the infant.[221] In many of these infants, no neurologic symptoms are present, and the hemorrhage is recognized on computed tomography of the head.[222]

Anemia Due to Blood Drawing for Laboratory Analysis

A major cause of anemia in critically ill neonates treated in neonatal intensive care units is frequent blood drawing for laboratory analysis. In very-low-birth-weight infants (<1500 g), a 1-mL blood draw represents 1% or more of the total blood volume (Fig. 2–10). In neonates weighing less than 1500 g, blood drawings during the first four weeks of hospitalization may range from 5% to 45% of the calculated total blood volume.[223] A study in 60 very-low-birth-weight infants (560 to 1450 g) showed an average of 4.8 punctures per day per infant, with a mean blood loss for diagnostic sampling of 50.3 mL/kg per 28-day period (range, 7 to 142 mL).[224] Increased blood loss was associated with increased number of transfusions.

Various approaches for limiting the amount of blood drawn for laboratory tests include the following:

1. Reducing the amount of blood discarded from central venous lines before blood for cultures is obtained. It has been shown that discarding only 0.3 mL in infants and 1.0 mL in children does not affect the accuracy of central venous line cultures.[225]

2. Use of micromethods that reduce blood loss from peripheral arterial catheters during sampling.[226]

3. Use of a closed method that allows return of the initial sample drawn to clear a line to the patient. This technique has been shown to reduce blood loss due to diagnostic sampling, even in adult patients.[227, 228]

4. Reducing the amount of blood drawn in excess of that needed for the analytic procedure (25% of the blood removed in neonatal intensive care unit settings is in excess of the analytic need[223]).

5. Reducing the need for blood drawing through the use of transcutaneous monitoring techniques (40% of the blood drawn in a neonatal intensive care unit setting is for analysis of blood gases and electrolytes[223]).

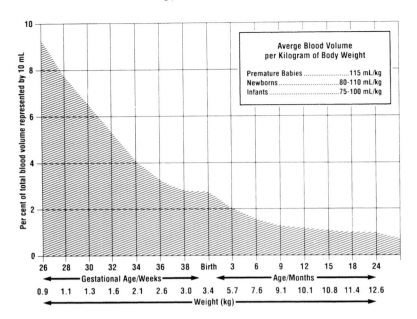

Averge Blood Volume per Kilogram of Body Weight

Premature Babies ....115 mL/kg
Newborns ....80-110 mL/kg
Infants ....75-100 mL/kg

Figure 2-10. Average blood volume per kilogram of body weight. (From Werner M (ed): Microtechniques for the Clinical Laboratory. New York, John Wiley & Sons, 1976, p 2. Copyright © 1976. Reprinted by permission of John Wiley & Sons, Inc.)

Recognition of the Infant with Blood Loss

The clinical manifestations of hemorrhage are dependent on the site of bleeding, the extent of the hemorrhage, and whether the blood loss is acute or chronic. The features that are useful in distinguishing infants with acute and chronic blood loss at the time of delivery are described in Table 2–13. Asphyxiated infants may also display pallor. Features that aid in distinguishing the infant with asphyxia from the infant with acute blood loss are presented in Table 2–14. In all circumstances associated with late third-trimester bleeding, multiple births, cesarean sections, a nuchal cord, any form of cord compression, or a difficult delivery, a hemoglobin determination should be obtained promptly in the infant. Even when the first value is normal, a repeat hemoglobin determination should be performed 6 to 12 hours after birth.

ANEMIA AS A RESULT OF A HEMOLYTIC PROCESS

A *hemolytic process* is generally defined as a pathologic process that results in a shortening of the normal red cell life span of 120 days. For neonates, a different definition that recognizes that the normal red cell life span of term infants is only 60 to 80 days (and may be as short as 20 to 30 days in infants born at 30 to 32 weeks of gestation) must be employed. A hemolytic process during the neonatal period is usually manifested by one of the following combinations of clinical and laboratory findings:

1. A persistent increase in the reticulocyte count, with or without an abnormally low hemoglobin concentration in the absence of current or previous hemorrhage.
2. A rapidly declining hemoglobin concentration without an increase in the reticulocyte count in the absence of hemorrhage.

Most infants with a hemolytic anemia have an accompanying hyperbilirubinemia; however, in the majority of infants in whom the bilirubin level exceeds 12 mg/dL, an increase in red cell destruction, as reflected by an increase in blood carboxyhemoglobin levels, cannot be demonstrated.[229] Approximately 30% of infants with an increase in carboxyhemoglobin levels have maximum bilirubin values of less than 8 mg/dL. The major causes of a shortened red cell life span in the neonatal period are listed in Table 2–15. Only the most salient features of those hereditary hemolytic anemias that manifest themselves in the neonatal period are discussed in this section. Extensive descriptions of these disorders appear in other portions of the text.

Table 2-14. DIFFERENTIAL DIAGNOSIS OF PALLOR IN THE NEWBORN

Asphyxia	Acute Severe Blood Loss	Hemolytic Disease
1. Respiratory findings: retractions, response to oxygen, cyanosis 2. Moribund appearance 3. Bradycardia 4. Stable Hb	1. Decrease in venous and arterial pressure 2. Rapid shallow respirations 3. Acyanotic 4. Tachycardia 5. Drop in Hb	1. Hepatosplenomegaly, jaundice 2. Positive result on Coombs' test 3. Anemia

Adapted from Kirkman HN, Riley HD, Jr: Posthemorrhagic anemia and shock in the newborn due to hemorrhage during delivery: report of 8 cases. Pediatrics 1959; 24:97. Copyright American Academy of Pediatrics, 1959.

Table 2-15. CAUSES OF A HEMOLYTIC PROCESS IN THE NEONATAL PERIOD

A. *Immune*
   Rh incompatibility
   ABO incompatibility
   Minor blood group incompatibility
   Maternal autoimmune hemolytic anemia
   Drug-induced hemolytic anemia
B. *Infection*
   Bacterial sepsis
   Congenital infections
      Syphilis
      Malaria
      Cytomegalovirus
      Adenovirus
      Rubella
      Toxoplasmosis
      Disseminated herpes
C. *Disseminated Intravascular Coagulation*
D. *Macro- and Microangiopathic Anemias*
   Cavernous hemangioma or hemangioendothelioma
   Large vessel thrombi
   Renal artery stenosis
   Severe coarctation of the aorta
E. *Galactosemia*
F. *Prolonged or Recurrent Metabolic or Respiratory Acidosis*
G. *Hereditary Disorders of the Red Cell Membrane*
   Hereditary spherocytosis
   Hereditary elliptocytosis
   Hereditary stomatocytosis
   Hereditary xerocytosis
   Other rare membrane disorders
H. *Pyknocytosis*
I. *Red Cell Enzyme Deficiencies*
   G6PD deficiency, pyruvate kinase deficiency,
      5'-nucleotidase deficiency, glucose phosphate
      isomerase deficiency
J. *Alpha-Thalassemia Syndromes*
K. *Alpha-Chain Structural Abnormalities*
L. *Gamma-Thalassemia Syndromes*
M. *Gamma-Chain Structural Abnormalities*

Hemoglobinopathies

Clinically significant hemoglobinopathies in the newborn may be categorized, as in the older child, as defects of structure or defects of synthesis (thalassemic syndromes). Because of the rapid evolutionary changes that occur in the fetus and newborn with respect to globin chain synthesis, a unique situation exists. Certain hereditary defects of hemoglobin may be seen at this age; some of these defects spontaneously resolve (e.g., γ chain defects), whereas other defects, clinically inapparent at birth, produce clinical problems at a later age (e.g., β chain disorders). Other defects that might be thought to be similar in their clinical manifestations throughout life, such as α chain defects, in fact may act differently in the newborn period when paired with a γ chain rather than with a β chain.

Defects of Hemoglobin Structure

Alpha Chain Structural Defects. When α chain variants of hemoglobin occur, they are present in significant concentration at birth; this is because the α chain is common to all forms of hemoglobin present at birth. In contrast, β chain variants such as Hb S become quantitatively significant only as β chain synthesis replaces γ chain production during the first months after birth. When the amino acid alteration is in the α chain, the concentration of the abnormal hemoglobin will remain fairly constant during infancy and adulthood; however, during infancy, the abnormal hemoglobin will be present primarily in a fetal form ($\alpha_2^x\gamma_2$), with a lesser amount in the adult form ($\alpha_2^x\beta_2$). An example of this is Hb D-St. Louis trait ($\alpha_2^{68\ Asn} \rightarrow {}^{Lys}\beta_2$), in which the total concentration of abnormal hemoglobin ($\alpha_2^x\gamma_2 + \alpha_2^x\beta_2$) was found to be 27% in neonates in comparison with adults, who averaged 28% Hb D in the heterozygous state.[230]

Fortunately, most α chain mutations do not cause clinically significant disorders in adults, and the same situation appears to exist in newborns. Most infants with α chain mutations are detected only as part of routine neonatal screening programs. Occasionally, the fetal form of an α chain mutation is clinically more significant than the adult form of the mutation. Neonates with Hb Hasharon ($\alpha_2^{\ 14\ Asp} \rightarrow {}^{His}\beta_2$) are an example of this phenomenon. Hb Hasharon is a mildly unstable hemoglobin. The unstable mutant hemoglobins have a greater tendency to dissociate into subunits, and this increased dissociation leads to hemolysis. Hb F is less stable than Hb A, presumably as a result of a 10-fold greater affinity between α and β chains than betweeen α and γ chains. As a mildly unstable hemoglobin, the interaction between Hasharon α chains and normal β chains must be minimally decreased, but the interaction between Hasharon α chains and γ chains in the fetal form of Hb Hasharon would be expected to be considerably less, resulting in an even more unstable form of the α chain variant. Levine and co-workers[231] described a 965-g newborn who was heterozygous for Hb Hasharon. This infant manifested a hemolytic anemia that resolved coincidentally with the transition from the fetal to the adult form of Hb Hasharon trait at several months of age.

Beta Chain Structural Defects. The β chain mutations generally produce no clinical symptomatology in the newborn period. This does not mean that chain variants are never a problem in the neonate, nor does it mean that these variants cannot be easily detected in the laboratory.

Although Hb A usually constitutes less than 30% of the normal hemoglobin at birth, it is possible that the amount may, under certain circumstances, be far greater. Because the $\gamma \rightarrow \beta$ chain switchover begins at about 32 weeks of gestation, any disorder that causes the fetus to destroy its existing red cell population will result in a replacement with red cells having a markedly different Hb F:Hb A ratio at the time of delivery. Fetomaternal blood group incompatibility and intrauterine blood loss may, for example, unmask a β chain defect earlier than it might otherwise be detected.

Sickle cell hemoglobinopathies are the most commonly encountered β chain variants in the newborn period. Several cases of homozygous sickle cell disease have presented clinically in the neonate. In patients with homozygous sickle cell disease, the Hb S concentration at birth is usually about 20%.

In infants who have been diagnosed with sickle cell anemia in the first 30 days of life because of some specific symptomatology, the most common findings are jaundice, fever, pallor, respiratory distress, and abdominal distention. Hyperbilirubinemia appears to be more common among newborns with sickle cell anemia.[232] Hegyi and co-workers[233] described a full-term newborn who developed abdominal distention during the first day of life. The cord bilirubin value was 3.1 mg/dL, the hemoglobin level was 12.7 g/dL, and the reticulocyte count was 13.3%. No evidence of glucose-6-phosphate dehydrogenase deficiency or blood group incompatibility was found, but hemoglobin electrophoresis demonstrated 20% Hb S and 80% Hb F. The child rapidly improved but was later found dead in her crib on the fifth day of life. Postmortem examination revealed sickle cells in multiple organs and histopathologic findings consistent with widespread vaso-occlusion, including multifocal enterocolitis.

Of special concern is the problem of "iatrogenic" sickle cell crisis—the exchange transfusion of neonates with respiratory distress syndrome with the use of blood from apparently healthy donors who happen to have sickle cell trait.[234] Such transfusions can produce death in the hypoxic infant.

Gamma Chain Structural Defects. Table 2–16 lists the most commonly observed γ chain structural hemoglobinopathies. These variants are quite interesting because they represent disorders that spontaneously resolve as γ chain production diminishes. The concentrations of these hemoglobins in cord blood average 10% to 20% of the total hemoglobin and appear to represent the heterozygous state of these γ chain hemoglobinopathies.[230] The structural γ defects generally present no hematologic disturbances and usually are found during newborn screening programs. Hb F-Poole is an exception to this rule. Hb F-Poole is an unstable hemoglobin that presents as a Heinz-body hemolytic anemia during the first weeks of life.[235]

Defects in Hemoglobin Synthesis

In newborn infants, defects in hemoglobin synthesis create a greater variety of thalassemia syndromes than may occur at any other time of life. Newborns may demonstrate all varieties of α-thalassemia, β-thalassemia, γ-thalassemia, or δ-thalassemia, or any combination of these.

Alpha-Thalassemia Syndromes in the Neonate. In the newborn period, hemolytic disease due to thalassemia has invariably been associated with homozygous α-thalassemia. A large spectrum of α-thalassemia syndromes may be observed in the newborn period.

Silent Carrier (One-Gene Defect). Thus far, no observations have been made of this disorder in the neonatal period. This entity would be suspected only if a parent were known to be a silent carrier.

Alpha-Thalassemia Trait (Two-Gene Defect). Although the α-thalassemia syndromes have been described for more than 20 years, the heterozygous state (trait) has been difficult to identify because of the mild hematologic changes that accompany this disorder. Older children and adults may demonstrate a very mild anemia and microcytosis in the presence of a normal hemoglobin electrophoresis. The diagnosis is more easily made in the neonatal period than at any other time of life. This is because of two unique occurrences. First, microcytosis is observed in the cord blood of newborns with α-thalassemia trait. Because other causes of microcytosis are rare at this age, infants who are born with a low MCV are more likely to have α-thalassemia trait than any other disease. Second, α-thalassemia in newborns is associated with the presence of Hb Bart's (γ_4), which is easily identified.

Hemoglobin values in neonates with thalassemia trait are no different from those of normal neonates (range, 15.2 to 18.5 g/dL).[236] The MCVs are significantly lower ($\pm 94\mu m^3$) than those of normal term infants ($106.4 \pm 5.7\mu m^3$). In addition, patients with the trait syndrome usually have a mean corpuscular hemoglobin of less than 29.3 pg. The determination of MCV and mean corpuscular hemoglobin appears to be an adequate screening test. The presence of Hb Bart's is the confirmatory finding.

Hemoglobin H Disease. This disorder appears to result from the inheritance of a three-gene deletion that results in sufficient α/β + γ chain imbalance to result in the presence of large quantities of Hb Bart's (γ_4) and some Hb H (β_4) in the newborn period. After the first few months of life, the Hb Bart's disappears, and the only remaining abnormal hemoglobin is Hb H.

Infants born with Hb H diseases have higher levels of Hb Bart's in their cord blood than do normal infants or individuals with α-thalassemia trait; however, they have lower levels than do homozygous infants with hydrops fetalis. Unlike infants with α-thalassemia trait, infants with Hb H disease are born with significant anemia. Microcytosis is present.[237] The hemolytic process may contribute to a somewhat increased incidence of neonatal jaundice.

Hydrops Fetalis. This four-gene deletion disease results in the death of the affected fetus. Because of the

Table 2-16. GAMMA CHAIN HEMOGLOBINOPATHIES Gγ OR Aγ

Hb	Substitution			136	% Abnormal Hb F/Total Hb F
F Malaysia	1 Gly	→	Cys	G	19
F Texas I	5 Glu	→	Lys	A	12
F Texas II	6 Glu	→	Lys	?	8
F Auckland	7 Asp	→	Asn	G	13
F Alexandria	12 Thr	→	Lys	?	10–15
F Melbourne	16 Gly	→	Arg	G	29
F Kuala Lumpur	22 Asp	→	Gly	A	16–18
F Jamaica	61 Lys	→	Glu	A	11–15
F Sardinia	75 Ile	→	Thr	?	10–35
F Victoria Jubilee	80 Asp	→	Tyr	A	7
F Malta I	117 His	→	Arg	G	20–27
F Hull	121 Glu	→	Lys	A	12.5
F Carlton	121 Glu	→	Lys	G	26
F Port Royal	125 Glu	→	Ala	G	14–19
F Poole	130 Trp	→	Gly	G	?
F Dickinson	97 His	→	Arg	A	?

Hb F = fetal hemoglobin.

virtual absence of α chain synthesis, affected infants are born with Bart's Hb only (occasionally, however, some Hb Portland may be found). The peripheral blood smear demonstrates marked hypochromia, poikilocytosis, and target cells. This disorder must be distinguished from other causes of hydrops fetalis with severe anemia. A negative result on Coombs' test and the demonstration of intracellular crystals of Hb Bart's with supravital staining rapidly confirm the high probability of the homozygous state as the correct diagnosis. If death does not occur *in utero*, it occurs within minutes following birth. Although infants with hydrops fetalis have been reported to have cord hemoglobin values as high as 11 g/dL, the usual levels are much lower.[238] Oxygen delivery is severely impaired even when hemoglobin levels are greater because of the profound leftward shift of the oxyhemoglobin dissociation curve for Hb Bart's. When this disorder is detected *in utero*, the fetus may be salvaged with intrauterine transfusion and maintained by a postdelivery transfusion program.[239, 240]

Beta-Thalassemias. In the β-thalassemia syndromes (both trait and homozygous states), the disorders become apparent only after 2 or 3 months of age. In β-thalassemia minor, hematologic findings at birth are entirely normal, with microcytosis being noted later in the first 6 months of life. Similarly, in β-thalassemia major, no clinical findings are present initially; the first sign of any abnormality is the presence of nucleated red cells on smear or the maintenance of high Hb F concentrations. Any disorder that significantly alters the survival of fetal red cells (e.g., intrauterine blood loss or blood group incompatibility) could make the β-thalassemia syndromes clinically obvious at an earlier age.

Erlandson and Hilgartner[241] recorded their observations of infants who were diagnosed as having thalassemia major during the first 3 months of life. In four infants in whom the disease was diagnosed between 1 and 2 months of age, the hemoglobin concentrations were abnormally low. Morphologic erythrocyte abnormalities were already present at 3 days of age in one infant who also was mildly anemic (Hb level, 12.7 g/dL). The earliest morphologic abnormalities were similar to those found in the heterozygous state; however, by 2 months of age, the presence of marked numbers of normoblasts, consistent with homozygous thalassemia, was noted in all infants. Splenomegaly was not present in the one infant who was examined at birth but was apparent in all infants between 1 and 3 months of age. The fetal hemoglobin levels were elevated at 1 to 2 months of age. It would seem then that at least some manifestations of thalassemia major may be present at birth.

Gamma-Thalassemias. Theoretically, a decrease in γ chain synthesis (γ-thalassemia) would produce symptoms *in utero*. Because there are multiple structural genes for γ chain synthesis, the severity of γ-thalassemia would depend on the extent to which these genes were involved. The condition would be lethal if no γ chains were formed; if only one or two genes were involved, only slight hypochromia or, at most, a mild anemia would ensue. If the diagnosis were not established in the neonatal period, it would be missed, because as β chain synthesis replaces γ chain synthesis, the red cell changes would disappear.[242]

Combinations of Thalassemia Syndromes. Kan and co-workers[243] described a full-term infant who had a hemolytic hypochromic anemia at birth associated with microcytosis and nucleated red cells on smear. Neither Hb H nor Hb Bart's was detected. Studies of globin chain synthesis in peripheral blood revealed a deficiency in the synthesis of γ and β chains. As the infant matured, the peripheral smear morphology improved and became identical with that of the subject's father, who had β-thalassemia trait. Since then, several such cases have been reported (see Chapter 21).

Methemoglobinemia in Neonates Treated with Nitric Oxide

Methemoglobinemia is discussed in detail in Chapter 19. A new form of drug-induced methemoglobin (MetHb) has special relevance for oxygen transport in neonates. Pulmonary vasoconstriction is characteristic of persistent pulmonary hypertension of the newborn and is frequently seen in neonatal respiratory distress syndromes. Inhaled nitric oxide (NO) acts as a potent vasodilator on the pulmonary vasculature, improves oxygenation, and lowers pulmonary vascular resistance.[244-246] A potentially serious side effect of the administration of inappropriately high NO concentrations is the oxidation of Fe^{2+} of hemoglobin to form Fe^{3+} and MetHb. Detection of MetHb formation is particularly problematic in neonates owing to the interference of Hb F on MetHb determination. However, a new multiwavelength Hb photometer can minimize spectral differences between Hb A and Hb F and allow determination of MetHb in samples with high Hb F.[247] It is advisable to monitor MetHb levels in all neonates treated with NO.

Hereditary Disorders of the Red Cell Membrane

Hereditary spherocytosis, hereditary elliptocytosis, hereditary stomatocytosis, and hereditary xerocytosis all may be manifest in the newborn period. If a hemolytic anemia is detected during evaluation of hyperbilirubinemia, a precise diagnosis generally is not established in most patients until they are older. Hereditary spherocytosis is a general exception to this rule. The morphologic abnormality, the laboratory findings, and a positive family history usually enable the physician to make this diagnosis during the first days of life.

The classic morphologic abnormalities of patients with hereditary elliptocytosis may not be present during the first few weeks of life. Patients with the hemolytic form of hereditary elliptocytosis may display pyknocytes rather than elliptocytes early in life, and only after several months are the typical elliptocytes observed. These membrane disorders are described in detail in Chapter 17.

Red Cell Enzyme Deficiencies

Inherited disorders of red cell metabolism also may be anticipated to produce a hemolytic anemia early in life. The most common of these abnormalities are glucose-6-phosphate dehydrogenase deficiency and pyruvate kinase deficiency. These and other disorders of red cell metabolism are described in Chapters 17 and 18.

IMPAIRED RED BLOOD CELL PRODUCTION

The Diamond-Blackfan syndrome (pure red cell anemia, erythrogenesis imperfecta, or chronic aregenerative anemia) is an uncommon condition characterized by a failure of erythropoiesis but normal production of white blood cells and platelets (see Chapter 7).

Two reviews of the subject suggest that as many as 25% of affected patients may be anemic at birth.[248, 249] Hemoglobin values as low as 9.4 g/dL, accompanied by reticulocytopenia, have been observed during the first days of life.[250]

Low birth weight occurs in approximately 10% of all affected patients, with about half of this group being small for gestational age. There appears to be a slight increase in the incidence of miscarriages, stillbirths, and complications of pregnancy among the mothers who have given birth to infants with this syndrome.

Physical anomalies are present in about 30% of patients with Diamond-Blackfan syndrome.[250] The most common abnormality is short stature. This finding is obviously of little clinical assistance in the newborn period. Other abnormalities include microcephaly, cleft palate, anomalies of the eye, web neck, and thumb deformity. Triphalangeal thumb, duplications of the thumb, and bifid thumb have been described in association with this syndrome.

The inheritance of the Diamond-Blackfan syndrome is unclear. In the majority of the reported cases, no other family members are affected; this suggests an autosomal recessive pattern of inheritance. This view is supported by the fact that in two reports parental consanguinity was present; in addition, in 13 families, more than one affected child was observed.

It would appear from a review of the reported cases that the earlier the diagnosis is established, the greater is the likelihood that the patient will respond to steroid therapy.

Another cause of impaired red cell production in the neonatal period is Pearson's syndrome.[251] This syndrome is characterized by vacuolization of bone marrow precursors, sideroblastic anemia, and exocrine pancreatic dysfunction. This syndrome may be associated with Leigh disease (subacute necrotizing encephalopathy)[252] or with Kearns-Sayre syndrome (bilateral ptosis and atypical retinitis pigmentosa).[253, 254] A deletion in mitochondrial DNA[255] has been found in Pearson's syndrome.* A case of pyridoxine-refractory congenital sideroblastic anemia with autosomal reces-

sive inheritance has also been described.[257] Neonatal anemia with macrocytosis has been described in some cases of cartilage-hair hypoplasia.[258]

Impaired red cell production resulting in anemia during the neonatal period may also be observed as a result of congenital infections such as rubella, cytomegalovirus, adenovirus, and human parvovirus.[259] Congenital leukemia, Down syndrome, and osteoporosis may also produce anemia during the early days of life as a result of inadequate erythropoiesis.

A DIAGNOSTIC APPROACH TO THE ANEMIC NEWBORN

In view of the great number of entities that may be responsible for anemia in the newborn period, a disciplined approach to diagnosis is essential. A detailed family history and obstetric history should be obtained. The placenta should be examined whenever possible.

During the physical examination of the infant, particular attention should be devoted to detection of congenital anomalies, stigmata of intrauterine infection, internal hemorrhages, and the presence of hepatosplenomegaly.

Initial laboratory studies should include a complete blood count, red cell indices, reticulocyte count, direct Coombs' test, and examination of a well-prepared peripheral blood smear. Other useful simple procedures include a Heinz body preparation and the performance of a "wet prep" of the infant's erythrocytes.

One approach that relies on the reticulocyte count and cellular indices in arriving at a diagnosis is illustrated in Figure 2–11.

This approach can be supplemented with specific diagnostic tests as indicated.

PHYSIOLOGIC ANEMIA OF PREMATURITY

The hemoglobin concentration of term infants normally decreases over the first weeks of life; this is known as the "physiologic anemia of infancy." Infants who are born prematurely but are otherwise healthy experience a more exaggerated decrease in hemoglobin concentration (see the following paragraph). This has been termed the "physiologic anemia of prematurity."[260] The factors that influence the magnitude of this physiologic anemia include the nutritional status of the infant and a variety of complex adaptations to changes in oxygen availability.[261]

Cord hemoglobin values do not change significantly during the last trimester of pregnancy. After birth, the rapidity with which the hemoglobin level declines and the magnitude of the actual decrease vary directly with the degree of immaturity of the newborn. Although the nadir in hemoglobin concentration for normal full-term infants may be as low as 11.4 ± 0.9 g/dL by the age of 8 to 12 weeks, the average hemoglobin value observed by Schulman[260] in premature infants weighing less than 1500 g was 8.0 g/dL at the age of 4 to 8 weeks. The overall changes observed in well infants weighing less than 1500 g are depicted in Figure

---

*For a recent review on mitochondrial syndromes, see reference 256.

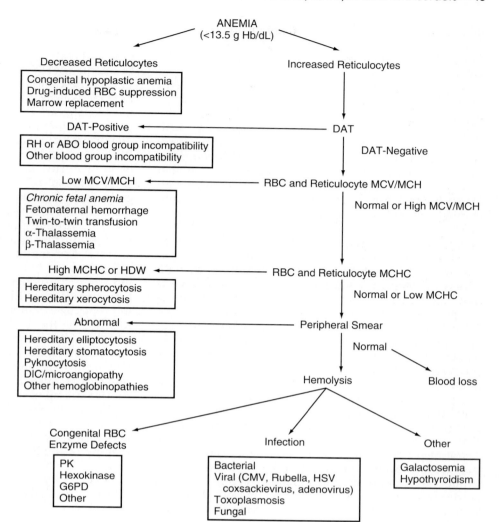

Figure 2-11. Diagnostic approach to anemia in the newborn. DAT = direct antiglobulin test; MCV/MCH = mean corpuscular volume/mean corpuscular hemoglobin; MCHC = mean corpuscular hemoglobin concentration; HDW = hemoglobin distribution width; DIC = disseminated intravascular coagulation; PK = pyruvate kinase; G6PD = glucose-6-phosphate dehydrogenase; CMV = cytomegalovirus; HSV = herpes simplex virus.

2–12. These data are consistent with the normal data found by others.[262]

It is generally agreed that this fall in hemoglobin concentration results in greatest part from a decrease

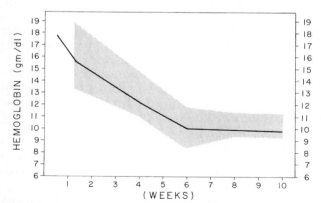

Figure 2-12. The relationship between Hb concentration and age from birth in a group of 40 infants with birth weights of less than 1500 g. *Dark line* indicates mean value; *shaded area* includes all values observed. All infants were vitamin E–iron sufficient.

in the red cell mass rather than a hemodilutional effect of an expanding plasma volume.[263] These changes occur at a time when the red cell survival of both term and premature infants is known to be shortened and when a striking decrease occurs in hematopoietic activity, as evidenced by a fall in reticulocyte count and a decrease in marrow erythroid elements.

Cord blood analysis generally demonstrates elevated levels of erythropoietin; these elevated levels are increased further in infants who experience transient hypoxemia at the time of delivery.[264, 265] One notable exception is seen in neonates with severe isoimmunization treated with intrauterine transfusion, who typically develop severe anemia postnatally. The anemia is due to a combination of continued immune-mediated hemolysis and suppressed erythropoiesis. Serum erythropoietin (EPO) in these neonates surged transiently at birth but did not reach "appropriate" levels until the hemoglobin level decreased to below 5 g/dL.[266] Otherwise, infants born anemic demonstrate a reticulocytosis. Increased erythropoiesis is generally seen in small-for-gestational-age infants who have suffered from intrauterine hypoxia.[267] The anemia of prematurity rarely occurs in association with cyanotic congenital heart disease or with respiratory insufficiency; this indicates that infants in the first few weeks of life can maintain higher oxygen-carrying capacities if the need arises.

An important insight into the ability of the preterm infant to adjust hemoglobin level adequately to his or her own specific requirements may be noted if the hematologic statuses of infants who are born with widely varying hemoglobin concentrations are compared in the first few months of life. Differences in initial hemoglobin levels greatly affect the hemoglobin concentration in the weeks after birth. Infants with lower hemoglobin levels at birth achieve minimum hemoglobin values more rapidly and their recovery phase occurs earlier when they are compared with infants born with higher hemoglobin levels.[261] It is interesting to note, however, that the minimum hemoglobin levels achieved are similar in infants born with widely discrepant hemoglobin values; this suggests that the signal for return of active erythropoiesis is roughly equivalent among infants.

Until recently, it was not clear how infants, particularly premature infants, could tolerate large declines in hemoglobin concentration while at the same time providing adequate supplies of oxygen to tissues. Adequate tissue oxygenation in the face of diminished oxygen-carrying capacity (lower hemoglobin concentration) can be accomplished only if oxygen demands are reduced or if one or more compensatory changes that are known to accompany anemia are observed. These responses include, in part, a higher cardiac output, an improved oxygen-unloading capacity, a redistribution of blood flow, and a greater oxygen extraction (a decrease in the oxygen tension in mixed central venous blood). Apparently, only some of these responses occur.

Cardiac output does not change significantly between the end of the first week of life and 3 months of age. Although the oxygen content of blood (milliliters of oxygen carried per 100 mL of blood) decreases to its lowest level in the first 2 to 3 months of life, this reflects nothing more than the overall decline in hemoglobin concentration. The oxygen-unloading capacity of blood—that is, the actual quantity of oxygen that is theoretically capable of being delivered to tissues—is constantly increasing from the moment of birth, even as the hemoglobin level falls.[268] This increase in oxygen unloading results from the gradual rightward shift in the oxyhemoglobin dissociation curve as the fetal hemoglobin levels decrease and the red cell 2,3-DPG level increases. The magnitude of this shift may be of profound physiologic significance for both term and premature infants.

Recombinant Human Erythropoietin and the Anemia of Prematurity

In 1977, Stockman and associates[269] observed EPO concentrations within or below the normal adult range in infants with anemia of prematurity. Very low levels for the degree of anemia have subsequently been observed and reported by others.[270, 271] EPO levels in neonates of different weight at birth vary over a wide range, but they seem to reach a nadir between days 7 and 50 independently of weight at birth; this is followed by the nadir in Hb concentration (between day 51 and 150).[272] These and other data indicate that the increase in EPO levels is insufficient for the degree of anemia when the neonates are compared with matched adults.[29, 273]

Investigation of *in vitro* erythroid colony growth has demonstrated normal numbers of both circulating BFU-Es[274] and bone marrow CFU-Es[275] in the anemia of prematurity. Both classes of erythroid progenitors show normal EPO dose-response curves. Taken together, the findings of low serum EPO concentrations, relative bone marrow erythroid hypoplasia, and a normal EPO dose-response curve suggest that inadequate EPO production is a major factor in the genesis of the anemia of prematurity.

The blunted EPO response to decreasing Hb levels[270] may be a consequence of the incomplete switch from liver to kidney as the major source of EPO production in premature infants and of the relative insensitivity to hypoxia of the liver-controlled EPO production. An additional factor may be related to a different clearance and volume of distribution of EPO in neonates that results in lower EPO levels.[276, 277] The anemia of prematurity also is due to blood loss related to the shorter life span of neonatal erythrocytes, and to the rapid growth observed in the first weeks of life, which is not accompanied by a parallel increase in red cell mass. Detailed reviews of the pathophysiology and therapy of the anemia of prematurity have been published.[174–176, 278, 279]

Table 2–17 presents a summary of studies published on the use of r-HuEPO in the anemia of prematurity. The use of r-HuEPO reduces the need for transfusions in premature infants weighing more than 1000 g,[280] a group that rarely undergoes transfusions. r-HuEPO may not be as effective in reducing transfusion requirements when it is used in infants weighing less than 1000 g or in neonates requiring artificial ventilation.[281] In a large, double-blind, placebo-controlled trial, r-HuEPO was shown to reduce blood transfusion in preterm infants (weight at birth, 924 ± 183 g).[282] Although the reduction in blood transfusions was statistically significant, the use of r-HuEPO resulted in only a small increase in the number of untransfused infants (from 31% to 43%). This disappointing result may be a function of poor EPO responsiveness, the variability in the r-HuEPO dosages used, or inconsistency in providing supplemental iron for sustaining the enhanced erythropoiesis induced by r-HuEPO. A detailed cost analysis of the use of EPO in the anemia of prematurity has recently been published.[282a]

Studies in adult subjects have identified a functional iron deficiency in normal iron-replete subjects treated with r-HuEPO and oral iron.[283] Oral iron administration is insufficient for sustaining the increased marrow activity in the presence of r-HuEPO, and intravenous iron supplementation should always be considered for premature infants, possibly in association with vitamin E supplementation.

Studies in adult patients have indicated that autolo-

Table 2-17. ERYTHROPOIETIN USE IN THE ANEMIA OF PREMATURITY

Reference	No. of Subjects, EPO	No. of Subjects, C	EPO Dose (U/kg per wk)	Iron Supplementation (mg/kg)	Reticulocyte Response	No. Transfused, EPO	No. Transfused, C	Iron Status, EPO	Neutropenia/ Infection	Thrombocytosis	Significant Effect
Halperin et al. (J Pediatr 1990; 116:776.)	7	—	75–300	2 per d	>Double	—	—	Decrease	5/no	Mild, transient	+
Obladen et al. (Contrib Nephrol 1991; 88:314.)	43	50	60	—	No change	23/43	21/50	No change	NA	No	—
Shannon et al. (J Pediatr 1991; 118:949.)	10	10	200	3 per d	Earlier increase	5/10	8/10	NA	No	—	—
Ohls et al. (J Pediatr 1991; 119:781.)	10	9	700	2 per d	>3-fold	0/10	9/9	NA	Mild/No	No	+
Shannon et al. (J Pediatr 1992; 120:586.)	4	4	500–1000	3–6 per d	2-fold	1/4	3/4	No change	No/no	No	+
Beck et al. (Eur J Pediatr 1991; 150:767.)	16	—	10–200	—	Variable	4/16	—	No change	5/no	Mild, transient	±
Halperin et al. (Eur J Pediatr 1992; 151:661.)	18	2	75–600	a. 2–5 per d b. 7–8 per d	3-fold	3/18	—	a. Decrease b. No change	No/no	Mild, transient	+
Mentzer et al. (Contrib Nephrol 1991; 88:306.)	10	10	200	3 per d	No change	Less	8/10	NA	No/no	No	±
Carnielli et al. (J Pediatr 1992; 121:98.)	11	11	1200	20 per wk, IV	Highly significant	0.8	3.1	NA	No/no	No	+
Emmerson et al. (Proc Int Soc Hematol 1992; 19a.)	16	8	100–450	NA	Highly significant	47%	88%	Decrease	NA	NA	+
Halvorsen et al. (Proc Int Soc Hematol 1992; 19a.)	14	13	300	18–36 per d	>2-fold	0/14	3/13	NA	No/NA	No	+
Soubasi et al. (Pediatr Res 1991; 30:645a.)	12	8	300	3 per d	2–4-fold	No differences		Decrease	No/no	Mild	±
Messer et al. (Pediatrics 1993; 92:519.)	21	10	300–600	NA	2-fold	3/21	5/10	NA	Mild, transient	NA	+
Attias et al. (Proc Am Soc Pediatr Hematol Oncol 1993; 2:23.)	12	11	900	6 per d	3-fold	0/12	6/11	Decrease	No/no	No	+
Meyer et al. (Pediatrics 1994; 93:918.)	40	40	600	3 per d	2-fold	7/40	21/40	Decrease	No/no	No	+
Maier et al. (N Engl J Med 1994; 330:1173.)	120	121	750	2 per d	2-fold	67/120	87/121	Decrease	No/no	NA	+
Shannon et al. (Pediatrics 1995; 95:1.)	77	80	500	3–6 per d	2–3-fold	33/77	25/80	Decrease	No/no	No	+

C = control; NA = not available; EPO = erythropoietin; IV = intravenous.
Modified from Attias MD: Pathophysiology and treatment of the anemia of prematurity. J Pediatr Hematol Oncol 1995; 17:13.

gous donation is not cost-effective when it is compared with allogeneic blood transfusion, mostly as a consequence of the high cost of collecting and discarding units that are not used.[284] However, reduction of allogeneic blood use by means of autologous blood donation (and the use of r-HuEPO) may be a prudent practice to follow, despite the associated additional cost.[285] Cost-benefit analysis does not indicate cost-effectiveness for the use of EPO in the neonatal settings.[286] However, this conclusion is based on the high cost of the product (to reach a break even point would require a 54% reduction in product cost) and on the way it is currently packaged (a 2000-U vial cannot be used more than once for the same patient, although it can be used for multiple patients on the same day). Changes in r-HuEPO price and packaging could make r-HuEPO therapy more similar in cost to allogeneic blood transfusion. r-HuEPO is a remarkably safe drug. No significant side effects have been reported with its use, with the exception of the occurrence of seizures and blood pressure elevation when the circulating red cell mass is increased too rapidly. r-HuEPO has been shown to increase total bilirubin production in premature infants without inducing clinically significant jaundice.[287] Use of r-HuEPO in preterm infants does not affect the ratio of HbF to HbA.[287a]

NEONATAL HYPERVISCOSITY

Neonates with hematocrits in excess of 65% are at some risk for *hyperviscosity syndrome,* which includes hypoglycemia, central nervous system injury,[288] and hypocalcemia with elevated plasma calcitonin gene–related peptide levels.[289] Infants with polycythemic hyperviscosity should undergo careful isovolumic partial plasma exchange transfusion, especially when abnormal results are obtained on cerebral blood flow velocity studies.[290] Although there is a good correlation between polycythemia and hyperviscosity, several infants with hyperviscosity syndrome have normal hematocrits and can be identified only with the use of viscosity measurements.[291] Several risk factors for neonatal polycythemia and hyperviscosity have been identified, such as maternal insulin-dependent diabetes,[292, 293] intrauterine growth retardation, perinatal asphyxia, twin-to-twin transfusion (recipient), delayed cord clamping, and Beckwith's syndrome.[294]

TRANSFUSIONS IN PREMATURE INFANTS

Red cell transfusion is discussed in Chapter 50; however, some of the problems unique to the neonatal setting are discussed in this section. For a more detailed discussion of issues relating to neonatal red cell transfusions, consult recent publications.[176, 295–298]

Decisions regarding the need for transfusion in low-birth-weight infants cannot be based on hemoglobin concentration or hematocrit alone. Wardrop and co-workers[299] have demonstrated that "available oxygen," and not absolute hemoglobin level, most closely correlates with the presence of symptoms and signs of hypoxemia such as tachycardia, tachypnea, easy fatigua-

bility, and poor feeding in low-birth-weight infants. Available oxygen is a reflection of the position of the oxyhemoglobin dissociation curve, the hemoglobin concentration, and the arterial oxygen saturation. Nomograms that illustrate the importance of these factors in making decisions regarding transfusion have been prepared.[300] These nomograms are based on assumptions regarding cardiac output and oxygen consumption that have been derived from serial measurements in low-birth-weight infants.[301] An example of the importance of the P_{50} and the arterial oxygen saturation in making decisions regarding the hemoglobin required for maintaining the central venous oxygen tension at 30 mm Hg is illustrated in Table 2–18.

As a general rule, hemoglobin values in otherwise healthy low-birth-weight infants should be maintained above 12 g/dL during the first 2 weeks of life. After that period, decisions regarding transfusion when determinations of "available oxygen" cannot be performed should be based on the infant's clinical condition. Factors to evaluate include the infant's weight gain, evidence of fatigue during feeding, tachycardia, tachypnea, and evidence of hypoxemia as reflected by an increase in blood lactic acid concentrations.[302] Infants with cardiac or pulmonary disease that reduces arterial oxygen saturation may require hemoglobin concentrations of at least 16 to 17 g/dL for their oxygen requirements to be adequately met. No guidelines for neonatal transfusions have been clearly defined. It is common practice to transfuse neonates for the following reasons[303]:

1. Replacement of blood drawn for testing when the cumulative blood loss reaches 5% or 10% of the total blood volume.
2. Maintenance of hematocrit greater than 40% in patients with severe respiratory distress or symptomatic heart disease.
3. Maintenance of hematocrit greater than 30% in neonates with cardiopulmonary problems or growth failure.

It has been estimated that more than 300,000 red blood cell transfusions are given annually to 38,000 premature neonates in the United States.[303] Most infants who weigh more than 1000 g do not receive transfusions in this country.[304] There has been a significant reduction in the prevalence of transfusions in the

Table 2–18. HEMOGLOBIN LEVELS REQUIRED IN LOW-BIRTH-WEIGHT INFANTS* TO MAINTAIN A CENTRAL VENOUS OXYGEN TENSION OF 30 mm Hg

P_{50} (mm Hg)	Arterial Oxygen Saturation (%)			
	95	90	85	80
20	10.0	13.0	20.0	>25.0
23	7.3	9.0	11.0	15.5
25	6.2	7.3	8.8	11.0
27	5.3	6.3	7.3	8.9

*Assumes a cardiac output of 250 mL/kg per minute and an oxygen consumption of 6.5 mL/kg per minute.

last 5 to 6 years owing to improved treatment and prevention of neonatal lung disease with surfactants, better ventilation, inhalation of NO, reduction in blood loss for analytical purposes, and less aggressive transfusion regimens. Neonatal transfusion practices in the United States have been studied in a national survey.[305, 306] Standards issued by the American Association of Blood Banks (AABB) require testing for ABO group and Rh type, as well as red cell antibody screening prior to the first transfusion. If the red cell antibody screen is negative and group O red cells are used, no additional testing is required for subsequent red cell transfusions. If cells other than group O are transfused, the initial sample should also be tested for passively acquired anti-A or anti-B immunoglobulins.[307] The survey indicated that a large number of institutions in the United States still perform unnecessary major antiglobulin crossmatches for neonatal transfusions. This practice leads to a greater amount of blood being drawn and, thus, more transfusions.

Traditionally, blood used for neonatal transfusion is less than 7 to 10 days old and is collected in anticoagulant citrate phosphate dextrose adenine (CPDA)-1 rather than in additive solutions, even though there is no good scientific evidence to support this practice with small-volume (10 mL/kg) red cell transfusions.[305, 308, 309] Use of specifically assigned units less than 14 days old and of sterile connecting devices allows reduction of donor exposure and has no adverse effects.[310] The exposure to different donors can be drastically reduced by the multiple use of a single unit of blood for a patient over 35 days.[311]

Low-risk cytomegalovirus blood products (cytomegalovirus-negative or leuko-depleted red cells) should be used only for neonates with weight at birth of less than 1200 g who are cytomegalovirus-negative or are of unknown cytomegalovirus status.[307]

Packed red cells should be adjusted to the desired hematocrit (60% to 79%) with normal saline or 5% albumin solution. However, a significant number of institutions still use fresh frozen plasma from the same donor or from a different donor for this purpose.[305] This practice is particularly widespread for exchange transfusions, in which red cells reconstituted in fresh frozen plasma from different donors are used—that is, each neonate is exposed to two different donors.

When RBCs are collected from direct donors, they should be irradiated to prevent graft-versus-host disease. Although there is no scientific evidence to support a benefit from the use of directed donors, this practice accounts for a significant number of blood transfusions in the neonatal settings.[305, 312]

A significant factor in determining different blood uses in the neonatal setting is related to existing institutional practice. Comparison of blood utilization in two neonatal intensive care units has revealed major differences in per cent of patients transfused and the number of transfusions, which cannot be accounted for by differences in disease severity.[313]

References

1. Wintrobe MM: Clinical Hematology. 5th ed. Philadelphia, Lea & Febiger, 1961, p 32.
2. Maximov AA: Relation of blood cells to connective tissue and endothelium. Physiol Rev 1924; 4:533.
3. Bloom W, Bartelmez GW: Hematopoiesis in young human embryos. Am J Anat 1940; 67:21.
4. Ehrlich P: De- und Regeneration roter Blutscheiben. Berhandl Gesellsch Charite Arzte, 1880.
5. Migliaccio G, Migliaccio AR, et al: Human embryonic hemopoiesis. Kinetics of progenitors and precursors underlying the yolk sac→liver transformation. J Clin Invest 1986; 78:51.
6. Thomas DB, Yoffey JM: Human foetal haematopoiesis. II. Hepatic haematopoiesis in the human foetus. Br J Haematol 1964; 10:193.
7. Fukuda A: Fetal hemopoiesis. II. Electron microscopic studies on human hepatic hemopoiesis. Virchows Arch B Zell Pathol 1974; 16:249.
8. Kimura N, Yamano Y, et al: Erythroid progenitors in human fetal liver. Nippon Ketsueki Gakkai Zasshi 1984; 47:1235.
9. Linch DC, Knott LJ, et al: Studies of circulating hemopoietic progenitor cells in human fetal blood. Blood 1982; 59:976.
10. Zauli G, Vitale M, et al: In vitro growth of human fetal CD34+ cells in the presence of various combinations of recombinant cytokines under serum-free conditions. Br J Haematol 1994; 86:461.
11. Lansdorp PM: Developmental changes in the function of hematopoietic stem cells. Exp Hematol 1995; 23:187.
12. Kalpaktsoglou PK, Emery JL: Human bone marrow during the last 3 months of intrauterine life. Acta Haematol 1965; 34:228.
13. Kelemen E, Calvo W, et al: Atlas of Human Hemopoietic Development. Berlin, Springer-Verlag, 1979.
14. Broxmeyer HE, Douglas GW, et al: Human umbilical cord blood as a potential source of transplantable hematopoietic stem/progenitor cells. Proc Natl Acad Sci U S A 1989; 86:3828.
15. Liang DC, Ma SW, et al: Granulocyte/macrophage colony-forming units from cord blood of premature and full-term neonates: its role in ontogeny of human hematopoiesis. Pediatr Res 1988; 24:701.
16. Forestier F, Daffos F, et al: Developmental hematopoiesis in normal human fetal blood. Blood 1991; 77:2360.
17. Valtieri M, Gabbianelli M, et al: Erythropoietin alone induces erythroid burst formation by human embryonic but not adult BFU-E in unicellular-serum-free culture. Blood 1989; 74:460.
18. Emerson S, Thomas S, et al: Developmental regulation of erythropoiesis by hematopoietic growth factors: analysis of populations of BFU-E from bone marrow, peripheral blood, and fetal liver. Blood 1989; 74:49.
19. Gardner D, Liechty KW, Christensen RD: Effects of interleukin-6 on fetal hematopoietic progenitors. Blood 1990; 75:2150.
20. Holbrook ST, Ohls RK, et al: Effect of interleukin-9 on clonogenic maturation and cell-cycle status of fetal and adult hematopoietic progenitors. Blood 1991; 77:2129.
21. Schibler KR, Yang YC, Christensen RD: Effect of interleukin-11 on cycling status and clonogenic maturation of fetal and adult hematopoietic progenitors. Blood 1992; 80:900.
22. Schibler KR, Li Y, et al: Possible mechanisms accounting for the growth factor independence of hematopoietic progenitors from umbilical cord blood. Blood 1994; 84:3679.
23. Traycoff CM, Abboud MR, et al: Rapid exit from G0/G1 phases of cell cycle in response to stem cell factor confers on umbilical cord blood CD34 + cells an enhanced *ex vivo* expansion potential. Exp Hematol 1994; 22:1264.
24. Pettengell R, Luft T, et al: Direct comparison by limiting dilution analysis of long-term culture-initiating cells in human bone marrow, umbilical cord blood, and blood stem cells. Blood 1994; 84:3653.
25. Gluckman E, Broxmeyer HE, et al: Hematopoietic reconstitution in a patient with Fanconi's anemia by means of umbilical-cord blood from an HLA-identical sibling. N Engl J Med 1989; 321:1174.
26. Gale RP: Cord-blood-cell transplantation—a real sleeper. N Engl J Med 1995; 332:392.
27. Wagner JE, Kerman NA, et al: Transplantation of umbilical cord blood in 50 patients: analysis of the registry data. Blood 1994; 84:395a.
28. Issaragrisil S, Visuthisakchai S, et al: Brief report: transplantation of cord-blood stem cells into a patient with severe thalassemia. N Engl J Med 1995; 332:367.

29. Halvorsen S: Plasma erythropoietin in cord blood during the first few weeks of life. Acta Pediatr Scand 1963; 52:425.
30. Matoth Y, Zaizov R: Regulation of erythropoiesis in the fetal rat. Proceedings of the Tel Aviv University Conference on Erythropoiesis, Petak Tikva, Israel. New York, Academic Press, 1970, p 24.
31. Jacobsen LO, Marks EK, et al: The effect of transfusion-induced polycythemia in the mother of the fetus. Blood 1959; 14:644.
32. Zanjani ED, Gidari AS, et al: Humoral regulation of erythropoiesis in the foetus. In Comline KS, Cross KW, et al (eds): Foetal and Neonatal Physiology. London, Cambridge University Press, 1973, p 448.
33. Orkin SH: Transcription factors and hematopoietic development. J Biol Chem 1995; 270:4955.
34. Simon MC, Pevny L, et al: Rescue of erythroid development in gene-targeted GATA-1-mouse embryonic stem cells. Nature Genet 1992; 1:92.
35. Perkins A, Sharpe AH, Orkin SH: Lethal beta-thalassemia in mice lacking the erythroid CACCC-transcription factor EKLF. Nature 1995; 375:318.
36. Stamatoyannopoulos G, Rosenblum BB, et al: Hb F and Hb A production in erythroid cultures from human fetuses and neonates. Blood 1979; 54:440.
37. Orkin SH: Regulation of globin gene expression in erythroid cells. Eur J Biochem 1995; 231:271.
38. Szelengi JG, Hollan SR: Studies on the structure of human embryonic haemoglobin. Acta Biochim Biophys Acad Sci Hung 1969; 4:47.
39. Hecht F, Motulsky AG, et al: Predominance of hemoglobin Gower 1 in early human embryonic development. Science 1966; 152:91.
40. Kamuzora H, Lehmann H: Human embryonic haemoglobins including a comparison by homology of the human ζ and α chains. Nature 1975; 256:511.
41. Ley T, Maloney K, et al: Globin gene expression in erythroid human fetal liver cells. J Clin Invest 1989; 83:1032.
42. Seip M: The reticulocyte level and the erythrocyte production judged from reticulocyte studies in newborn infants during the first week of life. Acta Paediatr (Stockholm)1955; 44:355.
43. Garby L, Sjoli S, et al: Studies on erythrokinetics in infancy. III. Plasma disappearance and red cell uptake of intravenously injected radioiron. Acta Paediatr (Stockh) 1963; 52:537.
44. Gairdner D, Marks J, et al: Blood formation in infancy. Normal erythropoiesis. Arch Dis Child 1952; 27:214.
45. Sturgeon P: Volumetric and microscopic pattern of bone marrow in normal infants and children. I. Volumetric pattern. Pediatrics 1951; 7:577.
46. Sturgeon P: Volumetric and microscopic pattern of bone marrow in normal infants and children. II. Cytologic pattern. Pediatrics 1951; 7:642.
47. Issaragrisil S: Correlation between hematopoietic progenitors and erythroblasts in cord blood. Am J Clin Pathol 1983; 80:865.
48. Man DL, Sites MD, et al: Erythropoietic stimulating activity during the first 90 days of life. Proc Soc Exp Biol Med 1965; 118:212.
49. Wranne L: Studies on erythrokinetics in infancy. Acta Paediatr Scand 1967; 56:381.
50. Perrine SP, Greene MF, Faller DV: Delay in the fetal globin switch in infants of diabetic mothers. N Engl J Med 1985; 327:569.
51. Little JA, Dempsey NJ, et al: Metabolic persistence of fetal hemoglobin. Blood 1995; 85:1712.
52. Bard H, Prosmanne J: Elevated levels of fetal hemoglobin synthesis in infants with chronic bronchopulmonary dysplasia. Pediatrics 1990; 86:193.
53. Bard H, Lachance C, et al: The reactivation of fetal hemoglobin synthesis during anemia of prematurity. Pediatr Res 1994; 36:253.
54. Bratteby E, Garby L: Development of erythropoiesis: infant erythrokinetics. In Nathan DG, Oski FA (eds): Hematology of Infancy and Childhood. 1st ed. Philadelphia, W.B. Saunders Co., 1974, p 56.
55. Landaw SA, Guancial RL: Shortened survival of fetal erythrocytes in the rat. Pediatr Res 1977; 11:1155.
56. Landaw SA: Decreased survival and altered membrane properties of red blood cells (RBC) in the newborn rat. Pediatr Res 1978; 12:395.
57. Serrani RE, Alonso D, Corchs JL: States of stability/lysis in human fetal and adult red blood cells. Arch Intern Physiol Biochim 1989; 97:309.
58. Pearson HA: Life span of the fetal red blood cell. J Pediatr 1967; 70:166.
59. Sjölin S: The resistance of red cells in vitro. A study of the osmotic properties, the mechanical resistance and the behavior of red cells of fetuses, children and adults. Acta Paediatr 1954; 43:1.
60. Goldbloom RB, Fischer E, et al: Studies on the mechanical fragility of erythrocytes. I. Normal values for infants and children. Blood 1953; 8:165.
61. Colombel L, Tchernia G, Mohandas N: Human reticulocyte maturation and its relevance to erythropoietic stress. J Lab Clin Med 1979; 94:467.
62. Thatte HS, Schrier SL: Comparison of transferrin receptor–mediated endocytosis and drug-induced endocytosis in human neonatal and adult RBCs. Blood 1988; 72:1693.
63. Colin FC, Schrier SL: Myosin content and distribution in human neonatal erythrocytes are different from adult erythrocytes. Blood 1991; 78:3052.
64. Zipursky A, Brown E, et al: The erythrocyte differential count in newborn infants. Am J Pediatr Hematol Oncol 1983; 5:45.
65. Maxwell DJ, Seshadri R, et al: Infantile pyknocytosis: a cause of intrauterine haemolysis in 2 siblings. Aust N Z J Obstet Gynaecol 1983; 23:182.
66. Holroyde CP, Oski FA, et al: The "pocked" erythrocyte. N Engl J Med 1969; 281:516.
67. Nathan DG, Gunn RB. Thalassemia: the consequences of unbalanced hemoglobin synthesis. Am J Med 1966; 41:815.
68. Pearson HA, Macintosh S, et al: Interference phase microscopic enumeration of pittet RBC and splenic function in sickle cell anemia. Pediatr Res 1978; 12:471.
69. Sills RH, Tamburlin JH, et al: Formation of intracellular vesicles in neonatal and adult erythrocytes: evidence against the concept of neonatal hyposplenism. Pediatr Res 1988; 24:703.
70. Matovcik LM, Junga IG, Schrier SL: Drug-induced endocytosis of neonatal erythrocytes. Blood 1985; 65:1056.
71. Dervichian D, Fournet C, et al: Structure submicroscopique des globules rouges contenant des hémoglobines abnormales. Rev Hematol 1952; 7:567.
72. Haberman S, Blanton P, et al: Some observations on ABO antigen sites of the erythrocyte membranes of adults and newborn infants. J Immunol 1967; 98:150.
73. Kurantsin-Mills J, Lessin LS: Freeze-etching and biochemical analysis of human fetal erythrocyte membranes. Pediatr Res 1984; 18:1035.
74. Schekman R, Singer SJ: Clustering and endocytosis of membrane receptors can be induced in mature erythrocytes of neonatal but not adult humans. Proc Natl Acad Sci 1976; 73:4075.
75. Kehry M, Yguerabid J, et al: Fluidity in the membranes of adult and neonatal human erythrocytes. Science 1977; 195:486.
76. Polychronakos C, Ruggere MD, et al: The role of cell age in the difference in insulin binding between adult and cord erythrocytes. J Clin Endocrinol Metab 1982; 55:290.
77. Funakoshi T, Morikawa H, et al: Insulin-like growth factor (IGF) receptor in human fetal erythrocytes and fetal rat liver. Nippon Naibunpi Gakkai Zasshi 1989; 65:728.
78. Bellussi G, Muccioli G, et al: Prolactin binding sites in human erythrocytes and lymphocytes. Life Sci 1987; 41:951.
79. Kearin M, Kelly JG: Digoxin "receptors" in neonates: an explanation of less sensitivity to digoxin than in adults. Clin Pharmacol Ther 1980; 28:346.
80. Koekebakker M, Barr RD: Acetylcholinesterase in the human erythron. I. Cytochemistry. Am J Hematol 1988; 28:252.
81. Neerhout RC: Erythrocyte lipids in the neonate. Pediatr Res 1968; 2:172.
82. Younkin S, Oski FA, et al: Observations on the mechanism of the hydrogen peroxide hemolysis test and its reversal with phenols. Am J Clin Nutr 1971; 24:7.
83. Mollison PL, Engelfriet CP, Contreras M: Blood Transfusion in Clinical Medicine. 9th ed. Oxford, Blackwell Scientific Publications, 1993, p 89.

84. Hollan SR, Szeleny JG, et al: Structural and functional differences between human foetal and adult erythrocytes. Haematology 1967; 4:409.

85. Serrani RE, Venera G, et al: Potassium influx in human neonatal red blood cells. Partition into its major components. Arch Intern Physiol Biochim 1990; 98:27.

86. Moore TJ, Hall N: Kinetics of glucose transfer in adult and fetal human erythrocytes. Pediatr Res 1971; 5:536.

87. Schettini F, Bratta A, et al: Acid lysis of red blood cells in normal children. Acta Paediatr Scand 1971; 60:17.

87a. Matsuo Y, Inoue F, et al: Changes of erythrocyte ouabain maximum binding after birth in neonates in relation to erythrocyte sodium and potassium concentrations. Early Hum Develop 1995; 43:59.

88. Brahm J, Wimberley PD: Chloride and bicarbonate transport in fetal red cells. J Physiol 1989; 419:141.

89. Linderkamp O, Hammer BJ, Miller R: Filterability of erythrocytes and whole blood in preterm and full-term neonates and adults. Pediatr Res 1986; 20:1269.

90. Colin FC, Gallois Y, et al: Impaired fetal erythrocyte's filterability: relationship with cell size, membrane fluidity, and membrane lipid composition. Blood 1992; 79:2148.

91. Buonocore G, Berni S, et al: Characteristics and functional properties of red cells during the first days of life. Biol Neonate 1991; 60:137.

92. Gross RT, Schroeder EA, et al: Energy metabolism in the erythrocytes of premature infants compared to full-term newborn infants and adults. Blood 1963; 21:755.

93. Konrad PN, Valentine WN, et al: Enzymatic activities and glutathione content of erythrocytes in the newborn: comparison with red cells of older normal subjects and those with comparable reticulocytosis. Acta Haematol 1972; 48:193.

94. Oski FA: Red cell metabolism in the newborn infant. V. Glycolytic intermediates and glycolytic enzymes. Pediatrics 1969; 44:84.

95. Witt I, Herdan M, et al: Vergleichende Untersuchungen von Enzymaktivitäten in Reticulocyten-reichen und Reticulocyten-armen Fraktionen aus Neugeborenen- und Erwachsenenblut. Klin Wochenschr 1968; 46:149.

96. Lestas AN, Rodeck CH, et al: Normal activities of glycolytic enzymes in the fetal erythrocytes. Br J Haematol 1982; 50:439.

97. Travis SF, Garvin JH Jr: *In vivo* lability of red cell phosphofructokinase in term infants. Pediatr Res 1977; 11:1159.

98. Vora S, Piomelli S: A fetal isozyme of phosphofructokinase in newborn erythrocytes. Pediatr Res 1977; 11:483.

99. Holmes EW Jr, Malone JL, et al: Hexokinase isoenzymes in human erythrocytes. Association of Type II with fetal hemoglobin. Science 1967; 156:646.

100. Schröter W, Tillman W: Hexokinase isoenzymes in human erythrocytes of adults and newborns. Biochem Biophys Res Commun 1968; 31:92.

101. Chen SH, Anderson JE, et al: Lysozyme patterns in erythrocytes from human fetuses. Am J Hematol 1977; 2:23.

102. Witt I, Witz D: Reinigung und Charakterisierung von Phosphopyruvatz-Hydratase (= Enolase; EC 4.2.1.11) aus Neugeborenen- und Erwachsenen-Erythrozyten. Hoppe Seylers Z Physiol Chem 1970; 351:1232.

103. Oski FA, Smith CA: Effect of pH on glycolysis in the erythrocytes of the newborn infant. Proc Soc Pediatr Res 1972; p 106.

104. Witt I, Müller H, Künzer W: Vergleichende biochemische Untersuchungen an Erythrocyten aus Neugeborenen- und Erwachsenen-Blut. Klin Wochenschr 1967; 45:262.

105. Bentley HP Jr, Alford CA Jr, et al: Erythrocyte glucose consumption in the neonate. J Lab Clin Med 1970; 76:311.

106. Oski FA, Travis SF: Effect of pH on glycolysis in the erythrocytes of the newborn infant. Proc Soc Pediatr Res 1972; p 106.

107. Oski FA: Red cell metabolism in the premature infant. II. The pentose phosphate pathway. Pediatrics 1967; 39:689.

108. Zipursky A, LaRue T, et al: The *in vitro* metabolism of erythrocytes from newborn infants. Can J Biochem Physiol 1960; 38:727.

109. Schröter W, Winter P: Der 2,3-Diphosphoglyceratstoffwechsel in den Erythrocyten Neugeborener und Erwachsener. Klin Wochenschr 1967; 45:255.

110. Trueworthy R, Lowman JT: Intracellular control of 2,3-diphosphoglycerate concentration in fetal red cells. Proc Soc Pediatr Res 1971, p 86.

111. Lestas AN, Bellingham AJ, Nicolaides KH: Red cell glycolytic intermediates in normal, anaemic and transfused human fetuses. Br J Haematol 1989; 73:387.

112. Jain SK: The neonatal erythrocyte and its oxidative susceptibility. Semin Hematol 1989; 26:286.

113. Shahal Y, Bauminger ER, et al: Oxidative stress in newborn erythrocytes. Pediatr Res 1991; 29:119.

114. Abbasi S, Ludomirski A, et al: Maternal and fetal plasma vitamin E to total lipid ratio and fetal RBC antioxidant function during gestational development. J Am Coll Nutr 1990; 9:314.

115. Glader BE, Conrad MD: Decreased glutathione peroxidase in neonatal erythrocytes: lack of relation to hydrogen peroxide metabolism. Pediatr Res 1972; 6:900.

116. Lestas AN, Rodeck CH: Normal glutathione content and some related enzyme activities in the fetal erythrocytes. Br J Haematol 1984; 57:695.

117. Gros RT, Bracci R, et al: Hydrogen peroxide toxicity and detoxification in the erythrocytes of newborn infants. Blood 1967; 29:481.

118. Whaun JM, Oski FA: Relation of red blood cell glutathione peroxidase to neonatal jaundice. J Pediatr 1970; 76:555.

119. Schröter W: Drug susceptibility and the development of erythrocyte enzyme systems. In Leiden, Stenfert, Krose: Nutricia Symposium: Metabolic Processes in the Fetus and Newborn Infant. 1971, p 73.

120. Aliakbar S, Brown PR, et al: Human erythrocyte superoxide dismutase in adults, neonates, and normal, hypoxaemic, anaemic and chromosomally abnormal fetuses. Clin Biochem 1993; 26:109.

121. Agostoni A, Gerli GC, et al: Superoxide dismutase, catalase, and glutathione peroxidase activities in maternal and cord blood erythrocytes. J Clin Chem Clin Biochem 1980; 18:771.

122. Bracci R, Martini G, et al: Changes in erythrocyte properties during the first hours of life: electron spin resonance of reacting sulfhydryl groups. Pediatr Res 1988; 24:391.

123. Haga P, Lunde G: Selenium and vitamin E in cord blood from preterm and full-term infants. Acta Paediatr Scand 1978; 67:735.

124. Schröter W, Bodemann H: Experimentally induced cation leaks of the red cell membrane. Biol Neonate 1970; 15:291.

125. Tillman W, Menke J, et al: The formation of Heinz bodies in ghosts of human erythrocytes of adults and newborn infants. Klin Wochenschr 1973; 51:201.

126. Kleihauer E, Bernau A, et al: Heinzkörperbildung in Neugeborenerythrozyten. 1. *In-vitro*-Studien über experimentelle Bedingungen und den Einfluss von Austauschtransfusionen. Acta Haematol 1970; 43:333.

127. Schröter W, Tillman W: Heinz body susceptibility of red cells and exchange transfusion. Acta Haematol 1973; 49:74.

128. Bracci R, Benedetti PA, et al: Hydrogen peroxide generation in the erythrocytes of newborn infants. Biol Neonate 1970; 15:135.

129. Lipschutz F, Lubin B, et al: Red cell oxygen consumption and hydrogen peroxide formation. Proc Soc Pediatr Res 1972, p 1051.

130. Löhr GW, Waller HD, et al: Quantitative Fermentbestimmungen in roten Blutzellen. Klin Wochenschr 1957; 35:871.

131. Oettinger L Jr, Mills WB: Simultaneous capillary and venous hemoglobin determinations in newborn infants. J Pediatr 1949; 35:362.

132. Moe PJ: Umbilical cord blood and capillary blood in the evaluation of anemia in erythroblastosis fetalis. Acta Paediatr Scand 1967; 56:391.

133. Linderkamp O, Versmold HT, et al: Capillary-venous hematocrit differences in newborn infants. I. Relationship to blood volume, peripheral blood flow, and acid-base parameters. Eur J Pediatr 1977; 127:9.

134. Usher R, Shepard M, et al: The blood volume of the newborn infant and placental transfusion. Acta Paediatr Scand 1963; 52:497.

135. Yao AC, Lind J, et al: Placental transfusion in the premature infant with observation on clinical course and outcome. Acta Paediatr Scand 1969; 58:561.

136. Gunther M: The transfer of blood between baby and placenta in the minutes after birth. Lancet 1957; 1:1277.

137. Ogata ES, Kitterman JA, et al: The effect of time of cord clamping and maternal blood pressure on placental transfusion with cesarean section. Am J Obstet Gynecol 1977; 128:197.

138. Linderkamp O, Nelle M, et al: The effect of early and late cord clamping on blood viscosity and other hemorheological parameters in full-term neonates. Acta Paediatr 1992; 81:745.

139. Nelle M, Zilow EP, et al: The effect of Leboyer delivery on blood viscosity and other hemorheological parameters in term neonates. Am J Obstet Gynecol 1993; 169:189.

140. Usher RH, Saigal S, et al: Estimation of red blood cell volume in premature infants with and without respiratory distress syndrome. Biol Neonate 1975; 26:241.

141. Kinmond S, Aitchison TC, et al: Umbilical cord clamping and preterm infants: a randomized trial. Br Med J 1993; 306:172.

142. Hofmeyr GJ, Gobetz L, et al: Periventricular/intraventricular hemorrhage following early and delayed umbilical cord clamping. A randomized controlled trial. Online J Curr Clin Trials Doc. No. 110 Dec 29, 1993.

143. Saigal S, Usher RH: Symptomatic neonatal plethora. Biol Neonate 1977; 32:62.

144. Saigal S, Wilson R, Usher R: Radiological findings in symptomatic neonatal plethora resulting from placental transfusion. Radiology 1977; 125:185.

145. Yao AC, Lind J: Effect of early and late cord clamping on the systolic time intervals of the newborn infant. Acta Paediatr Scand 1977; 66:489.

146. Erkkola R, Kero P, et al: Delayed cord clamping in cesarean section with general anesthesia. Am J Perinatol 1984; 1:165.

147. Mollison PL, Veall N, et al: Red cell and plasma volume in newborn infants. Arch Dis Child 1950; 25:242.

148. Jegier W, MacLaurin J, et al: Comparative study of blood volume estimation in the newborn infant using I 131–labeled human serum albumin (IHSA) and T-1824. Scand J Clin Lab Invest 1964; 16:125.

149. Usher R, Lind J: Blood volume of the newborn premature infant. Acta Paediatr Scand 1965; 54:419.

150. Sisson TRC, Lund CJ, et al: The blood volume of infants. I. The full-term infant in the first year of life. J Pediatr 1959; 55:163.

151. Cassady G: Plasma volume studies in low birth weight infants. Pediatrics 1966; 38:1020.

152. Russell SJM: Blood volume studies in healthy children. Arch Dis Child 1949; 24:88.

153. Brines JK, Gibson JG Jr, et al: Blood volume in normal infants and children. J Pediatr 1941; 18:447.

154. Brown E, Krouskop RW, et al: Blood volume and blood pressure in infants with respiratory distress. J Pediatr 1975; 87:1133.

155. Faxelius G, Raye J, et al: Red cell volume measurements and acute blood loss in high risk newborn infants. J Pediatr 1977; 90:273.

156. Shepherd AJ, Richardson CJ, et al: Nuchal cord as a cause of neonatal anemia. Am J Dis Child 1985; 139:71.

157. Forestier F, Daffos F, et al: Hematological values of normal fetuses between 18 and 30 weeks of gestation. Pediatr Res 1986; 20:342.

158. Dialio DH, Sidibe S, et al: Prévalence de l'anémie du nouveau-né au Mali. Cah Sante 1994; 4:341.

159. Forestier F, Daffos F, et al: Hematological values of 163 normal fetuses between 18 and 30 weeks of gestation. Pediatr Res 1986; 20:342.

160. Boyd PA, Keeling JW: Fetal hydrops. J Med Genet 1992; 29:91.

161. Saltzman DH, Frigoletto FD, et al: Sonographic evaluation of hydrops fetalis. Obstet Gynecol 1989; 74:106.

162. Oie BK, Hertel J, et al: Hydrops foetalis in 3 infants of a mother with acquired chronic pure red cell aplasia. Transitory red cell aplasia in 1 of the infants. Scand J Haematol 1984; 33:466.

163. Rejjal AL, Nazer H: Resolution of cystic hygroma, hydrops fetalis, and fetal anemia. Am J Perinatol 1993; 10:455.

164. Hirata GI, Masaki DI, et al: Color flow mapping and Doppler velocimetry in the diagnosis and management of a placental chorioangioma associated with non-immune fetal hydrops. Obstet Gynecol 1993; 81:850.

165. Panero C, Azzi A, et al: Fetoneonatal hydrops from human parvovirus B19. Case report. J Perinat Med 1994; 22:257.

166. Brabin B: Fetal anemia in malarious areas: its causes and significance. Ann Trop Paediatr 1992; 12:303.

167. Norton ME: Nonimmune hydrops fetalis. Semin Perinatol 1994; 18:321.

168. Lubin B: Neonatal anaemia secondary to blood loss. Clin Haematol 1978; 7:19.

169. Glader BE, Platt O: Haemolytic disorders of infancy. Clin Haematol 1978; 7:35.

170. Oski FA, Naiman JL: Hematologic Problems of the Newborn. 3rd ed. Philadelphia, W.B. Saunders Co. 1982, pp 56–86.

171. Blanchette VS, Zipursky A: Assessment of anemia in newborn infants. Clin Perinatol 1984; 11:489.

172. Dickerman JD: Anemia in the newborn infant. Pediatr Rev 1984; 6:131.

173. Anaemia in premature infants. Lancet 1987; 2:1371. Editorial.

174. Halperin DS: Use of recombinant erythropoietin in treatment of the anemia of prematurity. Am J Pediatr Hematol Oncol 1991; 13:351.

175. Dallman PR: Anemia of prematurity: the prospects for avoiding blood transfusions by treatment with recombinant human erythropoietin. Adv Pediatr 1993; 40:385.

176. Gallagher PG, Ehrenkranz RA: Erythropoietin therapy for anemia of prematurity. Clin Perinatol 1993; 20:169.

177. Kannourakis G: The biology of erythropoietin and its role in the anemia of prematurity. J Paediatr Child Health 1994; 30:293.

178. Faxelius G, Raye J, et al: Red cell volume measurements and acute blood loss in high-risk newborn infants. J Pediatr 1977; 90:273.

179. Zipursky A, Hull A, et al: Foetal erythrocytes in the maternal circulation. Lancet 1959; 1:451.

180. Ganshirt-Ahlert D, Borjesson-Stoll R, et al: Detection of fetal trisomies 21 and 18 from maternal blood using triple gradient and magnetic cell sorting. Am J Reprod Immunol 1993; 30:194.

181. Geifman-Holtzman O, Blatman RN, Bianchi DW: Prenatal genetic diagnosis by isolation and analysis of fetal cells circulating in maternal blood. Semin Perinatol 1994; 18:366.

182. Sebring ES, Polesky HF: Fetomaternal hemorrhage: incidence, risk factors, time of occurrence and clinical effects. Transfusion 1990; 30:344.

183. de Almeida V, Bowman JM: Massive fetomaternal hemorrhage: Manitoba experience. Obstetr Gynecol 1994; 83:323.

184. Pearlman MD, Tintinalli JE, Lorenz RP: A prospective controlled study of outcome after trauma during pregnancy. Am J Obstet Gynecol 1990; 162:1502.

185. Duleba AJ, Miller D, Taylor G: Expectant management of choriocarcinoma limited to placenta. Gynecol Oncol 1992; 44:277.

186. Kleihauer E, Hildegard B, et al: Demonstration von fetalem Hämoglobin in den Erythrocyten eines Blutausstrichs. Klin Wochenschr 1957; 35:637.

187. Patton WN, Nicholson GS, et al: Assessment of fetal-maternal hemorrhage in mothers with hereditary persistence of fetal hemoglobin. J Clin Pathol 1990; 43:728.

188. Bayliss KM, Kueck BD, et al: Detecting fetomaternal hemorrhage: a comparison of five methods. Transfusion 1991; 31:303.

189. Greenwalt TJ, Dumaswala UJ, Domino MM: The quantification of fetomaternal hemorrhage by an enzyme-linked antibody test with glutaraldehyde fixation. Vox Sang 1992; 63:268.

190. Garratty G, Arndt P: Applications of flow cytometry to transfusion science. Transfusion 1995; 35:157.

191. Benirschke K: Accurate recording of twin placenta. Obstetr Gynecol 1961; 18:334.

192. Rausen AR, London RD, et al: Generalized bone changes and thrombocytopenic purpura in association with intra-uterine rubella. Pediatrics 1965; 36:264.

193. Strong SJ, Comey G: The Placenta in Twin Pregnancy. New York, Pergamon Press, 1967.

194. Fries MH, Goldstein RB, et al: The role of velamentous cord insertion in the etiology of twin-twin transfusion syndrome. Obstet Gynecol 1993; 81:569.

195. Gonsoulin W, Moise KJ, et al: Outcome of twin-twin transfusion diagnosed before 28 weeks of gestation. Obstet Gynecol 1990; 75:214.

196. Blickstein I: The twin-twin transfusion syndrome. Obstet Gynecol 1990; 76:714.

197. Bruner JP, Rosemond RL: Twin-to-twin transfusion syndrome: a subset of the twin oligohydramnios-polyhydramnios sequence. Am J Obstet Gynecol 1993; 169:925.

198. Pinette MG, Pan Y, et al: Treatment of twin-twin transfusion syndrome. Obstet Gynecol 1993; 82:841.

199. Pochedly C, Musiker S: Twin-to-twin transfusion syndrome. Postgrad Med 1970; 47:172.

200. Tan KL, Tan R, et al: The twin transfusion syndrome. Clinical observations on 35 affected pairs. Clin Pediatr 1979; 18:111.
201. Klebe JG, Ingomar CJ: The fetoplacental circulation during parturition illustrated by the interfetal transfusion syndrome. Pediatrics 1972; 49:112.
202. Kirkman HN, Riley HD Jr: Posthemorrhagic anemia and shock in the newborn. A review. Pediatrics 1959; 24:97.
203. Weiner AS: Diagnosis and treatment of anemia of the newborn caused by occult placental hemorrhage. Am J Obstet Gynecol 1948; 56:717.
204. Novak F: Posthemorrhagic shock in newborns during labor and after delivery. Acta Med Iugoslav 1953; 7:280.
205. Clayton EM, Pryor JA, et al: Fetal and maternal components of third-trimester obstetric hemorrhage. Obstet Gynecol 1964 24:56.
206. Leonard S, Anthony B: Giant cephalohematoma of newborn. Am J Dis Child 1961; 101:170.
207. Robinson RJ, Rossiter MA: Massive subaponeurotic hemorrhage in babies of African origin. Arch Dis Child 1968; 43:684.
208. Packman DJ: Massive hemorrhage in the scalp of the newborn infant. Hemorrhagic caput succedaneum. Pediatrics 1962; 29:907.
209. Florentino-Pineda I, Ezhuthachan SG, et al: Subgaleal hemorrhage in the newborn infant associated with silicone elastomer vacuum extractor. J Perinatol 1994; 14:95.
210. Rausen AR, Diamond LK: Enclosed hemorrhage and neonatal jaundice. Am J Dis Child 1961; 101:164.
211. Potter EL: Fetal and neonatal deaths: a statistical analysis of 2000 autopsies. JAMA 1940; 115:996.
212. Henderson JL: Hepatic hemorrhage in stillborn and newborn infants; clinical and pathological study of 47 cases. J Obstet Gynaecol Br Emp 1941; 48:377.
213. Erakalis AJ: Abdominal injury related to the trauma of birth. Pediatrics 1967; 39:421.
214. Philipsborn HF Jr, Traisman HS, et al: Rupture of the spleen: a complication of erythroblastosis fetalis. N Engl J Med 1955; 252:159.
215. Leape LL, Bordy MD: Neonatal rupture of the spleen. Report of a case successfully treated after spontaneous cessation of hemorrhage. Pediatrics 1971; 47:101.
216. Yerby M: Epilepsy and pregnancy. New issues for an old disorder. Neurol Clin 1993; 4:777.
217. Abzug AJ, Levin MJ: Neonatal adenovirus infection: four patients and review of the literature. Pediatrics 1991; 87:890.
218. Hohlfeld P, Vial Y, et al: Cytomegalovirus fetal infection: prenatal diagnosis. Obstet Gynecol 1991; 78:615.
219. Nader PR, Margolin F: Hemangioma causing gastrointestinal bleeding. Case report and review of the literature. Am J Dis Child 1966; 111:215.
220. Svane S: Foetal exsanguination from hemangioendothelioma of the skin. Acta Paediatr Scand 1966; 55:536.
221. Rumack CM, Guggenheim MA, et al: Neonatal intracranial hemorrhage and maternal use of aspirin. Obstet Gynecol 1981; 58(Suppl):528.
222. Papile L, Burstein J, et al: Incidence and evolution of subependymal and intraventricular hemorrhage: study of infants with birth weights less than 1500 grams. J Pediatr 1978; 92:529.
223. Nexo E, Christensen NC, Olesen H: Volume of blood removed for analytical purposes during hospitalization of low-birthweight infants. Clin Chem 1981; 27:759.
224. Obladen M, Sachsenweger M, Stahnke M: Blood sampling in very low birth weight infants receiving different levels of intensive care. Eur J Pediatr 1988; 147:399.
225. Shulman RJ, Phillips S, et al: Volume of blood required to obtain central venous catheter blood cultures in infants and children. JPEN J Parenter Enteral Nutr 1993; 17:177.
226. Thorkelsson T, Hoath SB: Accurate micromethod of neonatal blood sampling from peripheral arterial catheters. J Perinatol 1995; 15:43.
227. Gleason E, Grossman S, Campbell C: Minimizing diagnostic blood loss in critically ill patients. Am J Crit Care 1992; 1:85.
228. Silver MJ, YH L, et al: Reduction of blood loss from diagnostic sampling in critically ill patients using a blood-conserving arterial line system. Chest 1993; 104:1711.
229. Necheles TF, Rai US, et al: The role of haemolysis in neonatal hyperbilirubinemia as reflected in carboxyhaemoglobin levels. Acta Paediatr Scand 1976; 65:361.
230. Minnich V, Cordonnier JK, et al: Alpha, beta and gamma hemoglobin polypeptide chains during the neonatal period with a description of a fetal form of hemoglobin D St. Louis. Blood 1962; 19:137.
231. Levine RL, Lincoln DR, et al: Hemoglobin Hasharon in a premature infant with hemolytic anemia. Pediatr Res 1975; 9:7.
232. van Wijgerden JA: Clinical expression of sickle cell anemia in the newborn. South Med J 1983; 76:478.
233. Hegyi T, Delphin ES, et al: Sickle cell anemia in the newborn. Pediatrics 1977; 60:213.
234. Veiga S, Varthianathan T: Massive intravascular sickling after exchange transfusion with sickle cell trait blood. Transfusion 1963; 3:387.
235. Lee-Potter JP, Deacon-Smith RA, et al: A new cause of hemolytic anemia in the newborn. J Clin Pathol 1975; 28:317.
236. Schmairer AH, Mauer HM, et al: Alpha thalassemia screening in neonates by mean corpuscular volume and mean corpuscular hemoglobin concentration. J Pediatr 1973; 83:794.
237. Koenig HM, Vedvidk TS, et al: Prenatal diagnosis of hemoglobin H disease. J Pediatr 1978; 92:278.
238. Thumasathit B, Nondasuta A, et al: Hydrops fetalis associated with Bart's hemoglobin in northern Thailand. J Pediatr 1968; 73:132.
239. Beaudry MA, Ferguson DJ, et al: Survival of a hydropic infant with homozygous alpha-thalassemia-l. J Pediatr 1986; 108:713.
240. Bianchi DW, Beyer EC, et al: Normal long-term survival with alpha-thalassemia. J Pediatr 1986; 108:716.
241. Erlandson ME, Hilgartner M: Hemolytic disease in the neonatal period. J Pediatr 1959; 54:566.
242. Stamatoyannopoulos G: Gamma-thalassemia. Lancet 1971; 2:192.
243. Kan YW, Forget BG, et al: Gamma-beta thalassemia: a cause of hemolytic disease of the newborn. N Engl J Med 1972; 286:129.
244. Abman SH, Griebel JL, et al: Acute effect of inhaled nitric oxide in children with severe hypoxemic respiratory failure. J Pediatr 1994; 124:881.
245. Journois D, Pouard P, et al: Inhaled nitric oxide as a therapy for pulmonary hypertension after operation for congenital heart defects. J Thorac Cardiovasc Surg 1994; 107:1129.
246. Winberg P, Lundell BP, Gustafsson LE: Effect of inhaled nitric oxide on raised pulmonary vascular resistance in children with congenital heart disease. Br Heart J 1994; 71:282.
247. Speakman ED, Boyd JC, Bruns DE: Measurement of methemoglobin in neonatal samples containing fetal hemoglobin. Clin Chem 1995; 41:458.
248. Alter BP, Nathan DG: Red cell aplasia in children. Arch Dis Child 1979; 54:263.
249. Diamond LK, Wang WC, et al: Congenital hypoplastic anemia. Adv Pediatr 1976; 22:349.
250. Diamond LK, Allen DM, et al: Congenital (erythroid) hypoplastic anemia. Am J Dis Child 1961; 102:149.
251. Pearson HA, Lobel JS, et al: A new syndrome of refractory sideroblastic anemia with vacuolization of marrow precursors and exocrine pancreatic dysfunction. J Pediatr 1979; 95:976.
252. Blatt J, Katerji A, et al: Pancytopenia and vacuolization of marrow precursors associated with necrotizing encephalopathy. Br J Haematol 1994; 86:207.
253. Simonsz HJ, Barlocher K, Rotig A: Kearns-Sayre's syndrome developing in a boy who survived Pearson's syndrome caused by mitochondrial DNA deletion. Doc Ophthalmol 1992; 82:73.
254. Fischel-Ghodsian N, Bohlman MC, et al: Deletion in blood mitochondrial DNA in Kearns-Sayre syndrome. Pediatr Res 1992; 31:557.
255. Rotig A, Colonna M, et al: A 13-bp direct repeat in mitochondrial DNA promotes deletions in Pearson's syndrome. Lancet 1989; 1:250.
256. Lestienne P, Bataille N: Mitochondrial DNA alterations and genetic diseases: a review. Biomed Pharmacol 1994; 48:199.
257. Jardine PE, Cotter PD, et al: Pyridoxine-refractory congenital sideroblastic anemia with evidence for autosomal inheritance: exclusions of linkage to ALAS2 at Xp11.21 by polymorphism analysis. J Med Genet 1994; 31:213.
258. Mäkitie O, Rajantie J, Kaitila I: Anemia and macrocytosis—unrecognized features in cartilage-hair hypoplasia. Acta Paediatr 1992; 81:1026.

259. Tugal O, Pallant B, et al: Transient erythroblastopenia of the newborn caused by human parvovirus. Am J Pediatr Hematol Oncol 1994; 16:352.

260. Schulman J: The anemia of prematurity. J Pediatr 1959; 54:633.

261. Stockman JA: The anemia of prematurity and the decision when to transfuse. Adv Pediatr 1983; 30:191.

262. Melhorn DK, Gross S: Vitamin E–dependent anemia in the preterm infant. I. Effects of large doses of medicinal iron. J Pediatr 1971; 79:569.

263. Bratteby LE: Studies on erythrokinetics in infancy. XI. The change in circulating red cell volume during the first five months of life. Acta Paediatr Scand 1968; 54:215.

264. Halvorsen S, Finne PH: Erythropoietin production in the human fetus and newborn. Ann N Y Acad Sci 1968; 149:516.

265. Rollins MD, Maxwell AP, et al: Cord blood erythropoietin, pH, PaO_2 and hematocrit following caesarean section before labour. Biol Neonate 1993; 63:147.

266. Willard DD, Gidding SS, et al: Effect of intravascular, intrauterine transfusion on prenatal and postnatal hemolysis and erythropoiesis in severe fetal isoimmunization. J Pediatr 1990; 117:447.

267. Humbert JR, Abelson H, et al: Polycythemia in small for gestational age infants. J Pediatr 1969; 75:812.

268. Cook CD, Brodie HR, et al: Measurement of fetal hemoglobin in newborn infants. Correlation with gestational age and intrauterine hypoxia. Pediatrics 1957; 20:272.

269. Stockman JA III, Garcia JF, et al: The anemia of prematurity. Factors governing the erythropoietin response. N Engl J Med 1977; 296:647.

270. Brown MS, Phibb RH, et al: Decreased response of plasma immunoreactive erythropoietin to "available oxygen" in anemia of prematurity. J Pediatr 1984; 105:793.

271. Stockman JA III, Graeber JE, et al: Anemia of prematurity. Determinants of erythropoietin response. J Pediatr 1984; 105:786.

272. Yamashita H, Kukita J, Ohga S: Serum erythropoietin levels in term and preterm infants during the first year of life. Am J Pediatr Hematol Oncol 1994; 16:213.

273. Emmerson AJB, Westwood NB, et al: Erythropoietin responsive progenitors in anemia of prematurity. Arch Dis Child 1991; 66:810.

274. Shannon KM, Naylor GS, et al: Circulating erythroid progenitors in the anemia of prematurity. N Engl J Med 1987; 317:728.

275. Rhondeau SM, Christensen RD, et al: Responsiveness to recombinant erythropoietin of marrow erythroid progenitors in infants with anemia of prematurity. J Pediatr 1988; 112:935.

276. Ruth V, Widness JA, et al: Postnatal changes in serum immunoreactive erythropoietin in relation to hypoxia before and after birth. J Pediatr 1990; 116:950.

277. Brown MS, Jones MA, et al: Single-dose pharmacokinetics of recombinant human erythropoietin in preterm infants after intravenous and subcutaneous administration. J Pediatr 1993; 122:655.

278. Strauss RG: Erythropoietin in the pathogenesis and treatment of neonatal anemia. Transfusion 1995; 35:68.

279. Attias D: Pathophysiology and treatment of the anemia of prematurity. J Pediatr Hematol Oncol 1995; 17:13.

280. Meyer M, Meyer JH, et al: Recombinant human erythropoietin in the treatment of the anemia of prematurity: results of a double-blind, placebo-controlled study. Pediatrics 1994; 93:918.

281. Soubasi V, Kremenopoulos G, et al: In which neonates does early recombinant human erythropoietin treatment prevent anemia of prematurity? Results of a randomized, controlled study. Pediatr Res 1993; 34:675.

282. Shannon KM, Keith JF, et al: Recombinant human erythropoietin stimulates erythropoiesis and reduces erythrocyte transfusions in very low birth weight preterm infants. Pediatrics 1995; 95:1.

282a. Fain J, Hilsenrath P, et al: A cost analysis comparing erythropoietin and red cell transfusions in the treatment of anemia of prematurity. Transfusion 1995; 35:936.

283. Brugnara C, Colella GM, et al: Effects of subcutaneous recombinant human erythropoietin in normal subjects: development of decreased reticulocyte hemoglobin content and iron-deficient erythropoiesis. J Lab Clin Med 1994; 123:660.

284. Etchason J, Petz L, et al: The cost effectiveness of preoperative autologous blood donations. N Engl J Med 1995; 332:719.

285. Rutherford CJ, Kaplan HS: Autologous blood donation—Can we bank on it? N Engl J Med 1995; 332:740.

286. Shireman TI, Hilsenrath PE, et al: Recombinant human erythropoietin vs. transfusions in the treatment of anemia of prematurity. Arch Pediatr Adolesc Med 1994; 148:582.

287. Baxter LM, Vreman HJ, et al: Recombinant human erythropoietin (r-HuEPO) increases total bilirubin production in premature infants. Clin Pediatr 1995; 34:213.

287a. Bechensteen AG, Refsum HE, et al: Effects of recombinant human erythropoietin on fetal and adult hemoglobin in preterm infants. Pediatr Res 1995; 38:729.

288. Black DB, Lubchenco LO, et al: Developmental and neurologic sequalae of neonatal hyperviscosity syndrome. Pediatrics 1982; 69:426.

289. Saggese G, Bertelloni S, et al: Elevated calcitonin gene–related peptide in polycythemic newborn infants. Acta Paediatr 1992; 81:966.

290. Bada HS, Korones SB, et al: Asymptomatic syndrome of polycythemic hyperviscosity: effect of partial plasma exchange transfusion. J Pediatr 1992; 120:579.

291. Drew JH, Guaran RL, et al: Cord whole blood hyperviscosity: measurement, definition, incidence and clinical features. J Paediatr Child Health 1991; 26:363.

292. Mimouni F, Miodovnik M, et al: Neonatal polycythemia in infants of insulin-dependent diabetic mothers. Obstet Gynecol 1986; 68:370.

293. Piacquadio K, Hollingsworth DR, Murphy H: Effects of in-utero exposure to oral hypoglycemic drugs. Lancet 1991; 338:866.

294. Oh W: Neonatal polycythemia and hyperviscosity. Pediatr Clin North Am 1986; 33:523.

295. Sacher R, Luban NLC, Strauss RG: Current practice and guidelines for the transfusion of cellular blood components in the newborn. Transfus Med Rev 1989; 3:39.

296. Yu VY, Gan TE: Red cell transfusion in the preterm infant. J Paediatr Child Health 1994; 30:301.

297. Dallman PR: Anemia of prematurity: the prospects for avoiding blood transfusions by treatment with recombinant human erythropoietin. Adv Pediatr 1993; 40:385.

298. Shannon K: Recombinant erythropoietin in anemia of prematurity: five years later. Pediatrics 1993; 92:614.

299. Wardrop CA, Holland BM, et al: Non physiological anemia of prematurity. Arch Dis Child 1978; 53:855.

300. Schneider AJ, Stockman JA III, Oski FA: Transfusion nomogram: an application of physiology to clinical decisions regarding the use of blood. Crit Care Med 1981; 9:469.

301. Stockman JA III, Levin E, et al: O_2 consumption of premature infants in the first 10 weeks of life: Response to transfusion. Pediatr Res 1979; 13:442.

302. Izraeli S, Ben-Sira L, et al: Lactic acid as a predictor for erythrocyte transfusion in healthy preterm infants with anemia of prematurity. J Pediatr 1993; 122:629.

303. Strauss RG: Transfusion therapy in neonates. Am J Dis Child 1991; 145:904.

304. Strauss RG: Erythropoietin and neonatal anemia. N Engl J Med 1994; 330:1227.

305. Levy GJ, Strauss RG, et al: National survey of neonatal transfusion practices: I. Red blood cell therapy. Pediatrics 1993; 91:523.

306. Strauss RG, Levy GJ, et al: National survey of neonatal transfusion practices: II. Blood component therapy. Pediatrics 1993; 91:530.

307. Standards for Blood Banks and Transfusion Services. 16th ed. Bethesda, MD, American Association of Blood Banks, 1994.

308. Luban NL, Strauss RG, Hume HA: Commentary on the safety of red cells preserved in extended-storage media for neonatal transfusions. Transfusion 1991; 31:229.

309. Patten E, Robbins M, et al: Use of red blood cells older than five days for neonatal transfusion. J Perinatol 1991; 11:37.

310. Cook S, Gunter J, Wissel M: Effective use of a strategy using assigned red cell units to limit donor exposure for neonatal patients. Transfusion 1993; 33:379.

311. Liu EA, Mannino FL, Lane TA: Prospective randomized trial of the safety and efficacy of a limited donor exposure transfusion program for premature neonates. J Pediatr 1994; 125:92.

312. Strauss RG, Sacher RA: Directed donations for pediatric patients. Transfus Med Rev 1988; 2:58.

313. Ringer SA, Richardson D, et al: Blood utilization in neonatal intensive care. Blood 1991; 78:353a.

Immune Hemolytic Disease

John M. Bowman

HISTORICAL ASPECTS

In 1609, a French midwife, Louyse Bourgeois, writing in the popular Paris press, was the first to describe hemolytic disease of the fetus and newborn (HDN). She reported the birth of twins: the first twin was bloated with fluid (hydropic) and died shortly after birth; the second appeared well but rapidly became jaundiced (icterus gravis), lay in a position of opisthotonos, and died (kernicterus). These two conditions, hydrops fetalis and kernicterus (yellow staining of the brain) were described in detail by pathologists at the turn of the century but were not thought to be the same entity until 1932. Diamond and co-workers[1] showed that hydrops fetalis, icterus gravis, and kernicterus were simply different spectra of the same disease characterized by hemolytic anemia, extramedullary erythropoiesis, hepatosplenomegaly, and the outpouring of immature nucleated red blood cells (RBCs) (erythroblasts, Fig. 3–1); they coined a new name for the disease: *erythroblastosis fetalis*. In 1938, Dr. Ruth Darrow, who had lost a baby to kernicterus, hypothesized that fetal RBCs, containing fetal hemoglobin, crossed the placenta into the maternal circulation, stimulating the mother to produce antifetal hemoglobin.[2] The antibody then crossed back into the fetal circulation and destroyed the fetal RBCs. Her hypothesis was correct except for the specific antigen and antibody involved.

In 1939, Levine and Stetson described a severe transfusion reaction in a woman following delivery of a hydropic stillborn infant.[3] The mother, who had a postpartum hemorrhage, received a transfusion of her husband's blood. She was determined to have an antibody that agglutinated her husband's RBCs. Levine postulated that she had become sensitized to an RBC antigen that the fetus had inherited from its father.

In 1940, Landsteiner and Wiener discovered the offending antigen.[4] They injected guinea pigs and rabbits with rhesus monkey RBCs. The animals obligingly produced rhesus monkey RBC antibodies. When they took blood samples from a group of Caucasians, they found that 85% had RBCs that were agglutinated by the rhesus RBC antisera—that is, these subjects were *rhesus (or Rh) positive*; 15% had RBCs that were not agglutinated—that is, these subjects were *rhesus (or Rh) negative*. This experiment was a major landmark in modern medicine. It provided the framework for modern immunohematology, unraveled the cause of immune hemolytic disease, provided the basis for the science of human anthropology, and allowed the development of relatively safe blood transfusion.

Levine and associates promptly obtained some of Landsteiner and Wiener's antiserum. They determined that Levine and Stetson's patient was Rh negative and her husband Rh positive and that her serum agglutinated the RBCs of Wiener and Landsteiner's Rh-positive individuals but did not agglutinate the RBCs of their Rh-negative subjects.[5] The monkey RBC antigen and antibody (L^W and anti-L^W) are not the same as the human D antigen and antibody; however, this difference does not detract from the importance of their discovery.

The cause of hemolytic disease of the fetus was established. A D-negative woman exposed to D-positive RBCs develops anti-D. The anti-D, if immunoglobulin G (IgG) in nature, traverses the placenta and coats the fetal D-positive RBCs, destroying them; this begins the chain of events leading to icterus gravis, kernicterus, and hydrops fetalis.

THE Rh BLOOD GROUP SYSTEM
Nomenclature and Inheritance

The *Rh blood group system* is still the most common cause of HDN. The system comprises a family of inherited antigens. Wiener and Wexler have proposed a single-gene locus occupied by a pair of complex agglutinogens,[6] and Rosenfield and colleagues have contributed a numbering nomenclature.[7] However, the theories of inheritance of Fisher and Race[8] appear the most

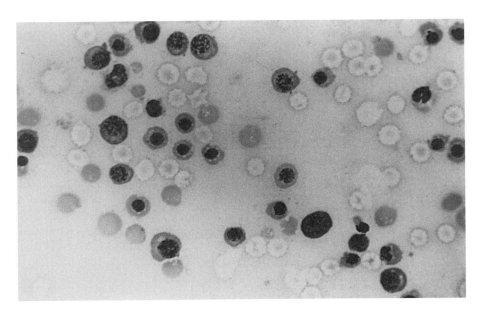

Figure 3-1. Cord blood of baby with severe Rh erythroblastosis fetalis who required multiple fetal transfusions and exchange transfusions. The smear was treated by Kleihauer's technique and Wright's staining. Note adult donor ghost red blood cells (RBCs), dark fetal RBCs, and early fetal erythroid series from erythroblasts through to normoblasts. (From Bowman JM: The management of Rh-isoimmunization. Obstet Gynecol 1978; 52:1. Reprinted with permission from The American College of Obstetricians and Gynecologists.)

Table 3–1. Rh GENE FREQUENCIES IN A CAUCASIAN CANADIAN POPULATION OF 2000 UNRELATED ADULTS

Gene Complex	Frequency (%)
CDe (R¹)	41.0
cde (r)	39.0
cDE (R²)	16.0
cDe (R⁰)	2.2
Cde (r')	1.1
cdE (r")	0.6
CDE (R²)	0.08
CdE (rʸ)	0.00

From Lewis M, Kaita H, Chown B: The inheritance of the Rh blood groups: Frequencies in 1000 unrelated Caucasian families consisting of 2000 parents and 2806 children. Vox Sang 1971; 20:502. Copyright S. Karger AG, Basel, Switzerland.

practical for clinical use and correspond well to the molecular cloning of the human blood group Rh polypeptides.[9] Fisher and Race proposed that there were three pairs of Rh antigens: Dd, Cc, and Ee. The presence or absence of the antigen D denotes Rh positivity or Rh negativity (the d antigen does not exist). The production of anti-D in D-negative women causes hemolytic disease in D-positive fetuses. The antigens are inherited in two sets of three (one set from each parent). CDe (R¹), c(d)e(r), cDE(R²) are the most common genotypes (Table 3–1).

About one half of D-positive individuals are homozygous for D, having inherited D from both parents. The other half are heterozygous for D, having inherited a D-containing set from one parent and a non–D-containing set from the other parent. The homozygous D-positive man paired with a D-negative woman can produce only D-positive fetuses, whereas the heterozygous D-positive man paired with the same woman can produce either a D-positive or D-negative fetus. Only D-positive fetuses can cause D immunization, and only D-positive fetuses are affected by the antibody produced.

The D and non-D polypeptides have been cloned. Jean-Pierre Cartron and co-workers have determined that the Rh blood group locus is the product of two homologous structural genes, one of which encodes the Cc/Ee polypeptide; the other (missing in D negative individuals) encodes the D antigen polypeptide.[9] The predicted translation of the D messenger ribonucleic acid is a 417–amino acid product having a molecular weight of 45,000. The D and Cc/Ee polypeptides differ by 36 amino acid substitutions (8.4% divergence). The similarity between the two genes supports the belief that they evolved by duplication of a common ancestral gene.

Because the d antigen does not exist, the heterozygosity of a man for D can only be determined if he fathers two infants who have received different sets of antigens from him. Because some sets are more common than others (see Table 3–1), the presence or absence of the other Rh antigens (C, c, E, e) will indicate the probable but not certain zygosity of the father for D (Table 3–2).

There are at least 43 more antigens in the Rh system than those already described. Cᵂ, an allele of C, and Dᵘ, an allele of D, are not uncommon. The majority of so-called Dᵘ individuals are genetically D-positive, the strength of the D antigen being depressed by the presence of C on the opposite chromosome. They are incapable of making anti-D. Rarely, so-called Dᵘ individuals are D variants, missing part of the D antigen. Rarely, a D-variant mother carrying a D-positive fetus may produce anti-D, which, on at least one occasion, produced hydrops fetalis.[10] Even more rarely, an Rh-negative mother carrying a Dᵘ fetus may become D immunized. D variants are more common in blacks than in those of other ethnicity.

Rh antigens are present only in the RBC membrane. A report that placental trophoblast may contain Rh antigenic determinants[11] has not been substantiated. Rare people without any Rh antigens (Rh null) have defective RBC membranes and some degree of hemolytic anemia.

The absence of the D antigen is a Caucasian trait. In most Caucasian groups, the incidence is 15% to 16%. In Finns, it is only 11% to 12%, and in the Basques about 35%. Millennia ago, races other than Caucasians were probably all D positive. They owe their present incidence of Rh negativity to the intermingling of Caucasian genes (North American Aborigines, 1% to 2%; American blacks, 7% to 8%; IndoEurasians, 4%; Asiatic Chinese and Japanese, almost zero).

Table 3–2. ZYGOSITY FOR Rh (D) OF D-POSITIVE FATHER (MOTHER D-NEGATIVE)*

Antigens Present in Father	Most Likely Rh Genotype	Less Likely Rh Genotype	Least Likely Rh Genotype
CDe CDee CDEee	CDe.CDe (R¹R¹) homozygous CDe.cde (R¹r) heterozygous CDe.cDE (R¹R²) homozygous	CDe.Cde (R¹r') heterozygous CDe.cDe (R¹R⁰) homozygous Cde.cDE (r'R²) CDe.cdE (R¹r") CDE.cde (R²r) heterozygous	Cde.cDe (r'R⁰) heterozygous CDE.cDe (R²R⁰) homozygous
DEc DEce Dce	cDE.cDE (R²R²) homozygous cDE.cde (R²r) heterozygous cDe.cde (R⁰r) heterozygous	cDE.cdE (R²r") heterozygous cDE.cDe (R²R⁰) homozygous cDe.cDe (R⁰R⁰) homozygous	cdE.cDe (r"R⁰) heterozygous

*Genotypes 1A and 4A can never be proved because a baby is of only one paternal genotype (CDe in 1 A and cDE in 4A). The remainder of the father's possible genotypes can be proved only if he produces children of two different genotypes.
From Bowman JM, Friesen RF: Rh-isoimmunization. In Goodwin JW, Godden JO, Chance G (eds): Perinatal Medicine. Baltimore, Williams & Wilkins, 1976.

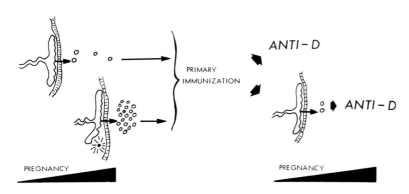

Figure 3-2. Diagrammatic representation of the hypothesis[2, 12] proved by Chown in 1954[13] that Rh-positive fetal RBCs traverse the placenta into the maternal circulation (small amounts during pregnancy, greater amounts at delivery). If the mother is Rh-negative, she responds by producing anti-D. The anti-D, if immunoglobulin G, traverses the placenta into the fetal circulation, coats the fetal D-positive RBCs, and hemolyzes them. (From Zipursky A, Pollock J, et al: Transplacental isoimmunization by fetal red blood cells. In Bergsma D (ed): Birth Defects Original Article Series. Symposium on the Placenta. The National Foundation. Vol. 1. No. 1. New York, Wiley-Liss, 1965, p 87. Copyright © 1965. Reprinted by permission of John Wiley & Sons, Inc.)

THE PATHOGENESIS OF MATERNAL Rh IMMUNIZATION

With the rapid institution of universal Rh-compatible blood transfusion, there was surprisingly very little reduction in the incidence of Rh immunization. It was noted, however, that Rh immunization almost exclusively appeared in parous D-negative women who had had at least one prior pregnancy. Because of this, Wiener, in 1948, resurrected Darrow's fetal transplacental hemorrhage (TPH) theory[12]—that is, D-positive fetal RBCs cross the placenta into the D-negative mother during pregnancy and at the time of delivery, and it is this mode of exposure that produces Rh immunization[12] (Fig. 3–2). Darrow and Wiener's TPH theory was proved by Chown in 1954.[13] A D-negative primigravida with no anti-D at the time of delivery gave birth to a very anemic infant with many circulating erythroblasts and with hepatosplenomegaly. However, the RBCs of the infant were direct antiglobulin test (DAT)–negative, and after delivery the woman appeared to be weakly D positive. Differential agglutination methods and quantitative fetal hemoglobin measurements from alkaline denaturation techniques showed that 8% of her circulating RBCs were D positive and of fetal origin, proving that a very large fetal TPH had occurred. Within 20 days after delivery, the woman produced a strong anti-D and subsequently had very severely affected erythroblastotic infants.

Although Chown's observation proved that Rh immunization occurred as a result of fetal TPH, knowledge regarding the frequency and size of fetal TPH had to await the development of the acid elution test of Kleihauer and associates in 1957.[14] This test, which depends on the resistance of fetal hemoglobin to acid elution (Fig. 3–3), can detect one fetal RBC in 200,000 adult RBCs. With this technique, the frequency and magnitude of fetal TPH have been determined (Table 3–3)[15]: 3% in the first trimester; 12% in the second trimester; 45% in the third trimester; and 64% immediately after birth. In 25% of pregnancies, no fetal RBCs can be detected at any time.[15] The magnitude of fetal TPH increases as pregnancy progresses. Fewer than 1% of women have hemorrhage exceeding 5 mL of fetal blood in their circulations; and fewer than 0.25% have hemorrhage greater than 30 mL. Certain obstetric situations increase the risk of TPH: antepartum hemorrhage, toxemia of pregnancy, external version, cesarean sec-

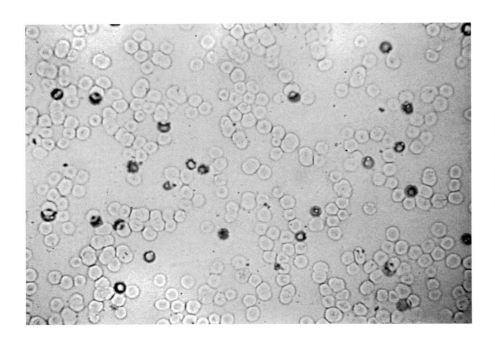

Figure 3-3. Acid elution technique of Kleihauer. Fetal RBCs stain with eosin and appear dark. Adult RBCs do not stain and appear as ghosts. This maternal blood smear contained 11.2% fetal RBCs, representing a transplacental hemorrhage of about 450 mL of blood. (From Bowman JM: Hemolytic disease of the newborn. In Conn HF, Conn RB (eds): Current Diagnosis 5. Philadelphia, W.B. Saunders Co., 1977, p 1103.)

Table 3-3. PREVALENCE OF FETAL TRANSPLACENTAL HEMORRHAGE IN 33 WOMEN DELIVERING ABO-COMPATIBLE BABIES

Gestation	No. with TPH (%)	No. Without TPH (%)
First trimester	1 (3)	32 (97)
Second trimester	4 (12)	29 (88)
Third trimester	15 (45)	18 (55)
After delivery	21 (64)	12 (36)
At any time during pregnancy and delivery	25 (76)	8 (24)

TPH = transplacental hemorrhage.
From Bowman JM, Pollock JM, Penston LE: Feto-maternal transplacental hemorrhage during pregnancy and after delivery. Vox Sang 1986; 100:567. Copyright 1986 S. Karger AG, Basel, Switzerland.

tion, and manual removal of the placenta. Amniocentesis, particularly if not carried out under ultrasound guidance, is a hazard (11.2% before ultrasound in one series).[16] Even with the use of ultrasound, TPH occurs in about 2.5% of cases after amniocentesis.[17]

A significant number of abortions, both spontaneous and therapeutic, are associated with fetal TPH. The Rh antigen is well developed by 30 to 45 days of gestation. After therapeutic abortion, about 4% of women may have TPH in excess of 0.2 mL of fetal blood.

THE PREVALENCE OF Rh IMMUNIZATION

Rh Immune Response

The Primary Immune Response

The primary immune response develops slowly. In experimental Rh immunization of male volunteers, an antibody may appear as early as 4 weeks after injection; usually, however, 8 to 9 weeks elapse before the response is apparent. Indeed, it may not be detectable for 6 months. The primary response is frequently weak and often IgM in nature. IgM anti-D does not traverse the placenta. The majority of D-negative women rapidly convert to IgG anti-D production. IgG anti-D traverses the placenta and produces fetal RBC hemolysis.

The Secondary Immune Response

Once the primary response has occurred, a second exposure to Rh-positive RBCs produces a rapid increase in anti-D, which is for the most part IgG in nature. Subsequent exposure may produce even higher levels. If the intervals between antigen exposure are great, the subsequent exposure is often associated with a marked increase in Rh antibody titer and increased avidity (binding constant) of the antibody for the Rh antigen. The greater the avidity of the Rh antibody for the Rh antigen (its binding constant), the greater will be the severity of Rh erythroblastosis.

The Dose of Rh Antigen Necessary for Producing Rh Immunization

Rh Immunizing Experiments

Amounts of D-positive blood required to produce Rh immunization may be small. In one study, 50% of volunteers were immunized by 10 mL of blood. In other experiments, two thirds were immunized by five injections of 3.5 mL; 80% by one injection of 0.5 mL of D-positive RBC[18]; and 30% by repeated injections of 0.1 mL of RBCs.[19] The prevalence of Rh immunization depends on the dose of D-positive RBCs, being 15% after administration of 1 mL and 65% to 70% after 250 mL. Secondary immune responses may occur after exposure to much smaller amounts (as little as 0.03 mL of D-positive RBCs).

Rh Immunization Clinical Studies

Serial fetal cell studies that use the Kleihauer technique during pregnancy and immediately after delivery allow the determination of the risk of Rh immunization in relation to the presence and size of fetal TPH. If the TPH is always less than 0.1 mL of RBCs, the prevalence of Rh immunization detectable up to 6 months after delivery is 3%[19]; when volumes exceed 0.4 mL, the prevalence is 22%.[18] Because in 75% to 80% of pregnancies the magnitude of TPH (if any) is always less than 0.1 mL, the majority of women are Rh immunized as a result of small or undetectable TPHs.

The Frequency of Rh Immunization

The prevalence of Rh immunization demonstrable within 6 months after delivery of the first Rh-positive, ABO-compatible infant is 8% to 9%. Nevanlinna noted that about the same number of mothers, who had no demonstrable Rh antibodies 6 months after delivery, indicated that they also were Rh immunized by the previous D-positive pregnancy by mounting a secondary immune response in the next D-positive pregnancy; a phenomenon that Nevanlinna called "sensitization."[20] The true prevalence of Rh immunization as a result of the first Rh-positive, ABO-compatible pregnancy is approximately 16%.

A woman not immunized by the first such pregnancy is at approximately the same risk in a second D-positive, ABO-compatible pregnancy. However, as parity increases and the number of women capable of an Rh immune response diminishes because they have become immunized, the number who mount a primary immune response decreases because of a greater residual number of "nonresponders." By the time an Rh-negative woman has completed her fifth ABO-compatible, Rh-positive pregnancy, the probability that she will be Rh immunized is about 50%. Before the Rh prevention era, 0.8% to 1.0% of pregnant women in Manitoba were Rh immunized.

About 25% to 30% of D-negative women are "nonresponders." They do not become Rh immunized, despite having many D-positive pregnancies; however, some may become Rh immunized following exposure to a very large amount of D-positive blood.

ABO incompatibility confers partial protection against Rh immunization. The incidence of Rh immunization 6 months after delivery of an ABO-incompatible, D-positive infant is 1.5% to 2%.[18] Partial protection is probably due to rapid intravascular hemolysis of the ABO-incompatible, D-positive, RBCs, with sequestration of D-positive stroma in the liver (an organ with poor antibody-forming potential) rather than in the spleen (the site of RBC stroma sequestration when extravascular RBC destruction occurs). Although ABO incompatibility confers substantial protection against the primary Rh immune response, it confers no protection against the secondary Rh immune response.[21]

Rh immunization during pregnancy, once considered to be a rare phenomenon, is not uncommon. In Winnipeg, 1.8% of Rh negative women (62 of 3533) without evidence of Rh immunization in early pregnancy were Rh immunized during pregnancy or within 3 days after delivery.[22] Rh immunization during pregnancy accounts for one eighth of Rh-negative women who will be Rh immunized by an Rh-positive pregnancy.

The risk of Rh immunization occurring after a spontaneous abortion is about 1.5% to 2%, increasing the later in gestation that abortion occurs. The risk is greater after therapeutic abortion, being 4% to 5%. Women who are Rh immunized after the small TPH that occurs at the time of abortion are good responders. They frequently have severely affected infants in subsequent pregnancies. Although the risk of immunization after abortion at 6 to 8 weeks of gestation is small, it becomes significant by the 10th to the 12th week.

PATHOGENESIS OF Rh HEMOLYTIC DISEASE

Erythropoiesis begins in the yolk sac of the human embryo by the third week of gestation. Rh antigen has been found in the RBC membrane by the sixth week. By 8 to 10 weeks' gestation, RBC production has begun in the liver and spleen. Normally, erythropoiesis has shifted to and is confined to the bone marrow by the sixth month. In the presence of fetal anemia due either to hemolysis or to blood loss, erythropoiesis may persist in the liver and spleen and may be extreme.

The fundamental cause of erythroblastosis is maternal D IgG antibody coating of D-positive fetal RBCs and their destruction. Hemolysis causes fetal anemia, which stimulates the production of erythropoietin. As a result, erythropoiesis increases. Fetal marrow RBC production cannot keep up with RBC destruction, and extramedullary erythropoiesis in the spleen, liver, kidneys, and adrenal glands recurs. Hepatosplenomegaly is a hallmark of erythroblastosis fetalis.

In the presence of extramedullary erythropoiesis, RBC maturation is poorly controlled. Immature nucleated RBCs, from normoblasts to early erythroblasts (see Fig. 3–1), are poured into the circulation.

Mechanism of Red Blood Cell Hemolysis

Complement-Mediated Hemolysis

When antibody fixes complement, such as anti-A and anti-B, severe RBC damage occurs. Large defects are produced in the RBC membrane. Intravascular hemolysis with hemoglobinemia and hemoglobinuria occurs. RBC debris is picked up for the most part in the liver, where it is phagocytized by the reticuloendothelial cells in the microcirculation.

Non–Complement-Mediated Hemolysis

When antibodies do not fix complement, such as anti-D (either IgG or IgM in nature), the mechanism of hemolysis is different. It is more subtle, but in the end it is as destructive as that of anti-A or anti-B. When anti-D attaches itself to the D antigen in the RBC membrane, the attraction of macrophages to the coated RBCs (chemotaxis) is increased. The coated RBCs adhere to the macrophages, forming rosettes. RBC adherence and the formation of rosettes occur particularly in the spleen, where the circulation slows and the hematocrit increases, bringing RBCs and macrophages into close apposition. Electron microscopy reveals macrophage pseudopods attaching to the RBC membrane, puckering and invaginating it.[23] A portion of the membrane may break off. The loss of membrane substance causes increased rigidity of the RBC with loss of deformability. Even if the RBC escapes the macrophage, it is damaged, with greater osmotic fragility and likelihood of lysis. In many other instances, phagocytosis of the antibody-coated RBC by macrophages occurs (Fig. 3–4).

A correlation has been established between lysis of RBCs sensitized in utero by killer lymphocytes and the severity of HDN.[24] When RBCs, sensitized with IgG antibodies, adhere to receptors for the Fc portion of IgG on killer cells, monocytes or macrophages, phagocytosis, and particularly cytotoxic RBC destruction occurs. Engelfriet and associates[25] have shown that phagocytosis and cytotoxic RBC lysis are independent mechanisms and that cytotoxicity is due to the release of lysosomal enzymes by monocytes-macrophages at their point of contact with the sensitized RBCs. This causes the RBCs to lyse.

Immunoglobulin G Subclasses and Severity of Hemolytic Disease

As already noted, the first stage in RBC destruction caused by non–complement-binding antibodies, such as anti-D, is adherence of the IgG-coated RBC to the Fc receptors of monocytes. The capacity of RBC-bound IgG3 antibodies to bind to these Fc receptors is greater than that of IgG1 antibodies. One might presume, therefore, that IgG3 anti-D is a more potent and lethal RBC antibody than IgG1 anti-D is; this is probably true, because clearance of Rh-positive RBCs is caused by fewer molecules of IgG3 anti-D than IgG1 anti-D.[26]

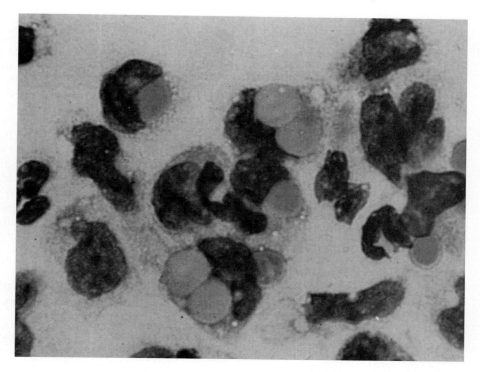

Figure 3–4. A Rebuck skin window preparation in which anti-D–sensitized erythrocytes have been ingested by macrophages. Note that neutrophil erythrophagocytosis is not seen. (From Zipursky A, Bowman JM: Isoimmune hemolytic disease. In Nathan DG, Oski FA (eds): Hematology of Infancy and Childhood, 4th ed. Philadelphia, W.B. Saunders Co., 1993, p 53.)

The increased potency of IgG3 compared with that of IgG1 is born out in studies that have shown that IgG1 and IgG3 anti-D in combination caused more severe hemolytic disease than did IgG1 anti-D alone.[27, 28]

IgG3 anti-D alone without accompanying IgG1 anti-D is observed much less frequently and is often of low titer. In one series,[27] IgG3 alone was invariably of low titer and produced mild disease only. In another series,[28] IgG3 alone produced Rh disease as severe as that caused by IgG1 alone but less severe than that caused by IgG1 and IgG3 in combination of equal titer.

In contradiction to the two observations of greater severity of hemolytic disease when IgG1 and IgG3 anti-D are both present,[27, 28] there is a report of greater severity of hemolytic disease when IgG1 alone was present with the Gm allotype Gm(4),[29] than when IgG1 and IgG3 were both present or when only IgG3 was present.[29] Taken on balance, it appears that IgG3 anti-D is a more dangerous antibody with respect to fetal D-positive RBC hemolysis than IgG1 anti-D, but it is usually found in significant concentration only when it is accompanied by IgG1 anti-D.

SEVERITY OF Rh HEMOLYTIC DISEASE

The degrees of severity of HDN are summarized in Table 3–4.

Mild (No Treatment Required)

The severity of HDN is determined by the amount of maternal IgG anti-D (titer), its binding constant (avidity for the Rh antigen), and the ability of the affected fetus to respond to hemolysis by erythropoiesis without the development of severe hepatocellular damage, portal obstruction, and hydrops fetalis.

One half of affected babies do not require treatment. They are only mildly anemic at birth (cord blood hemoglobin concentration greater than 120 to 130 g/L) and are not dangerously hyperbilirubinemic (cord serum bilirubin levels less than 50 to 60 μmol/L [3.0 to 3.5 mg/100 mL]). At the same time, their RBCs are coated with anti-D, yielding a positive direct antiglobulin (Coombs') test result.

In this group of affected babies, hemoglobin levels do not drop below 110 to 120 g/L, nor do serum indirect bilirubin levels exceed 340 μmol/L (20 mg/100 mL; in a premature infant, 210 to 305 μmol/L [15 to 18 mg/100 ml]) in the neonatal period. In the postneonatal period, hemoglobin levels do not drop below 70 to 80 g/L. No treatment is required. Such infants survive and develop normally, as they did 60

Table 3–4. DEGREES OF SEVERITY OF HEMOLYTIC DISEASE OF THE FETUS AND NEWBORN

Degree of Severity	Description	Incidence (%)
Mild	Indirect bilirubin level does not exceed 16–20 mg/100 mL; no anemia; no treatment needed	45–50
Moderate	Fetal hydrops does not develop; moderate anemia; severe jaundice with risk of kernicterus unless treated after birth	25–30
Severe	Fetal hydrops develops *in utero*	20–25
	Before 34 weeks	10–12
	After 34 weeks	10–12

years ago, before the discovery of the Rh system, when no treatment was available.

Moderate (Without Treatment, Icterus Gravis and Kernicterus Occur)

Intermediate disease is present in 25% to 30% of affected infants. Erythropoiesis is sufficient to maintain an adequate fetal hemoglobin level, but it is not so great that hepatic dysfunction and circulatory obstruction develop. The fetus is born in good condition at or near term. As long as the fetus is *in utero*, the products of blood destruction are transferred across the placenta and metabolized by the mother. After birth, the infant has to rely on its own resources to metabolize the products of hemolysis.

Following hemolysis, globin is split from the hemoglobin and is released, leaving the pigment heme. Heme is converted to *indirect* or *nonconjugated bilirubin*, which is neurotoxic. With increased hemolysis, there is increased production of indirect bilirubin. The ability of the newborn to metabolize indirect bilirubin is limited because his or her liver is deficient in both the transport protein Y and the microsomal enzyme glucuronyl transferase. These substances are responsible for intracellular binding of indirect bilirubin, its transport into the cytoplasm of the liver cell, and its conjugation into water-soluble, nontoxic bilirubin diglucuronide (*direct* or *conjugated bilirubin*); direct bilirubin is in turn excreted into the biliary canaliculi, travels down the bile ducts, and enters the small bowel.

Water-insoluble indirect bilirubin is lipid-soluble and can circulate only in plasma bound to a protein carrier albumin. When the bilirubin-binding capacity of albumin is exceeded, unbound "free" indirect bilirubin appears. The free bilirubin cannot remain in plasma, a watery medium, and so it diffuses into tissues with a high lipid content. Neuronal membranes have a high lipid content. "Free" indirect bilirubin passes into the neuron, interferes with mitochondrial function, and produces swelling and ballooning of the mitochondria, and neuron cell death ensues. Because of the accumulation of bilirubin within them, the dead neurons appear yellow at postmortem examination (kernicterus).

Babies who develop kernicterus (bilirubin encephalopathy) become severely jaundiced. On the third to fifth day, they manifest signs of cerebral dysfunction such as lethargy and hypertonicity. They lie in a position of opisthotonos, with the neck extended and the knees, wrists, and elbows flexed. They suck poorly, their grasp and Moro reflexes disappear, and they may have convulsions. Finally, they become apneic and die.

About 10% of babies with signs and symptoms of kernicterus do not die. Jaundice fades, and hypertonicity is reduced. Initially, they may appear to be normal. As they become older, they show signs of severe neural damage. Most are profoundly deaf. Cerebral palsy of the spastic choreoathetoid type is present. Some children are severely intellectually retarded; others are not but have difficulty learning and functioning because of their deafness and spasticity.

Severe (Without Treatment, Hydrops Fetalis Occurs)

Despite their utilization of all of their RBC production resources, the remaining 20% to 25% of affected fetuses become progressively more anemic. Ascites with generalized edema (anasarca)—that is, hydrops fetalis—occurs. One half of these unfortunate fetuses become hydropic between 18 and 34 weeks' gestation, and the other half between 34 and 40 weeks' gestation.

The original belief that hydrops was due to fetal heart failure is only partially tenable. Although heart failure does occur in some fetuses and occurs in others if they live long enough (Fig. 3–5), a significant number of infants are not hypervolemic or in heart failure at birth.[30] Hepatic enlargement and hepatocellular damage are significant factors in the causation of hydrops fetalis.[31]

With severe hemolysis and progressively greater extramedullary erythropoiesis, the hepatic cords and hepatic circulation are distorted by the islets of erythropoiesis. Portal and umbilical venous obstruction with portal hypertension occurs. The placenta becomes edematous, and cytotrophoblast persists. Placental perfusion diminishes, and ascites develops. Further distortion of hepatic cords by islets of erythropoiesis inter-

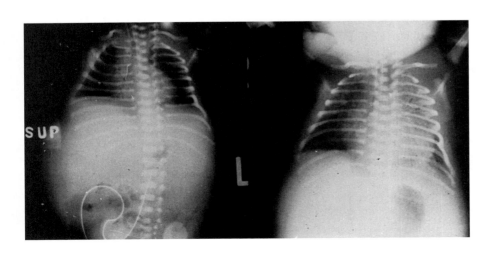

Figure 3–5. Radiograph of a hydropic newborn at birth and 6 hours later after exchange transfusion. Note the small size of the heart at the time of birth and the very marked increase in heart size and evidence of pulmonary congestion denoting heart failure 6 hours later. The fetus has extreme ascites. (From Bowman JM: Blood-group incompatibilities. In Iffy L, Kaminetzky HA (eds): Principles and Practice of Obstetrics and Perinatology, New York, John Wiley & Sons, 1981, p 1203. © Leslie Iffy, MD, Newark, NJ.)

Table 3–5. ALLOANTIBODIES REPORTED TO CAUSE HEMOLYTIC DISEASE

Within the Rh system	Anti-D, -c, -C, -C^w, -C^x, -e, -E, -E^w, -ce, -Ce^s, -Rh32, -Go^a, -Be^a, -Evans, -LW
Outside the Rh system	Anti-K, -k, -Ku, -Kp^a, -Kp^b, -Js^a, -Js^b, -Fy^a, -Fy3, -Jk^a, -Jk^b, -M, -N, -S, -s, -U, -Vw, -Far, -M^v -Mit, -Mt^a, -Mur, -Hil, -Hut, -En^a, PP$_1$P^k, -Lu^a, -Lu^b, -Lu9, -Di^b, -Di^b, -Yt^a, -Yt^b, -Do^a, -Co^a, -Wr^a
Antibodies to low-incidence antigens	Anti-Bi, -By, -Fr^a, -Good, -Rd, -Re^a, -Zd
Antibodies to high-incidence antigens	Anti-At^a, -Jr^a, -Lan, -Ge

feres with hepatocellular circulation and cell function. Albumin production drops, hypoalbuminemia develops, and generalized edema (anasarca) occurs. Pleural and pericardial effusions develop. In the most extreme cases, compression hypoplasia of the lungs makes oxygenation after birth impossible.

The hepatic damage theory of the pathogenesis of hydrops fetalis explains the inconsistent relationship of hydrops to the degree of anemia in some fetuses. Although most hydropic fetuses are severely anemic, some have hemoglobin levels well above 70 g/L; other fetuses are not hydropic even though they have much lower hemoglobin levels (in one instance, 25 g/L).

MATERNAL ALLOANTIBODIES CAUSING FETAL HEMOLYTIC DISEASE

Alloantibodies Other Than A and B

Anti-D in the Rh blood group system is still the most common antibody causing severe HDN. However, Rh preventive measures have produced a striking reduction in D alloimmunization.

In Manitoba (population, 1 million), the mean annual occurrence of D alloimmunization in pregnant women dropped from 194 in the 5-year period ending October 31, 1967 to 23 in the 5-year period ending October 31, 1994. In the same two periods, the mean annual occurrence of detected non-D alloimmunization in pregnant women, excluding ABO alloimmunization, increased from 14 to 108. This increase is partially the result of the increased screening of pregnant D-positive women. It also reflects a real increase in the occurrence of non-D alloimmunization because of the increased frequency of blood transfusion (transfused blood being only ABO and D compatible).

For this reason, non-D alloantibodies have assumed greater importance in the causation of hemolytic disease. The alloantibodies listed by Mollison and coworkers[32] as having been reported to cause HDN are listed in Table 3–5. They stated that of the multitude of antibodies implicated in the manifestation of HDN (see Table 3–5), those reported to produce moderate-to-severe hemolytic disease are all of those in the Rh blood group system, as well as anti-K, -Jk^a, -Js^a, -Js^b, -Ku, -Fy^a, -M, -N, -s, -U, -PP$_1$P^k, -Di^b, -Lan, -LW, -Far, -Good, -Wr^a, and -Zd.

This list appears intimidating, but it must be considered in conjunction with the frequency with which such antibodies occur and the frequency with which they cause significant HDN.

The increase in occurrence of non-D alloimmunization is reflected in the changing ratio of D to non-D alloimmunization in pregnant patients from outside Manitoba referred to the Rh Laboratory (Women's Hospital, Health Sciences Centre, Winnipeg, MB) for fetal treatment (Table 3–6). Although those with anti-D still predominate, the number of those referred with non-D alloimmunization has increased from 2 in the 10-year period ending December 31, 1973 to 25 in the 11-year period ending December 31, 1994. The non-D alloantibodies observed in pregnant Manitoban women during the 32-year period ending October 31, 1994 are listed in Tables 3–7 and 3–8. Although anti-E and anti-K were the most common (in 633 and 478 cases, respectively), only 18 of the 162 affected infants with disease due to anti-E and 8 of the 16 infants with disease due to anti-K required exchange transfusion or phototherapy, or both. Two infants with disease due to anti-Kell were very severely affected. Anti-c, when present, was more likely to cause HDN (54% versus 26% and 5.3% for anti-E and anti-K) and, in those affected, was more likely to cause disease requiring treatment than was anti-E (30% versus 11%). This was not the case for infants with disease due to anti-Kell, 50% of whom required treatment.[33] Anti-c, anti-Kell, and anti-Fy^a were the only non-D alloantibodies in the 32-year period that caused disease so severe that hydrops devel-

Table 3–6. NON-MANITOBA PATIENTS REFERRED TO THE WINNIPEG Rh LABORATORY WITH SEVERE FETAL HEMOLYTIC DISEASE*

5-Year Period	No. of Anti-D Patients	No. of Non–Anti-D Patients (%)	Non–Anti-D Specificity
1964–1968	57	0	
1969–1973	59	2 (3.3)	1K, 1E
1974–1978	24	1 (4.0)	1K
1979–1983	23	6 (20.7)	1K, 4c, 1Fy^a
1984–1988	60	13 (17.8)	6K, 3c, 1k, 1cE, 1Jk^a, 1CC^w
1989–1994†	64	12 (15.8)	9K, 2c, 1cE

*From January 1, 1964 to December 31, 1994: antibody specificity.
†Six-year period.

Table 3-7. SEVERITY OF HEMOLYTIC DISEASE IN MANITOBA OVER 32 YEARS*

Alloantibody Specificity	No. of Patients	Affected Patients (%)	No Treatment Required (%)	Phototherapy and/or Exchange Transfusion Required (%)	Stillborn Hydropic or Hb < 60 g/L (%)
D (19 y)	566	257 (47)	51	30	19
E	633	162 (26)	89	11	—
c, cE	302	164 (54)	70	23	7
C, Ce, Cᵂ, e	193	50 (36)	86	14	—
Kell	478	16 (3.3)	50	37	13
Kpᵃ	7	3 (43)	67	33	—
k	1	1 (100)	—	100	—
Fyᵃ	35	6 (17)	67	16	16
S	20	11 (55)	64	36	—

Hb = hemoglobin.
*From November 1, 1962 to October 31, 1994 except for Anti-D (November 1, 1975 to October 31, 1994).

oped, or fetuses required intrauterine transfusions, or infants were born with cord hemoglobin levels of less than 60 g/L.

Rarely, anti-C, -Ce, -Cᵂ, -Kpᵃ, -k, -Fyᵃ, and -S (see Table 3–7) have caused hemolytic disease severe enough to require treatment after birth, but only one, anti-Fyᵃ resulted in disease so severe that hydrops developed or that fetal transfusions were required. Other blood group antibodies in these pregnant Manitoban patients (see Table 3–8) demonstrated either no clinical disease or mild clinical disease that did not require treatment.

The experience of the Rh Laboratory over the past 31 years with 34 pregnant non-D alloimmunized women referred from *outside* Manitoba—a highly selected group with very severely affected fetuses drawn from a much greater population base—is somewhat different (see Table 3–6). In these referred women, there were examples of the following antibodies: anti-K (18 cases), -c (9 cases), -cE (2 cases) -k[34] (1 case), -Jkᵃ (1 case), -Fyᵃ (1 case), -CCᵂ (1 case), and -E (1 case); these antibodies produced HDN so severe that intrauterine treatment was required. There are rare instances of

other alloantibodies', usually benign ones, causing severe hemolytic disease (e.g., anti-Kpᵇ and anti-M).[35, 36]

ABO Hemolytic Disease

ABO HDN is quite different from HDN due either to anti-D or to other blood group antibodies. Anti-A and anti-B, which bind complement in adults, cause violent, life-threatening intravascular hemolysis after transfusion of ABO-incompatible blood. Fetal ABO HDN usually is much milder than Rh, c, K, and some other forms of "atypical" HDN. Although kernicterus may develop if the baby with ABO hemolytic disease is left untreated, hydrops rarely if ever occurs, and anemia at birth is usually moderate. There are very rare reports of hydrops fetalis due to ABO erythroblastosis,[37, 38] but in most reported cases, the possibility of nonimmune hydrops superimposed upon ABO erythroblastosis could not be excluded.

Several reasons can be listed for the paradoxical mildness of ABO HDN. First, there are fewer A and B antigenic sites on the fetal RBC membrane. Also, anti-A and anti-B do not bind complement on the fetal RBC membrane.[39] Second, anti-A and anti-B are mostly IgM, which does not cross the placenta. Third, the small amounts of IgG anti-A and anti-B that do traverse the placenta have myriad antigenic sites other than those on RBCs, other tissues, and secretions to which they may bind. Only a very small proportion of the minor amount of anti-A or anti-B that crosses the placenta adheres to antigen on the RBC membrane. Because there is very little antibody on the RBC, the cord blood DAT result in ABO hemolytic disease is only weakly positive and may be negative unless a sensitive test is used. Not infrequently, capillary blood taken when the infant is 2 or 3 days old yields a negative result no matter how sensitive the test used is.

In about 25% to 30% of ABO-incompatible babies, cord blood RBCs are weakly DAT-positive at delivery. Only a very small fraction of these infants develop clinical evidence of hemolytic disease (early and severe jaundice). In one hospital, of the 9000 ABO-incompatible babies delivered from 1954 to 1965, 2500 had

Table 3-8. ANTIBODIES ASSOCIATED WITH NO REQUIRED TREATMENT OR NO CLINICAL DISEASE (MANITOBA)

Not Affected	
Luᵃ	24
Luᵇ	2
P	25
Leᵃ (Leᵇ)	88
Wrᵃ	37
Multiple/rare	13
Nonspecific or high incidence	11
Affected but No Treatment Required	
Fyᵇ	1 of 4
Jkᵃ	5 of 14
Jkᵇ	1 of 4
s	3 of 4
M	3 of 129
LW	1 of 2
Kpᵃ	1 of 1
Autoantibodies	8 of 55

weakly DAT-positive RBCs, and only 41 (less than 2%) required exchange transfusion.[40]

ANTIBODY DETECTION AND MEASUREMENT

Saline Methods

Rh-positive RBCs suspended in isotonic saline are agglutinated only by IgM anti-D. IgG anti-D cannot bridge the gap between RBCs suspended in saline. Although it coats Rh-positive RBCs suspended in saline, it does not agglutinate them. Therefore, a maternal serum containing only IgG anti-D does not agglutinate Rh-positive RBCs suspended in saline. In the early 1940s, when saline-suspended RBC antibody screening techniques were the only ones in use, there was great confusion because many Rh-negative women giving birth to sick erythroblastotic babies had no demonstrable Rh antibodies in their sera.

Colloid Methods

Wiener[41] was the first to observe that Rh antibodies (IgG) that produce no agglutination of Rh-positive, saline-suspended RBCs promptly agglutinated the same RBCs if they were suspended in a more viscous medium such as albumin. The viscous media have higher dielectric constants; this property effects a reduction in the negative electrical potential of the RBC membrane, causing the RBCs to lie more closely together. IgG anti-D is then able to bridge the gaps between the RBCs and cause agglutination. Bovine serum albumin is the most frequently used colloid medium.[42]

Because IgM anti-D also agglutinates Rh-positive RBCs suspended in albumin, if saline and albumin titers of the same level are present, the albumin titer is not an accurate reflection of the amounts of IgG anti-D present. Mixing the serum that contains saline and albumin agglutinating anti-D with dithiothreitol causes disruption of IgM sulfhydryl bonds and destruction of IgM. Subsequent remeasurement of the serum anti-D titer in albumin gives a determination of the true IgG anti-D titer.

Indirect Antiglobulin Titer

When human serum (or specific human globulin) is injected into other animal species (e.g., rabbits, guinea pigs, or goats), the animals, recognizing the serum as foreign, produce antihuman globulin known as *Coombs' serum.*[43]

Rh-positive RBCs are incubated with the serum being tested for the presence of anti-D. If anti-D is present in the serum, the antibody adheres to the Rh-positive RBC membrane. The RBCs are then washed three or four times with isotonic saline to remove nonadherent human protein; they are then suspended in the antihuman globulin (Coombs') serum. If the RBCs are coated with anti-D, they are agglutinated by the antihuman globulin serum, reflecting a positive indirect antiglobulin (Coombs') test result. The reciprocal of the highest dilution of maternal serum that produces agglutination is the *indirect antiglobulin titer.* The indirect antiglobulin titer is a more sensitive screening and titration technique than the colloid method is. Titers of antibody in the same serum are usually one to three dilutions greater than albumin titers. The relationship between the two titers, however, varies greatly from laboratory to laboratory.

Enzyme Methods

Incubation of RBCs with enzymes such as papain, trypsin, and bromelin reduces the electrical potential of the RBC membranes. RBC treated with enzymes lie closer together when they are suspended in saline, and they are agglutinated by IgG anti-D. Enzyme screening methods are the most sensitive manual techniques available for detecting Rh immunization.[44]

Automated Analysis

AutoAnalyzer (AA) methods have been developed for the detection and measurement of Rh and other antibodies. The most commonly used techniques are the bromelin method[45] and the low ionic polybrene method,[46] as well as modifications of these two. AA techniques are the most sensitive methods for the detection of Rh antibody. An Rh antibody detected only by an AA method and not by any manual method must be viewed with caution. In 85% of instances of maternal serum Rh antibody identification by AA only and not confirmed by other methods, the mother may not be truly Rh immunized. The AA bromelin method has been modified to allow accurate quantitation of the amount of anti-D in serum.[47]

PREDICTIVE PARAMETERS DETERMINING THE SEVERITY OF FETAL HEMOLYTIC DISEASE

The problem of investigative and treatment measures in alloimmunized pregnant women is that they carry some risk to the fetus. Therefore, it is important that the severity of fetal disease be determined as accurately as possible, that investigative measures be restricted to pregnancies in which the fetus is at risk, and that treatment measures be confined to fetuses who require them in order to survive. The following investigative approaches may be used:

Eliciting a history indicating the severity of HDN in previous infants
Determination of maternal antibody titers
Cell-mediated maternal antibody functional assays
Amniotic fluid spectrophotometry
Fetal ultrasound
Percutaneous fetal blood sampling
Determination of D status of the fetus by polymerase chain reaction

Past Pregnancy History

Until 1961, the only measures available for predicting the severity of HDN were the severity of HDN in prior pregnancies and maternal antibody titers. Although it is usually true that the severity of HDN remains the same or increases during subsequent affected pregnancies, occasionally disease becomes less severe. With a past history of hydrops, a subsequent affected fetus has a 90% but not a 100% chance of becoming hydropic. If hydrops is going to develop, it does so usually at the same gestation or earlier, but occasionally it develops later. With a prior history of hydrops and a father heterozygous for the offending antigen, the physician is in a dilemma. The fetus may be D negative and unaffected or D positive and very severely affected. The resolution of this dilemma is addressed later in this chapter. In a first D-sensitized pregnancy, with no prior history of HDN, there is an 8% to 10% probability that hydrops will develop.

Maternal Alloantibody Titers

Although antibody titrations carried out in the same laboratory by the same experienced personnel using the same methods and test cells are reproducible and do give the physician some indication of risk, they are not of sufficient accuracy to allow potentially hazardous fetal treatment measures to be undertaken. In an 8-year period (1954 to 1961) in which 426 Rh-immunized women came for delivery at the Winnipeg General Hospital, 54 fetuses survived only because labor was induced and the fetuses delivered early. Sixty-seven perinatal deaths occurred. Of the 67 deaths, 34 were potentially salvageable with management measures available at that time (26 with earlier delivery, 8 with later delivery) if the degree of severity of disease had only been more accurately known. When these 121 most severely affected pregnancies were assessed, it was apparent that the accuracy of prediction of the severity of HDN was only 62%.[48]

Cell-Mediated Maternal Antibody Functional Assays

Because of the relatively poor correlation between blood group antibody titrations and the severity of HDN, various functional assays have been developed that reflect the binding constant or avidity of the antibody for the antigen on the RBC membrane and, therefore, its ability to produce severe HDN. These assays include the monocyte monolayer assay[28, 49] and antibody-dependent cellular cytotoxicity assay (ADCC) using lymphocytes,[50] monocytes,[51] and monocyte chemiluminescence.[52]

Each one of these assays has its proponents. Three papers have compared the functional assays. Hadley and associates[53] compared monocyte chemiluminescence, K cell lymphocyte ADCC, monocyte-macrophage ADCC, and a rosette assay using U937 cells. They found that monocyte-based (i.e., monocyte chemiluminescence and monocyte ADCC) functional assays predicted severity of disease better than did lymphocyte-based assays (i.e., rosette assay with U937 cells and K lymphocyte ADCC). Similarly, Zupanska and colleagues[28] found that the results of a monocyte-based assay (monocyte monolayer assay) correlated better with the clinical severity of hemolytic disease than did the results of rosette assays using lymphocytes. A survey by Mollison[54] of nine European laboratories carrying out functional assays, testing sera from mothers delivering babies with varying degrees of HDN, revealed correct results as follows: ADCC (monocytes), 60%; ADCC (lymphocytes), 57%; chemiluminescence, 51%; and rosetting and phagocytosis with peripheral monocytes, 41% (with U937 cells or cultured macrophages, 32%). The assays appeared to be more helpful in predicting mild or minimal disease than very severe disease. Obviously, because all of these assays measure the potential lethality of the maternal antibody, they are quite incapable of differentiating the unaffected antigen-negative fetus from the affected antigen-positive fetus.

A report has cast doubt on the ability of the monocyte-macrophage assay to predict the severity of HDN.[55] In sera from 41 pregnant women with potentially dangerous blood group antibodies who delivered affected babies, there was no correlation between the hematocrit of a fetal blood sample obtained at cordocentesis and the monocyte-macrophage assay.[55]

Thus, in summary, although the functional tests listed may be helpful in more accurately determining the fetus at risk and, therefore, in some pregnancies, precluding the need for invasive measures such as amniocentesis and fetal blood sampling, they in no way replace such invaluable perinatal management aids in the ultimate differentiation of the fetus who requires treatment *in utero* from the fetus who does not.

Amniotic Fluid Spectrophotometry

In 1961, Liley reported the use of amniotic fluid spectrophotometry as a means of determining the severity of HDN.[56] Although Bevis, in 1956, was the first to use amniotic fluid spectrophotometry,[57] Liley was the first to develop a method of measurement: the deviation from linearity at 450 nm, the absorption spectrum of bilirubin—that is, the ΔOD 450 reading (a measurement of the amniotic fluid bilirubin level). The method allowed communication from one center to another of an easily interpretable reading that readily gives an accurate determination of the severity of HDN. Readings falling into very high zone II or zone III (Fig. 3–6) indicate severe disease—that is, hydrops is present or will develop within 7 to 10 days; readings falling into zone I indicate either no disease or no anemia but reflect a 10% chance that exchange transfusion will be needed; readings in zone II indicate moderate disease that becomes more severe as readings approach the zone III boundary. The overall accuracy of prediction of hemolytic disease with the amniotic fluid technique is 95%; this accuracy can only be obtained with serial ΔOD 450 measurements. Amniotic fluid ΔOD 450 readings reflect the severity of disease more accurately in the third trimester than they do in the second trimester. In the second trimester, the zone boundaries have not been as accurately defined[58, 59]; again, this points to the need for serial measurements (often performed weekly

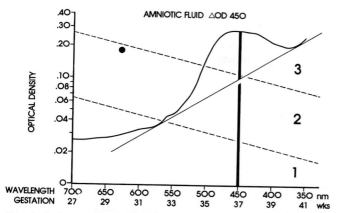

Figure 3–6. Amniotic fluid spectrophotometric reading (Liley's method) of ΔOD 450 (0.200 in this example) falls high in zone 2 at 29½ weeks' gestation, indicating severe Rh erythroblastosis. The *curved line* indicates results of analysis of OD on patient's liquor; the *full straight line* indicates the OD baseline. (From Bowman JM: Haemolytic disease of the newborn (erythroblastosis fetalis). In Roberton NRC (ed): Textbook of Neonatology. Edinburgh, Churchill Livingstone, 1986, p 473.)

for several weeks). Final readings falling in zone I and zone III have an accuracy of prediction rate of 98%, but final readings falling in zone II have an accuracy of prediction rate of only 90%.

The Liley zone boundaries before 24 weeks' gestation have been modified by inclining the boundaries downward at the same angle of declination as the angle of inclination after 24 weeks' gestation[33], this modification reflects the observation that ΔOD 450 readings (i.e., bilirubin levels) in pregnancies unaffected by HDN peak at 23 to 24 weeks' gestation[58] (Fig. 3–7).

Because fetal blood sampling, followed if necessary by intravascular fetal transfusions, is the most accurate means of determining the presence and severity of Rh hemolytic disease, amniotic fluid ΔOD 450 measurements are used for determining the need for fetal blood sampling. Specifically, fetal blood sampling should be carried out when a single or final ΔOD 450 reading is at the 65% to 75% level of zone II, modified before 24 weeks' gestation.

Amniocentesis is not without hazard. In the pre-ultrasound era, there was a 10% risk of placental trauma,[16] placing blood in the amniotic fluid; this produced 580-, 540-, and 415-nm oxyhemoglobin peaks, obscured the 450-nm peak, and made the fluid worthless for predicting the severity of hemolytic disease. Even more serious, placental trauma carries a great likelihood of producing a fetal-to-maternal TPH, exposing the mother to more fetal RBC antigen, increasing her antibody level, and increasing the severity of fetal hemolytic disease. With the advent of ultrasound placental localization, the risk of placental trauma at amniocentesis has been greatly reduced but not removed altogether (residual incidence, 2.5%[17]).

Perinatal Ultrasound

The development of ultrasound imaging techniques in the late 1970s was a major advance in the management of maternal blood group alloimmunization.[60] Ultrasound allows estimation of placental and hepatic size and determination of the presence or absence of edema, ascites, and other effusions (i.e., hydrops fetalis). It is of great benefit in assessing fetal well-being. It has increased the accuracy of placental localization and has reduced the prevalence of placental trauma at amniocentesis. It is essential in directing the transfusion needle with the least possible risk during both intraperitoneal and intravascular fetal transfusions.

Following intraperitoneal fetal transfusion, ultrasound confirms the presence of blood in the fetal peritoneal cavity, and serial examinations monitor its absorption. At the time of a direct fetal intravascular transfusion, ultrasound observation of turbulence within the fetal umbilical vessel as the blood is injected confirms that it is being transfused into the fetal circulation.

Although ultrasound makes the diagnosis of hydrops with great accuracy, unfortunately it may not make the diagnosis of impending hydrops until hydrops has developed. However, after fetal transfusions, ultrasound biophysical profile scoring provides an accurate assessment of fetal well-being and indicates whether improvement or deterioration is occurring.

Percutaneous Umbilical Blood Sampling

With the development of sophisticated ultrasound equipment and the availability of perinatologists skilled in its use, percutaneous fetal umbilical blood

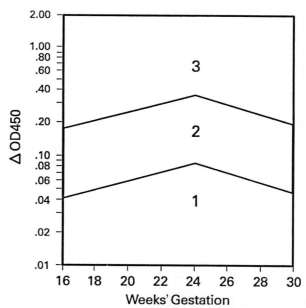

Figure 3–7. Modification of Liley's ΔOD 450 reading zone boundaries before 24 weeks' gestation. The zone boundary angle of declination before 24 weeks' gestation is the same as the zone boundary angle of inclination after 24 weeks' gestation. (From Bowman JM, Pollock JM, et al: Maternal Kell blood group alloimmunization. Obstet Gynecol 1992; 79:239. Reprinted with permission from the American College of Obstetricians and Gynecologists.)

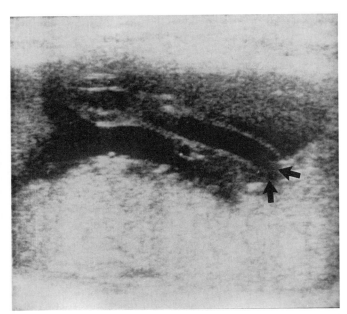

Figure 3–8. Real-time scan ultrasound view of the insertion of the umbilical vein into the placenta (arrows); the placenta is posterior. The lumen of the umbilical vein is sonar lucent. (From Bowman JM: Maternal blood group immunization. In Creasy RK, Resnik R (eds): Maternal-Fetal Medicine: Principles and Practice. 2nd ed. Philadelphia, W.B. Saunders Co., 1989, p 637.)

sampling became feasible in the mid 1980s[61] (Fig. 3–8). This procedure allows measurements of all blood parameters that can be measured after birth (hemoglobin, hematocrit, blood groups, DAT, serum bilirubin levels, platelet and leucocyte counts, serum protein levels, erythropoietin levels, and fetal blood gases). Fetal blood sampling is the most accurate means of determining the degree of severity of HDN in the absence of hydrops. The procedure is relatively benign, carrying with it a traumatic fetal mortality rate of a fraction of 1%.[61] Because the procedure does carry with it a great likelihood of fetal-to-maternal hemorrhage,[62] it should only be undertaken when serial amniotic fluid ΔOD 450 readings increase into the upper 65% to 75% of zone II or when an anterior placenta cannot be avoided at amniocentesis and maternal pregnancy history or maternal antibody titers place the fetus at risk. Fetal blood sampling may be possible as early as 18 weeks' gestation; it usually is feasible by 20 to 21 weeks' gestation. The preferred sampling site is the umbilical vessel (preferably the vein) at its insertion into the placenta. For this reason, the procedure is technically easier to perform if the placenta is implanted on the anterior uterine wall.

Determination of Fetal D Antigen Status by Polymerase Chain Reaction

As mentioned earlier, the Rh gene locus (which is on chromosome 1p36.2-p34), consists of two homologous genes designating the antigens CcEe and D. The sequences of the two genes are 96% identical, suggesting that they arose through the duplication of a single ancestral gene. The gene *RHCE* encodes the Cc and Ee proteins, probably by alternate splicing of a primary transcript.[9] The gene *RHD* encodes the D protein, which is absent on both chromosomes of D-negative individuals. The presence or absence of the *RHD* gene determines whether the fetus is D-positive or D-negative.

The cloning of the CcEe and D complementary deoxyribonucleic acid (DNA) has made it possible to determine the fetal D type in DNA obtained during chorionic villus biopsy or amniocentesis. Bennett and co-workers[63] were able to determine the D type using polymerase chain reaction assays on fetal cells obtained either from chorionic villus sampling or amniocentesis, with 100% accuracy in 30 samples tested. The Rh Laboratory at Women's Hospital has had 100% concordance in the testing of similar samples. It is now possible, therefore, to determine, with great accuracy, the D status of a fetus whose mother is Rh alloimmunized and whose father appears to be heterozygous for D by testing amniotic fluid or chorionic villus samples; the results support the diagnosis of a D-positive, affected fetus (indicating the need for further invasive diagnostic testing) or a D-negative, unaffected fetus (indicating that no further invasive tests are required).

Because fetal nucleated hematopoietic stem cells are present in the maternal circulation early in pregnancy, these cells are also subject to D antigen status determination by polymerase chain reaction methods. The ability to determine D antigen fetal status with a maternal blood sample PCR assay is now possible.[64] The method has not yet reached the level of accuracy required for applicability in clinical situations but will undoubtedly do so in the very near future. Once this accuracy has been achieved, a totally noninvasive method will be available for determining fetal D antigen status when the mother is D-alloimmunized.

MANAGEMENT OF MATERNAL ALLOIMMUNIZATION

Suppression of Alloimmunization

Since the mid-1940s, efforts have been made to suppress the strength of already developed maternal RBC immunization. Rh hapten has been shown to be worthless.[65] The value of Rh-positive RBC stroma as reported by Bierme and associates[66] has been disproven by Gold and colleagues.[67] The benefit of the administration of promethazine hydrochloride touted by Gusdon and co-workers[68] has been refuted by others. Administration of Rh immune globulin, of great value in Rh immunization prevention, has been shown to be quite ineffective in suppressing Rh immunization, no matter how weak, once Rh immunization has begun.[69, 70]

Two measures that probably are of benefit in reducing maternal antibody levels and ameliorating hemolytic disease are (1) intensive plasma exchange[71, 72] and (2) the administration of intravenous immune serum globulin (IGIV).[73, 74] With intensive plasma exchange, alloantibody levels can be lowered by as much as 75%. In the author's experience, after 6 to 8 weeks antibody

Immune Hemolytic Disease • 67

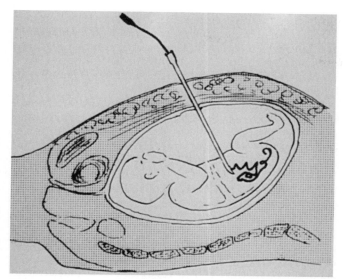

Figure 3-9. Diagram of intraperitoneal fetal transfusion (IPT). The Tuohy needle has been inserted across the maternal abdominal wall and uterine wall into the fetal peritoneal cavity, and an epidural catheter has been threaded into the peritoneal cavity of the fetus. The safest position for the fetus at IPT is not with the abdomen anterior (as shown in this diagram) because the umbilical fetal vessels will lie in the center of the target area. (From Bowman JM: Blood-group incompatibilities. In Iffy L, Kaminetzky HA (eds): Principles and Practice of Obstetrics and Perinatology. New York, John Wiley & Sons, 1981, p 1213. © Leslie Iffy, MD, Newark, NJ.)

Fc receptor saturation and reduction of IgG-coated RBC hemolysis by fetal reticuloendothelial Fc receptor saturation with the injected IGIV. If IGIV therapy is considered, it should be used in the same situation as intensive plasma exchange, beginning at 10 to 12 weeks' gestation. The recommended dose is 400 mg/kg of maternal body weight for 5 days, repeated at 3-week intervals, or 1 g/kg maternal body weight repeated at weekly intervals. Again, amniotic fluid or fetal blood sampling assessment of fetal disease at 18 to 20 weeks' gestation is essential.

Fetal Treatment

Induced Early Delivery

The primary problem since 1945 has been the management of the fetus destined to become hydropic *in utero*. In 1952, Chown hypothesized that induced early delivery might be the solution for the fetus destined to become hydropic after 32 to 34 weeks' gestation (50% of all hydrops); that is, accept the considerable risk from prematurity rather than the much greater risk of HDN. His conjecture was proved correct.[75] By 1961, the perinatal mortality from HDN in Manitoba was 16%. Until 1961, the major problem with early delivery was the inability to predict severity of hemolytic disease

levels tend to rebound, even with continued plasma exchange. Venous access becomes difficult, with the need for placement of arteriovenous shunts. The plasma must be replaced, partially with blood fractions (albumin and IGIV), in order to reduce antibody feedback rebound and to keep maternal serum albumin and IgG at adequate levels. Plasma exchange is tedious, costly, and uncomfortable. It is not without minor risk to the mother. The only expectation, with the use of intensive plasma exchange, is that fetal treatment measures may be delayed until the fetus is at greater than 22 to 24 weeks' gestation. The institution of plasma exchange does not obviate the need for investigative measures such as amniocentesis and fetal blood sampling. Plasma exchange should be reserved for the mother with a partner who is homozygous for the antigen to which she is immunized, and with a prior history of hydrops, at or before 24 to 26 weeks' gestation. Intensive plasma exchange should be started at 10 to 12 weeks' gestation when transfer of maternal IgG is beginning, with initial amniocentesis at 18 weeks' gestation or fetal blood sampling at 19 to 22 weeks' gestation.

The value of high-dose IGIV administration in the severely alloimmunized pregnant woman has been reported.[73, 74] Circulating maternal alloantibody levels can be halved subsequent to the negative feedback produced by total circulating maternal IgG levels of 25 to 30 g/L; this effect is readily achieved by a dose of 2 g/kg body weight. Further benefits of IGIV therapy may be a result of interference with the transfer of maternal antibody across the placenta by trophoblastic

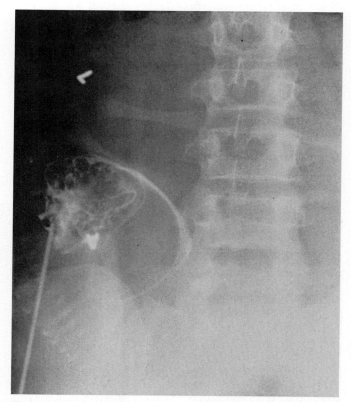

Figure 3-10. A successful catheterization of the fetal peritoneal cavity at IPT, as shown by the outlining of the diaphragm with radiopaque dye, the negative shadow of the fetal liver, and the negative shadows of the small bowel. (From Bowman JM: Maternal blood group immunization. In Creasy RK, Resnik R (eds): Maternal-Fetal Medicine: Principles and Practice. 2nd ed. Philadelphia, W.B. Saunders Co., 1989, p 634.)

accurately. With the introduction of amniotic fluid ΔOD 450 measurements by Liley in 1961,[56] this problem was partially solved. By 1964, the perinatal mortality from Rh hemolytic disease in Manitoba had been reduced to 13%.

Intrauterine Transfusions for Fetal Hemolytic Disease

Intraperitoneal Fetal Transfusions

In 1961, induced early delivery could not be undertaken before 31 to 32 weeks' gestation without encountering prohibitive mortality from prematurity and severe Rh disease. Eight per cent of fetuses become hydropic before 32 weeks' gestation. In 1963, the introduction of intraperitoneal fetal transfusions (IPT) by Liley[76] completely altered the prognosis for these most severely affected of all fetuses.

Since the turn of the century, it has been known that RBCs placed in the peritoneal cavity are absorbed and function normally. At one time, IPT was a favorite method for transfusing children with thalassemia. It was abandoned in favor of vascular transfusions because of the severe discomfort that it caused. Absorption is via the subdiaphragmatic lymphatic lacunae, up the right lymphatic duct, and into the venous circulation. Fetal breathing movements are necessary for absorption to occur.[77] In the absence of hydrops, 10% to 12% of infused RBCs are absorbed daily. Ascites *per se* does not prevent absorption, although the rate of absorption in its presence is more variable.[78] If the fetus is not breathing, absorption of RBCs does not occur.[77]

A 16-gauge, 18-cm Tuohy needle is directed under ultrasound guidance into the fetal abdomen (Fig. 3–9). An epidural catheter is then threaded down the needle, and the needle is withdrawn on to the maternal abdomen. The proper placement of the catheter tip is confirmed radiographically following the injection of 1 to 1.5 mL of radiopaque contrast medium by the demonstration of contrast under the diaphragm and around loops of small bowel (Fig. 3–10). Prior to the ultrasound era (before 1978), visualization of the contrast medium diffusing into a large volume of ascitic fluid (Fig. 3–11) was often the means by which the initial diagnosis of hydrops fetalis was made.

Although IPT was a major advance in the management of severe erythroblastosis fetalis, serious problems were associated with its application. The procedure is of no value for the nonbreathing moribund hydropic fetus.[77] The RBCs are not absorbed, and the fetus dies. If the placenta is implanted on the anterior uterine wall and must be transfixed by the Tuohy needle, the traumatic death rate per procedure is 7% (in Winnipeg). Following IPT, the spontaneous labor rate per patient is 30%. Fortunately, most of such deliveries occur after 30 weeks' gestation. Finally, although serial amniotic fluid ΔOD 450 measurements increase the accuracy of prediction of severity of HDN, inaccuracies do occur (e.g., the occasional only moderately affected fetus may have a zone III reading, and less commonly, the hydropic fetus may have a moderate zone II reading).

Direct Intravascular Fetal Transfusion

Attempts at direct intravascular transfusions (IVTs), either into a fetal or placental blood vessel approached via a hysterotomy incision, were attempted in the mid-1960s.[79–81] The results were poor because the women almost invariably went into labor. In 1981, Rodeck and co-workers reported direct fetal transfusions through a fetoscope.[82] Few others have achieved his skill with the fetoscope. Blood, meconium, or other turbid substances in the amniotic fluid makes fetoscopic visualization of the fetal blood vessels impossible.

With the introduction of fetal blood sampling, by the early to mid-1980s it became feasible to follow the sampling procedure with a direct IVT.[83–88] Under ultra-

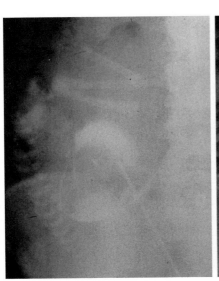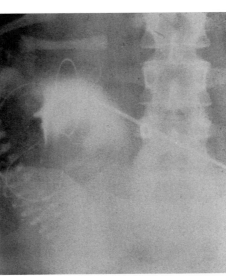

Figure 3–11. Hydrops fetalis at IPT. Note the gross ascites at both the first and second IPTs. The fetus, hydropic at birth with a cord hemoglobin of 9 g/100 mL (all donor RBCs) survived. (From Bowman JM: Maternal blood group immunization. In Creasy RK, Resnik R (eds): Maternal-Fetal Medicine: Principles and Practice. 2nd ed. Philadelphia, W.B. Saunders Co., 1989, p 636.)

sound guidance, the tip of a 22- or 20-gauge spinal needle is introduced into an umbilical blood vessel (preferably the vein, but occasionally the artery) at its insertion into the placenta or, rarely, at its insertion into the fetal abdomen.

Direct fetal IVT does not depend on diaphragmatic movement to increase hemoglobin levels. Therefore, it can be used for salvaging the moribund, nonbreathing fetus provided that the fetus still has umbilical blood flow. Direct IVT increases circulating hemoglobin levels in the fetus immediately, rather than in the 8 to 10 days required with IPT.

In Winnipeg, the venipuncturist, under the direction of the ultrasonographer, places the tip of a 22- or 20-gauge spinal needle in an umbilical blood vessel. Once the needle tip appears to be in the vessel, blood is aspirated; whether the blood is fetal is determined by a rapid alkaline denaturation test. The correct position of the needle tip is confirmed by the observation of turbulence coursing down the vessel following the injection of sterile isotonic saline. If fetal movements are likely to disturb the needle insertion, the fetus is paralyzed by the intravenous injection of pancuronium.

While the venipuncturist holds the needle hub and the blood transfusion tubing connector very firmly and the ultrasonographer watches the blood flow turbulence in the fetal blood vessel, the transfusionist (the third member of the team), transfuses compatible packed RBCs in 10 mL aliquots over 1 to 2 minutes until the desired transfusion volume is attained (mean, 40 to 50 mL/kg of estimated, nonhydropic fetal weight). If there is evidence of significant bradycardia or marked ventricular dilation, the transfusion is discontinued before the full volume has been administered.

IVT survival rates in Winnipeg (Table 3–9) are superior to IPT survival rates in every category: 88% versus 76% overall, 95% versus 87% in nonhydropic fetuses, and 73% versus 60% in hydropic fetuses, respectively.

Undoubtedly, if IVT is feasible, it is the procedure of choice. Only through IVT can the moribund, nonbreathing hydropic fetus be salvaged: 12 of 19 (63%) survived in Winnipeg. What is gratifying is the much lower overall risk attendant to IVT when it is compared with IPT (0.8% versus 3.5% per procedure).

Despite the great advantages of IVT, there are two situations in which IPT may be necessary and, therefore, the skill needed for carrying out IPT must be maintained. The first is a rare situation early in pregnancy (before 20 to 21 weeks' gestation), in which the cord vessels are too small for a successful venipuncture. The second and more common situation is the one, in which late in pregnancy (after 30 weeks' gestation and after several successful IVTs), increased fetal size obscures a posterior cord vessel insertion and makes venipuncture impossible.

Blood for Intrauterine Transfusion

The blood used for intrauterine transfusions, in either IPT or IVT, should have been drawn from the donor within 96 hours of its use. The author recommends that the unit have all plasma and buffy coat removed. RBCs for IPT or IVT are not washed and are not run through a leukocyte filter. Ideally, the packed RBC unit should be cytomegalovirus antibody negative.

For 28 years (from 1964 to 1992), packed RBCs used for fetal transfusions at the author's institution were not irradiated, initially because of the absence of the facilities for irradiation, and subsequently because it was believed that the normal, although immature, immune system of the fetus (as early as 20 weeks' gestation) was still sufficiently mature to prevent engraftment of any viable donor lymphocytes. This belief was borne out by the fact that, of 323 infants who survived after undergoing 1200 fetal transfusions in Winnipeg in that period, not one showed any evidence of graft-versus-host disease. Nevertheless, because of the very few instances of graft-versus-host disease following fetal transfusions[89, 90] and of the reassuring fact that γ-irradiation does not damage the viability of the RBCs if they are transfused promptly, the packed RBC unit is now irradiated just prior to the fetal transfusion.

Before the transfusion, 10 to 12 mL of sterile, isotonic saline are added to the packed RBC unit to render it slightly less viscous so that it may be transfused down the epidural catheter at IPT or down the 20- or 22-

Table 3–9. INTRAUTERINE FETAL TRANSFUSIONS (WINNIPEG): ULTRASOUND ERA

	Intraperitoneal Transfusions* from July 1980 to October 1986		Intravascular Transfusions† from May 1986 to February 1995	
	Total	Alive (%)	Total	Alive (%)
Fetuses, total	75	57 (76)	137	120 (88)
Nonhydropic	45	39 (87)	92	87 (95)
Hydropic	30	18 (60)	45	33 (73)
Moribund	8	0 (0)	19	12 (63)
Nonmoribund	22	18 (82)	26	21 (81)

*Total number, 204.
†Total number, 587.

gauge spinal needle used to make the cord venipuncture at IVT. The resultant hematocrit of the donor unit is 0.85 to 0.88.

Treatment of the Neonate with Hemolytic Disease

Exchange Transfusion

The key to the management of HDN is exchange transfusion, which was introduced by Wallerstein in 1945.[91] RBCs coated with antibody are replaced with RBCs negative for the antigen to which the mother is alloimmunized. Exchange transfusion corrects the anemia of the severely affected newborn, prevents hyperbilirubinemia by removing the infant's hemolysing erythrocytes, and removes some of the already formed bilirubin. Aliquots of 10 to 20 mL of the infant's blood are removed and replaced with antigen-negative donor blood. Generally, between 1.5 and 2 infant blood volumes are exchanged (130 to 170 mL/kg of body weight).

A two–blood volume exchange transfusion removes approximately 90% of the affected RBCs of the infant; 70% removal occurs after the first blood volume has been exchanged.

Bilirubin removal is not nearly as efficient as RBC removal because bilirubin bound to albumin is not only in the intravascular compartment but also in the extravascular compartment. Indeed, significantly more bilirubin is in the extravascular space. A two–blood volume exchange transfusion removes about 25% to 30% of the infant's total body bilirubin. Although the measured serum bilirubin immediately after exchange is usually about 50% of the pre-exchange serum bilirubin level, a rapid rebound of the serum bilirubin level to about 75% of the pre-exchange level occurs because of the influx of bilirubin from the extravascular compartment into the vascular compartment. If the indications for exchange transfusion are present, the procedure should be carried out promptly so that the hemolysing RBCs can be removed before they produce indirect bilirubin. The administration of albumin, 1 g/kg of body weight, prior to the exchange transfusion; or the addition of albumin, 4 to 6 g, to blood used for exchange transfusion increases the amount of bilirubin removed to about 35% of the total body bilirubin by drawing bilirubin into the vascular compartment. Albumin should not be administered in either fashion to the severely anemic infant. The increase in oncotic pressure and the increase in blood volume in the anemic infant may precipitate heart failure.

Exchange transfusion produces a significant drop in neutrophil levels; this drop is slowly compensated for but does not appear to have any clinical significance. A similar decrease in platelet levels (if the blood used is more than 24 hours old) also is of no clinical significance provided that the baby is not thrombocytopenic before the exchange transfusion.

Only very modest amounts of the offending antibody are removed by exchange transfusion because the antibody (IgG) is widely distributed, not only in the vascular space but also in the extravascular space.

Cord Blood Testing

A cord blood sample collected into anticoagulant (the author uses heparin) is obtained immediately after delivery. The RBCs are ABO and D tested and undergo DAT.[43] In all types of alloimmune HDN (with the exception of ABO HDN), the cord blood DAT result is strongly positive. In the author's experience, if cord blood is tested, then the DAT result is weakly but definitely positive in nearly all infants with ABO HDN. Hemoglobin and hematocrit measurements are carried out, and total and direct serum bilirubin levels are determined.

Indications for Exchange Transfusion

The hydropic infant who is born alive stresses all of the resources of the most highly developed tertiary-level neonatal unit. Once the infant has been intubated and stabilized, a single–blood volume exchange transfusion should be carried out as soon as possible. Further treatment measures for the hydropic infant are discussed later in this chapter.

Other than the presence of hydrops, indications for prompt exchange transfusion after delivery are appropriate cord hemoglobin and serum bilirubin findings. In the author's opinion, a hemoglobin level of 110 g/L or less is always an indication for exchange transfusion. In the prephototherapy era, a cord serum bilirubin level of 75 μmol/L (4.5 mg/dL) in the term infant, or 65 μmol/L (3.5 mg/dL) in the premature infant, also was an indication for prompt exchange transfusion. Now, in the phototherapy era, indications for exchange transfusion that are based on cord serum bilirubin levels are more relaxed. A prompt exchange transfusion should be carried out if the cord serum bilirubin is 95 μmol/L (5.5 mg/dL) (68 μmol/L (4 mg/dL) if the infant is premature). It should be understood that phototherapy (discussed in detail in Chapter 4) reduces bilirubin levels but does nothing to prevent the RBCs from hemolysing, with resultant anemia. The infant with immune HDN undergoing phototherapy should undergo serial hemoglobin estimations on at least a daily basis. If the cord hemoglobin and serum bilirubin levels do not meet the criteria for prompt exchange transfusion, then serum bilirubin level estimations should be carried out at 6- to 8-hour intervals. If, despite phototherapy, the serum bilirubin rises at a rate greater than 5 μmol/L per hour (0.3 mg/dL per hour), exchange transfusion should be undertaken.

Original studies of the risk of kernicterus in babies with HDN[92] showed that if indirect serum bilirubin levels in mature babies exceeded 340 μmol/L (20 mg/dL) but were less than 425 μmol/L (25 mg/dL), then the risk of kernicterus was approximately 10%. If the indirect bilirubin levels exceeded 510 μmol/L (30 mg/dL), then the risk of kernicterus was 50%. It was on the basis of these 1952 studies that 20 mg/dL was accepted as the indirect serum bilirubin level that should not be exceeded in babies with HDN, and this is still the generally accepted level. This level should be reduced significantly in the presence of prematurity or asphyxia and acidosis. Table 4–1 presents serum bilirubin concentrations (in milligrams per deciliter) at which exchange transfusions are indicated in the neonatal period. It should be noted that prevention of hyperbilirubinemia in the very premature infant by the aggressive use of phototherapy is more acceptable than allowing serum bilirubin to reach levels that require exchange transfusion. Although exchange transfusion in the relatively mature neonate who is in good condition carries with it a mortality rate of a fraction of 1%, this may not be the case in the sick, premature neonate.

Free Bilirubin and Reserve Albumin Binding Studies

It appears that the level of free unconjugated bilirubin is the determining factor in the pathogenesis of bilirubin encephalopathy (kernicterus; see Chapter 4). There is evidence that conjugated (direct) bilirubin and bilirubin bound to albumin do not penetrate the blood-brain barrier and do not cause kernicterus.[93] Efforts have been made to develop methods for measuring free unconjugated bilirubin in plasma and so-called "reserve albumin binding capacity" (RABC). The colorimetric hydroxybenzeneazobenzoic acid method has many detractors, but Johnson and Boggs[94] have shown that no nonacidotic infant whose RABC, as determined with this method, was kept above 50% developed kernicterus. Realizing that the RABC is a crude parameter that may not reflect the availability of residual bilirubin albumin binding sites accurately, the author does measure the RABC with this method whenever serum bilirubin levels exceed 315 μmol/L (18.5 mg/dL). If the RABC is below 50%, the author administers serum albumin, 1 g/kg of body weight, and carries out exchange transfusion with added albumin if the RABC is not promptly elevated above 50%, which it almost invariably is. Exchange transfusion with added albumin also is used if the serum bilirubin level continues to rise despite phototherapy and administration of albumin.

Other methods for measuring the amount of bilirubin bound to albumin[95, 96] are available, as are methods for determining free bilirubin levels.[97, 98] Although these methods were described as early as 1969, none has been universally accepted. It must be remembered that acidosis reduces bilirubin binding and that free fatty acids, some sulfamides, and benzoates compete for albumin binding sites and increase the risk of kernicterus.

Technique of Exchange Transfusion

The specific technical details of exchange transfusion have been reviewed elsewhere* and are only discussed briefly here. The blood should be ABO compatible and Rh negative. The author recommends that it also be Kell negative. If the mother is alloimmunized to an antigen other than D, the unit should be missing that antigen. It should be crossmatch compatible with the

---

*See reference 99.

mother's serum. If blood for exchange transfusion is to be made available before delivery, it should be group O blood. Although it is permissible to use ABO-specific blood for exchange transfusion, if the ABO status of the infant is known and there is no ABO incompatibility with the mother, the author tends to use group O blood for all exchange transfusions. Certainly, if the initial exchange transfusion is carried out using group O blood, any further exchange transfusions should be carried out with group O blood. Otherwise, jaundice due to ABO incompatibility may become a further complication.

Whether blood for exchange transfusion should be irradiated is a subject of controversy. There have been rare reports of graft-versus-host disease following exchange transfusion[89] and, in one instance, following exchange transfusion for ABO hemolytic disease.[100] When one considers the many thousands of exchange transfusions since 1945 and the relative paucity of such reports, it is apparent that graft-versus-host disease following exchange transfusion is exceedingly rare.

Nevertheless, if irradiation is available, blood for exchange transfusion should be irradiated, particularly if the infant is premature. If irradiation is not available, nonirradiated blood should be used because the risk of graft-versus-host disease following exchange transfusion in the erythroblastotic infant at greater than 30 weeks' gestation is very rare.

The author recommends that blood drawn into CPDA-1 (citrate phosphate dextrose adenine) anticoagulant be used for exchange transfusion. At the author's institution, heparinized blood has never been used, and its use is not recommended. Although the pH of CPDA-1–anticoagulated blood is modestly less than that of the infant's blood, the difference is easily compensated for by the infant. If the infant is acidotic, it is preferable to give sodium bicarbonate directly and never add it to the blood for exchange transfusion.

If the birth of a sick hydropic or prehydropic infant is expected, blood from an appropriate donor is collected within hours of the expected delivery so that it will be fresh and contains an adequate number of platelets. With the advent of fetal transfusions, the very ill anemic infants so often seen in the past are now rarely encountered. If the baby is not expected to be premature or very ill, blood that has been drawn 24 to 96 hours before the expected exchange transfusion is selected.

Before exchange transfusion, a plasma volume equivalent to the volume of anticoagulant present (60 mL for CPDA-1), or 80 to 90 mL if 25% albumin has been added, should be removed from the donor unit.

At the author's institution, blood warmers are not used during exchange transfusions. The blood in the administration set is exposed to heat in the infrared unit under which the infant is being exchanged and enters the infant's circulation at 25 to 30°C.

The original exchange transfusion technique of Wallerstein,[91] in which blood is removed from the sagittal sinus and infused into the saphenous vein, is not currently carried out. The umbilical vein transfusion technique described by Diamond and co-workers[101] is the universally accepted method. Briefly, under aseptic conditions and with the infant restrained on an infrared unit and connected to a heart and respiratory rate monitor, a size 5 or size 8 catheter is introduced into the umbilical vein and advanced until an obstruction is met. The catheter is then withdrawn about 5 mm and is adjusted until a free flow of blood is obtained. No attempt is made to pass the catheter across the ductus venosus. Depending on the size of the infant, a 10- to 20-mL aliquot of the infant's blood is removed and placed in a heparinized tube (the pretransfusion blood sample).

The exchange transfusion is then carried out in 10- to 20-mL aliquots until 170 mL/kg of the infant's body weight is reached or until the unit of partially packed, compatible blood (about 450 mL) is completely used up. Two units of blood are used only if 450 mL does not provide at least a 1.5–blood volume exchange transfusion. A 1.5–blood volume exchange transfusion provides 85% to 90% of the benefit of a two–blood volume exchange transfusion. Each infusion and withdrawal of blood is done gently and without undue haste. Otherwise, collapse of mesenteric blood vessels (if removal is too rapid) or sudden influx of unoxygenated blood (if infusion is too rapid) may lead to bowel wall ischemia, with the ever-present hazard of necrotizing enterocolitis.

At approximately each 150-mL mark of the exchange transfusion, the author infuses, slowly, 1.5 mL of 10% calcium gluconate. Although there is debate regarding the need for infusing calcium gluconate, since it may not raise ionized calcium levels, the author is convinced of its value and has used it safely for 40 years. As the exchange progresses, an increase in heart rate and irritability frequently is noted; this increase subsides when the calcium is infused.

Twenty to 30 seconds after the last volume of donor blood has been infused, 5 to 10 mL of blood are removed and placed in a heparinized tube (the postexchange transfusion sample). A pursestring suture is placed around the cord base (if the cord is fresh), or the roll of skin around the cord is approximated with a suture. The catheter is gently and slowly withdrawn, and the cord suture is tied. The exchange transfusion catheter is not left *in situ* because of the hazards of venous thrombosis. Once the umbilical vein has been catheterized, it is a simple matter to recatheterize the vein, if a further exchange transfusion is necessary.

Very rarely, catheterization of the umbilical vein is impossible, particularly if an initial exchange transfusion is required after 7 days (a rare event). A saphenous vein cutdown is the procedure of choice. Unless the operator is skilled in saphenous femoral cutdowns, the insertion of the catheter should be carried out by a surgical colleague. The operator cannulates the vein about 1 cm below its entrance into the femoral vein, using a catheter of the largest feasible diameter (size 18 to 20). The catheter is advanced 3 to 4 cm so that its tip lies free in the common iliac vein or the inferior vena cava. Exchange transfusion is carried out in the same manner. Although tedious because of the smaller size of the catheter, the procedure is usually just as

successful. Smaller transfusion aliquots may be necessary.

If an umbilical artery catheter is in place for any reason, it may be used for exchange transfusion provided that the arterial catheter is of an adequate diameter. Indeed, this is the preferred route of exchange transfusion for the very small premature infant.

Complications of Exchange Transfusion

The complications of exchange transfusion, listed in Table 3–10, may for the most part be avoided if the procedure is performed by an experienced and careful surgeon. Cardiac complications are rare if attention is devoted to umbilical venous blood pressures and the judicious use of deficit transfusions. Care must be taken to correct acidosis, if present; otherwise, umbilical venous pressure measurements may be falsely elevated. Cardiac arrest can be prevented with the use of blood that is less than 96 hours old and with the periodic administration of calcium gluconate. Similarly, embolic and thrombotic phenomena are entirely preventable by the operator with skill and experience in umbilical cannulation and exchange transfusion.

The risk of bleeding following the use of heparinized blood is one of the reasons that its use is not recommended. Severe thrombocytopenia is an ever-present problem in severe HDN and is aggravated by the invariable decrease in platelet levels after exchange transfusion, unless very fresh blood is used. Because donor blood must be subjected to various safety tests (e.g., screening for human immunodeficiency virus, HCV, hepatitis B surface antigen), which take several hours, very fresh blood may not be available. Platelet levels

Table 3–10. COMPLICATIONS OF EXCHANGE TRANSFUSION

Cardiac

Heart failure due to hypervolemia and transfusion overload

Cardiac arrest due to hyperkalemia, hypocalcemia, citrate toxicity

Emboli and Thrombosis

Air emboli due to negative umbilical venous pressure and faulty transfusion technique (care must also be taken when the umbilical vein is large and gaping because air may leak into the vein between the catheter and vein wall)

Portal thrombosis due to excess trauma during catheterization of the umbilical vein

Bleeding

Overheparinization of donor blood if heparinized blood is used

Thrombocytopenia, usually of moderate degree, but sometimes extreme in the presence of severe disease

Perforation of the umbilical vein at the time of catheterization

Sepsis

Bacterial, due to poor technique at exchange transfusion

Hepatitis due to donor blood-borne virus

Necrotizing enterocolitis with ileal or colonic perforation

---

must be monitored and platelet concentrates infused whenever the platelet count drops into the 30 to 40 × 10^9/L range.

Similarly, bacterial sepsis can be prevented if attention is devoted to very careful aseptic technique at the time of umbilical vein catheterization. Although the use of prophylactic antibiotics is frowned upon by many, the author uses them for 24 to 48 hours after both fetal and exchange transfusions and has encountered no problems with their use. It is believed that their use may have contributed to the low incidence of postexchange transfusion necrotizing enterocolitis.

Necrotizing enterocolitis is undoubtedly the most important major hazard that can occur after exchange transfusion.[99, 102, 103] It has occassionally been encountered in this author's experience. Prevention requires care and expertise in exchange transfusion. Every effort should be made to prevent wide pressure and volume variations during exchange transfusion. Blood injection and withdrawal should be carried out smoothly without undue haste. Marked negative or positive pressures should never be exerted with the exchange transfusion syringe. At the author's institution, babies are not fed for 8 to 12 hours after exchange transfusion; during this period, infusions of 10% glucose are used. Only when the infant's abdomen is soft with normal bowel sounds are feedings cautiously started.

General Measures

Breast feeding is strongly recommended. If the infant is mature and in good condition, he or she can be breast fed and be given phototherapy between feedings. Although Rh antibodies are present in breast milk, particularly in colostrum, very little antibody is absorbed,[104] and what is absorbed does not damage the antigen-negative RBCs present in the circulation after exchange transfusion. For these reasons, breast feeding should not be prohibited.

Phototherapy is discontinued once serum bilirubin levels decrease. As a rule, infants who have received transfusions can be discharged by the sixth or seventh day. Conversely, premature, very anemic, prehydropic or hydropic infants may extend the resources of the most highly developed tertiary-level neonatal intensive care unit and require many weeks of such care.

Ancillary Treatment Measures for Hyperbilirubinemia

Phototherapy, enzyme induction inhibition with phenobarbital, and the use of inhibitors of bilirubin production by the mesoporphyrins are discussed in Chapter 4. Only phototherapy has a place in the treatment of immune HDN.

MANAGEMENT OF SPECIAL PROBLEMS
Severe Anemia at Birth (Hemoglobin Level < 80 g/L)

Erythroblastotic babies with severe anemia usually are premature. Although most of them are not in heart failure at the time of birth, they may develop heart failure promptly after delivery. Paradoxically, this author has seen some very severely affected babies, particularly those in whom the cord was clamped late, who made no spontaneous respiratory effort until venesection and reduction of blood volume were carried out. Many of these infants require intubation and positive-pressure ventilation immediately after birth. Prompt clamping of the cord within 5 to 10 seconds after birth is important because the placental transfusion may precipitate heart failure.

Exchange transfusion should be carried out as soon as an adequate airway and ventilation have been established. Because infants requiring transfusion are small and may be in a precarious cardiovascular state, smaller volumes of blood (10 to 15 mL) are exchanged. The amount of reduction of the infant's blood volume, if any, is determined with frequent estimations of central venous pressure if the catheter has been passed through the ductus venosus. Central venous pressure should be maintained at between 3 and 5 cm H_2O. It is important that acidosis, if present, be corrected. Also, great care should be taken not to reduce the blood volume suddenly because the initial blood volume in the hydropic or prehydropic infant may not be grossly expanded. The risk of hypervolemia and heart failure becomes greater as the exchange transfusion progresses, when both hemoglobin and plasma protein levels are raised with increases in plasma osmotic pressure.

Heart Failure

Many of these infants, although not in heart failure at the time of birth, become so as evidenced by the occurrence of cardiomegaly and pulmonary congestion (see Fig. 3–5). In this situation, the infant may be digitalized as long as it is remembered that the premature infant may require very little digoxin for full digitalization. Also, a diuretic such as furosemide, 1 mg/kg of body weight, should be given once or twice daily.

Thrombocytopenia

Thrombocytopenia has already been discussed. Repeated platelet determinations are important. One unit of platelet concentrate should be given whenever the platelet count drops below 30 to 40 × 10^9/L.

The Syndrome of Hepatocellular Damage[99, 105]

Most severely anemic, erythroblastotic infants, particularly those who are hydropic or prehydropic, show signs of obstructive jaundice. There is extreme hepatomegaly due to the presence of islets of extramedullary erythropoiesis, which interfere with hepatocellular function and cause biliary canalicular obstruction. It is not unusual for peak bilirubin levels to reach 515 to 685 μmol/L (30 to 40 mg/dL) by the fifth or sixth day after birth; one half to two thirds of this amount may be direct-acting conjugated bilirubin.

The outlook for infants with the syndrome of hepato-cellular damage and their mode of management is similar to that outlined for severely anemic erythro-blastotic babies. Although direct bilirubin is nontoxic, its presence indicates severe disease and the involve-ment of other factors, such as heme pigment levels, anoxia, and acidosis, which increase the risk of kernict-erus. For this reason, exchange transfusion is carried out at indirect bilirubin levels that are somewhat lower than usual (290 to 325 μmol/L, or 17 to 19 mg/dL).

The syndrome of hepatocellular damage is often as-sociated with coagulation defects, making hemorrhage an ever-present risk. The blood used for transfusion of these babies preferably is less than 24 hours old. Again, if the baby is thrombocytopenic, platelet-rich blood should be used and a unit of platelets given after the exchange transfusion.

Although the use of corticosteroids has been advo-cated for the treatment of erythroblastotic infants with hepatocellular damage,[105] it is rarely necessary. Evi-dence of hepatic obstruction may persist for several weeks. In the author's experience, the syndrome invari-ably disappears and the infants are not left with any permanent hepatic damage or subsequent cirrhosis of the liver.

Infants Who Have Undergone Fetal Transfusions

Management of these very special infants does not differ from that of other erythroblastotic babies. Fortu-nately, severe respiratory distress is not a major prob-lem. Indications for exchange transfusion in these in-fants are the same as those for any other premature infants. Because these infants are often delivered with very little in the way of residual Rh-positive hemolyz-ing RBCs, their postdelivery management may be rela-tively simple. Nevertheless, because they may have very marked hepatosplenomegaly with residual in-tense erythropoiesis, they may require multiple ex-change transfusions. Conversely, a very significant number of babies born after intravascular fetal transfu-sions, usually at a relatively mature gestation (37 to 38 weeks), do not require exchange transfusion.

Persistent Hydrops Fetalis

The outlook for the hydropic fetus is much better if the fetus can be treated *in utero* and the condition reversed. However, the outlook for the severely hydropic neo-nate, although very guarded, is certainly not hopeless. Treatment does not differ greatly from that for the anemic nonhydropic infant, except that intubation and artificial positive-pressure ventilation are nearly always necessary and the problems of edema and residual ascites are ever-present.

Measures that are important in salvaging the baby with hydrops fetalis are immediate intubation, artificial ventilation, and abdominal paracentesis, with removal of some but not all of the residual ascitic fluid. Rapid and early repeated exchange transfusions with ade-quate control of venous pressure are necessary. Ancil-lary measures such as correction of acidosis, treatment of heart failure, maintenance of adequate platelet lev-els, and infusion of 10% dextrose and fresh frozen plasma are all important. It also is important to take care not to overload the already compromised circula-tion of these hydropic babies.

Management of ascites may be a problem. It would appear that removal of large volumes of ascitic fluid does not enchance the infant's chances of survival. The present recommended treatment is removal of only enough ascitic fluid to relieve respiratory distress and allow adequate oxygenation of the baby (about 100 to 200 mL). The rest should be allowed to remain, either to be absorbed and removed through further blood volume reduction and subsequent exchange transfu-sions or to be dissipated gradually through the para-centesis puncture wound.

Hypoglycemia

Severely affected erythroblastotic infants are hyperin-sulinemic and are at great risk of becoming hypogly-cemic, particularly after exchange transfusion with citrated blood. Immediately after delivery, an intrave-nous infusion of 10% dextrose should be started at 65 to 80 mL/kg of body weight daily and maintained until the oral intake is adequate and blood glucose levels remain above 2.2 mmol/L (40 mg/dL).

Follow-Up Care of the Infant with Hemolytic Disease

Whether or not the affected infant has required fetal transfusions or exchange transfusions, anemia in the first few weeks of life is very frequent. Hemoglobin levels should be checked at 10- to 14-day intervals until the infant is 8 to 12 weeks of age. The anemia is due to the gradual loss of transfused Rh-negative RBCs and to the failure of the infant's Rh-positive RBCs to replace them. This failure is initially due to hemolysis of any RBCs produced and to transient bone marrow hypopla-sia, which spontaneously resolves at 6 to 8 weeks of age.

In the interim, if hemoglobin levels drop into the 70 to 75 g/L range, a simple transfusion of 20 mL/kg of body weight of crossmatched, packed RBCs compatible with the infant's serum is administered. Because the infant is saturated with iron, the anemia is not due to iron deficiency, and iron supplementation is not indicated.

It is rarely necessary to give more than one booster transfusion. No effort should be made to raise the hemoglobin level above 110 to 120 g/L. After the infant is 6 to 8 weeks of age, bone marrow activity returns, reticulocytes appear in the circulation, and the hemo-globin level increases toward normal.

Recently, recombinant erythropoietin has been used with considerable success in the treatment of the ane-mia of prematurity, reducing or eliminating the need for erythrocyte transfusions in these infants.[106] One might conclude that treatment with erythropoietin might reduce the need for transfusion in the late anemia of infants with HDN. This author has not used recombinant erythropoietin for this purpose and would recommend caution in its use if there is a significant amount of residual passive antibody in the infant's circulation.

PREVENTION OF Rh IMMUNIZATION

About 16% of Rh-negative women who have delivered ABO-compatible, Rh-positive infants become Rh immunized as a result of the pregnancy. About 11% of the 16% (1.8% of the total) are Rh immunized by the time they deliver their babies.[22] The risk of Rh immunization is about 1.5% to 2% if the Rh-positive baby is ABO incompatible with his or her mother; it is about 2% if an Rh-negative woman has a spontaneous abortion and 4% to 5% if she has an interruption of her pregnancy.[107]

In 1900, Von Dungern proved the axiom that formed the basis for Rh prophylaxis 65 years later.[108] He injected a group of rabbits with RBCs from an ox. The rabbits obligingly produced ox RBC antibodies. When he injected a second group of rabbits with RBCs from the same ox and then gave them sera from the first group of rabbits (containing ox RBC antibodies), the second group of rabbits did not develop ox RBC antibodies. He proved that active immunization to an antigen is prevented by the presence of passive antibody to the antigen.

Trials of Prevention

More than 60 years after Von Dungern's report, the information he provided was first put to use almost simultaneously in New York[109] and Liverpool[110] and shortly thereafter in Winnipeg.[111] Initially, experiments involved giving Rh-negative male volunteers Rh-positive RBCs coated with Rh antibody.[112] When Rh immunization did not occur, volunteers were given Rh-positive RBCs followed by Rh antibody in the form of high-titer plasma or Rh immune globulin (RhIG or anti-D IgG). In every experiment, Rh immunization was prevented by administration of Rh antibody.[109-111] Clinical trials were then undertaken in which Rh-negative, unimmunized women were given RhIG intramuscularly following delivery of an Rh-positive infant.[113-115] All such Rh prevention trials were highly successful in preventing Rh immunization when RhIG was given within 72 hours post partum.

The licensure of RhIG in 1968 profoundly influenced the prevalence of Rh immunization. It should be administered to all Rh-negative pregnant women at 28 weeks' gestation; to all Rh-negative nonimmunized pregnant women who are likely to abort or are undergoing amniocentesis or chorionic villus sampling; or after any other invasive procedure. The dose during pregnancy should be 300 μg, repeated every 12 weeks until delivery.

RhIG should be given after delivery of an Rh-positive baby and after abortion. The usual dose after full-term delivery in the United States is 300 μg, although elsewhere 100 to 120 μg is administered with almost equal effectiveness. Following early first trimester abortion, a 50-μg minidose of RhIG, if available, is adequate; abortion later in pregnancy requires a dose of at least 100 μg.[116]

About 1 woman in 400 will have a fetal-to-maternal TPH of greater than 30 mL of fetal blood at the time of delivery. Prevention of Rh immunization in the presence of such a large dose of antigen requires the use of more than one dose of RhIG.

In the author's experience, careful attendance to all aspects of Rh prophylaxis as outlined has reduced the prevalence of Rh immunization by 96%.[117] Residual Rh immunization (failure of prophylaxis) is due to Rh immunization occurring before 28 weeks' gestation, undiagnosed prior abortion, and undiagnosed fetal transplacental bleeding during pregnancy sufficient to overwhelm the small amount of residual passive anti-D in the maternal circulation.[117]

CONCLUSIONS

Advances in prevention of Rh immunization and the management of immune HDN in the past 30 years have been dramatic. In Manitoba (population, 1 million), the prevalence of Rh immunization in pregnant women has been reduced by 92% (from 228 in 1962 to 18 in 1994); the number of exchange transfusions has also been decreased (from 226 in 1962 to 1 in 1994, carried out on an infant with anti-S immune hemolysis). The latter statistic has signaled a great problem in our education of pediatric residents and fellows, many of whom complete their training without ever having had the opportunity to see or carry out an exchange transfusion.

The reduction in the number of exchange transfusions carried out is primarily due not only to the reduction in the number of cases of immune HDN but also to the use of fetal transfusions in severely affected fetuses. The fetal transfusion neonate, after delivery, frequently does not require exchange transfusion but invariably requires one or more simple transfusions in the first few weeks of life.

These advances have also produced a very gratifying 98% reduction in perinatal deaths from immune HDN in Manitoba (from 141 in the 8-year period from 1962 to 1969 to 3 in the 8-year period 1987 to 1994).

References

1. Diamond LK, Blackfan KD, Baty JM: Erythroblastosis fetalis and its association with universal edema of the fetus, icterus gravis neonatorum and anemia of the newborn. J Pediatr 1932; 1:269.
2. Darrow RR: Icterus gravis (erythroblastosis neonatorum. An examination of etiologic considerations). Arch Pathol 1938; 25:378.
3. Levine P, Stetson RE: An unusual case of intra-group agglutination. JAMA 1939; 113:126.
4. Landsteiner K, Wiener AS: An agglutinable factor in human

blood recognized by immune sera for rhesus blood. Proc Soc Exp Biol Med 1940; 43:223.

5. Levine P, Katzin EM, Burnham L: Isoimmunization in pregnancy: Its possible bearing on the etiology of erythroblastosis fetalis. JAMA 1941; 116:825.

6. Wiener AS, Wexler IB: Heredity of the Blood Groups. New York, Grune & Stratton, 1958.

7. Rosenfield RE, Allan FH Jr, et al: A review of Rh serology and presentation of a new terminology. Transfusion 1962; 2:287.

8. Race RR: The Rh genotype and Fisher's theory. Blood 1948; 3:(special issue):27.

9. Le Van Kim C, Mouro I, et al: Molecular cloning and primary structure of the human blood group RhD polypeptide. Proc Natl Acad Sci U S A 1992; 89:10925.

10. Lacey PA, Caskey CR, et al: Fatal hemolytic disease of the newborn due to anti-D in an Rh-positive Dᵘ variant mother. Transfusion 1983; 23:91.

11. Goto S, Nishi H, Tomoda A: Blood group Rh-D factor in human trophoblast determined by immunofluorescent method. Am J Obstet Gynecol 1980; 137:707.

12. Wiener AS: Diagnosis and treatment of anemia of the newborn caused by occult placental hemorrhage. Am J Obstet Gynecol 1948; 56:717.

13. Chown B: Anemia from bleeding of the fetus into the mother's circulation. Lancet 1954; 1:1213.

14. Kleihauer E, Braun H, Betke K: Demonstration von fetalem Haemoglobin in den Erythrozyten eines Blutausstriches. Klin Wochenschr 1957; 35:637.

15. Bowman JM, Pollock JM, Penston LE: Fetomaternal transplacental hemorrhage during pregnancy and after delivery. Vox Sang 1986; 51:117.

16. Peddle LJ: Increase of antibody titer following amniocentesis. Am J Obstet Gynecol 1968; 100:567.

17. Bowman JM, Pollock JM: Transplacental fetal hemorrhage after amniocentesis. Obstet Gynecol 1985; 66:749.

18. Woodrow JC: Rh immunization and its prevention. The immune response in the mother. In Jensen KG, Killmann SA (eds): Series Hematologica III. Copenhagen, Munksgaard, 1970, p 3.

19. Zipursky A, Israels LG: The pathogenesis and prevention of Rh immunization. Can Med Assoc J 1967; 97:1245.

20. Nevanlinna HR: Factors affecting maternal Rh immunization. Ann Med Exp Fenn 1953; 31(Suppl 2):1.

21. Bowman JM: Fetomaternal ABO incompatibility and erythroblastosis fetalis. Vox Sang 1986; 50:104.

22. Bowman JM, Chown B, et al: Rh-isoimmunization during pregnancy: Antenatal prophylaxis. Can Med Assoc J 1978; 118:623.

23. Lobuglio AF, Cotran RS, Jandl JH: Red cells coated with immunoglobulin G: Binding and sphering by mononuclear cells in man. Science 1967; 158:1582.

24. Urbaniak SJ: Lymphoid cell dependent (K-cell) lysis of human erythrocytes sensitized with Rhesus alloantibody. Br J Haematol 1976; 33:409.

25. Engelfriet CP, Borne AEG, et al: Immune Destruction of Red Cells: A Seminar on Immune-Mediated Cell Destruction. Washington, DC, American Association of Blood Banks, 1981, p 113.

26. Thomson A, Contreras M, et al: Clearance of Rh D-positive red cells with monoclonal anti-D. Lancet 1990; 336:1147.

27. Pollock JM, Bowman JM: Anti-Rh(D) IgG subclasses and severity of Rh hemolytic disease of the newborn. Vox Sang 1990; 59:176.

28. Zupanska B, Brojer E, et al: Serological and immunological characteristics of maternal anti-Rh(D) antibodies in predicting the severity of haemolytic disease of the newborn. Vox Sang 1989; 56:247.

29. Parinaud J, Blanc M, et al: IgG subclasses and Gm allotypes of anti-D antibodies during pregnancy: Correlation with the gravity of the fetal disease. Am J Obstet Gynecol 1985; 151:1111.

30. Phibbs RH, Johnson P, Tooley WH: Cardio-respiratory status of erythroblastotic infants: II. Blood volume, hematocrit and serum albumin concentration in relation to hydrops fetalis. Pediatrics 1974; 53:13.

31. James LS: Shock in the newborn in relation to hydrops. In Robertson JG, Dambrosio F (eds): International Symposium on the Management of the Rh Problem. Ann Obstet Ginecol 1970; Special Number, p 193.

32. Mollison PL, Engelfriet CP, Contreras M: Hemolytic disease of the newborn. In Mollison PL (ed): Blood Transfusion in Clinical Medicine. 8th ed. Oxford, Blackwell Scientific Publications, 1987, p 639.

33. Bowman JM, Pollock JM, et al: Maternal Kell blood group alloimmunization. Obstet Gynecol 1992; 79:239.

34. Bowman JM, Harman CR, et al: Erythroblastosis fetalis produced by anti-k. Vox Sang 1989; 56:187.

35. Dacus JV, Spinnato JA: Severe erythroblastosis fetalis secondary to anti-Kpᵇ sensitization. Am J Obstet Gynecol 1984; 150:888.

36. MacPherson CR, Christiansen MJ, et al: Anti-M antibody as a cause of intrauterine death. Am J Clin Pathol 1961; 35:31.

37. Cox MT, Sheils L, et al: Fetal hydrops due to anti-B. Transfusion 1991; 31(Suppl):S29.

38. Miller DF, Petrie SJ: Fatal erythroblastosis fetalis secondary to ABO incompatibility: Report of a case. Obstet Gynecol 1963; 22:773.

39. Brouwers HAA, Overbeeke MAM, et al: Complement is not activated in ABO-haemolytic disease of the newborn. Br J Haematol 1988; 68:363.

40. Bowman JM: ABO hemolytic disease. In Creasy RK, Resnik R (eds): Maternal-Fetal Medicine: Principles and Practice. 2nd ed. Philadelphia, W.B. Saunders Co., 1989, p 652.

41. Wiener AS: Conglutination test for Rh sensitization. J Lab Clin Med 1945; 30:662.

42. Lewis M, Chown B: A short albumin method for the determination of isohemagglutinins, particularly incomplete Rh antibodies. J Lab Clin Med 1957; 50:494.

43. Coombs RRA, Mourant AE, Race RR: A new test for the detection of weak and "incomplete" Rh agglutinins. Br J Exp Pathol 1945; 26:255.

44. Lewis M, Kaita H, Chown B: Kell typing in the capillary tube. J Lab Clin Med 1958; 52:163.

45. Rosenfield RE, Haber GV: Detection and measurement of homologous human hemagglutinins. Presented at Automation in Analytical Chemistry–Technicon Symposia, Tarrytown, NY, 1965.

46. Lalezari P: A polybrene method for the detection of red cell antibodies. Fed Proc 1967; 26:756.

47. Moore BPL: Automation in the blood transfusion laboratory: I. Antibody detection and quantitation in the Technicon AutoAnalyzer. Can Med Assoc J 1969; 100:381.

48. Bowman JM, Pollock JM: Amniotic fluid spectrophotometry and early delivery in the management of erythroblastosis fetalis. Pediatrics 1965; 35:815.

49. Nance SJ, Nelson JM, et al: Monocyte monolayer assay: an efficient noninvasive technique for predicting the severity of hemolytic disease of the newborn. Am J Clin Pathol 1989; 92:89.

50. Urbaniak SJ, Greiss MA, et al: Prediction of the outcome of Rhesus haemolytic disease of the newborn: additional information using an ADCC assay. Vox Sang 1984; 46:323.

51. Engelfriet CP, Brouwers HAA, et al: Prognostic value of the ADCC with monocytes and maternal antibodies for haemolytic disease of the newborn (abstract). Book of Abstracts. Sydney, Australia, XXIst Congress of the International Society of Hematology and XIXth Congress of the International Society of Blood Transfusion, 1986, p 162.

52. Hadley AG, Kumpel BM, Merry AH: The chemiluminescent response of human monocytes to red cells sensitized with monoclonal anti-Rh(D) antibodies. Clin Lab Haematol 1988; 10:377.

53. Hadley AG, Kumpel BM, et al: Correlation of serological, quantitative and cell-mediated functional assays of maternal alloantibodies with the severity of haemolytic disease of the newborn. Br J Haematol 1991; 77:221.

54. Mollison P: Results of tests with different cellular bioassays in relation to severity of RhD haemolytic disease. Report from nine collaborating laboratories (collaborative study). Vox Sang 1991; 60:225.

55. Brown SJ, Perkins JT, et al: The monocyte-monolayer assay does not predict severity of hemolytic disease of the newborn. Transfusion 1991; 31(Suppl):S53.

56. Liley AW: Liquor amnii analysis in management of pregnancy complicated by rhesus immunization. Am J Obstet Gynecol 1961; 82:1359.

57. Bevis DCA: Blood pigments in haemolytic disease of the newborn. J Obstet Gynaecol Br Emp 1956; 63:68.

58. Nicolaides KH, Rodeck CH, et al: Have Liley charts outlived their usefulness? Am J Obstet Gynecol 1986; 155:90.

59. Ananth U, Queenan JT: Does midtrimester ΔO.D. 450 of amniotic fluid reflect severity of Rh disease? Am J Obstet Gynecol 1989; 161:47.

60. Chitkara U, Wilkins I, et al: The role of sonography in assessing severity of fetal anemia in Rh- and Kell-isoimmunized pregnancies. Obstet Gynecol 1988; 71:393.

61. Daffos F, Capella-Pavlovsky M, Forestier F: Fetal blood sampling during pregnancy with use of a needle guided by ultrasound: A study of 606 consecutive cases. Am J Obstet Gynecol 1985; 153:655.

62. Bowman JM, Pollock JM, et al: Fetomaternal hemorrhage following funipuncture: Increase in severity of maternal red-cell alloimmunization. Obstet Gynecol 1994; 84:839.

63. Bennett PR, Le Van Kim C, et al: Prenatal determination of fetal RhD type by DNA amplification. N Engl J Med 1993; 329:607.

64. Lo Y-MD, Bowel PJ, et al: Prenatal determination of fetal RhD status by analysis of peripheral blood of rhesus negative mothers. Lancet 1993; 341:1147. Letter.

65. Carter BB: Preliminary report on a substance which inhibits anti-Rh serum. Am J Clin Pathol 1947; 17:646.

66. Biermé SJ, Blanc M, et al: Oral Rh treatment for severely immunized mothers. Lancet 1979; 1:604.

67. Gold WR Jr, Queenan JT, et al: Oral desensitization in Rh disease. Am J Obstet Gynecol 1983; 146:980.

68. Gusdon JP Jr, Caudle MR, et al: Phagocytosis and erythroblastosis: 1. Modification of the neonatal response by promethazine hydrochloride. Am J Obstet Gynecol 1976; 125:224.

69. Bowman JM, Pollock JM: Reversal of Rh alloimmunization: Fact or fancy? Vox Sang 1984; 47:209.

70. De Silva M, Contreras M, Mollison PL: Failure of passively administered anti-Rh to prevent secondary Rh immune responses. Vox Sang 1985; 48:178.

71. Graham-Pole J, Barr W, Willoughby MLN: Continuous flow plasmapheresis in management of severe Rhesus disease. BMJ 1977; 1:1185.

72. Robinson EAE, Tovey LAD: Intensive plasma exchange in the management of severe Rh disease. Br J Haematol 1980; 45:621.

73. Berlin G, Selbing A, Ryden G: Rhesus haemolytic disease treated with high-dose intravenous immunoglobulin. Lancet 1985; 1:1153. Letter.

74. Margulies M, Voto LS, et al: High-dose intravenous IgG for the treatment of severe Rhesus alloimmunization. Vox Sang 1991; 61:181.

75. Chown B, Bowman WD: The place of early delivery in the prevention of fetal death from erythroblastosis. Pediatr Clin North Am 1958; May:279.

76. Liley AW: Intrauterine transfusion of fetus in hemolytic disease. BMJ 1963; 2:1107.

77. Menticoglou SM, Harman CR, et al: Intraperitoneal fetal transfusion: Paralysis inhibits red cell absorption. Fetal Ther 1987; 2:154.

78. Lewis M, Bowman JM, et al: Absorption of red cells from the peritoneal cavity of a hydropic twin. Transfusion 1973; 13:37.

79. Adamsons K Jr, Freda VJ, et al: Prenatal treatment of erythroblastosis fetalis following hysterotomy. Pediatrics 1965; 35:848.

80. Asensio SH, Figueroa-Longo JG, Pelegrina A: Intrauterine exchange transfusion. Am J Obstet Gynecol 1966; 95:1129.

81. Seelen J, Van Kessel H, et al: A new method of exchange transfusion in utero: Cannulation of vessels on the fetal side of the human placenta. Am J Obstet Gynecol 1966; 95:872.

82. Rodeck CH, Holman CA, et al: Direct intravascular fetal blood transfusion by fetoscopy in severe rhesus isoimmunization. Lancet 1981; 1:625.

83. De Crespigny LC, Robinson HP, et al: Ultrasound-guided blood transfusion for severe rhesus isoimmunization. Obstet Gynecol 1985; 66:529.

84. Berkowitz RL, Chikara U, et al: Intrauterine intravascular transfusions for severe red blood cell isoimmunization: Ultrasound-guided percutaneous approach. Am J Obstet Gynecol 1986; 155:574.

85. Nicholaides KH, Soothill PW, et al: Rh disease: Intravascular fetal blood transfusion by cordocentesis. Fetal Ther 1986; 1:185.

86. Seeds JW, Bowes WA: Ultrasound-guided intravascular transfusion in severe rhesus immunization. Am J Obstet Gynecol 1986; 154:1105.

87. Grannum PAT, Copel JA, et al: The reversal of hydrops fetalis by intravascular intrauterine transfusions in severe isoimmune fetal anemia. Am J Obstet Gynecol 1988; 158:914.

88. Harman CR, Bowman JM, et al: Intrauterine transfusion—Intraperitoneal versus intravascular approach: A case-control comparision. Am J Obstet Gynecol 1990; 162:1053.

89. Parkman R, Mosier D, et al: Graft-versus-host disease after intrauterine and exchange transfusions for hemolytic disease of the newborn. N Engl J Med 1974; 290:359.

90. Naiman JL, Punnett HH, et al: Possible graft-versus-host reaction after erythroblastosis fetalis. N Engl J Med 1969; 281:697.

91. Wallerstein H: Treatment of severe erythroblastosis by simultaneous removal and replacement of blood of the newborn. Science 1946; 103:583.

92. Hsia DYY, Allen FH Jr, et al: Erythroblastosis VIII. Studies of serum bilirubin in relation to kernicterus. N Engl J Med 1952; 247:668.

93. Chan G, Schiff D, et al: Competitive binding of free fatty acids and bilirubin to albumin: differences in HBABA dye versus Sephadex G-25 interpretation of results. Clin Biochem 1971; 4:208.

94. Johnson LH, Boggs TR: Failure of exchange transfusion to prevent cerebral damage when employed so as to maintain serum bilirubin concentrations below 18–20 mg/100 ml. Abstract 200. Presented at the 40th Annual Meeting of the Society for Pediatric Research, Atlantic City, 1970, p 107.

95. Lee KS, Gartner LM, Vaisman SL: Measurement of bilirubin albumin binding. I. Comparative analysis of four methods and four human serum albumin preparations. Pediatr Res 1978; 12:301.

96. Odell GB, Cohen SM, Kelly PC: Studies in kernicterus. II. The determination of the saturation of serum albumin with bilirubin. J Pediatr 1969; 74:214.

97. Chunga F, Lardinois R: Separation by gel filtration and microdetermination of unbound bilirubin. I. In vitro albumin and acidosis effects on albumin-bilirubin binding. Acta Paediatr Scand 1971; 60:27.

98. Cashore WJ, Monin PJ, Oh W: Serum bilirubin binding capacity and free bilirubin concentration: A comparison between Sephadex G-25 filtration and peroxidase oxidation techniques. Pediatr Res 1978; 12:195.

99. Bowman JM: Neonatal management. In: Queenan JT (ed): Modern Management of the Rh Problem. 2nd ed. Hagerstown, MD, Harper & Row, 1977, p 200.

100. Lauer BA, Githens JH, et al: Probable graft-vs-graft reaction in an infant after exchange transfusion and marrow transplantation. Pediatrics 1982; 70:43.

101. Diamond LK, Allen FH Jr, Thomas WO: Erythroblastosis fetalis. VII. Treatment with exchange transfusion. N Engl J Med 1951; 244:39.

102. Corkery JJ, Dubowitz V, et al: Colonic perforation after exchange transfusion. BMJ 1968; 4:345.

103. Castor WR: Spontaneous perforation of the bowel in the newborn following exchange transfusion. Can Med Assoc J 1968; 99:934.

104. Bowman JM: Gastro-intestinal absorption of iso-hemagglutinin. Am J Dis Child 1963; 105:352.

105. Dunn PM: Obstructive jaundice and haemolytic disease of the newborn. Arch Dis Child 1963; 38:54.

106. Ohis RK, Christensen RD: Recombinant erythropoietin compared with erythrocyte transfusion in the treatment of anemia of prematurity. J Pediatr 1991; 119:781.

107. Freda VJ, Gorman JG, et al: The threat of Rh immunization from abortion. Lancet 1970; 2:147.

108. Von Dungern F: Beiträge zur Immunitätslehr. Munch Med Wochenschr 1900; 47:677.

109. Freda VJ, Gorman JG, Pollack W: Successful prevention of experimental Rh sensitization in man with an anti-Rh gamma-2-globulin antibody preparation: A preliminary report. Transfusion 1964; 4:26.

110. Clarke CA, Donohoe WTA, et al: Further experimental studies in the prevention of Rh-haemolytic disease. BMJ 1963; 1:979.

111. Zipursky A, Israels LG: The pathogenesis and prevention of Rh immunization. Can Med Assoc J 1967; 97:1245.
112. Stern K, Goodman HS, Berger M: Experimental isoimmunization to hemoantigens in man. J Immunol 1961; 87:189.
113. Chown B, Duff AM, et al: Prevention of primary Rh immunization: First report of the Western Canadian Trial. Can Med Assoc J 1969; 100:1021.
114. Pollack W, Gorman JG, et al: Results of clinical trials with RhoGAM in women. Transfusion 1968; 8:151.
115. Combined study: Prevention of Rh-haemolytic disease: results of the clinical trial. A combined study from centres in England and Baltimore. BMJ 1966; 2:907.
116. Blajchman M, Zipursky A, et al: McMaster Conference on Prevention of Rh Immunization, September 28–30, 1977. Vox Sang 1979; 36:50.
117. Bowman JM, Pollock JM: Failures of intravenous Rh immune globulin prophylaxis: An analysis of the reasons for such failures. Transf Med Rev 1987; 1:101.

Disorders of Bilirubin Metabolism

Peter F. Whitington · Estella M. Alonso

Jaundice is among the most commonly observed clinical signs in the newborn, and thus an understanding of bilirubin metabolism is important for pediatricians. Bilirubin determination is a valuable tool in clinical evaluation because it represents the interaction between the hematologic and hepatobiliary systems. Pediatricians should understand the normal metabolism of bilirubin and the clinical conditions in which this metabolism is altered if they are to effectively manage the large number of jaundiced infants encountered in their practices. This chapter discusses the chemistry, synthesis, transport, metabolism, and disposal of bilirubin, both in health and in disease.

CHEMISTRY OF BILIRUBIN AND ANALYTIC CONSIDERATIONS
Structure and Physical Chemistry of Bilirubin

Bilirubin is a compound with a molecular weight of 584. It consists of four substituted pyrrole rings linked

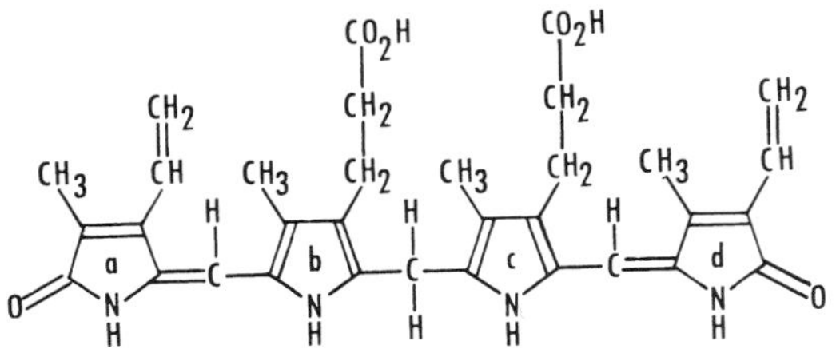

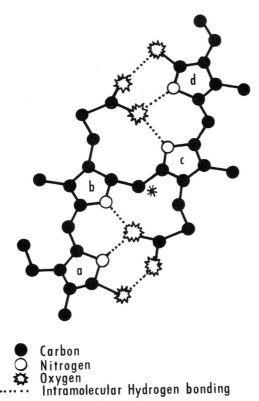

Figure 4–1. Standard chemical structure of bilirubin IXα.

by two methyne (—CH=) groups and one central methene (—CH₂—) group[1] (Fig. 4–1). It is derived entirely from the protoporphyrin in hemoglobin and other iron-containing heme proteins.[1, 2] The structure of bilirubin determines its physical characteristics.[3] Intramolecular hydrogen bonds between the propionic acid carboxyl groups and the opposing pyrrole lactam systems cause the molecule to fold on itself at the flexible central methene bridge; this folding renders the molecule nonpolar and almost insoluble in water at physiologic pH (Fig. 4–2).[4–8] Its aqueous solubility is less than 0.005 mg/dL (86 nmol/L) at pH 7.4.[6] It is highly soluble in relatively polar organic solvents (e.g., chloroform) and is essentially insoluble in nonpolar solvents (e.g., diethyl ether).[1, 6]

● Carbon
○ Nitrogen
✹ Oxygen
...... Intramolecular Hydrogen bonding

Figure 4–2. Naturally occurring structure of bilirubin IXα, demonstrating intramolecular hydrogen bonding (.....) and rotation of a–b and c–d dipyrroles around the central methene carbon (*). (From Bonnett R, Davies JE, Hursthouse MB: The structure of bilirubin. Nature 1976; 262:326. Reprinted by permission from *Nature*. Copyright © MacMillan Magazines Ltd.)

Isomers of Bilirubin

The asymmetry of the molecule, which determines bilirubin's peculiar physical chemistry, is caused by the specificity of heme oxygenase for cleaving heme (IX ferroprotoporphyrin) at the α-methyne linkage; this cleavage results in the production of only bilirubin IXα (see section on bilirubin synthesis).[9–12] Nonenzymatic cleavage of the β-, γ-, and δ-sites results in the production of trace amounts of the IXβ, γ, and δ bilirubin isomers.[13–15] Acid-catalyzed cleavage of the central methene bridge of bilirubin IXα and scrambling of the dissimilar dipyrrole halves can result in the formation of three α-isomers: bilirubin III, IX, and XIIIα.[16, 17] Trace quantities of all of these isomers of bilirubin can be found in bile.[15] The isomers of bilirubin that are formed during phototherapy are discussed in the section on this therapeutic technique.

Conjugated Bilirubin

The conjugation of bilirubin occurs at the C8 and C12 propionic acid carboxyl groups by the enzymatic formation of ester bonds, usually with a glycoside moiety. Glucuronide esters are the most common conjugates of bilirubin in humans.[18, 19] Conjugation abolishes internal hydrogen bonding by consuming one or both of the carboxyl groups and by introducing a bulky glycoside moiety that prevents the bilirubin molecule from folding on itself. As a consequence, conjugated bilirubin is much more water-soluble and more easily filtered by the kidney than bilirubin.[20] For this reason, urinalysis can be used to define the nature of bilirubin in blood. When a tube of urine obtained from a baby with unconjugated hyperbilirubinemia is shaken, the foam at the top is white. It turns yellow if small amounts of conjugated bilirubin are present in the urine. Thus, a positive "shake test" result suggests the presence of conjugated hyperbilirubinemia.

Bilirubin Covalently Bound to Albumin

Newer methods of measuring bilirubin in serum have resulted in the discovery of *delta bilirubin* or *biliprotein*, a fraction of serum bilirubin that is covalently bound to albumin (see section on measurement of bilirubin).[21–24] This fraction may account for a large proportion of the total bilirubin in patients with cholestatic jaundice, but it is absent in patients with unconjugated hyperbilirubinemia.[25, 26] This complex is formed in plasma by a nonenzymatic process that involves acyl migration of bilirubin from its glucuronide ester with the formation of an amide linkage between one propionic acid side chain and a lysine residue of plasma albumin.[27]

Measurement of Bilirubin in Serum

The diazo reaction is the basis for most clinical determinations of bilirubin. This reaction, which was discovered by Ehrlich in 1883 and fully described by van den Bergh in 1916,[1] involves the hydrolysis of bilirubin at the central methene bridge and the subsequent reaction of one dipyrrole with the diazonium to form an azo-dipyrrole. The second dipyrrole combines with the complementary half of another previously hydrolyzed bilirubin molecule to form bilirubin, which can react further. In stepwise fashion, all available bilirubin is converted to azo-dipyrroles, which are red and have an absorption maximum at 530 to 540 nm.[1, 28] The procedure calls for the dilution of serum with water and the addition of a diazotizing agent, usually diazo-sulfanilic acid. Some of the bilirubin, the *direct-reacting* fraction, reacts immediately with the diazotizing agent. The remainder does not react until an *accelerator*—usually alcohol or caffeine—is added, causing a conformational change in albumin that displaces bilirubin. In the presence of an accelerator, all serum bilirubin reacts, yielding the *total bilirubin value*. The total bilirubin value minus the direct-reacting bilirubin value is the *indirect-reacting bilirubin value*.

The measurement of total bilirubin by the van den Bergh reaction is very reproducible, but the determination of the direct-reacting bilirubin is not reproducible because of its dependence on the conditions of the assay and on time.[29] The direct-reacting fraction constitutes all bilirubin conjugates as well as delta bilirubin. A portion of unconjugated bilirubin also reacts; this reaction confounds the interpretation of results, particularly in patients with high levels of unconjugated bilirubin. The higher the total bilirubin level—even if it consists of only unconjugated bilirubin—the higher the direct-reacting bilirubin level; a useful rule of thumb is that a direct-reacting bilirubin value less than 10% of the total value is within the normal error of the test. Despite this problem, determination of direct-reacting bilirubin is still a standard clinical test in many hospitals. A value greater than 1 mg/dL or more than 10% of a total bilirubin level of above 10 mg/dL is considered abnormal. The presence of bilirubin covalently bound to albumin (delta bilirubin) presents another problem with interpretation; the concentration of the direct-reacting fraction remains high for a period equal to the life of circulating serum albumin, even if the level of conjugated bilirubin decreases to normal. Thus, after relief of extrahepatic bile duct obstruction, the direct-reacting bilirubin level remains increased even in the absence of conjugated bilirubin.

The introduction of the Kodak Ektachem system resulted in a significant improvement in the clinical measurement of bilirubin.[30] The system uses film technology to effect separation of the various species of bilirubin before they react with the diazotizing agent. It allows for the independent and extremely accurate measurement of total bilirubin, unconjugated bilirubin, and conjugated bilirubin. The quantity of delta bilirubin can also be calculated. The system precisely measures conjugated bilirubin in the physiologic range (less than 0.3 mg/dL), and the conjugated value is not affected by a high total bilirubin concentration. However, it does not permit the separate measurement of bilirubin monoglucuronide and diglucuronide. At present, only complex methods that employ high-performance liquid chromatography of azo-dipyrroles are able to distinguish mono- and diconjugated bilirubins.[31–33]

Some nurseries use the *bilirubinometer* for the measurement of bilirubin. This simple instrument provides an estimate of the serum bilirubin concentration that is based on the direct optical absorbance of bilirubin at 340 nm.[34] Although measurement with the bilirubinometer is simple and rapid, it is unreliable. Many substances in serum interfere with the test because they produce turbidity or have absorbances similar to that of bilirubin. Also, no measure of direct-reacting or conjugated bilirubin is provided by this instrument. The bilirubinometer can be used to follow the course of unconjugated hyperbilirubinemia during therapy if the values it provides are frequently confirmed by the van den Bergh method.

Cutaneous Bilirubinometry

The presence of jaundice correlates with an elevation of serum bilirubin concentration. In the newborn with an elevated unconjugated bilirubin level, icteric skin is generally perceptible at a serum bilirubin level of about 5 mg/dL. In the older child and adult, scleral icterus can be seen with bilirubin levels as low as 2.0 mg/dL. Cutaneous bilirubinometry using reflectance spectroscopy has been used for quantitating jaundice in the newborn.[35, 36] The technique involves the use of a probe that emits light at a wavelength of 465 nm perpendicular to the plane of the skin; the amount of light reflected back into a photodiode array is then measured. The device is placed tightly on a blanched area of skin, usually over the sternum. Because bilirubin absorbs light at this wavelength, the amount of light returning to the photodiode is inversely proportional to the amount of bilirubin in the skin. Cutaneous bilirubinometry is an inaccurate means of measuring serum bilirubin because the relationship between skin reflectance and serum bilirubin is complex. In an individual infant, cutaneous bilirubinometry correlates with serum bilirubin level; thus, the technique can be used to record change over time. The values obtained should be confirmed by serum bilirubin measurement at least once per day.

BILIRUBIN SYNTHESIS, TRANSPORT, AND METABOLISM

Serum concentrations of both bilirubin and its conjugates are determined by the rates of entry of the pigments into the circulation and their rates of removal.[37, 38] In the case of unconjugated bilirubin, two major sources of entry must be considered: new synthesis from heme, and reabsorption from the intestine after biliary excretion (Fig. 4–3).

Virtually all of the circulating bilirubin in the normal adult is derived from new synthesis, whereas a significant proportion of that in the newborn is contributed by the enteric pool.[38, 39] Clearance of bilirubin depends entirely on the liver. The minute amount of conjugated bilirubin in serum of healthy individuals (about 0.1 mg/dL) is evidently regurgitated from hepatocytes.

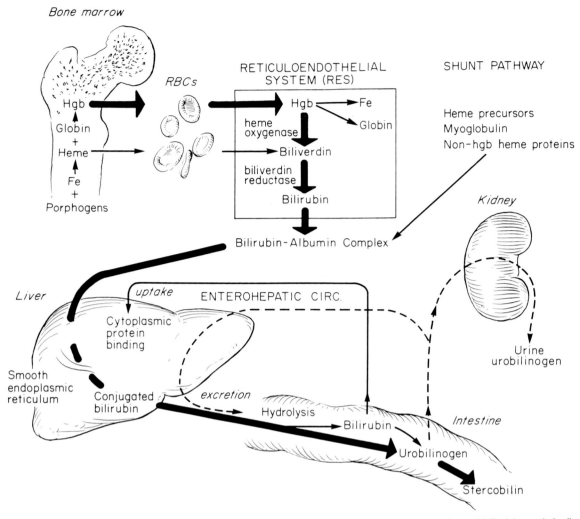

Figure 4–3. Pathways of bilirubin synthesis, transport, and metabolism. (From Gartner LM: Disorders of bilirubin metabolism. In Assali NS (ed): Pathophysiology of Gestation. Vol. III. New York, Academic Press, 1972, p 457.)

In patients with cholestasis, conjugated bilirubin can account for almost all serum bilirubin. Clearance of conjugated bilirubin can be hepatic or renal.[20, 40] In conditions of total hepatic excretory failure, such as total extrahepatic biliary atresia, renal clearance and other poorly understood disposal mechanisms usually maintain conjugated bilirubin concentrations below 20 mg/dL.

Bilirubin Synthesis

The normal adult makes 250 to 350 mg of bilirubin per day (on average, 4.4 mg/kg of body weight per day).[37] Approximately 70% to 80% of new bilirubin is derived from senescent circulating erythrocytes and is formed approximately 120 days after the original synthesis of the heme. The remainder is formed in the degradation of heme from immature erythrocyte precursors and tissue hemeproteins—in particular, hepatic cytochromes, catalase, and tryptophan pyrrolase.[2, 41, 42] The synthesis of bilirubin from these sources follows origi-

nal heme synthesis by only 1 to 5 days and is often referred to as *early-labeled bilirubin production*, as defined by studies in which isotopically labeled heme precursors are administered and bile pigment excretion is monitored over time.[42] Although nearly every tissue is capable of degrading heme to bilirubin, the reticuloendothelial organs, especially the spleen and the liver, are responsible for the majority of bilirubin synthesis.[43]

The conversion of heme to bilirubin requires two enzymatic steps, which may be closely linked. The first step involves heme oxygenase, which can be isolated from the microsomal fractions of macrophages in spleen, bone marrow, liver, and hepatocytes.[12, 44, 45] It functions in complex with reduced nicotinamide adenine dinucleotide phosphate (NADPH)–cytochrome-*c* reductase to remove the α-methyne bridge carbon, which is oxidized to carbon monoxide[46]; as a result, the cyclic tetrapyrrole heme is converted to the linear tetrapyrrole biliverdin, and one molecule of ferrous iron is released.[44, 47] Free hemoporphyrin is cleaved more rapidly than hemoglobin, so it seems that the iron-containing protoporphyrin IX molecule is first removed from the protein moiety before it reacts with heme oxygenase.[45] The process is stereospecific and yields only biliverdin IXα. Molecular oxygen and NADPH are required.

The heme oxygenase reaction is the rate-limiting step in bilirubin synthesis and can be upregulated three- to fivefold in response to hemolysis.[45] Substrate-mediated regulation occurs at the transcriptional level. Similarly, after splenectomy hepatic heme oxygenase activity increases two- to threefold in compensation. Fasting results in increased bilirubin production by temporarily increasing the activity of heme oxygenase.[48, 49] This is thought to be one reason why patients with Gilbert's syndrome exhibit increased serum bilirubin levels after fasting and may contribute to the jaundice observed in infants with pyloric stenosis.[50–52]

The carbon monoxide formed during heme degradation is excreted unchanged by the lung.[53] Although there are other potential endogenous sources of small amounts of carbon monoxide (e.g., lipid peroxidation),[46, 54] quantitative estimation of its excretion offers a reasonably accurate assessment of the rate of heme degradation from all sources and, therefore, of bilirubin synthesis.[55–57]

The second step of bilirubin synthesis involves biliverdin reductase, which is found in the cytosol of most cells. This enzyme catalyzes the conversion of biliverdin to bilirubin by reduction at the central methyne bridge, with NADPH as the hydrogen donor.[58–60] Biliverdin reductase is stereospecific for biliverdin IXα.[61] The three enzymes involved in bilirubin synthesis—heme oxygenase, cytochrome-*c* reductase, and biliverdin reductase—may exist as a ternary complex located at the cytosol–endoplasmic reticulum interface in tissues involved in bilirubin synthesis.[62] Such a configuration may account for the rapidity with which bilirubin is synthesized. Exogenously administered heme first appears in bile as conjugated bilirubin within 2 minutes, whereas administered biliverdin appears in less than 1 minute.[10, 63, 64]

The conversion of biliverdin—a green, water-soluble, and apparently nontoxic pigment—to the water-insoluble and toxic bilirubin seems to confer little biologic advantage.[58] One possible advantage is improvement of placental transport. Heme turnover occurs throughout gestation, and removal of the metabolic end-products is an important placental function. A specific transporter for bilirubin and passive diffusion are apparently important for bilirubin clearance. Biliverdin, with its increased water solubility, would not be cleared as well as bilirubin by the placenta.[65, 66] Bilirubin formation may, therefore, confer to mammals an advantage that is not shared by birds and reptiles, which do not reduce biliverdin to bilirubin.[58] Postnatally, bilirubin synthesis may serve to protect the kidneys and other tissues. If it were filtered in large amounts by a kidney capable of concentrating the urine, biliverdin could "salt out," forming crystals and producing obstruction of renal tubules and collecting ducts.

Bilirubin is an antioxidant that is potentially capable of protecting tissues against peroxidative injury.[67–70] Bilirubin, with its extended system of conjugated double bonds and a reactive hydrogen atom, could function as an important scavenger for peroxyl radicals. Both bilirubin and biliverdin function as effective antioxidants at micromolar concentrations in multilamellar liposomes.[68] This antioxidant activity increases as the oxygen concentration in the system decreases, and at low oxygen tensions bilirubin is more effective than α-tocopherol at suppressing lipid peroxidation.[71] In primary rat hepatocyte culture, bilirubin in solution with albumin has a cytoprotective effect on cells exposed to inducers of free radical stress.[72] This cytoprotection also was demonstrated for human erythrocytes and was significant at physiologic levels of bilirubin (3.4 to 26 μmol/L). Furthermore, an *in vivo* study examining rat liver chemiluminescence demonstrated that induction of heme oxygenase by cobalt chloride increased the level of reactive oxygen species, reduced intrahepatic glutathione content, and markedly decreased the activity of the important antioxidant enzymes superoxide dismutase, catalase, and glutathione peroxidase. Pretreatment of the animals with bilirubin infusion prevented the heme oxygenase induction, attenuated the increase in chemiluminescence, and prevented a decrease in the level of hepatic glutathione.[73] The results of both of these studies strongly suggest that the antioxidant properties of bilirubin are important under physiologic and stress conditions.[74] However, a protective effect has been difficult to demonstrate in human neonates.[75] Increased bilirubin production may, indeed, increase tissue lipid peroxidation.[76] Further work in this area is needed to determine the teleologic role of bilirubin in protecting the newborn animal during its transition to an oxygen-rich environment. Some similar protection may also be conferred by bilirubin excreted in bile into the intestine, which is particularly well endowed with mechanisms for producing oxidative tissue injury.[77, 78]

Bilirubin Transport in Plasma

Unconjugated bilirubin in plasma is tightly bound to albumin.[79] The primary binding site has a binding affinity of 10^8 mol^{-1}.[6, 80–83] A second binding site of somewhat lower affinity also exists, and the presence of a third, and additional, weaker binding sites has been postulated.[82, 84, 85] One gram of albumin can bind 8.3 mg of bilirubin at the primary binding site; thus, a patient with an albumin concentration of 3.5 g/dL can potentially bind 29 mg/dL of plasma. The second binding site could double the theoretic capacity to 58 mg/dL. Diminished albumin concentrations, the presence of substances competing with bilirubin for the same sites, and alterations in the configuration of albumin that diminish the affinity of the binding sites can reduce the binding capacity and affinity. Conjugates of bilirubin also are bound to albumin in serum, with less than 1% existing in their free form; however, the binding affinity for these conjugates is much less than that for bilirubin.[83]

Studies in analbuminemic rats have demonstrated

that plasma lipoproteins can serve as important carriers for bilirubin.[86-89] Serum bilirubin in analbuminemic rats is bound to a lipoprotein fraction; this binding effectively protects the animals from brain injury. Furthermore, exogenously administered bilirubin is transported to the liver, where uptake is undisturbed by the absence of albumin.[88] It is interesting that about 40% of bilirubin in hyperbilirubinemic Gunn rats, which have normal serum albumin, is bound to a similar protein fraction.[87] These data suggest that plasma lipoproteins have an important role in bilirubin transport, at least in the presence of low albumin or high bilirubin concentrations.

The binding capacity and affinity of albumin for bilirubin have been measured for both investigative and clinical purposes with a variety of techniques, including competitive dye binding, spectral characterization, assessment of binding of pigment to alternate artificial and natural ligands, fluorescence of bound bilirubin, quenching of albumin fluorescence, and enzymatic measurement of free or unbound bilirubin. Although these techniques have been used for almost 20 years, much uncertainty still remains about the interpretation of results in light of theories of binding, and even greater uncertainty surrounds the application of these techniques to clinical evaluation or prediction of toxicity. The concepts and methodology of determining binding capacity, constraints in interpreting results, and relationships of binding to bilirubin toxicity have been reviewed in detail elsewhere.[90-94]

Hepatic Uptake of Bilirubin

The liver is uniquely structured for the uptake of protein-bound metabolites from plasma. The hepatocyte has no basement membrane; its plasma membrane is separated from the blood within the hepatic sinusoids only by vascular endothelial cells that contain fenestrae large enough to permit access of plasma proteins to the perihepatocytic space (space of Disse). Furthermore, the hepatic cord structure permits contact with plasma by a large portion of the surface of each hepatocyte. Hepatic uptake of albumin-bound bilirubin is efficient and, under normal conditions, works at far less than capacity.[95-97] Even with extremely high rates of bilirubin production, hepatic uptake is probably not limiting to bilirubin clearance.

Bilirubin enters the hepatocyte from plasma by means of a non–energy-dependent process facilitated by a membrane transport protein; this process also is involved in the transport of several organic anions.[98-105] A variety of candidate organic anion transport proteins have been isolated.[105] In the rat, a 55-kd organic anion binding protein has been determined to be important in bilirubin uptake. Its function can be inhibited by an antibody to the purified protein.[100] Uptake is not enhanced or reduced by the binding of bilirubin to albumin; this supports the conclusion that the membrane receptor has an *in vivo* affinity that allows it to readily extract bilirubin from albumin.[106]

After uptake, bilirubin briefly accumulates in the cytosol of the hepatocyte. It is mainly bound to *ligandin*

or *Y protein*, a 47-kd basic protein that accounts for 10% of all liver cytoplasmic protein and that also is found in kidney and small intestinal mucosa. It can efficiently bind bilirubin, as well as a number of other organic anions.[107] It also possesses an enzymatic activity, glutathione s-transferase.[108, 109] The ligandin molecule consists of two subunits; one is required for binding of organic anions, and both are required for its enzymatic activity. A second smaller (12-kd) cytoplasmic protein designated as *Z protein* also binds bilirubin, although with less affinity than ligandin.[107, 110] Z protein is identical to fatty acid–binding protein of intestinal mucosa and liver.[111] Its major function appears to be the intracellular binding and trafficking of fatty acids, and its role in bilirubin metabolism is unclear.

Considerable data indicate that bilirubin flux across the hepatocyte basolateral membrane is bidirectional.[112] It has been estimated that in normal people up to 40% of bilirubin taken up by hepatocytes refluxes unchanged back into plasma. Ligandin appears not to be directly involved in bilirubin uptake, but it does limit the amount of reflux back into plasma. Although the binding affinity of ligandin for bilirubin is less than that of albumin, the total binding capacity of ligandin permits sufficient retention of bilirubin to make its overall uptake efficient. Induction of increased levels of ligandin, as occurs with the administration of phenobarbital and with thyroidectomy, increases the overall efficiency of bilirubin uptake. Decreased levels of ligandin correlate with a reduction in uptake in newborn monkeys.[113]

The current model of bilirubin uptake suggests that the rate-limiting event is its delivery to the sinusoidal membrane.[114] With increasing concentrations of bilirubin in plasma, the rate of bilirubin uptake by the liver increases; however, this process may be saturable in the presence of extremely high levels of bilirubin. The normal low level of serum bilirubin results from inefficient delivery at low concentrations and from reflux from hepatocytes. Chronic hemolytic states lead to increased synthesis and delivery of bilirubin to the liver and result in increases in uptake. An incremental increase in serum bilirubin level is seen with any major increase in production because of relatively inefficient delivery and increased reflux.

Bilirubin Conjugation

The conjugation process that results in the formation of bilirubin mono- and diglucuronide accounts for the disposal of essentially all bilirubin.[19] Small amounts are converted to water-soluble substances by conjugation with substances other than glucuronic acid,[18] and trivial amounts by other hepatic biotransformation reactions.[115-120] Bilirubin uridine diphosphate (UDP)–glucuronosyltransferase (bilirubin UGT) catalyzes the transfer of glucuronic acid from uridine diphosphoglucuronic acid (UDPGA) to form glucuronide esters at the C8 and C12 carboxyl groups of bilirubin.[121] UDPGA is derived from glucose and is synthesized from uridine diphosphoglucose by the soluble cytoplasmic enzyme uridine diphosphoglucose dehydrogenase. The products of the reaction are bilirubin monoglucuronide (BMG) and bilirubin diglucuronine (BDG).[122-124] Recent work has demonstrated the presence of β-glucuronidase within the endoplasmic reticulum and has provided evidence that it functions to deconjugate BDG and BMG. The resultant bilirubin can be reconjugated or can efflux from the endoplasmic reticulum.[125] The regulatory role that this reaction has is unknown.

Within the hepatocyte, bilirubin must be delivered to the endoplasmic reticulum, the site of conjugation. Ligandin may play a role in the intracellular trafficking of bilirubin, but growing evidence suggests that intracellular membranes primarily serve this function. Recent evidence suggests that the unique physical chemistry of bilirubin, which is neither water nor lipid soluble, causes it to adsorb to—rather than be solubilized in—the phospholipid bilayers of intracellular organelles.[126-128] Transfer of bilirubin molecules from donor lipid vesicles to acceptor vesicles occurs at very rapid rates (transfer being complete within 20 ms).[129] Also, the rate of glucuronidation by microsomal vesicles *in vitro* is enhanced by the delivery of bilirubin bound to phospholipid vesicles.[130] At present, the relative contributions of ligandin and membrane-to-membrane transfer to the transport of bilirubin from the plasma membrane to the endoplasmic reticulum is not known.

The cloning of the rat and human bilirubin UGT genes has resulted in major advances in the understanding of the function of this enzyme and the molecular genetics of disorders in which it is deficient (Crigler-Najjar syndrome, the Gunn rat; see section on disorders of hepatic bilirubin metabolism).[131-144] Data continue to indicate that bilirubin UGT is a member of a multigene family encoding for various UGTs that are more or less homologous and that have selective or overlapping substrate specificities.[145-150] Two isoforms of human bilirubin UGT (bilirubin UGT1A1 and UGT2B) that share a common functionally important 3' region with phenol-UGT (which functions in conjugating menthol) have been identified, but each has a unique functionally important 5' region. Two genetic defects in patients with Crigler-Najjar syndrome type 1—one a substitution resulting in a serine-to-phenylalanine change, and the other a substitution producing a premature stop codon—are in the common region and result in the production of defective bilirubin UGT and phenol-UGT.[142, 151-155] The bilirubin UGT complementary deoxyribonucleic acids (cDNAs) of several patients have been expressed in a bilirubin UGT–deficient cell line, and all resulted in the complete absence of active bilirubin UGT.[156] Two other affected individuals have been found to have defects in the unique 5' region of bilirubin UGT1A1. If both bilirubin UGT1A1 and bilirubin UGT2B function to conjugate bilirubin, these patients should not have been severely affected, but they were. Again, cDNAs were expressed in a bilirubin UGT–deficient cell line, demonstrating that only bilirubin UGT1A1 is active *in vivo* in the conjugation of bilirubin.[157]

Bilirubin UGT appears to be relatively selective for bilirubin and BMG as substrates.[158] Evidence suggests that the enzyme exists as a tetramer, with one subunit being required for the conjugation of bilirubin and all four for the further conjugation of BMG to BDG.[159] It is an integral membrane protein, and its activity is abolished by its removal from membranes.[160, 161] Latency experiments have demonstrated the functional moiety to be inside of the endoplasmic reticulum.[162] Sequencing data suggest that it is anchored in the membrane by a C-terminal hydrophobic domain and that most of the enzyme resides within the lumen of the endoplasmic reticulum.[134, 136] Although this enzyme is predominantly hepatic, it has been detected in the kidney, stomach, small bowel, colon, and skin.[163-166]

The total capacity of bilirubin UGT to form BMG has been estimated to be 100-fold greater than the normal load of bilirubin presented to the liver for disposal; thus, it does not work at saturation for bilirubin.[167] Bilirubin UGT catalyzes the formation of BMG nonpreferentially at either the C8 or the C12 position.[168, 169] The same active site catalyzes the formation of BDG from BMG.[168] The enzyme has a greater affinity for bilirubin ($K_m \approx 1$ μmol/L) than for BMG ($K_m \approx 10$ μmol/L).[118, 170, 171] Its affinity for UDPGA is lower ($K_m \approx 200$ to 600 μmol/L). Bilirubin UGT appears to function at below saturation for UDPGA, which is present in liver tissue at a concentration of 0.6 to 1.2 mmol/L.[169-172] This may explain why bilirubin conjugation is sensitive to factors that affect UDPGA concentration in the liver. Factors (e.g., ethanol intake) that affect the redox state of the hepatocyte toward NADH (a potent inhibitor of uridine diphosphoglucose dehydrogenase) reduce bilirubin UGT activity.[159] Also, depletion of UDPGA resulting from the administration of xenobiotics requiring glucuronidation can affect the conjugation of bilirubin.[170, 173] Reduced UDPGA formation probably contributes to hyperbilirubinemia in infants of diabetic mothers. As mentioned earlier, fasting decreases UDPGA concentration, and this may contribute to fasting hyperbilirubinemia observed in Gilbert's syndrome.[159]

For conjugation to occur, bilirubin and UDPGA must gain access to bilirubin UGT, which is located within the endoplasmic reticulum.[174, 175] How bilirubin gains access is unknown. It may simply partition into the membrane; however, this seems unlikely given the current understanding of the interaction of bilirubin with lipid bilayers. Nevertheless, the facts that delivery of bilirubin adsorbed to phospholipid vesicles increases the rate of conjugation and that conjugation occurs at either carboxyl group suggest the importance of membrane transport.[129, 130] A specific transport protein has not been identified, and the predicted structure of bilirubin UGT does not suggest the presence of a membrane pore.[176] Although a mechanism for bilirubin transport has not been identified, a specific transporter for UDPGA has.[177, 178] Another cytosolic sugar nucleotide, UDP-*N*-acetylglucosamine, greatly enhances conjugation, probably by means of allosteric interaction with bilirubin UGT that greatly increases its affinity for UDPGA.[179] Divalent cations may also have a role in the regulation of bilirubin UGT activity.[180]

Two patterns of UGT development have been demonstrated: a fetal pattern that results in adult levels of UGT activity at birth, and an adult pattern in which adult activity is reached a few weeks after birth.[181–184] Bilirubin UGT belongs to the group demonstrating the adult pattern of development.[185, 186] Bilirubin UGT activity at 17 to 30 weeks of gestation is about 0.1% of adult levels, and at 30 to 40 weeks of gestation is about 1% of adult values. Adult values are reached by about 14 weeks after birth. This accelerated development appears to be initiated by birth itself. It follows premature birth without delay, and postmaturity delays its onset.[182, 185, 187] Ultimately, female rats have greater bilirubin UGT activity than do male rats,[188] and women have lower serum bilirubin concentrations than do men; these findings suggest that sex hormones influence development.

At least two additional carbohydrate conjugates of bilirubin—a glucoside and a xyloside—can also be found in small amounts in human bile.[18] Other species, particularly the dog, produce much larger proportions of nonglucuronide conjugates and have a mixed glucuronide-glucoside diester as the predominant conjugate in bile.[189] Apparently, only one transferase enzyme mediates the formation of all of these conjugates,[158] and there is some debate regarding why bilirubin is selectively conjugated with glucuronic acid in man. One theory postulates that the limited entry of water-soluble UDP-glycosides into the smooth endoplasmic reticulum involves a transport mechanism that is substrate specific.[162, 177, 178, 190] Other potential substrates for the transferase enzyme are not transported into the smooth endoplasmic reticulum and are available to the transferase enzyme only in trace amounts as a result of nonspecific leakage. Opponents of this theory suggest there is a different enzyme affinity for each of the various UDP-glycosides,[172, 191, 192] but there is evidence to the contrary.[122, 193] The increased proportion of nonglucuronide conjugates in the bile of fetuses can be explained by either theory—developmentally reduced specificity of either the transporter or bilirubin UGT. Differences in the lipid microenvironment in which bilirubin UGT functions is thought to have some effect on substrate specificity.[126, 194–198] Changes in microsomal microviscosity that occur in fetal and early postnatal development[199] may explain the patterns of bilirubin conjugation that favor conjugation with xylose and glucose in the fetus and newborn.[33, 200, 201]

Although BMG is water soluble and capable of being excreted into bile without further alteration by the hepatocyte, 80% of bilirubin is excreted in normal adults as BDG.[18, 19] In the neonate and in conditions associated with reduced transferase activity, such as Gilbert's syndrome, BMG is the predominant bile pigment.[18, 19, 202–204] A direct correlation exists between the relative amounts of BDG and BMG in bile and the level of bilirubin UGT activity.[205, 206] Because the glucuronide esters are formed sequentially (not simultaneously) and because the affinity of bilirubin UGT for bilirubin is greater than that for BMG, BMG is the predominant product as the system approaches the maximum rate of conjugation (saturation kinetics). In severe hemolysis, a shift toward the excretion of BMG may occur.[207]

Bilirubin Excretion

Hepatic excretion into bile rapidly follows conjugation—so rapidly, in fact, that BDG cannot be recovered from the liver even after bilirubin loading. Furthermore, excretion proceeds against a large concentration gradient, as biliary bilirubin concentrations are 40 times greater than in serum and 100 times greater than in liver cytoplasm.[208, 209] Excretion involves two steps: the movement of bilirubin conjugates from the endoplasmic reticulum to the canalicular membrane, and their translocation across the membrane into canalicular bile.

Little is known about the movement of bilirubin conjugates within the hepatocyte. Obviously, some system directs the movement toward the canalicular domain because very little of the conjugates refluxes into serum. Evidence is mounting that the vectoring is accomplished by means of a microtubule-dependent membrane translocation mechanism.[63, 64, 210, 211] Bilirubin excretion is somewhat dependent on the rates of bile salt and biliary lipid excretion, which are dependent on the hepatocyte microtubular system.[212–216] Xenobiotics that interfere with lipid excretion reduce bilirubin excretion as well.[217–219] These findings have been interpreted as reflecting either a primary dependence of bilirubin excretion on the microtubular system or its association with lipids destined for excretion.[220–224] Binding to cytosolic proteins may also occur, but the role of these proteins in intracellular transport is not known.

Canalicular excretion appears to be a carrier-mediated, adenosine triphosphate–dependent process that transports a variety of endogenous and exogenous organic anions.[225–228] Evidence supports the existence of a family of carriers with overlapping substrate specificity for organic anions and that bilirubin transport is stimulated by the bicarbonate ion.[229] Patients with Dubin-Johnson syndrome, for example, have defective excretion of bilirubin but normal excretion of conjugated bromosulfophthalein. Vesicular translocation may also have a role in bilirubin excretion.

Bilirubin excretion is dependent to a degree on bile formation; thus, significant reductions in bile salt excretion and bile flow reduce bilirubin excretory capacity,[230–232] but bilirubin is in no way responsible for bile formation. Even though relatively soluble, bilirubin conjugates do not remain monomeric in bile but rather form dimers or highly aggregated multimers or enter mixed biliary micelles.[7, 233] Therefore, even at very high concentrations, bilirubin in bile exerts a minimal osmotic effect.

Excretion is considered to be the rate-limiting step of overall bilirubin clearance from plasma. In situations of markedly increased bilirubin production, the retention of bilirubin conjugates is a reflection of this normal physiologic limitation.[208] It is not unusual to observe moderate elevations of conjugated bilirubin (usually less than 2 mg/dL) during periods of brisk hemolysis, such as in Rh incompatibility. This should not raise concerns that liver disease is present. Severe or chronic hemolysis can result in combined conjugated and unconjugated hyperbilirubinemia. The unconjugated fraction may result from inefficient uptake and retention by hepatocytes or from intracellular deconjugation. Microsomal β-glucuronidase is possibly responsible for this phenomenon as well as the appearance of BMG as a small proportion of bile pigment.

Elevated serum concentration of conjugated bilirubin usually indicates hepatic excretory dysfunction or cholestasis. Cholestasis is defined as a reduction in bile formation or flow and results in the retention of the constituents of bile, including conjugated bilirubin, bile acids, cholesterol, and phospholipid.[234, 235] The liver of the newborn is capable of only limited response to injury, and cholestasis can result from a variety of hepatobiliary diseases and the effects of systemic diseases on the liver (see section on conjugated hyperbilirubinemia in the newborn).[236] Thus, conjugated hyperbilirubinemia is a common sign of a wide range of diseases in newborns.

Enterohepatic Circulation of Bilirubin

Although hepatic excretion is often viewed as the final event in the disposal of bilirubin, events occurring within the intestine and enterohepatic circulation significantly influence serum bilirubin concentrations, particularly in the newborn.[39, 84, 237] Bilirubin conjugates are relatively unstable ester glucuronides and are readily hydrolyzed to unconjugated bilirubin within the intestinal lumen. Beta-glucuronidase is the enzyme responsible for enzymatic deconjugation of bilirubin ester glucuronides. Mucosal β-glucuronidase is plentiful in fetal intestinal mucosa and persists in the newborn, whereas bacterial β-glucuronidase level increases with the establishment of the enteric microflora.[238] Nonenzymatic hydrolysis may also occur in the alkaline environment of the neonate's upper intestine. Once hydrolysis occurs, bilirubin can be reabsorbed across the intestinal mucosa, probably through passive mech-

anisms,[239] to return to the liver via the portal circulation.

Bilirubin reaching the distal bowel is converted to a series of urobilinoids by a hydroxylation-reduction process performed by intestinal bacteria, primarily *Clostridium perfringens* and *Escherichia coli*.[240–242] Urobilinoids include urobilins, urobilinogens, stercobilinogens, and stercobilin; each of these substances is produced at sequential steps in the reduction process. Urobilinoid formation occurs in the distal intestinal tract, primarily in the colon, except in the presence of purulent infection of the upper intestine. Urobilinoids formed in the intestine are partially absorbed and enter an enterohepatic recirculation. A small portion is excreted in the urine, forming the basis of a clinical test for the differential diagnosis of cholestasis. Complete obstruction of the flow of bile into the intestine, such as in the presence of a common duct stone, results in the complete absence of urobilinoids in urine. Patients with cellular cholestasis, in contrast, usually have elevated urine urobilinogen concentrations. The bilirubin passing into the intestine, even though it enters in reduced amounts, results in urobilinogen formation and absorption. However, because cholestasis exists, hepatic clearance is reduced, and excess urobilinogen is excreted into the urine. This test is not reliable in the neonate because the intestinal microflora may not yet be established.

DEVELOPMENTAL ASPECTS OF BILIRUBIN METABOLISM AND TRANSPORT

Normal human newborns regularly develop elevated serum unconjugated bilirubin concentrations during the first 1 to 2 weeks of life (Fig. 4–4). This pattern of hyperbilirubinemia, known as *physiologic jaundice of the newborn*, results from a complex interaction among several normal, developmentally determined disturbances in bilirubin metabolism and transport. Many of the mechanisms of bile formation are defective in the newborn of several species. This so-called *physiologic chole-*

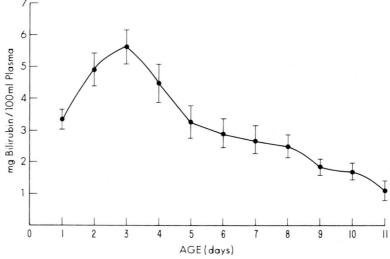

Figure 4–4. Mean total serum bilirubin concentrations from 29 normal-term human infants on days 1 through 11 after birth. *Vertical bars* illustrate one standard error of the mean. (From Gartner LM, Lee KS, et al: Development of bilirubin transport and metabolism in the newborn rhesus monkey. J Pediatr 1977; 90:513.)

stasis results in increased serum bile acid concentrations but does not contribute to physiologic jaundice. Physiologic jaundice results from the presentation of an increased load of bilirubin to an immature liver. The increased load results from increased synthesis and an overactive enterohepatic recirculation of bilirubin.

Bilirubin synthesis is normally increased in neonates. The technique most frequently utilized for indirect estimation of heme degradation in the newborn, carbon monoxide production, indicates that heme degradation and bilirubin formation are increased significantly.[57, 237, 243–245] The erythrocyte life span is diminished in the newborn (70 to 90 days in the neonate versus 120 days in the adult)[246, 247] and may be even briefer in the premature infant. In addition, in both mature and immature neonates, large pools of erythrocyte precursors that exist within the bone marrow, liver, and spleen may also contribute to excessive bilirubin production.

Direct measurement of bilirubin excretion in the bile of newborn rhesus monkeys has shown that the total load of bilirubin presented to the liver for excretion is at least fivefold greater in the neonate during the first 6 weeks of life than it is in older monkeys.[167] Diversion of bile away from the intestine in newborn rhesus monkeys has shown that nearly all of the increased bilirubin load after the first week of life is derived from intestinal reabsorption. Enteric bilirubin absorption also has a key role in physiologic jaundice of the human neonate. Evidence to this is the observation that oral administration of nonabsorbable substances that bind bilirubin, such as agar and activated charcoal, results in a significant reduction in peak serum bilirubin concentrations.[39, 248] Increased bilirubin absorption in the newborn probably results from the deconjugation of conjugated bilirubin by the action of mucosal β-glucuronidase. Studies in animals suggest that the colon may also serve as an effective site for bilirubin absorption if sufficient unconjugated bile pigment is present and the bacterial flora is minimal, as it may be in the newborn. Meconium is another source of bilirubin to be absorbed[249]; the amount of unconjugated bilirubin in meconium is estimated to be 80 to 180 mg, or 5- to 10-fold the normal amount of bilirubin produced in a day.[84] Unconjugated bilirubin absorbed from the bowel becomes a portion of the total bilirubin load that the liver must handle. No evidence suggests that increased enterohepatic recirculation of bilirubin is a major cause of the increase in physiologic jaundice of premature infants.

A somewhat limited capacity for bilirubin clearance also probably contributes to physiologic jaundice.[167, 185, 250, 251] A mature liver would handle the increased load with only slight elevation of serum bilirubin. In the full-term rhesus monkey, hepatic bilirubin UGT activity during the first 24 hours of life is approximately 5% of normal adult values, but it doubles by 24 hours of age. Peak serum bilirubin concentrations in the newborn monkey are reached at 24 hours and decline thereafter, coincident with the increase in transferase activity. Studies of autopsy material from aborted human fetuses, from infants, and from children have yielded similar information. Early in fetal development, there is a quantitative defect in bilirubin conjugation and a lack of specificity for conjugation with glucuronide. At 20 to 24 weeks of gestation, enzyme activity increases, and glucuronide monoconjugates appear in bile. At term, enzyme activity is 1% of adult activity, and BMG is the predominant bile pigment. Although this degree of reduction in conjugating capacity is not sufficient by itself to cause retention of bilirubin, the simultaneous sixfold increase in bilirubin load is sufficient to produce the observed increase in serum bilirubin.[167] As soon as bilirubin UGT activity increases sufficiently to accommodate the bilirubin load, the serum bilirubin concentration decreases. This occurs in the newborn monkey by 24 hours and in the human neonate by 72 to 96 hours.

Events that alter bilirubin UGT activity have an effect on physiologic jaundice. Prepartum induction of bilirubin UGT activity by the administration of phenobarbital to the mother in the last 2 weeks of gestation can eliminate physiologic jaundice in the newborn monkey. Administration of phenobarbital to pregnant women similarly reduces the severity of physiologic jaundice.[252, 253] In premature infants, delayed maturation of bilirubin UGT results in exaggerated physiologic jaundice.[167] In a rat model, this coincides with a reduction in the mass of endoplasmic reticulum.[187] Phenobarbital has little or no effect on serum bilirubin concentrations when it is administered to premature monkeys or to human premature neonates and is of little value in clinical management of the jaundiced premature infant.

A relatively stable but elevated serum unconjugated bilirubin concentration of approximately 2 mg/dL often persists for a time after jaundice has abated, normally until 12 to 14 days of life. In the premature infant, hyperbilirubinemia may persist for 4 or 5 weeks. The reasons for this are poorly understood, but evidence from the rhesus monkey indicates that it results from the simultaneous occurrence of defective hepatic uptake and a continued increased bilirubin load, primarily from enteric bilirubin absorption.[39, 167] Defective uptake may result from a developmental delay in production of ligandin, with increased reflux of bilirubin from hepatocytes,[113] or theoretically from a defect in the hepatocyte plasma membrane receptor for bilirubin. The uptake defect in the newborn is only relative, and an increased bilirubin load causes increased uptake, as it does in the adult. Bilirubin UGT has no role in this prolongation of hyperbilirubinemia because its activity matures earlier in life.

Fetal serum bilirubin is maintained at a low level (less than 2.0 mg/dL) exclusively by placental clearance, even though fetal hepatic bilirubin metabolism and excretion are established early in gestation. Placental transfer of unconjugated bilirubin results from active transport and passive diffusion.[65, 66] In the normal situation, there is a chemical gradient for bilirubin from fetus to mother, and bilirubin movement is favored by the higher albumin concentration in maternal plasma and the greater binding affinity of albumin relative to α-fetoprotein.[254, 255] In the rare circumstance that a mother has an elevated unconjugated bilirubin concentration, the fetus may exhibit a similar elevation.[84] Even in situations of markedly increased fetal bilirubin production, such as in Rh isoimmune hemolysis, fetal serum bilirubin concentrations rarely exceed 5 to 7 mg/dL; this explains the frequent absence of jaundice at birth in such babies. Immediately following cord clamping and placental clearance, serum bilirubin concentrations in these neonates rise rapidly, and clinical jaundice may be seen within 30 minutes after delivery. In contrast, fetal cholestatic liver diseases that cause retention of conjugated bilirubin are associated with jaundice at birth. The placenta is relatively impermeable to bilirubin conjugates because of their water solubility.[256] Cord serum direct-reacting bilirubin concentrations often exceed 7 mg/dL and at times are as high as 20 mg/dL. The presence of delta bilirubin in cord blood indicates prolongation of fetal cholestasis.

GENERAL CONCEPTS OF DISORDERED BILIRUBIN METABOLISM AND TRANSPORT IN THE NEWBORN

The processes that cause physiologic jaundice are present in virtually every neonate, so diseases that alter bilirubin metabolism must be diagnosed while superimposed on this background.[84, 237, 257] A difficult problem facing a clinician caring for a jaundiced newborn is distinguishing between simple physiologic jaundice and jaundice that is a manifestation of an additional pathologic process. In most infants, a superimposed disease such as hemolysis results in a serum bilirubin concentration above that expected in the normal newborn. Figure 4–5 provides guidelines regarding serum bilirubin and postpartum age that can be consulted in decision-making concerning the need for further evaluation. Sometimes, however, knowledge of serum bilirubin concentration alone does not permit differentiation between normal physiologic hyperbilirubinemia and pathologic conditions. The premature infant normally has a higher peak serum bilirubin level because of physiologic immaturity, but such an infant also exhibits hyperbilirubinemia more often as the result of pathologic conditions.[258] As a result, it is always wise to consider the possibility of a superimposed disease in premature infants with jaundice.

Elevated concentrations of conjugated or direct-reacting bilirubin always indicate disease and must be evaluated (see section on conjugated hyperbilirubinemia). In some hospitals, direct-reacting or conjugated fractions are not routinely determined when a serum bilirubin concentration is requested, particularly in a newborn. It should be standard practice to perform a measurement of the direct-reacting fraction at least every 1 to 2 days during the period of clinical jaundice. Examination of the urine visually and by dipstick also helps detect infants with cholestasis. In addition, direct-reacting bilirubin concentrations should always be determined prior to initiation of phototherapy because the infant with hepatocellular disease may develop the "bronze baby syndrome" when exposed to therapeutic

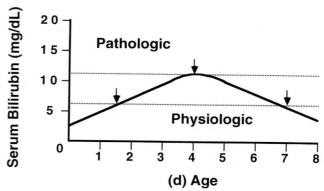

Figure 4–5. Defining pathologic jaundice. Infants whose total serum bilirubin level falls above the curve cannot be considered to have physiologic jaundice and deserve evaluation. The arrows indicate three points that deserve particular consideration. The *left arrow* indicates early jaundice; infants who are visibly jaundiced (having a serum bilirubin concentration of about 7 mg/dL *(lower broken line)*) at or before 36 hours of age probably have increased bilirubin production and should be evaluated for hemolysis. The *middle arrow* indicates exaggerated hyperbilirubinemia; infants with serum bilirubin concentrations above 12 mg/dL *(upper broken line)* require diagnostic study to determine the cause, as well as close monitoring to ensure that any further increase does not result in toxic levels (about 15 mg/dL in the healthy premature neonate, and approximately 20 mg/dL in the full-term neonate). These infants may have increased bilirubin production, reduced clearance, or increased enterohepatic circulation. The *right arrow* indicates prolonged jaundice; infants who are jaundiced for longer than 1 week probably have reduced clearance (hypothyroidism, hereditary hyperbilirubinemia) or increased enterohepatic circulation (breast-feeding). Any conjugated bilirubin level above 1 mg/dL or direct bilirubin level above 1 mg/dL, or 10% of the total bilirubin level, indicates possible hepatic dysfunction. (Adapted from Odell GB: Neonatal Hyperbilirubinemia. New York, Grune & Stratton, 1980, p 36.)

light.[259, 260] This is more fully discussed in the section on management of neonatal hyperbilirubinemia.

SPECIFIC DISEASES ASSOCIATED WITH UNCONJUGATED HYPERBILIRUBINEMIA OF THE NEWBORN
Hemolytic Disorders and Increased Bilirubin Production

The specific conditions causing increased erythrocyte destruction have been discussed in detail in the preceding chapter. In nearly all newborn infants with hemolytic disease, a major manifestation in addition to anemia is jaundice. Even mildly increased rates of hemolysis that may not cause anemia can lead to substantial increases in serum bilirubin levels, reflecting the delicate balance in the newborn between bilirubin load and hepatic clearance.[257]

Rh Isoimmune Hemolysis (Erythroblastosis Fetalis)

The most severe degrees of hyperbilirubinemia are seen in erythroblastosis[261] (see Chapter 3). Affected infants develop jaundice within the first few hours of life, and serum bilirubin concentrations routinely exceed safe limits within 48 hours. The magnitude of the peak serum bilirubin concentration may be crudely predicted from cord hemoglobin and bilirubin concentrations and reticulocyte and nucleated red blood cell counts, as well as from amniotic fluid bilirubin concentrations measured as the optical density at 450 nm.[262] These parameters also give an indication of anticipated need for exchange transfusion. Exceptions to these indications result from individual variations in infants' abilities to handle bilirubin loads.

Conjugated hyperbilirubinemia is occasionally observed in Rh erythroblastosis, particularly when intrauterine transfusions have effectively supported an infant with otherwise fatal intrauterine hemolysis.[207] This may be the result of exceeding the hepatic excretory capacity. However, true cholestasis may also result from hepatic congestion from extramedullary erythropoiesis and heart failure, or tissue hypoxia resulting from reduced hepatic blood flow and anemia.[263, 264] The development of secondary complications, including bacterial sepsis, biliary obstruction, and hepatic failure, can also contribute to cholestasis in infants with erythroblastosis fetalis.[261]

Infants with severe hyperbilirubinemia in association with Rh erythroblastosis appear to have a greater risk for bilirubin encephalopathy (kernicterus) than do infants with an equally high serum bilirubin level in the absence of severe hemolysis.[265] Circulating heme pigments or other erythrocyte components may interfere with albumin binding of bilirubin,[266] and complications of severe hemolytic disease such as cerebral hypoxia, acidosis, and infection may interrupt the defenses against bilirubin entry into brain cells[267–269] (see section on bilirubin encephalopathy). Therapy should be initiated at lower serum bilirubin concentrations in infants with Rh hemolysis than in infants with nonhemolytic hyperbilirubinemia.

Phototherapy and exchange transfusions are the major modes of therapy for hyperbilirubinemia in Rh erythroblastosis (see section on treatment of hyperbilirubinemia). With severe disease, exchange transfusions may be performed as emergency procedures almost immediately after delivery, but such transfusions are for treatment of anemia and heart failure, not for hyperbilirubinemia.[261] Theoretically, removal of sensitized red cells prior to their destruction should reduce the degree of hyperbilirubinemia, but indications for exchange transfusion should be based upon the need for immediate resuscitative treatment or the results of specific serum bilirubin concentration determinations. It should be kept in mind that serum bilirubin concentrations can rise extremely rapidly, and that therapy should be instituted in anticipation of the increase. Serum bilirubin concentrations should be determined at 4-hour intervals in infants with Rh erythroblastosis so that the rate of increase can be determined.

ABO Isoimmune Hemolysis (ABO Erythroblastosis)

Hemolysis is generally milder and briefer in ABO hemolytic disease and hyperbilirubinemia less extreme, although it occasionally can be severe.[270–274] Even in the absence of overt anemia, neonates with ABO incompatibility with the mother and a positive result on Coomb's test should be observed carefully, and serum bilirubin concentrations should be determined at the first sign of jaundice. ABO disease rarely causes hyperbilirubinemia beyond the fifth day of life.

Other Hemolytic Disorders

Glucose-6-phosphate dehydrogenase (G6PD) deficiency of erythrocytes is the most common enzyme deficiency of the red cells found to be associated with hyperbilirubinemia.[243, 275–277] African-American neonates with a mild form of disease usually only exhibit normal physiologic jaundice, but they may have exaggerated hyperbilirubinemia even in the absence of overt hemolysis. The reasons for this are unknown. In the Mediterranean and Oriental types of G6PD deficiency, severe hemolysis and jaundice may be seen.[278] Chemical exposure, such as to naphthalene vapors or high-dose synthetic vitamin K, and infection can incite brisk hemolysis and hyperbilirubinemia.[277] Mild hemolysis in the third or fourth week of life often does not produce jaundice because hepatic mechanisms for the disposal of bilirubin may have matured sufficiently by that time. Chronic brisk hemolysis may be associated with a mixed (conjugated and unconjugated) hyperbilirubinemia after hepatic uptake and conjugating mechanisms mature.

Structural abnormalities of red cells, such as spherocytosis, elliptocytosis, and pyknocytosis, also are rare causes of exaggerated neonatal hyperbilirubinemia and of chronic hyperbilirubinemia.[270]

Bacterial infection can increase the rate of erythrocyte destruction and jaundice. Congenital syphilis, rubella, and toxoplasmosis are infections that may be associated with increased hemolytic rates and hyperbilirubinemia.[279] In each of these diseases, hepatocellular damage and conjugated hyperbilirubinemia may also be present. Sequestered blood in hematomas and ecchymoses sometimes contributes to exaggerated hyperbilirubinemia. A hematoma may only slowly release bilirubin as macrophages gradually enter the mass and convert the heme to bilirubin, but a diffuse and widespread area of subcutaneous blood is more rapidly converted to bile pigment.[270] Red cell destruction may also be accelerated because of trapping in massive capillary and cavernous hemangiomas (so-called *Waring blender hemolysis*). If these involve the liver, a complex picture of anemia, heart failure, and mixed hyperbilirubinemia may be confused initially with severe isoimmune hemolytic disease.

Congenital erythropoietic porphyria is one of the rarest causes of hyperbilirubinemia due to hemolysis in the newborn period. Pink urine and neonatal onset of severe photosensitivity with formation of cutaneous bullae strongly suggest the diagnosis of congenital erythropoietic porphyria.[280, 281] It is important to identify this rare disorder before institution of phototherapy because intense light induces severe skin inflammation with bullae and may be fatal (see Chapter 12).

Hereditary Disorders of Hepatic Bilirubin Metabolism

Gilbert's Syndrome

This is a common disorder that is manifested by mild unconjugated hyperbilirubinemia. It usually presents in adolescence and early adulthood.[282-284] In various studies, it has been identified in 3% to 6% of the population. Clinically, the male-to-female ratio is 4:1.[285] This disparity is probably related to intrinsically better bilirubin clearance in females.[37] If the antimode for normal serum bilirubin is set at 1.4 mg/dL in males and at 0.7 mg/dL in females (serum bilirubin values above these levels are considered abnormal), there is no male predominance. Because molecular diagnosis is not available and because the disease has a marked variability in its expression, the mode of inheritance is not entirely certain. At least some cases appear to be inherited in an autosomal dominant fashion or possibly as the result of passage of one recessive gene defect.

The exact pathophysiology of the disease remains unclear, and Gilbert's syndrome seems to be a common manifestation of a variety of minor defects in the hepatic metabolism of organic anions. A universal defect appears to be a reduction in hepatic bilirubin UGT activity of 50% or more.[159, 284, 286-288] In one recent study, reduced transferase activity was related to a homozygous defect that introduced two extra bases in the TATAA element of the 5' promoter region of the bilirubin UGT gene (from A[TA]6TAA to A[TA]7TAA). This change resulted in reduced expression of a reporter gene expressed in a human hepatoma cell line and is assumed to have the same effect on bilirubin UGT activity *in vivo*.[288a] Further studies are required to determine whether this is a consistent defect in Gilbert's syndrome and how it contributes to hyperbilirubinemia. Although in general conflict with current thinking regarding the dependence of serum bilirubin on transferase activity, the 50% reduction in transferase activity observed in patients with Gilbert's syndrome is probably an important factor related to their jaundice. Although there is poor correlation between the activity of hepatic bilirubin UGT measured *in vitro* and bilirubin clearance capacity, administration of phenobarbital to these patients results in normalization of serum bilirubin activity.[289-291] This probably reflects the inadequacy of the measurement of transferase activity because no other tenable explanation exists for these observations. A significant proportion of these patients also have increased bilirubin production as a result of a slight increase in red cell turnover, dyserythropoiesis, or increased hepatic heme turnover.[291-293] These are not overt, pathologic defects and are only detected in the setting of reduced bilirubin clearance.

The heterogeneity of Gilbert's syndrome is best indicated by the variable defects in clearance of bilirubin, sulfobromophthalein (BSP), and indocyanine green that can be detected, indicating variable storage and transport defects.[284] Clearance of an intravenous bilirubin load test or of radiolabeled bilirubin is abnormal in patients with Gilbert's syndrome, who uniformly retain more than 15% after 4 hours (the normal amount retained is less than 5%).[203, 289, 294-297] Bile salt clearance is generally normal,[298, 299] but some subjects have shown abnormal clearance of ursodeoxycholic acid.[300] Based on the clearance of various organic anions, patients with phenotypic Gilbert's syndrome can be shown to have variable defects of anion clearance.[295, 301-303] It remains to be determined by molecular methods if Gilbert's syndrome is a single disease entity or a collection of disorders.

The serum bilirubin in patients with Gilbert's syndrome normally varies between 1 and 6 mg/dL; of this amount, 95% is unconjugated.[304, 305] The bile from patients with Gilbert's syndrome also contains an excess of BMG (23%); in normal individuals, the BMG level is much lower (7%).[203] Fasting and nicotinic acid infusion cause an increase in serum bilirubin level in patients with Gilbert's syndrome and may be helpful manipulations in establishing the diagnosis.[306, 307] Fasting causes an approximately three- to fourfold increase in the serum bilirubin from baseline, which may be related to reduced bilirubin clearance or to increased bilirubin production, or both.[48, 51, 308] Intravenous injection of 50 mg of nicotinic acid in adult subjects causes serum bilirubin level to increase more than threefold; this is in contrast to the less than twofold increase that occurs in the normal individual.[309] Evidence suggests that normal individuals and patients with Gilbert's syndrome experience equal degrees of increased bilirubin production after the injection of nicotinic acid, but serum bilirubin increases in inverse proportion to the clearance capacity, which is lower in Gilbert's syndrome.[310]

The diagnosis of Gilbert's syndrome rests on a combination of biochemical findings, examination of the family, and exclusion of other causes of hyperbilirubinemia. A presumptive diagnosis can be made in the individual with a mild increase in the serum level of unconjugated bilirubin (total, less than 6 mg/dL; unconjugated, greater than 95%) with no evidence of hemolytic disease (normal complete blood count, blood smear, and reticulocyte count), liver disease (normal concentrations of aminotransferases, alkaline phosphatase, γ-glutamyl transpeptidase, and serum bile acids), or other contributing factors (e.g., breast-feeding or intestinal disease). Finding Gilbert's syndrome in a parent or sibling of the patient provides important supporting evidence for the diagnosis. Follow-up over 1 to 2 years that demonstrates the same findings confirms the diagnosis. Invasive tests such as liver biopsy with measurement of bilirubin UGT activity are not necessary except in very unusual circumstances. No treatment is necessary.

The importance of Gilbert's syndrome in neonatal hyperbilirubinemia is unknown. Certainly, in the setting of isoimmune hemolytic disease, the patient with Gilbert's syndrome would be expected to exhibit greater than normal elevations of serum bilirubin.[311] Exaggerated jaundice in association with pyloric stenosis has also been observed and is consistent with the general effect of fasting in Gilbert's syndrome.[312] Finally, two patients in the authors' experience with apparent severe and prolonged breast milk–related jaundice have been diagnosed as also having Gilbert's syndrome.

Severe Familial Nonhemolytic Jaundice

Two genetically determined disorders with severe defects in hepatic bilirubin UGT activity have been described.[159, 283, 284] Both are associated with lifelong unconjugated hyperbilirubinemia with onset in the newborn period. Early in the newborn period, it may be extremely difficult to separate the two disorders from each other and from other causes of unconjugated hyperbilirubinemia.

Severe Familial Nonhemolytic Jaundice Type I (Crigler-Najjar Syndrome)

Severe familial nonhemolytic jaundice (SFNJ) type I is characterized by persistent unconjugated hyperbilirubinemia. If the patient remains untreated, bilirubin concentrations almost always are greater than 20 mg/dL and often exceed 30 mg/dL.[313] The disease is caused by an autosomal recessive inherited complete absence of bilirubin UGT. Several gene defects have been identified (see section on conjugation of bilirubin), and the disease seems to have major genetic heterogeneity.[314] Parents of affected patients have normal serum bilirubin levels but have transferase activity that is approximately 50% of normal. Affected individuals have a marked defect in bilirubin clearance to less than 1% of normal; the half-life of circulating bilirubin exceeds 156 hours.[289, 315] Bile contains markedly reduced amounts of bilirubin, of which about half is unconjugated bilirubin IXα. Other bile pigments include photoisomers of bilirubin, trace xylose and glucose conjugates of bilirubin, and diazonegative products of bilirubin oxidation. Most homozygous patients and heterozygous carriers have abnormalities in menthol conjugation,[284] which has been used in investigating patterns of inheritance.

The homozygous jaundiced (jj) Gunn rat is the animal equivalent of SFNJ type I.[316, 317] This animal has lifelong jaundice and a total absence of hepatic bilirubin UGT activity.[318] Small amounts of bilirubin can be identified in the bile of jaundiced (jj) rats, mainly as BMG,[119] despite the absence of bilirubin-specific transferase activity. These rats also excrete BMG and BDG when infused with bilirubin dimethyl ester.[205, 319] Together, these observations suggested that the conjugation defect could result from an abnormal microsomal membrane environment for transferase that alters its interaction with its natural substrate, bilirubin. However, when this was examined, microsomal membrane vesicles from jaundiced (jj) Gunn rats were found not to be different from those of outbred Wistar rats with regard to several measures of membrane order.[320] More recently, isoforms of glucuronosyltransferase have been isolated from the microsomal fraction from jaundiced (jj) and outbred (JJ) Wistar rats.[133] These studies have shown that jaundiced (jj) rats have transferase isoforms that are recognized by anti–rat liver UGT and have identical electrophoretic mobility to those from congenic Wistar rats. However, isoform V,

which is normally active in conjugation of bilirubin, has no activity in the jaundiced rats. Isoform I, which is normally active with *p*-nitrophenol as a substrate, is also partially defective. These data suggest that bilirubin UGT produced by the Gunn rat is defective, probably as the result of a single amino acid substitution, and that more than one transferase is affected, perhaps as the result of a repeated defective sequence in both proteins. A single base deletion resulting in a frameshift mutation that removes 115 amino acid residues from the carboxy terminus of the enzyme has been identified.[321] The identification of a gene defect has permitted accurate prenatal diagnosis in this model, a clear indication that prenatal diagnosis of SFNJ type I will soon be accomplished.[322]

The principal sign suggesting the presence of SFNJ type I is persistence of severe hyperbilirubinemia beyond the end of the first week of life. A family history of similar illness or of consanguineous mating further strengthens the suspicion. Collection of duodenal bile with analysis of the bilirubin and its azodipyrroles after the van den Bergh reaction by high-performance liquid chromatography is the preferred method of diagnosis.[284, 323] An indirect estimate of transferase activity can be obtained by the oral administration of menthol and measuring menthol glucuronide excretion in urine.[324, 325] Most homozygous patients have no menthol glucuronide in the urine, whereas both parents have amounts below 10% of normal. Neonatal liver biopsy with microassay for bilirubin UGT activity can be used to confirm the diagnosis but is rarely necessary. A trial of phenobarbital therapy demonstrates a failure to alter serum bilirubin concentrations, indicating a complete absence of inducible transferase activity; this is in contrast to the response in patients with the SFNJ type II (see later).[284]

The major complication resulting from the SFNJ type I is bilirubin encephalopathy (kernicterus).[313, 326–330] Before the advent of effective therapy, the majority of affected infants developed kernicterus in the newborn period. In recent years, the majority of affected infants have survived without clinical evidence of bilirubin encephalopathy. This probably reflects the general improvement of perinatal management and treatment. No specific treatment is available for this disorder. The goal of therapy is the maintenance of serum bilirubin concentrations at less than 20 mg/dL. Exchange transfusions and phototherapy are used to carry the infant past the second or third week of life, followed by home use of phototherapy for periods of 8 to 14 h/d.[331, 332] The response to phototherapy in some of these children diminishes over time, as evidenced by gradually rising serum bilirubin concentrations, from low levels of 12 to 15 mg/dL to levels higher than 25 mg/dL. Agar or other bilirubin-binding agents can be administered by mouth to augment the effect of phototherapy, but they are of limited value.[333] Alternative pathways for bilirubin catabolism may function in the setting of defective conjugation.[115–117, 119, 120] One alternate pathway is dependent on a specific cytochrome P-450 activity that can be induced by the administration of certain chemicals.[115, 120] Chlorpromazine in low doses is capable of inducing this activity and could be safely used in therapy of SFNJ type I, but it is not proven to be effective in any large number of patients. Anesthesia, infections, and other physiologic stresses have been associated with acute development of kernicterus and should be either avoided or treated promptly. Despite improved medical therapy, every known patient with SFNJ type I has ultimately developed neurologic disease during late adolescence or early adulthood unless he or she had undergone liver transplantation.[329, 334] The general treatment strategy involves medical therapy until serum bilirubin levels cannot be maintained in a safe range (less than 35 mg/dL in older children), at which time liver transplantation is performed.[335] Transplantation may entail replacing the entire liver or providing an auxiliary liver graft to provide the necessary bilirubin UGT activity.[336, 337]

Severe Familial Nonhemolytic Jaundice Type II (Arias Syndrome)

SFNJ type II presents in the newborn period as neonatal jaundice followed by persistence of elevated concentrations of serum unconjugated bilirubin.[284, 338] Serum bilirubin concentrations often exceed 20 mg/dL in the newborn, whereas in older children and adults they usually range from 6 to 20 mg/dL. SFNJ type II may be differentiated from SFNJ type I by the lower serum bilirubin concentrations after the newborn period[338, 339] and the response to phenobarbital administration.[290, 340, 341] Duodenal bile contains more than trace amounts of bilirubin, most of which is BMG.[342]

Genetic studies have suggested that this disorder may be inherited as an autosomal dominant trait with marked variability of penetrance.[343] One of the parents is often found to have unconjugated hyperbilirubinemia and profound reduction of hepatic transferase activity, and more distant relations from the affected parent's side also may be found to have the deficiency even though they do not have overt disease. Other studies have suggested that SFNJ type II may represent a homozygous state of a single type of Gilbert's syndrome or a compound of variants of Gilbert's syndrome.[284, 290, 344] Very recently, the defective cDNAs from two patients have been expressed in a bilirubin UGT–deficient cell line. In contrast to the complete inactivation that occurs in patients with SFNJ type I, bilirubin UGT was only partially inactivated in the two patients, with residual activity being about 4% of normal.[156] The major effect was a 10-fold decrease in the expressed enzyme's affinity for bilirubin. These data suggest a recessively inherited defect involving a gene mutation at a site that alters, but does not completely inactivate, the bilirubin binding domain of bilirubin UGT. SFNJ type II may, therefore, represent a common manifestation of several genetic defects.

Hepatic bilirubin UGT activity in patients with the SFNJ type II is just barely detectable,[202, 286, 338, 345] so low that measurement of transferase activity cannot be used reliably to differentiate SFNJ type II from type I.[340] Because only about 1% of normal enzyme activity is required for clearance of bilirubin, a very small shift in low level of enzyme activity in SFNJ type II can effect a marked change in serum bilirubin concentration. Small differences in enzyme activity in affected individuals apparently accounts for the variability of expression of the disorder. Administration of phenobarbital produces a significant decline in serum bilirubin concentration, often to less than 4 mg/dL.[290, 340, 341, 346–348] Continued administration of the drug maintains nearly normal serum bilirubin concentrations, but discontinuation of administration results in a return to pretreatment levels in 1 to 4 weeks. This suggests that the drug has induced increased bilirubin UGT activity, but the presence of such activity has been difficult to prove by enzyme assay, again probably because of the intrinsic difficulties of measuring activity at such low levels. Because patients with the SFNJ type I fail to respond to phenobarbital, its administration may be used in the differential diagnosis of severe nonhemolytic jaundice. Chronic phenobarbital administration is useful for maintaining cosmetically more acceptable skin color, but no patients with the type II syndrome have ever been shown to develop kernicterus beyond the immediate neonatal period.

Acquired Unconjugated Hyperbilirubinemia

Jaundice Associated with Breast-Feeding

A significant number of breast-fed infants develop exaggerated unconjugated hyperbilirubinemia, which in some cases persists through the first 3 or 4 months of life.[349, 350] Two separate periods of time must be considered when jaundice in the breast-fed infant is examined. During the first few days of life, breast-feeding is superimposed on the developmental factors that cause physiologic jaundice, which may cause it to be exaggerated. After the first week of life, physiologic jaundice should have abated; thus, breast-feeding is acting alone to cause jaundice, even though it is acting in a less than mature environment.

The concept that breast-feeding exaggerates physiologic jaundice is based on the observation that serum bilirubin levels exceed 12 mg/dL more frequently in breast-fed infants than in bottle-fed infants.[270, 351, 352] This is not a universal finding. At least two studies have failed to show any significant differences between serum bilirubin concentrations of breast-fed and bottle-fed infants during the first 3 days of life.[350, 353] The phenomenon may be related to inadequate caloric intake, which can increase bilirubin production[48, 49, 51, 354] and may reduce intestinal transit and enhance bilirubin absorption.[355] In some hospital settings, breast-feeding mothers are not encouraged to nurse with sufficient frequency to permit rapid and effective development of lactation. This may explain differences in the frequency and intensity of jaundice in breast-fed infants among hospitals. No therapy is needed beyond ensuring adequate caloric intake.[352, 356, 357] Attention should probably be given to ensuring the adequacy of breast-feeding, and if this cannot be accomplished, caloric supplementation should be provided.

Prolonged jaundice[358] is seen in approximately 1 in every 100 otherwise normal breast-fed infants throughout the world[351, 359]; up to 40% have abnormally high serum unconjugated bilirubin levels at 2 to 3 weeks of age.[360] Bilirubin concentrations rise to peak levels that may exceed 20 mg/dL by the end of the second week of life.[358, 361] With continued nursing, serum bilirubin concentrations typically decline gradually from their peak and approaching normal by 4 to 16 weeks of life. If one infant in a family has had breast milk–related jaundice, a recurrence rate of approximately 70% is to be anticipated in subsequently nursed infants.[361]

The mechanism by which breast milk causes infantile jaundice remains uncertain. Investigation has centered on the roles of two observed effects of breast milk on bilirubin metabolism: inhibition of bilirubin UGT, and enhancement of bilirubin absorption from the intestine. These may act alone or in conjunction to produce the breast milk–related jaundice syndrome. The earliest studies that implicated the presence in milk of the abnormal progesterone metabolite pregnane $3\alpha,20\beta$-diol[343, 362] or long-chain unesterified fatty acids,[363–365] both inhibitors *in vitro* of bilirubin UGT, have subsequently been discounted. To date, no factor in milk that inhibits bilirubin UGT has been identified as the cause of breast milk–related jaundice. It can be demonstrated in the laboratory that breast milks enhance the absorption of unconjugated bilirubin from the intestine of the rat.[360, 366] In one study, there was a good correlation between the absorption of bilirubin and the degree of infantile jaundice.[360] This effect, if expressed *in vivo* in the neonate, could increase the bilirubin load and produce jaundice. It has been suggested that β-glucuronidase activity in breast milk has a role in producing this syndrome.[367]

A clinical diagnosis of the breast milk–related jaundice syndrome may be established by the characteristic pattern of prolonged hyperbilirubinemia in a breast-feeding infant. The infants should be thriving, with good appetite, milk intake, and weight gain, and other definable causes of jaundice should be excluded. Any breast-fed baby with elevation of the conjugated bilirubin should be evaluated for liver disease. Tragically, the authors have seen several infants with biliary atresia and conjugated hyperbilirubinemia whose condition was dismissed as breast milk–related jaundice. A specific test for breast milk–related jaundice entails interruption of nursing, which results in a significant decline in serum bilirubin concentrations in 24 to 72 hours. Failure of serum bilirubin concentrations to decrease after 3 days of interruption indicates that the cause of jaundice was probably not related to breast milk. Resumption of nursing usually results in no more than a 2- to 3-mg/dL increase in serum bilirubin level. Temporary interruption of nursing is not recommended for diagnostic purposes alone because it may lead to detrimental biologic and psychologic effects and should be practiced only when the serum bilirubin concentration is at or close to the estimated toxic level.

Transient Familial Neonatal Hyperbilirubinemia (Lucey-Driscoll Syndrome)

Transient familial neonatal hyperbilirubinemia is an extremely rare disorder characterized by unconjugated hyperbilirubinemia during the first week of life.[368–370] A potent but unidentified inhibitor of bilirubin UGT can be found in the circulations of both the mother and infant; this inhibitor disappears from both by the end of the second postpartum week, and serum bilirubin concentrations in the infant decline to normal. The mother has no hyperbilirubinemia.

Intestinal Disorders

Disorders that reduce intestinal clearance are associated with an increased incidence of pathologic jaundice.[50, 371, 372] Up to 50% of infants with pyloric stenosis have elevated serum bilirubin concentrations, and about 10% develop jaundice. Pyloric stenosis has been shown to be associated with markedly suppressed levels of hepatic bilirubin UGT activity,[373] the mechanism of which is not known. Infants with pyloric stenosis also have reduced indocyanine green clearance, indicating an abnormality in hepatic clearance of organic anions that would also include bilirubin.[374] The cause of any clearance defect is not understood. Congenital intestinal obstruction usually presents with other signs, and the effect of obstruction on serum bilirubin concentrations is impossible to distinguish from the effects of general sickness and starvation. Hyperbilirubinemia also is occasionally associated with large bowel obstruction, as in Hirschsprung's disease.

Drugs and Unconjugated Hyperbilirubinemia

Xenobiotics potentially have broad-spectrum effects on bilirubin metabolism and transport. No drugs commonly used therapeutically for newborns are known to precipitate hemolytic disorders in otherwise normal infants, although some may in infants with G6PD deficiency.[277, 375] Novobiocin, an antibiotic that is an inhibitor of bilirubin UGT, is the only drug that has ever been demonstrated to produce unconjugated hyperbilirubinemia in the newborn and has been withdrawn from clinical use for many years.[376] All newly introduced drugs should be used in the newborn with great caution and with an awareness of potential detrimental metabolic effects, including induction of jaundice.

Endocrine Disorders

Congenital hypothyroidism is associated with prolonged unconjugated hyperbilirubinemia in approximately 10% of cases.[377–379] This probably results from the general depression of metabolism in the hypothyroid infant or from the dependence of the maturation of innumerable hepatic metabolic pathways on thyroxin. Infants of diabetic mothers likewise have an increased frequency of exaggerated and prolonged unconjugated hyperbilirubinemia.[380] One explanation is deficient production of UDPGA that results in reduced conjugation. Early feeding may help to alleviate the severity and duration of the jaundice.[381]

ETHNIC FACTORS IN NEONATAL JAUNDICE

Infants of Asian descent, including Chinese, Japanese, and Koreans, as well as Native American infants, have peak serum bilirubin levels that are approximately twice those of white or black infants during the first 3 or 4 days of life.[382–384] The pattern of hyperbilirubinemia and its universality suggest a genetically determined delayed maturation of the basic mechanisms responsible for physiologic jaundice. An increase in the endogenous carbon monoxide production suggests hemolysis in some cases, but in the majority of Asian and Native American infants, no hemolytic contribution can be demonstrated.[384, 385]

Individuals with exaggerated transient neonatal jaundice in more geographically localized areas also have been observed, the best studied being on the island of Lesbos in Greece.[386, 387] Although the island's population has a high incidence of G6PD deficiency, only about 5% of jaundiced infants have the enzyme deficiency.[375] A local environmental factor may contribute, but whether infants of Greek origin born outside of Greece are equally affected remains a subject of controversy.[387] Phenobarbital prophylaxis with treatment of both the pregnant mother and neonate ameliorates the severity of jaundice and the frequent need for exchange transfusions to prevent kernicterus.[388]

BILIRUBIN NEUROTOXICITY

Unconjugated bilirubin can, under certain conditions, enter the central nervous system and injure neurons in specific areas of the brain, resulting in the condition known as *kernicterus*.[237, 327] The pathophysiology of bilirubin neurotoxicity has not been established despite years of major investigative effort. The word *kernicterus* actually means "nuclear jaundice," which refers to the staining of dead neurons in the basal ganglia, hippocampal cortex, cerebellum, and subthalamic nuclei that fulfills the pathologist's definition of kernicterus.[327, 389] The clinical features include progressive lethargy, muscular rigidity, opisthotonos, high-pitched cry, fever, and convulsions that develop in an infant at risk.[390, 391] Fortunately, the full-blown clinical and pathologic syndrome of kernicterus is rarely encountered with modern nursery care, and the present focus of most clinical study is assessment of the risk of jaundiced infants for developing neurotoxicity that is manifested in more subtle ways, such as learning deficits.[392–396] It is probably safe to assume that bilirubin neurotoxicity includes a spectrum of clinical illness and pathologic injury that spans from full-blown kernicterus to minimally detectable learning deficits.

Pathogenesis of Bilirubin Neurotoxicity

Two major factors—albumin binding of bilirubin, and the blood-brain barrier—must be considered in the pathophysiology of bilirubin neurotoxicity.[393, 397] The protection conferred by albumin binding of bilirubin is clearly important in preventing neurotoxicity.[82, 398] The adequacy of binding is determined by the concentrations of albumin and bilirubin and by the binding affinity, which can be affected by substances that compete for bilirubin-binding sites. The theoretic binding capacity has been discussed earlier in the section dealing with bilirubin transport in plasma. In theory, the plasma albumin of a newborn can fully bind bilirubin at concentrations well above those that are considered to be unsafe. The theoretic situation is confounded in the clinical setting by variable binding affinity caused by circulating chemicals, whether xenobiotics or endogenous metabolites.

At present, the *in vivo* binding affinity of albumin for bilirubin cannot be accurately assessed.[90–94] A variety of methods for the measurement of albumin binding of bilirubin have been developed for both research and clinical purposes. These have been discussed earlier in this chapter in the section dealing with bilirubin transport. Although deficient albumin binding of bilirubin has been shown to be associated with development of kernicterus, these binding techniques have not been developed to the point of meriting broad clinical application. Several problems are associated with their use. The techniques are, in general, difficult to perform; furthermore, each yields somewhat different results, and this suggests that these tests measure different aspects of the binding relationship. The methods react differently to perturbations of the binding relationship as produced by the presence of drugs and metabolites. When performed *in vitro*, they may not reflect *in vivo* binding at all. At the present time, no binding method can be recommended for clinical use in the nursery, but further study of these techniques will perhaps provide a better understanding of the relationship between albumin binding and bilirubin encephalopathy.

The sick neonate may be exposed to many chemicals that have the potential for interfering with the albumin binding of bilirubin. Competition for binding at the high-affinity site is the mechanism by which sulfisoxazole and other sulfonamide drugs enhance the risk for kernicterus.[399, 400] This has provided a useful model for the study of kernicterus in animals, particularly with regard to the manipulation of a single limb of the complex equation that determines the movement of bilirubin into the central nervous system.[401, 402] Drugs known to reduce the affinity of albumin binding should be avoided, and new drugs should be considered as possible inhibitors when they are used for the clinical care of neonates.[403] Ceftriaxone and cefmenoxime have been shown to interfere with bilirubin binding to a significant degree and, thus, their use should be avoided in infants at risk for kernicterus.[404–406]

Elevated free fatty acids may have an effect on bilirubin binding, but the direction and the magnitude of the effect is not clear. Fatty acids bind to albumin in a region close to the high-affinity binding site for albumin. Various studies suggest that fatty acid binding to albumin interferes with or produces allosteric enhancement of bilirubin binding. In the clinical setting, conditions that produce elevated serum free fatty acid concentrations have been associated with an increased risk of neurotoxicity that is thought to be due to reduced binding affinity.[407–410] The major problem with this interpretation is the fact that conditions that increase fatty acid concentrations, such as fasting, cause many other changes that could affect binding or the blood-brain barrier. In infants without acute illness, moderate increases in serum free fatty acid concentration that can result from the administration of intravenous lipid and heparin probably do not significantly alter the bilirubin binding capacity of neonates.[85, 411–413]

Conjugated bilirubin does not enter the central nervous system but does bind to albumin and possibly competes with bilirubin for albumin binding. In clinical practice, it has been traditional to subtract the direct reacting fraction of bilirubin from the total serum bilirubin concentration in estimation of the risk for bilirubin neurotoxicity, but this method may not be completely accurate. Rather, conjugated bilirubin should be considered as an additional risk factor at any given level of unconjugated bilirubin.

The blood-brain barrier also is important in preventing bilirubin neurotoxicity.[392, 397, 398, 414] Certain clinical phenomena appear to enhance the risk for the development of kernicterus by interfering with the blood-brain barrier. These include prematurity, hypoxia, acidosis, hypoglycemia, hemolysis, and sepsis, with or without meningitis.[258, 414–417] Useful animal models have been developed to investigate the mechanisms by which the blood-brain barrier is breached in various clinical settings and are providing valuable insights.[418–424] Bacterial endotoxins and hypoxia appear to have particularly profound effects and increase the risk for kernicterus by damaging the endothelial lining cells of the cerebral capillaries or by altering the neuronal cell membranes to permit entry of bilirubin.

Some clinical conditions affect both binding and the blood-brain barrier, placing the jaundiced infant in double jeopardy. Acidosis is one of these conditions. Lowered pH weakens the binding affinity, and circulating organic acids compete with bilirubin for binding sites; at the same time, clinical acidosis is frequently encountered in settings in which the blood-brain barrier is impaired.[407, 425]

Once having gained entry into the neuron, bilirubin interferes with cellular function. In model systems, it can be shown to affect oxidative phosphorylation, cell respiration, protein synthesis, cell membrane transport, and glucose metabolism.[426–432] The particular affinity of bilirubin for the basal ganglia, hippocampal cortex, cerebellum, and subthalamic nuclei is not understood. Recent animal studies suggest that the clinical symptomatology of kernicterus may be produced by intravenous infusions of unconjugated bilirubin in the absence of staining of the brain and normal brain histology. Acute manipulations of bilirubin binding and the blood-brain barrier can be monitored by changes in auditory and visual evoked potentials in these animal models.

Clinical Manifestations of Bilirubin Neurotoxicity

The clinical manifestations correlating with bilirubin injury to brain range from complete absence of specific signs or symptoms to full-blown kernicterus. Approximately one half of infants demonstrating kernicterus die. Survivors of this clinical complex, as well as some infants who are essentially asymptomatic as newborns, demonstrate choreoathetoid cerebral palsy, high-frequency deafness, and less commonly, mental retardation.[433] Alterations in neurophysiologic studies such as auditory evoked potentials have been related to risk factors for bilirubin neurotoxicity.[434] Other epidemiologic studies have associated mild motor, cognitive, and behavioral disorders later in infancy and childhood with elevated neonatal serum bilirubin concentrations.[395, 435, 436] The importance of the effect of mild hyperbilirubinemia on neural development, however, remains to be determined.

Bilirubin is toxic to tissues other than brain. Infants found to have kernicterus at autopsy frequently have extraneural deposits of bilirubin, particularly in the intestinal mucosa, pancreas, and renal papillae.[437] Bilirubin nephropathy can be demonstrated in the jaundiced Gunn rat,[438] but the human clinical condition remains to be defined. However, the possibility of extraneural toxicity accounting for clinical disease cannot be ignored.

TREATMENT OF NEONATAL HYPERBILIRUBINEMIA AND PREVENTION OF BILIRUBIN NEUROTOXICITY

At the present time, the prevention of bilirubin injury to the brain is empirical and based on "safe" serum bilirubin concentrations adjusted according to birthweight or gestational age and clinical status. Although earlier studies indicated the critical importance of serum bilirubin concentrations in excess of 20 mg/dL in the causation of kernicterus, this value should not be considered as a "magic number" below which there is no danger. As previously discussed, many factors contribute to the risk for developing neurotoxicity, and kernicterus can occur in the sick neonate, even at serum unconjugated bilirubin concentrations as low as 5 mg/dL. Vigorous attention to the intensive care of small and sick neonates appears to be effective in preventing the development of kernicterus in high-risk infants if it is kept in mind that serum bilirubin represents a loaded gun that can be discharged by a variety of insults. The sicker the infant, the greater the risk at any given bilirubin level.

Exchange transfusion and phototherapy are the two treatment modalities most commonly used to lower serum bilirubin concentrations or maintain them in

Table 4–1. SERUM BILIRUBIN CONCENTRATIONS (mg/dL) AT WHICH EXCHANGE TRANSFUSIONS ARE INDICATED DURING THE NEONATAL PERIOD

	Birth Weight (g)					
	<1000	*1000–1249*	*1250–1499*	*1500–1999*	*2000–2499*	*>2500*
Healthy infants	10	13	15	17	18	20
High-risk infants*	10	10	13	15	17	18

*High-risk infants include those with perinatal asphyxia, hypoxia, acidosis, hypoalbuminemia, hemolysis, hypothermia, and septicemia.

a safe range. The recommended maximum allowable serum bilirubin concentrations before exchange transfusion should be performed for infants of various weights are listed in Table 4–1. The technique and complications of exchange transfusions are discussed in Chapter 3.

Phototherapy

Phototherapy is effective for the treatment of neonatal jaundice from a variety of causes.[439, 440] It has been adopted worldwide as the first-line treatment of unconjugated hyperbilirubinemia and is probably much overused. As many as 10% of newborns in the United States receive phototherapy for neonatal jaundice; this frequent application probably exceeds the actual need.[440]

Indications for Use. Phototherapy should be considered as the first-line therapy for all unconjugated hyperbilirubinemia deserving treatment. For example, in severe hyperbilirubinemia due to Rh hemolytic disease, it reduces the need for exchange transfusion, thereby decreasing morbidity.[441] In such a case, the benefit overwhelmingly outweighs the risk. On the other hand, phototherapy should not be used in patients with physiologic jaundice, in whom there is no risk of bilirubin-induced injury.

Phototherapy is limited with regard to its ability to acutely reduce serum bilirubin levels in states with markedly increased production. It is most effective when used prophylactically in anticipation of the potential requirement for exchange transfusion. At these authors' medical center, phototherapy is being used according to the policies outlined in Table 4–2. All infants weighing less than 1500 g at birth receive prophylactic phototherapy because of the excessive morbidity and mortality observed during exchange transfusions and because of the desire to completely avoid the procedure in this very-high-risk group of infants. It is used therapeutically for low-birth-weight infants weighing more than 1500 g at birth with moderate hyperbilirubinemia and for full-term infants having severe hyperbilirubinemia that could prompt the need for exchange transfusion if it remains untreated.

Mechanism of Action. Phototherapy reduces serum bilirubin mainly by the mechanism of photoisomerization of bilirubin.[439, 442–444] *Photoisomerization* is defined as a change in the configuration of the bilirubin molecule due to the absorption of light energy. This mechanism was first identified in Gunn rats, which lack the ability to conjugate bilirubin. When exposed to therapeutic light, these rats rapidly exhibit biliary excretion of bilirubin.[445, 446] A similar effect has been confirmed in jaundiced human infants and probably represents the major effect of therapeutic light.[447]

Bilirubin absorbs light energy mainly in the blue-green range. The energy is dissipated in the complex system of conjugated and double bonds of the molecule; this results in configurational changes, including the production of a class of compounds collectively called *photobilirubin* (Fig. 4–6). The folding that makes unconjugated bilirubin IXα insoluble in water is made possible by the flexibility of the central methene carbon bridge and the *Z configuration* (from *zusammen*, German for "together") of the 4- and 15-methyne carbon bridges. With the energy supplied by light, these relatively rigid bridges are converted to the *E configuration* (from *entgegen*, German for "opposite") with disruption of internal hydrogen bonds. The bilirubin molecule is unfolded, freeing the carboxyl groups to interact with the aqueous environment and making the compound much more soluble in water. Three configurational isomers are formed: 4E,15Z-photobilirubin; 4Z,15E-photobilirubin; and 4E,15E-photobilirubin. The first two are thermodynamically unstable and spontaneously revert to insoluble bilirubin in minutes; the 4E,15E-photobilirubin isomer is more stable but is formed only in small quantities.[443, 444, 448, 449] The configurational isomers are rapidly formed during phototherapy and are easily excreted by the liver without conjugation.[450–453] Another phototherapy-induced isomer of bilirubin called *cyclo-*

Table 4–2. GUIDELINES FOR THE USE OF PHOTOTHERAPY DURING THE NEWBORN PERIOD

Birthweight (g)	Indication for Phototherapy
<1500	Start phototherapy during first 24 h of life regardless of serum bilirubin concentration
1500–1999	Without hemolysis, start phototherapy at serum bilirubin level of 10 mg/dL
	With hemolysis, start phototherapy at serum bilirubin level of 8 mg/dL
2000–2499	Without hemolysis, start phototherapy at serum bilirubin levels of 12 mg/dL
	With hemolysis, start phototherapy at serum bilirubin level of 10 mg/dL
>2500	Without hemolysis, no indication for phototherapy in healthy baby
	With hemolysis, start phototherapy at serum bilirubin of 15 mg/dL

Phototherapy to be continued until serum bilirubin concentration has stabilized at or has fallen to less than one half of the exchange transfusion indication level listed in Table 4–1.

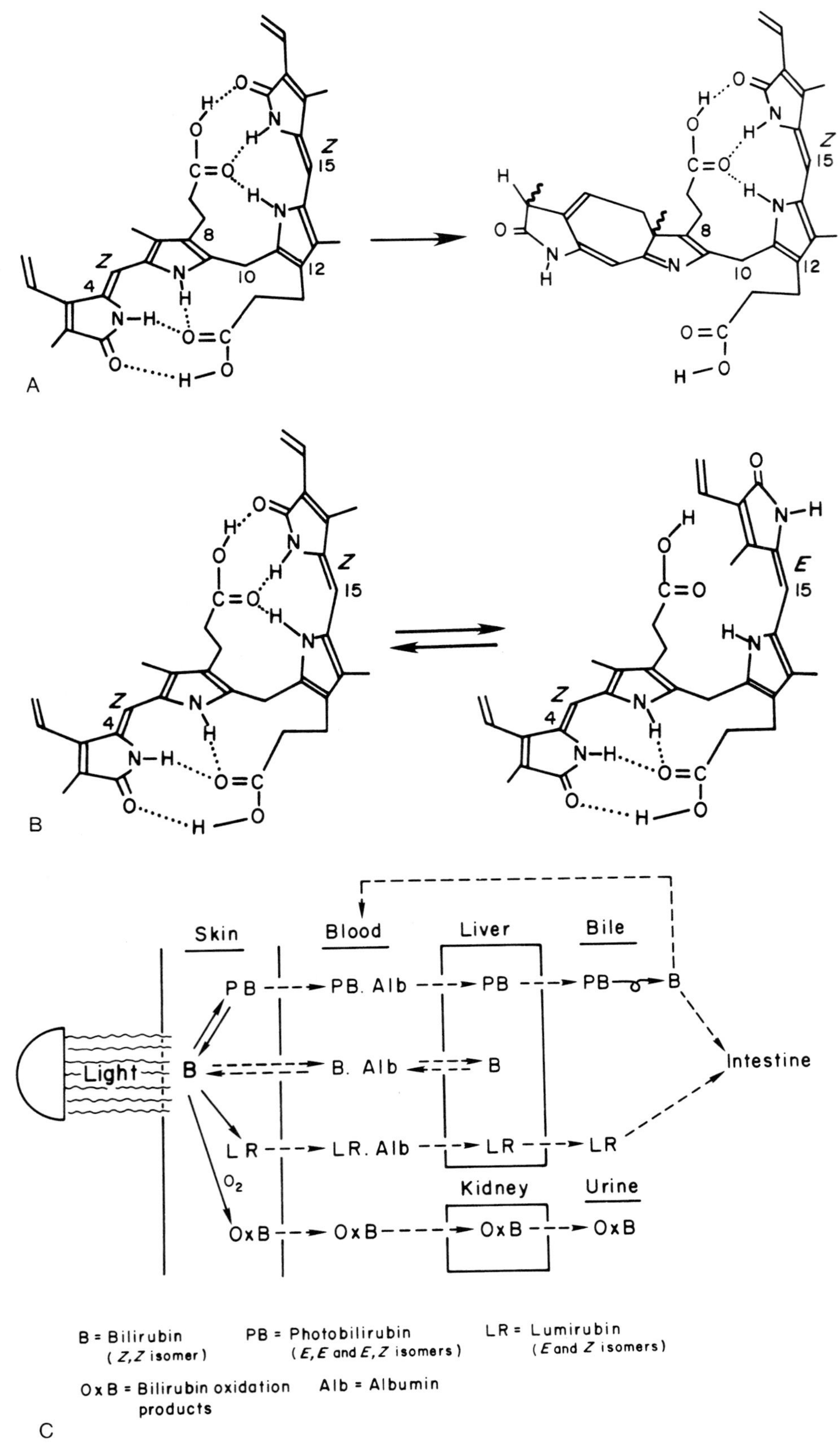

Figure 4-6. The mechanism of phototherapy. *A,* Z–E carbon double-bond configurational isomerization of bilirubin. *B,* Intramolecular cyclization of bilirubin in the presence of light to form lumirubin. *C,* General mechanism of phototherapy for neonatal jaundice. *Solid arrows* represent chemical reactions; *broken arrows* represent transport processes. Pigments may be bound to proteins in compartments other than blood. Some excretion of photoisomers in urine also occurs. (From McDonagh AF, Lightner DA: 'Like a shrivelled blood orange'—bilirubin, jaundice, and phototherapy. Pediatrics 1985; 75:443. Copyright American Academy of Pediatrics 1985.)

bilirubin or *lumirubin* is the product of intramolecular endovinyl cyclization of 4E,15Z-photobilirubin.[454] Although accounting for only a small percentage of photoisomers formed, it is perhaps the most important product of phototherapy because it is totally stable and cannot revert to bilirubin.[455] Cyclobilirubin is excreted less rapidly in the Gunn rat under phototherapy than are the configurational isomers.[456] However, the clearance of cyclobilirubin formed during phototherapy in premature infants appears to be more rapid than that of the configurational isomers, having a mean half-life of 111 minutes (compared with one of 15 hours for the isomers).[457] The extent to which the formation of cyclobilirubin contributes to the clearance of bilirubin during phototherapy, therefore, remains unclear. Overall, photoisomerization is responsible for more than 80% of the effect of phototherapy.[444]

The efficiency of phototherapy is reduced because the configurational isomers in the intestine revert to bilirubin, which is readily absorbed.[333] Adequate caloric intake and frequent feeding increase the effectiveness of phototherapy, whereas partial or complete starvation decreases the level of reduction of serum bilirubin by phototherapy. The efficacy of phototherapy can be enhanced by the simultaneous oral administration of agents that bind bilirubin.[333, 458]

Photodegradation also occurs to a small degree.[444] When bilirubin in the skin absorbs light energy and is elevated from its triplet (ground) energy state to the singlet state, the energy can be transferred to molecular oxygen. This produces singlet oxygen, which is capable of oxidizing compounds containing double bonds. Free radicals, which are capable of a wide variety of oxidizing reactions, also are generated. Bilirubin, in addition to sensitizing these reactions, is oxidized by them. The products formed by these reactions include biliverdin, dipyrroles, and monopyrroles, all of which are water soluble and can be excreted by the liver or kidney without conjugation. Evidence suggests that photodegradation is a minor mechanism of phototherapy, but significant amounts of water-soluble photodegradation products of bilirubin can be identified in the urine of infants receiving light therapy.[459] This class of reactions may account for up to 20% of the bilirubin excreted as a result of phototherapy.

In both mechanisms, bilirubin absorbs the energy of light to initiate the photodynamic reaction.[460] Only tissue bilirubin is subject to the photodynamic reaction, and light effectively penetrates only the outermost 2 mm of the skin.[461] It is imperative that as much skin as possible be exposed for the effect to be maximum. Newer methods of distributing light to greater areas of skin, such as fiberoptic blankets, have not been sufficiently tested to determine their effectiveness. Because the maximum absorption of bilirubin IXα is in the wavelength range of 425 to 475 nm, blue light has been considered to be the most effective for therapy.[462] Studies have shown that tissue and protein binding of bilirubin alters the absorption spectrum and that the maximum quantum yield for photoisomerization occurs at a wavelength of 520 nm (green light).[463] Light of longer wavelength would also be safer in theory, but would not penetrate skin as well.[464–467] Further study will be required to determine what role green light has in phototherapy.

Complications. High-energy light has considerable potential to cause toxicity in the developing neonate.[442, 444, 468, 469] Phototherapy has been shown to result in a number of physiologic changes and pathologic alterations in the newborn undergoing treatment for jaundice. The potential for injury from light is compounded by the fact that unconjugated bilirubin is a sensitizer of photodynamic reactions that result in the production of singlet oxygen. This, in turn, can result in the oxidation of a variety of compounds containing double bonds. Thus, cell membranes and other important organic compounds can be injured as a result of phototherapy. A few important complications of phototherapy have been recorded, but the full potential toxicity of this modality has yet to be determined.

Riboflavin, a vitamin that contains double bonds, can be oxidized during phototherapy. A deficiency state can develop with the use of prolonged phototherapy, which can be prevented by a daily riboflavin intake of 0.3 mg.[470, 471] Riboflavin is itself a sensitizer of photodynamic reactions and has been shown to accelerate the destruction of methionine, tryptophan, and histidine in amino acid solutions exposed to light. Likewise, oxidation of polyunsaturated, essential fatty acids is accelerated by exposure to light *in vitro*.[472] The binding of some fatty acids to albumin, however, increases the quantum yield of phototherapy for the production of bilirubin photoisomers.[472, 473] The innumerable possible interactions of light energy, bilirubin, and organic compounds must be considered in assessing the safety of this therapy.

Some infants treated with phototherapy exhibit increased bilirubin excretion but no reduction of serum bilirubin, suggesting that light may increase the rate of hemolysis. *In vitro*, blue light causes increased loss of erythrocyte potassium and membrane ATPase activity, lysis of resealed erythrocyte membranes, and cross-linking of erythrocyte membrane polypeptides.[474–476] The Gunn rat treated with blue light exhibits increased osmotic fragility of erythrocytes,[474–477] but no apparent alteration in red cell survival.[478] However, the human fetal erythrocyte membrane is quite susceptible to oxidative stress.[478a] A variety of erythrocyte membrane enzymes are inactivated, and the oxyhemoglobin dissociation curve of fetal blood is shifted by bilirubin sensitized photoreaction.[479] Finally, patients with inherited deficiency of G6PD of the Mediterranean type may develop significant hemolysis upon exposure to therapeutic light.[480]

The effect of phototherapy on the binding capacity of albumin for bilirubin has been investigated. Conflicting results have been obtained. *In vitro*, photooxidation of albumin can be demonstrated, but *in vivo*, there appears to be no reduction in the binding affinity or capacity of albumin during phototherapy.[481–483] Therapeutic light does decrease the concentration of serum albumin in treated infants, presumably because of photooxidation, but this reduction is not clinically significant.[483] Administering albumin increases the effectiveness of phototherapy in low-birth-weight infants.[484]

A number of potentially important alterations of physiology have been observed during phototherapy.[468] Retinal changes can result from prolonged exposure to intense light, but shielding the eyes from light, as is now common practice, prevents any long-term measurable optic injury.[485–488] Preterm infants demonstrate a reduced growth rate and an increased frequency of hypocalcemia.[489, 490] These effects may be due to the direct influence of light on hormone production or to the disruption of the circadian rhythm.[491, 492]

The large increase of unconjugated bilirubin delivered to the intestine causes a dramatic alteration in intestinal physiology.[447] Clinically apparent diarrhea occurs in 10% of treated infants.[493] Diarrhea is probably due to intestinal secretion induced by bilirubin,[494] which can be reversed by the administration of agar.[495] Transient lactase deficiency probably does not occur, as was previously thought.[496–498]

A specific, pathologic complication of phototherapy is the *bronze baby syndrome*. This rare disorder, which occurs in fewer than 1 in 1000 infants receiving phototherapy, is characterized by the development of brown-black discoloration of the serum, urine, and skin.[259, 260, 499–504] It appears after many hours of exposure to light and has almost always been associated with the presence of mild or moderate conjugated hyperbilirubinemia prior to phototherapy. The development of this complication probably requires the presence of pre-existing cholestatic liver disease in the infant; thus, it has been assumed that a pigment normally excreted into bile during phototherapy is retained. Based on chromatographic and spectroscopic data, the retained pigments are either polymers of photobilirubin[503] or photodegradation products of Cu(II)-porphyrin.[504, 505] It is not known at this time whether the bronze baby syndrome is simply a cosmetic defect or carries a risk for secondary tissue damage. It is generally recommended that infants with cholestasis not be exposed to phototherapy lights and that light therapy be promptly discontinued in all infants who develop cholestasis or bronzing. Discontinuation of phototherapy usually is associated with prompt disappearance of the pigment from the serum, urine, and skin.

Metalloporphyrins

The metalloporphyrins are substituted heme compounds in which other multivalent metals are chelated by protoporphyrin IX in the place of iron. The discovery that metalloporphyrins can inhibit bilirubin formation has led to their potential use in chemotherapy of neonatal hyperbilirubinemia.[506–509] They interact with the prosthetic site of heme oxygenase and have variable effects on enzyme activity, some acting as competitive inhibitors and others as inducers of the enzyme.[506]

The best studied has been Sn-protoporphyrin. Studies in animals have shown impressive reduction of bilirubin production and serum bilirubin levels in a variety of experimental conditions. Normal physiologic jaundice in newborn rats and monkeys can be prevented by the administration of Sn-protoporphyrin.[510, 511] The compound also inhibits carbon monoxide excretion in adult mice[512] and reduces endogenous bilirubin production in adult rats.[513] It has not shown serious toxicity in animals, but important questions remain about the potential for light-induced oxidative injury.[508, 514] Sn-Protoporphyrin is a potent photosensitizer, accepting light energy with a maximum absorption at a wavelength of 400 nm, elevating electrons to the triplet excited state. As it gives up energy, it elevates available oxygen to produce toxic singlet oxygen, which can injure cells and membranes, particularly the skin. This potential for toxicity must be studied in greater detail.

Sn-Protoporphyrin has been used in a clinical trial involving neonates.[507] Greek infants with ABO incompatibility received Sn-protoporphyrin. Some received low-dose, single injections and others higher-dose, multiple injections. The group treated with the higher doses had a significant reduction in serum bilirubin level and a reduced need for phototherapy, but the effect was small. The peak bilirubin value in the treated group was 5.2 mg/dL, as compared with 7.6 mg/dL in the control group. Toxic effects were few. Of 12 babies given both Sn-protoporphyrin and phototherapy, 2 developed mild skin sensitivity. The drug has also been used in a patient with Crigler-Najjar syndrome, in which it may have value in temporarily reducing serum bilirubin concentrations.[515]

At the present time, there remains considerable interest in the metalloporphyrins and their application to the treatment of neonatal jaundice. Improved methods for targeting the drugs to improve efficacy and reduce toxicity may increase their clinical usefulness.[516] It will probably be several years before they have general clinical application.

CONJUGATED HYPERBILIRUBINEMIA OF THE NEWBORN

Elevated serum concentrations of conjugated or direct-reacting bilirubin virtually always indicates the presence of liver dysfunction. Rarely, very brisk rates of bilirubin production and conjugation can overwhelm the excretory capacity of the liver and result in mild retention of conjugated bilirubin. This clinical situation is not likely to be confused with liver disease, but some systemic disease states, such as sepsis, can cause both hemolysis and hepatocyte dysfunction. The conditions of liver dysfunction to be considered here are the hereditary conjugated hyperbilirubinemias and cholestasis. The former is considered in some detail in this section. Only a conceptual overview of the latter is presented.

Hereditary Conjugated Hyperbilirubinemia

Two extremely rare hereditary disorders that affect the excretion of conjugated bilirubin by the hepatocyte have been described.[159, 284, 517, 518] These have the common characteristic of elevating serum concentrations of conjugated bilirubin; however, they vary in other respects.

Dubin-Johnson Syndrome

This is the more common of the two hereditary conjugated hyperbilirubinemias.[284] This benign condition is characterized by an excretory defect for several organic anions, including conjugated bilirubin.[518–520] Serum bilirubin varies from 1.5 to 6.0 mg/dL, over half of which is conjugated.[520, 521] Other routine liver function tests are normal, including serum bile salt concentrations. The liver is often grossly black in color, and histologically a dark pigment in hepatocyte lysosomes that is derived either from melanin or from catecholamines is retained.[522, 523] Oral cholecystography dye is not excreted normally, and this results in failure to visualize the gallbladder. Techniques employing the study of kinetics of excretion of scintigraphic dyes can now be used to confirm this diagnosis and differentiate it from Rotor's syndrome.[524, 525]

The Dubin-Johnson defect presumably involves the canalicular transport mechanism, although the exact defect has not been defined.[518] The BSP clearance study demonstrates an excretory defect. BSP is normally taken up by the hepatocyte and conjugated with glutathione before excretion. The normal plasma disappearance curve reflects uptake only because there is no regurgitation of conjugated BSP. The curve in a patient with Dubin-Johnson syndrome demonstrates normal early clearance; however, after 45 minutes, reflux of conjugated BSP causes a secondary rise in serum BSP concentration.[526] Further studies with BSP have demonstrated a normal storage capacity but a marked reduction in excretion.

Animal equivalents of Dubin-Johnson syndrome have permitted more careful investigation of possible defects.[518] The animals used are the Corriedale sheep and three rat strains—the Groningen yellow rat, the transport negative rat, and the Eisai hyperbilirubinemic rat.[225–228] Most work has utilized the rat models for obvious reasons. These rats are thought to have similar if not identical defects, and the defects are similar in most respects to those occurring in humans. Most studies have led to the conclusion that these rats—and by inference humans with Dubin-Johnson syndrome—have a genetic defect in a canalicular ATP-dependent organic anion transporter (see section on bilirubin excretion). This results in defective excretion of bilirubin conjugates (BMG and BDG). It should be emphasized that these rats and humans with Dubin-Johnson syndrome have normal concentrations of bilirubin in bile and that they depend almost exclusively on the liver for clearance of bilirubin. The defect is mild and results only in a different steady-state condition from the normal.

A hallmark of Dubin-Johnson syndrome is a defect in the clearance of coproporphyrin that results in an abnormal ratio of isomers in the urine of affected patients. The total excretion of coproporphyrin is normal. However, more than 80% of coproporphyrin in the urine of these patients is coproporphyrin I; in contrast, normal patients have 75% of coproporphyrin as coproporphyrin III.[527] The reason for this is unknown.

Dubin-Johnson syndrome is inherited as an autosomal recessive trait, and obligate heterozygotes have normal serum bilirubin concentrations. The diagnosis is established in the individual with a moderate degree of conjugated hyperbilirubinemia, without abnormal liver function test results, and with abnormal urinary coproporphyrin I excretion. Liver biopsy demonstrates hepatocyte pigment but is not necessary for establishing the diagnosis. No therapy is needed.

Rotor Syndrome

This very rare autosomal recessive familial disorder involves the storage capacity and excretion of conjugated bilirubin and results in elevated levels of conjugated and unconjugated bilirubin.[159, 284, 517, 518, 528] Results of other liver function tests are normal, and in contrast to the situation in Dubin-Johnson syndrome, the gallbladder is visualized with orally administered cholecystography dye and no abnormal hepatocyte pigment is present. The baseline serum bilirubin concentration varies from 2 to 7 mg/dL, but during illness can increase to 25 mg/dL. BSP clearance is delayed and does not manifest the secondary increase seen in Dubin-Johnson syndrome.[529] Urinary coproporphyrin excretion is two- to fivefold normal, and compared with in normal patients, coproporphyrin I preponderates (about 40%).[530] Obligate heterozygotes also excrete abnormal amounts of coproporphyrin in the urine, whereas serum bilirubin levels are normal. No treatment is needed.

The lack of an animal model has limited the investigation of the pathophysiology of Rotor syndrome. Since this disorder apparently results from a defect in the storage of conjugated bilirubin, a deficiency of ligandin, which may serve to shuttle both unconjugated and conjugated bilirubin through the hepatocyte, could be involved.[209] However, bilirubin uptake is normal and there is no apparent excess efflux of unconjugated bilirubin from the hepatocyte, which mitigates against a deficiency of ligandin. Current understanding of the postconjugation processing of bilirubin suggests that it involves vesicular storage and transport (see section on bilirubin excretion). The defect in Rotor's syndrome can be explained by a disordered vesicular transport system, but proof of this is lacking.[518]

Acquired Conjugated Hyperbilirubinemia (Cholestasis)

Cholestasis is defined as reduced bile formation or flow. The actual measurement of the rates of bile formation and flow is not possible, so a clinical definition of cholestasis is the presence of any condition that results in the abnormal retention of substances normally excreted into bile. In addition to conjugated bilirubin, other biliary components, such as bile salts, cholesterol, and phospholipids, are retained as a result of a generalized defect in hepatic biliary secretion.[234, 235] The pathologist's definition of cholestasis includes the retention of bile in the liver (a grossly green liver). Bile can be retained in various liver elements (bile ducts and ductules, canaliculi, and hepatocytes), depending on the disease causing cholestasis. The retention of bile results in secondary injury to hepatocytes—so-called *cholate injury*—which is seen to some degree in all cholestatic conditions. This injury and other cellular events result in increased serum concentrations of liver enzymes (aminotransferases, γ-glutamyltranspeptidase, alkaline phosphatase, and others). These markers are not disease-specific, but significant elevations of liver enzymes in association with elevated conjugated bilirubin strongly suggest primary liver disease.

Cholestasis can result from any alteration of hepatocyte function that interferes with canalicular bile formation (hepatocellular cholestasis) or mechanical obstruction of the intrahepatic or extrahepatic bile ducts (ductal cholestasis or obstructive jaundice).[234, 235] The division of cholestatic diseases into hepatocellular and ductal disorders is somewhat arbitrary because the mechanism of cholestasis in many diseases is not clearly understood. The mechanism of cholestasis in large duct obstruction is obvious: the impairment of bile hydraulics. On the other hand, the pathophysiology of hepatocellular cholestasis is poorly understood. Furthermore, it is not clear whether paucity of interlobular bile ducts, a pathologic finding in several chronic cholestasis syndromes, is the cause or effect of reduced bile flow. Although the events that lead to cholestasis may vary, the results are often the same. Secondary events, such as bile salt–induced injury to intracellular membranes, amplify the process, which "snowballs" into serious liver disease. It is often difficult to distinguish hepatocellular cholestasis from bile duct obstruction on clinical grounds. For example, the serum concentration of conjugated bilirubin is often higher in infants with hepatocellular cholestasis (idiopathic neonatal hepatitis) than in those with biliary obstruction (extrahepatic biliary atresia). As already mentioned, any elevation of serum conjugated bilirubin should be considered a sign of possible cholestatic liver disease and should be investigated appropriately.

The newborn's liver is relatively sensitive to the development of cholestasis in response to a wide variety of insults.[531] Several of the critical mechanisms for bile salt uptake and bile formation are underdeveloped at birth, which probably accounts for the cholestatic tendencies of neonates. Indeed, "physiologic cholestasis,"[532] in which serum bile salt concentrations are elevated to a level equal to that of the adult with pathologic cholestasis, is evident in the infant during the first several months of life. A wide variety of insults, such as gram-negative sepsis, heart failure, metabolic disease, or exposure to toxic substances, are capable of further compromising the mechanisms for bile formation and can cause clinical cholestasis in the neonate.

Generalized sepsis and urinary tract infection often are associated with the development of conjugated hyperbilirubinemia in newborns.[533] Bacterial infection appears to produce a toxic injury to the hepatocellular excretory apparatus without direct infection of the liver, resulting in retention of conjugated bilirubin. Often, serum transaminase or alkaline phosphatase levels are not elevated, although mild liver function test abnormalities indicating general liver cell injury may be seen in some patients. Histologic study reveals cholestasis, focal liver cell necrosis, and nonspecific liver damage.[279] Bacterial toxins have a direct cholestatic effect on liver,[534, 535] and release of such toxins into the circulation may be responsible for this disorder. In some affected individuals, hemolysis may also be induced by severe bacterial infection, and this may contribute further to the development of conjugated hyperbilirubinemia. In all cases of this syndrome, effective treatment of the infection results in prompt elimination of the hyperbilirubinemia and in the return of liver enzymes to normal. No long-term sequelae are recognized.

The more important causes of neonatal cholestasis are listed in Table 4–3. The relative frequencies of the various specific disorders that cause cholestasis in the newborn have changed over the last several decades because of changes in the precision of diagnosis, with resultant erosion of the size of the idiopathic group. Several secondary disorders related to medical management of sick newborns have emerged as important causes of cholestasis. Despite this, two idiopathic disorders continue to constitute the majority: biliary atresia and giant cell hepatitis. To attempt a discussion of the diagnosis and management of the diseases causing

Table 4–3. SHORT LIST OF DISORDERS THAT CAUSE MORE THAN 95% OF CASES OF NEONATAL CHOLESTASIS

Infectious

Sepsis, usually gram-negative enteric organisms
Other bacterial infections, particularly gram-negative enteric urinary tract infections
Syphilis
Congenital viral infections

Toxic

Total parenteral nutrition
Drug hepatotoxicity

Metabolic and Familial

Alpha₁-antitrypsin deficiency
Progressive familial intrahepatic cholestasis (Byler's disease)
Arteriohepatic dysplasia (Alagille's syndrome)
Errors of bile salt synthesis
Neonatal hemochromatosis
Galactosemia*
Hereditary fructose intolerance*
Tyrosinemia*
Zellweger's syndrome
Cystic fibrosis

Anatomic Obstruction

Choledochal cyst
Cholelithiasis

Idiopathic Neonatal Cholestasis

Neonatal giant cell hepatitis
Nonsyndromic ductal hypoplasia
Biliary atresia

*These fairly common diseases produce a toxic hepatopathy syndrome and rarely present with cholestasis.

neonatal cholestasis is beyond the scope of this chapter. The reader is referred to reviews on the subject.[531, 536]

References

1. With TK: Bile Pigments: Chemical, Biological, and Clinical Aspects. London, Academic Press, 1968.
2. Robinson SH: The origins of bilirubin. N Engl J Med 1968; 279:143.
3. Falk H: Molecular structure of bile pigments. In Ostrow JD (ed): Bile Pigments and Jaundice. New York, Marcel Dekker, 1986, p 7.
4. Bonnett R, Davies JE, et al: The structure of bilirubin. Nature 1976; 262:326.
5. Hutchinson DW, Johnson B, Knell AJ: Tautomerism and hydrogen bonding in bilirubin. Biochem J 1971; 123:483.
6. Brodersen R: Bilirubin. Solubility and interaction with albumin and phospholipid. J Biol Chem 1979; 254:2364.
7. Ostrow JD, Celic L, Mukerjee P: Molecular and micellar associations in the pH-dependent stable and metastable dissolution of unconjugated bilirubin by bile salts. J Lipid Res 1988; 29:335.
8. Hahm JS, Ostrow JD, et al: Ionization and self-association of unconjugated bilirubin, determined by rapid solvent partition from chloroform, with further studies of bilirubin solubility. J Lipid Res 1992; 33:1123.
9. Schmid R, McDonagh AF: The enzymatic formation of bilirubin. Ann N Y Acad Sci 1975; 244:533.
10. Brown SB, King RF: The mechanism of haem catabolism. Bilirubin formation in living rats by [180]oxygen labelling. Biochem J 1978; 170:297.
11. Brown SB, Troxler RF: Heme degradation and bilirubin formation. In Heirwegh KPM, Brown SB (eds): Bilirubin. Boca Raton, FL, CRC Press, 1982, p 1.
12. Tenhunen R: The enzymatic conversion of heme to bilirubin in vivo. Ann Clin Res 1976; 8(Suppl 17):2.
13. Bonnett R, McDonagh AF: Oxidative cleavage of the haem system: the four isomeric biliverdins of the IX series. J Chem Soc Chem Commun 1970; 4:237.
14. McDonagh AF, Assisi F: Commercial bilirubin: a trinity of isomers. FEBS Lett 1971; 18:315.
15. Blanckaert N, Heirwegh KPM, et al: Comparison of biliary excretion of the four isomers of bilirubin-IX in Wistar and homozygous Gunn rats. Biochem J 1977; 164:229.
16. McDonagh AF, Assisi F: Direct evidence for the acid-catalysed isomeric scrambling of bilirubin IX-α. J Chem Soc Chem Commun 1972; 1:117.
17. Wooldridge TA, Lightner DA: Separation of the III-α, and XIII-α isomers of bilirubin and bilirubin dimethyl ester by high performance liquid chromatography. J Liq Chromatogr 1978; 1:653.
18. Fevery J, Van Damme B, et al: Bilirubin conjugates in bile of man and rat in the normal state and in liver disease. J Clin Invest 1972; 51:2482.
19. Fevery J, Blankaert N: Bilirubin conjugates: formation and detection. In Popper H, Schaffner F (eds): Progress in Liver Disease. Vol. V. New York, Grune & Stratton, 1976, p 183.
20. Ullrich D, Tischler T, et al: Renal clearance of bilirubin conjugates in newborns of different gestational age. Eur J Pediatr 1993; 152:837.
21. Keunzle CC, Maier C, Ruttner JR: The nature of four bilirubin fractions from serum and three bilirubin fractions from bile. J Lab Clin Med 1966; 67:294.
22. Keunzle CC, Sommerhalder M, et al: Separation and quantitative estimation of four bilirubin fractions from serum and three bilirubin fractions from bile. J Lab Clin Med 1966; 67:294.
23. Lauff JJ, Kasper ME, et al: Isolation and preliminary characterization of a fraction of bilirubin in serum that is firmly bound to protein. Clin Chem 1982; 28:629.
24. Lauff JJ, Kasper ME, Ambrose RT: Quantitative liquid-chromatographic estimation of bilirubin species in pathologic serum. Clin Chem 1983; 29:800.
25. Weiss JS, Gautam A, et al: The clinical importance of a protein-bound fraction of serum bilirubin in patients with hyperbilirubinemia. N Engl J Med 1983; 309:147.
26. Blanckaert N, Servaes R, LeRoy P: Measurement of bilirubin-protein conjugates in serum and application to human and rat sera. J Lab Clin Med 1986; 108:77.
27. Wu T-W: Delta bilirubin: the fourth fraction of bile pigments in human serum. Isr J Chem 1983; 23:241.
28. Malloy HT, Evelyn KA: The determination of bilirubin within the photoelectric colorimeter. J Biol Chem 1937; 119:481.
29. Killenberg PG, Stevens RD, et al: The laboratory method as a variable in the interpretation of serum bilirubin fractionation. Gastroenterology 1980; 78:1011.
30. Wu T-W, Dappen GM, Powers DM, et al: The Kodak Ektachem clinical chemistry slide for measurement of bilirubin in newborns: principles and performance. Clin Chem 1982; 28:2366.
31. Spivak W, Carey MC: Reverse-phase h.p.l.c. separation, quantification and preparation of bilirubin and its conjugates from native bile. Quantitative analysis of the intact tetrapyrroles based on h.p.l.c. of their ethyl anthranilate azo derivatives. Biochem J 1985; 225:787.
32. Spivak W, Yuey W: Application of a rapid and efficient h.p.l.c. method to measure bilirubin and its conjugates from native bile and in model bile systems. Potential use as a tool for kinetic reactions and as an aid in diagnosis of hepatobiliary disease. Biochem J 1986; 234:101.
33. Rosenthal P, Blanckaert N, et al: Formation of bilirubin conjugates in human newborns. Pediatr Res 1986; 20:947.
34. Jackson SH, Hernandez AH: A new "Bilirubinometer" and its uses in estimating total and conjugated bilirubin in serum. Clin Chem 1970; 16:462.
35. Ballowitz L, Avery ME: Spectral reflectance of the skin. Biol Neonate 1970; 15:348.
36. Schreiner RL, Hannemann RE, et al: Relationship of skin reflectance and serum bilirubin: full-term Caucasian infants. Human Biol 1979; 51:31.
37. Berk PD, Howe RB, et al: Studies of bilirubin kinetics in normal adults. J Clin Invest 1969; 48:2176.
38. Berk PD, Martin JF, et al: Unconjugated hyperbilirubinemia: physiologic evaluation and experimental approaches to therapy. Ann Intern Med 1975; 82:552.
39. Poland RL, Odell GB: Physiologic jaundice: the enterohepatic circulation of bilirubin. N Engl J Med 1971; 284:1.
40. Fulop M, Sandson J, Brazeau P: Dialysability, protein binding and renal excretion of plasma conjugated bilirubin. J Clin Invest 1965; 44:666.
41. London IM, West R, et al: On origin of bile pigment in normal man. J Biol Chem 1950; 184:351.
42. Israels LG: The bilirubin shunt and shunt hyperbilirubinemia. In Popper H, Schaffner F (eds): Progress in Liver Disease. Vol. III. New York, Grune & Stratton, 1970, p 1.
43. Hughes-Jones NC, Cheney B: The use of ^{51}Cr and ^{39}Fe as red cell labels to determine the fate of normal erythrocytes in the rat. Clin Sci 1961; 20:323.
44. Tenhunen R, Marver HS, Schmidt R: Microsomal heme oxygenase. Characterization of the enzyme. J Biol Chem 1969; 244:6388.
45. Tenhunen R, Marver HS, Schmid R: The enzymatic catabolism of haemoglobin: stimulation of microsomal heme oxygenase by hematin. J Lab Clin Med 1970; 75:410.
46. Rodgers PA, Vreman HJ, et al: Sources of carbon monoxide (CO) in biological systems and applications of CO detection technologies. Semin Perinatol 1994; 18:2.
47. Tenhunen R, Ross ME, et al: Reduced nicotinamide-adenine dinucleotide phosphate dependent biliverdin reductase: partial purification and characterization. Biochemistry 1970; 9:298.
48. Bakken AF, Thaler MM, Schmid R: Metabolic regulation of heme catabolism and bilirubin production. 1. Hormonal control of hepatic heme oxygenase activity. J Clin Invest 1972; 51:530.
49. Kutz K, Egger G, et al: Effect of fasting on endogenous carbon monoxide production in normal subjects and those with constitutional hepatic dysfunction. In Berk PD, Berlin NI (eds): Chemistry and Physiology of Bile Pigments. Bethesda, MD, U.S. Department of Health, Education and Welfare, 1977, p 156.
50. Arias IM, Schorr JB, et al: Congenital hypertrophic pyloric stenosis with jaundice. Pediatrics 1959; 24:338.
51. Felsher BF, Richard D, Redeker AG: The reciprocal relation between caloric intake and the degree of hyperbilirubinemia in Gilbert's syndrome. N Engl J Med 1970; 283:170.

52. Felsher BF, Carpio NM: Calorie intake and unconjugated hyperbilirubinemia. Gastroenterology 1975; 69:42.

53. Coburn RF, Williams WJ, et al: Endogenous carbon monoxide production in patients with hemolytic anemia. J Clin Invest 1966; 45:460.

54. Engel RR. Alternative sources of carbon monoxide. In Berk PD, Berlin NI (eds): Chemistry and Physiology of Bile Pigments. Bethesda, MD, Department of Health Education and Welfare, 1977, p 148.

55. Berk PD, Rodkey FL, et al: Comparison of plasma bilirubin turnover and carbon monoxide production in man. J Lab Clin Med 1974; 83:29.

56. Stevenson DK, Ostrander CR, et al: Trace gas analysis in bilirubin metabolism: a technical review and current state of the art. Adv Pediatr 1982; 29:129.

57. Stevenson DK, Vreman HJ, et al: Bilirubin production in healthy term infants as measured by carbon monoxide in breath. Clin Chem 1994; 40:1934.

58. Colleran E, O'Carra P: Enzymology and comparative physiology of biliverdin reduction. In Berk PD, Berlin NI (eds): Chemistry and Physiology of Bile Pigments. Bethesda, MD, Department of Health, Education and Welfare, 1977, p 69.

59. Maines MD: Multiple forms of biliverdin reductase: function, multiplicity, regulatory mechanisms, and clinical applications. FASEB J 1988; 2:2557.

60. Maines MD: Multiple forms of biliverdin reductase: age-related change in pattern of expression in rat liver and brain. Mol Pharmacol 1990; 38:481.

61. Frydman RB, Bari S, et al: The enzymatic and chemical reduction of extended biliverdins. Biochem Biophys Res Commun 1990; 171:465.

62. Yoshinaga T, Sassa S, Kappas A: The occurrence of molecular interactions among NADPH-cytochrome c reductase, heme oxygenase, and biliverdin reductase in heme degradation. J Biol Chem 1982; 257:7786.

63. Crawford JM, Ransil BJ, et al: Hepatic disposition and biliary excretion of bilirubin and bilirubin glucuronides in intact rats: differential processing of pigments derived from intra- and extrahepatic sources. J Clin Invest 1987; 79:1172.

64. Crawford JM, Hauser SC, Gollan JL: Formation, hepatic metabolism, and transport of bile pigments: a status report. Semin Liver Dis 1988; 8:105.

65. Brandes JM, Berk PD, et al: Transport of bilirubin and glucose by the isolated perfused human placenta. Contrib Gynecol Obstet 1985; 13:147.

66. McDonagh AF, Palma LA, Schmid R: Reduction of biliverdin and placental transfer of bilirubin and biliverdin in the pregnant guinea pig. Biochem J 1981; 194:273.

67. Frei B, Stocker R, Ames BN: Antioxidant defenses and lipid peroxidation in human blood plasma. Proc Natl Acad Sci USA 1988; 85:9748.

68. Stocker R, Glazer AN, Ames BN: Antioxidant activity of albumin-bound bilirubin. Proc Natl Acad Sci USA 1987; 84:5918.

69. Farrera JA, Jauma A, et al: The antioxidant role of bile pigments evaluated by chemical tests. Bioorg Med Chem 1994; 2:181.

70. Krinsky NI. Mechanism of action of biological antioxidants. Proc Soc Exp Biol Med 1992; 200:248.

71. Neuzil J, Stocker R: Free and albumin-bound bilirubin are efficient co-antioxidants for alpha-tocopherol, inhibiting plasma and low density lipoprotein lipid peroxidation. J Biol Chem 1994; 269:16712.

72. Wu TW, Carey D, et al: The cytoprotective effects of bilirubin and biliverdin on rat hepatocytes and human erythrocytes and the impact of albumin. Biochem Cell Biol 1991; 69:828.

73. Llesuy SF, Tomaro ML: Heme oxygenase and oxidative stress. Evidence of involvement of bilirubin as physiological protector against oxidative damage. Biochim Biophys Acta 1994; 1223:9.

74. Pauly TH, Smith M, Gillespie M: Bilirubin as an antioxidant: effect on group B streptococci-induced pulmonary hypertension in infant piglets. Biol Neonate 1991; 60:320.

75. Fauchere JC, Meier-Gibbons FE, et al: Retinopathy of prematurity and bilirubin—no clinical evidence for a beneficial role of bilirubin as a physiological anti-oxidant. Eur J Pediatr 1994; 153:358.

76. Olinescu R, Alexandrescu R, et al: Tissue lipid peroxidation may be triggered by increased formation of bilirubin in vivo. Res Commun Chem Pathol Pharmacol 1994; 84:27.

77. Granger DN: Role of xanthine oxidase and granulocytes in ischemia-reperfusion injury. Am J Physiol 1988; 255:H1269.

78. Crissinger KD: Regulation of hemodynamics and oxygenation in developing intestine: insight into the pathogenesis of necrotizing enterocolitis. Acta Paediatr 1994; 396(Suppl):8.

79. Tiribelli C, Ostrow JD: New concepts in bilirubin chemistry, transport and metabolism. Hepatology 1993; 17:715.

80. Jacobsen J: Binding of bilirubin to human serum albumin—determination of the dissociation constants. FEBS Lett 1969; 5:112.

81. Jacobsen C, Jacobsen J: Dansylation of human serum albumin in the study of the primary binding sites of bilirubin and L-tryptophan. Biochem J 1979; 181:251.

82. Brodersen R: Bilirubin transport in the newborn infant, reviewed with relation to kernicterus. J Pediatr 1980; 96:349.

83. Jacobsen J, Brodersen R: Albumin-bilirubin binding mechanism. J Biol Chem 1983; 258:6319.

84. Odell GB: Neonatal jaundice. In Popper H, Schaffner F (eds): Progress in Liver Disease. Vol V. New York, Grune & Stratton, 1976, p 457.

85. Brodersen R: Free bilirubin in blood plasma of the newborn: effects of albumin, fatty acids, pH, displacing drugs and phototherapy. In Stern L, Oh W, et al (eds): Intensive Care of the Newborn. Vol II. New York, Masson, 1978, p 331.

86. Inoue M, Hirata E, et al: The role of albumin in the hepatic transport of bilirubin: studies in mutant analbuminemic rats. J Biochem 1985; 97:737.

87. Takahashi H, Sugiyama K, et al: Penetration of bilirubin into the brain in albumin-deficient and jaundiced rats (AJR) and Nagase analbuminemic rats (NAR). J Biochem 1984; 96:1705.

88. Yamashita M, Adachi Y, et al: Serum binding and biliary excretion of bilirubin after bilirubin loading in Nagase analbuminemic rats and heterozygous (Jj) Gunn rats. J Lab Clin Med 1988; 112:443.

89. Suzuki N, Yamaguchi T, Nakajima H: Role of high-density lipoprotein in transport of circulating bilirubin in rats. J Biol Chem 1988; 263:5037.

90. Lee KS, Gartner LM: Bilirubin binding by plasma proteins: a critical evaluation of methods and clinical implications. Rev Perinatal Med 1978; 2:319.

91. Cashore WJ, Gartner LM, et al: Clinical application of neonatal bilirubin binding determinations: current status. J Pediatr 1978; 93:827.

92. Wells R, Hammond K, et al: Relationships of bilirubin binding parameters. Clin Chem 1982; 28:432.

93. Gitzelmann-Cumarasamy N, Kuenzle CC: Bilirubin binding tests: living up to expectations. Pediatrics 1979; 64:375.

94. Ryahl RG, Peake MJ: Theoretical constraints in the measurement of serum bilirubin binding capacity. Clin Biochem 1982; 15:146.

95. Paumgartner G, Reichen J: Kinetics of hepatic uptake of unconjugated bilirubin. Clin Sci Mol Med 1976; 51:169.

96. Sorrentino D, Potter BJ, Berk PD: From albumin to the cytoplasm: the hepatic uptake of organic anions. Prog Liver Dis 1990; 9:203.

97. Sorrentino D, Berk PD: Mechanistic aspects of hepatic bilirubin uptake. Semin Liver Dis 1988; 8:119.

98. Wolkoff AW, Chung G: An organic anion binding protein isolated from rat liver cell plasma membrane. Gastroenterology 1978; 75:995.

99. Berk PD, Potter BJ, Stremmel W: Role of plasma membrane ligand-binding proteins in the hepatocellular uptake of albumin-bound organic anions. Hepatology 1987; 7:165.

100. Stremmel W, Berk PD: Hepatocellular uptake of sulfobromophthalein and bilirubin is selectively inhibited by an antibody to the liver plasma membrane sulfobromophthalein/bilirubin binding protein. J Clin Invest 1986; 78:822.

101. Stremmel W: What's new in the hepatocellular uptake mechanism of bilirubin and fatty acids? Pathol Res Pract 1988; 183:524.

102. Stremmel W, Diede HE: Cellular uptake of conjugated bilirubin and sulfobromophthalein (BSP) by the human hepatoma cell line Hep G2 is mediated by a membrane BSP/bilirubin binding protein. J Hepatol 1990; 10:99.

103. Adachi Y, Roy-Chowdhury J, et al: Hepatic uptake of bilirubin

diglucuronide: analysis by using sinusoidal plasma membrane vesicles. J Biochem 1990; 107:749.

104. Goeser T, Nakata R, et al: The rat hepatocyte plasma membrane organic anion binding protein is immunologically related to the mitochondrial F1 adenosine triphosphatase beta-subunit. J Clin Invest 1990; 86:220.

105. Weinman SA: Identifying the hepatic organic transporter: one of many? Hepatology 1994; 20:1642.

106. Stollman YR, Gartner U, et al: Hepatic bilirubin uptake in the isolated perfused rat liver is not facilitated by albumin binding. J Clin Invest 1983; 72:718.

107. Fleischner GM, Arias IM: Structure and function of ligandin and Z protein in the liver. A progress report. In Popper H, Schaffner F (eds): Progress in Liver Diseases. Vol. V. New York, Grune & Stratton, 1976, p 172.

108. Kaplowitz N: Physiological significance of glutathione S-transferases. Am J Physiol 1980; 239:439.

109. Ookhtens M, Lyon I, et al: Inhibition of glutathione efflux in the perfused rat liver and isolated hepatocytes by organic anions and bilirubin. Kinetics, sidedness, and molecular forms. J Clin Invest 1988; 82:608.

110. Theilmann L, Stollman YR, et al: Does Z-protein have a role in transport of bilirubin and bromosulfophthalein by isolated perfused rat liver? Hepatology 1984; 4:923.

111. Ockner RK, Manning JA, Kane JP: Fatty acid binding protein isolation from rat liver, characterization and immunochemical quantification. J Biol Chem 1982; 257:7872.

112. Farrell GC, Gollan JL, Schmid R: Efflux of bilirubin into plasma following hepatic degradation of exogenous heme. Proc Soc Exp Biol Med 1980; 163:504.

113. Levi AJ, Gatmaitan Z, et al: Deficiency of hepatic organic anion binding protein and impaired organic anion uptake by liver and "physiologic" jaundice in newborn monkeys. N Engl J Med 1970; 283:1136.

114. Weisiger RA: Dissociation from albumin: a potentially rate-limiting step in the clearance of substances by the liver. Proc Natl Acad Sci USA 1985; 82:1563.

115. Kapitulnik J, Ostrow JD: Stimulation of bilirubin catabolism in jaundiced Gunn rats by an inducer of microsomal mixed-function mono-oxygenases. Proc Natl Acad Sci USA 1978; 75:682.

116. Cardenas-Vazquez R, Yokosuka O, Billing BH: Enzymatic oxidation of unconjugated bilirubin by rat liver. Biochem J 1986; 236:625.

117. Berry CS, Zarembo JE, Ostrow JD: Evidence for conversion of bilirubin to dihydroxyl derivatives in the Gunn rat. Biochem Biophys Res Commun 1972; 49:1366.

118. Cuypers HT, Ter Haar EM, Jansen PL: Microsomal conjugation and oxidation of bilirubin. Biochim Biophys Acta 1983; 758:135.

119. Blanckaert N, Fevery J, Heirwegh KPM: Characterization of the major diazo-positive pigments in bile of homozygous Gunn rats. Biochem J 1977; 164:237.

120. DeMatteis F, Dawson SJ, et al: Inducible bilirubin-degrading system of rat liver microsomes: role of cytochrome P450IA1. Mol Pharmacol 1991; 40:686.

121. Burchell B, Coughtrie MW: UDP-glucuronosyltransferases. Pharmacol Ther 1989; 1989:125.

122. Burchell B, Blanckaert N: Bilirubin mono- and di-glucuronide formation by purified rat liver microsomal bilirubin UDP-glucuronyltransferase. Biochem J 1984; 223:461.

123. Blanckaert N, Gollan J, Schmid R: Bilirubin diglucuronide synthesis by a UDP-glucuronic acid-dependent enzyme system in rat liver microsomes. Proc Natl Acad Sci USA 1979; 76:2037.

124. Chowdhury JR, Chowdhury NR, et al: Bilirubin mono- and diglucuronide formation by human liver in vitro: assay by high-pressure liquid chromatography. Hepatology 1981; 1:622.

125. Whiting JF, Narciso JP, et al: Deconjugation of bilirubin-IX alpha glucuronides: a physiologic role of hepatic microsomal beta-glucuronidase. J Biol Chem 1993; 268:23197.

126. Whitmer DI, Russell PE, et al: Hepatic microsomal glucuronidation of bilirubin is modulated by the lipid microenvironment of membrane-bound substrate. J Biol Chem 1986; 261:7170.

127. Zucker SD, Storch J, et al: Mechanism of the spontaneous transfer of unconjugated bilirubin between small unilamellar phosphatidylcholine vesicles. Biochem 1992; 31:3184.

128. Zucker SD, Goessling W, et al: Membrane lipid composition

129. Whitmer DI, Russell PE, Gollan JL: Membrane-membrane interactions associated with rapid transfer of liposomal bilirubin to microsomal UDP-glucuronyltransferase. Relevance for hepatocellular transport and biotransformation of hydrophobic substrates. Biochem J 1987; 244:41.

130. Whitmer DI, Ziurys JC, Gollan JL: Hepatic microsomal glucuronidation of bilirubin in unilamellar liposomal membranes. Implications for intracellular transport of lipophilic substrates. J Biol Chem 1984; 259:11969.

131. Jackson MR, McCarthy LR, et al: Cloning of cDNAs coding for rat hepatic microsomal UDP-glucuronosyltransferases. Gene 1985; 34:147.

132. Jackson MR, McCarthy LR, et al: Cloning of a human liver microsomal UDP-glucuronosyltranferase cDNA. Biochem J 1987; 242:581.

133. Chowdhury NR, Gross F, et al: Purification of multiple normal and functionally defective isoforms of UDP-glucuronyltransferase from Gunn rat liver. J Clin Invest 1987; 79:327.

134. Burchell B, Jackson MR, et al: The molecular biology of UDP-glucuronosyltransferases. Biochem Soc Trans 1987; 15:581.

135. Burchell B, Coughtrie MW, et al: Genetic deficiency of bilirubin glucuronidation in rats and humans. Mol Aspects Med 1987; 9:429.

136. Mackenzie PI: Rat liver UDP-glucuronosyltranferase. Sequence and expression of cDNA encoding a phenobarbital-inducible form. J Biol Chem 1986; 261:6119.

137. Mackenzie PI, Rodbourn L: Organization of the rat UDP-glucuronosyltransferase, UDPGTr-2, gene and characterization of its promoter. J Biol Chem 1990; 265:11328.

138. Robertson KJ, Clarke D, et al: Investigation of the molecular basis of the genetic deficiency of UDP-glucuronosyltransferase in Crigler-Najjar syndrome. J Inherit Metab Dis 1991; 14:563.

139. Clarke DJ, Keen JN, Burchell B: Isolation and characterization of a new hepatic bilirubin UDP-glucuronosyltransferase. Absence from Gunn rat liver. FEBS Lett 1992; 299:183.

140. Ritter JK, Crawford JM, Owens IS: Cloning of two human liver bilirubin UDP-glucuronosyltransferase cDNAs with expression in COS-1 cells. J Biol Chem 1991; 266:1043.

141. Bosma PJ, Chowdhury NR, et al: Sequence of exons and the flanking regions of human bilirubin-UDP-glucuronosyltransferase gene complex and identification of a genetic mutation in a patient with Crigler-Najjar syndrome, type I. Hepatology 1992; 15:941.

142. Bosma PJ, Chowdhury JR, et al: Mechanisms of inherited deficiencies of multiple UDP-glucuronosyltransferase isoforms in two patients with Crigler-Najjar syndrome, type I. FASEB J 1992; 6:2859.

143. Chowdhury JR, Chowdhury NR: Unveiling the mysteries of inherited disorders of bilirubin glucuronidation. Gastroenterology 1993; 105:288.

144. Aono S, Yamada Y, et al: A new type of defect in the gene for bilirubin uridine 5'-diphosphate-glucuronosyltransferase in a patient with Crigler-Najjar syndrome type I. Pediatr Res 1994; 35:629.

145. Nagai F, Homma H, et al: Studies on the genetic linkage of bilirubin and androsterone UDP-glucuronyltransferases by cross-breeding of two mutant rat strains. Biochem J 1988; 252:897.

146. Mackenzie PI: Expression of chimeric cDNAs in cell culture defines a region of UDP glucuronosyltransferase involved in substrate selection. J Biol Chem 1990; 265:3432.

147. Brierley CH, Burchell B: Human UDP-glucuronosyltransferase: chemical defense, jaundice and gene therapy. Bioessays 1993; 15:749.

148. Burchell B, Nebert DW, et al: The UDP glucuronosyltransferase gene superfamily: suggested nomenclature based on evolutionary divergence. DNA Cell Biol 1991; 10:487.

149. Ritter JK, Chen F, et al: Two human liver cDNAs encode UDP-glucuronosyltransferases with 2 log differences in activity toward parallel substrates including hyodeoxycholic acid and certain estrogen derivatives. Biochemistry 1992; 31:3409.

150. Owens IS, Ritter JK: The novel bilirubin/phenol UDP-glucuron-

osyltransferase *UGT1* gene locus: implications for multiple non-hemolytic familial phenotypes. Pharmacogenetics 1992; 2:93.

151. Ritter JK, Yeatman MT, et al: A phenylalanine codon deletion at the *UGT1* gene complex locus of a Crigler-Najjar type I patient generates a pH-sensitive bilirubin UDP-glucuronosyltransferase. J Biol Chem 1993; 268:23573.

152. Ritter JK, Yeatman MT, et al: Identification of a genetic alteration in the code for bilirubin UDP-glucuronosyltransferase in the *UGT1* gene complex of a Crigler-Najjar type I patient. J Clin Invest 1992; 90:150.

153. Erps LT, Ritter JK, et al: Identification of two single base substitutions in the *UGT1* gene locus which abolish bilirubin uridine diphosphate glucuronosyltransferase activity in vitro. J Clin Invest 1994; 93:564.

154. Moghrabi N, Clarke DJ, et al: Cosegregation of intragenic markers with a novel mutation that causes Crigler-Najjar syndrome type 1: implication in carrier detection and prenatal diagnosis. Am J Hum Genet 1993; 53:722.

155. Moghrabi N, Clarke DJ, et al: Identification of an A-to-G missense mutation in exon 2 of the *UGT1* gene complex that causes Crigler-Najjar syndrome type 2. Genomics 1993; 18:171.

156. Seppen J, Bosma PJ, et al: Discrimination between Crigler-Najjar type I and II by expression of mutant bilirubin uridine diphosphate-glucuronosyltransferase. J Clin Invest 1994; 94:2385.

157. Bosma PJ, Seppen J, et al: Bilirubin UDP-glucuronosyltransferase 1 is the only relevant bilirubin glucuronidating isoform in man. J Biol Chem 1994; 269:17960.

158. Chowdhury NR, Arias IM, et al: Substrates and products of purified rat liver bilirubin UDP-glucuronosyltransferase. Hepatology 1986; 6:123.

159. Jansen PL, Oude Elferink RP: Hereditary hyperbilirubinemias: a molecular and mechanistic approach. Sem Liver Dis 1988; 8:168.

160. Erickson RH, Zakim D, Vessey DA: Preparation and properties of a phospholipid-free form of microsomal UDP-glucuronosyltransferase. Biochemistry 1978; 17:3706.

161. Jansen PLM, Arias IM: Delipidation and reactivation of UDP glucuronosyltransferase from rat liver. Biochim Biophys Acta 1975; 391:28.

162. Vanstapel F, Blanckaert N: Topology and regulation of bilirubin UDP-glucuronyltransferase in sealed native microsomes from rat liver. Arch Biochem Biophys 1988; 263:216.

163. Peters WH, Allebes WA, et al: Characterization and tissue specificity of a monoclonal antibody against human uridine 5′-diphosphate-glucuronosyltransferase. Gastroenterology 1987; 93:162.

164. Chowdhury JR, Novikoff PM, et al: Distribution of UDP-glycuronosyltransferase in rat tissue. Proc Natl Acad Sci USA 1985; 82:2990.

165. Peters WH, Nagengast FM, van Tongeren JH: Glutathione S-transferase, cytochrome P450, and uridine 5′-diphosphate-glucuronosyltransferase in human small intestine and liver. Gastroenterology 1989; 96:783.

166. Sutherland L, Ebner T, Burchell B: The expression of UDP-glucuronosyltransferases of the UGTI family in human liver and kidney and in response to drugs. Biochem Pharmacol 1993; 45:295.

167. Gartner LM, Lee KS, et al: Development of bilirubin transport and metabolism in the newborn rhesus monkey. J Pediatr 1977; 90:513.

168. Crawford JM, Ransil BJ, et al: Hepatic microsomal bilirubin UDP-glucuronosyltransferase. The kinetics of bilirubin mono- and diglucuronide synthesis. J Biol Chem 1992; 267:16943.

169. Vanstapel F, Blanckaert N: On the binding of bilirubin and its structural analogues to hepatic microsomal bilirubin UDP glucuronyltransferase. Biochemistry 1987; 26:6074.

170. Hjelle JJ: Hepatic UDP-glucuronic acid regulation during acetaminophen. J Pharmacol Exp Ther 1986; 237:750.

171. Peters WH, Jansen PL: Microsomal UDP-glucuronyltransferase–catalyzed bilirubin diglucuronide formation in human liver. J Hepatol 1986; 2:182.

172. Mackenzie PI: The effect of *N*-linked glycosylation on the substrate preferences of UDP glucuronosyltransferases. Biochem Biophys Res Commun 1990; 166:1293.

173. Kamisako T, Adachi Y, Yamamoto T: Effect of UDP-glucuronic acid depletion by salicylamide on biliary bilirubin excretion in the rat. J Pharmacol Exp Ther 1990; 254:380.

174. Hauser SC, Ziurys JC, Gollan JL: Subcellular distribution and regulation of hepatic bilirubin UDP-glucuronyltransferase. J Biol Chem 1984; 259:4527.

175. Hauser SC, Gollan JL: Mechanistic and molecular aspects of hepatic bilirubin glucuronidation. Prog Liver Dis 1990; 9:225.

176. Shepherd SR, Baird SJ, et al: An investigation of the transverse topology of bilirubin UDP-glucuronyltransferase in rat hepatic endoplasmic reticulum. Biochem J 1989; 259:617.

177. Hauser SC, Ziurys JC, Gollan JL: A membrane transporter mediates access of uridine 5′-diphosphoglucuronic acid from the cytosol into the endoplasmic reticulum of rat hepatocytes: implications for glucuronidation reactions. Biochim Biophys Acta 1988; 967:149.

178. Bossuyt X, Blanckaert N: Carrier-mediated transport of intact UDP-glucuronic acid into the lumen of endoplasmic-reticulum–derived vesicles from rat liver. Biochem J 1994; 302:261.

179. Vessey DA, Goldenberg J, Zakim D: Kinetic properties of microsomal UDP-glucuronosyltransferase. Evidence for cooperative kinetics and activation by UDP-*N*-acetylglucosamine. Biochim Biophys Acta 1973; 309:58.

180. Zakim D, Goldenberg J, Vessey DA: Effects of metals on the properties of hepatic microsomal uridine diphosphate glucuronosyltransferase. Biochemistry 1973; 12:4068.

181. Goldstein RB, Vessey DA, et al: Perinatal developmental changes in hepatic UDP-glucuronyltransferase. Biochem J 1980; 186:841.

182. Campbell MT, Wishart GJ: The effect of premature and delayed birth on the development of UDP-glucuronyltransferase activities towards bilirubin, morphine and testosterone in the rat. Biochem J 1980; 186:617.

183. Leakey JE, Hume R, Burchell B: Development of multiple activities of UDP-glucuronosyltransferase in human liver. Biochem J 1987; 243:859.

184. Burchell B, Coughtrie M, et al: Development of human liver UDP-glucuronosyltransferases. Dev Pharmacol Ther 1989; 13:70.

185. Kawade N, Onishi S: The prenatal and postnatal development of UDP glucuronyltransferase activity towards bilirubin and the effect of premature birth on this activity in the human liver. Biochem J 1981; 196:257.

186. Coughtrie MW, Burchell B, et al: The inadequacy of perinatal glucuronidation: immunoblot analysis of the developmental expression of individual UDP-glucuronosyltransferase isoenzymes in rat and human liver microsomes. Mol Pharmacol 1988; 34:729.

187. Cukier JO, Whitington PF, Odell GB: Bilirubin, UDP-glucuronyl transferase of liver in post-mature rats. A functional and morphologic comparison. Lab Invest 1981; 44:368.

188. Muraca M, Fevery J: Influence of sex and sex steroids on bilirubin uridine diphosphate-glucuronosyltransferase activity of rat liver. Gastroenterology 1984; 87:308.

189. Heirwegh KPM, Fevery J, et al: Separation by thin-layer chromatography and structure elucidation of bilirubin conjugates isolated from dog bile. Biochem J 1975; 145:185.

190. Berry C, Hallinan T: Summary of a novel three component regulatory model for uridine diphosphate glucuronyl transferase. Biochem Soc Trans 1976; 4:650.

191. Sommerer U, Gordon ER, Goresky CA: Microsomal specificity underlying the differing hepatic formation of bilirubin glucuronide and glucose conjugates by rat and dog. Hepatology 1988; 8:116.

192. Senafi SB, Clarke DJ, Burchell B: Investigation of the substrate specificity of a cloned expressed human bilirubin UDP-glucuronosyltransferase: UDP-sugar specificity and involvement in steroid and xenobiotic glucuronidation. Biochem J 1994; 303:233.

193. Gourley GR, Mogilevsky WM, et al: Effects of anesthetic agents on bile pigment excretion in the rat. Hepatology 1985; 5:610.

194. Eletr S, Zakim D, Vessey DA: A spin-label study of the role of phospholipids in the regulation of membrane-bound microsomal enzymes. J Mol Biol 1973; 78:351.

195. Hochman Y, Zakim D: Evidence that UDP-glucuronosyltransferase in liver microsomes at 37 degrees C is in a gel phase lipid environment. J Biol Chem 1983; 258:11758.

196. Hochman Y, Kelley M, Zakim D: Modulation of the number of ligand binding sites of UDP-glucuronosyltransferase by the gel to liquid-crystal phase transition of phosphatidylcholines. J Biol Chem 1983; 258:6509.

197. Magdalou J, Hochman Y, Zakim D: Factors modulating the catalytic specificity of a pure form of UDP-glucuronosyltransferase. J Biol Chem 1982; 257:13624.

198. Zakim D, Vessey DA: The effect of a temperature-induced phase change within membrane lipids on the regulatory properties of microsomal uridine diphosphate glucuronosyltransferase. J Biol Chem 1975; 78:351.

199. Kapitulnik J, Tshershedsky M, Barenholz Y: Fluidity of the rat liver microsomal membrane: increase at birth. Science 1979; 206:843.

200. Vaisman SL, Lee K-S, Gartner LM: Xylose, glucose and glucuronic acid conjugation of bilirubin in the newborn rat. Pediatr Res 1976; 10:967.

201. Blumenthal SG, Stucker T, et al: Changes in bilirubins in human prenatal development. Biochem J 1980; 186:693.

202. Fevery J, Blanckaert N, Heirwegh KPM: Unconjugated bilirubin and an increased proportion of bilirubin monoconjugates in the bile of patients with Gilbert's syndrome and Crigler-Najjar syndrome. J Clin Invest 1977; 60:970.

203. Goresky CA, Gordon ER, et al: Definition of a conjugation dysfunction in Gilbert's syndrome: studies of the handling of bilirubin loads and of the pattern of bilirubin conjugates secreted in bile. Clin Sci Mol Med 1978; 55:63.

204. Fevery J, Blanckaert N, LeRoy P, et al: Analysis of bilirubins in biological fluids by extraction and thin-layer chromatography of the intact tetrapyrroles: application to bile of patients with Gilbert's syndrome, hemolysis, or cholelithiasis. Hepatology 1983; 3:177.

205. Gourley GR, Arend R, Mogilevsky WS, et al: Bilirubin conjugate excretion and bilirubin uridine diphosphoglucuronyltransferase activity in nonjaundiced homozygous and heterozygous Gunn rats. J Lab Clin Med 1986; 108:436.

206. Adachi Y, Yamashita M, et al: Proportion of conjugated bilirubin in bile in relation to hepatic bilirubin UDP-glucuronyltransferase activity. Clin Biochem 1990; 23:131.

207. Muraca M, Rubaltelli FF, et al: Unconjugated and conjugated bilirubin pigments during perinatal development. II. Studies on serum of healthy newborns and of neonates with erythroblastosis fetalis. Biol Neonate 1990; 57:1.

208. Gartner LM, Lane DL, et al: Bilirubin transport by liver in adult *Macaca mulatta*. Am J Physiol 1971; 220:1528.

209. Wolkoff AW, Ketley JN, et al: Hepatic accumulation and intracellular binding of conjugated bilirubin. J Clin Invest 1977; 61:142.

210. Crawford JM, Berken CA, Gollan JL: Role of the hepatocyte microtubular system in the excretion of bile salts and biliary lipid: implications for intracellular vesicular transport. J Lipid Res 1988; 29:144.

211. Crawford JM, Gollan JL: Hepatocyte cotransport of taurocholate and bilirubin glucuronides: role of microtubules. Am J Physiol 1988; 255:G121.

212. Goresky CA, Haddad HH, et al: The enhancement of maximal bilirubin excretion with taurocholate-induced increments in bile flow. Can J Physiol Pharmacol 1974; 52:389.

213. Collado PS, Munoz ME, et al: Influence of bile acids on the biliary transport maximum of phenolsulfonphthalein in the rat. Clin Exp Pharmacol Phys 1988; 15:893.

214. Esteller A, Gonzalez J, et al: Enhancement of maximal bilirubin excretion by bile salts in the anesthetized rabbit. Q J Exp Physiol 1984; 69:217.

215. Garcia-Marin JJ, Gonzalez J, Esteller A: Influence of dehydrocholate on bilirubin transport into bile in the rat. Digestion 1986; 33:80.

216. Verkade HJ, Havinga R, et al: Mechanism of bile acid–induced biliary lipid secretion in the rat: effect conjugated bilirubin. Am J Physiol 1993; 264:G462.

217. Apstein MD: Inhibition of biliary phospholipid and cholesterol secretion by bilirubin in the Sprague-Dawley and Gunn rat. Gastroenterology 1984; 87:634.

218. Kohlhaw K, Christians U, et al: Cyclosporine and bilirubin metabolites compete for the hepatic excretory system. Transplant Proc 1994; 26:2798.

219. Roman ID, Monte MJ, et al: Inhibition of hepatocytary vesicular transport by cyclosporin A in the rat: relationship with cholestasis and hyperbilirubinemia. Hepatology 1990; 12:83.

220. Crawford JM, Crawford AR, Strahs DC: Microtubule-dependent transport of bile salts through hepatocytes: cholic vs. taurocholic acid. Hepatology 1993; 18:903.

221. Crawford JM, Crawford AR: Push me–pull you: the challenge of endocytic sorting. Hepatology 1993; 17:342.

222. Dubin M, Maurice M, et al: Influence of colchicine and phalloidin on bile secretion and hepatic ultrastructure in the rat. Possible interaction between microtubules and microfilaments. Gastroenterology 1980; 79:646.

223. Gregory DH, Vlahcevic ZR, et al: Mechanism of secretion of biliary lipids: role of a microtubular system in hepatocellular transport of biliary lipids in the rat. Gastroenterology 1978; 74:93.

224. Tazuma S, Holzbach RT: Transport of conjugated bilirubin and other organic anions in bile: relation to biliary lipid structures. Proc Natl Acad Sci U S A 1987; 84:2052.

225. Sathirakul K, Suzuki H, et al: Kinetic analysis of hepatobiliary transport of organic anions in Eisai hyperbilirubinemic mutant rats. J Pharmacol Exp Ther 1993; 265:1301.

226. Nishida T, Gatmaitan Z, et al: Two distinct mechanisms for bilirubin glucuronide transport by rat bile canalicular membrane vesicles. Demonstration of defective ATP-dependent transport in rats (TR⁻) with inherited conjugated hyperbilirubinemia. J Clin Invest 1992; 90:2130.

227. Kuronuma Y, Yoshida H, et al: Relationship between biliary excretion of bilirubin and glutathione disulfide. Gastroenterol Jpn 1993; 28:292.

228. Jansen PL, Peters WH, Meijer DK: Hepatobiliary excretion of organic anions in double-mutant rats with a combination of defective canalicular transport and uridine 5'-diphosphate-glucuronyltransferase deficiency. Gastroenterology 1987; 93:1094.

229. Adachi Y, Koyayashi H, et al: Bilirubin diglucuronide transport by rat liver canalicular membrane vesicles: stimulation by bicarbonate ion. Hepatology 1991; 14:1251.

230. Ricci GL, Cornelius M, et al: Maximal hepatic bilirubin transport in the rat during somatostatin-induced cholestasis and taurocholate-choleresis. J Lab Clin Med 1983; 101:835.

231. Ricci GL, Michiels R, et al: Enhancement by secretin of the apparently maximal hepatic transport of bilirubin in the rat. Hepatology 1984; 4:651.

232. Sieg A, Stiehl A, et al: Similarities in maximal biliary bilirubin output in the normal rat after administration of unconjugated bilirubin or bilirubin glucuronide. Hepatology 1984; 10:14.

233. Carey MC, Koretsky AP: Self-association of unconjugated bilirubin:IXα in aqueous solution at pH 10.0 and physical-chemical interactions with bile salt monomers and micelles. Biochem J 1979; 179:675.

234. Phillips MJ, Poucell S, Oda M: Mechanisms of cholestasis. Lab Invest 1986; 54:593.

235. Reichen J, Simon FR: Mechanisms of cholestasis. Int Rev Exp Pathol 1984; 26:231.

236. Balistreri WF: Neonatal cholestasis. J Pediatr 1985; 106:171.

237. Odell GB: Neonatal Hyperbilirubinemia. New York, Grune & Stratton, 1980.

238. Elder G, Gray CH, et al: Bile pigment fate in the gastrointestinal tract. Semin Hematol 1972; 9:71.

239. Lester R, Schmid R: Intestinal absorption of bile pigments. II. Bilirubin absorption in man. N Engl J Med 1963; 269:178.

240. Dhar GJ: Enterohepatic circulation and plasma transport of urobilinogen. In Berk PD, Berlin NI (eds): Chemistry and Physiology of Bile Pigments. Bethesda, MD, US Department of Health, Education and Welfare, 1977, p 526.

241. Watson CJ: Composition of the urobilin group in urine, bile and feces and the significance of variations in health and disease. J Lab Clin Med 1959; 1:54.

242. Watson CJ: The urobilinoids: milestones in their history and some recent developments. In Berk PD, Berlin NI (eds): Chemistry and Physiology of Bile Pigments. Bethesda, MD, US Department of Health, Education and Welfare, 1977, p 469.

243. Brown A: Erythrocyte metabolism and hemolysis in the newborn. Pediatr Clin North Am 1966; 13:879.

244. Maisels MJ, Pathak A, et al: Endogenous production of carbon monoxide in normal and erythroblastotic newborn infants. J Clin Invest 1971; 50:1.

245. Bartoletti AL, Stevenson DK, et al: Pulmonary excretion of

carbon dioxide in the human infant as an index of bilirubin production. I. Effects of gestational and postnatal age and some common neonatal abnormalities. J Pediatr 1979; 94:952.

246. Pearson H: Life-span of the fetal red blood cell. J Pediatr 1967; 70:166.

247. West MF, Grieder AR: Erythrocyte survival in newborn infants as measured by chromium and its relation to postnatal serum bilirubin level. J Pediatr 1961; 54:194.

248. Ustrom RA, Eisenklam E: The enterohepatic shunting of bilirubin in the newborn infant. I. Use of oral activated charcoal to reduce normal serum bilirubin values. J Pediatr 1964; 65:27.

249. Weisman LE, Merenstein GB, et al: The effect of early meconium evacuation on early-onset hyperbilirubinemia. Am J Dis Child 1983; 137:666.

250. Lathe GH, Walker MJ: The synthesis of bilirubin glucuronide in animal and human liver. Biochem J 1958; 70:705.

251. Brown AK, Zuelzer WW: Studies on the neonatal development of the glucuronide conjugating system. J Clin Invest 1958; 37:332.

252. Maurer HM, Wolff JA, et al: Reduction in concentration of total serum bilirubin in off-spring of women treated with phenobarbitone during pregnancy. Lancet 1968; 2:122.

253. Vaisman SL, Gartner LM: Pharmacologic treatment of neonatal hyperbilirubinemia. Clin Perinatol 1975; 2:37.

254. Rouslahti E, Estes T, Seppala M: Binding of bilirubin by bovine and human serum α-fetoprotein. Biochim Biophys Acta 1979; 578:511.

255. Hsia JC, Er SS, Tan CT: α-Fetoprotein binding specificity for arachidonate, bilirubin, docosahexaenoate, and palmitate. J Biol Chem 1980; 255:4224.

256. Wynn RM: The placental transfer of bilirubin. Am J Obstet Gynecol 1963; 86:841.

257. Gourley GR, Odell GB: Bilirubin metabolism in the fetus and neonate. In Lebenthal E (ed): Human Gastrointestinal Development. New York, Raven Press, 1989, p 581.

258. Ackerman BD, Dyer GY, et al: Hyperbilirubinemia and kernicterus in small premature infants. Pediatrics 1970; 45:918.

259. Gartner LM: The bronze baby syndrome. J Pediatr 1976; 88:465.

260. Kopelman AE, Brown RS, et al: The "bronze" baby syndrome: a complication of phototherapy. J Pediatr 1972; 81:466.

261. Grannum PA, Copel JA: Prevention of Rh isoimmunization and treatment of the compromised fetus. Semin Perinatol 1988; 12:324.

262. Gottvall T, Hilden JO, Selbing A: Evaluation of standard parameters to predict exchange transfusions in the erythroblastotic newborn. Acta Obstet Gynecol Scand 1994; 73:300.

263. Dunn PM: Obstructive jaundice and hemolytic disease of the newborn. Arch Dis Child 1963; 38:54.

264. Barss VA, Doubilet PM, et al: Cardiac output in a fetus with erythroblastosis fetalis: assessment using pulsed Doppler. Obstet Gynecol 1987; 70:442.

265. Maisels MJ: Bilirubin: on understanding and influencing its metabolism in the newborn infant. Pediatr Clin North Am 1972; 19:447.

266. Kirk JJ, Ritter DA, Kenny JD: The effect of hematin on bilirubin binding in bilirubin-enriched neonatal cord serum. Biol Neonate 1984; 45:53.

267. Nicolini U, Santolaya J, et al: Changes in fetal acid base status during intravascular transfusion. Arch Dis Child 1988; 63:710.

268. Soothill PW, Nicolaides KH, et al: The effect of replacing fetal hemoglobin with adult hemoglobin on blood gas and acid-base parameters in human fetuses. Am J Obstet Gynecol 1988; 66:158.

269. Grant EG, Schellinger D, et al: Intracranial hemorrhage in neonates with erythroblastosis fetalis: sonographic and CT findings. Am J Neuroradiol 1984; 5:259.

270. Palmer DD, Drew JH: Jaundice: a 10-year experience of 41,000 live born infants. Aust Paediatr J 1983; 19:86.

271. Orzalezi M, Gloria F, et al: ABO system incompatibility: relationship between direct Coombs' test positivity and neonatal jaundice. Pediatrics 1973; 51:288.

272. Bowman JM: Fetomaternal ABO incompatibility and erythroblastosis fetalis. Vox Sang 1986; 50:104.

273. Levine DH, Meyer HB: Newborn screening for ABO hemolytic disease. Clin Pediatr 1985; 24:391.

274. Sivan Y, Merlob P, et al: Direct hyperbilirubinemia complicating ABO hemolytic disease of the newborn. Clin Pediatr 1983; 22:537.

275. Doxiadis SA, Fessas P, et al: Glucose-6-phosphate dehydrogenase deficiency: new aetiologic factor of severe neonatal jaundice. Lancet 1961; 1:297.

276. Doxiadis SA, Valaes T, et al: Risk of severe jaundice in glucose-6-phosphate dehydrogenase deficiency of the newborn. Differences in population groups. Lancet 1964; 2:1210.

277. Owa JA: Relationship between exposure to icterogenic agents, glucose-6-phosphate dehydrogenase deficiency and neonatal jaundice in Nigeria. Acta Paediatr Scand 1989; 78:848.

278. Meloni T, Cutillo S, et al: Neonatal jaundice and severity of glucose-6-phosphate dehydrogenase deficiency in Sardinian babies. Early Hum Dev 1987; 15:317.

279. Bernstein J, Brown AK: Sepsis and jaundice in early infancy. Pediatrics 1962; 29:873.

280. Eriksen L, Hofstad F, et al: Congenital erythropoietic porphyria, the effect of light shielding. Acta Paediatr Scand 1973; 62:385.

281. Kappas A, Sassa S, et al: The porphyrias: congenital erythropoietic porphyria. In Scriver CR, Beaudet AL, et al (eds): The Metabolic Basis of Inherited Disease. 6th ed. New York, McGraw-Hill Book Co., 1989, p 1329.

282. Gilbert A, Lereboullet P: La cholemie simple familiale. Semaine Medicale 1901; 21:241.

283. Berk PD, Wolkoff AW, et al: Inborn errors of bilirubin metabolism. Med Clin North Am 1975; 59:803.

284. Odell GB, Gourley GR: Hereditary hyperbilirubinemia. In Lebenthal E (ed): Textbook of Gastroenterology and Nutrition in Infancy. New York, Raven Press, 1989, p 949.

285. Owens D, Evans J: Population studies on Gilbert's syndrome. J Med Genet 1975; 12:152.

286. Black M, Billing BH: Hepatic bilirubin UDP-glucuronyl transferase activity in liver disease and Gilbert's syndrome. N Engl J Med 1969; 280:1266.

287. Auclair C, Hakim J, et al: Bilirubin and paranitrophenol glucuronyl activities of the liver in patients with Gilbert's syndrome. Enzyme 1976; 21:97.

288. Felsher BF, Craig JR, Carpio N: Hepatic bilirubin glucuronidation in Gilbert's syndrome. J Lab Clin Med 1973; 81:829.

288a. Bosma PJ, Chowdhury JR, et al: The genetic basis of the reduced expression of bilirubin UDP-glucuronosyltransferase 1 in Gilbert's syndrome. N Engl J Med 1995; 333:1171.

289. Billing BH, Gray CH, et al: The metabolism of [14C]-bilirubin in congenital nonhaemolytic hyperbilirubinemia. Clin Sci 1964; 27:163.

290. Black M, Fevery J, et al: Effect of phenobarbitone on plasma [14C] bilirubin clearance in patients with unconjugated hyperbilirubinemia. Clin Sci Mol Med 1974; 46:1.

291. Metreau JM, Yvart J, et al: Role of bilirubin over production in revealing Gilbert's syndrome: is dyserythropoiesis an important factor? Gut 1978; 19:838.

292. Berk PD, Blaschke TF: Detection of Gilbert's syndrome in patients with hemolysis: a method using radioactive chromium. Ann Intern Med 1972; 77:527.

293. Powell LW, Billing BH, Williams HS: The assessment of red cell survival in idiopathic unconjugated hyperbilirubinemia (Gilbert's syndrome) by the use of radioactive diisopropylfluorophosphate and chromium. Aust Ann Med 1967; 16:221.

294. Berk PD, Bloomer JR, et al: Constitutional hepatic dysfunction (Gilbert's syndrome): a new definition based on kinetic studies with unconjugated radiobilirubin. Am J Med 1970; 49:296.

295. Berk PD, Blaschke TF, Waggoner JG: Defective BSP clearance in patients with constitutional hepatic dysfunction (Gilbert's syndrome). Gastroenterology 1972; 63:472.

296. Billing BH, Williams R, Richards TG: Defects in hepatic transport of bilirubin in congenital hyperbilirubinemia: an analysis of plasma bilirubin disappearance curves. Clin Sci 1964; 27:245.

297. Okoliesanyi L, Ghidini O, et al: An evaluation of bilirubin kinetics with respect to the diagnosis of Gilbert's syndrome. Clin Sci Mol Med 1978; 54:539.

298. Roda A, Roda E, et al: Serum primary bile acids in Gilbert's syndrome. Gastroenterology 1982; 82:77.

299. Vierling JM, Berk PD, et al: Normal fasting-state levels of serum cholyl-conjugated bile acids in Gilbert's syndrome: an aid to diagnosis. Hepatology 1982; 2:340.

300. Ohkubo H, Okuda K, et al: Ursodeoxycholic acid oral clearance test in patients with constitutional hyperbilirubinemia and effect of phenobarbital. Gastroenterology 1981; 81:126.

301. Nambu M, Namihisa T: Hepatic transport and metabolism of various organic anions in patients with congenital non-hemolytic hyperbilirubinemia, including constitutional indocyanine green excretory defect. J Gastroenterol 1994; 29:228.

302. Ohkubo H, Okuda K, Jida S: A constitutional unconjugated hyperbilirubinemia combined with indocyanine green intolerance: a new functional disorder. Hepatology 1981; 1:319.

303. Martin JF, Vierling JM, et al: Abnormal hepatic transport of indocyanine green in Gilbert's syndrome. Gastroenterology 1976; 70:385.

304. Ullrich D, Sieg A, et al: Normal pathways for glucuronidation, sulfation and oxidation of paracetamol in Gilbert's syndrome. Eur J Clin Invest 1987; 17:237.

305. Sieg A, Stiehl A, et al: Gilbert's syndrome: diagnosis by typical serum bilirubin pattern. Clin Chem Acta 1986; 154:41.

306. Thomsen HF, Hardt F, Juhl E: Diagnosis of Gilbert's syndrome. Reliability of the caloric restriction and phenobarbitone stimulation tests. Scand J Gastroenterol 1981; 16:699.

307. Olsson R, Lindstedt G: Evaluation of tests for Gilbert's syndrome. Acta Med Scand 1980; 207:425.

308. Owens D, Sherlock S: Diagnosis of Gilbert's syndrome: role of reduced caloric intake test. BMJ 1973; 3:559.

309. Rollinghoff W, Paumgartner G, Preisig R: Nicotinic acid test in the diagnosis of Gilbert's syndrome: correlation with the bilirubin clearance. Gut 1981; 22:663.

310. Gentile S, Tiribelli C, et al: Dose dependence of nicotinic acid–induced hyperbilirubinemia and its dissociation from hemolysis in Gilbert's syndrome. J Lab Clin Med 1986; 107:166.

311. Lake AM, Truman JT, et al: Marked hyperbilirubinemia with Gilbert's syndrome and immunohemolytic anemia. J Pediatr 1978; 93:812.

312. Labrune P, Myara A, et al: Jaundice with hypertrophic pyloric stenosis: a possible early manifestation of Gilbert syndrome. J Pediatr 1989; 115:93.

313. Crigler JF Jr, Najjar VA: Congenital familial non-hemolytic jaundice with kernicterus. Pediatrics 1952; 10:169.

314. Labrune P, Myara A, et al: Genetic heterogeneity of Crigler-Najjar syndrome type I: a study of 14 cases. Hum Genet 1994; 94:693.

315. Schmid R, Hammaker L: Metabolism and disposition of C14-bilirubin in congenital nonhemolytic jaundice. J Clin Invest 1963; 42:1720.

316. Gunn CH: Hereditary acholuric jaundice in a new mutant strain of rats. J Hered 1938; 29:137.

317. Schmid R, Axelrod J, et al: Congenital jaundice in rats due to a defect in glucuronide formation. J Clin Invest 1958; 37:1123.

318. Strebel L, Odell GB: Bilirubin uridine diphospho-glucuronyl transferase in rat liver microsomes: genetic variation and maturation. Pediatr Res 1971; 5:548.

319. Odell GB, Cukier JO, Gourley GR: The presence of a microsomal UDP-glucuronyl transferase for bilirubin in homozygous jaundiced Gunn rats and in the Crigler-Najjar syndrome. Hepatology 1981; 1:307.

320. Whitington PF, Black DD, et al: Evidence against an abnormal hepatic microsomal lipid matrix as the primary defect in the jaundiced Gunn rat. Biochim Biophys Acta 1985; 812:774.

321. Iyanagi T, Watanabe T, Uchiyama Y: The 3-methylcholanthrene-inducible UDP-glucuronosyltransferase deficiency in the hyperbilirubinemic rat (Gunn rat) is caused by a -1 frameshift mutation. J Biol Chem 1989; 264:21302.

322. Huang TJ, Chowdhury JR, et al: Prenatal diagnosis of bilirubin-UDP-glucuronosyltransferase deficiency in rats by genomic DNA analysis. Hepatology 1992; 16:756.

323. Sinaasappel M, Jansen PL: The differential diagnosis of Crigler-Najjar disease, types 1 and 2, by bile pigment analysis. Gastroenterology 1991; 100:783.

324. Childs B, Sidbury JB, Migeon CJ: Glucuronic acid conjugation by patients with familial nonhemolytic jaundice and their relatives. Pediatrics 1959; 23:903.

325. Szabo L, Ebrey P: Studies on the inheritance of Crigler-Najjar's syndrome by the menthol test. Acta Pediatr Hung 1963; 4:153.

326. Cowger ML: Bilirubin encephalopathy. In Gaull G (ed): Biology of Brain Dysfunction. New York, Plenum Press, 1973, p 265.

327. Odell GB, Schutta HS: Bilirubin encephalopathy. In McCandless DW (ed): Cerebral Energy Metabolism and Metabolic Encephalopathy. New York, Plenum Press, 1985, p 229.

328. Whitington GL: Congenital nonhemolytic icterus with damage to the central nervous system. Report of a case in a negro child. Pediatrics 1960; 25:437.

329. Wolkoff AW, Chowdhury JR, et al: Crigler-Najjar syndrome (Type 1) in an adult male. Gastroenterology 1979; 76:840.

330. Labrune PH, Myara A, et al: Cerebellar symptoms as the presenting manifestations of bilirubin encephalopathy in children with Crigler-Najjar type I disease. Pediatrics 1992; 89:768.

331. Arrowsmith WA, Payne RB, Littlewood JM: Comparison of treatment for congenital nonobstructive nonhaemolytic hyperbilirubinemia. Arch Dis Child 1974; 50:197.

332. Gorodischer R, Levy G, et al: Congenital nonobstructive, nonhemolytic jaundice: effect of phototherapy. N Engl J Med 1970; 282:375.

333. Odell GB, Gutcher GR, et al: Enteral administration of agar as an effective adjunct to phototherapy of neonatal hyperbilirubinemia. Pediatr Res 1983; 17:810.

334. Kaufman SS, Wood RP, et al: Orthotopic transplantation of type I Crigler-Najjar syndrome. Hepatology 1986; 6:1259.

335. Whitington PF, Emond JC, et al: Orthotopic auxiliary liver transplantation for Crigler-Najjar syndrome type I. Lancet 1993; 342:779.

336. Broelsch CE, Emond JC, et al: Application of reduced size liver transplants as split grafts, auxiliary orthotopic grafts and living related segmental transplants. Ann Surg 1990; 212:368.

337. Whitington PF, Alonso EM, Piper J: Liver transplantation for inborn errors of metabolism. Int Pediatr 1993; 8:30.

338. Arias IM, Gartner LM, et al: Chronic nonhemolytic unconjugated hyperbilirubinemia with glucuronyl transferase deficiency. Am J Med 1969; 47:395.

339. Gollan JL, Huang SN, et al: Prolonged survival in three brothers with severe type 2 Crigler-Najjar syndrome. Ultrastructure and metabolic studies. Gastroenterology 1975; 68:1543.

340. Bloomer JR, Berk PD, et al: Bilirubin metabolism in congenital nonhemolytic jaundice. Pediatr Res 1971; 5:256.

341. Ertel IJ, Newton WAJ: Therapy in congenital hyperbilirubinemia: phenobarbital and diethylnicotinamide. Pediatrics 1969; 44:43.

342. Gordon ER, Shaffer EA, Sass-Kortsak A: Bilirubin secretion and conjugation in the Crigler-Najjar syndrome type II. Gastroenterology 1976; 70:761.

343. Arias IM, Gartner LM, et al: Prolonged neonatal unconjugated hyperbilirubinemia associated with breast feeding and a steroid pregnane-3(αβ)-diol, in maternal milk which inhibits glucuronide formation in vitro. J Clin Invest 1964; 43:2037.

344. Hunter JO, Thompson PH, et al: Inheritance of type 2 Crigler-Najjar hyperbilirubinemia. Gut 1973; 14:46.

345. Duhamel G, Blanckaert N, et al: An unusual case of Crigler-Najjar disease in the adult. Classification of types I and II revisited. J Hepatol 1985; 1:47.

346. Crigler JF, Gold NI: Effect of sodium phenobarbital on bilirubin metabolism in an infant with congenital, nonhemolytic, unconjugated hyperbilirubinemia and kernicterus. J Clin Invest 1969; 48:42.

347. Kreek MJ, Sleisenger MH: Reduction of serum-unconjugated-bilirubin with phenobarbitone in adult nonhaemolytic unconjugated hyperbilirubinemia. Lancet 1968; 2:73.

348. Yaffe SJ, Levy G, et al: Enhancemant of glucuronide-conjugating capacity in a hyperbilirubinemic infant due to apparent enzyme induction by phenobarbital. N Engl J Med 1966; 275:1461.

349. Schneider AP: Breast milk jaundice in the newborn: a real entity. JAMA 1986; 255:3270.

350. Odievre M: L'ictère au lait de femme. Arch Fr Pediatr 1973; 30:569.

351. Clarkson JE, Cowan JO, Herbison GP: Jaundice in full term healthy neonates—a population study. Aust Paediatr J 1984; 20:303.

352. Lascari AD: "Early" breast-feeding jaundice: clinical significance. J Pediatr 1986; 108:156.

353. Dahms BB, Krauss AN, et al: Breast feeding and serum bilirubin values during the first 4 days of life. J Pediatr 1973; 83:1049.

354. Bloomer JR, Barrett PV, et al: Studies on the mechanisms of fasting hyperbilirubinemia. Gastroenterology 1971; 61:479.

355. De Charvalho M, Robertson S, Klaus M: Fecal bilirubin excretion and serum bilirubin concentrations in breast-fed and bottle-fed infants. J Pediatr 1985; 107:786.

356. Auerbach KG, Gartner LM: Breastfeeding and human milk: their association with jaundice in the neonate. Clin Perinatol 1987; 14:89.

357. Amato M, Howald H, von Muralt G: Interruption of breast-feeding versus phototherapy as treatment of hyperbilirubinemia in full-term infants. Helv Paediatr Acta 1985; 40:127.

358. Newman AJ, Gross S: Hyperbilirubinemia in breast-fed infants. Pediatrics 1963; 32:995.

359. Winnfield CR, MacFaul R: Clinical study of prolonged jaundice in breast and bottle-fed babies. Arch Dis Child 1978; 53:506.

360. Alonso EM, Whitington PF, et al: Enterohepatic circulation of non-conjugated bilirubin in rats fed human milk. J Pediatr 1991; 118:425.

361. Gartner LM, Arias IM: Studies of prolonged neonatal jaundice in the breast-fed infant. J Pediatr 1966; 68:54.

362. Arias IM, Gartner LM: Production of unconjugated hyperbilirubinemia in full-term newborn infants following administration of pregnane-3(αβ)-diol. Nature 1964; 203:1292.

363. Levillain P, Odievre M, et al: Possibilités d'inhibition de la glucuro-conjugaison de la bilirubine en fonction de la teneur en acides gras libres du lait maternel. Biochim Biophys Acta 1972; 264:538.

364. Bevan BR, Holton JB: Inhibition of bilirubin conjugation in rat liver slices by free fatty acids, with relevance to the problem of breast milk jaundice. Clin Chem Acta 1972; 41:101.

365. Hargreaves T: Effect of fatty acids on bilirubin conjugation. Arch Dis Child 1973; 48:446.

366. Gartner LM, Lee K, Moscioni AD: Effect of milk feeding on intestinal bilirubin absorption in the rat. J Pediatr 1983; 56:455.

367. Gourley GR, Arend RA: Beta-glucuronidase and hyperbilirubinemia in breast-fed and formula-fed babies. Lancet 1986; 1:644.

368. Lucey JF, Arias IM, et al: Transient familial neonatal hyperbilirubinemia. Am J Dis Child 1960; 100:787.

369. Lucey FF, Driscoll JJ: Physiological jaundice re-examined. In Sass-Kortsak A (ed): Kernicterus. Toronto, University of Toronto Press, 1961, p 29.

370. Arias IM, Wolfson S, et al: Transient familial neonatal hyperbilirubinemia. J Clin Invest 1965; 44:1442.

371. Boggs TR, Bishop H: Neonatal hyperbilirubinemia associated with high obstruction of the small bowel. J Pediatr 1965; 66:349.

372. Karp M, McCarthy R: Congenital hypertrophic pyloric stenosis with jaundice. Ann Paediatr 1962; 198:274.

373. Wooley MM, Felsher BF, et al: Jaundice, hypertrophic pyloric stenosis, and hepatic glucuronyl transferase. J Pediatr Surg 1974; 9:359.

374. Roth B, Statz A, et al: Elimination of indocyanine green by the liver in infants with hypertrophic pyloric stenosis and icteropyloric syndrome. J Pediatr 1981; 99:240.

375. Valaes T, Karaklis A, et al: Incidence and mechanism of neonatal jaundice related to glucose-6-phosphate dehydrogenase deficiency. Pediatr Res 1969; 3:448.

376. Lokietz H, Dowben RM, et al: Studies on the effect of novobiocin on glucuronyl transferase. Pediatrics 1963; 32:47.

377. Cristensen JF: Prolonged icterus neonatorum and congenital myxedema. Acta Paediatr Scand 1956; 45:367.

378. Akerren Y: Prolonged jaundice in the newborn associated with congenital myxedema. Acta Paediatr Scand 1954; 43:411.

379. MacGillivray MH, Crawford JD, et al: Congenital hypothyroidism and prolonged neonatal hyperbilirubinemia. Pediatrics 1967; 40:283.

380. Taylor PM, Wolfson JH, et al: Hyperbilirubinemia in infants of diabetic mothers. Biol Neonate 1963; 5:289.

381. Hubbell JP Jr, Drorbaugh JE, et al: "Early" versus "late" feeding of infants of diabetic mothers. N Engl J Med 1961; 265:835.

382. Brown WR, Boon WH: Ethnic group differences in plasma bilirubin levels of full-term healthy Singapore newborns. Pediatrics 1965; 36:745.

383. Lu T-C, Wei H: Increased incidence of severe hyperbilirubinemia among newborn Chinese infants with G-6-PD deficiency. Pediatrics 1966; 37:994.

384. Horiguchi T, Bauer C: Ethnic differences in neonatal jaundice: comparison of Japanese and Caucasian newborn infants. Am J Obstet Gynecol 1975; 121:71.

385. Johnson JD, Angelus P, et al: Exaggerated jaundice in Navajo neonates. The role of bilirubin production. Am J Dis Child 1986; 140:889.

386. Drew JH, Kitchen WH: Jaundice in infants of Greek parentage: the unknown factor may be environmental. J Pediatr 1976; 89:248.

387. Drew JH, Barrie J, et al: Factors influencing jaundice in immigrant Greek infants. Arch Dis Child 1978; 53:49.

388. Valaes T, Petmezaki S, et al: Effect on neonatal hyperbilirubinemia of phenobarbital during pregnancy or after birth: practical value of the treatment in a population with high risk of unexplained severe neonatal jaundice. In Bergsma D (ed): Bilirubin Metabolism in the Newborn. Baltimore, Williams & Wilkins, 1970, p 46.

389. Rose AL, Johnson A: Bilirubin encephalopathy: neuropathological and histochemical studies in the Gunn rat model. Neurology 1972; 22:420.

390. Sherwood AJ, Smith JF: Bilirubin encephalopathy. Neuropathol Appl Neurobiol 1983; 9:271.

391. Van Praagh R: Diagnosis of kernicterus in the neonatal period. Pediatrics 1961; 28:870.

392. Hansen TWR, Bratlid D: Bilirubin and brain toxicity. Acta Paediatr Scand 1986; 75:513.

393. Hansen TW: Bilirubin in the brain. Distribution and effects on neurophysiological and neurochemical processes. Clin Pediatr 1994; 33:452.

394. Scheidt PC, Mellits ED, et al: Toxicity of bilirubin in neonates: infant development during first year in relation to maximum neonatal serum bilirubin concentration. J Pediatr 1977; 91:292.

395. Rubin RA, Balow B, Fisch RO: Neonatal serum bilirubin levels related to cognitive development at ages 4 through 7 years. J Pediatr 1979; 94:601.

396. Odell GB, Storey GNB, et al: Studies in kernicterus. III. The saturation of serum proteins with bilirubin during neonatal life and its relationship to brain damage at five years. J Pediatr 1970; 76:12.

397. Cashore WJ: Kernicterus and bilirubin encephalopathy. Semin Liver Dis 1988; 8:163.

398. Wennberg RP, Hance AJ: Experimental bilirubin encephalopathy: importance of total bilirubin, protein binding, and blood-brain barrier. Pediatr Res 1986; 20:789.

399. Odell GB, Cohen SN, et al: Studies in kernicterus. II. The determination of the saturation of serum albumin with bilirubin. J Pediatr 1969; 74:214.

400. Silverman WA, Anderson DH, et al: A difference in mortality rate and incidence of kernicterus among premature infants allotted to two prophylactic antibacterial regimens. Pediatrics 1956; 18:614.

401. Shapiro SM: Brainstem auditory evoked potentials in an experimental model of bilirubin neurotoxicity. Clin Pediatr 1994; 33:460.

402. Shapiro SM: Acute brainstem auditory evoked potential abnormalities in jaundiced Gunn rats given sulfonamide. Pediatr Res 1988; 23:306.

403. Walker PC: Neonatal bilirubin toxicity. A review of kernicterus and the implications of drug-induced bilirubin displacement. Clin Pharmacokinet 1987; 13:26.

404. Martin E, Fanconi S, et al: Ceftriaxone–bilirubin-albumin interactions in the neonate: an in vivo study. Eur J Pediatr 1993; 1993:530.

405. Nerli B, Pico G: Identification of the cephalosporin human serum albumin binding sites. Pharmacol Toxicol 1993; 73:297.

406. Onks DL, Harris JF, Robertson AF: Cefmenoxime and bilirubin: competition for albumin binding. Pharmacol Toxicol 1991; 68:329.

407. Gartner LM, Lee KS: Bilirubin binding, free fatty acids and a new concept for the pathogenesis of kernicterus. In Bergsma DL, Blondheim SH (eds): Bilirubin Metabolism in the Newborn. New York, Elsevier, l976, p 265.

408. Stavinsky R, Shafrir E: Displacement of albumin-bound bilirubin by free fatty acids: implications for neonatal hyperbilirubinemia. Clin Chim Acta 1970; 29:311.

409. Wooley PV, Hunter M: Binding and circular dichroism data on

bilirubin albumin in the presence of oleate and salicylate. Arch Biochem 1970; 140:197.

410. Ostrea EM Jr, Bassel M, Fleury CA, et al: Influence of free fatty acids and glucose infusion on serum bilirubin and bilirubin binding to albumin: clinical implications. J Pediatr 1983; 102:426.

411. Whitington PF, Burckart GH, et al: Alterations in reserve bilirubin binding capacity of albumin by free fatty acids. II. In vitro and in vivo studies using difference spectroscopy. J Pediatr Gastroenterol Nutr l982; 1:495.

412. Soltys BJ, Hsia JC: Human serum albumin. I. On the relationship of fatty acid and bilirubin binding sites and the nature of fatty acid allosteric effects—a monoanionic spin label study. J Biol Chem 1978; 253:3023.

413. Spear ML, Stahl GE, et al: Effect of heparin dose and infusion rate on lipid clearance and bilirubin binding in premature infants receiving intravenous fat emulsions. J Pediatr 1988; 112:94.

414. Bratlid D, Cashore WJ, et al: Effect of serum hyperosmolality on opening of blood-brain barrier for bilirubin in rat brain. Pediatrics 1983; 71:909.

415. Gartner LM, Snyder RN, et al: Kernicterus: high incidence of premature infants with low serum bilirubin concentrations. Pediatrics 1970; 45:906.

416. Lucey JF: The unsolved problem of kernicterus in the susceptible low birth weight infant. Pediatrics 1972; 49:646.

417. Perlman MA, Gartner LM, et al: The association of kernicterus with bacterial infection in the newborn. Pediatrics 1980; 65:26.

418. Levine RL, Fredericks WR, Rappaport SI: Clearance of bilirubin from rat brain after reversible osmotic opening of the blood-brain barrier. Pediatr Res 1985; 19:1040.

419. Hansen TW, Sagvolden T, Bratlid D: Open-field behavior of rats previously subjected to short-term hyperbilirubinemia with or without blood-brain barrier manipulations. Brain Res 1987; 424:26.

420. Hansen TW, Maynard EC, et al: Endotoxemia and brain bilirubin in the rat. Biol Neonate 1993; 63:171.

421. Brann BS, Stonestreet BS, et al: The in vivo effect of bilirubin and sulfisoxazole on cerebral oxygen, glucose, and lactate metabolism in newborn piglets. Pediatr Res 1987; 22:135.

422. Jirka JH, Duckrow RB, et al: Effect of bilirubin on brainstem auditory evoked potentials in the asphyxiated rat. Pediatr Res 1985; 19:556.

423. Burgess GH, Stonestreet BS, et al: Brain bilirubin deposition and brain blood flow during acute urea-induced hyperosmolality in newborn piglets. Pediatr Res 1985; 19:537.

424. Ives NK, Bolas NM, Gardiner RM: The effects of bilirubin on brain energy metabolism during hyperosmolar opening of the blood-brain barrier: an in vivo study using ^{31}P nuclear magnetic resonance spectroscopy. Pediatr Res 1989; 26:356.

425. Meisel P, Jahrig D, et al: Bilirubin binding and acid-base equilibrium in newborn infants with low birthweight. Acta Paediatr Scand 1988; 77:496.

426. Odell GB: Influence of pH on the distribution of bilirubin between albumin and mitochondria. Proc Soc Exper Biol Med 1965; 120:352.

427. Cowger ML: Mechanisms of bilirubin toxicity on tissue culture cells; factors that affect toxicity, reversibility by albumin, and comparison with other respiratory poisons and surfactants. Biochem Med 1971; 5:1.

428. Noir BA, Boveris A, et al: Bilirubin: a multisite inhibitor of mitochondrial respiration. FEBS Lett 1972; 27:270.

429. Weil ML, Menkes JH: Bilirubin interaction with ganglioside: possible mechanism of kernicterus. Pediatr Res 1975; 9:791.

430. Gurba PE, Zand R: Bilirubin binding to myelin basic protein, histones and its inhibition in vitro of cerebellar protein synthesis. Biochem Biophys Res Commun 1974; 58:1142.

431. Amit Y, Chan G, et al: Bilirubin toxicity in a neuroblastoma cell line N-115: I. effects on Na$^+$/K$^+$ ATPase, [^{3}H]-thymidine uptake, L-[^{35}S]-methionine incorporation, and mitochondrial function. Pediatr Res 1989; 25:364.

432. Amit Y, Poznansky MJ, Schiff D: Bilirubin toxicity in a neuroblastoma cell line N-115: Delayed effects and recovery. Pediatr Res 1989; 25:369.

433. Hyman CB, Keaster J, et al: CNS abnormalities after neonatal hemolytic disease or hyperbilirubinemia. Am J Dis Child 1969; 117:395.

434. Hung KL: Auditory brainstem responses in patients with neonatal hyperbilirubinemia and bilirubin encephalopathy. Brain Dev 1989; 11:297.

435. Boggs TR Jr, Hardy JB, et al: Correlation of neonatal serum total bilirubin concentrations and developmental status at age 8 months. J Pediatr 1967; 71:553.

436. Naeye RL: Amniotic fluid infections, neonatal hyperbilirubinemia and psychomotor impairment. Pediatrics 1978; 62:497.

437. Bernstein J, Landing BJ: Extraneural lesions associated with neonatal hyperbilirubinemia and kernicterus. Am J Pathol 1961; 40:371.

438. Odell GB, Natzschka JC, Storey GNB: Bilirubin nephropathy in the Gunn strain of rat. Am J Physiol 1967; 212:931.

439. Ennever JF: Phototherapy in a new light. Pediatr Clin North Am 1986; 33:603.

440. Fetus and Newborn Committee, Canadian Pediatric Society: Use of phototherapy for neonatal hyperbilirubinemia. Can Med Assoc J 1986; 134:1237.

441. Ebbesen F: Superiority of intensive phototherapy—blue double light—in rhesus haemolytic disease. Eur J Pediatr 1979; 130:279.

442. Cohen AN, Ostrow JD: New concepts in phototherapy: photoisomerization of bilirubin IXa and potential toxic effects of light. Pediatrics 1980; 65:740.

443. McDonagh AF, Lightner DA: "Like a shrivelled blood orange"—bilirubin, jaundice, and phototherapy. Pediatrics 1985; 75:443.

444. McDonagh AF, Lightner DA: Phototherapy and the photobiology of bilirubin. Semin Liver Dis 1988; 8:272.

445. McDonagh AF, Ramonas LM: Jaundice phototherapy: micro flow-cellphotometry reveals rapid biliary response of Gunn rats to light. Science 1978; 201:829.

446. Ostrow JD: Photocatabolism of labeled bilirubin in the congenitally jaundiced (Gunn) rat. J Clin Invest 1971; 50:707.

447. Lund HT, Jacobsen J: Influence of phototherapy on unconjugated bilirubin in duodenal bile of newborn infants with hyperbilirubinemia. Acta Paediatr Scand 1972; 61:693.

448. Lightner DA, Wooldridge TA: Configurational isomerization of bilirubin and the mechanism of jaundice phototherapy. Biochem Biophys Res Commun 1979; 86:235.

449. Lightner DA, Wooldridge TA, et al: Photobilirubin: an early bilirubin photoproduct detected by absorbance difference spectroscopy. Proc Natl Acad Sci U S A 1979; 76:29.

450. Onishi S, Isobe K, et al: Demonstration of a geometric isomer of bilirubin-IXα in the serum of a hyperbilirubinaemic newborn infant and the mechanism of jaundice phototherapy. Biochem J 1980; 190:533.

451. Lamola AA, Blumberg WE, et al: Photoisomerized bilirubin in blood from infants receiving phototherapy. Proc Natl Acad Sci U S A 1981; 78:1882.

452. Isobe K, Onishi S: Kinetics of the photochemical interconversion among geometric photoisomers of bilirubin. Biochem J 1981; 193:1029.

453. Pellegrino JM, Roma MG, et al: Hepatic handling of photoirradiated bilirubin. A study in isolated perfused Wistar rat liver. Biochim Biophys Acta 1991; 1074:25.

454. Onishi S, Miura I, et al: Structure and thermal interconversion of cyclobilirubin IXα. Biochem J 1984; 218:667.

455. Onishi S, Isobe K, et al: Metabolism of bilirubin and its photoisomers in newborn infants during phototherapy. J Biochem 1986; 100:789.

456. Onishi S, Ogino T, et al: Biliary and urinary excretion rates and serum concentration changes of four bilirubin photoproducts in Gunn rats during total darkness and low or high illumination. Biochem J 1984; 221:717.

457. Ennever JF, Costarino AT, et al: Rapid clearance of a structural isomer of bilirubin during phototherapy. J Clin Invest 1987; 79:1674.

458. Maurer HM, Shumway CN, et al: Controlled trial comparing agar, intermittent phototherapy and continuous phototherapy for reducing neonatal hyperbilirubinemia. J Pediatr 1973; 73:115.

459. Lightner DA, Linnane WP, et al: Bilirubin photooxidation products in the urine of jaundiced neonates receiving phototherapy. Pediatr Res 1984; 18:696.

460. Lightner DA: The photoreactivity of bilirubin and related pyrroles. Photochem Photobiol 1977; 26:427.

461. Vogl TP: Phototherapy of neonatal hyperbilirubinemia: bilirubin in unexposed areas of the skin. J Pediatr 1974; 85:707.
462. Gutcher GR, Yen WM, et al: The in vitro and in vivo photoreactivity of bilirubin. I. Laser-defined wavelength dependence. Pediatr Res 1983; 17:120.
463. Vecchi C, Donzelli GP, et al: Green light in phototherapy. Pediatr Res 1983; 17:461.
464. Ennever JF, McDonagh AF, Speck WT: Phototherapy for neonatal jaundice: optimal wavelengths of light. J Pediatr 1983; 103:295.
465. Ennever JF, Sobel M, et al: Phototherapy for neonatal jaundice: in vitro comparison of light sources. Pediatr Res 1984; 18:667.
466. Romagnoli C, Marrocco G, et al: Phototherapy for hyperbilirubinemia in preterm infants: green versus blue or white light. J Pediatr 1988; 112:476.
467. Agati G, Fusi F, et al: Quantum yield and skin filtering effects on the formation rate of lumirubin. J Photochem Photobiol 1993; 18:197.
468. Wu P-Y, Hodgeman JE, et al: Metabolic aspects of phototherapy. Pediatrics 1985; 75:427.
469. Wurtman RJ, Cardinali DP: The effects of light on man. In Bergsma D (ed): Bilirubin Metabolism in the Newborn. White Plains, NY, Excerpta Medica Series, National Foundation–March of Dimes, 1976, p 100.
470. Tan KL, Chow MT, et al: Effect of phototherapy on neonatal riboflavin status. J Pediatr 1978; 93:494.
471. Gromisch DS, Lopez R, et al: Light (phototherapy)–induced riboflavin deficiency in the neonate. J Pediatr 1977; 90:118.
472. Ostrea EM, Fleury CA, et al: Accelerated degradation of essential fatty acids as a complication of phototherapy. J Pediatr 1983; 102:617.
473. Malhorta V, Greenberg JW, et al: Fatty acid enhancement of the quantum yield for the formation of lumirubin from bilirubin bound to albumin. Pediatr Res 1987; 21:530.
474. Odell GB, Brown RS, et al: The photodynamic action of bilirubin on erythrocytes. J Pediatr 1972; 81:473.
475. Ostrea EM Jr, Cepeda EE: Red cell membrane lipid peroxidation and hemolysis secondary to phototherapy. Acta Paediatr Scand 1985; 74:378.
476. Girotti AW: Bilirubin-photosensitized cross-linking of polypeptides in the isolated membrane of the human erythrocyte. J Biol Chem 1978; 253:7186.
477. Cukier JO, Maglalang AC, et al: Increased osmotic fragility of erythrocytes in chronically jaundiced rats after phototherapy. Acta Paediatr Scand 1979; 68:903.
478. Howe RB, Hadland CR, et al: Effect of phototherapy on serum bilirubin levels and red blood cell survival in congenitally jaundiced Gunn rats. J Lab Clin Med 1978; 92:221.
478a. Oski FA: The erythrocyte and its disorders. In Nathan DG, Oski FA (eds): Hematology of Infancy and Childhood. 4th ed. Philadelphia, W.B. Saunders Co., 1992, p 26.
479. Ostrea EM, Odell GB: Photosensitized shift in the O₂ dissociation curve of fetal blood. Acta Paediatr Scand 1974; 63:341.
480. Kopelman AE, Ey JL, et al: Phototherapy in newborn infants with glucose-6-phosphate dehydrogenase deficiency. J Pediatr 1978; 93:497.
481. Odell GB, Brown RS, et al: Dye sensitized photo-oxidation of albumin associated with a decreased capacity for protein-binding of bilirubin. Birth Defects 1970; 6:31.
482. Cashore WJ, Karotkin EH, et al: The lack of effect of phototherapy on serum bilirubin-binding capacity in newborn infants. J Pediatr 1975; 87:977.
483. Ebbesen F, Jacobsen J: Bilirubin-albumin binding affinity and serum albumin concentration during intensive phototherapy (blue double light) in jaundiced newborn infants. Eur J Pediatr 1980; 134:261.
484. Ebbesen F, Brodersen R: Albumin administration combined with phototherapy in treatment of hyperbilirubinemia in low-birth-weight infants. Acta Paediatr Scand 1981; 70:649.
485. Sisson TRC, Glauser SC, et al: Retinal changes produced by phototherapy. J Pediatr 1970; 77:221.
486. Dobson V, Riggs LA, et al: Electroretinographic determination of dark adaptation functions of children exposed to phototherapy as infants. J Pediatr 1974; 85:25.
487. Dobson V, Cowett RM, et al: Long-term effect of phototherapy on visual function. J Pediatr 1975; 86:555.
488. Valkeakari T, Anttolainen I, et al: Follow-up study of photo-treated fullterm newborns. Acta Paediatr Scand 1981; 70:21.
489. Romagnoli C: Phototherapy-induced hypocalcemia. J Pediatr 1979; 94:815.
490. Wu PYK, Lim RC, et al: Effect of phototherapy in preterm infants on growth in the neonatal period. J Pediatr 1974; 85:563.
491. Hakanson DO, Bergstrom WH. Phototherapy-induced hypocalcemia in newborn rats: prevention by melatonin. Science 1981; 214:807.
492. Lemaitre BJ, Toubas PL, et al: Increased gonadotropin levels in newborn premature females treated by phototherapy. Biochem Med 1979; 10:335.
493. John E: Complications of phototherapy in neonatal jaundice. Aust Pediatr J 1975; 11:53.
494. Whitington PF, Olsen WA, et al: The effect of bilirubin on the function of hamster small intestine. Pediatr Res 1981; 15:1009.
495. Li BUK, Whitington PF, et al: The reversal of bilirubin-induced intestinal secretion by agar. Pediatr Res 1984; 18:79.
496. Whitington PF: Effect of jaundice and phototherapy on intestinal mucosal bilirubin concentration and lactase activity in the congenitally jaundiced Gunn rat. Pediatr Res 1981; 15:345.
497. Bakken AF: Temporary intestinal lactase deficiency in light-treated jaundiced infants. Acta Paediatr Scand 1977; 66:91.
498. Dinari G, Cohen MI, et al: The effect of phototherapy on intestinal mucosal enzyme activity in the Gunn rat. Biol Neonate 1980; 38:179.
499. Sharma RK, Ente G, et al: A complication of phototherapy in the newborn: the "bronze baby." Clin Pediatr 1973; 12:231.
500. Clark CF, Torii S, et al: The "bronze baby" syndrome: postmortem data. J Pediatr 1976; 88:461.
501. Radermacher EH, Noirfalise A, et al: Das Bronze-Baby-Syndrom. Eine Komplikation der Fototherapie. Klin Pediatr 1977; 189:379.
502. Tan KL, Jacob E: The bronze baby syndrome. Acta Paediatr Scand 1982; 71:409.
503. Onishi S, Itoh S, et al: Mechanism of development of bronze baby syndrome in neonates treated with phototherapy. Pediatrics 1982; 69:273.
504. Rubaltelli FF, Jori G, et al: Bronze baby syndrome: a new porphyrin-related disorder. Pediatr Res 1983; 17:327.
505. Jori G, Reddi E, Rubaltelli FF: Bronze baby syndrome: an animal model. Pediatr Res 1990; 27:22.
506. Kappas A, Drummond GS, et al: Control of heme oxygenase and plasma levels of bilirubin by a synthetic heme analogue, tin-protoporphyrin. Hepatology 1984; 4:336.
507. Kappas A, Drummond GS, et al: Sn-protoporphyrin use in the management of hyperbilirubinemia in term infants with direct Coombs-positive ABO incompatibility. Pediatrics 1988; 81:485.
508. McDonagh AF: Purple versus yellow: preventing neonatal jaundice with tin-porphyrins. J Pediatr 1988; 113:777.
509. Stevenson DK, Rodgers PA, Vreman HJ: The use of metalloporphyrins for the chemoprevention of neonatal jaundice. Am J Dis Child 1989; 143:353.
510. Drummond GS, Kappas A: Chemoprevention of neonatal jaundice: potency of tin-protoporphyrin in an animal model. Science 1982; 217:1250.
511. Cornelius CE, Rodgers PA: Prevention of neonatal hyperbilirubinemia in rhesus monkeys by tin-protoporphyrin. Pediatr Res 1984; 18:728.
512. Milleville GS, Levitt MD, Engel RR: Tin protoporphyrin inhibits carbon monoxide production in adult mice. Pediatr Res 1985; 19:94.
513. Whitington PF, Moscioni AD, Gartner LM: The effect of tin(IV)-protoporphyrin-IX on bilirubin production and excretion in the rat. Pediatr Res 1987; 21:487.
514. McDonagh AF, Palma LA: Tin-protoporphyrin: a potent photosensitizer of bilirubin destruction. Photochem Photobiol 1985; 42:261.
515. Galbraith RA, Drummond GS, Kappas A: Suppression of bilirubin production in the Crigler-Najjar type I syndrome: studies with the heme oxygenase inhibitor tin-mesoporphyrin. Pediatrics 1992; 89:175.
516. Hamori CJ, Lasic DD, et al: Targeting zinc protoporphyrin liposomes to the spleen using reticuloendothelial blockade with blank liposomes. Pediatr Res 1993; 34:1.

517. Wolkoff AW: Inheritable disorders manifested by conjugated hyperbilirubinemia. Semin Liv Dis 1983; 3:65.

518. Zimniak P: Dubin-Johnson and Rotor syndromes: molecular basis and pathogenesis. Semin Liver Dis 1993; 13:248.

519. Dubin IN, Johnson FB: Chronic idiopathic jaundice with unidentified pigment in liver cells: a new clinicopathologic entity with a report of 12 cases. Medicine 1954; 33:155.

520. Dubin IN: Chronic idiopathic jaundice: a review of fifty cases. Am J Med 1958; 24:268.

521. Arias IM: Studies of chronic familial non-hemolytic jaundice with conjugated bilirubin in the serum with and without an unidentified pigment in the liver cells. Am J Med 1961; 31:510.

522. Swartz HM, Sarna T, Varma RR: On the nature and excretion of the hepatic pigment in the Dubin-Johnson syndrome. Gastroenterology 1979; 76:958.

523. Arias IM, Blumberg W: The pigment in Dubin-Johnson syndrome. Gastroenterology 1979; 77:820.

524. LeBouthillier G, Morais J, et al: Scintigraphic aspect of Rotor's disease with technicium-99m-mebrofenin. J Nucl Med 1992; 33:1550.

525. Pinos T, Constansa JM, et al: A new diagnostic approach to the Dubin-Johnson syndrome. Am J Gastroenterol 1990; 85:91.

526. Erlinger S, Dhumeaux D, Desjeux JF, et al: Hepatic handling of unconjugated dyes in the Dubin-Johnson syndrome. Gastroenterology 1973; 59:842.

527. Koskelo P, Toivonen I, Aldercreutz H: Urinary coproporphyrin isomer distribution in Dubin-Johnson syndrome. Clin Chem 1967; 13:1006.

528. Rotor AB, Manahan L, Florentin A: Familial nonhemolytic jaundice with direct van den Bergh reaction. Acta Med Phil 1948; 5:37.

529. Wolpert E, Pascasio FM, Wolkoff AW: Abnormal sulfobromophthalein metabolism in Rotor's syndrome and obligate heterozygotes. N Engl J Med 1977; 296:1099.

530. Shimizu Y, Naruto H, et al: Urinary coproporphyrin isomers in Rotor's syndrome: a study of eight families. Hepatology 1981; 1:173.

531. Watkins JB: Neonatal cholestasis: developmental aspects and current concepts. Semin Liver Dis 1993; 13:276.

532. Suchy FJ, Balistreri WF, et al: Physiologic cholestasis: elevation of the primary serum bile acid concentrations in normal infants. Gastroenterology 1981; 80:1037.

533. Escobedo MB, Barton LL, et al: The frequency of jaundice in neonatal bacterial infections. Clin Pediatr 1974; 13:656.

534. Utili R, Abernathy CO, et al: Cholestatic effects of *Escherichia coli* endotoxin on the isolated perfused rat liver. Gastroenterology 1976; 70:248.

535. Utili R, Abernathy CO, et al: Studies on the effects of *E. coli* endotoxin on canalicular bile formation in the isolated perfused rat liver. J Lab Clin Med 1977; 89:471.

536. Suchy FJ: Approach to the infant with cholestasis. In Suchy FJ (ed): Liver Disease in Children. St. Louis, Mosby-Year Book, 1994, p 349.

Developmental Hemostasis: Relevance to Newborns and Infants*

Maureen Andrew

*This work was supported by a grant-in-aid from the Medical Research Council of Canada.

Over the past century, the discovery of individual components of hemostasis and their interactions has been accompanied by the realization that hemostasis is a dynamic, evolving process that is age dependent and begins *in utero*. Recent studies have provided reference ranges that delineate age-dependent features of hemostasis and facilitate the evaluation of infants with hemostatic disorders. Although evolving, the hemostatic system in healthy fetuses and infants must be considered physiologic because neither hemorrhagic nor thromboembolic complications occur. However, the susceptibility of the young to hemostatic complications differs significantly from that of adults. For example, the prevalence of thromboembolic complications in hospitalized sick newborns is relatively rare compared with that in adults. In contrast, hemorrhagic complications are not uncommon in sick newborns and are most frequently due to events such as vitamin K (VK) deficiency and asphyxia.

The first week of life is a time when serious hemorrhagic and thrombotic complications occur from either hereditary or, more frequently, acquired pathologic disorders. The evaluation of newborns for hemorrhagic or thrombotic complications presents unique problems that are not encountered in older children and adults. For example, physiologic levels of many coagulation proteins in newborns are low, and this makes the diagnosis of some inherited and acquired hemostatic problems difficult to establish. Because the hemostatic system is dynamic, multiple reference ranges reflecting the gestational and postnatal age of infants are necessary.[1-3] The index of suspicion for severe congenital deficiencies of components of hemostasis must be increased in newborns, as most severe deficiencies present in the neonatal period.

After confirming the presence of a hemostatic problem, the clinician is faced with the challenge of providing a safe and effective form of therapy. Just as for adults, the efficacy and safety of therapeutic interventions for infants must undergo testing in randomized controlled trials, whenever feasible, and alternative study designs can be useful in dealing with rare or consistently life-threatening events. Guidelines for the classification of study design, and therefore the strength of the findings, have been established.[4] In this chapter, conclusions from studies with strong designs are given greater weight than conclusions from studies with weaker designs. When clinical data from studies in newborn infants are not available, extrapolations are made from data for adults in combination with results from *in vitro* studies and newborn animal models. An understanding of developmental hemostasis in the broadest sense optimizes the prevention, diagnosis, and treatment of hemostatic problems during childhood and undoubtedly provides new insights into the pathophysiology of hemorrhagic and thrombotic complications for all ages. In this chapter, platelet function, coagulation, and fibrinolysis are reviewed in the context of developmental hemostasis.

DEVELOPMENTAL HEMOSTASIS
Platelets
General Information

Platelets from cord blood have been extensively studied and compared with platelets from adults. Flow cytometry has facilitated the study of platelets directly from newborns because of the small sample volume required for extensive platelet function studies. Because cord and newborn platelets may have some differences in function, they are designated separately in this chapter. Differences in sample timing, method of collection, labor, concentrations, and compositions of platelet agonists, and laboratory testing likely contribute to apparently conflicting reports on cord platelet function.

Platelet Number, Size, and Survival

Platelet counts and mean platelet volumes in newborns are similar to those in adults, with values of 150,000 to 450,000 $\times 10^9$/L and 7 to 9 fL, respectively.[5-13] Platelet counts in fetuses between 18 and 30 weeks of gestation also fall within the adult range, with the average value being 250 $\times 10^9$/L.[14] Platelet survival has not been measured in healthy infants. However, the survival of ^{111}In oxine–labeled platelets is similar in adult and newborn rabbits,[10, 15] and in humans the platelet survivals are the longest in the least thrombocytopenic infants.[16] Together, these studies suggest that platelet survivals in newborns do not likely differ significantly from those in adults (i.e., 7 to 10 days).

Platelet Structure

Cord platelets have been examined for the presence of secretory granules and defects in release mechanisms. Electron microscopy studies have demonstrated normal numbers of granules; however, serotonin and adenosine diphosphate (ADP), which are stored in dense granules, are present at concentrations that are less than 50% of adult values.

Platelet Adhesion

When the endothelial lining of blood vessels is damaged or removed, platelets adhere to subendothelial layers, undergo changes in shape, and spread over the damaged surface. This process requires that *von Willebrand's factor (vWf)*, a plasma factor, binds to a specific component of the platelet membrane, glycoprotein Ib, forming a bridge between the subendothelial surface and platelet.[17] Platelet adhesion at birth has not been assessed with sensitive and reproducible assays; this may explain the conflicting *in vitro* results given in the literature.[18, 19] Glycoprotein Ib is present on fetal platelet membranes in adult quantities.[20] Both the plasma concentrations of vWf and the proportion of high-molecular-weight multimers (and therefore more active forms) of vWf are increased in newborns.[21, 22] The cord multimeric pattern of vWf appears similar to the forms released by endothelial cells; this similarity suggests that mechanisms for processing the multimeric structure of vWf may not be fully developed at birth. The quantitative and qualitative differences in vWf at birth are likely responsible for the enhanced cord platelet agglutination to low concentrations of ristocetin[21-23] and contribute to the short bleeding time in newborns.[18, 24-28]

Platelet Aggregation

Following activation of platelets, glycoproteins IIb and IIIa come together on platelet surfaces to form 1:1 complexes that are binding sites for fibrinogen and, to a lesser extent, vWf and fibronectin. Platelet-to-platelet adherence or aggregation is mediated by fibrinogen bound to glycoprotein IIb-IIIa. Glycoprotein IIb-IIIa complexes are expressed on platelet membranes early in gestation,[20] and fibrinogen is present in adult amounts by the time of viability.[1-3] The capacity of cord platelets to aggregate following exposure to a variety of agonists has been variable, with some observations being more consistent than others.

Epinephrine-induced aggregation of cord platelets is consistently decreased when compared with that of adult platelets because of the decreased availability of α-adrenergic receptors.[18, 19, 23, 29-36] This phenomenon is transient and is due to either delayed maturation of these receptors or occupation by catecholamines released during birth. Ristocetin-induced agglutination of cord platelets is consistently increased compared with that of adult platelets, likely because of quantitative and qualitative increases in the level of vWf.[1-3] Aggregation of cord platelets induced by ADP, collagen, thrombin, and arachidonic acid is variable and may be moderately decreased or similar to that of adult platelets.[29, 31, 32, 37-39]

Decreased aggregation of cord platelets implies either a storage pool deficiency or an abnormality in secretion. The modestly decreased aggregation with some platelet agonists was initially thought to be due to a physiologic storage pool deficiency.[19, 40, 41] However, differences from adult platelets are small, and following incubation of newborn platelets with radiolabeled adenine, normal specific radioactivities of platelet adenosine triphosphate (ATP) and ADP are measured.[19] The absence of a classic storage pool deficiency was further supported by normal studies of newborn platelet granules with electron microscopy.[23, 42]

An aspirin-like defect does not occur in newborn platelets because mixing studies of newborn and aspirin-treated platelets reveal normal platelet aggregation, production of arachidonic acid, and products of both the lipoxygenase and cyclooxygenase pathway.[19, 37, 41-46] Thus, neither a classic storage pool deficiency nor an aspirin-like platelet defect adequately explains the functional deficit of newborn platelets. Adult and newborn clots exhibit similar platelet-mediated clot retraction.[47]

Platelet Activation and Secretion

Studies of activation pathways leading to release have not identified specific abnormalities in cord platelets. Inositol phosphate production and protein phosphorylation are normal, as is production of arachidonic acid and its metabolites.[39] In fact, cord platelets release more arachidonic acid than adult platelets in response to stimulation by thrombin.[29] This increased release may be due to the greater reactivity of platelet membranes induced by low levels of vitamin E.[44, 48] Agonist receptors, with the exception of the α-adrenergic receptor discussed previously, do not appear to be decreased in number. Despite a poor response to collagen stimulation, cord platelets have normal numbers of the collagen receptor glycoprotein Ia-IIa present on platelet membranes.[20, 49] Coupling of agonist receptors to phospholipases may be the site of this transient activation defect in response to collagen.[50]

Studies of Platelets from Newborns

A few studies have assessed aggregation of newborn platelets obtained during the first few days of life; other studies have evaluated platelets of older neonates.[33, 36] In one study, abnormal platelet aggregation in response to ADP (decreased primary wave and absent secondary wave) was observed in cord platelet-rich plasma.[33] However, improved platelet aggregation was seen in newborn platelets drawn 2 hours after birth, with normalization of platelet aggregation at 48 hours.[36] Studies using whole-blood flow cytometry show that, compared with adult platelets, neonatal platelets are hyporeactive to thrombin, a combination of ADP and epinephrine, and a thromboxane A$_2$ analogue (Fig. 5–1).[29, 30, 34, 51] The clinical significance of these observations remains unknown.

Bleeding Time

Measurement of the bleeding time is currently the best *in vivo* test of platelet interaction with the vessel wall.[24] Automated devices modified for newborns and children are available and have been standardized.[25] Bleeding times in infants during the first week of life are

significantly shorter than those in adults.[18, 24–28] Several mechanisms contribute to this enhanced platelet/vessel wall interaction, including higher plasma concentrations of vWf,[1–3] enhanced function of vWf due to a disproportional increase in the high-molecular-weight multimeric forms,[21,22] active multimers, large red cells,[52] and high hematocrits.[53] The significance of mild platelet aggregation defects in cord platelets is uncertain when bleeding times in newborns are shorter than those in adults.

Activation During the Birth Process

There is strong evidence that platelets are activated during the birth process. Cord plasma levels of thromboxane B$_2$, β-thromboglobulin, and platelet factor 4 are increased,[44, 54, 55] the granular content of cord platelets is decreased, and epinephrine receptor availability is reduced, perhaps secondary to occupation.[54, 56] The mechanisms of activation are likely multifactorial and include thermal changes, hypoxia, acidosis, adrenergic stimulation, and the thrombogenic effects of amniotic fluid. Activation of the coagulation system may provide an explanation for the paradox that one-stage coagulation times are prolonged in the newborn but that various measures of whole-blood clotting duration are shortened relative to those in the adult.[18, 57, 58]

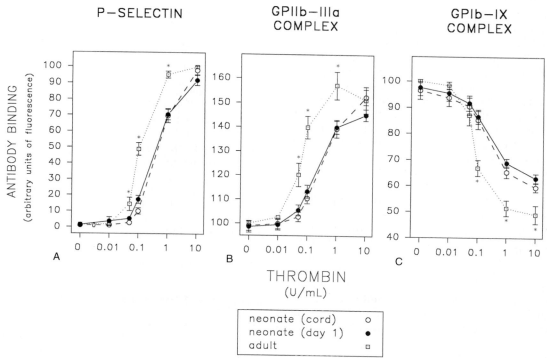

Figure 5–1. Effect of thrombin on the surface expression of P-selectin *(A)*, the glycoprotein IIb-IIIa complex *(B)*, and the glycoprotein Ib-IX complex *(C)* on neonatal and adult platelets in whole blood. Results were similar for cord and neonatal day one values. Expression of P-selectin and glycoprotein IIb-IIIa complexes was decreased in newborns, whereas glycoprotein Ib-IX expression was relatively preserved in newborns compared with adults following stimulation with thrombin. Data are expressed as mean ± SEM; n = 20. *Asterisks* indicate $P < .05$ for both cord blood and day one neonatal platelets compared with adult platelets. (From Rajasekhar D, Kestin A, et al: Neonatal platelets are less reactive than adult platelets to physiological agonists in whole blood. Thromb Haemost 1994; 72:957.)

Blood Vessel Wall: Age and Anticoagulant Properties

In the 1980s, it was established that the endothelium fulfills a complex role in hemostasis, preventing thrombotic complications under physiologic conditions and promoting fibrin formation when injured. One of the anticoagulant properties of endothelial cell surfaces is mediated by lipoxygenase and cyclooxygenase metabolites of unsaturated fatty acids. Prostacyclin (prostaglandin I_2) production by cord vessels exceeds that by vessels in adults.[59] A second endothelial cell–mediated antithrombotic property is the promotion of antithrombin III (AT-III) neutralization of thrombin by cell surface proteoglycans. Structurally, there is evidence that vessel wall glycosaminoglycans of the young differ from those of adults.[60, 61] Nitric oxide (NO), or endothelium-derived relaxing factor, is a labile humeral agent that modulates vascular tone in the fetal and postnatal lung and contributes to the normal decline in pulmonary vascular resistance at birth. Like prostacyclin, NO is a potent inhibitor of platelet activation and adhesion to the damaged vessel wall.[62] Cord plasma can generate less thrombin in the presence of human umbilical endothelial cells than it can against a plastic surface. This is owing to the cell surface promotion of AT-III inhibition of thrombin.[63]

THE COAGULATION SYSTEM

General Information

Our understanding of the physiology of hemostasis in newborns and infants is lacking compared with our knowledge of this subject as it pertains to adults. The reasons for this deficit are several: in newborns and infants, multiple reference ranges are required because these patients have rapidly evolving systems[1–3, 439]; blood sampling in the young is technically difficult; only small blood samples can be obtained; microtechniques are required[64]; and greater variability in plasma concentrations of coagulation proteins necessitates the use of large sample sizes.

Coagulation proteins do not cross the placental barrier but are independently synthesized by the fetus.[14, 65–76] Plasma concentrations of most coagulation proteins are measurable by a gestational age of 10 weeks, and they continue to increase gradually in parallel with the gestational age (Table 5–1). True reference ranges for extremely premature infants are not available because the majority of these infants have postnatal complications. Tables 5–2 to 5–5 provide reference ranges for coagulation proteins for premature (gestational age, 30 to 36 weeks) and full-term infants on day 1 of life as well as longitudinally, over the first 6 months of life.[1]

Screening Tests

The variable results for coagulation screening tests reflect the use of cord blood samples rather than samples from infants or differing ethnic populations, or the use of different reagents.[77, 78] Variation in prothrombin time (PT) results can be minimized by reporting the PT as

Table 5–1. REFERENCE VALUES FOR COMPONENTS OF THE COAGULATION SYSTEM IN HEALTHY FETUSES* AND PREMATURE INFANTS AT BIRTH†

Coagulation Tests	Gestational Age (wk)			
	19–27,		28–31,	
	M	(B)	M	(B)**
PT (s)	—		15.4	(14.6–16.9)
APTT (s)	—		108	(80.0–168)
Fibrinogen (g/L)	1.0	(±0.43)‡	2.56	(1.60–5.50)
Factor II (U/mL)	0.12	(±0.02)§	0.31	(0.19–0.54)
Factor V (U/mL)	0.41	(±0.10)‖	0.65	(0.43–0.80)
Factor VII (U/mL)	0.28	(±0.04)§	0.37	(0.24–0.76)
Factor VIII (U/mL)	0.39	(±0.14)‖	0.79	(0.37–1.26)
vWf (U/mL)	0.64	(±0.13)‖	1.41	(0.83–2.23)
Factor IX (U/mL)	0.10	(±0.01)§	0.18	(0.17–0.20)
Factor X (U/mL)	0.21	(±0.03)§	0.36	(0.25–0.64)
Factor XI (U/mL)	—		0.23	(0.11–0.33)
Factor XII (U/mL)	0.22	(±0.03)	0.25	(0.05–0.35)
PK (U/mL)	—		0.26	(0.15–0.32)
HMWK (U/mL)	—		0.32	(0.19–0.52)
AT-III (U/mL)	0.24	(±0.03)¶	0.28	(0.20–0.38)
HCII (U/mL)	0.27	(±0.05)¶	—	
Protein C (U/mL)	0.11	(±0.03)§	—	

All factors except fibrinogen are expressed as units per milliliter (U/mL) where pooled plasma contains 1.0 U/mL. All values are extrapolated from designated references and are expressed as a mean (M) followed by the lower and upper boundary (B).

PT = prothrombin time; APTT = activated partial thromboplastin time; vWf = von Willebrand's factor; PK = prekallikrein; HMWK = high-molecular-weight kininogen; AT-III = antithrombin III; HCII = heparin cofactor II.

*Gestational age, 19 to 27 weeks.
†Gestational age, 28 to 31 weeks.
‡From reference 68.
§From reference 72.
‖From reference 14.
¶From reference 74.
**From reference 599.

From Andrew M, Paes B, et al: Development of the human coagulation system in the full-term infant. Blood 1987; 70:165.

an *international normalized ratio (INR)* (see Tables 5–2 and 5–3).[79] The INR is calculated as the patient PT/control PT to the power of the *international sensitivity index.*[1–3] The international sensitivity index corrects for the large variation in sensitivity of thromboplastin reagents to plasma concentrations of coagulation proteins. The thrombin clotting time performed in the absence of calcium is prolonged because of the presence of the "fetal" form of fibrinogen at birth.[1–3] For Tables 5–2 and 5–3, the thrombin clotting time was measured in the presence of calcium, so that abnormal values secondary to the presence of heparin, as well as low levels of fibrinogen, could be detected.

Coagulant Proteins

The VK-dependent factors are the most extensively studied group of factors in infants. This attention reflects the importance of hemolytic disease of the newborn (HDN), an acquired bleeding disorder caused by pathologically low levels of the VK-dependent proteins.[80–82] Physiologically low levels of factors II, VII, IX, and X in Tables 5–2 and 5–3 are similar to those in other reports[1–3, 5, 83–92] and were measured in infants who received VK prophylaxis at birth. The levels of

Table 5–2. REFERENCE VALUES FOR COAGULATION TESTS IN HEALTHY FULL-TERM INFANTS DURING THE FIRST 6 MONTHS OF LIFE

Coagulation Tests	Day 1		Day 5		Day 30		Day 90		Day 180		Adult	
	M	(B)	M	(B)	M	(B)	M	(B)	M	(B)	M	(B)
PT (s)	13.0	(10.1–15.9)*	12.4	(10.0–15.3)*	11.8	(10.0–14.3)*	11.9	(10.0–14.2)*	12.3	(10.7–13.9)*	12.4	(10.8–13.9)
INR	1.00	(0.53–1.62)	0.89	(0.53–1.48)	0.79	(0.53–1.26)	0.81	(0.53–1.26)	0.88	(0.61–1.17)	0.89	(0.64–1.17)
APTT (s)	42.9	(31.3–54.5)	42.6	(25.4–59.8)	40.4	(32.0–55.2)	37.1	(29.0–50.1)*	35.5	(28.1–42.9)*	33.5	(26.6–40.3)
TCT (s)	23.5	(19.0–28.3)*	23.1	(18.0–29.2)	24.3	(19.4–29.2)	25.1	(20.5–29.7)*	25.5	(19.8–31.2)*	25.0	(19.7–30.3)
Fibrinogen (g/L)	2.83	(1.67–3.99)*	3.12	(1.62–4.62)*	2.70	(1.62–3.78)*	2.43	(1.50–3.79)*	2.51	(1.50–3.87)*	2.78	(1.56–4.00)
Factor II (U/mL)	0.48	(0.26–0.70)	0.63	(0.33–0.93)	0.68	(0.34–1.02)	0.75	(0.45–1.05)	0.88	(0.60–1.16)	1.08	(0.70–1.46)
Factor V (U/mL)	0.72	(0.34–1.08)	0.95	(0.45–1.45)	0.98	(0.62–1.34)	0.90	(0.45–1.32)	0.91	(0.55–1.27)	1.06	(0.62–1.50)
Factor VII (U/mL)	0.66	(0.28–1.04)	0.89	(0.35–1.43)	0.90	(0.42–1.38)	0.91	(0.39–1.43)	0.87	(0.47–1.27)	1.05	(0.67–1.43)
Factor VIII (U/mL)	1.00	(0.50–1.78)*	0.88	(0.50–1.54)*	0.91	(0.50–1.57)	0.79	(0.50–1.25)*	0.73	(0.50–1.09)	0.99	(0.50–1.49)
vWf (U/mL)	1.53	(0.50–2.87)	1.40	(0.50–2.54)	1.28	(0.50–2.46)	1.18	(0.50–2.06)	1.07	(0.50–1.97)	0.92	(0.50–1.58)
Factor IX (U/mL)	0.53	(0.15–0.91)	0.53	(0.15–0.91)	0.51	(0.21–0.81)	0.67	(0.21–1.13)	0.86	(0.36–1.36)	1.09	(0.55–1.63)
Factor X (U/mL)	0.40	(0.12–0.68)	0.49	(0.19–0.79)	0.59	(0.31–0.87)	0.71	(0.35–1.07)	0.78	(0.38–1.18)	1.06	(0.70–1.52)
Factor XI (U/mL)	0.38	(0.10–0.66)	0.55	(0.23–0.87)	0.53	(0.27–0.79)	0.69	(0.41–0.97)	0.86	(0.49–1.34)	0.97	(0.67–1.27)
Factor XII (U/mL)	0.53	(0.13–0.93)	0.47	(0.11–0.83)	0.49	(0.17–0.81)	0.67	(0.25–1.09)	0.77	(0.39–1.15)	1.08	(0.52–1.64)
PK (U/mL)	0.37	(0.18–0.69)	0.48	(0.20–0.76)	0.57	(0.23–0.91)	0.73	(0.41–1.05)	0.86	(0.56–1.16)	1.12	(0.62–1.62)
HMWK (U/mL)	0.54	(0.06–1.02)	0.74	(0.16–1.32)	0.77	(0.33–1.21)	0.82	(0.30–1.46)*	0.82	(0.36–1.28)*	0.92	(0.50–1.36)
Factor XIIIa (U/mL)	0.79	(0.27–1.31)	0.94	(0.44–1.44)*	0.93	(0.39–1.47)*	1.04	(0.36–1.72)*	1.04	(0.46–1.62)*	0.92	(0.50–1.36)
Factor XIIIb (U/mL)	0.76	(0.30–1.22)	1.06	(0.32–1.80)	1.11	(0.39–1.73)*	1.16	(0.48–1.84)*	1.10	(0.50–1.70)	0.97	(0.57–1.37)

All factors except fibrinogen are expressed as units per milliliter (U/mL) where pooled plasma contains 1.0 U/mL. All values are expressed as mean (M) followed by the lower and upper boundary encompassing 95% of the population (B). Between 40 and 77 samples were assayed for each value for the population.
INR = international normalized ratio; TCT = thrombin clotting time.
*Values indistinguishable from those of the adult.
From Andrew M, Paes B, Johnston M: Development of the hemostatic system in the neonate and young infant. Am J Pediatr Hematol Oncol 1990; 12:95.

Table 5–3. REFERENCE VALUES FOR COAGULATION TESTS IN HEALTHY PREMATURE INFANTS (30–36 WEEKS' GESTATION) DURING THE FIRST 6 MONTHS OF LIFE

Coagulation Tests	Day 1		Day 5		Day 30		Day 90		Day 180		Adult	
	M	(B)	M	(B)	M	(B)	M	(B)	M	(B)	M	(B)
PT (s)	13.0	(10.6–16.2)*	12.5	(10.0–15.3)*	11.8	(10.0–13.6)*	12.3	(10.0–14.6)	12.5	(10.0–15.0)*	12.4	(10.8–13.9)
INR	1.0	(0.61–1.70)	0.91	(0.53–1.48)	0.79	(0.53–1.11)	0.88	(0.53–1.32)	0.91	(0.53–1.48)	0.89	(0.64–1.17)
APTT (s)	53.6	(27.5–79.4)†	50.5	(26.9–74.1)	44.7	(26.9–62.5)	39.5	(28.3–50.7)	37.5	(27.2–53.3)	33.5	(26.6–40.3)
TCT (s)	24.8	(19.2–30.4)	24.1	(18.8–29.4)*	24.4	(18.8–29.9)	25.1	(19.4–30.8)	25.2	(18.9–31.5)	25.0	(19.7–30.3)
Fibrinogen (g/L)	2.43	(1.50–3.73)*, †	2.80	(1.60–4.18)*, †	2.54	(1.50–4.14)	2.46	(1.50–3.52)	2.28	(1.50–3.60)	2.78	(1.56–4.00)
Factor II (U/mL)	0.45	(0.20–0.77)	0.57	(0.29–0.85)†	0.57	(0.36–0.95)	0.68	(0.30–1.06)	0.87	(0.51–1.23)	1.08	(0.70–1.46)
Factor V (U/mL)	0.88	(0.41–1.44)*, †	1.00	(0.46–1.54)*	1.02	(0.48–1.56)*	0.99	(0.59–1.39)	1.02	(0.58–1.46)*	1.06	(0.62–1.50)
Factor VII (U/mL)	0.67	(0.21–1.13)	0.84	(0.30–1.38)	0.83	(0.21–1.45)	0.87	(0.31–1.43)	0.99	(0.47–1.51)*	1.05	(0.67–1.43)
Factor VIII (U/mL)	1.11	(0.50–2.13)	1.15	(0.53–2.05)*, †	1.11	(0.50–1.99)	1.06	(0.58–1.88)*, †	0.99	(0.50–1.87)*, †	0.99	(0.50–1.49)
vWf (U/mL)	1.36	(0.78–2.10)	1.33	(0.72–2.19)	1.36	(0.66–2.16)	1.12	(0.75–1.84)*, †	0.98	(0.54–1.58)*	0.92	(0.50–1.58)
Factor IX (U/mL)	0.35	(0.19–0.65)†	0.42	(0.14–0.74)*	0.44	(0.13–0.80)	0.59	(0.25–0.93)	0.81	(0.50–1.20)	1.09	(0.55–1.63)
Factor X (U/mL)	0.41	(0.11–0.71)	0.51	(0.19–0.83)	0.56	(0.20–0.92)	0.67	(0.35–0.99)	0.77	(0.35–1.19)	1.06	(0.70–1.52)
Factor XI (U/mL)	0.30	(0.08–0.52)†	0.41	(0.13–0.69)†	0.43	(0.15–0.71)†	0.59	(0.25–0.93)	0.78	(0.46–1.10)	0.97	(0.67–1.27)
Factor XII (U/mL)	0.38	(0.10–0.66)†	0.39	(0.09–0.69)†	0.43	(0.11–0.75)	0.61	(0.15–1.07)	0.82	(0.22–1.42)	1.08	(0.52–1.64)
PK (U/mL)	0.33	(0.09–0.57)	0.45	(0.25–0.75)	0.59	(0.31–0.87)	0.79	(0.37–1.21)	0.78	(0.40–1.16)	1.12	(0.62–1.62)
HMWK (U/mL)	0.49	(0.09–0.89)	0.62	(0.24–1.00)†	0.64	(0.16–1.12)†	0.78	(0.32–1.24)	0.83	(0.41–1.25)*	0.92	(0.50–1.36)
Factor XIIIa (U/mL)	0.70	(0.32–1.08)	1.01	(0.57–1.45)*	0.99	(0.51–1.47)*	1.13	(0.71–1.55)*	1.13	(0.65–1.61)*	1.05	(0.55–1.55)
Factor XIIIb (U/mL)	0.81	(0.35–1.27)	1.10	(0.68–1.58)*	1.07	(0.57–1.57)*	1.21	(0.75–1.67)	1.15	(0.67–1.63)	0.97	(0.57–1.37)

All factors except fibrinogen are expressed as units per milliliter (U/mL) where pooled plasma contains 1.0 U/mL. All values are given as a mean (M) followed by the lower and upper boundary encompassing 95% of the population (B). Between 40 and 96 samples were assayed for each value for the newborn. Some measurements were skewed owing to a disproportionate number of high values. The lower limits exclude the lower 2.5% of the population.
*Values indistinguishable from those of adults.
†Measurements are skewed owing to a disproportionate number of high values.
From Andrew M, Paes B, Johnston M: Development of the human coagulation system in the healthy premature infant. Blood 1988; 72:1651.

Table 5–4. REFERENCE VALUES FOR THE INHIBITORS OF COAGULATION IN INFANTS DURING THE FIRST 6 MONTHS OF LIFE

Inhibitor Levels	Day 1 M	(B)	Day 5 M	(B)	Day 30 M	(B)	Day 90 M	(B)	Day 180 M	(B)	Adult M	(B)
					Healthy Full-Term Infants							
AT (U/mL)	0.63	(0.39–0.87)	0.67	(0.41–0.93)	0.78	(0.48–1.08)	0.97	(0.73–1.21)*	1.04	(0.84–1.24)*	1.05	(0.79–1.31)
α₂M (U/mL)	1.39	(0.95–1.83)	1.48	(0.98–1.98)	1.50	(1.06–1.94)	1.76	(1.26–2.26)	1.91	(1.49–2.33)	0.86	(0.52–1.20)
C1E-INH (U/mL)	0.72	(0.36–1.08)	0.90	(0.60–1.20)*	0.89	(0.47–1.31)	1.15	(0.71–1.59)	1.41	(0.89–1.93)	1.01	(0.71–1.31)
α₁AT (U/mL)	0.93	(0.49–1.37)*	0.89	(0.49–1.29)*	0.62	(0.36–0.88)	0.72	(0.42–1.02)	0.77	(0.47–1.07)	0.93	(0.55–1.31)
HCII (U/mL)	0.43	(0.10–0.93)	0.48	(0.00–0.96)	0.47	(0.10–0.87)	0.72	(0.10–1.46)	1.20	(0.50–1.90)	0.96	(0.66–1.26)
Protein C (U/mL)	0.35	(0.17–0.53)	0.42	(0.20–0.64)	0.43	(0.21–0.65)	0.54	(0.28–0.80)	0.59	(0.37–0.81)	0.96	(0.64–1.28)
Protein S (U/mL)	0.36	(0.12–0.60)	0.50	(0.22–0.78)	0.63	(0.33–0.93)	0.86	(0.54–1.18)*	0.87	(0.55–1.19)*	0.92	(0.60–1.24)
TM (AU)[106]	10.55	(4.84–16.25)							7.26	(3.96–10.56)	4.60	(2.9–6.3)
TFPI (U/mL)‡	0.7331*										0.8270	
					Healthy Premature Infants (30–36 Weeks' Gestation)							
AT (U/mL)	0.38	(0.14–0.62)†	0.56	(0.30–0.82)	0.59	(0.37–0.81)†	0.83	(0.45–1.21)†	0.90	(0.52–1.28)†	1.05	(0.79–1.31)
α₂M (U/mL)	1.10	(0.56–1.82)†	1.25	(0.71–1.77)	1.38	(0.72–2.04)	1.80	(1.20–2.66)	2.09	(1.10–3.21)	0.86	(0.52–1.20)
C1E-INH (U/mL)	0.65	(0.31–0.99)	0.83	(0.45–1.21)	0.74	(0.40–1.24)†	1.14	(0.60–1.68)*	1.40	(0.96–2.04)	1.01	(0.71–1.31)
α₁AT (U/mL)	0.90	(0.36–1.44)*	0.94	(0.42–1.46)*	0.76	(0.38–1.12)†	0.81	(0.49–1.13)*, †	0.89	(0.45–1.40)*, †	0.93	(0.55–1.31)
HCII (U/mL)	0.32	(0.10–0.60)†	0.34	(0.10–0.69)	0.43	(0.15–0.71)	0.61	(0.20–1.11)	0.89		0.96	(0.66–1.26)
Protein C (U/mL)	0.28	(0.12–0.44)†	0.31	(0.11–0.51)	0.37	(0.15–0.59)†	0.45	(0.23–0.67)†	0.57	(0.31–0.83)	0.96	(0.64–1.28)
Protein S (U/mL)	0.26	(0.14–0.38)†	0.37	(0.13–0.61)	0.56	(0.22–0.90)	0.76	(0.40–1.12)†	0.82	(0.44–1.20)	0.92	(0.60–1.24)

AT = antithrombin; α₂M = α₂-macroglobulin; C1E-INH = C1 esterase inhibitor; α₁AT = α₁-antitrypsin; TM = thrombomodulin.
All values are expressed in units per milliliter (U/mL) where pooled plasma contains 1.0 U/mL. All values are given as a mean (M) followed by the lower and upper boundary encompassing 95% of the population (B). Between 40 and 75 samples were assayed for each value for the newborn. Some measurements were skewed owing to a disproportionate number of high values. The lower limits exclude the lower 2.5% of the population.
*Values indistinguishable from those of adults.
†Values different from those of full-term infants.
‡Cord blood.[108]
From Andrew M, Paes B, Johnston M: Development of the hemostatic system in the neonate and young infant. Am J Pediatr Hematol Oncol 1990; 12:95.

Table 5–5. REFERENCE VALUES FOR THE COMPONENTS OF THE FIBRINOLYTIC SYSTEM DURING THE FIRST 6 MONTHS OF LIFE

Fibrinolytic System	Day 1 M	(B)	Day 5 M	(B)	Day 30 M	(B)	Day 90 M	(B)	Day 180 M	(B)	Adult M (B)
					Healthy Full-Term Infants						
Plasminogen (U/mL)	0.58	(0.37–0.79)	0.65	(0.42–0.87)	0.59	(0.38–0.80)	0.74	(0.52–0.96)	0.90	(0.66–1.13)	1.00 (0.74–1.26)
TPA (ng/mL)	9.60	(5.00–18.9)	5.60	(4.00–10.0)*	4.10	(1.00–6.00)*	2.10	(1.00–5.00)*	2.80	(1.00–6.00)	4.90 (1.40–8.40)
α₂AP (U/mL)	0.85	(0.55–1.15)	1.00	(0.70–1.30)*	1.00	(0.76–1.24)*	1.08	(0.76–1.40)*	1.11	(0.83–1.39)*	1.02 (0.68–1.36)
PAI (U/mL)	6.40	(2.00–15.1)	2.30	(0.00–8.10)*	3.4	(0.00–8.80)*	7.20	(1.00–15.3)	8.10	(6.00–13.0)	3.6 (0.00–11.0)
					Healthy Premature Infants						
Plasminogen (U/mL)	0.51	(0.33–0.74)†	0.56	(0.36–0.78)†	0.54	(0.32–0.75)	0.71	(0.47–0.95)	0.82	(0.57–1.07)	1.00 (0.74–1.26)
TPA (ng/mL)	8.48	(3.00–16.70)	3.97	(2.00–6.93)*	4.13	(2.00–7.79)*	3.31	(2.00–5.07)*	3.48	(2.00–5.85)*	4.96 (1.46–8.46)
α₂AP (U/mL)	0.78	(0.40–1.16)	0.81	(0.49–1.13)†	0.89	(0.55–1.23)†	1.06	(0.64–1.48)*	1.15	(0.77–1.53)	1.02 (0.68–1.36)
PAI (U/mL)	5.40	(0.00–12.2)*, †	2.50	(0.00–7.10)*	4.30	(0.00–11.8)*	4.80	(1.00–10.2)*, †	4.90	(1.00–10.2)*, †	3.60 (0.00–11.0)
μ-PA (ng/mL)	0.18	(0.08–0.28)†									0.32 (0.18–0.46)
PAI-2 (ng/mL)	<1.6†										<1.6

TPA = tissue plasminogen activator; PAI = plasminogen activator inhibitor; μ-PA = urokinase plasminogen activator.
For α₂AP, values are expressed as units per milliliter (U/mL) where pooled plasma contains 1.0 U/mL. Plasminogen units are those recommended by the Committee on Thrombolytic Agents. Values for TPA are given as nanograms per milliliter. Values for PAI are given as units per milliliter where one unit of PAI-1 activity is defined as the amount of PAI-1 that inhibits one international unit of human single chain TPA. All values are given as a mean (M) followed by the lower and upper boundary encompassing 95% of the population (B).
*Values indistinguishable from those of adults.
†Values different from those of full-term infant.
‡Cord blood.
From Andrew M, Paes B, Johnston M: Development of the hemostatic system in the neonate and young infant. Am J Pediatr Hematol Oncol 1990; 12:95, and Reverdiau-Moalic P, Gruel Y, et al: Comparative study of the fibrinolytic system in human fetuses and in pregnant women. Thromb Res 1991; 61:489.

both the VK-dependent factors and the four contact factors (XI, XII, prekallikrein, and high-molecular-weight kininogen) gradually increase to values approaching those in the adult by 6 months of life.[1-3, 5] The prolonged activated partial thromboplastin time (APTT) during the first months of life is in large part due to the low levels of the four contact factors.[93]

Plasma levels of fibrinogen, factors V, VIII, and XIII, and vWf are not decreased at birth (see Tables 5-2 and 5-3).[1-3, 5, 83-92] Fibrinogen levels continue to increase after birth; this is important to recognize when an elevated fibrinogen level is used as a marker of sepsis.[94] Plasma levels of factor VIII are skewed toward the high measurements, necessitating an adjustment of the lower limit of normal (see Tables 5-2 and 5-3). Fewer than 1% of values for factor VIII are less than 0.40 units/mL, and all values are greater than 0.30 units/mL. Levels of both vWf and high-molecular-weight multimers are increased at birth and for the first 3 months of life.[29]

Inhibitors of Coagulation

Plasma concentrations of inhibitors of coagulation in newborns also differ from those in adults (see Table 5-4). Levels of C1 esterase inhibitor and α_2-macroglobulin are in the adult range at birth and increase to values well above adult levels by 6 months of age (see Table 5-4).[1] In contrast, levels of AT-III, protein C, protein S, and heparin cofactor II are low during the first week of life and in the range at which spontaneous thrombotic disorders occur in heterozygous adults. Only protein C levels remain low at 6 months of age and do not reach adult values until early childhood.[95] Tissue factor pathway inhibitor (TFPI) levels in newborns have been reported as 10.55 ± 5.7 AU (arbitrary units) or 64% of adult values.[96]

Regulation of Thrombin

Thrombin regulation, a key step in hemostasis, is both delayed and decreased in newborn plasma compared with adult plasma, and similar to plasmas from adults receiving therapeutic doses of warfarin or heparin (Fig. 5-2).[97] The amount of thrombin generated is directly proportional to the prothrombin concentration,[98] whereas the rate of thrombin generation reflects the concentration of other procoagulants. Thrombin generation in newborn plasma is further decreased in the presence of endothelial cell surfaces, but not to the same extent as adult plasma.[63]

Direct Inhibitors of Thrombin

Thrombin is directly inhibited by AT-III, heparin cofactor II, and α_2-macroglobulin. Alpha$_2$-macroglobulin is a more important inhibitor of thrombin in plasmas from newborns than it is in plasmas from adults.[99] Alpha$_2$-macroglobulin compensates, in part, for the low levels of AT-III in newborns, even in the presence of endothelial cell surfaces (Fig. 5-3).[99, 100] In addition, a circulating physiologic anticoagulant in cord blood has

properties similar to those of the glycosaminoglycan dermatan sulphate[61] and not to those of heparin.[61, 101] The fetal proteoglycan is present in plasma in concentrations of 0.29 μg/mL, has a molecular weight of 150,000 kd, and catalyzes thrombin inhibition by means of the natural inhibitor heparin cofactor II.[54, 56] The fetal anticoagulant also is present in plasmas from pregnant women and is produced by the placenta.[102] The length of time that the fetal anticoagulant circulates in newborns is not known; however, it is known that it is still present during the first week of life in sick premature infants with respiratory distress syndrome. Despite these differences, the rate of inhibition of thrombin is still slower in newborns than it is in adults.[99]

Protein C/Protein S System

A second mechanism for inhibiting thrombin coagulant activity is the *protein C/protein S system*. When thrombin binds to the endothelial cell surface receptor thrombomodulin, it no longer cleaves fibrinogen or factors V and VIII, nor does it activate platelets. However, it can change the VK-dependent inhibitor protein C to its

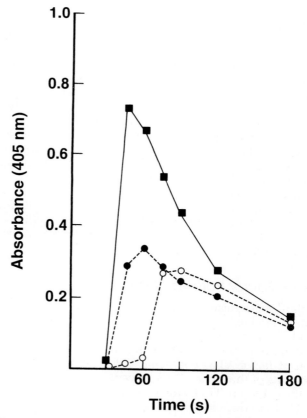

Figure 5-2. Thrombin generation following activation in the partial thromboplastin system was significantly decreased in plasma from full-term infants on day one of life (*solid circles*) and in that from premature infants on day one of life (*open circles*) compared with that from adults (*solid squares*). The amount of thrombin generated was determined on the basis of its ability to cleave a chromogenic substrate, which results in a change in the absorbance reading at 405 nm.

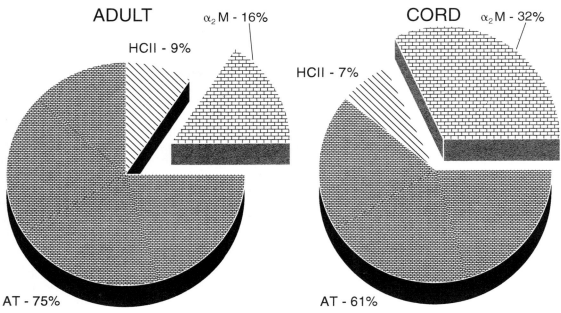

Figure 5–3. Percentage of ^{125}I-labeled thrombin complexed with inhibitors in pooled adult and newborn plasma. In adult plasma, antithrombin III (ATIII) inhibits 75% of the completed thrombin, whereas α_2 macroglobulin (α_2M) and heparin cofactor II (HCII) inhibit only 16% and 9%, respectively. In newborn plasma, α_2M inhibits 32% of the complexed thrombin, whereas ATIII and HCII inhibit 61% and 7%, respectively.

activated form, which, in the presence of protein S, inactivates factors Va and VIIIa by proteolytic degradation. At birth, plasma concentrations of protein C are very low, and they remain decreased during the first 6 months of life.[29] A "fetal" form of protein C differs from the adult form by a twofold increase in single-chain protein C.[103] Although total amounts of protein S are decreased at birth, functional activity is similar to that in the adult because protein S is completely present in the free, active form because of the absence of C4 binding protein.[104, 105] The influence of age on endothelial cell expression of thrombomodulin has not been determined; however, plasma concentrations of thrombomodulin are increased several-fold at birth and remain increased during early childhood.[106] Whether the overall activity of the protein C/protein S system varies with age is unknown.

Tissue Factor Pathway Inhibitor

A third mechanism regulating the generation of thrombin is effected by TFPI. A TFPI/factor Xa complex binds to factor VIIa/tissue factor (TF) in a factor Xa calcium-dependent reaction that results in the inhibition of factor VIIa. Following the generation of small amounts of thrombin, TFPI prevents further generation of thrombin via TF/FVIIa. Cord plasma concentrations of TFPI are decreased to 64% of adult values.[107, 108]

Regulation of Thrombin by Fibrin

The capacity of newborn fibrin clots to bind thrombin has been assessed through the measurement of fibrinopeptide A (FPA) production.[109] Cord plasma clots generate significantly less FPA than do adult plasma clots[109] because of the decreased plasma concentrations of prothrombin in cord plasma.[109] This observation suggests that thrombi in newborns may not have the same propensity to propagate as do thrombi in adult patients.

Physiologic Mechanisms

Potential mechanisms explaining the physiologically different plasma concentrations of coagulation proteins at birth include decreased production, accelerated clearance, and consumption at birth.

Production

Messenger ribonucleic acid (mRNA) levels have been measured for factors VII, VIII, IX, and X, fibrinogen, AT, and protein C in hepatocytes from 5 to 10-week-old human embryos and fetuses and in those from adults.[110] Embryonic-fetal transcripts and adult mRNAs are similar in size; and the nucleotide sequences of mRNA for factors IX and X were identical.[111] However, the expression of mRNA was variable, with adult values existing for some coagulation proteins but decreased expression for others (Fig. 5–4). Similar concentrations of prothrombin mRNA were found in the livers of newborn and adult rabbits[112]; another study reported lower prothrombin mRNA concentrations in sheep.[110]

Clearance

Fibrinogen, whether of fetal or adult origin, is cleared more rapidly in newborn lambs than it is in sheep.[113] Similarly, clearance of fibrinogen is accelerated in pre-

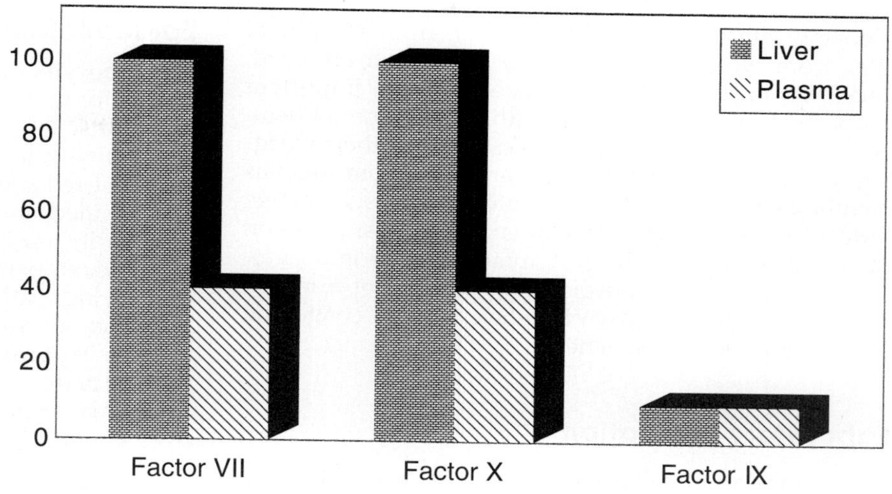

Figure 5–4. Concentrations of coagulation factors VII, IX, and X at 7 to 8 weeks' gestation in liver and plasma. Values are expressed as a percentage of adult levels. Interpretation: Liver and plasma values are similar for factor IX but are discordant for factors VII and X, indicating that multiple regulation mechanisms influence the ontogenic biologic availability of coagulation proteins.

mature infants with or without respiratory distress syndrome (RDS).[114, 115] AT-III survival times are shorter in healthy infants requiring exchange transfusion than they are in adults.[116] An increased basal metabolic rate in the young probably contributes to the accelerated clearance of proteins.[117] Although activation of the coagulation system occurs at birth,[66, 67, 118] it does not account for low concentrations of some coagulation proteins.[119–121]

Activation

Activation of coagulation *in vivo*, with the generation of thrombin, can be quantitated by specific activation peptides. Increased plasma concentrations of FPA and thrombin/antithrombin III complexes in cord plasma suggest that coagulation is activated at birth.[54, 56, 99, 122] However, this process seems to be well controlled and self limited. Indeed, activation of coagulation during the birth process does not result in significant consumption of circulating plasma coagulation proteins nor clinical morbidity.[66, 67]

THE FIBRINOLYTIC SYSTEM
Age and Components of the Fibrinolytic System

Although plasmin is generated and inhibited similarly in infants and adults, important differences do exist.[1] Plasma concentrations of fibrinolytic proteins differ in newborns and adults (see Table 5–5). In newborns, plasminogen levels are only 50% of adult values, α_2-antiplasmin levels are 80% of adult values, and plasma concentrations of PAI-1 and tissue plasminogen activator are significantly greater than adult levels.[1–3, 5, 83–91, 123–125] Increased levels of tissue plasminogen activator and PAI-1 on day 1 of life are in marked contrast to values from cord blood, in which concentrations of these two proteins are significantly lower than they are in adults.[123–125] The discrepancy between newborn and cord plasma concentrations of tissue plasminogen activator and PAI-1 can be explained by the enhanced release of tissue plasminogen activator and PAI-1 from the endothelium shortly following birth. PAI-2 levels are detectable in cord blood but are significantly lower than they are in pregnant women.[126] Plasminogen, like fibrinogen, has a fetal form. Fetal plasminogen exists in two glycoforms that have increased amounts of mannose and sialic acid.[127] The enzymatic activity of "fetal plasmin" as well as its binding to cellular receptors for fetal plasminogen are decreased. Cord levels of urokinase plasminogen activation have been measured in fetuses with activity levels of 0.18 ± 0.10 ng/mL, or 56% of adult values; and antigen levels of 0.23 ± 0.14, or 74% of adult values.[128] The plasma level of histidine-rich glycoprotein is 0.012 g/L (range, 0.005–0.020 g/L); this is in contrast to the adult level of 0.083 g/L (range, 0.05–0.12 g/L).[129–131]

Influence of Age on Endogenous Regulation of Fibrinolysis

Short whole-blood clotting times, short euglobulin lysis times, and increased plasma concentrations of the Bβ15-42 fibrin–related peptides all suggest that the fibrinolytic system is activated at birth.[2, 124] At the same time, the capacity of the fetal fibrinolytic system to generate plasmin in response to stimulation by a thrombolytic agent is decreased when compared with that of adults[132]; this reflects low levels of plasminogen.[29]

HEMORRHAGIC DISORDERS

Although acquired disorders are more frequent, severe forms of congenital factor deficiencies often first present in early infancy and should be seriously considered in otherwise healthy infants.[5, 84–89, 133]

Clinical Presentation

The clinical presentation of bleeding disorders is different in newborns than it is in children and adults. Bleeding may appear as oozing from the umbilicus, bleeding into the scalp, large cephalohematomas, bleeding after circumcision, bleeding from peripheral sites from which blood samples have been obtained, and bleeding into the skin. A small but important proportion of infants present with an intracranial hemorrhage (ICH) as the first manifestation of their bleeding tendency.[133–139] Sick infants can bleed from mucous membranes, the bladder, and sites of invasive procedures. Joint bleeding is infrequent. The most common causes of bleeding in healthy infants are thrombocytopenia secondary to transplacental passage of a maternal antiplatelet antibody, VK deficiency, and congenital coagulation factor deficiencies.

Laboratory Evaluation

The laboratory evaluation of infants with bleeding complications should include determination of PT, APTT, thrombin clotting time, fibrinogen level, platelet count, and in some patients, a bleeding time. Abnormalities in these tests usually prompt the selection of additional tests, such as specific factor assays and paracoagulation tests. For a male child in whom hemophilia A or B is suspected, specific factor assays should be performed regardless of the APTT value. Deficiencies of factor XIII and α_2-antiplasmin do not prolong the screening tests and must be measured directly if they are suspected.

Management

The appropriate management of an infant with a hemorrhagic disorder is dependent on the correct identification of the hemostatic defect. This information allows replacement therapy with specific factor concentrates, fresh frozen plasma (FFP), stored plasma, platelet concentrates, or cryoprecipitate. Other problems to consider are technical access, particularly if an exchange transfusion is planned, and the risk of graft-versus-host disease.

QUANTITATIVE PLATELET DISORDERS

General Information

Healthy infants have the same platelet counts as adults do,[5, 11] whereas premature infants have platelet counts that are slightly lower but still within the normal adult range (150×10^9 to 450×10^9/L).[5–9] The definition of thrombocytopenia in newborns is the same as that in adults: a platelet count less than 150×10^9/L. Studies of fetuses between 18 and 30 weeks' gestational age show a stable platelet count of approximately 250×10^9/L.[14] Consequently, platelet counts of less than 150×10^9/L are abnormal and indicate the need for investigation and, sometimes, treatment. Mean volumes of newborn platelets are similar to those of adult platelets, with values less than 10 fL (range, 7 to 9 fL).[9–11] Postnatally, mean platelet volumes increase slightly over the first 2 weeks of life, concomitantly with an increase in platelet count.[12, 13]

Epidemiology

Thrombocytopenia is the most common hemostatic abnormality in newborns admitted to neonatal intensive care units.[6, 8–10, 140] A single prospective cohort study[10, 27] and five retrospective reviews[9, 141–144] have provided the most reliable information on the frequency, natural history, mechanisms, and clinical impact of thrombocytopenia in newborns. There is general agreement that thrombocytopenia is indicative of the presence of an underlying pathologic process; however, the clinical relevance of mild thrombocytopenia remains to be proved. Approximately 22% of infants admitted into tertiary neonatal intensive care units develop thrombocytopenia.[10] For some infants, the thrombocytopenia is trivial, with platelet counts being between 100 and 150 $\times 10^9$/L. However, for 50% of affected infants, platelet counts decrease to less than 100×10^9/L, and for 20% of infants platelet counts are less than 50×10^9/L.[10] The natural history of thrombocytopenia in sick newborns is remarkably consistent[10]: it is present by day 2 of life in 75% of infants, reaches a nadir by day 4 in 75% of infants, and recovers to more than 150×10^9/L by day 10 of life in 86% of infants.[10, 143]

Pathogenesis

Thrombocytopenia can be caused by decreased platelet production, increased platelet destruction, or platelet pooling in an enlarged spleen, or by a combination of these mechanisms. Characterization of mechanisms responsible for thrombocytopenia is important because it has practical implications in assessing the risk of bleeding and management. Increased platelet destruction is the mechanism responsible for thrombocytopenia in most infants,[10, 15] whereas splenic sequestration contributes to thrombocytopenia in some infants.[15] The mean platelet volume at birth is similar to that of adults but increases significantly by day 7 of life in thrombocytopenic infants. Mean platelet volumes also increase by day 7 in sick nonthrombocytopenic infants in parallel with a decrease in their platelet count; this suggests that increased consumption of platelets occurs in many sick infants. Megakaryocytopoiesis differs in newborns and adults. There is an increased level of megakaryocyte progenitor cells in cord blood, particularly in premature infants.[145] Increased interleukin-11 expression and production in neonatal stromal cells may contribute to the increase in circulating thrombopoietic progenitors and increased progenitor proliferative rates observed in cord blood.[146]

At autopsy, thrombocytopenic infants have megakaryocyte numbers similar to those of nonthrombocytopenic infants with bone marrow biopsies.[10] The strongest evidence of platelet consumption comes from uniformly short survival times of radiolabeled platelets in thrombocytopenic infants.[10, 15, 26] Hypersplenism also is present in some infants.[15]

Increased Platelet Destruction

Thrombocytopenia due to increased platelet destruction can be considered as a nonimmune or an immune event. Frequent nonimmune causes of thrombocytopenia include disseminated intravascular coagulation (DIC) and exchange transfusion.[10] Exchange transfusions and intrauterine transfusions cause thrombocytopenia by a dilutional effect that depends on the amount of blood transfused.[143, 147] After an exchange transfusion, platelet counts increase within 3 days and reach pre-exchange levels by about 7 days.[84]

Immune Thrombocytopenia

Immune thrombocytopenia is defined as an increased rate of platelet clearance caused by platelet-associated immunoglobulin G (IgG) or complement. Elevated platelet-associated IgG levels are not diagnostic of idiopathic thrombocytopenic purpura but are associated with a variety of thrombocytopenic disorders. For reasons that are not clear, 50% of infants with platelet counts less than $100 \times 10^9/L$ have increased amounts of platelet-associated IgG on their platelets.[144, 148] Specific neonatal disorders associated with platelet-associated IgG are sepsis,[148] preeclampsia,[149] maternal idiopathic thrombocytopenic purpura, and neonatal alloimmune thrombocytopenia.

Disease States Associated with Platelet Consumption

Neonatal thrombocytopenia is associated with many pathologic states (Table 5–6).[6–8, 84] Acute asphyxia is a consistent cause of DIC and thrombocytopenia.[16] Chronic hypoxia, associated with placental dysfunction and intrauterine growth–retarded infants, also is associated with significant thrombocytopenia.[148] Both viral (rubella, herpes, echovirus, toxoplasma, cytomegalovirus, human immunodeficiency virus) and bacterial infections cause severe thrombocytopenia.[150] Mechanisms responsible for bacterial sepsis–induced thrombocytopenia are multifactorial and include consumption secondary to DIC, endothelial damage, platelet aggregation secondary to binding of bacterial products to platelet membranes, immune-mediated thrombocytopenia, and decreased production due to marrow infection.[151] Mechanisms responsible for thrombocytopenia caused by viruses include loss of sialic acid from platelet membranes due to viral neuraminidase, intravascular platelet aggregation, and degeneration of megakaryocytes. Congenital rubella causes thrombocytopenia in three quarters of infants with platelet counts ranging from 20 to $60 \times 10^9/L$ for the first 4 to 8 weeks of life. For premature infants, thrombocytopenia frequently complicates other disorders such as RDS, persistent pulmonary hypertension, necrotizing enterocolitis, preeclampsia, and hyperbilirubinemia treated with phototherapy.[147] Activation of coagulation with platelet consumption occurs in RDS, and mechanical ventilation may be an independent factor contributing to thrombocytopenia.[152] Persistent pulmonary hypertension in newborns may be due in part to intrapulmonary platelet aggregation and the release of platelet-derived vasoactive substances such as thromboxane A_2.[153] These infants are frequently thrombocytopenic and, at au-

Table 5–6. THE ETIOLOGY OF THROMBOCYTOPENIA

Increased Destruction

Immune-Mediated

Maternal idiopathic thrombocytopenic purpura
Maternal systemic lupus erythematosus
Maternal hyperthyroidism
Maternal drugs
Maternal preeclampsia
Neonatal alloimmune thrombocytopenia

Non–Immune-Mediated (Probably Related to DIC)

Asphyxia
Perinatal aspiration
Necrotizing enterocolitis
Hemangiomas
Neonatal thrombosis
Respiratory distress syndrome

Unknown

Hyperbilirubinemia
Phototherapy
Polycythemia
Rh hemolytic disease
Congenital thrombotic thrombocytopenic purpura
Total parenteral nutrition
Inborn errors of metabolism
Wiscott-Aldrich syndrome
Multiple congenital anomalies

Hypersplenism

Decreased Production of Platelets

Bone Marrow Replacement Disorders

Congenital leukemia
Congenital leukemoid reactions
Neuroblastoma
Histiocytosis
Osteopetrosis

Bone Marrow Aplasia

Thrombocytopenia with absence of the radius
Amegakaryocytic thrombocytopenia
Fanconi's anemia
Other marrow hypoplastic or aplastic disorders

DIC = disseminated intravascular coagulation.

topsy, have pulmonary microthrombi. Necrotizing enterocolitis is characterized by bloody stools, vomiting of bile-stained gastric residue, and abdominal distention. Approximately half of the affected infants are thrombocytopenic, with about 20% having laboratory evidence of DIC. Both hyperbilirubinemia and phototherapy are associated with mild thrombocytopenia in newborn humans and shortened platelet survival in rabbits.[15] When platelets are exposed to a broad-spectrum blue fluorescent light *in vitro*, aggregation is decreased and microscopic alterations in granules and external membranes occur.

Giant Hemangiomas

Giant hemangiomas, or Kasabach-Merritt syndrome[154–157] (see Chapter 46), cause a local consumptive coagulopathy characterized by hypofibrinogenemia, elevated levels of fibrinogen-fibrin degradation products, microangiopathic fragmentation of red cells, and thrombocytopenia.[158] The thrombocytopenia is usually severe, with platelet counts being less than $50 \times 10^9/$

L.[159] Approximately 50% of affected infants experience systemic bleeding during the first month of life.[159]

Drug-Induced Thrombocytopenia

Transplacental passage of drugs and drug-dependent antibodies can result in both maternal and neonatal thrombocytopenia.[19] However, these causes are rare and the evidence for them is weak.[160–164] Agents implicated are quinine, hydralazine, tolbutamide, and thiazide diuretics. Heparin has been identified as a cause of thrombocytopenia. If heparin-induced thrombocytopenia is suspected, heparin therapy should be discontinued immediately and alternative forms of anticoagulation therapy considered if necessary (see Chapter 43).

Other Associations

Thrombocytopenia is loosely associated with thromboembolic complications and polycythemia in infants with hematocrits greater than 0.70. However, the presence of thrombocytopenia may also reflect other concurrent disease processes. Infants with a familial form of hemolytic-uremic syndrome or thrombotic thrombocytopenic purpura have a schistocytic hemolytic anemia in association with transient neurologic or renal abnormalities.[165]

Decreased Platelet Production

Thrombocytopenia due to decreased platelet production is rare, accounting for less than 5% of thrombocytopenic infants (see Table 5–6).[6–8, 84] Causes in neonates include congenital leukemia, congenital leukemoid reactions with Down's syndrome, neuroblastoma, histiocytosis, some viral infections, osteopetrosis, and disorders of bone marrow failure (see Chapters 7, 33, 34, and 43).

Aplastic Disorders

Aplastic disorders include thrombocytopenia absent radius syndrome and amegakaryocytic thrombocytopenia[166, 167] (Chapter 7). Infants with aplastic disorders are at the greatest risk of serious bleeding in the form of ICH in the first months of life. Neither splenectomy nor steroids are of benefit for infants with this syndrome.[166, 167] Platelet transfusions are highly effective but should be reserved for symptomatic infants because prophylactic platelet transfusions could result in refractoriness due to alloimmunization.[167] By several months of age, increased numbers of megakaryocytes usually appear in the bone marrow, and platelet counts increase.[166, 167] A functional platelet defect may be present in some children with thrombocytopenia absent radius syndrome.[168] Isolated amegakaryocytic thrombocytopenia with normal radii and other rare reports of inherited forms of thrombocytopenia may present with bleeding during the newborn period.[169]

Hypersplenism

Decreased recovery of ^{111}In oxine–labeled platelets (fewer than 40% to 50%) indicates that increased splenic sequestration is a contributing cause of thrombocytopenia.[15] Thrombocytopenia secondary to hypersplenism is usually mild, with platelet counts ranging from 50×10^9 to $100 \times 10^9/L$.

Clinical Impact of Neonatal Thrombocytopenia

Clinically important bleeding is less likely to occur in patients with consumptive disorders than in patients with a regenerative thrombocytopenia. The bleeding risk is increased in patients who have both thrombocytopenia and a platelet function defect. Choosing a platelet count at which one should intervene, although simplistic, provides a guideline for therapy. A platelet count less than $50 \times 10^9/L$ places some otherwise healthy full-term newborns at risk for serious ICH.[166, 167, 170] The importance of "moderate" thrombocytopenia (platelet counts between 50×10^9 and $100 \times 10^9/L$) in sick premature infants has been a subject of controversy. The bleeding time, which reflects platelet number and function, is prolonged in about 60% of premature infants with "moderate" thrombocytopenia and is shortened when the platelet count increases above $100 \times 10^9/L$ following platelet transfusions.[27] A randomized controlled trial assessed the potential benefits of platelet concentrate transfusions in 154 premature thrombocytopenic infants during the first 72 hours of life.[171] Treated infants received platelet concentrates to maintain platelet counts above $150 \times 10^9/L$. No beneficial effect on ICH was shown in this study, which was designed to detect an effect of 25% or greater.[171] However, transfused infants had shortened bleeding times and required significantly less blood product support.

Treatment

The management of thrombocytopenic infants depends in part on the underlying disorder. If an infant is bleeding, a trial of platelet concentrates (10 to 20 mL/kg) is indicated. The increased platelet count usually shortens the bleeding time and is frequently clinically effective.[27] Autoimmune and alloimmune thrombocytopenias do not respond to random donor platelet concentrates and require specific forms of therapy.

Autoimmune and Alloimmune Thrombocytopenia

Immune thrombocytopenia should always be suspected in otherwise healthy infants with isolated severe thrombocytopenia. An IgG antiplatelet auto- or alloantibody is produced in mothers and crosses the placenta, causing fetal thrombocytopenia. Because the antibody is not autologous, the thrombocytopenia persists only as long as the maternal IgG antibody remains in the infant's circulation. Normally, this would be several months because the half-life of IgG is approximately 21 days. However, because the antibody binds to platelets, its life span is dependent on the life span of the sensitized platelets and thus can be very short. Therefore, immune thrombocytopenic disorders of neonates are usually short-lived but can cause serious bleeding, making the correct diagnosis and management of these disorders all the more important. The differentiation of autoimmune thrombocytopenia from alloimmune thrombocytopenia in neonates is critical because the management and severity of these disorders is quite different. Chapter 43 discusses these two forms of immune thrombocytopenia in detail.

Thrombocytosis

Elevated platelet counts are frequently observed in premature infants at approximately 4 to 6 weeks after birth.[172] There are no clinical manifestations of neonatal thrombocytosis, and therapeutic intervention is not indicated.

QUALITATIVE PLATELET DISORDERS

Despite the physiologic hyporeactivity of neonatal platelets in response to exposure to some agents, healthy infants do not have an increased risk of bleeding. Pathologic impairment of platelet function may occur, to a variable extent, secondary to the use of certain drugs or the presence of pathologic states in either mothers or infants. In mothers, these causative factors include the use of some drugs,[172] diabetes,[173–176] dietary abnormalities,[177–183] smoking,[184–186] and ethanol abuse[187]; in infants, they include the use of some drugs, perinatal aspiration syndrome,[143, 147, 188–190] hyperbilirubinemia,[191, 192] phototherapy,[192, 193] renal failure,[194] and hepatic failure.

Aspirin

Salicylate crosses the placenta and can be detected in fetuses following maternal ingestion.[160–163, 195–199] Clearance of salicylate is slower in newborns than it is in adults, and thus infants are potentially placed at risk for longer periods of time.[161] However, *in vitro* studies have not demonstrated an additive effect of aspirin on newborn platelets,[44, 197] and evidence linking maternal aspirin ingestion to clinically important bleeding in newborns is weak.[163, 200–203] There is little reason to have serious concerns about maternal ingestion of aspirin, but it is reasonable to advise mothers not to ingest aspirin unless specifically indicated by their physician.

Indomethacin

Indomethacin is an antiplatelet agent used for nonsurgical closure of a patent ductus arteriosus in premature infants.[204–206] Indomethacin, like salicylate, has a longer half-life in newborns than in adults (21 to 24 hours and 2 to 3 hours, respectively).[207] This is probably due to underdevelopment of hepatic drug metabolism, renal excretory function, or altered protein binding.[208, 209] Indomethacin inhibits platelet function in newborns, as evidenced by prolongation of bleeding times.[28, 210, 211] Randomized controlled trials have provided conflicting conclusions on the effect of indomethacin on intraventricular hemorrhage in premature infants.[212]

Maternal Diabetes

The reactivity of platelets from diabetic mothers and their infants is increased, with enhanced thromboxane B_2 production, enhanced platelet aggregation,[175, 213] and a lower threshold to many aggregating agents.[214] The enhanced platelet function in diabetes is associated with an increased synthesis of a prostaglandin E–like material that crosses the placenta and can affect the fetus.[215] The evidence linking enhanced platelet reactivity to thromboembolic complications in newborns is weak.[216, 217]

Diet

Alterations in the diet of mothers or infants during the postnatal period can affect newborn platelet function. Increases in the ratio of polyunsaturated fatty acids to saturated fatty acids in the diet of mothers breastfeeding their infants result in increases in the concentration of linoleic acid and enhance thromboxane B_2 production.[177] Infants receiving a diet deficient in essential fatty acids may have arachidonic acid depletion and platelet dysfunction.[179, 180, 218] Vitamin E functions as an antioxidant and as an inhibitor of platelet aggregation/release in humans.[181–183, 219, 220] Cases of vitamin E–deficient infants with increased platelet aggregation that reversed following vitamin E supplementation have been reported.[183, 221]

Amniotic Fluid

Amniotic fluid contains procoagulant activity that enhances the generation of thromboxane A_2 by platelets.[147, 188–190] Infants who develop a perinatal aspiration syndrome have pulmonary hypertension characterized by platelet thrombi in the pulmonary microcirculation. The exact mechanism or mechanisms leading to persistent pulmonary hypertension in these infants is unknown; however, alterations in prostaglandin synthesis,[183, 222] as well as thrombocytopenia, hypoxia, and acidosis, have been suggested.[9, 147, 188–190]

Nitric Oxide

Nitric oxide prevents adhesion of platelets to endothelial cells and inhibits ADP-induced aggregation of cord platelets in a manner similar to that in adults.[223–226]

CONGENITAL FACTOR DEFICIENCIES

For most hemostatic components, both severe and mild forms of deficiency can occur, with severe deficiencies frequently characterized by significant bleeding in newborns. Chapters 44 and 45 discuss congenital factor deficiencies in detail. Sixty-two reports describing 226 infants who bled because of a congenital factor deficiency at birth form the basis for the following discussion.

General Information

Inheritance

Deficiencies of factors II, V, VII, XI, and XII, prekallikrein, and high-molecular-weight kininogen are rare, autosomally inherited disorders, with consanguinity present in many families. Deficiencies of factor XII, prekallikrein, and high-molecular-weight kininogen do not result in hemorrhagic complications and thus are not considered further. Factors VIII and IX are sex-linked and are the most common congenital bleeding disorders in newborns. Rarely, combined deficiencies of factors II, VII, IX, and X or of factors V and VIII present in the neonatal period.[227, 228] Prenatal diagnosis of most congenital factor deficiencies is available, and tests may be performed so that either termination of pregnancy or management of affected infants can be planned (see Chapters 44 and 45).

Clinical Presentation

The majority of newborns with congenital coagulation factor deficiencies do not present with bleeding in the perinatal period unless a hemostatic challenge is present. On the other hand, unexplained bleeding in an otherwise healthy newborn should be carefully investigated because it may reflect the presentation of a congenital coagulation factor deficiency. With few exceptions, only severe forms of congenital coagulation factor deficiencies are manifested by bleeding in newborns. Table 5–7 summarizes the cases of newborns in the literature who bled at birth owing to a congenital coagulation protein deficiency. The most common sites of bleeding include the penis (i.e., after circumcision), umbilical cord, cranium (ICH), scalp, and heel (i.e., after peripheral heelsticks). The high prevalence of ICH may reflect a reporting bias, as clinically less important sites of hemorrhage may not be frequently reported. Although less common than ICH, subgaleal bleeding with concurrent shock and DIC may be the initial presentation of a congenital factor deficiency.[229]

ICH is rare in full-term infants[230] and usually occurs secondary to the presence of significant primary problems. Full-term infants with unexplained ICH should be carefully evaluated for congenital or acquired hemostatic defects.[133, 231–239] Unfortunately, the diagnosis of ICH may be delayed because of the nonspecific nature of the early clinical presentation, which includes lethargy, apnea, vomiting, and irritability. Further delays can occur when secondary coagulopathies such as DIC occur[240–243] and when plasma concentrations of the coagulation protein in question are physiologically low in newborns. The more extreme clinical presentation of ICH is usually recognized early and is characterized by seizures, meningismus, and a tense fontanelle.

Although severe deficiency of factor VIII is the most common cause of ICH from a coagulation factor deficiency,[244] severe congenital deficiencies of fibrinogen and factors II, V, VII, VIII, IX, X, XI, and XIII can cause ICH at birth. The incidence of ICH in newborns is unknown and likely is changing, reflecting improvement in perinatal care. The widespread use of ultrasound, a safe modality for the monitoring of fetuses at risk, has resulted in the detection of ICH *in utero*. *In utero* factor replacement has also been accomplished in several infants.[245]

Diagnosis

The diagnosis of a previously unexpected inherited coagulation protein deficiency is usually established on the basis of abnormal results on coagulation screening tests and subsequent specific coagulation protein assays. Studies of the parents are invaluable when physiologic levels overlap pathologic levels. Subsequently, or in already identified families, molecular techniques can be used for prenatal and postnatal diagnoses of most coagulation protein deficiencies (see Chapters 44 and 45).

Plasma concentrations of any coagulation protein must be interpreted in the context of age-specific physiologic values. Homozygous deficiencies of factors V, VII, and XIII result in levels of less than 0.01, 0.03, and 0.01 units/mL, respectively; these levels are easily distinguished from physiologic values. Similarly, the severe forms of both factor VIII and factor IX deficiencies are defined by the presence of levels less than 0.01 unit/mL. In contrast, homozygous deficiencies of

Table 5–7. CASES OF CONGENITAL FACTOR DEFICIENCIES PRESENTING WITH BLEEDING IN NEWBORNS

Factor	No. of Cases	ICH	Circumcision	Umbilicus	Hematoma	Puncture Site	Cephalohematoma	Subgaleal	GI
Fibrinogen	7	0	2	5	1	—	—	—	1
Factor II	1	0	—	—	—	—	—	—	1
Factor V	4	2	—	1	1	—	—	—	2
Factor VII	12	11	1	2	—	2	1	—	2
Factor VIII	144	23	75	3	4	17	9	10	—
Factor IX	27	3	16	2	3	3	1	1	—
vWf	4	1	—	1	2	1	—	—	—
Factor X	5	4	—	—	—	1	1	—	2
Factor XI	1	0	1	—	—	—	—	—	—
Factor XIII	25	4	—	24	4	13	—	—	—
Factors II, V, IX, and X	1	0	—	—	—	—	—	—	—
Factors V and VIII	1	0	—	—	—	—	—	—	—

ICH = intracranial hemorrhage; GI = gastrointestinal.
Note: All sites of bleeding are included for each patient.

factors II, X, and XI are defined by the presence of levels less than 0.20, 0.10, and 0.15 units/mL, respectively, all of which overlap physiologic levels. It seems probable that patients have values less than the physiologic range, but this conjecture has not been demonstrated.

Treatment

In the presence of active bleeding or a planned hemostatic challenge, the fundamental principle of management is to increase the plasma concentration of the deficient coagulation protein to a minimal hemostatic level. The minimal hemostatic level of a particular coagulation protein varies and is dependent on the protein and the nature of the hemostatic challenge (Table 5–8). Available treatment modalities include the use of plasma, cryoprecipitate, and factor concentrates.

Specific Coagulation Factor Deficiencies

(See Tables 5–7 and 5–8)

Fibrinogen Deficiency

Four publications identified seven newborns who bled due to afibrinogenemia, 2 of whom died.[246–249] Hemorrhagic events occurred at the umbilical cord, into soft tissues, and following circumcision. Replacement therapy consisted of the use of whole blood, cryoprecipitate, FFP, and fibrinogen concentrates. One infant, who presented with bleeding from the umbilicus following circumcision, was treated with Gelfoam and thrombin.[247]

Treatment. Although FFP can be used as initial therapy, cryoprecipitate and fibrinogen concentrates (virally inactivated, if available) are preferable.

Factor II Deficiency

Only one publication has reported a newborn with mild gastrointestinal bleeding due to severe factor II deficiency.[250] No replacement therapy was given. Reviews of adult patients have reported bleeding following invasive events such as circumcision and venipunctures or as soft tissue hematomas; umbilical cord bleeding or hemarthrosis was not reported.[247]

Treatment. Although FFP can be used as initial therapy, factor II concentrate or prothrombin complex concentrate (PCC) is preferable.

Factor V Deficiency

Three publications identified four newborns with bleeding due to severe factor V deficiency; one of these four newborns died.[245, 251, 252] Two infants presented with ICHs,[245, 252] one with umbilical bleeding,[251] and one with soft tissue bleeding.[251] Replacement therapy included whole blood, FFP, and the application of pressure on local sites of bleeding. One infant with ICH died at 6 days of age.[245] Although thrombotic complica-

Table 5–8. COAGULATION FACTOR PROTEINS

Factor	Plasma Concentration	Half-Life	Minimum Hemostatic Value	Replacement Therapy
Fibrinogen	1.56–4.00 g/L	3–5 d	0.5–1.0 g/L	Plasma Cryo C
Factor II	0.10 mg/mL	72 h	0.40 U/mL	Factor IIC PCC Plasma
Factor V	4–14 µg/mL	12–36 h	0.25 U/mL	FFP Cryo
Factor VII	300–500 ng/mL	3–7 h	0.15 U/mL	Factor VIIC PCC Plasma
Factor VIII	0.2 µg/mL	8–12 h	0.30 U/mL	Factor VIIIC
Factor IX	4 µg/mL	24 h	0.10 U/mL	Factor IXC PCC
vWf	3–12 µg/mL	1–4 h	0.25–0.50 U/mL	vWfC Cryo
Factor X	4–10 µg/mL	24–56 h	0.10 U/mL	PCC Plasma
Factor XI	2–7 µg/mL	40–80 h	0.20 U/mL	Factor XIC Plasma
Factor XIII	A: 15 µg/mL B: 21 µg/mL	4–14 d	0.10 U/mL	Factor XIIIC Cryo Plasma
AT-III	0.30 mg/mL	17–26 h	0.38–0.49 U/mL	AT-IIIC Plasma
Protein C	0.004 mg/mL	10 h	0.38–0.49 U/mL	Protein CC FFP
Protein S	25 µg/mL	24 h	0.40–0.55 U/mL	FFP

Cryo = cryoprecipitate; FFP = fresh frozen plasma; PCC = prothrombin complex concentrate; C = concentrate.

tions occur in some patients with factor V deficiency, they have not been reported in newborns.[253]

Treatment. Currently, only FFP is available as a replacement source for factor V.

Factor VII Deficiency

In general, patients with factor VII levels less than 1% have severe hemorrhages equivalent to those of severe hemophilia. Patients with factor VII levels of greater than 5% generally have mild hemorrhagic episodes. Congenital factor VII deficiency may occur in infants with Dubin-Johnson syndrome[254] or Gilbert's syndrome.[255] Eight publications identified 12 newborns who bled due to severe factor VII deficiency.[245, 256-262] The sites of bleeding were multiple; however, 11 of the 12 newborns had ICH, and all died as a result of ICH.[245, 256-261] Infants in the first year of life were also at an increased risk for ICH.[261]

Treatment. Replacement therapy consisted of exchange transfusion and the use of whole blood, FFP, serum, PCCs, and factor VII concentrates. In 1988, Daffos used fetal blood sampling to diagnose factor VII deficiency at 24 weeks of age, and the fetus was transfused *in utero* at 37 weeks with 200 units of factor VII concentrate.[245] The baby was born without hemorrhagic complications and did not bleed as a newborn. Although FFP or PCCs can be used as initial therapy, factor VII concentrate is the replacement product of choice.

Factor VIII Deficiency

The severity of factor VIII deficiency is determined by the plasma concentration of factor VIII, with a level of less than 1% being severe, 1% to 5% being moderate, and 5% to 50% being mild.[263] Severe factor VIII deficiency is the most common congenital disorder of the neonatal period. In addition, a small number of neonates with moderate and mild hemophilia present following a hemostatic challenge.[135, 139, 240, 264-268] Large cohort studies have revealed that approximately 10% of children with hemophilia are clinically symptomatic in the neonatal period.[244] An additional 40% present by 1 year of age; by 1.5 years, more than 70% have had a major bleeding event.[244] In less severe factor VIII deficiency, major hemorrhage occurs in only 2.5% of patients by the end of the neonatal period.[244]

Twenty publications identified 144 male infants with bleeding due to factor VIII deficiency in the neonatal period.[135, 139, 229, 240, 241, 264-278] Seventy-five infants (53%) presented with bleeding following circumcision, and 23 (16%) presented with ICH.* Eight infants died in the newborn period due to bleeding.[135, 240, 241, 275] In contrast to the case in older infants and children, bleeding into joints is extremely rare in neonates.[279] Severe factor VIII deficiency can, on rare occasion, occur in females with clinical presentation in the neonatal period. Three female infants have been reported to have bleeding from puncture sites and into the skin at birth. The

levels of factor VIII were less than 0.01 units/mL in two, and 0.04 unit/mL in the third.[280, 281] All three girls were diagnosed later in life, and they did not receive any form of replacement therapy at birth.

Treatment. Treatment was reported for only 47 of the 144 male infants and reflected the decade in which they were born. Since the 1980s, most infants have been treated with factor VIII concentrate or cryoprecipitate.[135, 229, 240, 241, 273-275, 277, 278] Recovery studies were reported for two infants.[267, 269] One infant received 80 units/kg followed by 40 units/kg every 12 hours. After 9 days, his factor VIII level exceeded 50% of normal.[269] The second infant had an ICH and received 60 to 100 units/kg every 24 hours to keep his factor VIII level greater than 50%.[267] Alternative therapy to factor VIII replacement has been used in newborns undergoing circumcision. In one study of 10 patients with severe bleeding, local fibrin glue was used instead of infusion of factor VIII concentrate.[282] Only two of three patients who bled postoperatively required factor VIII concentrate. Currently, factor VIII concentrates (recombinant or highly purified) are preferable to cryoprecipitate.

Factor IX Deficiency

The severity of factor IX deficiency is identical to that of factor VIII deficiency. Diagnosis of the milder forms of factor IX deficiency is complicated by physiologic levels of factor IX that can be as low as 0.15 unit/mL, and, in the rare infant, by the potential for concurrent VK deficiency. Ten publications identified 27 newborns with bleeding secondary to severe factor IX deficiency.* Twelve infants bled following circumcision, and three presented with ICH.[135, 139, 264, 276, 278, 283, 286] The 27 newborns also bled from diverse sites at presentation (see Table 5–7). Replacement therapy included the use of FFP (n = 4), PCC (n = 1), and factor IX concentrate (n = 1).

Treatment. Factor IX concentrates are the replacement product of choice and are preferable to PCC.

von Willebrand's Disease

Although von Willebrand's disease (vWD) is the most common congenital bleeding disorder, patients rarely present with the disease in the neonatal period. Plasma concentrations of vWf are increased, as is the proportion of high-molecular-weight multimers.[21, 22] Only three newborns with bleeding secondary to vWD have been identified.[287-289] One infant with type IIA vWD presented with umbilical bleeding and later with life-threatening epistaxis.[290] Two infants with type IIB vWD presented with bleeding at blood sampling sites, and soft tissue sites.[287] Repeat platelet counts were less than $50 \times 10^9/L$, and the bleeding time and APTT were prolonged. The vWf multimeric structure was characterized by the absence of the high-molecular-weight forms, and the patients' platelets aggregated at much lower ristocetin concentrations than did controls' platelets.[287] One infant presented on day seven of life with

---

*See references 135, 139, 240, 264, 267, 269, 271, 273, 275, 276, and 278.

*See references 135, 139, 264, 275, 276, 278, and 283 to 286.

an intracerebral and subdural hemorrhage.[289] The factor VIII level was 0.03 unit/mL, and the vWf:antigen (AG) and vWf:ristocetin cofactor (RCO) were undetectable. This infant was treated with a factor VIII concentrate of intermediate purity at a dose of 60 units/kg twice per day for 10 days, followed by once-per-day dosing for 10 days. The bleeding stopped, and the infant's neurologic status was normal.[289]

Treatment. Both type II and type III vWD can present in newborns and may require treatment. Until recently, cryoprecipitate was the treatment of choice because factor VIII concentrates contained very small amounts of the active high-molecular-weight multimers of vWf.[291] Some factor VIII concentrates now contain vWf and their use is an effective form of therapy (see Chapter 44).

Factor X Deficiency

Five newborns with bleeding due to severe factor X deficiency have been identified.[292–296] Four of the five infants had ICH; two subsequently died, and one remained in a coma.[292] One of the four with ICH was diagnosed *in utero* and, despite prophylactic administration of PCC in the first months of life, died as a result of ICH.[294] Other sites of bleeding were umbilical, gastrointestinal, and intra-abdominal.[292, 293, 295] Replacement therapy included whole blood, FFP, and PCC.

Treatment. If PCCs are not available, FFP can be used. When PCCs are available, they are the products of choice (see Chapter 45).

Factor XI Deficiency

Factor XI deficiency is different from other coagulation protein deficiencies in that symptoms of bleeding do not necessarily correlate with the factor XI level, nor do all patients with factor XI deficiency bleed. Bleeding often occurs following trauma or surgery, which in newborns is frequently circumcision.[297] Only one newborn with severe factor XI deficiency has been identified. The infant was a 3-day-old male with a factor XI level of 0.07 unit/mL who bled from the circumcision site.[297] He was successfully treated with FFP.

Treatment. Either FFP or cryoprecipitate can be used for the treatment of factor XI–deficient patients if factor XI concentrate is not available.

Factor XIII Deficiency

Twenty-five newborns with bleeding due to homozygous factor XIII deficiency have been identified.[136, 269, 298–305] Twenty-four of the 25 infants presented with the classic symptom of delayed bleeding from the umbilicus. Two infants had an ICH within 2 months of birth.[136, 305] One infant died in the neonatal period.[304] In later life, ICH occurs in 25% of reported cases.[304] Replacement therapy was administered with whole blood, FFP, cryoprecipitate, and factor XIII concentrate.

Treatment. Either cryoprecipitate or factor XIII concentrates can be used for the treatment of factor XIII–deficient patients. Newborns with factor XIII deficiency should be placed on a prophylactic regimen of factor XIII replacement because of the high incidence of ICH; plasma concentrations of factor XIII greater than 1% are effective, and the very long half-life of factor XIII permits once-per-month therapy.[286]

Familial Multiple Factor Deficiencies

Congenital deficiencies of two or more coagulation proteins have been reported for 16 different combinations of coagulation factors.[306] Bleeding in the neonatal period has only been reported for two infants with combined factor deficiencies. One infant had deficiencies of factor II, VII, IX, and X and presented with spontaneous bruising and umbilical stump bleeding; the bruising and bleeding continued until 3 months after birth, when the infant was treated with FFP.[228] A second infant who had deficiencies of factors V and VIII presented with serious bleeding (undescribed) in the first week of life.[227] FFP was administered without improvement.

Treatment. Initial therapy is usually with FFP. Subsequent treatment varies, depending on the specific factors affected.

ACQUIRED HEMOSTATIC DISORDERS
Disseminated Intravascular Coagulation

General Information. The term disseminated intravascular coagulation (DIC) was first used for describing the pathologic feature of diffuse fibrin deposition in the microvasculature.[307–309] Subsequently, a relationship between the clinico-pathologic findings and the decrease in the concentration of coagulation factors due to consumption was noted for both adults and infants.[310–314] Most recently, the term has been extended to include evidence of endogenous thrombin and plasmin generation on the basis of sensitive biochemical markers such as F1.2, thrombin/antithrombin III complex, and D-dimer. A database search of the literature identified 42 publications that focused on DIC in newborns: 19 case reports, 4 review articles, 12 case series, and 7 controlled trials. The following discussion reflects these studies.

Etiology. DIC is not a disorder in itself but a process that occurs secondary to a variety of underlying diseases in newborns.[94, 313, 315–325] Adverse events related to the fetal-placental unit may result in asphyxia and shock and thereby contribute to the release of tissue thromboplastin at the time of birth. Some of the common pathologic disorders related to prematurity, such as RDS, can be associated with DIC. A variety of other disorders such as viral or bacterial infections, hypothermia, and meconium or amniotic fluid aspiration syndromes may initiate DIC.[307–309, 326]

Clinical Presentation. The clinical spectrum of DIC is changing, reflecting the ever-improving perinatal care of sick infants. The intensity and duration of activation of the hemostatic system, the degree of blood flow impairment, and the functioning of the liver all influence the clinical severity of DIC.[325] In the past, infants who clinically manifested hemorrhagic or thrombotic complications from DIC frequently died.[307–309] Now the majority of infants with DIC survive, and for some DIC is of little clinical significance.[326]

Diagnosis. Historically, the laboratory diagnosis of DIC was characterized by a prolonged PT, a prolonged APTT, depletion of certain coagulation factors (fibrinogen, factor V, factor VIII), increased levels of fibrin degradation products, thrombocytopenia, and a microangiopathic hemolytic anemia.[94, 313, 315–325] Physiologic concentrations of fibrinogen and factors V and VIII are similar in newborns and adults; thus, pathologic decreases, as in DIC, are readily identified. The availability of sensitive markers for endogenous thrombin and plasmin generation has complicated the diagnosis of DIC in newborns. For example, plasma concentrations of thrombin/antithrombin III complexes are increased in healthy infants, probably as a reflection of activation of the coagulation system during birth.[54, 56, 99, 122] Positive results on these sensitive paracoagulation tests do not indicate the presence of DIC or the need for intervention. In practice, no single laboratory test can be used for confirming or excluding DIC.

Treatment. The cornerstone of the management of DIC remains the successful treatment of the underlying disorders. The decision to treat the hemostatic disorder often is difficult to make. In the absence of clinical manifestations, newborns probably do not require therapy for the hemostatic disorder itself. In the presence of clinically significant bleeding, therapeutic intervention with plasma products is indicated and often improves hemostasis. For infants between these two ends of the spectrum, treatment is dictated by the severity of the hemostatic impairment and the underlying problem. In general, the more pronounced the abnormalities detected in the laboratory, the greater the risk of bleeding or thrombotic complications. The argument that replacement therapy may "fuel the fire" is theoretic and has not been proven.

Therapeutic interventions given to improve hemostasis in infants with DIC have included the use of FFP, cryoprecipitate, factor concentrates (i.e., AT-III concentrates and PCCs), anticoagulants, and exchange transfusions. FFP is extensively used because it contains all of the coagulation proteins present in adult concentrations. Cryoprecipitate is used because of the increased concentrations of fibrinogen and factor VIII, two proteins that are frequently depleted in DIC. Exchange transfusions are occasionally used in severe DIC but their effects are transient unless the underlying problem resolves. PCCs have been used in newborns but are not generally recommended because of the potential for thrombotic and infectious side effects.[327]

Unfortunately, the timing and design of the available clinical studies do not permit the making of strong recommendations. In one study, mortality from DIC was evaluated in 33 infants who were randomized to a control group (n=11), treated by exchange transfusion (n=11), or treated with FFP (n=11).[328] The authors concluded that intervention did not affect survival; however, the sample size was too small and the sever-

ity of the illness (75% survival rate) too minimal for the hypothesis to be adequately tested. A further six controlled studies performed between 1968 and 1983 evaluated the effects of coagulation protein replacement on abnormal coagulation profiles, ICH, and death (Table 5–9).[327, 329–333] Three of these controlled studies focused on large groups of sick, low-birth-weight infants and full-term infants after asphyxia episodes.[327, 331, 332] One group reported a beneficial effect of FFP on the thrombotest as well as a decrease in mortality.[333] Another noted that the use of FFP in addition to cryoprecipitate and PCCs corrected the coagulation test results in 80% of infants.[330] The use of AT-III concentrates, which have been tested in small trials with the goal of decreasing the morbidity of DIC and RDS, cannot be recommended until further clinical trials have been carried out.[49, 334] Similarly, no clinical data support the use of heparin for most infants with DIC.[334–339] In the absence of definitive clinical trials, reasonable goals are maintaining platelet counts above $50 \times 10^9/L$, fibrinogen concentrations over 1.0 g/L, and PT values at levels normal for postnatal and gestational age.

Liver Disease

General Information. The coagulopathies of liver disease in newborns are similar to those of adults and reflect the failure of hepatic synthetic functions superimposed upon a physiologic immaturity, activation of the coagulation and fibrinolytic systems, poor clearance of activated coagulation factors, and the loss of hemostatic proteins into ascitic fluid.[340] The secondary effects of liver disease on platelet number and function also occur in newborns.[341–343] Thrombocytopenia is due to the impairment of platelet production, perhaps as a result of the direct invasion of megakaryocytes by the virus, splenic sequestration, and accelerated clearance.[344–347]

Only 28 reports in the literature have dealt with coagulopathies of liver disease in newborns, and all of these are case series.[348–357] Common causes of hepatic dysfunction in newborns include viral hepatitis, hypoxia, total parenteral nutrition, shock, and fetal hydrops.

The laboratory abnormalities induced by acute liver disease include prolongation of the PT and low plasma concentrations of several coagulation proteins, including fibrinogen.[358, 359] Chronic liver failure with cirrhosis is also characterized by a coagulopathy[360–363] and mild thrombocytopenia due to splenic sequestration.[364, 365] Secondary VK deficiency may occur owing to impaired absorption from the small intestine, particularly in intra- and extrahepatic biliary atresia.[366] Patients with clinical bleeding may benefit temporarily from replacement of coagulation proteins with FFP, cryoprecipitate, or exchange transfusion. However, without recovery of hepatic function, replacement therapy is futile. VK should be administered to infants suspected of cholestatic liver disease. PCCs containing factors II, VII, IX, and X should in general be avoided in newborns be-

Table 5-9. CLINICAL TRIALS ASSESSING THE BENEFITS OF PLASMA PRODUCTS

Author	No. of Subjects	Outcome		Comment
Beverley et al (1985)[329]		*IVH*		
Treatment (FFP)	36	5 (14%)		No effect on the PT or APTT
Control	37	15 (41%)		
Gross et al (1982)[328]		*Death*		
Treatment (ET)	11	4		No effect on the PT or fibrinogen level
Treatment (FFP)	11	5		
Control	11	3		
Turner (1981)[330]		*Death*		
Treatment (FFP, Cryo, Factor IXC)	39	23		PT, APTT, and fibrinogen level improved in treatment group
Control	39	22		
Watt et al (1973)[327]		*Death*	*ICH*	
Treatment (Factor IXC)	40	19 (47%)	12	TT lower in control group on day one
Control	40	16 (40%)	4*	
De Lemos et al (1973)[331]		*Death*		
Treatment (ET)	20	4 (25%)		Prolonged APTT associated with a poorer outcome
Control	20	16 (80%)*		
Hambleton and Appleyard (1973)[332]		*Death*	*ICH*	
Treatment (FFP)	33	9	2	Minor improvements on the PT and APTT
Control	33	10	3	
Gray et al (1968)[333]		*Death*		
Treatment (FFP)	26	1 (4%)		TT lower in infants who died
Control	48	9 (19%)		

ET = exchange transfusion; TT = thrombotest.
*A significant difference between groups of at least $P < .05$.

cause of the high risk of transmitting hepatitis and of thrombotic disease.[367]

Periventricular-Intraventricular Hemorrhage

The most frequent form of ICH in premature infants is *periventricular-intraventricular hemorrhage (PIVH)*.[368] The introduction of computed tomography and bedside ultrasound through the anterior fontanelle has permitted accurate detection of PIVH, determination of the natural history, and assessment of the effects of specific therapeutic interventions.[369–378] The incidence of PIVH in premature infants is decreasing, and this is likely a reflection of improvements in neonatal care.

Evolution of Periventricular-Intraventricular Hemorrhage

The hemorrhage, which usually begins within the first 6 hours of age,[377, 379–383] characteristically starts in the fragile microvasculature of the subependymal germinal matrix.[368] The germinal matrix hemorrhages rupture into the adjacent ventricle in approximately 80% of infants and may incite an arachnoiditis that obstructs cerebrospinal fluid flow. The consequences of PIVH include destruction of the germinal matrix with cyst formation, progressive posthemorrhagic ventricular dilation, and periventricular hemorrhagic infarction. Periventricular hemorrhagic infarction occurs in 15% to 20% of infants with IVH and is located in the periventricular white matter.[380, 381, 384–390] The hemorrhagic infarction is frequently asymmetric, is associated with an extensive IVH, and occurs late, with peak incidence on day four of life.[387, 388]

Etiology of Periventricular-Intraventricular Hemorrhage

The etiology of PIVH in premature infants is almost certainly multifactorial and is still incompletely understood. Fluctuation of cerebral blood flow is probably the mechanism of primary importance.[391–398] Other contributing mechanisms include increased fragility of the germinal matrix capillaries, oxidative damage to endothelium, and impairment of hemostasis.[329, 399–401]

Therapeutic Modalities

A variety of therapeutic modalities directed at decreasing the frequency and severity of PIVH have been tested.[402] In general, therapeutic interventions have included the use of agents that affect cerebral blood flow (phenobarbital before and after birth, indomethacin, pancuronium bromide), drugs that affect cell membranes (ethamsylate, vitamin E), and products that enhance hemostasis (ethamsylate, VK, FFP, tranexamic acid, platelet concentrates). Only the studies testing interventions directed at altering hemostasis are discussed in this section.

Trials of Coagulation Factor Replacement Before the 1980s

The immature physiologic state of hemostasis in premature infants and the association of pathologic alterations of hemostasis with PIVH form the rationale for intervention studies directed at enhancing hemostasis.* Six clinical trials with coagulation factor replacement were conducted between 1968 and 1981.[332, 333, 403, 405–407] The results of these early trials cannot be extrapolated to current practice because of the significant improvements in neonatal intensive care management and the availability of ultrasound for diagnosing PIVH. Since 1980, trials testing drugs or blood products that enhance specific aspects of hemostasis have been tested in infants at risk for PIVH (Table 5–10).

Antenatal Administration of Vitamin K

Beginning antenatally, VK was administered to mothers in order to increase plasma activities of VK-dependent coagulation proteins in premature infants (see Table 5–10). Of the three clinical trials conducted to test this hypothesis, two reported a benefit and one did not.[202, 203, 408] A placebo control group was not present in any study. Despite randomization, there were imbalances in the two positive studies between treatment and control groups that may have conferred a positive bias for the use of VK. Both positive studies reported an effect on coagulation tests that might reflect the administration of VK. The negative study did not iden-

*See references 27, 142, 171, 327 to 329, 333, 400, 403, and 404.

tify a positive effect on the infant's coagulation system. For all of these reasons, antenatal VK administration for the prevention of PIVH cannot be recommended at this time. This statement does not contradict the well-substantiated need for postnatal VK supplementation.

Trials of Replacement with Blood Products Since 1980

Three blood products have been tested in randomized controlled trials in PIVH (see Table 5–10). FFP was tested in one randomized controlled trial conducted in 1985. Treated newborns received 10 mL/kg of FFP on admission and at 24 hours of age.[329] Of the treated newborns, 5 of 36 developed ICH, whereas 15 of 37 control newborns did—a significant difference. However, without a placebo control group, it is possible that the beneficial effect observed was the result of "stabilizing the circulation" rather than improving hemostasis. In a second study of a blood product, factor XIII concentrates were given to premature infants to prevent ICH through enhancement of fibrin cross-linking.[409] Although this study reported a significant effect, the analysis was performed on a small subset of infants that was not balanced. Furthermore, there is no strong biological rationale to support the likely benefit of factor XIII concentrates because plasma concentrations of factor XIII at birth are well within the adult range (see

Table 5-10. PERIVENTRICULAR-INTRAVENTRICULAR HEMORRHAGE PREVENTION STUDIES

Study	No. of Subjects	Weight (kg)	Dose 1 (mg/kg)	Dose 2 (mg/kg)	PIVH
Vitamin K					
Pomerance et al (1987)[202]	53	1.5	10	10 × 2	↓
Morales et al (1988)[203]	100	1.5	10	10 mg for 5 d IM antenatally	↓
Kazzi et al (1989)[408]	98	2.5	10	20 mg/d orally antenatally	↔
Thorp et al (1994)[600]	164	1.3	10	10 × 1	↔
Blood Products					
Beverley et al (1985)[329] (FFP)	73	1.5	10 mL	10 mL × 2	↓
Shirahata et al (1990)[409] (FXIIIC)	21	—	100 U	None	↓
Andrew et al (1991)[404] (Platelet C)	154	1.5	10 mL	10 mL × 1–3	↔
Tranexamic Acid					
Hensey et al (1984)[410]	105	1.25	25 (U.IV)	25 × 20	↔
Ethamsylate					
Morgan et al (1981)[419]	73	1.5	12.5	12.5 × 16	↓
Benson et al (1986)[421]	330	1.5	12.5	12.5 × 16	↓
Indomethacin					
Hanigan et al (1988)[423]	111	1.3	0.1	0.4 × 3	↓
Ment et al (1988)[212]	36	1.25	0.1	0.1 × 3	↓
Bandstra et al (1988)[601]	199	1.3		0.1 × 2	↓
Bada et al (1989)[602]	141	1.5	0.2	0.1 × 2	↓
Mahony et al (1985)[603]	104	1.3	0.2	0.1 × 2	↓
Ment et al (1985)[422]	48	1.25	0.6	0.1 × 8	↓
Rennie et al (1986)[425]	50	1.75	0.2	0.2 × 2	↔
Vincer et al (1987)[604]	30	1.5	0.2	0.2 × 2	↔

↓ = The incidence of PIVH decreased with treatment.
↔ = The incidence of PIVH remaining the same with treatment.

Table 5–10). In a third study of a blood product, platelet concentrates were administered to thrombocytopenic infants because of the close association of PIVH and thrombocytopenia (see Table 15–10).[171, 404] One hundred and fifty-four premature infants who were thrombocytopenic during the first 72 hours of life were randomized to either a control or a treated group. Treated infants received platelet concentrates for maintaining platelet counts above $150 \times 10^9/L$. No beneficial effect on ICH was shown in this study, which was designed to detect an effect of 25% or greater.

Inhibition of Fibrinolysis

Tranexamic acid, an inhibitor of fibrinolysis, was tested in ICH because of increased fibrinolytic activity at birth (see Table 15–10).[401, 410] Tranexamic acid has been shown to reduce the incidence of recurrent subarachnoid hemorrhage in adults[411, 412] and to prevent bleeding after oral surgery in high-risk patients.[413, 414] In this study, 105 infants were randomized to receive tranexamic acid or placebo on day one of life and for 4 subsequent days. No significant effect was demonstrated.

Stabilization of Capillary Membranes

The microvasculature of the germinal matrix is fragile and thereby susceptible to rupture. Ethamsylate is a drug that may stabilize capillary membranes and increase platelet adhesiveness. Also, ethamsylate is an inhibitor of prostaglandin synthesis and may have effects on the cerebral vasculature. Ethamsylate reduces capillary bleeding during selected surgical interventions in humans (e.g., ear, nose, and throat surgery)[415–417] and decreases the incidence of PIVH in the beagle puppy model.[418] Two randomized controlled trials and one controlled trial have reported a reduction in PIVH with ethamsylate (see Table 5–10).[419–421] However, before ethamsylate can be generally recommended, neurodevelopmental follow-up is needed because of the remaining possibility that treatment could cause brain ischemia.[402]

Cerebral Blood Flow Regulation
(See Table 5–10)

Cerebral blood flow is regulated in part by prostaglandins such as prostacyclin and thromboxane A_2. Prostacyclin is a potent vasodilator that inhibits platelet aggregation, and thromboxane A_2 is a potent vasoconstrictor that promotes platelet aggregation. In the beagle puppy model, indomethacin, a drug that blocks the enzyme cyclooxygenase, significantly decreased the incidence of ICH. Indomethacin reduced plasma concentrations of 6-keto-prostaglandin $F_{1\alpha}$ and thromboxane B_2, the stable metabolites of prostacyclin and thromboxane A_2.[418] Four randomized controlled trials have been conducted with indomethacin, three of which demonstrated a beneficial effect[422–424] and one of which did not detect a change.[425]

Recommendations

Several confounding variables may have contributed to the differing results of the trials discussed. Of particular importance is the declining incidence of PIVH, which is likely a reflection of improvements in perinatal care. Ongoing clinical studies are necessary for testing potentially beneficial therapeutic agents within the context of improving clinical care. At this time, no firm recommendations can be made for any of the intervention modalities discussed because of a lack of consistent results and neurodevelopmental follow-up.[212]

Respiratory Distress Syndrome

RDS, an acute lung disorder that primarily affects premature infants, is characterized by diffuse atelectasis, hyaline membrane formation, permeability edema, and right-to-left shunting of pulmonary blood flow.[426–428] Increased pulmonary surface tension secondary to surfactant deficiency is an important mechanism that contributes to RDS.

Potential Role of Coagulation

One of the pathologic characteristics of RDS is fibrin deposition in both intra-alveolar and intravascular sites.[426–428] This observation has led several investigators to look for evidence of activation of coagulation in infants with RDS. Early studies reported decreased plasma concentrations of some coagulation proteins and inhibitors. However, these tests were neither sensitive nor specific for activation of coagulation with thrombin generation. The sensitive paracoagulation F1.2, thrombin/antithrombin III complex, and D-dimer tests have been measured in newborns with a spectrum of mild to severe RDS. A direct correlation among increasing thrombin generation, decreased AT-III levels, and the severity of RDS was observed. Furthermore, there is evidence to support that fibrin deposition within the lung likely contributes to the severity of lung disease.[429–432] In a piglet model of neonatal acute lung injury, increasing plasma concentrations of AT-III by means of the infusion of AT-III concentrates decreased the severity of the lung disease.[433]

Intervention Trials Influencing Hemostasis

The possible role of coagulation in acute neonatal lung disease has provided the rationale for four intervention studies directed at decreasing fibrin deposition through the use of anticoagulants, thrombolytic therapy, and AT-III concentrates (Table 5–11). In 1966, the value of urokinase-activated human plasmin was tested in a randomized, placebo-controlled, double-blind study of 60 infants with severe RDS; the study revealed that the plasmin effected a substantial increase in survival rate without toxicity.[434] In a second double-blind randomized study, 500 premature infants were treated with plasminogen or placebo intravenously within 60

Table 5-11. CLINICAL TRIALS ASSESSING THE POTENTIAL BENEFITS OF ANTICOAGULANT OR THROMBOLYTIC THERAPY IN NEWBORNS WITH RESPIRATORY DISTRESS SYNDROME

Reference	No. of Subjects	Outcome		
		Death	*RDS*	*ICH*
Markarian et al (1971)[339]				
Heparin	39	17 (44%)‡	26 (68.8%)‡	40% mild* 10% severe
Placebo	42	16 (38%)	22 (53.3%)	0% mild 61% severe
Ambrus et al (1966)[434]				
UK-Plasmin	32	9 (28%)*	—	7 (22%)‡
Placebo	28	17 (61%)		6 (21%)
Ambrus et al (1977)[435]				
Plasminogen C	251	6 (2%)*	35 (14%) mild‡ 19 (7%) severe†	1 (0.4%)‡
Placebo	249	20 (8%)	22 (9%) mild 31 (12%) severe	1 (0.4%)
Muntean and Rosseger (1989)[436]				
AT-IIIC	45	9 (20%)‡	23 (51%)‡	—
Control	53	8 (15%)	28 (53%)	

RDS = respiratory distress syndrome; UK = urokinase.
*Patients who were diagnosed with ICH at autopsy.
†Significantly different than placebo/control group.
‡Not significantly different than placebo/control group.

minutes of birth. There was a substantial decrease in severe clinical respiratory distress, in the number of deaths caused by hyaline membrane disease, and in the total mortality in the plasminogen-treated infants compared with the control subjects.[435] In a third trial, the effect of heparin on the development of RDS as well as its effect on the incidence of ICH was tested.[339] High-risk, low-birth-weight infants were randomized to receive heparin or placebo (saline), with nurses blinded to treatment. Eighty-one infants were included: 39 to the heparin group, and 42 to the placebo group. In the primary analyses, there was no difference in the number of deaths, incidence of RDS, or bleeding. However, on a subanalysis in which 7 moribund infants treated with heparin and 3 moribund infants treated with saline were excluded, the investigators suggested that there was a positive effect on mortality.[339] The fourth study was an open, randomized, controlled clinical trial that assessed the role of AT-III concentrates in 103 infants (45 receiving AT-III, and 53 receiving standard care alone).[436] There was no difference in duration of ventilation, ICH, or mortality.[436] Future clinical trials are needed for assessing the benefits of antithrombotic or thrombolytic therapy in RDS.

Vitamin K Deficiency

Historical View. The practice of delaying religious circumcision until day eight of life or later likely reflects the recognition that bleeding from VK deficiency can occur during the first week of life. The discovery of VK and its important role in hemostasis was intertwined with the role of VK in the treatment and subsequent prevention of hemorrhagic disease of the newborn (HDN). The controversy over the need for VK prophylaxis has continued throughout the 20th century and underscores the need for randomized controlled trials for evaluating potentially helpful intervention therapies.

HDN, as first described by Townsend in 1894, consisted of hemorrhaging from multiple sites in otherwise healthy infants in the absence of trauma, asphyxia, or infection on days one through five of life.[80] This report was followed by recognition that blood from newborns takes longer to clot than does adult blood.[5] Subsequently, a causal link between HDN and abnormal blood clotting was made.[5, 437–439] Initial treatment of patients with HDN consisted of the intravenous, intramuscular, or subcutaneous injection of blood or serum into infants. At this very early time, the difficulty of separating treatment response from spontaneous improvements was recognized. Later, a randomized controlled trial showed that the injection of intramuscular blood was not helpful in preventing the abnormalities in blood coagulation that occurred during the first week of life.[439] The link between VK deficiency and spontaneous hemorrhaging was first recognized in chicks in 1929.[440] The association between VK deficiency and HDN quickly followed, as did the subsequent treatment of infants with HDN.[5, 81, 82, 441]

The next historical step was the recognition of the link between decreased prothrombin activity and increased PTs on days two to four of life in the absence of prophylactic VK. Prothrombin activity was observed to return to normal by days 5 to 7 of life (Fig. 5–5).[5, 442–445] These observations led to the hypothesis that VK administered prophylactically could prevent HDN.[309, 442, 443, 446–451] There was uniform agreement that the prophylactic administration of VK to mothers or infants prevented the decrease in prothrombin activity during the first 3 to 4 days of life.[5, 441, 442, 447] On the basis of

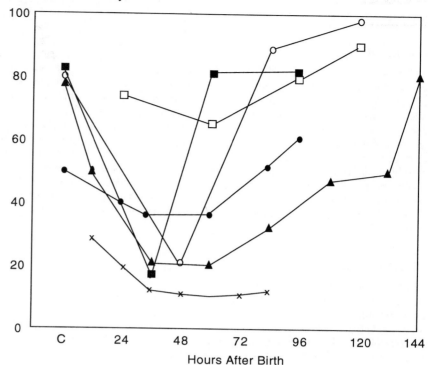

Figure 5-5. The plasma prothrombin activity in the neonatal period from various studies is shown.[5, 81, 442, 445, 621, 622] A consistent decrease in plasma prothrombin activity is demonstrated on days two and three of life; this is followed by an increase in activity.[5] The infants did not receive vitamin K.

these studies, VK prophylaxis was widely recommended. Subsequently, the scientific basis for this policy became less clear for several reasons. First, plasma concentrations of other coagulation proteins besides prothrombin were shown to be low in newborns. Second, there was increasing recognition that bleeding in neonates was often not due to VK deficiency.[5, 437, 438, 452, 453] Third, a water-soluble form of VK, when administered in high amounts (50 to 70 mg), resulted in a hemolytic anemia with resultant kernicterus in some infants.[5, 454, 455] Fourth, many clinicians suggested that VK prophylaxis was not needed for all healthy full-term infants.[453, 456–458] Consequently, VK prophylaxis was suspended in some countries, and this resulted in a recurrence of HDN.[5, 443, 459–471] Subsequently, numerous reports advocating or refuting the need for VK prophylaxis followed. Within the last 5 years, publications linking and refuting the link between prophylactic VK and cancer have been published.[89, 101, 439, 453, 458, 472–477] At this time, the author believes that the available evidence overwhelmingly supports the prophylactic administration of VK to all infants.

The following section critically analyzes the studies supporting or refuting the benefits and risks of prophylactic VK deficiency. In this discussion, the term vitamin-K-deficiency bleeding (VKDB) is used instead of HDN, because neonatal bleeding often is not due to VK deficiency and because VKDB may occur after the neonatal period.

Clinical Presentation. Infants are at greater risk for hemorrhagic complications from VK deficiency than are similarly affected adults because their plasma concentrations of VK-dependent factors are physiologi-

cally decreased.[1–3, 5, 462, 465] The clinical presentation of VKDB can be classified as classical, early, or late on the basis of the timing and type of complications (Table 5–12).[5, 460, 478–481] The *classical VKDB* presents on days two to seven of life in breast-fed, healthy, full-term infants.[5, 462, 466, 480–483] Causes include poor placental transfer of VK,[484–487] marginal VK content in breast milk (less than 20 μg/L), inadequate milk intake, and a sterile gut.[5] VKDB rarely occurs in formula-fed infants because commercially available formulas are supplemented with VK (approximately 830 mg/L).[488, 489] The frequency of occurrence of classical VKDB in the absence of VK prophylaxis depends on the population studied, the supplemental formula, and the frequency of breast-feeding. In the absence of prophylactic VK, the frequency of VKDB ranges from 0.25% to 1.7%.[5, 490] *Early VKDB* presents in the first 24 hours of life and is linked to maternal use of specific medications that interfere with VK stores or function.[491–493] *Late VKDB* presents between weeks two and eight of life and is linked to disorders that compromise the supply of VK.[494, 495]

Laboratory Diagnosis. Laboratory tests used to detect VK deficiency include screening tests, factor assays, determination of decarboxylated forms of VK-dependent factors, protein induced by vitamin K antagonists (PIVKA), and direct measurements of VK. The results of these tests must always be compared with values for age-matched, healthy, non–VK-deficient infants in order to distinguish physiologic and pathologic deficiencies.[496, 512] PIVKAs can be measured directly[86, 497–502] or as a discrepancy between coagulant activity and protein concentration measured immunologically or with an Echis assay.[501] Other tests have also been used to screen for VK deficiency.[503, 504]

Forms of Vitamin K

VK exists in three forms: VK_1 (phytonadione), which is present in leafy green vegetables; VK_2 (menaquinone), which is synthesized by intestinal bacterial flora; and VK_3 (menadione), which is a synthetic, water-soluble form. VK_3 is rarely used in newborns because in high doses it causes hemolytic anemia, resulting in jaundice and potential morbidity.[5, 454, 455] Newborn stores of VK are low, as evidenced by low levels of VK in cord blood and the livers of aborted fetuses.[213, 486, 487, 505] Recent studies measuring placental transport of VK show that only about 10% of maternally administered VK reaches the fetus.[506]

Prophylactic Vitamin K

Most of the controversy concerning the prophylactic use of VK can be explained by the design of the trials and the subsequent interpretation of their results. The strongest form of evidence comes from randomized controlled trials. Two randomized controlled trials have assessed the benefits of VK prophylaxis, using clinical bleeding as the outcome measure (Table 5–13).[490, 507] In the first study, 3338 full-term infants were randomized to receive either placebo, 100 μg of mena-

dione, or 5 mg of menadione intramuscularly.[490] The risk of ICH and of minor bleeding was significantly greater in the placebo group than in both of the treatment groups. These clinical results were supported by prolonged PTs in infants with hemorrhagic complications and by the correction of PT values following VK administration. A second study randomized 470 male infants who were undergoing circumcision to receive VK or nothing.[507] Infants who received prophylactic VK had significantly less bleeding than those who did not.[507] A subsequent smaller, non-blinded trial conducted by the same group produced similar results.[508]

A second level of support for the use of prophylactic VK comes from numerous studies in which laboratory evidence of VK deficiency was compared in infants who received VK at birth and in infants who did not receive VK (Table 5–14). These studies consistently indicate that biochemical evidence of VK deficiency is less frequently detected in infants who received VK prophylaxis than in those who did not.

A third level of support for prophylactic VK comes from cohort studies reporting biochemical indices of VK deficiency at birth[213, 482, 486, 487, 505]; large population based studies in which VK prophylaxis was never instituted; and studies in which VK prophylaxis was instituted and then withdrawn.[5, 443, 460-462, 483] In general, VKDB rarely occurred when VK prophylaxis was used but was observed when prophylactic VK therapy was withdrawn. Evidence also comes from numerous stud-

Table 5–12. FORMS OF VITAMIN-K-DEFICIENCY BLEEDING IN INFANCY

Early	Classical	Late
	Age	
<24 h	Days 2–7	0.5–6 mo
	Causes and Risk Factors	
Medications During Pregnancy		Marginal VK content in breast milk due to low VK intake and absorption
Anticonvulsants	Breast-feeding	Cystic fibrosis
Oral anticoagulants (rifampin, isoniazid)	Inadequate VK intake	Diarrhea
Antibiotics (rarely, idiopathic or hereditary)		α_1AT deficiency
		Hepatitis
		Celiac disease
	Localization in Order of Frequency	
ICH	ICH	ICH (>50%)
GI	GI	GI
Umbilicus	Umbilicus	Skin
Intra-abdominal	ENT region	ENT region
Cephalohematoma	Injection sites	Injection sites
	Circumcision	Urogenital tract
		Intrathoracic
	Frequency Without VK Prophylaxis	
Very rare	1.5% (1/10,000) births	4–10/10,000 births*
	Prophylaxis	
	Adequate VK supply	Adequate VK supply
Discontinue or replace offending medications	Early and adequate breast-feeding	Adequate breast-feeding
Maternal VK prophylaxis	Formula	Formula
	VK prophylaxis	VK prophylaxis†

VK = vitamin K; ENT = ear, nose, and throat.
*More common in Southeast Asia.
†Single intramuscular injection is better than single oral; repeated small doses are closer to physiologic conditions. Warning signs: neonatal icterus, poor feeding, failure to thrive, any form of bleeding.

Table 5-13. VITAMIN K PROPHYLAXIS: RANDOMIZED CONTROLLED TRIALS

Reference	All Bleeding*			Significant Bleeding†		Coagulation Studies†	
	n	*n*	%	*n*	%	*n*	*Abnormal*
Sutherland and Glueck (1967)[490]							
Vitamin K	2195	121	5.5	7	0.3	76	1
Control	1143	86	7.5	19	1.7§	60	18§
Vietti et al (1960)[507]							
Vitamin K	240	6	2.5	1	0.4	22	1
Control	230	32	13.9	14	6.0§	25	11§

n = number of subjects.
*Sutherland and Glueck, bleeding from any site; Vietti et al, any bleeding after circumcision.
†Sutherland and Glueck, bleeding in a significant site (central nervous system, adrenal glands) causing anemia, resuturing of a circumcision; Vietti et al, bleeding requiring resuturing of a circumcision.
†Prothrombin time in both studies.
§$P < .01$.

Table 5-14. EVIDENCE SUPPORTING THE BENEFITS OF VITAMIN K PROPHYLAXIS: LABORATORY SURROGATE OUTCOMES

Reference	No. of Patients	Coagulation Test	Other
Ogata et al (1988)[605]		PIVKA-II (day 7†)	
Control	23	15 (65%)	Affected infants responded to VK
VK	11	0 (0%)	
Widdershoven et al (1986)[499]		PIVKA-II	Days 1–4 Days 29–35
Control	12	5 (42%)	378 707
VK	13	0 (0%)	32,711* 698
Motohara et al (1987)[497]		PIVKA-II (1 mo)	
Control (Br)	5090	26 (0.51%)*	Affected infants responded to VK
VK (Br)	3206	6 (0.19%)	
Von Kries et al (1987)[606]		PIVKA-II	
Control	95	47 (48%)	Factor II <40% of adult level in 36% of control babies
VK	95	0* (0%)	and in 0% of treated
Garrow et al (1986)[504]		Thrombotest	
Control	24	15.2*	—
VK	24	39.1	
O'Connor and Addiego (1986)[607]		Factor II/Echis II	
Control	15	0.68	Similar results with oral VK
VK	15	0.96*	
Motohara et al (1985)[463]		PIVKA-II (day 3)	
Control	51	61.5%*	Affected infants responded to VK
VK	51	18.5%	
Aballi and de Lamerens (1978)[5]		Factor II (%)	
		Before *After*	
Control	57	23 20	4-h response to VK prophylaxis
VK	58	20 53*	
Keenan et al (1971)[608]		PT (s)	
Control	61	22	Affected infants responded to VK
VK	13	14*	
Wefring (1962)[609]		Thrombotest (<10%)	
Control	28	16 (57%)	Affected infants responded to VK
VK	83	2 (2%)	
Vietti et al (1961)[507]†		PT (s)	
Control	50	14 (28%)	Circumcised males bled in 0/39 (0%) cases in the control
VK	85	1 (1.1%)	group and in 4/15 (27%) cases in the VK group
Lehmann (1944)[462]†		PI (<30%)	
Control	90	55.5%	Death from bleeding occurred in 34 of 17,741
VK	122	0.8%	compared with 6 of 13,250 treated infants
Bruchsaler (1941)[441]		Prothrombin Index	
		Day 1 *Day 4*	
Control	30	58.3 55.4	—
VK	30	59.0 81.0	
Astrowe and Palmerton (1941)[610]		PT (s)	
		Birth *Day 3*	
Control	28	38.4 51.8	—
VK	18	46.0 34.0*	

VK = vitamin K; PT = prothrombin time; PI = prothrombin index; PIVKA-II = protein induced in vitamin K absence.
*Statistically significant differences ($P < .05$) between control and VK group.
†Control groups did not receive VK prophylaxis. The VK groups received prophylactic VK in differing amounts, by differing routes, and in some cases by formula supplementation.

ies reporting beneficial effects (either clinically or bio-chemically) following the administration of VK to mothers.[5, 446–448, 455, 509] The weakest supporting data come from comparisons of the incidence of VKDB in countries that do not provide prophylactic VK with that in countries that do administer VK prophylaxis.[5, 460] Finally, numerous cases of infants with VKDB who for a variety of reasons did not receive VK at birth have been reported.[468, 469, 510, 511]

Studies reported to refute the benefits of prophylactic VK use are also ranked by the strength of their study designs (Table 5–15). No randomized controlled trials have sample sizes sufficient to show that prophylactic VK does not prevent bleeding. Some small studies reported no clinical benefit from prophylactic VK. However, the strength of the conclusions from these studies is considerably reduced because of small sample sizes, sequential rather than concurrent controls, and the absence of information on feeding practices.[453] Some investigators studied cord blood only and did not demonstrate biochemical evidence of VK deficiency.* In other studies, mothers rather than infants received VK prophylaxis, which introduced the confounding variable of placental transport and delivery of VK to fetuses. Some of the latter studies did show a benefit of maternal VK prophylaxis on biochemical outcomes.

In 1990, a British study reported an unexpected association between childhood cancer and prophylactic VK use on the basis of a 1970 birth cohort.[513] Subsequently,

---

*See references 89, 101, 439, 453, 458, 472, 473, and 512.

Table 5-15. EVIDENCE AGAINST THE BENEFITS OF VITAMIN K PROPHYLAXIS

Reference	No. of Subjects	Coagulation Test			Other
Sanford et al (1942)[439]		*PT (%)*			
		Day 1	**Day 3**		No apparent difference in bleeding
Control	55	80	20*		
VK	40	82	75		
Potter (1945)[453]		*Mortality*			
Control	6630	90 (1.4%) ns			Death from all causes, not HDN; sequential study
VK	6004	89 (1.5%)			
Muller and Van Doorm (1977)[101]		*Prothrombin*			
		Activity	**Antigen**	**Echis**	
Cord Blood	43	51	53	54	—
Gobel et al (1977)[89]		*Factor II (%)*			
Control	15	20.8*			VK given as early feeds
VK	15	22.6			
Mori et al (1977)[473]		*Factor II (%)*			
		Day 1	**Day 2**		VK group had at least 10% increase in VK-dependent factors
Control	29	30.5	30.4		
VK	31	30.3	33.2		
Malia et al (1980)[458]		Similar values for activity and			—
Cord Blood	24	immunologic measurements for factors II, VII, IX, and X			
Corrigan and Kryc (1980)[472]		*Factor II Activity Ag Ratio:*			
Cord Blood	40	0.90			Similar results for prematures and adults
Pietersma-de Bruyer (1990)[512]		*Factor II (%)* **(act)**	*Factor II (%)* **(ant)**	*Factor X (%)* **(act)**	
Formula VK	8	58 ns	53 ns	74 ns	1 wk after birth
Breast milk	10	54	50	49	
Greer et al (1991)[611]		*Plasma Phylloquinone*			
Formula VK	11	5.19 ng/mL*			No apparent VK deficiency
Breast milk	23	<0.25 ng/mL			
Anai et al (1993)[612]		*Normotest (%)*			
Control	186	53.4 ± 9.9*			Maternal VK (oral)
VK	74	59.6 ± 10.0			
Dickson et al (1994)[613]		*PT* **(s)** *APTT* **(s)**	*Factor II (%)* **(act)**	*Factor II (%)* **(ant)**	
Control	16	17.0 53.4	35.7	39.8	Maternal VK (intramuscular) or placebo
VK	17	14.6 59.5	38.8	43.2	

ns = nonsignificant difference; HDN = hemolytic disease of the newborn.
*Statistically significant differences between control and VK groups, P < .05.

Table 5–16. STUDIES ASSESSING THE LINK BETWEEN VK PROPHYLAXIS AND CHILDHOOD CANCER

Reference	Study Design	No. of Subjects		Odds Ratio
Golding et al (1990)[474]	Case Control	Case Control	33† 99	7.8 —
Golding et al (1992)[475]	Case Control	Case Control	195† 558	1.97 (Ca)* (1.3–3.0)
Ekelund et al (1993)[476]	Cohort	Case Control	1,085,654‡ 272,080	1.01 (0.88–1.77)
Klebanoff (1993)[477]	Case Control	Case Control	44† 226	0.47 (L) 1.08 (Ca)

L = leukemia; Ca = cancer.
*Significant.
†Children who developed cancer versus children who did not.
‡Children given intramuscular VK versus children who received oral VK.

the same group conducted a case-control study designed to assess the risk of cancer associated with intramuscular VK among infants born in two hospitals between 1965 and 1987 and diagnosed with cancer between 1971 and 1989. They reported a significant association between intramuscular administration of VK and cancer, as compared with no VK prophylaxis or the oral administration of VK. Table 5–16 lists studies addressing the validity of the link. The link of VK prophylaxis to childhood cancer is weak, and the benefits of VK are clinically significant. At this time, the administration of prophylactic VK to newborns can be strongly recommended.

Prophylactic Vitamin K Administration

The recommendations for VK prophylaxis in many countries are reasonably similar.[506] Daily requirements of VK are approximately 1 to 5 μg/kg of body weight for newborns.[506] Most groups recommend a single dose of 0.5 to 1 mg intramuscularly or an oral dose of 2 to 4 mg at birth, with subsequent dosing for breast-fed infants. Oral VK prophylaxis is preferable to parenteral prophylaxis; studies have shown that oral administration of VK is as effective, less expensive, and less traumatic than intramuscular administration in preventing the classic presentation of VK deficiency.[506] However, orally administered VK_1 or VK_3 is not as effective as intramuscularly injected VK in the prevention of late VK deficiency (Table 5–17). In a 1990 randomized controlled trial in Thailand,[514] infants were given a single 2-mg dose of VK orally, 5 mg orally, or 1 mg intramuscularly. Although the mean levels of VK_1 were not significantly different in the treated infants given the various dosage forms, a trend toward the manifestation of higher levels was observed in intramuscularly treated infants. Strategies for preventing late VK deficiency include the repeat administration of oral VK in Germany[471] and Japan[515] or the continuous low-dose VK supplementation in the Netherlands.[471]

In addition to general prophylaxis at birth, patients in certain risk groups require additional VK prophylaxis (e.g., infants with α_1-antitrypsin deficiency, chronic diarrhea, cystic fibrosis, or celiac disease). Pregnant women receiving oral anticonvulsant therapy should receive about 5 mg of VK_1 daily during the third trimester for the prevention of overt VK deficiency in their infants at birth.

New Developments in Vitamin K Prophylaxis

A new mixed micelle oral VK_1 preparation that is readily absorbed has been tested in children.[506] Whether this preparation will negate the need for repeated dosing if the oral route is chosen requires further testing.

Treatment

An infant suspected of having VK deficiency should be treated immediately with VK while laboratory con-

Table 5–17. ORAL VITAMIN K VERSUS INTRAMUSCULAR VITAMIN K IN THE PREVENTION OF LATE VITAMIN K DEFICIENCY

Reference	Vitamin K	No. of Cases	Rate per 100,000	95% Clearance
United Kingdom (1991)[471]	nil	9	4.4	2.0–8.4
	oral: 1–2 mg	7	1.5	0.6–3.2
	IM: 1 mg	0	0	0.0–0.4
Sweden (1991)[614]	oral: 1–2 mg	16	6	3.7–9.8
	IM: 1 mg	0	0	0.0–5.6
Switzerland (1986)[615]	oral: 1–3 mg	7	6.4	2.5–13.1
	IM: 1 mg	0	0	0.0–5.3
Germany (1992)[515]	nil	10	7.2	3.5–13.3
	oral: 1–2 mg	2	1.4	0.2–5.2
	IM (SC): 1 mg	1	0.25	0.01–1.32
Japan (1992)[616]	nil	20.4*	10.5†	7.0–15.0
	MK-4 (2 mg: 1–3×)	29.5*	2.8†	2.0–3.78
United States (1995)[617]	oral: 2 mg	23,228	1.4–6.4	—
Germany (1995)[495, 618]	nil	89	5.31	2.81–29.58
	oral: 2 mg	10	1.21	0.97–11.52
	IM: 1 mg	2	0.36	—

IM = intramuscular injection.
*Estimated number of cases.
†Including strictly idiopathic cases and cases with recognized associated disease (almost all with ICH) but no cases of VK deficiency detected by mass screening; cases without clear information on VK prophylaxis were included in the VK prophylaxis group.

firmation is awaited. All infants with VKDB should be given VK either subcutaneously or intravenously, depending on the clinical problem. VK should not be given intramuscularly to infants with VKDN, as large hematomas may form at the site of the injection. The absorption of subcutaneously administered VK is rapid, and its effect is only slightly slower than that of systemically administered VK. Intravenous VK should be given slowly because it may induce an anaphylactoid reaction. Infants with major bleeding secondary to VK deficiency should also be treated with plasma products to rapidly increase levels of VK-dependent proteins. Plasma is the product of choice for the treatment of a non–life-threatening hemorrhagic event, whereas the use of PCCs should be considered for the management of life-threatening bleeding.

Extracorporeal Membrane Oxygenation

The use of extracorporeal membrane oxygenation (ECMO) began in the 1960s. Since then, thousands of infants have been treated, with a survival rate of those treated being approximately 60%. ECMO permits the transfer of oxygen into blood across a semipermeable membrane and is currently used for infants with life-threatening severe respiratory insufficiency. The underlying respiratory disorders include meconium aspiration syndrome, severe RDS, congenital diaphragmatic hernia, persistent pulmonary hypertension, and sepsis. Despite the widespread use of ECMO, few controlled trials assessing its efficacy have been published.[516–519] Clearly, more definitive trials are needed to validate the use of ECMO. The follow-up studies of the survivors of ECMO are most encouraging, with a majority of infants having normal developmental follow-up.

The most important side effect and leading cause of death in infants on ECMO is ICH. The cause of ICH is multifactorial, with vascular change, heparin, and thrombocytopenia all being contributing factors. It is unfortunate that there is no single predictor of ICH, although both low birth-weight and thrombocytopenia are associated with ICH. The latter has resulted in the clinical practice of maintaining platelet count at greater than $100 \times 10^9/L$. Data to date suggest that thrombin generation is impaired due to a consumptive coagulopathy and that a hyperfibrinolytic state exists along with impairment of platelet number and function.[520, 521] Heparin is used in full systemic doses, with a bolus of 100 to 150 U/kg followed by a continuous systemic infusion of heparin at 20 to 70 U/kg per hour. The laboratory goal is to maintain the activated clotting time at two- to threefold the baseline values (240 to 280 seconds). Although anticoagulation is required for ECMO, the optimal use of heparin has never been tested in clinical trials. Whether lower doses of heparin or the use of potentially safer anticoagulant drugs, such as low-molecular-weight heparins, have a role in ECMO remains to be determined.

THROMBOTIC DISORDERS
Congenital Prethrombotic Disorders

Patients with single-gene defects for recognized inherited prethrombotic disorders rarely present with their first thromboembolic complication during childhood unless another pathologic event unmasks the problem. In contrast, patients who are homozygotes or double heterozygotes for a congenital prethrombotic disorder usually present as newborns or young children. The following discussion is limited to the unique aspects of these inherited deficiencies in newborns. Chapter 46 discusses congenital prethrombotic disorders in detail. A database search of the literature from 1980 to 1995 identified infants who presented with thromboembolic complications in the first weeks of life and were subsequently shown to have an inherited prethrombotic disorder. No newborn cases of activated protein C resistance due to factor V Leiden were reported.

Homozygous Prethrombotic Disorders

General Information. Twenty-three reports have described 40 patients with homozygous protein C deficiency and one patient with homozygous protein S deficiency.[38, 96, 522–544] All patients presenting in the newborn period had undetectable levels of protein C (or protein S), whereas children with delayed presentation had detectable levels ranging between 0.05 and 0.20 units/mL.

Clinical Presentation. The classical clinical presentation of homozygous protein C/protein S deficiency consists of cerebral or ophthalmic damage (or both) that occurred *in utero*, purpura fulminans within hours or days of birth, and, on rare occasions, large vessel thrombosis. Purpura fulminans is an acute, lethal syndrome of DIC characterized by rapidly progressive hemorrhagic necrosis of the skin due to dermal vascular thrombosis.[263, 545, 546] The skin lesions start as small, ecchymotic sites that increase in a radial fashion, become purplish black with bullae, and then turn necrotic and gangrenous.[263, 546] The lesions occur mainly on the extremities but can occur on the buttocks, abdomen, scrotum, and scalp. They also occur at pressure points, at sites of previous punctures, and at previously affected sites. Affected infants also have severe DIC with secondary hemorrhagic complications.

Diagnosis. The diagnosis of infants with homozygous protein C/protein S deficiency is based on the appropriate clinical picture, a protein C/protein S level that is usually undetectable, heterozygous state in the parents, and, ideally, identification of the molecular defect. The presence of very low levels of protein C/protein S in the absence of clinical manifestations and of a family history cannot be considered diagnostic because physiologic plasma levels can be as low as 0.12 U/mL. The homozygous forms of AT-III (or heparin cofactor II) deficiency have not been confirmed in newborns, but one would anticipate that they would present with severe life-threatening thromboembolic complications. Molecular diagnosis is available for identified families (see Chapters 44 and 45).

Initial Treatment. The diagnosis of homozygous protein C/protein S deficiency is usually unanticipated and made at the time of the clinical presentation. Although numerous forms of initial therapy have been used, 10 to 20 mL/kg of FFP every 6 to 12 hours is usually the form of therapy that is most readily available.[547] Plasma levels of protein C achieved with these doses of FFP vary from 15% to 32% at 30 minutes after the infusion and from 4% to 10% at 12 hours.[532] Plasma levels of protein S (which was entirely bound to C4b) were 23% at 2 hours and 14% at 24 hours, with an approximate half-life of 36 hours.[544] Doses of protein C concentrate have ranged from 20 to 60 units/kg. In one study, a dose of 60 units/kg resulted in peak protein C levels of greater than 0.60 unit/mL.[548] Replacement therapy should be continued until all of the clinical lesions resolve, which is usually at 6 to 8 weeks. In addition to the clinical course, plasma D-dimer concentrations may be useful for monitoring the effectiveness of protein C replacement.[128]

Long-Term Therapy. The modalities used for the long-term management of infants with homozygous protein C/protein S deficiency included oral anticoagulation therapy, replacement therapy with either FFP or protein C concentrate, and liver transplantation.[543] When oral anticoagulation therapy is initiated, replacement therapy should be continued until the INR is therapeutic so that skin necrosis can be avoided. The therapeutic range for the INR can be individualized to some extent but is usually between 2.5 and 4.5. The risks of oral anticoagulation therapy include bleeding with high INRs and recurrent purpuric lesions with low INRs. Frequent monitoring of INR values is required if these complications are to be avoided. Bone development also should be monitored because the long-term effects of warfarin use on bones in young infants is unknown.

Heterozygote Prethrombotic Disorders

General Information. Thromboembolic events rarely occur in infants. When they do occur, a secondary, acquired insult is usually present. The few case reports in the literature described a diversity of clinical presentations that usually reflected the site of the thrombus. Purpura fulminans did not occur in any case. Although most infants died, many were left with residual complications secondary to the location of the thrombus, including the venous (systemic and central nervous system) and arterial systems (aorta, coronary arteries).[549–555] Low levels of proteins C and S have been described in Legg-Calvé-Perthes disease.[555]

Treatment. Treatments consisted of supportive therapy alone, anticoagulation with heparin, thrombolytic therapy, and replacement with specific factor concentrates.[556–558] For AT-III deficiency, AT-III concentrates were administered to 4 infants as either boluses or as continuous infusions. Boluses of 52 and 104 units/kg of AT-III concentrate increased AT-III levels from 0.10 unit/mL to 0.75 and 1.48 units/mL, respectively, at 1 hour.[558] At 24 hours, levels of AT-III had decreased to approximately 0.20 unit/mL.[558] A continuous infusion

of AT-III concentrate at a rate of 2.1 units/kg per hour maintained a plasma level of 0.40 to 0.50 unit/mL.[558]

ACQUIRED PROTHROMBOTIC DISORDERS

General Information

Reviews of the literature[90, 559, 560] and an international registry of neonatal thrombotic disease[561] have provided valuable information on the epidemiology of venous and arterial thrombotic disease in newborns. Symptomatic secondary thromboembolic complications occur more frequently in sick newborns than in children of any other age, with an incidence of approximately 2.4 per 1000 hospital admissions to the neonatal intensive care unit.[561] Catheters are responsible for over 80% of venous and 90% of arterial thrombotic complications.[561] Catheters are responsible for many of the factors that initiate thrombus formation (e.g., the presence of a foreign surface, endothelial cell damage, impairment of flow, and infusion of noxious substances).[561] Renal vein thromboses are the most frequent form of non–catheter-related thrombosis.[561] Other risk factors include increased blood viscosity, poor deformability of physiologically large red cells, polycythemia, dehydration, and activation of the coagulation and fibrinolytic systems secondary to a variety of medical problems. The following section discusses the epidemiology, diagnosis, and treatment of thromboembolic complications in newborns.

Venous Catheter–Related Thrombosis

The use of umbilical venous catheters and other forms of central venous catheters is associated with a significant risk of thrombosis.[562–564] According to autopsy studies, 20% to 65% of infants who die with an umbilical venous catheter in place have an associated thrombus. A database search of the literature from 1966 to 1995 identified 60 references to catheter-related thrombosis in infants. Of these, 44 were case reports or small case series. The appropriate placement of umbilical venous catheters is critical to the prevention of serious organ impairment, such as portal vein thrombosis and hepatic necrosis. Long-term sequelae of umbilical venous catheterization have not been rigorously studied but include portal vein thrombosis with portal hypertension, splenomegaly, gastric and esophageal varices, and hypertension. Until recently, pulmonary embolism was rarely diagnosed in sick newborns because its clinical signs were easily confused with those of RDS. The use of ventilation lung scintigraphy in newborns has facilitated the diagnosis of pulmonary embolism.[565]

Arterial Catheter–Related Thrombosis

General Information. Seriously ill infants require indwelling arterial catheters, which present a risk of thrombosis, regardless of the vessel and type of catheter chosen.[371, 566–570] Catheter-related thrombosis not only occludes catheters with loss of patency but also may obstruct major arterial vessels. In a retrospective examination of approximately 4000 infants who underwent umbilical artery catheterization, severe symptomatic vessel obstruction was observed in 1% of infants. Asymptomatic catheter-related thrombi occur more frequently, as evidenced by postmortem (3% to 59% of cases) and angiographic studies (10% to 90% of cases).

Diagnosis. Contrast angiography is considered the reference test for diagnosing arterial thrombosis. Noninvasive techniques such as Doppler ultrasound offer advantages, but their sensitivity and specificity are unknown. A review of 20 neonates with aortic thromboses treated in one institution revealed that ultrasound failed to identify thrombi in 4 patients, 3 of whom had complete aortic obstruction.[571]

Sequelae. The sequelae of catheter-related thrombosis can be immediate or long term. Acute symptoms reflect the location of the catheter and include renal hypertension, intestinal necrosis, and peripheral gangrene.[559] The long-term side effects of symptomatic and asymptomatic thrombosis of major vessels have not been studied but are likely significant.[559]

Prophylaxis with Heparin. A low-dose continuous heparin infusion (3 to 5 units/hour) is commonly used to maintain catheter patency. The effectiveness of heparin was assessed in seven studies focusing on three outcomes: patency, local thrombus, and ICH (Table 5–18).[566–570, 572] Patency, which is likely linked to the presence of local thrombus, is prolonged by the use of low-dose heparin.[567–570, 572] Local thromboses were assessed by ultrasound in two randomized studies. The sample sizes were too small to allow the forming of any meaningful conclusions.[566, 567] The evidence linking heparin to ICH in newborns is similarly weak.[570, 573] One study had a sample size of only 15 per arm,[570] and another case control study had a broad odds ratio that ranged from 1.4 to 11.0.[573] Thus, the magnitude of risk for ICH is uncertain.[573] Heparin is used in at least three quarters of American nurseries.[559]

Renal Vein Thrombosis

General Information. Renal vein thrombosis (RVT) occurs primarily in newborns and young infants. A database search of the literature identified 268 patients with renal vein thrombosis in 80 publications (67 case reports and 13 case series). Of the 268 evaluable cases, 79% presented within the first month, and usually within the first week of life. Some infants developed RVT *in utero*. The incidence among males and females was similar, and the left and right sides were affected equally. Bilateral RVT occurred in 24% of pediatric patients.

Clinical Presentation and Etiology. Presenting symptoms and clinical findings in neonates and older patients differ and are influenced by the extent and rapidity of thrombus formation. Neonates usually present with a flank mass, hematuria, proteinuria, thrombocytopenia, and nonfunction of the involved kidney. Clinical findings suggestive of acute inferior vena cava thrombosis include cold, cyanotic, and edematous lower extremities. RVTs result from pathologic states characterized by reduced renal blood flow, increased blood viscosity, hyperosmolality, or hypercoagulability.

Coagulation Abnormalities. The most common coagulation abnormality is thrombocytopenia, which is usually mild, having average values of $100,000 \times 10^9/$ L. Coagulation may be prolonged, and levels of fibrinogen-fibrin degradation products increased. Children with RVT should be evaluated for a congenital prothrombotic disorder.[574]

Diagnosis and Treatment. The diagnosis of RVT has changed from an autopsy finding to an antemortem diagnosis that requires confirmation with an objective test. Ultrasound is the radiographic test of choice owing to ease of testing and sensitivity to an enlarged kidney. Treatment options include supportive care, anticoagulation, and thrombolytic therapy. In the 1990s, there has been uniform agreement that aggressive sup-

Table 5-18. UMBILICAL ARTERY CATHETERIZATION

Reference	Level	Intervention	No. of Patients	Bleeding	Event (B or TE)
Jackson et al (1987)[566]	II	HB-PU	61	*	13 TE
		PVC	64	*	23 TE
Horgan et al (1987)[567]	II	Heparin	59	*	16 TE
		No Heparin	52	*	18 TE
Rajani et al (1979)[568]	I	Heparin	32	*	4 B‡
		Placebo	30	*	19 B
David et al (1981)[572]	II	Heparin	26	0†	3 B‡
		No Heparin	26	0†	15 B
Bosque and Weaver (1986)[569]	II	Heparin (C)	18	*	0 B‡
		Heparin (I)	19	*	8 B
Horgan et al (1987)[567]	II	Heparin	59	*	2 B‡
		No Heparin	52	*	10 B
Ankola and Atakent (1993)[570]	II	Heparin	15	4 ICH	2 B‡
		No Heparin	15	5 ICH	11 B

B = blocked; TE = thromboembolic event; HB-PU = heparin-bonded polyurethane; PVC = polyvinyl chloride; C = continuous; I = intermittent.
*Not reported.
†No hemorrhage.
‡$P < .05$.
From Michelson AD, Bovill E, Andrew M: Antithrombotic therapy in children. Chest 1995; 108:506S.

portive care is indicated. However, the use of anticoagulants and thrombolytic agents is controversial. One approach is to use supportive care for unilateral renal vein thrombosis in the absence of uremia and extension into the inferior vena cava. Heparin therapy should be considered for unilateral RVT that does extend into the inferior vena cava or for bilateral RVT owing to the risk of pulmonary embolism and complete renal failure. Thrombolytic therapy should be considered in the presence of bilateral renal vein thrombosis and renal failure. Thrombectomy, though a common therapeutic choice in the past, is rarely indicated.

Outcome. RVT has changed from a frequently lethal complication to one which over 85% of children survive. Unfortunately, no recent studies have assessed the long-term morbidity, such as hypertension and renal atrophy.

Spontaneous Venous and Arterial Thrombosis

Spontaneous venous thrombosis occurs in adrenal veins, the inferior vena cava, the portal vein, the hepatic veins, and the venous system of the brain.[559, 560] Spontaneous occlusion of arterial vessels in the absence of a catheter is unusual but can occur in ill infants. As in catheter-related thrombosis, the clinical presentation reflects the vessel that is occluded. Complete occlusion of a vessel can lead to gangrene and loss of the affected limb or to ischemic organ damage.[559, 560] The presence of systemic hypertension in newborns is frequently related to renal artery thrombosis, even in the absence of a catheter.

Heparin Therapy in Newborns

The lack of consensus for prophylaxis and treatment of thromboembolic complications in newborns reflects the lack of controlled trials in this area. Recommendations for adult patients provide useful guidelines but do not likely reflect optimal therapy for newborns. Current therapeutic options include supportive care alone, anticoagulant therapy, thrombolytic therapy, and thrombectomy. For most infants who develop thrombotic complications, the cause of thrombosis is a catheter-related thrombus that is clinically silent. In most nurseries, catheters are not routinely checked for associated thrombosis; thus, by exclusion, most infants with clinically silent thrombi receive supportive care alone.

Age-Dependent Features. Heparin's anticoagulant activities are mediated by catalysis of AT-III inhibition of thrombin and, secondarily, of other serine proteases. Although the dosing of heparin therapy in newborns differs from that in adults, optimal dosing cannot be predicted. Observations suggesting that the heparin requirements of neonates are decreased compared with those of adults are several. First, the capacity of plasmas from healthy newborns to generate thrombin is both delayed and decreased when compared with that of adult plasmas and is similar to that of plasmas from adults receiving therapeutic amounts of heparin.[97, 98] Second, at heparin concentrations in the therapeutic

range, the capacity of plasmas from healthy newborns to generate thrombin is barely measurable.[575] Third, the amount of clot-bound thrombin is decreased in newborns because low plasma concentrations of prothrombin likely reduce heparin requirements.[109] Observations that suggest that heparin requirements are increased in neonates compared with adults include the following: (1) the clearance of heparin is accelerated in newborns[576, 577]; (2) plasma concentrations of AT-III are decreased to levels frequently less than 0.40 in premature infants, which may limit heparin's antithrombotic activities[1–3]; and (3) studies in a newborn piglet model of venous thrombosis have shown that low AT-III levels limit the anticoagulant and antithrombotic effectiveness of heparin.[558, 578]

Indications, Therapeutic Range, and Dose. Indications for heparin therapy in newborns remain unclear. Although the benefits of heparin therapy in newborns are likely similar to those in adults, the relative risk that major bleeding will occur with its use is likely increased. Infants with extending thrombotic complications, or with threatened organ or limb viability may benefit from heparin therapy.

Therapeutic ranges reflect the optimal risk/benefit ratio of anticoagulant therapy with regards to recurrent thrombotic events and bleeding complications. In the absence of clinical trials in newborns, one approach is to use heparin in doses that achieve the lower therapeutic range for adults (see Chapter 46). Close monitoring of the thrombus with objective tests such as ultrasound is recommended.

Average doses of heparin required in newborns to achieve adult therapeutic APTT values are bolus doses of 75 to 100 units/kg and average maintenance doses of 28 units/kg per hour. The duration of heparin therapy required for the treatment of thromboembolic complications is uncertain. One approach is to treat for 10 to 14 days with heparin alone. If there is subsequent extension of the thrombus in the absence of anticoagulation therapy, treatment with oral anticoagulants should be considered. In general, the use of oral anticoagulants should be avoided whenever possible in newborns because of the risk of bleeding and difficulties in monitoring. There are clear exceptions to this approach, such as the infant with homozygous protein C/protein S deficiency or recurrent thrombotic events.

Adverse Effects. There are two clinically important adverse effects of heparin therapy: ICH, and heparin-induced thrombocytopenia.[579–581] In the absence of an alternative cause, thrombocytopenic patients should be evaluated for heparin-induced thrombocytopenia and treated with alternative therapy.

In the future, new anticoagulant drugs, such as low-molecular-weight heparin, offer significant therapeutic advantages over heparin for newborns.[559, 582] The potential advantages of the use of low-molecular-weight heparin include predictable bioavailability, the need for minimal monitoring, ease of administration, decreased bleeding, and equal or increased efficacy. Low-molecular-weight heparins are particularly helpful in patients who are vulnerable to bleeding complications, such as sick premature infants.

Oral Anticoagulant Therapy in Newborns

Age-Dependent Features. Chapter 46 discusses oral anticoagulation therapy in children in detail; thus, only specific issues related to newborns are discussed in this section. Oral anticoagulants function by reducing plasma concentrations of the VK-dependent proteins. At birth, levels of the VK-dependent proteins are similar to those found in adults receiving therapeutic amounts of oral anticoagulants for deep venous thrombosis/pulmonary embolism.[1-3, 575, 583-585] In addition, stores of VK are low, and a small number of newborns have evidence of functional VK-deficiency.[496] These features significantly increase the sensitivity of newborns to oral anticoagulants and potentially their risk of bleeding. Oral anticoagulant therapy should be avoided when possible during the first month of life.[496, 586] Unfortunately, a small number of infants require extended anticoagulation therapy, and heparin cannot be used for extended periods of time because of the risk of osteopenia. The use of low-molecular-weight heparin is an option that should be considered; however, studies of its use in newborns are limited.[559]

Indications, Therapeutic Range, Dose. The optimal therapeutic INR range is unknown for newborns and almost certainly differs from that for adults. Recommendations for oral anticoagulation therapy in adults can be used as a guideline for determining the lowest effective dose, which to some extent can be individualized. Maintenance doses for therapeutic amounts of oral anticoagulants are age-dependent, with infants requiring the highest doses (0.32 mg/kg).

Adverse Effects. Close monitoring of oral anticoagulation in newborns is required if both hemorrhagic and recurrent thrombotic complications are to be prevented. Unfortunately, infants have poor venous access as well as complicated medical problems.[587-595] Weekly or biweekly measurements of the INR and frequent dose adjustments are required[596] (see Chapter 46). Doses are affected by diet, medication, and intercurrent illnesses.

Breast-fed infants are very sensitive to oral anticoagulants because of the low concentrations of VK in breast milk.[5, 159, 213, 488, 505, 597] Daily supplementation of breast-fed infants with small amounts of commercial formulas reduces their sensitivity to oral anticoagulants and the risk of sudden increases in INR values. In contrast to breast-fed infants, infants receiving commercial formulas or total parenteral nutrition are resistant to oral anticoagulants because of VK supplementation.[334, 488] Reducing or removing VK supplementation in infants receiving total parenteral nutrition significantly reduces the dose requirements. Most infants requiring oral anticoagulants also require other medications on an intermittent and long-term basis. The effects of dosage changes and the introduction of new medications must be closely supervised.

Antiplatelet Agents in Newborns

Antiplatelet agents are rarely used in newborns for antithrombotic therapy. The hyporeactivity of neonatal platelets and the paradoxically short bleeding time suggest that optimal use of antiplatelet agents differs in newborns and in adults. Aspirin is the most commonly used antiplatelet agent. The use of empirical low doses of 1 to 5 mg/kg per day has been proposed as adjuvant therapy for patients with Blalock-Taussig shunts, some endovascular stents, and some cerebrovascular events.[598, 599]

Thrombolytic Therapy in Newborns

Age-Dependent Features. The activities of thrombolytic agents are dependent on the endogenous concentrations of plasminogen, which are physiologically decreased at birth.[132] Low plasminogen levels result in impairment of the capacity to generate plasmin[124] and a decrease in the capacity to thrombolyse fibrin clots.[132] Increasing plasma concentrations of plasminogen with purified plasminogen has resulted in fibrin clot lyses that were greater than those occurring in adult plasma, likely owing to the decreased levels of α_2-antiplasmin in the plasma of newborns. If an infant does not respond to thrombolytic therapy, replacement of plasminogen should be considered.

Indications, Therapeutic Range, and Dose. Infants who develop serious thrombotic complications, as defined by organ or limb impairment, may benefit from thrombolytic therapy. The clinical objective is removal of the clot as quickly and safely as possible. The surgical removal of a clot in a major vessel in infants can be curative; however, it is technically difficult and poses a considerable life-threatening risk to infants, who often are premature. In the absence of contraindications, the use of thrombolytic agents in these infants is a preferred approach. Doses, monitoring, and adverse effects are discussed in Chapter 46.

References

1. Andrew M, Paes B, et al: Development of the human coagulation system in the full-term infant. Blood 1987; 70:165.
2. Andrew M, Paes B, Johnston M: Development of the hemostatic system in the neonate and young infant. Am J Pediatr Hematol Oncol 1990; 12:95.
3. Andrew M, Paes B, et al: Development of the human coagulation system in the healthy premature infant. Blood 1988; 72:1651.
4. Cook D, Guyatt G, et al: Rules of evidence and clinical recommendations on the use of antithrombotic agents. Chest 1992; 102:305S.
5. Aballi A, de Lamerens S: Coagulation changes in the neonatal period and in early infancy. Pediatr Clin North Am 1962; 9:785.
6. Andrew M, Kelton JG: Neonatal thrombocytopenia. Clin Perinatol 1984; 11:359.
7. Pearson HA, McIntosh S: Neonatal thrombocytopenia. Clin Haematol 1978; 7:111.
8. Gill FM: Thrombocytopenia in the newborn. Semin Perinatol 1983; 7:201.
9. Mehta P, Vasa R, et al: Thrombocytopenia in the high-risk infant. J Pediatr 1980; 97:791.
10. Castle V, Andrew M, et al: Frequency and mechanism of neonatal thrombocytopenia. J Pediatr 1986; 108:749.
11. Beverley DW, Inwood MJ, et al: "Normal" haemostasis parameters: a study in a well-defined inborn population of preterm infants. Early Hum Dev 1984; 9:249.
12. Kipper S, Sieger L: Whole blood platelet volumes in newborn infants. J Pediatr 1982; 101:763.

13. Arad ID, Alpan G, et al: The mean platelet volume (MVP) in the neonatal period. Am J Perinatol 1986; 3:1.

14. Forestier F, Daffos F, et al: Hematological values of 163 normal fetuses between 18 and 30 weeks of gestation. Pediatr Res 1986; 20:342.

15. Castle V, Coates G, et al: [111]Indium oxine platelet survivals in the thrombocytopenic infant. Blood 1987; 70:652.

16. Castle V, Coates G, et al: The effect of hypoxia on platelet survival and site of sequestration in the newborn rabbit. Thromb Haemost 1988; 59:45.

17. Jenkins CS, Phillips DR, et al: Platelet membrane glycoproteins implicated in ristocetin-induced aggregation. J Clin Invest 1976; 57:112.

18. Mull MM, Hathaway WE: Altered platelet function in newborns. Pediatr Res 1970; 4:229.

19. Whaun JM, Smith GR, Sochor V: Effect of prenatal drug administration on maternal and neonatal platelet aggregation and PF4 release. Haemostasis 1980; 9:226.

20. Gruel Y, Boizard B, et al: Determinations of platelet antigens and glycoproteins in the human fetus. Blood 1986; 68:488.

21. Katz J, Moake J, et al: Relationship between human development and disappearance of unusually large von Willebrand factor multimers from plasma. Blood 1989; 73:1851.

22. Weinstein M, Blanchard R, et al: Fetal and neonatal von Willebrand factor (vWF) is unusually large and similar to the vWF in patients with thrombotic thrombocytopenia purpura. Br J Haematol 1989; 72:68.

23. Ts'ao C, Green D, Schultz K: Function and ultrastructure of platelets of neonates; enhanced ristocetin aggregation of neonatal platelets. Br J Haematol 1976; 32:225.

24. Harker LA, Slichter SJ: The bleeding time as a screening test for evaluation of platelet function. N Engl J Med 1972; 287:155.

25. Andrew M, Paes B, et al: Evaluation of an automated bleeding time device in the newborn. Am J Hematol 1990; 35:275.

26. Feusner JH: Normal and abnormal bleeding times in neonates and young children utilizing a fully standardized template technique. Am J Clin Pathol 1980; 74:73.

27. Andrew M, Castle V, et al: Clinical impact of neonatal thrombocytopenia. J Pediatr 1987; 110:457.

28. Andrew M, Castle V, et al: A modified bleeding time in the infant. Am J Hematol 1989; 30:190.

29. Stuart M, Dusse J, et al: Differences in thromboxane production between neonatal and adult platelets in response to arachidonic acid and epinephrine. Pediatr Res 1984; 18:823.

30. Corby D, O'Barr T: Decreased alpha-adrenergic receptors in newborn platelets. Cause of abnormal response to epinephrine. Dev Pharmacol Ther 1981; 2:215.

31. Barradas MA, Mikhailidis DP: An investigation of maternal and neonatal platelet function. Biol Res Pregnancy Perinatol 1986; 7:60.

32. Gader AMA, Bahakim H, et al: Dose-response aggregometry in maternal/neonatal platelets. Thromb Haemost 1988; 60:314.

33. Hicsomnez G, Prozorova-Zamani V: Platelet aggregation in neonates with hyperbilirubinemia. Scand J Haematol 1980; 24:67.

34. Alebouyeh M, Lusher J, et al: The effect of 5-hydroxytryptamine and epinephrine on newborn platelets. Eur J Pediatr 1978; 128:163.

35. Sadowitz PD, Walenga RW, et al: Decreased plasma arachidonic acid binding capacity in neonates. Biol Neonate 1987; 51:305.

36. Landolfi R, De Cristofaro R, et al: Placental-derived PGI$_2$ inhibits cord blood platelet function. Haematologica (Pavia) 1988; 73:207.

37. Ahlsten G, Ewald U, Tuvemo T: Arachidonic acid–induced aggregation of platelets from human cord blood compared with platelets from adults. Biol Neonate 1985; 47:199.

38. Andrews NP, Pipkin FB, Hepinstall S: Blood platelet behaviour in mothers and neonates. Thromb Haemost 1985; 53:428.

39. Israels S, Daniels M, McMillan E: Deficient collagen-induced activation in the newborn platelet. Pediatr Res 1990; 27:337.

40. Corby DG, Zuck TF: Newborn platelet dysfunction: A storage pool and release defect. Thromb Haemost 1976; 36:200.

41. Stuart MJ: A storage pool deficiency in neonatal platelets. Thromb Haemost 1976; 38:4. Abstract.

42. Koztalanyi G, Jobst K, et al: ADP-induced surface changes of adult and newborn platelets. Br J Haematol 1980; 46:257.

43. Stuart MJ: The neonatal platelet: Evaluation of platelet malonyl dialdehyde formation as an indicator of prostaglandin synthesis. Br J Haematol 1978; 39:83.

44. Stuart MJ, Dusse J: In vitro comparison of the efficacy of cyclooxygenase inhibitors on the adult versus neonatal platelet. Biol Neonate 1985; 47:265.

45. Walenga RW, Sunderji SG, Stuart MJ: Formation of hydroxyeicosatetraenoic acids (HETE) in blood from adults versus neonates: Reduced production of 12-HETE in cord blood. Pediatr Res 1988; 24:563.

46. Weiss JH, Aledort MK, Kochwa S: The effect of salicylate on the hemostatic properties of platelets in man. J Clin Invest 1968; 47:2169.

47. Israels SJ, Gowen B, Gerrard JM: Contractile activity of neonatal platelets. Pediatr Res 1987; 21:293.

48. Stuart MJ, Oski FA: Vitamin E and platelet function. Am J Pediatr Hematol Oncol 1979; 1:77.

49. Hanada T, Abe T, Takita H: Antithrombin III concentrates for treatment of disseminated intravascular coagulation in children. Am J Pediatr Hematol Oncol 1985; 7:3.

50. Corby DG, O'Barr TP: Neonatal platelet function: A membrane-related phenomenon? Haemostasis 1981; 10:177.

51. Jones CR, McCabe R, et al: Maternal and fetal platelet responses and adrenoreceptor binding characteristics. Thromb Haemost 1985; 53:95.

52. Aarts PAMM, Bolhuis PA, et al: Red blood cell size is important for adherence of blood platelets to artery subendothelium. Blood 1983; 62:214.

53. Fernandez F, Gaudable C, et al: Low hematocrit and prolonged bleeding time in uraemic patients: Effect of red cell transfusions. Br J Haematol 1985; 59:139. Abstract.

54. Suarez CR, Menendez CE, et al: Neonatal and maternal hemostasis. Value of molecular markers in the assessment of hemostatic status. Semin Thromb Haemost 1984; 10:280.

55. Kaplan KL, Owen J: Plasma levels of B-thromboglobulin and platelet factor IV as indices of platelet activation in vivo. Blood 1981; 57:199.

56. Suarez CR, Gonzalez J, et al: Neonatal and maternal platelets: Activation at time of birth. Am J Hematol 1988; 29:18.

57. Blifield C, Courtney JT, Gross JR: Assessment of neonatal platelet function using a viscoelastic technique. Ann Clin Lab Sci 1986; 16:373.

58. Saleem A, Blifield C, et al: Viscoelastic measurement of clot formation: a new test of platelet function. Ann Clin Lab Sci 1983; 13:115.

59. Jacqz EM, Barrow SE, Dollery CT: Prostacyclin concentrations in cord blood and in the newborn. Pediatrics 1985; 76:954.

60. Kumar V, Berenson G, et al: Acid mucopolysaccharides of human aorta. Part 1. Variations with maturation. J Atheroscler Res 1967; 7:573.

61. Andrew M, Mitchell L, et al: An anticoagulant dermatan sulphate proteoglycan circulates in the pregnant woman and her fetus. J Clin Invest 1992; 89:321.

62. Abman SH: Pathogenesis and treatment of neonatal and postnatal pulmonary hypertension. Curr Opin Pediatr 1994; 6:239.

63. Xu L, Delorme M, et al: Thrombin generation in newborn and adult plasma in the presence of an endothelial surface. Thromb Haemost 1991; 65:1230. Abstract.

64. Johnston M, Zipursky A: Microtechnology for the study of the blood coagulation system in newborn infants. Can J Med Technol 1980; 42:159.

65. Cade J, Hirsh J, Martin M: Placental barrier to coagulation factors: Its relevance to the coagulation defect at birth and to haemorrhage in the newborn. BMJ 1969; 2:281.

66. Kisker C, Robillard J, Clarke W: Development of blood coagulation—a fetal lamb model. Pediatr Res 1981; 15:1045.

67. Andrew M, O'Brodovich H, Mitchell L: The fetal lamb coagulation system during normal birth. Am J Hematol 1988; 28:116.

68. Holmberg L, Henriksson P, et al: Coagulation in the human fetus, comparison with term newborn infants. J Pediatr 1974; 85:860.

69. Jensen A, Josso S, et al: Evolution of blood clotting factors in premature infants during the first ten days of life: a study of 96 cases with comparison between clinical status and blood clotting factor levels. Pediatr Res 1973; 7:638.

70. Mibashan R, Rodeck C, et al: Plasma assay of fetal factors VIIIc and IX for prenatal diagnosis of haemophilia. Lancet 1979; 1:1309.

71. Forestier F, Cox WL, et al: The assessment of fetal blood samples. Am J Obstet Gynecol 1988; 158:1184. Abstract.

72. Forestier F, Daffos F, et al: Vitamin K dependent proteins in fetal hemostasis at mid trimester pregnancy. Thromb Haemost 1985; 53:401.

73. Forestier F, Daffos E, et al: Prenatal diagnosis of hemophilia by fetal blood sampling under ultrasound guidance. Haemostasis 1986; 16:346. Abstract.

74. Toulon P, Rainaut M, et al: Antithrombin III (ATIII) and heparin cofactor II (HCII) in normal human fetuses (21st-27th week). Thromb Haemost 1986; 56:237. Abstract.

75. Barnard DR, Simmons MA, Hathaway WE: Coagulation studies in extremely premature infants. Pediatr Res 1979; 13:1330.

76. Nossel HL, Lanzkowsky P, et al: A study of coagulation factor levels in women during labour and in their newborn infants. Thromb Diath Haemorrh 1966; 16:185.

77. Hirsh J, Ofosu F, Cairns J: Advances in antithrombotic therapy. In Hoffbrand AV (ed): Recent Advances in Hematology. New York, Churchill Livingstone, 1985, p 333.

78. Koepke JA: Partial thromboplastin time test—proposed performance guidelines. ICSH panel on the APTT. Thromb Haemost 1986; 55:143.

79. Hirsh J: Oral anticoagulant drugs. N Engl J Med 1991; 324:1865. Review article.

80. Townsend CW: The haemorrhagic disease of the newborn. Arch Pediatr 1894; 11:559.

81. Dam H, Tage-Hansen E, Plum P: K-avitaminose hos spaede born som aarag til hemorrhagisk diathese. Ugesk Laeger 1939; 101:896.

82. Brinkhous KM, Smith HP, Warner ED: Plasma prothrombin level in normal infancy and in hemorrhagic disease of the newborn. Am J Med Sci 1937; 193:475. Abstract.

83. Bleyer W, Hakami N, Shepard T: The development of hemostasis in the human fetus and newborn infant. J Pediatr 1971; 79:838.

84. Hathaway WE, Bonnar J: Bleeding disorders in the newborn infant. In Oliver TKJ (ed): Perinatal Coagulation. Monographs in Neonatology. New York, Grune & Stratton, 1978, p 115.

85. Gross S, Melhorn D: Exchange transfusion with citrated whole blood for disseminated intravascular coagulation. J Pediatr 1971; 78:415.

86. Buchanan G: Coagulation disorders in the neonate. Pediatr Clin North Am 1986; 33:203.

87. Montgomery R, Marlar R, Gill J: Newborn haemostasis. Clin Hematol 1985; 14:443.

88. Gibson B: Neonatal haemostasis. Arch Dis Child 1989; 64:503.

89. Gobel U, Voss HC, et al: Etiopathology and classification of acquired coagulation disorders in the newborn infant. Klin Wschr 1979; 57:81.

90. McDonald M, Hathaway W: Neonatal haemorrhage and thrombosis. Semin Perinatol 1983; 7:213.

91. Strothers J, Boulton F, et al: Neonatal coagulation. Lancet 1975; 1:408. Letter.

92. Bahakim H, Gader A, et al: Coagulation parameters in maternal and cord blood at delivery. Ann Saudi Med 1990; 10:149.

93. Andrew M, Karpatkin M: A simple screening test for evaluating prolonged partial thromboplastin times in newborn infants. J Pediatr 1982; 101:610.

94. Zipursky A, Jaber H: The hematology of bacterial infection in newborn infants. Clin Hematol 1978; 7:175.

95. Karpatkin M, Manucci PM, et al: Low protein C in the neonatal period. Br J Haematol 1986; 62:137.

96. Ozkutlu S, Saraclar M, et al: Two-dimensional echocardiographic diagnosis of tricuspid valve noninfective endocarditis due to protein C deficiency (lesion mimicking tricuspid valve myxoma). Jpn Heart J 1991; 32:139.

97. Schmidt B, Ofosu F, et al: Anticoagulant effects of heparin in neonatal plasma. Pediatr Res 1989; 25:405.

98. Andrew M, Schmidt B, et al: Thrombin generation in newborn plasma is critically dependent on the concentration of prothrombin. Thromb Haemost 1990; 63:27.

99. Schmidt B, Mitchell L, et al: Alpha-2-macroglobulin is an important progressive inhibitor of thrombin in neonatal and infant plasma. Thromb Haemost 1989; 62:1074.

100. Levine JJ, Udall JN, et al: Elevated levels of alpha 2--macroglobulin-protease complexes in infants. Biol Neonate 1987; 51:149.

101. Muller AD, Van Doorm JM: Heparin-like inhibitor of blood coagulation in normal newborn. Nature 1977; 267:616.

102. Delorme M, Xu L, et al: Anticoagulant dermatan sulfate proteoglycan in the term human placenta. J Clin Invest 1995 (in press).

103. Manco-Johnson MJ, Marlar R, Hathaway WE: Neonatal protein C: Evidence for a dysfunctional protein and for the predisposition to thrombosis. Thromb Haemost 1985; 54:838. Abstract.

104. Moalic P, Gruel Y, et al: Levels and plasma distribution of free and c_4b-BP-bound protein S in human fetuses and full-term newborns. Thromb Res 1988; 49:471.

105. Schwarz HP, Muntean W, et al: Low total protein S antigen but high protein S activity due to decreased c_4b-binding protein in neonates. Blood 1988; 71:562.

106. Aurousseau M, Amiral J, Boffa M: Level of plasma thrombomodulin in neonates and children. Thromb Haemost 1991; 65:1232. Abstract.

107. Buckell M: The effect of citrate on euglobin methods of estimating fibrinolytic activity. J Clin Pathol 1958; 11:403.

108. Weissbach G, Harenberg J, et al: Tissue factor pathway inhibitor in infants and children. Thromb Res 1994; 73:441.

109. Patel P, Weitz J, et al: Decreased thrombin activity of fibrin clots prepared in cord plasma compared with adult plasma. Pediatr Res 1996; 39:826.

110. Kisker CT, Perlman S, et al: Measurement of prothrombin mRNA during gestation and early neonatal development. J Lab Clin Med 1988; 112:407.

111. Hassan H, Leonardi C, et al: Blood coagulation factors in human embryonic-fetal development: Preferential expression of the FVII/tissue factor pathway. Blood 1990; 76:1158.

112. Karpatkin M, Blei F, et al: Prothrombin expression in the adult and fetal rabbit liver. Pediatr Res 1991; 30:266.

113. Andrew M, Mitchell L, et al: Fibrinogen has a rapid turnover in the healthy newborn lamb. Pediatr Res 1988; 23:249.

114. Feusner J, Slichter S, Harker L: Acquired haemostatic defects in the ill newborn. Br J Haematol 1983; 53:73.

115. Karitzky D, Kleine N, et al: Fibrinogen turnover in the premature infant with and without idiopathic respiratory distress syndrome. Acta Paediatr Scand 1971; 60:465.

116. Schmidt B, Wais U, et al: Plasma elimination of antithrombin III is accelerated in term newborn infants. Eur J Pediatr 1984; 141:225.

117. Esmon NL, Owen WG, Esmon CT: Isolation of a membrane bound cofactor for thrombin-catalyzed activation of protein C. J Biol Chem 1982; 257:859.

118. Andrew M, O'Brodovich H, Mitchell L: The fetal lamb coagulation system during birth asphyxia. Am J Hematol 1988; 28:201.

119. Witt I, Muller H, Kunter LJ: Evidence for the existence of fetal fibrinogen. Thromb Diath Haemorrh 1969; 22:101.

120. Hamulyak K, Nieuwenhuizen W, et al: Re-evaluation of some properties of fibrinogen purified from cord blood of normal newborns. Thromb Res 1983; 32:301.

121. Galanakis DK, Mosesson MW: Evaluation of the role of in vivo proteolysis (fibrinogenolysis) in prolonging the thrombin time of human umbilical cord fibrinogen. Blood 1976; 48:109.

122. Yuen PMP, Yin JA, Lao TTH: Fibrino-peptide A levels in maternal and newborn plasma. Eur J Obstet Gynecol 1989; 30:239.

123. Corrigan J: Neonatal thrombosis and the thrombolytic system. Pathophysiology and therapy. Am J Pediatr Hematol Oncol 1988; 10:83.

124. Corrigan J, Sluth J, et al: Newborn's fibrinolytic mechanism: Components and plasmin generation. Am J Hematol 1989; 32:273.

125. Kolindewala JK, Das BK, et al: Blood fibrinolytic activity in neonates: Effect of period of gestation, birth weight, anoxia and sepsis. Indian Pediatr 1987; 24:1029.

126. Lecander I, Astedt B: Specific plasminogen activator inhibitor of placental type PAI 2 occurring in amniotic fluid and cord blood. J Lab Clin Med 1987; 110:602.

127. Edelberg JM, Enghild JJ, et al: Neonatal plasminogen displays altered cell surface binding and activation kinetics. Correlation with increased glycosylation of the protein. J Clin Invest 1990; 86:107.

128. Reverdiau-Moalic P, Gruel Y, et al: Comparative study of the fibrinolytic system in human fetuses and in pregnant women. Thromb Res 1991; 61:489.

129. Corrigan J, Jeter M: Histidine-rich glycoprotein and plasminogen plasma levels in term and preterm newborns. Am J Dis Child 1990; 144:825.

130. Corrigan JJ, Jeter MA: Tissue type plasminogen activator, plasminogen activator inhibitor, and histidine-rich glycoproteins in stressed newborns. Pediatrics 1992; 89:43.

131. Caccamo ML, Rossi E, et al: The fibrinolytic system in the newborn: role of histidine-rich glycoprotein. Biol Neonate 1992; 61:281.

132. Andrew M, Brooker L, et al: Fibrin clot lysis by thrombolytic agents is impaired in newborns due to a low plasminogen concentration. Thromb Haemost 1992; 68:325.

133. Girolami A, De Marco L, et al: Rarer quantitative and qualitative abnormalities of coagulation. Clin Hematol 1985; 14:385.

134. Silverstein A: Intracranial bleeding in hemophilia. Arch Neurol 1960; 3:141.

135. Yoffe G, Buchanan G: Intracranial haemorrhage in newborn and young infants with hemophilia. J Pediatr 1988; 113:333.

136. Abbondanzo S, Gootenberg J, et al: Intracranial hemorrhage in congenital deficiency of factor XIII. Am J Pediatr Hematol Oncol 1988; 10:65.

137. Struwe F: Intracranial hemorrhage and occlusive hydrocephalus in hereditary bleeding disorders. Dev Med Child Neurol 1970; 12:165.

138. Mariani G, Mazzucconi M: Factor VII congenital deficiency. Clinical picture and classification of the variants. Haemostasis 1983; 13:169.

139. Baehner R, Strauss H: Hemophilia in the first year of life. N Engl J Med 1966; 275:524.

140. Pearson HA, Shulman NR, et al: Isoimmune neonatal thrombocytopenic purpura. Clinical and therapeutic considerations. Blood 1964; 23:154.

141. Gajl-Paczalska K: Plasma protein composition of hyaline membrane in the newborn as studied by immunofluorescence. Arch Dis Child 1964; 39:226.

142. Lupton BA, Hill A, et al: Reduced platelet count as a risk factor for intraventricular hemorrhage. Am J Dis Child 1988; 142:1222.

143. Austin N, Darlow BA: Transfusion-associated fall in platelet count in very low birthweight infants. Aust Paediatr J 1988; 24:354.

144. Samuels P, Main E, et al: Abnormalities in platelet antiglobulin tests in preeclamptic mothers and their neonates. Am J Obstet Gynecol 1987; 157:109.

145. Olson T, Levine R, et al: Megakaryocytes and megakaryocyte progenitors in human cord blood. Am J Pediatr Hematol Oncol 1992; 14:241.

146. Suen Y, Chang M, et al: Regulation of interleukin-11 protein and mRNA expression in neonatal and adult fibroblasts and endothelial cells. Blood 1994; 84:4125.

147. Stuart MJ, Wu J, et al: Effect of amniotic fluid on platelet thromboxane production. J Pediatr 1987; 110:289.

148. Tate DY, Carlton GT, et al: Immune thrombocytopenia in severe neonatal infections. J Pediatr 1981; 98:449.

149. Podolsak B: Thrombopoiesis in newborn infants after exchange blood transfusion. Z Kinderheilkd 1973; 114:13.

150. Patrick CH, Lazarchick J: The effect of bacteremia on automated platelet measurements in neonates. Am J Clin Pathol 1990; 93:391.

151. Weinblatt ME, Scimeca PG, et al: Thrombocytopenia in an infant with AIDS. Am J Dis Child 1987; 141:15.

152. Ballin A, Koren G, et al: Reduction of platelet counts induced by mechanical ventilation in newborn infants. J Pediatr 1987; 111:445.

153. Horgan MJ, Carrasco NJM, Risemberg H: The relationship of thrombocytopenia to the onset of persistent pulmonary hypertension of the newborn in the meconium aspiration syndrome. N Y State J Med 1985; 85:245.

154. Shim WK: Hemangiomas of infancy complicated by thrombocytopenia. Am J Surg 1968; 116:896.

155. Fost NC, Esterly NB: Successful treatment of juvenile hemangiomas with prednisone. J Pediatr 1968; 72:351.

156. Johnson DH, Vinson AM, Wirth FH: Management of hepatic hemangioendotheliomas of infancy by transarterial embolization: A report of two cases. Pediatrics 1984; 73:546.

157. Orchard PJ, Smith CMI, et al: Treatment of haemangioendotheliomas with alpha interferon. Lancet 1989; 2:565. Letter.

158. Larsen EC, Zinkham WH, et al: Kasabach-Merritt syndrome: therapeutic considerations. Pediatrics 1987; 79:971.

159. Andrew M: The hemostatic system in the infant. In Nathan D, Oski F (eds): Hematology of Infancy and Childhood. 4th ed. Philadelphia, W.B. Saunders Co., 1992, p 115.

160. Corby DG, Schulman I: The effects of antenatal drug administration on aggregation of platelets of newborn infants. J Pediatr 1971; 79:307.

161. Levy G, Garrettson LK: Kinetics of salicylate elimination by newborn infants of mothers who ingested aspirin before delivery. Pediatrics 1974; 53:201.

162. Ylikorkala O, Makila UM, et al: Maternal ingestion of acetylsalicylic acid inhibits fetal and neonatal thromboxane in humans. Am J Obstet Gynecol 1986; 155:345.

163. Haslam RR, Ekert H, Gillam GL: Hemorrhage in a neonate possibly due to maternal ingestion of salicylate. J Pediatr 1974; 84:556.

164. Cariou R, Toblem G, et al: Effect of lupus anticoagulant or antithrombogenic properties of endothelial cells—inhibition of thrombomodulin-dependent protein C activation. Thromb Haemost 1988; 60:54.

165. Murphy WG, Moore JC, Kelton JG: Calcium-dependent cysteine protease activity in the sera of patients with thrombotic thrombocytopenic purpura. Blood 1987; 70:1683.

166. Hall JG, Levin J, et al: Thrombocytopenia with absent radius. Medicine 1969; 48:411.

167. Hedberg VA, Lipton JM: Thrombocytopenia with absent radii. A review of 100 cases. Am J Pediatr Hematol Oncol 1988; 10:51.

168. Homans AC, Cohen JL, Mazur EM: Defective megakaryocytopoiesis in the syndrome of thrombocytopenia with absent radii. Br J Haematol 1988; 70:205.

169. Lecompte T: Hereditary thrombocytopenias. Curr Stud Hematol Blood Transfus 1988; 55:162.

170. Hegde UM: Immune thrombocytopenia in pregnancy and the newborn. Br J Obstet Gynaecol 1985; 92:657.

171. Andrew M, Caco C, et al: A randomized controlled trial of platelet transfusions in thrombocytopenic premature infants. J Pediatr 1993; 123:285.

172. Chan KW, Kaikov Y, Wadsworth LD: Thrombocytosis in childhood: A survey of 94 patients. Pediatrics 1989; 84:1064.

173. Ostermann H, van de Loo J: Factors of the hemostatic system in diabetic patients. A survey of controlled studies. Haemostasis 1986; 16:386.

174. Stuart MJ, Elrad H, et al: Increased synthesis of prostaglandin endoperoxides and platelet hyperfunction in infants of mothers with diabetes mellitus. J Lab Clin Med 1979; 94:12.

175. Kääpä P, Knip M, et al: Increased platelet thromboxane B_2 production in newborn infants of diabetic mothers. Prostaglandins Leukot Med 1986; 21:299.

176. Stuart MJ, Sunderji SJ, Allen JB: Decreased prostacyclin production in the infant of the diabetic mother. J Lab Clin Med 1981; 98:412.

177. Kääpä P, Uhari M, et al: Dietary fatty acid and platelet thromboxane production in puerperal women and their offspring. Am J Obstet Gynecol 1986; 155:146.

178. Friedman Z, Lamberth ELJ, Stahlman MT: Platelet dysfunction in the neonate with essential fatty acid deficiency. J Pediatr 1977; 90:439.

179. Friedman Z, Danon A, et al: Rapid onset of essential fatty acid deficiency in the newborn. Pediatrics 1976; 58:640.

180. Friedman Z, Seyberth H, et al: Decreased prostaglandin E turnover in infants with essential fatty acid deficiency. Pediatr Res 1978; 12:711.

181. Machlin LJ, Filipski R, et al: Influence of vitamin E on platelet aggregation and thrombocythemia in the rat. Proc Soc Exp Biol Med 1973; 149:275.

182. Stuart MJ: Vitamin E deficiency: Its effect on platelet-vascular interaction in various pathologic states. Ann N Y Acad Sci 1982; 393:277.

183. Lake AM, Stuart MJ, Oski FA: Vitamin E deficiency and enhanced platelet function: reversal following E supplementation. J Pediatr 1977; 90:722.

184. Ahlsten G, Ewald U, et al: Aggregation of and thromboxane B$_2$ synthesis in platelets from newborn infants of smoking and non-smoking mothers. Prostaglandins Leukot Med 1985; 19:167.

185. Ahlsten G, Ewald U, Tuvemo T: Maternal smoking reduces prostacyclin formation in human umbilical arteries. A study on strictly selected pregnancies. Acta Obstet Gynecol Scand 1986; 65:645.

186. Davis RB, Leuschen MP, et al: Evaluation of platelet function in pregnancy. Comparative studies in non-smokers and smokers. Thromb Res 1987; 46:175.

187. Ylikorkala O, Halmesmaki E, Viinikka L: Effect of ethanol on thromboxane and prostacyclin synthesis by fetal platelets and umbilical artery. Life Sci 1987; 41:371.

188. Segall ML, Goetzman BW, Schick JB: Thrombocytopenia and pulmonary hypertension in the perinatal aspiration syndromes. J Pediatr 1980; 96:727.

189. Levin DL, Weinberg AG, Perkin RM: Pulmonary microthrombi syndrome in newborn infants with unresponsive persistent pulmonary hypertension. J Pediatr 1983; 102:299.

190. Suzuki S, Wake N, et al: New neonatal problems of blood coagulation and fibrinolysis. II. Thromboplastic effect of amniotic fluid, and its relation to lung maturity. J Perinatal Med 1976; 4:221.

191. Kääpä P: Immunoreactive thromboxane B$_2$ and 6-keto-prostaglandin F$_1\alpha$ in neonatal hyperbilirubinemia. Prostaglandins Leukot Med 1985; 17:97.

192. Maurer HM, Haggins JC, Still WJS: Platelet injury during phototherapy. Am J Hematol 1976; 1:89.

193. Karim MAG, Clelland IA, et al: β-Thromboglobulin levels in plasma of jaundiced neonates exposed to phototherapy. J Perinatal Med 1981; 3:141.

194. Remuzzi G: Bleeding in renal failure. Lancet 1988; 1:1205.

195. Bleyer WA, Breckenridge RT: Studies on the detection of adverse drug reactions in the newborn. II. The effects of prenatal aspirin on newborn hemostasis. JAMA 1970; 213:2049.

196. Rumack CM, Guggenheim MA, et al: Neonatal intracranial hemorrhage and maternal use of aspirin. Obstet Gynecol 1981; 58(Suppl):52S.

197. Ts'ao CH: Comparable inhibition of PRP of neonates and adults by aspirin. Haemostasis 1977; 6:118.

198. Palmisano PA, Cassady G: Salicylate exposure in the perinate. JAMA 1969; 209:556.

199. Casteels-Van Daele M, Jaeken J, et al: More on the effects of antenatally administered aspirin on aggregation of platelets of neonates. J Pediatr 1972; 80:685.

200. Territo M, Finklestein J, et al: Management of autoimmune thrombocytopenia in pregnancy and in the neonate. Obstet Gynecol 1973; 41:579.

201. Peters M, Jansen E, et al: Neonatal antithrombin III. Br J Haematol 1984; 58:579.

202. Pomerance JJ, Teal JG, et al: Maternally administered antenatal vitamin K$_1$: Effect on neonatal prothrombin activity, partial thromboplastin time, and intraventricular hemorrhage. Obstet Gynecol 1987; 70:235.

203. Morales WJ, Angel JL, et al: The use of antenatal vitamin K in the prevention of early neonatal intraventricular hemorrhage. Am J Obstet Gynecol 1988; 159:774.

204. Heymann MA, Rudolph AM, Silverman NH: Closure of the ductus arteriosus in premature infants by inhibition of prostaglandin synthesis. N Engl J Med 1976; 295:530.

205. Friedman WF, Hirschklau MJ, et al: Pharmacologic closure of patent ductus arteriosus in the premature infant. N Engl J Med 1976; 295:526.

206. Gersony WM, Peckham GJ, et al: Effects of indomethacin in premature infants with patent ductus arteriosus: Results of a national collaborative study. J Pediatr 1983; 102:895.

207. Friedman Z, Whitman V, et al: Indomethacin disposition and indomethacin-induced platelet dysfunction in premature infants. J Clin Pharmacol 1978; 18:272.

208. Guignard JP, Torrado A, et al: Glomerular filtration rate in the first three weeks of life. J Pediatr 1975; 87:268.

209. Brown AK, Zeulzer WW, Burnett HH: Studies on the neonatal development of the glucuronide system. J Clin Invest 1958; 37:332.

210. Setzer ES, Webb IB, et al: Platelet dysfunction and coagulopathy in intraventricular hemorrhage in the premature infant. J Pediatr 1982; 100:599.

211. Corrazza MS, Davis RF, et al: Prolonged bleeding time in preterm infants receiving indomethacin for patent ductus arteriosus. J Pediatr 1984; 105:292.

212. Ment LR, Ehrenkranz RA, et al: Intraventricular hemorrhage of the preterm neonate: prevention studies. Semin Perinatol 1988; 12:359.

213. Shearer MJ, Barkhan P, et al: Plasma vitamin K$_1$ in mothers and their newborn babies. Lancet 1982; 2:460.

214. Sagel J, Colwell JA, et al: Increased platelet aggregation in early diabetes mellitus. Ann Intern Med 1975; 82:733.

215. Halushka PU, Lurie D, Colwell JA: Increased synthesis of prostaglandins-E-like material by platelets from patients with diabetes mellitus. N Engl J Med 1977; 297:1306.

216. Cowett RM, Schwartz R: The infant of the diabetic mother. Pediatr Clin North Am 1982; 29:1213.

217. Oppenheimer EH, Esterly JR: Thrombosis in the newborn: Comparison between infants of diabetic and non-diabetic mothers. J Pediatr 1965; 67:549.

218. Dixon RH, Rosse WF: Platelet antibody in autoimmune thrombocytopenia. Br J Haematol 1975; 31:129.

219. Cox AC, Rao GHR, et al: The influence of vitamin E quinone on platelet structure, function and biochemistry. Blood 1980; 55:907.

220. Steiner M, Anastasi J: Vitamin E—an inhibitor of the platelet thromboxane production. J Pediatr 1987; 110:289.

221. Khurshid M, Lee TJ, et al: Vitamin E deficiency and platelet functional defect in a jaundiced infant. BMJ 1975; 4:19.

222. Kääpä P: Platelet thromboxane B$_2$ production in neonatal pulmonary hypertension. Arch Dis Child 1987; 62:195.

223. Varela A, Runge A, et al: Nitric oxide and prostacyclin inhibit fetal platelet aggregation: A response similar to that observed in adults. Am J Obstet Gynecol 1992; 167:1599.

224. Radomski M, Palmer R, Moncada S: Endogenous nitric oxide inhibits human platelet adhesion to vascular endothelium. Lancet 1987; 2:1057.

225. Golino P, Capelli-Bigazzi M, et al: Endothelium-derived relaxing factor modulates platelet aggregation in an in vivo model of recurrent platelet activation. Circ Res 1992; 71:1447.

226. Bodzenta-Lukaszyk A, Gabryelewicz A, et al: Nitric oxide synthase inhibition and platelet function. Thromb Res 1994; 75:667.

227. Mazzone D, Fichera A, et al: Combined congenital deficiency of factor V and factor VIII. Acta Haematol 1982; 68:337.

228. McMillan C, Roberts H: Congenital combined deficiency of coagulation factors II, VII, IX and X. N Engl J Med 1966; 274:1313.

229. Rohyans J, Miser A, Miser J: Subgaleal hemorrhage in infants with hemophilia: Report of two cases and review of the literature. Pediatrics 1982; 70:306.

230. Hayden CK, Shattuck KE, et al: Subependymal germinal matrix hemorrhage in fullterm neonates. Pediatrics 1985; 75:714.

231. Scher MS, Wright FS, et al: Intraventricular hemorrhage in the fullterm neonate. Arch Neurol 1982; 39:769.

232. Jackson JC, Blumhagen JD: Congenital hydrocephalus due to prenatal hemorrhage. Pediatrics 1983; 72:344.

233. Serfontein GL, Rom S, Stein S: Posterior fossa subdural hemorrhage in the newborn. Pediatrics 1980; 65:40.

234. Gunn TR, Mok PM, Becroft DMO: Subdural hemorrhage in utero. Pediatrics 1985; 76:605.

235. Cartwright GW, Culbertson K, et al: Changes in clinical presentation of term infants with intracranial hemorrhage. Dev Med Child Neurol 1979; 21:730.

236. Palma PA, Miner ME, et al: Intraventricular hemorrhage in the neonate at term. Am J Dis Child 1979; 133:941.

237. Chaplin ER Jr, Goldstein GW, Norman D: Neonatal seizures, intracerebral hematoma, and subarachnoid hemorrhage in fullterm infants. Pediatrics 1979; 63:812.

238. Guckos-Thoeni U, Boltshauser E, Willi UV: Intraventricular hemorrhage in fullterm neonates. Dev Med Child Neurol 1982; 24:704.

239. Mackay RJ, Crespigny L, et al: Intraventricular hemorrhage in term neonates: Diagnosis by ultrasound. Aust Paediatr J 1984; 18:205.

240. Bray G, Luhan N: Hemophilia presenting with intracranial hemorrhage. Am J Dis Child 1987; 141:1215.

241. Schmidt B, Zipursky A: Disseminated intravascular coagulation masking neonatal hemophilia. J Pediatr 1986; 109:886.
242. Baugh R, Deemar K, Zimmerman J: Heparinase in the activated clotting time assay: monitoring heparin-independent alterations in coagulation function. Anesth Analg 1992; 74:201.
243. Karpatkin S, Strick N, et al: Cumulative experience in the detection of antiplatelet antibody in 234 patients with idiopathic thrombocytopenic purpura, systemic lupus erythematosus and other clinical disorders. Am J Med 1972; 52:776.
244. Smith P: Congenital coagulation protein deficiencies in the perinatal period. Semin Perinatol 1990; 14:384.
245. Daffos F, Forestier F, et al: Prenatal diagnosis and management of bleeding disorders with fetal blood sampling. Am J Obstet Gynecol 1988; 158:939.
246. Manios S, Schenck W, Kunzer W: Congenital fibrinogen deficiency. Acta Pediatr Scand 1968; 57:145.
247. Lewis J, Spero J, et al: Transfusion support for congenital clotting deficiencies other than hemophilia. Clin Hematol 1984; 13:119.
248. Zenny J, Chevrot A, et al: Lésions hémorragiques intra-osseuses des afibrinémies congénitales. A propos d'un nouveau cas. J Radiol 1981; 62:263.
249. Fried K, Kaufman S: Congenital afibrinogenemia in 10 offspring of uncle-niece marriages. Clin Genet 1980; 17:223.
250. Gill F, Shapiro S, Schwartz E: Severe congenital hypoprothrombinemia. J Pediatr 1978; 93:264.
251. Seeler R: Parahemophilia. Factor V deficiency. Med Clin North Am 1972; 56:119.
252. Whitelaw A, Haines M, Bolsover W, et al: Factor V deficiency and antenatal ventricular hemorrhage. Arch Dis Child 1984; 59:997.
253. Roberts H, Lefkowitz J: Inherited disorders of prothrombin conversion. In Colman R, Hirsh J, et al (eds): Hemostasis and Thrombosis. Basic Principles and Clinical Practice. 3rd ed. Philadelphia, J.B. Lippincott Co., 1994, p 200.
254. Seligsohn U, Shani M, Ramot B: Dubin-Johnston syndrome in Israel II. Association with factor VII deficiency. Q J Med 1970; 39:569.
255. Seligsohn U, Shani M, et al: Gilbert syndrome and factor VII deficiency. Lancet 1970; 1:1398.
256. Rabiner S, Winick M, Smith C: Congenital deficiency of factor VII associated with hemorrhagic disease of the newborn. Pediatrics 1960; 25:101.
257. Matthay K, Koerper M, Ablin A: Intracranial hemorrhage in congenital factor VII deficiency. J Pediatr 1979; 94:413.
258. van Creveld S, Veder H, Blans M: Congenital hypoproconvertinemia. Ann Pediatr 1956; 187:373.
259. Girolami A, Cattorozi Y, et al: Congenital factor VII deficiency: A case report. Blut 1973; 27:236.
260. van Creveld S, Veder H, Kleinherenbrink W: Congenital hypoproconvertinemia II. Ann Pediatr 1958; 190:316.
261. Ragni M, Lewis J, et al: Factor VII deficiency. Am J Hematol 1981; 10:79.
262. Schubert B, Schindera F: Congenital factor VII deficiency in a newborn. Hämophilie-Symposion 1988. Abstract.
263. Adcock D, Brozna J, Marlar R: Proposed classification and pathologic mechanisms of purpura fulminans and skin necrosis. Semin Thromb Haemost 1990; 16:333.
264. Schulman I: Pediatric aspects of the mild hemophilias. Med Clin North Am 1962; 46:93.
265. Kozinn P, Ritz N, et al: Massive hemorrhage—scalps of newborn infants. Am J Dis Child 1964; 108:413.
266. Kozinn P, Ritz N, Horowitz A: Scalp hemorrhage as an emergency in the newborn. JAMA 1965; 194:179.
267. McCarthy J, Coble L: Intracranial hemorrhage and subsequent communicating hydrocephalus in a neonate with classical hemophilia. J Pediatr 1973; 51:122.
268. Umetsu M, Chiba Y, et al: Cytomagalovirus-mononucleosis in a newborn infant. Arch Dis Child 1975; 50:396.
269. Volpe J, Manica J, et al: Neonatal subdural hematoma associated with severe hemophilia A. J Pediatr 1976; 88:1023.
270. Cohen D: Neonatal subgaleal hemorrhage in hemophilia. J Pediatr 1978; 93:1022.
271. Eyster M, Gill F, et al: Central nervous system bleeding in hemophiliacs. Blood 1978; 51:1179.
272. Koch J: Haemophilia in the newborn. A case report and literature review. South Afr Med J 1978; 53:721.
273. Pettersson H, McClure P, Fitz C: Intracranial hemorrhage in hemophilic children. Acta Radiol [Diagn] 1984; 25:161.
274. Bisset R, Gupta S, Zammit-Maempel I: Case report: Radiographic and ultrasound appearances of an intra-mural haematoma of the pylorus. Clin Radiol 1988; 39:316.
275. Kletzel M, Miller C, et al: Postdelivery head bleeding in hemophilic neonates. Am J Dis Child 1989; 143:1107.
276. Ljung R, Petrini P, Nilsson I: Diagnostic symptoms of severe and moderate haemophilia A and B. Acta Paediatr Scand 1990; 79:196.
277. Oski F: Blood coagulation and its disorders in the newborn. In Oski F, Naiman J (eds): Hematologic Problems in the Newborn. 3rd ed. Philadelphia, W.B. Saunders Co., 1982, p 137.
278. Hartmann J, Diamond L: Hemophilia and related hemorrhagic disorders. Practitioner 1957; 178:179.
279. Rosendaal F, Smit C, Briet E: Hemophilia treatment in historical perspective: A review of medical and social developments. Ann Hematol 1991; 62:5.
280. Stormorken H, Hessel B, et al: Severe factor VIII deficiency in a chromosomally normal female. Thromb Res 1986; 44:113.
281. Mannucci P, Coppola R, et al: Direct proof of extreme lyonization as a cause of low factor VIII levels in females. Thromb Haemost 1978; 39:544.
282. Martinowitz U, Varon D, et al: Circumcision in hemophilia: The use of fibrin glue for local hemostasis. J Urol 1992; 148:855.
283. Trotter C, Hasegawa D: Hemophilia B. Case study and intervention plan. JOGN Nurs 1983; 12:82.
284. Schwartz I, Root A: Hypercalcemia associated with normal I^{125}-dihydroxyvitamin D concentrations in a neonate with factor IX deficiency. J Pediatr 1989; 114:509.
285. Pegelow C, Borromeo Antigua M, et al: Plasma support for surgery in a premature infant with factor IX deficiency. Am J Dis Child 1989; 143:638. Letter.
286. Stowell K, Figueiredo M, et al: Haemophilia B Liverpool: A new British family with mild haemophilia B associated with a 6 G to A mutation in the factor IX promoter. Br J Haematol 1993; 85:188.
287. Donner M, Holmberg L, Nilsson IM: Type IIB von Willebrand's disease with probable autosomal recessive inheritance and presenting as thrombocytopenia in infancy. Br J Haematol 1987; 66:349.
288. Bignall P, Standen G, et al: Rapid neonatal diagnosis of von Willebrand's disease by use of the polymerase chain reaction. Lancet 1990; 336:638. Letter.
289. Gazengel C, Fischer A, et al: Treatment of type III von Willebrand's disease with solvent/detergent-treated factor VIII concentrates. Nouv Rev Fr Hematol 1988; 30:225.
290. Pasi K, Williams M, et al: Clinical and laboratory evaluation of the treatment of von Willebrand's disease patients with heat-treated factor VIII concentrate (BPL 8Y). Br J Haematol 1990; 75:228.
291. Goudemand J, Mazurier C, et al: Clinical and biological evaluation in von Willebrand's disease of a von Willebrand factor concentrate with low factor VIII activity. Br J Haematol 1992; 80:214.
292. Girolami A, Molaro G, et al: Severe congenital factor X deficiency in 5-month-old child. Thromb Diath Haemorrh 1970; 24:175.
293. Machin S, Winter M, et al: Factor X deficiency in the neonatal period. Arch Dis Child 1980; 55:406.
294. De Sousa C, Clark T, Bradshaw A: Antenatally diagnosed subdural haemorrhage in congenital factor X deficiency. Arch Dis Child 1988; 63:1168.
295. Sandler E, Gross S: Prevention of recurrent intracranial hemorrhage in a factor X deficient infant. Am J Pediatr Hematol Oncol 1992; 14:163.
296. Ruane B, McCord F: Factor X deficiency—A rare cause of scrotal haemorrhage. Ir Med J 1990; 83:163. Letter.
297. Kitchens C: Factor XI: A review of its biochemistry and deficiency. Semin Thromb Haemost 1991; 17:55.
298. Duckert F, Jung E, Shmerling D: Hitherto undescribed congenital haemorrhagic diathesis probably due to fibrin stabilizing factor deficiency. Thromb Diath Haemorrh 1960; 5:179.

299. Barry A, Delage M: Congenital deficiency of fibrin stabilizing factor: observation of a new case. N Engl J Med 1965; 272:943.

300. Vosburgh E: Rational intervention in von Willebrand's disease. Hosp Pract 1993; 28:31.

301. Fisher S, Rikover M, Naor S: Factor 13 deficiency with severe hemorrhage diathesis. Blood 1966; 28:34

302. Britten A: Congenital deficiency of factor XIII (fibrin-stabilizing factor). Am J Med 1967; 43:751.

303. Ozsoylu S, Altay C, et al: Congenital factor XIII deficiency: Observation of two cases in the newborn period. Am J Dis Child 1971; 122:541.

304. Francis J, Todd P: Congenital factor XIII deficiency in a neonate. BMJ 1978; 2:1532.

305. Merchant R, Agarwal B, et al: Congenital factor XIII deficiency. Indian Pediatr 1992; 29:831.

306. Mammen E, Murano G, Bick R: Combined congenital clotting factor abnormalities. Semin Thromb Haemost 1983; 9:55.

307. Boyd J: Disseminated fibrin thromboembolism among neonates dying more than 48 hours after birth. J Clin Pathol 1969; 22:663.

308. Boyd J: Disseminated fibrin thromboembolism among neonates dying within 48 hours of birth. Arch Dis Child 1967; 42:401.

309. Boyd J: Disseminated fibrin thromboembolism in stillbirths; a histological picture similar to one form of maternal hypofibrinogenemia. J Obstet Gynaecol Br Commonw 1966; 73:629.

310. Lascari A, Wallace P: Disseminated intravascular coagulation in newborns. Survey and appraisal as exemplified in two case histories. Clin Pediatr 1971; 10:11.

311. Phillips LL: Alterations in blood clotting system in disseminated intravascular coagulation. Am J Cardiol 1967; 20:174.

312. Rodriguez-Erdmann F: Bleeding due to increased intravascular blood coagulation. Hemorrhagic syndrome caused by consumption of blood clotting factors (consumption coagulates). N Engl J Med 1965; 273:1310.

313. Hathaway W, Mull M, Pechet G: Disseminated intravascular coagulation in the newborn. Pediatrics 1969; 43:233.

314. Dube B, Bhargava V, et al: Disseminated intravascular coagulation in neonatal period. Indian Pediatr 1986; 23:925.

315. Abildgaard C: Recognition and treatment of intravascular coagulation. J Pediatr 1969; 74:163.

316. Watkins M, Swan S, et al: Coagulation changes in the newborn with respiratory failure. Thromb Res 1980; 17:153.

317. Markarian M, Lindley A, et al: Coagulation factors in pregnant women and premature infants with and without the respiratory distress syndrome. Thromb Diath Haemorrh 1967; 17:585.

318. Appleyard W, Cottom D: Effect of asphyxia on thrombotest values in low birthweight infants. Arch Dis Child 1970; 45:705.

319. Anderson J, Brown J, Cockburn F: On the role of disseminated intravascular coagulation on the pathology of birth asphyxia. Dev Med Child Neurol 1974; 16:581.

320. Chessells J, Wigglesworth J: Coagulation studies in severe birth asphyxia. Arch Dis Child 1971; 46:253.

321. Chessells J, Wigglesworth J: Haemostatic failure in babies with rhesus isoimmunization. Arch Dis Child 1971; 46:38.

322. Chessells J, Wigglesworth J: Coagulation studies in preterm infants with respiratory distress and intracranial hemorrhage. Arch Dis Child 1972; 47:564.

323. Altstaff L, Dennis L, et al: Disseminated intravascular coagulation and hyaline membrane disease. Biol Neonate 1971; 19:227.

324. Edson J, Blaese R, et al: Defibrination syndrome in an infant born after abruptio placentae. J Pediatr 1968; 72:342.

325. Corrigan J: Activation of coagulation and disseminated intravascular coagulation in the newborn. Am J Pediatr Hematol Oncol 1979; 1:245.

326. Schmidt B, Vegh P, et al: Coagulation screening tests in high risk neonates: A prospective cohort study. Arch Dis Child 1992; 67:1196.

327. Waltt H, Kurz R, et al: Intracranial haemorrhage in low birth weight infants and prophylactic administration of coagulation factor concentrates. Lancet 1973; 1:1284.

328. Gross S, Filston H, Anderson J: Controlled study of treatment for disseminated intravascular coagulation in the neonate. J Pediatr 1982; 100:445.

329. Beverley D, Pitts-Tucker T, et al: Prevention of intraventricular haemorrhage by fresh frozen plasma. Arch Dis Child 1985; 60:710.

330. Turner T: Randomized sequential control trial to evaluate effect of purified factor II, VII, IX, and X concentrate, cryoprecipitate and platelet concentrate in management of preterm low birthweight and mature asphyxiated infants with coagulation defects. Arch Dis Child 1981; 51:810.

331. De Lemos R, McLaughlin G, et al: Abnormal partial thromboplastin time and survival in respiratory distress syndrome. Effect of exchange transfusion. Pediatr Res 1973; 7:396. Abstract.

332. Hambleton G, Appleyard W: Controlled trial of fresh frozen plasma in asphyxiated low birthweight infants. Arch Dis Child 1973; 48:31.

333. Gray O, Ackerman A, Fraser A: Intracranial hemorrhage and clotting defects in low birth weight infants. Lancet 1968; 1:545.

334. Von Kries R, Stannigel H, Gobel U: Anticoagulant therapy by continuous heparin-antithrombin III infusion in newborns with disseminated intravascular coagulation. Eur J Pediatr 1985; 114:191.

335. Yamada K, Shirahata A, et al: Therapy for DIC in newborn infants. Bibl Haematol 1983; 49:329.

336. Corrigan JJ: Heparin therapy in bacterial septicemia. J Pediatr 1977; 91:695.

337. Corrigan JJ, Jordan CM: Heparin therapy in septicemia with disseminated intravascular coagulation: Effect on mortality and on correction of hemostatic defects. N Engl J Med 1970; 283:778.

338. Gobel U, von Voss H, et al: Efficiency of heparin in the treatment of newborn infants with respiratory distress syndrome and disseminated intravascular coagulation. Eur J Pediatr 1980; 133:47.

339. Markarian M, Luchenco LO, Rosenblut E: Hypercoagulability in premature infants with special reference to the respiratory distress syndrome and hemorrhage. II. The effect of heparin. Biol Neonate 1971; 17:98.

340. Kelly D, Summerfield J: Hemostasis in liver disease. Semin Liver Dis 1987; 7:182.

341. von Breedin K: Hämorrhagische Diathesen bei Lebererkrankungen unter besonderer Berücksichtigung der Thrombocytenfunction. Acta Haematol 1962; 27:1.

342. Rubin M, Weston MJ, et al: Abnormal platelet function and ultrastructure in fulminant hepatic failure. Q J Med 1977; 46:339.

343. Weston M, Langley P, et al: Platelet function in fulminant hepatic failure and effect of charcoal haemoperfusion. Gut 1977; 18:897.

344. Osborn J, Shahidi N: Thrombocytopenia in murine cytomegalovirus infections. J Lab Clin Med 1973; 81:53.

345. Chesney P, Taher A, et al: Intranuclear inclusions in megakaryocytes in congenital cytomegalovirus infection. J Pediatr 1978; 92:957.

346. Zinkham W, Medearis D Jr, Osborn J: Blood and bone marrow findings in congenital rubella. J Pediatr 1967; 71:512.

347. Lafer C, Morrison A: Thrombocytopenic purpura progressing to transient hypoplastic anemia in a newborn with rubella syndrome. Pediatrics 1966; 38:499.

348. Bortolotti F, Vajro P, et al: Hepatitis C in childhood: epidemiological and clinical aspects. Bone Marrow Transplant 1993; 12(Suppl 1):21.

349. Kulhanjian J: Fever, hepatitis and coagulopathy in a newborn infant. Pediatr Infect Dis 1992; 11:1069.

350. Telfer M: Clinical spectrum of viral infections in hemophilic patients. Hematol Oncol Clin North Am 1992; 6:1047.

351. van Saene H, Stoutenbeek C, et al: Selective decontamination of the digestive tract contributes to the control of disseminated intravascular coagulation in severe liver impairment. J Pediatr Gastroenterol Nutr 1992; 14:436.

352. Kuhn W, Rath W, et al: The HELLP syndrome. Clinical and laboratory test results. Rev Franc Gynecol Obstet 1992; 87:323.

353. Meili E: Treatment of hemophilia. Schweiz Med Wochenschr 1991; 43:82.

354. Dresse M, David M, et al: Successful treatment of Kasabach-Merritt syndrome with prednisone and epsilon-aminocaproic acid. Pediatr Hematol Oncol 1991; 8:329.

355. Noseda G, Roy C, et al: Acute hepatic insufficiency disclosing congenital syphilis. Arch Fr Pediatr 1990; 47:445.

356. Rathgeber J, Rath W, Wieding J: Anesthesiologic and intensive care aspects of severe pre-eclampsia with HELLP syndrome. Anasth Intensivther Notfallmed 1990; 25:206.

357. Kurzel R: Can acetaminophen excess result in maternal and fetal toxicity? South Med J 1990; 83:953.

358. Dupuy J, Frommel D, Alagille D: Severe viral hepatitis B in infants. Lancet 1975; 1:191.

359. Mindrum G, Glueck H: Plasma prothrombin time in liver disease: Its clinical and prognostic significance. Ann Intern Med 1959; 50:1370.

360. Hope P, Hall M, et al: Alpha-1-antitrypsin deficiency presenting as a bleeding diathesis in the newborn. Arch Dis Child 1982; 57:68.

361. Olivera J, Elcarte R, et al: In Eguesx. Galactosemia of early diagnosis with psychomotor retardation. An Esp Pediatr 1986; 25:267.

362. Mercier J, Bourrillon A, et al: Hereditary fructose intolerance with early onset. Arch Fr Pediatr 1976; 10:945.

363. DiBattista C, Rossi L, et al: Hereditary tyrosinemia in acute form. Pediatr Med Chir 1981; 3:101.

364. Aster R: Pooling of platelets in the spleen: Role in the pathogenesis of "hypersplenic" thrombocytopenia. J Clin Invest 1966; 45:645.

365. Stein S, Harker L: Kinetic and functional studies of platelets, fibrinogen, and plasminogen in patients with hepatic cirrhosis. J Lab Clin Med 1982; 99:217.

366. Blanchard R, Furie B, et al: Acquired vitamin K–dependent carboxylation deficiency in liver disease. N Engl J Med 1981; 305:242.

367. Goldsmith J, Kasper C, et al: Coagulation factor IX: Successful surgical experience with a purified factor IX concentrate. Am J Hematol 1992; 40:210.

368. Volpe J: Intraventricular hemorrhage in the premature infant—Current concepts. Part I. Ann Neurol 1989; 25:3.

369. Volpe JJ: Neonatal intraventricular hemorrhage. N Engl J Med 1981; 304:886.

370. White L: CT brain scanning in neonates: indications and practices. Appl Radiol 1979; 8:58.

371. Bejar R, Curbelo V, et al: Diagnosis and follow-up of intraventricular and intracerebral hemorrhages by ultrasound studies of infant's brain through the fontanelles and sutures. Pediatrics 1980; 66:661.

372. Mack LA, Wright K, et al: Intracranial hemorrhage in premature infants: Accuracy of sonographic evaluation. Am J Roentgenol 1981; 137:245.

373. Pape KE, Bennett-Britton S, et al: Diagnostic accuracy of neonatal brain imaging: A postmortem correlation of computed tomography and ultrasound scans. J Pediatr 1983; 102:275.

374. Graziani LJ, Pasto M, et al: Cranial ultrasound and clinical studies in preterm infants. J Pediatr 1985; 106:269.

375. Sinha SK, Davies JM, et al: Relation between periventricular haemorrhage and ischaemic brain lesions diagnosed by ultrasound in very preterm infants. Lancet 1985; 2:1154.

376. Perlman JM, Nelson JS, et al: Intracerebellar haemorrhage in a premature newborn: Diagnosis by real-time ultrasound and correlation with autopsy findings. Pediatrics 1983; 71:159.

377. Dolfin T, Skidmore MB, et al: Incidence, severity and timing of subependymal and intraventricular hemorrhages in preterm infants born in a perinatal unit as detected by serial real-time ultrasound. Pediatrics 1983; 71:541.

378. Trounce JQ, Fagan D, Levene MI: Intraventricular haemorrhage and periventricular leucomalacia: ultrasound and autopsy correlation. Arch Dis Child 1986; 61:1203.

379. Ment LR, Duncan CC, Ehrenkranz RA: Intraventricular hemorrhage of the preterm neonate. Semin Perinatol 1987; 11:132.

380. Papile L, Burstein J, et al: Incidence and evolution of subependymal and intraventricular hemorrhage: A study of infants with birth weights less than 1,500 gm. J Pediatr 1978; 92:529.

381. Tsiantos A, Victorin L, Relier JP: Intracranial hemorrhage in the prematurely born infant: Timing of clots and evaluation of clinical signs and symptoms. J Pediatr 1974; 85:854.

382. Hambleton G, Wigglesworth JS: Origin of intraventricular hemorrhage in the preterm infant. Arch Dis Child 1976; 51:651.

383. Szymonowicz W, Yu VYH: Timing and evolution of periventricular haemorrhage in infants weighing 1250 g or less at birth. Arch Dis Child 1984; 59:7.

384. Shinnar S, Molteni A, et al: Intraventricular hemorrhage in the premature infant: a changing outlook. N Engl J Med 1982; 306:1464.

385. Ahmann PA, Lazzara A, et al: Intraventricular hemorrhage in the high-risk preterm infant: Incidence and outcome. Ann Neurol 1980; 7:118.

386. Levene MI, de Vries L: Extension of neonatal intraventricular hemorrhage. Arch Dis Child 1984; 59:631.

387. Guzzetta F, Shackelford G, et al: Periventricular intraparenchymal echodensities in the premature newborn: critical determinant of neurological outcome. Pediatrics 1986; 78:995.

388. Gould S, Howard S, et al: Periventricular intraparenchymal cerebral haemorrhage in preterm infants: the role of venous infarction. J Pathol 1987; 151:197.

389. Rushton D, Preston P, Durbin G: Structure and evolution of echo dense lesions in the neonatal brain. Arch Dis Child 1985; 60:798.

390. Takashima S, Mito T, Ando Y: Pathogenesis of periventricular white matter hemorrhages in preterm infants. Brain Dev 1986; 8:25.

391. Perlman JM, McMenamin JB, Volpe JJ: Fluctuating cerebral blood-flow velocity in respiratory distress syndrome. N Engl J Med 1983; 309:204.

392. Perlman JM, Hill A, Volpe JJ: The effect of patent ductus arteriosus on flow velocity in the anterior cerebral arteries: Ductal steal in the premature newborn infant. J Pediatr 1981; 99:767.

393. Lou HC: Perinatal hypoxic-ischaemic brain damage and intraventricular haemorrhage: A pathogenic model. Arch Neurol 1980; 37:585.

394. Sonesson S, Winberg P, Lundell BPW: Early postnatal changes in intracranial arterial blood flow velocities in term infants. Pediatr Res 1987; 22:461.

395. Tweed A, Cote J, et al: Impairment of cerebral blood flow autoregulation in the newborn lamb by hypoxia. Pediatr Res 1986; 20:516.

396. Greisen G, Johansen K, et al: Cerebral blood flow in the newborn infant: Comparison of Doppler ultrasound and ^{133}xenon clearance. J Pediatr 1984; 104:411.

397. Ment LR, Duncan CC, et al: Intraventricular hemorrhage in the preterm neonate: Timing and cerebral blood flow changes. J Pediatr 1984; 104:419.

398. Goddard J, Lewis R, et al: Moderate, rapidly induced hypertension as a cause of intraventricular hemorrhage in the newborn beagle model. J Pediatr 1980; 96:1057.

399. McDonald MM, Johnson ML, et al: Role of coagulopathy in newborn intracranial hemorrhage. Pediatrics 1984; 74:26.

400. Beverley DW, Chance GW, et al: Intraventricular haemorrhage and haemostasis defects. Arch Dis Child 1984; 59:444.

401. Gilles FH, Price RA, et al: Fibrinolytic activity in the ganglionic eminence of the premature human brain. Biol Neonate 1971; 18:426.

402. Horbar J: Prevention of periventricular-intraventricular hemorrhage. In Sinclair J, Bracken M (eds): Effective care of the newborn infant. Oxford, Oxford University Press, 1992, p 562.

403. Turner T, Prowse CV, et al: A clinical trial on the early detection and correction of haemostatic defects in selected high-risk neonates. Br J Haematol 1981; 47:65.

404. Andrew M, Caco C, et al: Benefits of platelet transfusions in premature infants: A randomized controlled trial. Thromb Haemost 1991; 65:721. Abstract.

405. Thomas D, Burnard E: Prevention of intraventricular haemorrhage in babies receiving artificial ventilation. Med J Aust 1973; 1:933.

406. Watl H, Fodisch N, et al: Intracranial haemorrhage in low–birth weight infants and prophylactic administration of coagulation-factor concentrate. Lancet 1973; 1:1284.

407. Gupta J, Starr H, et al: Intraventricular haemorrhage in the newborn. Med J Aust 1976; 2:338.

408. Kazzi NJ, Ilagen MB, Liang KC: Maternal administration of vitamin K does not improve the coagulation profile of preterm infants. Pediatrics 1989; 84:1045.

409. Shirahata A, Nakamura T, et al: Blood coagulation findings and the efficacy of factor XIII concentrate in premature infants with intracranial hemorrhages. Thromb Res 1990; 57:755.

410. Hensey OJ, Morgan MEI, Cooke RW: Tranexamic acid in the prevention of periventricular hemorrhage. Arch Dis Child 1984; 59:719.

411. Fodstad H, Forssell A, et al: Antifibrinolysis with tranexamic acid in aneurysmal subarachnoid haemorrhage: a consecutive controlled clinical trial. Neurosurgery 1981; 8:158.

412. Bartlett J: Subarachnoid haemorrhage. BMJ 1981; 283:1347.

413. Sindet-Pederson S, Stenbjerb S: Effect of local antifibrinolytic treatment with tranexamic acid in hemophiliacs undergoing oral surgery. J Oral Maxillofac Surg 1986; 44:703.

414. Sindet-Pederson S, Ramstrom G, et al: Hemostatic effect of tranexamic acid mouthwash in anticoagulant-treated patients undergoing oral surgery. N Engl J Med 1989; 320:840.

415. Papatheodossiou N: A double-blind clinical trial on dicynone in tonsillectomy. Med Hyg 1973; 31:1818.

416. Symes DM, Offen DN, et al: The effect of dicynene on blood loss during and after transurethral resection of the prostate. Br J Urol 1975; 47:203.

417. Harrison R, Campbell S: A double-blind trial of ethamsylate in the treatment of primary intrauterine-device menorrhagia. Lancet 1976; 2:283.

418. Ment L, Stewart W, et al: Beagle puppy model of intraventricular hemorrhage: Randomized indomethacin prevention trial. Neurology 1983; 33:179.

419. Morgan MEI, Ben JWT, Cooke RWI: Ethamsylate reduces the incidence of periventricular haemorrhage in very low birth weight babies. Lancet 1981; 2:830.

420. Cooke RWI, Morgan MEI: Prophylactic ethamsylate for periventricular haemorrhage. Arch Dis Child 1984; 59:82.

421. Benson JWT, Drayton MR, et al: Multicentre trial of ethamsylate for prevention of periventricular haemorrhage in very low birthweight infants. Lancet 1986; 2:1297.

422. Ment LR, Duncan CC, Ehrenkranz RA: Randomized indomethacin trial for prevention of intraventricular hemorrhage in very low birth weight infants. J Pediatr 1985; 107:937.

423. Hanigan WC, Kennedy G, et al: Administration of indomethacin for the prevention of periventricular-intraventricular hemorrhage in high-risk neonates. J Pediatr 1988; 112:941.

424. Ment LR, Duncan CC, Ehrenkranz RA: Randomized low dose indomethacin trial for prevention of intraventricular hemorrhage in very low birth weight neonates. J Pediatr 1988; 112:948.

425. Rennie JM, Doyle J, Cooke RWI: Early administration of indomethacin to preterm infants. Arch Dis Child 1986; 61:233.

426. Bachofen M, Weibel E: Structural alterations of lung parenchyma in the adult respiratory distress syndrome. Clin Chest Med 1982; 3:35.

427. Gajl-Peczalska K: Plasma protein composition of hyaline membrane in the newborn as studied by immunofluorescence. Arch Dis Child 1964; 39:226.

428. Gitlin D, Kumate J, et al: The selectivity of the human placenta in the transfer of plasma proteins from mother to fetus. J Clin Invest 1964; 43:1938.

429. Seeger W, Stohr G, Wolf H: Alteration of surfactant function due to protein leakage: special interaction with fibrin monomer. J Appl Physiol 1985; 58:326.

430. Saldeen T: Fibrin-derived peptides and pulmonary injury. Ann N Y Acad Sci 1982; 384:319.

431. Fukuda Y, Ishizaki M, et al: The role of intraalveolar fibrosis in the process of pulmonary structural remodelling in patients with diffuse alveolar damage. Am J Pathol 1987; 126:171.

432. Damiano V, Cherian P, et al: Intraluminal fibrosis induced unilaterally by lobar instillation of $CdCl_{22}$ into the rat lung. Am J Pathol 1990; 137:883.

433. Schmidt B, Davis P, et al: Efficacy of thrombin inhibition in a piglet model of neonatal acute lung injury. Thromb Haemost 1993; 69:1020. Abstract.

434. Ambrus C, Weintraub D, Ambrus J: Studies on hyaline membrane disease. III. Therapeutic trial of urokinase-activated human plasmin. Pediatrics 1966; 38:231.

435. Ambrus C, Choi T, et al: Prevention of hyaline membrane disease with plasminogen. A cooperative study. JAMA 1977; 237:1837.

436. Muntean W, Rosseger H: Antithrombin III concentrate in preterm infants with IRDS: An open, controlled, randomized clinical trial. Thromb Haemost 1989; 62:288. Abstract.

437. Kugelmass IN: The management of hemorrhagic problems in infancy and childhood. JAMA 1932; 99:895.

438. Clifford SH: Hemorrhagic disease of the newborn. A critical consideration. J Pediatr 1941; 18:333.

439. Sanford HN, Gasteyer TH, Wyat L: The substances involved in the coagulation of the blood of the newborn. Am J Dis Child 1932; 43:58.

440. Dam CPH: Cholesterinstoffwechsel in Hühnereierin und Hühnchen. Biochem Z 1929; 215:475.

441. Bruchsaler FS: Vitamin K and the prenatal and postnatal prevention of hemorrhagic disease in newborn infants. J Pediatr 1941; 18:317.

442. Nygaard KK: Prophylactic and curative effect of vitamin K in hemorrhagic disease of the newborn (hypothrombinemia hemorrhagica neonatorum). A preliminary report. Acta Obstet Gynecol Scand 1939; 19:361.

443. Waddell WW, Guerry D: The role of vitamin K in the etiology, prevention, and treatment of hemorrhage in the newborn infant. Part II. J Pediatr 1939; 15:802.

444. Dam H, Glavind J, et al: Investigations into the cause of the physiological hypoprothrombinemia in new-born children. IV. The vitamin K content of woman's milk and cow's milk. Acta Med Scand 1942; 112:211.

445. Quick AJ, Grossman AM: Prothrombin concentration in newborns. Proc Soc Exp Biol Med 1939; 41:227.

446. Fitzgerald JE, Webster A: Effect of vitamin K administered to patients in labor. Am J Obstet Gynecol 1940; 40:413.

447. Hellman LM, Shettles LB: The prophylactic use of vitamin K in obstetrics. South Med J 1942; 35:289.

448. Mull JW, Bill AH, et al: Effect on the newborn of vitamin K administered to mothers in labor. J Lab Clin Med 1941; 26:1305.

449. Sanford HN, Morrison HJ, et al: The substances involved in the coagulation of the blood of the newborn. III. The effect of with-holding protein and fat from the diet. Am J Dis Child 1932; 43:571.

450. Gellis SS, Lyon RA: The influence of the diet of the newborn infant on the prothrombin index. J Pediatr 1941; 19:495.

451. Motohara K, Matsukane I, et al: Relationship of milk intake and vitamin K supplementation to vitamin K status in newborns. Pediatrics 1989; 84:90.

452. Aballi AJ, Lopez Banus V, et al: The coagulation defect of fullterm infants. Pediatr Internaz 1959; 9:315.

453. Potter EL: The effect on infant mortality of vitamin K administered during labor. Am J Obstet Gynecol 1945; 50:235.

454. Committee on Nutrition A: Vitamin K compounds and water-soluble analogues: Use in therapy and prophylaxis in pediatrics. Pediatrics 1961; 28:501.

455. Lucey JF, Dolan RG: Hyperbilirubinemia of newborn infants associated with the parenteral administration of a vitamin K analogue to the mothers. Pediatrics 1959; 23:553.

456. Parks J, Sweet LK: Does the antenatal use of vitamin K prevent hemorrhage in the newborn infant? Am J Obstet Gynecol 1942; 44:432.

457. Waddell WW Jr, Whitehead BW: Neonatal mortality rates in infants receiving prophylactic doses of vitamin K. South Med J 1945; 38:349.

458. Malia RG, Preston FE, et al: Evidence against vitamin K deficiency in normal neonates. Thromb Haemost 1980; 44:159.

459. Dyggve H: The prophylactic use of vitamin K in obstetrics. South Med J 1942; 35:289.

460. MacElfresh ME: Coagulation during the neonatal period. Am J Med Sci 1961; 242:77.

461. Lawson RB: Treatment of hypoprothrombinemia (hemorrhagic disease) of the newborn infant. J Pediatr 1941; 18:224.

462. Lehmann J: Vitamin K as a prophylactic in 13,000 infants. Lancet 1944; 1:493.

463. Motohara K, Endo F, Matsuda I: Effect of vitamin K administration on acarboxy prothrombin (PIVKA-II) levels in newborns. Lancet 1985; 2:242.

464. Lane PA, Hathaway WE: Medical progress: Vitamin K in infancy. J Pediatr 1985; 106:351.

465. von Kries RV, Shearer MJ, Gobel U: Vitamin K in infancy. Eur J Pediatr 1988; 147:106.

466. Rose SJ: Neonatal hemorrhage and vitamin K. Acta Haematol 1985; 74:121.

467. O'Connor ME, Livingstone DS, et al: Vitamin K deficiency in breast feeding. Am J Dis Child 1983; 137:601.

468. Behrmann BA, Chan WK, Finer NN: Resurgence of hemorrhagic disease of the newborn, a report of three cases. Can Med Assoc J 1985; 133:884.

469. Binder L: Hemorrhagic disease of the newborn: An unusual etiology of neonatal bleeding. Ann Emerg Med 1986; 15:935.

470. Tulchinsky T, Patton M, et al: Mandating vitamin K prophylaxis for newborns in New York State. Am J Public Health 1993; 83:1166.

471. McNinch A, Tripp J: Haemorrhagic disease of the newborn in the British Isles: two year prospective study. BMJ 1991; 303:1105.

472. Corrigan J, Kryc JJ: Factor II (prothrombin) levels in cord blood. Correlation of coagulant activity with immunoreactive protein. J Pediatr 1980; 97:979.

473. Mori PG, Bisogni S, et al: Vitamin K deficiency in the newborn. Lancet 1977; 2:188. Letter.

474. Golding J, Paterson M, Kinlen L: Factors associated with childhood cancer in a national cohort study. Br J Cancer 1990; 62:304.

475. Golding J, Birmingham K, et al: Intramuscular vitamin K and childhood cancer. BMJ 1992; 305:341.

476. Ekelund H, Finnstrom O, et al: Administration of vitamin K to newborn infants and childhood cancer. BMJ 1993; 307:89.

477. Klebanoff MA, Read JS, et al: The risk of childhood cancer after neonatal exposure to vitamin K. N Engl J Med 1993; 329:905.

478. Fetus and Newborn Committee: Canadian Pediatric Society. The use of vitamin K in the perinatal period. Can Med Assoc J 1988; 139:127.

479. Hathaway WE: ICTH Subcommittee on Neonatal Hemostasis. Thrombos Haemost 1986; 55:145.

480. Hathaway WE: New insights on vitamin K. Hematol Oncol Clin North Am 1987; 1:367.

481. Shapiro AD, Jacobson LJ, et al: Vitamin K deficiency in the newborn infant: Prevalence and perinatal risk factors. J Pediatr 1986; 109:675.

482. Hall MA, Pairaudeau P: The routine use of vitamin K in the newborn. Midwifery 1987; 3:170.

483. Hanawa Y, Maki M, et al: The second nation-wide survey in Japan of vitamin K deficiency in infants. Eur J Pediatr 1988; 147:472.

484. Mandelbrot L, Guillaumont M, et al: Placental transfer of vitamin K1 and its implications in fetal haemostasis. Thromb Haemost 1988; 60:39.

485. Hamulyak K, de Boer–van den Berg MAG: The placental transport of [3H] vitamin K1 in rats. Br J Haematol 1987; 65:335.

486. Hiraike H, Kimura M, Itokawa Y: Determination of K vitamins (phylloquinone and menaquinones) in umbilical cord plasma by a platinum-reduction column. J Chromotogr 1988; 430:143.

487. Hiraike H, Kimura M, Itokawa Y: Distribution of K vitamins (phylloquinone and menaquinones) in human placenta and maternal and umbilical cord plasma. Am J Obstet Gynecol 1988; 158:564.

488. Haroon Y, Shearer MJ, et al: The content of phylloquinone (vitamin K1) in human milk, cow's milk and infant formula foods determined by high-performance liquid chromatography. J Nutr 1982; 112:1105.

489. von Kries R, Becker A, Gobel U: Vitamin K in the newborn: Influence of nutritional factors on acarboxy-prothrombin detectability and factor II and VII clotting activity. Eur J Pediatr 1987; 146:123.

490. Sutherland JM, Glueck HI: Hemorrhagic disease of the newborn; breast feeding as a necessary factor in the pathogenesis. Am J Dis Child 1967; 113:524.

491. Srinivasan G, Seeler RA, Tiruvury A, Pildes RS: Maternal anticonvulsant therapy and hemorrhagic disease of the newborn. Obstet Gynecol 1982; 59:250.

492. Mountain KR, Hirsh J, Gallius AS: Neonatal coagulation defect due to anticonvulsant drug treatment in pregnancy. Lancet 1970; 1:265.

493. Laosombat V: Hemorrhagic disease of the newborn after maternal anticonvulsant therapy: A case report and literature review. J Med Assoc Thai 1988; 71:643.

494. Martin-Bouyer G, Linh PD, Tuan LC: Epidemic of haemorrhagic disease in Vietnamese infants caused by warfarin-contaminated talcs. Lancet 1983; 1:230.

495. Sutor A, Dagres N, Neiderhoff H: Late form of vitamin K deficiency bleeding in Germany. Klin Padiatr 1995; 207:89.

496. Bovill E, Soll R, et al: Vitamin K1 metabolism and the production of des-carboxy prothrombin and protein C in the term and premature neonate. Blood 1993; 81:77.

497. Motohara K, Endo F, Matsuda I: Screening for late neonatal vitamin K deficiency by acarboxyprothrombin in dried blood spots. Arch Dis Child 1987; 62:370.

498. Motohara K, Kuroki Y, et al: Detection of vitamin K deficiency by use of an enzyme-linked immunosorbent assay for circulating abnormal prothrombin. Pediatr Res 1985; 19:354.

499. Widdershoven J, Kollee L, et al: Biochemical vitamin K deficiency in early infancy: diagnostic limitation of conventional coagulation tests. Helv Paediatr Acta 1986; 41:195.

500. Widdershoven J, Lambert W, et al: Plasma concentrations of vitamin K1 and PIVKA-II in bottle-fed and breast-fed infants with and without vitamin K prophylaxis at birth. Eur J Pediatr 1988; 148:139.

501. Fujimura Y, Okubo Y, et al: Studies on precursor proteins PIVKA-II, -IX, and -X in the plasma of patients with 'hemorrhagic disease of the newborn.' Haemostasis 1984; 14:211.

502. Kotohara K, Endo F: Effect of vitamin K administration on acarboxy prothrombin (PIVKA-II) levels in newborns. Lancet 1985; 2:243.

503. Shirahata A, Nojiri T, et al: Normotest screenings and prophylactic oral administration for idiopathic vitamin K deficiency in infancy. Nippon Ketsueki Gakkai Zasshai 1982; 45:867.

504. Garrow D, Chisolm M, Radford M: Vitamin K and thrombotest values in fullterm infants. Arch Dis Child 1986; 61:349.

505. Greer FR, Mummah-Schendel LL, et al: Vitamin K1 (phylloquinone) and vitamin K2 (menaquinone) status in newborns during the first week of life. Pediatrics 1988; 81:137.

506. von Kries R, Hanawa Y: Neonatal Vitamin K prophylaxis: Report of Scientific and Standardization Subcommittee on Perinatal Haemostasis. Thromb Haemost 1993; 69:293.

507. Vietti TJ, Murphy TP, et al: Observation on the prophylactic use of vitamin K in the newborn. J Pediatr 1960; 56:343.

508. Vietti TJ, Stephens JC, Bennett KR: Vitamin K-1 prophylaxis in the newborn. JAMA 1961; 176:791.

509. Fresh JW, Adams H, Morgan FM: Vitamin K—blood clotting studies during pregnancy and prothrombin and proconvertin levels in the newborn. Obstet Gynecol 1959; 13:37.

510. Chaou W, Chou M, Eitzman DV: Intracranial hemorrhage and vitamin K deficiency in early infancy. J Pediatr 1984; 105:880.

511. Lane PA, Hathaway WE, et al: Fatal intracranial hemorrhage in a normal infant secondary to vitamin K deficiency. Pediatrics 1983; 72:562.

512. Pietersma-de Bruyer AL, van Haard PM, et al: Vitamin K1 levels and coagulation factors in healthy term newborns until 4 weeks after birth. Haemostasis 1990; 20:8.

513. Butler NR, Golding J, et al: Recent findings of the 1970 Child Health and Education Study: preliminary communication. J R Soc Med 1982; 75:781.

514. Hathaway W, Isarangkura P, et al: Comparison of oral and parenteral vitamin K prophylaxis for prevention of late hemorrhagic disease of the newborn. J Pediatr 1991; 119:461.

515. von Kries R, Gobel U: Vitamin K prophylaxis and late haemorrhagic disease of newborn (HDN). Acta Pediatr Scand 1992; 81:655.

516. Zreik H, Bengur R, et al: Superior vena cava obstruction after extracorporeal membrane oxygenation. J Pediatr 1995; 127:314.

517. Truog R: Randomized controlled trials: Lessons from ECMO. Clin Res 1992; 40:519.

518. Bartlett R, Roloff D, et al: Extracorporeal circulation in neonatal respiratory failure: A prospective randomized study. Pediatrics 1985; 76:479.

519. Rosenburger WF, Lachin JM: The use of response-adaptive designs in clinical trials. Control Clin Trials 1993; 14:471.

520. Robinson T, Kickler T, et al: Effect of extracorporeal membrane oxygenation on platelets in newborns. Crit Care Med 1993; 21:1029.

521. Plotz F, van Oeveren W, et al: Blood activation during neonatal extracorporeal life support. J Thorac Cardiovasc Surg 1993; 105:823.

522. Pescatore P, Horellou H, et al: Problems of oral anticoagulation in an adult with homozygous protein C deficiency and late onset of thrombosis. Thromb Haemost 1993; 69:311.

523. Marlar R, Sills R, et al: Protein C survival during replacement therapy in homozygous protein C deficiency. Am J Hematol 1992; 41:24.

524. Deguchi K, Tsukada T, et al: Late-onset homozygous protein C deficiency manifesting cerebral infarction as the first symptom at age 27. Intern Med 1992; 31:922.

525. Yamamoto K, Matsushita T, et al: Homozygous protein C deficiency: identification of a novel missense mutation that causes impaired secretion of the mutant protein C. J Lab Clin Med 1992; 119:682.

526. Auberger K: Evaluation of a new protein C concentrate and comparison of protein C assays in a child with congenital protein C deficiency. Ann Hematol 1992; 64:146.

527. Grundy C, Melissari E, et al: Late-onset homozygous protein C deficiency. Lancet 1991; 338:575.

528. Marlar R, Neumann A: Neonatal purpura fulminans due to homozygous protein C or protein S deficiencies. Semin Thromb Haemost 1990; 16:299.

529. Tripodi A, Franchi F, et al: Asymptomatic homozygous protein C deficiency. Acta Haematol 1990; 83:152.

530. Petrini P, Segnestam K, et al: Homozygous protein C deficiency in two siblings. Pediatr Hematol Oncol 1990; 7:165.

531. Marlar R, Adcock D, Madden R: Hereditary dysfunctional protein C molecules (type II): assay characterization and proposed classification. Thromb Haemost 1990; 63:375.

532. Marlar R, Montgomery R, Broekmans A: Report on the diagnosis and treatment of homozygous protein C deficiency. Report of the working party on homozygous protein C deficiency of the ISTH—Subcommittee on protein C and protein S. Thromb Haemost 1989; 61:529.

533. Ben-Tal O, Zivelin A, Seligsohn U: The relative frequency of hereditary thrombotic disorders among 107 patients and thrombophilia in Israel. Thromb Haemost 1989; 61:50.

534. Burrows R, Kelton J: Low fetal risks in pregnancies associated with idiopathic thrombocytopenic purpura do not justify obstetrical interventions. Am J Obstet Gynecol 1990; 163:1147.

535. Hartman R, Manco-Johnson M, et al: Homozygous protein C deficiency: early treatment with warfarin. Am J Pediatr Hematol Oncol 1989; 11:395.

536. Vukovich T, Auberger K, et al: Replacement therapy for a homozygous protein C deficiency-state using a concentrate of human protein C and S. Br J Haematol 1988; 70:435.

537. Gladson C, Groncy P, Griffin J: Coumarin necrosis, neonatal purpura fulminans, and protein C deficiency. Arch Dermatol 1987; 123:1701a.

538. Casella J, Bontempo F, et al: Successful treatment of homozygous protein C deficiency by hepatic transplantation. Lancet 1988; 1:435.

539. Manco-Johnson M, Marlar R, et al: Severe protein C deficiency in newborn infants. J Pediatr 1988; 113:359.

540. Peters C, Casella J, et al: Homozygous protein C deficiency: observations on the nature of the molecular abnormality and the effectiveness of warfarin therapy. Pediatrics 1988; 81:272.

541. Miletich J, Sherman L, Broze G: Absence of thrombosis in subjects with heterozygous protein C deficiency. N Engl J Med 1987; 317:991.

542. Rappaport E, Speights V, et al: Protein C deficiency. South Med J 1987; 80:240.

543. Marlar R, Montgomery R, et al: Diagnosis and treatment of homozygous protein C deficiency. J Pediatr 1989; 114:528.

544. Mahasandana C, Suvatte V, et al: Homozygous protein S deficiency in an infant with purpura fulminans. J Pediatr 1990; 117:750.

545. Auletta M, Headington J: Purpura fulminans: a cutaneous manifestation of severe protein C deficiency. Arch Dermatol 1988; 124:1387.

546. Adcock D, Hicks M: Dermatopathology of skin necrosis associated with purpura fulminans. Semin Thromb Haemost 1990; 16:283.

547. Estelles A, Garcia-Plaza I, et al: Severe inherited protein C deficiency in a newborn infant. Thromb Haemost 1984; 52:53.

548. Dreyfus M, Magny J, et al: Treatment of homozygous protein C deficiency and neonatal purpura fulminans with a purified protein C concentrate. N Engl J Med 1991; 325:1565.

549. Dahlback B, Hildebrand B: Inherited resistance to activated protein C is corrected by anticoagulant cofactor activity found to be a property of factor V. Proc Natl Acad Sci U S A 1994; 91:1396.

550. Svensson P, Dahlback B: Resistance to activated protein C as a basis for venous thrombosis. N Engl J Med 1994; 330:517.

551. Rogers PC, Silva MP, et al: Renal vein thrombosis and response

552. Lobato-Mendizabal E, Ruiz-Arguelles GJ, Toquero-Franco O: Effect of danazol on heterozygous protein C coagulation deficiency exacerbated by Salmonella typhi sepsis. Bol Med Hosp Infant Mex 1989; 46:343.

553. Simioni P, de Ronde H, et al: Ischemic stroke in young patients with activated protein C resistance. A report of three cases belonging to three different kindreds. Stroke 1995; 26:885.

554. Cucuianu M, Blaga S, et al: Homozygous or compound heterozygous qualitative antithrombin III deficiency. Nouv Rev Fr Hematol 1994; 35:335.

555. Glueck CJ, Glueck HI, et al: Protein C and S deficiency, thrombophilia, and hypofibrinolysis: pathophysiologic causes of Legg-Perthes disease. Pediatr Res 1994; 35:383.

556. Schander K, Niesen M, et al: Diagnose und Therapie eines kongenitalen Antithrombin III Manglas in der neonatalen Periode. Blut 1980; 40:68.

557. Soutar R, Burrows P, et al: Overtight diaper precipitating iliac vein thrombosis in antithrombin III–deficient neonate. Arch Dis Child 1993; 69:599.

558. Shiozaki A, Arai T, et al: Congenital antithrombin III–deficient neonate treated with antithrombin III concentrates. Thromb Res 1993; 70:211.

559. Schmidt B, Andrew M: Neonatal thrombotic disease: Prevention, diagnosis and therapy. J Pediatr 1988; 113:407.

560. Schmidt B, Zipursky A: Thrombotic disease in newborn infants. Clin Perinatol 1984; 11:461.

561. Schmidt B, Andrew M: Neonatal thrombosis: Report of a prospective Canadian and International registry. Pediatrics 1995; 96:939.

562. David M, Andrew M: Venous thromboembolism complications in children: A critical review of the literature. J Pediatr 1993; 123:337.

563. Andrew M, David M, et al: Venous thromboembolic complications (VTE) in children: First analyses of the Canadian Registry of VTE. Blood 1994; 83:1251.

564. Schmidt B, Andrew A: A prospective international registry of neonatal thrombotic diseases. Pediatr Res 1994; 35:170a. Abstract.

565. O'Brodovich H, Coates J: Quantitative ventilation perfusion lung scans in infants and children: Utility of a submicronic radiolabeled aerosol to assess ventilation. J Pediatr 1984; 105:377.

566. Jackson J, Truog W, et al: Efficacy of thromboresistant umbilical artery catheters in reducing aortic thrombosis and related complications. J Pediatr 1987; 110:102.

567. Horgan M, Bartoletti A, et al: Effect of heparin infusates in umbilical arterial catheters on frequency of thrombotic complications. J Pediatr 1987; 111:774.

568. Rajani K, Goetzman B, et al: Effect of heparinization of fluids infused through an umbilical artery catheter on catheter patency and frequency of complications. Pediatrics 1979; 63:552.

569. Bosque E, Weaver L: Continuous versus intermittent heparin infusion of umbilical artery catheters in the newborn infant. J Pediatr 1986; 108:141.

570. Ankola P, Atakent Y: Effect of adding heparin in very low concentration to the infusate to prolong the patency of umbilical artery catheters. Am J Perinatol 1993; 10:229.

571. Vailas G, Brouillette R, et al: Neonatal aortic thrombosis: recent experience. J Pediatr 1986; 109:101.

572. David R, Merten D, et al: Prevention of umbilical artery catheter clots with heparinized infusates. Dev Pharmacol Ther 1981; 2:117.

573. Lesko S, Mitchell A, et al: Heparin use a risk factor for intraventricular hemorrhage in low birth weight infants. N Engl J Med 1986; 314:1156.

574. Rogers P, Silva M, et al: Renal vein thrombosis and response to therapy in a newborn due to protein C deficiency. Eur J Pediatr 1989; 149:124.

575. Andrew M, Mitchell L, et al: Thrombin regulation in children differs from adults in the absence and presence of heparin. Thromb Haemost 1994; 72:836.

576. Andrew M, Ofosu F, et al: Heparin clearance and ex vivo recovery in newborn piglets and adult pigs. Thromb Res 1988; 52:517.

to therapy in a newborn due to protein C deficiency. Eur J Pediatr 1989; 149:124.

577. McDonald MM, Jacobson LJ, et al: Heparin clearance in the newborn. Pediatr Res 1981; 15:1015.

578. Schmidt B, Buchanan M, et al: Antithrombotic properties of heparin in a neonatal piglet model of thrombin induced thrombosis. Thromb Haemost 1988; 60:289.

579. Murdoch I, Beattie R, Silver D: Heparin-induced thrombocytopenia in children. Acta Paediatr 1993; 82:495.

580. Spadone D, Clark F, et al: Heparin-induced thrombocytopenia in the newborn. J Vasc Surg 1992; 15:306.

581. Mocan H, Beattie T, Murphy A: Renal venous thrombosis in infancy: long-term follow-up. Pediatr Nephrol 1991; 5:45.

582. Hirsh J, Levine M: Low molecular weight heparin. Blood 1992; 79:1.

583. Hathaway W, Corrigan J: Report of scientific and standardization subcommittee on neonatal hemostasis. Thromb Haemost 1991; 65:323.

584. Corrigan J: Normal hemostasis in fetus and newborn: Coagulation. In Polin R, Fox W (eds): Fetal and Neonatal Physiology. Philadelphia, W.B. Saunders Co., 1992, p 1368.

585. Hathaway WE, Bonnar J: Hemostatic Disorders of the Pregnant Woman and Newborn Infant. New York, Elsevier Science Publishing Co., 1987.

586. Schmidt B, Andrew M: Report of scientific and standardization subcommittee on neonatal hemostasis diagnosis and treatment of neonatal thrombosis. Thromb Haemost 1992; 67:381.

587. El Makhlouf A, Friedli B, et al: Prosthetic heart valve replacement in children. J Thorac Cardiovasc Surg 1987; 93:80.

588. Sade R, Crawford F, et al: Valve prostheses in children: A reassessment of anticoagulation. J Thorac Cardiovasc Surg 1988; 95:553.

589. Rao S, Solymar L, et al: Anticoagulant therapy in children with prosthetic valves. Ann Thorac Surg 1989; 47:589.

590. Serra A, McNicholas K, et al: The choice of anticoagulation in pediatric patients with the St. Jude Medical valve prostheses. J Cardiovasc Surg 1987; 28:588.

591. McGrath L, Gonzalez-Lavin L, et al: Thromboembolic and other events following valve replacement in a pediatric population treated with antiplatelet agents. Ann Thorac Surg 1987; 43:285.

592. Spevak P, Freed M, et al: Valve replacement in children less than 5 years of age. J Am Cardiol 1986; 8:901.

593. Harada Y, Imai Y, et al: Ten-year follow-up after valve replacement with the St. Jude Medical prosthesis in children. J Thorac Cardiovasc Surg 1990; 100:175.

594. Stewart S, Cianciotta D, et al: The long-term risk of warfarin sodium therapy and the incidence of thromboembolism in children after prosthetic cardiac valves. J Thorac Cardiovasc Surg 1987; 93:551.

595. Woods A, Vargas J, et al: Antithrombotic therapy in children and adolescents. Thromb Res 1986; 42:289.

596. Andrew M, Marzinotto V, et al: Oral anticoagulant therapy in pediatric patients: A prospective study. Thromb Haemost 1994; 71:265.

597. von Kries R, Shearer MJ, et al: Vitamin K1 content of maternal milk: Influence of the stage of lactation, lipid composition, and vitamin K1 supplements given to the mother. Pediatr Res 1987; 22:513.

598. Hathaway WE: Use of antiplatelet agents in pediatric hypercoagulable states. Am J Dis Child 1984; 138:301.

599. Barnard D, Simmons M, Hathaway W: Coagulation studies in extremely premature infants. Pediatr Res 1979; 13:1330.

600. Thorp JA, Parriott J, et al: Antepartum vitamin K and phenobarbital for preventing intraventricular hemorrhage in the premature newborn: a randomized, double-blind, placebo-controlled trial. Obstet Gynecol 1994; 83:70.

601. Bandstra E, Montalvo BM, Goldberg RNE: Prophylactic indomethacin for prevention of intraventricular hemorrhage in premature infants. Pediatrics 1988; 82:533.

602. Bada H, Korones S, et al: Partial plasma exchange transfusion improves cerebral hemodynamics in symptomatic neonatal polycythemia. Am J Med Sci 1986; 291:11.

603. Mahony L, Caldwell R, et al: Indomethacin therapy on the first day of life in infants with very low birthweight. J Pediatr 1985; 106:801.

604. Vincer M, Allen A, et al: Early intravenous indomethacin prolongs respiratory support in very low birth weight infants. Acta Paediatr Scand 1987; 76:894.

605. Ogata T, Motohara K, et al: Vitamin K effect in low birth weight infants. Pediatrics 1988; 81:423.

606. von Kries R, Kreppel S, et al: Acarboxyprothrombin activity after oral prophylactic vitamin K. Arch Dis Child 1987; 62:938.

607. O'Connor ME, Addiego JE: Use of oral vitamin K1 to prevent hemorrhagic disease of the newborn infant. J Pediatr 1986; 108:616.

608. Keenan WJ, Jewett T, Glueck HI: Role of feeding and vitamin K in hypoprothrombinemia of the newborn. Am J Dis Child 1971; 121:271.

609. Wefring KW: Hemorrhage in the newborn and vitamin K prophylaxis. J Pediatr 1962; 61:686.

610. Astrowe PS, Palmerton ES: Clinical studies with vitamin K in newborn infants. J Pediatr 1941; 18:507.

611. Greer FR, Marshall S, et al: Vitamin K status of lactating mothers, human milk, and breast-feeding infants. Pediatrics 1991; 88:751.

612. Anai T, Hirota Y, et al: Can prenatal vitamin K1 (phylloquinone) supplementation replace prophylaxis at birth? Obstet Gynecol 1993; 81:251.

613. Dickson RC, Stubbs TM, Lazarchick J: Antenatal vitamin K therapy of the low birth weight infant. Am J Obstet Gynecol 1994; 170:85.

614. Ekelund H: Late haemorrhagic disease in Sweden 1987–1989. Acta Paediatr Scand 1991; 80:966.

615. Tonz O, Schubinger G: Neonatale Vitamin K Prophylaxe und Vitamin K Mangelblutungen in der Schweiz 1986–1988. Schweiz Med Wochenschr 1988; 118:1747.

616. Hanawa Y: Vitamin K deficiency in infancy: the Japanese experience. Acta Paediatr Jpn 1992; 34:107.

617. Clark F, James E: Twenty-seven years of experience with oral vitamin K1 therapy in neonates. J Pediatr 1995; 127:301.

618. Sutor A: Vitamin K deficiency bleeding in infants and children. Semin Thromb Haemost 1995; 21:317.

619. Michelson AD, Bovill E, Andrew M: Antithrombotic therapy in children. Chest 1995; 108:506S.

620. Rajasekhar D, Kestin A, et al: Neonatal platelets are less reactive than adult platelets to physiological agonists in whole blood. Thromb Haemost 1994; 72:957.

621. Sanford HN, Shmigelsky I, Chapin JM: Is administration of vitamin K to the newborn of clinical value? JAMA 1942; 118:697.

622. Jobes D, Nicolson S, et al: Coagulation defects in neonates during cardiopulmonary bypass. Ann Thorac Surg 1993; 55:1283.

III

Bone Marrow Failure

The Anatomy and Physiology of Hematopoiesis

The Bone Marrow Failure Syndromes

Principles of Bone Marrow and Stem
Cell Transplantation

The Anatomy and Physiology of Hematopoiesis

Colin A. Sieff • David G. Nathan • Steven C. Clark

A review of the anatomy and physiology of normal hematopoiesis is presented in this chapter to provide a basis of understanding of the marrow failure syndromes described at length in Chapter 7. The phylogeny of hematopoiesis is briefly discussed, and marrow anatomy and the egress of recognizable hematopoietic cells from the marrow into the peripheral blood are described. A more detailed analysis follows of the cellular bases of erythrocyte, granulocyte-macrophage, and megakaryocyte development, including discussions of the pluripotent stem cells, the more committed but still undifferentiated progenitor cells, and the differentiated precursors of the mature formed elements of the blood. Much of this chapter is devoted to the interactions of growth factors and the cells that produce them in the up-regulation of hematopoiesis. The mechanisms of down-regulation of hematopoiesis by cell interactions and cytokines are touched on here, but they are less well understood despite the fact that they are likely to influence the pathophysiology of aplastic anemia and other marrow failure syndromes.

HISTORY*

That "blood is life" was appreciated by Empedocles in the fifth century BC. The theory that the vasculature contains blood, phlegm, black bile, and yellow bile, all revealed when freshly let blood is permitted to separate, is attributed to Polibus, the son-in-law of Hippocrates. Servetus recognized the systemic and lesser circulations in the 16th century. He was burned at the stake, in part because he did not accept the dogma that blood must pass through the intraventricular cardiac septum.

In view of the present growth of knowledge of hematology, it is remarkable to realize that the concept of the circulation of the blood was finally established by Harvey only a little over 300 years ago. This began the clinical application of blood transfusion, of which Pepys wrote "it gave rise to many pretty wishes as of the blood of a Quaker to be let into an Archbishop and such like."

In the mid-17th century, Swammerdam observed red blood corpuscles in the microscope and Malpighi discovered the capillary circulation in the lung and in the omentum. But it was not until the 19th century that the source of blood cell production began to be successfully explored. Houston suggested that red cells were

derived from leukocytes in the lymphoid system. Zimmerman believed that erythrocytes were derived from platelets, an opinion shared by Hayem. Addison, perhaps not surprisingly, attributed red cell production to the adrenals, and Reikert finally suggested that red cells might be produced in the embryonic liver. In fact, it was not until 1868 that Neumann demonstrated that red cells arise from precursors in the marrow. The modern understanding of the physiology of hematopoiesis then began.

PHYLOGENY

Much can be learned about the physiology of hematopoiesis from study of the evolution of oxygen transport, a subject reviewed by Lehman and Huntsman.[1]

One of the major advantages of mammalian life over that of invertebrates is the capacity to package large amounts of hemoglobin within cells. This permits the delivery of oxygen to tissues without the enormous increase in oncotic pressure that would be induced by a similar concentration of high-molecular-weight hemoglobin free in the plasma. The renewal rate of red cells is a function of metabolic rate or basal heat production. This is illustrated dramatically in studies of the animal kingdom, ranging from the turtle to the pygmy shrew, and by comparisons of red cell renewal in marmots during periods at ambient and cold temperatures,[2] in rats,[3] and in frogs.[4]

The production of blood cells in bone marrow is a late development in phylogeny. Red cells are found in the coelomic cavity of the worm and are produced in the kidneys of the goldfish. The influence of oxygen demand on the production of red cells[5] is illustrated by the effects of hyperoxia on bled rats[6] and the behavior of the European eel, one of the few vertebrate forms that ordinarily lacks erythrocytes in its juvenile state. When the adult eel struggles against the current up the rivers of Europe, hemoglobin-containing nucleated cells appear in its plasma. This influence of oxygen demand on respiratory pigment production is also illustrated in non–red cell–producing organisms such as Daphnia, the English water flea, a creature that produces high-molecular-weight hemoglobin in its ovaries when it is exposed to low oxygen tension in stagnant ponds. The discovery of transcription factors that function as oxygen sensors provides a potential molecular explanation for these regulatory mechanisms.[7–9]

MARROW ANATOMY

The relative red (active) marrow space of a child is much greater than that of an adult, presumably because the high requirements for red cell production

---

*For an entertaining review from which this précis was in part drawn, see Robb-Smith AHT: The growth of knowledge of functions of the blood. In MacFarlane RG, Robb-Smith AHT (eds): Functions of the Blood. Oxford, Blackwell Scientific Publications, 1961. For more details, see also Wintrobe M: Blood Pure and Eloquent. New York, McGraw-Hill Book Company, 1980.

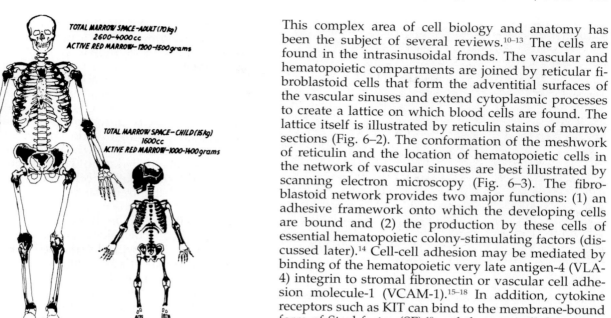

Figure 6–1. Comparison of active red marrow–bearing areas in the child and the adult. Note the almost identical amount of active red marrow in the child and adult despite a five-fold discrepancy in body weight. (From MacFarlane RC, Robb-Smith AHT (eds): Functions of the Blood. New York, Academic Press, 1961, p 357.)

during neonatal life demand the resources of the entire production potential of the marrow. During postnatal life the demands for red cell production ebb, and much of the marrow space is slowly and progressively filled with fat (Fig. 6–1). In certain disease states that are usually associated with anemia, such as myeloid metaplasia, hematopoiesis may return to its former sites in the liver, spleen, and lymph nodes and may also be found in the adrenals, cartilage, adipose tissue, thoracic paravertebral gutters, and even the kidneys.

The microenvironment of the marrow cavity is a vast network of vascular channels or sinusoids in which float fronds of hematopoietic cells, including fat cells.

This complex area of cell biology and anatomy has been the subject of several reviews.[10–13] The cells are found in the intrasinusoidal fronds. The vascular and hematopoietic compartments are joined by reticular fibroblastoid cells that form the adventitial surfaces of the vascular sinuses and extend cytoplasmic processes to create a lattice on which blood cells are found. The lattice itself is illustrated by reticulin stains of marrow sections (Fig. 6–2). The conformation of the meshwork of reticulin and the location of hematopoietic cells in the network of vascular sinuses are best illustrated by scanning electron microscopy (Fig. 6–3). The fibroblastoid network provides two major functions: (1) an adhesive framework onto which the developing cells are bound and (2) the production by these cells of essential hematopoietic colony-stimulating factors (discussed later).[14] Cell-cell adhesion may be mediated by binding of the hematopoietic very late antigen-4 (VLA-4) integrin to stromal fibronectin or vascular cell adhesion molecule-1 (VCAM-1).[15–18] In addition, cytokine receptors such as KIT can bind to the membrane-bound form of Steel factor (SF),[19] and the extracellular matrix proteins secreted by stromal cells may actually provide a binding site for some growth factors or for hematopoietic cells.[20–22]

A schema of the marrow circulation is shown in Figure 6–4. The central and radial arteries ramify in the cortical capillaries, which in turn join the marrow sinusoids and drain into the central sinus. Cells that egress from the marrow sinusoids then join the venous circulation through comitant veins. The inner, or luminal, surface of the vascular sinusoids is lined with endothelial cells, the cytoplasmic extensions of which overlap, or interdigitate, with one another. The escape of developing hematopoietic cells into the sinus for transport to the general circulation occurs through gaps that develop in this endothelial lining and even through endothelial cell cytoplasmic pores.

The location of the different hematopoietic cells is not random. Clumps of megakaryocytes are found adjacent to marrow sinuses. They shed platelets, the fragments of their cytoplasm, directly into the lumen. This reduces the requirement for movement of bulky

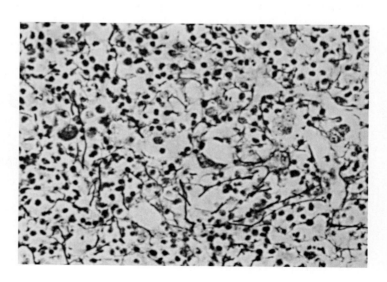

Figure 6–2. Bone marrow biopsy of a patient with mild myelofibrosis shows a slight increase in the number of reticulin fibers in a delicate discontinuous fiber network. (Gomori stain ×350.) (From Lennert K, Nagai K, et al: Pathoanatomical feature of the bone marrow. Clin Hematol 1975; 4:335.)

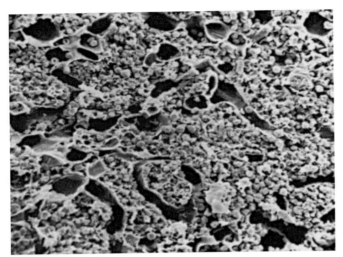

Figure 6-3. Scanning electron micrograph of rat femoral marrow. The hematopoietic cells are grouped between the interlacing network of vascular sinuses. Many cells are dislodged when the marrow is transected, and separate spaces are present where cells had been. (From Lichtman MA, Chamberlain JK, et al: Factors thought to contribute to the regulation of egress of cells from marrow. In Silber K, LoBue L, et al (eds): The Year in Hematology, 1978. New York, Plenum Medical Book Company, 1978, pp 243–279.)

mature megakaryocytes, a mobility characteristic of the granuloid- and erythroid-differentiated precursors as they approach the point at which they egress from the marrow. A schema that illustrates the transfer of hematopoietic cells into the sinus is shown in Figure 6–5. Disruption of the function of microenvironmental cells inhibits long-term murine marrow cultures.[23] Such disruptions may be responsible for certain cases of aplastic anemia.

HEMATOPOIETIC CELLS

Stem Cells

The concept that sustained hematopoiesis derives from pluripotent stem cells was first suggested by Jacobson and colleagues,[24] who showed that mice can be pro-

tected from the lethal affects of whole-body irradiation by exteriorization and shielding of the spleen. This protective effect was shown to be cell-mediated by the observation that the injection of spleen cells could initiate recovery and re-establish hematopoiesis in irradiated animals.[25] The clonal nature of hematopoiesis and the concept that a single pluripotent stem cell exhibits the capacity to repopulate the entire hematopoietic system was first demonstrated experimentally by Till and McCulloch,[26] who also used the mouse as an experimental system. They demonstrated that colonies of hematopoietic cells could be observed in the spleen of the transplanted, irradiated recipients within 10 days after the transplant. These colonies contained precursors to erythrocytes, granulocytes and macrophages, and megakaryocytes. Subsequent experiments using karyotypically marked donor cells confirmed the clonal origin of the differentiated cells in the colony, proving that a single pluripotent stem cell had given rise to these differentiated cells.[27] It was also shown that each colony contained a number of stem cells that could again form a colony of differentiated progeny in a second irradiated recipient, demonstrating their self-renewal capacity. This is true only of spleen colonies that are present on day 12 through 14 (spleen colony-forming units [CFU-S_{12}]). Colonies observed on days 7 to 8 after marrow infusion are transient, disappear by day 12, and are neither multipotential nor self-maintaining.[28] Under steady-state conditions no more than 10% of the CFU-S become committed to differentiation during any given 3-hour period. This can be demonstrated by removing murine marrow cells to *in vitro* culture for 3 hours. During this period, half the cells are exposed to an agent such as ^{3}H-thymidine or to hydroxyurea, which will kill cells undergoing a round of DNA replication, while the other half are not exposed to the toxic agent. The number of surviving CFU-S in the treated culture is then compared with the number of CFU-S in the control culture by titrating each cell population using irradiated recipients in the spleen colony assay. The demonstration of a stem cell that can differentiate to form progenitor cells for erythropoiesis, granulopoiesis, and megakaryopoiesis is completely consistent with subse-

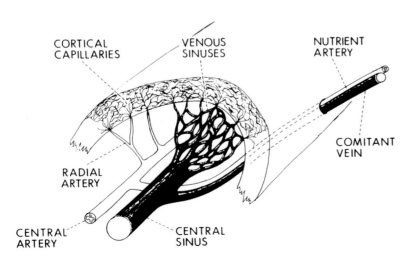

CORTICAL CAPILLARIES

VENOUS SINUSES

NUTRIENT ARTERY

RADIAL ARTERY

CENTRAL ARTERY

CENTRAL SINUS

COMITANT VEIN

Figure 6-4. A schematic representation of the circulation of the marrow. The nutrient artery, central arteries, and radial arteries feed the cortical capillaries. The cortical capillaries anastomose with the marrow sinuses, which drain into the large central sinus. The central sinus enters the comitant vein by which the marrow effluent enters the systemic venous circulation. An interesting feature of the circulation of marrow is the transit of nearly all arterial blood through cortical capillaries before entering the marrow sinuses. Not shown are the arterial communications from muscular arteries that feed the periosteum and penetrate the cortex to anastomose with intracortical vessels. (From Lichtman MA, Chamberlain JK, et al: Factors thought to contribute to the regulation of egress of cells from marrow. In Silber K, LoBue J, et al (eds): The Year in Hematology, 1978. New York, Plenum Medical Book Company, 1978, pp 243–279.)

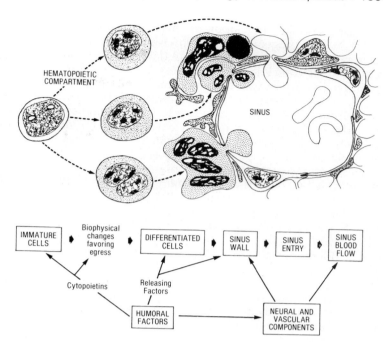

Figure 6–5. A schematic diagram of the factors that may be involved in controlling the release of marrow cells. The central relationship between the hematopoietic compartment and the marrow sinus is depicted. The drawing highlights the similarity of the egress process for the three major hematopoietic cells: reticulocytes in the top pathway, granulocytes and monocytes in the center pathway, and platelets in the lower pathway. Immature cells undergo biophysical changes under the influence of cytopoietins that favor egress. In the case of the reticulocyte, enucleation precedes egress. This is shown by the solid black inclusion in the perisinal macrophage representing nucleophagocytosis antecedent to digestion of the erythroblast nucleus. The cytoplasmic protrusion of the megakaryocyte presumably detaches itself from the cell and will further fragment into platelets in the circulation. (From Lichtman MA, Chamberlain JK et al: Factors thought to contribute to the regulation of egress of cell from marrow. In Silber K, LoBue J, et al (eds): The Year in Hematology, 1978. New York, Plenum Medical Book Company, 1978, pp 243–279.)

quent observations in disease states such as chronic myelogenous leukemia[29, 30] and polycythemia vera,[31, 32] in which a clonal origin of abnormal erythroid, granulocytic, and megakaryocytic precursor cells and lymphocytes can be demonstrated (see Chapter 34).

The demonstration of a pluripotent stem cell in adult bone marrow led to a systematic search for the ontogenic origins of hematopoietic stem cells (HSC). Experiments performed by Moore and Metcalf[33, 34] clearly demonstrated the presence of cells capable of repopulating the adult marrow in the yolk sac and the murine fetal liver. Subsequent work has confirmed and extended these observations,[35] although recent data show that HSC may arise simultaneously in the yolk sac and the intraembryonic aorta/gonad/mesonephros (AGM) region.[36] A difficulty here is that primordial germ cells also arise or migrate through this region and have been shown to have the potential to generate HSC.[37] A point of interest that arises is whether the stem cells observed in yolk sac, fetal liver, and adult marrow, and spleen are functionally equivalent in every respect. One experimental finding that suggests functional differences between CFU-S at different stages of development of the mouse was made by Micklem and Ross.[38] Their experimental approach was to transfer spleen cells sequentially from a repopulated recipient to an irradiated recipient. Experiments of this type had previously shown that the capacity for transfer of CFU-S from adult marrow or spleen was finite, and in fact only three serial transfers could be accomplished.[39] Micklem and Ross showed that cells transplanted from the yolk sac to the spleen of an irradiated recipient could be serially transplanted as many as seven times before further proliferative capacity was lost. CFU-S derived from fetal livers were capable of five to six serial transfers.

Studies of Hellman and co-workers[40] have provided a model of the stem cell compartment in which there is a continuum of cells with decreasing capacities for self-renewal, increasing likelihood for differentiation, and increasing proliferative activity. Cells progress in a unidirectional fashion in this continuum. It is the most primitive cells with the greatest self-renewal capacity that reconstitute long-term hematopoiesis after transfer into irradiated recipient mice. These cells, termed *long-term reconstituting hematopoietic stem cells* (LTR-HSC), were shown to be separable from CFU-S$_{12}$ in a limiting dilution assay designed to detect and enumerate "cobblestone areas."[41] This assay is derived from the original "Dexter" technique for long-term culture of murine marrow in which CFU-S, granulocyte-macrophage colony-forming units (CFU-GM), and erythrocyte burst-forming units (BFU-E) flourish for many months on and within an adherent stromal monolayer.[42] The areas of active hematopoiesis have a "cobblestone" appearance. In the limiting-dilution assay, different concentrations of bone marrow cells are plated onto a series of microwells that contain a pre-established stromal monolayer, and at 5 weeks the cobblestone areas that comprise proliferating blast cells within the stromal cell layer are counted.[41] In cell separation experiments, their numbers correlate with a cell fraction that is characterized by low mitochondrial mass per cell (minimal retention of the supravital fluorochrome rhodanine-123); this cell fraction is enriched for marrow repopulating cells but depleted of CFU-S$_{12}$.[41, 43] An even more impressive separation of pre–CFU-S from CFU-S$_{12}$ was obtained by counter-current elutriation.[44] Intermediate and rapidly sedimenting cells contained more than 99% CFU-S$_{12}$ as well as the cells responsible for short-term reconstitution. In contrast, long-term reconstituting cells (>60 days) came from a slowly sedimenting fraction that contained only 0.25% CFU-S$_{12}$.

In summary, LTR-HSC are cells capable of long-term

reconstitution of myelopoiesis and lymphopoiesis. More mature progenitor cells, represented by CFU-S$_{12}$, give rise to spleen colonies 12 to 14 days after injection into irradiated recipients, exhibit less self-renewal and proliferative capacity, and are generally limited to myeloid differentiation. The most mature compartment, represented by cells that give rise to spleen colonies 6 to 8 days after transplantation (CFU-S$_8$), have limited self-renewal and proliferative capacities. The relationship between the *in vivo* LTR-HSC assay and *in vitro* assays that measure blast cell colonies capable of forming additional colonies after replating,[45] high proliferative potential colony-forming cells (HPP-CFC) that form large monocyte colonies (up to 5×10^4 cells),[46] or cells that survive in long-term cultures[47] is at this point unresolved.

Considerations of stem cell heterogeneity are of clinical relevance, because any manipulations of human bone marrow before allogeneic or autologous transplantation requires preservation of the most primitive stem cell compartment. Morphologically, stem cells appear to be medium-sized mononuclear cells with a very high nuclear:cytoplasmic ratio, basophilic cytoplasm devoid of granules, and prominent nucleoli.

A cell with the characteristics of a self-renewing multipotential stem cell has not been clearly defined in humans for obvious reasons. However, the presence of stem cells capable of long-term hematopoietic reconstitution (LTR-HSC) is inferred from the success of bone marrow transplantation, using bone marrow or blood as a source of cells in humans[48, 49] and blood as a source of reconstituting cells in canine models.[50] However, these transplantation experiments do not prove that the LTR-HSC present in the marrow and blood of human and canine species are capable of self-renewal. More differentiated stem cells could have established the hematopoietic graft. Rigid proof of the presence of self-renewing stem cells requires the use of a secondary transfer assay, in which the primary transplanted cells themselves are used for reconstitution of second irradiated hosts. Colonies morphologically similar to CFU-S have been observed after careful examination of spleens from bone marrow transplant recipients who died early in the engraftment process, which then allowed analysis of their spleens at times similar to day 8 to 14 after transplant in the mouse.[51] Obviously, however, cells from such colonies cannot be used to attempt reconstitution of secondary hosts.

The growth of LTR-HSC in the marrow may require a microenvironmental "niche."[52, 53] Thus, isogeneic marrow infusions are not successful unless the recipient is irradiated or treated with sufficient doses of cytotoxic drugs to create an adequate number of "niches." Therefore, reports of failure of engraftment in aplastic anemia using identical twin donors do not necessarily suggest an immunologic basis for the disease but could just as well imply persistence of nonfunctional pluripotent progenitors in the aplastic marrow "niches." These abnormal cells must be destroyed, if present, to allow implantation of transfused normal progenitors.

Many *in vitro* assays have been proposed as "surrogate" stem cell assays, but until homogeneous populations can be evaluated in both *in vitro* and *in vivo* assays it will be impossible to determine the precise cell type measured by these methods. Fauser and Messner and others[30, 54–56] demonstrated colonies in semisolid media that contain granulocytes, erythrocytes, monocytes, and megakaryocytes (CFU-GEMM) in methylcellulose cultures of human bone marrow. A unique type of *in vitro* blast cell colony that comprises small numbers of blast cells with higher self-renewal capacity (secondary colonies on replating) than CFU-GEMM has been described.[45] Evidence for the presence of pluripotent HSC is also derived from the human "Dexter" technique for liquid culture of marrow in which myeloid progenitors (mostly CFU-GM) are sustained for about 2 months on and within an adherent stromal monolayer.[57, 58] The progenitors can be detected by replating into methylcellulose with several growth factors at 5 to 8 weeks, thereby demonstrating that unipotent and multipotent cells are generated in this culture system. Eaves and colleagues have adapted this long-term culture technique to a limiting dilution assay in which long-term culture initiating cells (LTC-IC) can be quantitated after culture at different concentrations on a stromal layer for 5 weeks followed by replating in methylcellulose to score for the number of wells that do not contain colonies.[59] The analogous cobblestone area–forming cell assay has also been adapted to human cells.[60] Last, an assay that measures the enormous proliferative capacity of primitive progenitor cells is the HPP-CFC assay, which gives rise to macroscopically (>5 mm) visible *in vitro* colonies.[46, 61] A tentative relationship of the cells measured in these different assays to the stem cell is shown in Figure 6–6.

Application of these assays and analysis of HSC, in general, have been hindered by the low frequency of the cell in the hematopoietic population and the lack of reagents to identify stem cells. However, it is now possible to purify murine stem cells by several methods. Murine HSC can be highly purified by density gradient centrifugation combined with labeling with antibodies, lectins, or intracellular dyes (alone or in combination) followed by separation using fluorescence-activated cell sorting (FACS), immuno-panning, or immuno-magnetic beads. Immunologic reagents that define murine stem cell populations include Thy-1, Sca-1, and Qa-m7. Spangrude and co-workers[62] used FACS in combination with negative expression of T-cell, B-cell, granulocyte, and monocyte lineage (lin)-specific markers; low expression of Thy-1; and expression of the stem cell antigen (Sca-1). As few as 30 lin−, Thy-1-low, Sca-1+ cells can ensure survival at 30 days of 50% of lethally irradiated syngeneic recipients. This cell fraction is highly enriched for CFU-S$_{12}$, but its content of long-term repopulating cells (pre–CFU-S, discussed earlier) is uncertain. Bertoncello and co-workers[63] used antibodies to the Qa-m7 antigen and immuno-magnetic bead separation to purify HPP-CFC. These cells are considered by some to be the equivalent of the reconstituting stem cell. In these studies, up to 30% of the final cell population were HPP-CFC. Visser and co-workers[64] used combinations of density gradient centrifugation and labeling with wheat germ agglu-

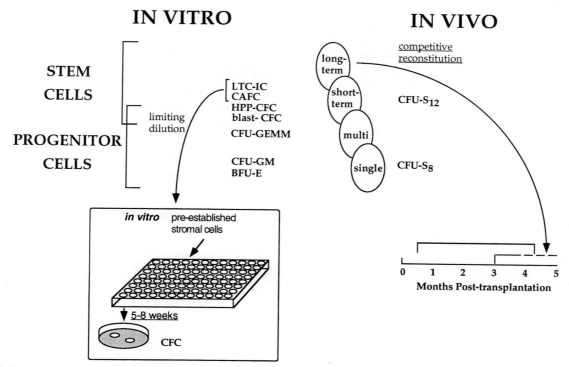

Figure 6–6. Schematic view of some general properties and assays for the heterogeneous cells that comprise the stem cell and progenitor cell compartments. Cells capable of permanently reconstituting *in vivo* hematopoiesis are separable from cells that give rise to CFU-S day 12 (CFU-S$_{12}$), but the precise developmental stage of *in vitro* long-term culture initiating cells (LTC-IC), cobblestone area–forming cells (CAFC), high proliferative potential colony-forming cells (HPP-CFC), and blast CFC is not established. In the progenitor compartment, mixed colonies of almost all lineage combinations have been described. CFU-GEMM = granulocyte-erythrocyte-monocyte-megakaryocyte colony-forming unit; CFU-GM = granulocyte-macrophage colony-forming unit; BFU-E = burst-forming unit–erythroid.

tinin and rhodanine-123 dye to purify stem cells capable of 30-day radioprotection after transplantation into lethally irradiated syngeneic murine recipients. Differences in physical properties and expression of the antigens CD34 and CD33 have been used to enrich for human stem cells. Although most colony-forming cells (CFC) express both the CD34 and CD33 antigens, cells that give rise to CFC in long-term bone marrow cultures (i.e., pre-CFC) can be separated by their expression of CD34, lack of expression of CD33, and intermediate forward light-scattering properties.[65] A G$_0$ CD34+ cell population has been isolated by exploiting the resistance of these cells to 5-fluorouracil (5-FU) in the presence of SF and interleukin (IL)-3.[66] The G$_0$ cells are also KIT, IL-6 receptor (IL-6R), and IL-1 receptor (IL-1R) positive; do not form progenitor-derived colonies on direct culture in methylcellulose; but, after 5 weeks in culture on stromal cells, do form primary colonies in methylcellulose, 40% of which are replatable. Furthermore, 89% of the cells (normalized for the maximum number of positive wells) score positive in an LTC-IC assay and, in long-term culture, myeloid and lymphoid cells can be derived. These data are unconfirmed but suggest that this cell population may represent a primitive resting multipotent HSC, possibly the LTR-HSC. The importance of CD34+ marrow cells is emphasized by *in vivo* simian studies. Similar to human bone marrow, the CD34 antigen is expressed by a minority of baboon cells, and infusion of these

cells isolated by immunoabsorption chromatography and FACS can reconstitute lymphohematopoiesis in lethally irradiated baboons.[67] The cloning of the murine CD34 complementary DNA (cDNA) has cast some doubt on expression of CD34 by LTR-HSC, at least in the mouse. A monoclonal antibody raised to murine CD34 was used to separate purified Sca-1+, KIT+, lin− bone marrow cells into CD34 low or negative (CD34-low/−), and CD34+ fractions. Interestingly, long-term multilineage reconstitution was observed after transplantation of the CD34-low/− cells, whereas the CD34+ fraction gave early but unsustained multilineage reconstitution.[68] It is possible that murine and primate LTR-HSC differ in their expression of CD34; however, the human and primate transplants have not used very highly purified cells, and so it is also possible that CD34-low/− cells could account for the long-term engraftment. Such data will therefore require careful evaluation.

Progenitor Cells

The pluripotent stem cells of the marrow slowly self-replicate while occasionally (and stochastically) differentiating into a stage of either lymphoid or myeloid commitment. The first step of myeloid commitment produces a progenitor capable of self-renewal and stochastic differentiation into all of the progenitors of the blood cells other than lymphoid cells. This is the myeloid stem cell. This cell, in turn, slowly self-replicates or stochastically enters a more committed progenitor stage such as the progenitors responsible for phagocytopoiesis or eosinophilopoiesis or those responsible for erythropoiesis, basophilopoiesis, and megakaryocytopoiesis.

Erythrocyte Colony-Forming Cells

The erythroid progenitor compartment is invisible to the light microscope. These committed progenitors of a single lineage are derived from the stochastic differentiation of bipotential or multipotential progenitors[69] that are, in turn, derived from a tiny population of totipotential stem cells (Fig. 6–7). In humans, the most primitive single lineage committed erythroid progenitors are erythrocyte burst-forming units. The BFU-E are so named because, in response to the combination of

erythropoietin (EPO) and either SF, IL-3, or granulocyte-macrophage colony-stimulating factor (GM-CSF) *in vitro* in semisolid (methylcellulose) cultures, they divide several times when still motile, thereby forming subpopulations of erythrocyte colony-forming units (CFU-E).[70] Then, each of the latter form a large colony of proerythroblasts that go on to form more mature erythroblasts and even reticulocytes. The burstlike morphology of the colony is responsible for the name of the progenitor. The entire process requires about weeks *in vitro*. Bone marrow also contains the more mature CFU-E that, under the influence of EPO, form small colonies of erythroblasts in 7 days.

Granulocyte and Macrophage Colony-Forming Cells

The first colony assays relevant to the study of the production of granulocytes and monocytes in the

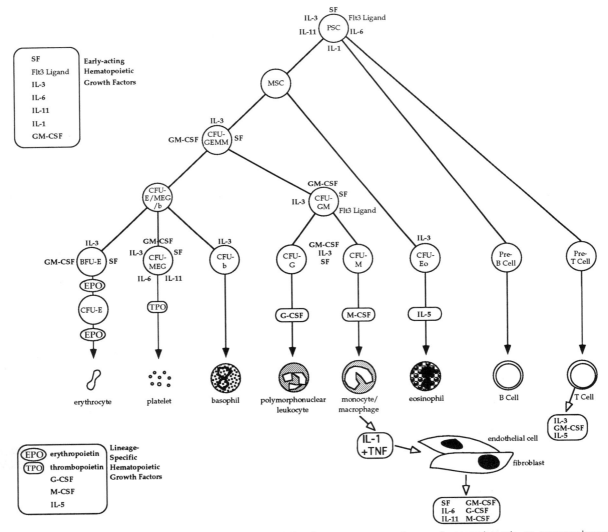

Figure 6–7. Major cytokine sources and actions. Cells of the bone marrow microenvironment such as macrophages (ma), endothelial cells (ec), and reticular fibroblastoid cells (fb) produce macrophage colony-stimulating factor (M-CSF), granulocyte-macrophage colony-stimulating factor (GM-CSF), granulocyte colony-stimulating factor (G-CSF), interleukin (IL-6), and probably Steel factor (SF: cellular sources not yet precisely determined) after induction with endotoxin (ma) or IL-1/TNF (ec, fb). T cells produce IL-3, GM-CSF, and IL-5 in response to antigenic and IL-1 stimulation. These cytokines have overlapping actions during hematopoietic differentiation, as indicated, and for all lineages optimal development requires a combination of early- and late-acting factors. PSC = pluripotent stem cells; MSC = myeloid stem cells; TNF = tumor necrosis factor.

mouse were described in 1965 by Pluznik and Sachs[71] and in 1966 by Bradley and Metcalf.[72] Analogous assays have been developed in the human system.[73] These groups demonstrated that individual cells derived from mouse spleen or bone marrow could give rise to colonies of up to several thousand differentiated granulocytes or macrophages in a soft agar medium. Seven to 8 days was required for full maturation of these colonies (12 to 14 days is required in humans). Appropriate studies were performed to demonstrate the single cell origin of the colonies. These studies also demonstrated that a single progenitor cell, which was termed the *colony-forming unit–culture* (or CFU-C), was capable of differentiation into both granulocytes and macrophages, thus the designation CFU-GM. Unit gravity sedimentation and other separation methods have been used to demonstrate that CFU-GM represent a cell population distinguishable from the pluripotent stem cell.[74] Long-term liquid bone marrow cultures have been particularly helpful in defining humoral and cell-cell interactions that induce myeloid differentiation.[75] CFU-GM give rise to the more mature granulocytes and macrophage colony-forming units, CFU-G and CFU-M, respectively.[71, 72] In addition, CFU-GM can be distinguished from the eosinophil progenitor (CFU-Eo), each arising independently from the myeloid stem cell. A progenitor more mature than CFU-GM, which differentiates to smaller clusters of mature myeloid cells earlier in culture than does CFU-GM, has been described.[46, 73, 76, 77] This is analogous to the erythroid system, in which BFU-E differentiate to a more mature progenitor, the CFU-E. A pre–CFU-GM similar to the most immature BFU-E with a slower sedimentation rate and lower cycling index than CFU-GM has been described in humans.[78–80] Thus, the myeloid progenitor population, like the erythroid, represents a continuum with respect to proliferative potential.

Megakaryocyte Colony-Forming Cells

Figure 6–7 provides an accepted if idealized schema of lineage-restricted megakaryocyte progenitor development. Evidence strongly suggests that the initial phase of differentiation into erythrocyte, basophil, and megakaryocyte (e/b/meg) commitment involves a single progenitor capable of giving rise to colonies of differentiated cells, all of which express a nuclear transcription factor known as GATA-1.[81, 82] Further evidence of a close developmental relationship between erythroid and megakaryocytic lineages comes from the *in vitro* cultures of progenitor-derived colonies in human erythroid leukemia cell lines. Studies of the erythroid colonies produced *in vitro* after culture of low density marrow cells in the presence of EPO reveal that a small but readily demonstrable fraction of the erythroid colonies are interspersed with megakaryocytes. Finally, human erythroid leukemia cells that express an erythroid phenotype constitutively become even more strikingly erythroid when incubated with δ-aminolevulinic acid, but express a megakaryocyte phenotype when they are exposed to low doses of phorbol myristate acetate.[83]

When the e/b/meg progenitor finally differentiates

to a stage called megakaryocyte-burst-forming units (BFU-meg), a restricted commitment to megakaryocyte differentiation is achieved. This is entirely analogous to the events previously described with respect to phagocyte and erythroid development. When driven by the appropriate growth factors (those that comprise megakaryocyte colony-stimulating activity [meg-CSA]), BFU-meg divide in culture for several days before they begin to differentiate into colonies that though few in number are relatively large and have a burstlike morphology. *In vivo*, BFU-meg mature to CFU-meg. When suitably stimulated by the growth factors in meg-CSA and by thrombopoietin, CFU-meg, which are found more frequently in human marrow than are BFU-meg, form relatively small single colonies. Both BFU-meg and CFU-meg express DR and CD3 antigens, whereas it is said that BFU-meg express only CD3.[84] This, of course, may be a matter of detection. Of great interest is the fact that at least one transcription factor, NF-E2, has been shown to regulate platelet production.[85] Mice rendered NF-E2 deficient die of bleeding due to absence of platelets. The thrombocytopenia is due to a block late in megakaryocyte maturation. Interestingly, these animals do not show an increase in thrombopoietin levels, suggesting that the megakaryocyte mass rather than the platelet count regulates thrombopoietin production.

Precursors and Mature Cells

The erythroid precursor or erythroblast pool represents about one third of the marrow cell population in the normal child older than age 3 or in the adult. Proerythroblasts are the earliest recognizable forms. These divide and mature through various stages that involve nuclear condensation and extrusion and hemoglobin accumulation. On average, each erythroblast can form about eight reticulocytes. Measurement of the total marrow proerythroblast content[86] and daily reticulocyte production shows that under normal conditions replicating proerythroblasts largely maintain the reticulocyte pool being renewed from the progenitor compartment at a rate of about 10% per day.[87]

Erythroid Development

Up to this point the nondescript *progenitors* of erythropoiesis have been discussed without reference to their physical appearance or to the appearance of their differentiated daughter cells. The best evidence suggests that hematopoietic progenitors or stem cells look like lymphoblasts,[88–90] and studies of peripheral blood have shown that BFU-E reside in the nonadherent "null" lymphocyte population.[91]

The pathway of erythroid *precursor* differentiation between the development of proerythroblasts and the mature red cell is known as the erythron and includes the functioning differentiated precursor cells observed in bone marrow aspirates and biopsy specimens. The morphology of erythroid precursor maturation is well described in several texts and is not repeated here. The salient features of the morphologic changes during cell development are related to biochemical and kinetic alterations that were reviewed by Granick and Levere[92] and are shown in Figure 6–8. The residence times spent in each morphologic compartment are shown at the bottom of the figure, but the average transit time from proerythroblast to emergence of the reticulocyte into the circulation is approximately 5 days.[93] In acute anemia, the transit time may decrease to as little as 1 or 2 days by means of skipped divisions.[94] The red cells that emerge are macrocytic and may bear surface i antigen and other fetal characteristics because the abbreviated time in the marrow compartment does not permit complete conversion of i antigen to I antigen or acquisition of certain other adult characteristics.[95] The cells also contain excessive burdens of the rubbish that normally accumulates during cell assembly,[96] because less time is available for the cleansing action of cell proteases and nucleases.[97] Thus, stress erythropoiesis is associated with circulating Pappenheimer bodies (iron granules), basophilic stippling (ribosomes), Heinz bodies (hemoglobin inclusions), and Howell-Jolly bodies (nuclear remnants).

The kinetics of erythropoiesis can be monitored by the use of radioactive iron and surface scanning. The various ferrokinetic patterns in human diseases are shown in Figure 6–9. The total distribution of erythroid marrow can be determined by scintigraphy using ^{111}InCl bound to transferrin, as shown in Figure 6–10.

Both iron-59 (^{59}Fe) kinetics and indium chloride-111 (^{111}InCl) scintigraphy can be useful in the diagnosis of marrow failure, but these techniques are rarely necessary. The initial uptake of ^{59}Fe in marrow is found primarily in proerythroblasts and early basophilic erythroblasts.[98] The same is true of ^{111}In if it is bound to transferrin before injection.[99] Otherwise, ^{111}In labels marrow reticulum cells.

Neutrophil Production

A model that describes the production and kinetics of neutrophils in humans is shown in Figure 6–11. It is highly compartmentalized. The relatively tiny peripheral blood pool is divided into two components in equilibrium; the circulating granulocyte pool (CGP) and the marginating granulocyte pool (MGP). These pools provide entrance into the tissues. The level of circulating cells is buffered by an immense narrow reserve of identifiable precursors, some of which are in the mitotic compartment and others in a maturing storage compartment. The transit times within each compartment are relatively long, so that a huge reserve remains available. The responses of these compartments to various diseases are detailed in Chapter 22. The kinetics of proliferation of recognizable cell precursors have been studied using labeled precursors of DNA. The so-called labeling indices from which mea-

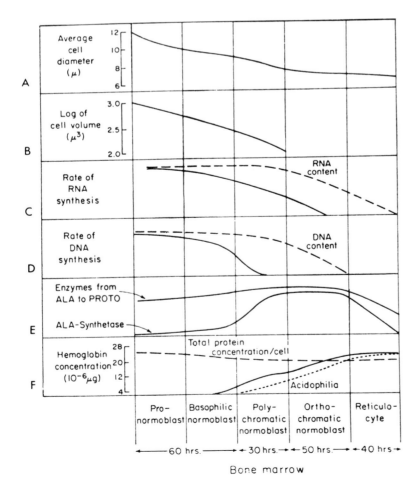

Figure 6–8. Erythroid maturation: alterations in cell size, rates of DNA and RNA synthesis, enzymes involved in heme synthesis, and hemoglobin concentration. Substances listed in the left-hand column are represented by corresponding solid black lines. Unless specified, graphs represent relative values. ALA = δ-aminolevulinic acid; PROTO = protoporphyrin. Considerable protein synthesis takes place during the earliest phase. After this, the nucleolus disappears but mitochondria remain. As the concentration of DNA decreases and the concentration of RNA starts to fall, hemoglobin begins to appear, increasing rapidly in amount. (From Granick S, Levere RD: Heme synthesis in erythroid cells. In Moore CV, Brown EB (eds): Progress in Hematology. Vol. IV. New York, Grune & Stratton, 1964, p 1.)

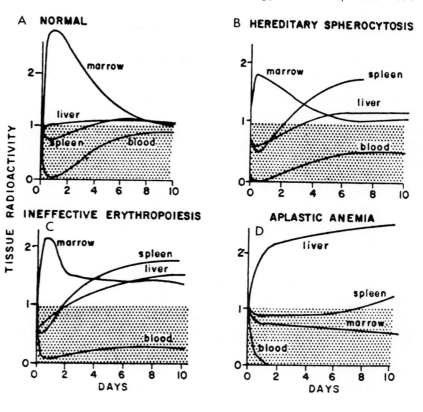

Figure 6-9. Pattern of radioactivity in blood and over sacrum (marrow), liver, and spleen during a ferrokinetic study. Representative data from patients with three different disorders and one normal individual are presented. (From Finch CA: Ferrokinetics in man. Medicine 1970; 49:17. Copyright 1970, The Williams & Wilkins Company, Baltimore.)

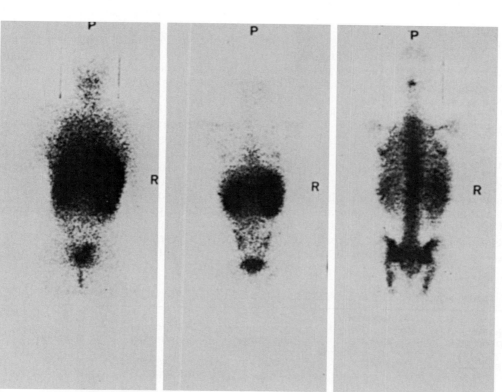

Figure 6-10. Spectrum of scintigraphic patterns in patients with idiopathic aplastic anemia. On the left is a scintigram of a patient before transplantation with renal but no marrow activity. In the middle is a scintigram of a patient with activity in the kidneys and borderline uptake within the marrow. On the right is a normal bone marrow scan in a patient after transplantation. Liver activity is seen in all three patterns, and splenic activity is seen in none. (From McNeil BJ, Rappeport JM, et al: Indium chloride scintigraphy: an index of severity in patients with aplastic anaemia. Br J Haematol 1976; 34:599.)

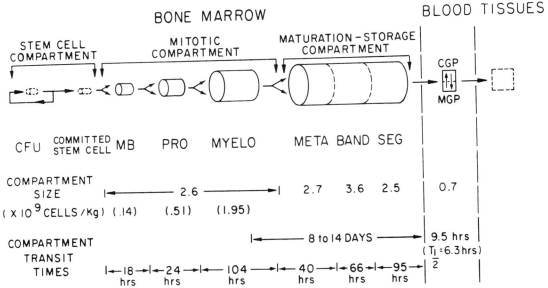

Figure 6-11. Model of the production and kinetics of neutrophils in humans. The marrow and blood compartments have been drawn to show their relative sizes. The compartment transit times, as derived from DF ^{32}P studies, are shown on the next to the last line. Values derived from titrated thymidine studies are shown on the last line. (From Wintrobe MM, Lee RG, et al: Clinical Hematology. Philadelphia, Lea & Febiger, 1975, p 244.)

surements of cell cycle times can be made have served as important approaches to the study of the pharmacology and toxicity of chemotherapy (see Chapter 31).

The final stages of granulocyte production, their release from the marrow, is also multifaceted.[100] At least four factors may influence granulocyte egress: (1) the organization and localization of the cells in relation to vascular channels; (2) the development of nuclear and cytoplasmic changes that increase cell deformability; (3) a hypothetical hormone called cell-releasing factor; and, finally, (4) the regulation of blood flow through vascular channels in the marrow.

Megakaryocyte Development

As shown in Figure 6–12, a morphologically detectable process of megakaryocyte formation begins with the development of an acetylcholinesterase-positive (ACHE+) cell (in the mouse) that is probably analogous to a megakaryoblast and remains capable of division in response to appropriate growth factors that must include the regulatory protein thrombopoietin (see later discussion of hematopoietic growth factors [HGFs]). Further differentiation of the ACHE+ cell into the mature megakaryocyte involves a unique process of cytoplasmic enlargement and nuclear endoreduplication, events that are also influenced by HGFs.

Levine and co-workers[101] and Williams and Levine[102] have provided some valuable cytologic characteristics of the megakaryocytic maturation process (Table 6–1 and Fig. 6–13). The progressive differentiation of megakaryocytes involves the curious endoreduplication phenomenon in which two episodes of chromosomal reduplication proceed apparently at the level of the late progenitor to produce the earliest recognizable megakaryoblast, an 8N cell.[103–105] The process of reduplication of chromosomes continues at the megakaryoblast level to produce 16N and 32N megakaryoblasts. The modal ploidy of the population is 16N. The endowment of DNA within each megakaryocyte is strongly correlated with the cytoplasmic volume of the cell and with the size of individual fragments that

Table 6-1. CYTOLOGIC CHARACTERISTICS OF MEGAKARYOCYTE MATURATION STAGES

Stage	Nuclear Morphology	Cytoplasmic Staining (Wright-Giemsa)	Approximate Size Range	Demarcation Membranes	Granules	Suggested Name
I	Compact (lobed)	Basophilic	6–24 μm	Present by electron microscopy	Few present by electron microscopy	Megakaryoblast
II	Horseshoe	Pink center	14–30 μm	Proliferating to center of cell	Starting to increase	Promegakaryocyte
III	Multilobed	Increasingly more pink than blue	15–56 μm	Extensive but asymmetric	Great numbers	Granular megakaryocyte
IV	Compact but highly lobulated	Wholly eosinophilic	20–50 μm	Evenly distributed	Organized into "platelet field"	Mature megakaryocyte

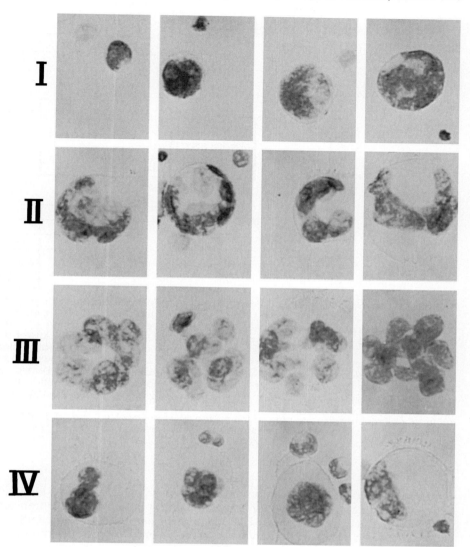

Figure 6-12. Photomicrographs of maturation stages of Feulgen-stained guinea pig megakaryocytes (magnification: ×760). Each row illustrates representative nuclear configurations of maturation stages I, II, III, and IV, respectively. (From Levine RF, Hazzard KC, et al: The significance of megakaryocyte size. Blood 1982; 60:1122.)

emerge from the extruded cytoplasm,[106, 107] but newly formed platelets are remodeled in the circulation to achieve a reasonably uniform size distribution. The spleen probably contributes significantly to the remodeling.

The process of endoreduplication of DNA ceases at the mature megakaryocyte stage, which is why sensitivity to cytotoxic agents is characteristic of early megakaryocyte precursors rather than the more mature precursors and why S-phase–specific cytotoxic agents destroy recognizable megakaryocytes if most of the megakaryocytes are relatively immature,[108, 109] such as in marrows recovering from previous insults or after an episode of thrombolytic thrombocytopenia.

Thus, increased platelet production seems to be derived from megakaryocytes with high ploidy,[110–112] whereas the megakaryocyte pool is replenished by division of cells with lower ploidy.[113, 114] In addition to its effects on platelet production, thrombopoietin appears to be largely responsible for endoreduplication, and thus for increased megakaryocyte ploidy[114–116] and for the general process of megakaryocyte morphogene-

sis.[117] In experimental thrombocytopenia, thrombopenic plasma contains increased thrombopoietin,[118–121] because platelets specifically bind thrombopoietin and remove it from the circulation.[122] When platelet levels fall, plasma levels of "free" thrombopoietin increase.[122] Thrombopoietin mRNA levels in some murine tissues are also inversely correlated with circulating platelet count.[123] Increased levels of circulating thrombopoietin also increase megakaryocyte ploidy.[124]

Bone Marrow Examination and Megakaryocytopoiesis. Despite the fact that the morphology of megakaryocyte development is fairly well established, bone marrow examinations can be of limited value in the various platelet disorders. Bone marrow smears and biopsy specimens provide insufficient data about thrombopoiesis because the final stage of platelet production, extrusion of cytoplasm into the sinusoid, and shedding of platelets (to be described later) is not appreciated by these techniques; only the relative numbers of megakaryocytes and their size and ploidy can be appreciated by routine morphologic methods. It is not surprising that such information is only loosely

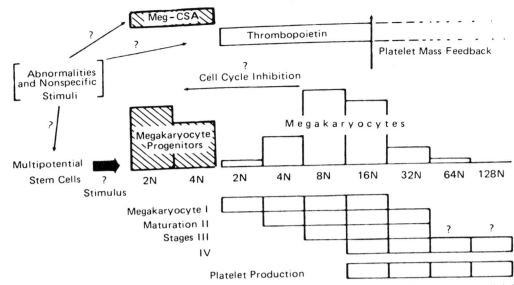

Figure 6-13. Thrombopoiesis. Shown horizontally in the center is the progression from uncommitted multipotential stem cells, through the proliferating progenitors detected in the *in vitro* clonogenic assays, to the spectrum of maturing megakaryocytes. The relative DNA levels of megakaryocytes and their precursors are given as ploidy values (N), where 2N is a diploid cell. The megakaryocytes are also presented vertically in terms of their maturation stages, ending in platelet shedding; a detailed classification of these stages is given in Table 6-1 and Figure 6-12. The columns show the maturation stages at particular ploidy ranges. Thus, 4N megakaryocytes are found at maturation stages I and II. The top row shows a postulated two-level regulatory process with megakaryocyte colony-stimulating activity (Meg-CSA) primarily influencing proliferation of progenitors and thrombopoietin required for megakaryocyte ploidy amplification and possibly for maturation. It is not certain that these regulators are completely exclusive in their target cell specificities as shown. Furthermore, no clear distinction is possible between the specific or nonspecific control of the two factors. Thrombopoietin production is sensitive to variations in platelet mass, as indicated in the figure; it is assumed that this feedback mechanism operates on the source of thrombopoietin. The progenitors might be controlled by cell cycle inhibition, perhaps as a consequence of normal numbers of megakaryocytes. (From Williams N, Levine RF: The origin, development and regulation of megakaryocytes. Br J Haematol 1982; 52:173.)

correlated with platelet production. Furthermore, sampling errors can be responsible for serious misinterpretations. This is a particular hazard in aspirates of neonatal marrow, in which megakaryocytes may be hard to detect whether platelet production is normal or not. Furthermore, megakaryocytes are not evenly distributed in marrow smears. They are more readily found around the edges of the particles, and they may be mistaken for broken cells by the untrained observer. Megakaryocyte nuclei are often found lying free in marrow smears, where they may be erroneously scored as tumor cells. Biopsy sections provide more accurate assessments of megakaryocyte number and distribution than smears, though the latter are usually sufficient (except in neonates) if examined carefully. Biopsies should not be attempted in neonates merely to define megakaryocytes; clinical judgment is a safer tool in these patients.

Examinations of routine marrow smears and biopsy specimens, though instructive, are limited by their two-dimensional views and the thickness of the sections. Megakaryocytes have a peculiar predilection to lie next to the endothelial cell lining of the fronds of developing marrow cells, perhaps because thrombopoietin is produced by these cells. In general, megakaryocytes are too large to squeeze through the sinusoidal meshwork so they merely push their cytoplasms through the fenestrations. The protruding cytoplasms form demarcation lines and then shatter into platelets, which are swept into the blood. The megakaryocyte nuclei rarely make the transfenestration journey into the sinusoids and thence the blood. If they do, they may be mistakenly interpreted by the unwary microscopist as tumor cells in the blood. Intact or partial megakaryocytes are regularly observed in the blood of patients with marrow-invasive diseases such as certain leukemias, metastatic cancers, granulomatous disorders, and fibrosis.

HEMATOPOIETIC GROWTH FACTORS

Beginning with the pioneering work in the early 1960s by Bradley and Metcalf[72] and Pluznik and Sachs,[71] it has been recognized that normal and leukemic blood progenitor cells can be propagated in culture in the presence of soluble growth factors. These factors were originally termed *colony-stimulating factors* (CSFs), based on their ability to support the formation of colonies of blood cells by bone marrow cells plated in semisolid medium.[125, 126] During the 1970s and 1980s, it was recognized that there exist multiple types of CSFs based on the different types of colonies that grow in the presence of the different factors, leading to the hypothesis that the growth and differentiation of blood cells are controlled, at least in part, by exposure of progenitor cells to CSFs having different lineage specificities.[125–127] With the molecular cloning of the genes for many of these factors and their receptors during the 1980s and 1990s it became possible to study in detail the structure, function, and biology of the recombinant CSFs as well as the molecular biology of their respective genes.[126–129] This analysis, along with similar work on the regulation of cells in the immune system, led to the realization that there exists a large family of interacting regulatory molecules now generally known as cytokines or lymphohematopoietic cytokines that together serve to control the hematopoietic and immune systems and to integrate the responses of these systems with those of other systems, perhaps most importantly, the nervous system.[129–132] This interacting network of cytokines includes the interferons,[133] interleukins,[134] tumor necrosis factors,[135] and HGFs (including the CSFs) (Table 6–2).[125, 126] Although certain members of each of these families can directly or indirectly influence hematopoiesis, here the focus is largely on molecules with major effects *in vitro* or *in vivo* in controlling hematopoietic cell growth. These molecules are referred to collectively as HGFs. This is not to imply that the only function or even necessarily that the major function of the factor is in regulation of hematopoiesis but rather that it is potentially significantly involved in regulating hematopoietic cell growth regardless of other functions that it might serve. The molecules selected as important HGFs for more detailed discussion are the colony-stimulating factors (granulocyte CSF [G-CSF],[136] GM-CSF,[126, 137] macrophage CSF [M-CSF, also known as CSF-1][138]), certain interleukins (IL-1[139, 140], IL-3[127, 141], IL-5[129, 142], IL-6[143], and IL-11[144–146]), and other HGFs (EPO,[147–149] thrombopoie-

Table 6–2. HUMAN HEMATOPOIETIC GROWTH FACTORS

Factor	Synonym	Chromosome	Protein (kd)	Source	Biologic Activities	
					Progenitors	**Mature Cells**
SF	Steel factor Stem cell factor Kit ligand	12q2-24	15–20 (×2) soluble and membrane forms	Stromal F, Vasc. Endo	Synergistic: IL-3, IL-11, IL-6 on blast CFC; Synergistic: IL-3, GM-CSF, G-CSF, Epo, Tpo on committed CFC	Mast cell growth
Flk2/Flt3 ligand				Spleen, lung	Synergistic: SF, IL-3, IL-11 on blast CFC; Synergistic: IL-3, GM-CSF, G-CSF on committed CFC; Synergistic: IL-7, SF on B cell progenitors	
IL-3	MultiCSF	5g23-31	15.14	T, mast	All CFC	eo, b, mo
GM-CSF	CSFα	5q23-31	14.4	T, Endo, F, M0	All CFC	n, mo, eo
G-CSF	CSFβ	17q11.2-21	18.6	M0, Endo, F	CFU-G	n
IL-5		5q31	13.2 (2)	T, mast	CFU-eo	eo
M-CSF	CSF-1	1p13-21	26 (×2)	F, Endo, F	CFU-M	m
EPO		7q11-22	18.4	Kidney	BFU-E, CFU-E,	eb
TPO		3q27-28	35	Liver, kidney, F, Endo	CFU-meg	meg
IL-1α		2q13	17	M0, F, Endo, Epi, K, SM	Synergistic: SF, IL-3, on blast CFU	Activates cytokine production
IL-1β		2q13	17	M0, F, Endo, Epi, K, SM		
IL-6		7p15	20.8	M0, T, B, F, Endo, K	Synergistic: SF, IL-3, on blast CFU	
IL-11		19q13.3-13.4	22	Stromal F	Synergistic: SF, IL-3 on blast CFC; IL-3, SF on CFU-meg	meg

eo = Eosinophil; n = polymorphonuclear neutrophil; mo = monocyte; b = basophil; eb = erythroblast; meg = megakaryocyte; Endo = endothelial cell; F = fibroblast; T = T cell; B = B cell; CFC = colony-forming cell; CFU = colony-forming unit; CFU-G = granulocyte CFU; CFU-M = monocyte/macrophage CFU; BFU-E = erythroid burst-forming unit; CFU-E = erythroid CFU; CFU-Eo = eosinophil CFU; CFU-Meg = megakaryocyte CFU; IL = interleukin; GM-CSF = granulocyte-macrophage colony-stimulating factor; G-CSF = granulocyte CSF; M-CSF = monocyte CSF; EPO = erythropoietin; SF = steel factor, TPO = thrombopoietin.

tin,[118] SF[150] [also known as KIT ligand or stem cell factor]), and Flk2/Flt3 ligand (generally known as Flt3 ligand).[151, 152]

Types of Factors

Although there are many ways to categorize the different cytokines and HGFs, for our purposes two different methods are most useful. The first is based on function and the second is through analysis of the sequences of the various HGFs and their receptors. Based on function, the HGFs to be discussed here fall into four groups: (1) lineage-specific factors, including G-CSF, M-CSF, EPO, thrombopoietin, and IL-5; (2) multilineage factors, including IL-3 and GM-CSF; (3) stem cell factors, including SF and Flt3 ligand; and (4) "synergistic" factors, including IL-1, IL-6, and IL-11. As an introduction to the HGFs, this is perhaps the most useful way of categorizing the molecules. However, from an evolutionary standpoint, it is interesting to note that these functionally related molecules largely fall into two gene families based on sequence similarities among themselves and their receptors. Most of the HGFs (and many other cytokines as well) signal through receptors known as "hematopoietin receptors," which are clearly related to each other at the amino acid sequence level.[132, 153–155] Although direct sequence similarity is often difficult to find among the HGFs themselves, the similarities in their three-dimensional structures, in the structures and linkages of their genes, and in the relatedness of their receptors argue that they are all members of a single gene family.[153] The HGFs discussed in detail here which do not use members of the hematopoietin receptor gene family (excluding IL-1) all signal through members of the receptor tyrosine kinase gene family, a large family of receptors that serve many different functions.[156] The HGFs that signal through receptor tyrosine kinases and thereby make up the second HGF gene family are SF,[150] M-CSF,[138] and Flt3 ligand.[151, 152, 157] In addition to the significance in the evolution of the two HGF gene families and their receptors, this classification into two gene families points to important differences in signal transduction triggered by the HGFs. The hematopoietin receptors, which have no intrinsic kinase activity,[155] transmit qualitatively different signals than do members of the receptor tyrosine kinase gene family.[158] Therefore, combinations of HGFs that trigger cells simultaneously through members of both receptor gene families can give very different signals than combinations that are restricted to triggering through one type of receptor. This classification, based on receptor type, should be kept in mind in the discussion of the different HGFs based on their function.

Lineage-Specific HGFs: G-CSF, M-CSF, IL-5, Thrombopoietin, and EPO

Early on, it was recognized that different CSFs could selectively support the growth of specific types of hematopoietic colonies.[125] Thus, when human bone marrow cells are cultured in semisolid medium in the presence of G-CSF, 7 to 8 days later colonies emerge that consist largely of mature neutrophilic granulocytes and their precursors.[125, 136] This led to the model that G-CSF, to a large degree, interacts with relatively late hematopoietic progenitors that have already committed to the neutrophil lineage (CFU-G) and serves to support their growth and final maturation into functional neutrophils.[136] Similar analysis has revealed that the other major hematopoietic cell lineages have analogous, lineage-specific late-acting factors and that these molecules frequently serve as important if not primary regulators of the respective pathways. Thus, M-CSF supports monocyte/macrophage colony growth and is important in supporting the growth and maturation of monocyte progenitors (CFU-M)[138]; IL-5 supports eosinophilic granulocyte colony formation and therefore supports the growth and maturation of eosinophil progenitors (CFU-Eo) as well as activating eosinophils[142, 159]; EPO is necessary for the growth and maturation of both earlier (BFU-E) and later (CFU-E) progenitors of the erythroid lineage[147]; and thrombopoietin directly supports the growth and maturation of megakaryocyte progenitors (CFU-meg) and the subsequent production of functional platelets.[118]

Although the regulation of the respective blood cell pathways by the lineage-specific HGFs is likely to be their major function, in no case is this lineage specificity absolutely maintained. G-CSF has been found to influence the migration and proliferation of endothelial cells, cells that express high-affinity receptors for this cytokine.[160] IL-5 serves as a growth factor for activated B cells, particularly in the mouse, and affects the type of immunoglobulin secreted by mature B cells.[161] EPO[162] and thrombopoietin[163] have been noted to interact with megakaryocyte and erythroid progenitors, respectively. M-CSF appears to be important in trophoblast development.[138] Finally, populations of early HSC have been found to express receptors for many cytokines; typically, these cells do not respond to single factors but require combinations of factors to trigger them into cycle.[164] "Lineage-specific" factors that have been reported to act in various combinations to trigger cycling of early "stem" cells include G-CSF,[165] M-CSF,[166] and thrombopoietin,[167] demonstrating that the molecules are not strictly "lineage-specific" even within the hematopoietic system. However, when administered in vivo, each of these molecules largely influences the growth and development of the expected lineage and the designation of lineage specificity seems warranted.

Multilineage HGFs: IL-3 and GM-CSF

Initial analysis of human bone marrow cell cultures grown in the presence of GM-CSF revealed that a variety of different colony types develop over a period of 10 to 14 days.[168] Mature blood cells that could be readily identified included neutrophils, monocytes/macrophages, and eosinophils. This led to the designation of the molecule as a "granulocyte-macrophage" colony-stimulating factor. In comparison with G-CSF, it was found that it took longer to produce colonies with identifiable neutrophils but the ultimate variety of cell types was greater. This led to a model in which GM-CSF acts on progenitors committed to produce either neutrophils or monocytes (CFU-GM), which is a precursor to the G-CSF–responsive CFU-G and the M-CSF–responsive CFU-M.[125, 168] These later progenitors apparently retain responsiveness to GM-CSF as well because mature monocytes and neutrophils can be observed in cultures supported by GM-CSF alone. That this model is not strictly correct was shown when recombinant GM-CSF was introduced into human bone marrow cultures in the presence of EPO and it was found that this combination of factors was very effective in supporting the development of erythroid colonies (murine GM-CSF is somewhat less effective in this regard).[125, 169, 170] Thus, despite its name, GM-CSF generally interacts with intermediate multilineage progenitors that yield neutrophils, eosinophils, monocytes, erythroid cells, and megakaryocytes (CFU-GEMM). At the time, these activities were similar to those ascribed to IL-3 in the murine system.[171] When human IL-3 was identified, it proved to have similar abilities to support multilineage colony formation, as does human GM-CSF, indicating that it interacts with slightly different but strongly overlapping subsets of progenitors.[172, 173] In comparison with GM-CSF, IL-3 is somewhat more effective in supporting multilineage, erythroid, and megakaryocyte colony formation and GM-CSF is slightly more effective with granulocyte and monocyte/macrophage colony formation.[172, 173] In serum-free conditions, the ability of IL-3 to support final neutrophil and monocyte maturation is significantly depressed, indicating that the later-acting factors, G-CSF or GM-CSF in the case of neutrophils or M-CSF or GM-CSF in the case of monocytes, are necessary for final end cell production.[174]

In addition to acting slightly earlier than GM-CSF, IL-3 is clearly distinguished in its activity by its ability to support the growth and maturation of mast cells and basophils.[175, 176] In the mouse, this was one of the first recognized activities of IL-3[171] and when first administered to primates, basophilia was one of the most prominent findings.[176, 177] Thus, IL-3 appears to be capable of supporting the growth and development of basophil and mast cell progenitors. GM-CSF appears to be important in the differentiation and development of dendritic cells from myeloid precursors, especially in combination with SF and tumor necrosis factor (TNF).[178]

IL-4 in mouse and humans has also been reported to support multilineage colony formation, including colonies that contain cells from the erythroid, megakaryocytic, neutrophilic, and monocytic lineages.[179–181] IL-4 in the mouse supports mast cell growth and therefore shares many activities with IL-3.[161] However, IL-4 plays very important roles in the development and maturation of T cells and B cells[161, 181, 182] and therefore on balance is likely to be more important in controlling immune cell development and function and is not discussed further here. IL-9 in both the murine and human systems has been shown to enhance erythroid colony formation in the presence of EPO[183] and appears to play a role in T-cell development as well,[184] but none of these activities have been very well characterized.

Early Acting HGFs: Steel Factor and Flt3 Ligand

Steel factor, also known as KIT ligand or stem cell factor,[150] and the Flt3 ligand,[152, 157] both receptor tyrosine kinase ligands, interact with a variety of hematopoietic progenitor cells, perhaps most importantly with very early stem cell populations. SF also plays an important role in melanocyte growth and development, which is reflected in the coat color effects of mutations in SF or its receptor, KIT.[150] Genetic analysis of mice clearly showed that mice defective in either SF (*Sl* mice) or in *KIT* (*W* mice) have serious hematopoietic defects, including macrocytic anemia, mast cell deficiencies, and deficiencies in the stem cell compartment.[150] These early studies had already indicated the critical importance of SF in the survival and development of stem cells. Mutations in the human *KIT* gene lead to a similar phenotype in melanocyte development in humans known as the piebald mutation; however, these patients do not have any hematologic problems, probably because severe mutations in this locus are likely to be lethal.[185] *In vitro*, the activities of SF are generally most evident when combined with other HGFs; its proliferative activity with hematopoietic cells in culture as a single factor is minimal.[150] In fact, culture of murine bone marrow cells in SF alone ultimately yields largely mast cells.[186] However, SF acts synergistically to enhance the activities of most of the other HGFs in culture and is particularly effective when combined with HGFs such as IL-3, IL-1, or IL-11 at promoting the expansion of "blast"-like cells that retain considerable potential for yielding multilineage colonies in secondary culture.[187–189] These colonies, when replated under conditions that support B-lymphocyte development or when transplanted into animals, also yield B and T lymphocytes, indicating that SF-responsive cells include primitive stem cells with both lymphoid and myeloid potential.[190, 191] SF has also been implicated in combination with IL-2 or IL-7 in early stages of T-cell development in the thymus,[192] with IL-7 in pre–B-cell growth,[193] and with IL-7 in enhancing natural killer (NK) cell responsiveness to IL-2.[150] However, that none of these lineages are dramatically affected in *W* or *Sl* mice indicates that SF-independent mechanisms can compensate in these lineages.

SF,[194] M-CSF,[195] and Flt3 ligand[196] are all expressed both as membrane-bound and soluble forms. In the case of SF, expression of membrane-bound forms of the molecule in the marrow microenvironment provides a nice model for how this growth factor might act locally. Indeed, cell lines that express exclusively membrane-associated SF are much more effective in supporting long-term hematopoiesis *in vitro* than cell lines that exclusively produce soluble forms of the molecule.[194] This interaction of membrane-associated SF with KIT provides one mechanism for the adherence of hematopoietic cells to stroma; binding of human megakaryocytes to fibroblasts can be blocked by antibodies to

KIT.[197] Finally, membrane-associated forms of SF in which the cytoplasmic domain is essentially missing result in male but not female sterility, suggesting that the cytoplasmic domain may have an as yet undetermined important biologic function.[150, 198]

As shown by the early genetic studies and confirmed through analysis of the recombinant protein, SF is not specific for the hematopoietic system. It is also an important growth factor for melanocytes and primordial germ cells, and it appears to play a role in development of the nervous system, perhaps as a neuronal guidance factor, although it has been difficult to demonstrate neurologic defects in W or Sl mice.[150]

The Flt3 receptor tyrosine kinase was originally identified as a novel receptor present in HSC; with human marrow, the expression is largely limited to the CD34+ cell population.[143, 199, 200] The Flt3 ligand alone yields low numbers of CFU-GM colonies from human bone marrow but acts synergistically with other cytokines, including IL-3, GM-CSF, EPO, and SF to yield enhanced colony formation, both in terms of size and numbers of colonies.[151, 152, 201] The synergy observed between Flt3 ligand and the other HGFs is comparable to that observed with SF in similar systems with the exception that Flt3 ligand has little effect on BFU-E.[157] Multifactor combinations with SF have been used for expansion of colony-forming cells in long-term cultures; Flt3 ligand has effects comparable to those of SF when combined with IL-1, IL-3, IL-6, and EPO in 4-week cultures.[202, 203] Like SF, Flt3 ligand in combination with other cytokines such as GM-CSF supports dendritic cell development from CD34+ bone marrow cells.[178] In contrast to SF, Flt3 ligand does not support the growth and development of mast cells.[151, 152] Despite this overlap in bioactivities, mice in which the Flt3 receptor tyrosine kinase has been disrupted appear to have normal hematopoiesis, with the only detectable defects observed within the B-lymphocyte lineage.[204] However, mice with both the KIT and Flt3 receptor tyrosine kinase genes disrupted display more severe hematologic complications than mice with either single mutation, suggesting that the two pathways can to some degree compensate for one another.[204] The importance of Flt3 ligand in B-cell growth has also been shown with cultures of primitive B-cell progenitors (CD34+/B220-low) in combination with either IL-7 or SF.[205] These findings argue for an important role for Flt3 ligand in hematopoiesis.

Synergistic Factors: IL-1, IL-6, and IL-11

Early in the 1980s, activities were identified that had the ability to enhance hematopoietic colony formation supported by other HGFs, particularly with early progenitor cells. One activity, designated hematopoietin 1, was subsequently purified and discovered to be IL-1.[166] In this fashion, IL-1 was recognized as having little ability on its own to stimulate hematopoietic colony formation but can act in synergy with other HGFs, notably IL-3, in increasing both the frequency of colony formation and the numbers of cells per colony.[206] Subsequent to the discovery of the synergistic activity of IL-

1, numerous other cytokines have emerged with similar activity, including IL-6,[207] IL-11,[208] leukemia inhibitory factor (LIF),[209] and IL-12.[210] Of these, IL-6, IL-11, and LIF all signal through a common signal transducing molecule, the gp130 component of the IL-6 receptor.[211] Because these molecules are likely to behave similarly in most systems and because IL-6 and IL-11 have been the most thoroughly studied, this discussion is limited to these two members of this family. IL-12, which signals through a distinct but perhaps similar pathway to gp130,[212] has interesting effects in combinations with other cytokines[210] but appears to be more important in regulating the development and activities of T and NK cells[213] and is not discussed further.

The effects of IL-1 on hematopoiesis have been highly complicated by the fact that this cytokine is a potent inducer of secondary cytokine production frequently by accessory cells in the culture.[214] The induction of other growth factors, notably IL-6, G-CSF, GM-CSF, and IL-11, is likely to contribute to the activity of IL-1 as a synergistic factor in hematopoietic colony formation. Nevertheless, combinations of IL-1 with other factors in cultures of highly purified hematopoietic cells typically yield synergistic effects, suggesting that at least some of the effects are direct.[215, 216] However, even with highly purified hematopoietic progenitor cell populations, the effects of IL-1 can be indirect. For example, Rodriguez and associates have reported that IL-1 can prevent apoptotic death of CD34+/lin− human bone marrow cells, but the effect is largely abrogated by antibodies to GM-CSF, suggesting that some progenitor cells in the population can produce their own GM-CSF.[217] Thus, the survival effect of IL-1 in some systems may also be indirectly mediated by induction of GM-CSF expression in CD34+/lin− bone marrow cells themselves.

IL-6 is an extremely pleiotropic cytokine with important effects on the growth and differentiation of T and B cells, on the induction of the hepatic acute phase response, and on enhancement of proliferation of hematopoietic progenitor cells.[143] IL-6 signaling, mediated by two members of the hematopoietin receptor gene family, IL-6R[218] and gp130,[219] was the first example of signaling through a commonly shared receptor subunit, gp130, which is now known to be involved in the signaling of LIF, IL-11, oncostatin M (OSM), ciliary neurotropic factor (CNTF), and cardiotrophin-1 (CT-1).[211, 220] Because most cells express gp130, the expression of other receptor components such as IL-6R or IL-11R generally determines whether a cell will respond to one of these family members; cells that express receptors for multiple members of this cytokine subgroup generally exhibit identical or nearly identical responses to each member whose receptor component is expressed by the cell.[211, 221]

The HGF activity of IL-6 was recognized when the cDNA for this cytokine was cloned by functional expression cloning from a human T-cell line that produced a weak colony-stimulating activity that supported modest CFU-GM colony formation with murine bone marrow target cells.[222] More detailed analysis in the murine system and subsequently the human system led to the realization that IL-6 has little if any ability to support colony formation on its own but can enhance colony formation supported by other HGFs, particularly IL-3 and SF.[188, 207] This effect was most prominent using bone marrow cells from mice isolated 2 days after treatment with 5-FU, a drug that enriches for primitive progenitors by selectively killing later, actively cycling cells in the bone marrow.[164] Bone marrow cells treated in this fashion generally yield significant numbers of colonies only when plated in the presence of multiple HGFs. In this system, IL-6 was found to enhance colony formation supported by IL-3 or SF. These early cells are typically quiescent in the G_0 phase of the growth cycle, and combined effects of cytokines, such as IL-3 and IL-6, are required to push them into active cycling.[164] Similar effects have been observed with cultures of purified early human hematopoietic progenitor cells.[223]

IL-11 was originally identified as a stimulatory activity for a murine hybridoma cell line,[224] but characterization in various hematopoietic cell culture systems soon revealed a much broader spectrum of biologic effects.[144, 225] Evaluation of various properties of IL-11 led to the realization that the IL-11 receptor complex employs the IL-6 gp130 signal transducing system. These two HGFs appear to have somewhat overlapping biologic activities.[226] In general, IL-6 has proved to have more effects on T and B cells than IL-11[143, 225] and similar effects in the hepatic acute phase response[227] and on osteoclast formation[228]; but IL-11 is somewhat more potent in megakaryocytopoiesis.[229] Like IL-6, the effects of IL-11 in hematopoietic cultures are largely only observed in combination with other factors. IL-11 in combination with SF or Flt3 ligand has proved to be very effective in supporting the growth of primitive hematopoietic progenitors.[201] In the murine system, the early targets of IL-11 in combination with SF include primitive stem cells that in secondary cultures yield hematopoietic cells and B lymphocytes and when transplanted into irradiated hosts yield T lymphocytes.[190] In combination with Flt3 ligand, IL-11 when plated with highly purified Sca-1+/lin− bone marrow cells in single cell per well cultures, 25% of the wells yielded colonies (75/300) and 23% of the colonies consisted of immature blastlike cells, a higher proportion than any of the other factor combinations tested.[201] Similarly, IL-11 in combination with Flt3 ligand or SF supports the expansion of CD34+ bone marrow cells *in vitro*.[202, 223, 230]

Early after its discovery, IL-11 was shown to have important effects on the growth and development of megakaryocyte progenitors.[224, 225, 229] Again, in this system, IL-11 had little effect on colony formation on its own but was found to act in synergy with IL-3, SF, or, more recently, with thrombopoietin in supporting CFU-meg colony formation.[231] When combined with IL-3, IL-11 increases the number as well as the size of the megakaryocyte colonies.[229] In human cell cultures, these effects are observed preferentially with earlier (BFU-meg) rather than later (CFU-meg) progenitor cell populations.[232] With more mature cells, IL-11 acts by itself in increasing the average ploidy of the mega-

karyocyes.[229] These effects of IL-11 on megakaryocytopoiesis have also been clear *in vivo*; administration of IL-11 to normal mice,[233] primates,[146] or patients[234] results in a significant increase in levels of circulating platelets and, in patients after myelosuppressive chemotherapy, in decreases in the numbers of patients needing platelet transfusions.[235] Finally, although thrombopoietin levels are likely to control the daily levels of platelets in circulation, circulating levels of IL-11 have been found to increase in patients undergoing severe myelosuppressive therapy,[235] suggesting that IL-11 may contribute to hematopoietic recovery after severe damage to the bone marrow.

IL-11 has also shown biologic effects in other systems as well. Within the erythroid lineage, IL-11 interacts with SF and EPO in supporting the formation of macroscopic erythroid bursts.[236] IL-11 appears to affect monocyte/macrophage development; secondary replating of blast colonies in IL-11 alone yields monocyte/macrophage colonies.[208] IL-11 more recently has been found to significantly inhibit production of inflammatory cytokines, including TNF by cultured macrophages.[237] This effect is likely to be a significant component of the anti-inflammatory properties of IL-11 that have been observed.[238] Other cell types that are affected by IL-11 include epithelial cells, which, at least *in vivo*, can be protected from radiation by treatment with IL-11,[239] and adipocyte progenitors, which are blocked from differentiation by exposure to IL-11.[240]

Cloning Hematopoietic Growth Factor Genes

Over the past 15 years, the cDNAs and genes for the HGFs and their receptors have been cloned. This work has provided an incredible array of tools for analysis of the molecular and cellular biology of hematopoiesis beginning with molecular clones for analysis of the expression of the HGF and HGF receptor (HGFR) genes as well as recombinant proteins for evaluation of the biology of the various factors *in vivo* and *in vitro* (see Table 6–2).

Although each cloning project is an important story in its own right, today, the more important information is what has been learned with these various tools. The interested reader is referred to the literature to learn the details of how cDNAs encoding each HGF were isolated. Essentially, the cloning efforts have followed four different strategies. The first to be used successfully was hybridization selection in which pools of candidate cDNAs are placed on nitrocellulose filters for testing for the ability to selectively enrich for messenger RNAs (mRNAs) that can be translated by microinjection into *Xenopus laevis* oocytes to yield the desired HGF biologic activity. This tedious strategy was successfully employed in identification of several cytokine genes in the early 1980s, including the gene for IL-6.[241] A second approach, which has been highly successful, is based on the purification to homogeneity of the protein to be molecularly cloned. By determination of amino acid sequences of peptides from the purified protein, it is possible to synthesize small (generally 13–25mer) DNA probes based on the genetic code that can be used directly to screen cDNA libraries for the desired clone. This methodology has been used by various laboratories to isolate the cDNAs for G-CSF,[242, 243] M-CSF,[244] EPO,[245] SF,[246, 247] and thrombopoietin.[124, 248] During the early 1980s, several laboratories developed methods for screening pools of cDNA clones for the ability to direct the expression of functionally active proteins after DNA transfection in mammalian COS cells. By testing the medium conditioned by the transfected COS cells for the bioactivity, it was possible to identify the desired cDNA clone. This methodology was effective in the identification of cDNA clones for GM-CSF,[249] IL-3,[250] IL-5,[161] and IL-11.[224] Finally, several HGFs have been identified through the use of their receptors when receptors with unknown ligands had been identified. This approach was used by various groups to identify cDNAs encoding SF,[251] Flt3 ligand,[151, 152] and, most recently, thrombopoietin.[248, 252, 253]

Structures of the Hematopoietic Growth Factor Proteins

One of the clear results of the analysis of the structures of the different cytokine genes was the realization that, despite generally low conservation of amino acid sequence, many of the lymphohematopoietic cytokines are distantly related in evolution. Perhaps not surprisingly, this also translates into similarities in protein structure. Together, these observations can be used to further subcategorize the cytokines into families, as proposed by Boulay and Paul.[153] In this scheme, the family can be subgrouped into the growth hormone subfamily (not relevant to this discussion); the IL-4 subfamily including IL-3, IL-4, IL-5, IL-13, and GM-CSF; the IL-6 family, including IL-6, IL-11, and G-CSF; the LIF subfamily, including LIF, OSM, CNTF, CT-1,[220] and IL-12p35; and the EPO subfamily, including EPO and thrombopoietin.[118, 153] Similarly, the receptor tyrosine kinase ligands SF, Flt3 ligand, and M-CSF are also clearly related structurally and evolutionarily.[196, 254]

The IL-4 subfamily consists of cytokine genes localized to chromosome 5 at 5q23-31, including *IL3, GM-CSF, IL4, IL5,* and *IL13*.[255] These cytokines are relatively small hematopoietins whose genes show similar intron/exon structures and whose proteins share several domains of low but significant sequence similarity.[132, 153, 155, 256] IL-4, IL-5, and GM-CSF, like many of the cytokines, have all been shown to have a four α-helical bundle structure in which the first and second helices and the third and fourth helices run parallel to one another, connected by long overhand loops.[153] Within the first helix (helix A) there is a conserved region that has been shown by mutational analysis to be important for receptor binding of IL-3, IL-5, and GM-CSF. This suggests that the different cytokines within this group may also preserve the mechanisms of binding to their respective receptors. Among these cytokines, IL-5 exists as a noncovalent dimer[142] whereas the others are all monomeric.

Members of the IL-6 subfamily, including IL-6, IL-11,

and G-CSF, show rather modest sequence similarity but display common gene organization and certain structural features that suggest evolutionary relatedness.[132, 153, 155] Sequence alignments of IL-6 and G-CSF show conservation of cysteine residues.[257] Interestingly, a cytokine identified in the chicken, myelomonocytic growth factor (MGF),[258] displays sequence similarities with G-CSF and IL-6, which suggests that all three are derived from a common ancestral gene; that corresponding G-CSF and IL-6 genes have not yet been found in chickens raises the possibility that MGF in birds might serve some or all of the functions of G-CSF and IL-6 in mammals. IL-11 shares a lower, but comparable sequence similarity with all of the other members of this gene family; this further divergence is also evident in the fact that IL-11 has lost all of the four cysteines found in the other members of the group.[153] The structure of G-CSF as determined by nuclear magnetic resonance spectroscopy has been reported to be a four α-helical bundle,[259] a structure likely to apply to other members of the group as well.

Before the discovery of thrombopoietin, EPO was the only member of the EPO subfamily. EPO shows some structural features similar to growth hormone and to G-CSF but at a very low level.[153] In contrast, the amino-terminal half of thrombopoietin shows strong sequence similarity with EPO whereas the carboxy-terminal half is unrelated to any known protein.[260–262] Like the other HGFs, EPO is predicted to have a four α-helical bundle structure, and this appears to have been preserved in the related domain of the thrombopoietin gene. The additional domain of thrombopoietin, which is heavily glycosylated, may serve to increase the serum half-life of the molecule. Both of these family members are believed to act as monomers.

The ligands for the receptor tyrosine kinase gene family members, SF, Flt3 ligand, and M-CSF share many common structural similarities.[150, 196, 263] All three contain transmembrane domains and are initially synthesized as dimeric integral membrane proteins. Although the membrane bound forms are functional, dimeric soluble forms are released from the cell by proteolysis and also display biologic activity. The extracellular domains display low but significant sequence similarity, including conservation of the positions of the cysteine residues involved in disulfide bridge formation.[196] Modeling of these extracellular domains indicates that they, too, are likely to form four α-helical bundle structures tethered to the membrane through variable spacer domains with dimerization through a cysteine located in the spacer domain.[196, 254]

Hematopoietic Growth Factor Gene Structures and Disruptions

Hematopoietin Receptor Ligands

G-CSF. The G-CSF gene, which has been localized to chromosome 17 at 17q11.2-q12,[264] consists of five exons spread over approximately 2.3 kb.[265] At the 5' end of the second intron there are two donor splice sites separated by 9 base pairs (bp); alternate splicing at these two different sites results in two forms of G-CSF differing by the insertion of three amino acids corresponding to the nine nucleotides present when the more distal splice donor is used.[265] However, no functional difference has been found between the two different forms of G-CSF, and it is not clear if differential splicing in the G-CSF gene serves a purpose. The chromosomal localization of the G-CSF gene initially led to speculation that it might be involved in the breakpoints of the t(15;17) translocation characteristic of acute promyelocytic leukemia. However, this proved not to be the case because the gene mapped proximal to the breakpoint and is not rearranged in the malignant clone that gives rise to this disorder.[265]

The combination of technology for regenerating mice from cultured embryonic stem cells and the ability to selectively disrupt genes in cultured mammalian cells has led to new methodology for studying gene function *in vivo* (mutants related to HGFs are summarized in Table 6–3).[266] Using this approach, Lieschke and colleagues[267] were able to generate mice with both copies of the G-CSF gene disrupted. These animals develop normally but as adults display 70% to 80% reduction in the levels of circulating neutrophils, a 50% reduction in the numbers of CFU-GM, and impaired resistance to challenge to infections with *Listeria monocytogenes*. These findings, which are in agreement with earlier

observations by Hammond and associates[268] in dogs that had developed cross-reacting antibodies to canine G-CSF, demonstrate the central role for G-CSF in controlling neutrophil levels.

Erythropoietin and Thrombopoietin. The erythropoietin gene *(EPO)*, which spans roughly 3000 bp and consists of five exons and four introns, has been mapped to chromosome 7q21.3-q22.1.[269, 270] Sequence similarity analysis indicated that *EPO* is a member of the cytokine gene family but is relatively distant from most of the other members.[153] However, this changed recently with the isolation of the gene for thrombopoietin. The thrombopoietin gene (THPO) has been localized to chromosome 3q27-28.[260–262] At the amino acid level, the first 153 residues (of a total of 353) show 23% identity to *EPO* (50% with conservative amino acid changes) whereas the remaining 181 residues of the carboxy-terminal domain of thrombopoietin are unrelated to any known proteins.[260] Even more compelling, the intron/exon junctions of the five protein-coding exons of thrombopoietin exactly match, in phase with the intron/exon boundaries of the five exons of the *EPO* gene.[260] Thus, the thrombopoietin and *EPO* genes have clearly evolved from a common ancestor and at some point the extra protein coding region found in the final coding exon of the thrombopoietin gene was either removed (in the case of the *EPO* gene) or added

Table 6–3. GENETIC DEFECTS IN RECEPTORS OR SIGNALING PROTEINS

Human Mutations			
Gene	**Mutation**	**Phenotype**	**Reference**
IL2RγC	Deletion	X-linked severe combined immunodeficiency (SCID)	873
JAK 3	Deletion	SCID	874
GCSFR	C-terminal deletion	Kostmann's disease	463
EPOR	C-terminal deletion	Benign erythrocytosis	534

Nonhuman Mutations				
Species	**Gene**	**Name**	**Phenotype**	**Reference**
Mouse	KIT	White-spotting	Macrocytic anemia, mast cell deficiency, lack of pigmentation, sterile	565, 566, 598
	Steel factor	Steel	Macrocytic anemia, mast cell deficiency, lack of pigmentation, sterile	565, 566, 598
	M-CSF	Osteopetrosis	Osteopetrosis due to decreased osteoclast function	292
	HCP	Motheaten	Immunodeficiency, autoimmune disease, and increased sensitivity to EPO	536
Drosophila	JAK homologue	Hopscotch	Tum^L allele is a gain-of-function mutation that causes leukemia	875, 876

Targeted Disruption in Murine Embryonic Stem Cells		
Gene	**Phenotype**	**Reference**
IL6	Decreased CFU-S and stem cell function	276
GM-CSF	Hematopoiesis normal; progressive accumulation of pulmonary surfactant	286, 287
G-CSF	Neutrophils 25% normal; impaired response to *Listeria monocytogenes* infection	267
EPO	Embryonic lethal—failure of definitive erythropoiesis	272
EPOR	Embryonic lethal—failure of definitive erythropoiesis	272
TPOR (MPL)	Platelets 15–20% normal	271
IL3Rβ	Normal hematopoiesis	714
IL3/5/GMRβc	Similar to *GM-CSF-/-* mice; also low eosinophils and impaired eosinophil response to *Nippostrongylus brasiliensis*	714
VAV	Not required for hematopoiesis	877

(in the case of the thrombopoietin gene) after the early duplication event. In analogy to the situation with IL-6 and G-CSF noted earlier, it may be interesting to analyze the corresponding gene structures in lower vertebrates to better understand how these important genes have evolved.

Although disruption of the thrombopoietin gene has not been reported, mice in which the *MPL* gene has been deleted have been described.[271] Although these animals develop normally and do not display significant abnormalities in bleeding times, they do have only 15% to 20% normal levels of circulating platelets. This result implies that thrombopoietin is very important for maintaining circulating levels of platelets but that other cytokines such as Steel factor, IL-3, and IL-11 are sufficiently redundant with thrombopoietin such that relatively normal hemostasis can be maintained in its absence. In the case of EPO, gene disruption results in embryonic lethality owing to failure of fetal liver erythropoiesis[272]; furthermore, immunization of sheep or rabbits with human EPO results in the development of cross-reacting antibodies that causes life-threatening anemia in the animals (Sklut P, Foster B: unpublished data, 1988). Thus, in the absence of functioning EPO, no other growth factors can sufficiently substitute for maintenance of homeostasis.

IL-6/gp130 Complex Ligands: IL-6 and IL-11. The genes for IL-6 *(IL6)* and IL-11 *(IL11)* have been localized to chromosomes 7p21 and 19q13.3-q13.4,[273, 274] respectively. Both genes consist of five exons and four introns. The gene for G-CSF *(CSF3)*, which has been mapped to chromosome 17q11.2-q12, has a similar structure and is almost certainly distantly related in evolution.[256]

Animals that have been engineered to lack the IL-6 gene develop normally but display significant deficiencies in various immune and inflammatory responses.[275] Interestingly, the hepatic acute-phase response in these animals is severely compromised after tissue damage but only moderately in response to lipopolysaccharide (LPS). The effects of disruption of the IL-6 gene on normal hematopoiesis are relatively minor: a slight decrease in peripheral blood leukocyte counts, 10% reduction in bone marrow cellularity, 50% reduction in CFU-S$_{d12}$, and a four- to five-fold reduction of pre–CFU-S.[276] These defects, plus possible defects in cellular maturation, result in impaired recovery and increased sensitivity to anemia induced by phenylhydrazine, suggesting an important role for IL-6 in hematopoiesis, particularly on early cell compartments. It will be interesting to compare these results with those from mice with homozygous IL-11 gene disruption when they are available.

GM-CSFR Complex Ligands: IL-3, GM-CSF, IL-5. The genes for each of these proteins comprise approximately 3000 bp divided among four (GM-CSF,[277, 278] IL-5,[161, 279]) or five (IL-3[278, 280]) exons with somewhat similar structures. All of these genes have been localized to the long arm of chromosome 5 at 5q23-q31,[255] a region commonly disrupted or deleted in patients with various malignant myeloid neoplasms.[281] This region also contains the genes for other important cytokines, including IL-4, IL-9, the gene for IL-12p40 (IL-12B) and

IL-13.[255, 281, 282] Despite this close clustering of important genes involved in various aspects of regulating the hematopoietic system, analysis of the defects in chromosome 5 from 135 patients has revealed that a minimal critical region at 5q31, deleted in every patient, does not contain any of these cytokine genes, suggesting that they are not generally involved in these malignancies.[281] Detailed mapping of the region has demonstrated that several of these genes are very closely linked: the GM-CSF and IL-3 genes are tandemly arrayed within 9 kb of one another (Fig. 6–14),[283] and the IL-4 and IL-13 genes are separated by only 12.5 kb.[255] This clustering of molecules with similar structures and functions, including sharing receptor components in the case of GM-CSF, IL-3, and IL-5,[284, 285] provides further strong support for the evolutionary relatedness of their respective genes.

Mice with homozygous disruption of GM-CSF develop normally and do not display any numerical defects in the levels of circulating granulocytes or monocytes nor in the levels of CFU-GM progenitors in marrow or spleen.[286, 287] However, these animals exhibit alveolar proteinosis with surfactant accumulation in the lungs based on defective alveolar macrophage function. Thus, GM-CSF plays an irreplaceable role in the function/development of certain macrophage populations but any function played by this cytokine in controlling basal or stimulated production of granulocytes or monocytes can be replaced by other factors. Engineering of mice with IL-3 gene disruptions has not been reported. However, many inbred mouse strains, including *A/J*, *Rf/J*, and *SJL/J* have a mutation that results in aberrant splicing of the specific IL-3α receptor subunit and selective loss of responsiveness to IL-3 without suffering any clear defects in hematopoiesis, suggesting that IL-3 may not serve any essential functions in hematopoiesis.[288, 289] However, these animals are not completely devoid of IL-3 function and, therefore, more complete disruption of the IL-3 gene is necessary to confirm these observations.

Receptor Tyrosine Kinase Ligands: M-CSF, Steel Factor, Flt3 Ligand

With the isolation of the genes encoding the *KIT* ligand (Steel factor) and the ligand for the Flt3 receptor, it has become clear that, like their receptor genes, the M-CSF, Steel factor, and Flt3 ligand genes are all evolutionarily related.[196, 254] The first of these to be identified was the gene for M-CSF *(CSF1)*, which proved to be a large gene (spanning more than 20 kb[290]) containing nine exons that has been localized to chromosome 1p13-21.[291] The gene for SF (the Steel gene) has a similar exon structure and has been localized to chromosome 12q22-q24.[263] The amino acid sequence identity shared by the external domains of these proteins is 16% (32% similarity with conservative changes),[254] and the disulfide structures have been preserved. The more recently cloned gene for Flt3 ligand also shows a similar gene structure with locations of introns reasonably well preserved with those of M-CSF and SF. However, if the sizes of exons are used as a measure of relatedness, the

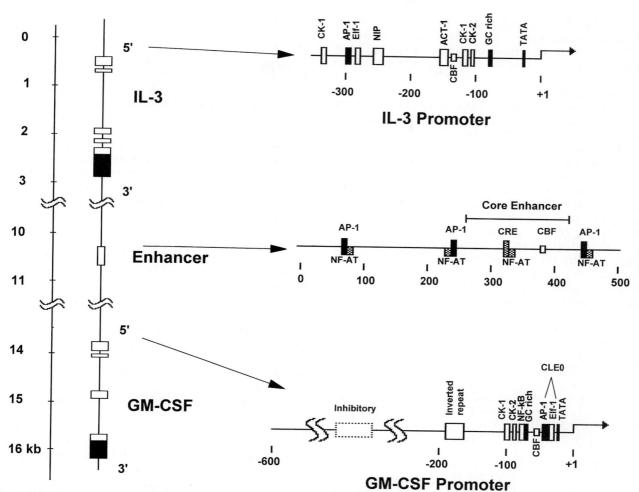

Figure 6-14. Genomic organization of the GM-CSF and IL-3 genes and regulatory elements in the GM-CSF/IL-3 locus of human chromosome 5. The 16-kb DNA map on the left illustrates the gene structures and orientations of the GM-CSF and IL-3 genes. The exons of the genes are shown as wide boxes with the darkened regions representing noncoding sequence. The approximate size and position of the intragenic enhancer is illustrated by a narrow box at approximately position 10.5 kb. The regulatory sequences from each region are illustrated on an expanded scale on the right. The positions of the individual elements are as indicated (see Table 6–4 and the text for definitions). TATA shows the positions of the TATA box in each promoter and +1 indicates the positions of the first nucleotide in the respective mRNAs.

corresponding exons of the latter two factors are more similar, suggesting that they might be more closely related to one another than to Flt3 ligand.[196]

The gene for M-CSF proved to be defective in the spontaneous osteopetrotic mutant mouse (*op/op*).[292] Female *op/op* mice are infertile, confirming the role of M-CSF in the biology of the pregnant uterus.[293] They also have a severe deficiency in the ability to develop osteoclasts derived from the monocytic lineage, resulting in the development of osteopetrosis and the failure to develop teeth.[294] However, the animals do develop some macrophage populations, indicating that M-CSF is important in many but not all macrophage-related lineages. The observation that some of the defects in the *op/op* mouse are corrected as the animals mature has led to speculation that alternative splicing of the mutant M-CSF transcript can lead to production of some functional M-CSF.[295] This raises the necessity of genetically engineering mice with substantial deletions in this gene to see if there is some redundancy in HGF function or if *op* is not a true null mutation.

Naturally occurring mutations in the Steel factor locus (*Sl* mice) or in the receptor for SF, *KIT* (*W* mice) result in profound effects on many stages of hematopoiesis, most notably in the stem cell, erythroid, and mast cell compartments.[150] These studies have clearly demonstrated the central role of SF in controlling hematopoietic cell function. Interestingly, disruption of the Flt3 receptor gene has relatively minor effects on hematopoiesis, the most notable being somewhat depressed levels of B lymphocyte precursors.[204] However, mice with both the *KIT* and Flt3 receptor tyrosine kinase genes disrupted display more severe hematologic complications than mice with either single mutation,[204] suggesting that the two factors do, at some level complement one another *in vivo*.

Hematopoietic Growth Factor Genes: Regulation of Expression

Many different cell types, including T and B cells, monocytes/macrophages, fibroblasts, epithelial cells, and endothelial cells, elaborate various HGFs, especially after stimulation.[127–129, 136] Indeed, Metcalf and associates have reported that conditioned media from murine organ cultures of lung, muscle, thymus, bone shaft, and heart all contain readily detectable levels of many different HGFs and cytokines.[296] However, serum levels of HGFs under steady-state conditions are very low but elevate rapidly after systemic administration of agents such as LPS.[296] Thus, it seems likely that normal hematopoiesis is maintained by low-level expression of HGFs locally in the microenvironment of the bone marrow, spleen, and thymus whereas systemic circulation of HGFs becomes more important after infection.[297] Because HGF production is closely regulated in most cell types, it may be that binding of hematopoietic cells to stromal cells also activates stromal HGF production analogous to the induction of IL-6 expression by binding of myeloma cells to stromal fibroblasts.[298]

Activation of HGF gene expression by various stimuli has been reported for many different cell types.[127–129, 136] This activation serves to accelerate blood cell production in times of stress, such as in response to infection, marrow damage, or severe bleeding. Among the many types of HGF-producing cells, the most prominent include T and B lymphocytes, monocytes/macrophages, and mesodermal cells, including fibroblasts, endothelial cells, and epithelial cells. Expression of some of the HGF genes, notably IL-3 and IL-5, is restricted largely to activated T cells.[161, 299, 300] Activated T cells also produce GM-CSF,[301] M-CSF,[302] and IL-6,[303] but these HGFs are produced by many other cells as well, including both monocytes/macrophages and the various mesodermally derived cells. G-CSF[136] is expressed by monocytes/macrophages and the various mesodermally derived cells whereas the expression of IL-11 is even further restricted because it does not appear to be made by T cells nor by monocyte/macrophages.[145, 225, 304] EPO expression is highly regulated by oxygen tension and is expressed during fetal development in the liver and in adults largely in the kidney.[148, 149] Thrombopoietin appears to be made constitutively in liver and kidney and at lower but inducible levels in the bone marrow.[118] SF[150] and Flt3[151, 152] ligand are broadly expressed in many mesodermal cell types but thus far little is known about the regulation of their expression.

The expression of the HGFs and other cytokines is often triggered in cells by exposure to other cytokines or growth factors, leading to the concept that there are complicated interacting networks of cytokines that serve to control and coordinate many physiologic responses.[130, 131] Finally, the circulating levels of blood cells are known to be directly controlled by production of the HGFs (e.g., EPO in the case of red cells),[148, 149] and therefore the control of expression of these genes is likely to be critically important for maintaining the appropriate numbers of cells. In this section, the expression and the regulation of expression of the different cytokine genes in different cell types are reviewed.

Regulation of mRNA Production

The activation of HGF gene expression is generally reflected by increases in the levels of the respective mRNAs. This is achieved either by enhancing the rate of transcription of the gene or by increasing the half-life of decay of the mRNA or by both mechanisms, as in the case of IL-11 expression in stromal cells.[304] Activators of gene expression, whether they are cytokines such as IL-1[139] or TNF[305] or bacterial products such as LPS,[139] interact with specific cellular receptors, resulting in activation of signal transduction cascades generally involving phosphorylation and dephosphorylation of specific intracellular proteins, calcium fluxes, and translocations of cytoplasmic proteins into the nucleus of the cell.[306] Transcriptional activation occurs through the activation and translocation into the nucleus of positive transcription factors that interact with sequences in the promoters or enhancers of the different genes.[307] These transcription factors are generally believed to stabilize the RNA polymerase II transcription complex that binds to the transcription initiation point in the promoter. This is accomplished either by interacting with the transcription complex or by displacing negative regulatory proteins from the promoter region.[307]

Stabilization of mRNAs inside cells is also a prominent regulatory mechanism for activation of gene expression.[308, 309] In many cell types, cytokine genes are continually transcribed but the resulting RNAs are rapidly degraded under steady-state conditions; in such cells, cytokine mRNA levels can be increased rapidly simply by inhibiting their degradation. This mechanism was first demonstrated in the case of GM-CSF when Shaw and Kamen[308] found that a conserved sequence element, AUUUA, in the 3' untranslated region of the mRNA served to decrease its stability, most likely through interaction with specific proteins.[310] They and others have shown that this destabilizer sequence is found in the mRNAs for most cytokine and transcription factor genes and is frequently important for regulating the levels of those particular mRNAs. The mechanism of increasing the mRNA half-life through interactions mediated by the destabilizer sequence is still poorly understood[311]; however, it is clear, for example, that stimulation of fibroblasts with IL-1 results both in activation of specific positive transcription factors and in activation of a pathway that blocks AUUUA-mediated mRNA degradation.[312] Perhaps not surprisingly, it has also been shown that multiple pathways are involved that can distinguish for example between Fos and various cytokine mRNAs in different cell types.[311, 312] Thus, regulation of gene expression through mRNA stabilization is gene and cell type specific analogous to the regulation through transcriptional activation, although the mechanisms involved are even more poorly understood.

As in other eukaryotic systems, considerable effort has been devoted to the analysis of the control of initiation of transcription of the HGF and cytokine genes in different cell types. This work typically begins with transfection of rather larger pieces of DNA into different cell types to identify regions in or near the gene that either enhance ("enhancers") or inhibit transcription of the gene from its promoter region. This type of analysis, for example, revealed the existence of an important enhancer located between the GM-CSF and IL-3 genes (see Fig. 6–14) that positively affects their expression.[313] More detailed analysis of the promoter function typically follows four approaches.[278] First, sequences flanking the 5' start site of transcription are compared between species and among the various promoters in search of conserved segments that might imply some important function. Second, the DNA flanking the gene is tested *in situ* for sensitivity to DNase because regulatory sequences are frequently "open" for interaction with transcription factors. Third, these and other sequences are evaluated for their abilities to bind to known transcription factors or to proteins found in nuclear extracts from the resting or activated cells of interest. This methodology has frequently been used to purify and molecularly clone genes encoding the different transcription factors. Finally, the promoter region sequences in normal or mutated form are connected to genes whose expression can readily be detected ("reporter genes") such as the enzymes β-galactosidase or luciferase in such a way that their function can be studied by transfection into various cell types. These promoter functional studies are critical for determining whether the transcription factors that bind to the different regulatory elements act in positive or negative fashion.

Comparative analysis of the nucleotide sequences of the various HGF and cytokine gene promoters with themselves and with other eukaryotic promoters has revealed the existence of many conserved sequence elements that serve in the regulation of cytokine gene expression.[299, 314] These sequences, which act as targets or "receptors" for the different transcription factors and transcription factor complexes, appear in different combinations in many of the different HGF promoters; most likely these combinations provide the basis for the unique regulation of each gene in each specific cell type. Some of the more important and more thoroughly characterized sequence elements and the transcription factors (or activation pathways) with which they interact are summarized in Table 6–4. In some cases, these sites have been implicated by homology and functional analysis as being important in regulation of HGF gene expression without definitive identification of the transcription factors involved. Two such sequences, designated cytokine 1 and cytokine 2 (CK-1 and CK-2 or CLE1 and CLE2), have been identified in the promoters of many different cytokine genes,[299, 315] but these sequences may interact with different transcription factors in different cell types and in different promoters.[316, 317] A third sequence, consensus lymphokine element 0 (CLE0), is found in the core of several different promoters; and it, too, interacts with multiple transcription factors.[318]

Functional studies of the various promoters has typically shown that transcriptional activation generally involves the activation of multiple transcription factors that interact in different combinations in different cell types to selectively and optimally induce transcription of the different genes.[319–321] As summarized in Table 6–4, many different transcription factors have been identified that play a role in the regulation of different HGF and other genes as well. Properties of some of the key factors are summarized below:

Table 6–4. REGULATORY ELEMENTS AND TRANSCRIPTION FACTORS INVOLVED IN HGF GENE REGULATION

Element	Sequence	Transcription Factor	Promoter/Enhancer
NF-kB	GGGpuNNPyPyCC	NF-kBp50, Rel A, Rel	IL-6, IL-3, IL-5, GM-CSF, G-CSF, M-CSF
AP-1	TGA(G/C)T(C/A)A	*fos/jun* family	IL-6, IL-3, IL-5, IL-11, GM-CSF, G-CSF
NF-AT	TGGAAGA	NF-ATp, NF-ATc, NF-ATx	IL-3, IL-6, IL-5, GM-CSF
C/EBP Family			
NF-IL6	ATTNNGNAAT	NF-IL, NF-IL6β	IL-5, IL-6, G-CSF
Ig/EBP	TTN(A/T)6(L/T)AAT	Ig/EBP	G-CSF
NF-IL-3a	TAATTACGTCTG	NF-IL3a/E4BP4	IL-3
NF-GMa	GPuGPuGTT(T/G)CAPy		GM-CSF
NF-GMb	TCAGPuTA		GM-CSF
OCT-1	ATGCAAAT	OCT-1	IL-3, IL-5, GM-CSF, G-CSF
CLE0	ATTAATCATTTCCTC		IL-3, IL-5, GM-CSF
CK-1	GAGATTCCAC	CD28 signaling, TNF response	IL-3, IL-5, IL-6, IL-11, GM-CSF, G-CSF
CK-2	TCAGGTA		IL-3, IL-5, GM-CSF, G-CSF
CBF/PEBP2	PuTACCPuCA	Heterodimers of PEBP2β with PEBP2αA or αB(AML-1)	GM-CSF
Ets family			
Ets-1	(G/C)(A/C)GGA(A/T)GPy	Ets-1	IL-5
Elfl	C(A/C)GGA(A/T)GPy	Elf1	IL-3, GM-CSF
PU.I	AGAGGAACT	PU.1	G-CSF
Sp1	(G/T)PuGGC(G/T)PuPu(G/T)	Sp1	IL-6
CRE	TGACGPy(C/A)Pu	CREB	IL-6, GM-CSF/IL-3 enhancer
HIF-1	TACGTGCT	HIF-1	Epo
Hormone receptor response element	(T/C)GACC(T/C) X2	HNF-4	Epo
GATA	(T/A)GATAPu	GATA-3	IL-5

NF-κB. Members of the nuclear factor κB (NF-κB) (also known as the *rel* family) family of transcription factors have been implicated in the inducible expression of many immune and inflammatory cytokines.[322, 323] Classic NF-κB consists of a heterodimeric complex (p50 and p65) that normally exists in the cytoplasm complexed with an inhibitory protein known as IκB. Activation by phosphorylation of IκB results in release of NF-κB and translocation into the nucleus where it binds to the regulatory sequence κB (GGGPuNNPyPyCC), resulting in enhanced transcription from that promoter.

AP-1 (Fos/Jun). In contrast to NF-κB, which pre-exists in cells, expression of transcription factors that interact with the activator protein-1 (AP-1) site (TGA(G/C)T(C/A)A)[324] is rapidly induced after a variety of extracellular stimuli.[319] The AP-1 transcription factors, originally recognized by the ability to interact with a specific sequence in SV40 enhancers have more recently been shown to consist of different complexes of members of the Fos gene family (*cFos, FOS, FRA1,* or *FRA2*) with members of the Jun gene family (cJun, JunB, or JunD). These proteins all contain a stretch of basic amino acids adjacent to a domain that forms an α-helical structure having five to seven leucines aligned along one face of the helix.[319, 325] The basic stretch has been shown to interact with DNA, whereas the leucine rich α-helix has been shown to interact hydrophobically with similar domains on other proteins to form heterodimers or homodimers,[319] leading to the designation "basic-leucine zipper" (bZIP) transcription factors. Many transcription factors have been found to contain such elements.[324]

NF-AT. Analysis of transcription factors induced in activated T cells led to the discovery of a complex designated nuclear factor of activated T cells (NF-AT).[320, 321] Induction of the NF-AT complex, which is sensitive to cyclosporine, proved to involve generation of a complex between members of a new transcription factor gene family, distantly related to NF-κB, designated NF-ATc and NF-ATp (110 to 115 kd) and an AP-1 transcription factor, often a Fos/Jun heterodimer.[321, 326] NF-ATc expression is relatively restricted to activated T cells, whereas NF-ATp is constitutively expressed in many cell types.[321] A third member of this family, designated NF-ATx, has been identified, suggesting that yet other members are to be found.[327] The active NF-AT complex (NF-ATp with Fos and Jun) was originally shown to play a key role in the induction of IL-2 gene expression[328] but is now known to be involved in the expression of many other genes in activated T cells.[320, 321] The minimum consensus sequence for the NF-AT complex is GGA((N)₉TCA.[329] This is a composite of an NF-ATp/c site (core GGAAA); an optimal site is TGGAAAAAT followed by either an AP-1 site (TGAGTCA) or a cyclic adenosine monophosphate response element (CRE) site (TGACGTCA).[329]

C/EBP Gene Family. The first member of the CCAAT/enhancer binding protein (C/EBP) gene family was identified as a bZIP enhancer binding protein related to *MYC* found in liver nuclear extracts.[330] This family, which has been enlarged by the discovery of

transcription factors involved in the activation of IL-6 gene expression, was designated nuclear factor IL-6 (NF-IL6)[331] and the related molecule, NF-IL6β.[332] NF-IL6 was originally identified as a nuclear factor induced by IL-1 expression that was required for activation of the IL-6 gene in response to IL-1. NF-IL6, in addition to regulating IL-6 gene expression, was found to be activated by IL-6 itself and to be important in regulating a number of other genes, including various hepatic acute-phase genes[333] and the G-CSF gene.[334] Another member of the C/EBP gene family, an immunoglobulin enhancer gene binding protein (Ig/EBP), has also been implicated in the transcription of the G-CSF gene.[335]

Ets Gene Family. The *Ets* genes (*ETS1* and *ETS2*) encode homologues of an avian leukemia virus oncogene and are transcription factors that often act cooperatively with Fos and Jun.[336] PU.1, a transcription factor identified from the nuclear extracts from a macrophage cell line as binding to a purine rich sequence (GAGGAA), proved to be related to the *Ets* gene product.[334] PU.1 is predicted to have a helix/loop/helix structure that has been implicated in DNA binding in a number of different proteins. Another member of this gene family, Elf-1, was identified as a transcription factor involved in activation of the IL-2 promoter[337] and has also been implicated in activation of the GM-CSF promoter in T cells.[338]

CRE Binding Proteins. Many promoters respond to activation by the nucleotide signaling molecule, cyclic adenosine monophosphate (AMP) through the cyclic AMP response element (CRE) (TGACGC/TC/AG/A). A family of transcription factors,[307, 324] part of the bZIP family, termed *CRE-binding proteins* (CREB) are nuclear proteins that are activated by phosphorylation that interact with CRE sites to induce gene transcription. Another protein, designated CREB-binding protein (CBP) has been identified that interacts with CREB in activating transcription.[337]

Core-Binding Factor/Polyomavirus Enhancer Binding Protein 2 (CBF/PEBP2). A heterodimeric (α and β chain) transcription factor recognizes the sequence Pu/TACCPuCA in the polyomavirus enhancer A core.[339] Two genes, *PEBP2αA* and *PEBP2αB*, have been identified that encode the α proteins (which bind DNA) and a single gene that encodes the β subunit (which does not bind DNA).[340, 341] Furthermore, *PEBP2aB* is expressed in two alternately spliced forms, leading to different proteins designated PEBP2αB1 and PEBP2αB2.[342] The human homologue of the PEBP2αB gene has been found to be *AML1*,[340] a gene mapped to the breakpoints of 8;21 and 3;21 translocations in certain myeloid leukemias,[343] whereas *PEBP2β* has been mapped to the breakpoint of inversion 16 translocations found in some acute myeloid leukemias.[344] The expression patterns of these genes are also consistent with a role in T cell–specific gene regulations.[345]

GATA Transcription Factors. The first member of this family of transcription factors was identified as an erythroid specific protein that bound the sequence (A/T)GATA(A/G).[346] Subsequently, two other members of the family have been found that are also generally important in hematopoiesis; GATA-3 has been implicated in activation of genes in T cells. These proteins contain DNA binding regions characterized by having multiple zinc atoms coordinated with cysteine and histidine residues known as "zinc fingers."[307]

Octamer Binding Proteins. The original members of this family, Oct-1 and Oct-2, were identified as transcription factors that bind an octamer sequence (ATTTGCAT) found in immunoglobulin gene promoters that were implicated in the activation of immunoglobulin genes.[307] These proteins contain a DNA binding domain known as a homeodomain, originally identified as conserved in several *Drosophila* regulatory proteins.[307] Multiple members of this family have now been reported.[324]

Sp1. Sp1 is a zinc finger–containing transcription factor that was originally identified as an activator of certain SV40 promoters.[307] It has subsequently proved to be involved in the activation of transcription of many different promoters.

Expression of HGFs by Activated T Cells: IL-3, IL-5, GM-CSF, IL-6, and M-CSF

Activation of T cells in response to antigens represents one of the key regulatory steps in controlling the immune system.[347] As part of this process, a variety of T-cell genes become transcriptionally active, including the genes for many cytokines, including GM-CSF,[278, 301] IL-3,[161, 278, 299, 300] IL-5,[161, 299, 348], IL-6,[303] and M-CSF.[302] Among these, expression of IL-3 and IL-5 is largely limited to activated T cells (but also mast cells activated through the IgE receptor[348]), at least in the mouse,[161, 299] whereas the expression of GM-CSF, IL-6, and M-CSF has been observed after activation of many different cell types. IL-6 expression has been commonly observed in murine T cells and T-cell clones, but with human cultures IL-6 expression by mitogen-stimulated T cells requires monocytes; the monocytes could be replaced by phorbol ester.[303] Hempel and co-workers have found that IL-10 interacts directly with T cells to inhibit IL-6 production, suggesting that IL-6 production may be controlled by important components of the cytokine network.[349] M-CSF, although not classically thought to be a T cell–derived HGF, has been shown to be expressed by normal T-cell populations in response to combined triggering of CD2 and CD28.[302] However, because of their relatedness yet differential expression, most attention is focused here on the control of the expression of GM-CSF and IL-3 in T cells.

In situ hybridization studies with purified human cell subsets suggest that CD4, CD8, and NK cells all express GM-CSF and IL-3; however, only a small fraction of T cells produce IL-3 or GM-CSF in response to phorbol 12-myristate 13-acetate (PMA) and the calcium ionophor ionomycin.[301] These studies indicated that only 1% and 10% of the activated T cells express IL-3 and GM-CSF, respectively, but this level could be increased substantially with the addition of IL-2 to the cultures. IL-3 expression is also limited to the CD28 + subset of human T cells.[350] Within helper T-cell subsets, GM-CSF and IL-3 are generally produced by both T_h1

and T_h2 helper T cells whereas IL-5 is largely produced by T_h2 cells.[351] As might be expected from their genetic linkage and similarities in function, the promoter regions of these three genes share numerous regulatory sequences but also display significant differences that likely contribute to the differential regulation of expression in different cell types.[278, 352, 353]

Antigen recognition by the T-cell receptor in combination with a co-stimulatory signal such as provided by CD28 interacting with B7 rapidly switches on intercellular signaling events, including protein phosphorylation, calcium mobilization, and inositol phospholipid hydrolysis. Signal transduction resulting in cytokine gene activation by the T-cell receptor can largely be bypassed by exposure of the cells to phorbol esters such as PMA that activate protein kinase C (PKC) and calcium ionophores (ionomycin) that mobilize calcium ions into the cell.[318, 347] Thus, triggering the T-cell receptor results in PKC activation and calcium mobilization, which ultimately leads to activation of transcription of various cytokine genes. This activation can be blocked by treatment with cyclosporine or FK506 (Tacrolimus).[320, 347] These findings have led to the study of cytokine gene expression in T-cell lines or clones following stimulation with phytohemagglutinin (PHA) to mimic T-cell receptor cross-linking, PMA to induce PKC activation/translocation, and ionomycin to induce calcium mobilization and in the presence of cyclosporine or Tacrolimus as a check for physiologic relevance.

The hGM-CSF promoter region, contained within a 650-bp fragment spanning the region −620 to +34 (relative to the start site of transcription) when linked to the reporter gene luciferase, is transcribed after transfection into PMA/ionomycin-stimulated human Jurkat T cells; this activation is cyclosporine sensitive.[278, 354] Systems such as this have been used to dissect the regulatory elements in the GM-CSF promoter and to identify the protein complexes involved in that regulation. The promoter region has been found to contain multiple DNA elements that together operate cooperatively in the activation of GM-CSF transcription (see Fig. 6–14). Although the nomenclature is not completely standardized, some of the important recognition sites include an inhibitory sequence (−600), a PMA/ionophor-responsive inverted repeat (−192 to −161),[355] two copies of the CK-1 sequence (one at −300 to −292 and the other at −101 to −92), a CK-2 site (−87 to −81) and a region designated CLE0 (−54 to 31).[354, 356] A consensus binding site for NF-κB partially overlaps with CK-2 (−85 to −76) and a GC rich (GC box) sequence (−76 to −71) that in the mouse has been found to bind constitutively expressed proteins in T cells.[357] The region spanned by CLE0 contains recognition sequences for AP-1 transcription complexes (−46 to −40), the transcription factor Ets (−39 to −33), and two repeats of another sequence, CATT(A/T) (−48 to −37), which has been found to be important in GM-CSF promoter function.[358] This complexity reflects the complex interactions of these elements in the GM-CSF promoter with multiple transcription factors in activated T cells, macrophages, and fibroblasts.

The CLE0 region of the murine and human GM-CSF gene (-54 to -31) is critical for promoter function and has been implicated in responses to T-cell receptor signals.[278, 354, 356] This region has been shown to bind the AP-1 (Fos/Jun) and NF-ATp/c, and Elf-1 transcription complexes with cooperative interactions.[338] Because activation of NF-ATp/c is sensitive to cyclosporine, involvement of this transcription complex in GM-CSF promoter function could at least partially account for the cyclosporine sensitivity of GM-CSF gene activation in T cells.[354] The CLE0 region in the mouse promoter has also been shown to bind cooperatively to the combinations of NF-AT, AP-1, and Elf-1, an Ets-related transcription factor expressed by activated T cells.[338, 354] The general picture that emerges is that multiple transcription factors individually bind weakly to their respective recognition sequences and interact cooperatively to form much more stable transcription complexes. Interactions with other transcription factors upstream may serve to further stabilize these complexes and activate the promoter. For example, mutations in the NF-κB site, which is upstream from CLE0, reduced the inducible expression of the GM-CSF promoter by 50%, indicating a role for NF-κB in mediating GM-CSF expression.[356] Thus, within the relatively small region from -85 to -31, the transcription factors NF-κB, NFAT, AP-1, and Elf-1 appear to interact synergistically in activating GM-CSF expression in T cells in a fashion similar to that described for the activation of the IL-2 promoter.[359] Most likely, these positive regulators serve to displace inhibitory, repressor proteins bound to the promoter in steady state. The requirement for multiple transcription factors activated through different pathways provides insurance against unwanted activation of the gene.

Data from several laboratories has implicated yet another transcription factor, CBF, in the regulation of GM-CSF gene expression. This is intriguing because one of the subunits of CBF (also known as PEBP2), PEBP2αB, is the gene *AML1*, a gene implicated in certain myeloid leukemias[340, 343] and another, PEBP2β, has been implicated in yet another subset.[344] A sequence between the NF-κB site and the CLE0 element (-58 to -52) (TGTGGTC) has been implicated as a potent inhibitory sequence, which is also the recognition sequence for CBF.[360] Takahashi and associates have clearly shown that the CBF transcription factor interacts with this region of the GM-CSF promoter, and, depending on which splice variant of the CBFα chain is expressed, the interaction can either stimulate (PEBP2αB1) or inhibit (PEBP2αB2) promoter function.[360] These observations would explain the potent negative regulation mediated by the CBF site in Jurkat cells if PEBP2αB2 were the predominant form of this subunit in the Jurkat cell line. It could also mean that the CBF sequence might be involved in positive regulation of the promoter in other cell types.

The levels of transcription from the core GM-CSF promoter region (-85 to -31) can be influenced by interactions of regulatory proteins with yet other sequences both nearby and somewhat farther away. A strong negative regulatory element has been identified around nucleotide -600[278] as well as a strong positive element around -194 that comprises an inverted repeat that enhances the rate of transcription of the first 150 bp of the promoter by approximately 10-fold.[355] However, this region is bound to a protein complex found in either resting or activated T cells, indicating that it might represent an enhancer sequence that is not specifically involved in activation of T-cell responses. In addition, either CK-1 sequence (found at positions -300 and -101) of the GM-CSF promoter has been shown to bind nuclear proteins and mediate responsiveness to CD28 signals in T cells.[316] CD28 stimulation can increase transcription by three- to six-fold (either CK-1 sequence is sufficient for this activity), and this pathway is not affected by PMA or ionomycin, indicating that NF-AT and AP-1 type transcription factor complexes are not involved. CK-1 has been shown in several promoters to be the response element for CD28-mediated signaling in T cells; however, the same sequence is involved in the responsiveness of the G-CSF promoter to TNF or IL-1 in fibroblasts.[316, 361] Thus, either CD28 and these cytokines share redundancy in their signal transduction pathways or the DNA sequence element CK-1 can interact with different transcription factor complexes in different cell types.

In addition to the regulatory regions immediately adjacent to the GM-CSF gene, an enhancer element has been identified 3 kb upstream from the GM-CSF gene (7 kb downstream from the IL-3 gene), which can upregulate GM-CSF (or IL-3) transcription by 10-fold in response to PMA and ionomycin.[329] This enhancer was initially identified as a PMA/ionomycin-inducible DNase hypersensitive site that was sensitive to cyclosporine treatment. Detailed mapping and sequencing of the region revealed that it contains four NF-AT sites, three of which function as enhancer elements when multimerized. These three sites all bind cooperatively with the NFAT$_p$ and AP-1 transcription factors to form NF-AT complexes. Interestingly, the NF-AT site in the "core" enhancer element (located at nucleotide 420 in Figure 6–14) contains an NFAT$_p$ binding site adjacent to a CRE instead of an AP-1 site.[313] Because this CRE site (TGACATCA) closely resembles the consensus AP-1 site (TGAGTCA), it may be that either AP-1 family members (Fos/Jun) or CREB/ATF proteins can interact with NF-AT family members to generate the NF-AT transcription complex at this site. This NF-AT element is also closely associated with a sequence that resembles the CBF binding site. The model that emerges is that early (within 15 minutes) after stimulation of T cells with PMA and ionophor, NF-AT$_{p/c}$ binds to its high affinity site in the core enhancer region, thereby facilitating AP-1 and CBF binding.[329] These interactions in turn would facilitate further interactions of NFAT$_{p/c}$ and AP-1 with adjacent, lower-affinity sites, thereby stabilizing and activating the entire enhancer region. This activated enhancer could then interact with specific transcription complexes bound to either the GM-CSF or IL-3 promoters to enhance their activities, respectively.

With the exception of the enhancer located between the IL-3 and GM-CSF genes, the regulatory sequences important in the control of IL-3 gene expression appear to lie within a 350-bp fragment upstream of the transcription start site.[278, 362] This region, as can be seen in Figure 6–14, contains sequence elements found in the GM-CSF promoter but also shows several significant differences in overall organization. The IL-3 promoter contains two CK1 sites (positions −333 to −324 and −126 to −117), 1 CK2 site (−115 to −108), an AP-1 site (−301 to −295), and an Ets site (−288 to −278). Masuda and associates[356] have identified a putative CLE0 element (−301 to −285) in the IL-3 promoter, but this region does not appear to be at the "core" of the IL-3 promoter and, therefore, it may not have the same importance that it appears to have in the GM-CSF, IL-4, and IL-5 promoters.[318, 363] In addition to these sites, footprint and functional analysis has identified other important positive elements designated NF-IL3A or ACT-1 (−156 to −147)[341] and IF-I^{IL-3} (for *in vivo* footprint-1) (−140 to −135)[364] and a potent negative regulatory site called nuclear inhibitory protein (NIP) site (−271 to −250).[365] Little is known about the function of the NIP site except that nuclear proteins can be identified that selectively bind to this region.[365] Perhaps regulation around the NIP site might account for the more restricted expression of IL-3 than GM-CSF because the latter promoter does not have an equivalent sequence.

Considerable effort has gone into understanding the interactions of transcription factors with the IL-3 promoter. Beginning at −301, an AP-1 site adjacent to an Ets site has been found to interact with Fos/Jun heterodimers in combination with the Elf-1 transcription factor.[363] This region is not sufficient for induction of IL-3 expression but serves to enhance expression in cooperation with other elements. A second critical region that contains multiple potential regulatory regions is located between −165 and −128. This region has been shown to bind to the constitutively expressed transcription factor Oct-1 (ATGAATAA) in cooperation with an inducible factor that shares properties with the octamer-1 (Oct-1)–associated protein (OAP^{40})[366, 367] originally identified as an inducible protein that cooperates with Oct-1 for binding to the antigen receptor response element (ARRE-1) in the IL-2 promoter.[368] Immediately adjacent to the ACT-1 site, the IF-1 site, identified by footprint analysis, has been found to bind to the transcription factor CBF (as noted earlier, the genes for the two subunits of CBF are related to genes implicated in certain forms of acute myeloid leukemia).[364] The IF-1 site has the sequence TGTGGT, which is closely related to the AML-1/CBF site (TGTGGTC) noted to be inhibitory in the GM-CSF promoter.[278] Presumably, CBF cooperates with the Oct-1/OAP^{40}-like complex bound to the ACT-1 site to enhance transcription of the IL-3 promoter. It will be interesting to compare the transcription complexes bound at the CBF sites in the IL-3 and GM-CSF promoters to understand why CBF acts positively[364] in the former case and negatively in the latter.[358] The 3' half of the ACT-1 sequence has been shown to bind to a transcription factor NF-IL3A, a factor whose expression was reported to be enhanced after activation at least in several T-cell

lines.[369] Clearly, this factor, which is a member of the bZIP transcription factor family, would be a candidate for the inducible OAP^{40}-like protein shown to be important in activation of IL-3 expression in T cells. However, NF-IL3A has proved to be identical to a transcriptional repressor protein, E4BP4, identified as a repressor of the adenovirus E4 promoter, which has been previously reported to be ubiquitously expressed.[370] Because of this complication, it remains to be seen whether NF-IL3A is the same as the OAP^{40}-like protein. IL-3 gene expression mediated by antigen tion of TCR, like that of GM-CSF, is also enhanced lation of CD28.[363] Although this has not been extensively investigated, the conserved CK-1 sequence (−126 in the IL-3 promoter) found in many cytokine genes has, in the case of IL-2 been shown to be the CD28 response element and most likely can account for the effects of CD28 stimulation on IL-3 expression.

Expression of the IL-5 gene, is largely restricted to activated T cells and mast cells (at least in the mouse).[353] In the mouse, IL-5 expression has been one of the defining characteristics of the T helper type 2 (T$_h$2) cell whereas IL-3 is made by both T$_h$1 and T$_h$2 helper T cells.[351] Cyclic AMP, which up-regulates the IL-5 promoter but down-regulates the IL-2 promoter in response to PMA, may contribute to these differences in expression.[371, 372] Many consensus transcription regulatory elements have been identified in the IL-5 promoter region, including Oct-1, NF-IL6, Ets-1, C/EBP, NFAT, CK-1, CK-2, CLE0, and GATA.[348, 353] In the D10 mouse T-cell clone system, the NF-AT site has been found to interact with an inducible NF-AT–related transcription complex involving AP-1.[372] This interaction was enhanced by the addition of cyclic AMP, opposite to its effect on NF-AT binding in the IL-2 promoter, perhaps contributing to the distinction between T$_h$1 and T$_h$2 cytokines. In murine mast cells, activation of the human IL-5 promoter (closely related to the murine) also involves an inducible NF-AT–like activity that interacts with the NFAT site in the absence of AP-1.[348] In this system, a constitutively expressed GATA-family transcription factor also interacts cooperatively with the NFAT factor to enhance expression of the IL-5 promoter.[348] Further work is necessary to determine the roles of the other regulatory elements and their corresponding transcription factors in IL-5 gene regulation.

Expression of HGFs by Monocytes/Macrophages and the Myeloid Leukemias: G-CSF, M-CSF, GM-CSF, IL-6, and Steel Factor

Monocytes/macrophages and related cells including dendritic cells, Kupfer cells in the liver, and Langerhans cells in the skin are key cells that serve many important functions in regulating the immune system.[373] Among the functions performed by these cells is the production of many cytokines, including TNF,[374] IL-1,[140] G-CSF,[136] M-CSF,[374] GM-CSF,[127] IL-6,[143] and IL-12,[373] in response to various stimuli, such as LPS,[373, 374]

IL-1,[130] IL-3,[375] GM-CSF,[376] and M-CSF.[377] Other cytokines, including IL-4,[378] IL-10,[379] and IL-11,[237] downregulate monocyte production of many of these cytokines. These interactions are key components of the interactions between T cells and monocytes in determining the nature and direction of the immune response. Different regulators have been found to induce different subsets of these cytokines. For example, LPS has been shown to induce expression of IL-1, IL-6, TNF, IL-1 receptor antagonist, GM-CSF, and G-CSF.[375] In contrast, IL-3 and GM-CSF failed to induce the expression of either GM-CSF or G-CSF but were found to induce M-CSF expression.[375] M-CSF has been shown to induce peritoneal macrophages to activate expression of GM-CSF and IL-6 at the transcriptional level, but additional signals are necessary to induce the release of the functional cytokine proteins from the cells.[380] Cooperative interactions between NF-κB and NF-IL6 have been implicated in the activation of IL-6 expression in the human monocytic U937 cells and murine P19 embryonic carcinoma cells.[381] Murine bone marrow–derived macrophages have been reported to constitutively express the mRNA for M-CSF and SF, and the level of expression can be enhanced by treating the cultures with pokeweed mitogen.[382]

The different HGF genes in monocytes can be upregulated by a variety of different mechanisms. In the case of IL-6, LPS and Mycobacterium tuberculosis activate gene expression at the transcriptional level through activation of the transcription factors NF-IL6 and NF-κB.[383] NF-IL6 expression increases during differentiation of myeloid leukemias and normal progenitors along monocyte pathways.[384] In contrast, activation of IL-1 and IL-6 expression by Salmonella typhimurium porins is largely mediated by mRNA stabilization.[385] Cytokine activation of monocyte IL-6 expression also occurs by various mechanisms, often involving interactions between NF-κB and NF-IL6.[381] However, LIF treatment of monocytes induces transcriptional activation of the IL-6 gene and this is largely mediated by NF-κB and not NF-IL6.[386] IL-2, IL-3, and GM-CSF have all been shown to induce monocyte expression of IL-6, and this expression is inhibited post-transcriptionally by treatment with IL-4.[375, 378] LPS-activated expression of IL-6 is potently inhibited at the transcriptional level by IL-10.[387] Activation of IL-6 expression by the combination of TNF and IFN-γ in the human THP-1 monocytic cell line involves the interactions of NF-κB, an interferon response element (IRF-1), and Sp1.[388] Activation of IL-6 expression by cyclic AMP or prostaglandins involves an AP-1 site at −280, a CRE at −160, the NF-IL6 element at −150, and the NF-κB site at −70 in a murine monocytic cell line.[389] In the same system, LPS induction is completely abolished by mutation of the NF-κB site with relatively little effect by mutation of the other sites. Perhaps surprisingly, treatment of monocytes with the anti-inflammatory cytokine transforming growth factor-β (TGF-β) also activates IL-6 expression.[390] In the case of G-CSF, expression can be activated by treatment of monocytes with either IL-1 or LPS (IFN-γ potentiates the LPS response)[391] and IL-4 given simultaneously can block this induction, an effect that is not mediated by mRNA stability but rather at the transcriptional level.[392] However, the IFN-γ enhancement effect appears to be largely at the level of mRNA stability; the mRNA half-life with LPS alone treatment is roughly 20 minutes but, after exposure to IFN-γ, the half-life increased to 120 minutes.[391] M-CSF gene expression can be activated in HL-60 cells, an event mediated by NF-κB.[393] These interactions between monocytes and T cells and the cytokines they produce, although complicated, are clearly important in determining the direction and extent of the resulting immune responses and are likely to play a key role in controlling the cytokine network.

Dendritic cells, which have been characterized as potent antigen-presenting cells, are also an important source of HGFs and other cytokines.[394] These cells, identified by morphology and ability to present antigen, may be derived from multiple hematopoietic lineages.[395] Originally believed to be largely of myeloid cell origin, at least some may in fact be derived from a progenitor common to the T, B, and NK cell lineages.[396] Dendritic cells, isolated from human peripheral blood, constitutively express many cytokines, including IL-6, IL-10, TNF, and TGF-β.[395] On activation with PMA they also elaborate IL-1, IL-9, GM-CSF, M-CSF, and G-CSF. In the case of IL-12, exposure of dendritic cells to Staphylococcus aureus or antigen-specific interaction with T cells alone resulted in activation of gene expression.[397] Thus, in the context of antigen presentation, dendritic cells can elaborate cytokines that are clearly important for regulating immune responses; it will be interesting to determine if the various HGFs elaborated by dendritic cells in response to PMA are also induced by direct interaction with T cells.

The growth factor responsiveness of primary leukemias and leukemic cell lines in culture raises the possibility that leukemogenesis might involve the disruption of the normal pathways of growth factor control of hematopoietic cell development.[398, 399] However, analysis of many primary samples of acute myeloid leukemia has revealed that in culture, most require exogenous growth factors, although occasionally the cells spontaneously produce G-CSF or GM-CSF.[398, 400, 401] In some of these cases, GM-CSF production is actually regulated through a paracrine loop in which the leukemic cells make and secrete IL-1, which in turn stimulates endogenous GM-CSF.[402] Thus, despite the commonly observed defects in chromosome 5 surrounding the genes for IL-3 and GM-CSF,[281] activation of the expression does not appear to be a primary event in leukemogenesis but as a secondary event may contribute to the severity of the leukemia.[401] A few cases have been reported in which there was frank overexpression of IL-3 genes by acute lymphocytic leukemic cells in which the IL-3 gene became activated through translocation into an immunoglobulin locus.[403, 404] At least one of these patients had eosinophilia, presumably due to increased levels of IL-3.[404] Both IL-3[405] and IL-11[406] have been reported to be autocrine growth factors for different megakaryoblastic leukemia cell lines, but it is not clear if this represents a property of the original leukemic cells or if selection of the cells in culture might have resulted in the activation of expression of these genes. The IL-3 promoter in megakaryoblastic leukemic cell lines uses many of the same transcription factors that it uses in activated T cells.[407] Finally, juvenile chronic myeloblastic leukemia was suspected of being the cause of autocrine expression of the GM-CSF gene, but more recently, it appears to be due to hyperresponsiveness to this HGF.[408, 409]

Expression of HGFs by Fibroblasts, Endothelial Cells, and Epithelial Cells: G-CSF, M-CSF, GM-CSF, IL-6, and IL-11

Different populations of fibroblasts, endothelial cells, and epithelial cells can be stimulated to produce cytokines by treatment with LPS,[410] phorbol esters,[278] or other cytokines, including IL-1,[139] TNF,[411] and platelet-derived growth factor (PDGF).[412] In many tissues, this is likely to be an integral part of the host response to infection: cytokine production at the site of infection should result in local activation of host defense effector cells and in the systemic recruitment of more effector cells until the infection is cleared.[296] In bone marrow, thymus, and spleen, these cell populations are likely to be critical components of the local microenvironment, which is involved in the normal proliferation, development, and differentiation of cells of the hematopoietic and lymphopoietic systems. The control of production of the various HGFs in the steady state is still poorly understood.[296]

Fibroblasts and endothelial cells are important sources of many of the HGFs, including G-CSF,[136] M-CSF,[138] GM-CSF,[278] IL-6,[413] IL-11,[225] SF,[150] and Flt3 ligand.[151, 152] This expression is regulated both transcriptionally and post-transcriptionally by exposure to LPS, phorbol esters, or cytokines such as IL-1, TNF, and interferon-γ (IFN-γ).[136, 414, 415] SF expression has been reported to be constitutive in human stromal bone marrow cultures, in endothelial cells, and in bone marrow–derived fibroblasts and is not responsive to IL-1.[416]

Although it is not clear that stromal fibroblasts from bone marrow are any more or less capable of cytokine production than fibroblasts from other tissues, because of their proximity to stem and progenitor cells they have long been studied for their ability to express HGFs. Many of these cells constitutively express the tyrosine kinase receptor ligands M-CSF and SF.[416, 417] IL-1 stimulation induces expression of G-CSF, GM-CSF, IL-6, and IL-11[304, 418, 419] and further up-regulates the M-CSF gene, a gene also further activated by IL-6.[411] Much of this induction is mediated by means of mRNA stability. In the case of G-CSF, despite the presence of an IL-1 response element in the promoter region,[361] most of the effect on marrow-derived stromal fibroblasts appears to be related to mRNA stability.[419] IL-6, GM-CSF, and IL-11 all behave similarly.[411] In the case of IL-11, several stromal cell lines have been found to express low constitutive levels of the cytokine and IL-1 induction results in enhanced mRNA stability. The constitutive expression and the activation of IL-11 expression by phorbol esters in the same cells is mediated through binding of a JunD/AP-1 complex to an AP-1 site in the promoter region. Expression of many cytokines, including GM-CSF and IL-6 but not M-CSF, by lung fibroblasts is down-regulated by glucocorticoid hormones such as dexamethasone and mediated by mRNA destablization.[420]

After myeloablation, circulating levels of many HGFs increase dramatically. In some cases this might result from mechanisms that sense low levels of the various blood cells. However, Hachiya and associates[421] have found that, in culture, TNF and IL-1 synergize with irradiation to up-regulate the expression of GM-CSF through both mRNA stabilization and activation of gene transcription. These observations raise the possibility that the myeloablative agents themselves may directly induce or enhance HGF production *in vivo* after various cancer therapy regimens.

IL-6 is expressed constitutively by thymic epithelial cells but is strongly further up-regulated by IL-1, LPS, or TNF.[422] IL-6 expression is also activated in normal bone marrow fibroblasts by myeloma cells, cells that generally require IL-6 for growth. This effect is at least partly transcriptionally regulated through NF-κB.[423] TNF and IL-1 induction of human fibroblasts is also at least in part mediated by NF-κB.[424] In bone marrow fibroblasts and in osteoblasts, IL-6 gene expression is down-regulated by the estrogen receptor, an effect mediated through interactions in the nucleus of the estrogen receptor with NF-κB and NF-IL6.[425] These effects of estrogen on IL-6 expression provide a possible explanation for the relationship between IL-6 and estrogen-deficiency–related bone loss osteoporosis.[426]

The regulation of the G-CSF promoter in fibroblasts shares some similarities and differences with those of the GM-CSF and IL-6 promoters.[361, 427] Regulation of transcription by TNF or IL-1 is mediated by a 330-bp 5' flanking sequence[335, 427]; this same sequence did not function in Jurkat T cells, nor did it mediate the phorbol ester induction of the promoter in fibroblasts.[335, 427] Mutations in any of the elements CK-1, NF-IL6 site, or octamer site abolished promoter function and responses to TNF and IL-1, whereas mutations in CK-2 and PU.1 had no effect.[335] Interestingly, the CK-1 sequence in the G-CSF promoter does not function in T cells, nor does the CK-1 sequence in the GM-CSF promoter mediate TNF induction of GM-CSF in fibroblasts.[317] Like the IL-6 promoter, cooperative interactions with NF-κB and NF-IL6 in binding to CK-1 and other nearby sequences are important in the TNF-mediated induction of promoter activity.[427] In addition, various other factors including Ig/EBP and two members of the activating transcription factor (ATF) family of transcription factors have been shown to interact with the G-CSF promoter in a region near the NF-IL6 site.[428]

Endothelial cells are another important source of HGFs. Human endothelial cells produce G-CSF, GM-CSF, and M-CSF in response to inflammatory cytokines such as IL-1 and TNF.[429, 430] In contrast to G-CSF and GM-CSF, SF mRNA is expressed constitutively by human umbilical vein endothelial cells.[431] The levels of SF mRNA are further increased in response to inflammatory mediators, including IL-1 and LPS. This induction results predominantly from mRNA stabilization by approximately three-fold. Increased expression of GM-CSF mRNA in human umbilical vein endothelial cells is also at least in part mediated by mRNA stabilization.[432] Possibly the induction of SF mRNA in endothelial cells contributes to the elevated plasma levels of this factor in patients with sepsis and patients with inflammatory diseases.[431] Finally, vascular endothelial cells express M-CSF in response to minimally modified low density lipoprotein through transcriptional activation mediated by NF-κB; however, it is not clear how this might contribute to the biology of the macrophage-derived foam cell in the atherosclerotic lesion.[433]

Regulation of Erythropoietin Expression by Hypoxia

Erythropoietin has long been recognized as the physiologic regulator of red cell production.[148, 149, 434] It is produced in the kidney and in the fetal liver in response to hypoxia or exposure to cobalt (II) chloride; the mechanism of the switch of production from predominantly fetal liver to predominantly kidney in adults is largely unknown.[435] Using a transgenic approach, Semenza and associates showed that EPO gene constructs containing 0.7 kb of 3' flanking sequences and 0.4 kb of 5' flanking sequence were inducible in the liver but not the kidneys of hypoxic mice; addition of 5.6 kb of additional 5' sequence suppressed the relatively high basal levels of improper expression and, finally, the further addition of 8 kb of 5' sequence resulted in proper, kidney-specific EPO gene expression.[436, 437] These studies mapped important negative regulatory elements between 0.4 and 6 kb upstream of the EPO gene and kidney-specific regulatory elements to an area between 6 and 14 kb 5' to the gene, indicating a complicated mechanism for regulation of its expression.

Given the complexity and large size of the EPO gene with its regulatory regions and the lack of kidney-derived cell lines, the study of the regulation of EPO expression has largely focused on two liver-derived cell lines, Hep G2 and Hep 3B in which expression is inducible by hypoxia or cobalt chloride.[148, 149] These studies have provided important basic information about the regulation of EPO gene expression in response to oxygen deprivation, but it should be remembered that this does not include the mechanism for kidney-specific expression in adults. Many proteins that react with molecular oxygen do so through a heme moiety, as best studied in the case of oxygen binding to hemoglobin. In hemoglobin, the oxygen binds reversibly to the ferrous iron atom in the center of the heme porphyrin. On oxygen binding, the conformation of the hemoglobin molecule changes. Cobalt or nickel can substitute for ferrous iron, but the poor binding of oxygen to cobalt and the lack of binding to nickel lock the hemoglobin molecule in the "deoxy" state.[148, 149] Finally, carbon monoxide competes with oxygen for binding to the ferrous iron atom. In Hep 3B cells, hypoxia, cobalt and nickel significantly stimulate EPO production whereas carbon monoxide inhibits hypoxia-

but not cobalt-induced EPO expression.[7] These results have been formulated into a model in which primary regulation of EPO gene expression is mediated by a heme protein–based oxygen sensor; binding of oxygen in equilibrium to this putative sensor would shift its conformation between an oxygenated (off) state and a deoxy (on) state; the deoxy form would activate a series of events leading to EPO gene transcription.[148, 149] In this model, cobalt substitution for ferrous iron would result in a failure to bind oxygen ("deoxy" state), thereby resulting in activation of EPO expression and, because carbon monoxide does not bind cobalt, it would not be expected to interfere with cobalt activation of EPO expression. However, cobalt should interfere with hypoxia-induced expression by binding ferrous iron and locking the putative heme protein in the "oxy" state. Further support for this model comes from the observation that inhibition of heme synthesis causes a five-fold reduction in hypoxia-induced EPO production.[148]

Downstream events from the oxygen sensor involved in activation of EPO gene expression require de novo protein synthesis, including the production of specific transcription factors.[438] One of these, a heterodimeric (subunits of 120 and 93 kd) basic helix-loop-helix transcription factor complex designated hypoxia-inducible factor 1 (HIF-1), has been purified and molecularly cloned.[8, 439] HIF-1 is induced in a variety of cell types in response to hypoxia or cobalt, indicating that, although it is important in activation of EPO expression, it is probably also important in the activation of other hypoxia-inducible genes.[8] HIF-1 has been shown to bind to an enhancer sequence located approximately 130 bp downstream from the poly-A addition signal of the EPO gene. This enhancer segment has been shown to render other promoter-reporter gene constructs responsive to hypoxia with typical inductions in the range of 4- to 15-fold, significantly less than the 50- to 100-fold induction observed with the chromosomal EPO gene in Hep 3B cells.[436]

In addition to HIF-1 and its role on the 3' EPO gene enhancer, other studies have identified a 53-bp sequence from the EPO promoter that confers oxygen sensitivity (6- to 10-fold inducibility) to a luciferase reporter gene.[440] Combination of the enhancer and promoter sequences together results in cooperative (50-fold) inducibility of transcription in response to hypoxia, approaching that observed in vivo. Because these sequence elements included the consensus hexanucleotide nuclear hormone receptor response elements, various orphan members of this gene family were examined for binding to the EPO promoter and enhancer and for their presence in transcription complexes isolated from Hep 3B nuclear extracts. One of these, hepatic nuclear factor 4 (HNF-4), proved to be present in these extracts and to play a critical role in hypoxia-induced activation of EPO gene expression in Hep 3B cells.[9] Together, HIF-1 and HNF-4, which are activated in response to hypoxia, have provided considerable insight into the transcriptional regulation of the EPO gene but thus far cannot account for the kidney restriction of expression in adults.

Regulation of Thrombopoietin Gene Expression

The cloning and expression of the gene for thrombopoietin[118] has provided new insight into the regulation of levels of platelets. Gene disruption studies of *MPL*, the receptor for thrombopoietin, in mice have shown that in the absence of the function of this pathway, mice have only 15% of the normal levels of circulating platelets.[271] Thus, whereas redundancy among the growth factors, perhaps including SF, IL-3, IL-6, and IL-11, can partially compensate for dysfunctional *MPL* signaling, thrombopoietin, like EPO in the erythrocyte lineage, appears to be the major regulator of circulating platelet levels.[118] However, in contrast to the control of EPO production, thrombopoietin gene expression does not seem to be transcriptionally regulated nor significantly influenced by platelet levels.[441] In adult mice, the major sources of thrombopoietin mRNA are the liver and kidney; in both organs, the gene is constitutively expressed and is not significantly up-regulated during thrombocytopenia. However, circulating levels of thrombopoietin increase rapidly during thrombocytopenia and decline as platelet counts return to normal.[122, 442] The observation that platelets can remove thrombopoietin from thrombocytopenic plasma *in vitro* has led to the model that thrombopoietin is constantly produced and released into circulation but, in normal circumstances, is rapidly removed by the circulating platelets.[122, 442] During thrombocytopenia, the platelet shortage fails to remove thrombopoietin as fast as it is made, resulting in elevated levels and stimulation of platelet production. This mechanism is similar to one proposed some years ago by Stanley and associates for the regulation of circulating M-CSF levels directly through consumption by the monocytes themselves.[443]

HEMATOPOIETIC GROWTH FACTOR RECEPTORS

Types of Receptors

Analysis of the actions of the HGFs on purified murine or human stem and progenitor cells (see later) has shown that there is considerable overlap in the action of the HGFs. Some insight into the apparent overlap in biologic activities of many cytokines has come from analysis of their structural homologies and from the cloning of many of their receptors. These receptors are all type 1 membrane glycoproteins with extracellular N-termini and single transmembrane domains and fall into two major classes. Receptors such as *KIT*, *FMS* (the M-CSF receptor), and Flt3 are characterized by a cytoplasmic tyrosine kinase domain, whereas most of the other receptors lack cytoplasmic tyrosine kinase activity and can be divided into four subclasses (Table 6–5). Most of the HGFRs (class 1) fall into a superfamily with structural features based on two or more linked fibronectin (FBN) type III domains (Fig. 6–15). Analogous FBN domains are found in the interferon (class 2) receptors, and the class 1 and 2 structures probably evolved from a common primitive adhesion molecule.[444] Whereas the TNF family of receptors (class 3) are characterized by an extracellular four-fold repeat of approximately 40 amino acids that contains six conserved cysteine residues (Cys repeat),[132] the IL-1 receptors (class 4) feature extracellular immunoglobulin-like repeats.

Structure and Binding Properties

Prototypes for the class 1 structure are the (nonhematopoietic) prolactin and growth hormone receptors.[445–447] All these polypeptides show no apparent homology to other known receptors and share a number of features (Fig. 6–16). The major homology lies in the extracellular domain, which is characterized by four conserved cysteine residues in the N-terminal FBN III repeat and a Trp-Ser-X-Trp-Ser (WSXWS) motif in the linked C-terminal FBN III repeat that forms a hydrophobic hinge between the two domains. In addition, the IL-6 family of receptors comprise members that each have an N-terminal immunoglobulin-like domain as well as extra FBN III repeats. The cytoplasmic regions of the receptor family show much less homology, although membrane proximal domains rich in prolines (box 1, within 20 amino acids of the membrane) and acidic residues (box 2), separated by a positionally conserved tryptophan, have been defined. Mutations within the box 1/2 domains have inactivated the mitogenic function of the receptors that have been examined,[448] whereas mutations of the conserved tryptophan inactivate some but not other receptors.[449] An additional interesting feature of many of the HGFRs is that receptor subunits are shared. GM-CSF, IL-3, and IL-5 all have receptors with unique α chains that bind their respective ligands with

Table 6–5. HEMATOPOIETIC GROWTH FACTOR RECEPTOR CLASSES

Type	Receptor	Cytokine
Tyrosine kinase (Ig repeats)	KIT, M-CSFR (FMS), Flt3	Four-α-helix bundle
Non–tyrosine kinase		
Class 1: HGFRs (FBN III domains)		Four-α-helix bundle
Shared βc	IL-3R, GM-CSFR, IL-5R	
Shared gp130	IL-6R, LIFR, IL-11R, IL-12R, OSMR	
Shared γc	IL-2R, IL-4R, IL-7R, IL-9R, IL-15R	
Single chain	G-CSFR, EPOR, TPOR (*MPL*)	
Class 2 (FBN III domains)	IFNα/βR, IFNγR	
Class 3 (Cys-repeats)	TNFR I, TNFR II, FAS, CD40	β-jellyroll wedge
Class 4 (Ig repeats)	IL-1R I and II	β-trefoil fold

TYROSINE KINASE **NON-TYROSINE KINASE**

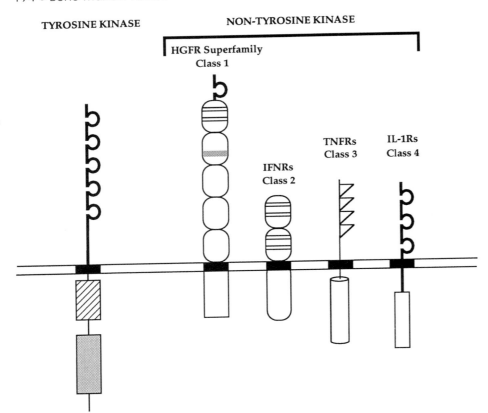

Figure 6–15. Receptors such as *KIT, FMS* (the M-CSFR), and Flt3 are characterized by a cytoplasmic tyrosine kinase domain, whereas most of the other receptors lack cytoplasmic tyrosine kinase activity and can be divided into four subclasses. Most of the hematopoietic growth factor receptors (HGFR) (class 1) fall into a superfamily with structural features based on at least two linked fibronectin (FBN) type III domains (five shown here); analogous FBN domains are found in the interferon (class 2) receptors (IFNRs); the tumor necrosis factor family of receptors (TNFRs) (class 3) are characterized by an extracellular four-fold repeat of approximately 40 amino acids that contains six conserved cysteine residues (Cys repeat); and the interleukin-1 receptors (IL-1Rs) (class 4) feature extracellular immunoglobulin-like repeats.

low affinity. They share a common β chain (βc) that converts ligand binding from low to high affinity in each case and is thought to be critical for signal transduction.[450] A similar arrangement is evident with the IL-6, LIF, OSM, IL-11, and CNTF receptors, all of which share a common β chain, namely gp130. An additional subunit, the low-affinity LIF receptor (LIFR), is shared by LIF, OSM, and CNTF. IL-6 and CNTF also use ligand specific α receptor components, and gp130 is thought to form homodimers when IL-6 binds the IL-6Rα and heterodimers with LIFR in the presence of LIF, OSM, or CNTF. The finding of shared subunits explains to a certain extent why the actions of GM-CSF and IL-3 overlap on many cells and why IL-6, LIF, and IL-11 all share pleiotropic actions on HSC and hepatic cells. The fact that IL-12 is a heterodimer of two polypeptides that are similar to IL-6 and the IL-6Rα provides an explanation for its biologic activities, at least on stem cells, falling into the IL-6 group.[257] The γ chain of the IL-2R is now known to be shared by the IL-4,[451, 452] IL-7,[453] IL-9,[454] and IL-15[455] receptors. Other members of the HGFR superfamily that act on lineage-restricted cells such as EPOR, G-CSFR, and thrombopoietin receptor appear not to require an additional subunit for ligand binding or signal transduction.

The binding properties of receptors for the murine and human HGFs have been characterized using iodinated purified natural or recombinant ligands.[125, 456] Distribution of receptors within the hematopoietic system is restricted to undifferentiated and maturing cells of the appropriate target cell lineages. Because lineage committed progenitor cells respond to more than one

factor, overlap in receptor expression occurs, as noted earlier. A major challenge is to determine whether the overlap represents functional redundancy or indicates subtle and complex control mechanisms that dictate the degree and perhaps localization of the hematopoietic response under different physiologic circumstances.[457] The number of IL-3, GM-CSF, G-CSF, and EPO receptors per cell is strikingly low (about 1000 sites per cell), whereas those for M-CSF are about 1 log higher. In all cases, affinity of a receptor for its ligand is high, with dissociation constants usually in the picomolar range. Stimulation of target cells can occur at concentrations of factor orders of magnitude lower than the equilibrium constant at which 50% of receptors are occupied, and therefore it is apparent that low receptor occupancy is sufficient to produce biologic effects.

Function

Selection Versus Instruction

A major issue is whether HGFs act merely by supporting the survival, proliferation, and differentiation of intrinsically programmed hematopoietic progenitor cells or whether they can recruit or direct differentiation along a particular pathway. If lineage-restricted receptors are important in directing the differentiation of multipotent cells to a particular lineage rather than acting merely as permissive factors, one might expect their expression on earlier multipotent cells or at least induction of expression very early in the sequence of commitment to that lineage. In the case of EPO for

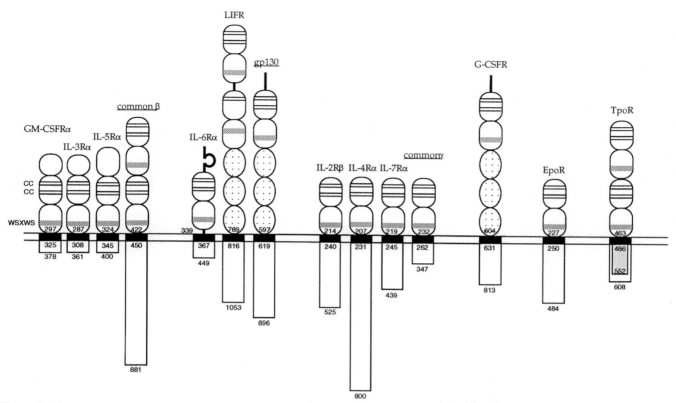

Figure 6-16. HGFR family. Diagram of some of the HGFRs that have been cloned. The extracellular domains are all characterized by one or two regions that contain four conserved cysteines and a tryptophan-serine-x-tryptophan-serine (WSXWS) motif, like the prolactin receptor. Unique features: IL-6Rα contains an immunoglobulin-like domain *(open circle)*; G-CSFR and LIFR contain three additional fibronectin type III–like regions *(dots)*. The intracellular domains show less homology. An additional interesting feature of many of the HGFRs is that receptor subunits are shared (in particular the IL-3R, IL-6R, and IL-2R groups). In contrast, lineage-restricted receptors such as the EPOR, G-CSFR, and thrombopoietin receptor (TpoR) appear not to require an additional subunit for ligand binding or signal transduction. LIFR = leukemia inhibitory factor receptor.

example, binding to EPOR would then lead to expression of other "downstream" erythroid lineage-specific proteins. Data on the expression of different receptors by the most primitive HSC from adults are very incomplete. The *KIT* receptor appears certainly to be expressed on stem cells, but whether receptors for other early-acting factors such as the IL-3 or IL-6 groups are expressed at this stage is uncertain. CD34 cells, a mixture of stem and progenitor cells, express IL-6, IL-3, GM-CSF, and a small number of EPO receptors,[458] whereas noncycling or "G_0" cells that survive 5-FU and are enriched for LTC-IC express KIT, IL-6Rα, gp130, and IL-1R, but interestingly not IL-3Rα or βc.[66] An attractive model, for which there is now both murine[459] and human[458] evidence, suggests that the early-acting synergistic HGFs such as IL-6 up-modulate IL-3R expression; IL-3 in turn up-modulates GM-CSFR and EPOR expression, and GM-CSF also up-modulates EPOR expression. Although these data on normal marrow cells do not show modulation of upstream HGFRs by downstream factors, some data suggest that in cell lines, any mitogenic stimulus, including EPO, can up-modulate IL-3R expression.[460]

Lineage-Specific Factors and the Induction of Differentiation

Do lineage-specific receptors direct differentiation or do intracellular proteins specific for lineage-restricted

cells have that function? With respect to receptor-driven events, a proximal cytoplasmic domain of the G-CSFR is essential for proliferation whereas a more distal domain is important for induction of acute-phase plasma protein expression when the receptor is transfected into hepatoma cell lines[461] or granulocyte specific proteins when it is introduced into murine IL-3-dependent FDC-P1 cells.[462] Support for a role for the G-CSFR in granulocyte differentiation comes from sequence analysis of the receptor in two patients with severe congenital neutropenia (Kostmann's disease) who developed acute myeloid leukemia.[463] Two different point mutations in the G-CSFR gene resulted in truncations of the C-terminal cytoplasmic region of the receptor and co-expression of both mutant and wild-type genes. The mutation was present in the neutropenic phase in one of the patients, suggesting that the mutation was not acquired along with the leukemia. Functional analysis by transfection of mutant or wild-type genes into murine 32D.C10 cells showed that the mutation acted as a "dominant negative" and prevented differentiation in response to G-CSF. Other evidence for an inductive role of receptors comes from murine long-term bone marrow cultures infected with a retroviral *FMS* vector that yielded a pre-B line with an immunoglobulin heavy chain gene rearrangement. This line grew in IL-7 or M-CSF; but interestingly, the switch to M-CSF led to macrophage maturation, suggesting that signals from this receptor can determine differentiation in these bipotent cells.[464] Last, transduction and stable expression of the EPOR in IL-3–dependent Ba/F3 cells results in cells that produce globin mRNA upon EPO but not IL-3 stimulation[465]; and a chimeric receptor that comprises the extracellular domain of GM-Rα and the cytoplasmic domain of the EPOR can induce increased glycophorin A expression in Ba/F3 cells, in contrast to the GM-Rα/βc control.[466] All of these experiments suggest that elements of the cytoplasmic domains of these receptors can direct both proliferation and differentiation.

Although it is intuitively easy to accept that the cytoplasmic domain of a receptor drives a specific response to its ligand, data with hybrid receptors appear to show just the opposite. These experiments show that the pattern of tyrosine phosphorylation induced by ligand binding is dictated more by the extracellular domain of the hybrid receptor than by the intracellular domain.[467–469] Although the pattern of tyrosine phosphorylation does not correlate with any specific differentiation response, these experiments are perhaps most easily explained by postulating that the extracellular domain of these receptors can interact with other proteins that dictate the phosphorylation response.

The view of lineage-specific receptors such as the G-CSFR or EPOR dictating differentiation signals has also been challenged by the introduction of the Bcl-2 gene (BCL2) into murine multipotent IL-3–dependent FDCP-Mix cells.[470] Parental FDCP-Mix cells continue to prolif-

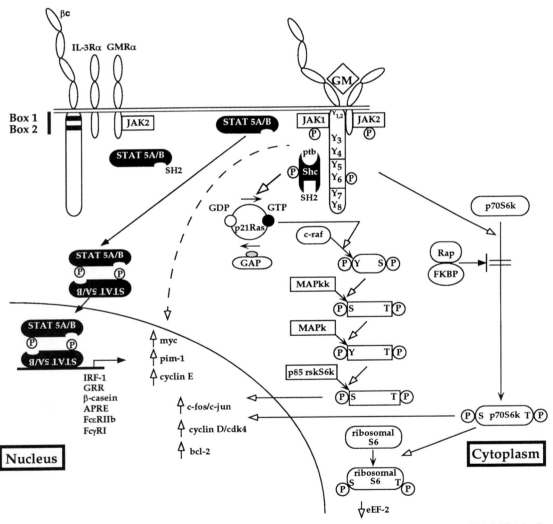

Figure 6–17. Signal transduction through the GM-CSF/IL-3 receptor. The figure illustrates that ligand (GM-CSF) binding (indicated as GM) induces the formation of GMRα/βc heterodimers. This is followed by recruitment of signaling molecules, many of which are shared by other receptors (see Table 6–6). Essential to a proliferative response are the box 1 and box 2 proximal cytoplasmic regions of βc and the proximal cytoplasmic domain of GMRα. JAK1 and JAK2 (Janus kinases) and other nonreceptor tyrosine kinases become phosphorylated, as does βc itself on Y_{750} (Y_6 in the diagram). At least four major pathways are activated: *MYC* and pim-1 induction by the proximal domain, essential for a proliferative response; JAK-mediated activation of STAT 5A and 5B, which translocate to the nucleus and activate transcription of genes with specific recognition sequences in their promoters; Shc phosphorylation and binding to βc, followed by RAS activation and phosphorylation of *RAF*, MAPkk, MAPk, p85S6k(rsk), and induction of Fos/Jun and probably BCL-2, important for cell proliferation and survival; and activation of p70S6k, also correlated with the cell proliferation and inhibited by rapamycin (Rap) bound to FK506 binding protein (FKBP).

erate as blasts in IL-3 and differentiate into myeloid or erythroid cells if the concentration of IL-3 is reduced and GM-CSF, G-CSF, or EPO are added; on withdrawal of IL-3, the cells die by apoptosis. The FDCP-Mix (Bcl-2) cells, however, show a delay in apoptosis in the absence of IL-3 and, remarkably, differentiate into granulocytes, monocytes, or erythroblasts in the absence of added growth factors. The horse serum used in these experiments was, however, able to modulate the differentiation outcome, which suggests that some factors present in serum do influence differentiation in this system.

Taken together, it is reasonable to conclude that the major role of HGF receptors is the survival, amplification, and, particularly in the case of the lineage-specific receptors, the completion of an intrinsic differentiation program of committed progenitor cells.

Signal Transduction

HGF-Induced Tyrosine Phosphorylation. More support for the notion that HGFRs merely amplify populations of intrinsically programmed differentiating hematopoietic cells comes from a wealth of data showing that several signaling proteins and pathways are common to many different receptor types. A paradigm common to receptors both with and without endogenous tyrosine kinase activity is that ligand binding induces homodimerization or heterodimerization of receptor subunits, and this is followed rapidly by transient tyrosine phosphorylation of the cytoplasmic domain of the receptor itself, of cytoplasmic tyrosine kinases, and of other cytoplasmic proteins involved in generating different signaling cascades (Fig. 6–17). In the case of the receptors with intrinsic tyrosine kinases, ligand-induced activation of their catalytic function leads to transphosphorylation or autophosphorylation of dimerized receptor subunits, but receptors that lack

a tyrosine kinase domain must recruit cytoplasmic tyrosine kinases. Data demonstrate that the family of Janus kinases (JAKs) may fulfill this role, but other nonreceptor kinases have been identified and may also be important. It is thought that tyrosine phosphorylation within the receptor cytoplasmic domain creates docking sites for substrates characterized by the presence of Src homology 2 (SH2) domains. These SH2 domains recognize phosphotyrosine in the context of specific short sequences of amino acids.[471]

There are four known members of the JAK family: JAK1, JAK2, JAK3, and TYK2.[472] All are 130- to 134-kd–related proteins that have a carboxy-terminal kinase domain immediately downstream of a pseudokinase domain (Fig. 6–18); three of them (JAK1, JAK2, and TYK2) were first cloned by cDNA rescue of mutagenized cells that failed to respond to interferon-α (IFN-α) or to IFN-γ. Thus, both the TYK2 and JAK1 genes could functionally reconstitute the cellular response to IFN-α in mutant cells that lack the TYK2 or JAK1 proteins, respectively.[473, 474]

Although it first appeared that HGFs activated JAK proteins in a rather promiscuous manner, some patterns have emerged (Table 6–6). Thus, receptors that comprise single chains, such as the EPOR, G-CSFR, and thrombopoietin receptor, associate with JAK2 (or to a lesser extent JAK1) in either a constitutive or ligand-dependent manner. Ligand binding and consequent clustering of receptor molecules lead to JAK2 aggregation and transphosphorylation at the lysine-glutamic acid-tyrosine-tyrosine (KEYY) site in the kinase activation loop (see Fig. 6–18). For example, EPO induces the rapid tyrosine phosphorylation of JAK2.[475] *In vitro* experiments show that JAK2 phosphorylation leads to activation of its kinase function, which, taken together with evidence of association of JAK2 with the EPOR, suggests that JAK2 may act as the "master" protein tyrosine kinase that mediates the biologic re-

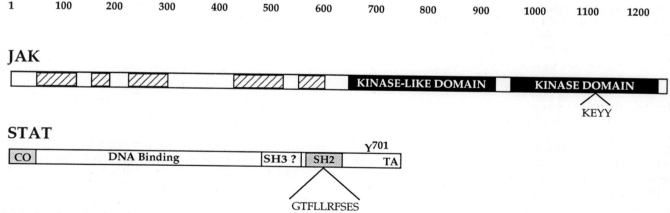

Figure 6–18. Structure of JAK and STAT (signal transducer and activator of transcription) proteins. The JAKs contain a carboxy-terminal tyrosine kinase domain and, immediately amino terminal, a kinase-like domain of unknown function. Blocks that are homologous among family members are indicated as black boxes. The STAT proteins contain an SH2 domain that contains the completely conserved GTFLLRFSS sequence; mutation of the arginine residue eliminates function. The SH2 domain is critical for recruitment to receptors and for STAT dimerization. The SH3-like domain is less conserved and is not known to bind to proline-containing proteins. The DNA binding domain is highly conserved, and after STAT dimerization binds similar symmetric dyad sequences (e.g., STAT 5: TTCC(A→T)GGAA). DNA binding is totally dependent on phosphorylation of a critical tyrosine (Y[701] in STAT 1). The carboxy terminus is required for transcriptional activation (TA). STAT 1β lacks this sequence and acts as a dominant negative. The amino terminus is conserved (CO) and is essential for function. (Data from Ihle.[907])

Table 6-6. JAK/STAT AND NONRECEPTOR PROTEIN TYROSINE KINASES (PTKs) ACTIVATED BY HEMATOPOIETIC GROWTH FACTOR RECEPTORS

Receptor	JAK Family	JAK Activated Stats	Other Nonreceptor PTKs
			PI3K[879-881]
KIT	JAK2[878]		
IFNRα/β	JAK1,[474, 497, 882] Tyk2[473]	STAT1,[883] STAT2,[883] STAT3[496]	
IFNRγ	JAK1,[474, 497, 882] JAK2[474, 497, 882]	STAT1[884]	
IL-3Rα(→βc)	JAK1,[484] **JAK2**[484]	STAT5,[506, 507] STAT6[885]	Lyn,[486, 487] Fyn,[487] Fes,[488] Tec[886]
GM-CSFRα(→βc)	**JAK1,**[485, 489] **JAK2**[485, 489]	STAT5[506, 507]	**Fes**[488]
IL-6Rα(→gp130)	**JAK1,**[499] **JAK2,**[499] **Tyk2**[499]	STAT1,[500, 501, 887] STAT3[499]	**Hck,**[888] **Btk,**[889] **Tec**[889]
IL-2Rα (→β,γC)	**JAK1,**[890, 891]	STAT3[892]	**Lck,**[895] **Fyn**[487]
IL-4,-7,-9,-15Rαs (→γC)	**JAK3**[890, 891]	STAT5,[893, 894] STAT6(IL-4[885])	**Lyn,**[487, 896] **Syk**[897]
EpoR	**JAK2**[475]	STAT5[507, 898, 899]	**Fes**[480]
G-CSFR	**JAK1,**[900] **JAK2**[901-903]	STAT3[901]	**Lyn,**[904] **Syk,**[904] c-rel[905]

Nonreceptor protein tyrosine kinases that associate with receptors are indicated in bold, and references are in superscript.
Adapted from a detailed review by Taniguchi T: Cytokine signaling through nonreceptor protein tyrosine kinases. Science 1995; 268:251. Copyright 1995, American Association for the Advancement of Science.

sponse to EPO. Support for this theory comes from observations that a kinase negative JAK2 acts as a dominant negative suppressor of the proliferative response to EPO[476] and that the box 1/box 2 proximal cytoplasmic domain of the EPOR is the region that both binds JAK2 and is essential for receptor function.[475] However, a number of other substrates are phosphorylated in response to EPO,[477-479] including nonreceptor kinases such as FES,[480] the p85 subunit of phosphatidylinositol 3-OH kinase (PI(3)K), and VAV, substrates such as phospholipase C-γ1 (PLC-γ1) and the adaptor molecule Shc and the tyrosine phosphatases hematopoietic cell phosphatase (HCP, SHPTPI, SHP, or PTP-1C) and Syp (also known as PTP-1D or SH-PTP2).

The other receptors that comprise more than one chain appear to associate with and activate several JAKs (see Table 6-6).[481] The β common component of the IL-3/GM-CSF receptor is tyrosine phosphorylated after IL-3 or GM-CSF stimulation.[482, 483] The tyrosine kinase that is responsible for ligand-induced receptor phosphorylation could be JAK2[484] or JAK1,[485] but the role of other recruited nonreceptor kinases such as lyn,[486] fyn,[487] or Fes[488] has not been clearly defined. Truncation mutants of βc show that the proximal cytoplasmic domain (amino acids 449 to 517) can induce JAK2 tyrosine phosphorylation and kinase activation,[489] and this truncated receptor also retains the capacity to induce MYC and pim-1 and to induce proliferation in serum-replete but not serum-free conditions.[482, 490-492] Both gp130 and LIFR can associate with and activate JAK1, JAK2, and Tyk2, but the pattern of such JAK family activation is distinct in different cell types.[493]

HGF-Induced Activation of STAT Proteins. The paradigm of the response to IFN has provided another major insight into a subsequent step in JAK family signal transduction. The kinase activities of Tyk2 and JAK1 that are activated after IFN-α binding lead to phosphorylation of 91/84-kd and 113-kd cytoplasmic proteins now referred to as STAT1α/STAT1β, and STAT2, respectively, where STAT stands for signal transducer and activator of transcription. STAT proteins are characterized by conserved carboxy-terminal SH2 domains and less conserved SH3 domains (see Fig. 6–18). Tyrosine phosphorylated STAT1α/β and STAT2 form heterodimers through their SH2 domains, bind to a 48-kd protein, translocate to the nucleus, and activate gene expression by binding to an interferon-stimulated response element (ISRE).[494-496] STAT1α is also tyrosine phosphorylated (at Y[701]) after IFN-γ binds to the IFN-γR, and this event is associated with tyrosine phosphorylation of JAK1 and JAK2.[497, 498] STAT1α homodimerizes, translocates to the nucleus, and binds to the IFN-γ activated sequence (GAS), thereby transcriptionally activating genes that contain this sequence in their promoters.

It was therefore no surprise that the JAK proteins activated by HGFRs also lead to phosphorylation and DNA binding of STAT proteins, and four additional members of the STAT family have been cloned: STAT 3, STAT 4, STAT 5, and STAT 6 (see Table 6–6). Thus, it has been shown that ligand-induced activation of gp130, the signal transducing component of the IL-6, LIF, IL-11, OSM, and ciliary neurotropic factor family of receptors, leads to tyrosine phosphorylation of the JAK-TYK family and activation of DNA binding of acute-phase response factor, an 89-kd phosphoprotein antigenically related to STAT1α.[493, 499] The gene for p89 has been cloned (STAT3).[500] Because of its relatedness to STAT1 and STAT2, STAT4 was cloned by low-stringency screening of a cDNA library[501] and by degenerate polymerase chain reaction.[502] Unlike the other STAT proteins, which are ubiquitously expressed, STAT4 expression is restricted to spermatogonia as well as thymic and myeloid cells. STAT4 mRNA levels appear to decline when 32Dcl1 cells differentiate in either G-CSF or EPO.[502] IL-12 has been shown to activate STAT4.[503] IL-3 and GM-CSF have been shown to activate a DNA binding protein of 80 kd that, like STAT1α, recognizes the IFN-γ response region located in the promoter of the Fcγ receptor gene.[504] An ovine DNA-binding activity induced by prolactin called mammary gland factor was cloned and is now named STAT5.[505] STAT5 is activated by EPO and growth hormone,[506] and the murine homologue has been shown to be activated by IL-3,

GM-CSF, and IL-5.[507] This 92-kd protein exists as two highly related proteins, STAT5A and STAT5B (96% identical), that are encoded by different genes. STAT6 is most closely related to STAT5 and is induced by IL-4.[508]

Do the JAK or STAT proteins account for the specificity of signaling through different receptors? The JAK family appears to be rather promiscuous in that any JAK appears capable of phosphorylating any STAT in co-expression studies in COS cells. However, studies of factor-dependent cells do show that there is some specificity in receptor recruitment of JAK and STAT proteins (see Table 6–6). Taking this together with the ability of STAT proteins to form homodimers and heterodimers with different affinities to GAS-like promoter elements might begin to explain the specific responses associated with distinct receptors.

HGF Signaling Through the Ras Pathway. Attention has focused on Ras as a "turnstile" through which signals from many receptors are routed.[509, 510] Ras guanosine triphosphate (GTP) can associate with and activate Raf-1 and mitogen-activated protein kinase (MAPK).[511] Ras is a 21-kd membrane-associated protein that cycles between the active GTP-bound and inactive guanosine diphosphate (GDP)-bound forms in response to extracellular signals from various HGF receptors, including KIT, IL-3, and GM-CSF receptors, T-cell receptor, IL-2R, and EPOR.[512–515] Activation of Ras is mediated by guanine-nucleotide releasing factors (GRFs) that catalyze the release of bound GDP and its exchange for GTP, whereas deactivation occurs by GTPase activating proteins (GAPs) such as p120^{GAP} and neurofibromin that accelerate the intrinsic activity of Ras, leading to hydrolysis of GTP to GDP. The mammalian prototype for GRF-mediated Ras activation is the epidermal growth factor receptor (EGFR), the cytoplasmic domain of which bears intrinsic tyrosine kinase activity. After ligand-mediated dimerization, the EGFR is activated through autophosphorylation or transphosphorylation of tyrosine 1068. An adaptor protein, Grb2, binds to this phosphotyrosine through its SH2 domain. This, in turn, leads to the formation of a ternary complex of EGFR, Grb2, and a GRF called SOS, which is analogous to the *Drosophila* son of sevenless (SOS) protein.[509, 510] SOS contains a proline-rich region that recognizes two SH3 domains of Grb2, and the complex then activates membrane-bound Ras GDP to Ras GTP. The proto-oncogene *VAV* also has Ras GDP/GTP nucleotide exchange activity[516] and is activated through tyrosine phosphorylation after cross-linking of the T-cell antigen receptor/CD3 complex. With respect to the HGF receptors, IL-2–mediated activation of the IL-2R leads to IL-2Rβ chain tyrosine phosphorylation and association of the receptor with Shc, another adaptor protein that is characterized by both an SH2 domain and a second recently described phosphotyrosine binding (PTB) domain.[517, 518] Shc itself becomes phosphorylated on tyrosine, and this in turn leads to recruitment of Grb2 and SOS.[519] The IL-3/GM-CSF–mediated signaling cascade involves phosphorylation of the β subunit itself as well as Shc, with subsequent increased levels of Ras GTP and activation of Raf-1, MAPK ki-

nase, and MAPK, followed by induction of *FOS* and *JUN* (see Fig. 6–17). Interestingly, this activity was mapped to the cytoplasmic domain of βc between amino acids 626 and 763, whereas a more proximal domain (amino acids 449 to 517) retains the capacity to induce *MYC* and pim-1.[491] The PTB domain of Shc has been shown to bind to tyrosine 577 of βc after JAK2-mediated phosphorylation of βc.[520] The C-terminal domain of βc, including the region that activates *RAS*, appeared not to be important for the proliferative response in experiments with receptor-transduced cell lines that were cultured in serum.[482, 490] However, serum can activate *RAS* independently of the receptor; and in serum-free cultures, *RAS* activation is important for both proliferative and survival (prevention of apoptosis) functions.[492, 521] In the case of the EPOR, ligand-induced phosphorylation of Shc and the association of Shc with the EPOR has also been demonstrated; phosphorylated Shc associates with Grb2, and *RAS* and the MAP kinase pathway are activated.[522–526] In summary, these three examples show that *RAS* is activated by a number of HGFRs and that the *RAS*-Raf-MAP kinase pathway may be important for proliferation and survival of hematopoietic cells.

The RAS pathway may also be important in certain leukemias. Neurofibromin, encoded by the NF-1 gene (*NF1*), is mutated in patients with autosomal dominant neurofibromatosis type 1 (NF-1). NF-1 shows sequence homology with yeast and mammalian GAP genes. Children with neurofibromatosis have an increased risk of juvenile chronic myeloid leukemia (JCML), monosomy 7 syndrome, and acute myeloid leukemia.[527, 528] Importantly, leukemic cells from children with NF-1 and myelodysplastic syndrome show loss of the normal NF-1 allele, thus implicating NF-1 as a tumor suppressor gene.[528] NF-1^{GAP} activity is significantly lower in cell lysates prepared from NF-1–associated leukemias than in normal bone marrow or non–NF-1 leukemic lysates.[529] Bone marrow mononuclear cells from patients with JCML show an increase in CFU-GM in response to GM-CSF but not IL-3. Interestingly, fetal liver cells from mice that are rendered null for the NF-1 gene show similar hypersensitivity to GM-CSF, indicating that NF-1^{GAP} may play a crucial and specific role in the response of myeloid cells to GM-CSF.[529, 530] NF-1$^{-/-}$ mice die *in utero* around day 13.5 to 14.5 of complex cardiac defects, but transplantation of day 11.5 to 13.5 fetal liver cells into lethally irradiated recipients produces a myeloproliferative syndrome similar to the human disease.[530] *BCR-ABL* is a chimeric oncogenic protein that shows dysregulated tyrosine kinase activity and is implicated in the pathogenesis of Philadelphia chromosome–positive chronic myeloid leukemia. A phosphorylated tyrosine (Y177) in the *BCR* first exon binds to the SH2 domain of Grb2 and activates *RAS*.[531] Mutation of the Y177 *BCR-ABL* to phenylalanine abolishes Grb2 binding and abrogates both *BCR-ABL*–induced *RAS* activation and transformation of primary bone marrow cultures.[531] In summary, *RAS* dysregulation may contribute to the increased proliferation that characterizes these two chronic leukemias.

Phosphatases and Receptor Signaling. The C-terminal domain of the EPOR has a negative regulatory role.[532] It is likely that this effect is mediated by a phosphatase that dephosphorylates kinase-associated tyrosines in this region, as has been shown for the IL-3R.[533] There is a fascinating report of a Finnish family with dominantly inherited benign erythrocytosis.[534] The proband, an Olympic cross-country skier, has a mutation in the EPOR that introduces a premature stop codon and generates a receptor lacking the C-terminal 70 amino acids. This mutation co-segregates with the disease phenotype in this large family. Data show that the non–transmembrane protein tyrosine phosphatase SH-PTP1 (also called HCP and PTP1C) associates by means of its SH2 domain with tyrosine-phosphorylated EPOR.[535] Mutational analysis mapped the binding site most probably to Y429, and this tyrosine is deleted with the C-terminal truncation of the EPOR in the Finnish family with benign erythrocytosis. Factor-dependent cells that express a Y429,431F mutant EPOR show increased sensitivity to EPO, as do cultured erythroid progenitors from patients with benign erythrocytosis.[535] CFU-E from mice that lack or have impaired SH-PTP1 activity (motheaten or motheaten viable) show a similar increased sensitivity to EPO.[536, 537] Therefore, a strong case can be made for postulating that EPO-induced activation and subsequent tyrosine phosphorylation of the EPOR leads to recruitment of SH-PTP1, which then plays a major role in terminating the EPO signal, possibly through dephosphorylation of JAK2[535] or other tyrosine kinases. Another nonreceptor protein, tyrosine phosphatase, called SH-PTP2 or Syp, has 50% to 60% identity with SH-PTP1 in both SH2 and catalytic domains. Despite this similarity, SH-PTP2 appears to be a positive regulator of some growth factor pathways.[538]

Hematopoietic Growth Factors and the Cell Cycle

To induce cell division, the HGF signaling cascade must eventually activate the cell cycle machinery, which is composed of cyclins, cyclin-dependent kinases, and other regulatory proteins. Data show that HGFs induce cell proliferation by acting during the G_1 phase of the cell cycle on a family of recently identified G_1 or D-type cyclins.[539] Unlike the A-, B-, and E-type cyclins, which periodically oscillate during the cell cycle and regulate the functions of p34cdc2 (cyclin B) and p33cdk2 (cyclins A and E), the D type cyclins (D1, D2, D3) are synthesized in G_1 as delayed early-response genes in response to growth factors (Fig. 6–19). Cyclin D1 associates only with p34cdk4, whereas cyclins D2 and D3 can associate with both p33cdk2 and p34cdk4. Overexpression of cyclin E leads to a reduction in the duration of the G_1 interval,[540] whereas interference with cyclin D1 function by either antibodies or antisense oligonucleotides can prevent entry into S phase.[541] Of great interest is the demonstration that D-type cyclins contain an amino-terminal LXCXE motif that binds to the retinoblastoma gene product pRb. This motif is shared by the oncoproteins SV40 large T antigen, adenovirus E1A, and papillomavirus E7 that also bind to

pRb. In overexpression experiments in insect Sf9 cells, complexes between pRb and D2 and D3 cyclins are destabilized when pRb is hyperphosphorylated.[542] Hypophosphorylated pRb binds to the transcription factor E2F, whereas hyperphosphorylation of pRb and its consequent dissociation from E2F allows E2F to promote the expression of target genes, some of which are expressed in S phase.[543] Further insight into the relationships between cyclins, HGFs, and proliferation versus differentiation comes from cyclin D overexpression studies in murine myeloid IL-3–dependent 32Dcl3 cells.[544] The parental cells, which normally express cyclins D2 and D3 but not D1, self-renew in IL-3 but growth arrest and differentiate into granulocytes if switched to G-CSF. p34cdk4, D2, and D3 cyclin levels correlate with the concentration of IL-3, whereas TGFβ1, which induces cell cycle arrest in mid G1, blocks IL-3–induced expression of p34cdk4 but not of cyclin D2 or D3.[545] In parallel, cyclin D2–associated kinase activity of pRb is induced by IL-3 in vitro and inhibited by TGFβ1 both in vitro and in vivo.[545] Cells that overexpress cyclins D2 and D3 (but not D1) show shortening of the G1 interval, compensatory lengthening of S phase, and inability to differentiate in G-CSF.[544, 546] Cells that express a mutant D2 that cannot bind to or hyperphosphorylate Rb are not blocked in differentiation, whereas the introduction of a kinase-defective mutant p34cdk4 into D2 overexpressors restores the G-CSF differentiation response.[544] Thus these data suggest that Rb (and/or related proteins) may play an important role in the regulation of differentiation, consistent with the observations that targeted disruption of the Rb-1 (RB1) gene results in death in utero with defects in neural development and erythroid differentiation.[547–549] Lethality is probably due to profound anemia that, similar to the GATA-1[550] and MYB[551] knockouts, develops during hepatic hematopoiesis. The control and mutant animals contain equivalent numbers of hepatic CFU-E at day 12.5, but those derived from mutant animals are defective in their differentiation capacity and generate fewer erythrocytes.

Several lines of evidence suggest a role for cyclins in oncogenesis. The proliferating cell nuclear antigen (PNCA) and p21 proteins normally associate with cyclin/cdk complexes. In cells transformed with DNA tumor viruses, p34cdk4 dissociates from cyclin D, PCNA, and p21 and associates instead with a novel 16-kd polypeptide.[552] Cyclin D1 has been implicated in oncogenesis as the putative oncogene (PRAD1) that is rearranged in parathyroid tumors, is translocated (as the BCL1 oncogene) to an immunoglobulin gene enhancer in some B-cell lymphomas and leukemias, and is amplified in other carcinomas (breast, head, and neck).[553–557]

BIOLOGY OF HEMATOPOIESIS

Stem Cells

The formed elements of the blood in vertebrates, including humans, continuously undergo replacement to maintain a constant number of red cells, white cells,

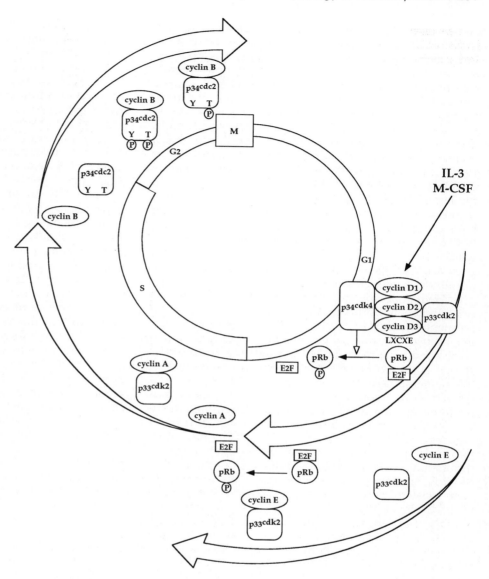

Figure 6-19. The cell cycle. The inner part of the figure shows the phases of the cell cycle. The arrows illustrate the approximate times and oscillating nature of the cyclin regulatory proteins. A, B, and E cyclins appear to oscillate as part of the intrinsic machinery of the cell cycle clock; and as levels increase, they bind to the kinases p33^{cdk2} and p34^{cdc2}. These kinases are activated through complex phosphorylation-dephosphorylation reactions mediated by other kinases and phosphatases (not shown). The G$_1$ or D cyclins are synthesized in response to HGF stimulation such as IL-3 or CSF-1 and bind to p34^{cdk4} (D1, D2, or D3 cyclins) or p33^{cdk2} (D2 and D3 cyclins). These cyclins bear an LXCXE motif that can hyperphosphorylate the retinoblastoma protein (pRb), dissociating it from the transcription factor E2F, which induces genes normally expressed in S phase. Cyclin E/p33^{cdk2} can also mediate this function. (In Sieff CA: Hematopoietic cell proliferation and differentiation. Curr Opin Hematol 1994; 1:310. Copyright 1994, Rapid Science Publishers.)

and platelets. The number of cells of each type is maintained in a very narrow range in the physiologically normal adult individual—approximately 5000 granulocytes, 5×10^6 red blood cells, and 150,000 to 300,000 platelets per microliter of whole blood (see Appendix for normal values in infancy and childhood). In this section the normal regulatory mechanisms that maintain a balanced production of new blood cells are examined. These regulatory systems are far from completely understood, but present evidence strongly supports the following basic principles, schematically depicted in Figure 6–7:

1. A single pluripotent stem cell is capable of giving rise to many committed progenitor cells. These committed progenitors are destined to form differentiated recognizable precursors of the specific types of blood cells.

2. The pluripotent stem cell is capable of self-renewal. The committed progenitor cells are limited in proliferative potential and are not capable of indefinite

self-renewal. In addition to their limited proliferative potential, committed progenitors also "die by differentiation,"[558] and their numbers depend on influx from the pluripotent stem cell pool.

3. The proliferative potential and differentiation of stem cells and committed progenitors may be influenced by adventitial cells or factors derived from them. Thymus-derived lymphocytes appear to contribute to the induction of spleen colony formation in irradiated recipients.[559–562] The hematopoietic role of thymus-derived cells is further supported by experiments demonstrating the defective restorative capacity of bone marrow from congenitally athymic[563] or neonatally thymectomized[564] mice.

4. Committed progenitor cells are capable of response to humoral or marrow stroma derived regulators, some produced in reaction to the circulating levels of a particular differentiated cell type. In this response, they proliferate and differentiate to form the recognizable blood cells. Under this type of control, amplification of production occurs at the committed progenitor

cell level. Most of the regulatory molecules are produced by hematopoietic accessory cells in close proximity to progenitor cells. These molecules are produced as part of an incompletely understood complex regulatory network operating at close range and may involve accessory cell/progenitor cell interactions. For most hematopoietic lineages studied, there appear to be at least two humoral regulators that work sequentially. The immature progenitor of a particular lineage has a greater requirement for a regulator that acts on all or many immature progenitors than do its more mature counterparts. As differentiation proceeds, sensitivity to the late-acting factor increases. This variable degree of response to late-acting regulators that are present at high concentrations during hematopoietic stress (e.g., EPO in anemia) may serve to protect the highly proliferative but numerically limited immature progenitor compartment from exhaustion or death by differentiation under these stress conditions.

5. Hematopoietic differentiation requires an appropriate microenvironment. In normal humans, this environment is confined to the bone marrow, whereas in the mouse the microenvironment includes both the spleen and bone marrow. The existence of the Steel (Sl) strains of mutant mice[565, 566] that exhibit a deficiency in the hematopoietic microenvironment (see later) suggests that the interactions between hematopoietic progenitors and the bone marrow microenvironment involve very specific molecular mechanisms, and recent data have shown that this is, in fact, so.[567] Progenitors may exist outside the marrow but do not normally differentiate in these extramedullary sites. A number of early hematopoietic cells including the pluripotent stem cells and certain committed progenitor cells have been demonstrated in the circulation of normal individuals or experimental animals.[50, 54, 568, 569] The capacity of HSC to negotiate nonhematopoietic tissues through the circulation is especially significant in relation to bone marrow transplantation, which is carried out by infusion of bone marrow or blood cells from the donor into the circulation of the recipient.[48] For example, blockade of hepatic asialoglycoprotein receptors enhances stem cell engraftment in murine spleen and marrow.[570] There is also convincing evidence that murine stem cells (CFU-S) and progenitors (CFU-GM) express "homing" or adhesive lectin receptors that bind to the mannose or galactose presented on stromal cells. For example, homing of transplanted mouse progenitors can be blocked by synthetic neoglycoproteins with these specificities, suggesting that stromal cells are likely to express these sugars.[571]

What controls the decision of CFU-S to undergo either self-replication or commitment to one of the many alternative differentiation pathways? In 1964, Till and co-workers,[558] in their seminal article, proposed that control of this process was "lax" and that any CFU-S could give rise to "colonies with widely differing characteristics." Careful analysis of CFU-S colonies revealed that whereas most colonies contained new CFU-S (self-replication), "their distribution among colonies was quite heterogeneous, with many colonies

containing few colony-forming cells and few containing very many." Over 20 years later, Suda and colleagues[69] analyzed the differentiation of murine hematopoietic colonies derived from paired progenitors (i.e., CFU-blast progenitors allowed to undergo one division) in culture and showed similar diversity in the colonies derived from each member of over 25% of the pairs. These observations lend further support for lax control or a "stochastic" mechanism of stem cell differentiation and indicate that, as well as amplification, control of differentiation must occur at the committed progenitor cell level.

If only 10% to 20% of stem cells are in cycle in the resting state, what is their role with regard to self-renewal versus differentiation and what is the role of the noncycling stem cells? The hypothesis that a series of stem cells may contribute clones successively to maintain hematopoiesis throughout the life span of an individual was first advanced by Kay.[572] Support for this hypothesis comes from transplant studies of recipients of small numbers of bone marrow cells[573, 574] and from experiments in which mixtures of fetal liver cells from different inbred mouse strains were introduced into W-mutant fetuses. W mutants exhibit a genetically determined deficiency of hematopoietic (as well as germ and follicle) stem cells (see later). Long-term monitoring showed clonal dominance followed by decline of cells of particular genotypes.[574]

The use of retroviral-mediated gene transfer to mark HSC has lent support to this hypothesis. Analysis of the viral integration patterns at intervals after transplantation has documented concurrent contributions of small numbers of stem cells to hematopoiesis, with changing patterns over time.[575, 576] Long-term analysis of female Safari cats (heterozygous for two G6PD isoforms) that were transplanted with small numbers (1 to 2×10^7/kg) of autologous marrow cells showed extensive variation in G6PD phenotype over a 4½-year period.[577] Computer modeling of the data was consistent with a stochastic model in which stem cells did not replicate more frequently than once every 3 weeks, which challenges many of the current strategies for inserting foreign genes into HSC. These conclusions are not supported by the work of Harrison and associates, who measured variances at successive intervals in recipients of marrow mixtures from two congenic donors. The high correlations observed in this study suggest that the transplanted stem cells continuously produce descendants.[578] However, if 10 to 20 (or more) clones are contributing to hematopoiesis simultaneously, then even with clonal succession one might expect variances between two alloenzymes at sequential samplings to be minimized. Furthermore, a longer-term analysis of viral integration patterns in multiple lineage progeny of stem cells transplanted into mice show that integration patterns are unstable initially but then stabilize and maintain a consistent pattern over many months.[579] Although this consistency does not appear to support the clonal succession hypothesis, the contributory role of unmarked stem cells in these experiments cannot be assessed. Furthermore, it is not possible to determine whether the immediate progeny of the transplanted (and retrovirally marked) stem cells might not all still have self-renewal capacity and subsequently contribute to hematopoiesis successively. Such clones would carry the same integration marker.

Although the factors that control the decision of stem cells to undergo either self-renewal or commitment to differentiate down one of the alternate lineage pathways are poorly understood, in recent years nuclear transcription factors have been characterized that play a role in stem or early progenitor cell proliferation and lineage commitment.[580] The tal-1/SCL, Rbtn2/LMO2, and GATA family of transcription factors are important in this regard. In particular, tal-1/SCL, a basic helix-loop-helix (bHLH) transcription factor, is expressed in bi-phenotypic (lymphoid/myeloid) and T-cell leukemias[581, 582] and in both early hematopoietic progenitors and more mature erythroid, mast, megakaryocyte, and endothelial cells.[583, 584] Targeted disruption of the tal-1/SCL gene leads to death *in utero* from absence of blood formation, and lack of *in vitro* myeloid colony formation suggests a role for this factor very early during hematopoiesis at the pluripotent or myeloid-erythroid stem cell level.[585, 586] Another transcription factor implicated in T-cell acute lymphoblastic leukemia is the LIM domain nuclear protein rhombotin 2 (rbtn2/LMO2).[587, 588] Mice that lack this factor die *in utero* and have the same bloodless phenotype as the *tal-1/SCL*[−/−] animals.[589] Interestingly, although rbtn2/LMO2 does not show sequence-specific DNA binding, immunoprecipitates in erythroid cells show that rbtn2/LMO2 exists in a complex with tal-1/SCL,[590, 591] suggesting a physiologic interaction *in vivo*. GATA-2 is expressed in the regions of the *Xenopus* and zebrafish embryos that are fated to become hematopoietic and is highly expressed in progenitor cells.[584, 592–594] Overexpression of GATA-2 in chicken erythroid progenitors leads to proliferation at the expense of differentiation.[595] Targeted disruption of the GATA-2 gene by homologous recombination in embryonic stem (ES) cells leads to reduced primitive hematopoiesis in the yolk sac and embryonic death by day 10 to 11.[596] Definitive hematopoiesis in liver and bone marrow is profoundly reduced with loss of virtually all lineages, and *in vitro* differentiation data show a marked deficiency of SF-responsive definitive erythroid and mast cell colonies and reduced macrophage colonies, suggesting that GATA-2 serves as a regulator of genes that control HGF responsiveness or proliferation of stem or early progenitor cells. These data contrast to the later time of embryonic death (day 15) from anemia during the mid fetal liver stage in mice with targeted disruption of *MYB*,[551] Rb,[547–549] and severe forms of *W* and *Sl* mutations (see later).[598] Similarly, loss of function of the AML-1 gene, which encodes one of the α subunits of the heterodimeric CBF, results in fetal death by day 12.5 owing to failure of production of all definitive hematopoietic lineages.[599] CBF recognition sequences are present in the IL-3, GM-CSF, M-CSFR, and T-cell antigen receptor promoters. The AML-1 gene is frequently rearranged in acute myeloid leukemia and childhood acute lymphoid leukemia and is expressed in myeloid and lymphoid cells.[588, 600]

HGFs also appear to influence at least some classes of stem cells. Analysis of the actions of HGFs on "purified" murine or human stem and progenitor cells has led to several major conclusions that should be interpreted in the light that, to date, even the most highly purified "stem cell" fractions are still heterogeneous with respect to content of LTR-HSC, HSC with short-term reconstituting potential, and lineage committed progenitors. HGFs such as SF and perhaps IL-3, granulocyte-macrophage colony-stimulating factor (GM-CSF), and granulocyte colony-stimulating factor (G-CSF) can independently support the survival of murine or human stem cell populations.[223, 601–603] However, of all these HGFs only SF has been shown to enhance the survival of murine LTR-HSC, and no single HGF or combination of HGFs has unequivocally shown the capacity to induce significant self-renewal of LTR-HSC.[604, 605] However, SF and SF + G-CSF have been shown to increase the murine HSC content approximately three-fold, as determined by competitive reconstitution measured 4 months after transplantation.[606, 607] IL-6–deficient mice show a reduction in CFU-S and failure of IL-6[−/−] bone marrow cells to contribute to long-term hematopoiesis after serial transfer.[276] In the human system, information on HSC self-renewal is not available because no human assay measures this property. Combinations of HGFs are necessary to induce or shorten the time to cell cycling of the most immature stem and progenitor cells. Examples are SF + IL-3 or either of these two factors + IL-6, IL-11, IL-12, LIF, or G-CSF.[164]

Analysis of mutations that affect the function of stem cells and the hematopoietic microenvironment through HGF interactions have provided important insights. Two murine mutations have been characterized in some detail, the Steel *(Sl)* and dominant white spotting *(W)* mutations.[565, 566, 598] Genetically affected mice that are defective at these loci have a severe macrocytic anemia associated with increased radiation sensitivity, lack of pigmentation, and sterility. Although phenotypically similar, these mutations map to different chromosomes (*W*–chromosome 5, *Sl*–chromosome 10) and have distinct hematologic characteristics. Best characterized at the molecular level, the *W* mutation results in a functional deficiency of HSC and particularly erythroid progenitors. Transplantation of normal bone marrow into homozygous *W* recipients completely corrects the hematopoietic abnormalities, whereas transplantation of W bone marrow into normal mice fails to reconstitute hematopoiesis.[566, 608] The *W* gene is allelic with the *KIT* proto-oncogene,[609, 610] which, as discussed earlier, is known to be a member of a tyrosine kinase receptor family,[611] as is *FMS*, the receptor for M-CSF. Several variants of the *W* mutation have been shown to be phenotypic expressions of specific mutations of the *KIT* gene, and the severity of the phenotypic changes associated with specific alleles correlates with the degree of functional impairment of kinase activity.[612]

In contrast, the Steel mutation affects the function of the cells of the microenvironment. *Sl/Sl*[d] bone marrow cells are capable of reconstituting hematopoiesis in irradiated normal mice, whereas transplantation of normal bone marrow into Sl/Sl^d animals fails to cure the defect.[613] A deeper insight into the molecular nature of this defect was provided by the purification of a factor that is active on mast cells and on post–5-FU mouse bone marrow (enriched for primitive stem cells but depleted of mature progenitors).[614, 615] This "stem cell factor" or "mast cell growth factor" was purified and its cDNA cloned. Labeling studies with the purified recombinant protein demonstrate that it is the ligand for KIT.[246, 251, 616, 617] Furthermore, administration of the factor to Sl/Sl^d mice corrects their macrocytic anemia and repairs their mast cell deficiency. The SF gene maps to the *Steel* locus on chromosome 10.[618] Confirmation for the hypothesis that SF is encoded by the Steel gene comes from Southern analysis of stromal lines from normal and Sl/Sl embryos (lethal).[247] Although multiple bands are present in the Eco R1 digested normal DNA hybridized with the SF probe, there is no hybridization with the Sl/Sl DNA. Moreover, less severe mutations at the Sl locus such as Sl^d are associated with smaller deletions at the Sl locus. The gene encodes a protein that exists in both transmembrane and secreted forms.[246, 619, 620] Thus, it is intriguing to speculate on a stromal cell/stem cell interaction role for the SF, whose biologic properties are characterized by lack of colony-stimulating activity alone but marked synergy with many CSFs specific for different cell lineages.

Two models have been proposed to explain the mechanisms that influence the choice of stem cells between self-renewal and commitment. A *stochastic model* was proposed by Till and colleagues.[558] In this model, self-renewal or differentiation are considered to occur in a random or stochastic manner, only dictated by a certain probability. Because no extrinsic source of stem cells exists, under steady-state conditions the overall probability of stem cell division resulting in self-renewal must be 0.5; probabilities less or greater than this value would lead to progressive stem cell depletion (aplasia) or expansion (leukemia), respectively. The commitment of stem cells could occur symmetrically, where overall, half the stem cells divide to produce progeny, both of which enter a differentiation pathway, whereas half the stem cells generate progeny that are both stem cells. Alternatively, asymmetric division would give rise to one stem cell and one cell committed to differentiate. Analysis of single cells from blast cell colonies has shown that hematopoietic cells can divide asymmetrically; these micromanipulated single cells give rise to colonies that comprise almost all possible lineage combinations.[69] Single cell analysis of purified human CD34+/CD45RA-low/CD71-low provides evidence for quiescent survival, self-renewal, and asymmetric division.[621] These data provide strong support for a stochastic mechanism to explain both commitment and restriction of differentiation potential. Differentiation of single blast cells into mature cells occurs in these methylcellulose cultures in the absence of an intact microenvironment. A source of HGFs is obligatory, however, as is the case for all colonies grown in semisolid media. It is important to recognize that while these random events occur with a given probability, it must be possible for that probability to be altered. For example, during the regeneration of hematopoietic tissues after injury by irradiation or cytotoxic drugs, the probability of generating stem cells must increase. How this probability is altered is one of the outstanding unanswered questions in hematopoiesis.

A contrasting model, proposed by Trentin,[622] postulates that the *hematopoietic microenvironment is inductive* (HIM) and is based on the observation that domains of a given lineage exist within single spleen colonies. Erythroid HIMs are thought to be more predominant in murine spleen, whereas granulocytic HIMs predominate in bone marrow. Transfer experiments showed that granulocytic cells predominate in the junctional region of bone marrow fragments implanted in spleen.[623] A major drawback of this model comes from an analysis of progenitors within these colonies. Correlations are not observed between mature cells and their respective committed progenitors.[624] The preponderance of differentiating cells of one or other type within colonies thus appears to result from events that affect maturation rather than lineage commitment. The nature of these events has not been established, but possibilities include the release of short-range lineage specific factors by stromal cells or perhaps the display of such growth factor molecules on the surface of their cell membranes. The Dexter culture system also lends powerful support to an essential role of stromal cells for stem cell survival, because the concentration of stem cells is highest within the adherent stromal layer itself. This and other observations related to the morphology of the focal development of hematopoietic islands attached to adherent cells has led to the postulate that HSC reside within stromal cell "niches" that play a vital role in supporting stem cell survival, perhaps by intimate cell contact.[52]

In summary, it appears likely that two types of extrinsic control can affect stem cell regulation; at one level is control by stromal cells, perhaps primarily on stem cell survival but also on their response to humoral factors; at a second level are the humoral growth factors, which appear to affect stem cells but probably have a greater affect on committed maturing progenitors and precursors.

Erythropoiesis

It is well established that the level of oxyhemoglobin and the rate of delivery of oxygen to the tissues is the fundamental stimulus of erythropoiesis.[5] In species that package hemoglobin in erythrocytes, EPO mediates the response to oxygen demand and does so by interacting with specific receptors[625] that are found on the surface of committed erythroid progenitor cells[626–628] and erythroblasts.[629] As discussed earlier, insight into the mechanism by which hypoxia induces a transcriptional increase in the expression *EPO* has come from the identification of the hypoxia-inducible transcription factors HIF-1α and HIF-1β.[439, 630]

It is believed that BFU-E do not ordinarily give rise to erythroblasts *in vivo* except under conditions of extreme anemic stress. Instead, they mature to single erythrocyte CFUs or CFU-E, which divide *in vivo*, and under the influence of lower concentrations of EPO form single, relatively small colonies of proerythroblasts at about 1 week *in vitro*. Many (at least half) CFU-E will form erythroid colonies *in vitro* in response to EPO alone. They do not require the additional presence of either GM-CSF or IL-3, having differentiated beyond this requirement.[631] All proerythroblasts can differentiate in the presence of EPO alone. In the steady state, the number of human CFU-E exceeds the number of BFU-E by a factor of 10. CFU-E are larger than BFU-E and because a higher fraction of CFU-E are in the S-phase of DNA synthesis than are BFU-E, the former exhibit a higher rate of "suicide" in response to exposure to tritiated thymidine. The membranes of mature BFU-E and CFU-E are CD34 + and HLA-DR +, and various negative and positive selection methods may be used to purify them from sources such as bone marrow and human fetal liver.[88, 632] They have the appearance of lymphoblasts.

The bone marrow of an adult mouse contains about 500 CFU-E per 10^5 nucleated cells. In response to anemic stress, as in hemorrhage or hemolysis, nearly the entire burden of accelerated reticulocyte production is born by the rapid EPO-dependent influx into the proerythroblast pool from the progenitor compartment.[87, 98] This produces an expanded proerythroblast pool. Little or no increase in the mitotic rate of recognizable erythroid precursors occurs.[87] Instead, the late BFU-E and CFU-E proliferate in response to the engagement of their EPO receptors by the hormone and, as well, differentiate to proerythroblasts and beyond. In normal murine marrow, the CFU-E frequency of about 500 per 10^5 nucleated cells increases to 1000 to 2000 CFU-E per 10^5 nucleated cells after experimental hemorrhage or hemolysis. In contrast, hypertransfused mice exhibit a reduced number of CFU-E per 10^5 nucleated marrow cells (values between 10% to 20% of normal have been reported).

During stress erythropoiesis induced by anemia, the orderly progression from immature BFU-E through CFU-E to proerythroblast is interrupted as high EPO levels appear to permit or induce differentiation of immature progenitors to proerythroblasts. In the rhesus monkey, this premature terminal differentiation may account for the marked increase in fetal hemoglobin content and F cells seen in simian stress erythropoiesis.[633] The ability of human progenitors to generate erythroblasts capable of synthesizing large quantities of fetal hemoglobin is less pronounced.[634] Thus, the accumulation of F cells in peripheral blood in response to anemia is relatively small.[635] Such red cells are usually macrocytic and carry the i antigen as well, but these two characteristics may relate to a short transit time through the marrow in response to EPO rather than to an intrinsic characteristic of fetal hemoglobin-containing cells themselves (see later). F cells are also present in very small numbers in the blood of normal individuals, but these cells are not macrocytic and do not bear i antigen. F cell progenitors can be detected

easily in the bone marrow of patients with various dyspoieses[636,637] and even in normal marrows.[638]

Transcription Factors and Erythropoiesis

As discussed earlier, targeted disruption of the tal-1/SCL, rbtn2/LMO-2, and GATA-2 genes lead to embryonic lethality owing to failure of blood production, probably at the level of HSC. GATA-1 expression is limited to multipotent progenitors and erythroid, megakaryocyte, mast, and eosinophil lineages.[81, 597, 639, 640] Analysis of chimeric mice injected at the blastocyst stage with GATA-1$^{-/-}$ ES cells shows a failure of a contribution of the GATA-1$^{-/-}$ cells to erythrocytes but development into other hematopoietic lineages, as well as other tissues.[550, 641] Differentiation assays *in vitro* show proerythroblast arrest and apoptosis of these cells.[642–644]

Growth Factors and Erythropoiesis

The regulation of the proliferation and maturation of erythroid progenitors depends on interaction with a number of growth factors. In recent years the availability of pure recombinant growth factors, the enrichment of target progenitor cells, and the use of defined "serum-free" culture conditions has provided insights into the role of these factors during hematopoiesis. Although much of the fundamental biology has been learned from traditional culture systems using fetal calf serum, conditioned medium, and unfractionated cells, the focus is on more recently obtained data.

EPO is essential for the terminal maturation of erythroid cells. Its major effect appears to be at the level of the CFU-E during adult erythropoiesis, and recombinant preparations[631] are as effective as the natural hormone.[645, 646] These progenitors do not require "burst-promoting activity"[647, 648] in the form of IL-3 or GM-CSF, and their dependence on EPO is emphasized by the observation that they will not survive *in vitro* in the absence of EPO. Because the majority of CFU-E are in cycle, their survival in the presence of EPO is probably tightly linked to their proliferation and differentiation to mature erythrocytes. EPO also acts on a subset of presumptive mature BFU-E, which also require EPO for survival and terminal maturation. A second subset of BFU-E, presumably less mature, survive EPO deprivation if burst-promoting activity is present, either as IL-3 or GM-CSF (IL-3 > GM-CSF). When EPO is added to these cultures on day 3, these BFU-E form typical colonies. Similar results are obtained in serum-deprived methylcellulose cultures in which the usual 30% fetal calf serum is substituted by bovine serum albumin (BSA)-adsorbed cholesterol, iron saturated transferrin, and insulin.[649] Under serum-deprived culture conditions the combination of IL-3 and GM-CSF results in more BFU-E than either factor alone when EPO is added on day 3.[649] Although EPO is crucial for the terminal differentiation of erythroid progenitors, data show that mice with homozygous null mutations of the *Epo* or *EpoR* genes form BFU-E and CFU-E normally, but they fail to differentiate into mature erythrocytes.[272] Both the $Epo^{-/-}$ and $EpoR^{-/-}$ mutations are embryonic lethal owing to failure of definitive (fetal liver) erythropoiesis. However, yolk sac erythropoiesis is only partially impaired, indicating the existence of a population of EPO-independent primary erythropoietic precursors. SF has marked synergistic effects on BFU-E cultured in the presence of EPO,[150, 650–652] although alone it has no colony-forming ability. SF is crucial for the normal development of CFU-E, because mice that lack SF (Sl mutants) or its receptor KIT (W mutants) are severely anemic and show a reduction in fetal liver CFU-E.[653] Studies of cell lines that express both KIT and EPOR (HCD57 cells) or are transduced with cDNAs for these two receptors (32D cells) showed that SF supports the proliferation of these cells only if the EPOR is also present.[654] Further studies showed that SF induces tyrosine phosphorylation of the EPOR and that KIT associates with the cytoplasmic domain of the tyrosine phosphorylated EPOR. Whether such an interaction between KIT and the EPOR occurs during normal erythropoiesis is not known.

Progenitors obtained from human fetal liver and cultured in serum-free conditions differ in their requirements for burst-promoting activity and EPO.[655, 656] Although adult BFU-E require IL-3 or GM-CSF and EPO for the development of maximal BFU-E colony number and size, embryonic BFU-E require only EPO for maximal BFU-E cloning efficiency; the addition of IL-3 or GM-CSF increases BFU-E size but not number. These results suggest that EPO receptors are expressed at an earlier stage of erythroid maturation in fetal cells and that during ontogeny expression of the EPO receptor (EPOR) becomes restricted to a subset of mature BFU-E and CFU-E. However, cord blood progenitors, in contrast to their adult counterparts, form "spontaneous" CFU-GM in the absence of HGFs, and this can be abrogated by the addition of antibodies to GM-CSF and IL-3; interestingly, GM-CSF and IL-3 transcripts were detected by RT-PCR in cord blood CD34+ cells and in the spontaneous colonies, suggesting that the progenitor cells or their immediate progeny may produce these two factors.[657] This provides an alternative explanation for the burst-promoting activity independence of primitive erythroid progenitors. During fetal development, the EPOR may be expressed by even more immature myeloid-erythroid progenitors such as CFU-Mix. Neonates with severe Rh hemolytic disease and very high EPO levels are born with neutropenia and thrombocytopenia.[658] Furthermore, premature infants who received recombinant EPO in a clinical trial developed neutropenia. In vitro, high concentrations of EPO reduce the number of CFU-GM colonies and decrease the number of granulocytes per colony, with newborn cells more sensitive to this effect than progenitors from adults.[659] These results do not appear to result from "crowding" in the culture dishes, because cord blood cells were plated at 10^4 cells/mL. In summary, the data are consistent with the hypothesis that the fetal EPOR is expressed on bi-potent progenitor cells and can influence the subsequent maturation of these cells.

Factors distinct from the classic CSFs may positively regulate erythropoiesis, either directly or indirectly. Limiting dilution studies of highly purified CFU-E in serum-free culture show that insulin and insulin-like growth factor I act directly on these cells.[660] The presence of EPO is essential in these studies, which contrast to earlier murine studies of unfractionated cells in which CFU-E respond to IGF-1 or insulin in the absence of EPO.[661] Another factor that enhances both BFU-E and CFU-E colony formation is activin. This protein dimer, also known as follicle-stimulating hormone-releasing protein, appears to have a lineage-specific effect on erythropoiesis that is indirect, because removal of monocytes or T lymphocytes abrogates its effect.[662] It is interesting that activin has been identified as the factor produced by vegetal cells during blastogenesis that induces animal ectodermal cells to form primary mesoderm.[663] Hepatocyte growth factor has also been shown to have synergistic effects on CFU-GEMM and BFU-E in EPO-containing cultures.[664]

Negative Regulation of Erythropoiesis

Observations that subsets of lymphocytes with an immunologic suppressor phenotype isolated from normal subjects can inhibit erythroid activity in vitro[665–667] correlate with reports of patients with a variety of disorders in whom anemia or granulocytopenia is associated with an expansion of certain T-lymphocyte populations.[668–672] In the rare disorder T lymphocytosis with cytopenia,[673] in vitro suppression of erythropoiesis has been correlated with the expansion of a T-lymphocyte population that may be the counterpart of the hematopoietic suppressor cells isolated from normal blood. The phenotype of these cells has been described in detail.[673, 674] The cell is a large granular lymphocyte that is both E rosette positive and CD8 (classic suppressor phenotype) positive. Suppressor T cells may also be involved in some cases of aplastic anemia[675, 676] or neutropenia[677] without an underlying immunologic disorder or an overt T-cell proliferation. Exactly how such suppressor T cells interact with hematopoietic progenitors, and what surface antigens are "seen" by the suppressors, are under intensive investigation. There is evidence to support the concept that suppression of erythroid colony expression in vitro is regulated by T cells and may be genetically restricted.[674, 678] Cell-cell interactions in immunologic systems have been well characterized with regard to surface determinants that allow for cellular recognition. That certain phenotypes of T cells "recognize" distinct classes of histocompatibility antigens on immunologic cell surfaces has been well described.[679] Thus, the observation that hematopoietic progenitors have a unique distribution of class II histocompatibility antigens on their cell surface[680–683] suggests a role for these antigens in the cell-cell interactions that regulate hematopoietic differentiation.

T cells may also inhibit erythropoiesis in a non-HLA restricted fashion by the production of inhibitory cytokines. Some lymphokines may inhibit erythropoiesis in vitro by a complex lymphokine cascade. Activation of T cells by the T-cell antigen receptor CD3 results in cell surface expression of the IL-2α chain (p55) and the acquisition of IL-2 responsiveness.[684] IL-2 inhibits BFU-E in the presence of these IL-2R+ cells, possibly by inducing their release of IFN-γ. CD2 can serve as an alternative pathway of T-cell activation and may do so through binding to its ligand LFA-3 on antigen-presenting cells. Blockade of CD2 with monoclonal antibody leads to abrogation of IL-2/IFN-γ mediated BFU-E suppression.[685] These data are difficult to reconcile with the observation that IL-2 incubation of PMA/calcium ionophor–activated CD4+ T cells leads to marked expansion of IL-3 and GM-CSF mRNA+ cells by *in situ* hybridization.[301] Most CD4+ T cells express CD28 as well, and there is evidence to suggest that IL-3 production is restricted to CD28+ T cells.[350] It thus appears paradoxical that both potent stimulating and inhibitory lymphokines can be produced by activating T cells through the same pathway.

TNF also suppresses erythropoiesis *in vitro*.[686, 687] The injection of peritoneal macrophages into a Friend murine leukemia virus–infected animal results in rapid but transient resolution of the massive erythroid hyperplasia associated with this disease. This may be due to elaboration by macrophages of IL-1α, which does not suppress erythropoiesis itself but acts by the induction of TNF. This effect is reversed by EPO.[688]

Myelopoiesis

Phagocyte Development

Although a clonogenic assay of granulocyte progenitors was developed almost a decade before the erythroid clonogenic assay, the various factors responsible for granulocyte macrophage development remain incompletely understood. Excellent reviews of early work in this field have been provided by Metcalf[76] and Moore.[73]

It is now accepted that CFU-GM is derived from the pluripotent progenitor and, under the influence of SF, IL-3, GM-CSF, G-CSF, and/or M-CSF, ultimately gives rise to mature granulocytes and monocytes. Monocytes irreversibly leave the circulation[689, 690] and differentiate further into fixed-tissue macrophages, a category comprising the alveolar macrophages,[691] hepatic Kupffer cells,[692] dermal Langerhans cells,[693] osteoclasts,[694] peritoneal and pleural macrophages, and perhaps brain microglial cells.[695] The enormous diversity of this system and the high turnover rate of granulocytes, as well as the necessity of maintaining splenic, marginated, and bone marrow granulocyte pools to meet sudden demands caused by infection, has led to the evolution of an extremely complex regulatory network. Indeed, although many of the factors that allow release of granulocytes from storage pools are distinct from CSF,[100] GM-CSF can inhibit granulocyte motility[696] as well as serve as an activator of granulocyte superoxide anion generation.[697] This complexity *in vivo* does not permit studies analogous to those in which erythropoiesis is influenced by hypertransfusion or hemorrhage[698, 699] and megakaryocytopoiesis is stimulated by induced thrombocytopenia.[700] Thus, investigators have relied heavily on *in vitro* progenitor assays to study the regulation of myelopoiesis.

Transcription Factors and Myelopoiesis

The PU.1(Spi-1) transcription factor is a member of the Ets family and is expressed principally in monocytes/macrophages and B lymphocytes and also in erythroid cells and granulocytes.[334, 701] Potential target genes include the integrin CD11b, M-CSFR, GM-CSFRα, G-CSFR, and the immunoglobulin λ light chain.[702–706] Mice that lack PU.1 die *in utero* with absence of monocytes, granulocytes, and T and B lymphocytes; anemia is variable and thus does not explain the prenatal mortality.[707] The C/EBP family of transcription factors bind to DNA through a basic region-leucine zipper domain (bZIP). There are several family members, C/EBPαβ (NF-IL-6), C/EBPγ, and C/EBPδ, that are differentially expressed during myelopoiesis, with an increase (C/EBPβ), or an increase followed by either a partial (C/EBPδ) or a marked (C/EBPα) reduction in level of expression during maturation of 32D.cl3 cells to terminally differentiated granulocytes.[708] C/EBPα has been implicated in the regulation of hepatocyte and adipocyte differentiation (levels are low in undifferentiated dividing cells but high in quiescent terminally differentiated cells) and also in myeloid CSF receptor promoter function.[709] Mice that lack C/EBPβ produce monocytes that are defective in bactericidal and tumoricidal function; and their macrophages and fibroblasts, but interestingly not their endothelial cells, fail to produce G-CSF in response to LPS.[710] Another family of transcription factors important for regulation of myeloid specific promoters such as those of the myeloperoxidase (MPO) and neutrophil elastase (NE) genes are factors that were first identified on the basis of their ability to bind to PEBP2/CBF. Two α subunits (PEBP2αA and PEBP2αB [the human homologue is known as AML-1]) bind DNA with low affinity, and affinity is strengthened in the presence of the non–DNA-binding β subunit (PEBP2β/CBFβ). AML-1 can act synergistically with C/EBPα to activate the M-CSFR promoter.[709] As noted earlier, *AML-1−/−* mice die *in utero* by day 12.5 owing to failure of production of all definitive hematopoietic lineages.[599]

Growth Factors and Myelopoiesis

Murine IL-3 stimulates a broad spectrum of myeloid progenitor cells, including pluripotent stem cells, granulocyte or macrophage colony-forming cells or units (CFU-GM, CFU-G, CFU-M), erythrocyte burst-forming units (BFU-E), eosinophil CFU (CFU-Eo), megakaryocyte CFU (CFU-meg) and mast cells. As its name implies, GM-CSF was initially shown to be more restricted as a stimulus of the proliferation and development of CFU-GM. However, murine studies with purified or recombinant factor have shown that it also stimulates the initial proliferation of other progenitors such as BFU-E as well (see earlier).[170, 711] The other murine factors, G-CSF and M-CSF, are more restricted and predominantly stimulate granulocyte and monocyte colony forming units (CFU-G and CFU-M), respectively.[712, 713]

With the possible exception of GM-CSF, the activities

of the human CSFs are similar to those of the corresponding murine factors. Both IL-3 and GM-CSF affect a similar broad-spectrum of human progenitor cells. This includes CFU-GEMM, CFU-GM, CFU-G, CFU-M, CFU-Eo and CFU-meg. In full serum cultures, IL-3 and GM-CSF alone stimulate the formation of colonies derived from CFU-GM, CFU-G, CFU-M, CFU-Eo, and CFU-meg. Data from serum free cultures suggest that in the presence of IL-3 or GM-CSF alone, myeloid colony-formation is much reduced and that optimal CFU-G or CFU-M proliferation requires the addition of G-CSF or M-CSF, respectively, to the cultures.[174, 649] Even in serum replete conditions, IL-3 acts additively or synergistically with G-CSF to induce more granulocyte colony formation than is observed with either factor alone.[173]

Insight into the *in vivo* role of GM-CSF comes from recent studies in which the GM-CSF was disrupted by homologous recombination in embryonic stem cells.[287] Mice that carried two null alleles of the GM-CSF gene showed normal basal hematopoiesis but developed progressive accumulation of surfactant lipids and proteins in the alveolar space, the defining characteristic of idiopathic human pulmonary alveolar proteinosis. Extensive lymphoid hyperplasia associated with lung airways and blood vessels was also found. Surfactant proteins and lipids are synthesized by type II pneumocytes and cleared from the alveolar space by type II cells and by alveolar macrophages. The lungs from the null animals showed normal surfactant synthetic capacity and no accumulation in type II pneumocytes. In contrast, the alveolar macrophages showed a marked increase of surfactant protein and lipid, suggesting strongly that these cells cannot process surfactant as a result of the lack of GM-CSF. Mice that were generated with null mutations of the common chain of the GM-CSF/IL-3/IL-5 receptor (β_c) show similar pulmonary pathology and also show low basal numbers of eosinophils and absence of blood and lung eosinophilia in response to infection with the parasite *Nippostrongylus brasiliensis*.[714] The G-CSF gene has also been disrupted by homologous recombination in ES cells.[267] $G\text{-}CSF^{-/-}$ mice have a chronic neutropenia (20% to 30% of normal levels) and reduced bone marrow myeloid precursors and progenitors. The animals also had a markedly impaired capacity to increase neutrophil and monocyte counts after infection with *Listeria monocytogenes*.

In addition to their effects on progenitor differentiation, the CSFs also induce a variety of functional changes in mature cells. GM-CSF inhibits polymorphonuclear neutrophil migration under agarose,[696] induces antibody-dependent cytotoxicity (ADCC) for human target cells,[697] and increases neutrophil phagocytic activity.[168] Some of these functional changes may be related to GM-CSF–induced increase in the cell surface expression of a family of antigens that function as cell adhesion molecules.[715] The increase in antigen expression is rapid and is associated with increased aggregation of neutrophils; both are maximal at the migration inhibitory concentration of 500 pM, and granulocyte-granulocyte adhesion can be inhibited by an antigen-specific monoclonal antibody. GM-CSF also acts as a potent stimulus of eosinophil ADCC, superoxide production, and phagocytosis.[716] G-CSF acts as a potent stimulus of neutrophil superoxide production, ADCC, and phagocytosis,[717] whereas M-CSF activates mature macrophages[718] and enhances macrophage cytotoxicity.

It is apparent then that the actions of the CSFs on mature cells parallel their spectrum of activity on immature progenitors. Murine IL-3, in contrast to human IL-3, does activate neutrophil function. The explanation for this species difference lies in the observation that murine neutrophils express the IL-3 receptor,[719] whereas it is undetectable on the surface of human neutrophils.

Megakaryocytopoiesis

The recent cloning of thrombopoietin has greatly clarified understanding of the regulation of megakaryocytopoiesis.[118] Before the discovery of thrombopoietin, several factors,[720] including IL-3,[721] IL-6,[722] IL-11,[723] SF,[724, 725] and even EPO,[726–728] were shown to stimulate megakaryocytopoiesis and thrombopoiesis *in vitro* and *in vivo*. IL-11 has even entered clinical trials.[235] IL-3, IL-6, and IL-11 engage heterodimeric receptors of the beta common (IL-3R) and gp130 families (IL-6R and IL-11R). SF engages a receptor the intracellular domain of which expresses tyrosine kinase activity on ligand binding. As already emphasized in this chapter, ligand engagements of these receptor families are known to induce early multipotent progenitors to proliferate and even differentiate toward lineage-specific progenitors, and SF, IL-3, and IL-11 participate in the induction of the proliferation and differentiation of lineage-specific progenitors. Hence, all of the just-mentioned HGFs, except EPO, can contribute collectively to what is known biologically as megakaryocyte colony-stimulating activity (meg-CSA).[727] EPO is probably not a functional component of meg-CSA. It induces only slight megakaryocyte differentiation and only at enormous concentrations.[729] It probably does so because the developing erythroid progenitor passes through a stage of trilineage restriction that includes erythroid, megakaryocytic, and basophil potential[81] and because, as previously mentioned, EPO and thrombopoietin share structural homology.

Meg-CSA is therefore a "soup" of growth factors that transduce three of the four classes of receptors that drive hematopoietic differentiation.[720] Three of these include the familiar beta common, tyrosine kinase, and gp130 families. All of these receptors, when engaged, drive early progenitor proliferation and partial differentiation to more mature progenitors, but the final steps of lineage-committed mature progenitor development into recognizable marrow precursors require a lineage-specific growth factor—G-CSF for the granulocyte, M-CSF for the macrophage, IL-5 for the eosinophil, and EPO for the erythrocyte.

The discovery of thrombopoietin provides the final step of understanding of megakaryocytopoiesis because this factor prominently induces lineage-restricted megakaryocyte progenitor proliferation, differentiation of those committed progenitors to megakaryoblasts, and, finally, differentiation of megakaryoblasts to the megakaryocytes that in turn produce platelets (see Fig. 6–13). However, this in no way implies that other meg-CSA components may not be useful in the therapy of hypoplastic thrombocytopenias. As is emphasized later, circulating thrombopoietin levels are high in those conditions just as EPO levels are elevated in the erythroid hypoplasias. Administration of high doses of EPO is usually of little benefit in the latter conditions. Thrombopoietin may be just as unsuccessful in certain megakaryocyte hypoplasias because those conditions are often associated with severe depletion of lineage-specific or multipotent progenitors. One or more of the growth factors that comprise meg-CSA, such as IL-11, may be more useful in such circumstances. Clinical trials now in progress will decide that issue.

Thrombopoietin

In 1993, Methia and co-workers performed what proved to be a critically important experiment.[730] They demonstrated that exposure of CD34 + progenitor cells in culture to oligonucleotides that were antisense to *MPL*, a proto-oncogene, inhibited the ability of these cells to form megakaryocyte, but not other hematopoietic colonies. This experiment, formed in the laboratory of Francoise Wendling, had its roots in Wendling's 1986 description of *MPL*, an oncogenic viral complex that produces a murine myeloproliferative and, ultimately, leukemic disease.[731] Four years later, Wendling's group cloned the virus and demonstrated that a gene transduced by the virus might be a cytokine receptor and was responsible for the transforming function.[732] Two years later, another French group, including one member of Wendling's laboratory, cloned the human homologue of *MPL* and demonstrated that it is a member of the HGFR superfamily. The physiologic ligand for this receptor was, as yet, unknown.[733, 734]

Wendling's 1993 experiment strongly suggested that the unknown ligand might be the long-sought thrombopoietin, and in 1994 several laboratories cloned or purified and sequenced the all-important growth factor[119, 248, 252, 735] and important physiologic studies of thrombopoietin were launched, particularly by Kaushansky and his co-workers.[118] As previously mentioned, thrombopoietin is localized on the long arm of chromosome 3. It contains five exons, the boundaries of which line up precisely with those of the *EPO* gene. The gene enjoys widespread tissue expression, including liver, kidney, smooth muscle, endothelial cells, and fibroblasts. Thus, thrombopoietin is produced at the site of hematopoiesis. Therefore, although its activity is increased in the blood during episodes of thrombopenia, it does not necessarily function as a hormone because it is produced directly at the site of thrombopoiesis. In this sense, it differs from EPO, which is not produced at all in marrow stroma. It is likely that the level of production of thrombpoietin is quite constant in all tissues. The blood levels may increase in thrombopenic states merely because circulating platelets and tissue megakaryocytes sop up the growth factor and carry it out of the circulation.[122, 736] This theory has received support from observations in mice with disruption of the murine transcription factor gene called *NF-E2*[85]; although these animals are thrombocytopenic they have an increase in megakaryocyte mass and no increase in serum thrombopoietin levels (Shivdasani R, Orkin S, de Sauvage F: unpublished observations, 1996).

As reviewed by Kaushansky,[118] the thrombopoietin molecule is considerably longer than the other HGF polypeptides. Its 5' half bears 23% sequence homology to EPO, whereas the 3' half bears no structural homology to any cytokine and may be removed by a proteolytic mechanism. Indeed, removal of this half does not ablate physiologic function. The resemblance of the 5' domain of the molecule to EPO may explain the synergy of thrombopoietin and EPO in megakaryocyte colony formation and platelet production.[118, 720] It is well-recognized that splenectomized individuals with persistent anemia usually have significant thrombocytosis and many individuals with red cell aplasia and high EPO levels also have thrombocytosis and megakaryocytosis.

The function of thrombopoietin has been studied carefully *in vivo* and *in vitro*. Although some of the *in vitro* experiments can be criticized because it is very difficult to achieve conditions in which only one factor at a time is studied, the model of megakaryocytosis discussed in the introduction to this section has been loosely confirmed.[118] Lineage specific CD34 + megakaryocyte progenitors bear receptors for SF, IL-3, IL-11, and thrombopoietin, the four major classes of hematopoietic cytokine receptors. Maximal megakaryocyte colony formation probably requires signaling by all four receptors, but thrombopoietin is the major factor involved in the final stages of megakaryocyte maturation, including maximal ploidy and cytoplasmic volume, and, therefore, platelet production.

Early therapeutic trials of thrombopoietin in mice have shown that thrombopoietin is species specific. Treatment of mice with murine thrombopoietin induces massive thrombocytosis, whereas human thrombopoietin is much less active in these animals. More importantly, thrombopoietin is active in reducing the platelet nadir in mice and primates rendered thrombopenic by chemotherapy or radiation. Whether it will be superior to IL-11 in this regard will likely depend on the extent of the progenitor depletion that occurs in human diseases. For example, repeated doses of chemotherapy in patients with cancer may so reduce the progenitor pool that drugs that induce proliferation of progenitors such IL-3 or IL-11 may be more effective than thrombopoietin or be required in addition to thrombopoietin for maximal restoration of megakaryocyte development.

Circulating Platelets

The differential diagnosis of thrombocytopenia rests first on evaluation of platelet morphology. In conditions in which megakaryocytopoiesis is accelerated, circulating platelet volume (and usually diameter) is increased. The reasons for this shift in volume are disputed. Some claim that young platelets are larger than old platelets.[737] Others suggest that large megakaryocytes give rise to large platelets.[738] Neither explanation satisfies all experimental and clinical conditions, but, in general, thrombocytopenia secondary to increased destruction of platelets is associated with platelets of large volume, and thrombocytopenia related to decreased production of platelets is associated with platelets of normal size. There are major exceptions to this rule. Patients with hyposplenism tend to have large platelets in their blood, whether thrombopoiesis is increased or not, and patients with primary abnormalities of platelet function, such as Wiskott-Aldrich syndrome or Bernard-Soulier syndrome, have platelet sizes that bear no relationship to platelet production. Thrombopoietin increases platelet production by increasing both the number and size of individual megakaryocytes. Though thrombopoietin is largely responsible for the later stages of recognizable megakaryocyte differentiation and proliferation of megakaryocyte progenitors, its function depends, at least in part, on the additional stimulation of megakaryocyte progenitors (and probably early megakaryocytes as well) with other growth factors, including IL-3, IL-11, and SF. As discussed earlier, the latter contribute, in combination, to what is known as "meg-CSA."

Down-Regulation of Megakaryocytes

There is great uncertainty about possible down-regulation of megakaryocytes. Platelet factor 4 seems to down-regulate colony formation in vitro,[739] which if active in vivo would provide an interesting feedback loop. TGF-β is also a potent inhibitor in vitro.[740] NK cells, which are thought by some to be general suppressors of hematopoiesis in vitro, actually enhance megakaryocyte colony formation in vitro.[739] In addition, an antibody to NK cells, when it is given intraperitoneally in massive doses to mice, abolishes the formation of colonies of megakaryocytes that can be grown in culture from murine marrow, suggesting that NK cells may actually play a stimulating role in vivo.[741] These are interesting studies that are, however, subject to varying interpretations.

Megakaryocyte Progenitors in Disease

A number of attempts have been made to relate diseases associated with elevated or depressed platelet counts to the number or the growth characteristics of megakaryocyte progenitors.[742] Most attempts have been relatively nonproductive, and very few have been carried out in childhood platelet disorders. Of particular interest is thrombocytosis, a generally benign condition in childhood.[743] Of greater import is essential thrombocythemia. Megakaryocyte progenitors in the latter condition are similar in their growth characteristics to the expanded numbers of erythroid progenitors in polycythemia vera. The latter develop into erythroid colonies without addition of EPO to the culture medium. The trace of EPO in the serum is sufficient to drive the sensitive receptor system in these progenitors. In a similar fashion, the numerous CFU-meg in essential thrombocythemia develop into megakaryocyte colonies in the absence of stimulation by aplastic anemia serum.[744] They are "thrombopoietin independent," and many produce endogenous thrombopoietin.

CLINICAL USE OF HEMATOPOIETIC GROWTH FACTORS

Correction or amelioration of marrow failure syndromes by administration of HGFs has been and continues to be the major practical goal of research in hematopoiesis. The goal could not be achieved, however, until recombinant DNA technology provided sufficient amounts of the hormones to permit interpretable investigations.

Animal Studies

IL-3

The discovery, cloning, and expression of the gene for murine multi-CSF or IL-3 presented the first opportunity to evaluate HGFs in an unambiguous fashion.[745, 746] Sublethally irradiated mice were infused for 7 days with recombinant multi-CSF or with control protein.[747] The spleens of the multi-CSF–treated marrow recipients were much larger than those of the controls, were more cellular, and contained more progenitors. The increase in progenitor cells affected erythroid and myeloid lineages. In contrast, bone marrow cellularity was unaffected and progenitor content was reduced. Metcalf and colleagues[748] injected mice with purified bacterially synthesized IL-3 by the intraperitoneal route and obtained similar results. In addition, 10-fold increases in blood eosinophil and 2- to 3-fold increases in neutrophil and monocyte levels were observed. The intraperitoneal injections also resulted in a 6- to 15-fold increase in peritoneal phagocytes with an increase in macrophage phagocytic activity.

These experiments clearly demonstrate that murine IL-3 influences the replication and growth potential of primitive hematopoietic progenitors and strongly suggest that whatever effect such hormones have on blood cell counts are related to their influences on progenitor function rather than to their effects on peripheral blood cell kinetics. They also suggest that the function of mature cells can be altered in vivo, an effect that would be expected to decrease rather than increase numbers of circulating phagocytes.

GM-CSF

The first indications that the human HGF GM-CSF could broadly stimulate hematopoiesis in vivo resulted from studies of the infusion of COS cell–produced GM-CSF into cynomolgus macaques.[749] Recombinant (r) human (h) GM-CSF acts on simian progenitors. The disappearance curve of intravenously injected metabolically labeled factor is complex and suggests a multicompartment turnover model, but the overall initial half-time of 15 to 20 minutes clearly demonstrated that infusion of the hormone at a concentration sufficient to maintain a functional blood level could be achieved.[749]

The effects of such infusions into normal *Macaca* fascicularis were striking. Large increments in all classes of leukocytes, including eosinophils and lymphocytes as well as reticulocytes, were observed during the hormone infusion. When the hormone treatment was terminated, the blood counts rapidly fell toward normal. A particularly striking reticulocytosis was observed in an animal with an acquired retroviral infection that was associated with secondary pancytopenia and an elevated EPO level. This "preclinical" trial in a severely ill monkey encouraged the conclusion that GM-CSF might play an important therapeutic role in various cytopenias, such as those observed in viral infections, including the acquired immunodeficiency syndrome (AIDS), or in autologous or allogeneic marrow transplantation.

The potential role of human recombinant GM-CSF in marrow transplantation was evaluated by the infusion of autologous marrow into rhesus monkeys (*Macaca mulatta*) 2 hours after lethal total body irradiation.[750] Recombinant hGM-CSF was administered at a daily dose of 50 units/min per kilogram continuously from 10 to 19 days before radiation or from 9 to 17 days beginning 2 or 3 days after irradiation. Both dosage schedules produced the same final results, although the blood counts of the animals that received the hormone before radiation were much higher at the onset of radiation than those who received the hormone only after radiation. In five separate studies, granulocytes recovered to a level greater than 1000/mm³ in 9 days rather than the minimum of 17 days observed in two untreated controls. In four of the five experiments, platelets recovered more rapidly as well.

G-CSF

Human G-CSF was also evaluated in simian preclinical trials. Cynomolgus monkeys treated with two daily subcutaneous injections of purified G-CSF for 14 to 28 days showed a dose-related increase in polymorphonuclear neutrophils, the plateau being reached after 1 week.[751] At the intermediate dose of 10 μg/kg per day, total white blood cell counts of 40,000 to 50,000/μL were observed. Neutrophil function was also enhanced. Encouraging results were also achieved in two cyclophosphamide-treated animals that received G-CSF either from 6 days before until 21 days after the cyclophosphamide treatment, or for 14 days from day 3 after cyclophosphamide administration. In both monkeys, the neutrophil count increased dramatically by day 6 to 7 after cyclophosphamide, reaching levels of 50,000/mL by the 10th day. The control animal remained pancytopenic for 3 to 4 weeks after treatment.

Human Clinical Studies

Several recombinant HGFs are under evaluation in a variety of clinical settings. Largely because of availability, initial studies focused on GM-CSF and G-CSF in both transient and long-standing bone marrow failure syndromes and on EPO in the anemia of chronic renal failure. More recently, other HGFs, such as M-CSF, SF, IL-1, IL-11, and thrombopoietin, are being evaluated. The availability of recombinant growth factors that stimulate myeloid progenitors raised several possibilities. First, they might shorten or prevent the hypoplasia that follows chemotherapy and make more intensive myeloablative chemotherapy regimens possible. However, because GM-CSF and IL-3 receptors are expressed by several nonhematopoietic cell types, malignancies of these cell lineages might also respond to growth factor therapy.

Malignant Disease

G-CSF. In the first phase I/II clinical studies in patients with malignant disease, administration of G-CSF by bolus or continuous intravenous infusion for 5 to 6 days before chemotherapy led to a dose-related increase in polymorphonuclear neutrophils.[752, 753] Rapid increases in neutrophil counts were observed, with maximal counts of 80 to 100×10^9/L at doses of 10 to 30 μg/kg per day. A transient depression in neutrophil counts was noted to precede this increase in one study.[754] In another study, rhG-CSF was given for 14 days after alternate cycles of intensive chemotherapy.[755] The period of neutropenia was reduced by a median of 80% (52%–100%) in the chemotherapy/G-CSF cycles, with a return to normal neutrophil counts within 2 weeks after chemotherapy. Infective episodes were observed during the cycles with chemotherapy that did not include G-CSF, whereas no infective episode occurred in those that did. G-CSF treatment after chemotherapy results in a significant reduction in the number of days per patient in which the neutrophil count is less than 1.0×10^9/L.[752] Antibiotic use to treat fever and neutropenia is also reduced, and all the patients could receive their next course of chemotherapy on schedule (vs. 29% of patients who did not receive G-CSF). The mature neutrophils produced in response to G-CSF have normal mobility and bactericidal capacity.[756] Preliminary analysis of a phase I/II study of G-CSF after intensive chemotherapy in children with advanced-stage neuroblastoma showed a reduction in the number of days with severe neutropenia as well as hospitalizations with neutropenia and fever compared with historical controls.[757]

The effect of G-CSF on progenitor cells is interesting. After melphalan and G-CSF, the absolute number of *circulating* progenitor cells of the granulocyte-macrophage, erythroid, mixed, and megakaryocyte lineages show a dose-related increase up to 100-fold after 4 days of treatment with rhG-CSF,[758] confirming earlier animal studies.[759, 760] The relative proportion of the early and late granulocyte progenitors and of early progenitors of different lineages remain unchanged; however, CFU-E, normally undetectable in blood, are markedly increased. In most patients there was a slight reduction in frequency of *bone marrow* progenitors, although this is difficult to interpret in view of the possibility of variable blood cell contamination of bone marrow samples. The mechanism for the increase in all progenitors in the blood is unclear; G-CSF has been shown to affect immature blast colony-forming cells, and it is possible that stem cells are stimulated *in vivo* to produce increased progenitors of all classes; alternatively, G-CSF may indirectly stimulate progenitors by induction of HGF production or by release into the circulation of bone marrow progenitor cells.

GM-CSF. Recombinant hGM-CSF has been administered in phase I/II studies to several adult groups of patients with advanced malignancy, both before and after chemotherapy.[761–763] Glycosylated GM-CSF produced in either mammalian (Chinese hamster ovary) cells or yeast and *Escherichia coli*–derived nonglycosylated GM-CSF have been evaluated with comparable results. A rapid, dose-related increase in polymorphonuclear neutrophils, monocytes, and eosinophils is observed in patients treated before chemotherapy. Neutrophils peak at 20 to 30 × 10⁹/L at doses from 4 to 32 μg/kg per day, and the substance is well tolerated at doses up to this level. A capillary leak syndrome and venous thrombi are observed at higher doses (64 μg/kg per day).[761] GM-CSF given after chemotherapy is associated with shorter periods of neutropenia (3.5 days vs. 7.4 days) and higher leukocyte nadirs.

Similar encouraging results have been obtained in children with solid tumors undergoing intensive chemotherapy.[764–766] Significantly shorter durations of severe neutropenia and thrombocytopenia were observed in a study of 25 children in whom yeast derived GM-CSF was given at 60 to 1500 μg/m² per day for 14 days after chemotherapy.[764]

Like G-CSF, GM-CSF also produced an increase in blood progenitor cells of both erythroid and myeloid lineages. Before chemotherapy, an 18-fold increase in blood CFU-GM and an 8-fold increase in BFU-E was noted; after chemotherapy, GM-CSF produced a much greater increase of progenitors (60-fold) when given during the recovery period.[767]

IL-3. A phase I/II study of the effect of rhIL-3 in patients with nonhematopoietic malignancies with normal marrow function, as well as lymphomas and bone marrow failure was reported.[768] Doses that ranged from 30 to 500 μg/m² were given for 15 days by daily subcutaneous injection. In the patients with normal hematopoiesis a dose-dependent increase (1.4 to 3.0 fold) in neutrophils was observed, with the major increase during the second week. This contrasts to the rapid neutrophil response that has been the experience with GM-CSF or G-CSF. Platelets and eosinophils also increased in a dose-dependent fashion up to the dose of 250 μg/m² per day (1.3–1.9-fold), and increases in basophil and lymphocytes were noted. Increases in reticulocytes that did not appear to be dose related were also observed in 70% of the patients. Similar results were observed in the patients with bone marrow failure, but stimulation of malignant B cells was seen in two patients with lymphoma. Examination of the bone marrow showed increases in cycling of CFU-GEMM, BFU-E, and CFU-GM, with increased bone marrow cellularity.[769] There was also an increase in blood CFU-GEMM and CFU-GM but a reduction in BFU-E.

In conclusion, results from this initial human IL-3 study indicate that IL-3 can induce a multilineage hematopoietic response.

Other Hematopoietic Growth Factors. Partially purified urinary M-CSF has been evaluated in patients with different malignancies who received myelotoxic chemotherapy. After treatment, patients received M-CSF for 5 days, but little, if any, effect was noted on the rate of neutrophil recovery. Monocytes and other hematopoietic lineages were also unaffected.[770] IL-11 has been shown to ameliorate the thrombocytopenia associated with chemotherapy for breast cancer.[771] IL-1, given at 0.03, 0.1, or 0.3 μg/kg per day for 5 days, was used in 43 adults with advanced neoplasms before or after carboplatin chemotherapy.[772] A third of the patients (5/15) given one of the higher two doses after chemotherapy had minimal thrombocytopenia (platelets >90,000/μL vs. median 19,000/μL without IL-1).

Bone Marrow Transplantation

GM-CSF, G-CSF, and M-CSF have been evaluated in clinical autotransplantation trials.

GM-CSF. Patients with nonhematopoietic malignancies were treated with high-dose combination chemotherapy, autologous bone marrow transplantation, and rhGM-CSF given by continuous intravenous infusion for 14 days beginning 3 hours after bone marrow infusion. There was a dose-related increase in the neutrophil count at day 14 (1411 cells/μL at 2 to 8 μg/kg per day, 2575 cells/μL at 16 μg/kg per day, and 3120 cells/μL at 32 μg/kg per day, compared with 863 cells/μL in 24 historical controls).[773] Although not statistically significant, there was an improved neutrophil response in patients who had not received previous chemotherapy compared with those who had (1832 vs. 833 cells/μL). A lower morbidity and mortality were also noted among the patients who received the GM-CSF; bacteremia occurred in 16% of treated patients compared with 35% of evaluable controls. Comparable results were reported in a study of patients with lymphoid malignancies who received rhGM-CSF as a 2-hour infusion daily for 14 days after chemotherapy, radiotherapy, and autologous bone marrow transplantation.[774] Neutrophil and platelet counts recovered more rapidly, there were fewer days with fever, and the extent of hospitalization was reduced in comparison with a historical control group. In the only reported pediatric study, nine patients received GM-CSF, 5 to 10 μg/kg per day, after bone marrow transplantation. Neutrophil recovery was accelerated, although there was no difference in fever, infection, or length of hospitalization when compared with historical controls.[775]

The response to GM-CSF after myelosuppression may be dependent on the infusion of sufficient progenitor cells. In an autotransplantation study of patients with acute lymphoid leukemia, bone marrows were purged with 4-hydroperoxycyclophosphamide and anti-T- or anti-B-cell lineage specific antibodies before transplantation.[776] Thirty per cent of the patients who received more than 64 μg/m² per day achieved an absolute neutrophil count of more than 1000/μL by day 21, whereas none of the nonresponders reached this level by day 27 post transplant. The responders required only one third as many platelet transfusions, and there was a trend to fewer red cell transfusions, higher M:E ratio, and earlier day of discharge in the responder group as well. Although bone marrow cell dose did not differ among the two groups, the number of CFU-GM progenitors infused per kilogram was significantly higher in the responders as compared with the nonresponders (17.5 [12–27] $\times$ 10³/kg vs. 2[0–7.2] $\times$ 10³/kg). Although it is possible that this accounts for the more rapid recovery rather than the rhGM-CSF infusion, the responder group all showed a rapid decrease in absolute neutrophil count within 48 to 72 hours of discontinuing GM-CSF; this is consistent with a stimulatory effect on bone marrow. One can conclude that GM-CSF is effective in this context provided that sufficient progenitor cells are present.

G-CSF. Recombinant human G-CSF was evaluated in patients with hematopoietic and nonhematopoietic malignancies after intensive chemotherapy and reinfusion of cryopreserved autologous bone marrow.[777] The rhG-CSF was given by continuous intravenous infusion from 24 hours after marrow infusion for a maximum of 28 days, beginning at 20 μg/kg per day and reducing the dose after the neutrophil count persistently exceeded 1 $\times$ 10⁹/L. The mean time to neutrophil recovery (>0.5 $\times$ 10⁹/L) occurred by day 11, 9 days earlier than in historical controls. This led to significantly fewer days of parenteral antibiotic therapy, but there was no effect on red cell or platelet recovery. Although the rate of recovery from neutropenia was faster than that reported for rhGM-CSF, the latter studies were phase I dose escalation evaluations, and many patients did not receive an optimal dose of GM-CSF. One study compared G-CSF with GM-CSF in exactly the same analogous bone marrow transplant protocol. The G-CSF group contained more patients with breast carcinoma who had received previous chemotherapy, and this group did not show a dose-related increase in neutrophil count after a 14-day continuous intravenous infusion at doses of 16, 32, and 64 μg/kg per day. Overall, however, total leukocyte recovery was slightly more rapid in the G-CSF group in comparison with the GM-CSF group. G-CSF administration resulted in two leukocyte peaks. The first at day 10 comprised lymphocytes, whereas the second at day 14 comprised mostly granulocytes; in contrast, GM-CSF produced a single peak at the end of the period of infusion. A major difference was observed with respect to neutrophil migration to an inflammatory site during CSF infusion after hematopoietic reconstitution.[778] Neutrophils did not migrate to skin chambers filled with autologous serum during GM-CSF treatment, a defect not encountered during the administration of G-CSF. There was, however, a similar reduction in the incidence of bacteremia with both GM-CSF and G-CSF (18% and 19%, respectively) in comparison with the historical controls (35%).

In conclusion, if neutrophil recovery is the goal after bone marrow transplantation, then G-CSF appears to be the factor of choice. It preserves neutrophil function

and is well tolerated. The inability to hasten platelet recovery is still the major challenge.

M-CSF. Human urinary M-CSF has been evaluated in a phase II study of patients with different malignancies who received cyclophosphamide, total-body irradiation, and either allogeneic or autologous bone marrow.[779] Human urinary CSF was given for 14 days by 2-hour intravenous infusion daily starting at day 1, day 4, or day 14. In patients who received CSF early, there was a significant reduction in the time to a neutrophil count > 1 $\times$ 10⁹/L when compared with a control group (16.7 vs. 25.4 days). However, the time to recovery of the control group is somewhat delayed in comparison with other reports (17 to 21 days).

Myelodysplasia

GM-CSF. Despite the theoretical risks of treating patients with myeloid stem cell clonal diseases with the CSFs, the factors have been evaluated in patients with refractory anemia (RA), RA with an excess of blasts (RAEB), RAEB in transformation (RAEBIT), and chronic myelomonocytic leukemia.[780–782] In an early study, GM-CSF was given by continuous infusion for 14 days and repeated after a 2-week rest period.[780] Five of the eight patients had received chemotherapy up to 4 weeks before study. Doses of 30 to 500 μg/m² were used. Blood leukocytes rose 5- to 70-fold and neutrophils rose 5- to 373-fold, and an absolute increase in monocytes, eosinophils, and lymphocytes was also noted. Three of the eight patients also had a 2- to 10-fold increase in platelet count and improvement in erythropoiesis, and two of the three became transfusion independent. Marrow cellularity increased, and there was a reduction in the proportion of blasts, although there was a transient and dose-related increase in the absolute number of circulating blasts. No patient developed overt leukemia during the period of follow-up (up to 32 weeks). There was no cytogenetic evidence for a reduction in abnormal clones, and it is likely that the stimulatory effect on hematopoiesis affects both normal and abnormal cells. A dose-related increase in neutrophils, monocytes, eosinophils, and lymphocytes was also noted in a study of 11 patients with myelodysplasia. However, four patients who presented with more than 14% blasts in the bone marrow showed an increase in blasts after therapy whereas an additional three patients showed an increase in blasts in the blood; five patients progressed to acute leukemia either during or within 4 weeks after treatment.[782] Unlike the earlier report, none of these patients had received previous chemotherapy.

G-CSF. A small number of patients have also been treated with G-CSF.[783, 784] Neutrophil responses were seen in 5 patients with myelodysplasia who received 50 to 1600 μg/m² per day by 30 minute infusion daily for 6 days. At the higher doses (400 μg/m² per day) the increase was sustained and associated with an increase in bone marrow cellularity. No reticulocyte or platelet increases were observed, and no patient progressed to an acute phase. Similar results were reported in a study of 12 patients given G-CSF by daily subcutaneous injection, with dose escalation from 0.1 to 3 µg/kg per day over an 8-week period.[784] Although 10 of the 12 patients showed elevations in neutrophils (5- to 40-fold), an increase in reticulocytes occurred in 5 patients with reduction in transfusion requirement in 2. There was no response in other cell lineages and no conversion to acute leukemia.

Aplastic Anemia

GM-CSF. Establishing a role for the CSFs in aplastic anemia will challenge investigators. Severe aplastic anemia is a heterogeneous disease that may result from either absent or defective stem cells, from microenvironmental defects, or from immunologically mediated suppression. Mortality is high and therapeutic options are limited to bone marrow transplantation if an appropriate donor is available or to immunosuppression (see Chapters 7 and 8). Whereas bone marrow transplantation can be curative, treatment with antithymocyte globulin (ATG) is sometimes effective but generally not curative. Other modalities such as cyclosporine and androgens may be partially effective in some patients. For these reasons, rhGM-CSF has been evaluated in a number of phase I/II studies. Administration of rhGM-CSF by bolus or continuous intravenous infusion for 7 or 14 days resulted in increased granulocytes, monocytes, and reticulocytes in six of eight cases.[781] In another small study, rhGM-CSF was given to cohorts of patients in escalating doses from 4 to 64 µg/kg per day by continuous intravenous infusion for 14 days. Although a dose-related effect was not observed, 10 of 11 evaluable patients had partial or complete responses in neutrophils, monocytes, and eosinophils, with increases in bone marrow cellularity. Importantly, the greatest increments occurred in patients with higher pretreatment neutrophil counts and more cellular marrows. Only 10% to 20% of patients show an increase in hemoglobin concentration and platelet count, and in all cases counts return to baseline after cessation of treatment.[785, 786] In the first report of rhGM-CSF treatment in childhood, three fourths of the evaluable patients responded with a significant rise in neutrophil count during the 28-day induction period.[787] Although neutrophil counts returned to baseline after cessation of treatment in all the responders with severe aplastic anemia, one patient with moderate aplasia maintained a trilineage response off therapy for more than 1 year. One cannot extrapolate from such a small experience, but the data underscore the point that responses are more likely in less severely affected cases.

Thus, in summary, it appears as though rhGM-CSF is palliative in aplastic anemia, with greater neutrophil responses evident in less severely affected patients. The most severely affected patients respond poorly.[788] No infections were observed during the study period in several reports, whereas infections were observed in others. Longer-term prospective comparative studies will be necessary to investigate morbidity.

G-CSF. Neutrophil responses have also been reported in a study of 20 children given 400 µg/m² per day G-CSF for 14 days.[789] Twelve patients responded by doubling their neutrophil counts, but other lineages were unaffected. In another pediatric study high doses of G-CSF (400 to 2000 µg/m² per day) induced neutrophil responses in 6 of 10 patients with very severe aplastic anemia.[790] Long-term treatment may be associated with multilineage responses when given alone[791] or in combination with cyclosporine.[792]

IL-3, IL-6, and EPO. Hematopoietic responses have been reported in a small phase I study of nine aplastic anemia patients given IL-3 250 to 500 µg/m² (five doubled their neutrophil counts; four showed an increase in reticulocyte counts but no reduction in transfusion requirement; and one increased platelet counts from 1 to 31 × 10⁹/L).[768] An increase in platelet count was reported in one of six patients entered in a phase I study of IL-6, although a dose-related decrease in neutrophils, monocytes, and lymphocytes was observed; and a proportion (about one third) of patients given EPO showed reduced transfusion requirement or an increase in hemoglobin.[793] Also promising preliminary results, including trilineage responses, have been reported in a small number of refractory aplastic anemia patients treated with low dose GM-CSF + EPO[794] or G-CSF + EPO.[795] The effects of EPO are unexpected because endogenous levels are very high in aplastic anemia.

Human Immunodeficiency Virus Infection

GM-CSF. HIV infection is associated with several hematologic abnormalities, including neutropenia, anemia, and thrombocytopenia. Anemia and neutropenia can be exacerbated by treatment with zidovudine, and rhGM-CSF has been evaluated in an effort to enhance immunologic and hematopoietic function and improve tolerance to therapeutic agents. In the first report of the use of rhGM-CSF in humans, cohorts of AIDS patients were treated with increasing doses of GM-CSF given by 14-day continuous intravenous infusion.[796] This resulted in a rapid, dose-related increase in neutrophils, bands, and eosinophils, with a slight increase in monocytes. A follow-up study with subcutaneous administration showed that these effects could be sustained for up to 6 months without evidence of tachyphylaxis.[797]

A concern with the use of GM-CSF in AIDS is possible enhancement of HIV replication. In one study of zidovudine given on an alternate-week schedule with GM-CSF, some patients showed increased viral p24 levels during therapy with GM-CSF. There is evidence, however, that GM-CSF may in fact augment zidovudine levels in monocytes, which suggests that the combination of zidovudine and GM-CSF might be advantageous.[798] This is not the case with newer nucleoside analogues such as dideoxycytidine and dideoxyinosine.[799] Two clinical studies have documented an increase in HIV p24 antigen while on GM-CSF,[800, 801] and therefore GM-CSF has been replaced by G-CSF for the treatment of neutropenia.

G-CSF. In a pilot study at the National Institutes of Health, G-CSF was evaluated in 19 pediatric AIDS patients who developed neutropenia while receiving zidovudine. The neutrophil count increased from a median of 1×10^9/L to 2.9×10^9/L at doses from 1 to 20 μg/kg per day, and in 17 of the 19 patients continued zidovudine therapy was well tolerated.[802] Of note was the development of thrombocytopenia in some patients; 2 patients developed G-CSF–dependent disseminated intravascular coagulation; and 1 patient developed an increase in myeloblasts that disappeared after stopping the G-CSF.[799]

Erythropoietin. EPO has been used in 12 anemic pediatric patients to determine if tolerance to zidovudine could be improved.[799] EPO was well tolerated, and at doses from 150 to 400 U/kg subcutaneously or intravenously three times a week all patients could be maintained on zidovudine with marked (4 patients) or moderate (4 patients) reduction in transfusion requirement.

Bone Marrow Failure Syndromes

The use of HGFs in the treatment of inherited bone marrow failure syndromes has been reviewed in detail.[803]

Fanconi's Anemia. GM-CSF has been studied in 7 patients with Fanconi's anemia,[804] and, more recently, trials of IL-3 and G-CSF are being evaluated.[803] Results show that all three HGFs can improve the neutrophil count in most pancytopenic patients, but platelet and hemoglobin levels are unaffected.

Diamond-Blackfan Anemia. Although there is no evidence that Diamond-Blackfan anemia is due to deficiency of EPO,[805] IL-3, or GM-CSF,[651] or an abnormality of *KIT* or its ligand SF,[806, 807] it is possible that pharmacologic doses of these factors might stimulate erythropoiesis. Niemeyer and colleagues[808] observed no reticulocyte or hemoglobin responses in 9 patients treated with rhEPO doses as high as 2000 U/kg per day. In contrast, 3 of 6 patients treated with IL-3 (60–125 μg/m² per day subcutaneously for 4 to 6 weeks) had reticulocyte increases, and 2 of the responders remained transfusion independent for 1.5 to 2 years off therapy.[809] Another IL-3 study[810] showed 4 responders of 18 patients treated with 0.5 to 10 μg/kg subcutaneously. Two responders developed deep vein thromboses necessitating discontinuation of treatment, whereas the other 2 patients sustained their responses, 1 on maintenance IL-3 for 31 months and 1 off treatment for 12 months after 30 months of therapy. In another study of 13 patients no responses were observed.[811] Thus, 6 patients have had significant erythroid responses to IL-3 of a total of 37 (14%), a rate similar to that reported by the European Working Group for Diamond-Blackfan anemia (3/25).[812]

Amegakaryocytic Thrombocytopenia. Amegakaryocytic thrombocytopenia is a rare disease that presents in infancy or early childhood as thrombocytopenia, frequent anemia, and progression to pancytopenia. Bone marrow megakaryocytes are absent or extremely scarce. A phase I/II IL-3 dose escalation study without or with sequential GM-CSF in five children with this disorder showed that IL-3 (but not IL-3/GM-CSF) in-

duced platelet responses in two patients and improvement in bruising, bleeding, and transfusion requirement in the other three.[721] The two platelet responders became unresponsive after several months of IL-3 maintenance (125–250 μg/m² per day), whereas another patient became platelet transfusion independent after 4 months of IL-3 and had a trilineage response sustained for almost 2 years. Five patients have been treated with PIXY321 (IL-3/GM-CSF fusion protein), and in two the platelet count increased.[803]

Kostmann's Disease. Severe congenital neutropenia or Kostmann's disease (see also Chapter 7) is a disorder of myelopoiesis characterized by impaired neutrophil differentiation and absolute neutrophil counts less than 200/μL. In contrast, monocytes and eosinophils are normal or increased. The bone marrow shows maturation arrest at the promyelocyte stage, and these cells are often atypical, with abnormal nuclei and vacuolated cytoplasm. The pathophysiology is uncertain. Reduced production or abnormal G-CSF is possible but unlikely in view of data that show that serum from these patients contain normal or elevated levels of G-CSF, as determined by Western blot and bioassay.[813] A progenitor defect is more likely, because *in vitro* cultures show normal CFU-M and CFU-Eo but impaired differentiation of CFU-G in the presence of either GM-CSF or G-CSF. Another possibility is that the GM-CSF or G-CSF receptor is abnormal. G-CSFRs show normal number and affinity in Kostmann's disease patients,[814] and a single-strand conformational polymorphism analysis of the cytoplasmic domain of the receptor showed no evidence for structural abnormality in six patients.[815] However, investigations have shown mutations in the C-terminal "differentiation" domain of the G-CSFR in two patients.[463]

The responses of these patients to exogenous G-CSF and GM-CSF are therefore of great interest. One study has compared the effects of GM-CSF and G-CSF in a small number of patients, and G-CSF alone was evaluated in other studies.[816–818] In these investigations *G-CSF produced a remarkable increase in neutrophils in all patients*. The dose necessary to maintain a neutrophil count greater than 1000/μL ranged from 3 to 15μg/kg per day. The monocyte count was also increased. In contrast, rhGM-CSF produced an increase in neutrophils in only one patient, whereas the others showed an increase in eosinophils and monocytes. Although the period of study was short, no new episodes of severe bacterial infection occurred during either GM-CSF or G-CSF treatment; this contrasts to the recurrent bacterial and fungal infections that occurred before treatment. A multicenter phase III study of G-CSF in 120 patients with severe chronic neutropenic disorders including Kostmann's disease, Shwachman-Diamond syndrome, and myelokathexis showed complete responses in 108 patients (absolute neutrophil count > 1.5×10^9/L), partial responses in 4 patients, and failure to respond in 8 patients.[819]

In the two G-CSF–treated patients with Kostmann's disease who developed acute myeloid leukemia,[463] two different point mutations in the G-CSF receptor resulted in truncations of the C-terminal cytoplasmic region of the receptor and co-expression of both mutant and wild-type genes. The mutation was present in the neutropenic phase in one of the patients, suggesting that the mutation was not acquired along with the leukemia. Functional analysis by transfection of mutant or wild-type genes into murine 32D.cl0 cells showed that the mutation acted as a "dominant negative" and prevented differentiation in response to G-CSF. These data raise the concern that treatment with G-CSF could accelerate the development of acute leukemia by stimulating the proliferation of precursor cells blocked in their capacity to differentiate. Three patients with Kostmann's disease developed acute myeloid leukemia without G-CSF treatment,[820] whereas four others have developed acute myeloid leukemia with or without monosomy 7 after treatment.[463, 821, 822] Acute myeloid leukemia with monosomy 7 developed in 5 of 6 patients with acquired severe aplastic anemia treated with G-CSF.[822, 823]

Cyclic Neutropenia. Cyclic neutropenia (see also Chapter 22) is a rare HSC disease characterized by regular 21-day cyclic fluctuations in numbers of neutrophils, monocytes, eosinophils, lymphocytes, platelets, and reticulocytes. Patients typically have recurrent episodes of fever, malaise, mucosal ulceration, and, occasionally, life-threatening infection during periods of neutropenia. Six patients were treated with intravenous or subcutaneous rhG-CSF for 3 to 15 months at doses ranging from 3 to 10 μg/kg per day.[824] The median neutrophil count increased from 0.7×10^9/L to 9.8×10^9/L. In five patients, cycling of blood counts continued, but the length of cycles decreased from 21 to 14 days. The number of days of severe neutropenia (< 200/μL) was reduced from a mean of 12.7 per month to less than 1 per month and, importantly, the nadir counts increased; neutrophil turnover increased almost four-fold; and migration to a skin window was normal. Average counts of other cells did not increase. One patient with disease of adult onset had a qualitatively different response with an increase in neutrophils and disappearance of the cyclic fluctuations in count. Therapy reduced the frequency of oropharyngeal inflammation, fever, and infections, demonstrating that treatment with rhG-CSF is effective management for such patients. These results have been confirmed in other studies and rhG-CSF is well tolerated.[825–827] GM-CSF has not been effective in two patients but eliminated severe neutropenia when given in low dose (0.3 μg/kg per day).[828–830]

Chronic Idiopathic Neutropenia. This disorder of myelopoiesis is characterized by maturation arrest of neutrophil precursors in the bone marrow, neutrophil counts of less than 1.5×10^9/L, and normal other cell lineages. Patients have mucosal ulcers, periodontal disease, and recurrent infections. The pathophysiology is uncertain; in vitro bone marrow culture shows normal numbers of myeloid progenitors; and antineutrophil antibodies are absent. A single patient who received 1 to 3 μg/kg per day rhG-CSF by subcutaneous injection showed normalization of the absolute neutrophil count with healing of chronic oral ulceration, reduction of episodes of recurrent infection, and minimal

side effects.[831] Cycling of neutrophils, monocytes, and platelets was induced with a 40-day periodicity; this contrasts to the normal 21-day cycle and out-of-phase fluctuation of neutrophils and monocytes seen in cyclic neutropenia.

Toxicity of Colony-Stimulating Factor Treatment

The CSFs tested in all these clinical trials have in general been well tolerated. Both GM-CSF and G-CSF induce a *transient leukopenia* in the first 30 minutes after administration by intravenous bolus injection. GM-CSF rapidly induces surface expression of the leukocyte adhesion protein CD11b (MO1) *in vitro*, and this is accompanied by an increase in neutrophil aggregation.[715] CD11a (LFA-1) and CD11c (gp 150, 95), two other members of this family of cell surface adhesion glycoproteins that have distinct α-chains but share a common β-chain (CD18) with CD11b, are unaffected by GM-CSF. These results have been corroborated by *in vivo* studies of sarcoma patients who received GM-CSF in a dose of 32 or 64 μg/kg per day. A marked increase of CD11b was noted that was evident by 30 minutes and persisted for 12 to 24 hours after treatment.[767] Radionuclide-labeled leukocytes are sequestered in the lungs after GM-CSF treatment,[754] probably due to the aggregability and adhesiveness induced by increased CD11b expression. Breathlessness and hypoxia have been observed in some patients, particularly after short-duration intravenous administration. CD11b is not modulated by G-CSF, and the reason for the transient leukopenia after treatment with G-CSF is at present unclear.

Both GM-CSF and G-CSF have been associated with *bone pain* coincident with or shortly after administration. Occasional increases in leukocyte alkaline phosphatase or lactate dehydrogenase have been noted. In contrast, GM-CSF has also induced *flulike symptoms*, including fever, flushing, malaise, myalgia, arthralgia, anorexia, and headache. Mild elevations of *transaminase levels* and *rash* are also reported. These effects are usually mild, are alleviated by antipyretics, and disappear with continued administration. More serious GM-CSF toxicity has been observed at higher dose levels (>32 μg/kg per day intravenously or >15 μg/kg per day subcutaneously). These include a capillary leak syndrome with weight gain due to fluid retention, manifested as pericardial or pleural effusions, ascites, or edema.[761, 773] Phlebitis was noted in initial studies when the GM-CSF was infused into small veins; large-vessel thrombosis has occurred with infusion of high doses into central veins.[761]

Antibodies to Recombinant Factors. rhGM-CSF that is produced in mammalian cells (Chinese hamster ovary cells) is variably glycosylated on both O-linked and N-linked sites. Production in *E. coli* results in nonglycosylated GM-CSF, and the yeast product is glycosylated at N-linked sites. All three products appear to be equally efficacious, but antibodies have been reported to 4 of 13 patients given the yeast-derived product in phase I/II studies.[832] The IgG antibodies developed by 7 days after the start of the infusion in all 4 patients, 3 of whom had received a bolus test dose; they were non-neutralizing as judged by bone marrow colony-forming assay, and they were directed at sites on the protein backbone of the GM-CSF molecule that are normally protected by *O*-linked glycosylation but that are exposed in the yeast and *E. coli*–derived products. No dose-limiting toxicity has been observed with G-CSF. However, one case of pathogenic neutrophil infiltration (acute febrile neutrophilic dermatosis or Sweet's syndrome) has been reported.[833] One patient with Kostmann's disease developed cutaneous necrotizing vasculitis (leukoclastic vasculitis) while on G-CSF treatment.[813, 817] As noted earlier, there is also concern that G-CSF will induce or accelerate the development of acute myeloid leukemia or myelodysplasia with monosomy 7 in aplastic anemia and Kostmann's disease, perhaps more likely in those patients with G-CSF receptor mutations that can transduce a proliferative but not a differentiation signal.

Fever is the most frequent side effect associated with administration of human urinary M-CSF.[770, 779] Malaise and headache and slight depression of blood pressure have also been observed. However, since this preparation is only partially purified, it is not clear which, if any, of these side effects are due to the M-CSF.

Anemia of Chronic Renal Failure

Erythropoietin. Anemia is a major complication of end-stage renal failure and is due primarily to a reduction in EPO production. Other mechanisms that may be involved are shortened red cell survival, iron deficiency, hypersplenism, possible circulating inhibitors of erythropoiesis, and aluminum-induced microcytosis. Several phase I, II, and III studies have documented that rhEPO can induce a dose-dependent increase in effective erythropoiesis.[834–836]

In a phase III study, patients received 150 or 300 units of rhEPO three times a week after hemodialysis and reached a target hematocrit of 35% by 8 to 12 weeks.[835, 836] The majority of patients required 50 to 125 units/kg intravenously three times a week after dialysis to maintain a hematocrit of about 35%. The increase in erythropoiesis required to normalize the hemoglobin requires mobilization of a considerable amount of iron; patients who improve, particularly rapidly, can develop absolute or relative iron deficiency. If iron is not given, the response to rhEPO becomes blunted; the standard corrective measure is intravenous administration of iron dextran or oral iron supplementation. Regular measurements of ferritin and transferrin saturation are necessary to ensure that iron stores are adequate.

EPO has been well tolerated, has resulted in elimination of transfusion dependency, and has not led to antibody formation. Hypertension, occasionally with encephalopathy, has been observed, particularly with rapid rises in hematocrit that lead to an increase in peripheral vascular resistance; induction with doses not greater than 150 units/kg is recommended to produce a gradual increase in hemoglobin levels. Some patients require either the initiation of antihypertensive medication or an adjustment of dose.

The effect of rhEPO in most studies appears to be restricted to the erythroid lineage. However, data from a phase III study of 303 patients show a significant increase in mean platelet count (224×10^9/L to 241×10^9/L at 6 months), which is not biologically meaningful. There is also a slight increase in blood urea nitrogen, creatinine, and serum potassium levels. The bone marrow progenitors from patients with end-stage renal failure were studied before and 2 weeks after rhEPO treatment. The concentration of BFU-E, CFU-E, and CFU-meg increased after therapy. Surprisingly, an increment in CFU-GM also occurred, and the number of progenitors of all classes in cell cycle almost doubled.[837]

Subjective improvement in appetite, energy, sleep pattern, and libido are also noted. A Canadian double-blind placebo controlled study of rhEPO treatment has provided objective evidence of benefit.

Extending this treatment to patients who do not yet require dialysis has met with similar success.[838] An issue that has yet to be resolved is financial; rhEPO is not inexpensive, and the National Kidney Foundation in the United States has issued guidelines for the use of rhEPO in which all patients with a hematocrit of less than 30% will be eligible. rhEPO is more effective when administered by the subcutaneous route, and this will be more convenient for patients and also allow a dose reduction.[839, 840] In predialysis patients, 100 units/kg subcutaneously provided a similar response to 150 units/kg given intravenously.[839] Evidence exists that the bioavailability of subcutaneous EPO is seven times greater than that of the intravenously administered drug.

Similar results have been obtained in several rhEPO studies in children.[841] Anemia was corrected within 3 to 4 months in 24 children with preterminal chronic renal failure treated with rhEPO and iron treatment, which was adjusted by careful monitoring of iron status. Hypertension is the most common side effect.[842–845] Interestingly, although the growth failure of children with terminal chronic renal failure is unaffected by rhEPO treatment, mean growth velocity in 22 children with preterminal chronic renal failure increased from −2.29 to −0.56 within the first 6 months of treatment.[841] Other possible benefits include reports of delay in progression of renal dysfunction in children with preterminal CRF and improvement in cognitive function.

Other Indications for Recombinant Erythropoietin Therapy. Several small clinical trials have evaluated the use of rhEPO in the anemia of prematurity.[846–853] These studies have been reviewed by Mentzer and Shannon,[854] and although study differences in patient population, transfusion criteria, rhEPO dose, and iron therapy make comparisons difficult, rhEPO treatment is safe and stimulates a reticulocyte response. An effect on hematocrit was observed only in the studies in which doses greater than 500 units/kg per week were used,[846, 847, 849, 852] and there appears to be a modest effect on transfusion requirement.

Preliminary data suggest that rhEPO may be useful

in the treatment of patients with the anemia of chronic disease associated with rheumatoid arthritis[855] and the anemia that complicates zidovudine treatment in patients with AIDS (see earlier).

In simian studies, hemoglobin F levels can be increased by administration of EPO.[856] If similar changes occur in humans, EPO may have a role in the management of sickle cell disease and thalassemia. Several small studies in sickle cell disease have shown that a hemoglobin F reticulocytosis can occur in some patients, while other patients show an increase in hemoglobin without a sustained hemoglobin F reticulocyte response, a finding that is of some concern because blood viscosity might be increased.[857] There are also data to suggest that hydroxyurea in combination with EPO can augment the hemoglobin F reticulocyte response, although the contribution of EPO is still uncertain.[858, 859] In patients with transfusion-dependent or untransfused thalassemia, variable responses to EPO alone have also been reported,[860–863] with some patients showing an increase in hemoglobin and F cells. The only report to show a consistent increase in fetal hemoglobin was a study of 10 untransfused thalassemic patients who received rhEPO (400–800 units/kg three times a week) as well as iron and hydroxyurea 4 days per week. Hemoglobin increased significantly in 8 of the 10 patients, with concomitant increases in fetal hemoglobin 5% to 20% above baseline.[863]

Finally, EPO can be used to increase the number of units of blood that can be obtained preoperatively in the context of autologous blood donation.[864]

Osteopetrosis

M-CSF. An interesting series of studies showed that osteopetrotic *op/op* mice do not produce M-CSF,[865, 866] that the *op* locus maps to the same region of chromosome 3 as the M-CSF gene, and that fibroblasts from the mice have a single base insertional mutation in the M-CSF gene that results in a premature stop codon.[292] Based on the observations that osteopetrosis in *op/op* mice can be corrected by M-CSF treatment,[867–869] a phase I/II study was designed to evaluate escalating doses of M-CSF in children with severe infantile osteopetrosis.[870] Preliminary results in one patient showed a partial response; in particular, growth velocity was maintained and relatively normal bone trabecular formation was observed on biopsy after 2 months of treatment. However, biochemical evidence of bone resorption was not seen.

Osteoclastic superoxide production and bone resorption can be stimulated by IFN-γ in osteopetrotic *mi/mi* mice,[871] and this cytokine has been evaluated in a phase I/II study in 14 patients with osteopetrosis.[872] An increase in leukocyte superoxide production, decrease in trabecular bone volume, and increase in hemoglobin and platelet counts after 6 months of treatment were measured.

CONCLUSION

Advances in molecular and cell biology have led to an unraveling of some of the most challenging and confusing aspects of the study of hematopoiesis. Therapeutic benefits are rapidly emerging from these discoveries. The field of hematopoiesis, once a jumble of unknown factors and activities, has come of age and is providing direct benefits to countless patients.

References

1. Lehmann H, Huntsman RG: Why are red cells the shape they are? The evolution of the human red cell. In MacFarlane RG, Robb-Smith AHT (eds): Function of the Blood. Oxford, Blackwell Scientific Publications, 1961, p 73.
2. Brace KC: Life span of the marmot erythrocyte. Blood 1953; 8:648.
3. Everett NB, Caffrey RW: Rate of red cell formation in rats at 24°C and 5°C. Anat Rec 1962; 143:339.
4. Cline MJ, Waldmann TA: Effect of temperature on erythropoiesis. Am J Physiol 1962; 203:401.
5. Grant WC, Root WS: Fundamental stimulus for erythropoiesis. Physiol Rev 1952; 32:449.
6. Necas E, Neuwirt J: Response of erythropoiesis to blood loss in hyperbaric air. Am J Physiol 1969; 216:800.
7. Goldberg MA, Dunning SP, et al: Regulation of the erythropoietin gene: evidence that the oxygen sensor is a heme protein. Science 1988; 242:1412.
8. Wang GL, Jiang BH, et al: Hypoxia-inducible factor 1 is a basic-helix-loop-helix-PAS heterodimer regulated by cellular O_2 tension. Proc Natl Acad Sci U S A 1995; 92:5510.
9. Galson DL, Tsuchiya T, et al: The orphan receptor hepatic nuclear factor 4 functions as a transcriptional activator for tissue-specific and hypoxia-specific erythropoietin gene expression and is antagonized by ear3/coup-tf1. Mol Cell Biol 1995; 15:2135.
10. Clark BR, Keating A: Biology of bone marrow stroma. Ann N Y Acad Sci 1995; 770:70. Review.
11. Muller-Sieburg CE, Deryugina E: The stromal cells' guide to the stem cell universe. Stem Cells 1995; 13:477. Review.
12. Wolf NS: The haemopoietic microenvironment. Clin Haematol 1979; 8:469.
13. Lichtman MA, Chamberlain JK, et al: Factors thought to contribute to the regulation of egress of cells from marrow. In Silber R, LoBue J, et al (eds): The Year in Hematology: 1978. New York, Plenum Publishing Corp., 1978, p 243.
14. Bagby GC: Production of multilineage growth factors by hematopoietic stromal cells: an intracellular regulatory network involving mononuclear phagocytes and interleukin-1. Blood Cells 1987; 13:147.
15. Simmons PJ, Masinovsky B, et al: Vascular cell adhesion molecule-1 expressed by bone marrow stromal cells mediates the binding of hematopoietic progenitor cells. Blood 1992; 80:388.
16. Miyake K, Weissman IL, et al: Evidence for the role of the integrin VLA-4 in lympho-hemopoiesis. J Exp Med 1991; 173:599.
17. Teixido J, Hemler ME, et al: Role of beta 1 and beta 2 integrins in the adhesion of CD34hi stem cells to bone marrow stroma. J Clin Invest 1996; 90:358.
18. Williams DA, Rios M, et al: Fibronectin and VLA-4 in hematopoietic stem cell–microenvironment interactions. Nature 1991; 352:438.
19. Kodama H, Nose M, et al: Involvement of the c-*kit* receptor in the adhesion of hematopoietic stem cells to stromal cells. Exp Hematol 1994; 22:979.
20. Gordon MY, Riley GP, et al: Compartmentalization of a haematopoietic growth factor. Nature 1987; 326:403.
21. Dexter TM, Coutinho LH, et al: Stromal cells in haemopoiesis. Ciba Found Symp 1990; 148:76. Review.
22. Baumheter S, Singer MS, et al: Binding of L-selectin to the vascular sialomucin CD34. Science 1993; 262:436.
23. Zuckerman KS, Rhodes RK, et al: Inhibition of collagen deposition in the extracellular matrix prevents the establishment of a stroma supportive of hematopoiesis in long-term murine bone marrow cultures. J Clin Invest 1985; 75:970.
24. Jacobson LO, Marks EK, et al: Role of the spleen in radiation injury. Proc Soc Exp Biol Med 1949; 70:7440.

25. Ford CE, Hamerton JL, et al: Cytological identification of radiation-chimaeras. Nature 1956; 177:452.
26. Till JE, McCulloch EA: A direct measurement of the radiation sensitivity of normal mouse bone marrow cells. Radiat Res 1961; 14:213.
27. Becker AJ, McCulloch EA, et al: Cytological demonstration of the clonal nature of spleen colonies. J Cell Physiol 1967; 69:65.
28. Magli MC, Iscove NN, et al: Transient nature of early haematopoietic spleen colonies. Nature 1982; 295:527.
29. Whang J, Frei E, et al: The distribution of the Philadelphia chromosome in patients with chronic myelogenous leukemia. Blood 1963; 22:644.
30. Fauser AA, Kanz L, et al: T cells and probably B cells arise from the malignant clone in chronic mylogenous leukemia. J Clin Invest 1985; 75:1080.
31. Raskind HS, Jacobson R, et al: Evidence for involvement of B lymphoid cells in polycythemia vera and essential thrombocythemia. J Clin Invest 1985; 75:1388.
32. Adamson JW, Fialkow PJ, et al: Polycythemia vera: stem cell and probable clonal origin of the disease. N Engl J Med 1976; 295:913.
33. Metcalf D, Moore MAS: Haematopoietic Cells. Amsterdam, North-Holland Publlishing Co., 1971, p 1.
34. Moore MAS, Metcalf D: Ontogeny of the haemopoietic system: yolk sac origin of in vivo and in vitro colony forming cells in the developing mouse embryo. Br J Haematol 1970; 18:279.
35. Huang H, Auerbach R: Identification and characterization of hematopoietic stem cells from the yolk sac of the early mouse embryo. Proc Natl Acad Sci U S A 1993; 90:10110.
36. Godin I, Dieterlen-Lievre F, et al: Emergence of multipotent hemopoietic cells in the yolk sac and paraaortic splanchnopleura in mouse embryos, beginning at 8.5 days postcoitus. Proc Natl Acad Sci U S A 1995; 92:773.
37. Rich IN: Primordial germ cells are capable of producing cells of the hematopoietic system in vitro. Blood 1995; 86:463.
38. Micklem HS, Ross E: Heterogeneity and aging of hematopoietic stem cells. Ann Immunol 1978; 129:367.
39. Siminovitch L, Till JE, et al: Decline in colony-forming ability of marrow cells subjected to serial transplantation into irradiated mice. J Cell Comp Physiol 1964; 64:23.
40. Hellman S, Botnick LE, et al: Proliferative capacity of murine hematopoietic stem cells. Proc Natl Acad Sci U S A 1978; 75:490.
41. Ploemacher RE, van der Sluijs JP, et al: An in vitro limiting-dilution assay of long-term repopulating hematopoietic stem cells in the mouse. Blood 1989; 74:2755.
42. Dexter TM: Cell interactions in vivo. Clin Haematol 1979; 8:453.
43. Ploemacher RE, Brons RHC: Separation of CFU-S from primitive cells responsible for reconstitution of the bone marrow hemopoietic stem cell compartment following irradiation: evidence for a pre-CFU-S cell. Exp Hematol 1989; 17:263.
44. Jones RJ, Wagner JE, et al: Separation of pluripotent haematopoietic stem cells from spleen colony-forming cells. Nature 1990; 347:188.
45. Nakahata T, Ogawa M: Identification in culture of a new class of hematopoietic colony forming units with extreme capability to self-renew and generate multipotential colonies. Proc Natl Acad Sci U S A 1982; 79:3943.
46. Bradley TK, Hodgson GS: Detection of primitive macrophage progenitor cells in mouse bone marrow. Blood 1979; 54:1446.
47. Harrison DE, Lerner CP, et al: Erythropoietic repopulating ability of stem cells from long-term marrow cultures. Blood 1987; 69:1021.
48. Thomas ED, Storb R, et al: Bone marrow transplantation. N Engl J Med 1975; 292:832.
49. To LB, Juttner CA: Peripheral blood stem cell autographing: a new therapeutic option for AML? Br J Haematol 1987; 66:285.
50. Calvo W, Fleidner TM, et al: Regeneration of blood-forming organs after autologous leukocyte transfusion in lethally irradiated dogs. II. Distribution and cellularity of bone marrow in irradiated and transfused animals. Blood 1976; 47:593.
51. Antin JH, Weinberg DS, et al: Evidence that pluripotent stem cells form splenic colonies in humans after marrow transplantation. Transplantation 1985; 39:102.
52. Schofield R: The relationship between the spleen colony-forming cell and the haemopoietic stem cell. Blood Cells 1978; 4:7.
53. Schofield R: The pluripotent stem cell. Clin Haematol 1979; 8:221.
54. Fauser AA, Messner HA: Granuloerythropoietic colonies in human bone marrow, peripherial blood, and cord blood. Blood 1978; 52:1243.
55. Fauser AA, Messner HA: Identification of megakaryocytes, macrophages and eosinophils in colonies of human bone marrow containing neutrophilic granulocytes and erythroblasts. Blood 1979; 53:1023.
56. Leary AG, Ogawa M, et al: Single cell origin of multilineage colonies in culture. J Clin Invest 1984; 74:2193.
57. Coulombel L, Kalousek DK, et al: Long-term marrow culture reveals chromosomally normal hematopoietic progenitor cells in patients with Philadelphia chromosome positive chronic myelogenous leukemia. N Engl J Med 1983; 308:1493.
58. Greenberg HM, Newberger PE, et al: Generation of physiologically normal human peripheral blood granulocytes in continuous bone marrow cultures. Blood 1981; 58:724.
59. Sutherland HJ, Lansdorp PM, et al: Functional characterization of individual human hematopoietic stem cells cultured at limiting dilution on supportive marrow stromal layers. Proc Natl Acad Sci U S A 1990; 87:3584.
60. Breems DA, Blokland EAW, et al: Frequency analysis of human primitive haematopoietic stem cell subsets using a cobblestone area forming cell assay. Leukemia 1994; 8:1095.
61. McNiece IK, Stewart FM, et al: Detection of human CFC with a high proliferative potential. Blood 1989; 74:609.
62. Spangrude GJ, Heimfeld S, et al: Purification and characterization of mouse hematopoietic stem cells. Science 1988; 241:58.
63. Bertoncello I, Bradley TR, et al: The concentration and resolution of primitive hemopoietic cells from normal mouse bone marrow by negative selection using monoclonal antibodies and Dynabead monodisperse magnetic microspheres. Exp Hematol 1989; 17:171.
64. Visser JWM, Bauman JGJ, et al: Isolation of murine pluripotent hemopoietic stem cells. J Exp Med 1984; 59:1576.
65. Andrews RG, Singer JW, et al: Precursors of colony-forming cells in humans can be distinguished from colony-forming cells by expression of the CD33 and CD34 antigens and light scatter properties. J Exp Med 1989; 169:1721.
66. Berardi AC, Wang A, et al: Functional isolation and characterization of human hematopoietic stem cells. Science 1995; 267:104.
67. Berenson RJ, Andrews RG, et al: Antigen CD34+ marrow cells engraft lethally irradiated baboons. J Clin Invest 1988; 81:951.
68. Osawa M, Hanada KI, et al: Long-term lymphohematopoietic reconstitution by a single CD34-low/negative hematopoietic stem cell. Science 1996; 273:242.
69. Suda T, Suda J, et al: Disparate differentiation in mouse hemopoietic colonies derived from paired progenitors. Proc Natl Acad Sci U S A 1984; 81:2520.
70. Axelrad AA, McLeod DL, et al: Properties of cells that produce erythrocytic colonies in vitro. In Robinson WA (ed): Hemopoiesis in Culture. DHEW publication NIH-74-205, Washington, DC, 1974, p 226.
71. Pluznik DH, Sachs L: The cloning of normal "mast" cells in tissues cultures. J Cell Comp Physiol 1965; 66:319.
72. Bradley TR, Metcalf D: The growth of mouse bone marrow cells in vitro. Aust J Exp Biol Med Sci 1966; 44:287.
73. Moore MAS: Humoral regulation of granulopoiesis. Clin Haematol 1979; 8:263.
74. Haskill JS, Moore MAS: Two-dimensional cell separation: a comparison of embryonic and adult haematopoietic stem cells. Nature 1970; 266:853.
75. Dexter TM, Allen TD, et al: Conditions controlling the proliferation of haemopoietic stem cells in vitro. J Cell Physiol 1977; 91:335.
76. Metcalf D: Detection and analysis of human granulocyte-monocyte precursors using semi-solid cultures. Clin Haematol 1979; 8:263.
77. Haskill JS, McNeil TA, et al: Density distribution analysis of in vivo and in vitro colony-forming cells in bone marrow. J Cell Physiol 1970; 75:167.
78. Jacobsen N, Broxmeyer HE, et al: Diversity of human granulopoietic percursor cells: separation of cells that form colonies in

diffusion chambers (CFU-d) from populations of colony-forming cells *in vitro* (CFU-c) by velocity sedimentation. Blood 1978; 52:221.

79. Jacobsen N, Broxmeyer HE, et al: Colony-forming units in diffusion chambers (CFU-d) and colony-forming units in agar culture (CFU-c) obtained from normal human bone marrow: a possible parent-progeny relationship. Cell Tissue Kinet 1979; 12:213.

80. Moore MAS, Broxmeyer HE, et al: Continuous human bone marrow culture: Ia antigen characterization of probable pluripotent stem cells. Blood 1980; 55:682.

81. Martin DIK, Zon LI, et al: Expression of an erythroid transcription factor in megakaryocytic and mast cell lineages. Nature 1990; 344:444.

82. Orkin SH: GATA-binding transcription factors in hematopoietic cells. Blood 1992; 80:575.

83. Long MW, Heffner CH, et al: Regulation of megakaryocyte phenotype in human erythroleukemia cells. J Clin Invest 1990; 85:1072.

84. Briddell RA, Brandt JE, et al: Characterization of the human burst-forming unit-megakaryocyte. Blood 1989; 74:145.

85. Shivdasani RA, Rosenblatt MF, et al: Transcription factor NF-E2 is required for platelet formation independent of the actions of thrombopoietin/MGDF in megakaryocyte development. Cell 1995; 81:695.

86. Duebelbeiss KA, Dancey JR, et al: Marrow erythroid and neutrophil cellularity in the dog. J Clin Invest 1975; 55:825.

87. Alpen EL, Cranmore D: Cellular kinetics and iron utilization in bone marrow as observed by Fe-59 radioautography. Ann Sci 1959; 77:753.

88. Emerson SG, Sieff CA, et al: Purification of fetal hematopoietic progenitors and demonstration of recombinant multipotential colony-stimulating activity. J Clin Invest 1985; 76:1286.

89. Duke KA, Van Nuord MJ, et al: Identification of cells in primate bone marrow resembling the hematopoietic stem cell in the mouse. Blood 1973; 42:195.

90. Rosse C: Small lymphocyte and transitional cell populations of the bone marrow: their role in the mediation of immune and hemopoietic progenitor cell functions. Int Rev Cytol 1976; 45:155.

91. Nathan DG, Chess L, et al: Human erythroid burst-forming unit: T-cell requirement for proliferation *in vitro*. J Exp Med 1978; 147:324.

92. Granick S, Levere RD: Heme synthesis in erythroid cells. Prog Hematol 1964; 4:1.

93. Finch CA: Ferrokinetics in man. Medicine 1970; 49:17.

94. Lord BI: Kinetics of the recognizable erythrocyte precursor cells. Clin Haematol 1979; 9:355.

95. Hillman RS, Giblett ER: Red cell membrane alteration associated with "marrow stress." J Clin Invest 1965; 44:1730.

96. Nathan DG: Rubbish in the red cell. N Engl J Med 1969; 281:558. Editorial.

97. Etlinger JD, Goldberg AL: Control of protein degradation in reticulocyte extracts by hemin. J Biol Chem 1980; 255:4563.

98. Alpen EL, Cranmore D: Observations on the regulation of erythropoiesis and on cellular dynamics by Fe-59 autoradiography. In Stohlman F Jr (ed): The Kinetics of Cellular Proliferation. New York, Grune & Stratton, Inc., 1959, p 290.

99. McNeil BJ, Rappeport JM, et al: Indium chloride scintigraphy: an index of severity in patients with aplastic anaemia. Br J Haematol 1976; 34:599.

100. Lichtman MA, Chamberlain JK, et al: The regulation of the release of granulocytes from normal marrow. In Greenwalt TJ, Jamieson GA (eds): The Granulocyte: Function and Clinical Utilization. New York, Alan R. Liss, Inc., 1977, p 53.

101. Levine RF, Hazzard KC, et al: The significance of megakaryocyte size. Blood 1982; 60:1122.

102. Williams N, Levine RF: The origin, development and regulation of megakaryocytes. Br J Haematol 1982; 52:173.

103. Odell TT Jr, Jackson CW, et al: Megakaryocytopoiesis in rats with special reference to polyploidy. Blood 1970; 35:775.

104. Odell TT Jr, Jackson CW: Polyploidy and maturation of rat megakaryocytes. Blood 1968; 32:102.

105. deLaval M, Paulus JM: Megakaryocytes, uninucleate polyploidy or plurinucleate cells. In Paulus JM (ed): Platelet Kinetics. Amsterdam, North-Holland Publishing Co., 1971, p 90.

106. Jackson CW: Cholinesterase as a possible marker for early cells of the megakaryocytic series. Blood 1973; 42:413.

107. Nakeff A, Floech DP: Separation of megakaryocytes from mouse bone marrow by density gradient centrifugation. Blood 1976; 48:133.

108. Feinendegen LE, Odartchenko N, et al: Kinetics of megakaryocyte proliferation. Proc Soc Exp Biol Med 1962; 111:177.

109. Ebbe S, Howard D, et al: Effects of vincristine on normal and stimulated megakaryopoiesis in the rat. Br J Haematol 1975; 29:593.

110. Odell TT Jr, Murphy JR: Effects of degree of thrombocytopenia on thrombocytopoietic response. Blood 1974; 44:147.

111. Levine RF: Culture *in vitro* of isolated guinea pig megakaryocytes in the rat. Blood 1977; 50:713.

112. Long MW, Henry RL: Thrombocytosis-induced suppression of small acetylcholinesterase-positive cells in bone marrow of rats. Blood 1979; 54:1338.

113. Mayer M, Schaefer J, et al: Identification of young megakaryocytes by immunofluorescence and cytophotometry. Blood 1978; 37:265.

114. Williams N, Eger RR, et al: Two-factor requirement for murine megakaryocyte colony formation. J Cell Physiol 1982; 110:101.

115. Levin J, Levin FC, et al: The effects of thrombopoietin on megakaryocyte-CFC, megakaryocytes, and thrombopoiesis: with studies of ploidy and platelet size. Blood 1982; 60:989.

116. Long MW, Williams N, et al: Immature megakaryocytes in the mouse: physical characteristics, cell cycle status, and *in vitro* responsiveness to thrombopoietic stimulating factor. Blood 1982; 59:569.

117. Leven RM, Yee MK: Megakaryocytes morphogenesis stimulated *in vitro* by whole and partially fractionated thrombocytopenic plasma: a model system for the study of platelet formation. Blood 1987; 69:1046.

118. Kaushansky K: Thrombopoietin: the primary regulator of platelet production. Blood 1995; 86:419. Review.

119. Kato T, Ogami K, et al: Purification and characterization of thrombopoietin. J Biochem 1995; 118:229.

120. Wendling F, Maraskovsky E, et al: c-Mpl ligand is a humoral regulator of megakaryocytopoiesis. Nature 1994; 369:571.

121. Hunt P, Hokom M, et al: Megakaryocyte growth and development factor (MGDF) is a potent, physiological regulator of platelet production in normal and myelocompromised animals. Blood 1994; 84(Suppl 1):390a. Abstract.

122. Kuter DJ, Rosenberg RD: The reciprocal relationship of thrombopoietin (c-Mpl ligand) to changes in the platelet mass during busulfan-induced thrombocytopenia in the rabbit. Blood 1995; 85:2720.

123. McCarty JM, Sprugel KH, et al: Murine thrombopoietin mRNA levels are modulated by platelet count. Blood 1995; 86:3668.

124. Kaushansky K, Lok S, et al: Promotion of megakaryocyte progenitor expansion and differentiation by the c-Mpl ligand thrombopoietin. Nature 1994; 369:568.

125. Metcalf D: The Molecular Control of Blood Cells. Cambridge, MA, Harvard University Press, 1988, p 1.

126. Metcalf D: Hemopoietic regulators and leukemia development: a personal retrospective. Adv Cancer Res 1994; 63:41.

127. Clark SC, Kamen R: The human hematopoietic colony-stimulating factors. Science 1987; 236:1229.

128. Metcalf D: The colony stimulating factors. Cancer 1990; 65:2185.

129. Moore MAS: Haemopoietic growth factor interactions: *in vitro* and *in vivo* preclinical evaluation. Cancer Surv 1990; 9:7.

130. Wong GG, Clark SC: Multiple actions of interleukin-6 within a cytokine network. Immunol Today 1988; 9:137.

131. Bazan JF: Neuropoietic cytokines in the hematopoietic fold. Neuron 1991; 7:197.

132. Bazan JF: Emerging families of cytokines and receptors. Curr Biol 1993; 3:603.

133. Pestka S, Langer JA, et al: Interferons and their actions. Annu Rev Biochem 1987; 56:727.

134. Strober W, James SP: The interleukins. Pediatr Res 1988; 24:549.

135. Shalaby MR, Pennica D, et al: An overview of the history and biologic properties of tumor necrosis factors. Springer Semin Immunopathol 1986; 9:33.

136. Demetri GD, Griffin JD: Granulocyte colony-stimulating factor and its receptor. Blood 1991; 78:2791.

137. Clark SC: Biological activities of human granulocyte-macrophage colony-stimulating factor. Int J Cell Cloning 1988; 6:365.

138. Roth P, Stanley ER: The biology of csf-1 and its receptor. Curr Top Microbiol Immunol 1992; 181:141.

139. Dinarello CA: The interleukin-1 family: 10 years of discovery. FASEB J 1994; 8:1314.

140. Dinarello CA: The biological properties of interleukin-1. Eur Cytokine Netw 1994; 5:517.

141. Yang YC, Clark SC: Interleukin-3: molecular biology and biologic activities. Hematol Oncol Clin North Am 1989; 3:441.

142. Sanderson CJ: Interleukin-5, eosinophils, and disease. Blood 1992; 79:3101.

143. Akira S, Taga T, et al: Interleukin-6 in biology and medicine. Adv Immunol 1993; 54:1.

144. Du XX, Williams DA: Interleukin-11: a multifunctional growth factor derived from the hematopoietic microenvironment. Blood 1994; 83:2023.

145. Yang YC: Interleukin 11: an overview. Stem Cells (Dayt) 1993; 11:474.

146. Goldman SJ: Preclinical biology of interleukin 11: a multifunctional hematopoietic cytokine with potent thrombopoietic activity. Stem Cells (Dayt) 1995; 13:462.

147. Goldwasser E, Beru N, et al: Erythropoietin. Immunol Ser 1990; 49:257.

148. Blanchard KL, Fandrey J, et al: Regulation of the erythropoietin gene. Stem Cells (Dayt) 1993; 11(Suppl 1):1.

149. Porter DL, Goldberg MA: Regulation of erythropoietin production. Exp Hematol 1993; 21:399.

150. Galli SJ, Zsebo KM, et al: The kit ligand, stem cell factor. Adv Immunol 1994; 55:1.

151. Lyman SD, James L, et al: Molecular cloning of a ligand for the flt3/flk-2 tyrosine kinase receptor: a proliferative factor for primitive hematopoietic cells. Cell 1993; 75:1157.

152. Hannum C, Culpepper J, et al: Ligand for FLT3/FLK2 receptor tyrosine kinase regulates growth of haematopoietic stem cells and is encoded by variant RNAs. Nature 1994; 368:643.

153. Boulay JL, Paul WE: Hematopoietin sub-family classification based on size, gene organization and sequence homology. Curr Biol 1993; 3:573.

154. Cosman D, Lyman SD, et al: A new cytokine receptor superfamily. Trends Biochem Sci 1990; 15:265.

155. Bazan JF: Haemopoietic receptors and helical cytokines. Immunol Today 1990; 11:350.

156. Hanks SK, Hunter T: Protein kinases 6. The eukaryotic protein kinase superfamily: kinase (catalytic) domain structure and classification. FASEB J 1995; 9:576.

157. Lyman SD, James L, et al: Cloning of the human homologue of the murine flt3 ligand: a growth factor for early hematopoietic progenitor cells. Blood 1994; 83:2795.

158. van der Geer P, Hunter T, et al: Receptor protein-tyrosine kinases and their signal transduction pathways. Annu Rev Cell Biol 1994; 10:251.

159. Lopez AF, Sanderson CJ, et al: Recombinant human interleukin-5 (IL-5) is a selective activator of human eosinophil function. J Exp Med 1988; 167:219.

160. Bussolino F, Wang JM, et al: Granulocyte- and granulocyte-macrophage-colony stimulating factors induce human endothelial cells to migrate and proliferate. Nature 1989; 337:471.

161. Yokota T, Arai N, et al: Molecular biology of interleukin 4 and interleukin 5 genes and biology of their products that stimulate B cells, T cells and hemopoietic cells. Immunol Rev 1988; 102:137.

162. Berridge MV, Fraser JK, et al: Effects of recombinant human erythropoietin on megakaryocytes and on platelet production in the rat. Blood 1988; 72:970.

163. Kobayashi M, Laver JH, et al: Recombinant human thrombopoietin (Mpl ligand) enhances proliferation of erythroid progenitors. Blood 1995; 86:2494.

164. Ogawa M: Differentiation and proliferation of hematopoietic stem cells. Blood 1993; 81:2844.

165. Ikebuchi K, Clark SC, et al: Granulocyte colony-stimulating factor enhances interleukin-3–dependent proliferation of multipotential hemopoietic progenitors. Proc Natl Acad Sci U S A 1988; 85:3445.

166. Stanley ER, Bartocci A, et al: Regulation of very primitive, multipotent, hemopoietic cells by hemopoietin-1. Cell 1986; 45:667.

167. Zeigler FC, de Sauvage F, et al: In vitro megakaryocytopoietic and thrombopoietic activity of c-mpl ligand (tpo) on purified murine hematopoietic stem cells. Blood 1994; 84:4045.

168. Metcalf D, Begley CG, et al: Biologic properties in vitro of a recombinant human granulocyte-macrophage colony-stimulating factor. Blood 1986; 67:37.

169. Metcalf D: Lineage commitment of hemopoietic progenitor cells in developing blast cell colonies: influence of colony-stimulating factors. Proc Natl Acad Sci U S A 1991; 88:11310.

170. Sieff CA, Emerson SG, et al: Human recombinant granulocyte-macrophage colony-stimulating factor: a multilineage hematopoietin. Science 1985; 230:1171.

171. Ihle JN, Keller J, et al: Biologic properties of homogeneous interleukin 3. I. Demonstration of WEHI-3 growth factor activity, mast cell growth factor activity, P cell–stimulating activity, and histamine-producing cell-stimulating activity. J Immunol 1983; 131:282.

172. Leary AG, Yang Y-C, et al: Recombinant gibbon interleukin 3 supports formation of human multilineage colonies and blast cell colonies in culture: comparison with recombinant human granulocyte-macrophage colony-stimulating factor. Blood 1987; 70:1343.

173. Sieff CA, Niemeyer CM, et al: Stimulation of human hematopoietic colony formation by recombinant gibbon multi-colony-stimulating factor or interleukin 3. J Clin Invest 1987; 80:818.

174. Sonoda Y, Yang Y-C, et al: Analysis in serum-free culture of the targets of recombinant human hemopoietic growth factors: interleukin 3 and granulocyte-macrophage colony-stimulating factor are specific for early developmental stages. Proc Natl Acad Sci U S A 1988; 85:4360.

175. Ottmann OG, Abboud M, et al: Stimulation of human hematopoietic progenitor cell proliferation and differentiation by recombinant human interleukin 3. Comparison and interactions with recombinant human granulocyte-macrophage and granulocyte colony-stimulating factors. Exp Hematol 1989; 17:191.

176. Mayer P, Valent P, et al: The in vivo effects of recombinant human interleukin-3: demonstration of basophil differentiation factor, histamine-producing activity, and priming of GM-CSF-responsive progenitors in nonhuman primates. Blood 1989; 74:613.

177. Donahue RE, Seehra J, et al: Human interleukin-3 and GM-CSF act synergistically in stimulating hematopoiesis in primates. Science 1988; 241:1820.

178. Szabolcs P, Moore MA, et al: Expansion of immunostimulatory dendritic cells among the myeloid progeny of human CD34+ bone marrow precursors cultured with c-kit ligand, granulocyte-macrophage colony-stimulating factor, and TNF-alpha. J Immunol 1995; 154:5851.

179. Keller U, Aman MJ, et al: Human interleukin-4 enhances stromal cell-dependent hematopoiesis: co-stimulation with stem cell factor. Blood 1994; 84:2189.

180. Sonoda Y, Okuda T, et al: Actions of human interleukin-4/B-cell stimulatory factor-1 on proliferation and differentiation of enriched hematopoietic progenitor cells in culture. Blood 1990; 75:1615.

181. Kishi K, Ihle JN, et al: Murine B-cell stimulatory factor-1 (BSF-1)/interleukin-4 (IL-4) is a multilineage colony-stimulating factor that acts directly on primitive hemopoietic progenitors. J Cell Physiol 1989; 139:463.

182. Paul WE: Interleukin-4: a prototypic immunoregulatory lymphokine. Blood 1991; 77:1859.

183. Donahue RE, Yang Y-C, et al: Human P40 T-cell growth factor (interleukin-9) supports erythroid colony formation. Blood 1993; 75:2271.

184. Renauld JC, Houssiau F, et al: Interleukin-9. Adv Immunol 1993; 54:79.

185. Spritz RA, Giebel LB, et al: Dominant negative and loss of function mutations of the c-kit (mast/stem cell growth factor receptor) proto-oncogene in human piebaldism. Am J Hum Genet 1992; 50:261.

186. Alexander WS, Lyman SD, et al: Expression of functional c-kit receptors rescues the genetic defect of W mutant mast cells. EMBO J 1991; 10:3683.

187. Tsuji K, Lyman SD, et al: Enhancement of murine hematopoiesis by synergistic interactions between steel factor (ligand for c-kit), interleukin-11, and other early acting factors in culture. Blood 1992; 79:2855.

188. Tsuji K, Zsebo KM, et al: Enhancement of murine blast cell colony formation in culture by recombinant rat stem cell factor, ligand for c-*kit*. Blood 1991; 78:1223.

189. Metcalf D, Nicola NA: Direct proliferative actions of stem cell factor on murine bone marrow cells *in vitro*: effects of combination with colony-stimulating factors. Proc Natl Acad Sci U S A 1991; 88:6239.

190. Hirayama F, Ogawa M: Negative regulation of early T lymphopoiesis by interleukin-3 and interleukin-1 alpha. Blood 1995; 86:4527.

191. Hirayama F, Shih JP, et al: Clonal proliferation of murine lymphohemopoietic progenitors in culture. Proc Natl Acad Sci U S A 1992; 89:5907.

192. Williams DE, de Vries P, et al: The steel factor. Dev Biol 1992; 151:368.

193. McNiece IK, Langley KE, et al: The role of recombinant stem cell factor in early B cell development. Synergistic interaction with IL-7. J Immunol 1991; 146:3785.

194. Toksoz D, Zsebo KM, et al: Support of human hematopoiesis in long-term bone marrow cultures by murine stromal cells selectively expressing the membrane-bound and secreted forms of the human homolog of the steel gene product, stem cell factor. Proc Natl Acad Sci U S A 1992; 89:7350.

195. Cerretti DP, Wignall J et al: Human macrophage-colony stimulating factor: alternative RNA and protein processing from a single gene. Mol Immunol 1988; 25:761.

196. Lyman SD, Stocking K, et al: Structural analysis of human and murine flt3 ligand genomic loci. Oncogene 1995; 11:1165.

197. Avraham H, Scadden D, et al: Interaction of human bone marrow fibroblasts with megakaryocytes: role of the c-kit ligand. Blood 1992; 80:1679.

198. Brannan CI, Lyman SD, et al: Steel-Dickie mutation encodes a c-kit ligand lacking transmembrane and cytoplasmic domains. Proc Natl Acad Sci U S A 1991; 88:4671.

199. Matthews W, Jordan C, et al: A receptor tyrosine kinase specific to hematopoietic stem and progenitor cell-enriched populations. Cell 1991; 65:1143.

200. Small D, Levenstein M, et al: STK-1, the human homolog of Flk-2/Flt-3, is selectively expressed in CD34+ human bone marrow cells and is involved in the proliferation of early progenitor/stem cells. Proc Natl Acad Sci U S A 1994; 91:459.

201. Hirayama F, Lyman SD, et al: The flt3 ligand supports proliferation of lymphohematopoietic progenitors and early B-lymphoid progenitors. Blood 1995; 85:1762.

202. McKenna HJ, de Vries P, et al: Effect of flt3 ligand on the ex vivo expansion of human CD34+ hematopoietic progenitor cells. Blood 1995; 86:3413.

203. Hudak S, Hunte B, et al: FLT3/FLK2 ligand promotes the growth of murine stem cells and the expansion of colony-forming cells and spleen colony-forming units. Blood 1995; 85:2747.

204. Mackarehtschian K, Hardin JD, et al: Targeted disruption of the flk2/flt3 gene leads to deficiencies in primitive hematopoietic progenitors. Immunity 1995; 3:147.

205. Hunte BE, Hudak S, et al: Flk2/flt3 ligand is a potent cofactor for the growth of primitive B cell progenitors. J Immunol 1996; 156:489.

206. Zhou YQ, Stanley ER, et al: Interleukin-3 and interleukin-1 alpha allow earlier bone marrow progenitors to respond to human colony-stimulating factor 1. Blood 1988; 72:1870.

207. Ikebuchi K, Wong GG, et al: Interleukin-6 enhancement of interleukin-3-dependent proliferation of multipotential hemopoietic progenitors. Proc Natl Acad Sci U S A 1987; 84:9035.

208. Musashi M, Yang Y-C, et al: Direct and synergistic effects of interleukin 11 on murine hemopoiesis in culture. Proc Natl Acad Sci U S A 1991; 88:765.

209. Leary AG, Wong GG, et al: Leukemia inhibitory factor/differentiation-inhibiting activity/human interleukin for DA cells augments proliferation of human hemopoietic stem cells. Blood 1990; 75:1960.

210. Hirayama F, Katayama N, et al: Synergistic interaction between interleukin-12 and steel factor in support of proliferation of murine lymphohematopoietic progenitors in culture. Blood 1994; 83:92.

211. Zhang XG, Gu JJ, et al: Ciliary neurotropic factor, interleukin 11, leukemia inhibitory factor, and oncostatin M are growth factors for human myeloma cell lines using the interleukin 6 signal transducer gp130. J Exp Med 1994; 179:1337.

212. Chua AO, Chizzonite R, et al: Expression cloning of a human IL-12 receptor component. A new member of the cytokine receptor superfamily with strong homology to gp130. J Immunol 1994; 153:128.

213. Trinchieri G: Interleukin-12: a proinflammatory cytokine with immunoregulatory functions that bridge innate resistance and antigen-specific adaptive immunity. Annu Rev Immunol 1995; 13:251.

214. Leary AG, Ikebuchi K, et al: Synergism between interleukin-6 and interleukin-3 in supporting proliferation of human hematopoietic stem cells: comparison with interleukin-1alpha. Blood 1988; 71:1759.

215. Srour EF, Brandt JE, et al: Relationship between cytokine-dependent cell cycle progression and MHC class II antigen expression by human CD34⁺HLA-DR⁻ bone marrow cells. J Immunol 1992; 148:815.

216. Jacobsen SE, Ruscetti FW, et al: Distinct and direct synergistic effects of IL-1 and IL-6 on proliferation and differentiation of primitive murine hematopoietic progenitor cells in vitro. Exp Hematol 1994; 22:1064.

217. Rodriguez C, Lacasse C, et al: Interleukin-1 beta suppresses apoptosis in CD34 positive bone marrow cells through activation of the type 1 IL-1 receptor. J Cell Physiol 1996; 166:387.

218. Yamasaki K, Taga T, et al: Cloning and expression of the human interleukin-6 (bsf-2/ifn beta 2) receptor. Science 1988; 241:825.

219. Hibi M, Murakami M, et al: Molecular cloning and expression of an IL-6 signal transducer, gp130. Cell 1990; 63:1149.

220. Pennica D, Shaw KJ, et al: Cardiotrophin-1. Biological activities and binding to the leukemia inhibitory factor receptor/gp130 signaling complex. J Biol Chem 1995; 270:10915.

221. Nishimoto N, Ogata A, et al: Oncostatin M, leukemia inhibitory factor, and interleukin 6 induce the proliferation of human plasmacytoma cells via the common signal transducer, gp130. J Exp Med 1994; 179:1343.

222. Wong GG, Witek-Giannotti JS, et al: Stimulation of murine hemopoietic colony formation by human IL-6. J Immunol 1988; 140:3040.

223. Leary AG, Zeng HQ, et al: Growth factor requirements for survival in G_0 and entry into the cell cycle of primitive human hematopoietic progenitors. Proc Natl Acad Sci U S A 1992; 89:4013.

224. Paul SR, Bennett F, et al: Molecular cloning of a cDNA encoding interleukin-11, a novel stromal cell-derived lymphopoietic and hematopoietic cytokine. Proc Natl Acad Sci U S A 1990; 87:7512.

225. Turner KJ, Clark SC: Interleukin-11: biological and clinical perspectives. In Mertelsmann R, Herrmann F (eds): Hematopoietic Growth Factors in Clinical Applications. New York, Marcel Dekker, 1995, p 315.

226. Yin T, Taga T, et al: Interleukin (IL)-6 signal transducer, gp130, is involved in IL-11 mediated signal transduction. Blood 1992; 80(Suppl 1):151a. Abstract.

227. Baumann H, Schendel P: Interleukin-11 regulates the hepatic expression of the same plasma protein genes as interleukin-6. J Biol Chem 1991; 266:20424.

228. Suda T, Udagawa N, et al: Modulation of osteoclast differentiation by local factors. Bone 1995; 17:87S.

229. Burstein SA, Mei R-L, et al: Leukemia inhibitory factor and interleukin-11 promote the maturation of murine and human megakaryocytes in vitro. J Cell Physiol 1992; 153:305.

230. van de Ven C, Ishizawa L, et al: IL-11 in combination with slf and G-CSF or GM-CSF significantly increases expansion of isolated CD34+ cell population from cord blood vs. adult bone marrow. Exp Hematol 1995; 23:1289.

231. Broudy V, Lin N, et al: Thrombopoietin (c-mpl ligand) acts synergistically with erythropoietin, stem cell factor, and interleukin-11 to enhance murine megakaryocyte colony growth and increases megakaryocyte ploidy in vitro. Blood 1995; 85:1719.

232. Bruno E, Briddell RA, et al: Effects of recombinant interleukin 11 on human megakaryocyte progenitor cells. Exp Hematol 1991; 19:378.

233. Neben TY, Loebelenz J, et al: Recombinant human interleukin 11 stimulates megakaryocytopoiesis and increases peripheral platelets in normal and splenectomized mice. Blood 1993; 81:901.

234. Gordon MS, Nemunaitis J, et al: A phase 1 trial of recombinant human interleukin-6 in patients with myelodysplastic syndromes and thrombocytopenia. Blood 1995; 85:3066.

235. Tepler I, Elias L, et al: A randomized placebo-controlled trial of recombinant human interleukin-11 in cancer patients with severe thrombocytopenia due to chemotherapy. Blood 1996; 87:3607.

236. Quesniaux VF, Clark SC, et al: Interleukin-11 stimulates multiple phases of erythropoiesis *in vitro*. Blood 1992; 80:1218.

237. Trepicchio WL, Bozza M, et al: Recombinant human interleukin-11 attenuation of the inflammatory response through downregulation of proinflammatory cytokine release and nitric oxide production. J Immunol 1996; 157:3627.

238. Keith JC Jr, Albert L, et al: IL-11, a pleiotropic cytokine: exciting new effects of IL-11 on gastrointestinal mucosal biology. Stem Cells (Dayt) 1994; 12(Suppl 1):79.

239. Potten CS: Interleukin-11 protects the clonogenic stem cells in murine small-intestinal crypts from impairment of their reproductive capacity by radiation. Int J Cancer 1995; 62:356.

240. Ohsumi J, Miyadai K, et al: Regulation of lipoprotein lipase synthesis in 3t3-l1 adipocytes by interleukin-11/adipogenesis inhibitory factor. Biochem Mol Biol Int 1994; 32:705.

241. Zilberstein A, Ruggieri R, et al: Structure and expression of cDNA and genes for human interferon-beta-2, a distinct species inducible by growth-stimulatory cytokines. EMBO J 1986; 5:2529.

242. Nagata S, Tsuchiya M, et al: Molecular cloning and expression of cDNA for human granulocyte colony-stimulating factor. Nature 1986; 319:415.

243. Souza LM, Boone TC, et al: Recombinant human granulocyte colony-stimulating factor: effects on normal and leukemic myeloid cells. Science 1986; 232:61.

244. Kawasaki ES, Ladner MB, et al: Molecular cloning of a complementary DNA encoding human macrophage-specific colony-stimulating factor (CSF-1). Science 1985; 230:291.

245. Jacobs K, Shoemaker B, et al: Isolation and characterization of genomic and cDNA clones of human erythropoietin. Nature 1985; 313:806.

246. Anderson DM, Lyman SD, et al: Molecular cloning of mast cell growth factor, a hematopoietin that is active in both membrane bound and soluble forms. Cell 1990; 63:235.

247. Zsebo KM, Williams DA, et al: Stem cell factor (SFC) is encoded at the Sl locus of the mouse and is the ligand for the c-*kit* tyrosine kinase receptor. Cell 1990; 63:213.

248. Bartley TD, Bogenberger J, et al: Identification and cloning of a megakaryocyte growth and development factor that is a ligand for the cytokine receptor Mpl. Cell 1994; 77:1117.

249. Wong GG, Witek JS, et al: Human GM-CSF: molecular cloning of the complementary DNA and purification of the natural and recombinant proteins. Science 1985; 228:810.

250. Yang Y-C, Ciarletta AB, et al: Human IL-3 (Multi-CSF): Identification by expression cloning of a novel hematopoietic growth factor related to murine IL-3. Cell 1986; 47:3.

251. Huang E, Nocka K, et al: The hematopoietic growth factor KL is encoded at the Sl locus and is the ligand of the c-*kit* receptor, the gene product of the W locus. Cell 1990; 63:225.

252. Lok S, Kaushansky K, et al: Cloning and expression of murine thrombopoietin cDNA and stimulation of platelet production *in vivo*. Nature 1994; 369:565.

253. de Sauvage FJ, Hass PE, et al: Stimulation of megakaryocytopoiesis and thrombopoiesis by the c-Mpl ligand. Nature 1994; 369:533.

254. Bazan JF: Genetic and structural homology of stem cell factor and macrophage colony-stimulating factor. Cell 1991; 65:9.

255. Dolganov G, Bort S, et al: Coexpression of the interleukin-13 and interleukin-4 genes correlates with their physical linkage in the cytokine gene cluster on human chromosome 5q23-31. Blood 1996; 87:3316.

256. Manavalan P, Swope DL, et al: Sequence and structural relationships in the cytokine family. J Protein Chem 1992; 11:321.

257. Merberg DM, Wolf SF, et al: Sequence similarity between NKSF and the IL-6/G-CSF family. Immunol Today 1992; 13:77.

258. Leutz A, Damm K, et al: Molecular cloning of the chicken myelomonocytic growth factor (cmgf) reveals relationship to interleukin 6 and granulocyte colony stimulating factor. EMBO J 1989; 8:175.

259. Zink T, Ross A, et al: Structure and dynamics of the human granulocyte colony-stimulating factor determined by NMR spectroscopy. Loop mobility in a four-helix-bundle protein. Biochemistry 1994; 33:8453.

260. Sohma Y, Akahori H, et al: Molecular cloning and chromosomal localization of the human thrombopoietin gene. FEBS Lett 1994; 353:57.

261. Foster DC, Sprecher CA, et al: Human thrombopoietin: gene structure, cDNA sequence, expression, and chromosomal localization. Proc Natl Acad Sci U S A 1994; 91:13023.

262. Gurney A, Kuang W, et al: Genomic structure, chromosomal localization, and conserved alternative splice forms of thrombopoietin. Blood 1995; 85:981.

263. Anderson DM, Williams DE, et al: Alternate splicing of mRNAs encoding human mast cell growth factor and localization of the gene to chromosome 12q22-q24. Cell Growth Differ 1991; 2:373.

264. Simmers RN, Webber LM, et al: Localization of the G-CSF gene on chromosome 17 proximal to the breakpoint in the t(15;17) in acute promyelocytic leukemia. Blood 1987; 70:330.

265. Nagata S, Tsuchiya M, et al: The chromosomal gene structure and two mRNAs for human granulocyte colony-stimulating factor. EMBO J 1986; 5:575.

266. Thomas KR, Capecchi MR: Site-directed mutagenesis by gene targeting in mouse embryo-derived stem cells. Cell 1987; 51:503.

267. Lieschke GJ, Grail D, et al: Mice lacking granulocyte colony-stimulating factor have chronic neutropenia, granulocyte and macrophage progenitor cell deficiency, and impaired neutrophil mobilization. Blood 1994; 84:1737.

268. Hammond WP, Csiba E, et al: Chronic neutropenia. A new canine model induced by human granulocyte colony-stimulating factor. J Clin Invest 1991; 87:704.

269. Shoemaker CB, Mitsock LD: Murine erythropoietin gene: cloning, expression, and human gene homology. Mol Cell Biol 1986; 6:849.

270. Law ML, Cai G-Y, et al: Chromosomal assignment of the human erythropoietin gene and its DNA polymorphism. Proc Natl Acad Sci U S A 1986; 83:6920.

271. Gurney AL, Carver-Moore K, et al: Thrombocytopenia in c-mpl-deficient mice. Science 1994; 265:1445.

272. Wu H, Liu X, et al: Generation of committed erythroid BFU-E and CFU-E progenitors does not require erythropoietin or the erythropoietin receptor. Cell 1995; 83:59.

273. Sutherland GR, Baker E, et al: Interleukin 4 is at 5q31 and interleukin 6 is at 7p15. Hum Genet 1988; 79:335.

274. McKinley D, Wu Q, et al: Genomic sequence and chromosomal location of human interleukin-11 gene (IL-11). Genomics 1992; 13:814.

275. Kopf M, Baumann H, et al: Impaired immune and acute-phase responses in interleukin-6-deficient mice. Nature 1994; 368:339.

276. Bernad A, Kopf M, et al: Interleukin-6 is required *in vivo* for the regulation of stem cells and committed progenitors of the hematopoietic system. Immunity 1994; 1:725.

277. Miyatake S, Otsuka T, et al: Structure of the chromosomal gene for granulocyte-macrophage colony stimulating factor: comparison of the mouse and human genes. EMBO J 1985; 4:2561.

278. Nimer SD, Uchida H: Regulation of granulocyte-macrophage colony-stimulating factor and interleukin 3 expression. Stem Cells 1995; 13:324.

279. Campbell HD, Tucker WQJ, et al: Molecular cloning, nucleotide sequence, and expression of the gene encoding human eosinophil differentiation factor (interleukin 5). Proc Natl Acad Sci U S A 1987; 84:6629.

280. Yang Y-C, Clark SC: Molecular cloning of a primate cDNA and the human gene for IL-3. Lymphokines 1988; 15:375.

281. Le Beau MM, Espinosa R III, Neuman WL, et al: Cytogenetic and molecular delineation of the smallest commonly deleted region of chromosome 5 in malignant myeloid diseases. Proc Natl Acad Sci U S A 1993; 90:5484.

282. Sieburth D, Jabs EW, et al: Assignment of genes encoding a unique cytokine (IL12) composed of two unrelated subunits to chromosomes 3 and 5. Genomics 1992; 14:59.

283. Yang Y-C, Kovacic S, et al: The human genes for GM-CSF and IL 3 are closely linked in tandem on chromosome 5. Blood 1988; 71:958.

284. Tavernier J, Devos R, et al: A human high affinity interleukin-5 receptor (IL5R) is composed of an IL5-specific α chain and a β chain shared with the receptor for GM-CSF. Cell 1991; 66:1175.

285. Kitamura T, Sato N, et al: Expression cloning of the human IL-3 receptor cDNA reveals a shared beta subunit for the human IL-3 and GM-CSF receptors. Cell 1991; 66:1165.

286. Stanley E, Lieschke GJ, et al: Granulocyte/macrophage colony-stimulating factor-deficient mice show no major perturbation of hematopoiesis but develop a characteristic pulmonary pathology. Proc Natl Acad Sci U S A 1994; 91:5592.

287. Dranoff G, Crawford AD, et al: Involvement of granulocyte-macrophage colony-stimulating factor in pulmonary homeostasis. Science 1994; 264:713.

288. Ichihara M, Hara T, et al: Impaired interleukin-3 (IL-3) response of the A/J mouse is caused by a branch point deletion in the IL-3 receptor α subunit gene. EMBO J 1995; 14:939.

289. Hara T, Ichihara M, et al: Interleukin-3 (IL-3) poor-responsive inbred mouse strains carry the identical deletion of a branch point in the IL-3 receptor α subunit gene. Blood 1995; 85:2331.

290. Ladner MB, Martin GA, et al: Human CSF-1: gene structure and alternative splicing of mRNA precursors. EMBO J 1987; 6:2693.

291. Morris SW, Valentine MS, et al: Reassignment of the human CSF1 gene to chromosome 1p13-p21. Blood 1991; 78:2013.

292. Yoshida H, Hayashi S-I, et al: The murine mutation osteopetrosis is in the coding region of the macrophage colony stimulating factor gene. Nature 1990; 345:442.

293. Pollard JW, Hunt JS, et al: A pregnancy defect in the osteopetrotic (op/op) mouse demonstrates the requirement for csf-1 in female fertility. Dev Biol 1991; 148:273.

294. Wiktor-Jedrzejczak W, Ratajczak MZ, et al: Csf-1 deficiency in the op/op mouse has differential effects on macrophage populations and differentiation stages. Exp Hematol 1992; 20:1004.

295. Hume DA, Favot P: Is the osteopetrotic (op/op mutant) mouse completely deficient in expression of macrophage colony-stimulating factor? J Interferon Cytokine Res 1995; 15:279.

296. Metcalf D, Willson TA, et al: Production of hematopoietic regulatory factors in cultures of adult and fetal mouse organs: measurement by specific bioassays. Leukemia 1995; 9:1556.

297. Quesenberry PJ, Crittenden RB, et al: In vitro and in vivo studies of stromal niches. Blood Cells 1994; 20:97.

298. Lokhorst HM, Lamme T, et al: Primary tumor cells of myeloma patients induce interleukin-6 secretion in long-term bone marrow cultures. Blood 1994; 84:2269.

299. Arai KI, Lee F, et al: Cytokines: coordinators of immune and inflammatory responses. Annu Rev Biochem 1990; 59:783.

300. Niemeyer CM, Sieff CA, et al: Expression of human interleukin-3 (multi-CSF) is restricted to human lymphocytes and T-cell tumor lines. Blood 1989; 73:945.

301. Wimperis JZ, Niemeyer CM, et al: Granulocyte-macrophage colony-stimulating factor and interleukin-3 mRNAs are produced by a small fraction of blood mononuclear cells. Blood 1989; 74:1525.

302. Cerdan C, Razanajaona D, et al: Contributions of the CD2 and CD28 T lymphocyte activation pathways to the regulation of the expression of the colony-stimulating factor (CSF-1) gene. J Immunol 1992; 149:373.

303. Horii Y, Muraguchi A, et al: Regulation of BSF-2/IL-6 production by human mononuclear cells. Macrophage-dependent synthesis of BSF-2/IL-6 by T cells. J Immunol 1988; 141:1529.

304. Yang L, Yang YC: Regulation of interleukin (IL)-11 gene expression in IL-1 induced primate bone marrow stromal cells. J Biol Chem 1994; 269:32732.

305. Yamato K, El-Hajjaoui Z, et al: Granulocyte-macrophage colony-stimulating factor: signals for its mRNA accumulation. Blood 1989; 74:1314.

306. Tjian R, Maniatis T: Transcriptional activation: a complex puzzle with few easy pieces. Cell 1994; 77:5.

307. Mitchell PJ, Tjian R: Transcriptional regulation in mammalian cells by sequence-specific DNA binding proteins. Science 1989; 245:371.

308. Shaw G, Kamen R: A conserved AU sequence from the 3' untranslated region of GM-CSF mRNA mediates selective mRNA degradation. Cell 1986; 46:659.

309. Sachs AB: Messenger RNA degradation in eukaryotes. Cell 1993; 74:413.

310. Nakamaki T, Imamura J, et al: Characterization of adenosine-uridine-rich RNA binding factors. J Cell Physiol 1995; 165:484.

311. Curatola AM, Nadal MS, et al: Rapid degradation of AU-rich element (ARE) mRNAs is activated by ribosome transit and blocked by secondary structure at any position 5' to the ARE. Mol Cell Biol 1995; 15:6331.

312. Falkenburg JH, Harrington MA, et al: Differential transcriptional and posttranscriptional regulation of gene expression of the colony-stimulating factors by interleukin-1 and fetal bovine serum in murine fibroblasts. Blood 1991; 78:658.

313. Cockerill P, Shannon M, et al: The granulocyte-macrophage colony-stimulating factor/interleukin 3 locus is regulated by an inducible cyclosporin A-sensitive enhancer. Proc Natl Acad Sci U S A 1993; 90:2466.

314. Jones NC, Rigby PW, et al: Trans-acting protein factors and the regulation of eukaryotic transcription: lessons from studies on DNA tumor viruses. Genes Dev 1988; 2:267.

315. Shannon MF, Gamble JR, et al: Nuclear proteins interacting with the promoter region of the human granulocyte/macrophage colony-stimulating factor gene. Proc Natl Acad Sci U S A 1988; 85:674.

316. Fraser JD, Weiss A: Regulation of T-cell lymphokine gene transcription by the accessory molecule CD28. Mol Cell Biol 1992; 12:4357.

317. Kuczek ES, Shannon MF, et al: A granulocyte-colony-stimulating factor gene promoter element responsive to inflammatory mediators is functionally distinct from an identical sequence in the granulocyte-macrophage colony-stimulating factor gene. J Immunol 1991; 146:2426.

318. Miyatake S, Shlomai J, et al: Characterization of the mouse granulocyte-macrophage colony-stimulating factor (GM-CSF) gene promoter: nuclear factors that interact with an element shared by three lymphokine genes–those for GM-CSF, interleukin-4 (IL-4), and IL-5. Mol Cell Biol 1991; 11:5894.

319. Curran T, Franza BR Jr: Fos and jun: the ap-1 connection. Cell 1988; 55:395.

320. Rao A: NF-ATp: a transcription factor required for the coordinate induction of several cytokine genes. Immunol Today 1994; 15:274.

321. Nolan GP: NF-AT-AP-1 and Rel-bZIP: hybrid vigor and binding under the influence. Cell 1994; 77:795.

322. Thanos D, Maniatis T: NF-kappa B: a lesson in family values. Cell 1995; 80:529.

323. Siebenlist U, Franzoso G, et al: Structure, regulation and function of NF-kappa B. Annu Rev Cell Biol 1994; 10:405.

324. Faisst S, Meyer S: Compilation of vertebrate-encoded transcription factors. Nucleic Acids Res 1992; 20:3.

325. Turner R, Tjian R: Leucine repeats and an adjacent DNA binding domain mediate the formation of functional cfos-cjun heterodimers. Science 1989; 243:1689.

326. Northrop JP, Ho SN, et al: Nf-AT components define a family of transcription factors targeted in T-cell activation. Nature 1994; 369:497.

327. Masuda ES, Naito Y, et al: NFATx, a novel member of the nuclear factor of activated T cells family that is expressed predominantly in the thymus. Mol Cell Biol 1995; 15:2697.

328. Flanagan WM, Corthesy B, et al: Nuclear association of a T-cell transcription factor blocked by FK-506 and cyclosporin A. Nature 1991; 352:803.

329. Cockerill PN, Bert AG, et al: Human granulocyte-macrophage colony-stimulating factor enhancer function is associated with cooperative interactions between AP-1 and NFATp/c. Mol Cell Biol 1995; 15:2071.

330. Johnson PF, Landschulz WH, et al: Identification of a rat liver nuclear protein that binds to the enhancer core element of three animal viruses. Genes Dev 1987; 1:133.

331. Akira S, Isshiki H, et al: A nuclear factor for IL-6 expression (NF-IL6) is a member of a C/EBP family. EMBO J 1990; 9:1897.

332. Kinoshita S, Akira S, et al: A member of the C/EBP family, NF-IL6 beta, forms a heterodimer and transcriptionally synergizes with NF-IL6. Proc Natl Acad Sci U S A 1992; 89:1473.

333. Poli V, Mancini FP, et al: IL-6DBP, a nuclear protein involved in interleukin-6 signal transduction, defines a new family of leucine zipper proteins related to C/EBP. Cell 1990; 63:643.

334. Klemsz MJ, McKercher SR, et al: The macrophage and B cell-specific factor PU.1 is related to the ets oncogene. Cell 1990; 61:113.

335. Nishizawa M, Wakabayashi-Ito N, et al: Molecular cloning of cDNA and a chromosomal gene encoding GPE1-BP, a nuclear protein which binds to granulocyte colony-stimulating factor promoter element 1. FEBS Lett 1991; 282:95.

336. Wasylyk B, Wasylyk C, et al: The c-ets proto-oncogenes encode transcription factors that cooperate with c-fos and c-jun for transcriptional activation. Nature 1990; 346:191.

337. Arany Z, Sellers WR, et al: E1a-associated p300 and CREB-associated CBP belong to a conserved family of coactivators. Cell 1994; 77:799. Letter.

338. Wang CY, Bassuk AG, et al: Activation of the granulocyte-macrophage colony-stimulating factor promoter in T cells requires cooperative binding of Elf-1 and AP-1 transcription factors. Mol Cell Biol 1994; 14:1153.

339. Wang S, Wang Q, et al: Cloning and characterization of subunits of the T-cell receptor and murine leukemia virus enhancer core-binding factor. Mol Cell Biol 1993; 13:3324.

340. Ogawa E, Maruyama M, et al: PEBP2/PEA2 represents a family of transcription factors homologous to the products of the *Drosophila* runt gene and the human *AML1* gene. Proc Natl Acad Sci U S A 1993; 90:6859.

341. Ogawa E, Inuzuka M, et al: Molecular cloning and characterization of PEBP2 beta, the heterodimeric partner of a novel *Drosophila* runt-related DNA binding protein PEBP2 alpha. Virology 1993; 194:314.

342. Bae SC, Ogawa E, et al: PEBP2 alpha B/mouse AML1 consists of multiple isoforms that possess differential transactivation potentials. Mol Cell Biol 1994; 14:3242.

343. Miyoshi H, Shimizu K, et al: T(8; 21) breakpoints on chromosome 21 in acute myeloid leukemia are clustered within a limited region of a single gene, *AML1*. Proc Natl Acad Sci U S A 1991; 88:10431.

344. Liu P, Tarle SA, et al: Fusion between transcription factor CBF beta/PEBP2 beta and a myosin heavy chain in acute myeloid leukemia. Science 1993; 261:1041.

345. Satake M, Nomura S, et al: Expression of the runt domain-encoding PEBP2 alpha genes in T cells during thymic development. Mol Cell Biol 1995; 15:1662.

346. Weiss MJ, Orkin SH: GATA transcription factors: key regulators of hematopoiesis. Exp Hematol 1995; 23:99.

347. Fraser JD, Straus D, et al: Signal transduction events leading to T-cell lymphokine gene expression. Immunol Today 1993; 14:357.

348. Prieschl EE, Gouilleux-Gruart V, et al: A nuclear factor of activated T cell-like transcription factor in mast cells is involved in IL-5 gene regulation after IgE plus antigen stimulation. J Immunol 1995; 154:6112.

349. Hempel L, Korholz D, et al: Interleukin-10 directly inhibits the interleukin-6 production in T-cells. Scand J Immunol 1995; 41:462.

350. Guba SC, Stella G, et al: Regulation of interleukin 3 gene induction in normal human T cells. J Clin Invest 1989; 84:1701.

351. Mosmann TR: Directional release of lymphokines from T cells. Immunol Today 1988; 9:306.

352. Tsuruta L, Lee HJ, et al: Regulation of expression of the IL-2 and IL-5 genes and the role of proteins related to nuclear factor of activated T cells. J Allergy Clin Immunol 1995; 96:11.

353. Lee HJ, Masuda ES, et al: Definition of *cis*-regulatory elements of the mouse interleukin-5 gene promoter. Involvement of nuclear factor of activated T cell-related factors in interleukin-5 expression. J Biol Chem 1995; 270:17541.

354. Jenkins F, Cockerill PN, et al: Multiple signals are required for function of the human granulocyte-macrophage colony-stimulating factor gene promoter in T cells. J Immunol 1995; 155:1240.

355. Staynov D, Cousins D, et al: A regulatory element in the promoter of the human granulocyte-macrophage colony-stimulating factor gene that has related sequences in other T-cell–expressed cytokine genes. Proc Natl Acad Sci U S A 1996; 92:3606.

356. Masuda ES, Tokumitsu H, et al: The granulocyte-macrophage colony-stimulating factor promoter *cis*-acting element CLE0 mediates induction signals in T cells and is recognized by factors related to AP1 and NFAT. Mol Cell Biol 1993; 13:7399.

357. Sugimoto K, Tsuboi A, et al: Inducible and non-inducible factors co-operatively activate the GM-CSF promoter by interacting with two adjacent DNA motifs. Int Immunol 1990; 2:787.

358. Nimer S, Fraser J, et al: The repeated sequence CATT(A/T) is required for granulocyte-macrophage colony-stimulating factor promoter activity. Mol Cell Biol 1990; 10:6084.

359. Hentsch B, Mouzaki A, et al: The weak, fine-tuned binding of ubiquitous transcription factors to the IL-2 enhancer contributes to its T cell-restricted activity. Nucleic Acids Res 1992; 20:2657.

360. Takahashi A, Satake M, et al: Positive and negative regulation of granulocyte-macrophage colony-stimulating factor promoter activity by AML1-related transcription factor, PEBP2. Blood 1995; 86:607.

361. Shannon MF, Coles LS, et al: Three essential promoter elements mediate tumour necrosis factor and interleukin-1 activation of the granulocyte-colony stimulating factor gene. Growth Factors 1992; 7:181.

362. Mathey-Prevot B, Andrews NC, et al: Positive and negative elements regulate human interleukin 3 expression. Proc Natl Acad Sci U S A 1990; 87:5046.

363. Gottschalk LR, Giannola DM, et al: Molecular regulation of the human IL-3 gene: inducible T cell-restricted expression requires intact AP-1 and ELF-1 nuclear protein binding sites. J Exp Med 1993; 178:1681.

364. Cameron S, Taylor DS, et al: Identification of a critical regulatory site in the human interleukin-3 promoter by *in vivo* footprinting. Blood 1994; 83:2851.

365. Engeland K, Andrews NC, et al: Multiple proteins interact with the nuclear inhibitory protein repressor element in the human interleukin-3 promoter. J Biol Chem 1995; 270:24572.

366. Ullman KS, Flanagan WM, et al: Activation of early gene expression in T lymphocytes by Oct-1 and an inducible protein, OAP40. Science 1991; 254:558.

367. Park JH, Kaushansky K, et al: Transcriptional regulation of interleukin 3 (IL-3) in primary human T lymphocytes. Role of AP-1- and octamer-binding proteins in control of IL-3 gene expression. J Biol Chem 1993; 268:6299.

368. Davies K, TePas EC, et al: Interleukin-3 expression by activated T cells involves an inducible, T-cell-specific factor and an octamer binding protein. Blood 1993; 81:928. Abstract.

369. Zhang W, Zhang J, et al: Molecular cloning and characterization of NF-IL3alpha, a transcriptional activator of the human interleukin-3 promoter. Mol Cell Biol 1995; 15:6055.

370. Cowell IG, Skinner A, et al: Transcriptional repression by a novel member of the bZIP family of transcription factors. Mol Cell Biol 1992; 12:3070.

371. Lee HJ, Koyano-Nakagawa N, et al: cAMP activates the IL-5 promoter synergistically with phorbol ester through the signaling pathway involving protein kinase A in mouse thymoma line EL-4. J Immunol 1993; 151:6135.

372. Stranick KS, Payvandi F, et al: Transcription of the murine interleukin 5 gene is regulated by multiple promoter elements. J Biol Chem 1995; 270:20575.

373. Trinchieri G: Interleukin-12: a cytokine produced by antigen-presenting cells with immunoregulatory functions in the generation of T-helper cells type 1 and cytotoxic lymphocytes. Blood 1994; 84:4008.

374. Dinarello CA: Interleukin-1 and its biologically related cytokines. Adv Immunol 1989; 44:153.

375. Cluitmans FH, Esendam BH, et al: Regulatory effects of T cell lymphokines on cytokine gene expression in monocytes. Lymphokine Cytokine Res 1993; 12:457.

376. Horiguchi J, Warren MK, et al: Expression of the macrophage-specific colony-stimulating factor in human monocytes treated with granulocyte-macrophage colony-stimulating factor. Blood 1987; 69:1259.

377. Warren MK, Ralph P: Macrophage growth factor CSF-1 stimulates human monocyte production of interferon, tumor necrosis factor, and colony stimulating activity. J Immunol 1986; 137:2281.

378. Cluitmans FH, Esendam BH, et al: IL-4 down-regulates IL-2-,

IL-3-, and GM-CSF-induced cytokine gene expression in peripheral blood monocytes. Ann Hematol 1994; 68:293.

379. Fiorentino DF, Zlotnik A, et al: IL-10 inhibits cytokine production by activated macrophages. J Immunol 1991; 147:3815.

380. Evans R, Kamdar SJ, et al: The potential role of the macrophage colony-stimulating factor, CSF-1, in inflammatory responses: characterization of macrophage cytokine gene expression. J Leukoc Biol 1995; 58:99.

381. Matsusaka T, Fujikawa K, et al: Transcription factors NF-IL6 and NF-kappa B synergistically activate transcription of the inflammatory cytokines, interleukin 6 and interleukin 8. Proc Natl Acad Sci U S A 1993; 90:10193.

382. Temeles DS, McGrath HE, et al: Cytokine expression from bone marrow derived macrophages. Exp Hematol 1993; 21:388.

383. Zhang Y, Broser M, et al: Activation of the interleukin 6 gene by Mycobacterium tuberculosis or lipopolysaccharide is mediated by nuclear factors NF IL-6 and NF-kappa B. Proc Natl Acad Sci U S A 1995; 92:3632.

384. Natsuka S, Akira S, et al: Macrophage differentiation-specific expression of NF-IL6, a transcription factor for interleukin-6. Blood 1992; 79:460.

385. Galdiero M, Cipollaro de L, et al: Interleukin-1 and interleukin-6 gene expression in human monocytes stimulated with Salmonella typhimurium porins. Immunology 1995; 86:612.

386. Gruss HJ, Brach MA, et al: Involvement of nuclear factor-kappa B in induction of the interleukin-6 gene by leukemia inhibitory factor. Blood 1992; 80:2563.

387. Wang P, Wu P, et al: IL-10 inhibits transcription of cytokine genes in human peripheral blood mononuclear cells. J Immunol 1994; 153:811.

388. Sanceau J, Kaisho T, et al: Triggering of the human interleukin-6 gene by interferon-gamma and tumor necrosis factor-alpha in monocytic cells involves cooperation between interferon regulatory factor-1, NF kappa B, and Sp1 transcription factors. J Biol Chem 1995; 270:27920.

389. Dendorfer U, Oettgen P, et al: Multiple regulatory elements in the interleukin-6 gene mediate induction by prostaglandins, cyclic AMP, and lipopolysaccharide. Mol Cell Biol 1994; 14:4443.

390. Moller A, Schwarz A, et al: Regulation of monocyte and keratinocyte interleukin 6 production by transforming growth factor beta. Exp Dermatol 1994; 3:314.

391. de Wit H, Dokter WH, et al: Interferon-gamma enhances the LPS-induced G-CSF gene expression in human adherent monocytes, which is regulated at transcriptional and posttranscriptional levels. Exp Hematol 1993; 21:785.

392. Vellenga E, Dokter W, et al: Interleukin-4 prevents the induction of G-CSF mRNA in human adherent monocytes in response to endotoxin and IL-1 stimulation. Br J Haematol 1991; 79:22.

393. Yamada H, Iwase S, et al: Involvement of a nuclear factor-kappa B-like protein in induction of the macrophage colony-stimulating factor gene by tumor necrosis factor. Blood 1991; 78:1988.

394. Steinman RM: The dendritic cell system and its role in immunogenicity. Annu Rev Immunol 1991; 9:271.

395. Zhou LJ, Tedder TF: A distinct pattern of cytokine gene expression by human CD83+ blood dendritic cells. Blood 1995; 86:3295.

396. Galy A, Travis M, et al: Human T, B, natural killer, and dendritic cells arise from a common bone marrow progenitor cell subset. Immunity 1995; 3:459.

397. Heufler C, Koch F, et al: Interleukin-12 is produced by dendritic cells and mediates T helper 1 development as well as interferon-gamma production by T helper 1 cells. Eur J Immunol 1996; 26:659.

398. Demetri GD, Griffin JD: Hemopoietins and leukemia. Hematol Oncol Clin North Am 1989; 3:535. Review.

399. Clark SC: Hematopoietic growth factors and the myeloid leukemias. In Brugge J, Curran T, et al (eds): Origins of Human Cancer: A Comprehensive Review. Plainview, NY, Cold Spring Harbor Laboratory Press, 1991, p 453.

400. Vellenga E, Young DC, et al: The effects of GM-CSF and G-CSF in promoting growth of clonogenic cells in acute myeloblastic leukemia. Blood 1987; 69:1771.

401. Rogers SY, Bradbury D, et al: Evidence for internal autocrine regulation of growth in acute myeloblastic leukemia cells. Exp Hematol 1994; 22:593.

402. Griffin JD, Rambaldi A, et al: Secretion of interleukin-1 by acute myeloblastic leukemia cells in vitro induces endothelial cells to secrete colony stimulating factors. Blood 1987; 70:1218.

403. Kishimoto H, Matsunaga T, et al: Leukemic erythroderma with elevated plasma IL-3 and hyperhistaminemia: in situ expression of IL-3 mRNA in leukemic cells. J Dermatol Sci 1995; 10:224.

404. Meeker TC, Hardy D, et al: Activation of the interleukin-3 gene by chromosome translocation in acute lymphocytic leukemia with eosinophilia. Blood 1990; 76:285.

405. Chen YZ, Gu XF, et al: Interleukin-3 is an autocrine growth factor of human megakaryoblasts, the DAMI and MEG-01 cells. Br J Haematol 1994; 88:481.

406. Kobayashi S, Teramura M, et al: Interleukin-11 acts as an autocrine growth factor for human megakaryoblastic cell lines. Blood 1993; 81:889.

407. Nimer S, Zhang J, et al: Transcriptional regulation of interleukin-3 expression in megakaryocytes. Blood 1996; 88:66.

408. Hess JL, Zutter MM, et al: Juvenile chronic myelogenous leukemia. Am J Clin Pathol 1996; 105:238.

409. Zecca M, Rosti V, et al: Juvenile chronic myelogenous leukemia: in vitro characterization before and after allogeneic bone marrow transplantation. Med Pediatr Oncol 1995; 24:166.

410. Watari K, Ozawa K, et al: Production of human granulocyte colony stimulating factor by various kinds of stromal cells in vitro detected by enzyme immunoassay and in situ hybridization. Stem Cells 1994; 12:416.

411. Mantovani L, Henschler R, et al: Regulation of gene expression of macrophage-colony stimulating factor in human fibroblasts by the acute phase response mediators interleukin (IL)-1beta, tumor necrosis factor-alpha, and IL-6. FEBS Lett 1991; 280:97.

412. Walther Z, May LT, et al: Transcriptional regulation of the interferon-beta 2/B cell differentiation factor bsf-2/hepatocyte-stimulating factor gene in human fibroblasts by other cytokines. J Immunol 1988; 140:974.

413. Sironi M, Sciacca FL, et al: Regulation of endothelial and mesothelial cell function by interleukin-13: selective induction of vascular cell adhesion molecule-1 and amplification of interleukin-6 production. Blood 1994; 84:1913.

414. Hirano T, Akira S, et al: Biological and clinical aspects of interleukin 6. Immunol Today 1990; 11:443.

415. Van Snick J: Interleukin-6: an overview. Annu Rev Immunol 1990; 8:253.

416. Heinrich MC, Dooley DC, et al: Constitutive expression of Steel factor gene by human stromal cells. Blood 1993; 82:771.

417. Cerretti DP, Wignall J, et al: Membrane bound forms of human macrophage colony stimulating factor (M-CSF, CSF-1). Prog Clin Biol Res 1990; 352:63.

418. Yang Y-C, Tsai S, et al: Interleukin-1 regulation of hematopoietic growth factor production by human stromal fibroblasts. J Cell Physiol 1988; 134:292.

419. Lilly M, Vo K, et al: Bryostatin 1 acts synergistically with interleukin-1alpha to induce secretion of G-CSF and other cytokines from marrow stromal cells. Exp Hematol 1996; 24:613.

420. Tobler A, Meier R, et al: Glucocorticoids downregulate gene expression of GM-CSF, NAP-1/IL-8, and IL-6, but not of M-CSF in human fibroblasts. Blood 1992; 79:45.

421. Hachiya M, Koeffler HP, et al: Tumor necrosis factor and interleukin-1 synergize with irradiation in expression of GM-CSF gene in human fibroblasts. Leukemia 1995; 9:1276.

422. Cohen-Kaminsky S, Delattre RM, et al: Synergistic induction of interleukin-6 production and gene expression in human thymic epithelial cells by LPS and cytokines. Cell Immunol 1991; 138:79.

423. Chauhan D, Uchiyama H, et al: Multiple myeloma cell adhesion-induced interleukin-6 expression in bone marrow stromal cells involves activation of NF-kappa B. Blood 1996; 87:1104.

424. Zhang YH, Lin JX, et al: Interleukin-6 induction by tumor necrosis factor and interleukin-1 in human fibroblasts involves activation of a nuclear factor binding to a kappa B-like sequence. Mol Cell Biol 1990; 10:3818.

425. Stein B, Yang MX: Repression of the interleukin-6 promoter by estrogen receptor is mediated by NF-kappa B and C/EBP beta. Mol Cell Biol 1995; 15:4971.

426. Poli V, Balena R, et al: Interleukin-6 deficient mice are protected from bone loss caused by estrogen depletion. EMBO J 1994; 13:1189.

427. Dunn SM, Coles LS, et al: Requirement for nuclear factor (NF)-kappa B p65 and NF-interleukin-6 binding elements in the tumor necrosis factor response region of the granulocyte colony-stimulating factor promoter. Blood 1994; 83:2469.

428. Nishizawa M, Nagata S: cDNA clones encoding leucine-zipper proteins which interact with G-CSF gene promoter element 1-binding protein. FEBS Lett 1992; 299:36.

429. Seelentag WK, Mermod J-J, et al: Additive effects of interleukin 1 and tumor necrosis factor α on the accumulation of the three granulocyte and macrophage colony-stimulating factor mRNAs in human endothelial cells. EMBO J 1987; 6:2261.

430. Zsebo KM, Yuschenkoff VN, et al: Vascular endothelial cells and granulopoiesis: interleukin-1 stimulates release of G-CSF and GM-CSF. Blood 1988; 71:99.

431. Koenig A, Yakisan E, et al: Differential regulation of stem cell factor mRNA expression in human endothelial cells by bacterial pathogens: an *in vitro* model of inflammation. Blood 1994; 83:2836.

432. Bagby GC, Shaw G, et al: Interleukin-1 stimulation stabilizes GM-CSF mRNA in human vascular endothelial cells: preliminary studies on the role of the 3' AU rich motif. Prog Clin Biol Res 1990; 352:233.

433. Rajavashisth TB, Yamada H, et al: Transcriptional activation of the macrophage-colony stimulating factor gene by minimally modified LDL. Involvement of nuclear factor-kappa B. Arterioscler Thromb Vasc Biol 1995; 15:1591.

434. Jelkmann W: Erythropoietin: structure, control of production, and function. Physiol Rev 1992; 72:449.

435. Eckardt KU, Ratcliffe PJ, et al: Age-dependent expression of the erythropoietin gene in rat liver and kidneys. J Clin Invest 1992; 89:753.

436. Semenza GL, Koury ST, et al: Cell-type-specific and hypoxia-inducible expression of the human erythropoietin gene in transgenic mice. Proc Natl Acad Sci U S A 1991; 88:8725.

437. Semenza GL, Nejfelt MK, et al: Hypoxia-inducible nuclear factors bind to an enhancer element located 3' to the human erythropoietin gene. Proc Natl Acad Sci U S A 1991; 88:5680.

438. Semenza GL: Regulation of erythropoietin production. New insights into molecular mechanisms of oxygen homeostasis. Hematol Oncol Clin North Am 1994; 8:863.

439. Wang GL, Semenza GL: Purification and characterization of hypoxia-inducible factor 1. J Biol Chem 1995; 270:1230.

440. Blanchard KL, Acquaviva AM, et al: Hypoxic induction of the human erythropoietin gene: cooperation between the promoter and enhancer, each of which contains steroid receptor response elements. Mol Cell Biol 1992; 12:5373.

441. Stoffel R, Wiestner A, et al: Thrombopoietin in thrombocytopenic mice: evidence against regulation at the mRNA level and for a direct regulatory role of platelets. Blood 1996; 87:567.

442. Chang M, Suen Y, et al: Differential mechanisms in the regulation of endogenous levels of thrombopoietin and interleukin-11 during thrombocytopenia: insight into the regulation of platelet production. Blood 1996; 88:3354.

443. Bartocci A, Mastrogiannis DS, et al: Macrophages specifically regulate the concentration of their own growth factor in the circulation. Proc Natl Acad Sci U S A 1987; 84:6179.

444. Bazan JF: Structural design and molecular evolution of a cytokine receptor superfamily. Proc Natl Acad Sci U S A 1990; 87:6934.

445. Boutin J-M, Jolicoeur C, et al: Cloning and expression of the rat prolactin receptor, a member of the growth hormone/prolactin receptor gene family. Cell 1988; 53:69.

446. Edery M, Jolicoeur C, et al: Identification and sequence analysis of a second form of prolactin receptor by molecular cloning of complementary DNA from rabbit mammary gland. Proc Natl Acad Sci U S A 1989; 86:2112.

447. Leung DW, Spencer SA, et al: Growth hormone receptor and serum binding protein: purification, cloning and expression. Nature 1987; 330:537.

448. Hatakeyama M, Mori H, et al: A restricted cytoplasmic region of IL-2 receptor beta chain is essential for growth signal transduction but not for ligand binding and internalization. Cell 1989; 59:837.

449. Miura O, Cleveland JL, et al: Inactivation of erythropoietin receptor function by point mutations in a region having homology with other cytokine receptors. Mol Cell Biol 1993; 13:1788.

450. Miyajima A, Mui AL-F, et al: Receptors for granulocyte-macrophage colony-stimulating factor, interleukin-3, and interleukin-5. Blood 1993; 82:1960.

451. Kondo M, Takeshita T, Iet al: Sharing of the interleukin-2 (IL-2) receptor γ chain between receptors for IL-2 and IL-4. Science 1993; 262:1874.

452. Russell S, Keegan AD, et al: Interleukin-2 receptor γ chain: a functional component of the interleukin-4 receptor. Science 1993; 262:1880.

453. Noguchi M, Nakamura Y, et al: Interleukin-2 receptor γ chain: a functional component of the interleukin-7 receptor. Science 1993; 262:1877.

454. Kimura Y, Takeshita T, et al: Sharing of the IL-2 receptor gamma chain with the functional IL-9 receptor complex. Int Immunol 1995; 7:115.

455. Giri JG, Ahdieh M, et al: Utilization of the beta and gamma chains of the IL-2 receptor by the novel cytokine IL-15. EMBO J 1994; 13:2822.

456. Nicola NA: Hemopoietic cell growth factors and their receptors. Annu Rev Biochem 1989; 58:45.

457. Metcalf D: Hemopoetic regulators—redundancy or subtlety? Blood 1993; 82:3515.

458. Testa U, Pelosi E, et al: Cascade transactivation of growth factor receptors in early human hematopoiesis. Blood 1993; 81:1442.

459. Jacobsen SEW, Ruscetti FW, et al: Induction of colony-stimulating factor receptor expression on hematopoietic progenitor cells: proposed mechanism for growth factor syngergism. Blood 1992; 80:678.

460. Liboi E, Jubinsky P, et al: Enhanced expression of interleukin-3 and granulocyte-macrophage colony-stimulating factor receptor subunits in murine hematopoietic cells stimulated with hematopoietic growth factors. Blood 1992; 80:1183.

461. Ziegler SF, Bird TA, et al: Distinct regions of the human granulocyte-colony-stimulating factor receptor cytoplasmic domain are required for proliferation and gene induction. Mol Cell Biol 1993; 13:2384.

462. Fukunaga R, Ishizaka-Ikeda E, et al: Growth and differentiation signals mediated by different regions in the cytoplasmic domain of granulocyte colony-stimulating factor receptor. Cell 1993; 74:1079.

463. Dong F, Brynes RK, et al: Mutations in the gene for the granulocyte colony-stimulating-factor receptor in patients with acute myeloid leukemia preceded by severe congenital neutropenia. N Engl J Med 1995; 333:487.

464. Borzillo GV, Ashmun RA, et al: Macrophage lineage switching of murine early pre-B lymphoid cells expressing transduced *fms* genes. Mol Cell Biol 1990; 10:2703.

465. Liboi E, Carroll M, et al: Erythropoietin receptor signals both proliferation and erythroid-specific differentiation. Proc Natl Acad Sci U S A 1993; 90:11351.

466. Jubinsky PT, Nathan DG, et al: A low-affinity human granulocyte-macrophage colony-stimulating factor/murine erythropoietin hybrid receptor functions in murine cell lines. Blood 1993; 81:587.

467. Sakamaki K, Wang H-M, et al: Ligand-dependent activation of chimeric receptors with the cytoplasmic domain of the interleukin-3 receptor beta subunit (betaIL3). J Biol Chem 1993; 268:15833.

468. Chiba T, Nagata Y, et al: Tyrosine kinase activation through the extracellular domains of cytokine receptors. Nature 1993; 362:646.

469. Chiba T, Nagata Y, et al: Induction of erythroid-specific gene expression in lymphoid cells. Proc Natl Acad Sci U S A 1993; 90:11593.

470. Fairbairn LJ, Cowling GJ, et al: Suppression of apoptosis allows differentiation and development of a multipotent hemopoietic cell line in the absence of added growth factors. Cell 1993; 74:823.

471. Songyang Z, Shoelson SE, et al: SH2 domains recognize specific phosphopeptide sequences. Cell 1993; 72:767.

472. Ihle JN, Witthuhn BA, et al: Signaling through the hematopoietic cytokine receptors. Annu Rev Immunol 1995; 13:369.

473. Velazquez L, Fellous M, et al: A protein tyrosine kinase in the interferon αβ signaling pathway. Cell 1992; 70:313.

474. Müller M, Briscoe J, et al: The protein tyrosine kinase JAK1

complements defects in interferon-αβγ signal transduction. Nature 1993; 366:129.

475. Witthuhn BA, Quelle FW, et al: JAK2 associates with the erythropoietin receptor and is tyrosine phosphorylated and activated following stimulation with erythropoietin. Cell 1993; 74:227.

476. Zhuang H, Patel SV, et al: Inhibition of erythropoietin-induced mitogenesis by a kinase-deficient form of Jak2. J Biol Chem 1994; 269:21411.

477. Linnekin D, Evans GA, et al: Association of the erythropoietin receptor with protein tyrosine kinase activity. Proc Natl Acad Sci U S A 1992; 89:6237.

478. Miura O, D'Andrea A, et al: Induction of tyrosine phosphorylation by the erythropoietin receptor correlates with mitogenesis. Mol Cell Biol 1991; 11:4895.

479. Yoshimura A, Lodish HF: *In vitro* phosphorylation of the erythropoietin receptor and an associated protein. Mol Cell Biol 1992; 12:706.

480. Hanazono Y, Chib S, et al: Erythropoietin induces tyrosine phosphorylation and kinase activity of the c-*fps/fes* proto-oncogene product in human erythropoietin-responsive cells. Blood 1993; 81:3193.

481. Ihle JN: Cytokine receptor signaling. Nature 1995; 377:591.

482. Sakamaki K, Miyajima I, et al: Critical cytoplasmic domains of the common beta subunit of the human GM-CSF, IL-3 and IL-5 receptors for growth signal transduction and tyrosine phosphorylation. EMBO J 1992; 11:3541.

483. Duronio V, Clark-Lewis I, et al: Tyrosine phosphorylation of receptor beta subunits and common substrates in response to interleukin-3 and granulocyte-macrophage colony-stimulating factor. J Biol Chem 1992; 267:21856.

484. Silvennoinen O, Witthuhn BA, et al: Structure of the murine JAK2 protein tyrosine kinase and its role in IL-3 signal transduction. Proc Natl Acad Sci U S A 1993; 90:8429.

485. Shikama Y, Barber DL, et al: A constitutively activated chimeric cytokine receptor confers factor-dependent growth in hematopoietic cell lines. Blood 1996; 88:455.

486. Torigoe T, O'Connor R, et al: Interleukin-3 regulates the activity of the LYN protein-tyrosine kinase in myeloid-committed leukemic cell lines. Blood 1992; 80:617.

487. Kobayashi N, Kono T, et al: Functional coupling of the *src*-family protein tyrosine kinases p59^{fyn} and p53/56^{lyn} with the interleukin 2 receptor: implications for redundancy and pleiotropism in cytokine signal transduction. Proc Natl Acad Sci U S A 1993; 90:4201.

488. Hanazono Y, Chiba S, et al: c-*fps/fes* protein-tyrosine is implicated in a signaling pathway triggered by granulocyte-macrophage colony-stimulating factor and interleukin-3. EMBO J 1993; 12:1641.

489. Quelle FW, Sato N, et al: JAK2 associates with the β$_c$ chain of the receptor for granulocyte-macrophage colony-stimulating factor, and its activation requires the membrane-proximal region. Mol Cell Biol 1994; 14:4335.

490. Weiss M, Yokoyama C, et al: Human granulocyte-macrophage colony-stimulating factor receptor signal transduction requires the proximal cytoplasmic domains of the αβ subunits. Blood 1993; 82:3298.

491. Sato N, Sakamaki K, et al: Signal transduction by the high-affinity GM-CSF receptor: two distinct cytoplasmic regions of the common β subunit responsible for different signaling. EMBO J 1993; 12:4181.

492. Kinoshita T, Yokota T, et al: Suppression of apoptotic death in hematopoietic cells by signalling through the IL-3/GM-CSF receptors. EMBO J 1995; 14:266.

493. Stahl N, Boulton TG, et al: Association and activation of Jak-Tyk kinases by CNTF-LIF-OSM-IL-6β receptor components. Science 1994; 263:92.

494. Fu X-Y: A transcription factor with SH2 and SH3 domains is directly activated by an interferon α-induced cytoplasmic protein tyrosine kinase(s). Cell 1992; 70:323.

495. Fu X-Y, Schindler C, et al: The proteins of ISGF-3, the interferon α-induced transcriptional activator, define a gene family involved in signal transduction. Proc Natl Acad Sci U S A 1992; 89:7840.

496. Darnell JE Jr, Kerr IM, et al: Jak-STAT pathways and transcriptional activation in response to IFNs and other extracellular signaling proteins. Science 1994; 264:1415.

497. Watling D, Guschin D, et al: Complementation by the protein tyrosine kinase JAK2 of a mutant cell line defective in the interferon-γ signal transduction pathway. Nature 1993; 366:166.

498. Shuai K, Stark GR, et al: A single phosphotyrosine residue of STAT91 required for gene activation by interferon γ. Science 1993; 261:1744.

499. Lütticken C, Wegenka UM, et al: Association of transcription factor APRF and protein kinase Jak1 with the interleukin-6 signal transducer gp130. Science 1994; 263:89.

500. Zhong Z, Wen Z, et al: Stat3: a STAT family member activated by tyrosine phosphoryation in response to epidermal growth factor and interleukin-6. Science 1994; 264:95.

501. Zhong Z, Wen Z, et al: Stat3 and Stat4: members of the family of signal transducers and activators of transcription. Proc Natl Acad Sci U S A 1994; 91:4806.

502. Yamamoto K, Quelle FW, et al: Stat4, a novel gamma interferon activation site-binding protein expressed in early myeloid differentiation. Mol Cell Biol 1994; 14:4342.

503. Jacobson NG, Szabo SJ, et al: Interleukin 12 signaling in T helper type 1 (Th1) cells involves tyrosine phosphorylation of signal transducer and activator of transcription (Stat)3 and Stat4. J Exp Med 1995; 181:1755.

504. Larner AC, David M, et al: Tyrosine phosphorylation of DNA binding proteins by multiple cytokines. Science 1993; 261:1730.

505. Wakao H, Gouilleux F, et al: Mammary gland factor (MGF) is a novel member of the cytokine regulated transcription factor gene family and confers the prolactin response. EMBO J 1994; 13:2182.

506. Gouilleux F, Pallard C, et al: Prolactin, growth hormone, erythropoietin and granulocyte-macrophage colony stimulating factor induce MGF-Stat5 DNA binding activity. EMBO J 1995; 14:2005.

507. Mui AL-F, Wakao H, et al: Interleukin-3, granulocyte-macrophage colony stimulating factor and interleukin-5 transduce signals through two STAT5 homologs. EMBO J 1995; 14:1166.

508. Hou J, Schindler U, et al: An interleukin-4-induced transcription factor: IL-4 Stat. Science 1994; 265:1701.

509. McCormick F: How receptors turn Ras on. Nature 1993; 363:15.

510. Feig L: The many roads that lead to Ras. Science 1993; 260:767.

511. Moodie SA, Willumsen BM, et al: Complexes of Ras-GTP with Raf-1 and mitogen-activated protein kinase kinase. Science 1993; 260:1658.

512. Satoh T, Nakafuku M, et al: Involvement of *ras* p21 protein in signal-transduction pathways from interleukin 2, interleukin 3, and granulocyte/macrophage colony-stimulating factor, but not from interleukin 4. Proc Natl Acad Sci U S A 1991; 88:3314.

513. Duronio V, Welham MJ, et al: p21^{ras} activation via hemopoietin receptors and c-kit requires tyrosine kinase activity but not phosphorylation of p21^{ras} GTPase-activating protein. Proc Natl Acad Sci U S A 1993; 89:1587.

514. Torti M, Marti KB, et al: Erythropoietin induces p21^{ras} activation and p120GAP tyrosine phosphorylation in human erythroleukemia cells. J Biol Chem 1992; 267:8293.

515. Downward J, Graves JD, et al: Stimulation of p21^{ras} upon T-cell activation. Nature 1990; 346:719.

516. Gulbins E, Coggeshall KM, et al: Tyrosine kinase-stimulated guanine nucleotide exchange activity of vav in T cell activation. Science 1993; 260:822.

517. Kavanaugh WM, Williams LT: An alternative to SH2 domains for binding tyrosine-phosphorylated proteins. Science 1994; 266:1862.

518. van der Geer P, Pawson T: The PTB domain: a new protein module implicated in signal transduction. Trends Biochem Sci 1996; 20:277.

519. Ravichandran KS, Burakoff SJ: The adapter protein Shc interacts with the interleukin-2 (IL-2) receptor upon IL-2 stimulation. J Biol Chem 1994; 269:1599.

520. Pratt JC, Weiss M, et al: Evidence for a physical association between the Shc-PTB domain and the β$_c$ chain of the granulocyte-macrophage colony stimulating receptor. J Biol Chem 1996; 271:12137.

521. Inhorn RC, Carlesso N, et al: Identification of a viablility domain in the granulocyte/macrophage colony-stimulating factor receptor β-chain involving tyrosine-750. Med Sci 1995; 92:8665.

522. Damen JE, Liu L, et al: Erythropoietin stimulates the tyrosine

phosphorylation of Shc and its association with Grb2 and a 145-Kd tyrosine phosphorylated protein. Blood 1993; 82:2296.

523. Cutler RL, Liu L, et al: Multiple cytokines induce the tyrosine phosphorylation of Shc and its association with Grb2 in hemopoietic cells. J Biol Chem 1993; 268:21463.

524. Komatsu N, Adamson JW, et al: Erythropoietin rapidly induces tyrosine phosphorylation in the human erythropoietin-dependent cell line, UT-7. Blood 1992; 80:53.

525. Carroll MP, Spivak JL, et al: Erythropoietin induces Raf-1 activation and Raf-1 is required for erythropoietin-mediated proliferation. J Biol Chem 1991; 266:14964.

526. Miura Y, Miura O, et al: Activation of the mitogen-activated protein kinase pathway by the erythropoietin receptor. J Biol Chem 1994; 269:29962.

527. Bader JL: Neurofibromatosis and cancer. Ann N Y Acad Sci 1986; 486:57.

528. Shannon KM, O'Connell P, et al: Loss of the normal *NF1* allele from the bone marrow of children with type 1 neurofibromatosis and malignant myeloid disorders. N Engl J Med 1994; 330:597.

529. Bollag G, Clapp DW, et al: Loss of NF1 results in activation of the Ras signaling pathway and leads to aberrant growth in haematopoietic cells. Nat Genet 1996; 12:144.

530. Largaespada DA, Brannan CI, et al: Nf1 deficiency causes Ras-mediated granulocyte/macrophage colony stimulating factor hypersensitivity and chronic myeloid leukaemia. Nat Genet 1996; 12:137.

531. Pendergast AM, Quilliam LA, et al: BCR-ABL-induced oncogenesis is mediated by direct interaction with the SH2 domain of the GRB-2 adaptor protein. Cell 1993; 75:175.

532. D'Andrea AD, Yoshimura A, et al: The cytoplasmic region of the erythropoietin receptor contains nonoverlapping positive and negative growth-regulatory domains. Mol Cell Biol 1991; 11:1980.

533. Yi T, Mui AL-F, et al: Hematopoietic cell phosphatase associates with the interleukin-3 (IL-3) receptor β chain and down-regulates IL-3-induced tyrosine phosphorylation and mitogenesis. Mol Cell Biol 1993; 13:7577.

534. de la Chapelle A, Traskelin A-L, et al: Truncated erythropoietin receptor causes dominantly inherited benign human erythrocytosis. Proc Natl Acad Sci U S A 1993; 90:4495.

535. Klingmüller U, Lorenz U, et al: Specific recruitment of SH-PTP1 to the erythropoietin receptor causes inactivation of JAK2 and termination of proliferative signals. Cell 1995; 80:729.

536. Van Zant G, Shultz L: Hematologic abnormalities of the immunodeficient mouse mutant, viable motheaten (me^v). Exp Hematol 1989; 17:81.

537. Schultz LD, Schweitzer PA, et al: Mutations at the murine motheaten locus are within the hematopoietic cell protein-tyrosine phosphatase *(Hcph)* gene. Cell 1993; 73:1445.

538. Sun H, Tonks NK: The coordinated action of protein tyrosine phosphatases and kinases in cell signaling. Trends Biochem Sci 1994; 19:480.

539. Sherr CJ: Mammalian G_1 cyclins. Cell 1993; 73:1059.

540. Ohtsubo M, Roberts JM: Cyclin-dependent regulation of G_1 in mammalian fibroblasts. Science 1993; 259:1908.

541. Baldin V, Lukas J, et al: Cyclin D1 is a nuclear protein required for cell cycle progression in G_1. Genes Dev 1993; 7:812.

542. Kato J-Y, Matsushime H, et al: Direct binding of cyclin D to the retinoblastoma gene product (pRb) and pRb phosphorylation by the cyclin-dependent kinase CDK4. Genes Dev 1993; 7:331.

543. Nevins JR: E2F: a link between the Rb tumor suppressor protein and viral oncoproteins. Science 1992; 258:424.

544. Kato J-Y, Sherr CJ: Inhibition of granulocyte differentiation by G_1 cyclins D2 and D3 but not D1. Proc Natl Acad Sci U S A 1993; 90:11513.

545. Ando K, Griffin J D: Cdk4 integrates growth stimulatory and inhibitory signals during G_1 phase of hematopoietic cells. Oncogene 1995; 10:751.

546. Ando K, Ajchenbaum-Cymbelista F, et al: Regulation of G_1/S transition by cyclins D2 and D3 in hematopoietic cells. Proc Natl Acad Sci U S A 1993; 90:9571.

547. Lee EY-HP, Chang C-Y, et al: Mice deficient for Rb are nonviable and show defects in neurogeneisis and haematopoiesis. Nature 1992; 359:288.

548. Clarke AR, Maandag ER, et al: Requirement for a functional *Rb-1* gene in murine development. Nature 1992; 359:328.

549. Jacks T, Fazeli A, et al: Effects of an *RB* mutation in the mouse. Nature 1992; 359:295.

550. Pevny L, Simon MC, et al: Erythroid differentiation in chimaeric mice blocked by a targeted mutation in the gene for transcription factor GATA-1. Nature 1991; 349:257.

551. Mucenski ML, McLain K, et al: A functional c-*myb* gene is required for normal murine fetal hepatic hematopoiesis. Cell 1991; 65:677.

552. Xiong Y, Zhang H, et al: Subunit rearrangement of the cyclin-dependent kinases is associated with cellular transformation. Genes Dev 1993; 7:1572.

553. Motokura T, Bloom T, et al: A novel cyclin encoded by a *bcl1*-linked candidate oncogene. Nature 1991; 350:512.

554. Rosenberg CL, Wong E, et al: PRAD1, a candidate BCL1 oncogene: mapping and expression in centrocytic lymphoma. Proc Natl Acad Sci U S A 1991; 88:9638.

555. Schuuring E, Verhoeven E, et al: Identification and cloning of two overexpressed genes, U21B31/PRAD1 and EMS1, within the amplified chromosome 11q13 region in human carcinomas. Oncogene 1992; 7:355.

556. Buckley MF, Sweeney KJ, et al: Expression and amplification of cyclin genes in human breast cancer. Oncogene 1993; 8:2127.

557. Callender T, el-Naggar AK, et al: PRAD-1 (CCND1)/cyclin D1 oncogene amplification in primary head and neck squamous cell carcinoma. Cancer 1994; 74:152.

558. Till JE, McCulloch EA, et al: A stochastic model of stem cell proliferation based on growth of spleen colony-forming cells. Proc Natl Acad Sci U S A 1964; 51:29.

559. Petrov RV, Khaitov RM, et al: Factors controlling stem cell recirculation. III. Effect of thymus on the migration and differentiation of hematopoietic stem cells. Blood 1977; 29:40.

560. Lord BI, Schofield R: The influence of thymus cells in hemopoiesis: stimulation of hemopoietic stem cells in a syngeneic, *in vivo* situation. Blood 1973; 42:395.

561. Trainin N, Resnitzky R: Influence of neonatal thymectomy on cloning capacity of bone marrow cells in mice. Nature 1963; 221:1154.

562. Prichard LL, Shinpock SG, et al: Augmentation of marrow growth by thymocytes separated by discontinuous albumin density-gradient centrifugation. Exp Hematol 1975; 3:94.

563. Zipori D, Trainin N: Defective capacity of bone marrow from nude mice to restore lethally irradiated recipients. Blood 1973; 42:671.

564. Zipori D, Trainin N: Impaired radioprotective capacity and reduced proliferative rate of bone marrow from neonatally thymectomized mice. Exp Hematol 1975; 3:1.

565. Pinkerton PH, Bannerman RM: The hereditary anemias of mice. Hematol Rev 1968; 1:119.

566. Bernstein SE, Russell ES, et al: Two hereditary mouse anemias (Sl/Sl^d and W/W^v) deficient in response to erythropoietin. Ann N Y Acad Sci 1968; 149:475.

567. Witte ON: Steel locus defines new multipotent growth factor. Cell 1990; 63:5.

568. Barr RD, Wang-Peng J, et al: Hematopoietic stem cells in human peripheral blood. Science 1975; 109:284.

569. Clarke BJ, Housman D: Characterization of an erythroid precursor cell of high proliferative capacity in normal human peripheral blood. Proc Natl Acad Sci U S A 1977; 74:1105.

570. Samlowski WE, Daynes RA: Bone marrow engraftment is enhanced by competitive inhibition of the hepatic asialoglycoprotein. Proc Natl Acad Sci U S A 1985; 82:2508.

571. Tavassoli M, Hardy C: Molecular basis of homing of intravenously transplanted stem cells to the marrow. Blood 1990; 76:1059.

572. Kay HEM: Hypothesis: how many cell-generations? Lancet 1965; II:418.

573. Micklem HS, Ansell JD, et al: The clonal organization of hematopoiesis in the mouse. Prog Immunol 1983; 5:633.

574. Mintz B, Anthony K, Litwin S: Monoclonal derivation of mouse myeloid and lymphoid lineages from totipotent hematopoietic stem cells experimentally transplanted in fetal hosts. Proc Natl Acad Sci U S A 1984; 81:7835.

575. Lemischka IR, Raulet DH, et al: Developmental potential and dynamic behavior of hematopoietic stem cells. Cell 1986; 45:917.

576. Capel B, Hawley R, et al: Clonal contributions of small numbers of retrovirally marked hematopoietic stem cells engrafted in unirradiated neonatal W/W^v mice. Proc Natl Acad Sci U S A 1989; 86:4564.

577. Abkowitz JL, Catlin SN, et al: Evidence that hematopoiesis may be a stochastic process *in vivo*. Nat Med 1996; 2:190.

578. Harrison DE, Astle CM, et al: Number and continuous proliferative pattern of transplanted primitive immunohematopoietic stem cells. Proc Natl Acad Sci U S A 1988; 85:822.

579. Jordan CT, Lemischka IR: Clonal and systemic analysis of long-term hematopoiesis in the mouse. Genes Dev 1990; 4:220.

580. Shivdasani RA, Orkin SH: The transcriptional control of hematopoiesis. Blood 1996; 87:4025.

581. Begley CG, Aplan PD, et al: Chromosomal translocation in a human leukemic stem-cell line disrupts the T-cell antigen receptor delta-chain diversity region and results in a previously unreported fusion transcript. Proc Natl Acad Sci U S A 1989; 86:2031.

582. Finger LR, Kagan J, et al: Involvement of the TCL5 gene on human chromosome 1 in T-cell leukemia and melanoma. Proc Natl Acad Sci U S A 1989; 86:5039.

583. Begley CG, Aplan PD, et al: The gene SCL is expressed during early hematopoiesis and encodes a differentiation-related DNA-binding motif. Proc Natl Acad Sci U S A 1989; 86:10128.

584. Mouthon MA, Bernard O, et al: Expression of tal-1 and GATA-binding proteins during human hematopoiesis. Blood 1993; 81:647.

585. Shivdasani RA, Mayer EL, et al: Absence of blood formation in mice lacking the T-cell leukaemia oncoprotein tal-1/SCL. Nature 1995; 373:432.

586. Robb L, Lyons I, et al: Absence of yolk sac hematopoiesis from mice with a targeted disruption of the scl gene. Proc Natl Acad Sci U S A 1995; 92:7075.

587. Boehm T, Foroni L, et al: The rhombotin family of cysteine-rich LIM-domain oncogenes: distinct members are involved in T-cell translocations to human chromosomes 11p15 and 11p13. Proc Natl Acad Sci U S A 1991; 88:4367.

588. Rabbitts TH: Chromosomal translocations in human cancer. Nature 1994; 372:143. Review.

589. Warren AJ, Colledge WH, et al: The oncogenic cysteine-rich LIM domain protein Rbtn2 is essential for erythroid development. Cell 1994; 78:45.

590. Valge-Archer VE, Osada H, et al: The LIM protein RBTN2 and the basic helix-loop-helix protein TAL1 are present in a complex in erythroid cells. Proc Natl Acad Sci U S A 1994; 91:8617.

591. Wadman I, Li J, et al: Specific *in vivo* association between the bHLH and LIM proteins implicated in human T cell leukemia. EMBO J 1994; 13:4831.

592. Dorfman DM, Wilson DB, et al: Human transcription factor GATA-2. Evidence for regulation of preproendothelin-1 gene expression in endothelial cells. J Biol Chem 1992; 267:1279.

593. Leonard M, Brice M, et al: Dynamics of GATA transcription factor expression during erythroid differentiation. Blood 1993; 82:1071.

594. Visvader J, Adams JM: Megakaryocytic differentiation induced in 416B myeloid cells by GATA-2 and GATA-3 transgenes or 5-azacytidine is tightly coupled to GATA-1 expression. Blood 1993; 82:1493.

595. Briegel K, Lim KC, et al: Ectopic expression of a conditional GATA-2/estrogen receptor chimera arrests erythroid differentiation in a hormone-dependent manner. Genes Dev 1993; 7:1097.

596. Tsai FY, Keller G, et al: An early haematopoietic defect in mice lacking the transcription factor GATA-2. Nature 1994; 371:221.

597. Sposi NM, Zon LI, et al: Cell cycle-dependent initiation and lineage-dependent abrogation of GATA-1 expression in pure differentiating hematopoietic progenitors. Proc Natl Acad Sci U S A 1992; 89:6353.

598. Russell ES: Hereditary anemias of the mouse: a review for geneticists. Adv Genet 1979; 20:357.

599. Okuda T, van Deursen J, et al: AML1, the target of multiple chromosomal translocations in human leukemia, is essential for normal fetal liver hematopoiesis. Cell 1996; 84:321.

600. Stegmaier K, Pendse S, et al: Frequent loss of heterozygosity at the TEL gene locus in acute lymphoblastic leukemia of childhood. Blood 1995; 86:38.

601. Bodine DM, Crosier PS, et al: Effects of hematopoietic growth factors on the survival of primitive stem cells in liquid suspension culture. Blood 1991; 78:914.

602. Itoh Y, Ikebuchi K, et al: Interleukin-3 and granulocyte colony-stimulating factor as survival factors in murine hemopoietic stem cells *in vitro*. Int J Hematol 1992; 55:139.

603. Katayama N, Clark SC, et al: Growth factor requirement for survival in cell cycle dormancy of primitive murine lympho-hematopoietic progenitors. Blood 1993; 81:610.

604. Neben S, Donaldson D, et al: Synergistic effects of interleukin-11 with other growth factors on the expansion of murine hematopoietic progenitors and maintenance of stem cells in liquid culture. Exp Hematol 1994; 22:353.

605. Li CL, Johnson GR: Stem cell factor enhances the survival but not the self-renewal of murine hematopoietic long-term repopulating cells. Blood 1994; 84:408.

606. Bodine DM, Seidel NE, et al: *In vivo* administration of stem cell factor to mice increases the absolute number of pluripotent hematopoietic stem cells. Blood 1993; 82:445.

607. Bodine DM, Orlic D, et al: Stem cell factor increases CFU-S number in vitro in synergy with interleukin-6, and *in vivo* in SL/SL^d mice as a single factor. Blood 1992; 79:913.

608. McCulloch EA, Siminovich L, et al: Spleen colony formation of anemic mice of genotype WW^v. Science 1964; 144:844.

609. Chabot B, Stephenson DA, et al: The proto-oncogenic c-*kit* encoding a transmembrane tyrosine kinase receptor maps to the mouse W locus. Nature 1988; 335:88.

610. Geissler EN, Ryan MA, et al: The dominant-white spotting (W) locus of the mouse encodes the c-*kit* proto-oncogene. Cell 1988; 55:185.

611. Yarden Y, Kuang W-J, et al: Human proto-oncogene c-*kit*: a new cell surface receptor tyrosine kinase for an unidentified ligand. EMBO J 1987; 6:3341.

612. Reith AD, Rottapel R, et al: W mutant mice with mild or severe developmental defects contain distinct point mutations in the kinase domain of the c-*kit* receptor. Genes Dev 1990; 4:390.

613. McCulloch EA, Siminovitch L, et al: The cellular basis of the genetically determined hemopoietic defect in anemic mice of genotype Sl/Sl^d. Blood 1965; 26:399.

614. Williams DE, Eisenman J, et al: Identification of a ligand for the c-*kit* proto-oncogene. Cell 1990; 63:167.

615. Zsebo KM, Wypych J, et al: Identification, purification, and biological characterization of hematopoietic stem cell factor from buffalo rat liver–conditioned medium. Cell 1990; 63:195.

616. Martin FH, Suggs SV, et al: Primary structure and functional expression of rat and human stem cell factor DNAs. Cell 1990; 63:203.

617. Nocka K, Buck J, et al: Candidate ligand for the c-*kit* transmembrane kinase receptor: KL, a fibroblast-derived growth factor stimulates mast cells and erythroid progenitors. EMBO J 1990; 9:3287.

618. Copeland NG, Gilbert DJ, et al: Mast cell growth factor maps near the steel locus on mouse chromosome 10 and is deleted in a number of steel alleles. Cell 1990; 63:175.

619. Flanagan JG, Leder P: The *kit* ligand: a cell surface molecule altered in steel mutant fibroblasts. Cell 1990; 63:185.

620. Flanagan JG, Chan DC, et al: Transmembrane form of the *kit* ligand growth factor is determined by alternative splicing and is missing in the Sl^d Mutant. Cell 1991; 64:1025.

621. Lansdorp PM, Dragowska W: Maintenance of hematopoiesis in serum-free bone marrow cultures involves sequential recruitment of quiescent progenitors. Exp Hematol 1993; 21:1321.

622. Curry JL, Trentin JJ: Hemopoietic spleen colony studies. I. Growth and differentiation. Dev Biol 1967; 15:395.

623. Trentin JJ: Influence of hematopoietic organ stroma (hematopoietic inductive microenvironments) on stem cell differentiation. In Gordon AS (ed): Regulation of Hematopoiesis. New York, Appleton-Century-Crofts, 1970, p 161.

624. Gregory CJ, McCulloch EA, et al: Repressed growth of C57BL marrow in hybrid hosts reversed by antisera directed against non-H-2 alloantigens. Transplantation 1972; 13:138.

625. D'Andrea AD, Lodish HF, et al: Expression cloning of the murine erythropoietin receptor. Cell 1989; 57:277.

626. Krantz SB, Goldwasser E: Specific binding of erythropoietin in spleen cells infected with the anemia strain of Friend virus. Proc Natl Acad Sci U S A 1984; 81:7574.

627. Sawyer ST, Krantz SB, et al: Receptors for erythropoietin in mouse and human erythroid cells and placenta. Blood 1989; 74:103.

628. Sawada K, Krantz SB, et al: Quantitation of specific binding of erythropoietin to human erythroid colony-forming cells. J Cell Physiol 1988; 137:337.

629. Akahane K, Tojo A, et al: Binding of iodinated erythropoietin to rat bone marrow cells under normal and anemic conditions. Exp Hematol 1989; 17:177.

630. Wang GL, Jiang B, et al: Hypoxia-inducible factor 1 is a basic-helix-loop-PAS heterodimer regulated by cellular $O_{2 \text{ tension}}$. Proc Natl Acad Sci U S A 1995; 92:5510.

631. Sieff CA, Emerson SG, et al: Dependence of highly enriched human bone marrow progenitors on hemopoietic growth factors and their response to recombinant erythropoietin. J Clin Invest 1986; 77:74.

632. Lansdorp PM, Dragowska W: Long-term erythropoiesis from constant numbers of CD34+ cells in serum-free cultures initiated with highly purified progenitor cells from human bone marrow. J Exp Med 1992; 175:1501.

633. Macklis RM, Javid J, et al: Synthesis of hemoglobin F in adult simian erythroid progenitor-derived colonies. J Clin Invest 1982; 70:752.

634. Friedman AD, Linch DC, et al: Determination of the hemoglobin F program in human progenitor-derived erythroid cells. J Clin Invest 1985; 75:1359.

635. Dover GJ, Boyer SH, et al: Production of erythrocytes that contain fetal hemoglobin in anemia: transient *in vivo* changes. J Clin Invest 1979; 63:173.

636. Kidoguchi K, Ogawa M, et al: Augmentation of fetal hemoglobin (HbF) synthesis in culture by human erythropoietin precursors in the marrow and peripheral blood: studies in sickle cell anemia and non-hemoglobinopathic adults. Blood 1978; 52:115.

637. Clarke BJ, Nathan DG, et al: Hemoglobin synthesis in human BFU-E and CFU-E–derived erythroid colonies. Blood 1979; 54:805.

638. Papayannopoulou T, Brice M, et al: Hemoglobin F synthesis *in vitro*: evidence for control at the level of primitive erythroid stem cells. Proc Natl Acad Sci U S A 1977; 74:2923.

639. Romeo P-H, Prandini M-H, et al: Megakaryocytic and erythrocytic lineages share specific transcription factors. Nature 1990; 344:447.

640. Zon LI, Yamaguchi Y, et al: Expression of mRNA for the GATA-binding proteins in human eosinophils and basophils: potential role in gene transcription. Blood 1993; 81:3234.

641. Simon MC, Pevny L: Rescue of erythroid development in gene targeted GATA-1 mouse embryonic stem cells. Nat Genet 1992; 1:92.

642. Weiss MJ, Keller G, et al: Novel insights into erythroid development revealed through *in vitro* differentiation of GATA-1-embryonic stem cells. Genes Dev 1994; 8:1184.

643. Pevny L, Lin C-S, et al: Development of hematopoietic cells lacking transcription factor GATA-1. Development 1995; 121:163.

644. Weiss MJ, Orkin SH: Transcription factor GATA-1 permits survival and maturation of erythroid precursors by preventing apoptosis. Proc Natl Acad Sci U S A 1995; 92:9623.

645. Eaves CJ, Eaves AC: Erythropoietin (Ep) dose-response curves for three classes of erythroid progenitors in normal human marrow and in patients with polycythemia vera. Blood 1978; 52:1196.

646. Eaves AC, Eaves CJ: Erythropoiesis in culture. Clin Haematol 1984; 13:371.

647. Iscove NN: Erythropoietin-independent stimulation of early erythropoiesis in adult bone marrow cultures by conditioned media from lectin stimulated mouse spleen cells. In Golde DW, Cline MJ, et al (eds): Hematopoietic Cell Differentiation. New York, Academic Press, Inc., 1978, p 37.

648. Li CL, Johnson GR: Stimulation of multipotential erythroid and other murine haematopoietic progenitor cells by adherent cell lines in the absence of detectable multi-CSF (IL3). Nature 1985; 316:633.

649. Sieff CA, Ekern SC, et al: Combinations of recombinant colony stimulating factors are required for optimal hematopoietic differentiation in serum-deprived culture. Blood 1989; 73:688.

650. Abkowitz JL, Sabo KM, et al: Diamond-Blackfan anemia: *in vitro* response of erythroid progenitors to the ligand for c-kit. Blood 1991; 78:2198.

651. Bagnara GP, Zauli G, et al: *In vitro* growth and regulation of bone marrow–enriched CD34+ hematopoietic progenitors in Diamond-Blackfan anemia. Blood 1991; 78:2203.

652. Olivieri NF, Grunberger T, et al: Diamond-Blackfan anemia: heterogeneous response of hematopoietic progenitor cells *in vitro* to the protein product of the *Steel* locus. Blood 1991; 78:2211.

653. Nocka K, Majumder S, et al: Expression of c-kit gene products in known cellular targets of W mutations in normal and W mutant mice–evidence for an impaired c-kit kinase in mutant mice. Genes Dev 1989; 3:816.

654. Wu H, Klingmüller U, et al: Interaction of the erythropoietin and stem-cell-factor receptors. Nature 1995; 377:242.

655. Migliaccio AR, Migliaccio G: Human embryonic hemopoiesis: control mechanisms underlying progenitor differentiation *in vitro*. Dev Biol 1988; 125:127.

656. Valtieri M, Gabbianelli M, et al: Erythropoietin alone induces erythroid burst formation by human embryonic but not adult BFU-E in unicellular serum-free culture. Blood 1989; 74:460.

657. Schibler KR, Li Y, et al: Possible mechanisms accounting for the growth factor independence of hematopoietic progenitors from umbilical cord blood. Blood 1994; 84:3679.

658. Koenig JM, Christensen RD: Neutropenia and thrombocytopenia in infants with Rh hemolytic disease. J Pediatr 1989; 114:625.

659. Christensen RD, Koenig JM, et al: Down-modulation of neutrophil production by erythropoietin in human hematopoietic clones. Blood 1989; 74:817.

660. Sawada K, Krantz SB, et al: Human colony-forming units-erythroid do not require accessory cells, but do require direct interaction with insulin-like growth factor I and/or insulin for erythroid development. J Clin Invest 1989; 83:1701.

661. Kurtz A, Jelkmann W: Insulin stimulates erythroid colony formation independently of erythropoietin. Br J Haematol 1983; 53:311.

662. Yu J, Shao L, et al: Characterization of the potentiation effect of activin on human erythroid colony formation *in vitro*. Blood 1989; 73:952.

663. Smith JC, Price BM, et al: Identification of a potent *Xenopus* mesoderm-inducing factor as a homologue of activin A. Nature 1990; 345:729.

664. Galimi F, Bagnara GP, et al: Hepatocyte growth factor induces proliferation and differentiation of multipotent and erythroid hemopoietic progenitors. J Cell Biol 1994; 127:1743.

665. Mangan KF, Chikkappa G, et al: Regulation of human blood erythroid burst-forming unit (BFU-E) proliferation by T lymphocyte subpopulations defined by Fc receptors and monoclonal antibodies. Blood 1982; 59:990.

666. Torok-Storb BJ, Martin PJ, et al: Regulation of in vitro erythropoiesis by normal T cells: evidence for two T cell subsets with opposing functions. Blood 1981; 58:171.

667. Lipton JM, Smith BR, et al: Suppression of *in vitro* erythropoiesis by a subset of large granular lymphocytes. Blood 1984; 64:337a.

668. Hoffman R, Kopel SD, et al: T cell chronic lymphocytic leukemia: presence in bone marrow and peripheral blood of cells that suppress erythropoiesis in vitro. Blood 1978; 52:255.

669. Bagby GC Jr: T lymphocytes involved in inhibition of granulopoiesis in two neutropenic patients are of the cytotoxic/suppressor (T3+T8+) subset. J Clin Invest 1981; 68:1597.

670. Abdou JI, NaPombejara C, et al: Suppressor cell-mediated neutropenia in Felty's syndrome. J Clin Invest 1978; 61:738.

671. Sugimoto M, Wakabayashi Y, et al: Effect of peripheral blood lymphocytes from systemic lupus erythematosus patients on human bone marrow granulocyte precursor cells (colony-forming units in culture). Stem Cells 1982; 2:164.

672. Bom-van Noorloos AA, Pegels JG, et al: Proliferation of T-gamma cells with killer-cell activity in two patients with neutropenia and recurrent infections. N Engl J Med 1980; 302:933.

673. Linch DC, Cawley JC, et al: Acquired pure red cell aplasia associated with an increase of T cells bearing receptors for the Fc of IgG. Acta Haematol 1981; 65:270.

674. Lipton JM, Nadler LM, et al: Evidence for genetic restriction

in the suppression of erythropoiesis by a unique subset of T lymphocytes in man. J Clin Invest 1983; 72:694.

675. Torok-Storb BJ, Sieff C, et al: *In vitro* tests for distinguishing possible immune-mediated aplastic anemia from transfusion-induced sensitization. Blood 1980; 55:211.

676. Bacigalupo A, Podesta M, et al: Immunosuppression of hematopoiesis in aplastic anemia: activity of T lymphocytes. J Immunol 1980; 125:1449.

677. Smith BR, Lipton JM, et al: Multiparameter flow cytometric characterization of a unique T-lymphocyte subclass associated with granulocytopenia and pure red cell aplasia. Blood 1984; 64:343a.

678. Torok-Storb BJ, Hansen JA: Modulation of *in vitro* BFU-E growth by normal Ia-positive T cells is restricted by HLA-DR. Nature 1982; 298:473.

679. Krensky AM, Reiss CS, et al: Long-term human cytolytic T-cell lines allospecific for HLA-DR6 antigen are OKT4+. Proc Natl Acad Sci U S A 1982; 79:2365.

680. Falkenburg JHF, Jansen J, et al: Polymorphic and monomorphic HLA-DR determinants on human hematopoietic progenitor cells. Blood 1984; 63:1125.

681. Sieff C, Bicknell D, et al: Changes in cell surface antigen expression during hemopoietic differentiation. Blood 1982; 60:703.

682. Greaves MF, Katz FE, et al: Selective expression of cell surface antigens on human haemopoietic progenitor cells. In Palek J (ed): Hematopoietic Stem Cell Physiology. New York, Alan R. Liss, Inc., 1985, p 301.

683. Sparrow RL, Williams N: The pattern of HLA-DR and HLA-DQ antigen expression on clonable subpopulations of human myeloid progenitor cells. Blood 1986; 67:379.

684. Burdach SEG, Levitt LJ: Receptor-specific inhibition of bone marrow erythropoiesis by recombinant DNA-derived interleukin-2. Blood 1987; 69:1368.

685. Burdach S, Shatsky M, et al: The T-cell CD2 determinant mediates inhibition of erythropoiesis by the lymphokine cascade. Blood 1988; 72:770.

686. Roodman DC, Bird A, et al: Tumor necrosis factor α and hematopoietic progenitors: effects of tumor necrosis factor on the growth of erythroid progenitors CFU-E and BFU-E and the hematopoietic cell lines K562, HL60, and HEL cells. Exp Hematol 1987; 15:928.

687. Broxmeyer HE, Williams DE, et al: The suppressive influences of human tumor necrosis factor on bone marrow hematopoietic progenitor cells from normal donors and patients with leukemia: synergism of tumor necrosis factor and interferon-gamma. J Immunol 1986; 136:4487.

688. Furmanski P, Johnson CS: Macrophage control of normal and leukemic erythropoiesis: identification of the macrophage-derived erythroid suppressing activity as interleukin-1 and the mediator of its *in vivo* action as tumor necrosis factor. Blood 1990; 75:2328.

689. Van Furth R, Raeburn JA, et al: Characteristics of human mononuclear phagocytes. Blood 1979; 54:485.

690. Meuret G: Human monocytopoiesis. Exp Hematol 1974; 2:238.

691. Thomas ED, Ramberg RE, et al: Direct evidence for a bone marrow origin of the alveolar macrophage in man. Science 1976; 192:1016.

692. Gale RP, Sparkes RS, et al: Bone marrow origin of hepatic macrophages (Kupffer cells) in humans. Science 1978; 201:937.

693. Katz SI, Tamaki K, et al: Epidermal Langerhans cells are derived from cells originating in bone marrow. Nature 1979; 282:324.

694. Ash P, Loutit JF, et al: Osteoclasts derived from haematopoietic stem cells. Nature 1980; 283:669.

695. Carr I: The biology of macrophages. Clin Invest Med 1978; 1:59.

696. Gasson JC, Weisbart RH, et al: Purified human granulocyte-macrophage colony-stimulating factor: direct action on neutrophils. Science 1984; 226:1339.

697. Weisbart RH, Golde DW, et al: Human granulocyte-macrophage colony-stimulating factor is a neutrophil activator. Nature 1985; 314:361.

698. Iscove NN: The role of erythropoietin in regulation of population size and cell cycling of early and late erythroid precursors in mouse bone marrow. Cell Tissue Kinet 1977; 10:373.

699. Udupa KB, Reissman KR: *In vivo* erythropoietin requirements of regenerating erythroid progenitors (BFU-e), CFU-e in bone marrow of mice. Blood 1979; 53:1164.

700. Odell TT Jr, McDonald TP, et al: Stimulation of platelet production by serum of platelet-depleted rats. Proc Soc Exp Biol Med 1961; 108:428.

701. Moreau-Gachelin F, Ray D, et al: The PU.1 transcription factor is the product of the putative oncogene *Spi-1*. Cell 1990; 61:1166.

702. Pahl HL, Scheibe RJ, et al: The proto-oncogene *PU.1* regulates expression of the myeloid-specific CD11b promotor. J Biol Chem 1993; 268:5014.

703. Pongubala JMR, Van Beveren C, et al: Effect of PU.1 phosphorylation on interaction with NF-EM5 and transcriptional activation. Science 1993; 259:1622.

704. Shin MK, Koshland ME: Ets-related protein PU.1 regulates expression of the immunoglobulin J-chain gene through a novel Ets-binding element. Genes Dev 1993; 7:2006.

705. Zhang DE, Fujioka K, et al: Identification of a region which directs the monocytic activity of the colony-stimulating factor 1 (macrophage colony-stimulating factor) receptor promoter and binds PEBP2/CBF (AML1). Mol Cell Biol 1994; 14:8085.

706. Hohaus S, Petrovick MS, et al: PU.1 (Spi-1) and C/EBP alpha regulate expression of the granulocyte-macrophage colony-stimulating factor receptor alpha gene. Mol Cell Biol 1995; 15:5830.

707. Scott EW, Simon MC, et al: Requirement of transcription factor PU.1 in the development of multiple hematopoietic lineages. Science 1994; 265:1573.

708. Scott LM, Civin CI, et al: A novel temporal expression pattern of three C/EBP family members in differentiating myelomonocytic cells. Blood 1992; 80:1725.

709. Zhang DE, Hetherington CJ, et al: CCAAT enhancer-binding protein (C/EBP) and AML1 (CBF alpha2) synergistically activate the macrophage colony-stimulating factor receptor promoter. Mol Cell Biol 1996; 16:1231.

710. Tanaka T, Akira S, et al: Targeted disruption of the NF-IL6 gene discloses its essential role in bacteria killing and tumor cytotoxicity by macrophages. Cell 1995; 80:353.

711. Metcalf D, Johnson GR, et al: Direct stimulation by purified GM-CSF of the proliferation of multipotential and erythroid precursor cells. Blood 1980; 55:138.

712. Metcalf D, Nicola NA: Proliferative effects of purified granulocyte colony-stimulating factor (G-CSF) on normal mouse hemopoietic cells. J Cell Physiol 1983; 116:198.

713. Metcalf D, Stanley ER: Haematological effects in mice of partially purified colony stimulating factor (CSF) prepared from human urine. Br J Haematol 1971; 21:481.

714. Nishinakamura R, Nakayama N, et al: Mice deficient for the IL-3/GM-CSF/IL-5 βc receptor exhibit lung pathology and impaired immune response while β_{IL3} receptor-deficient mice are normal. Immunity 1995; 2:211.

715. Arnaout MA, Wang EA, et al: Human recombinant granulocyte macrophage colony-stimulating factor increases cell-to-cell adhesion and surface expression of adhesion-promoting surface glycoproteins on mature granulocytes. J Clin Invest 1986; 78:597.

716. Lopez AF, To LB, et al: Stimulation of proliferation, differentiation, and function of human cells by primate interleukin 3. Proc Natl Acad Sci U S A 1987; 84:2761.

717. Lopez AF, Nicola NA, et al: Activation of granulocyte cytotoxic function by purified mouse colony stimulating factors. J Immunol 1983; 131:2983.

718. Hamilton JA, Stanley ER, et al: Stimulation of macrophage plasminogen activator activity by colony-stimulating factors. J Cell Physiol 1980; 103:435.

719. Nicola NA, Metcalf D: Binding of iodinated multipotential colony-stimulating factor (interleukin-3) to murine bone marrow cells. J Cell Physiol 1986; 128:180.

720. Debili N, Masse JM, et al: Effects of the recombinant hematopoietic growth factors interleukin-3, interleukin-6, stem cell factor, and leukemia inhibitory factor on the megakaryocytic differentiation of CD34+ cells. Blood 1993; 82:84.

721. Guinan EC, Lee YS, et al: Effects of interleukin-3 and granulocyte-macrophage colony-stimulating factor on thrombopoiesis in congenital amegakaryocytic thrombocytopenia. Blood 1993; 81:1691.

722. Hill RJ, Warren MK, et al: Stimulation of megakaryocytopoiesis in mice by human recombinant interleukin-6. Blood 1991; 77:42.

723. Neben S, Turner K: The biology of interleukin 11. Stem Cells 1993; 11(Suppl 2):156. Review.

724. Broudy VC, Lin NL, et al: Thrombopoietin (c-mpl ligand) acts synergistically with erythropoietin, stem cell factor, and interleukin-11 to enhance murine megakaryocyte colony growth and increases megakaryocyte ploidy *in vitro*. Blood 1995; 85:1719.

725. Briddell RA, Bruno E, et al: Effect of c-kit ligand on *in vitro* human megakaryocytopoiesis. Blood 1991; 78:2854.

726. Ishibashi T, Koziol JA, et al: Human recombinant erythropoietin promotes differentiation of murine megakaryocytes *in vitro*. J Clin Invest 1987; 79:286.

727. McDonald TP, Sullivan PS: Megakaryocytic and erythrocytic cell lines share a common precursor cell. Exp Hematol 1993; 21:1316.

728. Longmore GD, Pharr P, et al: Both megakaryocytopoiesis and erythropoiesis are induced in mice infected with a retrovirus expressing an oncogenic erythropoietin receptor. Blood 1993; 82:2386.

729. McDonald TP, Cottrell MB, et al: High doses of recombinant erythropoietin stimulate platelet production in mice. Exp Hematol 1987; 15:719.

730. Methia N, Louache F, et al: Oligodeoxynucleotides antisense to the proto-oncogene c-mpl specifically inhibit *in vitro* megakaryocytopoiesis. Blood 1993; 82:1395.

731. Wendling F, Varlet P, et al: A retrovirus complex including an acute myeloproliferative leukemia virus immortalizes hematopoietic progenitors. Virology 1986; 149:242.

732. Souyri M, Vigon I, et al: A putative truncated cytokine receptor gene transduced by the myeloproliferative leukemia virus immortalizes hematopoietic progenitors. Cell 1990; 63:1137.

733. Vigon I, Mornon J-P, et al: Molcular cloning and characterization of *MPL*, the human homolog of the v-*mpl* oncogene: identification of a member of the hematopoietic growth factor receptor superfamily. Proc Natl Acad Sci U S A 1992; 89:5640.

734. Cosman D: The hematopoietin receptor superfamily. Cytokine 1993; 5:95. Review.

735. Kuter DJ, Beeler DL, et al: The purification of megapoietin: a physiological regulator of megakaryocyte growth and platelet production. Proc Natl Acad Sci U S A 1994; 91:11104.

736. Emmons RV, Reid DM, et al: Human thrombopoietin levels are high when thrombocytopenia is due to megakaryocyte deficiency and low when due to increased platelet destruction. Blood 1996; 87:4068.

737. Karpatkin S: Heterogeneity of human platelets. I. Metabolic and kinetic evidence suggestive of young and old platelets. J Clin Invest 1969; 48:1073.

738. Paulus JM, Breton-Gorius J, et al: Megakaryocyte ultrastructure and ploidy in human macrothrombocytosis. In Baldini MG, Ebbe S (eds): Platelets, Production, Function, Transfusion and Storage. New York, Grune & Stratton, Inc., 1974, p 131.

739. Gewirtz AM, Calabretta B, et al: Inhibition of human megakaryocytopoiesis *in vitro* by platelet factor 4 (PF4) and a synthetic COOH-terminal PF4 peptide. J Clin Invest 1989; 83:1477.

740. Ishibashi T, Miller SL, et al: Type beta transforming growth factor is a potent inhibitor of murine megakaryocytopoiesis *in vitro*. Blood 1987; 69:1737.

741. Pantel K, Nakeff A: Differential effect of natural killer cells on modulating CFU-meg and BFU-E proliferation *in situ*. Exp Hematol 1989; 17:1017.

742. Hoffman R: Regulation of megakaryocytopoiesis. Blood 1989; 74:1196.

743. Chan KW, Kaikov Y, et al: Thrombocytosis in childhood: a survey of 94 patients. Pediatrics 1989; 84:1064.

744. Mazur EM, Cohen JL, et al: Growth characteristics of circulating hematopoietic progenitor cells from patients with essential thrombocythemia. Blood 1988; 71:1544.

745. Fung MC, Hapel AJ, et al: Molecular cloning for cDNA for murine interleukin-3. Nature 1984; 307:233.

746. Yokota T, Lee T, et al: Isolation and characterization of a mouse cDNA clone that expresses mast-cell growth factor activity in monkey cells. Proc Natl Acad Sci U S A 1984; 81:1070.

747. Kindler J, Thorens B, et al: Stimulation of hematopoiesis *in vivo* by recombinant bacterial murine interleukin 3. Proc Natl Acad Sci U S A 1986; 83:1001.

748. Metcalf D, Begley CG, et al: Effects of purified bacterially synthesized murine multi-CSF (IL-3) on hematopoiesis in normal adult mice. Blood 1986; 68:46.

749. Donahue RE, Wang EA, et al: Stimulation of hematopoiesis in primates by continuous infusion of recombinant human GM-CSF. Nature 1986; 321:872.

750. Nienhuis AW, Donahue RE, et al: Recombinant human granulocyte-macrophage colony stimulating factor (GM-CSF) shortens the period of neutropenia after autologous bone marrow transplantation in a primate model. J Clin Invest 1987; 80:573.

751. Welte K, Bonilla MA, et al: Recombinant human granulocyte-colony-stimulating factor: effects on hematopoiesis in normal and cyclophosphamide treated primates. J Exp Med 1987; 165:941.

752. Gabrilove J, Jakubowski A, et al: Effect of granulocyte colony-stimulating factor on neutropenia and associated morbidity due to chemotherapy for transitional-cell carcinoma of the urothelium. N Engl J Med 1988; 318:1414.

753. Morstyn G, Campbell L, et al: Effect of granulocyte colony stimulating factor on neutropenia induced by cytotoxic chemotherapy. Lancet 1988; 1:667.

754. Devereaux S, Linch DC, et al: Transient leucopenia induced by granulocyte-macrophage colony-stimulating factor. Lancet 1987; 2:1523.

755. Bronchud MH, Scarffe JH, et al: Phase I/II study of recombinant human granulocyte colony-stimulating factor in patients receiving intensive chemotherapy for small cell lung cancer. Br J Cancer 1987; 56:809.

756. Kodo H, Tajika K, et al: Acceleration of neutrophilic granulocyte recovery after bone-marrow transplantation by the administration of recombinant human granulocyte colony-stimulating factor. Lancet 1988; 2:38.

757. Santana VM, Bowman LC, et al: Trial of chemotherapy plus recombinant human granulocyte colony-stimulating factor on children with advanced neuroblastoma. Med Pediatr Oncol 1990; 18:395a.

758. Duhrsen U, Villeval J-L, et al: Effects of recombinant human granulocyte colony-stimulating factor on hematopoietic progenitor cells in cancer patients. Blood 1988; 72:2074.

759. Tamura M, Hattori K, et al: Induction of neutrophilic granulocytes in mice by administration of purified human native granulocyte colony-stimulating factor (G-CSF). Biochem Biophys Res Comm 1987; 142:454.

760. Shimamura M, Kobayashi Y, et al: Effect of human recombinant granulocyte colony-stimulating factor on hematopoietic injury in mice induced by 5-fluorouracil. Blood 1987; 69:353.

761. Antman KS, Griffin JD, et al: Effect of recombinant human granulocyte-macrophage colony-stimulating factor on chemotherapy-induced myelosuppression. N Engl J Med 1988; 319:593.

762. Herrmann F, Schulz G, et al: Hematopoietic responses in patients with advanced malignancy treated with recombinant human granulocyte-macrophage colony-stimulating factor. J Clin Oncol 1989; 7:159.

763. Steward WP, Scarffe JH, et al: Recombinant human granulocyte macrophage colony stimulating factor (rhGM-CSF) given as daily short infusions–a phase I dose-toxicity study. Br J Cancer 1989; 59:142.

764. Furman WL: Cytokine support following cytotoxic chemotherapy in children. Int J Pediatr Hematol/Oncol 1995; 2:163.

765. Saarinen UM, Hovi L, et al: Recombinant human granulocyte-macrophage colony-stimulating factor in children with chemotherapy-induced neutropenia. Med Pediatr Oncol 1992; 20:489.

766. Burdach S: Molecular regulation of hematopoietic cytokines: implications and indications for clinical use in pediatric oncology. Med Pediatr Oncol Suppl 1992; 2:10. Review.

767. Socinski MA, Cannistra SA, et al: Granulocyte-macrophage colony stimulating factor expands the circulating haemopoietic progenitor cell compartment in man. Lancet 1988; 1:1194.

768. Ganser A, Lindemann A, et al: Effects of recombinant human interleukin-3 in patients with normal hematopoiesis and in patients with bone marrow failure. Blood 1990; 76:666.

769. Ottmann OG, Ganser A, et al: Effects of recombinant human interleukin-3 on human hematopoietic progenitor and precursor cells *in vivo*. Blood 1990; 76:1494.

770. Motoyoshi K, Takaku F, et al: Protective effect of partially purified human urinary colony-stimulating factor on granulocytopenia after antitumor chemotherapy. Exp Hematol 1986; 14:1069.

771. Gordon MS, Battiato L, et al: Subcutaneously (SC) administered recombinant human interleukin-11 (neumega rhIL-11 growth factor; rhIL-11) prevents thrombocytopenia following chemotherapy (CT) with cyclophosphamide (C) and doxorubicin (A) in women with breast cancer. Blood 1993; 82:318a.

772. Smith JW, Longo DL, et al: The effects of treatment with interleukin-1 alpha in platelet recovery after high-dose carboplatin. N Engl J Med 1993; 328:756.

773. Brandt SJ, Peters WP, et al: Effect of recombinant human granulocyte-macrophage colony-stimulating factor on hematopoietic reconstitution after high-dose chemotherapy and autologous bone marrow transplantation. N Engl J Med 1988; 318:869.

774. Nemunaitis J, Singer JW, et al: Use of recombinant human granulocyte-macrophage colony-stimulating factor in graft failure after bone marrow transplantation. Blood 1990; 76:345.

775. Tapp H, Vowels M: Prophylactic use of GM-CSF in pediatric marrow transplantation. Transplant Proc 1992; 24:2267.

776. Blazar BR, Kersey JH, et al: In vivo administration of recombinant human granulocyte/macrophage colony-stimulating factor in acute lymphoblastic leukemia patients receiving purged autografts. Blood 1989; 73:849.

777. Sheridan WP, Morstyn G, et al: Granulocyte colony-stimulating factor and neutrophil recovery after high-dose chemotherapy and autologous bone marrow transplantation. Lancet 1989; 2:891.

778. Peters W, Stuart A, et al: Neutrophil migration is defective during recombinant human granulocyte-macrophage colony-stimulating factor infusion after autologous bone marrow transplantation in humans. Blood 1988; 72:1310.

779. Masaoka T, Motoyoshi K, et al: Administration of human urinary colony stimulating factor after bone marrow transplantation. Bone Marrow Transplant 1988; 3:121.

780. Vadhan-raj S, Keating M, et al: Effects of recombinant human granulocyte-macrophage colony-stimulating factor in patients with myelodysplastic syndromes. N Engl J Med 1987; 317:1545.

781. Antin JH, Smith BR, et al: Phase I/II study of recombinant human granulocyte-macrophage colony-stimulating factor in aplastic anemia and myelodysplastic syndrome. Blood 1988; 72:705.

782. Ganser A, Volkers B, et al: Recombinant human granulocyte-macrophage colony-stimulating factor in patients with myelodysplastic syndromes—a phase I/II trial. Blood 1989; 73:31.

783. Kobayashi Y, Okabe T, et al: Treatment of myelodysplastic syndromes with recombinant human granulocyte colony-stimulating factor: a preliminary report. Am J Med 1989; 86:178.

784. Negrin RS, Haeuber D, et al: Treatment of myelodysplastic syndromes with recombinant human granulocyte colony-stimulating factor: a phase I/II trial. Ann Intern Med 1989; 110:976.

785. Champlin RE, Nimer SD, et al: Treatment of refractory aplastic anemia with recombinant human granulocyte-macrophage-colony-stimulating factor. Blood 1989; 73:694.

786. Vadhan-raj S, Buescher S, et al: Stimulation of myelopoiesis in patients with aplastic anemia by recombinant human granulocyte-macrophage colony-stimulating factor. N Engl J Med 1988; 319:1628.

787. Guinan EC, Sieff CA, et al: A phase I/II trial of recombinant granulocyte-macrophage colony-stimulating factor for children with aplastic anemia. Blood 1990; 76:1077.

788. Nissen C, Tichelli A, et al: Failure of recombinant human granulocyte-macrophage colony-stimulating factor therapy in aplastic anemia patients with very severe neutropenia. Blood 1988; 72:2045.

789. Kojima S, Fukuda M, et al: Treatment of aplastic anemia in children with recombinant human granulocyte colony-stimulating factor. Blood 1991; 77:937.

790. Kojima S, Matsuyama T: Stimulation of granulopoiesis by high-dose recombinant human granulocyte colony-stimulating factor in children with aplastic anemia and very severe neutropenia. Blood 1994; 83:1474.

791. Sonoda Y, Yashige H, et al: Bilineage response in refractory aplastic anemia patients following long-term administration of recombinant human granulocyte colony-stimulating factor. Eur J Haematol 1992; 48:41.

792. Gluckman E, Esperou-Bourdeau H: Recent treatments of aplastic anemia. The International Group on SAA. Nouv Rev Fr Hematol 1991; 33:507.

793. Kojima S: Cytokine treatment of aplastic anemia. Int J Pediatr Hematol/Oncol 1995; 2:135.

794. Kurzrock R, Talpaz M, et al: Very low doses of GM-CSF administered alone with erythropoietin in aplastic anemia. Am J Med 1992; 93:41.

795. Hirashima K, Bessho M, et al: Successful treatment of aplastic anemia and refractory anemia by combination therapy with recombinant human granulocyte colony-stimulating factor and erythropoietin. Exp Hematol 1993; 21:1080a.

796. Groopman JE, Mitsuyasu RT, et al: Effects of recombinant human granulocyte-macrophage colony-stimulating factor on myelopoiesis in the acquired immunodeficiency syndrome. N Engl J Med 1987; 317:593.

797. Groopman JE, Molina J-M, et al: Hematopoietic growth factors: biology and clinical applications. N Engl J Med 1989; 321:1449.

798. Perno CF, Yarchoan R, et al: Replication of human immunodeficiency virus in monocytes: granulocyte/macrophage colony-stimulating factor (GM-CSF) potentiates viral production yet enhances the antiviral effect mediated by 3'-azido-2'3'-dideoxy-thymidine (AZT) and other dideoxynucleoside congeners of thymidine. J Exp Med 1989; 169:933.

799. Mueller BU: Role of cytokines in children with HIV infection. Int J Pediatr Hematol/Oncol 1995; 2:151.

800. Pluda JM, Yarchoan R, et al: Subcutaneous recombinant granulocyte-macrophage colony-stimulating factor used as a single agent and in an alternating regimen with azidothymidine in leukopenic patients with severe human immunodeficiency virus infection. Blood 1990; 76:463.

801. Kaplan LD, Kahn JO, et al: Clinical and virologic effects of recombinant human granulocyte-macrophage colony-stimulating factor in patients receiving chemotherapy for human immunodeficiency virus-associated non-Hodgkin's lymphoma: results of a randomized trial. J Clin Oncol 1991; 9:929.

802. Mueller BU, Jacobsen F, et al: Combination treatment with azidothymidine and granulocyte colony-stimulating factor in children with human immunodeficiency virus infection. J Pediatr 1992; 121:797.

803. Gillio AP, Guinan EC: Cytokine treatment of inherited bone marrow failure syndromes. Int J Pediatr Hematol/Oncol 1992; 2:123.

804. Guinan EC, Lopez KD, et al: Evaluation of granulocyte-macrophage colony-stimulating factor for treatment of pancytopenia in children with Fanconi anemia. J Pediatr 1994; 124:144.

805. Hammond D, Keighley G: The erythrocyte-stimulating factor in serum and urine in congenital hypoplastic anemia. Am J Dis Child 1960; 100:466.

806. Abkowitz JL, Broudy VC, et al: Absence of abnormalities of c-kit or its ligand in two patients with Diamond-Blackfan anemia. Blood 1992; 79:25. Abstract.

807. Sieff CA, Yokoyama CT, et al: The production of Steel factor mRNA in Diamond-Blackfan anaemia long-term cultures and interactions of Steel factor with erythropoietin and interleukin-3. Br J Haematol 1992; 82:640.

808. Niemeyer CM, Baumgarten E, et al: Treatment trial with recombinant human erythropoietin in children with congenital hypoplastic anemia. Contrib Nephrol 1991; 88:276.

809. Dunbar CE, Smith DA, et al: Treatment of Diamond-Blackfan anaemia with haematopoietic growth factors, granulocyte-macrophage colony stimulating factor and interleukin 3: sustained remissions following IL-3. Br J Haematol 1991; 79:316.

810. Gillio AP, Faulkner LB, et al: Treatment of Diamond-Blackfan anemia with recombinant human interleukin-3. Blood 1993; 82:744.

811. Olivieri NF, Feig SA, et al: Failure of recombinant human interleukin-3 therapy to induce erythropoiesis in patients with refractory Diamond-Blackfan anemia. Blood 1994; 83:2444.

812. Bastion Y, Bordigoni P, et al: Sustained response after recombinant interleukin-3 in patients with bone marrow failure. Blood 1994; 83:617.

813. Pietsch T, Buhrer C, et al: Blood mononuclear cells from patients with severe congenital neutropenia are capable of producing granulocyte colony-stimulating factor. Blood 1991; 77:1234.

814. Kyas U, Pietsch T, et al: Expression of receptors for granulocyte colony-stimulating factor on neutrophils from patients with severe congenital neutropenia and cyclic neutropenia. Blood 1992; 79:1144.

815. Guba SC, Sartor CA, et al: Granulocyte colony-stimulating factor (G-CSF) production and G-CSF receptor structure in patients with congenital neutropenia. Blood 1994; 83:1486.

816. Bonilla MA, Gillio AP, et al: Effects of recombinant human granulocyte colony-stimulating factor on neutropenia in patients with congenital agranulocytosis. N Engl J Med 1989; 320:1574.

817. Welte K, Zeidler C, et al: Differential effects of granulocyte-macrophage colony-stimulating factor and granulocyte-stimulating factor in children with severe congenital neutropenia. Blood 1990; 75:1056.

818. Boxer LA, Hutchinson R, et al: Recombinant human granulocyte-colony-stimulating factor in the treatment of patients with neutropenia. Clin Immunol Immunopathol 1992; 62:539.

819. Dale DC, Bonilla MA, et al: A randomized controlled phase III trial of recombinant human granulocyte colony-stimulating factor (filgrastim) for treatment of severe chronic neutropenia. Blood 1993; 81:2496.

820. Wong WY, Williams D, et al: Terminal acute myelogenous leukemia in a patient with congenital agranulocytosis. Am J Hematol 1993; 43:133.

821. Weinblatt ME, Scimeca P, et al: Transformation of congenital neutropenia into monosomy 7 and acute nonlymphoblastic leukemia in a child treated with granulocyte colony-stimulating factor. J Pediatr 1995; 126:263. Review.

822. Imashuku S, Hibi S, et al: Myelodysplasia and acute myeloid leukaemia in cases of aplastic anaemia and congenital neutropenia following G-CSF administration. Br J Haematol 1995; 89:188.

823. Kojima S, Tsuchida M, et al: Myelodysplasia and leukemia after treatment of aplastic anemia with G-CSF. N Engl J Med 1992; 326:1294. Letter.

824. Hammond WP IV, Price TH, et al: Treatment of cyclic neutropenia with granulocyte colony-stimulating factor. N Engl J Med 1989; 320:1306.

825. Sugimoto K, Togawal A, et al: Treatment of childhood-onset cyclic neutropenia with recombinant human granulocyte colony stimulating factor. Eur J Haematol 1990; 45:110.

826. Hanada T, Ono I, et al: Childhood cyclic neutropenia treated with granulocyte colony-stimulating factor. Br J Haematol 1990; 75:135.

827. Dale D, Bolyard A, et al: Cyclic neutropenia: natural history and effects of long-term treatment with recombinant human granulocyte colony-stimulating factor. Cancer Invest 1993; 11:219.

828. Wright D, Oette D, et al: Treatment of cyclic neutropenia with recombinant human granulocyte-macrophage colony-stimulating factor (rhGM-CSF). Blood 1989; 74:231a.

829. Freund M, Luft S, et al: Differential effect of GM-CSF and G-CSF in cyclic neutropenia. Lancet 1990; 336:313.

830. Kurzrock R, Talpaz M, et al: Treatment of cyclic neutropenia with very low-doses of GM-CSF. Am J Med 1991; 91:317.

831. Jakubowski AA, Souza L, et al: Effects of human granulocyte colony-stimulating factor in a patient with idiopathic neutropenia. N Engl J Med 1989; 320:38.

832. Gribben JG, Devereux S, et al: Development of antibodies to unprotected glycosylation sites on recombinant human GM-CSF. Lancet 1990; 335:434.

833. Glaspy JA, Baldwin GC, et al: Therapy for neutropenia in hairy cell leukemia with recombinant human granulocyte colony-stimulating factor. Ann Intern Med 1988; 109:789.

834. Winearls CG, Oliver DO, et al: Effect of human erythropoietin derived from recombinant DNA on the anemia of patients maintained by chronic haemodialysis. Lancet 1986; 11:1175.

835. Eschbach JW, Abdulhadi MH, et al: Recombinant human erythropoietin in anemic patients with end-stage renal disease. Ann Intern Med 1989; 111:992.

836. Adamson JW: The promise of recombinant human erythropoietin. Semin Hematol 1989; 26(Suppl 2):5.

837. Dessypris EN, Graber SE, et al: Effects of recombinant erythropoietin on the concentration and cycling status of human marrow hematopoietic progenitor cells *in vivo*. Blood 1988; 72:2060.

838. Laupacis A: Changes in quality of life and functional capacity in hemodialysis patients treated with recombinant human erythropoietin. Semin Nephrol 1990; 10(Suppl 1):11.

839. Eschbach JW, Kelly MR, et al: Treatment of the anemia of progressive renal failure with recombinant human erythropoietin. N Engl J Med 1989; 321:158.

840. Bommer J, Ritz E, et al: Subcutaneous erythropoietin. Lancet 1988; 2:406.

841. Muller-Wiefel DE, Amon O: Erythropoietin treatment of anemia associated with chronic renal failure in children. Int J Pediatr Hematol Oncol 1995; 2:87.

842. Offner G, Hoyer PF, et al: One year's experience with recombinant erythropoietin in children undergoing continuous ambulatory or cycling peritoneal dialysis. Pediatr Nephrol 1990; 4:498.

843. Scigalla P, Bonzel KE, et al: Therapy of renal anemia with recombinant human erythropoietin in children with end-stage renal disease. Contrib Nephrol 1989; 76:227.

844. Scharer K, Klare B, et al: Treatment of renal anemia by subcutaneous erythropoietin in children with preterminal chronic renal failure. Acta Pediatr 1993; 82:953.

845. Onkingco JRC, Ruley EJ, et al: Use of low-dose subcutaneous recombinant human erythropoietin in end-stage renal disease: experience with children receiving continuous cycling peritoneal dialysis. Am J Kidney Dis 1991; 18:446.

846. Ohls R, Christensen R: Recombinant erythropoietin compared with erythrocyte transfusion in the treatment of anemia of prematurity. J Pediatr 1991; 119:781.

847. Shannon KM, Mentzer WC, et al: Enhancement of erythropoiesis by recombinant human erythropoietin in low birth weight infants: a pilot study. J Pediatr 1992; 120:586.

848. Halperin D, Felix M, et al: Recombinant human erythropoietin in the treatment of infants with anemia of prematurity. Eur J Pediatr 1992; 151:661.

849. Carnielli V, Montini G, et al: Effect of high doses of human recombinant erythropoietin on the need for blood transfusions in preterm infants. J Pediatr 1992; 121:98.

850. Bechensteen AG, Haga P, et al: Erythropoietin, protein, and iron supplementation and the prevention of anaemia of prematurity. Arch Dis Child 1993; 69:19.

851. Perignon JL: Biochemical study of a case of hemolytic anemia with increased (85×) red cell adenosine deaminase. Adv Exp Med Biol 1984; 165:355.

852. Messer J, Haddad J, et al: Early treatment of premature infants with recombinant human erythropoietin. Pediatrics 1993; 92:519.

853. Soubasi V, Kremenopoulos G, et al: In which neonates does early recombinant human erythropoietin treatment prevent anemia of prematurity? Results of a randomized, controlled study. Pediatr Res 1993; 34:675.

854. Mentzer WC, Shannon KM: The use of recombinant human erythropoietin in preterm infants. Int J Pediatr Hematol Oncol 1995; 2:97.

855. Means RT, Olsen NJ, et al: Treatment of the anemia of rheumatoid arthritis with recombinant human erythropoietin: clinical and *in vitro* studies. Arthritis Rheum 1989; 32:638.

856. Umemura T, al-Khatti A, et al: Effects of interleukin-3 and erythropoietin on *in vitro* erythropoiesis and F cell formation in primates. Blood 1989; 74:1561.

857. al-Khatti A, Umemura T, et al: Erythropoietin stimulates F-reticulocyte formation in sickle cell anemia. Trans Assoc Am Physicians 1988; 101:54.

858. Goldberg MA, Brugnara C, et al: Treatment of sickle cell anemia with hydroxyurea and erythropoietin. N Engl J Med 1990; 323:366.

859. Rodgers GP, Dover GJ, et al: Augmentation by erythropoietin of the fetal-hemoglobin response to hydroxyurea in sickle cell disease. N Engl J Med 1993; 328:73.

860. Rachmilewitz EA, Goldfarb A, et al: Administration of erythropoietin to patients with β-thalassemia intermedia: a preliminary trial. Blood 1991; 78:1145.

861. Olivieri NF, Freedman MH, et al: Trial of recombinant human erythropoietin: three patients with thalassemia intermedia. Blood 1992; 80:3258. Letter.

862. Aker M, Dover G, et al: Sustained increase in the hemoglobin, hematocrit and RBC following long-term administration of recombinant human erythropoietin to patients with beta1-thalassemia intermedia. Blood 1993; 82:358a. Abstract.

863. Loukopoulos D, Voskaridou E, et al: Effective stimulation of erythropoiesis in thalassemia intermedia with recombinant human erythropoietin and hydroxyurea. Blood 1993; 82:357a.

864. Goodnough LT, Rudnick S, et al: Increased preoperative collection of autologous blood with recombinant human erythropoietin therapy. N Engl J Med 1989; 321:1163.

865. Felix R, Cecchini MG, et al: Impairment of macrophage colony-stimulating factor production and lack of resident bone marrow macrophages in the osteopetrotic op/op mouse. J Bone Miner Res 1990; 5:781.

866. Wiktor-Jedrzejczak W, Bartocci A, et al: Total absence of colony-stimulating factor 1 in the macrophage-deficient (op/op) mouse. Proc Natl Acad Sci U S A 1990; 87:4828. Published erratum appears in Proc Natl Acad Sci U S A 1991; 88:5937.

867. Felix R, Cecchini MG, et al: Macrophage colony stimulating factor restores in vivo bone resorption in the op/op osteopetrotic mouse. Endocrinology 1990; 127:2592.

868. Wiktor-Jedrzejczak W, Urbanowska E, et al: Correction by CSF-1 of defects in the osteopetrotic op/op mouse suggests local, developmental, and humoral requirements for this growth factor. Exp Hematol 1991; 19:1049.

869. Kodama H, Yamasaki A, et al: Congenital osteoclast deficiency in osteopetrotic (op/op) mice is cured by injections of macrophage colony-stimulating factor. J Exp Med 1991; 173:269.

870. Key LL Jr, Rodriguiz RM, et al: Cytokines and bone resorption in osteopetrosis. Int J Pediatr Hematol/Oncol 1995; 2:143.

871. Rodriguiz RM, Key LL Jr, et al: Combination macrophage-colony stimulating factor and interferon-gamma administration ameliorates the osteopetrotic condition in microphthalmic (mi/mi) mice. Pediatr Res 1993; 33:384.

872. Key LL, Ries WL, et al: Recombinant human interferon gamma therapy of osteopetrosis. J Pediatr 1992; 121:119.

873. Leonard WJ, Noguchi M, et al: The molecular basis of X-linked severe combined immunodeficiency: the role of the interleukin-2 receptor gamma chain as a common gamma chain, gamma c. Immunol Rev 1994; 138:61. Review.

874. Macchi P, Villa A, et al: Mutations of Jak-3 gene in patients with autosomal severe combined immune deficiency (SCID). Nature 1995; 377:65.

875. Luo H, Hanratty WP, et al: An amino acid substitution in the Drosophila hop^{Tum-l} Jak kinase causes leukemia-like hematopoietic defects. EMBO J 1995; 14:1412.

876. Harrison DA, Binari R, et al: Activation of a Drosophila Janus kinase (JAK) causes hematopoietic neoplasia and developmental defects. EMBO J 1995; 14:2857.

877. Zmuidzinas A, Fischer KD, et al: The vav proto-oncogene is required early in embryogenesis but not for hematopoietic development in vitro. EMBO J 1995; 14:1.

878. Brizzi MF, Zini MG, et al: Convergence of signaling by interleukin-3, granulocyte-macrophage colony-stimulating factor, and mast cell growth factor on JAK2 tyrosine kinase. J Biol Chem 1994; 269:31680.

879. Lev S, Givol D, et al: A specific combination of substrates is involved in signal transduction by the kit-encoded receptor. EMBO J 1991; 10:647.

880. Rottapel R, Reedijk M, et al: The Steel/W transduction pathway: kit autophosphorylation and its association with a unique subset of cytoplasmic signaling proteins is induced by the Steel factor. Mol Cell Biol 1991; 11:3043.

881. Herbst R, Lammers R, et al: Substrate phosphorylation specificity of the human c-kit receptor tyrosine kinase. J Biol Chem 1991; 266:19908.

882. Hunter T: Cytokine connections. Nature 1993; 366:114.

883. Leung S, Qureshi SA, et al: Role of STAT2 in the alpha interferon signaling pathway. Mol Cell Biol 1995; 15:1312.

884. Greenlund AC, Farrar MA, et al: Ligand-induced IFN gamma receptor tyrosine phosphorylation couples the receptor to its signal transduction system (p91). EMBO J 1995; 13:1591.

885. Quelle FW, Shimoda K, et al: Cloning of murine Stat6 and human Stat6, Stat proteins that are tyrosine phosphorylated in responses to IL-4 and IL-3 but are not required for mitogenesis. Mol Cell Biol 1995; 15:3336.

886. Mano H, Yamashita Y, et al: Tec protein-tyrosine kinase is involved in interleukin-3 signaling pathway. Blood 1995; 85:343.

887. Akira S, Nishio Y, et al: Molecular cloning of APRF, a novel IFN-stimulated gene factor 3 p91-related transcription factor involved in the gp130-mediated signaling pathway. Cell 1994; 77:63.

888. Ernst M, Gearing DP, et al: Functional and biochemical association of Hck with the LIF/IL-6 receptor signal transducing subunit gp130 in embryonic stem cells. EMBO J 1994; 13:1574.

889. Matsuda T, Takahashi-Tezuka M, et al: Association and activation of Btk and Tec tyrosine kinases by gp130, a signal transducer of the interleukin-6 family of cytokines. Blood 1995; 85:627.

890. Miyazaki T, Kawahara A, et al: Functional activation of Jak1 and Jak3 by selective association with IL-2 receptor subunits. Science 1994; 266:1045.

891. Johnston JA, Kawamura M, et al: Phosphorylation and activation of the Jak-3 Janus kinase in response to interleukin-2. Nature 1994; 370:151.

892. Nielsen M, Svejgaard A, et al: Interleukin-2 induces tyrosine phosphorylation and nuclear translocation of stat3 in human T lymphocytes. Eur J Immunol 1994; 24:3082.

893. Fujii H, Nakagawa Y, et al: Activation of Stat5 by interleukin 2 requires a carboxyl-terminal region of the interleukin 2 receptor beta chain but is not essential for the proliferative signal transmission. Proc Natl Acad Sci U S A 1995; 92:5482.

894. Beadling C, Guschin D, et al: Activation of JAK kinases and STAT proteins by interleukin-2 and interferon alpha, but not the T cell antigen receptor, in human T lymphocytes. EMBO J 1994; 13:5605.

895. Hatakeyama M, Kono T, et al: Interaction of the IL-2 receptor with the src-family kinase p56lck: identification of novel intermolecular association. Science 1991; 252:1523.

896. Torigoe T, Saragovi HU, et al: Interleukin 2 regulates the activity of the lyn protein-tyrosine kinase in a B-cell line. Proc Natl Acad Sci U S A 1992; 89:2674.

897. Minami Y, Nakagawa Y, et al: Protein tyrosine kinase Syk is associated with and activated by the IL-2 receptor: possible link with the c-myc induction pathway. Immunity 1995; 2:89.

898. Wakao H, Harada N, et al: Interleukin 2 and erythropoietin activate STAT5/MGF via distinct pathways. EMBO J 1995; 14:2527.

899. Gouilleux F, Wakao H, et al: Prolactin induces phosphorylation of Tyr694 of Stat5 (MGF), a prerequisite for DNA binding and induction of transcription. EMBO J 1994; 13:4361.

900. Nicholson SE, Oates AC, et al: Tyrosine kinase JAK1 is associated with the granulocyte-colony-stimulating factor receptor and both become tyrosine-phosphorylated after receptor activation. Proc Natl Acad Sci U S A 1994; 91:2985.

901. Tian SS, Lamb P, et al: Rapid activation of the STAT3 transcription factor by granulocyte colony-stimulating factor. Blood 1994; 84:1760.

902. Nicholson SE, Novak U, et al: Distinct regions of the granulocyte colony-stimulating factor receptor are required for tyrosine phosphorylation of the signaling molecules JAK2, Stat3, and p42, p44MAPK. Blood 1995; 86:3698.

903. Dong F, van Paassen M, et al: A point mutation in the granulocyte colony-stimulating factor receptor (G-CSF-R) gene in a case of acute myeloid leukemia results in the overexpression of a novel G-CSF-R isoform. Blood 1995; 85:902.

904. Corey SJ, Burkhardt AL, et al: Granulocyte colony-stimulating factor receptor signaling involves the formation of a three-component complex with Lyn and Syk protein-tyrosine kinases. Proc Natl Acad Sci U S A 1994; 91:4683.

905. Avalos BR, Hunter MG, et al: Point mutations in the conserved box 1 region inactivate the human granulocyte colony-stimulating factor receptor for growth signal transduction and tyrosine phosphorylation of p75^{c-rel}. Blood 1995; 85:3117.

906. Taniguchi T: Cytokine signaling through nonreceptor protein tyrosine kinases. Science 1995; 268:251.

907. Ihle JN: STATs: signal transducers and activators of transcription. Cell 1996; 84:331.

CHAPTER
7

The Bone Marrow Failure Syndromes

Blanche P. Alter • Neal S. Young

Bone marrow failure is characterized by a reduction in the effective production of mature erythrocytes, granulocytes, and platelets by the bone marrow that leads to peripheral blood pancytopenia. In some conditions, only one or two cell lines may be affected. Decreased transfer of mature *cells* from marrow to blood may be due to a reduction in the number or in the function of their *progenitors*. This results in a paucity of differentiated *precursors* in the marrow. Examples of such disorders include aplastic anemia (presumably involving the pluripotent hematopoietic progenitors) and Diamond-Blackfan anemia (involving the committed erythroid progenitors). In some disorders, there may be derangement of the development of the differentiated precursors, as occurs in many neutropenias. The number of differentiated precursors may be paradoxically increased in the marrow, whereas the number of their mature products is diminished in the blood; this state is referred to as *ineffective hematopoiesis*. It may be difficult to differentiate between primary progenitor abnormalities and environmental or nutritional insufficiency.

This chapter presents a review of the disorders associated with cytopenias due to bone marrow failure or ineffective hematopoiesis. Detailed discussion of neutropenias can be found in Chapter 22. Those disorders seen most frequently in the pediatric age group are emphasized.

APLASTIC ANEMIA

In aplastic anemia, peripheral blood pancytopenia results from reduced or absent production of blood cells in the bone marrow. The disorder may be acquired, inherited (genetic, but not necessarily expressed at birth), or congenital (present at birth), or any combination of these variants. The causes are multiple, and natural histories are diverse. Isolated single-cell deficiencies also may be acquired or inherited, and they may remain single cytopenias or be preludes to complete aplasia. Classifications of the aplastic anemias and the single cytopenias are presented in Tables 7–1 and 7–2.[1] Several reviews of these topics provide more detailed information than can be presented within the confines of this chapter[2, 3]; references to many earlier publications can be found in the previous edition of this book and in the authors' monograph.[2, 4]

The severity of aplastic anemia was classified by Camitta and co-workers in an effort to make possible the comparison of diverse groups of patients.[5] Diagnosis of *severe aplastic anemia* requires that the patient have at least two of the following anomalies: a granulocyte count below 500/μL, a platelet count below 20,000/μL, and a reticulocyte count below 1% after correction for hematocrit. In addition, the bone marrow biopsy must contain less than 25% of the normal cellularity. *Mild* or *moderate aplastic anemia*, sometimes called "hypoplastic anemia," is distinguished from the severe form by the presence of mild or moderate cytopenias and by normal or even increased bone marrow cellularity. These distinctions are more than semantic; they

Table 7-1. CLASSIFICATION OF THE APLASTIC ANEMIAS

Acquired

Secondary

  Radiation
  Drugs and chemicals:
    Regular: cytotoxic; benzene
    Idiosyncratic: chloramphenicol; anti-inflammatory drugs; antiepileptics; gold
  Viruses:
    Epstein-Barr virus (infectious mononucleosis)
    Hepatitis
    Parvovirus
    Human immunodeficiency virus
  Immune diseases:
    Eosinophilic fasciitis
    Hypoimmunoglobulinemia
  Thymoma
  Pregnancy
  Paroxysmal nocturnal hemoglobinuria
  Preleukemia

Idiopathic

Inherited

  Fanconi's anemia
  Dyskeratosis congenita
  Shwachman-Diamond syndrome
  Reticular dysgenesis
  Amegakaryocytic thrombocytopenia
  Familial aplastic anemias
  Preleukemia, myelodysplasia, monosomy 7
  Nonhematologic syndromes (e.g., Down, Dubowitz's and Seckel's syndromes)

Modified from Alter BP, Potter NU, Li FP: Classification and aetiology of the aplastic anaemias. Clin Haematol 1978; 7:431.

Table 7-2. CLASSIFICATION OF THE SINGLE CYTOPENIAS

Pure Red Cell Aplasia	Neutropenia	Thrombocytopenia
Acquired		
Idiopathic	Idiopathic	Idiopathic
Drugs, toxins	Drugs, toxins	Drugs, toxins
Immune		
Thymoma		
Transient erythroblastopenia of childhood		
Inherited		
Diamond-Blackfan anemia	Kostmann's syndrome	Amegakaryocytic
	Shwachman-Diamond syndrome	Thrombocytopenia with absent radii
	Reticular dysgenesis	

Modified from Alter B, Potter NU, Li FP: Classification and aetiology of the aplastic anaemias. Clin Hematol 1978; 7:431.

are critical for the prediction of outcome and the choice of therapy.

The first case of apparent bone marrow failure was described by Ehrlich in 1888, in a young pregnant woman (see later) who had an explosive fatal illness characterized by severe anemia, bleeding into skin and retina, and high fever.[6] At autopsy, the bone marrow was found to have been completely replaced by fat. The term *aplastic anemia* was apparently introduced by Vaquez and Aubertin in discussions of the Society of the Hospital of Paris in 1904.[7] The word *aplasia* is derived from the Greek verb πλαθω, meaning "to create, give shape," and thus emphasizes the functional abnormality in blood cell production.

The differential diagnosis of pancytopenia is extensive. Those disorders characterized by hypocellularity of the marrows include, in addition to aplastic anemia, myelodysplastic syndromes, preleukemias, some leukemias, and some lymphomas. Pancytopenia in primary marrow diseases with cellular marrow includes myelodysplastic syndromes, paroxysmal nocturnal hemoglobinuria (PNH), myelofibrosis, and some leukemias and lymphomas. Pancytopenia may occur secondary to systemic diseases, such as systemic lupus erythematosus, hypersplenism, vitamin B_{12} or folate deficiencies, metabolic diseases such as propionic acidemia,[8] alcohol abuse, and infections such as brucellosis, sarcoidosis, and tuberculosis. In addition, hypocellular marrow sometimes associated with pancytopenia may be due to Q fever, legionnaires' disease, anorexia nervosa, or starvation. Most of these entities are uncommon in children, and when pancytopenia is secondary, the systemic disease is usually obvious on evaluation of the patient's history and physical examination findings. The crucial differential diagnosis most often requires consideration of primary hematologic disorders and is resolved by the results of bone marrow aspirate and biopsy analysis.

Acquired Aplastic Anemia

Description

There are many large series of adult and pediatric patients with "acquired aplastic anemia," but the older literature is difficult to interpret because of the absence of strict diagnostic criteria. Cases are now included only if the bone marrow is hypocellular and if no evidence for inherited disease is apparent (see later). The distinction between acquired and inherited disease may present a clinical challenge, and the biologic separation may be subtle because acquired aplastic anemia may represent the outcome of an environmental insult in an individual of appropriate genetic background.

Physical Examination. The clinical appearance is related to the severity of the underlying pancytopenia. Hemorrhagic manifestations from thrombocytopenia are usually the first symptoms and include petechiae, ecchymoses, epistaxis, and bleeding from mucous membranes. Neutropenia causes oral ulcerations, bacterial infections, and fever; these signs are rarely present early. Erythropoietic failure leading to anemia and characterized by pallor, fatigue, and tachycardia is often late because the life span of the erythrocyte (120 days) far exceeds that of platelets (10 days) or white cells (variable, but measured in hours for granulocytes).

Epidemiology. The annual incidence of aplastic anemia has been established in Europe in large, formal epidemiologic studies as 2 per million per year. By comparison, the incidence of acute leukemia is about 50 per million per year. Higher figures for the rate of aplastic anemia have been obtained for smaller studies in the United States and earlier surveys in Europe, but these figures may have been inflated by the inclusion of cases of the more common syndrome myelodysplasia or by inaccuracy in defining the population catchment areas. Aplastic anemia is more common in the Orient than in the West. The incidence was accurately determined at 4 per million in Bangkok[9] and may be closer to 6 per million in rural areas of Thailand.[10] Geographic variance in prevalence is apparently due to environmental and not to genetic factors. For example, in Thailand, significant risk factors include low socioeconomic status, solvent exposure (in Bangkok), and rice farming (in the countryside).

The age distribution of mortality from aplastic anemia is relatively uniform until the age of 55 years; after this age, mortality increases substantially (Fig. 7-1).[11] A small peak in childhood is due to the inclusion of inherited cases. However, patterns of referral show peak incidences in those aged 20 to 25 years and in those older than 60 years. Again, the discrepancy is

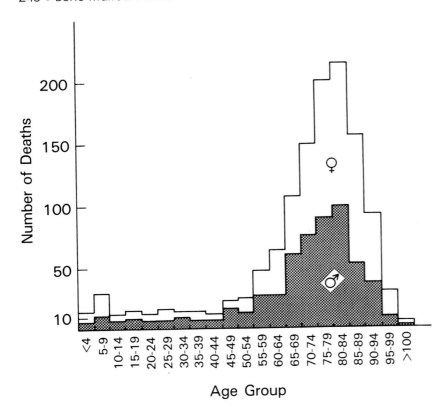

Figure 7-1. Age-adjusted mortality from aplastic anemia. In 1986, 1254 deaths were attributed to aplastic anemia; of these, 27 were "constitutional," 366 were "other," and 861 were "unspecified." (Data from Mortality. In Vital Statistics of the United States. 2nd ed. Washington, DC, US Department of Health and Human Services, 1986, p 122.)

likely the result of the inclusion of cases with myelodysplasia. The male-to-female ratio in acquired aplastic anemia is approximately 1:1.

Causal Factors

The actual cause of aplastic anemia is usually difficult to define in an individual patient. When no related factors are ascertained, the cases are classified as "idiopathic." Many patients have been exposed to several potentially myelosuppressive agents, and the number of possible associations depends in part on the intensity of the investigation. A drug or toxin is often implicated if the exposure to a previously implicated agent is appropriately extensive or temporally proximate; sometimes, a drug history is given significance only because all other factors are excluded. The course, management, and outcome are related more to the severity of the hematopoietic depression than to the cause, and they are similar for those cases with apparent cause and those that are idiopathic.

Genetic associations are discussed in detail later in this chapter. They often are underdiagnosed because of the lack of specific tests and the absence of overt abnormal phenotypes. There may be genetic abnormalities in DNA repair, drug metabolism, and immune response to viruses that are yet to be defined. Some of these possibilities are described in the following section. Families with higher-than-expected rates of aplastic anemia may represent undiagnosed Fanconi's anemia.

Drugs. The incidence of drug- and chemical-related aplastic anemia varies over time and from place to

place. Many drugs and toxins have been implicated by inferential and circumstantial evidence; the magnitude of the risk is usually unknown (Tables 7–3 and 7–4). Estimates have been made for a few agents but are based on extremely "soft" data regarding population-based utilizations. These agents and their prevalence of involvement are chloramphenicol, between 1:25,000 and 1:40,000; oxyphenylbutazone, 1:124,000; quinacrine, 1:40,000; cimetidine, 1:350,000; and carbamazepine, 1:200,000. Presence of an agent on this list suggests caution regarding its use, but no drug should be proscribed if there are strong clinical indications for its use. From a public health perspective, even drugs associated with an increased risk of marrow failure do not cause absolutely large numbers of cases of aplastic anemia.[12]

Note that even confirmed associations do not substantiate causality. Antibiotics may be administered for a viral infection that leads to aplastic anemia, or for symptoms from neutropenia in an undiagnosed case of aplastic anemia. Bleeding may be precipitated in undiagnosed thrombocytopenic patients who receive nonsteroidal anti-inflammatory drugs. There are known errors in associations: among 6 patients reported to have sniffed glue and become aplastic, 5 had sickle cell anemia and aplastic crises now known to be due to parvovirus infection.[13]

The relative frequencies of involvement of several presumed causative agents are shown in Table 7–4. The proportion of cases associated with particular drugs or chemicals has decreased with time, and a specific decline in the use of chloramphenicol is noted. Unexpectedly, chloramphenicol has not been associated with

Table 7-3. CLASSIFICATION OF DRUGS AND CHEMICALS ASSOCIATED WITH APLASTIC ANEMIA*

Agents That Regularly Produce Marrow Depression

Antibiotics: daunorubicin, doxorubicin hydrochloride (Adriamycin), chloramphenicol
Antimetabolites: antifolic compounds, nucleotide analogues
Antimitotics: vincristine, vinblastine, colchicine
Benzene and chemicals containing benzene: carbon tetrachloride, chlorophenols, kerosene, Stoddard's solvent
Cytotoxic cancer chemotherapy alkylating drugs: busulphan, melphalan, cyclophosphamide

Agents Possibly Associated, with Low Probability Relative to Use

Chloramphenicol
Insecticides: chlordane, chlorophenothane (DDT), gamma benzene hexachloride (lindane), parathion
Anticonvulsants: carbamazepine, hydantoins, phenacemide
Nonsteroidal anti-inflammatory agents: indomethacin, ibuprofen, oxyphenylbutazone, phenylbutazone, sulindac
Antihistamines: cimetidine, chlorpheniramine, ranitidine
Antiprotozoals: quinacrine, chloroquine
Sulfonamides: some antibiotics, antidiabetics (chlorpropamide, tolbutamide), antithyroids (methimazole, methylthiouracil, propylthiouracil), carbonic anhydrase inhibitors (acetazolamide, methazolamide)
Penicillamine
Metals: gold, arsenic, bismuth, mercury

Agents More Rarely Associated

Allopurinol (may potentiate marrow suppression by cytotoxic drugs)
Antibiotics flucytosine, mebendazole, methicillin, sulfonamides, streptomycin, tetracycline, trimethoprim/sulfamethoxazole
Carbimazole
Guanidine
Lithium
Methyldopa
Potassium perchlorate
Quinidine
Sedatives and tranquilizers: chlordiazepoxide, chlorpromazine, meprobamate, methyprylon, piperacetazine, prochlorperazine
Thiocyanate

*Agents are listed because they have been cited in the literature; inclusion in this list does not imply acceptance by the authors of a causal relationship.
Modified from Young NS, Alter BP: Aplastic Anemia: Acquired and Inherited. Philadelphia, W.B. Saunders Co., 1994, p 104.

aplastic anemia in the current epidemiologic study in Thailand.[10] However, much recent data may be incomplete because current reports of large numbers of cases focus more on therapy than on etiology. In general, for drug-related marrow suppression, particularly agranulocytosis, the rate of disease increases with age, tracking with increased medical drug use in older persons. The incidence of drug or chemical aplasia in pediatric cases is low, mainly because many of the drugs that may be related to aplasia are not used in childhood, with the exception of antiepileptic drugs.

Drug-related aplasia may occur in several ways. Myelosuppressive drugs, such as those used in cancer chemotherapy, lead to predictable and dose-related marrow suppression. Benzene, too, can be demonstrated to regularly suppress the bone marrow in animals in a dose-linked manner, and most individuals exposed to sufficient amounts of benzene would proba-

Table 7-4. RELATIVE FREQUENCIES OF ETIOLOGIC AGENTS

	Adult Cases										Pediatric Cases					
	1950–1959		1960–1969		1970–1979		Far East, 1970–1979		1980–1989		1960–1969		1970–1979		1980–1989	
Agent	No.	%	No.	%	No.	%	No.	%	No.	%	No.	%	No.	%	No.	%
Chloramphenicol	227	30	90	27	194	17	626	19	28	3	39	41	27	20	3	1
Phenylbutazone	1	<1	30	9	67	6	81	2	22	3	0	0	0	0	0	0
Sulfonamides	27	4	3	1	13	1	42	1	5	1	0	0	3	2	0	0
Anticonvulsants	15	2	8	2	16	2	35	1	4	<1	2	2	4	2	1	<1
Gold	0	0	3	1	12	1	11	<1	12	2	0	0	0	0	0	0
Benzene, solvents	24	6	14	4	37	3	95	3	21	3	1	1	4	3	3	1
Insecticides	9	1	29	9	15	1	122	4	11	1	2	2	1	1	5	2
Other drugs	118	16	26	8	169	13	451	12	60	7	11	11	3	2	13	6
Total drugs	427	57	203	60	523	45	1469	43	163	20	55	57	42	30	25	11
Total cases	756		339		1292		3391		811		96		138		225	

Data from Alter B, Potter NU, Li FP: Classification and aetiology of the aplastic anaemias. Clin Haematol 1978; 7:431; Young NS, Alter BP: Bone marrow failure. In Handin RI, Lux SE, Stossel TP (eds): Blood: Principles and Practice of Hematology. Philadelphia, J.B. Lippincott Co., 1991; and Alter BP: The bone marrow failure syndromes. In Nathan DG, Oski FA (eds): Hematology of Infancy and Childhood. 3rd ed. Philadelphia, W.B. Saunders Co., 1987, p 159.

bly suffer some type of marrow damage. In practice, most drug-related aplastic anemia is "idiosyncratic" and occurs unpredictably in only rare individuals who are prescribed the medication, sometimes weeks to months after its administration is discontinued. This last category of patients may possess a genetic propensity for this phenomenon. In the case of agents that can cause both dose-related and idiosyncratic aplastic anemia, the mechanisms may be different because both forms have not been reported in the same patient.

Chloramphenicol. This antibiotic was considered to be the commonest cause of aplastic anemia at the peak of its use, which began in 1949. It contains a nitrobenzene ring and thus resembles amidopyrine, a drug known to cause agranulocytosis. Recognition of the association of aplastic anemia and chloramphenicol has resulted in a decrease in the incidence of drug-related aplasia (see Table 7–4); studies have identified no cases to be associated with chloramphenicol among 135 patients with aplastic anemia, nor links in epidemiologic studies to the agent's use.[10, 15] However, the prevalence of aplastic anemia overall has not declined, suggesting that other agents may be relevant as well in populations with a genetic predisposition to marrow injury.

Chloramphenicol is the prime example of a drug that causes both dose-related marrow suppression and idiosyncratic aplastic anemia (Table 7–5).[16] The signs of dose-related toxicity appear more rapidly in patients with hepatic or renal disease because the drug must be inactivated by conjugation with glucuronide in the liver and excreted in the urine. High doses and high plasma levels correlate with the characteristic reversible erythroid depression. These effects on erythropoiesis have been blamed on inhibition of mitochondrial protein synthesis, suppression of ferrochelatase, blockage in heme synthesis, and reduced mitochondrial respiration caused by decreased synthesis of cytochromes. *In vitro,* chloramphenicol inhibits the growth of both colony-forming units–granulocyte macrophage (CFU-GMs) and colony-forming units–erythroid (CFU-Es) and also may inhibit the hematopoietic microenvironment.

Parenteral chloramphenicol is the succinate salt, whereas the oral drug is the free-base form (in pills) or palmitate (in oral suspensions); oral forms have greater bioavailability. Oral use far exceeds parenteral administration, and cases of aplastic anemia have now been reported after intravenous chloramphenicol administration.[17]

Chloramphenicol is the drug that was most frequently associated with idiosyncratic aplastic anemia in the past. A genetic predisposition may exist. Familial aplasia following chloramphenicol use was reported in an uncle-niece pair, as well as in two sets of identical twins. Also, some patients have the "chloramphenicol–hepatitis–aplastic anemia syndrome," first receiving oral or intravenous chloramphenicol, then having hepatitis 1 month later, and developing pancytopenia 1 month after that. Only 1 of 15 such patients survived. Because hepatitis itself is associated with aplastic anemia, the chloramphenicol link may have been only a coincidence.

Ocular administration also has been implicated (i.e., with the use of chloramphenicol-containing eyedrops or ointments). The "ocular" route may have in fact been oral, owing to passage of the agent through the lacrimal ducts into the nose, followed by the agent's being swallowed or absorbed across the nasal mucosa. A fatal case in a shepherd who sprayed sheep with the drug has also been reported; absorption in this case may have been transcutaneous or by inhalation.

The mechanism of the idiosyncratic aplasia remains unknown despite extensive investigation. In some studies, bone marrow cells from patients who have recovered were inhibited *in vitro* by chloramphenicol; however, in other studies, recovered marrows were resistant to the drug. The active component was hypothesized to be the p-NO_2 group. Transformation of this group to a nitroso group leads to toxic effects *in vitro.* Patients who develop aplastic anemia may have increased ability to reduce the drug to p-nitrosochloramphenicol. A derivative, thiamphenicol, in which the p-nitroso group is replaced with methylsulfoxyl, was not immediately linked to irreversible aplasia and in Europe appeared to be an effective alternative to chloramphenicol. However, aplastic anemia has been reported, perhaps in proportion to the use of thiamphenicol, and thus the use of this drug cannot be supported.[18] Yunis has studied the metabolism of

Table 7–5. CHARACTERISTICS OF TWO TYPES OF HEMATOLOGIC TOXICITY FROM CHLORAMPHENICOL

	Reversible Toxicity	Irreversible Aplasia
Incidence	Common	Rare
Bone marrow cellularity	Cellular	Aplastic
Relation to dose	Dose dependent	Not related to dose
Onset	Concurrent with drug therapy	3 wk to 5 mo from last dose
Bone marrow changes	Maturation arrest, erythroid; cytoplasmic and/or nuclear vacuolization	Aplasia
Peripheral blood	Reticulocytopenia, occasional leukopenia, and/or thrombocytopenia; anemia if treatment is prolonged; elevated serum iron	Pancytopenia
Presenting symptoms	None; pallor due to anemia (if treatment is prolonged)	Bleeding and/or infection
Outcome	Reversible	Usually fatal

From Yunis AA: Mechanisms underlying marrow toxicity from chloramphenicol and thiamphenicol. In Silber R, LoBue J, Gordon AS (eds): The Year in Hematology. New York, Plenum Medical Book Co., 1978, p 143.

chloramphenicol.[19] One finding was that gut bacteria can generate a highly toxic and short-lived intermediate compound capable of causing significant damage to DNA in cells *in vitro* and of inhibiting hematopoiesis; however, how this mechanism would account for rare aplasia is uncertain. There is one paradoxical report of a patient with chronic neutropenia who received chloramphenicol for infections; use was followed by an increase in neutrophil production that was drug dependent. Low doses of chloramphenicol may actually stimulate *in vitro* CFU-GM–derived colony formation.

Other Drugs. Nonsteroidal anti-inflammatory drugs, which are used more extensively in adults than in children, are associated with aplasia. A large case-control study found the risk for indomethacin to be 10.1, that for diclofenac sodium—6.8, and that for butazones—6.6 per million; an increased risk also was found for salicylates. Another drug associated with a risk of cytopenias in 2 per 100,000 patients is cimetidine. Sulfa-containing compounds, which appear as risk factors in most case-control studies of drugs and aplastic anemia, are used in a wide variety of clinical circumstances. Many of the drugs listed in Table 7–3 also have been associated with agranulocytosis. In general, only a minority of cases of aplastic anemia can be assigned a drug association, whereas most agranulocytosis is related to medication use.

Chemicals and Toxins

Benzene. Benzene is a particularly dangerous environmental contaminant. It is found in organic solvents, coal tar derivatives, and petroleum products. Fatal aplastic anemia or leukemia, or both, have been reported years later in factory workers who had benzene exposure. Benzene is concentrated in bone marrow fat, forms water-soluble intermediates, and damages DNA. It decreases the numbers of progenitors, and damages stroma as well. The risk of cytopenias is likely related to cumulative exposure.

Other Aromatic Hydrocarbons. Toxicity thought to be due to other organic solvents may in some instances be caused by benzene contaminants. Stoddard's solvent contains benzene. Neither pure toluene nor xylene, e.g., is a marrow toxin. Aromatic hydrocarbons are present in insecticides and herbicides and may comprise the solvents for these agents. Aplastic anemia has been linked by many case reports to insecticides, particularly γ-hexachlorobenzene (lindane) in children.[20] In Thailand, pesticides as a group are a risk factor for aplastic anemia.[10] Some organophosphate insecticides have been shown to inhibit *in vitro* hematopoietic colony formation, as has lindane.[21]

Ionizing Radiation. Marrow aplasia may occur as an acute toxic sequela of irradiation due to nuclear bomb explosion, fallout, reactor accidents, and accidental exposure in medicine and industry; however, radiation-related marrow aplasia is infrequent. Even in a restricted episode, such as the Chernobyl reactor accident in 1986, most immediate deaths were due to skin burns and damage to gastrointestinal and pulmonary systems. Bone marrow cells may be affected by high-energy γ-rays, which penetrate the viscera, as well as by ingested or absorbed lower-energy alpha particles. The radiation injury is to the actively replicating pool of precursor and progenitor cells and also to stem cells, in which DNA damage may have a more severe effect. Good supportive care, administration of hematopoietic growth factors, and marrow transplantation, when possible, may be helpful for patients with acute radiation-induced aplastic anemia (see below).

Chronic radiation-induced aplasia is dose related. Patients who were irradiated for ankylosing spondylitis had an increased risk of aplastic anemia, and American radiologists have been reported to have an increased death rate from aplasia (for both groups, the pathologic distinction of aplasia and myelodysplasia was not made). The incidence of late aplasia in atomic bomb victims was not increased, nor was it increased in patients receiving radiation therapy for malignancies. Knospe and co-workers suggested that irradiation with an exposure greater than 4.4 Gy was required for the development of aplasia; they also stated that low doses might damage only stem cells, whereas high doses would also damage the supportive hematopoietic stromal microenvironment.[22]

Infectious Agents. Patients with bacterial or viral illnesses frequently develop mild pancytopenia during or following the infection (see Chapter 54). Patients with bacterial or viral infections often receive antibiotics and other medications, and it is frequently not clear whether an ensuing aplastic anemia was caused by the infection, by the drug, or by the combination of the two—or even whether the infectious illness was the result, and not the cause, of the pancytopenia. However, several viruses do have specific hematopoietic effects (Fig. 7–2).[2, 23]

Parvovirus. Clinical aspects of parvovirus are discussed more completely in the section on pure red cell aplasia (PRCA). Human parvovirus B19 is a single-stranded DNA virus that causes the childhood exanthem fifth disease (erythema infectiosum).[24, 25] Fifth disease is a contagious febrile illness, with a characteristic facial erythema in children, and a rash with joint pain or frank arthritis observed in adults. In patients with hemolytic anemia, who have shortened red cell survival time and expanded marrow erythropoiesis, parvovirus infection leads to *transient aplastic crisis (TAC)*. TAC is an abrupt cessation of erythropoiesis, with reticulocytopenia, marrow erythroid aplasia, and severe anemia. This virus is now known to be the cause of aplastic crises in patients with sickle cell anemia,[26, 27] and it has been reported in patients with thalassemia, hereditary spherocytosis, red cell enzyme defects, and other types of erythroid stress (see later). Since TAC is by definition self-limited, red cell transfusion support should be provided for the acute anemia. Variable neutropenia and thrombocytopenia occasionally occur in TAC, as well as in normal individuals with parvovirus infection.

Hydrops fetalis may occur following *in utero* infection with parvovirus,[28] with fetal loss ensuing in approximately 5% of those infected in the first two trimesters. Hydrops can be detected by ultrasound, and intrauterine transfusions are offered for anemic fetuses.

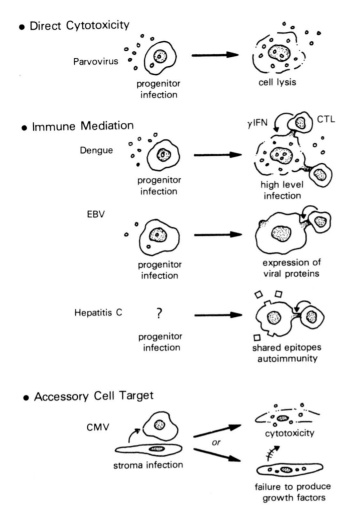

- **Direct Cytotoxicity**

  Parvovirus

  progenitor infection → cell lysis

- **Immune Mediation**

  Dengue

  progenitor infection → high level infection (γIFN, CTL)

  EBV

  progenitor infection → expression of viral proteins

  Hepatitis C ?

  progenitor infection → shared epitopes autoimmunity

- **Accessory Cell Target**

  CMV

  stroma infection → cytotoxicity *or* failure to produce growth factors

Figure 7–2. Mechanisms of virus-induced bone marrow failure. EBV = Epstein Barr virus; CMV = cytomegalovirus; CTL = cytotoxic lymphocyte; HGF = hematopoietic growth factor; HSC = hematopoietic stem cell. (With permission from Young NS, Alter BP: Bone marrow failure. In Handin RI, Lux SE, Stossel TP (eds): Blood: Principles and Practice of Hematology. New York, Lippincott-Raven, 1994. Illustrator, Joy D. Marlowe, M.A., A.M.I.)

Congenital parvovirus infection has been recorded after the treatment of *in utero* infection.[29] Surviving infants have a marrow picture of red cell aplasia or dysplasia. Virus has been detected in marrow but not in the circulation and only at low levels, and gene amplification techniques are required for measurement. Patients did not respond to immunoglobulin therapy.

Persistent parvovirus infection and *chronic PRCA* can occur in patients with immunodeficiency who cannot produce neutralizing antibody. This was found to be the cause of PRCA in an adult who was finally cured by infusion with immunoglobulins.[30] Patients with congenital immunodeficiency, acquired immunodeficiency syndrome,[31] and immune deficits following chemotherapy, starvation, or a bone marrow transplantation (BMT) may all be at risk. Parvovirus may account for as much as 15% of cases of PRCA.[32] Immunoglobulin therapy is effective in ameliorating or curing persistent parvovirus infection.

The mechanisms of parvovirus-induced aplasia are

outlined in Figures 7–2 and 7–3. Parvovirus replicates only in human erythroid progenitor cells.[33] Viral infection is directly cytotoxic. Giant pronormoblasts may be seen in the marrow. In normal individuals, the virus leads to antibody production—first, the production of immunoglobulin M (IgM), and then that of IgG; this, in turn, produces immune complexes that cause the rash symptoms of fifth disease in children and arthralgia in adults. Patients with an expanded erythron due to hemolytic anemia have a larger reservoir for viral replication; thus, they demonstrate viral excess, which leads to erythroid reinfection and transient aplastic crises, until they are able to produce sufficient antibody to clear the virus. Those with immune deficits, however, have viral persistence with continued marrow suppression; this cycle can be broken by treatment with commercial immunoglobulin, which contains antibody to parvovirus owing to the prevalence of this virus in the general population.

Tests for parvovirus include measurements of serum antibodies; detection of IgM indicates recent infection, but detection of IgG only past infection. Bone marrow examination for pathognomonic giant pronormoblasts is often rewarding. Parvovirus DNA must be measured to diagnose persistent infection; DNA may be detected in the marrow by direct *in situ* hybridization, and in the serum directly by hybridization, or following gene amplification by the polymerase chain reaction.

Hepatitis. As an identifiable clinical event, a prior episode of hepatitis is recognized in 2% to 5% of aplastic anemia patients in Western series[34]; the prevalence of prior hepatitis is about twofold this proportion in the Far East.[35] Among children with aplastic anemia in Taiwan, 24% had a history of recent acute hepatitis.[36] A previous episode of hepatitis was a significant risk factor in case-control studies of aplastic anemia in the United States and Bangkok.* In a far greater number, antecedent hepatitis may be subclinical, as about 50% of patients may have abnormally elevated hepatic transaminases on presentation, before their first transfusion. Although hepatitis is frequently associated with mild depression of blood cell counts, aplasia is a rare sequela, estimated to occur in fewer than 0.07% of the total number of pediatric hepatitis cases[37] and in fewer than 2% of those with non-A, non-B hepatitis.[38] In a report of 32 patients with liver transplantation for hepatic failure following non-A, non-B hepatitis, however, 28% developed aplastic anemia.[39] Aplasia has been reported following both hepatitis A and B virus infections,[40, 41] but the hepatitis/aplasia syndrome is clearly non-A, non-B and non-C in almost all cases.[42]

Aplastic anemia associated with hepatitis is particularly severe. More than 200 cases of aplastic anemia and hepatitis have been reported, with two thirds of those affected being male and three-quarters being younger than 20 years of age. In one series, more than 90% died within a year, and the mean survival was only 11 weeks.[43] BMT, antithymocyte globulin, and androgens have all been successful treatments.

Flaviviruses. Flaviviruses cause arbovirus hemor-

---

*Issaragrisil S: Personal communication, 1995.

INTERACTION AMONG PARVOVIRUS, TARGET CELL, AND IMMUNE RESPONSE

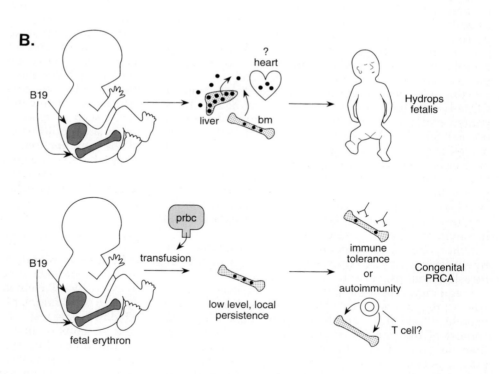

Figure 7–3. Pathogenesis of parvovirus disease. *A,* Etiology of acquired conditions: fifth disease, transient aplastic crisis, and pure red cell aplasia. *B,* Etiology of congenital conditions: hydrops fetalis and pure red cell aplasia. (Modified from Young NS, Alter BP: Bone marrow failure. In Handin RI, Lux SE, Stossel TP (eds): Blood: Principles and Practice of Hematology. New York, Lippincott-Raven, 1994. Illustrator, Joy D. Marlowe, M.A., A.M.I.)

rhagic fevers, dengue, and other hematodepressive syndromes. Dengue can propagate in bone marrow cultures without direct cytotoxicity, and dengue antigens induce lymphocyte activation and the release of suppressive cytokines.[44] Novel flavivirus-like viruses related to hepatitis C have recently been identified and are likely causative agents for non-A, non-B and non-C hepatitis cases.[45, 46]

Epstein-Barr Virus. Herpesviruses such as Epstein-Barr virus (EBV) are large, complex DNA viruses.[47] EBV causes infectious mononucleosis, which has pancytopenic complications in fewer than 1% of cases. More than 12 such cases have been reported; however, one half of these cases had a fatal outcome. EBV was demonstrated by immunologic and molecular methods in the bone marrow of six patients with aplastic anemia.[48] Only two had a history of typical mononucleosis, although all six had serologic evidence, suggesting that EBV may be an unrecognized cause of aplastic anemia. The EBV's target is obviously B cells, although T cells also may be infected.

Suppressor T cells may be activated in EBV infection, and this may be the mechanism for hematopoietic depression. Extreme examples of aberrant immune responses to EBV are the *X-linked lymphoproliferative syndrome* of immunoglobulin deficiency, chronic or fatal infectious mononucleosis, B cell lymphomas, and aplastic anemia.[49]

Cytomegalovirus and Human Herpesvirus 6. Cytomegalovirus, another herpesvirus, usually has a benign picture. However, it may lead to graft failure in immunosuppressed bone marrow transplant recipients.[50] CMV can infect marrow stromal cells *in vitro* and can inhibit their ability to produce growth factors[51]; direct progenitor cell infection by some CMV strains also has been documented.[51, 52] The recently discovered herpesvirus 6 is the cause of erythema subitum[53] and, like CMV, may be found in the marrow of patients with graft failure after transplantation,[54] as well as in hematopoietic progenitors infected *in vitro.*[55]

Human Immunodeficiency Virus. Patients with AIDS often have cytopenias,[56] but their marrow is much more commonly cellular and dysplastic than empty. Colony formation by marrow from patients may be diminished.[57–60] Hematologic problems could be due to opportunistic infections, neoplasms, or marrow suppression from the drugs used to treat AIDS and its complications. The action of human immunodeficiency virus-1 (HIV-1), a lentivirus, on hematopoietic cells remains a subject of controversy. HIV-1 infection of CD34+ cells has been difficult to detect *in vivo* from patient material[59, 61] or after tissue culture infection of normal cells.[59, 62] The virus apparently directly infects megakaryocytes, which bear the CD4 receptor present on T cells.[63] The virus also may affect stroma functions, at least *in vitro.*[64, 65] HIV-1 can act indirectly on hematopoiesis through inhibitory lymphokine production: the envelope glycoprotein can stimulate macrophages to produce tumor necrosis factor, which in turn inhibits hematopoietic colony formation.[66]

Other Viruses. Blood count abnormalities, which are rarely severe, may be observed in the course of rubella, measles, mumps, varicella, and influenza A.[2]

Pregnancy. The first patient with aplastic anemia was a pregnant woman.[6] Although this disease is not usually a "pediatric" problem, it may occur within the context of the practice of pediatric hematology. More than 60 cases of aplastic anemia have now been reported as being first diagnosed during pregnancy, and more than 30 cases of the disease were diagnosed before pregnancy.[67] Among those without known preceding aplasia, 25% died within the first 2 months following termination or delivery, and 50% eventually died from aplastic anemia. Although therapeutic termination is often recommended, only one of seven patients improved after termination. Among those with preexisting aplastic anemia, only seven died subsequent to delivery. Most fatal complications in both groups were due to bleeding. Red cell and platelet transfusion support should permit successful pregnancies, although clinical deterioration is possible. Estrogens, whose levels increase in pregnancy, may have a role in the associated aplastic anemia. Animal studies suggest that high doses of these hormones may be responsible for bone marrow suppression.[68] This may also be the mechanism for the worsening of hematopoiesis in pregnant patients with inherited bone marrow failure syndromes such as Fanconi's anemia (see later in this chapter).

Paroxysmal Nocturnal Hemoglobinuria. PNH is a disease characterized by variable combinations of mild to severe intravascular hemolysis, large venous thromboses, and aplastic anemia.[69] It is uncommon in adults and even rarer in children (see Chapter 14). There is a clear association of PNH with aplastic anemia: 20% to 30% of patients with PNH begin with pancytopenia and marrow hypoplasia, and 5% to 10% of patients with aplastic anemia develop PNH as they recover. According to flow cytometry results, a large proportion—as many as one half—of new aplastic anemia patients manifests the PNH defect, usually in granulocytes.[70] The selective advantage conferred on PNH progenitor cells may be intrinsically hematopoietic or related to immune system inhibition of marrow function.[71]

Immunologic Diseases. A rare collagen vascular syndrome, *eosinophilic fasciitis,* has been associated with aplastic anemia in 10% of cases.[72] This condition is usually found only in adults. The association of thymoma with hematopoietic failure is another rare immunologic condition, mostly but not exclusively with PRCA; only one child has been reported with this association.[73] Some of the adult cases had also received drugs such as chloramphenicol or sulfonamides, and the aplasia could have been due to the drugs alone, or to the combination. An iatrogenic aplasia can be induced by the transfusion of competent lymphocytes into immunodeficient hosts. In these cases, marrow failure is the cause of death in graft-versus-host disease.[74]

Laboratory Findings

Peripheral Blood. Blood counts are most often uniformly depressed. The fact that the circulation half-lives of blood elements are very different (granulocytes, 6 to 12 hours; platelets, 5 days; and erythrocytes, 60 days), suggests that bone marrow failure is not simultaneous or that compensatory mechanisms vary for the three different lineages. The blood smear shows a paucity of platelets and leukocytes but essentially normal red cell morphology. Automated counting indicates that the anemia is often macrocytic but sometimes normocytic and that the red cell distribution width (RDW), a numeric measure of anisocytosis, is normal.[75] Platelet size is not increased, as it is in most cases of immune thrombocytopenias. The absolute reticulocyte count is decreased. Granulocyte numbers are clearly diminished, as may be those of monocytes and lymphocytes.[76, 77]

Increases in fetal hemoglobin (Hb F) and red cell i antigen, along with macrocytosis, are manifestations of the fetal-like erythropoiesis seen in "stress" hematopoiesis,[78] but they have no prognostic value and often persist in recovered patients.

Results of the Ham or sucrose hemolysis tests may be positive if PNH is associated[79] (see earlier); more frequently, evidence of deficient glycophosphoinositol-linked protein expression on white cells may be found by flow cytometry.[70] Folate and vitamin B_{12} levels are normal or increased owing to lack of utilization; however, a folate-induced remission has been reported in one family.[80] Erythropoietin may be elevated to levels higher than those seen in comparable degrees of anemia due to iron deficiency or hemoglobinopathies.[81]

Serum transaminases may be high in patients with persistent hepatitis (see earlier). Immunoglobulin levels are occasionally decreased.[82] Peripheral blood or bone marrow chromosomes are normal; this finding is in contrast to the results in patients with Fanconi's anemia (see later) and myelodysplasia, including pediatric patients.[83]

Bone Marrow Morphology. Bone marrow examination must be done by aspiration and also by biopsy so that cellularity can be evaluated both qualitatively and quantitatively. These specimens are hypocellular, with empty spicules, fat, reticulum cells, plasma cells, and mast cells (Fig. 7–4). Aspirates alone may appear hypocellular owing to dilution with peripheral blood, or they may look hypercellular because of areas of focal

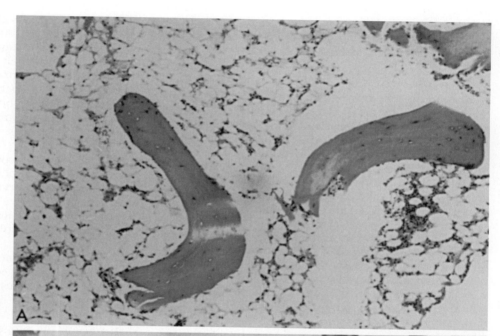

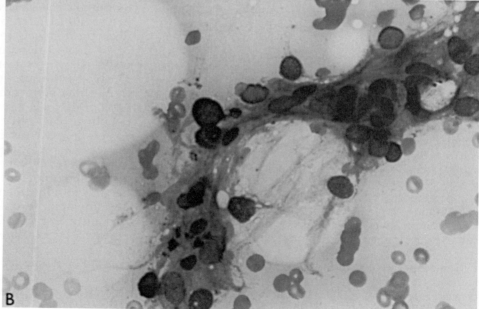

Figure 7–4. Bone marrow examination in severe aplastic anemia. *A,* Note hypocellularity in biopsy. *B,* Residual cells seen in aspirate are lymphocytes, stromal cells, plasma cells, and mast cells. (Courtesy of Dr. Gail Wolfe, Boston, MA.)

residual hematopoiesis. Biopsies provide larger, more reliable specimens for assessment of cellularity. Some dyserythropoiesis, with megaloblastosis and nuclear-cytoplasmic asynchrony, may be seen. An increase in the number of mast cells may be observed around the hypoplastic spicules. A proportion of marrow lymphocytes greater than 70% has been correlated with a poor prognosis.[84]

Bone Marrow Function. Marrow erythroid function can be derived from ferrokinetic studies. In hypoproliferative states, plasma iron concentration is increased, transferrin saturated, radiolabeled iron clearance prolonged, and plasma iron turnover decreased. Marrow scintigraphy using ^{111}In bound to transferrin documents the decreased erythron and may have prognostic value in aplastic anemia, PRCA, and myelofibrosis. Magnetic resonance imaging distinguishes bone marrow fat and cells by water content and may help to distinguish aplasia from myelodysplasia[85] as well as to follow recovery of hematopoiesis.[86]

Pathophysiology

Understanding the mechanism or the mechanisms for failure of hematopoiesis is predicated on our current knowledge of normal hematopoiesis (see Chapter 6). Disease could result from decreased numbers or defective function of the cellular or soluble components required for blood cell production, or from combinations of these factors. Conversely, observations of aplastic anemia in the clinic and in the laboratory also have provided insights into normal blood cell production.

There is no satisfactory animal model for the disease aplastic anemia. Nevertheless, treatment of animals with radiation and cytotoxic drugs and especially genetically defective mouse strains have illuminated relevant aspects of hematopoietic dysfunction. Marrow failure is produced after exposure to high doses of radiation in all species and by drugs that mimic the effects of radiation. In mice treated with busulfan, marrow failure is latent for many months; during this period, blood counts are maintained by very low numbers of progenitor and stem cells. In the congenitally anemic W/W^v mouse, stem cell numbers are small and the animals are cured by transplantation.[87] These mice have a mutation in the *KIT* gene, which codes for a transmembrane tyrosine kinase and is the receptor for stem cell factor (SCF). A similar disease phenotype is provided by the reciprocal defect in the Sl/Sl^d mouse, in which SCF production is defective; these animals can donate stem cells successfully but are inadequate as recipients in a transplant procedure. However, there is no evidence so far that either acquired aplastic anemia or inherited cytopenias in humans are due to similar mutations in genes for growth factors or their receptors. Lymphocytes can induce aplastic anemia after sublethal irradiation in certain murine strain combinations.[88]

Hematopoietic Stem and Progenitor Cells. Virtually all patients with aplastic anemia have greatly decreased numbers of blood and marrow committed progenitor cells, assayed as myeloid colony–forming cells (CFU-GMs); erythroid colony–forming cells (CFU-Es and BFU-Es); megakaryocytic progenitors (CFU-megas); and multipotent colony–forming cells (CFU-GEMMs). Until recently, true stem cells have not been assayable in humans; however, the *long-term culture-initiating cell* appears to be a surrogate test for this most primitive cell. These cells are severely reduced in number in both the marrow and blood in all cases of aplastic anemia.[89, 90] Hematopoietic cells can also be assessed phenotypically for the presence of the CD34 antigen, which defines a compartment of about 1% of marrow cells that includes progenitors and stem cells. CD34 + cells also are much diminished in aplastic anemia, and almost all patients show not only severe reduction in the numbers of these cells but also poor plating efficiency from purified CD34 + cells.[91, 92] Decreased stem cell numbers as measured *in vitro* have different implications clinically. The success of nonreplacement therapies, such as the administration of immunosuppressive drugs or androgens, suggests that, although quantitatively reduced, the number of stem cells remains sufficient to support adequate blood cell production in many patients. However, simple infusion of stem cells by BMT between identical twins, in which no conditioning or immunosuppression is provided, implies that stem cell replacement alone is sufficient for other cases. Low stem cell numbers persist even with hematologic recovery after immunosuppressive therapy, and a quantitative stem cell deficiency likely accounts for the observation of clonal hematopoiesis in aplastic anemia[93] as well as for the frequency of relapse and the late development of other hematologic diseases like PNH, myelodysplasia, and acute leukemia (see later).

There are a few examples of qualitatively abnormal pluripotent stem cells, which suggest a disordered stem cell that could be responsible for pancytopenia. Of course, in Fanconi's anemia, all hematopoietic cells share a defect in DNA repair (see later). In PNH, the stem cell and its progeny cannot present certain proteins at the cell surface; however, this defect alone may not be sufficient to produce the disease, as the clone does not dominate in cell culture, in transgenic mice, or, of course, in many patients. An odd example is a G6PD-AB heterozygous female who had stable pancytopenia and in whom only type B enzyme was found in all three peripheral blood cell types, as well as in most progenitors *in vitro*.[94] Although such tests are not definitive when very few cells are present, there has been little evidence for either gross cytogenetic abnormalities or specific oncogene mutations in aplastic anemia marrow on presentation of the disease.

Microenvironment. In theory, aplastic anemia could be due to a microenvironment that fails to support hematopoiesis—a lesion of "soil" rather than "seed."[22] The anemia of the Sl/Sl^d murine strain is an example of such a defect. Although defects in some stromal cell function have occasionally been measured in patients and although specific defects in growth factor production are shared by many patients, these defects do not appear to be causative for most cases. After marrow transplantation, most stroma cell elements remain of host origin,[95] yet these cells adequately support the donor's stem cells. In the laboratory, aplastic marrow usually provides normal adherent cell function in long-term or Dexter flask–type cultures; however, a patient's marrow is a poor source of clonogenic cells when grown on normal stroma, consistent with the defect in stem and progenitor cell numbers described earlier.[96] Some investigators have reported low fibroblast colony formation in aplastic anemia,[97] but this assay may not reflect stromal cell function.

Hematopoietic growth factor production and plasma levels are usually increased rather than decreased in patients with aplastic anemia. Erythropoietin level is even higher than anticipated for the degree of anemia.[81] In functional assays, burst-promoting activity (BPA), colony stimulating activity, and megakaryocyte-stimulating activity are all increased. Plasma levels of granulocyte colony-stimulating factor (G-CSF)[98, 99] and granulocyte-macrophage colony-stimulating factor (GM-CSF),[100] as well as *in vitro* production of GM-CSF and interleukin-3 (IL-3) by stromal cells or lymphocytes, are normal or high.[101, 102] Elevations of these factors may have some prognostic significance. Hematopoietic cells from aplastic anemia patients also appear to respond normally to growth factors *in vitro*.[103, 104] Two growth factors are abnormally low in aplastic anemia: IL-1, produced by monocytes[105, 106]; and SCF levels in blood.[107–109] Therapeutic trials with these factors have not been successful,[110, 111] casting doubt on the pathophysiologic significance of deficiency of these factors.

Immune Inhibition. Clinical data suggest that immune phenomena may be relevant in aplastic anemia. First, autologous recovery has been reported after either mismatched or matched transplants in patients prepared with antilymphocyte sera or cyclophosphamide. Second, one half or more of syngeneic (twin) BMTs require cytotoxic conditioning of the host.[112] Treatment with antilymphocyte globulins (without transplant) has a 50% success rate, patients who have failed antilymphocyte globulins may respond to cyclosporine, and intensification of immunosuppression by combination of these therapies has led to hematologic responses in 70% to 80% of cases (see later). Finally, histocompatibility studies conducted in Europe, Asia, and America have indicated an increased representation of HLA-DR2 among aplastic anemia patients, consistent with a genetically determined immune susceptibility to disease.[113–115] The immune pathophysiologic basis inferred from these clinical observations has been partly elucidated in detailed laboratory studies.

Lymphocytes. Equine antisera and cyclosporine are cytotoxic to lymphocytes and block T-cell function, respectively; they also perform many other activities. The inhibitory role of T cells was first implicated by studies in which myeloid colonies grew only after removal of the patients' lymphocytes; antilymphocyte serum improved growth, and patient cells inhibited colony growth from normal marrow. Inhibition in allogeneic mixtures might be due to allosensitization from transfusion of multiple blood products. A new approach to these studies was provided by Bacigalupo et al., who found that bone marrow from aplastic patients contained suppressor cells that produced a soluble inhibitor.[116] Lymphocytes with IgG receptors, *Tγ+ cells*, were reported in aplastic but not in normal bone marrow.[117] Later, these cells were characterized phenotypically as *activated cytotoxic lymphocytes*: CD8+ T cells expressing the antigens HLA-DR and the receptor for IL-2; activated cytotoxic T cells circulate,[118] but they may be present in the marrow when they are not detected in the blood.[119] Cell clones of this phenotype have been isolated from patients, and *in vitro* they overproduce inhibitory cytokines and inhibit hematopoiesis.[120–122] Notably, these more specific immune system abnormalities did not correlate with transfusion status,[123] and the number of activated lymphocytes decreases owing to immunosuppressive therapy.[119, 124]

Lymphokines. The soluble inhibitor produced by T cells was found to be γ-interferon.[125] This cytokine is produced at high levels in tissue cultures of patients' cells.[118, 124, 126] γ-Interferon gene expression, measured by reverse gene amplification of the specific mRNA, is found in the marrow of most patients with aplastic anemia but not in normal persons or in patients with other hematologic diseases who have undergone frequent transfusions.[127, 128] Other inhibitory cytokines, such as *tumor necrosis factor*[129, 130] and *macrophage inflammatory protein-1*,[106, 131] also are overexpressed in aplastic marrow. Both interferon and tumor necrosis factor directly and synergistically inhibit hematopoiesis *in vitro*.[132] In long-term bone marrow culture, constitutive low-level expression of γ-interferon is sufficient to markedly reduce the output of both committed progenitor cells and long-term culture-initiating cells, the stem cell surrogate.[133] Both interferon and tumor necrosis factor induce programmed cell death within the CD34+ compartment by increasing Fas antigen expression on target cells.[134] (Fas antigen is a cell surface molecule in the tumor necrosis factor receptor family; its activation signals apoptosis.) The fact that isolated and concentrated CD34 cells from patients with aplastic anemia formed colonies poorly (except in response to G-CSF) suggests that the disease may be due to an intrinsic defect rather than an increase in the level of a local cytokine.[135]

Natural Killer Cells. Natural killer cells have some features of cytotoxic-suppressor cells, such as lymphocyte origin, CD8 surface antigen, and the ability to produce γ-interferon, IL-2, and colony-stimulating activities. Natural killer cells are pathogenic in Tγ lymphoproliferative disease, in which patients have increased numbers of large granular lymphocytes and neutropenia or other single cytopenias.[136] However, the number of natural killer cells is most often decreased in the blood and marrow of patients with aplastic anemia; it returns to normal along with hematologic recovery.[137] Natural killer cells do not suppress *in vitro* hematopoiesis.

Antibodies. Involvement of an immunoglobulin-mediated mechanism is relatively clear in some of the single cytopenias, e.g., adult PRCA, transient erythroblastopenia of childhood, and immune neutropenias. These disorders are described in other sections. Only a few patients with idiopathic or drug-induced aplastic anemia have been shown to have antibodies, usually those associated with systemic lupus erythematosus. The antibodies inhibit *in vitro* colony formation and may be complement-dependent or independent.

Rarely, drug-dependent pancytopenia is antibody mediated, usually with antibody-drug complexes binding to progenitor cells that are "innocent bystanders." The antibodies may be to a drug's metabolites rather than to the drug itself. Autoantibodies may be an immune reaction to a damaged cell membrane or to the constituent of a lysed cell rather than to the normal progenitor cell.

Figure 7–5 depicts two models for bone marrow damage. In type I, irradiation, drugs, and chemicals such as benzene randomly cause damage to DNA. In type II aplasia, viruses or drugs or toxins incite an immune system reaction that in turn leads to cytotoxicity within the hematopoietic compartment. Recovery would occur if the stem cells could, in fact, repopulate adequately. In damage of both type I and type II, cell death among target cells occurs, probably by apoptotic mechanisms, and all proliferating cells are likely affected. Immune system attack may actually be more efficient than physical or chemical damage because of its high degree of specificity for hematopoietic cells and the lack of collateral effects on other organ systems.

Therapy and Outcome

Prognosis. Outcome depends on the types of treatments offered, the causes of the aplasias, and the eras and countries being analyzed. In a large series conducted before 1957, Wolff found a survival rate of only 3%.[138] In other series ending no later than 1965, complete recoveries were reported in 10% to 35% of

patients. In a series of 40 pediatric patients seen before 1958, Shahidi and Diamond found that only 2 patients recovered, 1 of whom later had recurrence.[139] The series summarized here may not have been rigorous with regard to the inclusion of only patients with severe disease.

The survival curve in aplastic anemia appears to be biphasic, with the mortality rate for the first 6 months being approximately 50% (Fig. 7–6).[140] Nathan calculated a mortality rate of 20% per month for those in the region with the steep slope, and a rate of 2% per month for the rest.[141] Many efforts have been made to determine criteria at presentation that identify those patients who are destined to do poorly. The most important indicator of the outcome in aplastic anemia is provided by the blood counts, and "moderate" and "severe" disease are now usually distinguished on the basis of the criteria of Camitta and co-workers.[5] An important addition to prognostic measurement is the category of "very severe," which designates the presence of an absolute neutrophil count below 200 cells/μL and identifies patients with the worst prognosis.[142] Also used in some series for predictive purposes is a marked reduction in the proportion of myeloid components of the bone marrow, usually stated as greater than 30% lymphocytes; however, this parameter is not universally accepted or widely applied in practice.[143] One study found that reduction of cell counts in the first 3 months was associated with death within 5 years; of course, almost one half of the patients died by the time of the 3-month assessment.[144]

Many of the prognostic algorithms were derived before current therapy was developed. The availability of platelet support (see below) has had a substantial impact; the major cause of death has now shifted from

PATHOPHYSIOLOGY OF APLASTIC ANEMIA

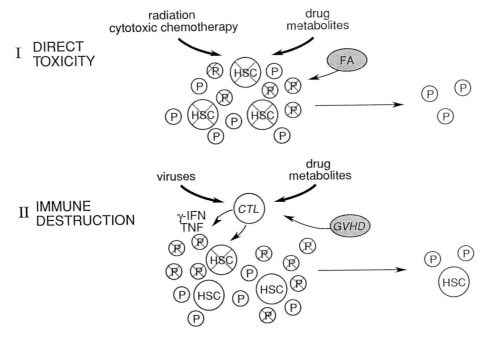

Figure 7–5. Two mechanisms of stem cell compartment damage. Type I involves DNA damaged by radiation and radiomimetic agents such as busulfan, as well as by other drugs (e.g., chloramphenicol). Fanconi's anemia is an example of inheritance of the inability to repair DNA damage. Type II is at the level of the more mature cell and involves the cell membrane or metabolism; such damage can be caused by many drugs, viruses, and immune mechanisms. P = progenitor; HSC = hematopoietic stem cell; IFN = interferon; TNF = tumor necrosis factor; CTL = cytotoxic T lymphocyte; GVHD = graft versus host disease.

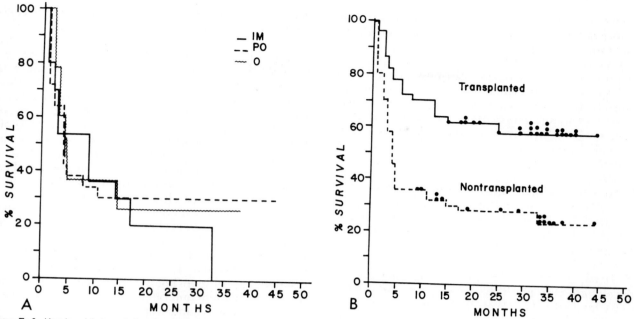

Figure 7-6. Kaplan-Meier plots of cumulative survival in severe aplastic anemia. Time is shown as months from diagnosis. *A,* The results of treatment with intramuscular (IM) or oral (PO) androgen compared with no treatment (O). *B,* The results of treatment with marrow transplantation. (From Camitta BM, Storb R, Thomas ED: Aplastic anemia (First of two parts). Pathogenesis, diagnosis, treatment, and prognosis. N Engl J Med 1982; 306:645. Modified, by permission, from the *New England Journal of Medicine.*)

bleeding to infection.[145] Identifying the patient with a poor prognosis is important for determining therapeutic choices. In general, if a young patient fits into the "severe" category, the first choice should be BMT from a matched sibling; "immunotherapy" is the next choice, with hematopoietic growth factors being the choice after that, and androgen treatment and other therapies the last options. Whether immunotherapy is effective because it attacks lymphocytes is unknown. Appropriate supportive care is, of course, critical no matter which primary treatment is selected.

Spontaneous Recovery. Spontaneous recovery has been reported anecdotally, although most cases were probably of moderate rather than of severe aplastic anemia. Supportive care (see later) may contribute to this; in one series, 14 of 33 children recovered,[146] and children with moderate aplastic anemia have been found to have an excellent prognosis even without specific treatment.[147] A study of immunosuppressive therapy in which 21 patients were randomized (some to receive only supportive care) found no improvement in the control group after 3 months.[148] If it does occur, spontaneous recovery nevertheless is sufficiently rare in severe aplastic anemia that all modalities of current therapy must be employed.

Supportive Care. One of the first and most important decisions to be made is whether a patient should receive a bone marrow transplant. If so, blood product support should be used sparingly, to avoid sensitization, and blood product donors should never be from the patient's family, for the same reason. HLA blood group typing of the patient and his or her family members should be initiated immediately. Complete red cell phenotyping should be done because erythro-

cyte antibodies may develop in patients who receive long-term blood product support. In addition, any exposure to potentially hazardous drugs or toxins should be eliminated.

Bleeding. Platelet (and red cell) support has probably had the greatest impact on survival in aplastic anemia and has changed the cause of death from bleeding to infection. Platelets can be provided from several individual units of blood or, preferably, by platelet pheresis from a single donor (which reduces antigenic exposure). A unit of platelets (equivalent to a single unit of blood) contains 5.5×10^{10} platelets, whereas a pheresis pack would contain from 3 to 6×10^{11}. Each unit should increase the platelet count by 10,000 cells/ μL per m² when measured at 1 hour. Poor responses may be due to allosensitization, infection, or poorly prepared platelets. If necessary, one or a few donors who are HLA compatible with the patient and whose platelets do provide a therapeutic increment should be identified. Filtration of platelets to remove white cells is more efficient than centrifugation.

The main role of prophylactic platelet support is reduction of the risk of intracranial hemorrhage, which is a rare but devastating event. For children with leukemia, the threshold platelet count has long been 20,000 cells/μL; however, this figure and the entire practice of prophylactic administration of platelet transfusions has recently been questioned.[149–151] Specific data are not available for aplastic anemia. Chronic platelet transfusions for aplastic anemia are not used as frequently as they are in leukemia, and they are usually given when there are symptoms of bleeding or when the platelet count is less than 10,000 cells/μL.

Other measures to reduce bleeding include maintenance of good dental hygiene, use of a soft toothbrush, avoidance of trauma, and avoidance of vasoconstrictive drugs. Intramuscular injections can be given and should be followed by 15 minutes of firm pressure to the injection site. Local oozing can be managed with topical agents such as Gelfoam, collagen, or thrombin. Antifibrinolytic agents such as ε-aminocaproic acid (Amicar) and tranexamic acid may decrease bleeding but have not been proved effective in a small controlled trial.[152] For ε-aminocaproic acid, the dose is approximately 0.1 g/kg every 6 hours orally. Low doses of steroids (e.g., prednisone, 5 to 10 mg every other day) may promote vascular integrity, although the scanty experimental data for this practice are from animals treated with higher doses. Drugs that may interfere with platelet function, such as aspirin or nonsteroidal anti-inflammatory drugs, should be avoided in thrombocytopenia.

Infections. Studies of infection in aplastic anemia specifically are very few.[145, 153] Severe granulocytopenia may last for years. However, the immune systems of granulocytopenic patients remain intact; this is in contrast to the situation of patients with malignancies who receive chemotherapy and who experience immunosuppression. In aplastic anemia, neutropenia (and perhaps monocytopenia) increases the risk of bacterial infection. In leukemic patients, the risk of infection increases as the number of granulocytes falls, with the risk being 20% at 500 to 1000 cells/μL, and 50% at less than 100 cells/μL. Because neutropenia precludes the development of an inflammatory response, identification of an infected locus is often difficult. The bacterial organisms may be gram-negative bacilli such as *Escherichia coli, Klebsiella pneumoniae,* and *Pseudomonas aeruginosa,* as well as gram-positive cocci, including *Staphylococcus aureus* and *S. epidermidis* and streptococci. Immunosuppression due to preparation for BMT or as primary therapy for the aplastic anemia may lead to unusual bacterial, fungal, viral, and protozoan infections. Recommendations for specific antibiotics and other anti-infection agents are beyond the scope of this chapter, and regimens are changing rapidly as new generations of treatments are developed.

The use of prophylactic antibiotics has no role in the "well" patient with aplastic anemia. In the context of fever and neutropenia, complete evaluation and cultures of all possible sites should be followed by the administration of broad-spectrum parenteral antibiotics. The recommendation from the oncology experience is to use triple antibiotics: cephalosporin, a semisynthetic penicillin, and an aminoglycoside; therapy with a third-generation cephalosporin, ceftazidime, may be equivalent. Treatment is best continued for a full 14 days, even if culture results are negative. Fungal infections occur frequently in patients who have received repeated or extended courses of antibiotics; candidiasis and especially aspergillosis, which lead to sinusitis, lung disease, or disseminated infection, are distressingly frequent causes of death in aplastic anemia.[145] Aggressive introduction of amphotericin B treatment is indicated in the persistently febrile patient who is unre-

sponsive to antibiotics or in the appropriate clinical setting.

Prophylactic granulocyte transfusions are not used. The life span of granulocytes in the circulation or in tissues is a matter of hours, and thus appropriate transfusions cannot be sustained. Similarly, with the development of modern antibiotics, granulocyte transfusions are no longer generally provided for the febrile patient, even though they may have some efficacy.[154] Alloimmunization may jeopardize platelet transfusion, and the granulocytes may fail to get to the infected sites.[155] Prevention of infection is clearly important. Hand washing and maintenance of good dental hygiene are simple but effective. Total gnotobiotic environments can be achieved with the use of laminar air filters, sterilized food, and oral nonabsorbable antibiotics. The availability of such environments is limited, as is their acceptance by patients, and they are not standard care in aplastic anemia. Less extensive isolation has the disadvantage of reducing contact between medical personnel and patient and often provides little more benefit than extensive hand washing.

Anemia. Red cells should be provided as needed (in the form of packed washed red cells or after they have been passed through a filter to remove white blood cells to decrease the risk of sensitization to white cell antigens). The hemoglobin should be maintained at a level consistent with normal activities (probably greater than 9 g/dL) if routine transfusions are to be used. Severe anemia also can contribute to the bleeding diathesis secondary to chronic thrombocytopenia. However, chronic anemia is well tolerated once adaptation has occurred, and a child who can sustain a hemoglobin level greater than 6 g/dL without transfusions (i.e., a child who is not bleeding) should be permitted to do so. Long-term transfusions lead to iron overload, with accumulation in critical organs. Liver iron stores can be directly and noninvasively assayed by magnetic techniques, which yield a much more accurate measurement than the serum determination of ferritin.[156] Permanent damage to heart, liver, and endocrine glands can be prevented by iron chelation therapy.[157] Desferrioxamine therapy, which is self-administered by the patient subcutaneously, should be instituted in the chronically transfused patient before significant hemosiderosis occurs, usually after the infusion of about 50 units of red blood cells. If the patient is also severely thrombocytopenic, subcutaneous therapy may be difficult. Oral iron chelators may be as effective[158, 159]; however, neutropenia has occurred with the use of these agents, and their application has not yet been approved in the United States. (See Chapter 21 for details regarding chelation.)

Bone Marrow Transplantation. The general topic of BMT is described in Chapter 8; because of its important role in the management of aplastic anemia, it is discussed briefly here.

The earliest transplants involved twins. Subsequent definition of the human histocompatibility gene complex, development of immunosuppressive regimens, and improved support of severely pancytopenic patients led to more general application of this form of therapy. Figure 7–6 shows the initial controlled trial of the International Aplastic Anemia Study Group, in which patients who received transplants had a clear advantage over those who received no treatment or androgens (see later).

Outcomes for BMT have been reported by large registries, which combine the results of many contributing centers, or in single-center studies by the largest referral centers[160–173] (Table 7–6). From the most recent data reported to the International Bone Marrow Transplant Registry and the European Group for Bone Marrow Transplantation, long-term survival rates (5-year actuarial rates) are projected to be 60% to 70%.[172, 173] The most recent figures from some individual hospitals are even better: at Johns Hopkins Hospital in Baltimore, the projected survival rate is 80%[169]; at the University of Washington Medical Center in Seattle, it is 92%.[170]

Mortality and morbidity in marrow transplant for aplastic anemia are due to graft rejection, graft-versus-host disease, and the serious infections that frequently accompany these complications. Successful engraftment is linked to the number of donor stem cells provided, with more than 4×10^8 cells/kg being recommended. Graft rejection is linked to a history of transfusions and subsequent allosensitization. Virtually untransfused recipients have outcomes similar to those of syngeneic twins who have undergone transplants (Fig. 7–7).[174] In registry studies, modest numbers of blood transfusions (40 units or less) also did not adversely affect outcomes. The detrimental role of transfusions may have been decreased through the routine use of leukocyte-free products, as well as by the strict avoidance of the use of family members as donors.[175] Hematologic chimerism is highly associated with graft

rejection, and second transplants for graft failure are often unsuccessful.[176]

More aggressive immunosuppression, although improving engraftment, leads to increases in the rates of graft-versus-host disease. This disease occurs when donor T cells recognize minor histocompatibility antigens; it is more frequent in older than in younger patients, perhaps owing to defective thymic function and lymphocyte maturation. In general, as many as 50% of patients develop some degree of chronic graft-versus-host disease; 20% experience it as a serious complication, 5% as a fatal sequela. The rate of graft-versus-host disease increases with age. In one series, the incidence rose from 19% for those younger than 10 years of age, to 46% for those 11 to 30 years of age, and to 90% for those older than 31 years of age.[177] Children have a much lower rate of graft-versus-host disease than do adults (between 10%[178] and 30%[179]); this lower rate translates into improved survival for those younger than 20 or 30 years of age. Improved prophylaxis and management of graft-versus-host disease with cyclosporine has decreased both the rate and severity of this complication in older patients in more recent studies (see Table 7–6; see also Chapter 8).

The prior discussion refers to transplants from HLA-matched sibling donors. However, 75% of transplant patients do not have such a donor. Alternative donors include phenotypically but not genotypically matched relatives, partially matched (mismatched) relatives, and histocompatible but unrelated volunteers. Success has been reported in the occasional instance in which a family member is a phenotypic match as a result of, for example, haplotype sharing between parents.[180]

Unrelated donors must be located through registries

Table 7-6. RECENT RESULTS OF ALLOGENEIC BONE MARROW TRANSPLANTATION IN APLASTIC ANEMIA*

Institution	Years	N	Age in y (mean)	Conditioning Rx	GVHD Px	Graft Rejection/ Failure (%)	AGVHD (%)	CGHVD (%)	Actuarial Survival (%)	F/U (y)
Hôpital St. Louis	1980–1989	107	5–46 (19)	CY + TAI	MTX, CSA, or MTX + CSA	3	36	35	68 ± 10 (at 5 y)	1–10 (3.75)
UCLA	1984–1988	290	0.7–41 (19)	CY + TLI	MTX ± CSA	17	21	12	78 ± 15 (at 5 y)	0.5–5 (2.3)
Johns Hopkins	1984–1991	24	4–53 (21)	CY + CSA	CSA	29	5	0	79 ± 8	2–5 (3)
Hutchinson	1988–1993	39	2–52 (24.5)	CY + ATG	MTX + CSA	5	15	34	92 (at 3 y)	0.8–5 (2.5)
IBMTR	1980–1987	595	1–>40	CY ± TLI, TAI, or TBI	MTX, CSA, or MTX + CSA	10	40	45	63 (at 5 y)	—
IBMTR	1985–1991	737	—	—	—	—	—	—	64 ± 4 (at 5 y)	—
EGBMT	1980–1989	540	—	—	—	—	—	—	63 (at 5 y)	—
	1990–1994	165	—	—	—	—	—	—	72 (at 3.5 y)	—

Px = prophylaxis; Rx = therapy; GVHD = graft-versus-host disease; AGVHD = acute GVHD; CGVHD = chronic GVHD; F/U = follow-up; CY = cyclophosphamide; MTX = methotrexate; CSA = cyclosporine; TBI = total body irradiation; TAI = total abdominal irradiation; TLI = total lymphoid irradiation; ATG = antithymocyte globulin; UCLA = University of California at Los Angeles; IBMTR = International Bone Marrow Transplant Registry; EGBMT = European Group for Bone Marrow Transplantation.
*Especially when results are reported early, Kaplan-Meier estimates may be higher than ultimate actual survival figures. For late complications such as chronic GVHD, prevalence in the susceptible population is the relevant figure, to correct for censoring due to death; for the first four studies quoted, the percentages represent the actual prevalence in the population at risk (either explicit in the publication or extracted from the results), and for the Seattle study (Hutchinson), the stated actuarial risk is quoted.
From Young NS, Barrett AJ: The treatment of severe acquired aplastic anemia. Blood 1995; 85:3367.

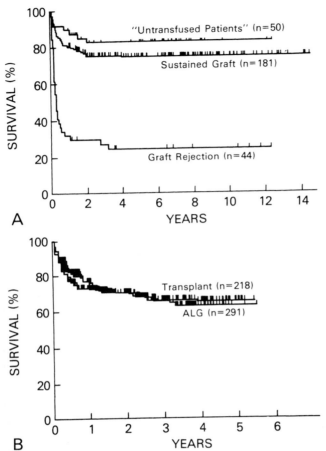

Figure 7-7. Actuarial survivals in severe aplastic anemia. A, Bone marrow transplantation (BMT), showing the critical role of graft acceptance in the determination of outcome. (From Deeg HJ, Self S, et al: Decreased incidence of marrow graft rejection in patients with severe aplastic anemia: Changing impact of risk factors. Blood 1986; 68:1363.) B, BMT compared with immunosuppression. (From Gordon-Smith EC: Treatment of severe aplastic anemia by bone marrow transplantation. Hematol Oncol 1987; 5:255.)

of volunteers, which are now sufficiently large that matches can readily be found for common HLA types. However, those with rare genotypes and members of ethnic minorities are still not well served.[181] Transplants from unrelated donors have been successful, but they have also been associated with a high rate of early mortality due to graft failure and frequently fatal graft-versus-host disease. The European Bone Marrow Transplant Group found an actuarial survival of 45% for those with phenotypically identical donors, one of 25% for a single locus mismatch, and a rate of 11% for a mismatch of two to three loci.[182] In the American National Donor Marrow Program, survival for aplastic anemia was 29% at 2 years, and almost one half these patients appeared not to have achieved engraftment.[183] In the European International Marrow Unrelated Search and Transplant (IMUST) trial, the survival rate after transplantation from an unrelated donor was about one-half that after conventional transplantation, mainly as a consequence of the high rate of graft

rejection or failure.[184] The best results have been obtained in young children who are treated with a very intensive conditioning program (one that would not be tolerated by adults); in the Milwaukee series, survival and late complications have been similar to those occurring after conventional transplantation.[185, 186] The logistics of arranging an unrelated donor transplant currently require about 4 months of preparation—time enough to conduct a trial of immunosuppressive treatment before a commitment to this high-risk procedure is made.

Immunosuppression. *Antilymphocyte globulin (ALG)* and *antithymocyte globulin (ATG)*, or the sera produced by immunization of horses or rabbits with human thoracic duct lymphocytes or thymocytes, are highly cytotoxic reagents with activity against all blood and marrow cells, including progenitors. These reagents were initially used to decrease the rate of rejection of HLA-matched bone marrow. They also were employed with androgens to permit at least temporary engraftment with haploidentical marrow in aplastic patients without a matched donor. Autologous recoveries occurred in some of these patients; they encouraged several groups to examine the use of ATG or ALG with and without haploidentical marrow and androgens.

Table 7–7 summarizes the data from several of the larger studies of this type,[4] and Figure 7–7 compares results of ALG therapy with those of marrow transplantation.[187] The overall hematologic response rate (transfusion independence) is 45%, and the survival rate is 60%. These rates compare favorably with the 25% to 30% survival rates obtained with supportive care alone (see Figs. 7–6 and 7–7) and are similar to outcomes of marrow transplantation when a matched donor is available. The results shown in Table 7–7 include only adults or adults plus children. For children, outcomes for transplant have generally been superior (if not always statistically better) than those for immune therapy, perhaps because children do so well after transplantation.

The authors recommend doses of ATG at 40 mg/kg per day for 4 days. Treatment for longer periods may result in substantial serum sickness and no significant additional benefit. The patient begins to make antibodies to horse protein about 1 week after first exposure; at this point, equine antibodies are rapidly cleared from the circulation, and this reduces the effective dose and enhances immune complex formation.

Concomitant administration of androgens has worked better at some institutions than at others, and androgens generally are not used in the United States. Corticosteroids are usually given (prednisone, 1 mg/kg) to reduce the symptoms from serum sickness. High-dose methylprednisolone (see later) is sometimes added by European clinicians, but direct comparisons have revealed no difference in outcome between low and high doses.[188] High doses of steroids also entail the risk of irreversible and painful avascular necroses, usually of femora or humeri.[189]

Immediate allergic reactions to ALG are rare and can be predicted by skin testing followed by desensitization in those who are allergic.[190] *Serum sickness* due to

Table 7-7. ANTITHYMOCYTE GLOBULIN/ANTILYMPHOCYTE GLOBULIN TREATMENT OF APLASTIC ANEMIA

Center	Other Therapy	N	Improvement (%)	Survival (%)	F/U (y)	Reference
EGBMT	BMT ± androgens	126	33	50	1	207
Leiden	± BMT	20	35	55	5	966
Cleveland	Steroids	11	54	50	3	967
UCLA	Steroids	33	53	62	2	148
Aplastic Anemia Study Group	BMT, androgens	29	69	76	2	968
Minnesota	Steroids	19	63	71	1	969
Basel	Androgens ± BMT	72	61	75	1.5	263
Austria	Steroids	15	79	80	1	126
Seattle	Steroids, androgens	46	41	65	3	970
NHLBI	Steroids	77	48	58	1	192
United Kingdom*	Steroids	64	40	53	6	971
Vanderbilt*	± Androgens	22	44	62	2	972
Mexico	Steroids	22	42	51	1.5	973

BMT = bone marrow transplant; NHLBI = National Heart, Lung and Blood Institute.
*Some patients received two courses of antilymphocyte globulin. Improvement means transfusion-independence. Steroids are listed when they were the sole concomitant therapy.

immune complex deposition occurs in almost all patients who are treated for 10 days or longer. It manifests as fever, a serpiginous rash at the volar-dorsal border of the hands and feet, arthralgia, myalgia, lassitude, and changes in urine sediment. Shorter ATG treatment courses are less often associated with serum sickness, and serum sickness is not a prerequisite for hematologic recovery. Thrombocytopenia may be a major problem and requires intensive support; ATG binds to determinants on all cell types in blood and marrow.[191]

Responses usually occur within the first 3 months, if at all, and some degree of blood count improvement by 3 months may correlate with survival.[192] All ATG and ALG preparations are lytic of T lymphocytes and recognize a broad range of human cell-surface antigens. There is no good *in vitro* evidence for clinically ineffective lots.

The antilymphocyte preparations contain heterogeneous mixtures of antibodies to lymphocytes and are clearly immunosuppressive as well as generally cytotoxic. They lead to rapid lymphopenia during and immediately following treatment, and reduced levels of activated lymphocytes persist for months. Monoclonal antibodies are inadequately immunosuppressive and do not appear to be effective as primary treatment for aplastic anemia. ATG and ALG also can stimulate lymphocyte function and lead to production of lymphokines *in vitro*; however, no correlation may exist between these observations and clinical responses.[193]

The *in vitro* studies suggesting that cellular suppression of hematopoiesis is relevant in aplastic anemia are reviewed earlier in this chapter in the section on pathophysiology. Although several laboratories suggested that *in vitro* T cell depletion, the addition of ALG, or co-culture results reflect *in vivo* responses to ALG treatment, other studies failed to confirm these results.[2, 4] One group observed an increase in the number of peripheral blood BFU-Es 48 hours after ATG treatment in those destined to respond, if they were treated with a single course within a month of the diagnosis of aplastic anemia.[194] This test is obviously useless in the determination of which patients should

be given ATG. There is probably no basis for deciding who will respond to ALG or why it may be effective, but it is recommended as a first-line therapy for those patients who are not candidates for marrow transplant because it can induce a remission even though the marrow remains abnormal.[195]

Cyclosporine (formerly cyclosporin A) is a fungal cyclic undecapeptide and an effective immunosuppressive agent.[196] It is a specific T-cell inhibitor, preventing production of IL-2 and γ-interferon but not of CSFs.[197] Initial reports suggested that cyclosporine could be effective even in patients who had failed other treatments.[2] Reports of larger series of patients suggested that about one half of patients who had failed ATG or ALG treatment subsequently experienced remission with cyclosporine.[198, 199] The recommended oral dose is 12 mg/kg per day in adults and 15 mg/kg per day in children (disparity attributable to differences in drug metabolism), so as to maintain blood trough levels between 100 and 250 ng/mL as measured by radioimmunoassay. One randomized trial comparing ALG with cyclosporine as initial therapy found equivalent but low responses.[200]

Toxic effects from cyclosporine use are not insignificant and include hypertension, azotemia, hirsutism, gingival hypertrophy, immunodeficiency, increase in serum creatinine levels, irreversible nephrotoxicity, and *Pneumocystis carinii* pneumonia.[196] As with ATG, *in vitro* tests of the effect of cyclosporine on progenitor cells do not predict responses.[201] Because cyclosporine is thought to be more specific than ATG, it further implicates T-cell mediation in the pathophysiology of aplastic anemia; however, cyclosporine therapy has a broad range of effects, and conclusions about pathophysiology derived from therapy are usually unsatisfactory.

Intensive Immunosuppression. The combination of ALG and ATG with cyclosporine is based on the clinical efficacy of each agent individually and on their separate and potentially complementary modes of action. Three recent trials have strongly suggested that their combination is more effective at inducing hematologic responses than either drug alone, producing transfusion independence in 70% to 80% of patients with severe aplastic anemia (Table 7–8).[202–204] In a large German multicenter trial, patients randomized to receive ALG plus cyclosporine had higher response rates and better survival than did those receiving only ALG, a difference most notable in those with severe disease.[205] In a National Institutes of Health (NIH) study, the response rate at 1 year for ATG plus cyclosporine was also about twice that of historical controls treated with ATG alone.[204] In a recent European collaboration, which combined ALG, cyclosporine, and G-CSF, survival in severe aplastic anemia was 92% at about 3 years.[203] Importantly, intensive immunosuppression has greatly improved the results of therapy in two groups notoriously refractory to ALG or ATG alone—patients with very severe disease, as determined by extremely low neutrophil counts; and children. In the NIH Clinical Center trial, survival curves of those older and younger than 35 years of age were superimposable; also, there was no significant difference when the division was made at 20 years.

Corticosteroids. Very high doses of corticosteroids led to a 40% response in a small series.[206] Methylprednisolone is given as intravenous boluses: 20 mg/kg per day on days 1 to 3, 10 mg/kg per day on days 4 to 7, 5 mg/kg per day on days 8 to 11, 2 mg/kg per day on days 12 to 20, 1 mg/kg per day until day 30, and maintenance with 0.1 to 0.2 mg/kg per day thereafter. In a comparative trial, the initial results with ALG were the same as with methylprednisolone,[207] and many patients who failed corticosteroid treatments subsequently responded to ALG. This steroid protocol is associated with substantial toxicities, including hypertension, hyperglycemia, fluid retention, potassium wasting, and increased susceptibility to fungal infections, as well as masking of fever, psychosis, and aseptic necroses of femoral and humeral heads. High-dose methylprednisolone should be restricted to circumstances in which ATG is unavailable or prohibitively expensive.

Late Complications. Immunosuppression can result in long-term survival that is very similar to that with marrow transplantation[160]; the most recent retrospective analysis of the European data suggests that immunosuppressive therapy is superior to marrow transplantation by this criterion for patients of all ages and degrees of severity except children for whom there was a slight advantage for transplant. However, immunosuppression is associated with problems not observed in marrow transplantation, in which survival at 6 months can be reliably construed as evidence of hematologic cure. In contrast, a large proportion of patients who were successfully treated by immunosuppression—about 30%—will experience relapse[204, 208]; fortunately, relapses often respond to reinstitution of cyclosporine or retreatment with ALG or ATG. More serious and more mysterious is the late development of clonal hematologic diseases, especially PNH, myelodysplasia, and acute myelogenous leukemia, often years after stable blood count recovery was induced. Laboratory evidence of PNH developed in 13% of patients in one large series: about 10% acquired myelodysplasia, and 7% acute leukemia.[195] Other malignant diseases (solid tumors) also develop in about 2% to 3% of patients who are treated with either immunosuppression or transplantation.[209] Clonal hematologic disease may occur more rarely in children than in adults, but the probability of late complications should be considered in choosing definitive therapy in aplastic anemia.

Hematopoietic Growth Factors. Although patients with aplastic anemia do not have a deficiency of most hematopoietic growth factors (see earlier), pharmacologic levels might stimulate hematopoiesis of one or more cell lines.[210, 211] Published trials in aplastic anemia have appeared for GM-CSF, G-CSF, IL-3, IL-1, and IL-6; the total number of patients treated in these protocols is not large, and because of their experimental nature, only a minority of participants have been children. Growth factors have been administered at a variety of doses by continuous or intermittent IV injection or by daily or alternate-day SC injection. The initial report of the use of GM-CSF, which suggested broad hematologic responses in the majority of patients,[212] has not been confirmed in subsequent series[213, 214]; furthermore, the factor has been ineffective in infected, severely neutropenic patients.[215] The white cell count usually increases promptly because of an increase in the number of neutrophils, eosinophils, and monocytes. Bone marrow myelopoiesis can appear, but the CFU-GM response is variable.[212, 216] The myeloid response tends to correlate with the pretreatment neutrophil count: residual myelopoiesis may be necessary for a significant effect. In general, continued growth factor treatment is required for sustaining the white blood cell count, and neutrophil numbers may decrease even despite chronic therapy. Reticulocyte and platelet responses have rarely been noted.[214, 217]

Table 7–8. INTENSIVE IMMUNOSUPPRESSION IN SEVERE APLASTIC ANEMIA

Study, Year	Regimen	N	Median Age (y (range))	Median ANC/μL (% of cases with < 200/μL)	Response	Survival	Relapse	Median F/U (d)
German multicenter, 1992	ALG + CSA	43	32 (7–80)	480 (19)	70% at 6 mo	64% at 41 mo	11%	516 (183–1295)
EGBMT, 1995	ALG + CSA + G-CSF	40	16 (2–72)	190 (50)	82% at 1 y	92% at 34 mo	3%	428 (122–1005)
NIH, 1995	ATG + CSA	51	28 (3–79)	340 (42)	78% at 1 y	86% at 1 y, 72% at 2 y	18% at 1 y, 36% at 2 y	912 (218–1714)

ANC = absolute neutrophil counts; G-CSF, granulocyte colony–stimulating factor; NIH, National Institutes of Health.
From Young NS, Barrett AJ: The treatment of severe acquired aplastic anemia. Blood 1995; 85:3367.

G-CSF has shown the most promise in aplastic anemia, especially among younger patients. In a study of Japanese children with mainly severe aplastic anemia, 2 weeks of intravenous G-CSF administration led to an increase in neutrophil counts in 12 of 20 patients; additionally, 3 of 5 patients responded to the administration of higher doses.[218] Patients who were recently diagnosed or who had extremely low starting neutrophil counts were less likely to respond, although 6 of 10 with very severe neutropenia did have increased neutrophil counts.[219] As with GM-CSF therapy, responses were restricted to the myeloid series and were transient, with all patients returning to their initial white cell values with discontinuation of treatment. Bilineage and trilineage responses to G-CSF therapy also have been reported.[220–222] Responses may be delayed.[223] Another Japanese multicenter trial tested chronic G-CSF therapy in a mixed group of adults (including those with moderate and severe as well as treated and untreated disease) who received variable doses of factor by a variety of routes.[224] Marked increases in neutrophil count were seen in almost all patients, although only a few had very severe depression of granulocytes at the start of therapy; 10 of 27 patients also showed improvement in anemia, and 3 of these 10 had higher platelet counts as well. Blood count findings were paralleled by marrow progenitor results. G-CSF can be administered subcutaneously at 5 to 10 μg/kg per day, and the dose and frequency of injection titered to the neutrophil count.

First use of IL-3 in aplastic anemia was reported in a German study of 9 patients.[225, 226] Hematologic responses were modest and largely restricted to the granulocyte series. IL-3 has appeared to be less effective in increasing neutrophil counts in aplastic anemia than it does in myelodysplasia, less effective for neutropenia than GM-CSF or G-CSF, and disappointing in its action on platelet counts.[227–229] Combined therapy with IL-3 and GM-CSF has not produced results better than those obtained with either factor alone[230]; however, in one patient who had failed G-CSF treatment, administration of IL-3 followed by G-CSF use led to a marked increase in neutrophil count.[231]

IL-1 is one of only a few growth factors known to be underproduced by cells in patients with aplastic anemia,[105, 232] but IL-1 was without hematologic effect in two small series of refractory patients,[111, 233] and toxicity was substantial.

Erythropoietin levels in plasma are very high in aplastic anemia, but some patients have apparently responded to prolonged administration of extremely high doses of recombinant erythropoietin.[107] Bilineage and trilineage responses to combinations of erythropoietin and G-CSF[234] or GM-CSF[235] have been reported in a few cases.

Even transient elevations in neutrophil number early in the course of aplastic anemia might prolong survival sufficiently to allow recovery with immunosuppression or until a BMT can be performed; thus, these factors logically could be added to conventional regimens, as prophylaxis or at the first infectious episode. Case reports have suggested success with addition of a growth factor to conventional immunosuppression,[236] G-CSF, and cyclosporine therapy.[237, 238] Small numbers of patients have been treated with GM-CSF before or during immunosuppressive therapy; neutrophil counts have been raised, and patients may have fared better in their long-term outcome.[239–241] The best results with immunosuppression have been achieved when G-CSF was routinely added to a regimen of ALG and cyclosporine.[203] Randomized trials will be required to establish the benefit of G-CSF in this setting.

Toxicities of recombinant human growth factors vary. GM-CSF is generally well-tolerated except at very high doses. Symptoms of "cytokine flu"—fever, headache, and myalgia—are common but do respond to acetaminophen or resolve with the passage of time. Bone pain may be a symptom of increased marrow activity. At higher doses, the severity of symptoms increases, and there may be evidence of visceral engorgement and fluid retention, probably secondary to "capillary leakage." The toxic effects of IL-3 are similar, usually including fever, chills, and headache. Hypotension is the dose-limiting toxicity of IL-1. The use of G-CSF is virtually without side effects. Myelodysplasia and leukemia have been reported in aplastic children treated with hematopoietic growth factors[242] and acute myeloid leukemia in an elderly woman with aplastic anemia.[243]

SCF is only beginning to be used in phase I clinical trials, but it did increase marrow stem cell numbers in patients with advanced breast cancer.[244]

Androgens. Androgens no longer have a primary role in the management of aplastic anemia, unless all of the therapies discussed above are unavailable or unsuccessful. As described earlier, androgens also have been used as adjuncts to immunosuppression. Their use over a few months was not helpful in a randomized American trial,[245] and in a more recent randomized European study, they enhanced the response rate in severely neutropenic women only, but without improving survival.[246]

The mechanism of action was reviewed extensively by Gardner and Besa.[247] Androgens increase erythropoietin production,[248] stimulate erythroid stem cells,[249] and increase hemoglobin levels in normal males at puberty and in patients treated for arthritis, breast cancer, or in old age. Shahidi and Diamond were the first to report success with testosterone[250] and large confirmatory series were published from France[144] and Mexico.[251] However, later critical evaluations revealed no evidence supporting the use of androgens. Li and associates[84] reported greater than 75% mortality in children despite the use of androgens; Davis and Rubin observed a similar result in adults.[252] Androgen-treated patients often did not do as well as those who were not treated with these hormones.[253, 254] The older publications often failed to distinguish moderate from severe patients. Camitta and co-workers performed a prospective, multicenter analysis beginning in 1974 and concluded that androgens (whether oral or intramuscular) were no more effective than supportive care alone for *severe* aplastic anemia (see Fig. 7–6).[140, 255]

The apparent success of androgens may be an artifact

in some series: because one half of the patients die within 3 to 6 months of diagnosis, the result of the treatment of a patient who was referred after that period of time is already biased toward survival.[144] Patients with *moderate* aplastic anemia may indeed do well on androgens. In one small series, an increase in marrow CFU-Es when androgens were added *in vitro* correlated with an *in vivo* response.[256] A few reports of androgen-dependent patients have been published.[4]

Several androgens have been used, including methyltestosterone, testosterone enanthate, testosterone propionate, oxymetholone, etiocholanolone, and danazol. The oral dose is 2 to 5 mg/kg per day, and the intramuscular dose is usually 1 to 2 mg/kg per week; nandrolone decanoate is administered at a dose of 5 mg/kg per week. The orally given 17α-alkylating agents present a risk of liver toxicity. Cholestatic jaundice and hepatomegaly are usually reversible. Peliosis hepatis (blood lakes) have been reported.[257] Hepatic tumors are a serious risk, although the pathologic picture is usually that of a benign adenoma; such tumors may be reversible when use of the androgen is discontinued. Other side effects of anabolic steroids include masculinization with hirsutism, baldness, deepening of the voice, and enlargement of the genitalia. Acne, flushing of the skin, nausea, and sodium and fluid retention also occur. The appetite is stimulated, and there is weight gain with increased muscular development. There may be an increase in the rate of skeletal maturation, with eventual premature fusion and ultimate short stature. However, treatment for up to 1 year may be insufficient for this problem to develop.[258] All patients who receive androgens should be monitored with frequent liver function testing, annual liver ultrasound examinations, and annual bone age determinations. Four adults who received oxymetholone for aplastic anemia developed acute myeloblastic leukemia (AML).[259] However, no leukemias were found among 100 children treated with androgens for aplastic anemia or other indications.[260]

Other Therapies

Cyclophosphamide. A few patients who received high-dose cyclophosphamide as preparation for marrow transplant rejected their grafts and had autologous recoveries, leading to treatment with this drug without transplant. A survey of the members of the American Society of Hematology identified only 2 responders in 73 patients; clearly, these two patients could have had spontaneous recoveries.[261] Administration of high doses of cyclophosphamide is an effective immunosuppressive therapy and is not myeloablative; this treatment may be reasonable in refractory or failed cases of severe aplastic anemia. In fact, a recent report indicated a complete response in 7 of 10 patients treated with 45 mg/kg per day for 4 days.[261a]

Splenectomy. Splenectomies were often performed until recently, perhaps for want of something better to offer to patients. A review in 1957 indicated improvements in 20 of 35 patients.[262] More recently, the operation has been performed to facilitate supportive care.[263] Unless there are clear indications of hypersplenism impacting on platelet and red cell transfusion support,

the operation does not seem warranted in patients at risk of bleeding and infections. Occasionally, patients with persistent or recurrent thrombocytopenia may improve following splenectomy.

Response to Treatment. Whichever therapy is selected, the earliest response may be heralded by the appearance of a few granulocytes and nucleated red cells in the circulation. Red-cell size distribution histograms show a macrocytic shoulder.[264] Reticulocytes appear, transfusions decline, and the hemoglobin level increases slowly. The white cell count rises next. The last cell line to return is often the platelets, whose numbers may remain low for months or even years. The recovering red cells are not normal; in addition to macrocytosis, Hb F level is increased and fetal membrane antigens may remain present (Fig. 7–8).[265] Long-term survivors (except those with successful transplants) often have residual abnormalities, such as thrombocytopenia, red cell macrocytosis, and elevated Hb F levels.[266]

Inherited Bone Marrow Failure Syndromes

The term *constitutional aplastic anemia* was defined by O'Gorman Hughes as "chronic bone marrow failure associated with other features, such as congenital anomalies, a familial incidence, or thrombocytopenia at birth."[267] Although these disorders are "inherited bone marrow failure syndromes," their hematologic components are often not evident at birth. The subdivisions in the older literature are confusing and no longer relevant:

> *Type I*, or aplastic anemia with physical abnormalities, is now diagnosed if clastogen-induced chromosomal breaks are present; physical abnormalities may be absent.
>
> *Type II*, or familial aplastic anemia without physical anomalies, is now known to be a subset of type I.
>
> *Type III*, or amegakaryocytic thrombocytopenia, also is now more stringently defined.

All of the specific disorders, both included and ignored by the above terminology, are referred to by their eponyms, until more specific information becomes available.

One hypothesis regarding "acquired" aplastic anemia is that it occurs in rare individuals (homozygotes or heterozygotes) who are genetically predisposed to marrow damage. In this section, homozygotes for autosomal recessive bone marrow failure genes (and hemizygotes for X-linked genes) who can be identified by their phenotype are discussed. Heterozygotes are identified from family studies, but molecular biology approaches may soon permit testing of the hypothesis. The phenotypes of patients with genes for aplastic anemia vary widely, and the categories may inadvertently include patients with congenital (i.e., present at birth) but not necessarily inherited phenocopies. Detailed references not provided here can be found in previous editions of this book,[4] as well as in the authors' monograph.[2]

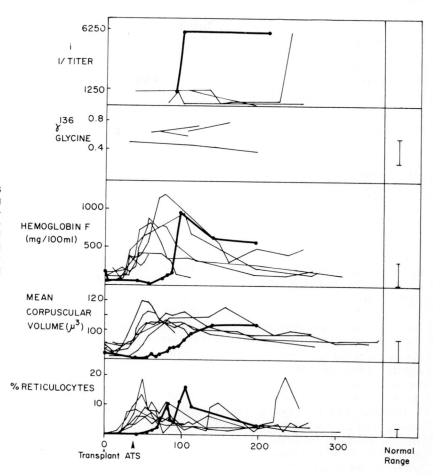

Figure 7–8. Time course of fetal-like erythropoiesis during recovery from aplastic anemia following BMT. The *thin lines* represent patients who recovered with transplanted cells; the *heavy line* represents a patient who rejected transplant, received further treatment with antithymocyte serum, and had an autologous recovery. (From Alter BP, Rappeport JM, et al: Fetal erythropoiesis following bone marrow transplantation. Blood 1976; 48: 843.)

The incidence of these inherited conditions is difficult to ascertain. Among 134 children with aplastic anemia seen at the Children's Hospital Medical Center in Boston from 1958 to 1977, 40 were diagnosed with inherited diseases from birth to the age of 17 years.[1] Twenty-six had Fanconi's anemia (FA), 10 familial aplasia without physical or cytogenetic evidence for FA, and 4 developed pancytopenia following amegakaryocytic thrombocytopenia. In a similar interval at the Prince of Wales Hospital in Australia from 1964 to 1984, 12 of 34 children had inherited syndromes, and 8 of these had FA.[268] The authors estimate that at least 25% of childhood aplastic anemia occurs in the presence of known marrow failure genes. The genetic syndromes must be sought in all patients with aplastic anemia, because the inherited and acquired disorders differ in treatment and prognoses.

PANCYTOPENIAS

Fanconi's Anemia

Description

In 1927, Fanconi described three brothers who had pancytopenia as well as physical abnormalities; he called their macrocytic anemia "perniziosiforme."[269] Uehlinger soon described a similar condition in a patient with abnormalities of the thumb and kidney.[270]

According to Fanconi,[271] Naegeli suggested in 1931 that the term "Fanconi's anemia" be used for patients with familial aplastic anemia and congenital physical anomalies. Patients are diagnosed as having FA if they have characteristic chromosome breaks following clastogenic stress; the presence of physical anomalies or aplastic anemia is not required for diagnosis. Useful reviews of FA can be found in several sources.[2, 4, 272, 273]

More then 1000 cases have been reported in varying detail, and many of the older cases are reviewed elsewhere.[2, 4, 274] Table 7–9 summarizes these cases according to the decade of the report, and the ages at diagnosis are shown in Figure 7–9. The ratio of males to females is 1.3:1. Before the 1980s, diagnoses were made when aplastic anemia (or leukemia or cancer) had developed; more recent diagnoses also are made on the basis of positive results on chromosome breakage studies in siblings of affected individuals or in patients with "characteristic" physical anomalies without aplastic anemia. The mean age at diagnosis in males was 7.8 years, and in females was 8.8 years, with ranges for these two groups being from birth to 30 years of age and from birth to 48 years of age, respectively. Seventy-five per cent were between 4 and 14 years of age at diagnosis.

There are two extremes in the FA patient groups. Four per cent were diagnosed between birth and 1 year of age (nine in their first month), and at least one half

Table 7-9. FANCONI'S ANEMIA LITERATURE

	1927-1960	1961-1970	1971-1980	1981-1990	1991-1994	Total
No. of patients	118	119	261	290	167	955
Male:female	1.4	1.7	1.4	1.1	1.2	1.3
Male, age* at diagnosis, mean	7.5	7.8	7.6	7.9	8.5	7.8
Median	6	7	6	6.5	6	8
Range	0.5–30	0.6–21	0–28	0–29	0–34	0–34
Female, age* at diagnosis, mean	7.6	9.4	8.9	8.7	9.3	8.8
Median	7	8	7.5	8	7	6.5
Range	1–14	0–35	0–48	0–32	0–36	0–48
No. of males ≤ 1 y	1	1	9	8	5	24
No. of females ≤ 1 y	2	1	3	4	5	15
No. of males ≥ 16 y	5	5	14	14	11	49
No. of females ≥ 16 y	0	5	11	16	9	41

*Ages are in years.

of these had hematologic signs at diagnosis. Thus, FA cannot be excluded from the differential diagnosis of aplastic anemia during infancy. Ten per cent were diagnosed at the age of 16 years or older. This rate of diagnosis is deceptively low, because the diagnosis of FA must be actively sought in adult patients who are normal on physical examination or who have only subtle abnormalities (see later). FA is undoubtedly more common than it was thought to be before the development of specific chromosome testing.

Physical Examination. Until recently, patients were recognized only by the presence of some of the characteristic physical findings summarized in Tables 7–10 and 7–11. A higher proportion of patients diagnosed in infancy had major characteristic anomalies, e.g., those involving the thumbs and radii, kidneys, head, eyes, and ears, as well as areas of the gastrointestinal tract. Conversely, those who were diagnosed when they were older had fewer of these anomalies. Short stature and skin pigmentary problems are only apparent with age,

and thus did not distinguish patients belonging to either of the two age extremes.

The patient shown in Figure 7–10 exhibits the "classic" anomalies of FA, including short stature, abnormality of the thumbs, microcephaly, café au lait and hypopigmented spots, and a characteristic facial appearance (a broad nasal base, epicanthal folds, and micrognathia). FA and *thrombocytopenia absent radii* (TAR; see later) can be distinguished from each other: in FA, if the radii are affected, the thumbs are always abnormal; in TAR, in which radii are absent, the thumbs are always present. The list in Table 7–11 includes both common and very rare findings, in approximate order of frequency. Skin involvement is the most frequent sign, followed by poor growth, anomalies of the upper arms, and structural renal abnormalities. Some patients have been misdiagnosed as having *VATER syndrome* because of the specific types of anomalies that they had (*v*ertebral defects, *a*nal atresia, *tr*acheoesophageal fistula, *r*enal defects, and *r*adial limb defects).[275–277] The malformations described in the 1993 International Fanconi Anemia Registry (IFAR) report are similar to those outlined in this chapter.[276]

The IFAR used a stepwise multivariate analysis to identify eight variables that discriminated between patients who were chromosome breakage–positive ("FA homozygotes") and those who were chromosome breakage–negative ("non-FA").[278] One point was given for each of the following: microphthalmia, birthmarks, genitourinary anomalies, growth retardation, absence of radius or thumb, and thrombocytopenia; one point was subtracted for learning disabilities and other skeletal abnormalities. Higher scores indicated an increased probability of having FA. Of course, this scoring system does not detect the large group of FA patients without anomalies and only provides a probability determination for those who do have such findings.

The proportion of FA homozygotes with normal apperances is underestimated by literature review. Two families that included such homozygotes were first described by Estren and Dameshek in 1947.[279] Subsequently, Li and Potter[280] reported that a cousin of one of the original families had typical FA with chromosome breaks. The results of chromosome breakage studies in patients with the "Estren-Dameshek" disorder are

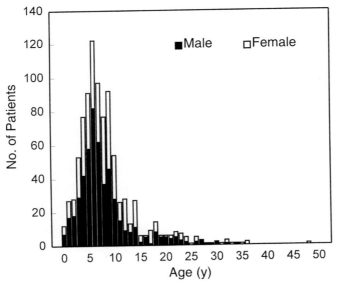

Figure 7-9. Age at diagnosis in more than 900 published cases with Fanconi's anemia. *Shaded bars* represent males, and *open bars*, females. (See text for definition of ``diagnosis.'')

Table 7-10. PHYSICAL ABNORMALITIES IN FANCONI'S ANEMIA*

Abnormality	All Patients	Age ≤1 y at Diagnosis	Age ≥16 y at Diagnosis
No. of patients	955	40	91
Male:female	1.3	1.5	1.2
Skin	60%	35%	66%
Short stature	57%	50%	59%
Upper limb anomalies	48%	68%	37%
Hypogonads, male	37%	42%	47%
Hypogonads, female	3%	19%	5%
Head	27%	38%	16%
Eyes	26%	33%	22%
Renal	23%	45%	19%
Birth-weight ≤2500 g	12%	50%	7%
Developmental delay	13%	5%	7%
Lower limbs	8%	15%	4%
Ears	10%	25%	10%
Increased reflexes	7%	3%	3%
Other skeletal anomalies	6%	8%	13%
Cardiopulmonary	6%	18%	3%
Gastrointestinal	4%	30%	0%
Other anomalies	5%	3%	2%
None, or not reported	20%	15%	20%
Short stature only	1%	0%	0%
Skin only	3%	0%	3%
Short stature and skin only	4%	3%	5%
Short stature and/or skin	8%	3%	9%

*Data represent percentage of patients with the abnormality. The proportions are underestimates because some reports did not provide physical descriptions. Many patients had multiple anomalies.

indistinguishable from those in patients with classic FA with anomalies. Thus, patients without anomalies represent just one end of the spectrum of FA. Literature reports of patients who were identified because they had affected siblings indicate that at least 25% of patients do not have anomalies.[281, 282] Our own review (see Table 7–10) identified 28% of patients who fit into this category. Twenty per cent were entirely normal, whereas the others were short or had skin abnormalities. Close to 40% of the 370 patients analyzed in the IFAR were reported to be physically "normal."[276]

Inheritance and Environment. FA is an autosomal recessive disorder, despite the slight preponderance of males described in the literature (see Table 7–9). The IFAR reported a male-to-female ratio of 1.06:1.0. In a large single study,[283] 30% of families had two affected children, with consanguinity in 10%. Our survey identified at least 70 families with consanguinity, 170 with affected siblings, and 11 with affected cousins. Twenty-eight mothers of FA patients had miscarriages; some of these fetuses had significant physical anomalies and are presumed homozygotes. Segregation analysis of the 86 cases reported by Schroeder et al.[283] and 88 patients in the IFAR confirmed the monogenic autosomal recessive inheritance pattern.[284] All races and ethnic groups have been reported, including Caucasians, Blacks, Asians, and Native Americans.

The heterozygote frequency may be 1 in 300 in the United States and in Europe,[283, 285] and 1 per 100 in South African Afrikaans, owing to a founder effect.[286] In some families, siblings had physical abnormalities without hematologic disease. In other families, some siblings had pancytopenia and normal physical findings, whereas other siblings had classical malformations. In one family, one brother had typical short stature, horseshoe kidney, and aplastic anemia, and another had aplastic anemia followed by PNH, and a cousin died of aplastic anemia.[287] The brother with PNH was later proved to have FA on the basis of chromosome breakage studies and died from lung cancer at the age of 67 years.* All of the variations may reflect incomplete expression of the homozygous state, or they may occur in heterozygotes; testing for chromosome breakage would be helpful. The varied expression might also be the result of allelic but different gene defects or of nonallelic mutations; it also might be related to different environmental influences.

Patients with characteristic malformations or with affected siblings can be diagnosed on the basis of chromosome studies in the *preanemic phase* (see references 2 and 4). They can avoid drugs that are implicated in acquired aplastic anemia (see Table 7–3). Follow-up may permit definition of the reason for development of aplastic anemia or malignancy in FA and may provide more accurate data on the proportion of FA homozygotes who "escape" such complications.

The environment may explain aplasia in some cases. In one FA family, one sister with aplastic anemia died at the age of 16 years (this individual had a history of treating skin infections with topically applied coal tar).[288] The other two, whose FA was confirmed by detection of chromosome breakage, had only mild pancytopenia for longer than 20 years. One died at the age of 38 years (with refractory anemia as well as

*Dacie J, Gordon-Smith EC: Personal communication, 1995.

Table 7-11. SPECIFIC TYPES OF ANOMALIES IN FANCONI'S ANEMIA*

Skin
Generalized hyperpigmentation on trunk, neck, and intertriginous areas; café au lait spots; hypopigmented areas; gray or bronze color; large freckles

Microsomia
Short stature; delicate features; small size; underweight

Upper Limbs
Thumbs: absent or hypoplastic; supernumerary, bifid, or duplicated; rudimentary or vestigial; short, low set, attached by a thread, triphalangeal, tubular, stiff, hyperextensible
Radii: absent or hypoplastic (only with abnormal thumbs); absent or weak pulse
Hands: clinodactyly; hypoplastic thenar eminence; six fingers; absent first metacarpal; enlarged, abnormal fingers; short fingers, transverse crease
Ulnae: dysplastic

Gonads
Males: hypogenitalia; undescended testes; hypospadias; abnormal genitalia; absent testis; atrophic testes; azoospermia; phimosis; abnormal urethra; micropenis; delayed development
Females: hypogenitalia; bicornuate uterus; abnormal genitalia; aplasia of uterus and vagina; atresia of uterus, vagina, and ovary

Other Skeletal
Head and face: microcephaly; hydrocephalus; micrognathia; peculiar face; bird face; flat head; frontal bossing; scaphocephaly; sloped forehead; choanal atresia
Neck: Sprengel's deformity; short, low hair line; web
Spine: spina bifida (thoracic, lumbar, cervical, occult sacral); scoliosis; abnormal ribs; sacrococcygeal sinus; sacral agenesis; Klippel Feil syndrome; vertebral anomalies; extra vertebrae

Eyes
Small eyes; strabismus; epicanthal folds; hypertelorism; ptosis; slanting; cataracts; astigmatism; blindness; epiphora; nystagmus; proptosis; small iris; hypotelorism; anophthalmia

Ears
Deafness (usually conductive); abnormal shape; atresia; dysplasia; low set, large, or small; infections; abnormal middle ear; absent drum; dimples; rotated; canal stenosis

Renal
Kidneys ectopic or pelvic; abnormal, horseshoe, hypoplastic, or dysplastic; absent; hydronephrosis or hydroureter; infections; duplicated; rotated; reflux; hyperplasia; no function; abnormal artery

Gastrointestinal
High arched palate; atresia (esophagus, duodenum, jejunum); imperforate anus, tracheoesophageal fistula; Meckel's diverticulum; umbilical hernia; hypoplastic uvula; abnormal biliary ducts; megacolon; abdominal diastasis; Budd-Chiari syndrome; anterior anus; persistent cloaca; annular pancreas

Lower Limbs
Feet: toe syndactyly; abnormal toes; flat feet; short toes; club feet; six toes; supernumerary toe; abnormal
Legs: congenital hip dislocation; Perthes' diseases; coxa vara; abnormal femur; thigh osteoma; abnormal legs

Cardiopulmonary
Patent ductus arteriosus; ventricular septal defect; abnormal; peripheral pulmonic stenosis; aortic stenosis; coarctation; absent lung lobes; vascular malformation; aortic atheromas; atrial septal defect; tetralogy of Fallot; pseudotruncus; hypoplastic aorta; abnormal pulmonary drainage; double aortic arch; cardiac myopathy

Other
Slow development; hyperreflexia; Bell's palsy; central nervous system arterial malformation; moyamoya syndrome; absent corpus callosum; stenosis of the internal carotid artery; small pituitary gland; accessory spleen; absent breast buds

*Abnormalities are listed in approximate order of frequency within each category.

precancerous skin and cervical findings), whereas the other remains well at the age of 42 years. Thus, the same FA genes in different external or internal (other gene) environments resulted in different phenotypes.

Aplastic anemia in FA homozygotes developed following several environmental events,[2, 4] such as viral illnesses, hepatitis, and primary tuberculosis. Several patients received chloramphenicol before the onset of aplasia. These examples also suggest an environmental role. Several sets of siblings developed aplastic anemia at the same age. This observation supports the involvement of a genetic component, and thus the relative roles of environment and genes may vary.

Laboratory Findings

Patients often have mild or moderate thrombocytopenia or leukopenia before pancytopenia, but severe aplasia eventually develops in most cases. Even in the FA patient with normal blood cell counts (preanemic, or treatment-responsive), erythrocytes often are macrocytic. Examination of the blood smear shows large red cells with mild poikilocytosis and anisocytosis, as well as decreased numbers of platelets and leukocytes (Fig. 7–11). In FA, the red cells may be larger than they are in acquired aplastic anemia, and Hb F levels may be higher. When aplastic, the FA bone marrow is hypocel-

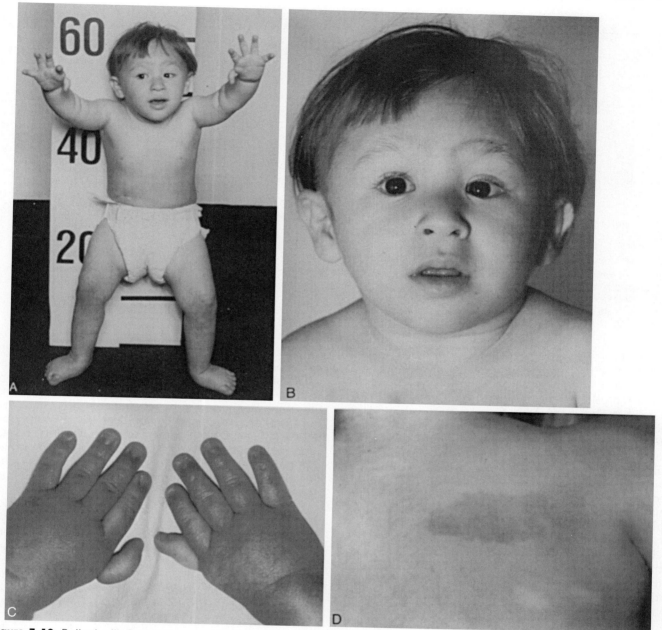

Figure 7-10. Patient with Fanconi's anemia, with several classic phenotypic features. The patient is a 3 year old male. *A,* Front view. *B,* Face. *C,* Hands. *D,* Back right shoulder. The features to be noted include short stature, dislocated hips, microcephaly, broad nasal base, epicanthal folds, micrognathia, thumbs attached by threads, and café au lait spots with hypopigmented areas beneath.

lular and fatty, demonstrating few hematopoietic elements and a relative increase in the numbers of lymphocytes, reticulum cells, mast cells, and plasma cells; the marrow appears identical to that observed in acquired aplasia (see Fig. 7–4). Areas of hypercellular marrow disappear as the aplasia progresses.[271]

FA patients have "stress erythropoiesis," producing erythrocytes with fetal characteristics[78] as do patients with acquired aplastic anemia during recovery. This "fetal-like" erythropoiesis, present in preanemic, anemic, or remission FA patients, is characterized by macrocytosis and increased levels of Hb F (as determined by alkali denaturation and Kleihauer-Betke acid elu-

tion) and i antigen. These features also identify nonanemic FA siblings. The Hb F is distributed unevenly (not clonally), and there is no single-cell concordance of the fetal-like features. The level of Hb F or the degree of macrocytosis does not provide prognostic information. Serum erythropoietin in FA patients is increased to levels that are much higher than those expected for the degree of anemia in children with hemolytic anemias.[2]

Table 7–12 summarizes our clinical classification of FA,[289] utilizing the hematologic information to determine whether a patient is asymptomatic (group 6) or has very severe aplastic anemia (group 1). The classification may permit better interpretation of laboratory

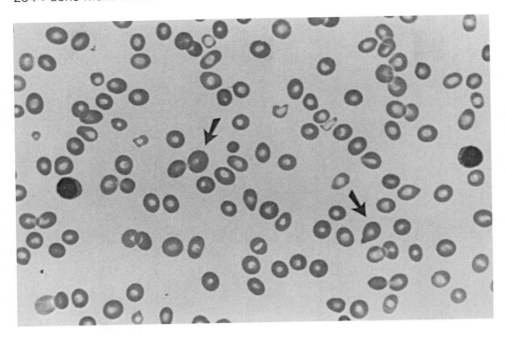

Figure 7-11. Peripheral blood from a patient with Fanconi's anemia. Note anisocytosis, macrocytes *(arrows)*, thrombocytopenia, and neutropenia. (Courtesy of Dr. Gail Wolfe; with permission from Alter BP: The bone marrow failure syndromes. In Nathan DG, Oski FA (eds): Hematology of Infancy and Childhood. 3rd ed. Philadelphia, W.B. Saunders Co., 1987, p 159.)

information, including the findings of hematopoietic cultures (see below) or other research data of potential relevance.

The red cell survival is slightly short, but hemolysis is not a major component. Ferrokinetics indicate ineffective erythropoiesis as well as relative marrow failure. Dyserythropoiesis has been noted, with fragmentation and multinuclearity. Marrow imaging with ^{99m}Tc sulfur colloid in FA showed paradoxical and irregular tracer distribution that was distinct from the uniform reduction seen in acquired aplastic anemia.[290] This may relate to the varied and irregular development of aplasia in FA.

Although red cell hexokinase level was reported as decreased by Löhr and co-workers,[291] later studies by others did not substantiate this finding.[292, 293] Several other glycolytic enzymes also were found to be normal, although Jalbert and colleagues reported elevated enzyme levels resembling findings in myelodysplasias.[294]

The small size of FA patients was ascribed to *growth hormone deficiency* in 17 of 23 cases in which growth hormone was measured (the remaining 6 had normal levels of growth hormone).[2, 4] Treatment with the hormone was reported to increase growth in 5 patients but not in 3 others, and hematologic improvement did not occur in any. In some families, growth hormone deficiency and FA segregated independently. The role of recombinant growth hormone in growth and hematopoiesis requires evaluation, and a potential association between growth hormone therapy and leukemia needs careful consideration.[295, 296]

The diagnostic laboratory test is chromosome breakage analysis that uses metaphase preparations of phytohemagglutinin-stimulated cultured peripheral blood lymphocytes. A high proportion of cells from FA patients have breaks, gaps, rearrangements, exchanges, and endoreduplications (Fig. 7–12). Although the breakage rate is increased in baseline cultures,[2, 4] it is more dramatically increased when clastogenic agents such as diepoxybutane (DEB) or mitomycin C (MMC)

Table 7-12. CLINICAL CLASSIFICATION OF FANCONI'S ANEMIA

Group	Transfusions	Androgen or Cytokine Treatment	Status
1	Yes	No	Severe aplastic anemia; failed or never received androgens
2	Yes	Yes	Severe aplastic anemia; currently on but not responding to androgens
3	No	Yes	Previously severe or moderate aplasia; responding to androgens or cytokines
4	No	No	Severe or moderate aplastic anemia, needs treatment
5	No	No	Stable, with some sign of marrow failure (e.g., mild anemia, neutropenia, thrombocytopenia, high mean corpuscular volume, high Hb F)
6	No	No	Normal hematology ± normal Hb F

Hb F = hemoglobin F.
From Alter BP, Knobloch ME, Weinberg RS: Erythropoiesis in Fanconi's anemia. Blood 1991; 78:602.

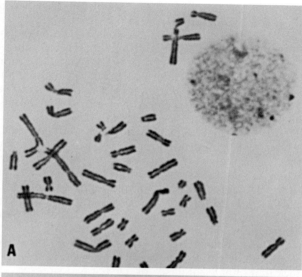

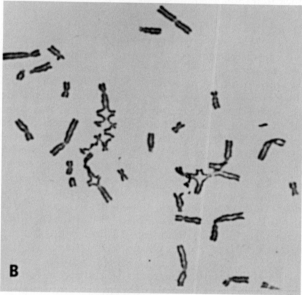

Figure 7–12. Cytogenetic findings in peripheral blood lymphocytes in Fanconi's anemia. *A,* Spontaneous chromatid breakage. *B,* Multiple breakage following culture with diepoxybutane. (From Auerbach AD, Adler B, Changati RSK: Prenatal and postnatal diagnosis and carrier detection of Fanconi anemia by a cytogenetic method. Pediatrics 1981; 67:128. Copyright American Academy of Pediatrics 1981.)

are used (see later). Breakage is infrequent when direct preparations of bone marrow are examined because cells with significant abnormalities may divide slowly or may not survive *in vivo.* Cultured skin fibroblasts also have abnormal chromosomes. The "spontaneous" aberrations seen in culture may be artifacts, induced by unknown factors in the medium; because marrow cells are not cultured, these abnormalities would not be evident. No apparent relationship exists between hematologic status or clinical course and chromosome findings. Some FA patients may not have spontaneous breaks even though they have a positive result when DEB or MMC is used. *Bona fide* FA patients may not have increased breaks even with DEB.[296a] Similar spon-

taneous but not induced chromosomal changes are seen in Bloom's syndrome and ataxia telangiectasia[297] (see below). However, cells in Bloom's syndrome show increased sister chromatid exchange following treatment with BUdR, whereas cells in FA do not.[298]

Another approach to the diagnosis of FA involves flow cytometry rather than the counting of chromosomal aberrations. FA cells grow slowly owing to prolongation of the G2 phase of the cell cycle.[2, 4] Cells treated with alkylating agents fail to divide but do undergo DNA replication and accumulate in the G2 phase, during which they are detected because of the increased amount of DNA that they contain.[299–302]

According to the IFAR, FA homozygotes have a mean of 8.96 breaks per cell following culture of blood lymphocytes with DEB, compared with a mean of 0.06 in normal persons.[303] Ten per cent of the IFAR patients had clonal rather than uniform breakage, with breaks present in 10% to 40% of their cells[304]; others have also observed clonality.[305] The number of breaks per cell with breaks remains very high, and fibroblasts show uniform breakage. However, there remain patients with some of the phenotypic features of FA whose chromosome breakage is not increased with DEB or MMC[272, 296a]; do these patients indeed have extremely clonal FA, or do they have FA-like gene mutations?

Prenatal diagnosis was done by chorionic villus sampling at 9 to 12 weeks' gestation, or amniocentesis was performed at approximately 16 weeks' gestation in more than 120 fetuses. In one series, 10 of 58 chorionic villus samples and 10 of 64 amniocentesis samples had an increase in the number of DEB-induced breaks.[306] One false-negative diagnosis was made on the basis of chorionic villus sampling, and no confirmatory amniocentesis sample was obtained. The cultured cells grew more slowly in the positive cases than in the negative ones. Three cases were also examined by prenatal fetal blood sampling, either solely[307] or for confirmation of an abnormal chorionic villus or amniotic fluid sampling result.[308, 309] Only one third of the affected cases had physical anomalies; this finding supports the suggestion that many homozygotes may lack malformations. Increased breakage was reported in two cases not known to be at risk for FA.[308, 310] Prenatal diagnosis can now be performed with direct analysis of DNA for known mutations in families in which the genetic defect is known[311] (see later).

Laboratory evaluation of patients in whom FA is suspected should include complete blood counts, red cell size analysis, and Hb F determination. Skeletal radiography and renal ultrasound can be done in those with physical anomalies or after the diagnosis has been proved. The specific test is chromosome breakage analysis, both without and following clastogenic stress. Such tests have identified FA in patients with physical anomalies who were not anemic,[312–314] (see Fig. 7–10) and have been used for diagnosing FA in patients with aplastic anemia without malformations.[315, 316] Patients with malformations who *may not* have FA also can be identified and the possibility of their having FA excluded. Fanconi's "anemia" is redefined to include patients who have the characteristic chromosomal response to clastogenic stress, may have normal findings on physical examination, and may not have hematologic disease.

Fanconi's Anemia Heterozygotes

Congenital malformations, particularly anomalies of the genitourinary system and those of the hand, are found more frequently in FA relatives than in the general population (possible heterozygotes).[317] Some parents had physical abnormalities such as short stature but did not have hematologic disease.[318–320] Petridou and Barrett noted that obligate heterozygotes had increased Hb F levels, decreased natural killer cell counts, and poor responses to mitogens.[320] FA heterozygotes may also be detected as a group by chromosome breakage analysis, but for individuals there is an overlap with the normal range.

Pathophysiology

The underlying defect in FA is unknown, and the relationship among birth defects, hematopoietic failure, malignancies, and chromosome breakage is elusive. Development of hematopoiesis and the areas generally affected in FA occurs at 25 to 34 days' gestation, and a common toxic insult has been implicated.[321] The FA genotype presumably increases susceptibility to agents that may cause aplastic anemia in "normal" individuals (see Table 7–3). The oncogenic compounds that damage DNA *in vitro* also may be toxic *in vivo*. This section provides a brief review of this topic; more details can be found elsewhere.[2, 273]

Clastogenic agents that cause chromosome breakage include radiation and bifunctional cross-linkers such as MMC, nitrogen mustard, DEB, and cyclophosphamide. Monofunctional agents are not toxic; this suggests that interstrand cross-links cannot be repaired. Table 7–13 lists several of the biochemical defects described in FA; more details can be found elsewhere.[2] The variable and sometimes contradictory results might now be ascribed to the fact that different cell lines were used in each study; some of these lines have now been classified as to their complementation group (see later).

One theory proposes that FA cells are damaged by accumulated oxygen free radicals, which are produced by mutagenic factors such as high oxygen tension, γ-radiation, near-ultraviolet radiation, clastogens, and drugs that generate the reactive hydroxyl radical $HO^{\bullet}$.[322, 323] Red cell levels of superoxide dismutase (SOD) were low,[2] whereas white cell concentrations of SOD were normal. Normal levels of red cell SOD, catalase, and glutathione peroxidase also were reported, although the concentration of glutathione transferase was increased. Normal levels of SOD were found in FA fibroblasts, which had increased Mn-SOD, catalase, and glutathione peroxidase concentrations; thus, the suggestion was made that oxidant effects may be restricted to the hematopoietic system. The addition of SOD or catalase to FA lymphocyte cultures decreased the numbers of breaks. Other investigators found that SOD, catalase, or cysteine decreased the number of MMC-induced breaks, but in similar proportions in normal fibroblasts as in FA fibroblasts. Culture of lymphocytes in the presence of increased oxygen tension resulted in an increase in the number of spontaneous breaks in some FA cells and not in normal cells, and in all FA cells following inclusion of MMC. SOD increased the survival of FA fibroblasts cultured with MMC. Low oxygen tension or antioxidants were used to improve growth and decrease spontaneous and induced chromosome breaks in FA cells. A handful of FA patients were treated with intravenous SOD, which resulted in transient decreases in the number of spontaneous chromosome breaks and, in one patient, in an increase in the number of marrow progenitors.[324, 325]

FA cells grow slowly and have a prolonged G2 phase (see earlier). They are susceptible to transformation by simian virus 40 or adenovirus 12 and express simian virus 40 T antigen.[2] Sister chromatid exchange is generally not increased in FA cells, either spontaneously or after treatment with mutagens. FA cells were found to be hypomutable by *in vitro* cross-linkers, and mutations in FA were primarily deletions rather than point mutations, as are seen in normal cells.[326, 327]

Table 7–13. BIOCHEMICAL DEFECTS IN FANCONI'S ANEMIA

Feature	Group A	Group B*	References
Spontaneous chromosome breakage	High	Less high	332
MMC-induced chromosome breakage	High	Moderate	332, 974
Growth inhibition by MMC	Yes	—	975
Recovery of DNA synthesis after 8MOP/UVA	No	Yes	332, 976
Cross-link repair	Deficient	Efficient	977–979
Incision of interstrand cross-links	Decreased	—	980, 981
Endonuclease that repairs interstrand cross-links	Decreased	—	982
Incision of monoadducts	—	Decreased	980, 983
Endonuclease that recognizes monoadducts	—	Decreased	982
DNA double-strand break repair	Reduced	Normal	984
DNA ligase	Reduced	—	985
	Reduced	—	986–988
ADPRT	Normal	Normal	
Thymine-dimer excision	Normal	—	989

MMC = mitomycin C; 8-MOP/UVA = 8-methoxypsoralen/ultraviolet; ADPRT = adenosine diphosphate–ribosyl transferase.
*Group B is now known to include C, D and E (see text).
Adapted from Young NS, Alter BP: Aplastic Anemia: Acquired and Inherited. Philadelphia, W.B. Saunders Co., 1994, p 313.

Co-culture of FA cells with other FA or normal human or CHO cells suggested correction of FA by diffusible factors in some studies but not others.[328] Consistent correction was found in hybrid cells of different complementation groups.[329, 330] Duckworth-Rysiecki and co-workers[331] defined groups A and B, and Digweed and associates[332] noted that the reported biochemical variations might be ascribed to such groupings, with group A being more severe (see Table 7–13). It now appears that there are at least five complementation groups.[333, 334] The complementation group does not appear to correlate with clinical status, which can range from extremely mild to very severe, even within group C.[306, 335]

DNA. Investigators at the Buchwald laboratory cloned the gene for FA complementation group C (*FAC*) by functional complementation using an Epstein-Barr virus shuttle vector.[336] The complementary DNA has 4566 base pairs, codes for a 557–amino acid protein, and is located at 9q22.3.[333] Normal *FAC* corrected MMC sensitivity in cells mutant in *FAC*,[336] an antisense oligonucleotide inhibited growth of normal hematopoietic progenitors,[337] and the hematopoietic growth defect from progenitors of group C patients was corrected with a recombinant adenovirus-associated vector.[338] The FAC protein is found in the cytoplasm in normal cells; this suggests that its role for regulating DNA repair must be indirect.[339, 340]

FAC is mutated in approximately 10% to 15% of patients with FA.[335, 341] A mutation common to only Ashkenazi Jews is IVS4 +4 A→T,[342] which is associated with a severe phenotype of multiple birth defects.[335] The carrier frequency in Ashkenazi Jews is close to 1%, and it was not found in non-Jewish controls.[343] A milder phenotype is seen in those of European ancestry who have other *FAC* mutations, such as 322delG, Q13X, R185X, and D195V.[335, 344] These mutations produce truncated proteins with some activity.[344a]

Genetic linkage analysis suggested that the gene for complementation group A might be on 20q.[345] Transfection with mouse DNA led to identification of a DNA fragment that partially corrects the group D cellular defect and localizes to 11q23.[346] More recent studies suggested that group A maps to 16q[346a] and group D to 3p.[346b] In 1996, the FAA gene was finally cloned.[346c]

Hematopoietic Defect. The hematopoietic defect in FA is evident at the progenitor cell level. Colonies from bone marrow CFU-GM, CFU-E, and BFU-E, as well as from blood BFU-E, were all decreased in aplastic FA patients,[289] as they were in a very small number who did not have aplastic FA.[289, 347] Only one patient had a level of progenitor cells that was even close to normal.[348] Prospective studies of nonanemic FA patients may be helpful in prediction of outcome; the authors' results suggest a correlation between erythroid progenitor-derived colonies and clinical status as defined in Table 7–12.[289, 349] Erythroid colony growth was improved with hematopoietic growth factors such as SCF or low oxygen tension,[349] although the effect of SCF was not found in all studies.[350] Although long-term marrow culture stromal layers were formed with the use of FA bone marrow, Stark et al. found that the

stroma did not generate CFU-GM[351]; however, Butturini and Gale did find myelopoiesis in long-term marrow cultures.[352] Most of the culture data, however, as well as cures with BMT (see below), suggest a defect in the pluripotent stem cell in FA aplasia. In addition, Segal and co-workers inhibited *in vitro* hematopoiesis in normal cells treated with an antisense oligonucleotide to the *FAC* gene.[337] Although the DNA repair defect is in all cells, hematopoietic failure is what usually leads the patient to seek medical attention.

The level of tumor necrosis factor-α was increased in FA plasma, whereas that of interferon-γ was not.[353] Production of IL-6 was decreased by FA lymphoblasts or fibroblasts,[354–358] although some cell lines did produce increased levels of some cytokines.[358] Addition of IL-6 corrected MMC cytotoxicity.[354] Tumor necrosis factor-α was overproduced by lymphoblasts from patients in four complementation groups, the addition of IL-6 decreased the overproduction of TNF-α, and antibodies to TNF-α improved MMC sensitivity.[359] SCF production was normal[355] or low,[357, 358] as was that of IL-1,[355] whereas GM-CSF and G-CSF production was low, variable,[355, 357, 358] or even high.[356] The complementation groups were not known, and thus the cytokine heterogeneity may have a genetic basis.

One study suggested that tumor suppressor gene *p53* was not mutated in 13 FA patients,[360] although neither *p53* expression nor apoptosis—perhaps related events—was induced by irradiation.[361] MMC-induced apoptosis was normal in FA, suggesting that apoptosis is not involved in MMC hypersensitivity.[362]

Animal Model. There is no good animal model for FA. A candidate mouse is the genetically anemic mouse, an/an, Hertwig's anemia, with mild macrocytic anemia, decreased progenitors, and a cytogenetic abnormality caused by unequal segregation at mitosis.[363] The murine *FAC* gene has been cloned[364] and mapped to mouse chromosome 17, in the region of flexed-tail; however, the data do not demonstrate *FAC* mutation in these mice.[365]

Therapy and Outcome

Prognosis. The cumulative survival for the FA patients reported in the literature by decades is shown in Figure 7–13. The predicted median age of survival is 19 years; 25% are projected to live beyond age of 29. The median survival improved from 10 years in those reported before 1960 to 30 years in those reported within the past 5 years. Initially, when the only treatment was blood transfusion, 80% died within 2 years after the onset of aplastic anemia,[366] and almost all died within 4 years, with extended survivals occurring only rarely.[367, 368] Patients with birth defects had a median survival age of 16 years; in those without birth defects, the age was 20 years. In the IFAR, in which diagnosis may have preceded aplastic anemia, the projected median survival was reported to be 25 years of age.[369]

Older Patients. Older females have delayed menarche, irregular menses, and early menopause, which can result in hypoestrogenemia and osteoporosis. Of more

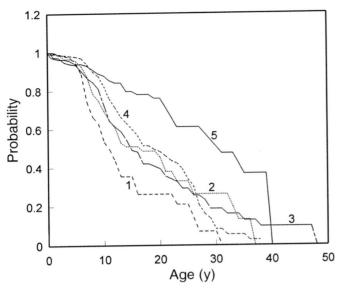

Figure 7–13. Kaplan-Meier plot of cumulative survival age in years in Fanconi's anemia, according to dates of literature reports. Line 1 = 1927 to 1960; line 2 = 1961 to 1970; line 3 = 1971 to 1980; line 4 = 1981 to 1990; line 5 = 1991 to 1994.

than 100 females cited in the literature or reported to the IFAR, 19 FA females who reached at least 16 years of age have been pregnant.[2, 67] FA was diagnosed before pregnancy in nine, during pregnancy in five, and after delivery in five. Twenty-nine pregnancies resulted in 7 miscarriages, 22 births, and 21 surviving children. Nine patients required red cell and/or platelet transfusions during the pregnancies or at delivery, six had cesarean sections for failure of labor to progress, and four had preeclampsia or eclampsia. FA pregnancy has complications but can be managed with high-risk obstetric and intensive hematologic care. None of the FA mothers died peripartum, although nine died at ages 24 to 45; seven deaths were attributed to malignancies. The risk of any type of malignancy (not just gynecologic) is more than threefold greater in females than in males (see later).

Older males are small, with underdeveloped gonads and abnormal spermatogenesis.[370] Four FA males were reported to have fathered children.[67, 283, 371] Fewer than 5% of the males who reached the age of 16 years were reported to have fathered children, but this figure may be low because paternity is less often noted in medical histories than is maternity. Several males whose FA diagnosis was made when they were adults did have a prior history of infertility.

Androgen Therapy. Androgen therapy for the aplastic anemia of FA was initiated by Shahidi and Diamond in 1959, who observed improvement in the first six patients treated.[139, 372] In larger series, Sanchez-Medal[373] and Najean[374] found that 75% of patients showed some degree of initial response. Responses usually begin with reticulocytosis, with a rise in hemoglobin level occurring within 1 to 2 months. White cell counts may increase next; in contrast, the platelet response usually is incomplete and may take 6 to 12 months to reach its maximum.

Almost all patients relapse with the termination of androgen therapy; fewer than a dozen have successfully discontinued treatment, often at the time of puberty.[2] Many eventually became resistant to the androgen that they were receiving, and changing to another only occasionally provided another response. For the more than 300 patients reported to have received androgens, the predicted median survival age is 18 years; for the more than 600 not treated, it is 16 years. Responders to androgens had a projected median survival age of 20 years, compared with one of 14 years for the nonresponders. Late complications may be seen in some FA patients because their life expectancy has been extended by the androgens (see later).

Although some reports suggest that the use of androgens alone is as effective as the use of androgens combined with corticosteroids,[374] the general recommendation is that combination therapy be administered. Growth acceleration due to the androgens may be counterbalanced by growth retardation due to the corticosteroids.[375] Corticosteroids also may decrease bleeding at a given platelet count, perhaps by promoting vascular stability.[376] The androgen most frequently used is oxymetholone, an oral 17-α alkylated androgen, at a dose of 2 to 5 mg/kg per day. Prednisone is used at a dose of 5 to 10 mg every other day. If an injectable androgen is desired because of the decreased risk of hepatotoxicity, the usual form is nandrolone decanoate, 1 to 2 mg/kg per week intramuscularly; in this situation, ice packs and pressure are used to prevent hematomas. Etiocholanolone has been used with success in an otherwise refractory patient.* The first sign of response to androgens may be the appearance of macrocytic red cells and an increase in the proportion of red cells containing Hb F. Potential side effects of androgens include obstructive liver disease, peliosis hepatitis, and liver tumors (see later). Patients on androgens should be monitored frequently with liver chemistry studies and ultrasound. Responders should have their androgen dose tapered very slowly but probably not discontinued. The only group of patients in whom discontinuation might be considered is the South African Afrikaaners, who may be genetically distinct.[377] In most of the experiences elsewhere, relapses occur when androgen therapy is stopped, and subsequent remissions in a patient receiving the same or different preparations are sometimes elusive.

Bone Marrow Transplantation. BMT offers the only possibility of cure for aplastic anemia in FA and possibly a cure for or prevention of leukemia. There is a risk, however, that chemotherapy or irradiation—or both—may accelerate the appearance of secondary malignancies. Four tongue cancers were reported among more than 50 long-term survivors[378–381]; this exceeds the reported 3% after BMT for aplastic anemia.[209]

Survival curves for the more than 170 transplanted FA patients in whom sufficient detail was reported are shown in Figure 7–14. Thirty received a standard cyclophosphamide preparation, 50 mg/kg per day over 4 days,[2, 382] and 14 of these survived (47%). Studies

*Gardner FH: Unpublished data.

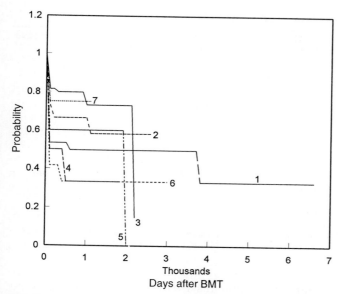

Figure 7–14. Kaplan-Meier plot of cumulative survival interval in Fanconi's anemia following BMT. Time is shown as days from transplant. Line 1 = cyclophosphamide 200 mg/kg; line 2 = various preparations; line 3 = cyclophosphamide 20 mg/kg in combination with TAI; line 4 = unrelated donor; line 5 = mismatched family member donor; line 6 = patient had leukemia or MDS pre-transplant; line 7 = cord transplant.

showing that a metabolite of cyclophosphamide is toxic to FA cells[383, 384] explain the frequent clinical symptoms of severe mucositis with intestinal malabsorption and hemorrhages, fluid retention, cardiac failure, and hemorrhagic cystitis.[385] Various other protocols included procarbazine, antithymocyte globulin, and fractionated total lymphoid irradiation or thoracoabdominal irradiation, and T-cell depletion[2, 382, 386–388]; 66% survived. Gluckman and co-workers then reduced the cyclophosphamide dose to 20 mg/kg divided over 4 days and administered 5 Gy of thoracoabdominal irradiation.[389] Among 71 patients treated with this protocol, 53 survived (75%)[2, 390, 391]; a recent report from another center indicates 100% survival in 18 patients.[392] Graft rejection and graft-versus-host disease were no more frequent in these FA patients than in those with transplants for acquired aplastic anemia. Among 13 FA patients who had leukemia or myelodysplastic syndromes, only 5 survived (see later).[2, 382, 391, 393]

Many patients do not have an HLA-compatible sibling. There is some parental sharing of haplotypes, leading to an unexpectedly high rate of HLA identity between patients and parents, who may be used as donors.[394, 395] Partially mismatched family members were donors in 10 cases[2, 388, 391] (the modified cyclophosphamide–thoracoabdominal irradiation preparation was used); 5 patients survived. Unrelated computer-matched donors also were recorded in 12 cases, with 5 patients surviving.[2, 391, 396] All of these mismatched transplants are particularly at risk for rejection or graft-versus-host disease. Use of molecular tools for HLA genotyping may decrease the risks of these transplants.[397]

HLA-matched sibling donors need to be screened for occult FA homozygosity with thorough physical examinations, complete blood counts (including determination of red cell size and Hb F level), and clastogen-induced chromosome breakage. In one unsuccessful transplant, the donor had undiagnosed FA.[398] Umbilical cord blood contains hematopoietic progenitor cells and can be cryopreserved from a sibling diagnosed *in utero* to not have FA for use in a later transplantation.[399] Three of four such cases were reconstituted at later than 6 months.[392, 400, 401]

Other Treatment. Supportive care must be provided as for any patient with aplastic anemia. ε-Aminocaproic acid, 0.1 g/kg per 6 hours orally, may be used for symptomatic bleeding. No family member should be used as a blood product donor until it has been determined that transplantation will not be performed (whether the transplant donor is related or unrelated); this approach decreases the chance of sensitization. Blood products filtered free of the leukocytes should be used to reduce reactions and HLA sensitization from white cells. The possibility of BMT must be considered early. Although androgens and transfusions do not preclude BMT, the best results are obtained in those with minimal medical complications. Drugs and chemicals that may be implicated as causal in acquired aplastic anemia (see Table 7–3) should be avoided. Medications that interfere with platelet function should not be given to thrombocytopenic patients; such medications include aspirin, antihistamines, nonsteroidal anti-inflammatory drugs, glycerol guaiacolate, vitamin E, and cod liver oil. However, if a severe allergic reaction occurs during a blood transfusion, diphenhydramine can be used emergently.

Splenectomy is not indicated unless hypersplenism is clearly present. Thirty-eight cases were reported as resulting in no apparent long-term benefit. There was some transient improvement of pancytopenia, but at a time when bone marrow was not yet hypocellular.[2] The use of immunotherapy has no basis. Although high-dose methylprednisolone[402] and ATG[403] were used in FA, many patients in whom these modalities as well as cyclosporine therapy were unsuccessful have gone unreported. Approximately 10% of adults who failed to respond to any of these approaches were shown subsequently to have previously undiagnosed FA on clastogenic stress–induced chromosome breakage studies.*

The use of lithium was reported to improve blood counts in 2 of 5 FA patients—presumably in those whose marrow reserve was still present.[404]

Hematopoietic growth factors are an area of current investigation. GM-CSF, 2.5 to 10 μg/kg per day, was used in 10 patients; in 8 of these, absolute neutrophil counts improved, but no impact on hemoglobin or platelet counts was observed.[405–407] G-CSF given at 2.5 to 5 μg/kg per day or every other day increased the absolute neutrophil counts in 10 of 10 patients, with increased hemoglobin levels observed in 4 patients and augmented platelet counts in 3.[408] Although such factors may also predispose to leukemia,[409] these and oth-

---

*Auerbach AD, Young NS: Unpublished data.

Table 7-14. COMPLICATIONS IN FANCONI'S ANEMIA

	Leukemia	MDS	Cancer	Liver Disease
No. of patients	83	31	46	37
Percentage of total	9%	3%	5%	4%
Male:female	1.3	1.1	0.5	1.6
Age* at diagnosis of FA, mean	10	13	12	9
Median	9	12	10	6
Range	0.1–28	1–31	0.1–32	1–48
Percentage ≥16 y	20%	32%	30%	11%
Age at complication, mean	14	17	23	16
Median	14	17	26	13
Range	0.1–29	5–31	0.3–38	3–48
No. without pancytopenia (%)	20 (24%)	13 (42%)	7 (16%)	1 (3%)
No. without androgens (%)	39 (47%)	19 (61%)	18 (39%)	1 (3%)
No. reported deceased (%)	65 (78%)	23 (74%)	28 (61%)	32 (86%)

MDS = myelodysplastic syndrome; FA = Fanconi's anemia.
*Ages are in years. One hundred forty-seven patients had one or more malignancy; the number of malignancies was 155. MDS cases include six who developed leukemia; the others are not included in the total. Four patients with tumors after BMT are not included.

ers, such as IL-3 and erythropoietin, still need to be adequately tested in FA. In preliminary studies, it was found that IL-3 produced a myeloid response in 3 of 5 patients with FA.[410]

Complications

The *in vitro* data regarding defects in DNA repair and cellular damage suggest that FA might be a premalignant condition; this conjecture is supported by the *in vivo* observations. More than 150 leukemias or tumors have been reported, for an overall incidence of greater than 15%. Because this incidence value reflects the biased reporting of interesting cases, the true figure may be greater, and thus long-term prospective analysis is necessary. Among 388 patients registered in the IFAR by 1994, 60 (15%) had leukemia or myelodysplastic syndrome (MDS) (the numbers were not reported separately); solid tumors were not described.[411] In a detailed literature review conducted by the authors, more than 80 patients had leukemia, more than 40 had solid tumors, and approximately 30 had liver tumors (Table 7–14). Up to 25% never had aplastic anemia, and approximately one half never received androgens prior to ascertainment of a malignant disorder. The male-to-female ratio is greater than 1 for all categories except that for solid tumors, in which females far outnumber males; removal of those women with gynecologic cancer still leaves an unexplained threefold excess of females (Table 7–15; see also Table 7–14).

Even a single gene for FA was thought to confer a risk of malignancy. Garriga and Crosby found an increased incidence of leukemia in FA families,[412] and Swift reported a predisposition to cancer in heterozygotes.[413, 414] These analyses were later extended from the original 8 families to 25 families by Swift and colleagues,[415] and to 15 families by Potter and associates[416]; both groups found no increase in cancer. (Another disorder thought to be present at increased frequency in FA heterozygotes is diabetes mellitus.[417, 418]) The erroneous conclusions were attributed to small numbers, incorrect assignment of heterozygotes, and biased selection.

Leukemia. Leukemia was reported in more than 80 cases of FA, affecting close to 10% of the FA patients in the literature. In one series of 44 patients, 9 developed leukemia (20%) and 5 more were preleukemic.[419] In 20 patients, FA was diagnosed only when these patients presented with leukemia without a preceding aplastic anemia. These 20, in addition to 19 who did have

Table 7-15. TYPES OF CANCER IN FANCONI'S ANEMIA

Type	No. of Patients*	Males	Females
Oropharyngeal	15	7	10
Cricoid	1	—	1
Gingiva	4	2	2
Gingiva, tongue	1	1	—
Jaw, benign	1	—	1
Mandible	1	—	1
Pharynx	1	1	—
Tongue	6	3	5
Gastrointestinal	16	4	12
Anus	4	—	4
Anus (Bowen's)	1	—	1
Colon, anus	1	—	1
Esophagus	8	2	6
Gastric adenoma	2	2	—
Gynecologic	11	—	11
Breast	3	—	3
Cervix	1	—	1
Cervix, vulva	1	—	1
Vulva	6	—	6
Brain	4	1	3
Astrocytoma	2	—	2
Medulloblastoma	2	1	1
Other	8	1	7
Bone marrow lymphoma	1	—	1
Bronchopulmonary	1	1	—
Eyelid (Bowen's)	1	—	1
Renal	1	—	1
Skin	2	—	2
Bowen's	1	—	1
Wilms'	1	—	1

*Number of tumors (54) exceeds number of patients (44). Eleven patients had >2 primaries, including 2 with liver cancer and 1 with leukemia.

pancytopenia, never received androgens, and thus androgens cannot be considered causative. A recent communication cites two patients who presented with acute myelomonocytic leukemia in whom the diagnosis of FA was not made until after BMT; these two patients developed toxicity from the preparation. In retrospect, these patients had increased chromosome breakage.[420]

The characteristics of the leukemic patients are summarized in Table 7–14. The male-to-female ratio is 1.3:1. FA was diagnosed at a mean age of 10 years, and leukemia itself was diagnosed at a mean age of 14 years. The proportion of patients older than 16 years of age at diagnosis was greater in the leukemic group (20% compared with 10% of the total) and included nine patients in their twenties whose FA was first diagnosed when they presented with leukemia.

Because the most common leukemia in children is lymphocytic, it is noteworthy that until 1989 all leukemias were myeloid. Older references are cited elsewhere.[2, 421–423] Three cases of acute lymphoblastic leukemia (ALL) have been reported[424] and three mentioned,[411] although it is not entirely clear whether these cases are in fact ALL. Twenty-nine of the leukemias were acute myeloblastic,[425, 426] 20 were acute myelomonocytic, 9 acute monocytic,[426] 7 were erythroleukemia,[427] 6 were acute unspecified, 5 were acute nonlymphocytic,[428, 429] 2 were chronic myelomonocytic,[430] and 1 was acute megakaryoblastic. Several patients were discussed in more than one publication, and thus the number of literature reports exceeds the actual number of cases. Five patients with leukemia had coincidental hepatic tumors discovered at postmortem examination,[429, 431–434] and one had an astrocytoma.[425]

Treatment of the leukemia was less than satisfactory, and death occurred on average within the first 2 months following diagnosis. FA patients with leukemia are exquisitely sensitive to the toxic effects of chemotherapy, as predicted by the discussion earlier regarding agents that increase damage to DNA. The combination of leukemias that are difficult to treat (i.e., myeloid), abnormal DNA repair, and lack of marrow reserve does not afford a good prognosis. Long-term remissions are very rare.[427] BMT from an unrelated donor was attempted unsuccessfully in one patient.[435] Figure 7–15 shows the Kaplan-Meier plots for survival in patients with malignancies. Although the median survival age for leukemia and that for FA overall were similar, the slope of the survival curve was steeper for those with leukemia. Almost 80% of those with leukemia had died by the time of the reports, and follow-up was not available for most of the rest. Will all patients develop leukemia if they do not die from aplastic anemia first? Probably not, because the older patients are at the additional risk for other malignancies (see later). However, only long-term prospective studies can be used to answer this question properly.

Preleukemia/Myelodysplastic Syndrome. Several FA patients had syndromes that were called "myelodysplastic," "refractory anemia," or "preleukemia." Some of these patients developed full-blown leukemia,

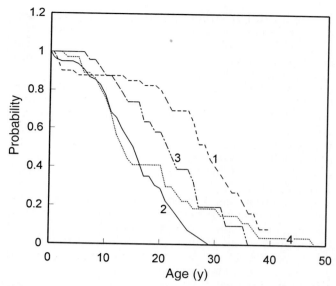

Figure 7–15. Kaplan-Meier plot of cumulative survival in Fanconi's anemia following complications. Time is shown as age in years. Line 1 = cancer; line 2 = leukemia; line 3 = myelodysplastic syndrome (MDS); line 4 = liver disease.

whereas others died or were reported only in their preleukemic phase. Thirty had clonal cytogenetic abnormalities in bone marrow but did not yet have leukemia.[423] Chromosome 7 was involved in 52% of those with AML, but in only 16% of those with MDS; chromosome 1 was involved in 24% of AML. Some details of the cytogenetic findings are in a summary by Berger and Le Coniat[436]; others have been provided by Alter.[436a] Six (19%) developed leukemia within 2 years and died soon thereafter, whereas 15 died at up to 12 years later without leukemia; 10 were alive at up to 3 years, also without leukemia. Approximately 30% or more FA patients develop a clonal cytogenetic abnormality, but whether this is in fact a true marker for "preleukemia" is not yet clear. The IFAR data suggest an actuarial probability of the development of clonal abnormalities of greater than 60% by the age of 30 years.[411] The clones may be transient, and their presence suggests population of the bone marrow by a small number of stem cells, which at another time may have no or different marker chromosomes.[423] Clonal hematopoiesis at the molecular level was identified in 1 of 3 with aplastic anemia, in 3 of 3 with MDS, and in 1 with AML; neither *N-ras* nor *p53* were mutant in those clones.[437]

Three patients had Sweet's syndrome (acute neutrophilic infiltration of skin, which is associated with malignancy in 20% of cases).[438] All had myelodysplastic bone marrows, and two had clonal chromosome abnormalities. The skin infiltrates responded to prednisone, but sustained treatment was required. This outcome differs from responses in non-FA patients with Sweet's syndrome, in whom permanent resolution of symptoms may occur.

Cancer. Forty-six patients (5%) were reported with cancers other than leukemia or liver. The group with cancer differs from the entire FA population (see Tables

7–14 and 7–15) in several categories.[436a] The preponderance of females is large, even following exclusion of those with gynecologic malignancies. The age at diagnosis of FA was on average 12 years in the cancer group, with 30% being 16 years of age or older when diagnosed. Seven never had aplastic anemia, and these in addition to nine more never received androgen therapy. The majority of the tumors developed in patients who were at least 13 years old, and the average age was 23 years. The younger patients were a 4-month-old who had a bone marrow lymphoma,[439] a 1.5-year-old who had a Wilms' tumor and a medulloblastoma,[440] 1.8- and 4.9-year-old cousins with an astrocytoma and a medulloblastoma,[277] and a 1.5-year-old with leukemia and an astrocytoma[425]; all but one of the tumors was not diagnosed ante mortem. These recent reports of brain tumors indicate that signs of increased intracranial pressure such as headache and vomiting should prompt a high index of suspicion for central nervous system malignancy.

Most of the tumors were gastrointestinal and of squamous cell type, and their locations ranged from the oropharynx to the anus (see Table 7–15).[2, 436a] One fourth were gynecologic, including vulvar and breast tumors. All four patients with brain tumors were younger than 5 years of age (see earlier). The "other" category included only one or two patients with each type of cancer. Eleven patients had multiple primary tumors, including two with liver tumors[441, 442] and one with leukemia.[425] In several patients, more than one area was involved, and it was not always clear which was the primary tumor. Reported combinations include Wilms' tumor and medulloblastoma; anal and vulvar tumors; gingival and tongue tumors; colonic, anal, and vulvar tumors; gingival and esophageal tumors; cervical and vulvar tumors; anal and vulvar tumors; tongue and vulvar tumors; anal and eyelid tumors; and skin, cervical, tongue, and breast tumors. A few patients have been reported more than once, further complicating identification of the actual number of cases with tumors.

The survival curves in Figure 7–15 show that cancer is a disease of the older FA patients who do not die first from aplastic anemia, leukemia, or liver disease. The predicted median survival for those with cancer is 28 years, at which age 70% of the total group of FA patients have already died. This risk is a particular concern for the older female FA patient. Recommended surveillance for cancers includes biannual gynecologic examinations and Pap smears, yearly rectal examinations, frequent dental and oropharyngeal evaluations, as well as yearly esophageal endoscopy and, less frequently, radiography with barium swallow (because of radiation exposure).

Once the diagnosis of a malignancy has been made, duration of survival averages less than 8 months. In one patient, a bronchogenic carcinoma was not detected until death from bleeding.[443] Another patient developed breast cancer at age 26 and died from metastatic disease 3 years later.[444] Treatment of the tumors is difficult because of increased toxicity imposed by chemotherapy or radiotherapy. Surgery is performed whenever possible. More than 60% of the patients had died by the time that their tumors were reported.

Liver Disease. Liver disease, mostly hepatic tumors, was reported in almost 40 patients (5%).[2, 436a] The male-to-female ratio of 1.6:1 and the mean age at diagnosis of FA of 9 years (see Table 7–14) indicate that this group resembles the total FA group. The age at which liver complications were detected was on average 16 years; however, the range was broad and encompassed the oldest patients. Only one patient did not have antecedent androgen treatment,[445] and thus it is likely that androgen treatment increases the risk of liver disease in FA patients. Twenty tumors were called "hepatocellular carcinomas" or "hepatomas." Two of these were called "benign"; two also had adenomas, and only one (the only one who had increased α-fetoprotein levels) had metastases. Six adenomas were reported, and two tumors were not specified. One of the adenomas had metastasized. One might speculate that the distinction between adenoma and hepatoma is not entirely clear, just as the interpretation of a bone marrow malignancy as myelodysplastic is at times subjective. One patient also had tongue cancer,[442] another had esophageal cancer,[441] and 5 had leukemia.[429, 431–434] In at least four patients, the liver tumors were found only at postmortem examination.[446–449] One patient had unexplained hepatic coma.[283] Seven had peliosis hepatitis, and six had peliosis with a tumor.

In five patients, discontinuation of therapy with androgens, alone or combined with BMT, led to resolution of the tumors or peliosis.[436a, 450–453] Surgical removal of tumors was undertaken occasionally. The prognosis was very poor: more than 85% had died by the time of reporting. However, the deaths were not due to the liver tumors, but rather to the underlying hematologic conditions. The projected survivals shown in Figure 7–15 further indicate that the patients with liver disease do poorly. The average survival was less than 4 months; only one patient lived for longer than 6 months after the diagnosis of liver tumor was made.[454, 455]

Summary of Malignancy in Fanconi's Anemia. The absolute risk of FA patients' developing leukemia, liver tumor, or other cancer is at least 15% in the literature; however, the true incidence may be obscured by over- or under-reporting. The 1994 IFAR report cited an actuarial risk of approximately 50% for development of leukemia or MDS by the age of 40 years, but it did not address the development of solid tumors.[411] Thus, risk of malignancy is particularly important in older patients. Prolongation of survival by a combination of androgens, better supportive care, BMT, and perhaps gene therapy may delay the appearance of malignancies. In addition, FA may be diagnosed by chromosome breakage analysis in patients with malignancies but without any other stigmata of FA. Concerns about the development of malignancies in older patients should not be considered contraindications to aggressive management, such as BMT, although cytoreductive chemotherapy and irradiation themselves may increase the risk of malignancies. To some degree, aplastic anemia may now be considered to be the least of the problems of the FA patient, who also is at risk for the development of liver tumors, leukemia, MDS, and solid tumors.

Dyskeratosis Congenita

Description

Dyskeratosis congenita (DC; also known as Zinsser-Cole-Engman syndrome) is a rare form of ectodermal dysplasia. Dermatologic manifestations and nail dystrophies begin in the first decade of life and leukoplakia in the second; both disorders become more extreme with increasing age. The diagnostic triad includes reticulated hyperpigmentation of the face, neck, and shoulders; dystrophic nails; and mucous membrane leukoplakia. Aplastic anemia occurs in one half of patients with DC, usually in the second decade of life, and cancer develops in 10% in the third and fourth decades.

Inheritance and Environment. More than 200 cases of DC have been reported, and all ethnic groups are represented in its distribution.[2, 4, 456, 457] Despite the general impression that DC is an X-linked recessive disorder, the male-to-female ratio of occurrence is 4.3:1.0. In fact, DC appears to have three patterns of inheritance (Table 7–16):

1. *X-linked recessive:* Single-case males or male-only families provide more than 160 cases, including the single-case males, male sibling pairs, uncle-nephew families, and males with maternal male cousins.

2. *Autosomal recessive:* Includes 26 cases, with 17 sporadic females, 5 consanguineous families, and 5 brother-sister sets.

3. *Autosomal dominant:* Seven families had two or three generations of males and females, with passage through both sexes and consanguinity in one family.

The apparently autosomal families might in fact be X-linked with X-inactivation, but this is less likely than the model of three different genes producing similar phenotypes. The X-linked recessive group also might include sporadic males who actually have autosomal mutations. Some X-linked males may now be identified with Xq28 restriction fragment length polymorphisms.[458] Caucasians, blacks, and Asian patients are represented in all groups. The dominant group seems to have the mildest disease, with a lower incidence of findings in the diagnostic triad and a lessened frequency of occurrence of cancer or aplastic anemia (see Table 7–16). The age at diagnosis is also higher in the dominant group, but this may reflect the biased retrospective ascertainment in family studies.

Physical Examination. In Table 7–17, the frequencies of occurrence of the major physical abnormalities in DC are compared with those in FA. Complete details are provided in the references cited earlier. Reticulated hyperpigmentation involves the face, neck, shoulders, and trunk. Nail dystrophy involves both hands and feet, and nail plates are small, develop longitudinal ridges, and disappear with age (Fig. 7–16; see color section at front of this volume). Ocular findings include epiphora (excessive tearing due to blockage of lacrimal ducts), blepharitis, cataracts, loss of eyelashes, conjunctivitis, ectropion, glaucoma, strabismus, ulcers, and Coats' retinopathy. Multiple dental caries and early tooth loss are common. Osteoporosis, fractures, aseptic necroses (most of these patients had been on prednisone), and scoliosis occur. Intracranial calcifications have been reported. Patients commonly have a small, delicate appearance. Hyperhidrosis of the palms and soles is reported. Premature graying and early loss of the hair are noted. Predominantly mucosal urinary tract disorders include urethral stenoses, phimosis, hypospadias, pyelonephritis, penile leukoplakia, and horseshoe kidney. Esophageal strictures, diverticula, spasms, duodenal ulcers, anal leukoplakia, bifid uvula, and umbilical hernia have all been reported, as have hypoplastic testes in males and vaginal constriction and vulvar leukoplakia in females. A few females

Table 7–16. DYSKERATOSIS CONGENITA LITERATURE

Characteristic	X-Linked Males† (%)	Autosomal Recessive (%)	Autosomal Dominant (%)
No. of patients	162	26	28
Male:female	162	8:26 = 0.3	12:16 = 0.75
Age* at diagnosis, mean	19	14	29
Median	16	11	26
Range	0.3–68	1.2–42	7–50
No. with nails abnormal	147 (91)	27 (79)	12 (43)
Mean age at nails abnormal	9	6	10
No. with skin abnormal	151 (93)	28 (82)	18 (64)
Mean age at skin abnormal	9	7	14
No. with leukoplakia	115 (71)	21 (58)	8 (29)
Mean age at leukoplakia	12	6	15
No. with aplastic anemia	76 (47)	20 (59)	4 (14)
Mean age at aplastic anemia	14	12	16
No. with cancer	17 (11)	4 (12)	2 (7)
Mean age at cancer	32	30	33
No. reported deceased	44 (27)	8 (24)	1 (4)
Mean age at deaths	21	21	39
Projected 50% survival age	33	33	>50

*Ages are in years.
†See text for definition of X-linked males.

Table 7-17. COMPARISON OF DYSKERATOSIS CONGENITA AND FANCONI'S ANEMIA

Feature	Dyskeratosis Congenita	Fanconi's Anemia
No. of patients	224	955
Male:female	4.3	1.3
Nail dystrophy	83%	0%
Skin pigmentation	88%	60%
Leukoplakia	64%	0%
Eyes	45%	26%
Teeth abnormal	21%	0%
Developmental delay	16%	13%
Skeletal (including hands)	17%	62%
Hair abnormal	17%	0%
Short stature	15%	57%
Gastrointestinal	13%	4%
Hyperhidrosis	12%	0%
Birth-weight <2500 g	8%	12%
Renal	8%	23%
Hypogonadism, male	4%	37%
Head	2%	27%
Ears	2%	10%
Cardiopulmonary	0.4%	6%
Other anomalies	0.4%	5%
Increased reflexes	0%	7%
Age at aplastic anemia, mean	14 y	9 y
Cancer	10%	8%*
Leukemia	0.4%	9%
Chromosome breaks	13%	100%

*Includes tumors of all tissues, including liver.

(four) did have successful pregnancies. Interstitial pneumonitis was reported in four patients.

DC has sometimes been confused with FA. In a series of five patients with FA, one patient probably had DC.[368] Table 7–17 indicates that both disorders may involve skin, hematopoiesis, and malignancies; however, the ages and types of involvement are quite different. FA can now be specifically diagnosed with chromosome breakage analysis (see earlier).

Aplastic Anemia. Approximately one half of the patients with known X-linked or autosomal recessive DC developed aplastic anemia (see Table 7–16) at an aver-

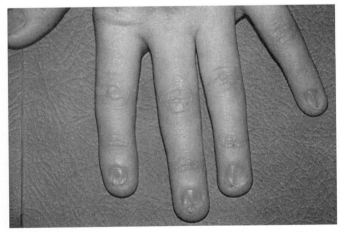

Figure 7-16. Dystrophic nails in dyskeratosis congenita (see color section at front of this volume). (From Drachtman RA, Alter BP: Dyskeratosis congenita. Dermatol Clin 1995; 13:33.)

age age of the midteens (Fig. 7–17). Often, the diagnosis of DC was only made after the onset of hematologic changes, although in retrospect the manifestations of DC usually occurred first.

Laboratory Findings

Blood and Marrow

In most patients with DC, the first hematologic findings are thrombocytopenia or anemia, followed by pancytopenia. Bone marrow examinations often reveal increased cellularity at the outset, suggesting an element of hypersplenism. However, hypocellularity then ensues, consistent with the diagnosis of aplastic anemia. Macrocytosis and elevation of Hb F levels ("stress erythropoiesis") are common.[459] Ferrokinetics are consistent with aplasia. Decreased immunoglobulin levels or cellular immunity is found inconsistently.[460]

The results of chromosome breakage studies were normal in more than 35 patients, including more than a dozen examined with DEB, MMC, or nitrogen mustard.[2, 4, 461–466] However, an increase in the number of chromosome breaks and rearrangements[2, 4, 461, 467–469] and sister chromatid exchanges (SCEs)[2, 4, 468, 470] also was reported. DC can be clearly distinguished from FA if clastogen-induced chromosome breakage is negative.

Pathophysiology

DC probably has at least three genotypes that lead to the DC phenotype (see earlier). The Xq28 restriction fragment length polymorphism[458, 471] might be used for prenatal diagnosis,[472] but the diagnosis of the propositus may not be possible until adolescence. All germ layers are affected: the ectoderm by dyskeratosis and pigmentation; the endoderm by leukoplakia; and the mesoderm by aplastic anemia. DC also is premalignant.

A detailed review of DC as a chromosomal instability disorder has been provided by Dokal and Luzzatto[473]; however, findings are not always consistent. Evidence for a defect in DNA cross-link repair has not been confirmed, nor was an increase in SCEs found consistently. Simian virus 40 transformation was not increased as it is in FA. The plating efficiency of fibroblasts in DC was decreased, MMC sensitivity was increased, and growth was improved with SOD; fibroblasts also grew more rapidly than normal and had chromosomal rearrangements. Increased G2 phase sensitivity with decreased repair of chromatid breaks was reported in response to X-irradiation and bleomycin.[474, 475] This sensitivity was in both X-linked males and autosomal recessive families and was present in heterozygotes.[476]

Hematopoietic Defect. Hematopoietic cultures were usually done from patients who already had hematologic signs, and the number of progenitors was reduced or zero in all.[2, 349, 461, 464–466, 477, 478] *In vitro*, GM-CSF or IL-3 increased the number of colonies in one study[479] but not in another,[466] and SCF did so in the culture from one patient.[349] Long-term marrow cultures suggested that the defect was in the stem cells, not in the microenvironment.[477]

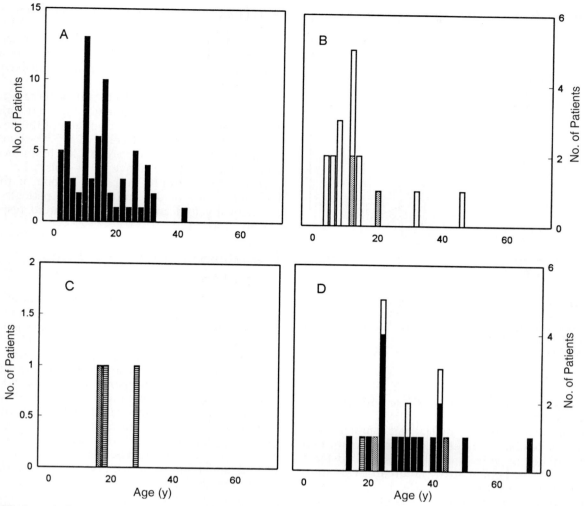

Figure 7–17. Age at diagnosis of aplastic anemia (*A–C*) and cancer (*D*) in published cases of dyskeratosis congenita from 1910 to 1995. *A,* X-linked males (see text for definition). *B,* Autosomal recessive. *C,* Autosomal dominant. *D,* Cancer. Solid bars = X-linked males; stippled bars = autosomal recessive males; open bars = autosomal recessive females; diagonally crosshatched bars = dominant males; horizontally crosshatched bars = dominant females.

One patient developed pancytopenia following chloramphenicol treatment.[480] As in other inherited syndromes, the combination of environment and genes for marrow failure may be required for aplastic anemia to appear.

Therapy and Outcome

Prognosis. The prognosis for patients with DC is not good; however, it is possible that hematologists know about only the cases with complications. Forty-four deaths were reported in 162 X-linked cases (27%), 8 in 26 autosomal recessive cases (31%), and 1 in 28 dominant cases (4%) (see Table 7–16). The mean age at death was in the twenties. The predicted median ages of survival are 33 years for X-linked and autosomal recessive patients (Fig. 7–18). The actual number of deaths for those with aplastic anemia was 28 of 76 in X-linked patients (37%), 6 of 20 in autosomal recessive patients (30%), and 1 of 4 in dominant patients (25%). The interval from the occurrence of hematologic signs to

death averaged 4 years, as in untreated FA. Deaths from cancer (see later) occurred in 11 of 17 X-linked patients (65%) and in 2 of 4 autosomal recessive patients (50%) in the third and fourth decades of life. Eight of 10 patients with both aplastic anemia and cancer died.[2] The remaining deaths were from infection or causes not described.

Cancer. Sixteen X-linked males had cancers, and two of these had more than one. Most of these cancers were squamous cell carcinomas, with some adenocarcinomas also occurring.[2] There were eight oropharyngeal tumors, involving the nasopharynx, lip, mouth, palate, tongue, and cheek. Seven tumors were gastrointestinal and included esophageal, gastric, and rectal cancers. The other cancers include bronchial adenocarcinoma,[481] Hodgkin's disease, pancreatic adenocarcinoma, and a plantar tumor. Four autosomal recessive patients had squamous cell tumors involving the cervix and vagina, nose and tongue, buccal mucosa, and hand. Two autosomal dominant patients had a skin carcinoma *in situ* and a tongue epidermoid squamous cell carcinoma.[482]

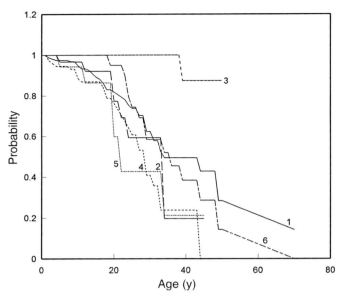

Figure 7-18. Kaplan-Meier plot of cumulative survival age in years in dyskeratosis congenita. Line 1 = X-linked males; line 2 = autosomal recessives; line 3 = autosomal dominants; line 4 = X-linked males with aplastic anemia; line 5 = autosomal recessives with aplastic anemia; line 6 = all patients with cancer.

The predicted median survival for those with cancer is 33 years (see Fig. 7–18).

Leukemia. Two X-linked males had acute myelomonocytic leukemia,[477] consistent with the type of leukemia anticipated in patients with a "stem cell" defect.*

Treatment for the bone marrow failure in DC is similar to that in FA. Androgens, usually in combination with prednisone, were given to 26 patients; 12 of these patients demonstrated improvements (46%). Death occurred 3 years after the onset of aplasia without androgen treatment, and 5 years after onset with this treatment. Androgen responders must continue treatment, and subsequent treatment failures may occur. Eight patients had only temporary responses to splenectomy. Supportive care consisting of the administration of blood products, antibiotics, and ε-aminocaproic acid should be provided as described earlier. Therapy with ALG or cyclosporine is not likely to be effective (they did not work in one of the authors' patients treated at another institution).[456]

Bone Marrow Transplantation. More than a dozen BMTs have been done in patients with DC, but only five patients survived until the time of reporting or later follow-up.[170, 461–465, 468, 483–489]† Deaths were from graft-versus-host disease; veno-occlusive disease, renal failure, and thrombotic microangiopathic syndrome; fungal pneumonia; graft failure (from a matched unrelated donor)[465]; and idiopathic pulmonary fibrosis. Because the clinical manifestations of DC appear late, it is possible that sibling donors may be undetected patients with DC. In three cases, BMT preceded the diagnosis of DC, and the skin and oral manifestations were initially thought to be graft-versus-host disease.[462, 487, 488, 490] BMT may also increase the risk of secondary tumors in DC, as it does in FA. Transplantation in DC requires caution, and irradiation may not have a role in preparation.[484]

Hematopoietic growth factors may have a role that has been, as of yet, inadequately explored. Brief trials of GM-CSF therapy led to a doubling of the neutrophil count (but not above 1000 cells/μL),[463, 491] whereas brief treatment with G-CSF at 5 μg/kg led to an increase in neutrophil counts to above 5000 cells/μL.[465, 466] IL-3 produced a neutrophil response in one of three DC patients.[410] One of the authors' own patients had an excellent myeloid and transient erythroid response to G-CSF.

Shwachman-Diamond Syndrome

Description

Shwachman-Diamond syndrome (SD; also known as Bodian-Shwachman syndrome) consists of exocrine pancreatic insufficiency combined with neutropenia. More than 200 cases of SD have been reported (Table 7–18).[2, 4] Signs of pancreatic insufficiency are apparent early in infancy and include malabsorption, steatorrhea, and failure to thrive. Neutropenia usually is detected in infancy or early childhood and is associated with skin infections or pneumonia. Many patients have anemia or thrombocytopenia, which may precede the neutropenia. Approximately 25% develop full-blown aplastic anemia. The male-to-female ratio of occurrence is 1.7 overall, and 1.3 in those with pancytopenia. More than 40 families had more than 1 affected child, and the inheritance is thought to be autosomal recessive, despite the absence of reports of consanguinity. Patients with SD have been reported among all racial and ethnic groups. Pregnancies and birth histories are unremarkable, with the exception that about 10% of SD patients are born with low birth-weight.

The most prominent findings on physical examina-

Table 7-18. SHWACHMAN-DIAMOND SYNDROME LITERATURE

	Total (%)	Pancytopenia (%)
No. of patients	200	44
Male:female	1.7	1.3
Number with metaphyseal dysostosis	68 (34)	12 (27)
Age at malabsorption		
Mean	9 mo	7 mo
Median	4 mo	2 mo
Range	0–15 y	0–9 y
Number with leukemia	10 (5)	6 (14)
Number of deaths	38 (19)	14 (32)
Age at death		
Mean	6 y	10 y
Median	3 y	9 y
Range	0.4–35 y	1.7–35 y
Projected 50% survival age	>35 y	24 y

---

*Hows J: Personal communication, 1994.

†Julius R: Personal communication, 1990; Kato S: Personal communication, 1990.

tion are malnourishment and short stature in more than 50% of patients, the majority of whom have metaphyseal dysostosis. Mental retardation was reported in 15%. Other common physical findings include protuberant abdomen and an ichthyotic skin rash. Patients have had microcephaly, hypertelorism, retinitis pigmentosa, syndactyly, cleft palate, dental dysplasia, ptosis, strabismus, short neck, coxa valga, and skin pigmentation.

The combination of pancreatic dysfunction and bone marrow failure was noted by Ozsoylu and Argun,[492] who found decreased duodenal trypsin levels in patients with acquired aplastic anemia or FA. However, patients with SD have decreased levels of amylase and lipase as well as of trypsin. In addition, patients with acquired aplasia or FA do not have malabsorption.

Laboratory Findings

In SD, total white counts are often less than 3000 cells/μL, and neutrophil counts are less than 1500 cells/μL on at least one occasion. Neutropenia may be chronic, intermittent, or cyclic and is usually evident early in childhood. Anemia occurs in more than one third of patients but may be mild (hemoglobin level between 7 and 10 g/dL); however, transfusions are sometimes necessary. Thrombocytopenia with counts less than 100,000 cells/μL is seen in over 20% of cases. The bicytopenic combination of neutropenia and anemia or thrombocytopenia also is common. Pancytopenia occurred in 44 patients (22%), was manifest after the onset of neutropenia, and appeared at a mean age of 9 years, at a median age of 6 years, and within an age range of 1 to 35 years. A possible defect in neutrophil mobility may explain the occurrence of infections, even when the neutrophil count is not extremely low.

Bone marrow cellularity is decreased in one half of patients, with other marrows showing a myeloid maturation arrest or appearing normal. The erythroid series is normal or hyperplastic. Hb F levels often are increased even without anemia, suggesting the presence of marrow stress. Low levels of immunoglobulins were reported in a few patients. Hepatic dysfunction and fibrosis have been noted occasionally. Pancreatic insufficiency is documented as low levels or absence of duodenal trypsin, amylase, and lipase. SD patients do not have cystic fibrosis, and sweat chloride levels are normal. Radiologic evidence of metaphyseal dysostosis was recorded in 34%. Chromosomes are normal, without increased breakage following clastogenic stress.

Pathophysiology

The inheritance appears to be autosomal recessive, despite the prevalence among males. Although the exocrine pancreas and bone marrow hematopoiesis develop at approximately the same time *in utero*, familial cases as well as SD in only one of a pair of twins militate against an intrauterine insult as the cause. A stem cell deficit was suggested by a decrease in the number of marrow CFU-GMs and CFU-Es in most patients, without evidence for humoral or cellular inhibitors of granulopoiesis. The reduction in the number of hematopoietic progenitor cells is similar to that in other inherited bone marrow failure syndromes.

Therapy and Outcome

The malabsorption in patients with SD responds to treatment with oral pancreatic enzymes. Infections resulting from neutropenia are treated with the appropriate antibiotics, and anemia and thrombocytopenia are managed with transfusions of red cells or platelets as needed. Fewer than a dozen patients were treated with corticosteroids, with hematologic improvement occurring in one half. Even fewer received androgens in combination with steroids (see section on FA), with some improvement; one patient required the addition of cyclosporine to the regimen.[493]

More than 20% of the SD patients developed pancytopenia, and 5% developed leukemia (see later). Deaths were reported (see Table 7–18) in 19% of all patients in the SD group—32% of those who had pancytopenia, and 80% of those who had leukemia. The projected median survival age is more than 35 years for all, 24 years for those with aplastic anemia, and 10 years for those with leukemia. Those without these complications reach a survival rate plateau of greater than 80% by the age of 6 years (Fig. 7–19). Infection or bleeding were the causes of most deaths. As with most of the patients with inherited bone marrow failure disorders, the number of mild or asymptomatic cases in the literature is underestimated, and the overall prognosis may not be as bad as is implied in this text.

Leukemia. Leukemia was reported in 10 patients (9 males) at a mean age of 13 years (range, 2 to 38 years). Two patients had SD siblings. There were 3 cases of

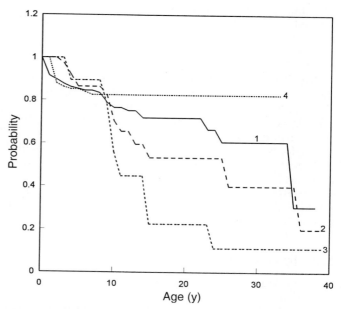

Figure 7-19. Kaplan-Meier plot of cumulative survival age in years in Shwachman-Diamond Syndrome. Line 1 = total; line 2 = pancytopenia; line 3 = leukemia; line 4 = other.

ALL, 3 cases of AML, and 1 case each of acute myelo-monocytic leukemia, monocytic leukemia, erythroleu-kemia, and juvenile chronic myelocytic leukemia.[2, 4, 494] Only one patient had received treatment with predni-sone combined with androgen for aplastic anemia. One patient with ALL and one with AML were still alive after 1 year, whereas the others died at 1 month to 2 years following the diagnosis of leukemia. Four pa-tients had cytogenetic abnormalities: two with addi-tional G group chromosomes, one with monosomy 7 plus a marker, and one with translocation 18. One had an apparent 8-month preleukemic phase.[495] In one series, four patients were reported to have MDS (one with refractory anemia, two with refractory anemia with excess blasts, and one with refractory anemia with excess blasts in transformation) at 4 to 10 years of age[83]; only one was still alive 6 years later, but none were reported to have developed leukemia. In another re-view of 21 SD patients, 6 developed MDS, and in 4 of these MDS transformed to leukemia.[496] Thus, SD resembles most of the other inherited bone marrow failure syndromes in that it is characterized by a pro-pensity for malignancy.

Bone Marrow Transplantation. One patient died from cyclophosphamide cardiotoxicity,[497] whereas an-other was cured following the same preparative regi-men of 50 mg/kg per day for 4 days.[498]

Hematopoietic Growth Factors. Six of seven patients treated with G-CSF had an elevation of neutrophil counts[499–502]; one patient failed to respond to GM-CSF.[503]

Cartilage-Hair Hypoplasia

Description

Cartilage-hair hypoplasia (CHH) is an autosomal reces-sive chondrodysplasia characterized by short stature and fine, sparse hair. More than 300 patients, primarily of Amish and Finnish background, have been de-scribed.[504, 505] Patients with CHH resemble those with SD, with more than 80% having metaphyseal dys-ostosis, some malabsorption, and hematologic abnor-malities.[506]

Physical Examination. The short stature in CHH is due to short-limbed dwarfism.[505] More than 90% of CHH patients have hypoplastic hair that lacks the cen-tral pigment core.[507] Ligament laxity is common. Other skeletal findings include chest deformity, varus lower limbs, lordosis, and scoliosis. Gastrointestinal problems include aganglionic megacolon (Hirschsprung's dis-ease) and other anatomic anomalies.

Inheritance and Environment. The majority of CHH patients are Amish (a founder effect[504]) and Finnish, but other Caucasians with the disease have been reported.

Laboratory Findings

Anemia and macrocytosis with or without anemia were observed frequently in the Finnish patients, as were increased Hb F levels, which are consistent with stress erythropoiesis.[506, 508] For only about 25 patients was anemia described in any detail. Bone marrow findings ranged from erythroid hypoplasia to maturation arrest to normal. Some patients were initially reported as having Diamond-Blackfan anemia.[509–511] Lymphopenia was seen in over 60% and neutropenia in 25% of cases; both cellular and soluble immunodeficiency are often a part of this syndrome.[512]

Pathophysiology

DNA. High-resolution linkage-disequilibrium map-ping in Amish and Finnish families localized the gene for CHH to 9p21-p13.[513] Prenatal diagnosis correctly identified one affected in four fetuses examined.[514]

Hematopoietic Defect. As in other inherited marrow failure anemias, the numbers of CFU-Es were low and those of BFU-Es almost zero in eight patients.[508] Pro-genitor counts for myeloid and megakaryocytic lin-eages were also low. Some of the patients had normal blood counts, despite a reduction in progenitor counts. Serum erythropoietin levels were higher than predicted from the hemoglobin level, as in other marrow failure patients.[2] Increased red cell adenosine deaminase level, common in Diamond-Blackfan anemia (see later), was reported in a boy with CHH who was not anemic.[515]

Therapy and Outcome

Transfusions and steroids were employed for the ane-mia, and many of the patients tended to outgrow their marrow failure. Among 108 Finnish patients, 16 deaths included 3 from anemia, 4 with pneumonia, 2 with sepsis, and 2 from Hirschsprung's disease.[505]

Complications

Cancer. Malignancies occur at increased frequency in CHH. Hodgkin's disease was reported in 3 pa-tients,[516, 517] and the Finnish series included 6 patients with pulmonary lymphoma at age 10, intestinal lymph-osarcoma at 22, malignant testis tumor at 6 months, and 3 patients with skin basal cell carcinomas at 33, 35, and 48 years of age.[505]

Pearson's Syndrome

Pearson's syndrome (refractory sideroblastic anemia with vacuolization of bone marrow precursors and exocrine pancreatic dysfunction) was astutely recognized and reported by Pearson in four patients in 1979.[518] The pathognomonic deletion of mitochondrial DNA was described by Rotig and co-workers in 1990,[519] provid-ing a molecular diagnostic test as well as an explana-tion for the clinical features, which include anemia and metabolic acidosis. More than 40 cases have been reported.[2,*] The male-to-female ratio of occurrence is 0.9. The inheritance is maternal because mitochondria are found in ova but not sperm. No affected siblings have been reported. One family was consanguineous,[520] and in another the mother had Kearns-Sayre syn-

---

*Arkin S, Alter BP: Unpublished data.

drome.[521] All racial and most ethnic groups have been affected.

Physical Examination. Seven term infants had a history of low birth-weight, although only one patient[522] was premature by dates. Nineteen patients were described as being short or as having malabsorption or failure to thrive. Physical anomalies are not common; however, one patient was reported with hypoplastic mandible and large ears, and another with abnormal arm skin pigmentation. One of our patients had metopic synostosis, inguinal hernias, and hypospadias.[522]

Laboratory Findings

Anemia was diagnosed before 1 month of age in 25% and by 6 months of age in 70% of affected infants. The mean hemoglobin level was 5.5 g/dL (range, 2.1 to 9.1 g/dL). Three patients had hydrops.[519, 522] Nineteen had absolute neutrophil counts below 1000 cells/μL, and 20 had platelet counts below 150,000 cells/μL (15 below 100,000 cells/μL). Most patients had macrocytic red cells. The bone marrows of essentially all patients had vacuolated myeloid or erythroid precursors; many had a decreased number of erythroblasts, and all but one had sideroblasts; and most had ringed sideroblasts (Fig. 7–20).

Pathophysiology

The mitochondrial deletion was reported in 26 patients, the length of which ranged from 2.7 to 7.767 kb; 15 patients had a 4.977-kb deletion. The respiratory enzymes involved in the deletions are relevant to oxidative phosphorylation and include nicotinamide-adenine dinucleotide (reduced form), cytochrome oxidase and adenosine triphosphatase, as well as transfer RNAs and ribosomal RNAs.[523] Patients have organs and cells with variable numbers of deleted and normal mitochondria. Fluctuations over time (e.g., owing to marrow improvement) might relate to selective expansion of normal or abnormal clones, explaining both interpatient and intrapatient variability in phenotype. De Vivo has prepared an excellent review of mitochondrial diseases.[524]

CFU-E numbers were decreased in three patients,[518, 522, 525] and those of BFU-Es were reduced in two.[522, 526] The number of CFU-GMs was normal in two[518] and was zero in one.[526] Thus, the number of committed progenitors is usually low, at least at the time when the patients have cytopenias.

Therapy and Outcome

The clinical problems can be separated into those that are hematologic and those that are metabolic. Although 75% of the patients received transfusions, all who did not die from other causes had an increase in hemoglobin level at a mean of 2 and at a maximum of 4 years. Neutropenia and thrombocytopenia were usually not of major significance. G-CSF and erythropoietin were given to 2 patients,[522, 527] with possible response to the G-CSF. The role of growth factors has not been substan-

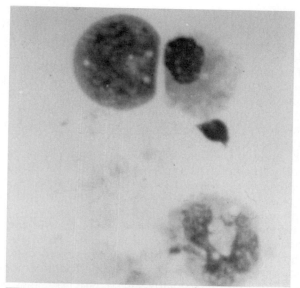
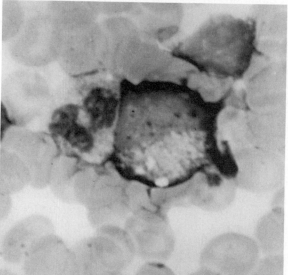
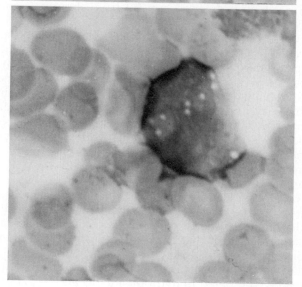

Figure 7–20. Bone marrow myeloid precursors in Pearson's syndrome, showing cytoplasmic vacuoles.

tiated, but their use on an investigative basis is probably warranted. In general, the hematologic problems are not fatal, and good supportive care should be provided.

The major problem is acidosis. Specific therapy is aimed at bypass of the deleted respiratory enzymes through the use of thiamine, riboflavin, levocarnitine, and coenzyme Q. The small numbers of patients treated and the variability of the disease do not yet permit any conclusions.

The rate of mortality is high, and death occurs early. Twenty-three died at a mean age of 2.4 years (range, 2 months to 9 years), and 19 were alive at a mean age of 6.7 years (range, 0 to 19 years). The 50% survival rate is projected at 3 years of age; the 5-year survival rate is estimated at 39%. Deaths were primarily due to acidosis, sepsis, and liver or renal failure. Five patients outgrew their hematologic problems but did develop symptoms of Kearns-Sayre syndrome (ophthalmoplegia, pigmentary retinopathy, ataxia, and heart block) at ages 7 to 13 years.[528–532] Diabetes mellitus was noted in 10%. Autopsies revealed pancreatic fibrosis in a few patients. So far, none have developed leukemia, nor has any undergone BMT or other organ transplantation.

Prenatal testing of fetal blood, chorionic villi, or amniocytes might be offered, but such testing would be low yield (few affected mothers and no siblings were reported). The mother's DNA should be examined, however. In one family, the mother had Kearns-Sayre syndrome, with the same mitochondrial DNA deletion as her child with Pearson's syndrome.[521]

Pearson's syndrome should be added to the differential diagnosis of refractory anemia in children, especially of those without a clonal cytogenetic abnormality. For example, Bader-Meunier and associates reported two children having refractory anemia with ringed sideroblasts; both had bone marrow vacuoles, one had a mitochondrial DNA deletion, and the other did not have a deletion but did have abnormal mitochondrial enzyme activities.[533]

Pearson's syndrome can now be redefined as refractory sideroblastic anemia (or refractory anemia with ringed sideroblasts) with vacuolated marrow precursors and with deletion of mitochondrial DNA. Other dysfunctions in this syndrome, such as pancreatic insufficiency, acidosis, and renal tubular insufficiency, are commonly seen but not mandatory for diagnosis. DNA deletion is complicated: patients with Kearns-Sayre syndrome may have identical deletions but not have hematologic signs; alternatively, patients with bone marrow findings as in Pearson's syndrome may not have DNA deletions, but they may have abnormal mitochondrial enzymes. Still other mitochondrial disorders may be due to point mutations or to deletions smaller than those that can be detected by the Southern blot technique.

Pearson's syndrome is probably underdiagnosed and must be considered in hydropic infants and in patients with cytopenias associated with renal or liver disease, sepsis, or acidosis, as well as in children with refractory anemia or myelodysplasia, particularly those with ringed sideroblasts.

Reticular Dysgenesis

The term *reticular dysgenesis* (thymic alymphoplasia with aleukocytosis) is used to describe infants with congenital agranulocytosis, lymphopenia, and absent cellular and humoral immunity. Since it was first reported by de Vaal and Seynhaeve in 1959,[534] almost two dozen cases have been reported,[2, 535–537] including one set of twins and three sets of siblings. Despite a fourfold preponderance among males, the number of cases is too low to prove that it is an X-linked disorder. The identification of three sets of siblings and one set of twins, as well as one family with consanguinity, is also consistent with an autosomal recessive inheritance. These cases include one with a similar phenotype in which the mother received azathioprine for renal disease; however, this case may have been acquired rather than inherited.[538, 539]

Patients usually present with signs of infection at birth or early in infancy. The mean age was 14 days, the median age 1 day, and the range from 0 to 105 days. The birth-weights of eight infants were less than 2500 g. On radiography, no lymph nodes or tonsils were seen, and no thymic shadow was observed. At autopsy, the thymuses were extremely small, the lymph nodes absent, and the spleens without follicles.

Blood counts showed severe lymphopenia and granulocytopenia. Anemia was reported in nine patients, and thrombocytopenia in only one. Bone marrows were hypocellular, with no myeloid or lymphoid precursors; sometimes, a reduction in erythropoiesis was observed as well. One patient had dyserythropoietic erythroid precursors, one had a promyelocyte arrest, and one had aplastic marrow. Bone marrow cultures from four patients contained no or very few hematopoietic colonies,[2] a finding that supports the stem cell model. Although the majority of the patients did not have complete aplastic anemia, they certainly do serve as examples of neutropenia and lymphopenia.

Most of the patients died from infection (8 in the first month) at a mean age of 2 months, a median age of 1 month, and a range in age of 3 days to 5 months. One infant who survived for 17 weeks was maintained in a gnotobiotic environment.[540] Five had BMTs; two of these survived, one for more than 4 months and the other for more than 1 year.[535, 536, 541–543] One patient who successfully underwent transplantation without immunosuppression became a complete chimera, with donor erythrocytes; this patient was unlike patients with severe combined immunodeficiency, in whom only the lymphocytes become donor. This suggests that the defect is in the pluripotential hematopoietic stem cell. However, another patient had only lymphoid reconstitution without immunosuppression.[535]

Reticular dysgenesis is an example of a defect of an earlier stem cell that is involved in most of the other inherited aplastic anemias (i.e., affecting the lymphoid as well as the myeloid series).

Amegakaryocytic Thrombocytopenia

Description

A small number of patients with inherited aplastic anemia present with thrombocytopenia in infancy and develop pancytopenia later. This syndrome was called *type III constitutional aplastic anemia* by O'Gorman Hughes,[544] but the term *amegakaryocytic thrombocytopenia* is more helpful. The differential diagnosis of neonatal thrombocytopenia is lengthy; the disorder discussed here excludes those with increased bone marrow megakaryocyte counts, as well as those due to congenital infection (particularly a viral infection, such as rubella). Immune thrombocytopenias also are excluded, despite the occasional development of amegakaryocytosis, presumably due to the reactivity of antiplatelet antibodies with megakaryocytes.[545] TAR syndrome, as well as acquired amegakaryocytic thrombocytopenia, is discussed in the section on single cytopenias. FA, which can begin with thrombocytopenia, was discussed earlier in this chapter. Children with known associated trisomies, such as trisomies 13 and 18, also have been excluded.

The authors are aware of 21 reports of thrombocytopenia in the first year of life (15 in the first week) and of 5 other cases with onset at 2 to 9 years of age associated with no physical anomalies but with the absence of or a reduction in the number of bone marrow megakaryocytes (Table 7–19).[2, 546] The male-to-female ratio is 1.1. In addition, 17 children were described with amegakaryocytic thrombocytopenia in the first year (11 in the first week) and 1 at 3 years whose physical abnormalities fit no other syndrome. The male-to-female ratio is 3.3. Contained within this group is a subset of patients with microcephaly and cerebellar or cerebral atrophy who were first described by Hoyeraal and colleagues, and later addressed by other investigators.[547–549] Additional abnormalities include cardiac disease, abnormal facies, retarded development, abnormal hips or feet, kidney abnormalities, eye anomalies, and cleft or high arched palate. Some of the physical findings resemble those seen in FA, which cannot always be excluded retrospectively from the reports.

Eleven families with males without anomalies could be X-linked, and 10 could be autosomal recessive (i.e., they included females). Two families included patients with and without anomalies,[550, 551] and thus separation into the two categories is somewhat arbitrary. One family included an anencephalic sibling and relatives with missing fingers[544]; in another family, one brother died with leukemia.[552] Eight of the families with anomalies could be X-linked, and three could be autosomal recessive (i.e., they included females). One family had parental consanguinity.[553]

Pregnancies and deliveries were essentially unremarkable, although the frequency of spontaneous abortions was increased in both groups (reported in eight families). Low birth-weight was reported in three families without and in five with anomalies.

Bleeding in the skin, mucous membranes, or gastrointestinal tract was usually the presenting sign. Eleven patients with no anomalies and six with anomalies developed pancytopenia.

Laboratory Findings

The first abnormality noted is thrombocytopenia. Although white blood cell counts and hemoglobin levels are normal, the red cells are macrocytic and levels of Hb F and i antigen are increased, findings that suggest a broader level of marrow failure. One 5-year-old boy with amegakaryocytic thrombocytopenia had increased mean cell volume and Hb F level but had not yet developed aplastic anemia.[554] Platelet counts ranged

Table 7–19. AMEGAKARYOCYTIC THROMBOCYTOPENIA LITERATURE

	No Anomalies (%)	Anomalies (%)	Total (%)
No. of patients	26	18	44
Male:female	1.1	3.3	1.6
Age at thrombocytopenia			
Mean	11 mo	5 mo	9 mo
Median	7 d	7 d	7 d
Range	0–9 y	0–3 y	0–9 y
No. with aplastic anemia*	11 (42)	6 (33)	17 (39)
Mean	3.7 y	3.1 y	3.5 y
Median	3 y	3 y	3 y
Range	0.4–12.5 y	1.1–6 y	0.4–12.5 y
No. with leukemia/MDS	2 (8)	—	2 (5)
No. of deaths, thrombocytopenia	7 (27)	9 (50)	16 (36)
Age at death, thrombocytopenia			
Mean	2.9 y	6 mo	1.6 y
Median	2 wk	2 mo	2 mo
Range	0.01–9 y	0–1.9 y	0.01–9 y
No. of deaths, aplastic anemia	8 (31)	6 (30)	14 (32)
Age at death, aplastic anemia			
Mean	7.9 y	4.1 y	6.3 y
Median	5 y	3 y	3.6 y
Range	0.6–21 y	1.9–10 y	0.6–21 y
Projected 50% survival age	6 y	1 y	3 y

*Aplastics include two with leukemia or myelodysplasia.

from 0 to 80,000/µL at diagnosis. Bone marrow examination reveals normal cellularity with absence or decreased numbers of megakaryocytes. Those mega-karyocytes that are present are small and appear to be inactive. Homologous platelet survival is normal because the defect is underproduction, not increased destruction.[552] Evolution into pancytopenia is associ-ated with the development of hypocellular marrow with increased lymphocyte and plasma cell counts, as in any aplastic anemia. Peripheral blood chromosomes do not have the increase in the number of breaks characteristic of FA. In one patient who had myelodys-plasia, the absence, partial deletion, or trisomy of chro-mosome 19 was observed in 11 of 55 marrow cells.[555]

Prenatal diagnosis may be based on platelet counts in midtrimester fetal blood. Mibashan and Millar de-tected thrombocytopenia in one of three fetuses at risk.[556]

Pathophysiology

The disease appears to be either or both X-linked reces-sive and autosomal recessive. The thrombocytopenia is associated with a decrease in or absence of megakaryo-cytes. The number of megakaryocyte progenitors was reduced in five patients, with improvement occurring in the presence of the combination of IL-3 and GM-CSF.[546] In those with aplastic anemia, myeloid and ery-throid progenitor cells are decreased in number or absent[2]; progenitors also were decreased in one patient who was studied during the thrombocytopenic phase.[349] Because all of the inherited aplastic anemias can begin with thrombocytopenia, this anomaly may represent only a phase in the evolution of aplasia.

Therapy and Outcome

Thrombocytopenia Alone. Fifteen of those without anomalies did not develop aplastic anemia; one was alive with macrocytosis and elevated Hb F level.[554] The seven reported deaths were due to bleeding or infec-tion, or to both. Twelve of those with anomalies did not develop pancytopenia. Nine patients died; hemor-rhage or infection was responsible for the deaths, even though many of these babies also had complex cardio-vascular or cerebral problems. Most cases were de-scribed before 1980, and systematic platelet support was not reported. Treatment with IL-3 decreased bleed-ing in five patients who did not respond to GM-CSF.[546]

Aplastic Anemia. Aplastic anemia developed at a mean of 3.7 years in 11 of the 26 with normal findings on physical examination. Eight died, from bleeding and/or sepsis. One patient whose brother died from aplastic anemia not responsive to androgen therapy received a bone marrow transplant from his sister and is the only long-term survivor.[557,*] Six of those with physical anomalies also developed aplastic anemia at a mean age of 6 months, and none survived past the age of 10 years.

Leukemia. One male with normal physical appear-ance developed aplastic anemia at the age of 5 years,

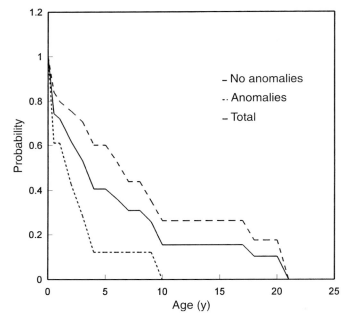

Figure 7-21. Kaplan-Meier plot of cumulative survival age in years in amegakaryocytic thrombocytopenia.

failed to improve on androgens in combination with steroids, and had acute myelomonocytic leukemia at age 16: this patient died at age 17.[544,*] One female had thrombocytopenia at 2 months and pancytopenia at 5 months of age, as well as myelodysplasia with abnor-malities of chromosome 19.[555] Amegakaryocytic throm-bocytopenia is thus another of the marrow failure syn-dromes that predisposes to malignancy.

Treatment. Steroids alone were effective in fewer than one third of cases. Steroids in combination with androgens led to temporary or partial responses in rare patients with normal physical appearances and aplastic anemia, but all of these patients subsequently died. None of those with anomalies responded to steroid treatment. Four patients underwent splenectomies that were ineffective.

The projected median survival ages are 6 years for those without and 1 year for those with anomalies (Fig. 7-21); the average age at time of death among the reported cases was 6 and 2 years, respectively. The mean ages at time of death for those with pancytopenia were 8 and 4.1 years, those with only thrombocyto-penia died at mean ages of 2.9 and 0.5 years, respec-tively.

Platelet support might prevent early death from thrombocytopenia and perhaps be associated with a higher rate of evolution to aplastic anemia. BMT may offer the only possibility for cure, although hematopoi-etic growth factors should be tested as they become available.

Familial Marrow Dysfunction
Description

A large group of apparently familial marrow failure syndromes do not fit any of the classifications de-

---

*Gelfand E: Personal communication, 1984.

*Potter NU, Alter BP: Unpublished data.

Table 7–20. FAMILIAL APLASTIC ANEMIA AUTOSOMAL DOMINANT, WITH ANOMALIES

	Age Group	No. Affected	No. of Generations
IVIC syndrome: radial hypoplasia, deaf, thrombocytopenia	Children, adults	24 3 2	5 2 2
WT syndrome: hand anomalies, leukemia	Children, adults	4 8 10	3 5 3
Aplasia, leukemia, pigmentation, warts, immunodeficiency	Adults	4	2
Radial-ulnar fusion	Adults	6 10	4 2
Ataxia, acute nonlymphocytic leukemia, monosomy 7, immunodeficiency	Children	5 3	1 2
Abnormal thumbs	Child, adult	2	2

scribed so far (Tables 7–20 to 7–25). Some partially resemble FA, SD, or DBA. In many cases, diseases in other family members include aplastic anemia, leukemia, and immunodeficiency. The age of onset is from childhood to adulthood. The inheritance patterns are dominant, recessive, and X-linked. Sporadic cases of aplastic anemia with physical anomalies that are not FA also are observed.

Autosomal Dominant with Physical Anomalies (see Table 7–20). The *IVIC syndrome*, named with the initials of the institution at which it was first reported (Instituto Venezolano de Investigaciónes Científicas), is characterized by radial ray hypoplasia with absent thumbs or hypoplastic radial carpal bones, hearing impairment, strabismus, imperforate anus, and thrombocytopenia. Twenty-nine people in three multigenerational families had anomalies.[558–560] Mild thrombocytopenia and leukocytosis appeared before the age of 50 years in 13 individuals in the first family. The incidence of hematologic abnormalities is unknown because many patients are still young. Baseline chromosome breakage was normal. Despite the absence of complete aplastic

Table 7–21. FAMILIAL APLASTIC ANEMIA AUTOSOMAL RECESSIVE, WITH ANOMALIES

	Age Group	No. Affected	No. of Generations
Microcephaly, short stature, immunodeficiency, increase in sister chromatid exchanges	Children, adults	3 siblings	1
Central nervous system anomalies	Children	2 siblings	1
Oculocutaneous albinism, immunodeficiency	Children	2 cousins	1
Facial dysmorphia, steatorrhea	Children	3 siblings	1
Diaphyseal dysplasia	Children	5 1 2 siblings	1 1 1

Table 7–22. FAMILIAL APLASTIC ANEMIA AUTOSOMAL DOMINANT, WITHOUT ANOMALIES

	Age Group	No. Affected	No. of Generations
Vascular occlusions	Children, adults	19	5
Neutropenia	Adults	2	2
Idiopathic aplastic anemia	Child, adult	2	2
Leukemia, MDS	Children, adults	5	2
Leukemia, monosomy 7	Adults	8 siblings, cousins	1
Acquired aplastic anemia	Adults	9 in 4 families	2

anemia, the physical findings do resemble those seen in FA. It has been suggested that this syndrome be renamed "oculo-oto-radial syndrome."[561]

Members of three families were reported to have disease resembling FA, but with an autosomal dominant inheritance pattern. It was called the *WT syndrome*, after the first initials of the first two families in which the disorder was identified.[562, 563] The patients had radial-ulnar hypoplasia, abnormal thumbs, short fingers, clinodactyly of the fifth finger, pancytopenia or thrombocytopenia, or leukemia, or any combination of these features. These physical findings were subtly different from those of classical FA, and baseline chromosome breaks were not seen. The authors suggested that several cases of "atypical FA" might instead be WT syndrome. Chromosome studies following clastogenic stress might now help to resolve this confusion.

Members of one family had dominant bone marrow failure, acute nonlymphocytic leukemia, hyperpigmented skin, warts, immune dysfunction, and multiple spontaneous abortions.[564] DEB-induced chromosome breakage was not increased; thus, this disorder loosely resembles FA clinically but not genetically. Dokal and co-workers reported two families with dominant proximal fusion of the radius and ulna in which two members of each had aplastic anemia or leukemia.[565] One family was reported in which the son had finger-like thumbs, and he and his mother had pancytopenia; DEB-induced chromosome breakage was normal.[566]

Li and co-workers described a family with *ataxia-pancytopenia syndrome*. Four brothers plus the father had cerebellar atrophy and ataxia. The surviving sister has ataxia and mild unexplained anemia.[567, 568] Two brothers died from aplastic anemia, and a third from

Table 7–23. FAMILIAL APLASTIC ANEMIA AUTOSOMAL RECESSIVE, WITHOUT ANOMALIES

	Age Group	No. Affected	No. of Generations
Immunodeficiency, cutaneous malignancies	Children	2 siblings	1
Immunodeficiency	Adults	4 siblings	1*
Thrombocytopenia, t(13;14)	Adults	2 siblings	1
Xeroderma pigmentosum	Children	5 in 5 families	1
Acquired aplastic anemia	Adults	10 in 4 families	1

*Consanguineous.

Table 7-24. FAMILIAL APLASTIC ANEMIA X-LINKED RECESSIVE, WITHOUT ANOMALIES

	Age Group	No. Affected	No. of Generations
Leukemia, MDS	Children, adults	8 males	3
Lymphoproliferative syndrome	Children	17 males	4 in 25 families
Acquired aplastic anemia	Adults	2 males	2

acute myelogenous leukemia; the fourth brother was followed through hypoplastic anemia, immune deficiency, preleukemia, and monosomy 7 until he died from acute myelomonocytic leukemia. In a second family with similar features, one brother with monosomy 7 died at the age of 5 years from acute nonlymphocytic leukemia that had been preceded by pancytopenia; the sister and the mother have cerebellar ataxia.[569] The inheritance appears to be autosomal dominant with variable expression.

Autosomal Recessive with Anomalies (see Table 7–21). Three siblings in a consanguineous family had microcephaly, short stature, immunodeficiency, skin abscesses, anemia, and increased spontaneous but not DEB-induced chromosome breaks, as well as increased sister chromatid exchange.[570] Another sibling pair had central nervous system malformations and hypocellular marrows, but normal results on chromosome breakage analysis.[571] Two cousins (male and female) had oculocutaneous albinism, microcephaly, facial dysmorphia, immunodeficiency, neutropenia, and thrombocytopenia.[572] Three siblings with consanguineous parents had facial dysmorphia, steatorrhea, increased skin folds, congenital heart disease, vesicoureteral reflux, decreased cellular immunity, and severe neutropenia, with normal chromosomes.[573] This family might belong in the SD category, despite the absence of metaphyseal dysplasia (see earlier).

Seven families with a specific pattern of inheritance have been reported: five sporadic, one consanguineous, and one with affected siblings. Diaphyseal dysplasia and anemia were observed in all and thrombocytopenia in one of the families.[574–576] The anemia re-

Table 7-25. SPORADIC APLASTIC ANEMIA WITH ANOMALIES

	Age Group	No. Affected	No. of Generations
Friedreich's ataxia, short stature, hypogonadism	Child	1 male	1
Cerebellar ataxia	Child	1 male	1
Short, web neck, proximal thumbs	Child	1 female	1
Skin pigmentation	Child	1 female	1
de Lange's syndrome	Child	2 males 1 female	1
Various anomalies reported to the IFAR	Children	11	1

IFAR = International Fanconi Anemia Registry.

sponded to prednisone, suggesting that these patients might also have been classified as having Diamond-Blackfan anemia (see earlier).

Autosomal Dominant Without Physical Anomalies (see Table 7–22). Aufderheide described a family in which 14 patients representing 5 generations developed mild to profound single cytopenias or pancytopenia by the third decade of life.[577] Vascular occlusions were present in 9 members. One patient did have chromosome breaks in 20% of his cells, whereas his father, who also had aplastic anemia, had intact chromosomes. Kato and colleagues reported a mother with aplastic anemia and her son with adult-onset neutropenia and thrombocytopenia.[578] A mother and child pair with idiopathic aplastic anemia also was reported.[579] Kaur and associates described 5 members of a family with acute myeloid leukemia or MDS; other family members had hypoplastic anemia.[580] Chitambar and co-workers described 8 out of 14 family members (both sexes) with aplastic anemia, acute nonlymphocytic leukemia, and monosomy 7 in one generation of a large maternal kindred.[581] In a report on 19 members of 8 families with "acquired aplastic anemia," 4 families with 9 patients had a vertical pattern—that is, a parent or aunt or uncle also had aplasia.[582] These cases could be due to common environmental factors or to a genetic propensity for bone marrow failure.

Autosomal Recessive Without Anomalies (see Table 7–23). Abels and Reed reported two brothers who were short, had macrocytosis, and developed pancytopenia at about 10 years of age.[583] One had immune deficiency and multiple cutaneous squamous and basal cell carcinomas. He also had oral telangiectasias and neck and chest poikiloderma; these findings suggested but were insufficient to diagnose DC. Because both patients were male, the inheritance might also be X-linked recessive. Linsk and colleagues described a consanguineous family with associated immune disorders in which 4 out of 6 siblings had PRCA or neutropenia, as well as unusual crystalloid structures in their neutrophils, as demonstrated by electron microscopy.[584] Two adult siblings had thrombocytopenia and a Robertsonian translocation t(13;14); however, other siblings with the translocation were hematologically normal.[585] In the Scandinavian report on "acquired aplastic anemia" with multiple family members (mentioned earlier),[582] 10 patients in 4 families belonged to sibships.

A clearly autosomal recessive DNA repair disorder, *xeroderma pigmentosum*, has been reported to be associated with aplastic anemia,[586] as well as with MDS[587] and acute myeloid leukemia.[588, 589] Marrow failure is not usually associated with xeroderma pigmentosum, in which skin cancer is the major problem because of ultraviolet light–sensitivity.

X-Linked Recessive Without Anomalies (see Table 7–24). In an X-linked recessive family described by Li and associates, 8 males in 3 generations had adult-onset pancytopenia, acute myelogenous leukemia, light chain disease, or acute lymphocytic leukemia (in 1).[590] In one of the Scandinavian families, a man and his maternal uncle had aplastic anemia.[582] The *X-linked lymphoproliferative syndrome* has more than 25 kindreds.[49] At least 17 of the boys developed fatal aplastic anemia during or before malignant infectious mononucleosis.[591] Other components of this syndrome include hypoproliferative disorders, agranulocytosis, hypogammaglobulinemia, and proliferative disorders associated with the Epstein-Barr virus (American Burkitt's lymphoma, immunoblastic B cell sarcoma, plasmacytoma, and fatal mononucleosis). Restriction fragment length polymorphisms localized this gene to the region of Xq24-q27.[592]

Sporadic cases characterized by aplastic anemia and physical abnormalities are summarized in Table 7–25. A 16-year-old male with Friedreich's ataxia, short stature, hypogonadism, and hyperreflexia had macrocytic hypoplastic anemia that was responsive to testosterone.[593] Peripheral blood but not marrow chromosomes showed baseline increased breakage. A 3-year-old boy had cerebellar ataxia, translocation (1;20), and aplasia, without increased baseline chromosome breakage.[594] A girl had short stature, dysmorphic facies, web neck, and proximal thumbs, as well as pancytopenia without increased chromosome breakage.[595] A 12-year-old girl had skin pigmentation and marrow failure; results of DEB-induced chromosome breakage testing were normal.[596] Three patients with the Brachmann-de Lange syndrome had thrombocytopenia that, in two of the patients, progressed to aplastic anemia.[597, 598] Eleven children with aplastic anemia and anomalies were reported to the IFAR; in these, chromosome breakage was not increased by DEB.[304] Many patients who in fact did not have FA may have been called FA in the older literature and are included in our own analyses (see earlier). Only modern testing for clastogen-induced chromosome breakage facilitates proper categorization of all of these.

Several cases do not fit into any categories.[2] In 3 of the 8 families having 19 members with aplastic anemia cited earlier,[582] the anemia might have been related to drug use. Four families had more than one patient with chloramphenicol-related aplastic anemia. Two families had siblings with aplastic anemia following hepatitis. Gold, methyprylon (piperidine) and idiopathic aplastic anemia have also each been reported in sets of siblings.

It would appear that aplastic anemia may be associated with familial (genetic) predisposition to specific adverse environments. In some cases, physical abnormalities may direct attention to the possibly inherited nature of the condition. The familial and inherited marrow failure syndromes are clearly heterogeneous, representing a large variety of phenotypes and inheritance patterns. Only diligent investigation elucidates the relevant genetic and environmental factors.

Laboratory Findings

The patients in this heterogeneous group have variable degrees of pancytopenia, macrocytosis, Hb F level elevation, and hypocellular bone marrows. Only those whose families show additional features, such as immune deficiencies, novel chromosomes, or monosomy 7, may be distinguished from those with nonfamilial aplastic anemia. Those with familial disease but without characteristic findings are more difficult to detect. Baseline chromosome breakage is usually normal in the non-FA familial cases, but examination with clastogenic agents is required for definitive differentiation. Those patients who have hypoplastic or aplastic anemia also have reduced numbers of hematopoietic stem cells, another nonspecific finding.[557]

Pathophysiology

The aplastic anemia is the result of combinations of genetic and environmental factors that are unique to each family. The inheritance patterns are autosomal dominant, autosomal recessive, and X-linked recessive, as well as multifactorial. Because some of the families have features resembling those found in FA, it can be speculated that some of the genes may be allelic. The defects may be multiple, even at the hematopoietic level, because some of the patients have only single cytopenias. Thus, pluripotent or specific committed progenitor cells may be defective.

Therapy and Outcome

Many of the patients discussed in this section died from their aplastic anemia. Several were treated with transfusions, antilymphocyte globulin, androgens, or BMT, with some limited success being achieved. Since each case is practically unique, the only suggestion is that androgens might be more effective than immunosuppression. However, because immune dysfunction is part of some of the syndromes, even this statement is overly simplistic. In general, drug treatment and supportive care should be the same as described earlier for FA or for acquired aplastic anemia. BMT is risky because the potential donor may have the same condition. In several families, aplastic anemia is just the first step to preleukemia and leukemia. The overall prognosis for patients with familial bone marrow failure is poor.

Down Syndrome

Down syndrome (trisomy 21) infants often have a neonatal transient myeloproliferative syndrome. Later, there also is an increased risk of leukemia.[599] Five patients with aplastic anemia were reported.[2] A 17-year-old boy with "idiopathic" aplastic anemia and trisomy 21 apparently responded to androgen therapy. A newborn with trisomy 21, cystic fibrosis, and amegakaryocytic thrombocytopenia died at 49 days; this infant had pancytopenia shortly before death. A 12-year-old boy developed aplastic anemia that was unresponsive to androgen treatment and died within 10 weeks[600]; another patient with aplastic anemia at 19 months responded to androgen therapy. A fifth patient developed aplastic anemia at 9 months and died at 26 months with gastroenteritis. Bone marrows were hypocellular. The last patient had increased numbers of CFU-GMs with both cellular and serum inhibitors of hematopoiesis. Because of the small number of cases of trisomy 21 and aplastic anemia, it is not clear whether this is a true association or merely a coincidence.

Dubowitz's Syndrome

Dubowitz's syndrome is a rare, apparently autosomal recessive condition in which aplastic anemia has been reported in about 10% of the approximately 50 cases. The major features include intrauterine and postnatal growth retardation, microcephaly, moderate mental retardation, hyperactivity, eczema, and facial anomalies such as hypertelorism, epicanthal folds, blepharophimosis, broad nose, and abnormal ears. Autosomal recessive inheritance was suggested by a recent summary of 17 males and 21 females,[601] with one set of twins, four sibling pairs, and one consanguineous family. Seven patients had bone marrow failure noted at the ages of 3 to 12 years, with pancytopenia, macrocytosis, increased Hb F levels, and hypoplastic marrow or marrow with myeloid maturation arrest.[602–605] One of two who received oxymetholone experienced a response to treatment. Chromosome breakage was normal in three, and increased with the use of MMC and DEB in two. Three patients had malignancies—namely, lymphoma, ALL, and neuroblastoma.[606, 607] This syndrome is another that is characterized by growth defects and is associated with hematopoietic disorders and malignancies.

Seckel's Syndrome

Seckel's syndrome is another rare autosomal recessive condition with aplastic anemia. The term *Seckel's syndrome* may have been overused in the characterization of a heterogeneous group of more than 60 reported microcephalic dwarfs, and thus the true number of those affected is uncertain. The stringent definition includes severe intrauterine and postnatal growth retardation, severe microcephaly, severe mental retardation, typical face with receding forehead and chin, antimongoloid slant of palpebral fissures, a prominently curved nose, relatively large eyes and teeth, highly arched palate, hirsutism, and clinodactyly.[608] At least 25% developed aplastic anemia[2, 609] or malignancies (Hodgkin's disease, lymphosarcoma and neuroblastoma, ALL (n = 2),[610] acute myeloid leukemia,[611] and hepatoma[612]). The aplasias were noted at the ages of 4 to 16 years. Three patients died from sepsis (or causes not reported) at 7, 9, and 12 years of age, 2 to 5 years after diagnosis. Two failed to respond to androgen treatment, and all required transfusions. One died 2 weeks after BMT, and one was alive 1.5 years after BMT. The cancers were diagnosed at ages 1 to 26 years, and the patients did not survive. The diagnosis of FA was considered in many patients because they were small, microcephalic, retarded, and had pancytopenia. Actually, patients with Seckel's syndrome are much smaller and more severely microcephalic and retarded than those with FA. Results of chromosome studies were normal in five patients[609, 613, 614]; endogenous breakage was increased in one patient and was in-

creased further with MMC testing in a sibling.[615] However, the diagnosis of FA could not be firmly established. Two patients with Seckel's syndrome without aplastic anemia had normal endogenous chromosomes and normal SCEs.[616] Seckel's syndrome is another autosomal recessive syndrome characterized by growth retardation, occasional aplastic anemia, and, probably, chromosome breakage that is not increased.

Noonan's Syndrome

Patients with Noonan's syndrome have characteristic facies, with hypertelorism, ptosis, low-set ears, and short necks, as well as short stature and congenital heart defects; these patients resemble those with Turner's syndrome (45,XO). Inheritance is autosomal dominant in one half of the cases, and genetic linkage has localized the gene to chromosome 12q.[617] Three patients with amegakaryocytic thrombocytopenia diagnosed from birth to the age of 30 years have been reported[618–620]; another patient was diagnosed with pancytopenia and hypocellular marrow at the age of 4 years.[621] As in the other syndromes, the incidence of marrow failure is unknown.

SINGLE CYTOPENIAS

Bone marrow failure disorders in which only one cell line is involved are called *single cytopenias*. Most patients with these disorders do not go on to develop pancytopenias, unlike those described above. White cell and platelet disorders are discussed at length in other chapters of this text (see Chapters 22 and 43).

Red Blood Cells
Acquired Pure Red Cell Aplasia

This disorder is associated with isolated failure of erythropoiesis. Patients with PRCA have anemia, reticulocytopenia, and bone marrow erythroblastopenia, with normal white blood cell and platelet counts.[2, 4, 622] The differential diagnosis is shown in Table 7–26. Those disorders that are uniquely pediatric—namely, inherited PRCA (Diamond-Blackfan anemia) and transient erythroblastopenia of childhood (TEC)—are described at length later in this section. The other conditions listed in Table 7–26 occur in both children and adults or primarily in adults; a few of these conditions are discussed briefly here.

Description

This specific anemia is a rare acquired disease that occurs at a mean age of 60 years[2, 4, 622]; however, 10% of the cases reported in one review were teenagers.[623] Rare familial cases have been reported.[624, 625] The male-to-female ratio of occurrence is 2:1 in those without and 1:2 in those with a thymoma, which was present in 50% of patients in one analysis.[626] There is no racial predilection.

Table 7–26. DIFFERENTIAL DIAGNOSIS OF PURE RED CELL APLASIA*

Inherited

Diamond-Blackfan anemia

Acquired

Thymoma and Malignancy

Thymoma
Lymphoid malignancies: chronic lymphocytic leukemia, lymphoma, malignant histiocytosis, Kaposi's sarcoma, acute lymphocytic leukemia, Hodgkin's disease, multiple myeloma
Other hematologic diseases: myelodysplasia, chronic myelogenous leukemia, myelofibrosis
Paraneoplastic to solid tumors: carcinomas of bronchus, breast, stomach, thyroid, bile duct, skin

Collagen Vascular Disease

Systemic lupus arythematosus
Juvenile rheumatoid arthritis
Rheumatoid arthritis
Multiple endocrine gland insufficiency

Autoantibodies **(dark type)**

Anti erythroblast
Anti erythroid progenitor
Anti erythropoietin

Virus

Human parvovirus B19
Hepatitis
Adult T-cell leukemia virus
Epstein-Barr virus
Human immunodeficiency virus (HIV)

Pregnancy

Drugs

Probably Associated

Antiepileptics (diphenylhydantoin, carbamazepine, sodium dipropylacetate, sodium valproate)
Azathioprine
Chloramphenicol and thiamphenicol
Sulfonamides (salicylazosulfapyridine, sulfathalazine, methazolamide (and hepatitis)), chlorpropamide, sulfathiazole, co-trimoxazole
Isoniazid
Procainamide

Occasional, Possibly Coincidentally Associated

Nonsteroidal anti-inflammatory drugs (aminopyrine, phenylbutazone, fenoprofen, sulindac)
Allopurinol
Halothane (and hepatitis)
D-Penicillamine
Dapsone
Quinidine and quinacrine
Gold
Benzene and compounds with benzene (pentachlorophenol, arsenicals, insecticides)

Idiopathic

---

*Some drugs have been linked to pure red cell aplasia (PRCA) in patients with diseases that may predispose to PRCA; some drugs have been given to patients who may have had acute parvovirus infection.

From Young NS, Alter BP: Bone marrow failure. In Handin RI, Lux SE, Stossel TP (eds): Blood: Principles and Practice of Hematology. New York, Lippincott-Raven, 1994. Illustrator, Joy D. Marlowe, M.A., A.M.I.

Most cases of acquired PRCA are probably primary and occur without obvious associations with any of the factors listed in Table 7–26. Many of these patients have soluble or, more frequently, cellular inhibitors of erythropoiesis. Still others do not have inhibitors or known associations and thus have truly idiopathic disease.

Laboratory Findings

The anemia usually is normochromic and normocytic, although macrocytosis has been seen. White cell and platelet counts are only rarely decreased. Bone marrow cellularity is normal, with decreased numbers or absence of erythroid precursors. Serum iron concentration is increased and iron binding saturated, and ferrokinetic studies show prolonged clearance of ^{59}Fe, reduced plasma iron turnover, and very low iron utilization. Bone marrow imaging with ^{111}In shows diminished uptake.

Chest radiography may identify a mediastinal mass, but thymomas should be sought with computed tomography. Immune deficits and hypogammaglobulinemia occur. Autoimmune disease can be documented with antibodies to red cells, acetylcholinesterase (myasthenia), smooth muscle, intrinsic factor, and nuclei (collagen vascular disease), as well as with the finding of paraproteins. In any patient determined to have autoimmune disease, only one or two of these abnormalities are found.

Clinical Associations

Immune Diseases. Thymoma is the most familiar association, although the over-reporting of interesting observations has probably exaggerated this lesion's actual prevalence, which may be much lower.[627] Among all patients with thymomas, 5% to 10% develop PRCA. Only one case was reported in a child; this child had a thymoma and later developed pancytopenia.[73] Thymoma and even thymectomy may precede the onset of PRCA by several years. The thymomas are usually spindle cell type and encapsulated, although malignant metastatic tumors can occur. The tumors must be excised, but hematologic improvement need not follow their removal.

Many PRCA patients, with or without thymomas, have evidence of other autoimmune dysfunction, such as myasthenia gravis, collagen vascular diseases (e.g., systemic lupus erythematosus), multiple endocrinopathies, and immunologic abnormalities. Among patients with lymphoid neoplasms, the incidence of PRCA may be as high as 6%[628] (see Table 7–26).

Drugs. PRCA has occurred during treatment with some drugs or after exposure to some chemicals (see Table 7–26), and it has responded to removal of the causative agent. In a few instances, rechallenge with the agent led to recurrence of the reversible anemia. One example of such a drug is phenytoin, which has been reported several times as causing PRCA and which has been associated with a drug-dependent antibody in at least one case.[629] Another antiepileptic that has rarely caused PRCA in children is sodium valproate.[630]

Viruses. Viral hepatitis is presumed to be a cause of PRCA[624] and has been ascribed to humoral[631] or cellular[632] inhibitors of erythropoiesis. PRCA has occurred in the setting of infectious mononucleosis[633] and human T-cell lymphotropic virus type I infection.[634] A virus of interest that may cause PRCA is the human immunodeficiency virus (HIV),[635] although this virus is unlikely to have a direct role. One virus of specific hematologic relevance is parvovirus, which is discussed later in this chapter. (Viruses can cause PRCA in animals; such viruses include feline leukemia virus[636] and simian parvovirus.[637])

Nutrition. PRCA was documented in children with malnutrition, and it is associated with protein deficiency.[2, 4] The aplasia sometimes develops during refeeding of the marasmic patient, who may respond to treatment with riboflavin or prednisone. Baboons who were made riboflavin deficient developed erythroid aplasia that responded to riboflavin or prednisone. Humans who were made experimentally riboflavin deficient also developed PRCA that responded to treatment with this vitamin. Some patients with kwashiorkor developed transient PRCA during refeeding despite administration of folic acid and riboflavin. The specific roles of hematinics during the refeeding of malnourished patients are undoubtedly complex. Thiamine-responsive anemia, diabetes, and deafness occur in beriberi, as well as in patients whose thiamine stores are normal and yet respond to high-dose thiamine treatment. This condition may be autosomal recessive.

Other Factors. A few cases of PRCA have appeared during pregnancy and resolved post partum.[638] Occasionally, patients with apparent autoimmune hemolytic anemia have also had bone marrow erythroblastopenia.[639] Infants with immune hemolytic anemia due to Rh incompatibility may have transient marrow erythroblastopenia, presumably due to antibody reaction with erythroid precursors, as well as with mature erythrocytes.

Pathophysiology

Gasser was the first to suggest that PRCA might be an "allergic reaction" due perhaps to antibody to bone marrow cells.[640] The hypothesis was supported by several studies: some plasmas inhibited heme production in bone marrow suspensions; fluorescent marker–labeled purified γ-globulin was found to be specific for erythroblast nuclei; some plasmas led to complement-mediated erythroblast cytolysis; and a few patients were found to have antibody to erythropoietin.[623, 641, 641a] Assays of erythroid colony formation[2, 4] have shown serum inhibitors in almost one half of patients (without lymphoid malignancies). Autologous colony growth was often exuberant in the absence of the patient's sera. Purified IgG was inhibitory in several cases. Inhibitory T cells are detected in 75% of all patients.[2, 4, 642] Patients with chronic T-cell lymphocytosis have a T8 phenotype, with genetic restriction of marrow suppression. Patients with T-cell chronic lymphocytic leukemia had inhibitory T cells, as did patients with B-cell chronic lymphocytic leukemia.

Lacombe and co-workers correlated erythroid colony growth *in vitro* with outcome in 22 patients with idiopathic PRCA.[643] Thirteen type I patients were demonstrated to have normal or increased numbers of CFU-E–derived colonies in fetal calf or normal AB sera, and 4 also had normal blood BFU-E frequencies. Most of these patients did well with immunosuppressive therapy. Five type II patients had decreased frequencies of marrow CFU-Es and blood BFU-Es and did poorly. Four type III patients had total absence of erythroid progenitors and failed immunotherapy; this outcome suggests that these patients might have had a stem cell defect. Erythroid cultures have a role in the management of PRCA: colony growth is predictive of a response to immunosuppressive therapy, and a cellular or humoral mechanism may be demonstrated by cell depletion or serum addition experiments.

Therapy and Outcome

Response may occur in drug-mediated PRCA when use of the drug is discontinued. Remission occurs following thymectomy in 25% of those with a thymoma. The next therapeutic step is some form of "immunosuppression."[2, 4] Prednisone induces remission in about one third of cases. Cytotoxic drugs such as 6-mercaptopurine, azathioprine, or cyclophosphamide can be used if prednisone is ineffective. Alternatively, many patients respond to antilymphocyte globulins or cyclosporine.[644] Plasmapheresis was useful in a few patients who clearly had antibodies to erythroid progenitors. Less effective treatments include splenectomy and danazol therapy. Responses to intravenous immunoglobulin administration may represent successful treatment of occult parvovirus infection (see next section). Fortunately, most patients eventually improve; in one series, spontaneous remissions occurred in 14% of patients, whereas all modalities failed in 34% of patients.[645] Supportive care may be needed for the anemia (e.g., periodic red cell transfusions and iron chelation therapy), as described earlier for patients with aplastic anemia. Deaths in patients with PRCA are due to autoimmune diseases, pancytopenia, or complications from transfusion support. Evolution to leukemia in these patients is rare (<5%).[646]

Parvovirus

Description

Transient Aplastic Crises. Human parvovirus B19 has direct effects on hematopoiesis and causes several hematologic syndromes.[25, 647] B19 parvovirus is the causative agent in fifth disease, the common childhood exanthem, and polyarthropathy in adulthood. Parvovirus infection is common in children and adults, and the rate of IgG seropositivity increases with age, so that most elderly individuals have evidence of past infection. Most frequently, infection is asymptomatic.[648]

The virus was first associated with disease when it was detected in the sera of children with sickle cell anemia during aplastic crises.[26] Virtually all community-acquired transient aplastic crises are secondary to acute parvovirus infection.[27] Transient aplastic crisis due to parvovirus occurs in other hemolytic anemias, in compensated hemolysis, with iron deficiency or bleeding, and under conditions of erythropoietic "stress."[2, 4] Transient aplastic crisis appears as a severe worsening of chronic anemia or as the abrupt onset of anemia in compensated hemolysis; the anemia may be life threatening. Reticulocytes are absent in the blood and erythroid precursor cells in the marrow; giant pronormoblasts, the pathognomonic feature of B19 parvovirus infection, may be scattered throughout the aspirate. Rarely, marrow necrosis can occur. The disease is self-limited, and anemia resolves over the course of 1 to 2 weeks as antibodies against the virus are produced.

There is little evidence of involvement of human parvovirus B19 in acquired aplastic anemia.[2, 4] Only occasional cases of transient erythroblastopenia of childhood have been linked to the virus.[649, 650] Suppression of other cell lines can occur,[651, 652] and viral infection has been suggested to be causative in some cases of childhood neutropenia, as well as in idiopathic thrombocytopenic purpura.[653] The parvovirus has also been implicated in some vasculitides[654] and as a cause of hemophagocytic syndrome.[655]

Pure Red Cell Aplasia. Chronic anemia due to persistent parvovirus infection occurs in the context of immunodeficiency: in congenital immunodeficiency syndromes, in acquired immunodeficiency secondary to HIV type 1 infection, and with iatrogenic immunosuppression during chemotherapy for cancer, for autoimmune disease, or after transplantation.[25, 656] The underlying immunodeficiency state (which, when congenital, usually is termed *Nezelof's syndrome*) may be clinically subtle, and chronic infection has been described in apparently normal persons.[657] In acquired immunodeficiency syndrome (AIDS), PRCA due to parvovirus may be the presenting syndrome.[31] About 15% of "idiopathic" PRCA is probably due to persistent parvovirus infection.[32] As in transient aplastic crisis, marrow studies show the absence of erythroid cells except for the presence of rare giant early erythroid forms.[31]

Hydrops Fetalis. *In utero* infection with parvovirus, particularly during the second trimester, may lead to nonimmune hydrops fetalis, which can be detected by ultrasound.[658–660] The risk of death due to hydrops when the mother has documented parvovirus infection has been estimated from epidemiologic studies to be about 9%, and infection earlier in pregnancy may result in spontaneous abortions in about 5% of cases.[661–664] Maternal blood shows evidence of recent parvovirus infection with IgM antibody or IgG seroconversion and may have elevated α-fetoprotein levels. Fetal blood sampling may demonstrate anemia. Treatment can be provided with intrauterine simple or exchange transfusions performed by skilled perinatal obstetricians.

Congenital Infection. Three cases of congenital parvovirus infection that resulted in a clinical picture resembling Diamond-Blackfan anemia or constitutional dyserythropoiesis were described in infants who survived hydrops because they received a transfusion.[29] Establishing the diagnosis is difficult because the virus is restricted to the marrow and detectable only with the use of gene amplification methods. In case reports, congenital parvovirus infection has been associated with myocarditis,[659] advanced liver disease,[665] and thrombocytopenia.[666]

Laboratory Findings

The presence of giant pronormoblasts, when observed on analysis of a marrow aspirate, strongly suggests the diagnosis of parvovirus infection. Antibodies to parvovirus may be detected in commercial assays that use classic serologic techniques. Viremia usually lasts a week and is followed by an increase in IgM and, later, IgG titers. Normal volunteer studies demonstrated that marrow suppression occurs during the period of viremia and that fifth disease symptoms accompany antibody production and are likely immunecomplex mediated.[667] Marrow recovery follows antibody synthesis. Demonstration of increased IgG levels indicates past infection. Examination for viral DNA can be performed with serum by direct hybridization, or following gene amplification by the sensitive technique of polymerase chain reaction.[30]

Pathophysiology

The DNA virus infects mature erythroid progenitors (CFU-Es), preventing further replication and maturation; BFU-Es also are affected, but neither stem cells nor CFU-GMs are viral targets.[668, 669] *In vitro*, growth of erythroid colonies is prevented. The virus replicates in cell cultures that contain erythroid progenitors and erythropoietin, whether the cells are derived from marrow, blood, or fetal liver.[33, 670–672] The viral nonstructural protein effects direct cytotoxicity on the host cell. Phenotypically, the target cell has erythroid characteristics, including glycophorin expression.[673] The basis of erythroid tropism lies in the cellular receptor for the virus, globoside, or erythrocyte P antigen[674]; a glycolipid present on erythroid cells and some megakaryocytes; and endothelial cells, as well as placenta, fetal liver, and heart cells. Individuals of the unusual P erythrocyte phenotype are not susceptible to parvovirus B19 infection.[675] The clinical consequence of parvovirus infection is the arrest of erythropoiesis; however, in normal persons, the duration of erythropoietic failure is sufficiently brief that significant anemia does not occur. If the red cell survival is short, usually as a result of hemolysis, symptomatic anemia rapidly develops. Persistent infection is due to the immunocompromised host's inability to produce neutralizing antibody to the virus.[676]

Therapy and Outcome

The aplasia in hemolytic anemias is transient; however, supportive transfusions may be needed (usually, only on one occasion) until the marrow recovers, within 1 to 2 weeks. Fetal transfusions have been employed to treat hydrops *in utero* or at birth. Therapy with commercial immunoglobulins breaks the cycle of viral replication in the erythron and can be curative or ameliorative in persistent parvoviremia and chronic anemia.

Diamond-Blackfan Anemia

Description

Josephs first mentioned red cell aplasia in infancy in two cases reported in 1936.[677] Two years later, four more cases were presented by Diamond and Blackfan.[678] Synonyms and eponyms have included "congenital hypoplastic anemia," "chronic congenital aregenerative anemia," "erythrogenesis imperfecta," "chronic idiopathic erythroblastopenia with aplastic anemia (type Josephs-Diamond-Blackfan)," and "Diamond-Blackfan anemia." Diamond and Blackfan called it "congenital hypoplastic anemia" because they thought it differed from complete aplastic anemia (pancytopenia) only in degree. The term "hypoplastic" is now used when marrow depression is only partial and thus is not appropriate for describing a single cytopenia. "Erythrogenesis imperfecta" is probably the most descriptive appellation, but the term "Diamond-Blackfan anemia (DBA)" is used here because this is the term most frequently encountered in the literature.

The current diagnostic criteria for DBA are as follows: (1) normochromic, usually macrocytic but occasionally normocytic anemia developing early in childhood; (2) reticulocytopenia; (3) normocellular bone marrow with selective deficiency of red cell precursors; (4) normal or slightly decreased leukocyte counts; and (5) normal or often increased platelet counts. These criteria distinguish DBA from aplastic anemia (see earlier) but may not always distinguish it from TEC (see later in this chapter).

The data regarding the incidence of DBA are limited. A 7-year study in northern England found an annual incidence of one child per million children per year.[679] National DBA registries are developing, with 19 patients identified in Holland from 1963 to 1989,[680] more than 150 registered in North America,[681] and 66 found in the United Kingdom.[682] More than 500 cases of DBA have been described in the literature (Table 7–27), and many of the references are cited in previous reviews.[2, 4, 550, 683–685] The anemia is usually noted in infancy, but DBA has been diagnosed in patients as old as 34 years of age (Fig. 7–22). Males with DBA were diagnosed

slightly younger than females with the disease. Ten per cent were severely anemic at birth, 25% by 1 month, 50% by 2 months, 75% by 6 months, and almost 90% by 1 year of age. Seven per cent were diagnosed between the ages of 1 and 2 years. In total, however, 13% were diagnosed at an age of 1 year or older. The male-to-female ratio is 1.1. Although most reported cases are in Caucasians, DBA has been diagnosed in more than 20 blacks, more than a dozen Japanese, 4 Asian Indians, and 1 Navajo.

One case presented at an older age. A 34-year-old male with anemia had an anemic daughter and, subsequently, a grandson with classic DBA.[686, 687] Two adults with long-standing anemia who were short and had features typical of DBA, including web neck and thenar atrophy, responded to prednisone therapy.[688]

Inheritance and Environment. The inheritance of DBA is not clear and may have more than one pattern. *Dominant inheritance* is apparent in 20 families in which 1 parent had childhood anemia requiring transfusions or steroid therapy, or both, and one or more children have classic DBA.[2, 4, 689, 690] In these dominant families, involvement among fathers and mothers is equal. In one family, the maternal grandfather, mother, and a son all had DBA[686, 687]; in another, the patients were the grandfather, father, uncle, and son. In a family with two affected DBA children, the grandfather had refractory sideroblastic anemia.[691, 692] There are two reports of three-generation families with seven and six patients, respectively.[693, 694] Four families with affected stepchildren also were reported. In three, the father was the link; in the fourth family, it was the mother. In all four families, the carrier parent had increased Hb F levels and macrocytosis without significant anemia. The numbers of males and females in the dominant group are equal, the incidence of physical abnormalities low, and the clinical course generally milder than in the overall DBA population.

Recessive inheritance might be invoked in another 32 families, of whom 9 had consanguinity[2, 4, 695–697] and 23 had more than 1 affected child with normal parents. Details were provided for 54 cases and the sex of the affected siblings were given for several more. In this small group, twice as many males were affected as females. Twelve sibling or cousin sets consist of males only, two sets are females, and five sets are males and females. One set of male twins was reported in a

Table 7-27. DIAMOND-BLACKFAN ANEMIA LITERATURE

	1927–1960	1961–1970	1971–1980	1981–1990	1991–1995	Total
No. of patients	78	110	91	109	139	527
Male:female	0.8	1.2	1.1	1.3	1.2	1.1
Male, age* at diagnosis, mean	3.6	5.4	7.6	12.9	18.6	10.1
Median	2	2	2	2	3	2
Range	0–24	0–48	0–54	0–48	0–164	0–408
Female, age* at diagnosis mean	6.2	5.4	8.2	15.2	22	11.6
Median	3	2	3	3	3	3
Range	0–28	0–46	0–48	0–264	0–420	0–420
No. of males >1 y	1	6	8	2	8	25
No. of females >1 y	6	4	7	5	11	33

*Ages are in months.

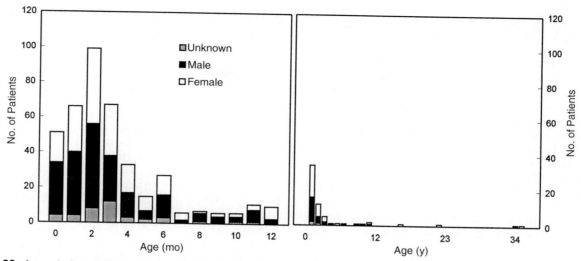

Figure 7-22. Age at diagnosis in more than 500 published cases with Diamond-Blackfan anemia (DBA). Shaded bars = males; open bars = females; Crosshatched bars = sex not reported.

siblingship with three affected males[698]; one set of affected identical twins has also been reported.[699] Anomalies occurred more frequently in the recessives than in the overall group, but the anemia was milder and more responsive.

The recessive cases are presumably autosomal, although X-linked inheritance might explain the families in which only males were affected. The "recessive" families might also be dominant with variable expression, but consanguinity makes this possibility less likely. Approximately 75% of cases are sporadic, suggesting new mutations, acquired disease, or variable penetrance.

Although data in the literature regarding pregnancies are often incomplete, more than a dozen mothers of children with DBA had previous stillbirths or miscarriages. Problems during pregnancy include preeclampsia, toxemia, rashes, premature placental separation, placental infarcts, hemorrhage, spotting, and positive test results for syphilis. Exposures during pregnancy involved stilbestrol, x-rays, chlorothiazide, reserpine, thyroid hormones, prednisone, phenylbutazone, chloramphenicol, and anagyrine. More than 30 patients weighed less than 2500 g at birth. Of these, only a dozen were premature by date, and the rest were small for gestational age (intrauterine growth retardation). Although birth-lengths were rarely recorded, several were below 45 cm. The low birthweights might reflect pregnancy problems or poor growth intrinsic to DBA itself.

Most patients were pale at birth or soon thereafter. Jaundice due to hemolytic disease of the newborn from Rh or ABO incompatibility occurred occasionally, leading to prolonged anemia that became chronic or that sometimes resolved after a few months. Antecedent illnesses were reported, including diarrhea, respiratory infections, urinary tract infections, measles, mumps, or a reaction to smallpox vaccination. One child was treated with chloramphenicol.[700] In most children, the illness was more likely to be due to the anemia or

unrelated rather than the cause of the anemia. Signs of anemia included pallor, lethargy, irritability, and heart failure. Three infants were born following intrauterine infection with parvovirus and had B19 DNA in bone marrow cells (as detected with PCR),[29] but none responded to intravenous immunoglobulin therapy. Another patient had a parvovirus-induced relapse from a spontaneous remission of his DBA.[701] The role of parvovirus in DBA needs to be examined more closely.

Physical Examination. Physical appearances were abnormal in more than 100 patients (24%) and more frequently in females than in males (28% and 22%, respectively; Table 7–28). Abnormalities of the head and face were the most common. The typical face was described by Cathie as "tow coloured hair, snub nose, wide set eyes, thick upper lip, and an intelligent expression"[702]; these features were observed in many of the children, who resembled each other more than

Table 7-28. PHYSICAL ABNORMALITIES IN DIAMOND-BLACKFAN ANEMIA

Abnormality	Males	Females	Total
No. of patients	254	226	527
Birth-weight, ≤2500 g	6%	11%	7%
Head, face, palate	7%	14%	10%
Upper limbs	7%	10%	8%
Short stature	12%	14%	13%
Eyes	6%	7%	6%
Renal	4%	4%	4%
Neck	0.4%	2%	1%
Hypogonadism	5%	0%	3%
Retardation	2%	4%	2%
Lower limbs	0%	1%	1%
Cardiopulmonary	2%	2%	2%
Nose	1%	1%	1%
Other skeletal	4%	6%	4%
Other anomalies	6%	5%	5%
At least one abnormality*	22%	28%	24%

*Excludes low birth-weight as the only finding. Several patients had more than one birth defect.

they did their own family members. Cleft lip or palate occurred in 3%. Other findings included micrognathia, microcephaly or macrocephaly, macroglossia, wide fontanelle, and dysmorphic features.

A specific comment must be made regarding upper limb anomalies, which are found in about 50% of FA patients (see earlier) and at least 8% of DBA patients. The most frequent feature in DBA is flattening of the thenar eminences or weakness of radial pulses, but other radial hand anomalies also are common. Triphalangeal thumbs were reported in 19 patients (bilateral in 14, and unilateral in 5) in whom the course of anemia was not different from that of the entire DBA group.[2, 4, 697, 703] Although this association has been separated by some into the *Aase syndrome*, it is probably an inappropriate example of splitting rather than lumping.[704] Almost two dozen patients had bifid, supernumerary, absent, or subluxated thumbs,[2, 4, 704–706] also both unilaterally or bilaterally.

At least two dozen patients were short, unrelated to corticosteroid therapy. Four of 8 short DBA patients were growth hormone deficient and two were borderline, and growth hormone treatment did improve growth.[707] There were several reports of dwarfism,[2, 4] including achondroplasia, metaphyseal dysostosis, and cartilage-hair hypoplasia. Almost two dozen cases had short or web necks and included both Klippel-Feil syndrome (fused cervical vertebrae) and Sprengel's deformity (elevation of the scapula). A "Turner-like" phenotype was sometimes mentioned.

Eye anomalies in 30 patients included hypertelorism, blue sclerae, glaucoma, epicanthal folds, microphthalmos, cataracts, and strabismus. Kidney abnormalities such as horseshoe, duplicated, and absent kidneys also were noted in a few patients. Five per cent of males had hypogonadism, and a dozen patients were retarded. Lower limb problems included hip dislocation, achondroplasia, and club foot. Congenital heart disease was seen occasionally. The presence of anomalies serves more to confirm the diagnosis of DBA than to provide any prognosis regarding the course of the disease.

Laboratory Findings

All patients with DBA are by definition anemic. Although limited, data regarding hemoglobin levels at birth range from 2.6 to 14.8 g/dL, with a median hemoglobin level of 7 g/dL. In those infants diagnosed within the first 2 months of life, the range was from 1.5 to 10 g/dL and the median was 4 g/dL. In those diagnosed after 2 months, the hemoglobin level was also usually in the 4 g/dL range. Macrocytosis was frequent (but often not reported), and reticulocyte counts were decreased or zero. The representative blood smear in Figure 7–23 shows macrocytes, anisocytosis, and teardrops. White cell counts are usually normal, although they do often decrease with age. Twenty per cent of patients had counts of 5000 cells/μL or less at some time, and 5% had counts below 3000 cells/μL. Two heavily transfused older patients

developed significant neutropenia.* Platelet counts, although usually normal, were below 150,000 cells/μL at least once in 25% of patients and above 400,000 cells/μL in 20% of patients. Buchanan and co-workers noted elevated platelet counts in one half of 38 patients and decreased counts in one fourth on at least one occasion. Platelet function was normal.[708]

The level of Hb F is usually increased in DBA. It is distributed heterogeneously (Fig. 7–24), a factor indicating that the patients do not have a single clone of completely fetal cells. The Hb F has a fetal composition, with the ratio of $^G\gamma$ to $^A\gamma$ exceeding 60:40. The titer of red cell membrane antigen i also is increased, as in fetuses, whereas the adult counterpart, antigen I, remains at adult levels. These "fetal-like" erythrocyte features are seen in newly diagnosed patients and following treatment, and they persist even in spontaneous remissions. They are not unique to DBA but are characteristic of the "stress erythropoiesis" seen in any bone marrow failure.[78]

Bone marrow aspirates and biopsies demonstrate normal cellularity, myeloid cells, and megakaryocytes. Lymphocyte counts are often increased and were initially thought to be "hematogones."[709] Although eosinophilia was pointed out by Gasser,[640] it is not a common feature. Bernard and associates described three patterns of erythroid development.[710] The most common pattern is erythroid hypoplasia or total aplasia (Fig. 7–25), which is seen in 90% of patients. When present, the few erythroid precursors seen are immature proerythroblasts. The next most frequent pattern, seen in 5% of cases, is one of normal numbers and maturation of erythroblasts. The remaining 5% have erythroid hyperplasia but also a maturation arrest, with increased numbers of immature precursors.

Despite the variable bone marrow picture, all patients with DBA have reticulocytopenia. Thus, some patients have a form of ineffective erythropoiesis. In addition, dyserythropoietic morphology has been seen occasionally (see section on congenital dyserythropoietic anemia, later in this chapter). Two patients were reported to have ringed sideroblasts that later disappeared.[711, 712] Patients who have received multiple transfusions accumulate iron in marrow (see Fig. 7–25) and other organs.

Serum levels of iron, ferritin, folic acid, vitamin B_{12}, and erythropoietin[713] are all elevated. DBA is not due to a deficiency of any of the usual hematinic agents. Patients do not have antibodies to erythropoietin. Results of routine urinalyses are normal. A suggestion of an abnormality in tryptophan metabolism was not substantiated.[714] Hypocalcemia was observed, and mild hypogammaglobulinemia was noted in several patients. These parameters are normal in many other patients, however. Low numbers of T lymphocytes and a reduction in the ratio of helper cells to suppressor cells were reported by Finlay and co-workers, but abnormalities of T-cell function were not observed.[715] Ferrokinetic studies showed the expected delay in plasma iron clearance and low red cell utilization. Autologous

*Young NS: Unpublished data.

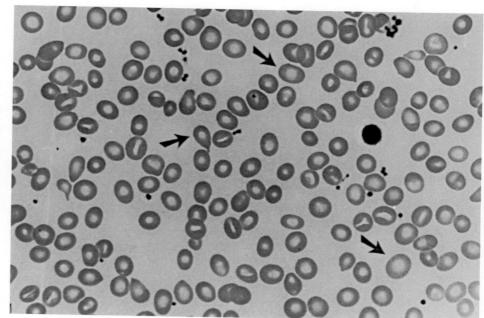

Figure 7-23. Peripheral blood from a patient with DBA. Note anisocytosis, with both microcytosis and macrocytosis, as well as teardrop erythrocytes *(arrows)*. (Courtesy of Dr. Gail Wolfe; with permission from Alter BP: The bone marrow failure syndromes. In Nathan DG, Oski FA (eds): Hematology of Infancy and Childhood. 3rd ed. Philadelphia, W.B. Saunders Co., 1987, p 159.)

red cell survival times were slightly shortened and haptoglobin levels were low; these findings suggest a mild hemolytic anemia. Patients with DBA have negative results on direct antiglobulin (Coombs') tests; their disease is not due to red cell autoantibodies, although alloantibodies may develop after many transfusions. Results of bone marrow cultures and erythropoietic inhibitor assays are described in the section on pathophysiology.

Abnormalities involving purine or pyrimidine metabolism were observed in red cell enzymes. Giblett and colleagues reported one patient with atypical DBA who also had lymphopenia and nucleoside-phosphorylase deficiency,[716] whereas other DBA patients had normal nucleoside-phosphorylase levels.[717] Zielke and co-workers found increased erythrocyte levels of the pyrimidine enzymes orotate phosphoribosyl transferase and orotidine monophosphate decarboxylase in 5 patients.[718] Increased orotidine monophosphate decarboxylase was observed in 5 of 10 patients in another study.[719] Because orotidine monophosphate decarboxylase level is age-dependent and is increased in cord blood cells, its elevation is consistent with the presence of young, fetal-like erythrocytes, as noted earlier.

Glader and colleagues noted increased red cell adenosine deaminase levels in 26 of 29 DBA patients[720] and in 2 of 12 parents.[717] Adenosine deaminase is a critical enzyme in the purine salvage pathway, and it is not

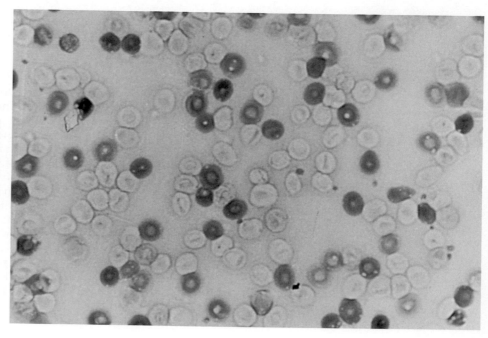

Figure 7-24. Kleihauer-Betke acid elution study of blood from a patient with DBA, showing the heterogeneous distribution of the fetal hemoglobin. (From Alter BP: The bone marrow failure syndromes. In Nathan DG, Oski FA (eds): Hematology of Infancy and Childhood. 3rd ed. Philadelphia, W.B. Saunders Co., 1987, p 159.)

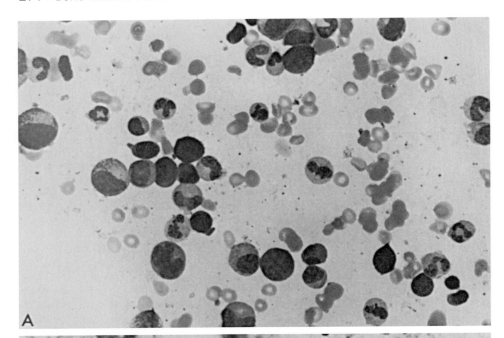

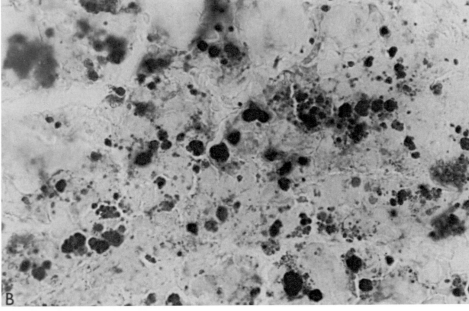

Figure 7-25. *A,* Bone marrow aspirate from a patient with DBA, showing normal cellularity with erythroid hypoplasia. *B,* Iron stain of bone marrow aspirate from a 2-year-old child with transfusion-dependent DBA. (Courtesy of Dr. Gail Wolfe; with permission from Alter BP: The bone marrow failure syndromes. In Nathan DG, Oski FA (eds): Hematology of Infancy and Childhood. 3rd ed. Philadelphia, W.B. Saunders Co., 1987, p 159.)

elevated in erythrocytes from cord blood or patients with hemolytic or other aplastic anemias. Whitehouse and co-workers also found an increase in adenosine deaminase level in 9 of 19 patients and in 2 of 15 relatives.[721] The significance of the elevation in adenosine deaminase level is not clear because this enzyme's level also is increased in some children with leukemia[720]; this increase may indicate disordered erythropoiesis that is not fetal-like. Detection of increased adenosine deaminase levels may be useful in distinguishing acute DBA from TEC (see later).[720]

Peripheral blood lymphocyte chromosomes are essentially normal in patients with DBA.[683] One patient had an achromatic area in chromosome 1,[722] and another had a pericentric inversion in chromosome 1.[723] Three of six patients in one series had an enlarged chromosome 16,[724] and one patient had breaks and endoreduplication of chromosome 16.[725] One patient had increased spontaneous and x-ray–induced chromosome breakage without increased breakage due to MMC.[726] Some investigators found no increased breakage to DEB.[566, 727] More than 50 patients have had normal chromosomes, including 20 of our own.[683] Sister chromatid exchange is also normal. Although some DBA patients may have physical features resembling those of FA, the chromosome studies are clearly distinctive.

Prenatal Diagnosis. One fetus with two DBA siblings apparently had high-output cardiac failure detected with two-dimensional fetal Doppler echocardiography.[728] The specificity of this assay has been questioned, however.[729] An untested hypothesis proposes that erythrocyte adenosine deaminase level would be increased in a fetus with DBA. Similarly, the number of BFU-Es in DBA fetal blood might be decreased (see below), but this too has not been examined. Because only approximately 10% of the DBA cases are familial, the opportunities for prenatal testing are limited.

Pathophysiology

Because the genetics, time of onset of anemia, and physical appearances of patients with DBA are varied, the disease may have multiple causes. Most *in vitro* studies of erythropoiesis were limited to small numbers of patients. Differing results may be due to true variability of the disease. The consensus is that there is an intrinsic abnormality in the erythroid progenitor cell, although a few studies have suggested extrinsic abnormalities in accessory cells or serum.

The level of the major erythropoietic hormone erythropoietin in DBA is higher than would be expected for the level of anemia.[2, 713] Transient improvements were seen in 6 of 10 patients given plasma infusions.[713, 730] The mechanism of response is unknown, and this observation has not been corroborated. The response was probably not due to provision of erythropoietin because the plasmas were from normal individuals.

Early case reports suggested that DBA might be due to red cell alloantibodies.[2, 4] The patients had neonatal jaundice and ABO or Rh incompatibility, and anemia persisted longer than expected; in a few patients, true DBA was eventually diagnosed. Antibody specificity may have included erythroblasts or progenitors; blood group sensitization may have been real but unrelated. The majority of patients did not have blood group incompatibility.

Ortega and co-workers[731] have proposed the existence of a circulating inhibitor of erythropoiesis, but this conjecture has not been confirmed.[732, 733] Treatment of patient serum with an antibody to erythropoietin failed to unmask an inhibitor of erythropoiesis. In erythroid progenitor cultures in semisolid media, only one patient was found to have a serum erythroid blocking factor that was seen only in allogeneic and not autologous cultures.[734]

Cellular inhibitors have also been proposed. Peripheral blood lymphocytes from six DBA patients who had received multiple transfusions inhibited erythroid colony formation by normal bone marrow cells.[735] However, Nathan and co-workers were unable to detect inhibitory lymphocytes from one of those patients using HLA-identical marrow as the target.[736] Another DBA patient had normal erythroid progenitor cells and no cellular inhibitors.[511] Suppressor T cells in the blood of two adults who had undergone frequent transfusion as children[734] were suggested to have been overcome by a serum blocking factor.[737] Finlay and associates observed T-cell suppression of normal erythroid colony growth in one of five patients.[715] Inhibitory monocytes were proposed by Zanjani and Rinehart.[738] One adult had normal bone marrow colonies, but heme synthesis was inhibited by her bone fragments; this implied the presence of a microenvironmental defect.[739]

Nathan and associates found no inhibition of normal or autologous marrow CFU-Es by lymphocytes from four transfusion-dependent patients and no inhibition of normal or autologous blood BFU-Es by lymphocytes from 8 other patients, some of whom were transfusion-dependent and others in steroid-independent remissions.[740] Patients' T cells stimulated normal blood null cell BFU-Es, as did normal T cells.[741] The cellular suppression phenomenon may relate to transfusion sensitization, and not to the pathophysiology of DBA.

Cumulative evidence indicates that the erythroid stem cell is defective in DBA. Cultures of bone marrow and blood mononuclear cells in plasma clot or methyl cellulose showed a decrease in or absence of CFU-Es or BFU-Es, or both, in most patients.[2, 4, 742–744] Normal numbers tended to be seen in younger, previously untreated patients.[742, 744] Those who subsequently responded to prednisone may have had better *in vitro* erythroid growth. The addition of steroids to cultures from a few patients increased colony growth and correlated with clinical response.

In some patients, unusually high concentrations of erythropoietin improved erythroid colony growth.[2, 4] Nathan and associates studied two relapsed patients who improved clinically with prednisone treatment and whose progenitors then responded to the usual levels of erythropoietin.[740] Crude erythropoietin, which may have contained other erythroid growth–promoting factors, was used for these experiments. Lipton and colleagues added "burst-promoting activity" and demonstrated increased erythroid growth and increased erythropoietin sensitivity in DBA bone marrow cultures.[745] They then enriched for erythroid progenitors by removing monocytes and lymphocytes and enhanced the burst-promoting activity effect; this suggested that burst-promoting activity acts directly on progenitors and not through accessory cells.[746] The burst-promoting activity probably involves specific growth factors and erythroid activity, such as GM-CSF and IL-3. Halpérin and colleagues reported that the size and number of marrow BFU-Es was enhanced with IL-3 *in vitro*.[747] The previously reported insensitivity to erythropoietin may have reflected insensitivity to burst-promoting activity or specifically to IL-3.

Mice with mutations at the *W* or *Sl* loci have macrocytic anemia, as well as absence of hair pigment, mast cell deficiency, and sterility.[87] Homozygote *W* mutants have a defect in their hematopoietic stem cells, whereas the defect in *Sl* mice is in the microenvironment. The *W* mutation is in the *KIT* protooncogene, a transmembrane tyrosine kinase receptor,[748] whereas the *Sl* mutation is in the *KIT* ligand, SCF.[749] These mice provide attractive models for human DBA. In fact, the human disease due to a mutation in *KIT* is piebaldism, a dominant disorder with a white forelock, but the rare homozygotes are not anemic.[750, 751] The anemia of *W* but not of *Sl* mice was improved with high doses of erythropoietin,[752] but neither anemia was responsive to steroid treatment[753] or IL-3[754] (see later). The genes for KIT and SCF did not demonstrate structural abnormalities in 30 patients,[755–758] suggesting that the DBA defect is not present in those genes. Despite this, SCF is an effective agent *in vitro* and leads to improvement or even normalization of growth of marrow BFU-Es (Fig. 7–26),[349, 742, 744, 756, 759, 760] and thus SCF remains a candidate for potential treatment trials.

Perdahl and associates have described an acceleration in programmed cell death (apoptosis) in DBA marrow.[761] They showed that progenitors were abnormally sensitive to deprivation of erythropoietin and that the typical DNA oligosomes appeared rapidly. These findings further indicate that the DBA defect is intrinsic to the erythroid progenitor cell.

Therapy and Outcome

Transfusions. Initially, the only available treatment for DBA was blood transfusion; without this treatment, affected children died of anemia.[677] Blood transfusion remains the mainstay for the steroid-resistant patient. Leukocyte-depleted packed red cells should be given every 3 to 6 weeks to keep hemoglobin levels above 6 g/dL. Crossmatching for minor blood groups is only necessary if sensitization leads to the appearance of alloantibodies. The major complication of transfusion is hemosiderosis, which was the cause of death in at least 20% of the more than 50 patients whose deaths were reported. The side effects of iron overload in DBA are identical to those seen in thalassemia major and include diabetes, cardiac failure, liver disease, growth failure, and failure to enter puberty. These complications do develop more slowly in DBA than in thalassemia, in which a hemolytic rather than an aplastic process is involved. Chelation of iron with subcutaneous desferrioxamine should begin as soon as patients have increased iron stores.

Splenectomy was reported in two dozen patients and had no beneficial effect except in those who had hypersplenism related to transfusions. One half of the splenectomy patients died, often from infections. Splenectomy is no longer recommended unless hypersplenism is present.

Corticosteroids. The use of corticosteroids was first proposed by Gasser, who noted erythroblastopenia in patients with transient allergic disorders and observed increased eosinophil counts in the marrows of patients with DBA.[640, 762] The drugs used initially were cortisone or adrenocorticotropic hormone,[763] but prednisone or prednisolone are now the drugs of choice. Allen and Diamond were the first to treat large numbers of patients, reporting remission in 12 of 22.[764]

Currently, the recommended initial dosage of prednisone is 2 mg/kg per day, given in 3 or 4 divided doses. Reticulocytes usually appear within 1 to 2 weeks. Some of the new erythropoiesis is apparently ineffective, because a sustained increase in hemoglobin level may not occur for several weeks; however, it is often seen within a month. The high, divided dose protocol should be continued until the hemoglobin level is greater than 10 g/dL. The prednisone dose should then be tapered slowly, by sequential elimination of the divided doses, until the patient is on a single daily dose that still maintains the hemoglobin level. This dose is then doubled and administered on alternate days; this is followed by a very slow decrease in the amount of the alternate-day dose, so that side effects are minimized. One group managed to give their patients prednisone daily for 1 week, followed by 1 or 2 weeks without the drug, to promote better growth[765]; this agenda failed in the authors' own attempts. Using alternate-day treatment, the prednisone dose varies from as little as 1 mg to as much as 40 mg, and patients can be extremely sensitive to small changes in dose. Side effects of steroids include growth retardation (seen in more than one half of patients),[684] osteoporosis, weight gain, cushingoid appearance, hypertension, diabetes, fluid retention, and gastric ulcers. A few patients had steroid-related cataracts or glaucoma.

The patterns of response to steroid therapy are numerous and include the following:

1. Rapid response, followed by steroid-independent remission, which occurs in less than 5% of patients.

2. Intermittent response, also seen in fewer than 5% of patients.

3. Response followed by steroid dependence, which was seen in 60% of patients. Up to 20% of these patients may eventually be able to maintain their hemoglobin levels without steroids.

4. Steroid response and dependence, followed by later failure to respond to the same or higher doses, seen in 5% of patients.

5. Requirement for very large daily doses with relapse when the dose is decreased, seen in fewer than 5% of patients. This usually means that transfusions must be resumed because of the side effects of the steroids.

6. No response, seen in 30% to 40% of patients.

Overall, steroid nonresponders, high-dose responders, and subsequent failures represent up to 50% of pa-

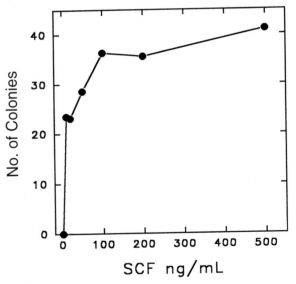

Figure 7-26. Stem cell factor (SCF) increases the numbers of erythroid progenitor-derived colonies from DBA bone marrow. This figure shows a representative study. (From Young NS, Alter BP: Aplastic Anemia. Acquired and Inherited. Philadelphia, W.B. Saunders Co., 1994, p 373.)

tients. In the total group, 15% to 20% may eventually have a spontaneous remission, regardless of their treatment response category. These remissions occurred at mean and median ages of 7 and 6 years, respectively, with the range being 1 month to 21 years of age.[2]

Failure to induce remission with prednisone therapy at 2 mg/kg per day should be followed by a trial of 4 to 6 mg/kg per day or by therapy with a different preparation such as prednisolone or dexamethasone. Use of marrow-suppressing drugs or those that might affect the metabolism of prednisone, such as phenytoin and phenobarbital, should be discontinued. Allen and Diamond[764] found that the response was better if the interval between diagnosis and treatment was short. A long interval might mean large numbers of transfusions were given with resultant hemochromatosis. Actually, steroid-induced remissions have been seen after 10 years of transfusions, and a history of transfusions should not preclude an adequate trial of steroid therapy coupled with iron chelation.

Several other therapeutic approaches have also been attempted.[2, 4] Androgens (see section on FA) were employed in more than 50 patients, but responses are rare. An attenuated androgen (danazol) was effective in two patients.[766] Treatment with 6-mercaptopurine was effective in 1 of 2 patients. Two patients had a transient reticulocytosis following cyclophosphamide and antilymphocyte globulin treatment,* whereas others did not respond to cyclophosphamide alone.[705] Vincristine also has been ineffective. Ozsoylu reported the successful use of high doses of intravenous or oral methylprednisolone, as described earlier for severe acquired aplastic anemia.[767] A few patients responded transiently to a combination of cyclosporine and prednisone, with reduction in dose but not elimination of prednisone.[2, 4, 29, 689, 696, 742, 768, 769] Intravenous immuno-

*Young NS: Unpublished data.

globulin also was ineffective.[29, 705, 768, 769] The rare anecdotal responses to immunosuppressive agents suggest that DBA might be an autoimmune disease, but the *in vitro* data do not support a role for such a mechanism (see earlier).

BMT is a possibility for those who do not respond to reasonable doses of steroids. Among 29 patients who received transplants from HLA-matched sibling donors and 1 unrelated donor, 19 survived.[2, 4, 770–773] Ages at transplantation ranged from 1 to 31 years, and all patients were steroid nonresponders or had relapse while on steroid therapy. Deaths were due to infection and graft-versus-host disease. The patients were prepared with various combinations of antilymphocyte globulin, procarbazine, total lymphoid irradiation, busulfan, and cyclophosphamide. Making the decision to carry out BMT in DBA is complicated because up to 20% of patients may eventually (but unpredictably) have a spontaneous remission; also, BMTs are generally more successful in young, relatively untransfused (and unsensitized) patients.

The survival data on more than 500 cases in the literature are shown in Figures 7–27 and 7–28. The predicted median survival ages have increased with time, exceeding 54 years in the cases reported in the last 5 years and averaging 42 years overall. Initially, those who did not receive steroids died if transfusions were not provided or died from iron overload if transfusions were not accompanied by iron chelation. Steroid treatment resulted in improvement of the survival curves, from a median of 19 years for those untreated to one of 42 years for those receiving steroids. Separate analyses of males and females, those with dominant or recessive inheritance, and those with abnormal thumbs did indicate differences in survival. However, the projected median survival following BMT is only 13 years of age, which suggests that older patients may not be good candidates for BMT.

Figure 7-27. Kaplan-Meier plot of cumulative survival age in years in DBA, according to dates of literature reports. Line 1 = 1936 to 1960; line 2 = 1961 to 1970; line 3 = 1971 to 1980; line 4 = 1981 to 1990; line 5 = 1991 to 1995.

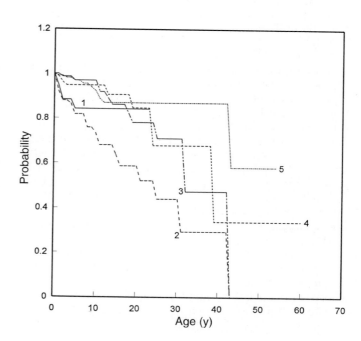

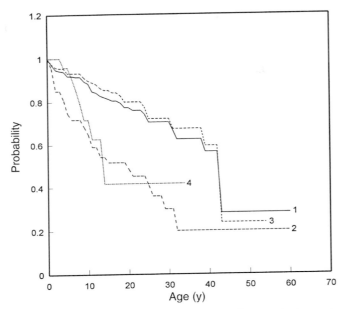

Figure 7-28. Kaplan-Meier plot of cumulative survival age in years in DBA, according to type of treatment. Line 1 = all patients; line 2 = no steroid; line 3 = steroid; line 4 = BMT.

Deaths were reported for more than 60 patients (approximately 15%); death occurred at a mean age of 10 years and median age of 5 years. Among those with "dominant" DBA, four (10%) died at the ages of 9, 10, 39, and 43 years. None of those with "recessive" disease were reported as deceased; this suggests that recessive disease may be milder (however, the authors are aware of two unreported deaths in this category). Two of 40 patients with thumb anomalies, including 1 of 19 years with triphalangeal thumbs, died at the ages of 2 and 31 years. Deaths were from complications of iron overload, as well as from pneumonia or sepsis, or both. Less frequent causes were BMT complications, leukemia (see later), renal disease, anesthesia, pulmonary emboli, and undefined central nervous system disorders.

Approximately 75 patients have participated in trials of hematopoietic growth factors. Ten patients failed to respond to low to moderate doses of erythropoietin[774, 775]; there are theoretic reasons to examine very high doses, however (see Pathophysiology, earlier in this section). Nine of more than 60 patients responded to IL-3 (14%).[776–780] A few of those remained in remission while off IL-3, whereas others were IL-3–dependent. *In vitro* growth of erythroid colonies in the presence of IL-3 was not predictive of response.[777] The use of GM-CSF was ineffective in 6 patients.[776] Cytokine treatment remains experimental, and the most effective agent used *in vitro*, SCF, is not yet being tested in clinical trials for DBA.

The long-term prognosis remains uncertain. The group with the best prognosis are those who respond to steroid therapy, approximately 50% of patients. Those who do not respond to steroids or those who eventually fail steroid treatment need transfusions and chelation therapy, BMT (if a donor is available), and

perhaps hematopoietic growth factors. The quality of life is usually quite good, particularly for those experiencing spontaneous remission and for steroid responders who can be maintained on low doses. Transfusion-dependent patients can be chelated as are patients with thalassemia major. Many DBA patients are now adults, and some have had normal children. Temporary worsening of anemia was noted during pregnancy in a few DBA patients, perhaps because of hormonal inhibition of erythropoiesis.[2]

Leukemia and Cancer. Leukemia was described in 9 patients, or 2% of the literature reports. One girl developed ALL at the age of 13 years and had a history of a spontaneous remission of her DBA at the age of 5 years.[781] The ALL also remitted completely, and the patient had neither DBA nor leukemia at the age of 17 years.* A female and a male from Diamond's original series[691] had intermittent remissions of DBA but died from AML at the ages of 31 and 43 years.[782]† The male had received irradiation to his thymus and to his long bones in order to "stimulate the bone marrow." One girl who had received cyclophosphamide died from acute promyelocytic leukemia at the age of 13 years.[783] A boy developed acute megakaryoblastic leukemia at the age of 14 months; the anemia present from 2 months of age might in fact have been a long preleukemic phase.[784] One male died at the age of 25 years from metastatic hepatocellular carcinoma that developed in a hemosiderotic liver.[785] Glader and colleagues reported three male steroid nonresponders who developed MDS at the ages of 13, 21, and 22 years.[786] The disease of one evolved into acute myelomonocytic and that of another into myeloid leukemia; the third died from complications of MDS. Two became transfusion independent and had nucleated red cells in the circulation when the myelodysplasia appeared. Another male who had DBA from age 7 months developed AML at 2 years of age.[773] Five of the 9 with leukemia died at 2 to 43 years of age. In a review of 72 patients seen in Boston, 4 had AML; it was predicted that 23% would have AML by age 30 to 40 years.[787]

One boy with hemochromatosis died with a hepatoma.[785] A female with DBA from birth developed breast cancer at the age of 22 years and responded to chemotherapy. She received a BMT at the age of 31 years for the DBA (not for the breast cancer) and was alive 3 years later.[771] Additional solid tumors reported in DBA include two patients with Hodgkin's disease, and one each with hepatocellular carcinoma, stomach cancer, osteogenic sarcoma, and vaginal melanoma,[787, 787a, 787b] as well as lung cancer‡ and lymphoma.§ Although the incidence of malignancies is not very high in DBA, it is above normal.

There are no well documented DBA cases that evolved into complete aplastic anemia, except following severe iron overload, perhaps associated with hepatitis, or during terminal sepsis. One pancytopenic pa-

---

*Schaison G: Personal communication, 1982.
†Gardner FH: Personal communication, 1977.
‡Nathan DG: Personal communication, 1996.
§Potter NU: Personal communication, 1996.

tient was mentioned without details by Najean.[788] In general, DBA remains a single cytopenia, and the prognosis for patients with it is better than that for those with many of the other marrow failure disorders.

Transient Erythroblastopenia of Childhood

Description

Acute erythroblastopenia in previously hematologically normal children was first described by Gasser in 1949.[762] Gasser reported 12 children in whom erythroblastopenia followed toxic, allergic, or infectious episodes. Because these children recovered rapidly, they did not develop anemia. Later, Baar evaluated red cell life span in an 8-year-old with "complete transient aplasia of the erythropoietic tissue."[789] In 1970, Wranne described 4 cases of temporary red cell aplasia as "erythroblastopenia of childhood."[790] More than 600 cases of TEC have been reported since 1970, as detailed case reports as well as series of cases without individual data.[2, 4, 679, 791, 792] These children have temporary peripheral blood reticulocytopenia and usually have anemia and bone marrow erythroblastopenia, with normal white blood cell and platelet counts. Young

patients with TEC were sometimes initially diagnosed as DBA; Table 7–29 distinguishes the two conditions. An English regional study found that the annual incidence of DBA was 1 and that of TEC was 5 per million children[679]; the comparable figure in Sweden was 4.3 per 100,000—the same as that for acute lymphocytic leukemia, but 10-fold greater than that found in England![791]

TEC is an acquired anemia in a previously healthy child, for whom prior normal blood counts are sometimes available. The male-to-female ratio of occurrence is 1.2:1, and the mean and median ages at diagnosis are 40 and 23 months, respectively (Fig. 7–29). More than 80% were 1 year of age or older; in contrast, fewer than 15% of those with DBA were of this age. However, only 10% of TEC patients were older than 3 years of age, with the oldest male being 10 and the oldest female being 16 years of age. There was a history of a preceding viral illness (upper respiratory or gastrointestinal) in approximately one half of patients, at a mean age of 1 year and an age range of 0 to 4 months. Because viral illnesses are common in young children, it is difficult to determine their relevance, although a viral etiology for TEC does have appeal (see Pathophysiology, earlier in this section). Neurologic manifestations of anemia—either seizures or transient ischemic attacks—were reported in 10 patients.[2, 4, 793–795] Drugs and toxins to which patients were exposed included piperazine, organic phosphates, penicillin, aspirin, sulfonamides, valproic acid, phenytoin, phenobarbital, and insecticides.[2, 4, 794, 795]

Familial TEC has been described in only three reports. One set of identical twins and a set of fraternal twins had simultaneous onset of anemia,[796, 797] and a pair of siblings had TEC at similar ages, 21 and 19

Table 7–29. COMPARISON OF DIAMOND-BLACKFAN ANEMIA AND TRANSIENT ERYTHROBLASTOPENIA OF CHILDHOOD

	DBA	TEC
No. of patients	527	608
Male:female	1.1	1.2
Male, age* at diagnosis, mean	10	40
Median	2	23
Range	0–408	1–120
Female, age* at diagnosis, mean	12	40
Median	3	23
Range	0–420	2–192
Males >1 y	10%	85%
Females >1 y	15%	82%
Etiology	Inherited?	Acquired
Antecedent history	None	Viral illness
Physical examination findings abnormal	24%	<1%
Hemoglobin (g/dL)	1.5–10	2.2–12.5
WBC < 3000/μL, or ANC < 1000/μL	5%	19%
Platelets > 400,000/μL	20%	60%
Red cell ADA	Increased	Normal
MCV increased at diagnosis	~80%	8%
During recovery	~100%	~90%
In remission	~100%	0%
Hb F increased at diagnosis	~100%	~25%
During recovery	~100%	~100%
In remission	~85%	0%
i Antigen increased at diagnosis	~100%	~20%
During recovery	~100%	~60%
In remission	~90%	0%

DBA = Diamond-Blackfan anemia; TEC = transient erythroblastopenia of childhood; WBC = white blood cell count; ADA = adenosine deaminase.
*Ages are in months.
Adapted with permission from Alter BP, Young NS: The bone marrow failure syndromes. In Nathan DG, Oski FA (eds): Hematology of Infancy and Childhood. 4th ed. Philadelphia, W.B. Saunders Co., 1993, p 216; and Alter BP: Childhood red cell aplasia. Am J Pediatr Hematol Oncol 1980; 2:121.

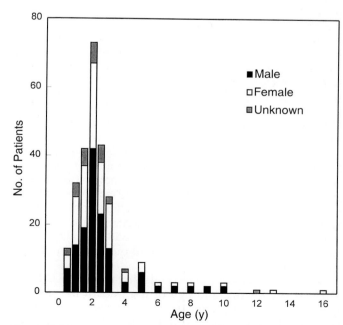

Figure 7–29. Age at diagnosis in more than 500 published cases of transient erythroblastopenia of childhood. Shaded bars = males; open bars = females; crosshatched bars = sex not reported.

months, but 2 years apart.[798] These familial occurrences suggest that TEC may result from the combination of an environmental factor (e.g., an infection) and a genetic propensity. All ethnic groups have been represented, including blacks and Japanese. Most of the reports have been of persons from temperate climates.

Seasonal TEC was suggested by the reports of apparent clusters, mostly from June to October (from November to March in one series).[2] All but one of these reports was from North America. However, the temporal clustering is not statistically significant. The number of cases is sufficiently small that the reported monthly variations may have been guided by chance. Clusters may be due to specific local viral epidemics, but until the putative virus is identified, this possibility remains speculation.

Findings on physical examinations are essentially normal in TEC, except for pallor and signs of anemia, such as tachycardia. The onset is gradual, and the pallor often is not noticed by the parents until the anemia is substantial.

Laboratory Findings

Hemoglobin levels ranged from 2.2 to 12.5 g/dL, with mean and median values of 5.7 g/dL. Reticulocyte counts were below 1% in most of the children, except those who were already recovering. White blood counts were often normal, but the absolute neutrophil count was below 1000 cells/μL in 19% of patients.[2, 4] In two large series, 5 of 24 and 12 of 64 patients had neutrophil counts below 1000 cells/μL. Platelet counts below 100,000 cells/μL were reported in only five patients, three of whom were also neutropenic. It is possible that whatever suppresses the marrow affects all cell lines in a few patients. Two dozen white blood counts were above 10,000 cells/μL, perhaps as a result of intercurrent infections. Platelet counts were above 400,000 cells/μL in 75 patients (60% of those with platelet counts reported), as was seen in 20% of DBA children. The mean cell volumes were usually normal when corrected for age. The mean and median were 81 fL, and the range was from 63 fL to 112 fL. Hb F levels ranged from 0.2% to 9.2%, but were usually normal. One small study reported an excess of patients with blood group A,[799] but this finding was not observed in another small study.[800] More than 90% had significant to profound marrow erythroblastopenia. The erythroblasts that were seen usually had a maturation arrest. Increased marrow lymphocyte counts led to the erroneous diagnosis of acute leukemia at least once.[801] Five per cent to 10% of patients presented with reticulocytosis or erythroid hyperplasia, or with both, and they presumably were recovering without the benefit of medical attention.[2, 4, 792]

Several features of the red cells distinguish TEC from DBA, if the history and age of the patient are insufficient. Wang and Mentzer pointed out that the erythrocytes in TEC have normal "adult" (or at least child and not fetal) mean cell volumes and levels of Hb F, i antigen, and red cell enzymes[802]; in contrast, values for these parameters are more "fetal" in DBA. These distinctions are only relevant if the TEC patient is studied while reticulocytopenic. During the recovery phase, patients with TEC undergo "stress erythropoiesis," as do any patients demonstrating bone marrow recovery. They produce a transient cohort of "fetal-like" erythrocytes that can be detected as soon as reticulocytes appear, by means of a sensitive immunologic assay for F reticulocytes.[2, 4] The authors documented that this cohort of fetal-like erythrocytes subsequently evolves into normal red cells.[800] Interpretation of the mean cell volume and the Hb F, i antigen, and red cell enzyme levels depends on the stage of the illness. The ultimate distinction between TEC and DBA often is only clear after the fact. However, macrocytosis, elevated Hb F level, and reticulocytopenia with marrow erythroblastopenia in a child younger than 1 year of age are most likely indicative of DBA. Red cell adenosine deaminase concentration is elevated in most cases of DBA and is normal in TEC (elevation of the level of this enzyme may be helpful; see earlier discussion of DBA).

Two patients also had another transient condition, called "transient hyperphosphatasemia of infancy," characterized by temporary and unexplained elevation of alkaline phosphatase levels in the absence of liver or bone disease.[794]

Pathophysiology

The history of an antecedent (usually viral) illness 2 months before TEC diagnosis suggests a viral cause. Total suppression of normal erythropoiesis would lead to symptomatic anemia in 1 to 2 months, but it is not clear why patients would then recover within another month. The prime viral suspect is parvovirus (see earlier in chapter), but analyses of specific antibody in more than 50 cases yielded positive results in only 7 patients,[2, 4, 792, 803–806] one of whom was infected in utero in the third trimester.[806] One case had echovirus 11.[793] Another also had Kawasaki's syndrome.[807] The role of a virus that inhibits growth of CFU-Es in patients with normal erythropoiesis[668, 808, 809] has not yet been proved, and confirmation will require sensitive assays for antigen or parvoviral DNA. (See earlier in this chapter for a more detailed discussion of viruses and aplastic anemia).

Erythropoietin levels are high, as expected for anemic patients.[810] More than a dozen laboratories examined erythroid progenitor cell cultures in approximately 50 patients (Table 7–30). One half of 35 patients analyzed had decreased numbers of CFU-Es, and one third had decreased numbers of BFU-Es; these findings suggest that the defect might be in CFU-Es.[2, 4, 811] Koenig and colleagues found serum or IgG inhibitors of normal progenitors in 4 patients and autologous inhibition in 1.[812] Forty patients had assays for autologous or allogeneic serum inhibitors; positive results were obtained in more than 60% of these patients.[2, 4, 793] Autologous or allogeneic cellular inhibitors were also reported in up to one third of 17 patients.[2, 4, 811] Only a few parameters were examined in any single patient. TEC may be due to an unknown virus that infects

Table 7-30. ERYTHROID CULTURES IN TRANSIENT ERYTHROBLASTOPENIA OF CHILDHOOD*

Assay	No. Studied	Result	N	%
Marrow	35			
Progenitor Cells				
Decreased				
CFU-E	33		17	52
BFU-E	27		8	30
Both	26	Both	8	31
	26	Only CFU-E	4	15
Serum Inhibitors	40			
Autologous	21	IgG, 9/9; IgM, 1/1	13	62
Allogeneic	29	IgG, 9/15	19	66
Both	10		5	50
Cellular Inhibitors	17			
Autologous MNC	8		2	25
Allogeneic MNC	6		2	33
Both MNC	4		1	25
Autologous T cells	9		2	22
Allogeneic T cells	2		0	0
Both T cells	2		0	0

CFU-E = colony-forming unit–erythroid; BFU-E = burst–forming unit–erythroid; MNC = mononuclear cells.
*A total of 50 patients had cultures performed for some or all of the following: bone marrow cells, serum, IgG, IgM, peripheral blood MNC, and T cells. See text for references.

CFU-Es and is not cleared until specific antibodies develop. An IgG directed against erythroid progenitors may develop and appear as a "serum" inhibitor. Recovery in these cases might require the development of anti-idiotype antibodies.

Therapy and Outcome

As indicated by the word "transient," all patients with TEC recover. TEC recurred in only two cases, and both within 1 year.[810, 813] Most patients are usually well within 1 to 2 months from diagnosis, and 5% to 10% have already begun to recover by the time they present for medical care. Eight months was the longest interval to recovery without recurrence, and only 10 patients took 4 months or more. No treatment was necessary for almost one half of those for whom the clinical course was described. Most patients had already reached their lowest hemoglobin level by the time they received medical attention. Transfusions were given to 60% of patients, and a single transfusion was sufficient in 90%. Prednisone was administered to 20%; reticulocytes often appeared within 1 day, but this was clearly unrelated to the steroid therapy.

The current recommendation is to observe patients with TEC and to transfuse only if they develop cardiovascular compromise from their anemia. It is amazing how well these children cope with hemoglobin levels of 5 g/dL, and it is often the cardiovascular or mental state of the physician rather than the patient's condition that leads to transfusion. Prednisone, anabolic steroids, or other immunosuppressive agents have no apparent role in the management of TEC. The prognosis is excellent, and the retrospective distinction of TEC from DBA is simple.

Congenital Dyserythropoietic Anemia
Introduction

The term *dyserythropoiesis* is used to describe ineffective, morphologically abnormal erythropoiesis. Conditions characterized by this dysfunction are not precisely bone marrow failure syndromes; however, they sometimes are congenital or inherited marrow disorders that may result in anemia without reticulocytosis. Ineffective erythropoiesis results from a discrepancy between erythroid output from marrow to circulation (anemia) and erythroid marrow content (erythroid hyperplasia). It implies intramedullary destruction, combining quantitative and qualitative decreases in erythropoiesis. The prefix *dys-* indicates qualitative abnormalities of the stem cell or the microenvironment. In aplastic anemia, erythropoiesis is quantitatively abnormal in the same compartments.

Approximately 1 in 1000 bone marrow erythroblasts is abnormal in normal individuals.[814] Multinucleated erythroblasts and karyorrhexis are occasionally seen in megaloblastic anemia, iron deficiency, leukemia, and hemolytic anemia, and are indicative of bone marrow stress. The frequency of dyserythropoietic erythroblasts may be substantial in both acquired and inherited aplastic anemia. In one study of aplastic anemia, 5% to 90% of erythroblasts were megaloblastic or showed nucleus-to-cytoplasm asynchrony, 1% to 3% were binucleate, and up to 5% had cytoplasmic connections or chromatin bridges.[815] During recovery from BMT, all patients had a transient wave of up to 30% dyserythropoietic erythroblasts.[816] These morphologic abnormalities are more extreme in *congenital dyserythropoietic anemia (CDA)* than in aplastic anemia or recovery from BMT.

In 1977, Lewis and Verwilghen reviewed CDA in detail in a book that remains a valuable resource.[817] The various types are characterized by anemia with insufficient reticulocytosis and ineffective erythropoiesis. All ethnic groups are affected. The major types are (Table 7–31):

Type I, macrocytosis, with bone marrow megaloblastoid changes and internuclear chromatin bridges

Type II, normocytosis or macrocytosis, with bi- and multinucleated marrow erythroblasts, pluripolar mitoses, and karyorrhexis

Type III, macrocytosis, with erythroblastic multinuclearity of up to 12 nuclei (gigantoblasts)

The morphologic features are the major diagnostic factors for types I and III. Type II is also known by the acronym *HEMPAS*, for *h*ereditary *e*rythroblastic *m*ultinuclearity with a *p*ositive *a*cidified *s*erum test, because of the positive reaction to some acidified normal sera described initially by Crookston and associates.[818] Almost 50 other cases that do not fit clearly into types I to III have been reported.

Type I

Approximately 70 cases of Type I CDA have been reported (the first 20 by Heimpel[2, 4, 819, 820]). The age of

Table 7–31. TYPES OF CONGENITAL DYSERYTHROPOIETIC ANEMIAS

Feature	Type I	Type II	Type III
No. of patients	70	130	40
Anemia	Mild to moderate	Mild to severe	Mild to moderate
Red cell size	Macrocytic	Normo- to macrocytic	Macrocytic
Marrow erythroblasts	Megaloblastoid, ~5% binucleated, chromatin bridges	10–40% bi- and multinucleated, karyorrhexis	10–40%, gigantoblasts
Inheritance	Recessive	Recessive	Dominant
Acid serum hemolysis	Negative	Positive	Negative
Reaction with			
Anti-i	Negative or slight	Strong	Negative or slight
Anti-I	Negative or slight	Strong	Negative or slight
Role of splenectomy	No improvement	Some improvement	Insufficient data
Transfusion dependence	15%	15%	2%

onset of anemia or jaundice ranged from infancy to old age, with a mean age of 15 years and a median age of 5 years. The male-to-female ratio was 1.2, and the inheritance was autosomal recessive. Nine families had consanguinity, and 10 families had affected siblings or cousins, or both. Physical examination shows slight icterus and moderate splenomegaly. Almost a dozen patients had brown skin pigmentation, toe syndactyly, or abnormal fingers.

CDA type I patients have a mild macrocytic anemia, with a mean hemoglobin level of 9 g/dL and a range of 3 to 15 g/dL. Reticulocyte levels range from 0.2% to 7%. The mean cell volume was 99 fL, and the range was 66 to 121 fL. Peripheral blood analysis showed anisocytosis, poikilocytosis, punctate basophilia, and occasional Cabot's rings. White blood cells and platelets were normal. Indirect bilirubin level was elevated (1 to 4 mg/dL), as was serum lactate dehydrogenase concentration; haptoglobin level was low, and transferrin was saturated. Further evidence for ineffective erythropoiesis was derived from the plasma iron turnover, which was as much as 10-fold normal, whereas red cell utilization was reduced to below 30%. Red cell survival was slightly shortened, and ^{51}Cr half-lives ranged from 14 to 30 days (mean, 21 days). Globin synthesis studies usually showed non-α/α ratios of 1, although imbalance of 0.5 to 0.8 was observed occasionally. Normal results were seen with the acidified serum test, and the i antigen titer was usually in the adult (low) range; this is in contrast to the situation in type II CDA (see later).

Bone marrow examination showed marked erythroid hyperplasia, with 25% to 80% erythroid precursors. The abnormalities were confined to the polychromatophilic and orthochromatic (i.e., mature) erythroblasts (Fig. 7–30). There was dissociation of nuclear and cytoplasmic maturation, with immature megaloblastoid nuclei and more mature cytoplasms. As many as 2% of the erythroblasts were large cells with incomplete nuclear division. Approximately 1% had double nuclei, with one component more mature than the other. Up to 2% of cells demonstrated thin chromatin bridges connecting the nuclei of two cells. Electron microscopy confirmed that the proerythroblasts were normal. The more mature erythroblasts had widening of nuclear membrane pores, with condensation, vacuolization, and disinte-

gration of nuclear chromatin, with cytoplasmic penetrance. There were also structural changes of the nucleolus, the appearance of microtubules, and the presence of siderotic material in the cytoplasm.

The defect is apparently at the stem cell level. The numbers of CFU-Es and BFU-Es were normal, but electron microscopy showed that the colonies contained a mixture of normal and abnormal cells.[821] This suggests that the abnormality is expressed variably in the mature progeny of each stem cell.

Treatment with the usual hematinics, such as vitamins, metals, and steroids, is without effect. Fifteen per cent of patients needed several or even chronic transfusions. Although splenomegaly was common, splenectomy did not improve the anemia in 10 cases. Some patients developed gallstones from the hemolytic anemia. Hemosiderosis was the most important long-term complication and was due to increased intestinal absorption of iron, ineffective erythropoiesis, and mild hemolysis; phlebotomy and iron chelation warrant consideration (see Chapters 11 and 21 for details). One patient received α-interferon for hepatitis C and became transfusion independent.[822] Deaths were reported in two cases, one at age 10 years from complications of splenectomy, and the other at 84 years from old age.

Type II

Type II CDA has been reported in approximately 130 patients. Many of the early cases were summarized by Verwilghen and associates[823, 824]; the molecular basis is the subject of an excellent review by Fukuda.[825] Twenty-five cases were in sibships, and 9 were in consanguineous families. The male-to-female ratio was 1:1, and the inheritance was autosomal recessive. The age at diagnosis ranged from infancy to adulthood, with an average age of 15 years and a median age of 13 years. The anemia varied from mild to sufficiently severe, such that regular transfusions were required in 15% of patients. Jaundice, hepatosplenomegaly, and gallstones were more common and the anemia generally greater in type II than type I CDA.

The hemoglobin levels varied widely (mean, 9 g/dL; range, 3 to 15 g/dL), whereas reticulocyte counts were normal or inadequately elevated and averaged 4%. Red cells were normochromic and normocytic in one half

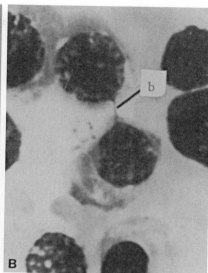

Figure 7-30. Bone marrow from a patient with congenital dyserythropoietic anemia type I. *A,* Small letter *a* indicates binucleate erythroblast, with nuclei of different size and maturity. *B,* Small letter *b* indicates internuclear chromatin bridges connecting two erythroblasts. (From Lewis SM, Verwilghen RL (eds): Dyserythropoiesis. London, Academic Press, 1977.)

of patients, and macrocytic in the other; the average mean cell volume was 93 fL, and the range 73 to 114 fL. Analysis of smears showed anisocytosis, poikilocytosis, teardrops, and basophilic stippling—all nonspecific findings. The red cell life span was shorter in type II CDA than in type I; the ^{51}Cr half-life averaged 18 days (range, 7 to 34 days). Electron microscopy demonstrated an excess of endoplasmic reticulum parallel to the cell membrane that led to the appearance of a characteristic "double membrane," or cistern, in late erythroblasts and some erythrocytes. Some bone marrow reticuloendothelial cells resembled Gaucher's cells, with birefringent, para-aminosalicylic acid–positive, needle-like inclusions; these cells may be the products of the catabolism of erythroblasts undergoing rapid turnover. The marrow showed erythroid hyperplasia, with 45% to 90% erythroid precursors; binucleate and multinucleated mature erythroblasts comprised 10% to 70% of the erythroid precursors (Fig. 7–31). The internuclear chromatin bridges of type I CDA were not present, and the multinuclearity was not as extreme as in type III CDA.

The pathognomonic findings in type II CDA are serologic.[818] In type II CDA, red cells are lysed by approximately 30% of acidified sera from normal individuals but not by the patient's own serum. By contrast, in PNH, the patient's cells are lysed by his or her own acidified serum. In type II CDA, the red cells have a specific type II CDA antigen, and many normal sera contain an anti–type II CDA IgM antibody. In some cases, up to 30 normal sera must be examined before the acidified test yields positive results; some of the patients in which this is necessary were called "type II variants" until the right serum was found.[826] Type II CDA erythrocytes also are more strongly agglutinated by anti-i antibody than are the cells of newborn infants or those of patients with stress erythropoiesis.[827] Studies with fluorescent labels demonstrated i antigen on every red cell in type II CDA. Heterozygotes also had increased expression of i antigen. Type II CDA cells are strongly agglutinated as well as lysed by anti-I anti-

body. Rosse and associates found that type II CDA cells bind a normal amount of complement 1 (C1) but more antibody and more C4 than do normal individuals.[828] This causes binding of an excess of C3, with resultant hemolysis. The red cell plasma membrane abnormality in type II CDA is related to decreased *N*-acetylglucosaminyltransferase levels. Bands 3 and 4.5 lack glycosylation with lactosaminoglycans.[829] The gene, *CDAN3*, has been localized to 15q21-q25.[830]

The numbers of erythroid progenitors in marrow and blood are probably normal in type II CDA. One study revealed only normal morphology of the erythroblasts produced by cultured CFU-Es,[831] but others reported multinuclearity similar to that seen *in vivo* in the bone marrow.[832, 833] As in type I, the defect appears to be at the level of the erythroid stem cell, with variable expression in the mature erythroblasts.

Patients with severe anemia require blood transfusions. Unlike the situation in type I, splenectomy has been effective in type II because of an apparent increase in red cell life span and abrogation of the need for transfusions. Iron accumulation does occur, both from transfusions and from increased intestinal absorption, even in patients who have not received transfusions. Death may result from cardiac compromise. Prophylactic phlebotomy or iron chelation, or both, have a definite role in the management of this disorder. Two patients died from hemochromatosis at the ages of 25 and 30 years.

Type III

Approximately 40 patients with type III CDA have been reported.[834, 835] Three families with two generations of involvement had dominant CDA, and there were two sets of affected siblings. The male-to-female ratio was 1.3. The average age at diagnosis was 21 years; the age at diagnosis ranged from birth to old age, as in types I and II CDA. The anemia was usually macrocytic and mild to moderate. The mean hemoglobin level was 10 g/dL, and the range from 5 to 14 g/

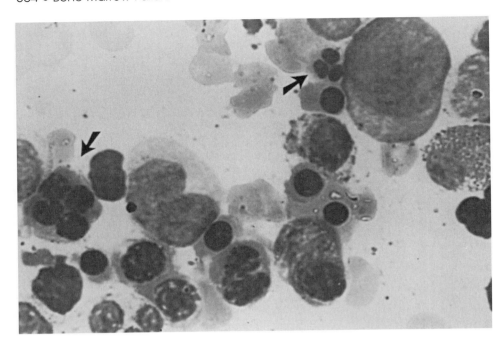

Figure 7-31. Bone marrow from a patient with congenital dyserythropoietic anemia type II, showing bi- and multinucleate erythroblasts. (Courtesy of Dr. Gail Wolfe; with permission from Alter BP: The bone marrow failure syndromes. In Nathan DG, Oski FA (eds): Hematology of Infancy and Childhood. 3rd ed. Philadelphia, W.B. Saunders Co., 1987, p 159.)

dL. Bone marrow erythroid hyperplasia was observed, with up to 75% erythroblasts, multinuclearity in 10% to 40% of erythroblasts, and the presence of unique "gigantoblasts" with up to 12 nuclei (Fig. 7–32). The acid serum lysis test always yielded negative results, and reactions with anti-i antibody were at the level seen in stress erythropoiesis and were weaker than in type II CDA. Red cell survival was slightly short, with ^{51}Cr half-lives being of 21 days' duration. As in the other CDAs, *in vitro* culture led to formation of colonies containing both normal and abnormal erythroblasts—indications of a stem cell abnormality.[836]

Transfusions or splenectomy were infrequently performed in these patients. As in the other CDAs, the major problem was hemosiderosis, which led to one death at age 42 years.

Variants

Almost 50 patients cannot be diagnosed as having any of the CDA types already described. The authors have attempted to classify these patients into discrete categories.[2, 4] *Type IV CDA* is the classification used in reports in which the bone marrow morphology resembles that of type II. The results of acidified serum tests were negative, although an insufficient number of sera may have been examined; also, the level of i antigen was not increased. One family had dominant inheritance; thus, at least some of these cases might indeed belong to a type different than type II, in which inheritance is autosomal recessive. Anemia appeared from infancy to adulthood and was mild in all but one patient. Ten per cent to 40% of the marrow erythroblasts were binucle-

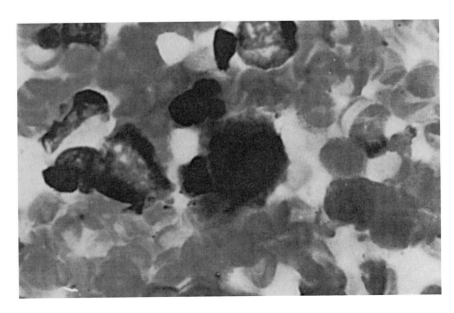

Figure 7-32. Bone marrow from a patient with congenital dyserythropoietic anemia type III, showing multinucleate erythroblast. (Photograph courtesy of Dr. Gail Wolfe; with permission from Alter BP: The bone marrow failure syndromes. In Nathan DG, Oski FA (eds): Hematology of Infancy and Childhood. 3rd ed. Philadelphia, W.B. Saunders Co., 1987, p 159.)

ate, as in type II. The clinical course was relatively benign, with splenectomy required in one case.

CDA with thalassemia is the term that has been used for 1 group of 12 patients in 5 families. One family had dominant inheritance, and one had three affected siblings. The age at diagnosis of mild to moderate anemia ranged from infancy to old age. Red cell size ranged from microcytic to macrocytic, and 5% to 35% of the marrow erythroblasts were multinuclear. The acid serum lysis tests yielded negative results, although i antigen was found in 2 of the families. Globin chain synthesis was imbalanced, with β/α ratios of 0.5, or similar to those seen in β-thalassemia trait. Although there may have been a coincidence of thalassemia trait and CDA, two of the families were from ethnic groups that did not have a high incidence of thalassemia.

More than 24 other families had CDAs that were even more difficult to classify. Two families had an affected parent and child, two had consanguinity, and three had affected siblings; all of the families may have different disorders. The proportion of binucleate or multinucleated erythroblasts was always between 1% to 15%. Some erythroblasts resembled type I cells with rare internuclear bridges, as well as type II cells, with symmetric binuclearity, karyorrhexis, and even double membranes (as seen with electron microscopy). The ages at diagnosis of the mild to severe anemia ranged from birth to adulthood, and red cell size from small to large. Six infants had intrauterine hydrops; one of these infants died.[2, 4, 837, 838] The results of acidified serum tests were usually negative, the level of i antigen varied, and red cell ^{51}Cr survival half-lives were of 5 to 29 days' duration. One case was associated with deficiency of erythroid CD44 and phenotypes In(a−b−) and Co(a−b−).[839] Six patients had splenectomy and did experience some improvement. Erythroid cultures from one case demonstrated multinuclearity in some cells within each colony[840]; this finding suggested a stem cell disorder, as in the other CDAs. The clinical variability suggests that these cases represent several types of CDA; perhaps they are double heterozygotes rather than homozygotes for recessive CDA genes.

White Cells

Acquired Agranulocytosis

This topic is discussed in detail in Chapter 22.

Kostmann's Syndrome

Description

The eponym *Kostmann's syndrome (KS)* is used to describe infants with extreme neutropenia (usually in the first year of life), severe pyogenic infections, and, until recently, early deaths. "Infantile genetic agranulocytosis" was first described by Kostmann in 1956.[841, 842] The syndrome that now bears his name also is called "severe chronic neutropenia," a term that does not totally distinguish all of the neutropenias of childhood (see Chapter 22 for a complete discussion of neutro-

penia). Almost 200 cases of KS have been reported in the literature (Table 7–32). The male-to-female ratio of occurrence is approximately 1:1, and the inheritance is autosomal recessive. Most of Kostmann's original 14 and subsequent 10 cases belonged to a very large intermarried kinship in northern Sweden.[843] Despite this founder effect, all ethnic groups are affected by KS, including blacks, Native Americans, and Asians. At least 11 patients were in consanguineous families, and more than 20 had affected siblings.

One half of the patients were symptomatic within the first month, and 90% by 6 months; the few who were diagnosed later may not have had KS. Birthweights were generally normal, as were findings on the physical examinations, except for signs of infection (e.g., skin abscesses). Four patients were short, four had mental retardation, three had cataracts, and two had microcephaly.

Laboratory Findings

Neutropenia is marked, although in several infants absolute neutrophil counts were close to normal in the first week; however, thereafter they declined rapidly. The average absolute neutrophil count was less than 200 cells/μL, and neutropenia was often total. Eosinophil and monocyte counts were sometimes very high (up to 80% monocytes in some patients), but these cells are not as effective phagocytes as are neutrophils. Increased immunoglobulin levels were often seen. KS is a single cytopenia, and patients with KS usually have normal hemoglobin levels and normal or increased platelet counts. Bone marrow examinations reveal normal cellularity, with absence of or marked decreases in the number of myeloid precursors and, often, a maturation arrest at the myelocyte or promyelocyte stage.

Pathophysiology

KS is an autosomal recessive disorder that primarily affects the neutrophil series. Numbers of bone marrow colony-forming units have been reported as decreased,

Table 7–32. KOSTMANN'S SYNDROME LITERATURE

Feature	Total	No G-CSF	G-CSF
No. of patients	173	133	40
Male:female	0.95	0.83	1.5
Age* at diagnosis, mean	2.8	2.7	2.9
Median	1	1	0–12
Range	0–48	0–48	
No. with leukemia (%)	8 (5%)	3 (2%)	5 (13%)
No. of deaths (%)	65 (38%)	64 (49%)	1 (3%)
Age† at death, mean	2.4	2.2	15
Median	0.8	0.8	15
Range	0.05–20	0.05–20	15
Projected 50% survival age†	13	3	>21

G-CSF = granulocyte colony–stimulating factor.
*Ages are in months.
†Ages are in years.

increased, or, most often, normal. The colonies rarely contain neutrophils[844] and more commonly comprise eosinophils, monocytes, and abnormal or arrested myeloid precursors.[845] Addition of SCF did lead to normal myeloid maturation.[846, 847] Long-term cultures from some patients also showed a block in myeloid differentiation.[844] Thus, in some patients, the *in vivo* defect in myeloid differentiation was duplicated *in vitro*.

The receptor for G-CSF appeared to be normal in most patients,[848, 849] but a nonsense mutation was found in one case[850] whose *in vivo* response pattern was identical to those of other patients with KS (see later). Two patients who developed leukemia while receiving G-CSF treatment also had mutations in the G-CSF receptor.[851, 852] The production of G-CSF and GM-CSF mRNA by the patients' mononuclear cells was normal.[853] Serum levels of G-CSF usually were increased,[854] a finding consistent with a receptor problem or a possible intracellular signaling defect in response to G-CSF.

Therapy and Outcome

In the era before G-CSF availability, the prognosis for patients with KS was very poor, with one half of patients reported to have died at a mean age of 2.2 years, at a median age of 9 months, and at ages ranging from 2 weeks to 20 years. Most of the deaths were from sepsis or pneumonia. Infections required antibiotics, which many patients received prophylactically. The projected median survival was 3 years, with 15% survivors older than 20 years of age (Fig. 7–33). BMT cured 3 of the 4 patients in whom it was reported.[846, 855–857] The use of lithium was proposed because it raises white cell counts in hematologically normal individuals, but it was relatively ineffective in KS.[858, 859] No cases

developed pancytopenia, and thus KS is a true single cytopenia.

The application of recombinant growth factors is an exciting but risky prospect for patients with KS (see later). Subcutaneously administered G-CSF raised neutrophil counts in children with KS in a dose-related manner. The factor must be administered chronically, is without major side effects, and markedly decreases the number and severity of infections.[2, 4, 502, 860, 861] The use of GM-CSF is associated with more side effects and predominantly increases eosinophil counts rather than neutrophil counts[862]; thus, G-CSF is the agent of choice. The dose of G-CSF is 5 to 10 µg/kg per day, subcutaneously; some patients do respond to much higher doses. The response rate is greater than 90%, and the median projected survival is more than 20 years of age. Osteoporosis has been observed in patients treated with G-CSF, either as a side effect or related to longer survival with KS.[861, 863]

Prenatal diagnosis using fetal blood obtained in the mid-trimester has been considered,[864] but the absolute neutrophil count is less than 200 cells/µL in normal fetuses,[865] and absolute neutropenia would be required for establishing a diagnosis of KS *in utero*.

Leukemia. At least three patients developed acute myeloid leukemia at 12, 14, and 14 years of age (two monocytic, and one myelomonocytic); all three died within 6 months.[861, 866, 867] In one family, one child had KS and a sibling died with acute lymphocytic leukemia.[868] Of concern is the observation that at least 5 patients developed leukemia, monosomy 7, or MDS (or combinations of these) within 1 to 5 years after they began receiving treatment with G-CSF; leukemia was not noted in concurrently treated patients with SD, cyclic, or benign neutropenias.[861, 869–871] Furthermore, two KS patients who did develop leukemia while receiving G-CSF had mutations in the G-CSF receptor.[851, 852] KS is due to an abnormality in the myeloid stem cell that causes ineffective myelopoiesis or dysmyelopoiesis; KS predisposes to malignancy, as do many of the other bone marrow stem cell disorders. The potential increase of this risk associated with cytokine treatment appears real, but its magnitude is unknown. Many of the patients who received G-CSF were already "older" and perhaps already at increased risk. Only careful prospective studies will clarify this issue.

Platelets

Acquired Amegakaryocytic Thrombocytopenia

Less than 50 patients have been reported with *acquired amegakaryocytic thrombocytopenia*.[2, 4, 872, 873] Females with the disease outnumber males at a ratio of 2.6:1. Although most patients are older than 55 years of age, the disease does occur in childhood.[874] The symptoms are related to the thrombocytopenia. Bone marrow examination distinguishes this disorder from immune thrombocytopenia (i.e., diagnosis is based on the absence rather than the presence of megakaryocytes). Confusion with and progression to aplastic anemia do

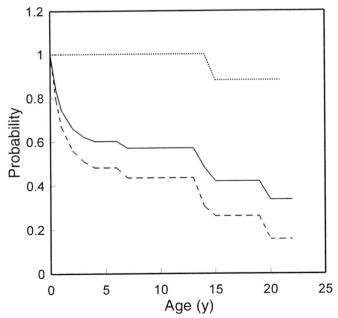

Figure 7-33. Kaplan-Meier plot of cumulative survival age in years in Kostmann's syndrome. Solid line = all patients; dashed line = no G-CSF; dotted line = G-CSF.

occur. Some patients with preleukemia may present with thrombocytopenia, including cytogenetic abnormalities of marrow cells.[875] Amegakaryocytic thrombocytopenia may be associated with the same conditions that are seen with pancytopenia, such as lupus erythematosus, hepatitis, and drug use. Red cell macrocytosis attests to the possibility that the lesion may involve an earlier-stage stem cell than the megakaryocyte progenitor.

In vitro studies showed decreased or absent megakaryocyte colony formation. Megakaryocyte CSF and thrombopoietin were increased in some patients but not all. Both T-cell and serum inhibitors have been observed. Clinical responses to treatment with ATG,[876] cyclosporine, cyclophosphamide, lithium, danazol, and prednisone have been reported.

Thrombocytopenia with Absent Radii

Description

Almost 200 cases of *thrombocytopenia with absent radii (TAR)* have been reported and summarized in reviews[2, 877–879] (Table 7–33). Diagnoses usually are made at birth because of the characteristic physical appearance combined with thrombocytopenia. The pathognomic physical finding is bilateral absence of the radii with presence of the thumbs (Fig. 7–34); this feature distinguishes TAR from FA and from trisomy 18, in which the thumbs are absent if the radii are absent. Babies with TAR often have hemorrhagic manifestations at birth, with 60% of those affected having petechiae or bloody diarrhea within the first week and

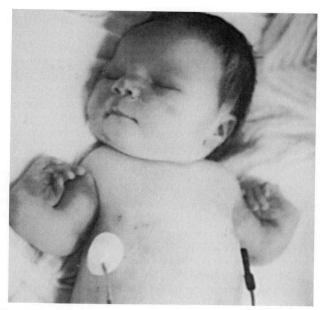

Figure 7–34. Newborn infant with thrombocytopenia with absent radii. Note that thumbs are present. (Photograph courtesy of Dr. Jeffrey Lipton; with permission from Alter BP: The bone marrow failure syndromes. In Nathan DG, Oski FA (eds): Hematology of Infancy and Childhood. 3rd ed. Philadelphia, W.B. Saunders Co., 1987, p 159.)

more than 95% by 4 months. Inheritance is autosomal recessive, and more than 20 families had affected siblings. In one case study, each in a set of identical twins had TAR,[880] whereas in another only one of a pair of fraternal twins was affected[881]; these findings are consistent with a genetic rather than an acquired cause. However, only three patients were reported to have consanguinity,[882–884] which suggests that TAR patients may be double heterozygotes for genes with similar effects, rather than true homozygotes. Parents usually are normal, and affected mothers have had normal children. At least four families involved more than one generation (aunts or uncles and nephews or nieces, with only one example of parent-to-child transmission), and four had affected cousins[2, 4]; one set of affected half-siblings was reported, suggesting dominant (or perhaps pseudodominant) inheritance in a few families. All ethnic groups are affected, including blacks; however, reports of the disease in Asians are rare, and this may reflect a reporting rather than a genetic bias. Other inherited hematologic conditions with radial ray anomalies include FA and DBA; however, only the platelet, and no other lineage, is significantly affected in TAR.

Table 7–33 compares the features of TAR with those of FA. All TAR patients had absence of radii but presence of thumbs (see Fig. 7–34). Most were bilateral; only four apparently *bona fide* cases had a typical hematologic pattern but absence of only one radius.[885–888] FA patients were even smaller than those with TAR. The hands of TAR patients often had shortening of the middle phalanx of the fifth finger (clinodactyly), finger syndactyly, and sometimes thumb hypoplasia. Almost one half had other forearm abnormalities, such as ab-

Table 7–33. COMPARISON OF THROMBOCYTOPENIA ABSENT RADII WITH FANCONI'S ANEMIA

Feature	TAR	FA
No. of patients	200	1000
Age* at diagnosis, mean	0	8.5
Male:female	0.7	1.3
Inheritance	Recessive	Recessive
Low birth-weight	10%	12%
Skeletal deformities		
Absent radii, thumbs present	100%	0%
Hand anomalies	45%	50%
Shoulders, neck, etc.	15%	6%
Lower limbs	40%	8%
Cardiac defects	10%	6%
Skin		
Hemangiomas	10%	0%
Pigmentation	0%	60%
Blood disease	Thrombocytopenia	Pancytopenia
Bone marrow	Megakaryocytes absent	Aplastic
Bone marrow colonies decreased	CFU-Meg	CFU-GM, CFU-E, BFU-E
Hb F level	Normal	Increased
Chromosome breaks	Absent	Present
Malignancies	0%	15%
No. of deaths	23%	38%
Projected 50% survival age*	>55	19

TAR = thrombocytopenia absent radii; CFU-meg = colony-forming unit–megakaryocyte; CFU-GM = colony-forming unit–granulocyte macrophage; CFU-E = colony-forming unit–erythroid; BFU-E = burst-forming unit–erythroid.
*Ages are in years.

sence of ulnae (more than 15%) and ulnar shortening or bowing (30%). Upper arms were abnormal in one third of patients, who had either short humeri (15%) or absence of humeri (10%). The ulnar or humeral lesions were bilateral in 90% of patients. Fifteen per cent had scapular hypoplasia and webbing of the neck, which resulted in abnormal upper body appearances. Micrognathia and occasional brachycephaly or microcephaly also were seen, as were hypertelorism, epicanthal folds, strabismus, and low set ears. Ten per cent had facial hemangiomas. Lower limb abnormalities in 40% included deformity, subluxation, or hypoplasia of the knees, dislocation of the hips or patellae, and varus or valgus rotation at the hips, knees, or feet, as well as shortness of the legs and absence of tibiae or fibulae. Ten per cent had congenital heart disease, such as atrial or ventricular septal defects, tetralogy of Fallot, dextrocardia, and ectopia cordis. Six patients had gonadal anomalies, including undescended testes, hypoplasia, unicornuate uterus, vaginal atresia, and absence of the cervix. Low birth-weight was noted at term in 10%. A detailed summary of the anomalies can be found elsewhere in the literature.[2]

In contrast, FA patients have absence of thumbs when radii are abnormal. Also, patients with TAR have only thrombocytopenia, whereas those with FA usually develop pancytopenia. Four patients with trisomy 18 had absence or hypoplasia of radii or thrombocytopenia (or both)[2, 4]; however, trisomy 18 is characterized by other findings in addition to the cytogenetic abnormality. Robert's syndrome and SC phocomelia may have a phenotype similar to that of TAR. Other syndromes that involve radial anomalies are beyond the scope of this analysis.

Bloody diarrhea in infancy ascribed specifically to cow's milk allergy was reported in 20%. Removal of milk from the diet alleviated the diarrhea and perhaps improved the thrombocytopenia.

Laboratory Findings

Platelet counts were below 50,000 cells/μL at the time of diagnosis in more than 80% of patients. Anemia occurred secondary to bleeding and was accompanied by reticulocytosis. Leukocytosis was above 15,000 cells/μL in more than 80%, above 20,000 cells/μL in 60%, and above 40,000 cells/μL in one third of the infants; occasionally, the leukocyte count exceeded 100,000 cells/μL. Circulating immature myeloid precursors were reported in more than a dozen infants, but none had true leukoerythroblastosis (see later). This leukemoid reaction has been mistaken for congenital leukemia, but usually it subsides during infancy. Extramedullary hematopoiesis may lead to splenomegaly. Eosinophilia was not uncommon. Bone marrow cellularity was normal, and myeloid and erythroid cell lines were normal or increased in number. The majority had absence of megakaryocytes; in the rest, these precursors were decreased in number, hypoplastic, or immature.

Normal laboratory tests include determination of mean cell volume, Hb F, and chromosome breakage,

the results of which clearly distinguish TAR from FA. Karyotyping also rules out trisomy 18. Hypogammaglobulinemia was reported only in a group of Nigerian patients.[887] Small platelets were reported only once.[889] Platelet function is generally normal, although a few patients did have abnormal platelet aggregation and storage pool defects.[2, 4] However, clinical symptoms are more likely related to quantitative rather than to qualitative defects.

Pathophysiology

Hematopoietic progenitor cell assays indicated normal myeloid and erythroid lineages. Some investigators found no growth of megakaryocytic progenitors, whereas others reported essentially normal growth.[2, 4] The plasma of one patient contained a unique megakaryocyte CSF. Because TAR is a true single cytopenia, without evolution to aplastic anemia or leukemia, the defect presumably involves only the megakaryocytic lineage.

Therapy and Outcome

Most patients with TAR bleed in infancy and then demonstrate improvement after the first year. More than 40 deaths were reported (23%), 85% of which occurred within the first year of life. Only one child died beyond the age of 3 years. The projected survival curve (Fig. 7–35) shows a plateau of 72% survival at 44 months. These data encompass over 40 years of TAR case reports. During this 40-year period, treatment may have been of limited scope, most of the deaths were from intracranial or gastrointestinal bleeding. Patients who survived the perilous first year had an increase

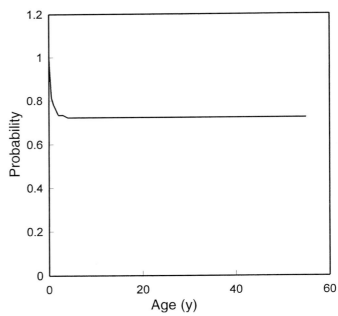

Figure 7–35. Kaplan-Meier plot of cumulative survival age in years in thrombocytopenia with absent radii. Note the plateau of 72% survival at the age of 4 years.

in platelet count to above 100,000 cells/µL, which is adequate for the necessary orthopedic procedures. Although thrombocytopenia sometimes recurred during illnesses, it was usually no longer severe. Those with milk allergy benefited from dietary modification.

The most important modern therapeutic advance has been platelet transfusion. Platelet transfusion is needed during bleeding episodes or operations and should provide prophylaxis for infants with severe symptomatic thrombocytopenia. Single donors reduce the risk of sensitization, and HLA-matched platelets can be used, if necessary. The platelet count should be maintained above 10,000 to 15,000 cells/µL. The duration of platelet support usually is shorter than 1 year. Other treatments, including splenectomy and corticosteroid and androgen therapies, were without apparent benefit; however, one adult had shown a transient increase in the platelet count following splenectomy.[890] A small dose of prednisone might decrease the bleeding tendency at a given platelet count, and ε-aminocaproic acid may also be useful (see the section on FA for details).

The leukemoid reaction and eosinophilia diminish after the first year. There have been no reports of aplastic anemia and only one of[890a] leukemia, although the high white cell count has led some infants to have socalled "congenital leukemia." Spontaneous improvement does occur, and heroic treatments such as myelotoxic drug regimens or BMT are usually not indicated, even though one patient with a life-threatening central nervous system hemorrhage underwent a successful BMT.[891] After infancy, TAR patients have a very good prognosis, and comprise the only bone marrow failure disorder with a plateau on the survival curve.

Prenatal diagnosis was performed in approximately two dozen cases. Absence of radii was diagnosed with the use of radiography or ultrasound.[2,4] Because unilateral radial aplasia has been reported, both forearms must be examined. In one case, micrognathia was detected on ultrasound. Patients not known to be at risk demonstrated characteristic limb abnormalities on ultrasound; also, cordocentesis revealed fetal thrombocytopenia.[892–894] Nine of the 16 fetuses known to be at risk were found to have TAR (more than the expected 25%); however, this result might represent reporting bias.

LEUKOERYTHROBLASTOSIS

Leukoerythroblastosis is observed in diverse disorders. The term was proposed by Vaughan in 1936 to describe "an anemia with the presence in the peripheral blood of immature red cells and a few immature white cells of the myeloid series"[895]—that is, erythroblasts and leukoblasts. The blood film shows normochromic and normocytic erythrocytes, with poikilocytes, teardrops, fragments, and target cells (Fig. 7–36). Giant platelets may also be seen. Leukoerythroblastosis must be distinguished from a *leukemoid reaction,* which is a reactive leukocytosis characterized by an orderly progression of myeloid cells from immaturity through maturity. The term *leukemic hiatus* applies when immature and mature white cells are seen without intermediate forms, producing a gap, or "hiatus."

The disorders that may be characterized by leukoerythroblastosis are outlined in Table 7–34.[896, 897] Many of these involve bone marrow invasion, particularly from metastatic solid tumors; hematologic malignancies; infections; or other marrow components, with the crowding of cells out of the marrow prematurely ("myelophthisis"). Hypoxia also might stimulate premature release. In myeloproliferative disorders, the premature release of nucleated cells may be related to their intrinsic abnormality. Several other chapters in this textbook discuss many of the diseases associated with leukoerythroblastosis.

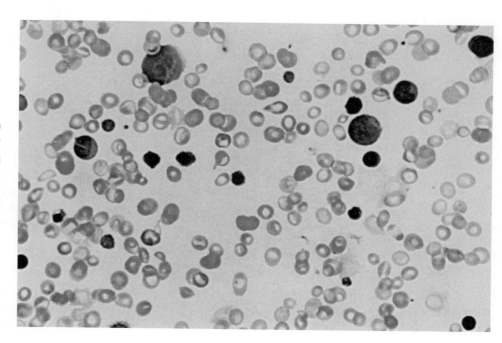

Figure 7-36. Peripheral blood from a patient with leukoerythroblastosis, in this case due to osteopetrosis. (Photograph courtesy of Dr. Gail Wolfe; with permission from Alter BP: The bone marrow failure syndromes. In Nathan DG, Oski FA (eds): Hematology of Infancy and Childhood. 3rd ed. Philadelphia, W.B. Saunders Co., 1987, p 159.)

Table 7-34. CONDITIONS ASSOCIATED WITH LEUKOERYTHROBLASTOSIS

Marrow Invasion

Tumor
Solid tumor with bone marrow metastases
Lymphoma
Hodgkin's disease
Multiple myeloma
Leukemia
Neuroblastoma
Preleukemia

Infection
Osteomyelitis
Sepsis
Tuberculosis
Congenital

Marrow Components
Osteopetrosis
Storage disease
Histiocytosis
Vasculitis, including rheumatoid arthritis

Myeloproliferative Disorders
Polycythemia vera
Myelofibrosis, myeloid metaplasia
Down syndrome transient myeloproliferative disease
Chronic myelogenous leukemia
Erythroleukemia
Thrombocythemia

Hematologic Disease
Erythroblastosis fetalis
Pernicious anemia
Thalassemia major
Other hemolytic anemias

Hypoxia
Cyanotic congenital heart disease
Congestive heart failure
Respiratory disease

Osteopetrosis

Description

Osteopetrosis, also known as "marble bone disease" or "Albers-Schönberg disease," was first described in 1904.[2, 4, 898] The variants include infantile-malignant autosomal recessive, intermediate autosomal recessive, and relatively benign autosomal dominant.[899–901] The milder dominant variety is diagnosed in late childhood and is characterized by dense bones that fracture easily; patients with this variant usually do not have hematologic problems. In contrast, the more severe recessive disorder is diagnosed in infancy and early childhood and is characterized by dense bones that fracture easily owing to a defect in bone resorption. These patients have large heads, sclerotic bones, and hepatosplenomegaly, and they develop blindness, deafness, and cranial nerve palsies because of bony scleroses, as well as pancytopenia. Many cases are familial, and the degree of consanguinity is high. The disease may be severe *in utero*, as there is often a history of stillbirths and spontaneous abortions. The intermediate recessive form, which is diagnosed in the first decade of life, is less severe than the infantile form. A subset of patients with this variant have a deficiency of carbonic anhydrase II.[902]

Laboratory Findings

Patients with infantile recessive osteopetrosis have severe macrocytic anemia, reticulocytosis, teardrop red cells, circulating erythroblasts, and leukocytosis with immature myeloid elements—all of which are components of leukoerythroblastosis due to myelophthisis. High levels of Hb F are a sign of stress erythropoiesis. The bone diploic spaces are small, and the marrow cavity is narrow. Bone marrow aspiration is difficult, and needles may break in attempts to penetrate the sclerotic bone. Biopsies show narrow medullary cavities, hypocellularity, fibrosis, and spindle cell stroma. Osteoblasts and osteoclasts are abundant. Hepatosplenomegaly develops because of extramedullary hematopoiesis. Hypersplenism ensues, leading to thrombocytopenia, leukopenia, and hemolytic anemia due to extracorpuscular destruction of intrinsically normal erythrocytes.

Pathophysiology

The osteoclasts are abnormal and are unable to resorb bone and perform normal remodeling. In an osteopetrotic mouse model, Walker showed that bone marrow or spleen cells from normal mice led to bone remodeling in osteopetrotic littermates, and spleen cells from affected mice led to osteopetrosis in normal mice.[903] A cytoplasmic marker (giant lysosomes in Chédiak-Higashi mice) was used to show that marrow transplants that cured osteopetrotic mice resulted in replacement of recipient osteoclasts with donor osteoclasts.[903] Similar studies using donor mice with defective erythropoiesis (W^e/W^v) suggested that the osteoclast stem cell may be more primordial than the colony-forming unit-spleen (CFU-S).[904] The defective donor erythrocytosis was replaced by the recipient's normal erythropoiesis even though the osteopetrosis was cured and the leukocytes and platelets were from the donor. *In vitro* studies indicate that osteoclasts are derived from hematopoietic stem cells that are in the mononuclear light-density fraction.[905] In humans as well, marrow transplantation is curative (see later), a fact indicating that the osteoclast is contained within the transplantable stem cell population.

Hematopoiesis itself is intrinsically normal. The peripheral blood has increased numbers of CFU-GMs, BFU-Es, and even CFU-Es. The last of these are normally found only in marrow and may migrate from the crowded bone marrow to sites of extramedullary hematopoiesis. Osteoclasts are numerically normal, morphologically normal or abnormal, and functionally abnormal.

Therapy and Outcome

Most patients with malignant osteopetrosis die in infancy or early childhood, and none were reported to have survived beyond 20 years of age. In a longitudinal study of 33 patients, the probability of survival at age 6 was 30%, and the median projected survival was 4 years.[900] Deaths were from the complications of bone marrow failure, infection, and hemorrhage. Host resistance may be impaired because circulating phagocytes, derived from the same lineage as osteoclasts, are defective in the generation of superoxide. Symptomatic anemia and thrombocytopenia can be treated with transfusions of red cells and platelets, but hypersplenism decreases the efficacy of such treatment. Splenectomy offers only temporary improvement because the rest of the reticuloendothelial system remains active and the primary bone disorder is not cured. Some patients responded to prednisone therapy, again with transient improvement because of decreased hypersplenism and reticuloendothelial suppression.[906, 907] Calcitriol was not consistently effective at stimulating bone resorption.[908, 909] The use of interferon-γ, which stimulates superoxide generation in chronic granulomatous disease, led to a decrease in trabecular bone area and significantly improved blood counts and superoxide production in 11 patients treated for 18 months.[910] In one adult with dominant disease, erythropoietin and corticosteroids were used successfully for treating myelophthisic pancytopenia.[911]

BMT was reported in more than 70 patients, with a 5-year survival of 79% in those who underwent the procedure with an HLA-identical donor.[912] The osteoclasts and hematopoietic cells were of donor origin, whereas the osteoblasts remained host. Restoration of normal hematopoiesis, improvement of radiographic findings, and stabilization of physical changes did occur; early transplantation offers the only hope for cure.

Prenatal diagnosis was first performed in 1943 with the use of radiography,[913] but errors were made.[914] Today, ultrasound is used to detect increased bone density, fractures, macrocephaly, and hydrocephaly, which can be confirmed with radiography.[915]

PRELEUKEMIA AND MYELODYSPLASTIC SYNDROME

Most of the syndromes of bone marrow failure (both acquired and inherited, and both pancytopenias and single cytopenias) are associated with the subsequent appearance of leukemia in at least a few patients[916] (Table 7–35). Several examples have been discussed earlier in this chapter, and many are presented elsewhere in this textbook. In this section, a few of the conditions in which pancytopenia is followed by leukemia that are not addressed elsewhere are briefly described. Specific genetic syndromes that may superficially resemble FA and in which leukemia may occur also are mentioned.

Bloom's Syndrome

Bloom's syndrome is a rare chromosome breakage syndrome. It may resemble FA at the physical and cytogenetic levels, and it is associated with the development of leukemia and other malignancies. The Bloom's Syndrome Registry contained 165 case reports at the time

Table 7–35. PRELEUKEMIC BONE MARROW DISORDERS

Acquired	Inherited
Aplastic anemia	Fanconi's anemia
Irradiation	Dyskeratosis congenita
Drugs	Shwachman-Diamond
Toxins	syndrome
Pure red cell aplasia	Kostmann's agranulocytosis
Thrombocytopenia	Diamond-Blackfan anemia
Neutropenia	Amegakaryocytic
Paroxysmal nocturnal	thrombocytopenia
hemoglobinuria	Familial marrow failure
Refractory sideroblastic anemia	Familial myeloproliferative
Preacute lymphocytic leukemia	disease
Myelodysplastic syndromes	Trisomy 21
Myeloproliferative disorders	Bloom's syndrome
	Ataxia telangiectasia
	Poland's syndrome

of its most recent update in 1993.[917] Bloom's syndrome is an autosomal recessive disorder with a male-to-female ratio of occurrence of 1.5. Although it has been reported in all ethnic groups, Bloom's syndrome is found predominantly among Ashkenazi Jews. Homozygotes are born at term, but their birth-weight and -length are substantially less than normal. Infants with the disease have feeding difficulties and grow slowly, developing into short, delicate individuals with fine-featured (bird-like) faces and small heads. The diagnostic triad includes stunted growth, telangiectatic erythema of the face, and sensitivity to the sun; all of these features may not be apparent in infancy. Almost all patients have café au lait spots. Additional physical findings include hypertrichosis, toe syndactyly, absence of toes, supernumerary digits, clinodactyly, prominent ears, hypospadias, and cryptorchidism. Some of the physical findings, particularly microsomia, café au lait spots, and hypogonadism, also are seen in FA.

Mild anemia has been reported occasionally. One patient had macrocytosis, dyserythropoietic features, 6% multinucleated erythroblasts in the marrow, and elevated Hb F level.[918] Several patients had low immunoglobulin levels. Patients' chromosomes are abnormal, with breaks, rearrangements, and quadriradii. The sister chromatid exchange rate is increased in Bloom's syndrome, whereas it is low in FA.[298] There is only one complementation group, even among patients of diverse ethnic origins.[919] The Bloom syndrome mutation was assigned to chromosome band 15q26.1 through the use of homozygosity mapping.[920]

Long-term follow-up identified 86 cancers in 60 patients: the first malignancy occurred at a mean age of the midtwenties, and secondary and subsequent primaries in the thirties.[917] The prevalence was the same in both sexes, unlike in FA (see earlier in chapter). Twenty-one leukemias or myelodysplasias were identified at a mean age of 17 years; of these, 6 were lymphocytic, and 7 were myelocytic. Among the five with MDS, two had primary malignancies (1 developed acute myelomonocytic leukemia [AMML]), and three developed carcinomas following chemotherapy for ALL or Hodgkin's disease. The tumors included 18 lymphomas, 2 cases of Hodgkin's disease, 41 carcinomas (10 large intestinal, 9 skin, 7 breast, 4 oropharyngeal, 3 laryngeal, 3 cervical, 2 squamous esophageal, 1 adenocarcinoma of the esophagus, 1 lung, and 1 metastatic), 2 osteogenic sarcomas, 1 Wilms' tumor, and 1 medulloblastoma. More than 40% of the patients had died by the time of reporting. Several patients have had bone marrow cryopreserved; autologous reinfusion might temporarily rescue a patient with leukemia or one who receives aggressive chemotherapy.

Prenatal diagnosis for Bloom's syndrome should be possible by means of detection of chromosomal breaks and increases in sister chromatid exchanges in amniocytes or chorionic villi. So far, the only positive diagnosis was made in a chorionic biopsy from a pregnancy that was soon followed by a spontaneous abortion.[921]

Ataxia Telangiectasia

The third syndrome characterized by chromosome breakage and malignancy (after FA and Bloom's syndrome) is *ataxia telangiectasia* (AT). Ataxia telangiectasia is an autosomal recessive disorder in which progressive cerebellar ataxia appears in early childhood along with telangiectases and multiple infections.[922] The patients have decreased numbers of T cells, particularly T helper cells, and reduced levels of IgA. Chromosome breaks are seen in T cells and fibroblasts but not in B cells, and the cells that do show breakage also have increased sensitivity to γ-irradiation. Breakpoints are nonrandom, involving rearrangements of chromosome 14 and other chromosomes in the areas of immune system genes. There are several complementation groups in ataxia telangiectasia, and the gene for one of these was localized to 11q22-23.[923] In fact, all complementation groups have recently been found to have mutations at this locus in the *ATM* gene, the product of which resembles phosphatidylinositol-3' kinases; these kinases are involved in mitogenic signal transduction, meiotic recombination, and cell cycle control.[924]

Close to 300 American patients were summarized by Morrell and co-workers in 1986[925]; of these, more than one half had died at a median age of less than 19 years. The leading cause of death in ataxia telangiectasia was pulmonary disease followed by cancer.[926] More than 100 ataxia telangiectasia patients were reported to have cancers, 41% of which were non-Hodgkin's lymphomas, 23% leukemia (all apparently lymphocytic), and the rest a variety of solid tumors (predominantly gastrointestinal or gynecologic). Although aplastic anemia has not been reported in ataxia telangiectasia, this disease is a chromosome breakage syndrome associated with malignancies, and in this regard it resembles FA.

Poland's Syndrome

Poland's syndrome is included in this discussion because of the association of hand deformities and malignancies. More than 150 cases have been reported. The major features are the absence of one pectoralis major muscle (75% on the right), syndactyly or brachydactyly of the ipsilateral hand, and hypoplasia of the ipsilateral arm. The male-to-female ratio of occurrence is 3:1, and

the incidence is 1 in 32,000. The condition may be sporadic and not genetic.[927, 928] Absence of the pectoralis major muscle alone occurs most frequently. Eleven patients with Poland's syndrome had leukemia (7 with acute lymphocytic, and 2 with AML) and 3 lymphoma; 5 of these 11 had only absence of a pectoralis major muscle. The ages of those with leukemia or lymphoma were between 3 and 15 years, except for two patients who were 25 and 28 years old. The association of malignancy with Poland's syndrome may be solely coincidental.[929]

Aplastic Anemia Preceding Acute Leukemia

Description

The term *preleukemia* usually is used to refer to adults with refractory anemia and MDS, more than half of whom go on to develop leukemia. However, a small number of both children and adults who eventually develop leukemia appear to have aplastic anemia without myelodysplastic features. In a meta-analysis of several large series, 3% of children with aplastic anemia developed leukemia, and 1.5% of those with ALL began with a hypoplastic phase.[2, 4, 930–933] More than 100 such cases have been reported in detail (Table 7–36). The male-to-female ratio of occurrence was 1:1. The average age at diagnosis of aplastic anemia was 6.1 years, the median age was 4.5 years, and ages ranged from 6 months to 19 years (Fig. 7–37). The average interval from aplasia to leukemia was 7 months, and the median interval was 3 months. Although the range was from 2 weeks to 6 years, only 12% of patients had an interval of longer than 1 year.

Laboratory Findings

Most patients had pancytopenia, but a few had PRCA, neutropenia, or bicytopenias. Bone marrows were hypocellular. Unlike in classic acquired aplastic anemia, megakaryocytes were normal in 15% of the cases. Bone marrow karyotypes also were normal. Most patients did not meet criteria for severe aplastic anemia (see above).

Clues to leukemia might derive from radiographic studies. Shackelford and colleagues[934] described generalized bony rarefaction, transverse metaphyseal radiolucent lines at the ends of the long bones, osteolytic lesions, subperiosteal new bone formation, and osteosclerosis. Another great pretender among the pancytopenias, rheumatoid arthritis, may also be diagnosed with radiography.

Pathophysiology

In hypoplastic preleukemia, the leukemia may have been present during the period of hypoplasia but not detected in the randomly sampled bone marrow aspirate. Biopsies would provide a better assessment of overall cellularity. Because bone marrows from young children, as well as those from patients with aplastic

Table 7-36. COMPARISON OF THE PRELEUKEMIAS OF CHILDHOOD

Feature	Hypoplastic	MDS, Normal Chromosome	MDS, Chromosome 7	MDS, Other Chromosome
No. of patients	110	85	103	43
Male:female	0.98	1.4	2.1	1.3
Age* at diagnosis, mean	6.1	6.9	5.5	8.5
Median	4.5	6	3.5	8.1
Range	0.5–19	0–18	0–19	0–18
No. developing leukemia	110 (100%)	33 (39%)	52 (50%)	21 (49%)
Interval† to leukemia				
Mean	7	14	24	27
Median	3	5	16	12
Range	0.5–68	0–100	0–168	0–240
No. of deaths (%)	45 (41%)	43 (51%)	76 (74%)	28 (65%)
Projected 50% survival age*	13	12	8	12
Projected 50% survival interval* from AA or MDS diagnosis	4	1	2	2
5-year survival from AA or MDS diagnosis (%)	48%	35%	21%	24%

*Ages are in years.
†Intervals are in months.
AA = aplastic anemia.

anemia, may have increased proportions of lymphocytes, the proportion of lymphoblasts may have been overlooked. The apparent rapid recoveries from aplastic anemia following treatment with corticosteroids may really have been early remissions in ALL. All of these possibilities may explain the short interval from the hypoplastic phase to frank leukemia in children.

The first step in stem cell malignant transformation may be hypoproliferation, with further evolution to hyperproliferation. In one patient there was an identical clonal immunoglobulin heavy chain gene rearrangement in the hypoplastic marrow cells as in the leukemic cells.[935] Another possibility is that aplasia and leukemia share a common cause, such as drug, chemical, radiation, virus, or other environmental hazard.[936] Exposure to drugs or toxins that might cause aplasia

or leukemia is less common in children than in adults. However, at least five children had received chloramphenicol, one had PNH, two had hepatitis, and one was positive for EBV—all of which are conditions that may have been related to aplasia or leukemia.

Therapy and Outcome

Almost one half of the cases were reported before 1981. The patients received transfusions as needed, and half received corticosteroids (combined with androgens in 20 cases). Remissions were frequent and usually occurred within 1 month. Leukemia was then diagnosed within a median of 3 months. Eighty-five per cent were ALL, 10% AML, and the rest myelodysplasia or lymphoma. Perhaps because ALL has a better progno-

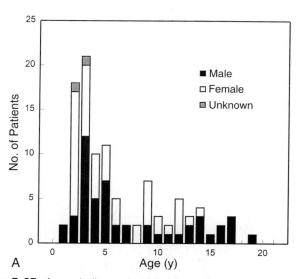

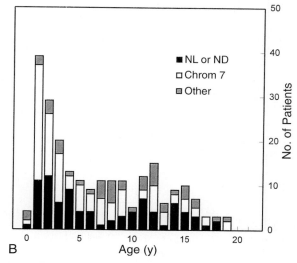

Figure 7-37. Age at diagnosis of first hematologic problem in patients with cytopenias followed by leukemia. *A,* Children with hypoplastic preleukemia. *B,* Children with myelodysplastic preleukemia. Shaded bars = males; open bars = females; crosshatched bars = sex not reported.

sis than AML, 60% of the children were still alive when reported. The average age at death was 9 years, or 2 years after the diagnosis of leukemia; the projected median survival was 4 years after detection of the first hematologic problem (Fig. 7–38). The predicted survival at 5 years after hypoplasia is 48%. The only possibility of cure might be BMT during leukemic remission. One patient who received a BMT for her aplastic anemia with only cyclophosphamide (in 1982) developed monosomy 7 ALL in host cells 11 months later[937]; this supports the conjecture that the leukemic clone caused the aplasia and emphasizes the need for adequate marrow suppression for BMT.

Myelodysplastic Preleukemia

Description

More than 200 pediatric patients[2, 4, 938–942] who resembled adults with "preleukemia" have been reported.[916] These patients have peripheral blood cytopenias with hypercellular bone marrows (i.e., ineffective hematopoiesis). The literature on adult patients uses the terms "myelodysplasia" or "refractory anemia." In 1982, Bennett and co-workers classified the syndrome for the French-American-British Co-operative Group[943] as follows:

1. Refractory anemia, anemia and reticulocytopenia, with normal or hypercellular marrow, erythroid hyperplasia or dyserythropoiesis, and a proportion of blast cells less than 5%.
2. Refractory anemia with ringed sideroblasts representing more than 15% of the total cell count.
3. Refractory anemia with excess blasts, hypercellular marrow with dysgranulopoiesis, dyserythropoiesis, or dysmegakaryocytopoiesis, in combination with a 5% to 20% proportion of marrow blasts and a less than 5% proportion of circulating blasts.
4. Chronic myelomonocytic leukemia, absolute monocytosis, increased marrow monocytes, less than 5% circulating blasts.
5. Refractory anemia with excess blasts in transformation, with a proportion of blasts in the blood greater than 5% and in the marrow from 20% to 30%, the presence of Auer rods, and nonconformity with any of the AML types M1 to M7 (see Chapter 33 for details). The abbreviation for myelodysplastic syndromes, MDS, is used generically.

The incidence of MDS resulting in acute nonlymphocytic leukemia in children was estimated as 17%,[944, 945] which is similar to the 5% to 20% incidence range seen in adults. The MDS-preleukemia patients are distinguished from the hypoplastic preleukemic patients discussed in the previous section on the basis of bone marrow hypercellularity and dysmyelopoietic changes. Half of the reported cases had clonal abnormalities involving chromosome 7 (usually monosomy 7; see Table 7–36). Because this may be a distinct syndrome that resembles CML, affected patients are analyzed separately,[2, 4] as are those with other clonal abnormalities and those with normal chromosomes.

Within the first year, a larger proportion of those with MDS than those with hypoplasia were symptomatic (see Fig. 7–38). Those with monosomy 7 were younger (see Table 7–36). There were several cases of siblings with MDS,[2, 4] with normal chromosomes or not reported, including one case of identical twins. Monosomy 7 occurred in siblings,[946] consanguineous families,[947] and dominant families.[567] Other clonal chromosome patterns also were seen in siblings and the other identical twin.[948, 949] There were twice as many males with monosomy 7 than females.

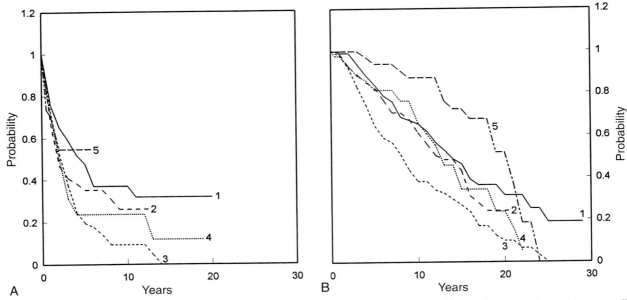

Figure 7–38. Kaplan-Meier plot of cumulative survival in years in preleukemia. *A*, Survival interval in years from the recognition of the initial hematologic problem. *B*, Survival age in years. Line 1 = hypoplastic; line 2 = MDS, normal chromosomes; line 3 = MDS, chromosome 7; line 4 = MDS, other chromosomes; line 5 = MDS after BMT.

Diagnosis was made on the basis of the presence of cytopenias in combination with a cellular bone marrow with dysplastic features (see later). Hepatosplenomegaly and extramedullary hematopoiesis are common. The cases summarized here include some of those who resembled those with leukemia even though they may not yet have developed this complication.

Laboratory Findings

The cytopenias varied from any of the single cytopenias to the bi- or pancytopenias. Leukoerythroblastosis, with a few nucleated red cells and left-shifted myeloid cells, often occurred. Stress erythropoiesis was manifested by increased levels of Hb F and i antigen and by fetal red cell enzyme patterns.[950, 951] Bone marrows were basically hypercellular and dyshematopoietic, with micromegakaryocytes, decreased nuclear segmentation in megakaryocytes, hypogranular myeloid maturation, dyserythropoiesis, and ringed sideroblasts (very rare in children). Half of the patients' marrows had deletion or abnormality of chromosome 7. Twenty per cent had other clonal abnormalities, such as trisomy 8 or 21; 5q− was rare in children compared with in adults.

Pathophysiology

Study has shown that the presence of glucose-6-phosphate dehydrogenase isoenzymes indicates that preleukemia in adults is a clonal hemopathy[952]; a similar study has not been done in children. Clonal cytogenetic abnormalities that are present in the preleukemic phase often persist in the leukemia, indicating a direct evolution. Myeloid and erythroid progenitors share the same clonal abnormality,[953] whereas lymphoid cells are excluded.[954] Hematopoiesis is ineffective *in vivo*, and the number of CFU-GMs is decreased, as is that of blood and marrow BFU-Es.[955, 956] It is presumed that a single stem cell mutation leads to myelodysplasia that evolves into leukemia. One immunodeficient patient had MDS due to chronic parvovirus infection, and improved with intravenous immunoglobulin.[957]

Therapy and Outcome

The interval from the onset of cytopenias to frank leukemia was on average between 14 and 26 months in children with MDS-leukemia, compared with 7 months in those with hypoplastic preleukemia (see Table 7–36). Disease in those without clonality appeared to evolve faster (or their MDS was not diagnosed as early because of the lack of a chromosomal marker). One apparent spontaneous remission of monosomy 7–MDS has been reported,[958] but in most cases the disease progressed (e.g., from refractory anemia to refractory anemia with excess blasts, or from refractory anemia with excess blasts to refractory anemia with excess blasts in transformation). Approximately 50% of patients developed leukemia, mostly acute nonlymphocytic leukemia; only 2 cases of ALL were recorded.[959, 960] More than 60% died within a mean of 2

years after their initial presentation. The projected median interval of survival is 1 to 2 years, and the 5-year survival is 21% to 24%, depending on the clonal pattern (see Fig. 7–38); these results are worse than those in patients with hypoplastic preleukemia.

Treatment for childhood myelodysplasia is less than satisfactory, with supportive transfusions as the mainstay of treatment. Splenectomy in a dozen patients led to only transient improvement in blood counts. Thirty per cent of those treated with steroids improved temporarily, perhaps owing to chemical shrinkage of the reticuloendothelial system. Cytoreductive agents were generally ineffective.[961] Experimental protocols such as those used in adults, which included low-dose cytosine arabinoside or 5-azacytidine, were used infrequently in children.[939, 962] Because of the high risk of leukemia, BMT was the treatment of choice for those patients with a donor.[962, 963] The 5-year survival rate was approximately 50%, and median projected survival interval from the time of BMT was longer than 6 years in more than 40 patients who received transplants while still myelodysplastic (see Fig. 7–38). Trials of recombinant human hematopoietic growth factor treatments are in progress in adults but not yet in children with MDS. Use of both GM-CSF and G-CSF may lead to dose-dependent increases in neutrophils; however, improvements in platelet counts and transfusion requirements are rare, and the number of blasts may increase.[964, 965] Erythropoietin improved hemoglobin levels in adults with refractory anemia and in those with refractory anemia with ringed sideroblasts, particularly patients with serum erythropoietin levels less than 100 mU/mL. There is concern, but no supporting data, that these factors may accelerate the leukemic transformation.

SUMMARY

The major inherited bone marrow failure disorders are summarized in Table 7–37. The diagnosis of "acquired" aplastic anemia or single cytopenia should not be made without serious consideration of these conditions. Physical anomalies may be subtle or absent, but family histories or specific laboratory investigations (e.g., chromosome breakage) may provide clues. The numbers of cases and the proportions in whom complications occur are not true incidence figures. They are based on literature reports, not on epidemiologic studies. Despite under-reporting and underdiagnosis, the numbers do provide some perspective about relative frequencies.

Most of these conditions are expressed in probable homozygotes (for autosomal recessives) or hemizygotes (X-linked). Because heterozygotes usually cannot be identified (except as parents), patients with multiple bone marrow failure genes or with "acquired" diseases that may in fact be inherited cannot be identified at this time.

Treatment of marrow failure depends on the specific diagnosis. Androgens may be effective in patients with pancytopenia due to Fanconi's anemia, DC, amegakaryocytic thrombocytopenia, or SD syndrome. Patients

Table 7-37. INHERITED BONE MARROW FAILURE SYNDROMES

Feature	Fanconi's Anemia	Dyskeratosis Congenita	Shwachman-Diamond Syndrome	Amega-karyocytic Thrombocyto-penia	Diamond-Blackfan Anemia	Kostmann's Syndrome	Thrombocyto-penia with Absent Radii
Approximate No. of patients	1000	225	200	45	550	200	200
Male:female	1.3	4.3	1.7	1.6	1.1	1	0.7
Genetics	AR	X	AR	X, AR	AR, AD, sporadic	AR	AR
Birth defects (%)	80	100	60	40	25	0	100
Upper limb (%)	48	15	<2	0	8	0	100
Median age at diagnosis	7.5 y	16 y	4 mo	7 d	2 mo	1 mo	Birth
First hematologic sign	Pancytopenia	Pancytopenia	Neutropenia	Thrombocyto-penia	Anemia	Neutropenia	Thrombocyto-penia
Bone marrow	Aplastic	Aplastic	Hypocellular, myeloid arrest	Absent or small megakaryo-cytes	Erythroid hypoplasia	Myeloid arrest	Absent or immature megakaryo-cytes
Aplastic anemia (%)	95	50	20	40	0	0	0
Leukemia/MDS (%)	12	0.4	5	5	2	2% pre–G-CSF; 13% on G-CSF	0
Cancer (%)	5	10	0	—	0.4	0	0
Liver disease (%)	4	0	0	—	0.2	0	0
Hb F level	Increased	Increased	Increased	Increased	Increased	Normal	Normal
Chromosomes	Breaks with clastogens	Bleomycin sensitive	Normal	Normal	Normal	Normal	Normal
Spontaneous remissions (%)	Very rare	0	Rare	0	20	0	75
Treatment	BMT, androgens	Androgens	G-CSF, BMT	BMT	Steroids, BMT, ?IL-3	G-CSF	Platelets
Response (%)	50, transient	50, transient	80	—	50	95	—
Prognosis	Poor	Poor	Fair	Poor	Good	Good	Good
Chromosome	Group C = 9q	Xq	—	—	—	—	—
Prenatal diagnosis	Chromosome breaks, FAC	Xq28 RFLP	Neutropenia	Thrombocyto-penia	?ADA, ?BFU-E	Neutropenia	Absent radii, thrombocyto-penia
Projected 50% survival age (y)	30	33	35	3	40	>20	>55

AR = autosomal recessive; AD = autosomal dominant; X = X-linked recessive; FAC = Fanconi's anemia complementation group C; RFLP = restriction fragment length polymorphism.

with Diamond-Blackfan anemia should receive cortico-steroids. G-CSF is particularly effective in Kostmann's syndrome. Platelets provide necessary (and necessarily temporary) support for patients with TAR. BMT for FA requires modification of preparative protocols; patients with DC need protocols that have not yet been developed; patients with SD may be able to undergo transplantation; and patients with DBA and TAR—which might and will improve spontaneously, respectively—may not need transplantation at all. The donor must be known to be unaffected by the familial disease. Immunotherapy and growth factor treatment may be provided for specific diseases. All treatments and diseases may evolve into leukemia or other malignancies, and high-risk therapies must be considered very carefully in patients whose underlying condition is prema-

lignant. Treatment of malignant complications is difficult in these inherited disorders, in which abnormalities involve more than just hematopoietic tissues.

Prenatal diagnosis is available for many of the inherited marrow failure disorders. Families are usually identified through a propositus, and monitoring is offered for subsequent pregnancies. Early diagnosis of an affected fetus may eventually lead to treatment *in utero* or at birth. Diagnosis of an unaffected HLA-identical fetus may provide placental blood for treatment of the propositus.

Clearly, much remains to be understood about the genetics, pathophysiology, and treatment of both "inherited" and "acquired" bone marrow failure syndromes. This understanding requires correct diagnoses as well as proper treatment and careful follow-up. The prognoses for most of these disorders have improved with recent therapeutic advances, and it is anticipated that this improvement will accelerate as greater knowledge of the specific molecular and cellular defects is attained.

References

1. Alter BP, Potter NU, Li FP: Classification and aetiology of the aplastic anaemias. Clin Haematol 1978; 7:431.
2. Young NS, Alter BP: Aplastic Anemia: Acquired and Inherited. Philadelphia, W.B. Saunders Co., 1994.
3. Gordon-Smith EC: Baillière's Clinical Haematology. Aplastic Anaemia. London, Baillière Tindall, 1989, p 194.
4. Alter BP, Young NS: The bone marrow failure syndromes. In Nathan DG, Oski FA (eds): Hematology of Infancy and Childhood. Philadelphia, W.B. Saunders Co., 1993, p 216.
5. Camitta BM, Thomas ED, et al: Severe aplastic anemia: A prospective study of the effect of early marrow transplantation on acute mortality. Blood 1976; 48:63.
6. Ehrlich P: Über einen Fall von Anämie mit Bemerkungen über regenerative Veränderungen des Knochenmarks. Charité-Annalen 1888; 13:300.
7. Vaquez MH, Aubertin C: L'anémie pernicieuse d'après les conceptions actuelles. Bull Mem Soc Med Hop Paris 1904; 21:288.
8. Wolf B, Hsia YE, et al: Propionic acidemia: A clinical update. J Pediatr 1981; 99:835.
9. Issaragrisil S, Sriratanasatavorn C, et al: Aplastic Anemia Study Group. Incidence of aplastic anemia in Bangkok. Blood 1991; 77:2166.
10. Issaragrisil S, Kaufman D, Young NS: The epidemiology of aplastic anemia in Thailand. Blood 1995; 86(Suppl 1):478a.
11. U.S. Public Health Service: Mortality. In Vital Statistics of the United States. 2nd ed. Washington, DC, U.S. Department of Health and Human Services, 1986, p 122.
12. Kaufman DW, Kelly JP, et al: The drug etiology of agranulocytosis and aplastic anemia. New York, Oxford University Press, 1991, p 259.
13. Powars D: Aplastic anemia secondary to glue sniffing. N Engl J Med 1965; 273:700.
14. International Agranulocytosis and Aplastic Anemia Study: Anti-infective drug use in relation to the risk of agranulocytosis and aplastic anemia. A report from the International Agranulocytosis and Aplastic Anemia Study. Arch Intern Med 1989; 149:1036.
15. Kaufman DW, Kelly JP, et al: Drugs in the aetiology of agranulocytosis and aplastic anaemia. Eur J Haemotol 1996; 57(Suppl):23.
16. Yunis AA: Mechanisms underlying marrow toxicity from chloramphenicol and thiamphenicol. In Silber R, LoBue J, Gordon AS (eds): The Year in Hematology. New York, Plenum Medical Book Co., 1978, p 143.
17. West BC, DeVault GA Jr, et al: Aplastic anemia associated with parenteral chloramphenicol: Review of 10 cases, including the second case of possible increased risk with cimetidine. Rev Infect Dis 1988; 10:1048.
18. DeRenzo A, Formisano S, Rotoli B: Bone marrow aplasia and thiamphenicol. Haematologica (Pavia) 1981; 66:98.
19. Yunis AA: Chloramphenicol toxicity: 25 years of research. Am J Med 1989; 87(3N):44N.
20. Brahams D: Lindane exposure and aplastic anaemia. Lancet 1994; 343:1092.
21. Parent-Massin D, Thouvenot D, et al: Lindane haematotoxicity confirmed by *in vitro* tests on human and rat progenitors. Hum Exp Toxicol 1994; 13:103.
22. Knospe WH, Crosby WH: Aplastic anaemia: A disorder of the bone-marrow sinusoidal microcirculation rather than stem-cell failure? Lancet 1971; 1:20.
23. Kurtzman G, Young N: Virus-associated bone marrow failure. Baillières Clin Haematol 1989; 2:51.
24. Young NS: Parvoviruses. In Fields BM, Knipe DM (eds): Virology. 3rd ed. New York, Raven Press, 1995.
25. Young NS: B19 parvovirus. In Young NS (ed): Baillière's Clinical Haematology. 8th ed. London, Baillière Tindall, 1995, p 25.
26. Pattison JR, Jones SE, et al: Parvovirus infections and hypoplastic crisis in sickle-cell anaemia. Lancet 1981; 1:664.
27. Serjeant GR, Topley JM, et al: Outbreak of aplastic crises in sickle cell anaemia associated with parvovirus-like agent. Lancet 1981; 2:595.
28. Anand A, Gray ES, et al: Human parvovirus infection in pregnancy and hydrops fetalis. N Engl J Med 1987; 316:183.
29. Brown KE, Green SW, et al: Congenital anaemia after transplacental B19 parvovirus infection. Lancet 1994; 343:895.
30. Kurtzman G, Frickhofen N, et al: Pure red-cell aplasia of 10 years' duration due to persistent parvovirus B19 infection and its cure with immunoglobulin therapy. N Engl J Med 1989; 321:519.
31. Frickhofen N, Abkowitz JL, et al: Persistent B19 parvovirus infection in patients infected with human immunodeficiency virus type 1 (HIV-1): A treatable cause of anemia in AIDS. Ann Intern Med 1990; 113:926.
32. Frickhofen N, Chen ZJ, et al: Parvovirus B19 as a cause of acquired chronic pure red cell aplasia. Br J Haematol 1994; 87:818.
33. Ozawa K, Kurtzman G, Young N: Productive infection by B19 parvovirus of human erythroid bone marrow cells *in vitro*. Blood 1987; 70:384.
34. Böttiger LE, Westerholm B: Aplastic anaemia. III. Aplastic anaemia and infectious hepatitis. Acta Med Scand 1972; 192:323.
35. Young NS, Issaragrisil S, et al: Aplastic anemia in the Orient. Br J Haematol 1986; 62:1.
36. Liang D-C, Lin K-H, et al: Post-hepatitic aplastic anaemia in children in Taiwan, a hepatitis prevalent area. Br J Haematol 1990; 74:487.
37. Pikis A, Kavaliotis J, Manios S: Incidence of aplastic anemia in viral hepatitis in children. Scand J Infect Dis 1988; 20:109.
38. Perrillo RP, Pohl DA, et al: Acute non-A, non-B hepatitis with serum sickness-like syndrome and aplastic anemia. JAMA 1981; 245:494.
39. Tzakis AG, Arditi M, et al: Aplastic anemia complicating orthotopic liver transplantation for non-A, non-B hepatitis. N Engl J Med 1988; 319:393.
40. Smith D, Gribble TJ, et al: Spontaneous resolution of severe aplastic anemia associated with viral hepatitis A in a 6-year-old child. Am J Hematol 1978; 5:247.
41. Kindmark C-O, Sjölin J, et al: Aplastic anaemia in a case of hepatitis B with a high titer of hepatitis B antigen. Acta Med Scand 1984; 215:89.
42. Hibbs JR, Frickhofen N, et al: Aplastic anemia and viral hepatitis. Non-A, non-B, non-C? JAMA 1992; 267:2051.
43. Hagler L, Pastore RA, Bergin JJ: Aplastic anemia following viral hepatitis: Report of two fatal cases and literature review. Medicine 1975; 54:139.
44. Nakao S, Lai C-J, Young NS: Dengue virus, a flavivirus, propagates in human bone marrow progenitors and hematopoietic cell lines. Blood 1989; 74:1235.
45. Simons JN, Leary TP, et al: Isolation of novel virus-like sequences associated with human hepatitis. Nat Med 1995; 1:564.
46. Simons JN, Pilot-Matias TJ, et al: Identification of two flavivirus-like genomes in the GB hepatitis agent. Proc Natl Acad Sci U S A 1995; 92:3401.
47. Tosato G, Taga K, et al: Epstein-Barr virus as an agent of haematological disease. In Young NS (ed): Baillière's Clinical Haematology. 8th ed. London, Baillière Tindall, 1995, p 165.
48. Baranski B, Armstrong G, et al: Epstein-Barr virus in the bone marrow of patients with aplastic anemia. Ann Intern Med 1988; 109:695.
49. Purtilo DT, Sakamoto K, et al: Epstein-Barr virus-induced diseases in boys with the X-linked lymphoproliferative syndrome (XLP). Update on studies of the registry. Am J Med 1982; 73:49.
50. Sing GK, Ruscetti FW: The role of human cytomegalovirus in haematological diseases. In Young NS (ed): Baillière's Clinical Haematology. 8th ed. London, Baillière Tindall, 1995, p 149.
51. Simmons P, Kaushansky K, Torok-Storb B: Mechanisms of cytomegalovirus-mediated myelosuppression: Perturbation of stromal cell function versus direct infection of myeloid cells. Proc Natl Acad Sci U S A 1990; 87:1386.

52. Maciejewski JP, Bruening E, et al: Infection of hematopoietic progenitor cells by human cytomegalovirus. Blood 1992; 80:170.

53. Carrigan DR, Knox KK: Human herpesvirus 6 (HHV-6) isolation from bone marrow: HHV-6-associated bone marrow suppression in bone marrow transplant patients. Blood 1994; 84:3307.

54. Lusso P, Gallo RC: Human herpesvirus 6. In Young NS (ed): Baillière's Clinical Haematology. 8th ed. London, Baillière Tindall, 1995, p 201.

55. Knox KK, Carrigan DR: In vitro suppression of bone marrow progenitor cell differentiation by human herpesvirus 6 infection. J Infect Dis 1992; 165:925.

56. Davis BR, Zauli G: Effect of human immunodeficiency virus infection on hematopoiesis. In Young NS (ed): Baillière's Clinical Haematology. 8th ed. London, Baillière Tindall, 1995, p 113.

57. Stella CC, Ganser A, Hoelzer D: Defective in vitro growth of the hemopoietic progenitor cells in the acquired immunodeficiency syndrome. J Clin Invest 1987; 80:286.

58. Bagnara GP, Zauli G, et al: Early loss of circulating hemopoietic progenitors in HIV-1–infected subjects. Exp Hematol 1990; 18:426.

59. de Luca A, Teofili L, et al: Haemopoietic CD34 + progenitor cells are not infected by HIV-1 in vivo but show impaired clonogenesis. Br J Haematol 1993; 85:20.

60. Zauli G, Re MC, et al: Impaired in vitro growth of purified (CD34 +) hematopoietic progenitors in human immunodeficiency virus-1 seropositive thrombocytopenic individuals. Blood 1992; 79:2680.

61. Von Laer D, Hufert FT, et al: CD34 + hematopoietic progenitor cells are not a major reservoir of the human immunodeficiency virus. Blood 1990; 76:1281.

62. Molina J-M, Scadden DT, et al: Lack of evidence for infection of or effect on growth of haematopoietic progenitor cells after in vivo or in vitro exposure to human immunodeficiency virus. Blood 1990; 76:2476.

63. Zucker-Franklin D, Seremetis S, Zheng ZY: Internalization of human immunodeficiency virus type I and other retroviruses by megakaryocytes and platelets. Blood 1990; 75:1920.

64. Cen D, Zauli G, et al: Effect of different human immunodeficiency virus type-1 (HIV-1) isolates on long-term bone marrow haemopoiesis. Br J Haematol 1993; 85:596.

65. Schwartz GN, Kessler SW, et al: Inhibitory effects of HIV-1 infected stromal cell layers on the production of myeloid progenitor cells in human long-term bone marrow cultures. Exp Hematol 1994; 22:1288.

66. Maciejewski JP, Weichold FF, Young NS: HIV-1 inhibition of hematopoiesis in vitro mediated by envelope glycoprotein and TNF-α. J Immunol 1994; 153:4303.

67. Alter BP, Frissora CL, et al: Fanconi's anemia and pregnancy. Br J Haematol 1991; 77:410.

68. Dukes PP, Goldwasser E: Inhibition of erythropoiesis by estrogens. Endocrinology 1961; 69:21.

69. Yeh ETH, Rosse WF: Paroxysmal nocturnal hemoglobinuria and the glycosylphosphatidylinositol anchor. J Clin Invest 1994; 93:2305.

70. Schrenzenmeier H, Hertenstein B, et al: A pathogenetic link between aplastic anemia and paroxysmal nocturnal hemoglobinuria is suggested by a high frequency of aplastic anemia with a deficiency of phosphatidylinositol glycan proteins. Exp Hematol 1995; 23:81.

71. Schubert J, Alvarado M, et al: Diagnosis of paroxysmal nocturnal haemoglobinuria using immunophenotyping of peripheral blood cells. Br J Haematol 1991; 79:487.

72. Hoffman R, Dainiak N, et al: Antibody-mediated aplastic anemia and diffuse fasciitis. N Engl J Med 1979; 300:718.

73. Talerman A, Amigo A: Thymoma associated with aregenerative and aplastic anemia in a five-year-old child. Cancer 1968; 21:1212.

74. Ferrara JLM, Deeg HJ: Graft-versus-host disease. N Engl J Med 1991; 324:667.

75. Bessman JD, Gilmer PR, Gardner FH: Improved classification of anemias by MCV and RDW. Am J Clin Pathol 1983; 80:322.

76. Twomey JJ, Douglass CC, Sharkey O Jr: The monocytopenia of aplastic anemia. Blood 1973; 41:187.

77. Elfenbein GJ, Kallman CH, et al: The immune system in 40 aplastic anemia patients receiving conventional therapy. Blood 1979; 53:652.

78. Alter BP: Fetal erythropoiesis in stress hematopoiesis. Exp Hematol 1979; 7:200.

79. Rosse WF: Paroxysmal nocturnal haemoglobinuria in aplastic anaemia. Clin Haematol 1978; 7:541.

80. Branda RF, Moldow CF, et al: Folate-induced remission in aplastic anemia with familial defect of cellular folate uptake. N Engl J Med 1978; 298:469.

81. Jelkmann W, Wiedenmann G: Serum erythropoietin level: Relationships to blood hemoglobin concentration and erythrocytic activity of the bone marrow. Klin Wochenschr 1990; 68:403.

82. Mir MA, Geary CG, Delamore IW: Hypoimmunoglobulinemia and aplastic anaemia. Scand J Haematol 1977; 19:225.

83. Passmore SJ, Hann IM, et al: Pediatric myelodysplasia: A study of 68 children and a new prognostic scoring system. Blood 1995; 85:1742.

84. Li FP, Alter BP, Nathan DG: The mortality of acquired aplastic anemia in children. Blood 1972; 40:153.

85. Negendank W, Weissman D, et al: Evidence for clonal disease by magnetic resonance imaging in patients with hypoplastic marrow disorders. Blood 1991; 78:2872.

86. McKinstry CS, Steiner RE, et al: Bone marrow in leukemia and aplastic anemia: MR imaging before, during, and after treatment. Radiology 1987; 162:701.

87. Russell ES: Hereditary anemias of the mouse: A review for geneticists. Adv Genet 1979; 20:357.

88. Knospe WH, Husseini SG, et al: Immunologically mediated aplastic anemia in mice: evidence of hematopoietic stromal injury and injury to hematopoietic stem cells. Exp Hematol 1994; 22:573.

89. Schrezenmeier H, Gerok M, Heimpel H: Assessment of frequency of hematopoietic stem cells in aplastic anemia by limiting dilution type long term marrow culture. Exp Hematol 1992; 20:806.

90. Maciejewski JP, Selleri C, et al: A severe and consistent deficit in marrow and circulating primitive hematopoietic cells (long-term-culture-initiating cells) in acquired aplastic anemia. Blood 1996; 88:1983.

91. Maciejewski JP, Anderson S, et al: Phenotypic and functional analysis of bone marrow progenitor cell compartment in bone marrow failure. Br J Haematol 1994; 87:227.

92. Scopes J, Bagnara M, et al: Haemopoietic progenitor cells are reduced in aplastic anaemia. Br J Haematol 1994; 86:427.

93. Young NS: The problem of clonality in aplastic anemia: Dr. Dameshek's riddle, restated. Blood 1992; 79:1385.

94. Abkowitz JL, Fialkow PJ, et al: Pancytopenia as a clonal disorder of a multipotent hematopoietic stem cell. J Clin Invest 1984; 73:258.

95. Athanasou NA, Quinn J, et al: Origin of marrow stromal cells and haemopoietic chimaerism following bone marrow transplantation determined by in situ hybridisation. Br J Cancer 1990; 61:385.

96. Marsh JCW, Chang J, et al: In vitro assessment of marrow 'stem cell' and stromal cell function in aplastic anemia. Br J Haematol 1991; 78:258.

97. Juneja HS, Lee S, Gardner FH: Human long-term bone marrow cultures in aplastic anemia. Int J Cell Cloning 1989; 7:129.

98. Kawakami M, Tsutsumi H, et al: Levels of serum granulocyte colony-stimulating factor in patients with infections. Blood 1990; 76:1962.

99. Omori F, Okamura S, et al: Levels of human serum granulocyte colony-stimulating factor and granulocyte-macrophage colony-stimulating factor under pathological conditions. Biotherapy 1992; 4:147.

100. Schrezenmeier H, Raghavachar A, Heimpel H: Granulocyte-macrophage colony-stimulating factor in the sera of patients with aplastic anemia. Clin Invest 1993; 71:102.

101. Kawano Y, Takaue Y, et al: Production of interleukin 3 and granulocyte-macrophage colony-stimulating factor from stimulated blood mononuclear cells in patients with aplastic anemia. Exp Hematol 1992; 20:1125.

102. Migliaccio AR, Migliaccio G, et al: Production of granulocyte colony-stimulating factor and granulocyte/macrophage-colony-stimulating factor after interleukin-1 stimulation of marrow stromal cell cultures from normal or aplastic anemia donors. J Cell Physiol 1992; 152:199.

103. Bacigalupo A, Piaggio G, et al: Response of CFU-GM to increasing doses of rhGM-CSF in patients with aplastic anemia. Exp Hematol 1991; 19:829.
104. Gibson FM, Scopes J, et al: *In vitro* response of normal and aplastic anemia bone marrow to mast cell growth factor and in combination with granulocyte-macrophage colony-stimulating factor and interleukin-3. Exp Hematol 1994; 22:302.
105. Nakao S, Matsushima K, Young N: Deficient interleukin 1 production by aplastic anemia monocytes. Br J Haematol 1989; 71:431.
106. Holmberg LA, Seidel K, et al: Aplastic anemia: Analysis of stromal cell function in long-term marrow cultures. Blood 1994; 84:3685.
107. Wodnar-Filipowicz A, Yancik S, et al: Levels of soluble stem cell factor in serum of patients with aplastic anemia. Blood 1993; 81:3259.
108. Holmberg LA, Yancik S, et al: Circulating levels of kit ligand (KL) in serum of patients with aplastic anemia, myelodysplasia or following allogeneic bone marrow transplantation. Exp Hematol 1992; 20:775.
109. Nimer SD, Leung DHY, et al: Serum stem cell factor levels in patients with aplastic anemia. Int J Hematol 1994; 60:185.
110. Walsh CE, Liu JM, et al: A trial of recombinant human interleukin-1 in patients with severe refractory aplastic anaemia. Br J Haematol 1992; 80:106.
111. Nemunaitis J, Ross M, et al: Phase I study of recombinant human interleukin-1b (rhIL-1b) in patients with bone marrow failure. Bone Marrow Transplant 1994; 14:583.
112. Hinterberger W, Raghavachar A, et al: Bone marrow transplantation from genotypically identical twins with aplastic anemia. In Raghavachar A, Schrezenmeier H, Frickhofen N (eds): Aplastic Anemia: Current Perspectives on the Pathogenesis and Treatment. Vienna, Blackwell-MZV, 1993, p 102.
113. Chapuis B, Von Fliedner VE, et al: Increased frequency of DR2 in patients with aplastic anaemia and increased DR sharing in their parents. Br J Haematol 1986; 63:51.
114. Nakao S, Yamaguchi M, et al: HLA-DR2 predicts a favorable response to cyclosporine therapy in patients with bone marrow failure. Am J Haematol 1992; 40:239.
115. Nimer SD, Ireland P, et al: An increased HLA DR2 frequency is seen in aplastic anemia patients. Blood 1994; 84:923.
116. Bacigalupo A, Podesta M, et al: T-derived colony-inhibiting activity (Td/CIA) in aplastic anemia (SAA) and in normal donors. In Young NS, Levine AS, Humphries RK (eds): Aplastic Anemia: Stem Cell Biology and Advances in Treatment. New York, Alan R. Liss, 1984, p 173.
117. Koller U, Hinterberger W, et al: Identification of activated T cells and the suppressor/inducer subset in patients suffering from severe aplastic anemia. Blut 1989; 58:21.
118. Zoumbos NC, Gascón P, et al: Circulating activated suppressor T lymphocytes in aplastic anemia. N Engl J Med 1985; 312:257.
119. Maciejewski JP, Hibbs JR, et al: Bone marrow and peripheral blood lymphocyte phenotype in patients with bone marrow failure. Exp Hematol 1994; 22:1102.
120. Herrmann F, Griffin JD, et al: Establishment of an interleukin 2–dependent T cell line derived from a patient with severe aplastic anemia, which inhibits *in vitro* hematopoiesis. J Immunol 1986; 136:1629.
121. Tong J, Bacigalupo A, et al: *In vitro* response of T cells from aplastic anemia patients to antilymphocyte globulin and phytohemagglutinin: Colony-stimulating activity and lymphokine production. Exp Hematol 1991; 19:312.
122. Nakao S, Takamatsu H, et al: Establishment of a CD4+ T cell clone recognizing autologous hematopoietic progenitor cells from a patient with immune-mediated aplastic anemia. Exp Hematol 1995; 23:433.
123. Hinterberger W, Adolf G, et al: Lymphokine overproduction in severe aplastic anemia is not related to blood transfusions. Blood 1989; 74:2713.
124. Laver J, Castro-Malaspina H, et al: *In vitro* interferon-gamma production by cultured T-cells in severe aplastic anaemia: correlation with granulomonopoietic inhibition in patients who respond to anti-thymocyte globulin. Br J Haematol 1988; 69:545.
125. Zoumbos NC, Gascón P, et al: Interferon is a mediator of hematopoietic suppression in aplastic anemia *in vitro* and possibly *in vivo*. Proc Natl Acad Sci U S A 1985; 82:188.
126. Hinterberger-Fischer M, Hinterberger W, et al: Treatment of severe aplastic anemia with combined immunosuppression (antithymocyte globulin and high-dose methylprednisolone). Acta Haematol 1986; 76:196.
127. Nakao S, Yamaguchi M, et al: Interferon-γ gene expression in unstimulated bone marrow mononuclear cells predicts a good response to cyclosporine therapy in aplastic anemia. Blood 1992; 79:2532.
128. Nistico A, Young NS: γ-Interferon gene expression in the bone marrow of patients with acquired aplastic anemia. Ann Intern Med 1994; 120:463.
129. Katevas P, Maciejewski J, et al: Increased expression of TNF-beta in patients with aplastic anemia. Blood 1993; 82:345a.
130. Schultz JC, Shahidi NT: Detection of tumor necrosis factor-α in bone marrow plasma and peripheral blood plasma from patients with aplastic anemia. Am J Hematol 1994; 45:32.
131. Maciejewski JP, Liu JM, et al: Expression of stem cell inhibitor (SCI) gene in patients with bone marrow failure. Exp Hematol 1992; 20:1112.
132. Selleri C, Young NS, Maciejewski J: Interferon-gamma and tumor necrosis factor-alpha broadly suppress human hematopoiesis and induce apoptosis in purified hematopoietic cells. J Cell Physiol 1995; 165:538.
133. Selleri C, Maciejewski J, Young NS: Interferon-γ constitutively expressed in the stromal microenvironment of human marrow cultures mediates hematopoietic inhibition. Blood 1996; 87:4149.
134. Maciejewski J, Selleri C, Young NS: Fas antigen expression on CD34+ human marrow cells is induced by interferon-gamma and tumor necrosis factor-alpha and potentiates hematopoietic suppression *in vitro*. Blood 1995; 85:3183.
135. Bacigalupo A, Piaggio G, et al: Collection of peripheral blood hematopoietic progenitors (PBHP) from patients with severe aplastic anemia (SAA) after prolonged administration of granulocyte colony-stimulating factor. Blood 1993; 82:1410.
136. Reynolds CW, Foon KA: Tg-lymphoproliferative disease and related disorders in humans and experimental animals: A review of the clinical, cellular, and functional characteristics. Blood 1984; 64:1146.
137. Gascon P, Zoumbos N, Young N: Analysis of natural killer cells in patients with aplastic anemia. Blood 1986; 67:1349.
138. Wolff JA: Anemias caused by infections and toxins, idiopathic aplastic anemia and anemia caused by renal disease. Pediatr Clin North Am 1957; 4:469.
139. Diamond LK, Shahidi NT: Treatment of aplastic anemia in children. Semin Hematol 1967; 4:278.
140. Camitta BM, Storb R, Thomas ED: Aplastic anemia. (First of two parts). Pathogenesis, diagnosis, treatment, and prognosis. N Engl J Med 1982; 306:645.
141. Nathan DG: "Myelophrenia": Its contribution to the management of aplastic anemia. In Young NS, Levine AS, Humphries RK (eds): Aplastic Anemia: Stem Cell Biology and Advances in Treatment. New York, Alan R. Liss, 1984, p xxi.
142. Bacigalupo A, Hows J, et al: Bone marrow transplantation (BMT) versus immunosuppression for the treatment of severe aplastic anaemia (SAA): a report of the EBMT SAA working party. Br J Haematol 1988; 70:177.
143. de Planque MM, van Krieken JHJM, et al: Bone marrow histopathology of patients with severe aplastic anaemia before treatment and at follow-up. Br J Haematol 1989; 72:439.
144. Najean Y, Pecking A: Prognostic factors in acquired aplastic anemia. A study of 352 cases. Am J Med 1979; 67:564.
145. Weinberger M, Elattar I, et al: Patterns of infection in patients with aplastic anemia and the emergence of aspergillus as a major cause of death. Medicine 1992; 71:24.
146. Heyn RM, Ertel IJ, Tubergen DG: Course of acquired aplastic anemia in children treated with supportive care. JAMA 1969; 208:1372.
147. Khatib Z, Wilimas J, Wang W: Outcome of moderate aplastic anemia in children. Am J Pediatr Hematol Oncol 1994; 16:80.
148. Champlin R, Ho W, Gale RP: Antithymocyte globulin treatment in patients with aplastic anemia. A prospective randomized trial. N Engl J Med 1983; 308:113.
149. Herman JH, Kamel HT: Platelet transfusion. Current techniques, remaining problems, and future prospects. Am J Pediatr Hematol Oncol 1987; 9:272.

150. Heyman MR, Schiffer CA: Platelet transfusion therapy for the cancer patient. Semin Oncol 1990; 17:198.

151. Patten E: Controversies in transfusion medicine. Prophylactic platelet transfusion revisited after 25 years: con. Transfusion 1992; 32:381.

152. Fricke W, Alling D, et al: Lack of efficacy of tranexamic acid in thrombocytopenic bleeding. Transfusion 1991; 31:345.

153. Keidan AJ, Tsatalas C, et al: Infective complications of aplastic anaemia. Br J Haematol 1986; 63:503.

154. DiNubile MJ: Therapeutic role of granulocyte transfusions. Rev Infect Dis 1985; 7:232.

155. Dutcher JP, Schiffer CA, et al: Alloimmunization prevents the migration of transfused indium-111–labeled granulocytes to sites of infection. Blood 1983; 62:354.

156. Brittenham GM, Cohen AR, et al: Hepatic iron stores and plasma ferritin concentration in patients with sickle cell anemia and thalassemia major. Am J Hematol 1993; 42:81.

157. Brittenham GM, Griffith PM, et al: Efficacy of deferoxamine in preventing complications of iron overload in patients with thalassemia major. N Engl J Med 1994; 331:567.

158. Olivieri NF, Matsui D, Berkovitch M: Superior effectiveness of the oral iron chelator L1 vs subcutaneous deferoxamine in patients with homozygous beta-thalassemia (HBT): the impact of patient compliance during two years of therapy. Blood 1992; 80:344a.

159. Kontoghiorghes GJ: Advances in oral iron chelation in man. Int J Hematol 1992; 55:27.

160. Young NS, Barrett AJ: The treatment of severe acquired aplastic anemia. Blood 1995; 85:3367.

161. Storb R: Bone marrow transplantation for aplastic anemia. Cell Transplant 1994; 2:365.

162. Gajewski JL, Champlin RE: How to manage severe aplastic anemia. Contemp Oncol 1994; 4:69.

163. Stewart FM: Hypoplastic/aplastic anemia. Role of bone marrow transplantation. Med Clin North Am 1992; 76:683.

164. Armitage JO: Bone marrow transplantation. N Engl J Med 1994; 330:827.

165. Deeg HJ, Klingemann H-G, Phillips GL: A Guide to Bone Marrow Transplantation. 2nd ed. Berlin, Springer-Verlag, 1992, p 310.

166. Treleaven J, Barrett J: Bone marrow transplantation in practice. Edinburgh, Churchill Livingstone, 1992, p 399.

167. Gluckman E, Socie G, et al: Bone marrow transplantation in 107 patients with severe aplastic anemia using cyclophosphamide and thoraco-abdominal irradiation for conditioning: Long-term follow-up. Blood 1991; 78:2451.

168. Champlin RE, Ho WG, et al: Bone marrow transplantation for severe aplastic anemia. Transplantation 1990; 49:720.

169. May WS, Sensenbrenner LL, et al: BMT for severe aplastic anemia using cyclosporine. Bone Marrow Transplant 1993; 11:459.

170. Storb R, Etzioni R, et al: Cyclophosphamide combined with antithymocyte globulin in preparation for allogeneic marrow transplants in patients with aplastic anemia. Blood 1994; 84:941.

171. Gluckman E, Horowitz MM, et al: Bone marrow transplantation for severe aplastic anemia: influence of conditioning and graft-versus-host disease prophylaxis regimens on outcome. Blood 1992; 79:269.

172. Bortin MM, Horowitz MM, Rowlings PA: 1993 progress report from the International Bone Marrow Transplant Registry. Bone Marrow Transplant 1993; 12:97.

173. Bacigalupo A: Severe aplastic anaemia working party. In: EBMT Working Parties Reports. London, Harrogate, 1994, p 49.

174. Deeg HJ, Self S, et al: Decreased incidence of marrow graft rejection in patients with severe aplastic anemia: Changing impact of risk factors. Blood 1986; 68:1363.

175. Bordin JO, Heddle NM, Blajchman MA: Biologic effects of leukocytes present in transfused cellular blood products. Blood 1994; 83:1703.

176. McCann SR, Bacigalupo A, et al: Graft rejection and second bone marrow transplants for aplastic anemia: a report from the Aplastic Anaemia Working Party of the European Bone Marrow Transplant Group. Bone Marrow Transplant 1994; 13:233.

177. Deeg HJ, Storb R, Thomas ED: Bone marrow transplantation: A review of delayed complications. Br J Haematol 1984; 57:185.

178. Sanders JE, Storb R, et al: Marrow transplant experience for children with severe aplastic anemia. Am J Pediatr Hematol Oncol 1994; 16:43.

179. McGlave PB, Haake R, et al: Therapy of severe aplastic anemia in young adults and children with allogeneic bone marrow transplantation. Blood 1987; 70:1325.

180. Vowels MR, Lam PT, et al: Bone marrow transplantation in children using closely matched related and unrelated donors. Bone Marrow Transplant 1991; 8:87.

181. Beatty PG, Dahlberg S, et al: Probability of finding HLA-matched unrelated marrow donors. Transplantation 1988; 45:714.

182. Bacigalupo A, Hows J, et al: Bone marrow transplantation for severe aplastic anemia from donors other than HLA identical siblings: a report of the BMT Working Party. Bone Marrow Transplant 1988; 3:531.

183. Kernan NA, Bartsch G, et al: Analysis of 462 transplantations from unrelated donors facilitated by the National Marrow Donor Program. N Engl J Med 1993; 328:593.

184. Downie TR, Hows JM, et al: A survey of use of unrelated volunteer donor bone marrow transplantation at 46 centres worldwide, 1989–93. International Marrow Unrelated Search and Transplant (IMUST) Study. Department of Transplantation Sciences, University of Bristol, Southmead Health Services, Westbury-on-Trym, UK. Bone Marrow Transplant 1995; 15:499.

185. Camitta B, Ash R, et al: Bone marrow transplantation for children with severe aplastic anemia: Use of donors other than HLA-identical siblings. Blood 1989; 74:1852.

186. Camitta B, Casper J, et al: Unrelated donor marrow transplantation (BMT) for children with severe aplastic anemia. Blood 1993; 82:344a.

187. Gordon-Smith EC: Treatment of severe aplastic anemia by bone marrow transplantation. Hematol Oncol 1987; 5:255.

188. Doney K, Pepe M, et al: Immunosuppressive therapy of aplastic anemia: Results of a prospective, randomized trial of antithymocyte globulin (ATG), methylprednisolone, and oxymetholone to ATG, very high-dose methylprednisolone, and oxymetholone. Blood 1992; 79:2566.

189. Marsh JCW, Zomas A, et al: Avascular necrosis after treatment of aplastic anaemia with antilymphocyte globulin and high-dose methylprednisolone. Br J Haematol 1993; 84:731.

190. Bielory L, Wright R, et al: Antithymocyte globulin hypersensitivity in bone marrow failure patients. JAMA 1988; 260:3164.

191. Greco B, Bielory L, et al: Antithymocyte globulin reacts with many normal human cell types. Blood 1983; 62:1047.

192. Young N, Griffith P, et al: A multicenter trial of antithymocyte globulin in aplastic anemia and related diseases. Blood 1988; 72:1861.

193. Kawano Y, Nissen C, et al: Immunostimulatory effects of different antilymphocyte globulin preparations: a possible clue to their clinical effect. Br J Haematol 1988; 68:115.

194. Torok-Storb B, Doney K, et al: Correlation of two in vitro tests with clinical response to immunosuppressive therapy in 54 patients with severe aplastic anemia. Blood 1984; 63:349.

195. Tichelli A, Gratwohl A, et al: Morphology in patients with severe aplastic anemia treated with antilymphocyte globulin. Blood 1992; 80:337.

196. Kahan BD: Cyclosporine. N Engl J Med 1989; 321:1725.

197. Bickel M, Tsuda H, et al: Differential regulation of colony-stimulating factors and interleukin 2 production by cyclosporin A. Proc Natl Acad Sci U S A 1987; 84:3274.

198. Leonard EM, Raefsky E, et al: Cyclosporine therapy of aplastic anaemia, congenital and acquired red cell aplasia. Br J Haematol 1989; 72:278.

199. Hinterberger-Fischer M, Hocker P, et al: Oral cyclosporin-A is effective treatment for untreated and also for previously immunosuppressed patients with severe bone marrow failure. Eur J Haematol 1989; 43:136.

200. Esperou H, Devergie A, et al: A randomized study comparing cyclosporin A and antithymocyte globulin for treatment of severe aplastic anemia. Nouv Rev Fr Hematol 1989; 31:65.

201. Bacigalupo A, Frassoni F, et al: Cyclosporin A (CyA) does not enhance CFU-c growth in patients with severe aplastic anaemia. Scand J Haematol 1985; 34:133.

202. Frickhofen N, Kaltwasser JP, et al: Treatment of aplastic anemia

with antilymphocyte globulin and methylprednisolone with or without cyclosporine. N Engl J Med 1991; 324:1297.

203. Bacigalupo A, Broccia G, et al: Antilymphocyte globulin, cyclosporin, and granulocyte colony-stimulating factor in patients with acquired severe aplastic anemia (SAA): A pilot study of the EBMT SAA working party. Blood 1995; 85:1348.

204. Rosenfeld S, Kimball J, et al: Intensive immunosuppression with antithymocyte globulin and cyclosporin as treatment for severe acquired aplastic anemia. Blood 1995; 85:3058.

205. Frickhofen N, Kaltwasser JP: Immunosuppressive treatment of aplastic anemia: a prospective, randomized multicenter trial evaluating antilymphocyte globulin (ALG) versus ALG and cyclosporine A. Blut 1988; 56:191.

206. Marmont AM, Bacigalupo A, et al: Treatment of severe aplastic anemia with high-dose methylprednisolone and antilymphocyte globulin. In Young NS, Levine AS, Humphries RK (eds): Aplastic Anemia: Stem Cell Biology and Advances in Treatment. New York, Alan R. Liss, 1984, p 271.

207. Gluckman E, Devergie A, et al: Results of immunosuppression in 170 cases of severe aplastic anaemia. Br J Haematol 1982; 51:541.

208. Schrezenmeier H, Marin P, et al: Relapse of aplastic anaemia after immunosuppressive treatment: a report from the European Bone Marrow Transplantation Group SAA Working Party. Br J Haematol 1993; 85:371.

209. Socie G, Henry-Amar M, et al: Malignant tumors occurring after treatment of aplastic anemia. N Engl J Med 1993; 329:1152.

210. Smith DH: Use of hematopoietic growth factors for treatment of aplastic anemia. Am J Pediatr Hematol Oncol 1990; 12:425.

211. Rowe JM, Rapoport AP: Hemopoietic growth factors: a review. J Clin Pharmacol 1992; 32:486.

212. Vadhan-Raj S, Buescher S, et al: Stimulation of myelopoiesis in patients with aplastic anemia by recombinant human granulocyte-macrophage colony-stimulating factor. N Engl J Med 1988; 319:1628.

213. Champlin RE, Nimer SD, et al: Treatment of refractory aplastic anemia with recombinant human granulocyte-macrophage colony-stimulating factor. Blood 1989; 73:694.

214. Antin JH, Smith BR, et al: Phase I/II study of recombinant human granulocyte-macrophage colony-stimulating factor in aplastic anemia and myelodysplastic syndrome. Blood 1988; 72:705.

215. Nissen C, Tichelli A, et al: Failure of recombinant human granulocyte-macrophage colony-stimulating factor therapy in aplastic anemia patients with very severe neutropenia. Blood 1988; 72:2045.

216. Champlin RE, Nimber SE, et al: Effects of recombinant human granulocyte-macrophage colony-stimulating factor as treatment for aplastic anemia and agranulocytosis. Prog Clin Biol Res 1990; 338:143.

217. Guinan EC, Sieff CA, et al: Granulocyte macrophage colony stimulating factor (GM-CSF) in aplastic anemia (AA). Pediatr Res 1989; 25:151A.

218. Kojima S, Fukada M, et al: Treatment of aplastic anemia in children with recombinant human granulocyte colony-stimulating factor. Blood 1991; 77:937.

219. Kojima S, Matsuyama T: Stimulation of granulopoiesis by high-dose recombinant human granulocyte colony-stimulating factor in children with aplastic anemia and very severe neutropenia. Blood 1994; 83:1474.

220. Sonoda Y, Yashige H, Fujii H, et al: Bilineage response in refractory aplastic anemia patients following long-term administration of recombinant human granulocyte colony-stimulating factor. Eur J Haematol 1992; 48:41.

221. Takahashi M, Yoshida Y, et al: Phase II study of recombinant human granulocyte-macrophage colony-stimulating factor in myelodysplastic syndrome and aplastic anemia. Acta Haematol 1993; 89:189.

222. Ashihara E, Shimazaki C, et al: Trilineage response in severe aplastic anemia following long-term therapy with recombinant human granulocyte colony-stimulating factor. Acta Haematol 1993; 90:159.

223. Higuchi T, Shimizu T, et al: Delayed granulocyte response to G-CSF in aplastic anemia. Am J Hematol 1994; 46:164.

224. Sonoda Y, Ohno Y, et al: Multilineage response in aplastic ane-mia patients following long-term administration of filgrastim (recombinant human granulocyte colony stimulating factor). Stem Cells (Dayt) 1993; 11:543.

225. Ganser A, Lindemann A, et al: Effects of recombinant human interleukin-3 in aplastic anemia. Blood 1990; 76:1287.

226. Ganser A: Clinical results with recombinant human interleukin-3. Cancer Invest 1993; 11:212.

227. Kurzrock R, Talpaz M, et al: Phase I study of recombinant human interleukin-3 in patients with bone marrow failure. J Clin Oncol 1991; 9:1241.

228. Gillio AP, Castro-Malaspina H, et al: A phase I trial of recombinant human interleukin-3 in patients with myelodysplastic syndrome and aplastic anemia. Blood 1990; 76:145a.

229. Nimer SD, Paquette RL, et al: A phase I/II study of interleukin-3 in patients with aplastic anemia and myelodysplasia. Exp Hematol 1994; 22:875.

230. Ganser A, Ottmann OG, Hoelzer D: Interleukin 3 and interleukin 3/GM-CSF combination therapy—Clinical implications. Stem Cells (Dayt) 1993; 11:465.

231. Geissler K, Fortinger C, et al: Effect of interleukin-3 on responsiveness to granulocyte-colony-stimulating factor in severe aplastic anemia. Ann Intern Med 1992; 117:223.

232. Gascon P, Scala G: Decreased interleukin-1 production in aplastic anemia. Am J Med 1988; 85:668.

233. Walsh CE, Liu JM, et al: A trial of recombinant human interleukin-1 in patients with severe refractory aplastic anaemia. Br J Haematol 1992; 80:106.

234. Bessho M, Toyoda A, et al: Trilineage recovery by combination therapy with recombinant human granulocyte colony-stimulating factor (rhG-CSF) and erythropoietin (rhEpo) in severe aplastic anemia. Br J Haematol 1992; 80:409. Letter.

235. Kurzrock R, Talpaz M, Gutterman JU: Very low doses of GM-CSF administered alone or with erythropoietin in aplastic anemia. Am J Med 1992; 93:41.

236. Potter MN, Mott MG, Oakhill A: The successful treatment of a case of very severe aplastic anaemia with granulocyte-macrophage colony stimulating factor and anti-lymphocyte globulin. Br J Haematol 1990; 75:618.

237. Kojima S, Fukuda M, et al: Cyclosporine and recombinant granulocyte colony-stimulating factor in severe aplastic anemia. N Engl J Med 1990; 323:920.

238. Weide R, Lyttelton M, et al: Sustained trilineage response in a patient with ALG-resistant severe aplastic anaemia after treatment with G-CSF, erythropoietin and cyclosporin A: association of recovery with marked elevation of serum alkaline phosphatase. Br J Haematol 1993; 85:608.

239. Gordon-Smith EC, Yandle A, et al: Randomised placebo controlled study of RH-GM-CSF following ALG in the treatment of aplastic anemia. Bone Marrow Transplant 1991; 7:78.

240. Doney K, Storb R, et al: Recombinant granulocyte-macrophage colony stimulating factor followed by immunosuppressive therapy for aplastic anaemia. Br J Haematol 1993; 85:182.

241. Rodgers GP, Kim BK, et al: Effect of GM-CSF as first therapy for severe aplastic anemia. Blood 1992; 80(Suppl 1):289a.

242. Kojima S, Tsuchida M, Matsuyama T: Myelodysplasia and leukemia after treatment of aplastic anemia with G-CSF. N Engl J Med 1992; 326:1294.

243. Izumi T, Muroi K, et al: Development of acute myeloblastic leukaemia in a case of aplastic anaemia treated with granulocyte colony-stimulating factor. Br J Haematol 1994; 87:666.

244. Tong J, Gordon MS, et al: *In vivo* administration of recombinant methionyl human stem cell factor expands the number of human marrow hematopoietic stem cells. Blood 1993; 82:784.

245. Champlin RE, Ho WG, et al: Do androgens enhance the response to antithymocyte globulin in patients with aplastic anemia? A prospective randomized trial. Blood 1985; 66:184.

246. Bacigalupo A, Chaple M, et al: Treatment of aplastic anemia (AA) with antilymphocyte globulin (ALG) and methylprednisolone (MPred) with or without androgens: a randomized trial from the EBMT SAA working party. Br J Haematol 1993; 83:145.

247. Gardner FH, Besa EC: Physiologic mechanisms and the hematopoietic effects of the androstanes and their derivatives. Curr Top Hematol 1983; 4:123.

248. Alexanian R: Erythropoietin and erythropoiesis in anemic man following androgens. Blood 1969; 33:564.

249. Singer JW, Adamson JW: Steroids and hematopoiesis. II. The effect of steroids on *in vitro* erythroid colony growth: evidence for different target cells for different classes of steroids. J Cell Physiol 1976; 88:135.

250. Shahidi NT, Diamond LK: Testosterone-induced remission in aplastic anemia of both acquired and congenital types. Further observations in 24 cases. N Engl J Med 1961; 264:953.

251. Sanchez-Medal L, Gomez-Leal A, et al: Anabolic androgenic steroids in the treatment of acquired aplastic anemia. Blood 1969; 34:283.

252. Davis S, Rubin AD: Treatment and prognosis in aplastic anaemia. Lancet 1972; 1:871.

253. Lynch RE, Williams DM, et al: The prognosis in aplastic anemia. Blood 1975; 45:517.

254. Williams DM, Lynch RE, Cartwright GE: Prognostic factors in aplastic anaemia. Clin Haematol 1978; 7:467.

255. Camitta BM, Storb R, Thomas ED: Aplastic anemia. (Second of two parts). Pathogenesis, diagnosis, treatment, and prognosis. N Engl J Med 1982; 306:712.

256. Kamamoto T, Ohkubo T, et al: Correlation between *in vitro* and *in vivo* response to androgens in patients with aplastic anemia. Int J Cell Cloning 1984; 2:173.

257. McGiven AR: Peliosis hepatitis: Case report and review of pathogenesis. J Pathol 1970; 101:283.

258. Bourliere B, Najean Y: Influence of long-term androgen therapy on growth: An analysis of 18 cases of aplastic anemia in children. Am J Dis Child 1987; 141:718.

259. Delamore IW, Geary CG: Aplastic anaemia, acute myeloblastic leukaemia, and oxymetholone. Br Med J 1971; 1:743.

260. Li FP, Nathan DG, Walker AN: Therapy-linked leukaemia. BMJ 1971; 3:765.

261. Griner PF: A survey of the effectiveness of cyclophosphamide in patients with severe aplastic anemia. Am J Hematol 1980; 8:55.

261a. Brodsky RA, Sensenbrenner LL, Jones RJ: Complete remission in severe aplastic anemia after high-dose cyclophosphamide without bone marrow transplantation. Blood 1996; 87:491.

262. Heaton LD, Crosby WH, Cohen A: Splenectomy in the treatment of hypoplasia of the bone marrow. With a report of twelve cases. Ann Surg 1957; 146:637.

263. Speck B, Gratwohl A, et al: Treatment of severe aplastic anemia. Exp Hematol 1986; 14:126.

264. Bessman JD, Gardner FH: Persistence of abnormal red cell and platelet phenotype during recovery from aplastic anemia. Arch Intern Med 1985; 145:293.

265. Alter BP, Rappeport JM, et al: Fetal erythropoiesis following bone marrow transplantation. Blood 1976; 48:843.

266. Freedman MH, Saunders EF, et al: Residual abnormalities in acquired aplastic anemia of childhood. JAMA 1974; 228:201.

267. O'Gorman Hughes DW: The varied pattern of aplastic anaemia in childhood. Aust Paediatr J 1966; 2:228.

268. Windass B, Vowels MR, et al: Aplastic anaemia in childhood: prognosis and approach to therapy. Med J Aust 1987; 146:15.

269. Fanconi G: Familiäre infantile perniziösaartige Anämie (perniziöses Blutbild und Konstitution). Jahrbuch Kinder 1927; 117:257.

270. Uehlinger E: Konstitutionelle infantile (perniziösaartige) Anämie. Klin Wochenschr 1929; 32:1501.

271. Fanconi G: Familial constitional panmyelocytopathy, Fanconi's Anemia (F.A.). I. Clinical aspects. Semin Hematol 1967; 4:233.

272. Alter BP: Annotation: Fanconi's anaemia and its variability. Br J Haematol 1993; 85:9.

273. Liu JM, Buchwald M, et al: Fanconi anemia and novel strategies for therapy. Blood 1994; 84:3995.

274. Alter BP, Potter NU: Long-term outcome in Fanconi's anemia: description of 26 cases and review of the literature. In German J (ed): Chromosome Mutation and Neoplasia. New York, Alan R. Liss, 1983, p 43.

275. Porteous MEM, Cross I, Burn J: VACTERL with hydrocephalus: One end of the Fanconi anemia spectrum of anomalies? Am J Med Genet 1992; 43:1032.

276. Giampietro PF, Adler-Brecher B, et al: The need for more accurate and timely diagnosis in Fanconi anemia: A report from the International Fanconi Anemia Registry. Pediatrics 1993; 91:1116.

277. Alter BP, Tenner MS: Brain tumors in patients with Fanconi's Anemia. Arch Pediatr Adolesc Med 1994; 148:661.

278. Auerbach A, Schroeder T: First announcement of the Fanconi Anemia International Registry. Blood 1982; 60:1054.

279. Estren S, Dameshek W: Familial hypoplastic anemia of childhood. Report of eight cases in two families with beneficial effect of splenectomy in one case. Am J Dis Child 1947; 73:671.

280. Li FP, Potter NU: Classical Fanconi anemia in a family with hypoplastic anemia. J Pediatr 1978; 92:943.

281. Glanz A, Fraser FC: Spectrum of anomalies in Fanconi anaemia. J Med Genet 1982; 19:412.

282. Riley E, Caldwell R, Swift M: Comparison of clinical features in Fanconi anemia probands and their subsequently diagnosed siblings. Am J Hum Genet 1979; 31:82A.

283. Schroeder TM, Tilgen D, et al: Formal genetics of Fanconi's anemia. Hum Genet 1976; 32:257.

284. Rogatko A, Auerbach AD: Segregation analysis with uncertain ascertainment: Application to Fanconi anemia. Am J Hum Genet 1988; 42:889.

285. Swift M: Fanconi anaemia: cellular abnormalities and clinical predisposition to malignant disease. In Congenital Disorders of Erythropoiesis. Ciba Foundation Symposium 37. Amsterdam, Elsevier North-Holland, 1976, p 115.

286. Rosendorff J, Bernstein R, et al: Fanconi anemia: Another disease of unusually high prevalence in the Afrikaans population of South Africa. Am J Med Genet 1987; 27:793.

287. Dacie JV, Gilpin A: Refractory anaemia (Fanconi type). Its incidence in three members of one family, with in one case a relationship to chronic haemolytic anaemia with nocturnal haemoglobinuria (Marchiafava-Micheli disease or 'nocturnal haemoglobinuria'). Arch Dis Child 1944; 19:155.

288. Shahidi NT, Gerald PS, Diamond LK: Alkali-resistant hemoglobin in aplastic anemia of both acquired and congenital types. N Engl J Med 1962; 266:117.

289. Alter BP, Knobloch ME, Weinberg RS: Erythropoiesis in Fanconi's anemia. Blood 1991; 78:602.

290. Chu J-Y, Ho JE, et al: Technetium colloid bone marrow imaging in Fanconi's anemia. Pediatrics 1979; 64:635.

291. Löhr GW, Waller HD: Hexokinasemangel in Blutzellen bei einer Sippe mit familiärer Panmyelopathie (Typ Fanconi). Klin Wochenschr 1965; 43:870.

292. de Grouchy J, de Nava C, et al: Études cytogénétique et biochimique de huit cas d'anémie de Fanconi. Ann Genet 1972; 15:29.

293. Magnani M, Novelli G, et al: Red blood cell hexokinase in Fanconi's anemia. Acta Haematol 1984; 71:341.

294. Jalbert PP, Leger J, et al: L'anémie de Fanconi: aspects cytogénétiques et biochimiques. À propos d'une famille. Nouv Rev Fr Hematol 1975; 15:551.

295. Fisher DA, Job J-C, et al: Leukaemia in patients treated with growth hormone. Lancet 1988; 1:1159.

296. Fradkin JE, Mills JL, et al: Risk of leukemia after treatment with pituitary growth hormone. JAMA 1993; 270:2829.

296a. Dokal I, Chase A, et al: Positive diepoxybutane test in only one of two brothers found to be compound heterozygotes for Fanconi's anaemia complementation group C mutations. Br J Haematol 1996; 93:813.

297. Schroeder TM, Kurth R: Spontaneous chromosomal breakage and high incidence of leukemia in inherited disease. Blood 1971; 37:96.

298. Chaganti RSK, Schonberg S, German J: A manyfold increase in sister chromatid exchanges in Bloom's syndrome lymphocytes. Proc Natl Acad Sci U S A 1974; 71:4508.

299. Kaiser TN, Lojewski A, et al: Flow cytometric characterization of the response of Fanconi's anemia cells to mitomycin C treatment. Cytometry 1982; 2:291.

300. Miglierina R, le Coniat M, et al: Diagnosis of Fanconi's anemia by flow cytometry. Nouv Rev Fr Hematol 1991; 32:391.

301. Arkin S, Brodtman D, et al: Cell cycle analysis in Fanconi anemia: a diagnostic test. Pediatr Res 1994; 35:157A.

302. Seyschab H, Friedl R, et al: Comparative evaluation of diepoxybutane sensitivity and cell cycle blockage in the diagnosis of Fanconi anemia. Blood 1995; 85:2233.

303. Auerbach AD, Alter BP: Prenatal and postnatal diagnosis of aplastic anemia. In Alter BP (ed): Methods in Hematology: Perinatal Hematology. Edinburgh, Churchill Livingstone, 1989, p 225.

304. Auerbach AD, Rogatko A, Schroeder-Kurth TM: International Fanconi Anemia Registry: Relation of clinical symptoms to diepoxybutane sensitivity. Blood 1989; 73:391.

305. Arwert F, Kwee ML: Chromosomal breakage in response to cross-linking agents in the diagnosis of Fanconi anemia. In Schroeder-Kurth TM, Auerbach AD, Obe G, (eds): Fanconi Anemia: Clinical, Cytogenetic and Experimental Aspects. Berlin, Springer-Verlag, 1989, p 83.

306. Auerbach AD: Fanconi anemia. Dermatol Clin 1995; 13:41.

307. Shipley J, Rodeck CH, et al: Mitomycin C induced chromosome damage in fetal blood cultures and prenatal diagnosis of Fanconi's anaemia. Prenat Diagn 1984; 4:217.

308. Trunca C, Watson M, et al: Prenatal diagnosis of Fanconi anemia in a fetus not known to be at risk. Am J Hum Genet 1984; 36:198S.

309. Boué PJ, Deluchat C, et al: Diagnostic prénatal des maladies géniques sur villosites choriales. J Genet Hum 1986; 34:221.

310. Hirsch-Kauffmann M, Schweiger M: Prenatal recognition of a defect in DNA repair. Mol Gen Genet 1981; 184:17.

311. Murer-Orlando M, Llerena JC Jr, et al: FACC gene mutations and early prenatal diagnosis of Fanconi's anaemia. Lancet 1993; 342:686.

312. Varela MA, Sternberg WH: Preanaemic state in Fanconi's anaemia. Lancet 1967; 2:566.

313. Pignatti CB, Bianchi E, Polito E: Fanconi's anaemia in infancy: Report of a case diagnosed in the pre-anaemic stage. Helv Paediatr Acta 1977; 32:413.

314. McIntosh S, Breg WR, Lubiniecki AS: Fanconi's anemia. The pre-anemic phase. Am J Pediatr Hematol Oncol 1979; 1:107.

315. Auerbach AD, Sagi M, Adler B: Fanconi anemia: Prenatal diagnosis in 30 fetuses at risk. Pediatrics 1985; 76:794.

316. Cohen MM, Simpson SJ, et al: The identification of Fanconi anemia genotypes by clastogenic stress. Am J Hum Genet 1982; 34:794.

317. Welshimer K, Swift M: Congenital malformations and developmental disabilities in ataxia-telangiectasia, Fanconi anemia, and xeroderma pigmentosum families. Am J Hum Genet 1982; 34:781.

318. Skikne BS, Lynch SR, et al: Fanconi's anaemia, with special reference to erythrokinetic features. S Afr Med J 1978; 53:43.

319. Altay C, Sevgi Y, Pirnar T: Fanconi's anemia in offspring of patient with congenital radial and carpal hypoplasia. N Engl J Med 1975; 293:151.

320. Petridou M, Barrett AJ: Physical and laboratory characteristics of heterozygote carriers of the Fanconi aplasia gene. Acta Paediatr Scand 1990; 79:1069.

321. Althoff H: Zur Panmyelopathie Fanconi als Zustandsbild multipler Abartungen. Z Kinderheilk 1953; 72:267.

322. Imlay JA, Linn S: DNA damage and oxygen radical toxicity. Science 1988; 240:1302.

323. Pritsos CA, Sartorelli AC: Generation of reactive oxygen radicals through bioactivation of mitomycin antibiotics. Cancer Res 1986; 46:3528.

324. Izakovic V, Strbakova E, et al: Bovine superoxide dismutase in Fanconi anaemia. Therapeutic trial in two patients. Hum Genet 1985; 70:181.

325. Liu JM, Auerbach AD, et al: A trial of recombinant human superoxide dismutase in patients with Fanconi anaemia. Br J Haematol 1993; 85:406.

326. Papadopoulo D, Guillouf C, et al: Hypomutability in Fanconi anemia cells is associated with increased deletion frequency at the HPRT locus. Proc Natl Acad Sci U S A 1990; 87:8383.

327. Papadopoulo D, Laquerbe A, et al: Molecular spectrum of mutations induced at the HPRT locus by a cross-linking agent in human cell lines with different repair capacities. Mutat Res 1993; 294:167.

328. Rugman FP, Ashby D, Davies JM: Does HLA-DR predict response to specific immunosuppressive therapy in aplastic anaemia? Br J Haematol 1990; 74:545.

329. Berger R, Bernheim A, et al: Bone marrow graft of a Fanconi's anemia patient. Cytogenetic study. Cancer Genet Cytogenet 1980; 2:127.

330. Zakrzewski S, Sperling K: Genetic heterogeneity of Fanconi's anemia demonstrated by somatic cell hybrids. Hum Genet 1980; 56:81.

331. Duckworth-Rysiecki G, Cornish K, et al: Identification of two complementation groups in Fanconi anemia. Somat Cell Mol Genet 1985; 11:35.

332. Digweed M, Zakrzewski-Ludcke S, Sperling K: Fanconi's anaemia: correlation of genetic complementation group with psoralen/UVA response. Hum Genet 1988; 78:51.

333. Strathdee CA, Duncan AMV, Buchwald M: Evidence for at least four Fanconi anaemia genes including FACC on chromosome 9. Nat Genetics 1992; 1:196.

334. Joenje H, Lo Ten Foe JR, et al: Classification of Fanconi anemia patients by complementation analysis: Evidence for a fifth genetic subtype. Blood 1995; 86:2156.

335. Verlander PC, Lin JD, et al: Mutation analysis of the Fanconi anemia gene FACC. Am J Hum Genet 1994; 54:595.

336. Strathdee CA, Gavish H, et al: Cloning of cDNAs for Fanconi's anaemia by functional complementation. Nature 1992; 356:763.

337. Segal GM, Magenis E, et al: Repression of Fanconi anemia gene (FACC) expression inhibits growth of hematopoietic progenitor cells. J Clin Invest 1994; 94:846.

338. Walsh CE, Nienhuis AW, et al: Phenotypic correction of Fanconi Anemia in human hematopoietic cells with a recombinant adeno-associated virus vector. J Clin Invest 1994; 94:1440.

339. Yamashita T, Barber DL, et al: The Fanconi anemia polypeptide FACC is localized to the cytoplasm. Proc Natl Acad Sci U S A 1994; 91:6712.

340. Youssoufian H: Localization of Fanconi anemia C protein to the cytoplasm of mammalian cells. Proc Natl Acad Sci U S A 1994; 91:7975.

341. Gibson RA, Ford D, et al: Genetic mapping of the FACC gene and linkage analysis in Fanconi anaemia families. J Med Genet 1994; 31:868.

342. Whitney MA, Saito H, et al: A common mutation in the FACC gene causes Fanconi anaemia in Ashkenazi Jews. Nat Genet 1993; 4:202.

343. Whitney MA, Jakobs P, et al: The Ashkenazi Jewish Fanconi anemia mutation: Incidence among patients and carrier frequency in the at-risk population. Hum Mutat 1994; 3:339.

344. Gibson RA, Hajianpour A, et al: A nonsense mutation and exon skipping in the Fanconi anaemia group C gene. Hum Mol Genet 1993; 2:797.

344a. Yamashita T, Wu N, et al: Clinical variability of Fanconi anemia (type C) results from expression of an amino terminal truncated Fanconi anemia complementation group C polypeptide with partial activity. Blood 1996; 87:4424.

345. Mann WR, Venkatraj VS, et al: Fanconi anemia: Evidence for linkage heterogeneity on chromosome 20q. Genomics 1991; 9:329.

346. Diatloff-Zito C, Duchaud E, et al: Identification and chromosomal localization of a DNA fragment implicated in the partial correction of the Fanconi anemia group D cellular defect. Mutat Res 1994; 307:33.

346a. Pronk JC, Gibson RA, et al: Localisation of the Fanconi anaemia complementation group A gene to chromosome 16q24.3. Nat Genet 1995; 11:338.

346b. Whitney M, Thayer M, et al: Microcell mediated chromosome transfer maps the Fanconi anaemia group D gene to chromosome 3p. Nat Genet 1995; 11:341.

346c. Lo Ten Foe JR, Rooimans MA, et al: Expression cloning of a cDNA for the major Fanconi anaemia gene, FAA. Nat Genet 1996; 14:320.

347. Daneshbod-Skibba G, Martin J, Shahidi NT: Myeloid and erythroid colony growth in non-anemic patients with Fanconi's anaemia. Br J Haematol 1980; 44:33.

348. Claustres M, Margueritte G, Sultan C: In vitro CFU-E and BFU-E responses to androgen in bone marrow from children with primary hypoproliferative anaemia—a possible therapeutic assay. Eur J Pediatr 1986; 144:467.

349. Alter BP, Knobloch ME, et al: Effect of stem cell factor on in vitro erythropoiesis in patients with bone marrow failure syndromes. Blood 1992; 80:3000.

350. Bagnara G, Strippoli P, et al: Effect of stem cell factor on colony growth from acquired and constitutional (Fanconi) aplastic anemia. Blood 1992; 80:382.

351. Stark R, Thierry D, et al: Long-term bone marrow culture in Fanconi's anaemia. Br J Haematol 1993; 83:554.

352. Butturini A, Gale RP: Long-term bone marrow culture in persons with Fanconi anemia and bone marrow failure. Blood 1994; 83:336.

353. Schultz JC, Shahidi NT: Tumor necrosis factor-α overproduction in Fanconi's anemia. Am J Hematol 1993; 42:196.

354. Rosselli F, Sanceau J, et al: Abnormal lymphokine production: a novel feature of the genetic disease Fanconi anemia. I. Involvement of interleukin-6. Hum Genet 1992; 89:42.

355. Stark R, Andre C, et al: The expression of cytokine and cytokine receptor genes in long-term bone marrow culture in congenital and acquired bone marrow hypoplasias. Br J Haematol 1993; 83:560.

356. Bagnara GP, Bonsi L, et al: Production of interleukin 6, leukemia inhibitory factor and granulocyte-macrophage colony stimulating factor by peripheral blood mononuclear cells in Fanconi's anemia. Stem Cells 1993; 11:137.

357. Wunder E, Mortensen BT, et al: Anomalous plasma concentrations and impaired secretion of growth factors in Fanconi's anemia. Stem Cells 1993; 11:144.

358. Bagby GC, Segal GM, et al: Constitutive and induced expression of hematopoietic growth factor genes by fibroblasts from children with Fanconi anemia. Exp Hematol 1993; 21:1419.

359. Rosselli F, Sanceau J, et al: Abnormal lymphokine production: A novel feature of the genetic disease Fanconi anemia. II. *In vitro* and *in vivo* spontaneous overproduction of tumor necrosis factor. Blood 1994; 5:1216.

360. Jonveaux P, Le Coniat M, et al: Lack of mutations in the *TP53* tumor suppressor gene exons 5 to 8 in Fanconi's anemia. Nouv Rev Fr Hematol 1991; 33:343.

361. Rosselli F, Ridet A, et al: P53-dependent pathway of radio-induced apoptosis is altered in Fanconi anemia. Oncogene 1995; 10:9.

362. Rey JP, Scott R, Muller H: Apoptosis is not involved in the hypersensitivity of Fanconi Anemia cells to mitomycin C. Cancer Genet Cytogenet 1994; 75:67.

363. Barker JE, Bernstein SE: Hertwig's anemia: Characterization of the stem cell defect. Blood 1983; 61:765.

364. Wevrick R, Clarke CA, Buchwald M: Cloning and analysis of the murine Fanconi anemia group C cDNA. Hum Mol Genet 1993; 2:655.

365. Wevrick R, Barker JE, et al: Mapping of the murine and rat *FACC* genes and assessment of flexed-tail as a candidate mouse homolog of Fanconi anemia group C. Mamm Genome 1993; 4:440.

366. Bernard J, Mathé G, Najean Y: Contribution à l'étude clinique et physiopathologique de la maladie de Fanconi. Rev Franc Etudes Clin Biol 1958; 3:599.

367. Dawson JP: Congenital pancytopenia associated with multiple congenital anomalies (Fanconi type). Pediatrics 1955; 15:325.

368. McDonald R, Goldschmidt B: Pancytopenia with congenital defects (Fanconi's anaemia). Arch Dis Child 1960; 35:367.

369. Auerbach AD, Frissora CL, Rogatko A: International Fanconi anemia registry (IFAR): Survival and prognostic factors. Blood 1989; 74:43a.

370. Bargman GJ, Shahidi NT, et al: Studies of malformation syndromes of man XLVII: Disappearance of spermatogonia in the Fanconi anemia syndrome. Eur J Pediatr 1977; 125:163.

371. Liu JM, Auerbach AD, Young NS: Fanconi anemia presenting unexpectedly in an adult kindred with no dysmorphic features. Am J Med 1991; 91:555.

372. Shahidi NT, Diamond LK: Testosterone-induced remission in aplastic anemia. Am J Dis Child 1959; 98:293.

373. Sanchez-Medal L: The hemopoietic action of androstanes. Prog Hematol 1971; 7:111.

374. Najean Y: Androgen therapy in aplastic anaemia in childhood. In: Congenital Disorders of Erythropoiesis. Ciba Foundation Symposium 37. Amsterdam, Elsevier, 1976, p 354.

375. Shahidi NT, Crigler JF Jr: Evaluation of growth and of endocrine systems in testosterone-corticosteroid–treated patients with aplastic anemia. J Pediatr 1967; 70:233.

376. Kitchens CS: Amelioration of endothelial abnormalities by prednisone in experimental thrombocytopenia in the rabbit. J Clin Invest 1977; 60:1129.

377. Smith S, Marx MP, et al: Clinical aspects of a cluster of 42 patients in South Africa with Fanconi anemia. In Schroeder-Kurth TM, Auerbach AD, Obe G (eds): Fanconi Anemia: Clinical, Cytogenetic and Experimental Aspects. Berlin, Springer-Verlag, 1989, p 34.

378. Flowers MED, Doney KC, et al: Marrow transplantation for Fanconi anemia with or without leukemic transformation: an update of the Seattle experience. Bone Marrow Transplant 1992; 9:167.

379. Bradford CR, Hoffman HT, et al: Squamous carcinoma of the head and neck in organ transplant recipients: Possible role of oncogenic viruses. Laryngoscope 1990; 100:190.

380. Socie G, Henry-Amar M, et al: Increased incidence of solid malignant tumors after bone marrow transplantation for severe aplastic anemia. Blood 1991; 78:277.

381. Murayama S, Manzo RP, et al: Squamous cell carcinoma of the tongue associated with Fanconi's anemia: MR characteristics. Pediatr Radiol 1990; 20:347.

382. Zanis-Neto J, Ribeiro RC, et al: Bone marrow transplantation for patients with Fanconi anemia: A study of 24 cases from a single institution. Bone Marrow Transplant 1995; 15:293.

383. Berger R, Bernheim A, et al: *In vitro* effect of cyclophosphamide metabolites on chromosomes of Fanconi anaemia patients. Br J Haematol 1980; 45:565.

384. Auerbach AD, Adler B, et al: Effect of procarbazine and cyclophosphamide on chromosome breakage in Fanconi anemia cells: Relevance to bone marrow transplantation. Cancer Genet Cytogenet 1983; 9:25.

385. Gluckman E, Devergie A, Dutreix J: Bone marrow transplantation for Fanconi anemia. In Schroeder-Kurth TM, Auerbach AD, Obe G (eds): Fanconi Anemia: Clinical, Cytogenetic and Experimental Aspects. Berlin, Springer-Verlag, 1989, p 60.

386. Shinohara O, Kato S, et al: Growth after bone marrow transplantation in children. Am J Pediatr Hematol Oncol 1991; 13:263.

387. Howell RT: Evaluation of chromosomal damage following allogeneic bone marrow transplant in a patient with Fanconi's anemia. J Med Genet 1992; 29:203.

388. Yabe M, Yabe H, et al: Bone marrow transplantation for Fanconi anemia. Adjustment of the dose of cyclophophamide for preconditioning. Am J Pediatr Hematol Oncol 1993; 15:377.

389. Gluckman E, Devergie A, Dutreix J: Radiosensitivity in Fanconi anaemia: application to the conditioning regimen for bone marrow transplantation. Br J Haematol 1983; 54:431.

390. Di Bartolomeo P, Girolamo GD, et al: Allogeneic bone marrow transplantation for Fanconi anemia. Bone Marrow Transplant 1992; 10:53.

391. Socié G, Gluckman E, et al: Bone marrow transplantation for Fanconi anemia using low-dose cyclophosphamide/thoracoabdominal irradiation as conditioning regimen: chimerism study by the polymerase chain reaction. Blood 1993; 82:2249.

392. Kohli-Kumar M, Morris C, et al: Bone marrow transplantation in Fanconi anemia using matched sibling donors. Blood 1994; 84:2050.

393. Philpott NJ, Marsh JCW, et al: Successful bone marrow transplant for Fanconi anaemia in transformation. Bone Marrow Transplant 1994; 14:151.

394. Hansen JA, Good RA, Dupont B: HLA-D compatibility between parent and child. Transplantation 1977; 23:366.

395. O'Reilly RJ, Pollack MS, et al: HLA histocompatibility between parent and affected child in Fanconi's anemia. Pediatr Res 1982; 16:210A.

396. Minchinton RM, Waters AH, et al: Selective thrombocytopenia and neutropenia occurring after bone marrow transplantation—evidence of an auto-immune basis. Clin Lab Haematol 1984; 6:157.

397. Begovich AB, Erlich HA: HLA typing for bone marrow transplantation. New polymerase chain reaction–based methods. JAMA 1995; 273:586.

398. Deeg HJ, Storb R, et al: Fanconi's anemia treated by allogeneic marrow transplantation. Blood 1983; 61:954.

399. Broxmeyer HE, Douglas GW, et al: Human umbilical cord blood as a potential source of transplantable hematopoietic stem/progenitor cells. Proc Natl Acad Sci U S A 1989; 86:3828.

400. Gluckman E, Broxmeyer HE, et al: Hematopoietic reconstitution in a patient with Fanconi's anemia by means of umbilical-cord blood from an HLA-identical sibling. N Engl J Med 1989; 321:1174.

401. Gluckman E, Devergie A, et al: Transplantation of umbilical cord blood in Fanconi's anemia. Nouv Rev Fr Hematol 1991; 32:423.

402. Ozsoylu S: Treatment of aplastic anemia. J Pediatr 1983; 102:484.

403. Speck B, Gratwohl A, et al: Treatment of severe aplastic anaemia with antilymphocyte globulin or bone-marrow transplantation. BMJ 1981; 282:860.

404. Boggs DR, Joyce RA: The hematopoietic effects of lithium. Semin Hematol 1983; 20:129.

405. Ferguson L, Hoots K, et al: Long-term bone marrow (BM) cultures with recombinant human granulocyte-macrophage colony stimulating factor (rhGM-CSF) in children with cytopenias: A correlation with clinical response. Blood 1988; 72(Suppl 1):115a.

406. Guinan EC, Lopez ED, et al: Evaluation of granulocyte-macrophage colony-stimulating factor for treatment of pancytopenia in children with Fanconi anemia. J Pediatr 1994; 124:144.

407. Kemahli S, Canatan D, et al: GM-CSF in the treatment of Fanconi's anaemia. Br J Haematol 1994; 87:871.

408. Rackoff WR, Orazi A, et al: Prolonged administration of granulocyte colony-stimulating factor (Filgrastim) to patients with Fanconi anemia: A pilot study. Blood 1996; 88:1588.

409. Nathan DG: Hope for hematopoietic hormones. N Engl J Med 1987; 317:626.

410. Gillio AP, Gabrilove JL: Cytokine treatment of inherited bone marrow failure syndromes. Blood 1993; 81:1669.

411. Butturini A, Gale RP, et al: Hematologic abnormalities in Fanconi anemia: An International Fanconi Anemia Registry study. Blood 1994; 84:1650.

412. Garriga S, Crosby WH: The incidence of leukemia in families of patients with hypoplasia of the marrow. Blood 1959; 24:1008.

413. Swift M: Fanconi's anaemia in the genetics of neoplasia. Nature 1971; 230:370.

414. Swift M: Malignant disease in heterozygous carriers. Birth Defects 1976; 12:133.

415. Swift M, Caldwell RJ, Chase C: Reassessment of cancer predisposition of Fanconi anemia heterozygotes. J Natl Canc Inst 1980; 65:863.

416. Potter NU, Sarmousakis C, Li FP: Cancer in relatives of patients with aplastic anemia. Cancer Genet Cytogenet 1983; 9:61.

417. Swift M, Sholman L, Gilmour D: Diabetes mellitus and the gene for Fanconi's anemia. Science 1972; 178:308.

418. Morrell D, Chase CI, et al: Diabetes mellitus in ataxia-telangiectasia, Fanconi anemia, xeroderma pigmentosum, common variable immune deficiency, and severe combined immune deficiency families. Diabetes 1986; 35:143.

419. Schaison G, Leverger G, et al: L'anémie de Fanconi. Fréquence de l'évolution vers la leucémie. Presse Med 1983; 12:1269.

420. Gyger M, Perrault C, et al: Unsuspected Fanconi's anemia and bone marrow transplantation in cases of acute myelomonocytic leukemia. N Engl J Med 1989; 321:120.

421. Hanscombe O, Vidal M, et al: High-level, erythroid-specific expression of the human α-globin gene in transgenic mice and the production of human hemoglobin in murine erythrocytes. Genes Dev 1989; 3:1572.

422. Alter BP: Leukemia and preleukemia in Fanconi's anemia. Cancer Genet Cytogenet 1992; 58:206.

423. Alter BP, Scalise A, et al: Clonal chromosomal abnormalities in Fanconi's anemia: What do they really mean? Br J Haematol 1993; 85:627.

424. Yetgin S, Tuncer M, et al: Acute lymphoblastic leukemia in Fanconi's anemia. Am J Hematol 1994; 45:94.

425. Griffin TC, Friedman DJ, et al: Fanconi anemia complicated by acute myelogenous leukemia and malignant brain tumor. Blood 1992; 80(Suppl 1):382a.

426. Berger R, le Coniat M, Schaison G: Chromosome abnormalities in bone marrow of Fanconi anemia patients. Cancer Genet Cytogenet 1993; 65:47.

427. Russo CL, Zwerdling T: Recognition of Fanconi's anemia eight years following treatment for acute nonlymphoblastic leukemia. Am J Hematol 1992; 40:78. Letter to the editor.

428. Athale UH, Rao SR, et al: Fanconi's anemia: a clinico-hematological and cytogenetic study. Indian Pediatr 1992; 28:1003.

429. Touraine RL, Bertrand Y, et al: Hepatic tumours during androgen therapy in Fanconi anaemia. Eur J Pediatr 1993; 152:691.

430. Kohli-Kumar M, Harris R, Morris C: Bone marrow transplantation in Fanconi anemia with non-sibling donors or following leukemia transformation. Blood 1992; 80(Suppl 1):527a.

431. Sarna G, Tomasulo P, et al: Multiple neoplasia in two siblings with a variant form of Fanconi's anemia. Cancer 1975; 36:1029.

432. Perrimond H, Juhan-Vague I, et al: Évolution médullaire et hépatique après androgènothérapie prolongée d'une anémie de Fanconi. Nouv Rev Fr Hematol 1977; 18:228.

433. Obeid A, Hill FGH, et al: Fanconi anemia: oxymetholone hepatic tumors, and chromosome aberrations associated with leukemic transition. Cancer 1980; 46:1401.

434. Bessho F, Mizutani S, et al: Chronic myelomonocytic leukemia with chromosomal changes involving 1p36 and hepatocellular carcinoma in a case of Fanconi's anemia. Eur J Haematol 1989; 42:492.

435. Gingrich RD, Ginder GD, et al: Allogeneic marrow grafting with partially mismatched, unrelated marrow donors. Blood 1988; 71:1375.

436. Berger R, Le Coniat M: Cytogenetic studies in Fanconi anemia induced chromosomal breakage and cytogenetics. In Schroeder-Kurth TM, Auerbach AD, Obe G (eds): Fanconi Anemia: Clinical, Cytogenetic and Experimental Aspects. Berlin, Springer-Verlag, 1989, p 93.

436a. Alter BP: Fanconi's anemia and malignancies. Am J Hematol 1996; 53:99.

437. Venkatraj VS, Gaidano G, Auerbach AD: Clonality studies and N-ras and p53 mutation analysis of hematopoietic cells in Fanconi anemia. Leukemia 1994; 8:1354.

438. Baron F, Sybert VP, Andrews RG: Cutaneous and extracutaneous neutrophilic infiltrates (Sweet syndrome) in three patients with Fanconi anemia. J Pediatr 1989; 115:726.

439. van Niekerk CH, Jordaan C, Badenhorst PN: Pancytopenia secondary to primary malignant lymphoma of bone marrow as the first hematologic manifestation of the Estren-Dameshek variant of Fanconi's anemia. Am J Pediatr Hematol Oncol 1987; 9:344.

440. de Chadarevian J-P, Vekemans M, Bernstein M: Fanconi's anemia, medulloblastoma, Wilms' tumor, horseshoe kidney, and gonadal dysgenesis. Arch Pathol Lab Med 1985; 109:367.

441. Linares M, Pastor E, et al: Hepatocellular carcinoma and squamous cell carcinoma in a patient with Fanconi's anemia. Ann Hematol 1991; 63:54.

442. Guy JT, Auslander MO: Androgenic steroids and hepatocellular carcinoma. Lancet 1973; 1:148.

443. Schroeder TM: Genetically determined chromosome instability syndromes. Cytogenet Cell Genet 1982; 33:119.

444. Jacobs P, Karabus C: Fanconi's anemia. A family study with 20-year follow-up including associated breast pathology. Cancer 1984; 54:1850.

445. Cattan D, Kalifat R, et al: Maladie de Fanconi et cancer du foie. Arch Fr Mal App Dig 1974; 63:41.

446. Farrell GC: Fanconi's familial hypoplastic anaemia with some unusual features. Med J Aust 1976; 1:116.

447. Evans DIK: Aplastic anaemia in childhood. In Geary CG (ed): Aplastic Anaemia. London, Baillière Tindall, 1979, p 161.

448. Moldvay J, Schaff Z, Lapis K: Hepatocellular carcinoma in Fanconi's anemia treated with androgen and corticosteroid. Zentralbl Pathol 1991; 137:167.

449. Cap J, Ondrus B, Danihel L: Focal nodular hyperplasia of the liver and hepatocellular carcinoma in children with Fanconi's anemia after long-term treatment with androgens. Bratisl Lek Listy 1983; 79:73.

450. Kew MC, Van Coller B, et al: Occurrence of primary hepatocellular cancer and peliosis hepatis after treatment with androgenic steroids. S Afr Med J 1976; 50:1233.

451. Maves CK, Caron KH, et al: Splenic and hepatic peliosis: MR findings. Am J Roentgenol 1992; 158:75.

452. Schmidt E, Deeg HJ, Storb R: Regression of androgen-related hepatic tumors in patients with Fanconi's anemia following marrow transplantation. Transplantation 1984; 37:452.

453. Ortega JJ, Olive T, et al: Bone marrow transplant in Fanconi's anemia. Results in five patients. Sangre 1990; 35:433.

454. Recant L, Lacy P: Fanconi's anemia and hepatic cirrhosis. Am J Med 1965; 39:464.

455. Johnson FL, Feagler JR, et al: Association of androgenic-anabolic steroid therapy with development of hepatocellular carcinoma. Lancet 1972; 2:1273.

456. Drachtman RA, Alter BP: Dyskeratosis congenita: Clinical and genetic heterogeneity. Report of a new case and review of the literature. Am J Pediatr Hematol Oncol 1992; 14:297.

457. Drachtman RA, Alter BP: Dyskeratosis congenita. Dermatol Clin 1995; 13:33.

458. Connor JM, Gatherer D, et al: Assignment of the gene for dyskeratosis congenita to Xq28. Hum Genet 1987; 72:348.

459. Reichel M, Grix A, Isseroff R: Dyskeratosis congenita associated with elevated fetal hemoglobin, X-linked ocular albinism, and juvenile-onset diabetes mellitus. Pediatr Dermatol 1992; 9:103.

460. Ortega JA, Swanson VL, et al: Congenital dyskeratosis. Zinsser-Engman-Cole syndrome with thymic dysplasia and aplastic anemia. Am J Dis Child 1972; 124:701.

461. Dokal I, Bungey J, et al: Dyskeratosis congenita fibroblasts are abnormal and have unbalanced chromosomal rearrangements. Blood 1992; 80:3090.

462. Phillips RJ, Judge M, et al: Dyskeratosis congenita: delay in diagnosis and successful treatment of pancytopenia by bone marrow transplantation. Br J Dermatol 1992; 127:278.

463. Putterman C, Safadi R, et al: Treatment of the hematological manifestations of dyskeratosis congenita. Ann Hematol 1993; 66:209.

464. Forni G, Melevendi C, et al: Dyskeratosis congenita: Unusual presenting features within a kindred. Pediatr Hematol Oncol 1993; 10:145.

465. Pritchard SL, Junker AK: Positive response to granulocyte-colony-stimulating factor in dyskeratosis congenita before matched unrelated bone marrow transplantation. Am J Pediatr Hematol Oncol 1994; 16:186.

466. Oehler L, Reiter E, et al: Effective stimulation of neutropoiesis with rh G-CSF in dyskeratosis congentia: a case report. Ann Hematol 1994; 69:325.

467. Kehrer H, Krone W, et al: Cytogenetic studies of skin fibroblast cultures from a karyotypically normal female with dyskeratosis congenita. Clin Genet 1992; 41:129.

468. Kajtar P, Mehes K: Bilateral Coats retinopathy associated with aplastic anaemia and mild dyskeratotic signs. Am J Med Genet 1994; 49:374.

469. Kehrer H, Krone W: Chromosome abnormalities in cell cultures derived from the leukoplakia of a female patient with dyskeratosis congenita. Am J Med Genet 1992; 42:217. Letter to the editor.

470. Carter DM, Pan M, et al: Psoralen-DNA cross-linking photoadducts in dyskeratosis congenita: delay in excision and promotion of sister chromatid exchange. J Invest Dermatol 1979; 73:97.

471. Arngrimsson R, Dokal I, et al: Dyskeratosis congenita: three additional families show linkage to a locus in Xq28. J Med Genet 1993; 30:618.

472. Mann WR, Venkatraj VS, et al: Use of a polymorphic DNA probe for diagnosis of dyskeratosis congenita. Clin Res 1990; 38:627A.

473. Dokal I, Luzzatto L: Dyskeratosis congenita is a chromosomal instability disorder. Leuk Lymphoma 1994; 15:1.

474. Pai GS, Yan Y, et al: Bleomycin hypersensitivity in dyskeratosis congenita fibroblasts, lymphocytes, and transformed lymphoblasts. Cytogenet Cell Genet 1989; 52:186.

475. DeBauche DM, Pai GS, Stanley WS: Enhanced G2 chromatid radiosensitivity in dyskeratosis congenita fibroblasts. Am J Hum Genet 1990; 46:350.

476. Ning Y, Yongshan Y, et al: Heterozygote detection through bleomycin-induced G2 chromatid breakage in dyskeratosis congenita families. Cancer Genet Cytogenet 1992; 60:31.

477. Marsh JCW, Will AJ, et al: "Stem cell" origin of the hematopoietic defect in dyskeratosis congenita. Blood 1992; 79:3138.

478. Navarro JT, Ribera JM, et al: Hipoplasia medular asociada a disqueratosis congenita. Sangre 1994; 39:207.

479. Michalevicz R, Baron S, et al: Granulocytic macrophage colony stimulating factor restores in vitro growth of granulocyte-macrophage bone marrow hematopoietic progenitors in dyskeratosis congenita. Isr J Med Sci 1989; 25:193.

480. Georgouras K: Dyskeratosis congenita. Aust J Dermatol 1965; 8:36.

481. Morrison D, Rose EL, et al: Dyskeratosis congenita and nasopharyngeal atresia. J Laryngol Otol 1992; 106:996.

482. Anil S, Beena VT, et al: Oral squamous cell carcinoma in a case of dyskeratosis congenita. Ann Dent 1994; 53:15.

483. Lemarchand-Venencie F, Gluckman E, et al: Syndrome de Zinsser-Cole-Engmann. Ann Dermatol Venereol 1982; 109:783.

484. Berthou C, Devergie A, et al: Late vascular complications after bone marrow transplantation for dyskeratosis congenita. Br J Haematol 1991; 79:335.

485. Mahmoud HK, Schaefer UW, et al: Marrow transplantation for pancytopenia in dyskeratosis congenita. Blut 1985; 51:57.

486. Chessells J, Harper J: Bone marrow transplantation for dyskeratosis congenita. Br J Haematol 1992; 81:314.

487. Ivker RA, Woosley J, Resnick SD: Dyskeratosis congenita or chronic graft-versus-host disease? A diagnostic dilemma in a child eight years after bone marrow transplantation for aplastic anemia. Pediatr Dermatol 1993; 10:362.

488. Ling NS, Fenske NA, et al: Dyskeratosis congenita in a girl simulating chronic graft-vs-host disease. Arch Dermatol 1985; 121:1424.

489. Conter V, Johnson FL, et al: Bone marrow transplantation for aplastic anemia associated with dyskeratosis congenita. Am J Pediatr Hematol Oncol 1988; 10:99.

490. Esterly NB: Nail dystrophy in dyskeratosis congenita and chronic graft-vs-host disease. Arch Dermatol 1986; 122:506.

491. Russo CL, Glader BE, et al: Treatment of neutropenia associated with dyskeratosis congenita with granulocyte-macrophage colony-stimulating factor. Lancet 1990; 336:751.

492. Ozsoylu S, Argun G: Tryptic activity of the duodenal juice in aplastic anemia. J Pediatr 1967; 70:60.

493. Barrios NJ, Kirkpatrick DV: Successful cyclosporin A treatment of aplastic anaemia in Shwachman-Diamond syndrome. Br J Haematol 1990; 74:540.

494. Seymour JF, Escudier SM: Acute leukemia complicating bone marrow hypoplasia in an adult with Shwachman's syndrome. Leuk Lymphoma 1993; 12:131.

495. Huijgens PC, Van der Veen EA, et al: Syndrome of Shwachman and leukaemia. Scand J Haematol 1977; 18:20.

496. Smith OP, Chessells JM, et al: Haematologic abnormalities in Shwachman-Diamond syndrome: A review of twenty one patients. Br J Haematol 1995; 89:2.

497. Tsai PH, Sahdev I, et al: Fatal cyclophosphamide-induced congestive heart failure in a 10-year-old boy with Shwachman-Diamond syndrome and severe bone marrow failure treated with allogeneic bone marrow transplantation. Am J Pediatr Hematol Oncol 1989; 12:472.

498. Barrios N, Kirkpatrick D, et al: Bone marrow transplant in Shwachman Diamond syndrome. Br J Haematol 1991; 79:337.

499. Bonilla MA, Gilmore B, et al: In vivo administration of recombinant human G-CSF corrects the neutropenia associated with Schwachman-Diamond syndrome. Blood 1989; 74(Suppl 1):324a.

500. Adachi N, Tsuchiya H, et al: rhG-CSF for Shwachman's syndrome. Lancet 1990; 336:1136.

501. Paley C, Murphy S, et al: Treatment of neutropenia in Shwachman Diamond syndrome (SDS) with recombinant human granulocyte colony stimulating factor (RH-GCSF). Blood 1991; 78(Suppl 1):3a.

502. Dale DC, Bonilla MA, et al: A randomized controlled phase III trial of recombinant human granulocyte colony-stimulating factor (filgrastim) for treatment of severe chronic neutropenia. Blood 1993; 81:2496.

503. Ferguson L, Hoots K, et al: Long-term bone marrow (BM) cultures with recombinant human granulocyte-macrophage colony stimulating factor (rhGM-CSF) in children with cytopenias: A correlation with clinical response. Blood 1988; 72:115a.

504. McKusick VA, Eldridge R, et al: Dwarfism in the Amish. II. Cartilage-hair hypoplasia. Bull Johns Hopkins Hosp 1965; 116:285.

505. Makitie O, Kaitila I: Cartilage-hair hypoplasia—Clinical manifestations in 108 Finnish patients. Eur J Pediatr 1993; 152:211.

506. Mäkitie O, Rajantie J, Kaitila I: Anaemia and macrocytosis—unrecognized features in cartilage-hair hypoplasia. Acta Paediatr 1993; 81:1026.

507. Lux SE, Johnston RB Jr, et al: Chronic neutropenia and abnormal cellular immunity in cartilage-hair hypoplasia. N Engl J Med 1970; 282:231.

508. Juvonen E, Makitie O, et al: Defective in-vitro colony formation of haematopoietic progenitors in patients with cartilage-hair hypoplasia and history of anaemia. Eur J Pediatr 1995; 154:30.

509. Sacrez R, Levy J, et al: Anémie de Blackfan-Diamond associée à des malformations multiples. Med Inf 1965; 72:493.

510. L'Hirondel J, Caen J, et al: Anémie de Blackfan-Diamond et dyostose métaphysaire récessive autosomique. Ouest Med 1967; 20:1152.

511. Harris RE, Baehner RL, et al: Cartilage-hair hypoplasia, defective T-cell function, and Diamond-Blackfan anemia in an Amish child. Am J Med Genet 1981; 8:291.

512. Virolainen M, Savilahti E, et al: Cellular and humoral immunity in cartilage-hair hypoplasia. Pediatr Res 1978; 12:961.

513. Sulisalo T, Francomano CA, et al: High-resolution genetic mapping of the cartilage-hair hypoplasia (CHH) gene in Amish and Finnish families. Genomics 1994; 20:347.

514. Sulisalo T, Sillence D, et al: Early prenatal diagnosis of cartilage-hair hypoplasia (CHH) with polymorphic DNA markers. Prenat Diagn 1995; 15:135.

515. Sanchez-Corona J, Garcia-Cruz D, et al: Increased adenosine deaminase activity in a patient with cartilage-hair hypoplasia. Ann Genet 1990; 33:99.

516. Roberts MA, Arnold RM: Hodgkin's lymphoma in a child with cartilage-hair hypoplasia: case report. Mil Med 1984; 149:280.

517. Gorlin RJ: Cartilage-hair-hypoplasia and Hodgkin disease. Am J Med Genet 1992; 44:539.

518. Pearson HA, Lobel JS, et al: A new syndrome of refractory sideroblastic anemia with vacuolization of marrow precursors and exocrine pancreatic dysfunction. J Pediatr 1979; 95:976.

519. Rotig A, Cormier V, et al: Pearson's marrow-pancreas syndrome. A multisystem mitochondrial disorder in infancy. J Clin Invest 1990; 86:1601.

520. Gurgey A, Rotig A, et al: Pearson's marrow-pancreas syndrome in 2 Turkish children. Acta Haematol 1992; 87:206.

521. Bernes SM, Bacino C, et al: Identical mitochondrial DNA deletion in mother with progressive external ophthalmoplegia and son with Pearson marrow-pancreas syndrome. J Pediatr 1993; 123:598.

522. Oblender MG, Richardson CJ, Alter BP: Pearson syndrome (PS) presenting as nonimmune hydrops fetalis. Clin Res 1993; 41:803A.

523. Sano T, Ban K, et al: Molecular and genetic analyses of two patients with Pearson's marrow-pancreas syndrome. Pediatr Res 1993; 34:105.

524. De Vivo D: The expanding clinical spectrum of mitochondrial diseases. Brain Dev 1993; 15:1.

525. Blaw ME, Mize CE: Juvenile Pearson syndrome. J Child Neurol 1993; 5:186.

526. Favareto F, Caprino D, et al: New clinical aspects of Pearson's syndrome. Report of three cases. Haematologica 1989; 74:591.

527. Fleming WH, Trounce I, et al: Cytokine treatment improves the hematologic manifestations of Pearson's syndrome. Blood 1994; 84(Suppl 1):27a.

528. Larsson N-G, Holme E, Kristiansson B, et al: Progressive increase of the mutated mitochondrial DNA fraction in Kearns-Sayre syndrome. Pediatr Res 1990; 28:131.

529. McShane MA, Hammans SR, et al: Pearson syndrome and mitochondrial encephalomyopathy in a patient with a deletion of mtDNA. Am J Hum Genet 1991; 48:39.

530. Baerlocher KE, Feldges A, et al: Mitochondrial DNA deletion in an 8-year-old boy with Pearson syndrome. J Inherit Metab Dis 1992; 15:327.

531. Simonsz HJ, Bärlocher K, Rötig A: Kearns-Sayre's syndrome developing in a boy who survived Pearson's syndrome caused by mitochondrial DNA deletion. Doc Ophthalmol 1992; 82:73.

532. Nelson I, Bonne G, et al: Kearns-Sayre syndrome with sideroblastic anemia: Molecular investigations. Neuropediatrics 1992; 23:199.

533. Bader-Meunier B, Rotig A, et al: Refractory anaemia and mitochondrial cytopathy in childhood. Br J Haematol 1994; 87:381.

534. De Vaal OM, Seynhaeve V: Reticular dysgenesia. Lancet 1959; 2:1123.

535. Bujan W, Ferster A, et al: Use of recombinant human granulocyte colony stimulating factor in reticular dysgenesis. Br J Haematol 1992; 81:128.

536. Bujan W, Ferster A, et al: Effect of recombinant human granulocyte colony-stimulating factor in reticular dysgenesis. Blood 1993; 82:1684.

537. Azcona C, Alzina V, et al: Use of recombinant human granulocyte-macrophage colony stimulating factor in an infant with reticular dysgenesis. Eur J Pediatr 1994; 153:164.

538. DeWitte DB, Buick MK, et al: Neonatal pancytopenia and severe combined immunodeficiency associated with antenatal administration of azathioprine and prednisone. J Pediatr 1984; 105:625.

539. Alter BP: Neonatal pancytopenia after maternal azathioprine therapy. J Pediatr 1985; 106:691.

540. Haas RJ, Niethammer D, et al: Congenital immunodeficiency and agranulocytosis (reticular dysgenesia). Acta Paediatr Scand 1977; 66:279.

541. Levinsky RJ, Tiedeman K: Successful bone-marrow transplantation for reticular dysgenesis. Lancet 1983; 1:671.

542. Roper M, Parmley RT, et al: Severe congenital leukopenia (reticular dysgenesis). Am J Dis Child 1985; 139:832.

543. Chin TW, Plaeger-Marshall S, et al: Lymphokine-activated killer cells in primary immunodeficiency and acquired immunodeficiency syndrome. Clin Immunol Immunopathol 1989; 53:449.

544. O'Gorman Hughes DW: Aplastic anaemia in childhood. III. Constitutional aplastic anaemia and related cytopenias. Med J Austr 1974; 1:519.

545. Bizzaro N, Dianese G: Neonatal alloimmune amegakaryocytosis. Vox Sang 1988; 54:112.

546. Guinan EC, Lee YS, et al: Effects of interleukin-3 and granulocyte-macrophage colony-stimulating factor on thrombopoiesis in congenital amegakaryocytic thrombocytopenia. Blood 1993; 81:1691.

547. Hoyeraal HM, Lamvik J, Moe PJ: Congenital hypoplastic thrombocytopenia and cerebral malformations in two brothers. Acta Paediatr Scand 1970; 59:185.

548. Berthet F, Caduff R, et al: A syndrome of primary combined immunodeficiency with microcephaly, cerebellar hypoplasia, growth failure and progressive pancytopenia. Eur J Pediatr 1994; 153:333.

549. Aalfs CM, Van den Berg H, et al: The Hoyeraal-Hreidarsson syndrome: the fourth case of a separate entity with prenatal growth retardation, progressive pancytopenia and cerebellar hypoplasia. Eur J Pediatr 1995; 154:304.

550. Alter BP: The bone marrow failure syndromes. In Nathan DG, Oski FA (eds): Hematology of Infancy and Childhood. 3rd ed. Philadelphia, W.B. Saunders Co., 1987, p 159.

551. Griffiths AD: Constitutional aplastic anaemia: a family with a new X linked variety of amegakaryocytic thrombocytopenia. J Med Genet 1983; 20:361.

552. Buchanan GR, Scher CS, et al: Use of homologous platelet survival in the differential diagnosis of chronic thrombocytopenia in childhood. Pediatrics 1977; 59:49.

553. Hreidarsson S, Kristjansson K, et al: A syndrome of progressive pancytopenia with microcephaly, cerebellar hypoplasia and growth failure. Acta Paediatr Scand 1988; 77:773.

554. Van Oostrom CG, Wilms RHH: Congenital thrombocytopenia, associated with raised concentrations of haemoglobin F. Helv Paediatr Acta 1978; 33:59.

555. Harris MB, Najfeld V, et al: Congenital amegakaryocytic thrombocytopenia: a case report with chromosomal abnormalities. Unpublished, 1984.

556. Mibashan RS, Millar DS: Fetal haemophilia and allied bleeding disorders. Br Med Bull 1983; 39:392.

557. Freedman MH: Congenital failure of hematopoiesis in the newborn infant. Clin Perinatol 1984; 11:417.

558. Arias S, Penchaszadeh VB, et al: The IVIC syndrome: A new autosomal dominant complex pleiotropic syndrome with radial ray hypoplasia, hearing impairment, external ophthalmoplegia, and thrombocytopenia. Am J Med Genet 1980; 6:25.

559. Sammito V, Motta D, et al: IVIC syndrome: report of a second family. Am J Med Genet 1988; 29:875.

560. Czeizel A, Goblyos P, Kodaj I: IVIC Syndrome: Report of a third family. Am J Med Genet 1989; 32:282.

561. Neri G, Sammito V: Re: IVIC Syndrome report by Czeizel et al. Am J Med Genet 1989; 33:284.

562. Gonzalez CH, Durkin-Stamm MV, et al: The WT syndrome—A "new" autosomal dominant pleiotropic trait of radial/ulnar hypoplasia with high risk of bone marrow failure and/or leukemia. Birth Defects 1977; 8:31.

563. Smith ACM, Hays T, et al: WT syndrome: a third family. Am J Hum Genet 1987; 41:A84.

564. Alter CL, Levine PH, et al: Dominantly transmitted hematologic dysfunction clinically similar to Fanconi's anemia. Am J Hematol 1989; 32:241.

565. Dokal I, Ganly P, et al: Late onset bone marrow associated with proximal fusion of radius and ulna: a new syndrome. Br J Haematol 1989; 71:277.

566. McFarland G, Say B, et al: A condition resembling congenital hypoplastic anemia occurring in a mother and son. Clin Pediatr 1982; 12:755.

567. Li FP, Potter NU, et al: A family with acute leukemia, hypoplastic anemia and cerebellar ataxia. Association with bone marrow C-monosomy. Am J Med 1978; 65:933.

568. Li FP, Hecht F, et al: Ataxia-pancytopenia: Syndrome of cerebellar ataxia, hypoplastic anemia, monosomy 7, and acute myelogenous leukemia. Cancer Genet Cytogenet 1981; 4:189.

569. Daghistani D, Curless R, et al: Ataxia-pancytopenia and monosomy 7 syndrome. J Pediatr 1989; 115:108.

570. Yanabe Y, Nunoi H, et al: A disease with immune deficiency, skin abscesses, pancytopenia, abnormal bone marrow karyotype, and increased sister chromatid exchanges: An autosomal recessive chromosome instability syndrome? Jpn J Human Genet 1990; 35:263.

571. Drachtman R, Weinblatt M, et al: Marrow hypoplasia associated with congenital neurologic anomalies in two siblings. Acta Paediatr Scand 1990; 79:990.

572. Kotzot D, Richter K, Gierth-Fiebig K: Oculocutaneous albinism, immunodeficiency, hematological disorders, and minor anomalies: A new autosomal recessive syndrome? Am J Med Genet 1994; 50:224.

573. Stoll C, Alembik Y, Lutz P: A syndrome of facial dysmorphia, birth defects, myelodysplasia and immunodeficiency in three sibs of consanguineous parents. Genet Couns 1994; 5:161.

574. Ghosal SP, Mukherjee AK, et al: Diaphyseal dysplasia associated with anemia. J Pediatr 1988; 113:49.

575. Ozsoylu S: High-dose intravenous methylprednisolone therapy for anemia associated with diaphyseal dysplasia. J Pediatr 1993; 114:904.

576. Gumruk F, Besim A, Altay C: Ghosal haemato-diaphyseal dysplasia: a new disorder. Eur J Pediatr 1993; 152:218.

577. Aufderheide AC: Familial cytopenia and vascular disease: a newly recognized autosomal dominant condition. Birth Defects 1972; 8:63.

578. Kato J, Niitsu Y, et al: Chronic hypoplastic neutropenia. A case of familial occurrence of chronic hypoplastic neutropenia and aplastic anemia. Rinsho Ketsueki 1986; 27:407.

579. Keiser G: Erworbene Panmyelopathien. Schweiz Med Wochenschr 1970; 100:1938.

580. Kaur J, Catovsky D, et al: Familial acute myeloid leukaemia with acquired Pelger-Huet anomaly and aneuploidy of C group. BMJ 1972; 11:327.

581. Chitambar CR, Robinson WA, Glode LM: Familial leukemia and aplastic anemia associated with monosomy 7. Am J Med 1983; 75:756.

582. Sleijfer DT, Mulder NH, et al: Acquired pancytopenia in relatives of patients with aplastic anaemia. Acta Med Scand 1980; 207:397.

583. Abels D, Reed WB: Fanconi-like syndrome. Immunologic deficiency, pancytopenia, and cutaneous malignancies. Arch Dermatol 1973; 107:419.

584. Linsk JA, Khoory MS, Meyers KR: Myeloid, erythroid, and immune system defects in a family. A new stem-cell disorder? Ann Intern Med 1975; 82:659.

585. Nowell P, Besa E, et al: Two adult siblings with thrombocytopenia and a familial 13;14 translocation. Cancer Genet Cytogenet 1984; 11:169.

586. Salob SP, Webb DKH, Atherton DJ: A child with xeroderma pigmentosum and bone marrow failure. Br J Dermatol 1992; 126:372.

587. Berbis P, Beylot C, et al: Xeroderma pigmentosum and refractory anaemia in two first cousins. Br J Dermatol 1989; 121:767.

588. Berlin C, Tager A: Xeroderma pigmentosum—Report of eight cases of mild to moderate type and course: A study of response to various irradiations. Dermatologica 1958; 116:27.

589. Reed WB, Landing B, et al: Xeroderma pigmentosum. Clinical and laboratory investigation of its basic defect. JAMA 1969; 207:2073.

590. Li FP, Marchetto DJ, Vawter GR: Acute leukemia and preleukemia in eight males in a family: An X-linked disorder? Am J Hematol 1979; 6:61.

591. Grierson H, Purtilo DT: Epstein-Barr virus infections in males with the X-linked lymphoproliferative syndrome. Ann Intern Med 1987; 106:538.

592. Skare JC, Milunsky A, et al: Mapping the X-linked lymphoproliferative syndrome. Proc Natl Acad Sci U S A 1987; 84:2015.

593. Samad FU, Engel E, Hartmann RC: Hypoplastic anemia, Friedreich's ataxia and chromosomal breakage: Case report and review of similar disorders. South Med J 1973; 66:135.

594. Nagata M, Hara T, et al: Aplastic anemia associated with ataxia and chromosome translocation (1;20). Acta Haematol 1990; 84:198.

595. Sackey K, Sakati N, et al: Multiple dysmorphic features and pancytopenia: a new syndrome? Clin Genet 1985; 27:606.

596. Muroi K, Amemiya Y, et al: Long-term bone marrow failure accompanied by skin pigmentation. Int J Hematol 1991; 54:281.

597. Froster UG, Gortner L: Thrombocytopenia in the Brachmann-de Lange syndrome. Am J Med Genet 1993; 46:730.

598. Fryns JP, Vinken L: Thrombocytopenia in the Brachmann-de Lange syndrome. Am J Med Genet 1994; 49:360.

599. Weinstein HJ: Congenital leukemia and the neonatal myeloproliferative disorders associated with Down's syndrome. Clin Haematol 1978; 7:147.

600. Weinblatt ME, Higgins G, Ortega JA: Aplastic anemia in Down's syndrome. Pediatrics 1981; 67:896.

601. Kuster W, Majewski F: The Dubowitz syndrome. Eur J Pediatr 1986; 144:574.

602. Walters TR, Desposito F: Aplastic anemia in Dubowitz syndrome. J Pediatr 1985; 106:622.

603. Berthold F, Fuhrmann W, Lampert F: Fatal aplastic anaemia in a child with features of Dubowitz syndrome. Eur J Pediatr 1987; 146:605.

604. Ilyina HG, Lurie IW: Dubowitz syndrome: Possible evidence for clinical subtype. Am J Med Genet 1990; 35:561.

605. Thuret I, Michel G, et al: Chromosomal instability in two siblings with Dubowitz syndrome. Br J Haematol 1991; 78:124.

606. Grobe H: Dubowitz syndrome and acute lymphatic leukemia. Monatsschr Kinderheilkd 1983; 131:467.

607. Sauer H, Spelger G: Dubowitz syndrome with immunodeficiency and solid malignant tumor in two siblings. Monatschr Kinderheilkd 1977; 125:885.

608. Majewski F, Goecke T: Studies of microcephalic primordial dwarfism I: Approach to a delineation of the Seckel syndrome. Am J Med Genet 1982; 12:7.

609. Espérou-Bourdeau H, Leblanc T, Schaison G, et al: Aplastic anemia associated with "bird-headed" dwarfism (Seckel syndrome). Nouv Rev Fr Hematol 1993; 35:99.

610. Seemanova E, Passarge E, et al: Familial microcephaly with normal intelligence, immunodeficiency, and risk for lymphoreticular malignancies: A new autosomal recessive disorder. Am J Med Genet 1985; 20:639.

611. Hayani A, Suarez CR, et al: Acute myeloid leukaemia in a patient with Seckel syndrome. J Med Genet 1994; 31:148.

612. Sall MG, Badiane M, et al: Seckel's nanism: concerning one case. Dakar Med 1990; 35:46.

613. Lilleyman JS: Constitutional hypoplastic anemia associated with familial "bird-headed" dwarfism (Seckel syndrome). Am J Pediatr Hematol Oncol 1984; 6:207.

614. Dohlsten M, Carlsson R, et al: Immunological abnormalities in a child with constitutional aplastic anemia. Pediatr Hematol Oncol 1986; 3:89.

615. Butler MG, Hall BD, et al: Do some patients with Seckel syndrome have hematological problems and/or chromosome breakage? Am J Med Genet 1987; 27:645.

616. Cervenka J, Tsuchiya H, et al: Seckel's dwarfism: Analysis of chromosome breakage and sister chromatid exchanges. Am J Dis Child 1979; 133:555.

617. Jamieson CR, Van Der Burgt I, et al: Mapping a gene for Noonan syndrome to the long arm of chromosome 12. Nat Genet 1994; 8:357.

618. Noonan JA: Hypertelorism with Turner phenotype. A new syndrome with associated congenital heart disease. Am J Dis Child 1968; 116:373.

619. Char F, Caralis DG, Voigt GC: Noonan syndrome in 30-year-old male with cyanotic congenital heart disease. Birth Defects 1972; 8:243.

620. Evans DGR, Lonsdale RN, Patton MA: Cutaneous lymphangioma and amegakaryocytic thrombocytopenia in Noonan syndrome. Clin Genet 1991; 39:228.

621. Feldman KW, Ochs HD, et al: Congenital stem cell dysfunction associated with Turner-like phenotype. J Pediatr 1976; 88:979.

622. Freedman MH: Pure red cell aplasia in childhood and adolescence: Pathogenesis and approaches to diagnosis. Br J Haematol 1993; 85:246.

623. Krantz SB, Zaentz SD: Pure red cell aplasia. In Gordon AS, Silber R, LoBue J (eds): The Year in Hematology. New York, Plenum Press, 1977, p 153.

624. Sears DA, George JN, Gold MS: Transient red blood cell aplasia in association with viral hepatitis. Occurrence four years apart in siblings. Arch Intern Med 1975; 135:1585.

625. Loeb VJ, Moore CV, Dubach R: The physiological evaluation and management of chronic bone marrow failure. Am J Med 1953; 15:499.

626. Hirst E, Robertson TI: The syndrome of thymoma and erythroblastopenic anemia. A review of 56 cases including 3 case reports. Medicine 1967; 46:225.

627. Dessypris EN: Pure Red Cell Aplasia. Baltimore, The Johns Hopkins University Press, 1988.

628. Chikkappa G, Zarrabi MH, Tsan M-F: Pure red-cell aplasia in patients with chronic lymphocytic leukemia. Medicine 1986; 65:339.

629. Dessypris EN, Redline S, et al: Diphenylhydantoin-induced pure red cell aplasia. Blood 1985; 65:789.

630. MacDougall LG: Pure red cell aplasia associated with sodium valproate therapy. JAMA 1982; 247:53.

631. Zaentz SD, Krantz SB, Sears DA: Studies on pure red cell aplasia. VII. Presence of proerythroblasts and response to splenectomy: a case report. Blood 1975; 46:261.

632. Wilson HA, McLaren GD, et al: Transient pure red-cell aplasia: cell-mediated suppression of erythropoiesis associated with hepatitis. Ann Intern Med 1980; 92:196.

633. Purtilo DT, Zelkowitz L, et al: Delayed onset of infectious mononucleosis associated with acquired agammaglobulinemia and red cell aplasia. Ann Intern Med 1984; 101:180.

634. Levitt LJ, Reyes GR, et al: Human T cell leukemia virus-1-associated T-suppressor cell inhibition of erythropoiesis in a patient with pure red cell aplasia and chronic TG-lymphoproliferative disease. J Clin Invest 1988; 81:538.

635. Berner YN, Berrebi A, et al: Erythroblastopenia in acquired immunodeficiency syndrome (AIDS). Acta Haematol 1983; 70:273. Letter.

636. Linenberger ML, Abkowitz JL: Haematological disorders associated with feline retrovirus infections. In Young NS (ed): Baillière's Clinical Haematology. 8th ed. London, Baillière Tindall, 1995, p 73.

637. O'Sullivan MG, Anderson DC, et al: Identification of a novel simian parvovirus in cynomolgus monkeys with severe anemia. A paradigm of human B19 parvovirus infection. J Clin Invest 1994; 93:1571.

638. Baker RI, Manoharan A, et al: Pure red cell aplasia of pregnancy: a distinct clinical entity. Br J Haematol 1993; 85:619.

639. Eisemann G, Dameshek W: Splenectomy for "pure red-cell" hypoplastic (aregenerative) anemia associated with autoimmune hemolytic disease. Report of a case. N Engl J Med 1954; 251:1044.

640. Gasser C: Aplastische Anämie (chronische Erythroblastophthise) und Cortison. Schweiz Med Wochenschr 1951; 81:1241.

641. Peschle C, Marmont AM, et al: Pure red cell aplasia: Studies on an IgG serum inhibitor neutralizing erythropoietin. Br J Haematol 1975; 30:411.

641a. Casadevall N, Dupuy E, et al: Brief report: Autoantibodies against erythropoietin in a patient with pure red-cell aplasia. N Engl J Med 1996; 334:630.

642. Murase T: Bilineage hematopoietic inhibitor and T lymphocyte dysfunction in a patient with pure red cell aplasia, myasthenia gravis and thymoma. Exp Hematol 1993; 21:451.

643. Lacombe C, Casadevall N, et al: Erythroid progenitors in adult chronic pure red cell aplasia: Relationship of in vitro erythroid colonies to therapeutic response. Blood 1984; 64:71.

644. Chikkappa G, Pasquale D, et al: Cyclosporine and prednisone therapy for pure red cell aplasia in patients with chronic lymphocytic leukemia. Am J Hematol 1992; 41:5.

645. Clark DA, Dessypris EN, Krantz SB: Studies on pure red cell aplasia. XI. Results of immunosuppressive treatment of 37 patients. Blood 1984; 63:277.

646. Dessypris EN, Fogo A, et al: Studies on pure red cell aplasia. X. Association with acute leukemia and significance of bone marrow karyotype abnormalities. Blood 1980; 56:421.

647. Young NS, Fields BM, Knipe DM: Virology. New York, Raven Press, 1995.

648. Woolf AD, Campion GV, et al: Clinical manifestation of human parvovirus B19 in adults. Arch Intern Med 1989; 149:1153.

649. Wodzinski MA, Lilleyman JS: Transient erythroblastopenia of childhood due to human parvovirus B19 infection. Br J Haematol 1989; 73:127.

650. Guillot M, Lefrere JJ, et al: Acute anaemia and aplastic crisis without haemolysis in human parvovirus infection. J Clin Pathol 1987; 40:1264.

651. Potter CG, Potter AC, et al: Variation of erythroid and myeloid precursors in the marrow and peripheral blood of volunteer subjects infected with human parvovirus (B19). J Clin Invest 1987; 79:1486.

652. Srivastava A, Bruno E, et al: Parvovirus B19–induced perturbation of human megakaryocytopoiesis in vitro. Blood 1990; 76:1997.

653. McClain K, Estrov Z, et al: Chronic neutropenia of childhood: frequent association with parvovirus infection and correlations with bone marrow culture studies. Br J Haematol 1993; 85:57.

654. Finkel TH, Torok TJ, et al: Chronic parvovirus B19 infection and systemic necrotising vasculitis: opportunistic infection or aetiological agent? Lancet 1994; 343:1255.

655. Shirono K, Tsuda H: Parvovirus B19–associated haemophagocytic syndrome in healthy adults. Br J Haematol 1995; 89:923.

656. Kurtzman GJ, Ozawa K, et al: Chronic bone marrow failure due to persistent parvovirus infection. N Engl J Med 1987; 317:287.

657. Faden H, Gary GWJ, Anderson LJ: Chronic parvovirus infection in a presumably immunologically healthy woman. Clin Infect Dis 1992; 15:595.

658. Anderson MJ, Khousam MN, et al: Human parvovirus B19 and hydrops fetalis. Lancet 1988; 1:535.

659. Porter HJ, Khong TY, et al: Parvovirus as a cause of hydrops fetalis: detection by in situ DNA hybridisation. J Clin Pathol 1988; 41:381.

660. van Elsacker-Niele AMW, Salimans MMM, et al: Fetal pathology in human parvovirus B19 infection. Br J Obstet Gynaecol 1989; 96:768.

661. Anderson LJ, Hurwitz ES: Human parvovirus B19 and pregnancy. Clin Perinatol 1988; 15:273.

662. Kinney JS, Anderson LJ, et al: Risk of adverse outcomes of pregnancy after human parvovirus B19 infection. J Infect Dis 1988; 157:663.

663. Hall SM, Cohen BJ, et al: Prospective study of human parvovirus (B19) infection in pregnancy. BMJ 1990; 300:1166.

664. Rodis JF, Quinn DL, et al: Management and outcomes of pregnancies complicated by human B19 parvovirus infection: A prospective study. Am J Obstet Gynecol 1990; 163:1168.

665. Metzman R, Anand A, et al: Hepatic disease associated with intrauterine parvovirus B19 infection in a newborn premature infant. J Pediatr Gastroenterol Nutr 1989; 9:112.

666. Wright IMR, Williams ML, Cohen BJ: Congenital parvovirus infection. Arch Dis Child 1991; 66:253.

667. Anderson MJ, Higgins PG, et al: Experimental parvoviral infection in humans. J Infect Dis 1985; 152:257.

668. Mortimer PP, Humphries RK, et al: A human parvovirus–like virus inhibits haematopoietic colony formation in vitro. Nature 1983; 302:426.

669. Takahashi T, Ozawa K, et al: Susceptibility of human erythropoietic cells to B19 parvovirus in vitro increases with differentiation. Blood 1990; 75:603.

670. Ozawa K, Kurtzman G, Young N: Replication of the B19 parvovirus in human bone marrow cell cultures. Science 1986; 233:883.

671. Morey AL, Patou G, Myint S, et al: In vitro culture for the detection of infectious human parvovirus B19 and B19-specific antibodies using foetal haematopoietic precursor cells. J Gen Virol 1992; 73:3313.

672. Schwarz TF, Serke S, et al: Replication of parvovirus B19 in

hematopoietic progenitor cells generated *in vitro* from normal human peripheral blood. J Virol 1992; 66:1273.

673. Morey AL, Fleming KA: Immunophenotyping of fetal haemopoietic cells permissive for human parvovirus B19 replication *in vitro*. Br J Haematol 1992; 82:302.

674. Brown KE, Anderson SM, Young NS: Erythrocyte P antigen: Cellular receptor for B19 parvovirus. Science 1993; 262:114.

675. Brown KE, Hibbs JR, et al: Resistance to parvovirus B19 due to lack of virus receptor (erythrocyte P antigen). N Engl J Med 1994; 330:1192.

676. Kurtzman GJ, Cohen BJ, et al: Immune response to B19 parvovirus and an antibody defect in persistent viral infection. J Clin Invest 1989; 84:1114.

677. Josephs HW: Anaemia of infancy and early childhood. Medicine 1936; 15:307.

678. Diamond LK, Blackfan KD: Hypoplastic anemia. Am J Dis Child 1938; 56:464.

679. Kynaston JA, West NC, Ried MM: A regional experience of red cell aplasia. Eur J Pediatr 1993; 152:306.

680. Bresters D, Bruin MCA, van Dijken PJ: Congenital hypoplastic anemia in the Netherlands. Tijdschr Kindergeneeskd 1991; 59:203.

681. Vlachos A, Alter BP, et al: The Diamond-Blackfan anemia registry (DBAR). Pediatr Res 1994; 35:171A.

682. Ball SE, McGuckin C, et al: The Diamond Blackfan Anemia Registry. Br J Haematol 1994; 86:18.

683. Alter BP: Childhood red cell aplasia. Am J Pediatr Hematol Oncol 1980; 2:121.

684. Diamond LK, Wang WC, Alter BP: Congenital hypoplastic anemia. Adv Pediatr 1976; 22:349.

685. Alter BP, Nathan DG: Red cell aplasia in children. Arch Dis Child 1979; 54:263.

686. Wallman IS: Hereditary red cell aplasia. Med J Aust 1956; 2:488.

687. Gray PH: Pure red-cell aplasia. Occurrence in three generations. Med J Aust 1982; 1:519.

688. Balaban EP, Buchanan GR, et al: Diamond-Blackfan syndrome in adult patients. Am J Med 1985; 78:533.

689. Splain J, Berman BW: Cyclosporin A treatment for Diamond-Blackfan anemia. Am J Hematol 1992; 39:208.

690. Gojic V, Van't Veer-Korthof ET, et al: Congenital hypoplastic anemia: Another example of autosomal dominant transmission. Am J Med Genet 1994; 50:87.

691. Diamond LK, Allen DM, Magill FB: Congenital (erythroid) hypoplastic anemia. Am J Dis Child 1961; 102:403.

692. Gardner FH, Nathan DG: Hypochromic anemia and hemochromatosis—response to combined testosterone, pyridoxine, and liver extract therapy. Trans Am Clin Climatol Assoc 1961; 73:121.

693. Krivit W, Nelson E, Sundberg D: Erythrogenesis imperfecta in seven individuals in three generations. Pediatr Res 1978; 12:467.

694. Viskochil DH, Carey JC, et al: Congenital hypoplastic (Diamond-Blackfan) anemia in seven members of one kindred. Am J Med Genet 1990; 35:251.

695. Bertolani MF, Baroncini A, et al: Malattia di Blackfan-Diamond con genitali ambigui. Pediatr Med Chir 1993; 15:589.

696. Madanat F, Arnaout M, et al: Red cell aplasia resembling Diamond-Blackfan anemia in seven children in a family. Am J Pediatr Hematol Oncol 1994; 16:260.

697. Yetgin S, Balci S, et al: Aase-Smith syndrome: Report of a new case with unusual features. Turk J Pediatr 1994; 36:239.

698. Bello A, Dorantes S, Alvarez-Amaya C: La anemia hipoplastica en la edad pediatrica. Bol Med Hosp Infant Mex 1983; 40:718.

699. Waterkotte GW, McElfresh AE: Congenital pure red cell hypoplasia in identical twins. Pediatrics 1974; 54:646.

700. Schorr JB, Cohen ES, et al: Hypoplastic anemia in childhood. Jewish Mem Hosp Bull 1962; 6:126.

701. Tchernia G, Morinet F, et al: Diamond Blackfan anaemia: apparent relapse due to B19 parvovirus. Eur J Pediatr 1993; 152:209.

702. Cathie IAB: Erythrogenesis imperfecta. Arch Dis Child 1950; 25:313.

703. D'Avanzo M, Pistoia V, et al: Heterogeneity of the erythropoietic defect in two cases of Aase-Smith syndrome. Pediatr Hematol Oncol 1994; 11:189.

704. Alter BP: Thumbs and anemia. Pediatrics 1978; 62:613.

705. Sumimoto S-I, Kawai M, et al: Intravenous c-globulin therapy in Diamond-Blackfan anemia. Acta Paediatr Jpn 1992; 34:179.

706. Hing AV, Dowton SB: Aase syndrome: Novel radiographic features. Am J Med Genet 1993; 45:413.

707. Becker RE, Maurer H, et al: Growth hormone deficiency (GHD) in Diamond-Blackfan anemia (DBA). Pediatr Res 1991; 29:74A.

708. Buchanan GR, Alter BP, et al: Platelet number and function in Diamond-Blackfan anemia. Pediatrics 1981; 68:238.

709. Vogel P, Bassen FA: Sternal marrow of children in normal and in pathologic states. Am J Dis Child 1939; 57:245.

710. Bernard J, Seligmann M, et al: Anémie de Blackfan-Diamond. Nouv Rev Fr Hematol 1962; 2:721.

711. Boxer LA, Hussey L, Clarke TL: Sideroblastic anemia following congenital erythroid hypoplasia. J Pediatr 1971; 79:681.

712. Girot R, Griscelli C: Érythroblastopénie à rechutes. À propos d'un cas suivi pendant 22 ans. Nouv Rev Fr Hematol 1977; 18:555.

713. Hammond D, Shore N, Movassaghi N: Production, utilization and excretion of erythropoietin. I. Chronic anemias. II. Aplastic crisis. III. Erythropoietic effects of normal plasma. Ann N Y Acad Sci 1968; 149:516.

714. Price JM, Brown RR, et al: Excretion of urinary tryptophan metabolites by patients with congenital hypoplastic anemia (Diamond-Blackfan syndrome). J Lab Clin Med 1970; 75:316.

715. Finlay JL, Shahidi NT, et al: Lymphocyte dysfunction in congenital hypoplastic anemia. J Clin Invest 1982; 70:619.

716. Giblett ER, Ammann AJ, et al: Nucleoside-phosphorylase deficiency in a child with severely defective T-cell immunity and normal B-cell immunity. Lancet 1975; 1:1010.

717. Glader BE, Backer K, Diamond LK: Elevated erythrocyte adenosine deaminase activity in congenital hypoplastic anemia. N Engl J Med 1983; 309:1486.

718. Zielke HR, Ozand PT, et al: Elevation of pyrimidine enzyme activities in the RBC of patients with congenital hypoplastic anaemia and their parents. Br J Haematol 1979; 42:381.

719. Glader BE, Backer K: Comparative activity of erythrocyte adenosine deaminase and orotidine decarboxylase in Diamond-Blackfan anemia. Am J Hematol 1986; 23:135.

720. Glader BE, Backer K: Elevated red cell adenosine deaminase activity: a marker of disordered erythropoiesis in Diamond-Blackfan anaemia and other haematologic diseases. Br J Haematol 1988; 68:165.

721. Whitehouse DB, Hopkinson DA, et al: Adenosine deaminase activity in a series of 19 patients with the Diamond-Blackfan syndrome. Adv Exp Med Biol 1986; 195(Pt A):85.

722. Tartaglia AP, Propp S, et al: Chromosome abnormality and hypocalcemia in congenital erythroid hypoplasia (Blackfan-Diamond syndrome). Am J Med 1966; 41:990.

723. Heyn R, Kurczynski E, Schmickel R: The association of Blackfan-Diamond syndrome, physical abnormalities, and an abnormality of chromosome 1. J Pediatr 1974; 85:531.

724. Philippe N, Requin C, Germain D: Études chromosomiques dans 6 cas d'anémie de Blackfan-Diamond. Pediatrie 1971; 26:47.

725. Brizard CP, Fayard C, et al: Anémie par anerythroblastose (Type Blackfan-Diamond) chez une enfant porteuse d'anomalies chromosomiques constitutionnelles. Pediatrie 1971; 26:305.

726. Iskandar O, Jager MJ, et al: A case of pure red cell aplasia with high incidence of spontaneous chromosome breakage: a possible x-ray sensitive syndrome. Hum Genet 1980; 55:337.

727. Pfeiffer RA, Ambs E: The Aase syndrome: Autosomal-recessive hereditary, connatal erythroid hypoplasia and triphalangeal thumbs. Monatsschr Kinderheilkd 1983; 131:235.

728. Visser GHA, Desmedt MCH, Meijboom EJ: Altered fetal cardiac flow patterns in pure red cell anaemia (the Blackfan-Diamond syndrome). Prenat Diagn 1988; 8:525.

729. Van der Mooren K: Fetal anemia. Prenat Diag 1989; 9:450.

730. Gurney CW, Pierce MI, et al: The stimulatory effect of "anemic plasma" in congenital hypoplastic anemia. J Lab Clin Med 1957; 50:821.

731. Ortega JA, Shore NA, et al: Congenital hypoplastic anemia inhibition of erythropoiesis by sera from patients with congenital hypoplastic anemia. Blood 1975; 45:83.

732. Geller G, Krivit W, et al: Lack of erythropoietic inhibitory effect of serum from patients with congenital pure red cell aplasia. J Pediatr 1975; 86:198.

733. Freedman MH, Amato D, Saunders EF: Haem synthesis in the Diamond-Blackfan syndrome. Br J Haematol 1975; 31:515.

734. Steinberg MH, Coleman MF, Pennebaker JB: Diamond-Blackfan syndrome: Evidence for T-cell mediated suppression of erythroid development and a serum blocking factor associated with remission. Br J Haematol 1979; 41:57.

735. Hoffman R, Zanjani ED, et al: Diamond-Blackfan syndrome: Lymphocyte-mediated suppression of erythropoiesis. Science 1976; 193:899.

736. Nathan DG, Hillman DG, Breard J: The influence of T cells on erythropoiesis. In Stamatoyannopoulos G, Nienhuis AW (eds): Cellular and Molecular Regulation of Hemoglobin Switching. New York, Grune & Stratton, 1979, p 291.

737. Steinberg MH, Coleman MB, Pennebaker JB: Diamond-Blackfan anemia: The role of immunoglobulin blocking factor in remission. Am J Hematol 1980; 8:213.

738. Zanjani EM, Rinehart JJ: Role of cell-cell interaction in normal and abnormal erythropoiesis. Am J Pediatr Hematol Oncol 1980; 2:233.

739. Ershler WB, Ross J, et al: Bone-marrow microenvironment defect in congenital hypoplastic anemia. N Engl J Med 1980; 302:1321.

740. Nathan DG, Clarke BJ, et al: Erythroid precursors in congenital hypoplastic (Diamond-Blackfan) anemia. J Clin Invest 1978; 61:489.

741. Nathan DG, Hillman DG, et al: Normal erythropoietic helper T cells in congenital hypoplastic (Diamond-Blackfan) anemia. N Engl J Med 1978; 298:1049.

742. McGuckin CP, Ball SE, Gordon-Smith EC: Diamond-Blackfan anaemia: three patterns of in vitro response to haemopoietic growth factors. Br J Haematol 1995; 89:457.

743. Sieff CA, Yokoyama CT, et al: The production of steel factor mRNA in Diamond-Blackfan anaemia long-term cultures and interactions of steel factor with erythropoietin and interleukin-3. Br J Haematol 1992; 82:640.

744. Casadevall N, Croisille L, et al: Age-related alterations in erythroid and granulopoietic progenitors in Diamond-Blackfan anaemia. Br J Haematol 1994; 87:369.

745. Lipton JM, Kudisch M, et al: Defective erythroid progenitor differentiation system in congenital hypoplastic (Diamond-Blackfan) anemia. Blood 1986; 67:962.

746. Tsai PH, Arkin S, Lipton JM: An intrinsic progenitor defect in Diamond-Blackfan anemia. Br J Haematol 1989; 73:112.

747. Halperin DS, Estrov Z, Freedman MH: Diamond-Blackfan anemia: Promotion of marrow erythropoiesis in vitro by recombinant interleukin-3. Blood 1989; 73:1168.

748. Geissler EN, Ryan MA, Housman DE: The dominant-white spotting (W) locus of the mouse encodes the c-kit proto-oncogene. Cell 1988; 55:185.

749. Zsebo KM, Wypych J, et al: Identification, purification, and biological characterization of hematopoietic stem cell factor from Buffalo rat liver–conditioned medium. Cell 1990; 63:195.

750. Spritz RA, Giebel LB, Holmes SA: Dominant negative and loss of function mutations of the c-kit (mast/stem cell growth factor receptor) proto-oncogene in human piebaldism. Am J Hum Genet 1992; 50:261.

751. Spritz RA: Lack of apparent hematologic abnormalities in human patients with c-kit (stem cell factor receptor) gene mutations. Blood 1992; 79:2497.

752. Cynshi O, Satoh K, et al: Effects of recombinant human erythropoietin on anaemic W/Wv and Sl/Sld mice. Br J Haematol 1990; 75:319.

753. Alter BP, Gaston T, Lipton JM: Lack of effect of corticosteroids in W/Wv and Sl/SlD mice: These mice are not a model for steroid-responsive Diamond-Blackfan anemia. Eur J Haematol 1993; 50:275.

754. Ody C, Kindler V, Vassalli P: Interleukin 3 perfusion in W/Wv mice allows the development of macroscopic hematopoietic spleen colonies and restores cutaneous mast cell number. J Exp Med 1990; 172:403.

755. Abkowitz JL, Broudy VC, et al: Absence of abnormalities of c-kit or its ligand in two patients with Diamond-Blackfan anemia. Blood 1992; 79:25.

756. Olivieri NF, Grunberger T, et al: Diamond-Blackfan anemia: Heterogenous response of hematopoietic progenitor cells in vitro to the protein product of the Steel locus. Blood 1991; 78:2211.

757. Drachtman RA, Geissler EN, Alter BP: The SCF and c-kit genes in Diamond-Blackfan anemia. Blood 1992; 79:2177.

758. Spritz RA, Freedman MH: Lack of mutations of the MGF and KIT genes in Diamond-Blackfan anemia. Blood 1993; 81:3165.

759. Abkowitz JL, Sabo KM, et al: Diamond-Blackfan anemia: In vitro response of erythroid progenitors to the ligand for c-kit. Blood 1991; 78:2198.

760. Bagnara GP, Zauli G, et al: In vitro growth and regulation of bone marrow enriched CD34+ hematopoietic progenitors in Diamond-Blackfan anemia. Blood 1991; 78:2203.

761. Perdahl EB, Naprstek BL, et al: Erythroid failure in Diamond-Blackfan anemia is characterized by apoptosis. Blood 1994; 83:645.

762. Gasser C: Akute Erythroblastopenie. Schweiz Med Wochenschr 1949; 79:838.

763. Hill JM, Hunter RB: ACTH therapy in refractory anemias. In JR Mote (ed): Proceedings of the Second Clinical ACTH Conference, Volume II—Therapeutics. New York, Blakiston, 1951, p 181.

764. Allen DM, Diamond LK: Congenital (erythroid) hypoplastic anemia. Am J Dis Child 1961; 102:416.

765. Sjölin S, Wranne L: Treatment of congenital hypoplastic anaemia with prednisone. Scand J Haematol 1970; 7:63.

766. Gomez-Almaguer D, Gonzalez-Llano O: Danazol in the treatment of Blackfan-Diamond anemia. Blood 1993; 80:382a.

767. Ozsoylu S: Oral megadose methylprednisolone for the treatment of Diamond-Blackfan anemia. Pediatr Hematol Oncol 1994; 11:561.

768. Bejaoui M, Fitouri Z, et al: Failure of immunosuppressive therapy and high-dose intravenous immunoglobulins in four transfusion-dependent, steroid-unresponsive Blackfan-Diamond anemia patients. Haematologica 1993; 78:38.

769. Monteserin MC, Garcia Vela JA, et al: Cyclosporin A for Diamond-Blackfan anemia: A new case. Am J Hematol 1993; 42:406.

770. Saunders EF, Olivieri N, Freedman MH: Unexpected complications after bone marrow transplantation in transfusion-dependent children. Bone Marrow Transplant 1993; 12:88.

771. Greinix HT, Storb R, et al: Long-term survival and cure after marrow transplantation for congenital hypoplastic anaemia (Diamond-Blackfan syndrome). Br J Haematol 1993; 84:515.

772. Mugishima H, Gale RP, et al: Bone marrow transplantation for Diamond-Blackfan anemia. Bone Marrow Transplant 1995; 15:55.

773. Mori PG, Haupt R, et al: Pentasomy 21 in leukemia complicating Diamond-Blackfan anemia. Cancer Genet Cytogenet 1992; 63:70.

774. Niemeyer CM, Baumgarten E, et al: Treatment trial with recombinant human erythropoietin in children with congenital hypoplastic anemia. Contrib Nephrol 1991; 88:276.

775. Fiorillo A, Poggi V, et al: Unresponsiveness to erythropoietin therapy in a case of Blackfan Diamond anemia. Am J Hematol 1991; 37:65. Letter to the editor.

776. Dunbar CE, Smith DA, et al: Treatment of Diamond-Blackfan anaemia with haematopoietic growth factors, granulocyte-macrophage colony stimulating factor and interleukin 3: sustained remissions following IL-3. Br J Haematol 1991; 79:316.

777. Gillio AP, Faulkner LB, et al: Treatment of Diamond-Blackfan anemia with recombinant human interleukin-3. Blood 1993; 82:744.

778. Bastion Y, Bordigoni P, et al: Sustained response after recombinant interleukin-3 in Diamond Blackfan anemia. Blood 1994; 83:617.

779. Olivieri NF, Feig SA, et al: Failure of recombinant human interleukin-3 therapy to induce erythropoiesis in patients with refractory Diamond-Blackfan anemia. Blood 1994; 83:2444.

780. Krsnik I, Arribalzaga K, et al: Interleukin-3 (IL-3) is not effective in all cases of Blackfan-Diamond anemia. Br J Haematol 1994; 87:156.

781. D'Oelsnitz M, Vincent L, et al: À propos d'un cas de leucémie aiguë lymphoblastique survenue après guérison d'une maladie de Blackfan-Diamond. Arch Fr Pediatr 1975; 32:582.

782. Wasser JS, Yolken R, et al: Congenital hypoplastic anemia (Diamond-Blackfan syndrome) terminating in acute myelogenous leukemia. Blood 1978; 51:991.

783. Krishnan EU, Wegner K, Garg SK: Congenital hypoplastic anemia terminating in acute promyelocytic leukemia. Pediatrics 1978; 61:898.

784. Basso G, Cocito MG, et al: Congenital hypoplastic anaemia developed in acute megakaryoblastic leukaemia. Helv Paediatr Acta 1981; 36:267.

785. Steinherz PG, Canale VC, Miller DR: Hepatocellular carcinoma, transfusion-induced hemochromatosis and congenital hypoplastic anemia (Blackfan-Diamond syndrome). Am J Med 1976; 60:1032.

786. Glader BE, Flam MS, et al: Hematologic malignancies in Diamond Blackfan anemia. Pediatr Res 1990; 27:142A.

787. Janov A, Leong T, et al: Diamond-Blackfan anemia. Natural history and sequelae of treatment. Medicine 1996; 75:77.

787a. Haupt R, Dufour C, et al: Diamond-Blackfan anemia and malignancy: A case report and a review of the literature. Cancer 1996; 77:1961.

787b. Van Dijken PJ: Diamond-Blackfan anemia and malignancy: A case report and a review of the literature. Cancer 1996; 77:1962.

788. Hardisty RM: Diamond-Blackfan anaemia. In: Congenital Disorders of Erythropoiesis. Ciba Foundation Symposium 37 (new series). Amsterdam, Elsevier, 1976, p 89.

789. Baar HS: The life span of red blood corpuscles in erythronophthisis. Acta Haematol 1952; 7:17.

790. Wranne L: Transient erythroblastopenia in infancy and childhood. Scand J Haematol 1970; 7:76.

791. Skeppner G, Wranne L: Transient erythroblastopenia of childhood in Sweden: incidence and findings at the time of diagnosis. Acta Paediatr 1993; 82:574.

792. Cherrick I, Karayalcin G, Lanzkowsky P: Transient erythroblastopenia of childhood. Am J Pediatr Hematol Oncol 1994; 16:320.

793. Elian JC, Frappaz D, et al: Transient erythroblastopenia of childhood presenting with echovirus 11 infection. Acta Paediatr 1993; 62:492.

794. Hefelfinger DC: Simultaneous hyperphosphatasemia and erythroblastopenia of childhood. Clin Pediatr 1993; 32:175.

795. Chabali R: Transient erythroblastopenia of childhood presenting with shock and metabolic acidosis. Pediatr Emerg Care 1994; 10:278.

796. Labotka RJ, Maurer HS, Honig GR: Transient erythroblastopenia of childhood. Review of 17 cases, including a pair of identical twins. Am J Dis Child 1981; 135:937.

797. Glader BE: Diagnosis and management of red cell aplasia in children. Hematol Oncol Clin North Am 1987; 1:431.

798. Seip M: Transient erythroblastopenia in siblings. Acta Paediatr Scand 1982; 71:689.

799. Wegelius R, Weber TH: Transient erythroblastopenia in childhood. A study of 15 cases. Acta Paediatr Scand 1978; 67:513.

800. Link MP, Alter BP: Fetal erythropoiesis during recovery from transient erythroblastopenia of childhood (TEC). Pediatr Res 1981; 15:1036.

801. Gerrits GPJM, van Oostrom CG, de Vaan GAM: Severe anemia caused by transient erythroblastopenia in children (TEC). Tijdschr Kindergeneeskd 1982; 50:97.

802. Wang WC, Mentzer WC: Differentiation of transient erythroblastopenia of childhood from congenital hypoplastic anemia. J Pediatr 1976; 88:784.

803. Nagai K, Morohoshi T, et al: Transient erythroblastopenia of childhood with megakaryocytopenia associated with human parvovirus B19 infection. Br J Haematol 1992; 80:131.

804. Nikkari S, Meurman O, Wanne O: Parvovirus B19 and transient erythroblastopenia of childhood. Br J Haematol 1993; 83:679.

805. Miyata H, Yagi K, et al: Transient erythroblastopenia due to human parvovirus B19 infection: a case report of a boy suffering from purpura. Acta Paediatr Jpn 1994; 36:217.

806. Tugal O, Pallant B, et al: Transient erythroblastopenia of the newborn caused by human parvovirus. Am J Pediatr Hematol Oncol 1994; 16:352.

807. Frank GR, Cherrick I, et al: Transient erythroblastopenia in a child with Kawasaki syndrome: A case report. Am J Pediatr Hematol Oncol 1994; 16:271.

808. Young NS, Mortimer PP, et al: Characterization of a virus that causes transient aplastic crisis. J Clin Invest 1984; 73:224.

809. Mortimer PP: A virological perspective on bone marrow failure. In Young NS, Levine AS, Humphries RK (eds): Aplastic Anemia: Stem Cell Biology and Advances in Treatment. New York, Alan R. Liss, 1984, p 121.

810. Lovric VA: Anaemia and temporary erythroblastopenia in children. A syndrome. Aust Ann Med 1970; 1:34.

811. Tamary H, Kaplinsky C, et al: Transient erythroblastopenia of childhood. Evidence for cell-mediated suppression of erythropoiesis. Am J Pediatr Hematol Oncol 1993; 15:386.

812. Koenig HM, Lightsey AL, et al: Immune suppression of erythropoiesis in transient erythroblastopenia of childhood. Blood 1979; 54:742.

813. Freedman MH: 'Recurrent' erythroblastopenia of childhood. An IgM-mediated RBC aplasia. Am J Dis Child 1983; 137:458.

814. Lewis SM, Verwilghen RL: Dyserythropoiesis: definition, diagnosis and assessment. In Lewis SM, Verwilghen RL (eds): Dyserythropoiesis. London, Academic Press, 1977, p 3.

815. Frisch B, Lewis SM: The bone marrow in aplastic anaemia: Diagnostic and prognostic features. J Clin Pathol 1974; 27:231.

816. Rozman C, Feliu E, et al: Transient dyserythropoiesis in repopulated human bone marrow following transplantation: an ultrastructural study. Br J Haematol 1982; 50:63.

817. Lewis SM, Verwilghen RL: Dyserythropoiesis. London, Academic Press, 1977.

818. Crookston JH, Crookston MC, et al: Hereditary erythroblastic multinuclearity associated with a positive acidified-serum test: a type of congenital dyserythropoietic anaemia. Br J Haematol 1969; 17:11.

819. Heimpel H: Congenital dyserythropoietic anaemia type I: clinical and experimental aspects. In: Congenital Disorders of Erythropoiesis. CIBA Foundation Symposium 37. Amsterdam, Elsevier, 1976, p 135.

820. Heimpel H: Congenital dyserythropoietic anaemia, Type I. In Lewis SM, Verwilghen RL: Dyserythropoiesis. London, Academic Press, 1977, p 55.

821. Vainchenker W, Guichard J, et al: Congenital dyserythropoietic anaemia type I: Absence of clonal expression in the nuclear abnormalities of cultured erythroblasts. Br J Haematol 1980; 46:33.

822. Lavabre-Bertrand T, Blanc P, et al: Alpha-interferon therapy for congenital dyserythropoiesis type I. Br J Haematol 1995; 89:929.

823. Verwilghen RL, Lewis SM, et al: HEMPAS: Congenital dyserythropoietic anaemia (Type II). Q J Med 1973; 42:257.

824. Verwilghen RL: Congenital dyserythropoietic anaemia type II (HEMPAS). In: Congenital Disorders of Erythropoiesis. CIBA Foundation Symposium 37. Amsterdam, Elsevier, 1976, p 151.

825. Fukuda MN: Congenital dyserythropoietic anaemia type II (HEMPAS) and its molecular basis. Baillières Clin Haematol 1993; 6:493.

826. Seip M, Skrede S, et al: A case of variant congenital dyserythropoietic anemia revisited. Scand J Haematol 1982; 28:278.

827. Giblett ER, Crookston MC: Agglutinability of red cells by anti-i in patients with thalassaemia major and other haematological disorders. Nature 1964; 201:1138.

828. Rosse WF, Logue GL, et al: Mechanisms of immune lysis of the red cells in hereditary erythroblastic multinuclearity with a positive acidified serum test and paroxysmal nocturnal hemoglobinuria. J Clin Invest 1974; 53:31.

829. Fukuda MN, Dell A, Scartezzini P: Primary defect of congenital dyserythropoietic anemia type II. Failure in glycosylation of erythrocyte lactosaminoglycan proteins caused by lowered N-acetylglucosaminyltransferase II. J Biol Chem 1987; 262:7195.

830. Lind L, Sandstrom H, et al: Localization of the gene for congenital dyserythropoietic anemia type III, CDAN3, to chromosome 15q21-q25. Hum Mol Genet 1995; 4:109.

831. Tebbi K, Gross S: Absence of morphological abnormalities in marrow erythrocyte colonies (CFU-E) from a patient with HEMPAS-II. J Lab Clin Med 1978; 91:797.

832. Vainchenker W, Guichard J, Breton-Gorius J: Morphological abnormalities in cultured erythroid colonies (BFU-E) from the blood of two patients with HEMPAS. Br J Haematol 1979; 42:363.

833. Roodman GD, Clare CN, Mills G: Congenital dyserythropoietic anemia type II (CDA-II): chromosomal banding studies and adherent cell effects on erythroid colony (CFU-E) and burst (BFU-E) formation. Br J Haematol 1982; 50:499.

834. Wolff JA, Von Hofe FH: Familial erythroid multinuclearity. Blood 1951; 6:1274.

835. Goudsmit R: Congenital dyserythropoietic anaemia, type III. In

Lewis SM, Verwilghen RL (eds): Dyserythropoiesis. London, Academic Press, 1977, p 83.

836. Vainchenker W, Breton-Gorius J, et al: Congenital dyserythropoietic anemia type III. Studies on erythroid differentiation of blood erythroid progenitor cells (BFUE) *in vitro*. Exp Hematol 1980; 8:1057.

837. Sansone G, Masera G, et al: An unclassified case of congenital dyserythropoietic anaemia with a severe neonatal onset. Acta Haematol 1992; 88:41.

838. Roberts DJ, Nadel A, et al: An unusual variant of congenital dyserythropoietic anaemia with mild maternal and lethal fetal disease. Br J Haematol 1993; 84:549.

839. Parsons SF, Jones J, et al: A novel form of congenital dyserythropoietic anemia associated with deficiency of erythroid CD44 and a unique blood group phenotype [In(a−b−), Co(a−b−)]. Blood 1994; 83:860.

840. Brochstein JA, Siena S, et al: Congenital dyserythropoietic anemia (CDA) with karyorrhexis. Pediatr Res 1985; 19:258A.

841. Kostmann R: Infantile genetic agranulocytosis. A new recessive lethal disease in man. Acta Paediatr Scand 1956; 45:1.

842. Kostmann R: Infantile genetic agranulocytosis. A review with presentation of ten new cases. Acta Paediatr Scand 1975; 64:362.

843. Iselius L, Gustavson KH: Spatial distribution of the gene for infantile genetic agranulocytosis. Hum Hered 1984; 34:358.

844. Coulombel L, Morardet N, et al: Granulopoietic differentiation in long-term bone marrow cultures from children with congenital neutropenia. Am J Hematol 1988; 27:93.

845. Zucker-Franklin D, L'Esperance P, Good RA: Congenital neutropenia: An intrinsic cell defect demonstrated by electron microscopy of soft agar colonies. Blood 1977; 49:425.

846. Hestdal K, Welte K, et al: Severe congenital neutropenia: Abnormal growth and differentiation of myeloid progenitors to granulocyte colony-stimulating factor (G-CSF) but normal response to G-CSF plus stem cell factor. Blood 1993; 82:2991.

847. Shitara T, Ijima H, et al: Increased cytokine levels and abnormal response of myeloid progenitor cells to granulocyte colony-stimulating factor in a case of severe congenital neutropenia. *In vitro* effects of stem cell factor. Am J Pediatr Hematol Oncol 1994; 16:167.

848. Guba SC, Sartor CA, et al: Granulocyte colony-stimulating factor (G-CSF) production and G-CSF receptor structure in patients with congenital neutropenia. Blood 1994; 83:1486.

849. Sandoval C, Parganas E, et al: Lack of alterations in the cytoplasmic domains of the granulocyte colony-stimulating factor receptors in eight cases of severe congenital neutropenia. Blood 1995; 85:852.

850. Dong F, Hoefsloot LH, et al: Identification of a nonsense mutation in the granulocyte-colony-stimulating factor receptor in severe congenital neutropenia. Proc Natl Acad Sci U S A 1994; 91:4480.

851. Dong F, Brynes RK, et al: Mutations in the gene for the granulocyte colony-stimulating-factor receptor in patients with acute myeloid leukemia preceded by severe congenital neutropenia. N Engl J Med 1995; 333:487.

852. Naparstek E: Granulocyte colony-stimulating factor, congenital neutropenia, and acute myeloid leukemia. N Engl J Med 1995; 333:516.

853. Bernhardt TM, Burchardt ER, Welte K: Assessment of G-CSF and GM-CSF mRNA expression in peripheral blood mononuclear cells from patients with severe congenital neutropenia and in human myeloid leukemic cell lines. Exp Hematol 1993; 21:163.

854. Mempel K, Pietsch T, et al: Increased serum levels of granulocyte colony-stimulating factor in patients with severe congenital neutropenia. Blood 1991; 77:1919.

855. Pahwa RN, O'Reilly RJ, et al: Partial correction of neutrophil deficiency in congenital neutropenia following bone marrow transplantation (BMT). Exp Hematol 1977; 5:45.

856. Rappeport JM, Parkman R, et al: Correction of infantile agranulocytosis (Kostmann's syndrome) by allogeneic bone marrow transplantation. Am J Med 1980; 68:605.

857. Zintl F, Hermann J, et al: Bone marrow transplantation (BMT) in the treatment of genetic disease, Part 2. Kinderarztl Prax 1991; 59:10.

858. Barrett AJ: Clinical experience with lithium in aplastic anemia and congenital neutropenia. Adv Exp Med Biol 1980; 127:305.

859. Chan HSL, Freedman MH, Saunders EF: Lithium therapy of children with chronic neutropenia. Am J Med 1981; 70:1073.

860. Donadieu J, Boutard P, et al: A phase II study of recombinant human granulocyte colony-stimulating factor (rHuG-CSF, lenograstim) in the treatment of agranulocytosis in children. Nouv Rev Fr Hematol 1994; 36:441.

861. Bonilla MA, Dale D, et al: Long-term safety of treatment with recombinant human granulocyte colony-stimulating factor (r-metHuG-CSF) in patients with severe congenital neutropenias. Br J Haematol 1994; 88:723.

862. Welte K, Zeidler C, et al: Differential effects of granulocyte-macrophage colony-stimulating factor and granulocyte colony-stimulating factor in children with severe congenital neutropenia. Blood 1990; 75:1056.

863. Bishop NJ, Williams DM, et al: Osteoporosis in severe congenital neutropenia treated with granulocyte colony-stimulating factor. Br J Haematol 1995; 89:927.

864. Cividalli G, Yarkoni S, et al: Can infantile hereditary agranulocytosis be diagnosed prenatally? Prenat Diagn 1983; 3:157.

865. Millar DS, Davis LR, et al: Normal blood cell values in the early mid-trimester fetus. Prenat Diagn 1985; 5:367.

866. Gilman PA, Jackson DP, Guild HG: Congenital agranulocytosis: Prolonged survival and terminal acute leukemia. Blood 1970; 36:576.

867. Rosen RB, Kang S-J: Congenital agranulocytosis terminating in acute myelomonocytic leukemia. J Pediatr 1979; 94:406.

868. Lui V, Ragab AH, et al: Infantile genetic agranulocytosis and acute lymphocytic leukemia in two sibs. J Pediatr 1978; 92:1028.

869. Dale DC: Hematopoietic growth factors for the treatment of severe chronic neutropenia. Stem Cells 1995; 13:94.

870. Weinblatt ME, Scimeca P, et al: Transformation of congenital neutropenia into monosomy 7 and acute nonlymphoblastic leukemia in a child treated with granulocyte colony-stimulating factor. J Pediatr 1995; 126:263.

871. Imashuku S, Hibi S, et al: Myelodysplasia and acute myeloid leukaemia in cases of aplastic anaemia and congenital neutropenia following G-CSF administration. Br J Haematol 1995; 89:188.

872. Hoffman R: Acquired pure amegakaryocytic thrombocytopenic purpura. Semin Hematol 1991; 28:303.

873. Young NS: Acquired pure red cell aplasia and amegakaryocytic thrombocytopenia. In Young NS, Alter BP (eds): Aplastic Anemia: Acquired and Inherited. Philadelphia, W.B. Saunders Co., 1994, p 216.

874. Scarlett JD, Williams NT, McKellar WJD: Acquired amegakaryocytic thrombocytopaenia in a child. J Paediatr Child Health 1992; 28:263.

875. Xue Y, Zhang R, et al: Acquired amegakaryocytic thrombocytopenis purpura with a Philadelphia chromosome. Cancer Genet Cytogenet 1993; 69:51.

876. Dharmasena F, Galton DAG: Remission of amegakaryocytic thrombocytopenia induced by antilymphocyte globulin (ALG). Br J Haematol 1986; 63:205.

877. Hall JG, Levin J, et al: Thrombocytopenia with absent radius (TAR). Medicine 1969; 48:411.

878. Hall JG: Thrombocytopenia and absent radius (TAR) syndrome. J Med Genet 1987; 24:79.

879. Hedberg VA, Lipton JM: Thrombocytopenia with absent radii. A review of 100 cases. Am J Pediatr Hematol Oncol 1988; 10:51.

880. Messen S, Vargas L, et al: Congenital thrombocytopenia and absent radius syndrome in identical twins. Rev Chil Pediatr 1986; 57:559.

881. Dodesini G, Frigerio G, Cocco E: La trombocitopenia congenita ipoplastica con aplasia bilaterale del radio. Minerva Pediatr 1979; 31:1023.

882. Teufel M, Enders H, Dopfer R: Consanguinity in a Turkish family with thrombocytopenia with absent radii (TAR) syndrome. Hum Genet 1983; 64:94.

883. Shalev E, Weiner E, et al: Micrognathia-prenatal ultrasonographic diagnosis. Int J Gynaecol Obstetr 1983; 21:343.

884. Ceballos-Quintal JM, Pinto-Escalante D, Gongora-Biachi RA: TAR-like syndrome in a consanguineous Mayan girl. Am J Med Genet 1992; 43:805.

885. Nilsson LR, Lundholm G: Congenital thrombocytopenia associated with aplasia of the radius. Acta Paediatr 1960; 49:291.

886. Whitfield MF, Barr DGD: Cow's milk allergy in the syndrome of thrombocytopenia with absent radius. Arch Dis Child 1976; 51:337.

887. Adeyokunnu AA: Radial aplasia and amegakaryocytic thrombocytopenia (TAR syndrome) among Nigerian children. Am J Dis Child 1984; 138:346.

888. Fromm B, Niethard FU, Marquardt E: Thrombocytopenia and absent radius (TAR) syndrome. Int Orthop 1991; 15:95.

889. Bessman JD, Harrison RL, et al: The megakaryocyte abnormality in thrombocytopenia-absent radius syndrome. Blood 1983; 62:143.

890. Armitage JO, Hoak JC, et al: Syndrome of thrombocytopenia and absent radii: Qualitatively normal platelets with remission following splenectomy. Scand J Haematol 1978; 20:25.

890a. Camitta BM, Rock A: Acute lymphoidic leukemia in a patient with thrombocytopenia/absent radii (TAR) syndrome. Am J Pediatr Hematol Oncol 1993; 15:335.

891. Brochstein JA, Shank B, et al: Marrow transplantation for thrombocytopenia-absent radii syndrome. J Pediatr 1992; 121:587.

892. Donnenfeld AE, Wiseman B, et al: Prenatal diagnosis of thrombocytopenia absent radius syndrome by ultrasound and cordocentesis. Prenat Diagn 1990; 10:29.

893. Labrune P, Pons JC, et al: Antenatal thrombocytopenia in three patients with TAR (thrombocytopenia with absent radii) syndrome. Prenat Diagn 1993; 13:463.

894. Weinblatt M, Petrikovsky B, et al: Prenatal evaluation and *in utero* platelet transfusion for thrombocytopenia absent radii syndrome. Prenat Diagn 1994; 14:892.

895. Vaughan JM: Leuco-erythroblastic anaemia. J Pathol Bacteriol 1936; 42:541.

896. Weick JK, Hagedorn AB, Linman JW: Leukoerythroblastosis. Diagnostic and prognostic significance. Mayo Clin Proc 1974; 49:110.

897. Sills RH, Hadley RAR: The significance of nucleated red blood cells in the peripheral blood of children. Am J Pediatr Hematol Oncol 1983; 5:173.

898. Albers-Schönberg H: Roentgenbilder einer seltenen Knochenerkrankung. Munch Med Wochenschr 1904; 51:365.

899. Shapiro F: Osteopetrosis. Current clinical considerations. Clin Orthop Rel Res 1993; 294:34.

900. Gerritsen EJA, Vossen JM, et al: Autosomal recessive osteopetrosis: Variability of findings at diagnosis and during the natural course. Pediatrics 1994; 93:247.

901. Bollerslev J, Mosekilde L: Autosomal dominant osteopetrosis. Clin Orthop Rel Res 1993; 294:45.

902. Sly WS, Hewett-Emmett D, et al: Carbonic anhydrase II deficiency identified as the primary defect in the autosomal recessive syndrome of osteopetrosis with renal tubular acidosis and cerebral calcification. Proc Natl Acad Sci U S A 1983; 80:2752.

903. Walker DG: Spleen cells transmit osteopetrosis in mice. Science 1975; 190:785.

904. Marshall MJ, Nisbet NW, et al: Tissue repopulation during cure of osteopetrotic (mi/mi) mice using normal and defective (W^e/W^v) bone marrow. Exp Hematol 1982; 10:600.

905. Scheven BAA, Visser JWM, Nijweide PJ: *In vitro* osteoclast generation from different bone marrow fractions, including a highly enriched haematopoietic stem cell population. Nature 1986; 321:79.

906. Moe PJ, Skjaeveland A: Therapeutic studies in osteopetrosis. Report of 4 cases. Acta Paediatr Scand 1969; 58:593.

907. Reeves J, Huffer W, et al: The hematopoietic effects of prednisone therapy in four infants with osteopetrosis. J Pediatr 1979; 94:210.

908. Key L, Carnes D, et al: Treatment of congenital osteopetrosis with high-dose calcitriol. N Engl J Med 1984; 310:409.

909. van Lie Peters EM, Aronson DC, et al: Failure of calcitriol treatment in a patient with malignant osteopetrosis. Eur J Pediatr 1993; 152:818.

910. Key LL, Rodriguiz RM, et al: Long-term treatment of osteopetrosis with recombinant human interferon gamma. N Engl J Med 1995; 332:1594.

911. Meletis J, Samarkos M, et al: Correction of anaemia and thrombocytopenia in a case of adult type I osteopetrosis with recombinant human erythropoietin (rHuEPO). Br J Haematol 1995; 89:911.

912. Gerritsen EJA, Vossen JM, et al: Bone marrow transplantation for autosomal recessive osteopetrosis: A report from the working part on inborn errors of the European Bone Marrow Transplantation Group. J Pediatr 1994; 125:896.

913. Jenkinson EL, Pfisterer WH, et al: A prenatal diagnosis of osteopetrosis. Am J Roentgenol 1943; 49:455.

914. Golbus MS, Koerper MA, Hall BD: Failure to diagnose osteopetrosis *in utero*. Lancet 1976; 2:1246.

915. Khazen NE, Faverly D, et al: Lethal osteopetrosis with multiple fractures *in utero*. Am J Med Genet 1986; 23:811.

916. Pierre RV: Preleukemic states. Semin Hematol 1974; 11:73.

917. German J: Bloom Syndrome: A Mendelian prototype of somatic mutational disease. Medicine 1993; 72:393.

918. Freeman AI, Edwards JA, et al: Morphologic studies in a recently described dyserythropoietic state. Blood 1972; 40:473.

919. Weksberg R, Smith C, et al: Bloom syndrome: A single complementation group defines patients of diverse ethnic origin. Am J Hum Genet 1988; 42:816.

920. German J, Roe AM, et al: Bloom syndrome: An analysis of consanguineous families assigns the locus mutated to chromosome band 15q26.1. Proc Natl Acad Sci U S A 1994; 91:6669.

921. Howell RT, Davies T: Diagnosis of Bloom's syndrome by sister chromatid exchange evaluation in chorionic villus cultures. Prenat Diagn 1994; 14:1071.

922. Gatti RA: Ataxia-telangiectasia. Dermatol Clin 1995; 13:1.

923. Gatti RA, Berkel I, et al: Localization of an ataxia-telangiectasia gene to chromosome 11q22–23. Nature 1988; 336:577.

924. Savitsky K, Bar-Shira A, et al: A single ataxia telangiectasia gene with a product similar to P1–3 kinase. Science 1995; 268:1749.

925. Morrell D, Cromartie E, Swift M: Mortality and cancer incidence in 263 patients with ataxia-telangiectasia. J Natl Cancer Inst 1986; 77:89.

926. Hecht F, Hecht BK: Cancer in ataxia-telangiectasia patients. Cancer Genet Cytogenet 1990; 46:9.

927. David TJ: Nature and etiology of the Poland anomaly. N Engl J Med 1972; 287:487.

928. McGillivray BC, Lowry RB: Poland syndrome in British Columbia: Incidence and reproductive experience of affected persons. Am J Med Genet 1977; 1:65.

929. Gilman PA, Miller RW: No link between Poland syndrome and leukemia? Am J Dis Child 1982; 136:176.

930. Choudhry VP, Adhikari RK, Saraya AK: Aplastic anemia—An early phase preceding acute lymphatic leukemia. Indian J Pediatr 1982; 49:343.

931. Reid MM, Summerfield GP: Distinction between aleukaemic prodrome of childhood acute lymphoblastic leukaemia and aplastic anaemia. J Clin Pathol 1992; 45:697.

932. Armata J, Grzeskowiak-Melanowska J, et al: Prognosis in acute lymphoblastic leukemia (ALL) in children preceded by an aplastic phase. Leuk Lymphoma 1994; 13: 517.

933. Hasle H, Heim S, et al: Transient pancytopenia preceding acute lymphoblastic leukemia (pre-ALL). Leukemia 1995; 9:605.

934. Shackelford GD, Bloomberg G, McAlister WH: The value of roentgenography in differentiating aplastic anemia from leukemia masquerading as aplastic anemia. Am J Roentgenol Radiol Ther 1972; 116:651.

935. Liang R, Cheng G, et al: Childhood acute lymphoblastic leukaemia presenting with relapsing hypoplastic anaemia: progression of the same abnormal clone. Br J Haematol 1993; 83:340.

936. Dameshek W: Riddle: What do aplastic anemia, paroxysmal nocturnal hemoglobinuria (PNH) and "hypoplastic" leukemia have in common? Blood 1967; 30:251.

937. Klingemann H, Storb R, et al: Acute lymphoblastic leukaemia after bone marrow transplantation for aplastic anaemia. Br J Haematol 1986; 63:47.

938. Wegelius R: Bone marrow dysfunctions preceding acute leukemia in children: a clinical study. Leuk Res 1992; 16:71.

939. Tuncer MA, Pagliuca A, et al: Primary myelodysplastic syndrome in children: the clinical experience in 33 cases. Br J Haematol 1992; 82:347.

940. Castro-Malaspina H, Schaison G, et al: Subacute and chronic myelomonocytic leukemia in children (juvenile CML). Clinical and hematologic observations, and identification of prognostic factors. Cancer 1984; 54:675.

941. Hasle H: Myelodysplastic syndromes in childhood—classifi-

cation, epidemiology, and treatment. Leuk Lymphoma 1994; 13:11.

942. Gadner H: Experience in pediatric myelodysplastic syndromes. Hematol Oncol Clin North Am 1992; 6:655.

943. Bennett JM, Catovsky D, et al: Proposals for the classification of the myelodysplastic syndromes. Br J Haematol 1982; 51:189.

944. Blank J, Lange B: Preleukemia in children. J Pediatr 1981; 98:565.

945. Niebrugge DJ: Preleukemia in children. J Pediatr 1982; 100:507.

946. Hirose M, Kawahito M, Kuroda Y: Myelodysplastic syndrome in two young brothers. Br J Haematol 1995; 89:211.

947. Sheffer R, Cividalli G, et al: Disturbed patterns of globin chain synthesis in childhood monosomy 7 myeloproliferative syndrome. Br J Haematol 1988; 68:357.

948. Paul B, Reid MM, et al: Familial myelodysplasia: progressive disease associated with emergence of monosomy 7. Br J Haematol 1987; 65:321.

949. Svarch E, de la Torres E: Myelomonocytic leukaemia with a preleukaemic syndrome and Ph1 chromosome in monozygotic twins. Arch Dis Child 1977; 52:72.

950. Rochant H, Dreyfus B, et al: Refractory anemias, preleukemic conditions, and fetal erythropoiesis. Blood 1972; 39:721.

951. Valentine WN, Konrad PN, Paglia DE: Dyserythropoiesis, refractory anemia, and "preleukemia": Metabolic features of the erythrocytes. Blood 1973; 41:857.

952. Raskind WH, Tirumali N, et al: Evidence for a multistep pathogenesis of a myelodysplastic syndrome. Blood 1984; 63:1318.

953. Hogge DE, Shannon KM, et al: Juvenile monosomy 7 syndrome: Evidence that the disease originates in a pluripotent hemopoietic stem cell. Leuk Res 1987; 11:705.

954. Gerritsen W, Donohue J, et al: Clonal analysis of myelodysplastic syndrome: Monosomy 7 is expressed in the myeloid lineage, but not in the lymphoid lineage as detected by fluorescent in situ hybridization. Blood 1992; 80:217.

955. Koeffler HP, Golde D: Human preleukemia. Ann Intern Med 1980; 93:347.

956. Chui DHK, Clarke BJ: Abnormal erythroid progenitor cells in human preleukemia. Blood 1982; 60:362.

957. Hasle H, Kerndrup G, et al: Chronic parvovirus infection mimicking myelodysplastic syndrome in a child with subclinical immunodeficiency. Am J Pediatr Hematol Oncol 1994; 16:329.

958. Benaim E, Hvizdala EV, et al: Spontaneous remission in monosomy 7 myelodysplastic syndrome. Br J Haematol 1995; 89:947.

959. Horsman DE, Massing BG, et al: Unbalanced translocation (1;7) in childhood myelodysplasia. Am J Hematol 1988; 27:174.

960. Anonymous: Case records of the Massachusetts General Hospital. Weekly clinicopathological exercises. Case 16-1987. A 14-year-old boy with fluctuating pancytopenia and a nasopharyngeal mass. N Engl J Med 1987; 316:1008.

961. Creutzig U, Cantu-Rajnoldi A, et al: Myelodysplastic syndromes in childhood. Am J Pediatr Hematol Oncol 1987; 9:324.

962. Appelbaum FR, Storb R, et al: Treatment of preleukemic syndromes with marrow transplantation. Blood 1987; 69:92.

963. Guinan EC, Tarbell NJ, et al: Bone marrow transplantation for children with myelodysplastic syndromes. Blood 1989; 73:619.

964. Vadhan-Raj S, Keating M, et al: Effects of recombinant human granulocyte-macrophage colony-stimulating factor in patients with myelodysplastic syndromes. N Engl J Med 1987; 317:1545.

965. Negrin RS, Haeuber DH, et al: Treatment of myelodysplastic syndromes with recombinant human granulocyte colony-stimulating factor. Ann Intern Med 1989; 110:976.

966. Jansen J, Zwaan FE, et al: Anti-thymocyte globulin treatment for aplastic anemia. Scand J Haematol 1982; 28:341.

967. Rothmann SA, Streeter RR, et al: Treatment of severe aplastic anemia with antithymocyte globulin. Exp Hematol 1982; 10:809.

968. Camitta B, O'Reilly RJ, et al: Antithoracic duct lymphocyte globulin therapy of severe aplastic anemia. Blood 1983; 62:883.

969. Miller WJ, Branda RF, et al: Antithymocyte globulin treatment of severe aplastic anaemia. Br J Haematol 1983; 55:17.

970. Doney K, Storb R, et al: Treatment of aplastic anemia with antithymocyte globulin, high-dose corticosteroids, and androgens. Exp Hematol 1987; 15:239.

971. Marsh JCW, Hows JM, et al: Survival after antilymphocyte globulin therapy for aplastic anemia depends on disease severity. Blood 1987; 70:1046.

972. Means RT Jr, Krantz SB, et al: Re-treatment of aplastic anaemia with antithymocyte globulin or antilymphocyte serum. Am J Med 1988; 84:678.

973. Delgado-Lamas JL, Lopez-Karpovitch X, et al: Low doses of high-potency antithymocyte globulin (ATG) in severe aplastic anemia: Experience with the Mexican ATG. Acta Haematol 1989; 81:70.

974. Digweed M, Zakrzewski-Ludcke S, Sperling K: Complementation studies in Fanconi anemia using cell fusion and microinjection of mRNA. In Schroeder-Kurth TM, Auerbach AD, Obe G (eds): Fanconi Anemia: Clinical, Cytogenetic and Experimental Aspects. Berlin, Springer-Verlag, 1989, p 236.

975. Duckworth-Rysiecki G, Cornish K, et al: Identification of two complementation groups in Fanconi anemia. Somat Cell Mol Genet 1985; 11:35.

976. Moustacchi E, Papadopoulo D, et al: Two complementation groups of Fanconi's anemia differ in their phenotypic response to a DNA-crosslinking treatment. Hum Genet 1987; 75:45.

977. Gruenert DC, Cleaver JE: Repair of psoralen-induced crosslinks and monoadducts in normal and repair-deficient human fibroblasts. Cancer Res 1985; 45:5399.

978. Kaye J, Smith CA, Hanawalt PC: DNA repair in human cells containing photoadducts of 8-methoxypsoralen or angelicin. Cancer Res 1980; 40:696.

979. Matsumoto A, Vos J-M, Hanawalt PC: Repair analysis of mitomycin C–induced DNA crosslinking in ribosomal RNA genes in lymphoblastoid cells from Fanconi's anemia patients. Mutat Res 1989; 217:1985.

980. Moustacchi E, Averbeck D, et al: Phenotypic and genetic heterogeneity in Fanconi anemia, fate of cross-links, and correction of the defect by DNA transfection. In Schroeder-Kurth TM, Auerbach AD, Obe G (eds): Fanconi Anemia: Clinical, Cytogenetic and Experimental Aspects. Berlin, Springer-Verlag, 1989, p 196.

981. Papadopoulo D, Averbeck D, Moustacchi E: The fate of 8-methoxypsoralen-photoinduced DNA intrastrand crosslinks in Fanconi's anemia cells of defined genetic complementation groups. Mutat Res 1987; 184:271.

982. Lambert MW, Tsongalis GJ, et al: Defective DNA endonuclease activities in Fanconi's anemia cells, complementation groups A and B. Mutat Res 1992; 273:57.

983. Averbeck D, Papadopoulo D, Moustacchi E: Repair of 4,5'-trimethylpsoralen plus light-induced DNA damage in normal and Fanconi's anemia cell lines. Cancer Res 1988; 48:2015.

984. Coquerelle TM, Weibezahn KF: Rejoining of DNA double-strand breaks in human fibroblasts and its impairment in one ataxia telangiectasia and two Fanconi strains. J Supramol Struct Cell Biochem 1981; 17:369.

985. Hirsch-Kauffmann M, Schweiger M, et al: Deficiency of DNA ligase activity in Fanconi's anemia. Hum Genet 1978; 45:25.

986. Klocker H, Auer B, et al: DNA repair dependent NAD+ metabolism is impaired in cells from patients with Fanconi's anemia. EMBO J 1983; 2:303.

987. Schweiger M, Auer B, et al: The Fritz-Lipmann Lecture. DNA repair in human cells. Biochemistry of the hereditary diseases Fanconi's anaemia and Cockayne syndrome. Eur J Biochem 1987; 165:235.

988. Scovassi AI, Stefanini M, et al: The basal and the mutagen-induced levels of ADP-ribosyl transferase activity are not modified in Fanconi's anemia cells. Mutat Res 1989; 225:65.

989. Klocker H, Burtscher HJ, et al: Fibroblasts from patients with Fanconi's anemia are not deficient in excision of thymine dimer. Eur J Cell Biol 1985; 37:240.

Principles of Bone Marrow and Stem Cell Transplantation

Eva C. Guinan • Barbara E. Bierer

Bone marrow and stem cell transplantation has become the accepted therapeutic modality for a wide variety of diseases, including hematologic malignancies, aplastic anemia, immunodeficiency disorders, other congenital hematologic defects, and a number of solid tumors. Preparation for stem cell transplantation (SCT) involves delivery of lethal chemotherapy or radiation therapy or both that ablates normal (and abnormal) hematopoiesis, creates "space" in the microenvironment to allow the donor marrow to proliferate, and provides sufficient immunosuppression to allow engraftment. Such intensive preparation renders the host immunocompromised and at risk for a wide variety of bacterial, viral, and fungal infections for a protracted period of time. Other complications, including graft

rejection, graft-verus-host disease (GVHD), and the risk of relapse of initial disease, limit the wide applicability of bone marrow transplantation (BMT). However, important advances in the mechanistic understanding of BMT coupled with advances in the supportive care and clinical management of SCT recipients render this approach an important therapy for a number of patients for whom no other therapeutic alternative is available.

The first report detailing infusion of bone marrow in an effort to initiate hematopoiesis was in 1939: a patient with aplastic anemia was treated by regular transfusions as well as the infusion of a small aliquot of bone marrow from his brother.[1] Subsequently, Jacobson and colleagues demonstrated that lethally irradiated mice could recover normal murine hematopoiesis by shielding the spleen from radiation.[2, 3] Later, it became clear that the protective effect was conferred by hematopoietic elements in the bone marrow or spleen that could reconstitute hematopoiesis in an irradiated recipient.[4] The stem cells in the marrow could be cryopreserved in glycerol and could be shown to reconstitute hematopoiesis when thawed.[5] The animal did well if histocompatible stem cells were infused but suffered from GVHD, then termed *secondary disease,* if given cells from a histoincompatible or allogeneic donor.[6] Furthermore, genetic factors influenced the severity of GVHD.[7] The administration of methotrexate was effective prophylaxis against or treatment of GVHD.[8] These findings, coupled with an increased understanding of the biology of the immune response, paved the way for human marrow transplant studies.

HISTORY AND OVERVIEW

The first attempt at human BMT was carried out in 1957 by E. Donnall Thomas, for which he was awarded a Nobel Prize. These first experiments demonstrated that chemotherapy followed by intravenous marrow infusion could result in a transient graft, although all the patients died of progressive disease.[9] In 1959, lethal doses of total-body irradiation (TBI) and bone marrow from an identical twin were used to transplant two patients with advanced acute lymphoblastic leukemia.[10] Hematopoiesis was established within weeks, although the patients died of progressive disease later. The first successful allogeneic transplants were performed in 1968 and 1969; three patients with different congenital immunodeficiencies underwent transplantation and survived.[11–15]

Bone marrow and SCT are currently applied to a number of malignant and nonmalignant disorders in which replacement of bone marrow–derived populations of cells is necessary or may be beneficial. A number of sources of pluripotent hematopoietic stem cells exist, and the choice of stem cells depends in large part on the indications for transplantation. Although bone marrow was initially considered the only source of pluripotent hematopoietic stem cells, more recently it has become clear that peripheral blood stem cells (PBSC) contain self-renewing stem cells as well. The proportion of stem cells in the peripheral blood increases after chemotherapy or administration of growth factors (e.g., granulocyte colony-forming factor [G-CSF] or granulocyte-macrophage colony-stimulating factor [GM-CSF]) or both, termed *mobilized PBSC.* Because G-CSF can be administered to normal donors, both autologous and allogeneic PBSC transplants can now be performed. More recently, umbilical cord blood (UCB) cells have been used as a source of stem cells, as reviewed later.

Autologous BMT involves reinfusion of a patient's own hematopoietic stem cells after administration of high-dose chemotherapy, radiation therapy, or both. Clearly, however, the harvested cells must be free of contaminating tumor. Although techniques for "purging" tumor cells and for "positively selecting" stem cells away from tumor cells are improving, the requirement that the graft be free of tumor limits the applicability of autologous transplantation. In addition, failure of autologous immunologic response against any residual or recurrent tumor may limit success. Allogeneic SCT involves the infusion of marrow cells from a related or unrelated donor (UD) to a recipient; in the event that the patient and donor are identical twins, the transplant is termed *syngeneic.* Complications of the transplant, such as graft rejection and GVHD, increase, however, with increasing human leukocyte antigen (HLA) disparity between donor and host; and a genotypically HLA-identical sibling, if available, is generally the preferred donor.[16, 17] However, because of current socioeconomic and other norms leading to limitation of nuclear family size, it is estimated that only 15% to 40% of patients will have an HLA-identical family-related donor.[18, 19] For all other patients, there remain more novel alternatives. The patient may undergo SCT from a family-related donor that is mismatched (haploidentical).[16, 17] Alternatively, the patient may find a donor from a volunteer UD pool.[20–22] In general, the degree of HLA disparity increases the toxicity and complications of the transplant. A registry of stored UCB products has been initiated, rendering unrelated UCB a potential alternative as well.[23–25] Finally, the patient may undergo autologous transplant if the bone marrow or PBSC is spared of tumor infiltration.

The specific conditioning regimen used to prepare the patient is reviewed in detail in the next section. In brief, the preparative regimen must reduce or eliminate tumor burden from the patient, should provide sufficient immunosuppression to permit engraftment, and should create "space" within the hematopoietic microenvironment for the infused cells. These directives must obviously be modified in the case of congenital immunodeficiencies and congenital hematopoietic disorders. After conditioning, the stem cells are infused into the host; the day of stem cell infusion is generally referred to as day 0. Neutrophil engraftment occurs at day 10 to 24 after infusion, with red cell and platelet recovery somewhat more delayed. A number of peritransplant and post-transplant complications contribute not only to long-term survival but also to quality of life after transplant (Table 8–1). There is a risk of early graft rejection and of late graft failure. Early complications of transplantation relate to profound pancytopenia, including thrombocytopenia with bleeding and hemorrhage and neutropenia with infection; toxicity of the regimen, including veno-occlusive disease of the liver (VOD); and the immunologic reaction of the graft against the host tissues (acute GVHD). Chronic GVHD is a late sequela of allogeneic transplantation. Finally, the transplant may not be successful: there is a risk of disease relapse. Each of these factors and complications is considered in detail in this chapter.

The evolution of BMT into a practical and curative therapy has depended on a number of important advances. These include an appreciation of the human histocompatibility system and methods to type the do-

Table 8-1. COMPLICATIONS OF BONE MARROW
TRANSPLANTATION

Short Term
Graft rejection
Infection
Bleeding
Acute graft-versus-host disease
Veno-occlusive disease of the liver
Idiopathic pneumonitis
Side effects of radiation therapy, chemotherapy, and
    immunosuppressive therapy (e.g., radiation nephritis,
    azotemia)

Long Term
Late graft failure
Chronic graft-versus-host disease and its sequelae (e.g.,
    bronchiolitis obliterans)
Pulmonary disorders
Infection
Altered intellectual and growth development in children
Reduced stamina
Endocrine dysfunction
    Hypothyroidism
    Growth retardation (children)
    Pubertal delay; gonadal failure
    Sexual dysfunction (both sexes)
Complications secondary to radiation therapy (e.g.,
    cataracts, radiation nephritis)
Complications secondary to immunosuppressive therapy
    (e.g., aseptic necrosis of bone (hips, ankles,
    shoulders), hemolytic uremic syndrome)
Dental problems
Psychosocial problems
Increased risk of second malignancies

nor and recipient first serologically and, more recently, using molecular probes. The preparative regimen for BMT involving either TBI plus chemotherapy or combination chemotherapy alone had to be delivered effectively but without fatal toxicity. Thus the ability to deliver uniform TBI by high-energy linear accelerators, with the concomitant control of dose rate, paved the way for many current antileukemic preparative regimens. Meticulous attention to the needs of the patient in the early post-transplant period has promoted developments in supportive care. The early and aggressive use of antibiotics, antifungal agents, and antiviral agents is important during the early neutropenic period and during the period of profound and persistent immunosuppression that follows successful engraftment. Advances in transfusion support of the BMT patient have occurred, including irradiation of the blood product, the availability of leukopheresed platelet products and viral (hepatitis, cytomegalovirus [CMV]) typing of the product. Nutritional needs of the patient are now addressed with parenteral nutrition if necessary. The ability to establish long-term vascular access with indwelling lines has significantly changed the experience and comfort of BMT recipients. At one time BMT was offered only to the rare patient with end-stage disease. Continued research and improvements in the techniques and outcome of BMT, however, have impacted on the indications for which the procedure is recommended.

In addition, interest and evolution of current research in gene transfer may result in alternative cura-tive treatment strategies for stem cell disorders, particularly those characterized by single gene defects, such as thalassemias, sickle cell disease, Gaucher's disease, Fanconi's anemia, and others. To be clinically successful, gene transfer needs to be safe, to result in stable infection of a substantial number of long-term repopulating stem cells, and to result in permanent expression of the transferred gene at a level that is sufficient to eliminate disease symptoms. Although the first demonstrations of gene transfer into murine hematopoietic stem and progenitor cells occurred more than a decade ago, these endpoints have been difficult to achieve in larger animals. Nonetheless, substantial clinical experience has accumulated regarding the retroviral transduction of human cells. Brenner and colleagues marked bone marrow cells with a retrovirus carrying the *Neo*-resistance gene in patients with acute myeloblastic leukemia (AML) or neuroblastoma in first remission to identify the origin of relapse after auto-transplant.[26–30] An additional use of gene marking or insertion has been explored in other auto-transplant settings for hematologic malignancies.[31] In other settings, Wilson and Grossman have used retroviruses to replace the missing gene in patients with a severe form of familial hypercholesterolemia[32] and Culver and colleagues have introduced the *tk* gene into brain tumors to sensitize them to ganciclovir.[33] The early-generation trials have demonstrated only limited efficiency of either viral integration or gene expression. It is too early to determine if there will be long-term complications, such as an appreciable rate of insertional mutagenesis.

The first steps have also been taken in gene therapy for patients with congenital diseases of the hematopoietic stem cells. In efforts from multiple groups, the cells of immunodeficient patients with adenosine deaminase (ADA) deficiency have been transduced with retroviral vectors containing a normal ADA gene.[34–36] This procedure was carried out repetitively over several years with clinical stability/improvement and improvement in laboratory parameters of T-cell function. However, maintenance use of an intravenous source of ADA confounds interpretation of these results and limited detection of virus has been reported. These experiments suggest that current methodologies do not result in sufficient efficiency of gene transfer and that long intervals may be necessary to assess the potential success of a given approach. Thus, despite the potential of gene transfer as a therapeutic modality, actual reduction of this procedure to practice has been extremely difficult and its value as an adjunct or competitor to hematopoietic SCT depends on further development and evaluation.

CONDITIONING REGIMENS

The first attempts at human marrow transplantation carried out by Thomas and colleagues in 1957,[10] and a subsequent experience using UD bone marrow to treat victims of a radiation accident in Belgrade reported by Mathé and associates in 1959,[37] established the basic principle of TBI-based conditioning despite demonstration of only transient donor hematopoiesis. Work initiated by Santos, Owens, and Sensenbrenner in the 1960s delineated the potential role of cyclophosphamide in recipient conditioning.[38] However, preparation of patients with advanced leukemia with cyclophosphamide alone resulted in a universal relapse rate in survivors and relapse was also frequently observed in patients prepared with TBI alone.[38–42] Spurred by inadequate access to costly radiation facilities, the use of busulfan as a alternative ablative agent was developed in the early to mid-1970s.[43]

A variety of conditioning regimens were evaluated over the next decade with little overall success secondary both to leukemic relapse and what was later recognized to be GVHD. However, the desired effects of a conditioning regimen were generally defined to be threefold: (1) hematopoietic ablation of recipient bone marrow to create space or competitive advantage for donor cells, (2) host immunosuppression to prevent graft rejection, and (3) eradication of diseased cells. It became clear that the relative importance of these ends differed between patient populations. For example, attempts to increase antileukemic efficacy in TBI-based regimens by the use of high-dose cytarabine or etoposide in place of or in addition to cyclophosphamide stemmed from persistently significant relapse rates after SCT. In contrast, T-cell depletion and alternative donor SCT protocols defined graft failure/rejection as a prominent limitation, resulting in new chemotherapeutic and radiation schedules designed to increase recipient immunosuppression. Preparative regimens for patients with aplastic anemia and children with severe combined immunodeficiency (SCID) capitalized on, respectively, their relative aplasia and immunosuppression. In addition, as autologous stem cell support for high-dose chemotherapy became increasingly used for a variety of hematopoietic and nonhematopoietic malignancies, many new conditioning regimens were developed emphasizing potential antitumor effects. Although individual studies have demonstrated acceptable or even favorable outcomes related to some of these changes, no consensus as to optimal preparation of the recipient for either autologous or allogeneic SCT has emerged. Some key issues are highlighted in the next sections.

Total-Body Irradiation. Total dose, dose rate, fraction size, interfraction interval, and shielding are among the TBI parameters most manipulated in SCT conditioning. An ideal schedule would maximize malignant cell kill, hematopoietic ablation, and, in the case of allogeneic SCT, immunosuppression while limiting both acute and chronic toxicity. The first Seattle studies were conducted with single-fraction treatment, and, in 1982[44] and 1986,[45] results were also reported of the first randomized trial of single fraction (1000 cGy) versus fractionated (200 cGy daily for 6 days) radiation. The short- and long-term survival advantage rested with the fractionated schedule. TBI toxicity in general increases with total dose but is very dependent on fractionation and dose rate. In general, higher total dose, higher dose rate, and larger fraction size are associated with greater hematopoietic ablative effect (and therefore potentially greater antileukemic efficacy) and with

better immunosuppression. Studies from Seattle have demonstrated increased antileukemic efficacy with increased total dose, but lung, liver, and kidney tolerances were limiting.[46, 47] Fractionation yields the theoretical advantage of improved tissue tolerance, leading to decreased acute toxicity and reduced late effects, but carries the risk of decreased antileukemic efficacy. Just as the relative requirements for immunosuppression and ablation differ between types of SCT (e.g., immunosuppression is inconsequential in auto-transplant), toxicity considerations vary considerably depending on the condition and age of the recipient. It may be that alternative TBI approaches should be used for children, but the relative merits of divergent approaches are incompletely explored. For example, fractionated TBI preceding cyclophosphamide, etoposide, or cytarabine has been successfully used in children but no direct comparison with drug-first regimens has been conducted.[48–50] Overall, the issues of total dose, fractionation, dose rate, and schedule are far from resolved.

Busulfan. Developed in the mid-1970s, busulfan/cyclophosphamide (BU/CY) rapidly became an established regimen for patients with AML for either allogeneic[51] or autologous SCT.[52–54] The original regimen, BU/CY4 (big BU/CY, BU 4 mg/kg per day for 4 days followed by CY 50 mg/kg per day for 4 days) was joined by BU/CY2 (little BU/CY, in which the CY was delivered as 60 mg/kg per day for 2 days),[52–56] and utilization has expanded to include patients with acute lymphoblastic leukemia (ALL) and chronic myelogenous leukemia (CML). The BU/CY regimen has been used extensively in pediatric patients in an effort to avoid radiation-mediated toxicity. In particular, pediatric patients with storage disorders and with immunodeficiency disorders such as Wiskott-Aldrich syndrome and familial erythrophagocytic lymphohistiocytosis as well as patients with thalassemia have been conditioned with this regimen.[57–61]

Total-Body Irradiation Versus Busulfan. Several randomized studies have compared BU/CY and TBI-based regimens.[62–66] Overall results are similar although suggestive that both relapse rates and regimen-related toxicity, particularly VOD of the liver, may be decreased in the TBI-containing regimens. However, variability of the chemotherapy component of TBI-based regimens and potential differences in the antileukemic efficacy of BU/CY4 and BU/CY2 regimens[67] render definitive generalizations from these reports difficult. Furthermore, reports in which decreased bioavailability, increased volume of distribution, and increased clearance rate of busulfan in children have been suggested as mechanisms of treatment failure raise the question of how to interpret studies in which such data are unavailable.[68–71] Alternative busulfan dosing, based on plasma levels, has been suggested,[72] and comparison of "optimal" BU/CY with CY/TBI has not been reported. However, because busulfan-containing regimens have often been reported to result in increased toxicity in comparison with TBI-based regimens, increases in busulfan dose may further increase regimen-related morbidity.[64, 73, 74] Monitoring of busulfan pharmacokinetics has suggested that increased area under the curve may be associated with increased VOD.[75] Individualizing busulfan dosing may therefore increase the risk/benefit ratio. The relative differences in late toxicity in pediatric patients receiving either TBI or busulfan are not completely understood. This literature is reviewed in the section on late complications (see later).

Alternative Regimens. The addition or substitution of a variety of chemotherapeutic agents to the backbone of CY/TBI, and less commonly BU/CY, has met with mixed success. Etoposide, cytarabine, and busulfan have been added to or substituted for cyclophosphamide in TBI-based regimens in multiple trials.[50, 76–83] Etoposide has also replaced cyclophosphamide in busulfan-based protocols.[84, 85] Autologous transplant programs, free from the constraints of achieving immunosuppression, have also developed a multitude of conditioning regimens, of which the most common are referred to by the acronyms CBV (cyclophosphamide, carmustine [BCNU], etoposide [VP-16]); BACT (carmustine [BCNU], cytarabine [Ara-C], cyclophosphamide, 6-thioguanine); BEAM (carmustine [BCNU], etoposide [VP-16], cytarabine [Ara-C], melphalan); and CBP (cyclophosphamide, carmustine [BCNU], cisplatin). In addition, fluorouracil, high-dose methotrexate, doxorubicin, cisplatin, carboplatin, thiotepa, melphalan, and many other agents have been used in a variety of high-dose chemotherapeutic regimens supported by autologous stem cell infusion. In the allogeneic setting, alternative regimens have often shown equivalent benefit in terms of disease control to "conventional" regimens. Some show an increase in toxicity, but no regimen has established unequivocal superiority in terms of disease-free or overall survival. Given the more limited follow-up and the extraordinary diversity of diseases and regimens in use, establishment of relative efficacy in the realm of autologous SCT is likely to be a prolonged process.[86–88]

SOURCES OF STEM CELLS

Selection of an appropriate source of stem cells for the patient undergoing SCT has become a more complex undertaking in recent years. For each disease entity, the clinician must consider what sources of stem cells are available and what are the relative risks and benefits associated with each potential stem cell source.

Autologous Stem Cell Transplantation

Over the past decade, increasing numbers of cancer patients with either hematologic malignancies or solid tumors have elected to undergo autologous SCT. In fact, the number now ranges in the tens of thousands worldwide. The fundamental hypothesis supporting this therapeutic approach is the belief that tumor cells are responsive to very high doses of cytotoxic agents (dose intensification) and that a high-dose treatment regimen can be devised in which the major dose-limiting toxicity resides in marrow aplasia. This toxicity can be ameliorated by autologous stem cells obtained either by bone marrow harvest or by apheresis of peripheral blood to collect PBSC. Utilization of autologous cells to support and reconstitute the host after aggressive ablative or near-ablative therapy is best explored in both Hodgkin's and non-Hodgkin's lymphomas, less well developed in acute and chronic leukemias, and still considered experimental, albeit relatively widely applied, for a growing number of pediatric and adult solid tumors. As well, the relative merits and demerits of each autologous cell source are still not firmly established.

Method of Collection. Bone marrow is harvested under general or regional anesthesia in an operating room. Most often, the entire volume can be aspirated from the posterior iliac crests but aspiration of the anterior iliac crests and even sternum may be required to obtain an adequate cell concentration. Prior radiation to the pelvis or severe myelofibrosis may significantly limit the yield of marrow cells. Multiple aspirations are performed, usually through a limited number of skin holes (two to three per side), under general or spinal anesthesia, to a total volume of 10 to 15 mL/kg recipient body weight. The marrow is filtered through a fine wire mesh to rid the product of aggregates and bony spicules. Bone marrow harvest is a very safe and well-tolerated procedure with an extremely low probability of complications reported,[89] although the heavily pretreated autologous donor may have increased potential operative morbidity secondary to end-organ compromise and may also be more difficult to harvest owing to either underlying disease or prior therapy. PBSC are collected by leukapheresis; and in the pediatric patient, special attention must be paid to volume and access issues.[90] Leukapheresis in children often requires the placement of a specialized pheresis catheter. Thus, the patient still requires an operative procedure, which in pediatrics in almost always performed with the use of general anesthesia. Although PBSC can be collected from individuals without prior intervention, the yield is low and many hours of collection over many days are required. Optimization of yield is achieved by collection after cytoreduction, most frequently high-dose cyclophosphamide, or use of the hematopoietic growth factors G-CSF or GM-CSF. The best schedules of both priming and collection are not yet established for children or adults. However, successful engraftment using a single apheresis product has been reported.[91] In the future, UCB cells collected and cryopreserved at the time of delivery may provide a source of autologous stem cells for both hematopoietic reconstitution and, potentially, gene therapy.

Contamination by Tumor Cells. A major limitation of autologous SCT remains contamination of the stem cell product with residual malignant cells. Although the relative contributions of either residual tumor within the host or tumor reinfused with stem cells to subsequent relapse remain unknown, increasing evidence from gene-marking studies suggests that reinfused cells contribute to relapse. In addition, *in vitro* assays of tumor cell colony formation and minimal residual disease detection by polymerase chain reaction suggest that contamination of the stem cell source by tumor cells is associated with an increased relapse rate after SCT. No randomized clinical trial of PBSC versus bone marrow with respect to disease-free survival (DFS) has been reported. However, paired samples of PBSC and bone marrow have been examined in a variety of settings (e.g., breast cancer, non-Hodgkin's lymphoma) in which PBSC have revealed lower levels of tumor cell contamination.[92, 93] PBSC may still have significant numbers of tumor cells present.[92] PBSC contamination with neuroblastoma may exceed that of bone marrow.[94] Priming with growth factors does not appear to increase the circulating tumor cell concentration.[95]

A variety of methodologies have been developed to eliminate, or purge, tumor cells from stem cell collections. These are based on either positive or negative selection. The major clinically applied positive selection strategy is that of stem cell enrichment, most often selection of CD34+ cells. Negative selection is based on technologies that deplete tumor cells to a greater degree than normal stem cells. Strategies include the use of pharmacologic agents (e.g., mafosfamide), immunologic reagents targeting tissue specific antigens (e.g., neural crest antigens in neuroblastoma), and manipulation of physical or culture properties of cells. Combinations of both negative and positive selection strategies may improve both the yield and purity of stem cell collections. Increasing evidence in multiple clinical settings demonstrates an association between minimal residual tumor contamination and relapse and, conversely, suggests that more effective purging strategies may be associated with improved DFS. However, randomized studies comparing purged and unpurged stem cells have yet to be reported.

Engraftment. Trilineage hematologic reconstitution has been achieved after the infusion of autologous bone marrow, bone marrow and PBSC, and PBSC alone. The most mature studies are of patients reconstituting hematopoiesis with autologous marrow. Engraftment after bone marrow infusion is both reliable and durable, whereas durability of PBSC-reconstituted hematopoiesis, undertaken more recently, is less fully evaluated. The best predictor of engraftment and rate of hematologic recovery has not been established. Although CD34 number, colony-forming unit–granulocyte-macrophage (CFU-GM), CFU-GEMM (CFU–granulocyte-erythroid-monocyte-macrophage), burst forming units–erythroid (BFU-E), nucleated cell count, and other measures have correlated with time to engraftment in some studies, correlations have not been universal and may additionally depend on the patient population, method of cell procurement, and subsequent cell manipulation.[96]

Reconstitution of hematopoiesis after autologous bone marrow infusion has shown some tendency to be delayed when compared with the allogeneic setting. This delay is presumed due to the extent, nature, and duration of prior therapy. In addition, cell manipulation *ex vivo* (purging) may also contribute to delayed engraftment. Reconstitution after SCT with autologous bone marrow can be hastened somewhat by the addition of hematopoietic growth factors to the post-SCT supportive care regimen, although the extent and nature of prior therapy may limit response to growth factors. Preliminary information in both the preclinical and clinical arenas suggests that prior aggressive chemotherapy may limit potential for hematologic recovery.[97–99] Prior intensive chemotherapy supported by use of growth factors may also contribute to poor engraftment after autologous transplantation.[100] In fact, despite recovery of peripheral blood counts, hematologic marrow reserves as assessed by *in vitro* measures of hematopoiesis may be blunted for many years after autologous SCT.[101]

Addition of mobilized PBSC to bone marrow has resulted in a dramatic decrease in days of neutropenia and thrombocytopenia in most series with or without subsequent growth factor support. Further, use of mobilized PBSC as the sole stem cell source has been almost universally associated with more rapid hematologic recovery, particularly of the peripheral platelet count. It is still debatable whether the use of hematopoietic growth factors in this setting further enhances the rate of engraftment, but available data suggest that it may. Whether the process of PBSC transplantation will result in durable hematopoiesis over decades is not yet evaluable, but graft failure has not been reported as a frequent complication. Most studies suggest that the increased rate of engraftment observed with PBSC results in decreased days in hospital, use of antibiotics, and associated supportive services. The overall impact of PBSC versus bone marrow as a stem cell source on the efficacy, toxicity, and cost of transplantation has yet to be determined.

Myelodysplasia as a Late Complication. It has long been appreciated that intensive chemotherapy, particularly with alkylating agents, may result in an increased risk of subsequent myelodysplasia (MDS). Many patients who come to autologous transplantation have received treatment with such agents. Over the past several years, increasing numbers of patients developing MDS after autologous transplantation have been reported.[102–104] In some series of autologous SCT for non-Hodgkin's lymphoma, the actuarial incidence is predicted to be as high as 5% to 10%. Strikingly, most of the cases are in patients who have received TBI-based conditioning. Whether the MDS results from previously damaged reinfused hematopoietic cells or from residual hematopoietic cells sustaining further injury during conditioning is unresolved.[105] Resolution of this issue will have a major impact on the future conduct of autologous transplantation programs.

Allogeneic Stem Cell Transplantation

Since the first allogeneic transplants executed in 1957, tens of thousands of patients have undergone SCT from an allogeneic donor. The stem cell source has overwhelmingly been from a matched sibling donor. However, with improvements in immunosuppression and ability to prevent or treat GVHD, alternative increasing disparate allogeneic stem cell sources have been utilized. These include mismatched family members, so called haploidentical SCT, as well as UD SCT.

A number of international registries, many able to reference each other's files, facilitate the identification and evaluation of potential UDs. There are almost 2 million donors listed in the National Marrow Donor Program (NMDP) and approximately 3.4 million worldwide. In addition, increasing interest has been focused on the cryopreservation of UCB for autologous, conventional allogeneic, and UD SCT. Registries of banked UD UCB collections are being established and expanded.

The selection of an allogeneic stem cell source is dependent on many variables, including the aggressiveness of the underlying disorder, the accessibility of a donor, and, particularly, the degree of histocompatibility between host and potential donor. Increasing histoincompatibility has historically contributed to both an increased rate of graft rejection and severe acute and chronic GVHD. The best results are reported when fully histocompatible sibling donors are used, but only approximately 25% of patients will have such a donor available. Even in this matched setting, selection can be further refined according to gender, history of donor parity, donor infectious disease status, donor age, and other variables. For the majority of patients who do not have a matched sibling donor, potential sources include a phenotypically matched but genotypically distinct family member, a more disparate family member, or a volunteer UD donor. The likelihood of the first is low while more mismatched family members are available to the vast majority of the population. The likelihood of locating an appropriate UD bone marrow donor is dependent both on the patient's ethnicity (in as much as it determines histocompatibility antigen and haplotype frequency) and on the composition of the donor pool. For example, for whites of mid and northern European descent the likelihood of finding a six-antigen matched UD approaches 50%. In contrast, the extreme genetic heterogeneity of the African-American population coupled with under-representation of this population in volunteer registries makes the likelihood of finding a similar donor approximately 10%. Thus, additional strategies to broaden the donor base by using increasingly disparate donors or alternative stem cell sources, such as PBSC and UCB, which may have different biologic properties, have become more prevalent. The success of these attempts will rest on better definition of the most important major and minor histocompatibility elements and cellular interactions governing allorecognition in the SCT setting as well as further refinement of clinical approaches to these problems.

Typing. The initial identification of antigens involved in allograft rejection or acceptance resulted from experimentation in inbred mouse strains. The genes encoding for the antigens most associated with allograft rejection became known as the major histocompatibility complex (MHC). In humans, the MHC maps to a region of the short arm of chromosome 6, which is known as the HLA system. The MHC codes for many genes, and the identification and exploration of the functional importance of some of these gene products is still ongoing. Among the best characterized gene products are the class I and class II antigens. The

MHC class I antigens are expressed on nearly all human cells (with rare exceptions such as the erythrocyte and corneal endothelium). MHC class II proteins have a much more restricted expression. They are constitutively expressed on "professional" antigen-presenting cells, including dendritic cells, B cells, and monocytic cells, including monocytes, macrophages, and Langerhans cells, and may be induced on a variety of human cells, most notably activated T cells and endothelium. These genes are highly polymorphic, and both MHC class I and II play a central role in the presentation of antigen to T lymphocytes. In the human, MHC class I molecules include HLA-A, B, and C molecules whereas MHC class II are the so called HLA-D molecules. Classically, MHC class I molecules are identified serologically whereas MHC class II antigens are both serologically and cellularly defined (see later). It is generally accepted that antigen-presenting cells present peptide antigens in the groove of the MHC class II molecules to the T-cell receptor complex on CD4+ helper T cells. In contrast, all nucleated cells are capable of presenting peptide antigens in the groove of the MHC class I molecule to the T-cell receptor complex on CD8+ cytotoxic/suppressor T cells. In addition to MHC class I and class II, ever-increasing evidence demonstrates the existence of minor histocompatibility antigens in humans.[106, 107] Although these antigens may not be directly responsible for organ and bone marrow rejection, human typing studies suggest that these minor antigens may be critical in the generation of GVHD.[106, 107]

Historically, HLA typing has been performed by using antibodies derived from postpartum sera, from persons who have undergone transplants or transfusions, or even from persons immunized for the purpose of generating specific serologic reagents. These antibodies have been used in a standardized complement-dependent, microcytotoxicity assay with purified T or B lymphocytes as their target cell.[108] The extensive cross-reactivity among products coded by the alleles of the HLA-A and HLA-B loci, known as cross-reactive groups, makes precise delineation of the MHC class I antigens by this technique difficult. In contrast, HLA-D specificities were originally defined by their ability to stimulate T-lymphocyte proliferation in a mixed leukocyte culture.[109] It has become increasing clear that the HLA-D region is a complex region composed of many loci that in aggregate induce the mixed leukocyte culture reaction.[110] There are at least five subregions, including DR, DQ, and DP, but the number of genes transcribed differs between different HLA class II haplotypes. Serologic reagents have been developed that define 14 HLA-DR loci.

Considering the importance of major and minor histocompatibility antigens in the generation of graft rejection and GVHD as well as subsequent immunocompetence, the development of increasingly sophisticated methods to identify distinct alleles encoding both class I, class II, and, in the future, minor antigens is not surprising. Among the techniques developed is one-dimensional isoelectric focusing gel electrophoresis, which is especially informative for determination of class I alleles.[111] The first attempts to use molecular genetic techniques were based on application of restriction fragment length polymorphism analysis of genomic DNA by Southern blotting using HLA region probes. This rapidly gave way to current technology in which sequence-specific oligonucleotide probes and, in some cases, direct sequence analysis are performed. Generation of appropriate probes and sequence data has resulted in more accurate and detailed description of MHC class I and II alleles. This has already led to a great multiplication in the known HLA specificities. This fine analysis is increasingly being used to determine the haplotypes of individuals. The implications of more exact typing in the family setting, where the haplotypes are "conserved," are probably confined to the potential identification of minor histocompatibility antigen differences, allowing for better selection between possible donors. In the UD setting, it is yet to be established which antigens and what degree of matching are most likely to lead to good outcome, but these tools should enable such an analysis.

Methods of Collection. The physical methodology of bone marrow collection is identical to that described earlier for autologous SCT. If there is ABO incompatibility, the red cells may be removed before infusion.[112, 113] The marrow may be manipulated *ex vivo* to remove donor T lymphocytes (see later) or tumor cells. It is estimated that only 1% of the total pluripotent hematopoietic stem cell population is removed in a typical bone marrow harvest. Risks to the donor are minimized by the fact that the donor is generally a healthy individual undergoing an elective procedure. Potential short- and long-term complications include risks of anesthesia, blood loss and potential transfusion, pain, neurologic deficits, and psychosocial complications. In the most truly altruistic setting, UD bone marrow harvest, only 5% to 8% of donors expressed any ambivalence about their participation. This was most marked if the transplant was subsequently unsuccessful.[114]

Although the overwhelming majority of allogeneic SCT has employed bone marrow as the stem cell source, during the past several years a number of centers have reported early results of allogeneic PBSC transplants.[115] Donor stem cells have generally been mobilized with G-CSF and pheresis performed with peripheral access. Complications have included bone pain, as a side effect of G-CSF, and inability to use the peripheral access, resulting in central line placement.[116, 117] The implications of mobilizing and harvesting PBSC from pediatric donors have not been fully explored.

Since the first description of its use in a child with Fanconi's anemia in 1988,[118] UCB has become an increasingly investigated stem cell source. Placental blood is recovered from the umbilical vein by drainage or catheterization, and techniques to optimize the volume, sterility, and quality of UCB cells are being investigated.[24, 119] If indicated, in the related setting, determination of the HLA type of the fetus can be performed before delivery. Otherwise, typing and analysis is performed on samples from the UCB collection.

Selection of a UD, whether bone marrow or UCB, is facilitated by the availability of epidemiologic information (e.g., age, sex, parity) as well as HLA typing stored in a database that can be accessed rapidly and efficiently through electronic mail. Complementary databases exist on frequently updated CD/ROM. By comparing a potential patient's HLA type with those listed and categorized in the registries, one can estimate the likelihood of a successful search, devise search strategies for patients with relatively unique HLA types, and sort among potential bone marrow versus UCB sources. Although the UCB cell source can be readily supplied after confirmatory typing, the completion of a UD bone marrow donor search is more involved. Potential donors, once identified, must be contacted and give consent to proceed, and the donor center must arrange for appropriate confirmatory laboratory studies and medical and other evaluations and schedule the harvest. The time from formal search to BMT averages 4 to 5 months, although in some cases the time is much shorter.

Engraftment. Donor hematopoietic engraftment after allogeneic SCT can be documented both by analysis of chimerism as well as by the recovery of peripheral blood cell counts. Whereas crude techniques suggested that complete reconstitution with donor cells was the norm, current, more sensitive DNA amplification technologies have demonstrated residual host hematopoiesis for variable periods of time, certainly up to 1 year.[120–122] Mixed lymphoid chimerism is also well documented.[120–123] The implications of mixed chimerism with respect to subsequent relapse remain controversial, probably because the current extremely sensitive assays generate data that are difficult to interpret uniformly, and because outcome may well differ by disease type.[124] For example, chimerism after BMT for CML is quite reliably related to subsequent relapse and this may not be true for other diseases.[123–125]

The rate of engraftment after allogeneic BMT varies somewhat with the GVHD prophylactic regimen used. In general, neutrophil recovery is achieved within 2 to 3 weeks and platelet recovery occurs 1 to 2 weeks thereafter. The use of methotrexate in the prophylactic regimen is associated with delay in count recovery; conversely, recovery after T cell–depleted BMT is more rapid. Use of colony-stimulating factors after BMT is associated with more rapid neutrophil recovery after related BMT, a finding confirmed in small pediatric series.[126–131] No change in platelet recovery has been noted. Interestingly, preliminary data do not show any colony-stimulating factor–mediated acceleration of engraftment in patients undergoing UD BMT.[132]

Less is known about engraftment using alternative allogeneic stem cell sources. With the use of allogeneic PBSC, a multifold increment in CD34+ cell dose can be achieved.[116, 117, 133] Although platelet recovery may be accelerated, the rate of neutrophil engraftment may not be different from that seen with BMT and CSF support.[117] Full chimerism has been documented after allogeneic PBSC transplantation. In the relatively limited experience to date, neutrophil recovery following related UCB transplantation is perhaps slightly delayed in comparison to that expected with other SCT and time to platelet recovery is prolonged.[23] The use of hematopoietic growth factors after UCB transplantation has not been associated with accelerated hematopoietic reconstitution.[23] Follow-up is insufficient to allow evaluation of the durability of UCB grafts.

PERITRANSPLANT SUPPORTIVE CARE

The intensive myeloablative preparative regimen given to ensure tumor eradication and a successful graft leads to an extended period of aplasia that lasts until robust engraftment occurs. After engraftment and despite freedom from neutropenia and platelet and red cell transfusions, the patient remains profoundly immunocompromised for a prolonged period of time after allogeneic SCT. Some immunologic compromise, less well understood, also follows autologous SCT.

Transfusion Support

Virtually all patients require red cell and platelet transfusions during transplant. All blood products should be irradiated to prevent transfusion-induced GVHD from lymphocyte contamination of the blood product.[134–136] In addition, it is recommended that blood products be administered through an in-line filter to remove potentially deleterious lymphocytes and leukocytes that may harbor latent viruses such as CMV.[137] The use of leukocyte-poor blood products has been shown to be essentially equivalent to using CMV-seronegative blood products to prevent CMV infection.[138] In addition, one prospective, randomized trial demonstrated the efficacy of leukocyte-poor blood products over CMV-unscreened, infused blood products,[139] although this remains debatable. It is generally recommended that all SCT recipients receive irradiated, leukocyte-poor blood products regardless of the interval after transplant. Furthermore, patients should wear a Medical Alert bracelet detailing their transfusion requirements in case of emergency.

Whether platelet and red cell transfusions should be given prophylactically during the period of pancytopenia remains an area of controversy. No recommendations can supplant the need for clinical judgment in every situation, and only guidelines are proferred. There is a clear increase in clinical and occult bleeding in patients with platelet counts less than $10 \times 10^9/L$; the risk of bleeding was increased in the setting of fever and decreasing counts in patients with leukemia.[140] Many caregivers use prophylactic platelet transfusions if the platelet count falls below some threshold, often 5 to 20 $\times$ $10^9/L$, if there is clinical evidence of bleeding, or as prophylaxis against bleeding in advance of a minor or major surgical procedure.[141] The desire to prevent untoward bleeding complications is balanced by the risk of platelet alloimmunization, the lack of compatible donors for an allosensitized patient, the finite risk of transfusion-associated infection, and the cost of blood products.

Infection Prophylaxis and Treatment

Susceptibility to infections is a major complication of SCT, and one that resolves only with complete and sustained immune reconstitution of the host. Advances in our understanding of the prevention and treatment of infectious complications of SCT have improved the immediate peritreatment outcome. However, infectious complications are increased in patients with both acute and chronic GVHD and are therefore an important comorbid variable in the outcome of these disorders. The deficits in the host immune response vary with time after transplant, as does susceptibility to infection. A complete review of susceptibility to, prophylaxis against, and treatment of infections associated with SCT and the immunodeficiency that follows SCT is obviously beyond the scope of this chapter, and only principles of management are discussed here.

Early after preparative cytoreductive chemotherapy and continuing for a number of weeks after marrow infusion, patients are severely neutropenic. In addition, the preparative regimen damages the mucosal and epithelial barriers, which normally provide important defenses against microbial invasion. Exposure to potentially infectious individuals or environments is minimized. Meticulous hand washing by all caregivers and visitors is essential. The use of laminar air flow environments with gut decontamination has been shown to increase survival in a series of patients with aplastic anemia.[142, 143] Gut decontamination and either laminar air flow or high-efficiency particulate air (HEPA)-filtered rooms are widely used in the allogeneic setting, but the contributions of each to outcome are unknown.

Early after transplant, neutropenic patients are at risk for viral, bacterial, and fungal infections. Reactivation of herpes simplex virus 1 and 2 infection occurs in approximately 70% of seropositive patients; seropositive patients are, therefore, often given prophylactic acyclovir therapy.[144–146] Gram-positive bacteria are now more common pathogens than gram-negative bacteria (of culture positive isolates) since the introduction of indwelling central venous lines.[147–149] In addition, the risk of gram-negative sepsis has decreased secondary to the prompt initiation of broad-spectrum antibiotics at the first onset of fever. Intravenous γ-globulin replacement appears to decrease gram-negative sepsis after transplant.[150] Because fungal, and particularly candidal, infection is common during neutropenia, many patients receive antifungal prophylaxis, including low-dose amphotericin B[151–153] and, more recently, fluconazole.[154] Enthusiasm for prophylactic antifungal treatment is tempered by the observation that patients may be more likely to suffer from fluconazole-resistant fungal organisms as a consequence of prophylactic therapy.[155]

After engraftment, patients continue to have depressed T-cell function and decreased antibody production and remain at risk for a variety of infections. This risk is particularly prolonged in recipients of allogeneic transplants, who, despite phenotypically normal circulating lymphocytes continue to have depressed cellular immunity for at least 1 year after transplant. The degree of host immunoincompetence depends on a number of factors, including the source of stem cells (allogeneic versus autologous), degree of HLA disparity between the donor and host, whether the bone marrow was depleted of T cells or otherwise manipulated, pharmacologic immunosuppressive therapy after transplant, and, importantly, occurrence and severity of GVHD after transplant. Indwelling central venous catheters and mucosal breakdown secondary to GVHD remain sources of infection. However, viral infection, and particularly CMV infection, presents a major risk to patients. Both seropositive patients and seronegative patients who have received grafts from seropositive donors are at the greatest risk for CMV; these patients and seropositive recipients are often treated prophylactically with regimens to prevent reactivation of CMV, such as ganciclovir with immune globulin. In addition, patients are at risk of varicella-zoster virus reactivation. Fungal infection remains a common source of infection in the immunocompromised individual; recurrent and persistent fever of unknown origin may respond to a prolonged course of antifungal agents for occult infection. This risk is higher in patients with GVHD who remain on corticosteroids and other immunosuppressive therapy. All patients are at risk for the development of *Pneumocystis carinii* after transplant; allogeneic recipients usually receive appropriate prophylaxis (e.g., trimethoprim-sulfamethoxazole, dapsone, pentamidine) for 1 year after transplant, whereas autologous recipients may only receive prophylaxis for 6 months.

The risk of infection decreases with enhanced cellular immunity after transplant. The notable exceptions are patients with chronic GVHD (see later) and patients who remain on chronic immunosuppressive therapy who remain at risk for recurrent bacterial infections, notably with encapsulated organisms; for viral infections, notably varicella-zoster virus; for *P. carinii*; and for fungal infections. They, therefore, should receive appropriate prophylaxis.

Nutrition Support

Provision of nutritional support during SCT requires an appreciation of the metabolic needs of the individual patient that are, in turn, influenced by comorbid complications of transplant. Cytoreductive therapy induces gastrointestinal damage that may progress further with the onset of GVHD. Several studies have demonstrated the efficacy of total parenteral nutrition (TPN) when enteral nutrition is no longer possible.[156, 157] In addition, a prospective randomized trial demonstrated a survival advantage to patients given TPN during SCT compared with control subjects.[157] However, in addition to expense, TPN has attendant potential complications, including vascular access difficulties, abnormal liver function, and episodes of hyperglycemia and hyperlipidemia. Some patients may be able to maintain their nutritional needs orally throughout transplant, and both enteral and TPN routes may be used on occasion. Resumption of enteral feeding should be encouraged, and continued monitoring of nutritional intake is necessary not only after engraftment and through the period of GVHD but also after discharge from the hospital.

EARLY COMPLICATIONS OF STEM CELL TRANSPLANTATION

Graft Rejection

Failure of hematopoietic recovery is a rare event after matched sibling SCT for hematologic malignancy.[16] Although graft failure and graft rejection are not always easy to separate, failure to recover hematopoiesis ("graft failure") appears to increase with increasing genetic disparity, with presence of a positive crossmatch for anti–donor lymphocytotoxic antibody, and with the use of T-cell depletion as GVHD prophylaxis.[16, 17, 158–164] In addition, patients with aplastic anemia, particularly if previously transfused, have a high rate of apparent graft rejection.[165–168] Patients with storage disorders and osteopetrosis (see discussions of specific diseases later in the chapter) may also have an increased failure rate, presumably due in part to disordered microenvironment and perhaps to their immunocompetence. Adjustments to both chemotherapy and radiotherapy components of conditioning regimens, the use of monoclonal antibodies targeting selected effector cell populations, and increases in cell dose (including the use of PBSC in addition to bone marrow) are among the manipulations that have shown some promise in reducing graft failure.[133, 158, 165, 167, 169–173] The increased risk of graft failure after T-cell depletion of the marrow suggests that mature donor T cells facilitate alloengraftment; the immunologic mechanism by which this occurs is not clear. Mature donor T cells may themselves secrete or induce the secretion by bone marrow stromal cells of essential cytokines that promote engraftment. A number of approaches have been explored to overcome graft failure associated with T-cell depletion. First, simply increasing the number of cells in the graft decreases the risk of graft failure.[173] Second, intensification of the conditioning regimen has been successful, implying that residual host hematopoietic elements are involved in mediating graft rejection.[158] However, such intensification is associated with increased transplant-related morbidity and mortality. Third, because the risk of graft failure appears to increase with more exhaustive T-cell depletion, less extensive T-cell removal from the graft has been attempted.[159, 174] Removal of selective T-cell subsets, defined either phenotypically or functionally, is now being explored.

Veno-occlusive Disease of the Liver

The syndrome of VOD of the liver occurs in a variety of clinical settings. In SCT, it follows cytoreductive therapy.[175–179] It has been reported to occur with essentially all preparative regimens and in recipients of both autologous and allogeneic transplants.[175–180] VOD is characterized by liver enlargement and pain, fluid retention and weight gain, and an increase in serum bilirubin level. The signs and symptoms of VOD usually present before day 20 after SCT but may present considerably later. Other explanations for these signs and symptoms should be excluded as fully as possible.

Histologic changes in the liver that accompany the

clinical diagnosis are characteristic.[175, 181, 182] Typically, the hepatic venules are occluded and there is eccentric luminal narrowing of the hepatic venules. With increasing disease severity, sinusoidal fibrosis and hepatocyte necrosis are present. The primary cytopathic event appears to be damage to the sinusoidal endothelium and hepatocytes caused by cytotoxic drugs and their metabolites. Secondary pathophysiologic changes include microthromboses in the hepatic venules and later sinusoidal fibrosis with portal hypertension.

The severity of VOD is best predicted not by pathology, however, but by the severity and day of onset of weight gain and elevation of serum bilirubin level. Treatment options for patients with severe VOD remain limited.[175] Meticulous fluid management must be maintained; whether minimizing fluid retention with the use of diuretics and hemodialysis is of benefit or predisposes to hepatorenal syndrome remains controversial. Thrombolytic therapy using recombinant human tissue plasminogen activator has been tried,[183–187] although not in a randomized trial. Prostaglandin E_1 has been variably reported to be ineffective[188] or effective in a small series of patients[189]; whether these latter patients would have resolved their VOD spontaneously cannot be known. Although liver transplantation may be curative,[190, 191] it is difficult to perform emergently. Surgical approaches to relieve portacaval pressure using a variety of shunts may be lifesaving.[192, 193] Finally, a number of experimental approaches, including the use of defibrotide (a polydeoxyribonucleotide derived from mammalian tissues that acts on vascular endothelium and has antithrombotic, anti-ischemic, and thrombolytic properties),[194] are now being explored. Unfortunately, despite recognition of the clinical syndrome and efforts to prevent and treat the disease, it remains a major source of morbidity and mortality after transplantation. Patients with severe VOD die of multiorgan failure, with renal, cardiac, and respiratory compromise.

Because treatment of VOD is largely supportive, the focus has turned to prevention of its occurrence.[175, 177, 178, 195, 196] Patients with elevated results of liver function tests, a history of hepatitis, or fever immediately before transplant are at an increased risk for VOD.[175, 177, 178, 195, 196] Recognition of patients at highest risk may serve to identify patients in whom alternative approaches should be employed or SCT can be delayed or declined for patients at high risk. The lowest doses of cytoreductive therapy should be used that do not compromise efficacy.[175–178, 195, 196] With a greater understanding of individual variations of chemotherapy pharmacokinetics, individualized treatment programs, doses, and schedules can be devised. Recipients of T cell–depleted marrow appear to have a decreased incidence of VOD,[197] but whether this reflects a true decrease or simply elimination of patients with methotrexate toxicity or hepatic GVHD from the numerator is unclear. A number of alternative prophylactic strategies have been piloted, although few have been studied extensively. Use of the methylxanthine analogue pentoxifylline as prophylaxis against the development of VOD has failed to show efficacy in prospective, randomized trials,[198, 199] although its use was associated with decreased proinflammatory cytokines (i.e., tumor necrosis factor-α) both *in vivo*[200] and *in vitro*.[201] Vasodilator therapy with prostaglandin E_1 has been attempted without clear success.[202] Prevention of microthromboses by prophylactic use of heparin has not been shown to have any effect.[175, 203, 204] The use of low-molecular-weight heparin appears to decrease bleeding incidence and duration and may decrease the incidence and severity of VOD[205]; this treatment awaits prospective, double-blind analysis for confirmation of the promising initial results. A pilot study[206] followed by a prospective, randomized trial[207] reported that patients treated with prophylactic ursodiol therapy had a decreased incidence of VOD than patients receiving placebo. Repleting glutathione stores appears to prevent endothelial damage secondary to metabolism of a number of chemotherapeutic agents; whether glutathione will also protect tumor cells from the cytotoxic effects of these agents is a theoretical but real concern.

Acute Graft-Versus-Host Disease

First reported by Barnes and Loutit in 1954,[6] the syndrome of acute GVHD (then termed *secondary disease* because it followed radiation sickness, which occurred first) was observed in lethally irradiated animals given allogeneic spleen cells. The animals developed skin abnormalities and diarrhea and eventually succumbed to a wasting illness. Criteria for the development of GVHD were presented by Billingham,[208] who asserted that (1) "the graft must contain immunologically competent cells"; (2) "the host must possess important transplantation alloantigens that are lacking in the donor graft, so that the host appears foreign to the graft and is, therefore, capable of stimulating it antigenically" and (3) "the host itself must be incapable of mounting an effective immunological reaction against the graft, at least for sufficient time for the latter to manifest its immunological capabilities; that is, it must have the security of tenure." The observation that GVHD is caused by donor alloreactivity in an immunoincompetent host has now been shown to be due to T lymphocytes contained in the marrow graft that proliferate and differentiate in the host. These T cells then recognize host alloantigens as foreign and, through direct effector mechanisms and by inflammatory mediators released by both T cells and host tissues, mediate tissue damage.[209, 210] Animal studies and later trials in human transplant recipients demonstrated that T-cell depletion from the marrow inocula can abrogate the development of GVHD, albeit at an increased risk of graft rejection and of relapse of initial disease.[211] Donor cells contain T (or other) cells capable of recognizing malignant cells and mediating a graft-versus-leukemia and, perhaps, a graft-versus-tumor effect.[212] Indeed, patients with hematologic malignancies who develop mild to moderate GVHD have a decreased risk of disease relapse.[212–215] Efforts to distinguish the populations of T cells that mediate GVHD from those that mount a graft-versus-leukemia response is a topic of current research.

Table 8–2. GLUCKSBERG CRITERIA FOR STAGING AND GRADING OF ACUTE GRAFT-VERSUS-HOST DISEASE

Organ	Stage	Extent of Organ Involvement
Skin	1	<25%
	2	25–50%
	3	Generalized erythema
	4	Desquamation, bullous
Liver	1	2–3 mg/dL*
	2	3.1–6 mg/dL
	3	6.1–15 mg/dL
	4	>15 mg/dL
Gastrointestinal (children)	1	10–15 mL stool/kg/d
	2	16–20 mL stool/kg/d
	3	21–25 mL stool/kg/d
	4	>25 mL stool/kg/d. Severe pain with or without ileus
Gastrointestinal (adult)	1	500–1000 mL stool/d; nausea, anorexia
	2	1000–1500 mL stool/d; histologic diagnosist of upper gastrointestinal GVHD
	3	1500–2000 mL stool/d
	4	>2000 mL stool/d; ileus, severe pain

Overall Clinical Grade	Organ System	Clinical Stage
I (mild)	Skin	1–2
	Liver	1
	Gastrointestinal	0
II (moderate)	Skin	1–3
	Liver	1–2
	Gastrointestinal	1
III (severe)	Skin	2–4
	Liver	2–4
	Gastrointestinal	2–4
IV (life threatening)‡	Skin	2–4
	Liver	2–4
	Gastrointestinal	2–4

*Modified Glucksberg scale[216] to prevent overlap in categories.
†Data from Weisdorf DJ, Snover DC, et al: Acute upper gastrointestinal graft-versus-host disease: clinical significance and response to immunosuppressive therapy. Blood 1990; 76:624.
‡With severe constitutional symptoms.

The clinical syndrome of acute GVHD develops within 100 (and usually within 60) days of allogeneic SCT. Chronic GVHD is a distinctive clinical syndrome that occurs after day 100 and is discussed later. Acute GVHD classically involves the skin, liver, and gastrointestinal tract, although the severity of involvement of each organ may vary. For that reason, the severity of acute GVHD is graded based on staging the involvement of individual organs and then determining the overall grade of the disease. Table 8–2 presents the modified Glucksberg criteria[216] used most commonly for historical reasons; further modifications have been and are being introduced[42, 217, 218]; and, more recently, a severity index (Table 8–3) developed by the International Bone Marrow Transplant Registry (IBMTR) has been used.[219]

The first manifestation of GVHD is often a rash, presenting as a maculopapular eruption, often initially

Table 8–3. INTERNATIONAL BONE MARROW TRANSPLANT REGISTRY (IBMTR) SEVERITY INDEX FOR ACUTE GRAFT-VERSUS-HOST DISEASE

Severity Index	Maximum Organ Stage	RR Treatment-Related Mortality (95% CI)	RR Treatment Failure (95% CI)	Glucksberg
0	No GVHD	1.00	1.00	
A	Skin 1 only	0.84 (0.6, 1.18)	0.85 (0.68, 1.05)	0
B	Any organ stage 2*	1.90 (1.5, 2.42)	1.21 (1.02–1.43)	I
C	Any organ stage 3	4.34 (3.33, 5.67)	2.19 (1.78, 2.71)	I, II, III, IV
D	Any organ stage 4	11.9 (9.12, 15.5)	5.68 (4.57, 7.08)	II, III, IV
				IV

*Any organ stage 1 other than skin alone (e.g., skin 1, gut 1 = Severity Index B).
CI = confidence interval; RR = relative risk.

involving the palms and soles, back of neck and ears, and later the trunk and extremities. Biopsy specimens from involved areas often demonstrate epidermal basal cell vacuolization, followed by epidermal basal cell apoptotic death with lymphoid infiltration.[220] Characteristic eosinophilic bodies may be seen. With increasing severity, bullous formation with epidermal separation and necrosis is observed.[221] Hepatic GVHD often presents as cholestatic jaundice, which must be differentiated from VOD, infection, and drug toxicity.[222, 223] Although not without attendant risks of bleeding and pain, liver biopsy may be helpful in that characteristic pathologic changes[197, 224] are often observed that aid in the differential diagnosis. Gastrointestinal involvement classically presents as watery, often "seedy" diarrhea and may progress to include crampy abdominal pain, bleeding, and ileus.[222, 223] By convention, stool volume is used to quantitate the severity of gut involvement, and rectal or colonic biopsy may reveal crypt cell necrosis with lymphocytic infiltration, and, with increasing severity, crypt abscess or loss and mucosal denudation.[222, 223, 225] These three organs are staged individually for severity of involvement, after which an overall grade of GVHD is assigned, according to criteria developed by Glucksberg and co-workers (see Table 8–2) or the IBMTR (see Table 8–3). However, other symptoms and findings may suggest acute GVHD. Involvement of the upper gastrointestinal tract is suggested by symptoms of anorexia, inanition, and vomiting.[218] Endoscopy with biopsy is minimally invasive and may reveal crypt cell apoptosis with dropout. The differential diagnosis of upper gastrointestinal GVHD includes viral or fungal infection, dyspepsia, and gastritis, all common conditions in the immunosuppressed SCT recipient. Lastly, fever, thrombocytopenia, anemia, pulmonary involvement, and vascular leak may accompany acute GVHD.

There are several risk factors for the development of acute GVHD. Increasing genetic disparity between the donor and host increases the incidence and severity of GVHD[226–229] and is the most important single predictor of acute GVHD. Increasing age of the recipient increases the risk of acute GVHD.[227, 229, 230] The use of a female donor for a male recipient and female donor history of parity also appear to increase the risk of acute GVHD.[227–229] The source of allogeneic cells may also color the risk for subsequent GVHD. For example, the number of T cells collected during pheresis is significantly greater than during bone marrow harvest. Early reports suggest that the rate of severe acute GVHD in patients receiving such T cell-rich PBSC with standard GVHD prophylaxis may not be greater than that seen after similar BMT.[116, 117, 231] There is some suggestion that the rate of chronic GVHD is increased.[232] Insufficient data are available to comment definitively on the alloreactivity and GVHD potential of UCB, matched or mismatched. Early results suggest that there may be a decrease in acute GVHD severity.[23, 25, 233–235]

Therapeutic strategies are aimed at either prevention (prophylaxis) of acute GVHD or its treatment. Clearly, selection of the best available donor based on HLA determinants by molecular techniques is the single most important factor in preventing severe GVHD,[16, 17] and considerations of donor sex and parity are advisable if there is a choice of donors. If the patient is seronegative for CMV, selection of a CMV-negative donor appears to reduce the risk of GVHD as well as of CMV after transplant.[227] Whether the source of hematopoietic stem cells (i.e., bone marrow, PBSC, UCB) modifies the risk of acute GVHD is an area of controversy. In addition, other supportive care measures such as the use of intravenous immunoglobulin[150] and the use of protective isolation with gut decontamination have decreased the incidence of GVHD.[236–238]

Conventional prophylactic approaches have attempted to inhibit T-cell responses by relying on *in vivo* immunosuppression. Essentially all current pharmacologic regimens employ combinations of immunosuppressive agents that target different molecular intermediates of T-cell signaling. Cyclosporine (Sandimmune) and tacrolimus (Prograf) both inhibit calcineurin activity, a serine-threonine phosphatase whose activity is essential for T-cell cytokine transcription.[239] Methotrexate prevents T-cell proliferation,[240] whereas high-dose corticosteroids are lympholytic. Current combinations utilize cyclosporine or tacrolimus plus methotrexate and/or prednisone.[241] A common prophylactic regimen includes cyclosporine given intravenously at a dose of 1.5 mg/kg every 12 hours until oral administration at a dose of 6.25 mg/kg every 12 hours is tolerated. Doses are adjusted to achieve desired blood levels. Cyclosporine is continued on a tapering schedule through day 180 after transplant. Methotrexate is given at 15 mg/m^2 on day 1 and at 10 mg/m^2 on days 3, 6, and 11 after marrow infusion. This regimen has been shown to reduce the incidence and severity of acute GVHD and improves long-term survival in some patient groups in comparison to single-agent therapy.[166, 242–246] Note that cyclosporine levels must be closely followed to prevent toxicity, and one study has shown that cyclosporine doses can be decreased in the first 2 weeks after transplant with decreased hepatotoxicity and without a concurrent increase in the incidence of acute GVHD.[247] More recently, continuous infusion cyclosporine has been used in an attempt to decrease further cyclosporine-associated toxicity without compromising efficacy, and a number of novel agents and approaches are being tested.[248]

As discussed earlier, selective depletion of T lymphocytes from the donor marrow inocula effectively prevents GVHD. T cells can be removed by a variety of techniques, including lectin depletion or anti–T-cell monoclonal antibodies plus complement, coupled to immunotoxin derivatives, or purged using magnetic beads. Each of these techniques may effect up to a 3 log or more depletion of T cells. Unfortunately, T-cell depletion is associated with an increased risk of graft failure and, for patients with hematologic malignancies, of leukemic relapse. Thus, the long-term survival rates of patients who have undergone T cell–depleted grafts are similar to those of patients who have received conventional *in vivo* immunosuppression after transplantation.[213, 244, 249, 250]

The outcome and long-term survival of patients with

acute GVHD vary directly with the grade of GVHD and response to treatment. The mainstay of treatment of established, acute GVHD remains the administration of glucocorticoids. Glucocorticoids (generally methylprednisolone) have been used in a variety of schedules and doses.[241, 251] The lympholytic effects of very high dose corticosteroids must be balanced by the increased risk of infections.[252–254] Patients failing or progressing on corticosteroid therapy have been tried on a number of agents but secondary treatment of GVHD is often unsuccessful.[255] Generally, cyclosporine is continued at therapeutic levels in patients who develop acute GVHD, and it may be initiated in patients who have never received the drug. Antithymocyte globulin and methods targeting CD5, CD3, interleukin-2 receptor, and tumor necrosis factor-α and its receptor have all been attempted with varying, incomplete, or unpredictable responses. Novel methods of approaching the treatment of patients with corticosteroid-resistant acute GVHD that do not compromise the ability to mount an immune response against infection are needed.

LATE COMPLICATIONS OF TREATMENT

The increased frequency of allogeneic and autologous transplantation coupled with improvements in supportive care and selection of patients with improved performance status and less advanced disease has resulted in a substantial number of long-term survivors. Thus, delayed complications secondary to both the chemoradiotherapy used to prepare patients for SCT and the transplant process itself (e.g., GVHD and propensity to infection) are just now being better defined with regard to incidence, severity, and outcome.

Chronic Graft-Versus-Host Disease

GVHD was initially characterized as occurring in two phases; acute GVHD generally presented within the first 100 days after transplant, whereas chronic GVHD occurred after day 100 (Table 8–4). It has become evident that certain cases of chronic GVHD can present as early as day 50 to 60 after marrow infusion, defined by both clinical and histopathologic criteria.[256] Chronic

GVHD may occur *de novo* or in patients who have experienced acute GVHD. The morbidity and mortality of chronic GVHD is most severe in patients who have progressive chronic GVHD after acute GVHD, followed by patients who have quiescent chronic GVHD, followed by patients in whom chronic GVHD is diagnosed *de novo* without antecedent acute GVHD.[257] The pathogenesis of chronic GVHD may involve T-cell recognition of minor histocompatibility antigens or loss of peripheral T-cell tolerance leading to symptoms resembling autoimmune disorders.

Risk factors for development of chronic GVHD include HLA disparity between donor and host, prior acute GVHD, increasing patient age, and possibly latent donor viral infection.[258–260] In addition, the use of female donors for male recipients and the use of sensitized donors (by prior pregnancy or transfusions) may increase the risk of chronic GVHD.[258–260] Rapid taper of cyclosporine after SCT, the use of T-cell infusions, and infection may increase the risk of chronic GVHD as well.[261]

The diagnosis of chronic GVHD is made by a combination of clinical and pathologic features. The syndrome resembles autoimmune systemic collagen vascular diseases with protean manifestations involving essentially every organ (Table 8–5). Pathologic changes in the skin involve epithelial cell damage characterized by basal cell degeneration and necrosis, and, later, epidermal atrophy and dermal fibrosis.[262, 263] Skin involvement may present as lichen planus, areas of local erythema, and areas of hyperpigmentation or hypopigmentation. The skin may be dry, freckling, or ulcerated and aggravated by exposure to sunlight. Sclerodermatous changes may evolve to flexion contractures. Hair follicles may be involved, and areas of alopecia may develop. Eye involvement is common; decreased tearing is quantitated by a Schirmer test. Sicca syndrome is a common presenting complaint, and tongue depapillation is evident on examination. There is often scalloping of the lateral margins of the tongue. The tongue, buccal mucosa, and gums may have lichen planus–like lesions, which should not be confused with, but may co-occur with, oral candidiasis. A biopsy specimen typically shows lichenoid changes with mononuclear infiltrates, epithelial cell necrosis, and salivary gland inflammation, lymphocytic infiltrate, and fibrosis. Involvement of the liver with chronic GVHD is manifest by obstructive jaundice, which may progress, if untreated, to bridging necrosis and cirrhosis. Gastrointestinal signs include inanition with progressive weight loss, chronic malabsorption, diarrhea, anorexia, nausea, and vomiting. Biopsy demonstrates single cell apoptosis with crypt destruction and may show fibrosis of the lamina propria. Early chronic GVHD may present as diffuse myositis and tendonitis. Progressive joint involvement, which may result from the myositis and tendonitis or simply from overlying skin fibrosis, results in decreased range of motion and flexion contractures. Chronic GVHD may involve the lungs with signs and symptoms of obstructive lung disease progressing to bronchiolitis obliterans (see later). Persistent immunodeficiency with pro-

Table 8–4. COMPARISON OF ACUTE AND CHRONIC GRAFT-VERSUS-HOST DISEASE

	Acute GVHD	Chronic GVHD
Incidence	40–60%	20–40%
Onset	Day 7–60 (up to 100)	Day >100 (often >60)
Manifestations:		
Skin	Erythematous rash	Sclerodermatous changes
Gut	Secretory diarrhea	Dry mouth; sicca
Liver	Hepatitis	Esophagitis, malabsorption, cholestasis
Other	Fever	Pulmonary dysfunction
	?Diffuse alveolar hemorrhage	Contractures
		Alopecia
		Thrombocytopenia

Table 8–5. CLINICOPATHOLOGIC FEATURES OF CHRONIC GRAFT-VERSUS-HOST DISEASE

System	Features
Systemic	Recurrent infections with immunodeficiency Weight loss Sicca syndrome Debility

Skin	Lichen planus, scleroderma, hyperpigmentation or hypopigmentation
	Dry scale, ulcerated, erythema, freckling
	Flexion contractures
	   Biopsy: Epithelial cell damage
	       Basal cell degeneration and necrosis
	       Epidermal atrophy and dermal fibrosis

Hair	Alopecia

Mouth	Sicca syndrome, depapillation of tongue with variegations
	Scalloping of lateral margins
	Lichen planus and ulcer, angular tightness
	   Biopsy: Lichenoid changes with mononuclear infiltrates
	       Epithelial cell necrosis
	       Salivary gland inflammation, lymphocytic infiltrate, fibrosis

Joints	Decreased range of motion, diffuse myositis/tendonitis
Eyes	Decreased tearing, injected sclerae, conjunctivae

Liver	↑ Alkaline phosphatase > transaminases and bilirubin
	Cholestasis, cirrhosis
	   Biopsy: Focal portal inflammation with bile ductule obliteration
	       Chronic aggressive hepatitis
	       Bridging necrosis
	       Cirrhosis

Gastrointestinal	Failure to thrive (children), weight loss (adults)
	Esophageal strictures, malabsorption, chronic diarrhea
	   Biopsy: Crypt destruction, single cell dropout
	       Fibrosis of lamina propria

Lung	Bronchiolitis obliterans, chronic rales Cough, dyspnea, wheezing Pneumothorax *Pulmonary function tests:* Decreased forced expiratory volume
Heme	Refractory thrombocytopenia Eosinophilia
Spleen	Howell-Jolly bodies

foundly depressed B- and T-cell responses predisposes to recurrent and severe infections. Patients may have reduced IgG2 and IgG4, decreased mucosal IgA, diminished delayed-type hypersensitivity, and hyposplenism. They are susceptible to opportunistic infections with encapsulated organisms (primarily pneumococcus), *P. carinii*, varicella-zoster, and herpes simplex and may have a variety of chronic infections, including sinusitis, bronchitis, and conjunctivitis.

Staging of chronic GVHD is based on degree of organ involvement (Table 8–6). Limited chronic GVHD is based on localized skin involvement with or without hepatic dysfunction. All other manifestations of chronic GVHD are classified as extensive chronic GVHD. Limited chronic GVHD may resolve spontaneously without specific therapy,[257] and patients with limited chronic GVHD have a favorable outcome.[257]

The best prophylactic treatment for chronic GVHD is prevention of acute GVHD, because *de novo* chronic GVHD is less common when compared with the incidence in patients who have had acute GVHD.[260] Treatment involves corticosteroids (usually oral prednisone), which may be used simultaneously or on an alternate-day schedule with cyclosporine.[264] The addition of azathioprine may be corticosteroid sparing in patients unable to taper primary therapy without re-

crudescence of disease. The hydrophilic bile acid ursodeoxycholic acid may be added in patients with cholestatic liver involvement. A number of other therapies are being tested, including psoralen plus ultraviolet radiation,[265–267] thalidomide,[268] and clofazimine.[269]

Equally important as immunosuppressive therapy for chronic GVHD is supportive care and symptomatic management of the patient. These therapies are directed to the specific organ or symptom. Patients with sicca syndrome are advised to use artificial tears with

Table 8–6. STAGING OF CHRONIC GRAFT-VERSUS-HOST DISEASE

Limited Chronic GVHD
  Localized skin involvement and/or
  Hepatic dysfunction due to chronic GVHD
Extensive Chronic GVHD
  Generalized skin involvement, or
  Localized skin involvement and/or hepatic dysfunction
    due to chronic GVHD, plus:
    Liver histology showing chronic aggressive hepatitis,
      bridging necrosis, or cirrhosis, or
    Eye involvement: Schirmer test (<5 mm wetting), or
    Involvement of minor salivary glands or oral mucosa
      demonstrated by buccal biopsy, or
    Involvement of any other target organ

careful ophthalmologic follow-up and artificial saliva with periodic dental examinations. Oral pilocarpine hydrochloride may relieve the symptoms of xerostomia.[270, 271] Regular and aggressive physical therapy with range of motion exercises is essential to prevent flexion contractures. Finally, immunoglobulin replacement and infection prophylaxis against *P. carinii* (trimethoprim/sulfamethoxazole, dapsone, others) and against encapsulated bacterial organisms (penicillin or equivalent) should be continued until 6 months after cessation of immunosuppressive agents.

Ophthalmologic Problems

A number of different ophthalmologic complications may attend SCT. Decreased lacrimation secondary to chronic GVHD may contribute to chronic ophthalmologic problems, including punctate keratopathy, scar formation, and corneal perforation.[272–274] At any time, patients may develop infectious complications (particularly with herpes simplex viruses). Cyclosporine usage is associated with a number of eye complaints, including an increasingly well-described syndrome of headache, hypertension, seizures, or visual impairment (see Neurologic Complications for a detailed description).[275–277] In addition, there are numerous reports of what can be grouped loosely as transplant-related retinopathy. Optic disc edema, either asymptomatic or presenting with visual blurring, has been described in patients who received cyclosporine for GVHD prophylaxis after either busulfan or TBI-based conditioning but not in patients who did not receive cyclosporine.[278, 279] Ischemic fundal lesions, detected as so-called cotton-wool spots, and, in some patients, optic disc edema, have been reported in 13% of patients treated with both TBI and cyclosporine and were not observed in patients who did not have concordance for these risk factors.[279] Lesions appeared 3 to 6 months after SCT, and the majority of patients had complaints of decreased visual acuity or other visual disturbance. Most discontinued cyclosporine, and half were treated with systemic corticosteroids. The majority of patients recovered visual acuity and resolved their ischemic lesions over time, but little further information is available about the course or prognosis of this complication. Occlusive microvascular retinopathy has also been described after autologous SCT after high-dose cytarabine and TBI,[280] suggesting that particular high-dose chemotherapy regimens may predispose to vascular injury at otherwise safe radiation doses,[280] an argument analogous to that for the development of post-SCT hemolytic-uremic syndrome.[281, 282]

A substantial risk of cataract development has been described. Although this incidence is increased in patients given single-dose TBI to approximately 80%, patients receiving fractionated TBI or chemotherapy-only regimens still have a 20% to 50% incidence of cataracts at 5 to 6 years.[283–285] Higher dose rate is also associated with an increased incidence.[286] The relative risk of cataracts and the need for subsequent cataract surgery may also be related to prior therapy or to glucocorticoid use for prophylaxis or management of GVHD.[284, 285]

Dental Problems

Disturbances in dental development have been described in children conditioned for SCT with TBI, particularly if SCT took place before age 6.[287] Characteristic findings include short dental roots, absence of root development, and microdontia. Subsequent decreased alveolar bone growth may lead to additional compromise of dental development. In addition, oral sicca syndrome (occurring as a complication of either TBI or chronic GVHD or both) may result in chronic oral mucosal injury, poor oral hygiene, and subsequent dental decay. The effects of prophylactic interventions are not well reported.

Pulmonary Complications

Pulmonary dysfunction of both restrictive and obstructive character may follow autologous and allogeneic SCT in children. Obstructive lung disease, characterized by either interstitial fibrosis or bronchiolitis obliterans pathologically,[288] has been reported in up to 20% of children after allogeneic SCT.[289] Whereas an estimated rate of obstructive lung disease of 2% to 3% has been reported in adults,[290, 291] more recent data suggest that the rate in adults and children is comparable.[292, 293] Rarely described after autologous SCT, obstructive lung disease has been associated most firmly with chronic GVHD, although associations with hypogammaglobulinemia, concurrent viral infections, and gastroesophageal reflux have also been reported.[288–292, 294–298] There is no clear association of TBI-based conditioning with obstructive lung disease. Obstructive lung disease may not be permanent or progressive because "transient" cases have been reported.[289] Poor survival of affected patients is suggested,[290] although symptomatic and radiographic improvement with immunosuppression has been described.[289, 299]

The etiology of restrictive abnormalities described after SCT is unclear. Modest decreases in total lung capacity, vital capacity, and forced expiratory volume in 1 second at 6 months after SCT have been described in cohorts of both adults and children.[298, 300, 301] These findings reverted to normal or near normal over time. Excluding patients with GVHD, no difference in autologous and allogeneic patients has been described. There may be a relationship to TBI-based conditioning, and fractionation may be sparing. The specific effects of prior drug exposure, particularly to nitrosoureas and bleomycin, and underlying pulmonary disease (e.g., asthma) on long-term pulmonary functioning in patients who underwent transplants as children are unknown.

Hematologic Complications

Patients who undergo ABO-incompatible allogeneic SCT are at risk for immune hemolytic anemias attributed to donor lymphocyte–produced antibodies. This type of hemolysis is seen most commonly in patients having received minor ABO-mismatched sibling or UD bone marrow.[302, 303] In this latter setting, hemolysis of transfused group O erythrocytes was also observed. This type of hemolysis is usually seen within weeks of SCT but may be prolonged or occasionally later in onset. A relationship to post-transplant immunosuppression with cyclosporine without methotrexate has been suggested.[302] Prolonged red cell aplasia lasting up to 8 months after ABO major mismatched SCT, also presumably on an immune basis, has been reported.[304] Cytopenias with demonstrable antiplatelet and antineutrophil antibodies have been identified after both autologous and allogeneic SCT.[305–308] These autoimmune cytopenias may present early after transplant or up to several years later and may respond to corticosteroids, intravenous γ-globulin, or other therapy. Pancytopenia, unrelated to graft rejection or graft failure, has been noted to occur with increased frequency in patients with histories of either acute or chronic GVHD.[257, 309] In addition, peripheral blood cell function may be aberrant. For example, neutrophil chemotaxis, superoxide production, and phagocytic capacity have been demonstrated to be abnormal for up to 12 months after SCT.[310] These defects may predispose to bacterial infections.

Coagulation factor deficiencies, specifically deficiencies of factors VII, XII, protein C, and antithrombin III, have been reported after autologous SCT.[311–313] A variety of microangiopathic syndromes have also been described after SCT, of which some have delayed onset. The use of cyclosporine for GVHD prophylaxis or treatment has been associated with both thrombotic thrombocytopenic purpura and hemolytic-uremic syndromes, which can occur either acutely or after periods of cyclosporine exposure.[314, 315] Specific therapeutic maneuvers have not been shown to be efficacious in either circumstance nor do the syndromes necessarily resolve with discontinuation of cyclosporine. A hemolytic-uremic syndrome, apparently related to the use of TBI in the conditioning regimen, may also occur (see Renal and Urinary Tract Complications).[281, 282, 316, 317]

Renal and Urinary Tract Complications

Patients may develop a hemolytic-uremic syndrome occurring from 4 to 9 months after SCT.[281, 282, 316, 317] This disorder generally presents as moderate hemolysis and renal dysfunction, although some patients have a more aggressive presentation with hypertension and seizures. The majority of reported cases appear to have resolved spontaneously over time, although modest persistent anemia as well as defects in renal function have been reported. Occasional patients have protracted and severe hematologic and renal manifestations, and the long-term sequelae with respect to renal function in pediatric patients remain unknown.

Chronic nephropathy is occasionally observed. This is most often related to nephrotoxic drugs delivered in the peritransplant period. It is widely appreciated that patients may develop acute, reversible renal insufficiency related to cyclosporine (often in the setting of elevated blood levels).[314, 318] Much more infrequently, patients receiving cyclosporine may develop chronic,

irreversible renal insufficiency.[318, 319] Patients who have received cyclophosphamide as part of their conditioning regimen, and potentially those having received ifosfamide, may have continuous or recurrent episodes of hemorrhagic cystitis for up to 10 years after treatment.[320, 321] Such patients may also experience dysuria, develop bladder fibrosis, and may have an increased risk for the development of bladder cancer.[320–322]

Neurologic Complications

Patients undergoing SCT may experience a variety of neurologic complications either directly or more indirectly related to their treatment. Acyclovir is used in many post-transplant settings for either prophylaxis or treatment of infection with herpes simplex viruses. Confusion, tremors, delusion, and frank psychosis have been associated with the use of this drug.[323] Similarly, mental status changes, paresthesias, and, uncommonly, seizures have been reported with the antiviral agents ganciclovir and foscarnet.[324–326] Impaired renal function, often seen in SCT patients, may potentiate the occurrence of these symptoms. Both prednisone and cyclosporine may have neurologic side effects. Psychosis or mood swings accompanying high-dose corticosteroid therapy are well described in the general medical literature. Cyclosporine administration may be associated with depression, tremors, seizures, and visual impairment.[275–277, 327] It has been postulated that both seizures and acute visual loss arise from hydrostatic changes accompanying cyclosporine-associated hypertension. These changes affect white matter, most commonly in the occipital area, and are accompanied by characteristic radiologic findings on magnetic resonance imaging. In general, symptoms abate rapidly on discontinuation or decreases in the dose of cyclosporine. Less commonly, hallucinations and ataxia have been observed.[328, 329] It has been suggested that hypomagnesemia potentiates or predisposes to cyclosporine-mediated neurotoxicity.[329] Thalidomide, under investigation for treatment of chronic GVHD, may produce sedation and, less commonly, severe peripheral neuropathy.[330]

Cerebrovascular accidents may also be observed after SCT. These are most common secondary to thrombocytopenia.[331] Decreased production of the clotting factor protein C, referred to in the section on hematologic complications, may also be a risk factor for intracranial hemorrhage, and one such case has been reported.[313]

Central nervous system (CNS) infectious complications related to either immunosuppression, chronic GVHD, or both also occur after SCT. Several autopsy series in the 1970s to 1980s demonstrated an incidence of CNS infection ranging from 5% to 7%.[331–333] A significant proportion (30%–50%) of these infections were due to *Aspergillus* species. Mortality from CNS aspergillosis is more than 94%.[334] Increased immunosuppression and GVHD accompanying many current SCT regimens, especially T cell–depleted or alternative donor, may well exacerbate this problem.[335] Infection with *Toxoplasma gondii* also occurs after SCT, although its overall incidence is still low. Patients may experience additional infectious neurologic complications, including bacterial meningitis. Presentation of meningitis, or indeed any CNS infection, may differ from that in an immunocompetent patient in that localizing signs and symptoms may be less dramatic. Patients may also develop encephalitis or meningoencephalitis with a variety of viruses, including cytomegalovirus, herpes simplex types 1 and 6, adenovirus, and varicella zoster.[336]

Leukoencephalopathy 4 to 5 months after SCT has been described, presenting as lethargy, slurred speech, ataxia, seizures, confusion, decreased sensorium, dysphagia, spasticity, or decerebrate posturing with consistent objective findings (on magnetic resonance imaging or biopsy). In a series of 415 patients from Seattle, a 7% incidence was described.[337] Leukoencephalopathy was observed only in patients who had received CNS radiation or intrathecal therapy or both before SCT and methotrexate intrathecal therapy after SCT.

The effects of different conditioning regimens on neuropsychological functioning have been incompletely investigated. In particular, analysis of very young patients is limited. Nonetheless, it is clear that many very young children, including those younger than 2 years of age, can undergo SCT with high doses of preparatory chemotherapy or radiotherapy and subsequently perform well in areas such as sensorimotor and cognitive functioning,[338–340] social development,[341] and school performance.[342] Preliminary identification of risk factors that may predict negative neuropsychological sequelae has been initiated. Potential factors include prior cranial radiation, radiation dose rate and cumulative dose, cumulative methotrexate dosing before and after SCT, exposure to other chemotherapeutic agents, age, and sex.

Endocrine Disorders

Significant endocrine toxicity is associated, although not exclusively, with radiation and is attenuated in both incidence and severity when radiation is fractionated. Endocrine evaluation of children having received BU/CY-containing regimens is less well reported. Adrenocortical function has been described as modestly deficient in one study and normal in another.[343, 344] Thyroid dysfunction is well documented. In radiation-containing regimens, the incidence of compensated hypothyroidism ranges from 13% to 39% and that of overt hypothyroidism from 3% to 20%.[344, 345] Both are reduced when children received fractionated rather than single-fraction TBI.[345] Normal thyroid function 1 year after SCT has been reported in a small cohort of patients after treatment with BU/CY.[345] The incidence of thyroid dysfunction increases over time after SCT.

Children undergoing SCT for underlying malignancy are at risk for both growth failure and growth hormone deficiency.[344–351] Concomitant factors such as prior treatment and chronic disease, corticosteroid use, chronic GVHD, and renal disease may complicate both the assessment of linear growth and the determination of etiology. In some studies, the relationship of low growth hormone to observed poor growth is unclear, and it is possible that direct radiation effects on bone and cartilage affect subsequent growth.[350] Fractionation of TBI may have a relative sparing effect whereas prior cranial radiation seems to be a particularly strong predictor of poor growth.[344–347, 352] The linear growth of children after BU/CY has been reported to be both no better than or significantly better than that of patients receiving fractionated TBI and cyclophosphamide.[350, 351] It is interesting that in the study in which significant growth failure was not noted in the BU/CY group overall, both growth hormone deficiency and poor linear growth were observed in the two BU/CY patients with higher busulfan levels than the others. Thus, the greater systemic busulfan exposure currently being pursued through the use of surface-area dosing and monitoring of levels may result in changes in the toxicity profile of this regimen.[350]

Gonadal failure has also been described after SCT. In both male and female prepubertal patients, delayed puberty associated with hypergonadotropic hypogonadism is frequent.[345] Primary gonadal failure has been described in approximately three fourths of postpubertal females after TBI-containing regimens, and such findings have also been noted in the same population after receiving BU/CY and other chemotherapy only regimens.[343–345, 353] Reduced uterine size and ovarian volume have been observed.[343, 353, 354] Other abnormalities noted in a majority of females who undergo transplants after puberty include reduced vaginal elasticity, pallor, decreased vaginal and cervical size, atrophic vulvovaginitis, introital stenosis, and loss of pubic hair.[354] These findings appear to be more frequent in but are not confined to patients having received radiation. No comparable data are published for the population prepubertal at SCT. Thus, female patients should be followed closely for gynecologic complications, and hormone replacement should be considered for alleviation of discomfort as well as for chemical indications.[354, 355] In postpubertal males, SCT with or without radiation-based conditioning often results in azoospermia while significant Leydig cell damage with decreased testosterone, decreased testicular volume, and decreased libido appear less frequently.[343–345, 353, 356] In both sexes, spontaneous recovery of gonadal function has occurred years after SCT. Fertility resulting in liveborn infants has been reported for both male and female SCT patients, including those who had received radiation.[345, 356]

Bone Problems

The most prominent bony complication of SCT, aseptic (avascular) necrosis, is a known complication of corticosteroid therapy and therefore is most likely to be seen after allogeneic SCT when corticosteroids are used as part of a GVHD prophylaxis or treatment schedule.[357–359] The incidence of aseptic necrosis and the percentage of patients who go on to require joint replacement are unreported. Patients receiving corticosteroids on a chronic basis may also be prone to osteoporosis. In addition, gonadal failure and hypoestrogenism related to conditioning therapy may place female patients at particular risk for early onset and severe osteoporosis.* Again, the incidence and severity of this potential complication and the long-term consequences for children are unclear. Growth of craniofacial bones in children undergoing SCT may be impaired, particularly those treated with TBI.[287] Patients developing chronic obstructive airway disease (bronchiolitis obliterans) may develop a pronounced pectus carinatum.

TRANSPLANTATION IN ACQUIRED DISEASES

Aplastic Anemia

Severe aplastic anemia (SAA) is a syndrome characterized by peripheral pancytopenia and marrow hypoplasia (see Chapter 7). Mortality associated with this disorder in children can be as high as 50% in the first 6 months.[360] Although a number of immunosuppressive and marrow stimulatory therapies have shown reasonable activity, the only curative treatment remains SCT. The potential efficacy of allogeneic SCT for patients with SAA was established with the initial publication in 1972 of results achieved in 4 patients.[361] Randomized studies have since established the superiority of matched allogeneic SCT over supportive care (androgens in the 1970s, immunosuppressive therapy with antithymocyte globulin in the 1980s and 1990s) in both children and, more recently, adults.[362–365] The actuarial survival of previously untransfused patients with SAA undergoing matched family SCT has been reported to be 82% at 10 years.[366] In another series of patients with more diverse characteristics, survival is approximately 70%.[367]

Notwithstanding its demonstrated efficacy, application of SCT to SAA has been fraught with problems. Most prominent of these has been the high rate of graft rejection.[166, 167, 367–369] In fact, the patterns of graft failure observed in syngeneic twins undergoing SCT for SAA suggested that there may be three general pathophysiologic bases for SAA: (1) stem cell abnormality (twin engrafts without conditioning), (2) immune-mediated defect (twin rejects simple infusion but accepts graft if conditioned with immunosuppressive therapy), and (3) microenvironmental defect (complete failure of engraftment despite aggressiveness of approach).[370] Previously transfused patients have a graft rejection rate as high as 40% when prepared with cyclophosphamide alone.[371] Risk factors identified for graft failure after SCT include low cell dose, positive crossmatch of recipient against donor in lymphocytotoxicity assay, previous transfusion, a non–radiation-containing regimen, a noncyclosporine GVHD prophylaxis regimen, or the use of T-cell depletion. The addition of buffy coat cells as well as the inclusion of additional immunosuppressive medications such as antithymocyte globulin in chemotherapy-only conditioning regimens, use of alternative radiotherapy schedules such as total lymphoid irradiation or low-dose TBI or thoracoabdominal

irradiation, more widespread use of cyclosporine, and more conservative transfusion practices have led to more successful outcomes.[165, 166, 169, 172, 367, 372] The potential impact of decreased transfusion-associated allosensitization associated with depletion of leukocytes through filters has not yet been assessed. No randomized trials of different conditioning regimens are reported. Approximately 600 patients who underwent transplantation in the 1980s have been analyzed in aggregate through the IBMTR.[166] Although the incidence of graft failure differed markedly among the different approaches used, overall survival did not.

Causes of treatment failure after allogeneic SCT for SAA thus vary significantly depending on patient and disease-related variables as well as the regimen chosen.[166, 167] Multivariate analyses also support the impression that children with SAA do particularly well after SCT.[166] The administration of donor buffy coat cells at the time of SCT decreases graft rejection but is associated with increased chronic GVHD.[169] Use of a conditioning regimen containing radiation also appears to be associated with less graft rejection but with more interstitial pneumonitis and GVHD.[166, 167] The impact of GVHD prophylaxis on outcome is pronounced. In several large analyses, use of cyclosporine is associated with a significant improvement in overall survival.[166, 167, 373, 374] In SAA (in which the dose of radiation is often low), radiation-based regimens may also be associated with a substantially increased risk of secondary solid malignancy when compared with chemotherapy-only regimens.[375–377]

The overall good outcome, coupled with the paucity of other therapeutic options, frequency of relapse, and growing concern over the evolution of MDS and AML in long-term survivors of immunosuppression has encouraged use of SCT in patients without a matched family donor.[378–380] Results have been mixed. Survival has ranged from 0% to 54% when mismatched family and matched and mismatched UDs are used.[21, 381–383] Unless the unique issues of SAA and graft failure prove too difficult, one would expect these outcomes to improve as patients are moved to SCT earlier and as overall alternative donor technology improves. Nonetheless, SCT for SAA has also been successfully extended to another unique setting, that of SAA complicating orthotopic liver transplantation for fulminant non-A, non-B hepatitis.[384, 385]

Myelodysplasia

Myelodysplasia has been estimated as accounting for about 3% of childhood hematologic malignancies and some additional percentage of patients first diagnosed with AML (see Chapter 34). Allogeneic SCT has been used successfully as therapy for pediatric MDS.[386–391] Both busulfan- and TBI-based regimens have been used successfully. In combined adult and pediatric series, prognostic variables most often associated with good outcome are younger age, shorter duration of disease, and SCT before the appearance of excess blasts/transition.[389, 390, 392] Marrow fibrosis and secondary AML have been reported to correlate with poor outcome.[386–390,]

---

*See references 343–346, 353–355, 357, and 358.

[392, 393] Although prior reports have implicated marrow fibrosis as a particular risk for poor hematologic recovery, more recent analyses do not substantiate this concern and fibrosis should not preclude consideration of SCT.[389, 390, 392–395] Alternative donors have been used with widely variable success.[21, 389, 396] Whereas the indolent course and good 5-year survival of adult patients with certain karyotypic abnormalities have made the decision to offer SCT to patients with MDS controversial (particularly for older individuals), these data may be less pertinent to children. On the other hand, ongoing studies of the response of pediatric patients with MDS to aggressive chemotherapy may color the triage of therapy, particularly for the patient without a matched donor.

Acute Lymphoblastic Leukemia

Although it is generally accepted that approximately two thirds of children with newly diagnosed ALL treated with aggressive, multiagent combination therapy will survive disease-free for prolonged periods of time, the management of patients with certain high-risk features, primary induction failure, or relapse remains controversial. In particular, the optimal treatment of second clinical remission childhood ALL remains unsettled. Numerous reports have demonstrated the success of allogeneic SCT for patients with second or greater remission ALL; however, the relative superiority of allogeneic SCT over autologous SCT or chemotherapy is a matter of debate.[397–402] DFS after matched-sibling allogeneic SCT ranges from 40% to 75% for children in secondary or subsequent remission.[49, 81, 403–408] Poor outcome after allogeneic SCT is predicted by a number of factors, including high initial white blood cell count, short initial remission, relapse on treatment, and previous CNS leukemia.[405–407, 409] A review in 1987 of 36 published reports concluded that SCT is never inferior to chemotherapy and is superior if relapse occurred within 18 months from diagnosis.[397] Subsequently, long-term follow-up reports of ALL patients treated by the Genoa and the St. Jude's/Seattle groups concluded that SCT was superior to chemotherapy.[408, 410] In contrast, Henze and associates reported that approximately one third of children with relapsed ALL who were treated with very aggressive chemotherapy achieved a long-lasting second clinical remission.[411] Moreover, the German cooperative group reported a trial of 51 children that corroborated that SCT is superior to conventional therapy for children who experience relapse early on aggressive primary therapy whereas children who have late relapses have an event-free survival (EFS) of approximately 40% with chemotherapy alone, thus concluding that SCT was not indicated for this later group.[406]

For ALL patients who are refractory to primary induction or reinduction therapy, the most likely potentially curative modality is allogeneic SCT. The presence and predictive value of poor prognostic factors and availability of an allogeneic donor are critical to the decision of whether to pursue additional conventional treatment or alternatively allogeneic or autologous

SCT. For example, children with Philadelphia chromosome–positive ALL (Ph[1]) appear to have a particularly poor prognosis. The IBMTR has reported the results of 67 HLA-matched sibling allografts for Ph[1]-positive ALL. The probability of 2-year DFS was approximately 38% if SCT was performed in first clinical remission and 41% if performed thereafter.[412, 413] Another sizable series reported 46% DFS if SCT was performed in the first clinical remission and 28% if performed after first relapse.[76] This suggests that allogeneic SCT is an effective treatment that may be advantageous to pursue in first clinical remission, although there is still likely to be efficacy after relapse. Such data have encouraged the use of UD SCT.[414] Insufficient data exist to perform similar analyses of outcome for patients with other high-risk features such as t(4;11) and t(8;14). Some centers pursue aggressive chemotherapy for such patients whereas others uniformly attempt SCT in first clinical remission.

A major obstacle to SCT remains the availability of appropriate donors, which autologous SCT can overcome. In ALL, obstacles to autologous SCT include the amount of prior therapy and resultant damage of bone marrow as well as bone marrow contamination by leukemic cells. Techniques to purge leukemic cells using either pharmacologic or immunologic methodologies are long established and relatively safe.[415] Billet and colleagues reported an EFS of 53% at 3 years for 51 children who underwent this procedure.[416, 417] As has been suggested with other modalities, the most important prognostic variable was the length of the first clinical remission. The relative merits of allogeneic versus autologous SCT are debatable.[418–420] Kersey and colleagues compared 91 patients, half receiving antibody-purged autologous and half receiving allogeneic BMT.[419] Patients receiving autografts reconstituted earlier, had shorter hospital courses and significantly fewer peritransplant deaths but experienced relapse earlier and more frequently. Although cause of treatment failure differed, no difference in long-term DFS was observed. In contrast, Blaise and co-workers reported 47 high-risk patients who received either allogeneic or autologous BMT in first clinical remission. Although acute mortality was higher for patients receiving allografts, only 9% of those receiving allografts versus 52% of those receiving autografts experienced relapse. These authors noted that patients who underwent allogeneic BMT did so much earlier and with less consolidation therapy. Nonetheless, they concluded that BMT was an effective form of consolidation for high-risk ALL in the first clinical remission and that allogeneic SCT was superior, similar to results of a randomized study in adult ALL in first clinical remission that also concluded that early allogeneic SCT is more effective consolidation treatment.[421] These data suggest that allogeneic SCT is superior to autologous SCT with respect to disease control but that the differences in cause of failure as well as scrutiny of prognostic variables may suggest subgroups for whom autologous SCT is an equivalent choice. The relative outcomes after alternative donor, matched sibling, and autologous SCT have not been analyzed.

Acute Myeloblastic Leukemia

The still controversial issue of whether to treat patients with AML with transplants in first clinical remission was first addressed in a series of prospective trials in the mid 1980s. In 111 consecutive patients, the Seattle group undertook matched sibling allogeneic SCT for patients who had a donor whereas the remaining patients received conventional intensification. The probability of 5-year DFS was 49% for SCT compared with 20% for chemotherapy alone.[422] A prospective randomized trial of young adults in first clinical remission resulted in an actuarial rate of relapse of 40% in the SCT group compared with 71% with chemotherapy alone. However, actuarial survival at greater than 4 years was not statistically different, suggesting that although SCT was more effective in preventing relapse there was increased treatment-related toxicity.[423] There have been two sizable, prospective pediatric AML clinical trials attempting to compare chemotherapy and allogeneic SCT in first clinical remission. The results of the first Children's Cancer Study Group (CCG) study showed that patients receiving matched sibling SCT fared significantly better than children who received chemotherapy alone (49% versus 36%).[424] The CCG has just completed another randomized phase III trial of the optimum treatment for 450 newly diagnosed patients achieving clinical remission in which patients were assigned to allogeneic SCT if there was a matched sibling donor or randomized to autologous SCT with 4-hydroperoxycyclophosphamide (4-HC)-purged bone marrow versus chemotherapy.[425] Preliminary analysis suggests that DFS with allogeneic SCT is superior to that achieved with intensive chemotherapy or autologous SCT and that chemotherapy alone is either equivalent to or likely better than autologous SCT. The same hierarchy pertains to overall survival. Nonetheless, the role of autologous SCT, the value of purging, and the best timing of its use remain unresolved issues. With the advent of alternative donor SCT, where limited reported data suggest approximately a 50% DFS at 2 years for patients in first or second clinical remission, the role of autologous SCT is likely to become even more controversial.[21, 414] Autologous remission bone marrow has been unmanipulated or purged with either chemotherapy (4-HC or related compounds) or alternatively with one or more combinations of antimyeloid monoclonal antibodies.[53, 78, 84, 426–428] Several comparative trials have examined the success of purged autografting versus allografts for both relapsed and first clinical remission patients. In a design similar to that of the CCG study cited earlier, Zittoun and co-workers reported on 623 patients, approximately 25% children, assigned to undergo allogeneic BMT or randomized to either autologous BMT or continued intensive chemotherapy after achieving first clinical remission.[429] DFS (55%) was greatest in the allogeneic SCT arm, followed by autologous BMT (48%) and intensive chemotherapy (30%). Unlike the CCG study, in which allogeneic BMT resulted in improved DFS and overall survival, overall survival was not significantly different in the BMT arms. In one recent pediatric single-arm study, DFS

after unpurged autologous BMT using melphalan was equivalent to that reported elsewhere after allogeneic SCT.[430] Autologous BMT has also been performed successfully with bone marrow harvested in the second clinical remission or later, and bone marrow cryopreserved in the first clinical remission has been used to perform BMT in the second clinical remission or untreated first relapse.[53, 78] In aggregate, despite DFS of 45% to 60% achieved with chemotherapy, the use of allogeneic BMT for patients in first clinical remission with a matched donor seems indicated whereas the roles and triage of alternative donor and autologous BMT remain controversial.

One strategy that would minimize exposure to the acute toxicities of SCT for the group as a whole might be to treat all patients with chemotherapy alone and to reserve BMT for children who experience relapse after an initial clinical remission. Data as to whether BMT in first clinical remission is more effective than in advanced AML is controversial.[431] DFS of patients transplanted in second clinical remission has most often been significantly less than that obtained after BMT in first clinical remission, although equivalent results were reported in one study.[55, 432–434] DFS of patients transplanted in untreated first ("early") relapse is 25% to 30%, including patients experiencing relapse after current intensive regimens.[55, 77, 432–434] Greater than 40% DFS has also been reported for patients undergoing BMT after primary induction failure.[435] Management would also be aided by identification of prognostic factors such as French-American-British (FAB) classification type or cytogenetics directing selection among post-remission treatments. This has been stymied by the fact that many high-risk populations do equally poorly with any modality.[82]

Chronic Myelogenous Leukemia and Juvenile Chronic Myelomonocytic Leukemia

Chronic myelogenous leukemia is a relatively uncommon disorder in children, but its clinical course and outcome with allogeneic SCT seem indistinguishable from the adult setting (see Chapter 34). The DFS and overall outcome of patients transplanted in chronic phase are excellent.[436–438] BMT in either accelerated phase or blast crisis is less effective.[438, 439] Transplant within a year of diagnosis is associated with better outcome.[438, 440, 441] The relevance of splenectomy, although controversial, appears minimal regarding most outcomes.[442] Use of T-cell depletion has been associated with a marked rate of relapse, suggesting a very significant role for allogeneic effect in control of this disorder, and post-BMT relapse has been successfully treated with infusion of donor lymphocytes.[440, 443–445]

There is no curative chemotherapy for juvenile chronic myelomonocytic leukemia (JCML) (see Chapter 34). Allogeneic SCT from both conventional and alternative donors has been used successfully.[446–449] Longer follow-up of larger patient cohorts suggests that the relapse rate is high and that relapse often occurs soon after SCT. Alternative pre- or post-SCT approaches are needed to successfully use SCT as a curative modality in this disorder.

Hodgkin's and Non-Hodgkin's Lymphoma

SCT has been utilized in children as well as adults with Hodgkin's disease (HD) or aggressive non-Hodgkin's lymphoma (NHL) who either relapse or have refractory disease after initial treatment with conventional chemotherapy. The most efficacious conditioning regimen remains uncertain, as DFS appears equivalent among series using either TBI-based or chemotherapy-only approaches. There has been increasing consensus about the use of autologous PBSC as a favored hematopoietic stem cell (HSC) source based on the favorable engraftment characteristics reviewed earlier. The potential for salvage of pediatric patients with Burkitt's lymphoma was established in 1986, when a 5-year French experience demonstrated approximately 50% DFS with the use of high-dose chemotherapy followed by autologous BMT.[449a] Similar results in children with a broader array of histologies have been reported more recently from other European centers and in larger combined pediatric and adult series.[449b–449e] Paralleling the findings in adult patients with lymphoma, DFS is most consistently predicted by the presence of lymphoma that demonstrates responsiveness to pre-SCT chemotherapy, with virtually no long-term survivors among patients who have chemotherapy-resistant disease prior to conditioning. There has also been interest in the role of allogeneic BMT in the treatment of NHL and HD. Retrospective case-controlled studies in adult/pediatric series suggest comparable results.[449f, 449g] A prospective trial revealed a lower relapse rate in those undergoing allogeneic BMT but no overall survival advantage.[449h] Whether this decrease in relapse rate reflects a graft-versus-lymphoma effect or merely the infusion of uncontaminated marrow is not clear. Characterization of patients at particularly high risk for failure after autologous SCT may serve to identify those most appropriate for alternative treatment approaches.

Neuroblastoma and Other Solid Tumors

The biology and treatment of pediatric solid tumors are treated elsewhere in this book (see Chapters 28 and 37). The most extensive SCT experience in pediatric solid tumors is in patients with advanced-stage neuroblastoma. Early studies documented long-term survival of a very small subset of patients undergoing autologous SCT.[450] Nonetheless, the contributions of autologous SCT to overall survival of high-risk patients has not yet been established.[451] The impact of purging the bone marrow or PBSC, type of conditioning regimen used, and use of biologic markers to select patients is being evaluated.[452–457] Small numbers of patients have also undergone allogeneic BMT with no clear improvement in outcome over that achieved with autologous SCT.[453, 455, 457]

Little has been published on the use of either allogeneic or autologous SCT for other nonhematologic malignancies. Some promise in terms of response rate has been observed for patients with sarcomas who have both minimal residual and chemosensitive disease, but the generalizability and durability of these responses will need to be established before widespread application can be supported.[454, 458]

TRANSPLANTATION IN GENETIC DISEASES

Allogeneic SCT has increasingly been evaluated as the major modality to cure children with inherited diseases. The most common inherited diseases that have been treated with SCT are reviewed, and the experience with rarer diseases is summarized in Table 8–7.

Immunodeficiency Disorders

Severe Combined Immunodeficiency Syndromes

Since the late 1960s, allogeneic BMT has been successfully employed to cure children with a number of lethal immunodeficiency diseases (Table 8–7), including severe combined immunodeficiency disease (SCID) and Wiskott-Aldrich syndrome. Mounting evidence demonstrates that SCID is a clinical syndrome resulting from one or more defects in molecules responsible for T-cell signaling. Depending on whether the critical defect resides in early or late T-cell ontogeny defines whether the patient will suffer from classic SCID, characterized by B and T lymphocytopenia and resulting agammaglobulinemia; common SCID, characterized by T lymphocytopenia and variable abnormal immunoglobulin profiles; or SCID secondary to ADA deficiency (which may have either of the above phenotypes). Without question, conventional, matched sibling allogeneic SCT for SCID is one of the major success stories of SCT. Unlike most other forms of SCT, transplantation in patients with SCID does not necessarily require conditioning. After conventional matched SCT without cytoreduction, phenotypic immune reconstitution will

Table 8–7. IMMUNODEFICIENCY DISORDERS TREATED WITH STEM CELL TRANSPLANTATION

Classic severe combined immunodeficiency disease (B⁻)
Common severe combined immunodeficiency disease (B⁺)
Adenosine deaminase deficiency
Reticular dysgenesis
Omenn's syndrome
Severe combined immunodeficiency disease associated with short-limbed dwarfism and ectodermal dysplasia
Familial erythrophagocytic lymphohistiocytosis
HLA class II deficiency (bare lymphocyte syndrome)
Purine nucleoside phosphorylase deficiency
X-linked lymphoproliferative disease
Leukocyte adhesion deficiency (CD11/18 deficiency)
Wiskott-Aldrich syndrome

take place within several weeks and evidence of good lymphocyte function will be evident by 2 to 3 months.[459] Grade II or greater acute GVHD is infrequently observed and contributes little to treatment-related mortality.[460] Similarly, chronic GVHD is uncommon. Dramatically improved long-term survivorship from the range of approximately 50% in the 1970s to nearly 90% by the end of the 1980s appears attributable to more rapid and precise diagnosis, followed by SCT at a younger age and in better condition, and to improved supportive care for infectious complications.[460, 461]

In the context of the remarkable successes observed in SCID and other severe immunodeficiency disorders treated with matched sibling SCT, increasing numbers of investigators have attempted to treat patients with SCID with marrows from mismatched family donors and UDs.[460–469] Early experience with haploidentical SCT was rife with graft rejection, frequent severe GVHD, and opportunistic infection, resulting in poor long-term survival. The development of T-cell depletion protocols combined with modified conditioning regimens significantly reduced the rate of graft rejection and significantly improved both hematopoietic and immunologic engraftment in the majority of patients. The majority of patients develop functional donor T lymphocytes, although reconstitution of B-cell immunity is much less frequent and (if present) delayed, particularly if cytoreduction is not used.[461, 462, 464, 470] This has led, particularly in Europe, to the more frequent adoption of complete cytoreduction to encourage the evolution of a fully-functional donor immune and hematopoietic system.[470] The most widely accepted criterion for complete cytoreduction is the diagnosis of ADA deficiency.[460] Overall, survival of patients with HLA-disparate donors after T cell–depleted SCT has risen substantially, to the range of 60% to 80%.[460, 461, 470] Nonetheless, treatment failure continues to be due to a different spectrum of problems than those seen in other SCT settings. Infection, graft failure, and post-SCT B-cell lymphoproliferative disease remain significant problems.[461, 468, 470, 471]

Alternative sources of stem cells including UD human fetal liver or thymus grafts have also been evaluated in the treatment of patients with SCID. Less than a third of these patients demonstrated durable engraftment, and even fewer achieved durable immunologic reconstitution.[468] Although intriguing, these studies did not significantly contribute to the treatment of patients with SCID and have been superseded by T cell–depleted haploidentical SCT.

Wiskott-Aldrich Syndrome

Wiskott-Aldrich syndrome is an X-linked recessive disorder in which progressive T-cell immunodeficiency is associated with eczema, small platelets, and absolute thrombocytopenia. The pathogenesis of this disorder is associated with aberrant expression of the CD43 molecule.[472] This disorder is reviewed in detail in Chapters 25 and 43. Like SCID, matched sibling allogeneic SCT was first undertaken in children with SCID in the late 1960s, and full correction of the disorder was reported in 1978.[473] Both TBI- and busulfan-based regimens have successfully been used in conditioning patients with Wiskott-Aldrich syndrome.[59, 460, 474–476] The overall outcome (almost 90% DFS) of this group of patients is among the best of any patient cohort undergoing allogeneic SCT.[59, 460, 474–476] This has led to extension of this approach to the use of mismatched family donors and UDs. Although it clearly offers an option for patients without an appropriate sibling donor, this experience has been less successful, with significant problems related to graft rejection and the development of post-transplant B-cell lymphoproliferative disease.[474, 477] Nonetheless, the salutary effects of splenectomy on quality of life and survival suggest that careful attention must be paid to such conservative treatment until outcome after alternative donor improves.[476]

Inherited Hematopoietic Disorders

Thalassemia

Until 20 years ago, Cooley's anemia was managed solely by red cell transfusion (see Chapter 21) Only 50% of patients survived to age 15, and few, if any, survived beyond age 25.[478] Although hypertransfusion regimens initiated in the 1960s virtually abolished both mortality directly related to severe anemia and bony deformity due to marrow expansion, fatality due to iron overload persisted.[478] Acquisition of blood-borne infection became an additional risk. The advent of subcutaneously administered iron chelation with desferrioxamine in the 1970s substantially altered the fatal course of transfusional hemosiderosis. Hypertransfusion and chelation have been demonstrated to prolong cardiac DFS in patients with effective iron chelation.[479–483] Although strongly suggestive that patients with thalassemia who comply with routine self-administration of desferrioxamine will remain free of cardiac and other iron-related toxicity for at least 1 to 2 decades, follow-up is insufficient to assess either the long-term efficacy or toxicity.

The successful application of SCT as an alternative treatment for thalassemia major was first reported in 1982.[484,485] Subsequently, a very large experience reported by Lucarelli and coworkers has unquestionably established the feasibility of SCT for thalassemia, with EFS hovering around 75%.[57] Portal fibrosis,[58, 486, 487] hepatomegaly, and history of inadequate chelation have been used to define a class of patients with poor outcome, although the generalizability of these findings is unclear because of the highly selected patient groups analyzed.[58, 486, 487] Nonetheless, older patients, those with more extensive hepatic damage, and those with more frequent transfusions appear to fare worse.[486, 488, 489] Both TBI- and busulfan-based conditioning have been employed successfully.[57] In addition to common causes of morbidity and mortality, rejection followed by persistence or recurrence of host (thalassemic) hematopoiesis remains a cause of treatment failure. Thus, although matched SCT is undoubtedly efficacious, the decision to pursue conservative chelation programs versus allogeneic BMT remains difficult for individual patients with suitable matched sibling donors. Only two cases of matched UD BMT have been reported. In both cases, the graft was rejected and thalassemia recurred.[57]

Sickle Cell Disease

Because the clinical course of SCD is highly variable, application of SCT as a treatment modality has been relatively slow to gain widespread acceptance. Debate about the factors necessary to identify candidates is vigorous and centers on defining markers of severity, delineating prognostic factors, evaluating potential synergistic damage to end organs already damaged by SCD, and the relative merits of alternative treatments such as hydroxyurea.[490, 491] In addition, the frequency with which parental consent for such a procedure would be given has been assessed, and it is clear that there is significant resistance to such a potentially morbid approach.[492] Furthermore, probability calculations applied to a review of the records of 143 children with SCD suggests, based on sibling number and exclusion of affected siblings, that only 18% of patients would have an appropriate sibling donor.

Nonetheless, several substantial series, as well as case reports, of BMT for SCD are found in the literature.[493-499] Overall, survival is good with resolution of vascular crises, with hemolysis, and with evidence of correction of prior splenic reticuloendothelial dysfunction.[495, 500] Expected rates of both acute and chronic GVHD have been observed. Neurologic complications, both hemorrhage and seizure, have been reported and may be increased in frequency particularly in patients with antecedent history of CNS complications.[497-499] Insufficient data exist to address long-term end organ function and survival of transplanted SCD patients.

Fanconi's Anemia

Fanconi's anemia is an autosomal recessive disorder clinically characterized by a highly variable physical phenotype, progressive marrow failure, and a marked propensity to develop AML and certain solid tumors (see Chapter 7). Although patients with Fanconi's anemia may exhibit excessive toxicity after exposure to alkylating agents, including cyclosporine and irradiation, development of specialized conditioning regimens has spurred the application of SCT as a treatment option.[501-508] In addition to successful BMT, the first reported UCB transplant was successfully undertaken for a child with Fanconi's anemia using UCB cells of an HLA-identical sibling.[118] A large retrospective of 199 patients reported to the IBMTR demonstrates a 2-year probability of survival of 66% after HLA-identical sibling BMT and 29% after alternative donor BMT.[507] The prognostic factors examined suggested that earlier intervention resulted in improved outcome. This suggestion is supported by single center data on 18 children with Fanconi's anemia transplanted from HLA-matched siblings relatively early in their disease course, with a DFS at 2 years of 95%.[504] In contrast, this center had very poor outcome using alternative donors (Harris

RE: personal communication, 1996). Because other data also support this poor outcome when alternative donors are selected, the best course of therapy for patients lacking an unaffected, matched sibling donor remains unclear.[381, 505, 507, 508] The advent of potential gene therapy options further muddies this issue (see Chapter 6). In addition, long-term follow-up to assess the effect of both radiation-based and non–radiation-based regimens on subsequent chimerism, hematologic malignancy, and risk for nonhematologic malignancy will define the true success of SCT as a therapy.

Diamond-Blackfan Anemia

Diamond-Blackfan anemia is a rare, heritable marrow failure syndrome. Patients are generally diagnosed in the first months of life, often exhibit macrocytosis and reticulocytopenia, and most frequently have a bone marrow exhibiting a selective decrease in erythroid precursors (see Chapter 7). Although approximately two thirds of patients initially respond to corticosteroids, significant numbers either fail to respond or lose response over time.[509] The toxicity of treatment, whether the sequelae of chronic transfusion or corticosteroid use, is significant.[509] In addition, the potential for development of leukemia in early to mid adulthood appears significant.[509] For these reasons, allogeneic SCT has been explored as a therapeutic option. Eighteen of 23 patients (78%) reported individually or to registries engrafted and are long-term survivors.[510-514]

Granulocyte and Platelet Disorders

Limited numbers of patients with many different disorders of myeloid function and number have had successful reconstitution of hematopoietic function by allogeneic SCT (Table 8–8 and specific diseases in Chapter 22). In general, patients were transplanted with BU/CY, although TBI-based regimens have also been used. The decision to transplant has resided in evaluation of the relative toxicity and benefit profiles of available treatment options.[515] For example, symptomatic improvement of patients with chronic granulomatous disease treated with γ-interferon, as well as potential for gene therapy, will decrease the already limited numbers of such patients considering SCT. The advent of cytokine therapy has also changed the outlook for many of the neutropenic disorders, most dramatically for patients with Kostmann's syndrome.[516] Nonetheless, both matched and mismatched SCT remain options for patients with high-risk diseases such as CD11/18 deficiency and Chédiak-Higashi syndrome or

Table 8–8. WHITE BLOOD CELL DISORDERS TREATED WITH STEM CELL TRANSPLANTATION

Chédiak-Higashi syndrome
Kostmann's syndrome
Chronic granulomatous disease
CD11/18 deficiency (leukocyte adhesion deficiency)
Neutrophil actin defects
Shwachman-Diamond syndrome

who have poor response to more conservative treatment.[21, 460, 515, 517]

Similarly, but in even smaller numbers, allogeneic SCT has successfully corrected platelet number and function in patients with congenital platelet disorders (see specific diseases in Chapter 43). Because other therapeutic options are limited, consideration of both matched and alternative donor SCT for disorders such as amegakaryocytic thrombocytopenia and Glanzmann's thrombasthenia is warranted.[382, 518, 519]

Osteopetrosis

This rare disorder results from dysfunction of osteoclasts with resulting inability to resorb and remodel bone and subsequent formation of excessive mineralized osteoid and cartilage. In addition to encroachment on optic and other cranial nerve foramina, eradication of the marrow space ensues. Thus, progressive neurologic and hematologic dysfunction develop early in childhood.[520] Studies in osteopetrotic mice revealed that the phenotype was reversed by engraftment of marrow from normal animals.[521] These and other studies confirmed that osteoclasts were macrophages with specialized functions, thus explaining the potential efficacy of SCT, demonstrated in subsequent human trials.[460, 520] Both busulfan- and TBI-based regimens have been used, and significant problems in engraftment have been described, attributed in part to disruption of the underlying marrow microenvironment. However, most failures have been associated with the use of T cell–depleted, histoincompatible grafts, which are themselves risk factors for graft failure.[460, 520] Several cases of hypercalcemia occurring in the first months after SCT have been described, and appropriate monitoring and plans for treatment of this complication should be part of any SCT for this disorder.[520, 522] Trials of novel therapeutics such as interferon-γ and macrophage colony-stimulating factor have suggested that they may have some activity in this disease but have not shown true reversal of the phenotype.[523] Because neurologic damage occurs early and is rarely reversible, the decision to proceed to SCT should be made rapidly. Depending on the future success of the ongoing efforts to explore the efficacy of cytokines, such a decision may include a prior trial of alternative therapy.

Storage Disorders

Disruption of cellular and then organ function secondary to substrate accumulation from an underlying enzymatic deficiency characterize the storage disorders (see Chapter 38). The rationale for SCT as a therapeutic maneuver rests on the belief that the most affected cell population (e.g., macrophages in Gaucher's disease) can be replaced by normal cells or that sufficient transfer of enzyme/enzyme-replete cells to affected cells and tissues will reverse existing and prevent subsequent damage. Historically, few treatment options other than palliative and supportive modalities have been available. More recently, availability of alglucer-

Table 8–9. STORAGE DISORDERS TREATED WITH STEM CELL TRANSPLANTATION

Hurler's syndrome
Hunter's syndrome
Sanfilippo's syndrome
Adrenoleukodystrophy
Metachromatic leukodystrophy
Globoid cell leukodystrophy (Krabbe's disease)
Maroteaux-Lamy syndrome
Gaucher's disease
Niemann-Pick disease
Wolman's disease
Glycogen storage disease (type II, Pompe's disease)
Farber's disease
Fucosidosis
I-cell disease
Mannosidosis
Morquio's disease
Batten disease

ase (Ceredase) enzyme infusion has dramatically altered the course of patients with Gaucher's disease.[524] Although similar inroads have not yet been made in other diseases, the concepts of gene transfer and somatic cell therapy as well as infusion of enzymes produced by recombinant techniques are being investigated in various animal models of such diseases.

Several excellent reviews of the results of SCT for specific storage disorders have been published.[60, 525–531] The rationale for SCT remains debatable for most of these diseases (Table 8–9). First, the capacity for repair or arrest of damage to affected organ systems, especially the CNS, remains unproven for many disorders. Evidence of efficacy in this regard is accumulating for some disorders, such as Maroteaux-Lamy syndrome, Sanfilippo's syndrome type B, metachromatic leukodystrophy, and globoid cell leukodystrophy.[60, 525–527, 532, 533] Second, availability of donors is a significant issue in all genetic issues, because siblings may also be homozygotes and heterozygotes for the defective gene. Although transplantation from a heterozygote for β-thalassemia is therapeutic, transplantation from a donor with limited enzyme levels may be less effective in patients with storage disorders. Acceptable levels of heterozygosity have not been well defined.[527, 529, 531] Third, the degree of damage present at the time of SCT will also color outcome. Attempts to define the appropriate evaluation of the patient before and after SCT are also underway.[60, 526, 527, 529, 531] Fourth, the relative risks of allogeneic SCT are more difficult to measure against the uncertain therapeutic gain of SCT for many of these disorders, making decisions, especially regarding the use of alternative donors, particularly difficult. Alternative donors have been used for patients with a variety of storage disorders.[21, 527] In general, the peri-SCT mortality has been significantly greater.

References

1. Osgood EE, Riddle MC, Mathews TJ: Aplastic anemia treated with daily transfusions and intravenous marrow; case report. Ann Intern Med 1939; 13:357.
2. Jacobson LO, Marks EK, et al: Role of the spleen in radiation injury. Proc Soc Exp Biol Med 1949; 70:7440.

3. Jacobson LO, Simmons EL, et al: Recovery from radiation injury. Science 1951; 113:510.

4. Ford CE, Hamerton JL, et al: Cytological identification of radiation-chimaeras. Nature 1956; 177:452.

5. Barnes DWH, Loutit JF: The radiation recovery factor: preservation by the Polge-Smith-Parkes techniques. J Natl Cancer Inst 1955; 15:901.

6. Barnes DWH, Loutit JF: Spleen protection: the cellular hypothesis. In Bacq ZM, Alexander P (eds): Radiobiology Symposium 1954. New York, Academic Press, 1954, pp 134–135.

7. Uphoff DE: Genetic factors influencing irradiation protection by bone marrow: I. The F1 hybrid effect. J Natl Cancer Inst 1958; 19:123.

8. Uphoff DE: Alteration of homograft reaction by A-methopterin in lethally irradiated mice treated with homologous marrow. Proc Soc Exp Biol Med 1958; 99:651.

9. Thomas ED, Lochte HL, Jr, et al: Intravenous infusion of bone marrow in patients receiving radiation and chemotherapy. N Engl J Med 1957; 257:491.

10. Thomas ED, Lochte HL, Jr., et al: Supralethal whole body irradiation and isologous marrow transplantation in man. J Clin Invest 1959; 38:1709.

11. Bach FH, Albertini RJ, et al: Bone marrow transplantation in a patient with the Wiskott-Aldrich syndrome. Lancet 1968; 2:1364.

12. de Koning J, van Bekkum DW, et al: Transplantation of bone marrow cells and fetal thymus in an infant with lymphopenic immunological deficiency. Lancet 1969; 1:1223.

13. Good RA, Meuwissen HJ, et al: Bone marrow transplantation: correction of immune deficit in lymphopenic immunologic deficiency and correction of an immunologically induced pancytopenia. Trans Assoc Am Physicians 1969; 82:278.

14. Good RA, Gatti A, et al: Successful marrow transplantation for correction of immunological deficit in lymphopenic agammaglobulinemia and treatment of immunologically induced pancytopenia. Exp Hematol 1969; 19:4.

15. Bortin MM, Bach FH, et al: 25th anniversary of the first successful allogeneic bone marrow transplants. Bone Marrow Transplant 1994; 14:211.

16. Beatty PG, Clift RA, et al: Marrow transplantation from related donors other than HLA-identical siblings. N Engl J Med 1985; 313:765.

17. Anasetti C, Amos D, et al: Effect of HLA compatibility on engraftment of bone marrow transplants in patients with leukemia or lymphoma. N Engl J Med 1989; 320:197.

18. Armitage JO: Bone marrow transplantation. N Engl J Med 1994; 330:827.

19. Mentzer WC, Heller S, et al: Availability of related donors for bone marrow transplantation in sickle cell anemia. Am J Hematol Oncol 1994; 16:27.

20. Champlin R, Coppo P, Howe C: National marrow donor program: progress and challenges. Bone Marrow Transplant 1993; 33:567.

21. Kernan NA, Bartsch G, et al: Analysis of 462 transplantation from unrelated donors facilitated by the national marrow donor program. N Engl J Med 1993; 328:593.

22. Anasetti C, Etzioni R, et al: Marrow transplantation from unrelated volunteer donors. Annu Rev Med 1995; 46:169.

23. Wagner JE, Kernan NA, et al: Allogeneic sibling umbilical-cord-blood transplantation in children with malignant and nonmalignant disease. Lancet 1995; 346:214.

24. Rubinstein P, Rosenfield RE, et al: Stored placental blood for unrelated bone marrow reconstitution. Blood 1993; 81:1679.

25. Kurtzberg J, Laughlin M, et al: Placental blood as a source of hematopoietic stem cells for transplantation into unrelated recipients. N Engl J Med 1996; 335:157.

26. Bradstock KF, Coles R, et al: Fatal obstructive airways disease after bone marrow transplantation. Transplant Proc 1984; 16:1034.

27. Brenner MK, Rill DR, et al: Gene-marking to trace origin of relapse after autologous bone-marrow transplantation. Lancet 1993; 341:85.

28. Brenner MK, Rill DR, et al: Gene marking to determine whether autologous marrow infusion restores long-term haemopoiesis in cancer patients. Lancet 1993; 342:1134.

29. Rill DR, Buschle M, et al: Retrovirus-mediated gene transfer as an approach to analyze neuroblastoma relapse after autologous bone marrow transplantation. Hum Gene Ther 1992; 3:129.

30. Rill DR, Moen RC, et al: An approach for the analysis of relapse and marrow reconstitution after autologous marrow transplantation using retrovirus-mediated gene transfer. Blood 1992; 79:2694.

31. Deisseroth AB, Kantarjian H, et al: Use of two retroviral markers to test relative contribution of marrow and peripheral blood autologous cells to recovery after preparative therapy. The University of Texas M.D. Anderson Cancer Center, Division of Medicine. Hum Gene Ther 1993; 4:71.

32. Wilson JM, Grossman M: Therapeutic strategies for familial hypercholesterolemia based on somatic gene transfer. Am J Cardiol 1993; 72:59D. Review.

33. Culver KW: Clinical applications of gene therapy for cancer. Clin Chem 1994; 40:510. Review.

34. Blaese RM, Culver KW: Gene therapy for primary immunodeficiency. Immunodefic Rev 1992; 3:329.

35. Kohn DB, Weinberg KI, et al: Gene therapy for neonates with ADA-deficient SCID by retroviral-mediated transfer of the human ADA cDNA into umbilical cord CD34+ cells. Blood 1993; 82:315a.

36. Hoogerbrugge PM, Beusecchem VV, et al: Gene therapy in 3 children with adenosine deaminase deficiency. Blood 1993; 82:315a.

37. Mathé G, Jammet H, et al: Transfusions et greffes de moelle osseuse homologue chez des humains irradiés à haute dause accidentellement. Rev Fr Etudes Clin Biol 1959; 4:226.

38. Santos GW: History of bone marrow transplantation. Clin Haematol 1983; 12:611.

39. Thomas ED, Buckner CD, et al: Allogeneic marrow grafting for hematological malignancy using HLA-A matched donor-recipient sibling pairs. Blood 1971; 38:267.

40. Santos GW, Sensenbrenner LL, et al: Marrow transplantation in man following cyclophosphamide. Transplant Proc 1971; 3:400.

41. Graw RG Jr, Yankee RA, et al: Bone marrow transplantation from HL-A matched donors to patient with acute leukemia: toxicity and antileukemic effect. Transplantation 1972; 14:79.

42. Thomas ED, Storb R, et al: Bone marrow transplantation. N Engl J Med 1975; 16:832–843, 895–902.

43. Tutschka PJ, Santos GW, Elfenbein GJ: Marrow transplantation in acute leukemia following busulfan and cyclophosphamide. Blut 1980; 25:375.

44. Thomas E, Clift R, et al: Marrow transplantation for acute nonlymphoblastic leukemia in first remission using fractionated or single dose irradiation. Int J Radiat Oncol Biol Phys 1982; 8:817.

45. Deeg H, Sullivan K, et al: Marrow transplantation for ANLL in first remission: Toxicity and long-term follow-up of patients conditioned with single dose or fractionated total body irradiation. Bone Marrow Transplant 1986; 1:151.

46. Buckner C, Clift R, et al: A randomized trial of 12 or 15.75 Gy of total body irradiation (TBI) in patients with ANLL and CML followed by marrow transplantation. Exp Hematol 1989; 17:522.

47. Clift R, Buckner C, et al: Allogeneic marrow transplantation in patients with chronic myeloid leukemia in the chronic phase: a randomized trial of two irradiation regimens. Blood 1991; 77:1660.

48. Kamani N, Bayever E, et al: Fractionated total-body irradiation preceding high-dose cytosine arabinoside as a preparative regimen for bone marrow transplantation in children with acute leukemia. Med Pediatr Oncol 1995; 25:179.

49. Brochstein JA, Kernan NA, et al: Allogeneic bone marrow transplantation after hyperfractionated total-body irradiation and cyclophosphamide in children with acute leukemia. N Engl J Med 1987; 317:1618.

50. Blume KG, Forman SJ, et al: Total body irradiation and high dose etoposide: a new preparatory regimen for bone marrow transplantation in patients with advanced hematologic malignancies. Blood 1987; 69:1015.

51. Santos GW, Tutschka PJ, et al: Marrow transplantation for acute nonlymphocytic leukemia after treatment with busulfan and cyclophosphamide. N Engl J Med 1983; 309:1347.

52. Santos GW: Antonio Raichs lecture. Autologous bone marrow transplantation. Sangre 1992; 37:471.

53. Yeager AM, Kaizer H, et al: Autologous bone marrow transplantation in patients with acute nonlymphocytic leukemia using *ex vivo* marrow treatment with 4-hydroperoxycyclophosphamide. N Engl J Med 1986; 315:141.

54. Beelen DW, Quabeck K, et al: Acute toxicity and first clinical results of intensive postinduction therapy using a modified busulfan and cyclophosphamide regimen with autologous bone marrow rescue in first remission of acute myeloid leukemia. Blood 1989; 74:1507.

55. Copelan EA, Biggs JC, et al: Treatment for acute myelocytic leukemia with allogeneic bone marrow transplantation following preparation with BuCy2. Blood 1991; 78:838.

56. Tutschka PJ, Copelan EA, Klein JP: Bone marrow transplantation for leukemia following a new busulfan and cyclophosphamide regimen. Blood 1987; 70:1382.

57. Lucarelli G, Clift RA: Bone marrow transplantation in thalassemia. In Forman SJ, Blume KG, Thomas ED (eds): Bone Marrow Transplantation. Boston, Blackwell Scientific Publications, 1994, pp 829–838.

58. Lucarelli G, Galimberti M, et al: Bone marrow transplantation in patients with thalassemia. N Engl J Med 1990; 322:417.

59. Rimm IJ, Rappeport JM: Bone marrow transplantation for the Wiskott-Aldrich syndrome. Transplantation 1990; 50:617.

60. Hoogerbrugge PM, Brouwer OF, et al: Allogeneic bone marrow transplantation for lysosomal storage diseases. Lancet 1995; 345:1398.

61. Blanche S, Caniglia M, et al: Treatment of hemophagocytic lymphohistiocytosis with chemotherapy and bone marrow transplantation: a single-center study of 22 cases. Blood 1991; 78:51.

62. Blume KG, Kopecky KJ, et al: A prospective randomized comparison of total body irradiation etoposide versus busulfan-cyclophosphamide as preparatory regimens for bone marrow transplantation in patients with leukemia who were not in first remission: a Southwest Oncology Group study. Blood 1993; 81:2187.

63. Clift RA, Buckner CD, et al: Marrow transplantation for chronic myeloid leukemia: a randomized study comparing cyclophosphamide and total body irradiation with busulfan and cyclophosphamide. Blood 1994; 84:2036.

64. Ringden O, Ruutu T, et al: A randomized trial comparing busulfan with total body irradiation as conditioning in allogeneic marrow transplant recipients with leukemia: a report from the Nordic Bone Marrow Tranplantation Group. Blood 1994; 83:2723.

65. Devergie A, Blaise D, et al: Allogeneic bone marrow transplantation for chronic myeloid leukemia in first chronic phase: a randomized trial of busulfan-cytoxan versus cytoxan-total body irradiation as preparative regimen: a report from the French Society of Bone Marrow Graft (SFGM). Blood 1995; 85:2263.

66. Blaise D, Maraninchi D, et al: Allogeneic bone marrow transplantation for acute myeloid leukemia in first remission: a randomized trial of a busulfan-cytoxan versus cytoxan-total body irradiation as preparative regimen: a report from the Groupe d'Etudes de la Greffe de Moelle Osseuse. Blood 1992; 79:2578.

67. Michel G, Gluckman E, et al: Allogeneic bone marrow transplantation for children with acute myeloblastic leukemia in first complete remission: impact of conditioning regimen without total-body irradiation—a report from the Société Francaise de Greffe de Moelle. J Clin Oncol 1994; 12:1217.

68. Hassan M, Ljungman P, et al: Busulfan bioavailability. Blood 1994; 84:2144.

69. Grochow LB, Krivit W, et al: Busulfan disposition in children. Blood 1990; 75:1723.

70. Yeager AM, Wagner JE, Jr., et al: Optimization of busulfan dosage in children undergoing bone marrow transplantation: a pharmacokinetic study of dose escalation. Blood 1992; 80:2425.

71. Vassal G, Deroussent A, et al: Is 600 mg/m² the appropriate dosage of busulfan in children undergoing bone marrow transplantation? Blood 1992; 79:2475.

72. Shaw PJ, Scharping CE, et al: Busulfan pharmacokinetics using a single daily high-dose regimen in children with acute leukemia. Blood 1994; 84:2357.

73. Shank B: Can total body irradiation be supplanted by busulfan in cytoreductive regimens for bone marrow transplantation. Int J Radiat Oncol Biol Phys 1994; 31:195.

74. Spitzer TR, Peters C, et al: Etoposide in combination with cyclophosphamide and total body irradiation or busulfan as conditioning for marrow transplantation in adults and children. Int J Radiat Oncol Biol Phys 1994; 29:39.

75. Grochow LB, Jones RJ, et al: Pharmacokinetics of busulfan: correlation with veno-occlusive disease in patients undergoing bone marrow transplantation. Cancer Chemother Pharmacol 1989; 25:55.

76. Chao NJ, Forman SJ, et al: Allogeneic bone marrow transplantation for high-risk acute lymphoblastic leukemia during first complete remission. Blood 1991; 78:1923.

77. Brown RA, Wolff SN, et al: High-dose etoposide, cyclophosphamide, and total body irradiation with allogeneic bone marrow transplantation for patients with acute myeloid leukemia in untreated first relapse: a study by the North American Marrow Transplant Group. Blood 1995; 85:1391.

78. Petersen FB, Lynch MHE, et al: Autologous marrow transplantation for patients with acute myeloid leukemia in untreated first relapse or in second complete remission. J Clin Oncol 1993; 11:1353.

79. Petersen FB, Buckner CD, et al: Etoposide, cyclophosphamide and fractionated total body irradiation as a preparative regimen for marrow transplantation in patients with advanced hematological malignancies: a phase I study. Bone Marrow Transplant 1992; 10:83.

80. Krance RA, Forman SJ, Blume KG: Total-body irradiation and high-dose teniposide: a pilot study in bone marrow transplantation for patients with relapsed acute lymphoblastic leukemia. Cancer Treat Rep 1987; 71:645.

81. Coccia PF, Strandjord SE, et al: High-dose cytosine arabinoside and fractionated total-body irradiation: an improved preparative regimen for bone marrow transplantation of children with acute lymphoblastic leukemia. Blood 1988; 71:888.

82. Bostrom B, Brunning RD, et al: Bone marrow transplantation for acute nonlymphocytic leukemia in first remission: analysis of prognostic factors. Blood 1985; 65:1191.

83. Petersen FB, Deeg HJ, et al: Marrow transplantation following escalating doses of fractionated total body irradiation and cyclophosphamide—a phase I trial. Int J Radiat Oncol Biol Phys 1992; 23:1027.

84. Chao NJ, Stein AS, et al: Busulfan/etoposide—initial experience with a new preparatory regimen for autologous bone marrow transplantation in patients with acute nonlymphoblastic leukemia. Blood 1993; 81:319.

85. Linker CA, Ries CA, et al: Autologous bone marrow transplantation for acute myeloid leukemia using busulfan plus etoposide as a preparative regimen. Blood 1993; 81:311.

86. Ayash LJ, Antman K, Cheson BD: A perspective on dose-intensive therapy with autologous bone marrow transplantation for solid tumors. Oncology 1991; 5:25.

87. Dicke KA, Spitzer G: Evaluation of the use of high-dose cytoreduction with autologous marrow rescue in various malignancies. Transplantation 1986; 41:4.

88. Cheson BD, Lacerna L, et al: Autologous bone marrow transplantation. Ann Intern Med 1989; 110:51.

89. Jin NR, Hill RS, et al: Marrow harvesting for autologous marrow transplantation. Exp Hematol 1985; 13:879.

90. Lasky LC, Bostrom B, et al: Clinical collection and use of peripheral blood stem cells in pediatric patients. Transplantation 1989; 47:613.

91. Negrin RS, Kusnierz-Glaz CR, et al: Transplantation of enriched and purged peripheral blood progenitor cells from a single apheresis product in patients with non-Hodgkin's lymphoma. Blood 1995; 85:3334.

92. Ross AA, Cooper BW, et al: Detection and viability of tumor cells in peripheral blood stem cell collections from breast cancer patients using immunocytochemical and clonogenic assay techniques. Blood 1993; 82:2605.

93. Gribben JG, Neuberg D, et al: Detection by polymerase chain reaction of residual cells with the bcl-2 translocation is associated with increased risk of relapse after autologous bone marrow transplantation for B-cell lymphoma. Blood 1993; 81:3449.

94. Moss TJ, Cairo M, et al: Clonogenicity of circulating neuro-

blastoma cells: implications regarding peripheral blood stem cell transplantation. Blood 1994; 83:3085.

95. Passos-Coelho JL, Ross AA, et al: Absence of breast cancer cells in a single-day peripheral blood progenitor cell collection after priming with cyclophosphamide and granulocyte-macrophage colony-stimulating factor. Blood 1995; 85:1138.

96. Hoffman R, Murray L: Biology and mobilization of peripheral blood mononuclear cell grafts. Hematol Oncol Ann 1994; 2:21.

97. Haas R, Mohle R, Fruhauf S, et al: Patient characteristics associated with successful mobilizing and autografting of peripheral blood progenitor cells in malignant lymphoma. Blood 1994; 83:3787.

98. Tricot G, Jagannath S, et al: Peripheral blood stem cell transplants for multiple myeloma: identification of favorable variables for rapid engraftment in 255 patients. Blood 1995; 85:588.

99. O'Day SJ, Rabinowe SN, et al: A phase II study of continuous infusion recombinant human granulocyte-macrophage colony-stimulating factor as an adjunct to autologous bone marrow transplantation for patients with non-Hodgkin's lymphoma in first remission. Blood 1994; 83:2707.

100. Freedman A, Neuberg D, et al: CHOP dose intensification with G-CSF in untreated advanced follicular lymphoma patients markedly depletes stem cell reserve for ABMT. Blood 1995; 86(Suppl 1):212a.

101. Domenech J, Linassier C, et al: Prolonged impairment of hematopoiesis after high-dose therapy followed by autologous bone marrow transplantation. Blood 1995; 85:3320.

102. Traweek ST, Slovak ML, et al: Clonal karyotypic hematopoietic cell abnormalities occurring after autologous bone marrow transplantation for Hodgkin's disease and non-Hodgkin's lymphoma. Blood 1994; 84:957.

103. Stone RM: Myelodysplastic syndrome after autologous transplantation for lymphoma: the price of progress? Blood 1994; 83:3437.

104. Miller JS, Arthur DC, et al: Myelodysplastic syndrome after autologous bone marrow transplantation: an additional late complication of curative cancer therapy. Blood 1994; 83:3780.

105. Chao NJ, Nademanee AP, et al: Importance of bone marrow cytogenetic evaluation before autologous bone marrow transplantation for Hodgkin's disease. J Clin Oncol 1991; 9:1575.

106. den Haan JM, Sherman NE, et al: Identification of a graft versus host disease–associated human minor histocompatibility antigen. Science 1995; 268:1476.

107. Goulmy E, Schipper R, et al: Mismatches of minor histocompatibility antigens between HLA-identical donors and recipients and the development of graft-versus-host disease after bone marrow transplantation. N Engl J Med 1996; 334:281.

108. Terasaki PI, McClelland JD: Microdroplet assay of human serum cytotoxins. Nature 1964; 204:998.

109. Yunis EJ, Amos DB: Three closely linked genetic systems relevant to transplantation. Proc Natl Acad Sci U S A 1971; 68:3031.

110. Dupont B, Hansen JA, et al: Typing for MLC determinants by means of LD-homozygous and LD-heterozygous test cells. Transplant Proc 1973; 5:1543.

111. Yang SY, Morishima Y, et al: Comparison of one dimensional IEF patterns for serologically detectable HLA-A and HLA-B allotypes. Immunogenetics 1984; 19:217.

112. Gale RP, Feig S, et al: ABO blood group system and bone marrow transplantation. Blood 1977; 50:185.

113. Jin N-R, Hill R, Segal G: Preparation of red-blood-cell–depleted marrow for ABO-incompatible marrow transplantation by density-gradient separation using the IBM 2991 blood cell processor. Exp Hematol 1987; 15:93.

114. Butterworth VA, Simmons RG, et al: Psychosocial effects of unrelated bone marrow donation: experiences of the national marrow donor program. Blood 1993; 81:1947.

115. Goldman J: Peripheral blood stem cells for allografting. Blood 1995; 85:1413.

116. Schmitz N, Dreger P, et al: Primary transplantation of allogeneic peripheral blood progenitor cells mobilized by filgrastim (granulocyte colony-stimulating factor). Blood 1995; 85:1666.

117. Korbling M, Przepiorka D, et al: Allogeneic blood stem cell transplantation for refractory leukemia and lymphoma: potential advantage of blood over marrow allografts. Blood 1995; 85:1659.

118. Gluckman E, Broxmeyer HE, et al: Hematopoietic reconstitution in a patient with Fanconi's anemia by means of umbilical cord blood from an HLA-identical sibling. N Engl J Med 1989; 321:1174.

119. Bertolini F, Lazzari L, et al: Comparative study of different procedures for the collection and banking of umbilical cord blood. J Hematother 1995; 4:29.

120. van Leeuwen JEM, van Tol MJD, et al: Persistence of host-type hematopoiesis after allogeneic bone marrow transplantation for leukemia is significantly related to the recipient's age and/or the conditioning regimen, but it is not associated with an increased risk of relapse. Blood 1994; 83:3059.

121. Hill RS, Petersen FB, et al: Mixed hematologic chimerism after allogeneic marrow transplantation for severe aplastic anemia is associated with a higher risk of graft rejection and a lessened incidence of acute graft-versus-host disease. Blood 1986; 67:811.

122. Petit T, Raynal B, et al: Highly sensitive polymerase chain reaction methods show the frequent survival of residual recipient multipotent progenitors after non–T-cell–depleted bone marrow transplantation. Blood 1994; 84:3575.

123. Mackinnon S, Barnett L, et al: Minimal residual disease is more common in patients who have mixed T-cell chimerism after bone marrow transplantation for chronic myelogenous leukemia. Blood 1994; 83:3409.

124. Bertheas MF, Lafage M, et al: Influence of mixed chimerism on the results of allogeneic bone marrow transplantation for leukemia. Blood 1991; 78:3103.

125. Roux E, Helg C, et al: Evolution of mixed chimerism after allogeneic bone marrow transplantation as determined on granulocytes and mononuclear cells by the polymerase chain reaction. Blood 1992; 79:2775.

126. Locatelli F, Zecca M, et al: Pilot trial of combined administration of erythropoietin and granulocyte colony-stimulating factor to children undergoing allogeneic bone marrow transplantation. Bone Marrow Transplant 1994; 14:929.

127. Tsuchiya S, Minegishi M, et al: Allogeneic bone marrow transplantation for malignant hematologic disorders in children. Tohoku J Exp Med 1992; 168:345.

128. Masaoka T, Takaku F, et al: Recombinant human granulocyte colony-stimulating factor in allogeneic bone marrow transplantation. Exp Hematol 1989; 17:1047.

129. Powles R, Smith C, et al: Human recombinant GM-CSF in allogeneic bone marrow transplant for leukemia: double blind placebo controlled trial. Lancet 1990; 336:1417.

130. Schriber JR, Chao NJ, et al: Granulocyte colony-stimulating factor after allogeneic bone marrow transplantation. Blood 1994; 84:1680.

131. Nemunaitis J, Buckner CD, et al: Phase I/II trial of recombinant granulocyte-macrophage colony stimulating factor following allogeneic bone marrow transplantation. Blood 1991; 77:2065.

132. Nemunaitis J, Anasetti C, et al: Phase II trial of recombinant human granulocyte-macrophage colony-stimulating factor in patients undergoing allogeneic bone marrow transplantation from unrelated donors. Blood 1992; 79:2572.

133. Aversa F, Tabilio A, et al: Successful engraftment of T-cell–depleted haploidentical "three-loci" incompatible transplants in leukemia patients by addition of recombinant human granulocyte colony-stimulating factor–mobilized peripheral blood progenitor cells to bone marrow inoculum. Blood 1994; 84:3948.

134. Anderson KC, Goodnough LT, Sayers M: Variation in blood component irradiation practice: implications for prevention of transfusion-associated graft-versus-host disease. Blood 1991; 77:2096.

135. Leitman SF, Holland PV: Irradiation of blood products. Indications and guidelines. Transfusion 1985; 25:293.

136. Greenbaum BH: Transfusion-associated graft-versus-host disease: historical perspectives, incidence, and current use of irradiated blood products. J Clin Oncol 1991; 9:1889.

137. Adler SP: Cytomegalovirus and transfusions. Transfus Med Rev 1988; 2:235.

138. Slichter SJ: Principles of transfusion support before and after bone marrow transplantation. In Forman SJ, Blume KG, Thomas ED (eds): Bone Marrow Transplantation. Cambridge, Mass., Blackwell Scientific Publications, Inc., 1994, p 273.

139. Bowden RA, Slichter SJ, et al: Use of leukocyte-depleted plate-

lets and cytomegalovirus-seronegative red blood cells for prevention of primary cytomegalovirus infection after marrow transplant. Blood 1991; 78:246.

140. Aderka D, Praff G, et al: Bleeding due to thrombocytopenia in acute leukemias and re-evaluation of the prophylactic platelet transfusion policy. Am J Med Sci 1986; 291:147.

141. Gmur J, Burger J, et al: Safety of stringent prophylactic platelet transfusion policy for patients with acute leukemia. Lancet 1991; 338:1223.

142. Navari RM, Buckner CD, Clift RA: Prophylaxis of infection in patients with aplastic anemia receiving allogeneic marrow transplants. Am J Med 1984; 76:564.

143. Schimpff SC, Hahn DM, et al: Comparison of basic infection prevention techniques, with standard room reverse isolation or with reverse isolation plus added air infiltration. Leuk Res 1978; 2:231.

144. Meyers JD, Flournoy N, Thomas ED: Infection with herpes simplex virus and cell-mediated immunity after marrow transplantation. J Infect Dis 1980; 142:338.

145. Elfenbein GJ, Saral R: Infectious disease during immune recovery after bone marrow transplantation. In Allen JC (ed): Infection and the Compromised Host. Baltimore, Williams & Wilkins, 1981, pp 157–196.

146. Hann IM, Prentice HG, et al: Acyclovir prophylaxis against herpes virus infections in severely immunocompromised patients: randomized double-blind trial. BMJ 1983; 287:384.

147. Rubin M, Hathorn JW, et al: Gram-positive infections and the use of vancomycin in 550 episodes of fever and neutropenia. Ann Intern Med 1988; 108:30.

148. Lowder JN, Lazarus HM, Herzig RH: Bacteremias and fungemias in oncologic patients with central venous catheters: changing spectrum of infection. Arch Intern Med 1982; 142:1456.

149. Karp JE, Dick JD, et al: Empiric use of vancomycin during prolonged treatment-induced granulocytopenia. Randomized, double-blind, placebo-controlled clinical trial in patients with acute leukemia. Am J Med 1986; 81:237.

150. Sullivan KM, Kopecky KJ, et al: Immunomodulatory and antimicrobial efficacy of intravenous immunoglobulin in bone marrow transplantation. N Engl J Med 1990; 323:705.

151. Tam JY, Blume KG, Prober CG: Fluconazole and Candida krusei fungemia. N Engl J Med 1992; 325:1315. Letter.

152. Perfect JR, Klotman ME, et al: Prophylactic intravenous amphotericin B in neutropenic autologous bone marrow transplant recipients. J Infect Dis 1992; 165:891.

153. O'Donnell MR, Schmidt GM, et al: Prophylactic low dose amphotericin B (AM-B) decreases systemic fungal infection (SFT) in allogeneic bone marrow transplant (BMT) recipients. Blood 1990; 76:558.

154. Goodman JL, Winston DJ, Greenfield RA: A controlled trial of fluconazole to prevent fungal infections in patients undergoing bone marrow transplantation. N Engl J Med 1992; 326:845.

155. Wingard JR, Merz WG, et al: Increase in Candida krusei infection among patients with bone marrow transplantation and neutropenia treated prophylactically with fluconazole. N Engl J Med 1991; 325:1274.

156. Szeluga DJ, Stuart RK, et al: Nutritional support of bone marrow transplant recipients: a prospective, randomized clinical trial comparing total parenteral nutrition to an enteral feeding program. Cancer Res 1987; 47:3309.

157. Weisdorf SA, Lysne J, Wind D: Positive effect of prophylactic total parenteral nutrition on long-term outcome of bone marrow transplantation. Transplantation 1987; 43:833.

158. Bozdech MJ, Sondel PM, et al: Transplantation of HLA-haploidentical T-cell–depleted marrow for leukemia: addition of cytosine arabinoside to the pretransplant conditioning prevents rejection. Exp Hematol 1985; 13:1201.

159. Antin J, Bierer N, et al: Selective depletion of bone marrow T lymphocytes with anti-CD5 monoclonal antibodies: effective prophylaxis for graft-versus-host disease in patients with hematologic malignancies. Blood 1991; 76:1464.

160. Mitsuyasu RT, Champlin RE, et al: Treatment of donor bone marrow with monoclonal anti–T-cell antibody and complement for the prevention of graft-versus-host disease. Ann Intern Med 1986; 105:20.

161. O'Reilly RJ, Collins NH, et al: Soybean lectin agglutination and E-rosette depletion for removal of T-cells from HLA identical marrow grafts: results in 60 consecutive patients transplanted for hematologic malignancy. In Hagenbeck A, Lowenberg B (eds): Minimal Residual Disease in Acute Leukemia. Dordrecht, The Netherlands, Nijhoff, 1986, p 37.

162. Hale G, Cobbold S, Waldmann H: T cell depletion with campath-1 in allogeneic bone marrow transplantation. Transplantation 1988; 45:753.

163. Martin PJ, Hansen JA, et al: Effects of in vitro depletion of T cells in HLA-identical allogeneic marrow grafts. Blood 1985; 66:664.

164. O'Reilly RJ, Collins NH, et al: Transplantation of marrow-depleted T cells by soybean lectin agglutination and E-rosette depletion: major histocompatibility complex–related graft resistance in leukemic transplant recipients. Transplant Proc 1985; 17:455.

165. Smith BR, Guinan EC, et al: Efficacy of a cyclophosphamide procarbazine antithymocyte serum regimen for prevention of graft rejection following marrow transplantation of transfused patients with aplastic anemia. Transplantation 1985; 39:671.

166. Gluckman E, Horowitz MM, et al: Bone marrow transplantation for severe aplastic anemia: influence of conditioning and graft-versus-host disease prophylaxis regimens on outcome. Blood 1992; 79:269.

167. Champlin RE, Horowitz MM, et al: Graft failure following bone marrow transplantation for severe aplastic anemia: risk factors and treatment results. Blood 1989; 73:606.

168. Champlin RE, Feig SA, Gale RP: Case problems in bone marrow transplantation: I. Graft failure in aplastic anemia: its biology and treatment. Exp Hematol 1984; 12:728.

169. Storb R, Doney KC, et al: Marrow transplantation with or without donor buffy coat cells for 65 transfused aplastic anemia patients. Blood 1982; 59:236.

170. Fischer A, Friedrich W, et al: Reduction of graft failure by a monoclonal antibody (anti-LFA-1-CD11a) after HLA nonidentical bone marrow transplantation in children with immunodeficiencies, osteopetrosis, and Fanconi's anemia: a European Group for Immunodeficiency/European Group for Bone Marrow Transplantation report. Blood 1991; 77:249.

171. Ganem G, Kuentz M, et al: Additional total-lymphoid irradiation in preventing graft failure of T-cell–depleted bone marrow transplantation from HLA-identical siblings. Transplantation 1988; 45:244.

172. Storb R, Etzioni R, et al: Cyclophosphamide combined with antithymocyte globulin in preparation for allogeneic marrow transplants in patients with aplastic anemia. Blood 1994; 84:941.

173. Shizuru JA, Jerabek L, et al: Transplantation of purified hematopoietic stem cells: requirements for overcoming the barriers of allogeneic engraftment. Biol Blood Marrow Transplant 1996; 2:3.

174. Soiffer RJ, Ritz J: Selective T cell depletion of donor allogeneic marrow with anti-CD6 monoclonal antibody: rationale and results. Bone Marrow Transplant 1993; 12:S7.

175. Bearman SI: The syndrome of hepatic veno-occlusive disease after marrow transplantation. Blood 1995; 85:3005.

176. Bearman SI, Appelbaum FR, et al: Regimen-related toxicity in patients undergoing bone marrow transplantation. J Clin Oncol 1988; 6:1562.

177. McDonald GB, Hinds MS, et al: Veno-occlusive disease of the liver and multiorgan failure after bone marrow transplantation: a cohort study of 355 patients. Ann Intern Med 1993; 118:255.

178. Jones RJ, Lee KSK, et al: Venocclusive disease of the liver following bone marrow transplantation. Transplantation 1987; 44:778.

179. Ayash LJ, Hunt M, et al: Hepatic veno-occlusive disease in autologous bone marrow transplantation of solid tumors and lymphomas. J Clin Oncol 1990; 8:1699.

180. Dulley FL, Kanfer EJ, et al: Venocclusive disease of the liver after chemoradiotherapy and autologous bone marrow transplantation. Transplantation 1987; 43:870.

181. Soiffer RJ, Dear K, et al: Hepatic dysfunction following T-cell depleted allogeneic bone marrow transplantation. Transplantation 1991; 52:1014.

182. Shulman HM, Fisher LB, et al: Venoocclusive disease of the liver after marrow transplantation: histological correlates of clinical signs and symptoms. Hepatology 1994; 19:1171.

183. Baglin TP, Harper P, Marcus RE: Veno-occlusive disease of the

liver complicating ABMT successfully treated with recombinant tissue plasminogen activator. Bone Marrow Transplant 1990; 5:439.

184. Bearman SI, Shuhart MC, et al: Recombinant human tissue plasminogen activator for the treatment of established severe veno-occlusive disease of the liver after bone marrow transplantation. Blood 1992; 80:2458.

185. Laporte JP, Lessage S, et al: Alteplase for hepatic veno-occlusive disease complicating bone marrow transplantation. Lancet 1992; 339:1057.

186. Rosti G, Bandini G, et al: Alteplase for hepatic veno-occlusive disease after bone-marrow transplantation. Blood 1992; 339:1481.

187. Ringden O, Wennberg L, et al: Alteplase for hepatic veno-occlusive disease after bone marrow transplantation. Lancet 1992; 340:546.

188. Gluckman E, Jolivet I, et al: Use of prostaglandin E$_1$ for prevention of liver veno-occlusive diseases in leukaemic patients treated by allogeneic bone marrow transplantation. Br J Haematol 1990; 74:277.

189. Ibrahim A, Pico JL, et al: Hepatic veno-occlusive disease following bone marrow transplantation treated by prostaglandin E$_1$. Bone Marrow Transplant 1991; 7:53.

190. Nimer SD, Milewicz AL, et al: Successful treatment of hepatic veno-occlusive disease in a bone marrow transplant patient with orthotopic liver transplantation. Transplantation 1990; 49:819.

191. Rapoport AP, Doyle HR, et al: Orthotopic liver transplantation for life-threatening veno-occlusive disease of the liver after allogeneic bone marrow transplantation. Bone Marrow Transplant 1991; 8:421.

192. Murray JA, LaBrecque DR, et al: Successful treatment of hepatic veno-occlusive disease in a bone marrow transplant patient with side-to-side portacaval shunt. Gastroenterology 1987; 92:1073.

193. Jacobson BK, Kalayoglu M: Effective early treatment of hepatic veno-occlusive disease with a central splenorenal shunt in an infant. J Pediatr Surg 1992; 27:531.

194. Ulutin ON: Antithrombotic effect and clinical potential of defibrotide. Semin Thromb Hemostas 1993; 19:186.

195. McDonald GB, Sharma P, et al: Venocclusive disease of the liver after bone marrow transplantation: diagnosis, incidence, and predisposing factors. Hepatology 1984; 4:16.

196. Ganem G, Saint-Marc Girardin M-F, et al: Venocclusive disease of the liver after allogeneic bone marrow transplantation in man. Int J Radiat Oncol Biol Phys 1988; 14:879.

197. Shulman HM, Sharma P, et al: A coded histologic study of hepatic graft-versus-host disease after human bone marrow transplantation. Hepatology 1988; 8:463.

198. Attal M, Huguet F, et al: Prevention of regimen-related toxicities after bone marrow transplantation by pentoxifylline: a prospective, randomized trial. Blood 1993; 82:732.

199. Clift RA, Bianco JA, et al: A randomized controlled trial of pentoxifylline for the prevention of regimen-related toxicities in patients undergoing allogeneic marrow transplantation. Blood 1993; 82:2025.

200. Bianco JA, Appelbaum FR, et al: Phase I–II trial of pentoxifylline for the prevention of transplant-related toxicities following bone marrow transplantation. Blood 1991; 78:1205.

201. Han J, Thompson P, Beutler B: Dexamethasone and pentoxifylline inhibit endotoxin-induced cachectin/tumor necrosis factor synthesis at separate points in the signaling pathway. J Exp Med 1990; 172:391.

202. Bearman SI, Shen DD, et al: A phase I/II study of prostaglandin E$_1$ for the prevention of hepatic veno-occlusive disease after bone marrow transplantation. Br J Haematol 1993; 84:724.

203. Attal M, Huguet F, et al: Prevention of hepatic veno-occlusive disease after bone marrow transplantation by continuous infusion of low-dose heparin: a prospective, randomized trial. Blood 1992; 79:2834.

204. Cahn JY, Flesch M, et al: Prevention of veno-occlusive disease of the liver after bone marrow transplantation: heparin or no heparin? Blood 1992; 80:2149.

205. Or R, Nagler A, et al: Low molecular weight heparin for the prevention of veno-occlusive disease of the liver in bone marrow transplantation patients. Transplantation 1996; 61:1067.

206. Essell JH, Thompson JM, et al: Pilot trial of prophylactic ursod-

iol to decrease the incidence of veno-occlusive disease of the liver in allogeneic bone marrow transplant patients. Bone Marrow Transplant 1994; 10:367.

207. Essell JH, Schroeder M, et al: A randomized double-blind trial of prophylactic ursodeoxycholic acid vs placebo to prevent veno-occlusive disease of the liver in patients undergoing allogeneic bone marrow transplantation. Blood 1994; 84:250a.

208. Billingham RE: The biology of graft-versus-host disease. In The Harvey Lectures. Vol. 62. New York, Academic Press, Inc., 1966, pp 21–78.

209. Ferrara JLM, Deeg HJ: Graft-versus-host disease. N Engl J Med 1991; 324:667.

210. Ferrara JLM, Deeg HJ, Burakoff SJ: Graft-vs.-Host Disease. New York, Marcel Dekker, Inc., 1997.

211. Martin PJ, Kernan NA: T-cell depletion for GVHD prevention in humans. In Ferrara JLM, Deeg HJ, Burakoff SJ (eds): Graft-vs.-Host Disease. New York, Marcel Dekker, Inc., 1997, pp 615–637.

212. Truitt RL, Johnson BD, et al: Graft versus leukemia. In Ferrara JLM, Deeg HJ, Burakoff SJ (eds): Graft-vs.-Host Disease. New York, Marcel Dekker, Inc., 1997, pp 385–423.

213. Horowitz MM, Truitt RL: Graft-versus-leukemia effects of bone marrow transplantation. In Atkinson K (ed): Clinical Bone Marrow Transplantation. Cambridge, England, Cambridge University Press, 1994, pp 704–714.

214. Horowitz MM, Gale RP, et al: Graft-versus-leukemia reactions after bone marrow transplantation. Blood 1990; 75:555.

215. Sullivan KM, Weiden PL, et al: Influence of acute and chronic graft-versus-host disease on relapse and survival after bone marrow transplantation from HLA-identical siblings as treatment of acute and chronic leukemia. Blood 1989; 73:1720.

216. Glucksberg H, Storb R, et al: Clinical manifestations of graft-versus-host disease in human recipients of marrow from HLA-matched sibling donors. Transplantation 1974; 18:295.

217. Przepiorka D, Weisdorf D, et al: Consensus conference on acute GVHD grading. Bone Marrow Transplant 1995; 15:825.

218. Weisdorf DJ, Snover DC, et al: Acute upper gastrointestinal graft-versus-host disease: clinical significance and response to immunosuppressive therapy. Blood 1990; 76:624.

219. Rowlings PA, Przepiorka D, et al: A revised grading system for acute graft-versus-host disease. Blood 1994; 84:539a.

220. Sale GE, Lerner KG, et al: The skin biopsy in the diagnosis of acute graft-versus-host disease in man. Am J Pathol 1977; 89:621.

221. Peck GL, Elias PM, Graw RG: Graft-versus-host reaction and toxic epidermal necrolysis. Lancet 1972; 2:1151.

222. McDonald GB, Shulman HM, et al: Intestinal and hepatic complications of human bone marrow transplantation: II. Gastroenterology 1986; 90:770.

223. McDonald GB, Shulman HM, et al: Intestinal and hepatic complications of human bone marrow transplantation: I. Gastroenterology 1986; 90:460.

224. Snover DC, Weisdorf SA, et al: Hepatic graft-versus-host disease: a study of the predictive value of liver biopsy in diagnosis. Hepatology 1984; 4:123.

225. Sale GE, McDonald GB, et al: Gastrointestinal graft-versus-host disease in man: a clinicopathologic study of the rectal biopsy. Am J Surg Pathol 1979; 3:291.

226. Beatty PG, Hansen JA, et al: Marrow transplantation from HLA-matched unrelated donors for treatment of hematologic malignancies. Transplantation 1991; 51:443.

227. Weisdorf D, Hakke R, Blazar B: Risk factors for acute graft versus host disease in histocompatible donor bone marrow transplantation. Transplantation 1991; 51:1197.

228. Nash RA, Pepe MS, et al: Acute graft-versus-host disease: analysis of risk factors after allogeneic marrow transplantation and prophylaxis with cyclosporine and methotrexate. Blood 1992; 80:1838.

229. Gale RP, Bortin MM, et al: Risk factors for acute graft-versus-host disease. Br J Haematol 1987; 67:397.

230. Klingemann HG, Storb R, et al: Bone marrow transplantation in patients aged 45 years and older. Blood 1986; 67:770.

231. Bensinger WI, Weaver CH, et al: Transplantation of allogeneic peripheral blood stem cells mobilized by recombinant human granulocyte colony-stimulating factor. Blood 1995; 85:1655.

232. Majolino I, Saglio G, et al: High incidence of chronic GVHD after primary allogeneic peripheral blood stem cell transplantation in patients with hematologic malignancies. Bone Marrow Transplant, 1996; 17:55.

233. Waber DP, Urion DK, et al: Late effects of CNS treatment of acute lymphoblastic leukemia in childhood are sex dependent. Dev Med Child Neurol 1990; 32:238.

234. Wagner JE, Kernan NA, et al: Transplantation of umbilical cord blood in 50 patients: analysis of the registry data. Blood 1994; 84:395a.

235. Wagner JE, Rosenthal J, et al: Successful transplantation of HLA-matched and HLA-mismatched umbilical cord blood from unrelated donors: analysis of engraftment and acute graft versus host disease. Blood 1996; 88:795.

236. Storb R, Prentice RL, et al: Graft-versus-host disease and survival in patients with aplastic anemia treated by marrow grafts from HLA-identical siblings: beneficial effect of a protective environment. N Engl J Med 1983; 308:302.

237. Vossen JM, Heidt PJ: Gnotobiotic measures for the prevention of acute graft-vs.-host disease. In Burakoff SJ, Deeg HJ, et al (eds): Graft-vs.-Host Disease: Immunology, Pathophysiology, and Treatment. New York, Marcel Dekker, Inc., 1990, pp 403–413.

238. Petersen FB, Buckner CD, et al: Laminar air flow isolation and decontamination: a prospective randomized study of the effects of prophylactic systemic antibiotics in bone marrow transplant patients. Infection 1986; 14:115.

239. Crum Vander Woude A, Bierer BE: Immunosuppression and immunophilin ligands: cyclosporin A, FK506, and rapamycin. In Ferrara JLM, Deeg HJ, Burakoff SJ (eds): Graft-vs.-Host Disease. New York, Marcel Dekker, Inc., 1997, pp 111–149.

240. Jolivet J, Cowan KH, et al: The pharmacology and clinical use of methotrexate. N Engl J Med 1983; 309:1094.

241. Chao NJ, Deeg HJ: In vivo prevention and treatment of GVHD. In Ferrara JLM, Deeg HJ, Burakoff SJ (eds): Graft-vs.-Host Disease. New York, Marcel Dekker, Inc., 1997, pp 639–666.

242. Storb R: Graft-versus-host disease after marrow transplantation. Prog Clin Biol Res 1986; 224:139.

243. Storb R, Deeg HJ, et al: Methotrexate and cyclosporine compared with cyclosporine alone for prophylaxis of acute graft-versus-host disease after marrow transplantation for leukemia. N Engl J Med 1986; 314:729.

244. Storb R, Deeg HJ, et al: Methotrexate and cyclosporine versus cyclosporine alone for prophylaxis of graft-versus-host disease in patients given HLA-identical marrow grafts for leukemia: long-term follow-up of a controlled trial. Blood 1989; 73:1729.

245. Storb R, Deeg HJ, et al: Graft-versus-host disease prevention by methotrexate combined with cyclosporin compared to methotrexate alone in patients given marrow grafts for severe aplastic anaemia: long-term follow-up of a controlled trial [see comments]. Br J Haematol 1989; 72:567.

246. Storb R, Sanders JE, et al: Graft-versus-host disease prophylaxis with methotrexate/cyclosporine in children with severe aplastic anemia treated with cyclophosphamide and HLA-identical marrow grafts. Blood 1991; 78:1144. Letter.

247. Stockschlaeder M, Storb R, et al: A pilot study of low-dose cyclosporin for graft-versus-host disease in patients given methotrexate/cyclosporine prophylaxis. Br J Haematol 1992; 80:49.

248. Beelen DW, Quabeck K, et al: Six weeks of continuous intravenous cyclosporine and short-course methotrexate as prophylaxis for acute graft-versus-host disease after allogeneic bone marrow transplantation. Transplantation 1990; 50:421.

249. Blaise D, Gravis G, Maraninchi D: Long-term follow-up of T-cell depletion for bone marrow transplantation. Lancet 1993; 341:51.

250. Maraninchi D, Blaise D, et al: Impact of T-cell depletion on outcome of allogeneic bone-marrow transplantation for standard-risk leukaemias. Lancet 1987; 2:175.

251. Sullivan KM: Graft-versus-host disease. In Forman SJ, Blume KG, Thomas ED (eds): Bone Marrow Transplantation. Cambridge, Mass, Blackwell Scientific Publications, Inc., 1994, pp 339–362.

252. Kanojia MD, Anagnostou AA, et al: High dose methylprednisolone treatment for acute graft-versus-host disease after bone marrow transplantation in adults. Transplantation 1984; 37:246.

253. Deeg HJ, Henslee-Downey PJ: Management of acute graft-versus-host disease. Bone Marrow Transplant 1990; 6:1.

254. Sayer HG, Longton G, et al: Increased risk of infection in marrow transplant patients receiving methylprednisolone for graft-versus-host disease prevention. Blood 1994; 84:1328.

255. Martin PJ, Schoch G, et al: A retrospective analysis of therapy for acute graft-versus-host disease: secondary treatment. Blood 1991; 77:1821.

256. Atkinson K, Horowitz MM, et al: Consensus among bone marrow transplanters for diagnosis, grading and treatment of chronic graft-versus-host disease. Bone Marrow Transplant 1989; 4:247.

257. Sullivan KM, Shulman HM, et al: Chronic graft-versus-host disease in 52 patients: adverse natural course and successful treatment with combination immunosuppression. Blood 1981; 57:267.

258. Storb R, Prentice RL, et al: Predictive factors in chronic graft-versus-host disease in patients with aplastic anemia treated by marrow transplantation from HLA-identical siblings. Ann Intern Med 1983; 98:461.

259. Niederwieser D, Pepe M, et al: Factors predicting chronic graft-versus-host disease and survival after marrow transplantation for aplastic anemia. Bone Marrow Transplant 1989; 4:151.

260. Atkinson K, Horowitz MM, et al: Risk factors for chronic graft-versus-host disease after HLA-identical sibling bone marrow transplantation. Blood 1990; 75:2459.

261. Ringden O, Deeg HJ: Clinical spectrum of graft-versus-host disease. In Ferrara JLM, Deeg HJ, Burakoff SJ (eds): Graft-vs.-Host Disease. New York, Marcel Dekker, Inc., 1997, pp 525–559.

262. Shulman HM, Sale GE, et al: Chronic cutaneous graft-versus-host disease in man. Am J Pathol 1978; 91:545.

263. Shulman HM, Sullivan KM, et al: Chronic graft-versus-host syndrome in man: a long-term clinicopathologic study of 20 Seattle patients. Am J Med 1980; 69:204.

264. Sullivan KM, Witherspoon RP, et al: Alternating-day cyclosporine and prednisone for treatment of high-risk chronic graft-v-host disease. Blood 1988; 72:555.

265. Kapoor N, Pelligrini AE, et al: Psoralen plus ultraviolet A (PUVA) in the treatment of chronic graft versus host disease: preliminary experience in standard treatment resistant patients. Semin Hematol 1992; 29:108.

266. Deeg HJ, Storb R, et al: Photoinactivation of lymphohemopoietic cells: studies in transfusion medicine and bone marrow transplantation. Blood Cells 1992; 18:151.

267. Thompson D, Sullivan K, et al: PUVA as adjuvant primary or salvage treatment for chronic graft-versus-host disease (GVHD). Blood 1995; 86:1581a.

268. Vogelsang GB, Farmer ER, et al: Thalidomide for the treatment of chronic graft-versus-host disease. N Engl J Med 1992; 326:1055.

269. Lee SJ, Wegner SA, et al: Treatment of chronic graft-versus-host disease with clofazimine. Blood 1997; 89:2298.

270. Johnson JT, Ferretti GA, et al: Oral pilocarpine for post-irradiation xerostomia in patients with head and neck cancer. N Engl J Med 1993; 329:390.

271. Singhal S, Mehta J, et al: Oral pilocarpine hydrochloride for the treatment of refractory xerostomia associated with chronic graft-versus-host disease. Blood 1995; 85:1147.

272. Jack MK, Jack GM, et al: Ocular manifestations of graft-v-host disease. Arch Ophthalmol 1983; 101:1080.

273. Livesey SJ, Holmes JA, Whittaker JA: Ocular complications of bone marrow transplantation. Eye 1989; 3:271.

274. Hirst WL, Jabs DA, et al: The eye in bone marrow transplantation: I. Clinical study. Arch Ophthalmol 1983; 101:580.

275. Rubin AM, Kang H: Cerebral blindness and encephalopathy with cyclosporine A toxicity. Neurology 1987; 37:1072.

276. Truwit CL, Denaro CP, et al: MR imaging of reversible cyclosporin A–induced neurotoxicity. Am J Neuroradiol 1991; 12:651.

277. Schwartz RB, Bravo SM, et al: Cyclosporine neurotoxicity and its relationship to hypertensive encephalopathy. AJR 1995; 165:627.

278. Avery R, Jabs DA, et al: Optic disc edema after bone marrow transplantation. Ophthalmology 1991; 98:1294.

279. Bernauer W, Gratwohl A, et al: Microvasculopathy in the ocular fundus after bone marrow transplantation. Ann Intern Med 1991; 115:925.

280. Lopez PF, Sternberg P, et al: Bone marrow transplant retinopathy. Am J Ophthalmol 1991; 112:635.

281. Guinan EC, Tarbell NJ, et al: Intravascular hemolysis and renal insufficiency after bone marrow transplantation. Blood 1988; 72:451.

282. Rabinowe SN, Soiffer RJ, et al: Hemolytic-uremic syndrome following bone marrow transplantation in adults for hematologic malignancies. Blood 1991; 77:1837.

283. Deeg HJ, Flournoy N, et al: Cataracts after total body irradiation and marrow transplantation: a sparing effect of dose fractionation. Int J Radiat Oncol Biol Phys 1984; 10:957.

284. Benyunes MC, Sullivan KM, et al: Cataracts after bone marrow transplantation: long-term follow-up of adults treated with fractionated total body irradiation. Int J Radiat Oncol Biol Phys 1995; 32:661.

285. Fife K, Milan S, et al: Risk factors for requiring cataract surgery following total body irradiation. Radiother Oncol 1994; 33:93.

286. Ozsahin M, Belkacemi Y, et al: Total-body irradiation and cataract incidence: a randomized comparison of two instantaneous dose rates. Int J Radiat Oncol Biol Phys 1993; 28:343.

287. Dahllof G, Forsberg C-M, et al: Facial growth and morphology in long-term survivors after bone marrow transplantation. Eur J Orthodont 1989; 11:332.

288. Johnson FL, Stokes DC, et al: Chronic obstructive airways disease after bone marrow transplantation. J Pediatr 1984; 105:370.

289. Schultz KR, Green GJ, et al: Obstructive lung disease in children after allogeneic bone marrow transplantation. Blood 1994; 84:3212.

290. Holland HK, Wingard JR, et al: Bronchiolitis obliterans in bone marrow transplantation and its relationship to chronic graft-v-host disease and low serum IgG. Blood 1988; 72:621.

291. Clark JG, Crawford SW, et al: Obstructive lung disease after allogeneic marrow transplantation: clinical presentation and course. Ann Intern Med 1989; 111:368.

292. Chan CK, Hyland RH, et al: Small-airways disease in recipients of allogeneic bone marrow transplants: an analysis of 11 cases and a review of the literature. Medicine 1987; 66:327.

293. Crawford SW, Clark JG: Bronchiolitis associated with bone marrow transplantation. Clin Chest Med 1993; 14:741.

294. Schultz KR, Fernandez CV, et al: Association of gastroesophageal reflux with obstructive lung diseases in children after allogeneic bone marrow transplantation. Blood 1995; 85:3763. Letter.

295. Clark JG, Schwartz DA, et al: Risk factors for airflow obstruction in recipients of bone marrow transplants. Ann Intern Med 1987; 107:648.

296. Atkinson K, Bryant D, et al: Obstructive airways disease: a rare but serious manifestation of chronic graft-versus-host disease after allogeneic marrow transplantation in humans. Transplant Proc 1984; 16:1030.

297. Beschorner WE, Saral R, et al: Lymphocytic bronchitis associated with graft-versus-host disease in recipients of bone-marrow transplants. N Engl J Med 1978; 299:1030.

298. Tait RC, Burnett AK, et al: Subclinical pulmonary function defects following autologous and allogeneic bone marrow transplantation: relationship to total body irradiation and graft-versus-host disease. Int J Radiat Oncol Biol Phys 1991; 20:1219.

299. Raschko JW, Cottler-Fox M, et al: Pulmonary fibrosis after bone marrow transplantation responsive to treatment with prednisone and cyclosporine. Bone Marrow Transplant 1989; 4:201.

300. Arvidson J, Bratteby L-E, et al: Pulmonary function after autologous bone marrow transplantation in children. Bone Marrow Transplant 1994; 14:117.

301. Kaplan EB, Wodell RA, et al: Late effects of bone marrow transplantation on pulmonary function in children. Bone Marrow Transplant 1994; 14:613.

302. Gajewski JL, Petz LD, et al: Hemolysis of transfused group O red blood cells in minor ABO-incompatible unrelated-donor bone marrow transplants in patients receiving cyclosporine without posttransplant methotrexate. Blood 1992; 79:3076.

303. Hows J, Beddow K, et al: Donor-derived red blood cell antibodies and immune hemolysis after allogeneic bone marrow transplantation. Blood 1986; 67:177.

304. Gmur JP, Burger J, et al: Pure red cell aplasia of long duration complicating major ABO-incompatible bone marrow transplantation. Blood 1990; 75:290.

305. Minchinton RM, Waters AH, et al: Platelet and granulocyte specific antibodies after allogeneic and autologous bone marrow grafts. Vox Sang 1984; 46:215.

306. Klumpp TR, Block CC, et al: Immune-mediated cytopenia following bone marrow transplantation: Case reports and review of the literature. Medicine 1992; 71:73.

307. Klumpp TR, Herman JH, et al: Autoimmune neutropenia following peripheral blood stem cell transplantation. Am J Hematol 1992; 41:214.

308. Bashey A, Owen I, et al: Late onset immune pancytopenia following bone marrow transplantation. Br J Haematol 1991; 78:268.

309. Peralvo J, Bacigalupo A, et al: Poor graft function associated with graft-versus-host disease after allogeneic marrow transplantation. Bone Marrow Transplant 1987; 2:279.

310. Zimmerli W, Zarth A, et al: Neutrophil function and pyogenic infections in bone marrow transplant recipients. Blood 1991; 77:393.

311. Kaufman PA, Jones RB, et al: Autologous bone marrow transplantation and factor XII, factor VII, and protein C deficiencies. Cancer 1990; 66:515.

312. Gordon B, Haire W, et al: High frequency of antithrombin 3 and protein C deficiency following autologous bone marrow transplantation and lymphoma. Bone Marrow Transplant 1991; 8:497.

313. Gordon BG, Saving KL, et al: Cerebral infarction associated with protein C deficiency following allogeneic bone marrow transplantation. Bone Marrow Transplant 1991; 8:323.

314. Shulman H, Striker G, et al: Nephrotoxicity of cyclosporin A after allogeneic marrow transplantation. N Engl J Med 1981; 305:1392.

315. Holler E, Kolb HJ, et al: Microangiopathy in patients on cyclosporine prophylaxis who developed acute graft-versus-host disease after HLA-identical bone marrow transplantation. Blood 1989; 73:2018.

316. Bergstein J, Andreoli SP, et al: Radiation nephritis following total-body irradiation and cyclophosphamide in preparation for bone marrow transplantation. Transplantation 1986; 41:63.

317. Spruce WE, Forman SJ, et al: Hemolytic uremic syndrome after bone marrow transplantation. Acta Haematol 1982; 67:206.

318. Hows JM, Chipping PM, et al: Nephrotoxicity in bone marrow transplant recipients treated with cyclosporin A. Br J Haematol 1983; 54:69.

319. Feutren G, Mihatsch J: Risk factors for cyclosporine-induced nephropathy in patients with autoimmune diseases. N Engl J Med 1992; 326:1654.

320. Stillwell TJ, Benson RCJ: Cyclophosphamide-induced hemorrhagic cystitis. A review of 100 patients. Cancer 1988; 61:451.

321. Jerkins GR, Noe HN, Hill D: Treatment of complications of cyclophosphamide cystitis. J Urol 1988; 139:923.

322. Fairchild W, Spence C, et al: The incidence of bladder cancer after cyclophosphamide therapy. J Urol 1979; 122:163.

323. Wade JC, Meyers JD: Neurologic symptoms associated with parenteral acyclovir treatment after marrow transplantation. Ann Intern Med 1983; 98:921.

324. Davis CL, Springmeyer S, Gmerek BJ: Central nervous system side effects of ganciclovir. N Engl J Med 1990; 322:933.

325. Chrisp P, Clissold SP: Foscarnet: a review of its antiviral activity, pharmacokinetic properties and therapeutic use in immunocompromised patients with cytomegalovirus retinitis. Drugs 1991; 41:104.

326. Jacobsen N, Badsberg JH, et al: Graft-versus-leukaemia activity associated with CMV-seropositive donor, post-transplant CMV infection, young donor age and chronic graft-versus-host disease in bone marrow allograft recipients. The Nordic Bone Marrow Transplantation Group [see comments]. Bone Marrow Transplant 1990; 5:413.

327. Schwartz RB, Jones KM, et al: Hypertensive encephalopathy: findings on CT, MR imaging, and SPECT imaging in 14 cases. AJR 1992; 159:379.

328. Noll RB, Kulkarni R: Complex visual hallucinations and cyclosporine. Arch Neurol 1984; 41:329.

329. Thompson CB, June CH, et al: Association between cyclosporine neurotoxicity and hypomagnesaemia. Lancet 1984; 2:1116.

330. Parker PM, Chao N, et al: Thalidomide as salvage therapy for chronic graft-versus-host disease. Blood 1995; 86:3604.

331. Mohrmann R, Mah V, Vinters HV: Neuropathologic findings after bone marrow transplantation: an autopsy study. Hum Pathol 1990; 21:630.

332. Patchell RA, White CL, et al: Neurologic complications of bone marrow transplantation. Neurology 1985; 35:300.

333. Winston DJ, Gale RP, et al: Infectious complications of human bone marrow transplantation. Medicine 1979; 58:1.

334. Denning DW, Stevens DA: Antifungal and surgical treatment of invasive aspergillosis: review of 2,121 published cases. Rev Infect Dis 1990; 12:1147.

335. Pirsch JD, Maki DG: Infectious complications in adults with bone marrow transplantation and T-cell depletion of donor marrow: increased susceptibility to fungal infections. Ann Intern Med 1986; 104:619.

336. Openshaw H, Slatkin NE: Neurological complications of bone marrow transplantation. In Forman SJ, Blume KG, Thomas ED (eds): Bone Marrow Transplantation. Oxford, Blackwell Scientific Publications, Inc., 1994, pp 482–484.

337. Thompson CB, Sanders JE, et al: The risks of central nervous system relapse and leukoencephalopathy in patients receiving marrow transplants for acute leukemia. Blood 1986; 67:195.

338. Smedler A-C, Ringden K, Bergman H, Bolme P: Sensory-motor and cognitive functioning in children who have undergone bone marrow transplantation. Acta Paediatr Scand 1990; 79:613.

339. Kaleita TA, Shields WD, Tesler A, Feig SA: Normal neurodevelopment in four young children treated with bone marrow transplantation for acute leukemia or aplastic anemia. Pediatrics 1989; 83:753.

340. Van Den Berg H, Gerritsen EJA, et al: Major complications of the central nervous system after bone marrow transplantation in children with acute lymphoblastic leukemia. Radiother Oncol 1990; 1:94.

341. Van Weel-Sipman MH, Van't Veer-Korthof ET, et al: Late effects of total body irradiation and cytostatic preparative regimen for bone marrow transplantation in children with hematological malignancies. Radiother Oncol 1990; 1:155.

342. Johnson FL, Rubin CM: Allogeneic marrow transplantation in the treatment of infants with cancer. Br J Cancer Suppl 1992; 18(Suppl):576.

343. Liesner RJ, Leiper AD, et al: Late effects of intensive treatment for acute myeloid leukemia and myelodysplasia in childhood. J Clin Oncol 1994; 12:916.

344. Sanders JE, Pritchard S, et al: Growth and development following marrow transplantation for leukemia. Blood 1986; 68:1129.

345. Sanders JE: Endocrine problems in children after bone marrow transplant for hematologic malignancies. Bone Marrow Transplant 1991; 8:2.

346. Sanders JE, Buckner CD, et al: Growth and development after bone marrow transplantation. Prog Clin Biol Res 1989; 309:375.

347. Huma Z, Boulad F, et al: Growth in children after bone marrow transplantation for acute leukemia. Blood 1995; 86:819.

348. Sklar CA: Growth following therapy for childhood cancer. Cancer Invest 1995; 13:511.

349. Shinohara O, Kato S, et al: Growth after bone marrow transplantation in children. Am J Pediatr Hematol Oncol 1991; 13:263.

350. Giorgiani G, Bozzola M, et al: Role of busulfan and total body irradiation on growth of prepubertal children receiving bone marrow transplantation and results of treatment with recombinant human growth hormone. Blood 1995; 86:825.

351. Wingard JR, Plotnick LP, et al: Growth in children after bone marrow transplantation: busulfan plus cyclophosphamide versus cyclophosphamide plus total body irradiation. Blood 1992; 79:1068.

352. Brauner R, Fontoura M, et al: Growth and growth hormone secretion after bone marrow transplantation. Arch Dis Child 1993; 68:458.

353. Chatterjee R, Mills W, Katz M, et al: Germ cell failure and Leydig cell insufficiency in post-pubertal males after autologous bone marrow transplantation with BEAM for lymphoma. Bone Marrow Transplant 1994; 13:519.

354. Schubert MA, Sullivan KM, et al: Gynecological abnormalities following allogeneic bone marrow transplantation. Bone Marrow Transplant 1990; 5:425.

355. Chiodi S, Spinelli S, et al: Cyclic sex hormone replacement therapy in women undergoing allogeneic bone marrow transplantation: aims and results. Bone Marrow Transplant 1991; 8:47.

356. Sanders JE, Buckner CD, et al: Late effects on gonadal function of cyclophosphamide total-body irradiation and marrow transplantation. Transplantation 1983; 36:252.

357. Mascarin M, Giavitto M, et al: Avascular necrosis of bone in children undergoing allogeneic bone marrow transplantation. Cancer 1991; 68:655.

358. Atkinson K, Cohen M, Biggs J: Avascular necrosis of femoral head secondary to corticosteroid therapy for graft-versus-host disease after marrow transplantation: Effective therapy with hip arthroplasty. Bone Marrow Transplant 1987; 2:421.

359. Russel JA, Blaley WB, et al: Avascular necrosis of bone in bone marrow transplant patients. Med Pediatr Oncol 1989; 17:140.

360. Li FP, Alter BP, Nathan DG: The mortality of acquired aplastic anemia in children. Blood 1972; 40:153.

361. Thomas ED, Buckner CD, et al: Aplastic anaemia treated by marrow transplantation. Lancet 1972; 1:284.

362. Camitta BM, Thomas ED, et al: A prospective study of androgens and bone marrow transplantation for treatment of severe aplastic anemia. Blood 1979; 53:504.

363. Bayever E, Champlin R, et al: Comparison between bone marrow transplantation and antithymocyte globulin in treatment of young patients with severe aplastic anemia. Pediatrics 1984; 105:920.

364. Paquette RL, Tebyani N, et al: Long-term outcome of aplastic anemia in adults treated with antithymocyte globulin: comparison with bone marrow transplantation. Blood 1995; 85:283.

365. Werner EJ, Stout RD, et al: Immunosuppressive therapy versus bone marrow transplantation for children with aplastic anemia. Pediatrics 1989; 83:61.

366. Anasetti C, Doney KC, et al: Marrow transplantation for severe aplastic anemia. Long-term outcome in fifty "untransfused" patients. Ann Intern Med 1986; 104:461.

367. Gluckman E, Socie G, et al: Bone marrow transplantation in 107 patients with severe aplastic anemia using cyclophosphamide and thoraco-abdominal irradiation for conditioning: long-term follow-up. Blood 1991; 78:2451.

368. Storb R, Prentice RL, Thomas ED: Marrow transplantation for treatment of aplastic anemia. An analysis of factors associated with graft rejection. N Engl J Med 1977; 296:61.

369. Storb R, Prentice RL, et al: Marrow transplantation from HLA-identical siblings for treatment of aplastic anemia: is exposure to marrow donor blood products 24 hours before high-dose cyclophosphamide needed for successful engraftment? Blood 1983; 61:672.

370. Champlin RE, Feig SA, et al: Bone marrow transplantation from identical twins in the treatment of aplastic anemia: implication for the pathogenesis of the disease. Br J Haematol 1984; 56:455.

371. Storb R, Longton G, et al: Changing trends in marrow transplantation for aplastic anemia. Bone Marrow Transplant 1992; 10:45.

372. Shank B, Brochstein JA, et al: Immunosuppression prior to marrow transplantation for sensitized aplastic anemia patients: comparison of TLI with TBI. Int J Radiat Oncol Biol Phys 1988; 14:1133.

373. Storb R, Deeg HJ, et al: Marrow transplantation for severe aplastic anemia: methotrexate alone compared with a combination of methotrexate and cyclosporine for prevention of acute graft-versus-host disease. Blood 1986; 68:119.

374. Storb R, Champlin RE: Bone marrow transplantation for severe aplastic anemia. Bone Marrow Transplant 1991; 8:69.

375. Socie G, Gluckman E, et al: Bone marrow transplantation (BMT) for acquired severe aplastic anaemia (SAA): long term follow-up of 107 consecutive patients. Bone Marrow Transplant 1991; 7:102.

376. Witherspoon RP, Storb R, et al: Cumulative incidence of secondary solid malignant tumors in aplastic anemia patients given marrow grafts after conditioning with chemotherapy alone. Blood 1992; 79:289.

377. Pierga J-Y, Socie G, et al: Secondary solid malignant tumors occurring after bone marrow transplantation for severe aplastic anemia given thoraco-abdominal irradiation. Radiother Oncol 1994; 30:55.

378. Young NS: The problem of clonality in aplastic anemia. Dr. Damshek's riddle, restated. Blood 1992; 79:1385.

379. Tichelli A, Gratwohl A, et al: Late haematological complications in severe aplastic anaemia. Br J Haematol 1988; 69:413.

380. Socie G, Henry-Amar M, et al: Malignant tumors occurring after treatment of aplastic anemia. N Engl J Med 1993; 329:1152.

381. Hows JM: Unrelated donor bone marrow transplantation for severe aplastic anaemia and Fanconi's anaemia. Bone Marrow Transplant 1989; 4:126.

382. Camitta B, Ash R, et al: Bone marrow transplantation for children with severe aplastic anemia: use of donors other than HLA-identical siblings. Blood 1989; 74:1852.

383. Margolis D, Camitta B, et al: Unrelated donor bone marrow transplantation to treat severe aplastic anemia in children and young adults. Br J Haematol 1996; 94:65.

384. Kawahara K, Storb R, et al: Successful allogeneic bone marrow transplantation in a 6.5-year-old male for severe aplastic anemia complicating orthotopic liver transplantation for fulminant non-A-non-B hepatitis. Blood 1991; 78:1140.

385. Dugan MJ, Rouch DA, et al: Successful allogeneic bone marrow transplantation in an adult with aplastic anemia following orthotopic liver transplantation for non-A, non-B, non-C hepatitis. Bone Marrow Transplant 1993; 12:417.

386. Ratanatharathorn V, Karanes C, et al: Busulfan-based regimens and allogeneic bone marrow transplantation in patients with myelodysplastic syndromes. Blood 1993; 81:2194.

387. Guinan EC, Tarbell NJ, et al: Bone marrow transplantation for children with myelodysplastic syndromes. Blood 1989; 73:619.

388. Nichols K, Parsons SK, Guinan EC: Long-term follow-up of twelve pediatric patients with primary myelodysplastic syndrome treated with HLA-identical sibling donor bone marrow transplantation. Blood 1996; 87:4020.

389. Anderson JE, Appelbaum FR, et al: Allogeneic marrow transplantation for refractory anemia: a comparison of two preparative regimens and analysis of prognostic factors. Blood 1996; 87:51.

390. De Witte T, Zwaan F, et al: Allogeneic bone marrow transplantation for secondary leukaemia and myelodysplastic syndrome: a survey by the European Bone Marrow Transplantation Group (EBMTG). Br J Haematol 1990; 74:151.

391. Tricot G, Van Hoof A, et al: Bone marrow transplantation performed as first-time treatment in two cases of secondary acute myeloid leukemia. Leuk Res 1984; 8:93.

392. Appelbaum FR, Barrall J, et al: Bone marrow transplantation for patients with myelodysplasia. Ann Intern Med 1990; 112:590.

393. Longmore G, Guinan EC, et al: Bone marrow transplantation for myelodysplasia and secondary acute nonlymphoblastic leukemia. J Clin Oncol 1990; 8:1707.

394. Soll E, Massumoto C, et al: Relevance of marrow fibrosis in bone marrow transplantation: a retrospective analysis of engraftment. Blood 1995; 86:4667.

395. Rajantie J, Sale GE, et al: Adverse effect of severe marrow fibrosis on hematologic recovery after chemoradiotherapy and allogeneic bone marrow transplantation. Blood 1986; 67:1693.

396. Bunin NJ, Casper JT, et al: Partially matched bone marrow transplantation in patients with myelodysplastic syndromes. J Clin Oncol 1988; 6:1851.

397. Butturini A, Rivera GK, et al: Which treatment for childhood acute lymphoblastic leukemia in second remission? Lancet 1987; 1:429.

398. Chessells JM, Rogers DW, et al: Bone-marrow transplantation has a limited role in prolonging second marrow remission in childhood lymphoblastic leukaemia. Lancet 1986; 1:1239.

399. Chessells JM: A reply to D. Pinkel. Allogeneic bone marrow transplantation in childhood leukemia: another form of intensive treatment. Leukemia 1989; 3:543.

400. Chessells JM: Treatment of childhood acute lymphoblastic leukaemia: present issues and future prospects. Blood Rev 1992; 6:193.

401. Chessells JM, Leiper AD, Richards SM: A second course of treatment for childhood acute lymphoblastic leukaemia: long-term follow-up is needed to assess results. Br J Haematol 1994; 86:48.

402. Ramsay NKC, Kersey JH: Indications for marrow transplantation in acute lymphoblastic leukemia. Blood 1990; 75:815.

403. Johnson FL, Thomas ED, et al: A comparison of marrow transplantation with chemotherapy for children with acute lymphoblastic leukemia in second or subsequent remission. N Engl J Med 1981; 305:846.

404. Sanders JE, Thomas ED, et al: Marrow transplantation for children with acute lymphoblastic leukemia in second remission. Blood 1987; 70:324.

405. Weisdorf DJ, Woods WG, et al: Allogeneic bone marrow transplantation for acute lymphoblastic leukaemia: risk factors and clinical outcome. Br J Haematol 1994; 86:62.

406. Dopfer R, Henze G, et al: Allogeneic bone marrow transplantation for childhood acute lymphoblastic leukemia in second remission after intensive primary and relapse therapy according to the BFM- and CoAll-protocols: results of the German cooperative study. Blood 1991; 78:2780.

407. Woods WG, Nesbit ME, et al: Intensive therapy followed by bone marrow transplantation for patients with acute lymphocytic leukemia in second or subsequent remission: determination of prognostic factors (a report from the University of Minnesota bone marrow transplantation team). Blood 1983; 61:1182.

408. Bacigalupo A, Van Lint M, et al: Allogeneic bone marrow transplantation versus chemotherapy for childhood acute lymphoblastic leukemia in second remission: an update. Bone Marrow Transplant 1990; 6:353.

409. Barrett AJ, Horowitz MM, et al: Marrow transplantation for acute lymphoblastic leukemia: factors affecting relapse and survival. Blood 1989; 74:862.

410. Johnson FL, Thomas ED: Treatment of relapsed acute lymphoblastic leukemia in childhood. N Engl J Med 1984; 310:263.

411. Henze G, Fengler R, et al: Six-year experience with a comprehensive approach to the treatment of recurrent childhood acute lymphoblastic leukemia (ALL-REZ BFM 85). A relapse study of the BFM group. Blood 1991; 78:1166.

412. Barrett AJ, Pollock B, et al: Chemotherapy versus bone marrow transplantation for children with acute lymphoblastic leukemia in second remission. Blood 1993; 82:194a.

413. Barrett AJ, Horowitz MM, et al: Bone marrow transplantation for Philadelphia chromosome–positive acute lymphoblastic leukemia. Blood 1992; 79:3067.

414. Camitta B, Truitt R, et al: Unrelated bone marrow donor transplants for children with leukemia or myelodysplasia. Blood 1995; 85:2354.

415. Ramsay N, LeBien T, et al: Autologous bone marrow transplantation for patients with acute lymphoblastic leukemia in second or subsequent remission: results of bone marrow treated with monoclonal antibodies BA-1, BA-2, and BA-3 plus complement. Blood 1985; 66:508.

416. Billett AL, Sallan SE: Autologous bone marrow transplantation in childhood acute lymphoid leukemia with use of purging. Am J Pediatr Hematol Oncol 1993; 15:162.

417. Billett A, Tarbell N, et al: Autologous bone marrow transplantation for relapsed childhood acute lymphoblastic leukemia after a short remission. Blood 1992; 80:24a.

418. Ohira M, Takayama J: Comparison of autologous and allogeneic bone marrow transplantation in children with acute leukemia. Acta Paediatr Jpn 1991; 33:558.

419. Kersey JH, Weisdorf D, et al: Comparison of autologous and allogeneic bone marrow transplantation for treatment of high-risk refractory acute lymphoblastic leukemia. N Engl J Med 1987; 317:461.

420. Blaise D, Gaspard MH, et al: Allogeneic or autologous bone marrow transplantation for acute lymphoblastic leukemia in first complete remission. Bone Marrow Transplant 1990; 5:7.

421. Attal M, Blaise D, et al: Consolidation treatment of adult acute lymphoblastic leukemia: A prospective, randomized trial comparing allogeneic versus autologous bone marrow transplantation and testing the impact of recombinant interleukin-2 after autologous bone marrow transplantation. Blood 1995; 86:1619.

422. Appelbaum FR, Dahlberg S, et al: Bone marrow transplantation or chemotherapy after remission induction for adults with acute nonlymphoblastic leukemia. Ann Intern Med 1984; 101:591.

423. Champlin RE, Ho WG, et al: Treatment of acute myelogenous leukemia. Ann Intern Med 1985; 102:285.

424. Nesbit M, Buckley J, et al: Comparison of allogeneic bone marrow transplantation (BMT) with maintenance chemotherapy in previously untreated childhood acute nonlymphocytic leukemia (ANLL). Proc Am Soc Clin Oncol 1987; 6:163. Abstract 640.

425. Woods WG, Neudorf S, et al: Aggressive post-remission (REM) chemotherapy is better than autologous bone marrow trans-

plantation (BMT) and allogeneic BMT is superior to both in children with acute myeloid leukemia (AML). Annu Meet Am Soc Clin Oncol 1996; 15:A1091.

426. Ball ED, Mills LE, et al: Autologous bone marrow transplantation for acute myeloid leukemia using monoclonal antibody-purged bone marrow. Blood 1990; 75:1199.

427. Robertson MJ, Soiffer RJ, et al: Human bone marrow depleted of CD33-positive cells mediates delayed but durable reconstitution of hematopoiesis: clinical trial of MY9 monoclonal antibody-purged autografts for the treatment of acute myeloid leukemia. Blood 1992; 79:2229.

428. Dusenbery KE, Daniels KA, et al: Randomized comparison of cyclophosphamide–total body irradiation versus busulfan-cyclophosphamide conditioning in autologous bone marrow transplantation for acute myeloid leukemia. Int J Radiat Oncol Biol Phys 1995; 31:119.

429. Zittoun RA, Mandelli F, et al: Autologous or allogeneic bone marrow transplantation compared with intensive chemotherapy in acute myelogenous leukemia. N Engl J Med 1995; 332:217.

430. Tiedemann K, Waters KD, et al: Results of intensive therapy in childhood acute myeloid leukemia, incorporating high-dose melphalan and autologous bone marrow transplantation in first complete remission. Blood 1993; 82:3730.

431. Gale RP, Butturini A: Is transplantation in first remission AML more effective than in advanced leukemia? Leuk Res 1989; 13:1035.

432. Bortin MM, Gale RP, et al: Bone marrow transplantation for acute myelogenous leukemia. JAMA 1983; 249:1166.

433. Appelbaum FR, Clift RA, et al: Allogeneic marrow transplantation for acute nonlymphoblastic leukemia after first relapse. Blood 1983; 61:949.

434. Dinsmore R, Kirkpatrick D, et al: Allogeneic bone marrow transplantation for patients with acute nonlymphocytic leukemia. Blood 1984; 63:649.

435. Forman SJ, Schmidt GM, et al: Allogeneic bone marrow transplantation as therapy for primary induction failure for patients with acute leukemia. J Clin Oncol 1991; 9:1570.

436. Thomas ED, Clift RA, et al: Marrow transplantation for the treatment of chronic myelogenous leukemia. Ann Intern Med 1986; 104:155.

437. Goldman JM: Bone marrow transplantation for chronic myeloid leukaemia. Leukemia 1992; 6:22.

438. Thomas ED, Clift RA: Indications for marrow transplantation in chronic myelogenous leukemia. Blood 1989; 73:861.

439. Martin PJ, Clift RA, et al: HLA-Identical marrow transplantation during accelerated-phase chronic myelogenous leukemia: analysis of survival and remission duration. Blood 1988; 72:1978.

440. Goldman JM, Szydlo R, et al: Choice of pretransplant treatment and timing of transplants for chronic myelogenous leukemia in chronic phase. Blood 1993; 82:2235.

441. Clift RA, Appelbaum FR, Thomas ED: Treatment of chronic myeloid leukemia by marrow transplantation. Blood 1993; 82:1954.

442. Kahls P, Schawrzinger I, et al: A retrospective analysis of the long-term effect of splenectomy on late infections, graft-versus-host disease, relapse, and survival after allogeneic marrow transplantation for chronic myelogenous leukemia. Blood 1995; 86:2028.

443. Kolb H-J, Schattenberg A, et al: Graft-versus-leukemia effect of donor lymphocyte transfusions in marrow grafted patients. Blood 1995; 86:2041.

444. Porter DL, Roth MS, et al: Induction of graft-versus-host disease as immunotherapy for relapsed chronic myeloid leukemia. N Engl J Med 1994; 330:100.

445. Mackinnon S, Papadopoulos EB, et al: Adoptive immunotherapy evaluating escalating doses of donor leukocytes for relapse of chronic myeloid leukemia after bone marrow transplantation: separation of graft-versus-leukemia responses from graft-versus-host disease. Blood 1995; 86:1261.

446. Rassam SMB, Katz F, et al: Successful allogeneic bone marrow transplantation in juvenile CML: conditioning or graft-versus-leukaemia effect? Bone Marrow Transplant 1993; 11:247.

447. Sanders JE, Buckner CD, et al: Allogeneic marrow transplantation for children with juvenile chronic myelogenous leukemia. Blood 1988; 71:1144.

448. Smith FO, Sanders JE, et al: Allogeneic marrow transplantation (BMT) for children with juvenile chronic myelogenous leukemia (JCML). Blood 1994; 84:201. Abstract 790.

449. Locatelli F, Niemeyer C, et al: Allogeneic bone marrow transplantation (BMT) for chronic myelomonocytic leukemia (CMML) in childhood: a report of the European Working Group on Childhood Myelodysplastic Syndrome (EWOG-MDS). Blood 1995; 86:93. Abstract 357.

449a. Philip T, Biron P, et al: Massive therapy and autologous bone marrow transplantation in pediatric and young adults: Burkitt's lymphoma (30 courses on 28 patients: a 5-year experience. Eur J Cancer Clin Oncol 1986; 22:1015.

449b. Loiseau HA, Hartmann O, et al: High-dose chemotherapy containing busulfan followed by bone marrow transplantation in 24 children with refractory or relapsed non-Hodgkin's lymphoma. Bone Marrow Transplant 1991; 8:465.

449c. Bureo E, Ortega JJ, et al: Bone marrow transplantation in 46 pediatric patients with non-Hodgkin's lymphoma. Bone Marrow Transplant 1995; 15:353.

449d. Vose JM, Anderson JR, et al: High-dose chemotherapy and autologous hematopoietic stem-cell transplantation for aggressive non-Hodgkin's lymphoma. J Clin Oncol 1993; 11:1846.

449e. Petersen FB, Appelbaum FR, et al: Autologous marrow transplantation for malignant lymphoma: a report of 101 cases from Seattle. J Clin Oncol 1990; 8:638.

449f. Chopra R, Goldstone AH, et al: Autologous versus allogeneic bone marrow transplantation for non-Hodgkin's lymphoma: a case-controlled analysis of the European Bone Marrow Transplant Group registry data. J Clin Oncol 1992; 10:1690.

449g. Milpied N, Fielding AK, et al: Allogeneic bone marrow transplant is not better than autologous transplant for patients with relapsed Hodgkin's disease. J Clin Oncol 1996; 14:1291.

449h. Ratanatharathorn V, Uberti J, et al: Prospective comparative trial of autologous versus allogeneic bone marrow transplantation in patients with non-Hodgkin's lymphoma. Blood 1994; 84:1050.

450. Seeger RC, Reynolds CP: Neuroblastomas. In Forman SJ, Blume KG, Thomas ED (eds): Bone Marrow Transplantation. Boston, Blackwell Scientific Publications, Inc., 1994, pp 814–826.

451. Shuster JJ, Cantor AB, et al: The prognostic significance of autologous bone marrow transplant in advanced neuroblastoma. J Clin Oncol 1991; 9:1045.

452. Treleaven JG, Ugelstad J, et al: Removal of neuroblastoma cells from bone marrow with monoclonal antibodies conjugated to magnetic microspheres. Lancet 1984; 1:70.

453. August CS, Serota FT, et al: Treatment of advanced neuroblastoma with supralethal chemotherapy, radiation, and allogeneic or autologous marrow reconstitution. J Clin Oncol 1984; 2:609.

454. Graham-Pole J, Lazarus HM, et al: High-dose melphalan therapy for treatment of children with refractory neuroblastoma and Ewing's sarcoma. Am J Pediatr Hematol Oncol 1984; 6:17.

455. Graham-Pole J, Gee A, et al: Myeloablative chemoradiotherapy and autologous bone marrow infusions for treatment of neuroblastoma: factors influencing engraftment. Blood 1991; 78:1607.

456. Kushner BH, O'Reilly RJ, et al: Myeloablative combination chemotherapy without total body irradiation for neuroblastoma. J Clin Oncol 1991; 9:274.

457. Dopfer R, Berthold F, et al: Bone marrow transplantation in children with neuroblastoma. Fol Haematol (Leipzig) 1989; 116:427.

458. Miser JS: Autologous bone marrow transplantation for the treatment of sarcomas. In Johnson FL, Pochedly C (eds): Bone Marrow Transplantation in Children. New York, Raven Press, Inc., 1990.

459. Wijnaendts L, Le Deist F, et al: Development of immunologic functions after bone marrow transplantation in 33 patients with severe combined immunodeficiency. Blood 1989; 74:2212.

460. Fischer A, Friedrick W, Levinsky R: Bone marrow transplantation for immunodeficiencies and osteopetrosis: European survey, 1968–1985. Lancet 1986; 2:1080.

461. Fischer A, Landais P, et al: Bone marrow transplantation (BMT) in Europe for primary immunodeficiencies other than severe combined immunodeficiency: a report from the European Group for BMT and the European Group for Immunodeficiency. Blood 1994; 83:1149.

462. Dror Y, Gallagher R, et al: Immune reconstitution in severe combined immunodeficiency disease after lectin-treated, T-cell–depleted haplocompatible bone marrow transplantation. Blood 1993; 81:2021.

463. Fischer A, Durandy A, et al: HLA-haploidentical bone marrow transplantation for severe combined immunodeficiency using E rosette fractionation and cyclosporine. Blood 1986; 67:444.

464. Buckley RH, Schiff SE, et al: Development of immunity in human severe primary T cell deficiency following haploidentical bone marrow stem cell transplantation. J Immunol 1986; 136:2398.

465. Reisner Y, Kappor N, et al: Transplantation for severe combined immunodeficiency with HLA-A, B, D, DR incompatible parental marrow cells fractionated by soybean agglutinin and sheep red blood cells. Blood 1983; 61:341.

466. Reinherz EL, Geha R, et al: Reconstitution after transplantation with T lymphocyte-depleted HLA haplotype-mismatched bone marrow for severe combined immunodeficiency. Proc Natl Acad Sci U S A 1982; 79:6047.

467. O'Reilly RJ, Keever CA, et al: The use of HLA-non-identical T-cell–depleted marrow transplants for correction of severe combined immunodeficiency disease. Immunodefic Rev 1989; 1:279.

468. O'Reilly RJ, Friedrich W, Small TN: Transplantation approaches for severe combined immunodeficiency disease, Wiskott-Aldrich syndrome, and other lethal genetic, combined immunodeficiency disorders. In Forman SJ, Blume KG, Thomas ED (eds): Bone Marrow Transplantation. Boston, Blackwell Scientific Publications, Inc., 1994, pp 849–873.

469. O'Reilly RJ, Dupont B, et al: Reconstitution of severe combined immunodeficiency by transplantation of marrow from an unrelated donor. N Engl J Med 1977; 297:1311.

470. Friedrich W: Marrow transplantation for primary immunodeficiency diseases. Marrow Transplant Rev 1994; 4:17, 19.

471. Fischer A, Blanche S, et al: Anti-B-cell monoclonal antibodies in the treatment of severe B-cell lymphoproliferative syndrome following bone marrow and organ transplantation. N Engl J Med 1991; 324:1451.

472. Remold-O'Donnell E, Rosen FS: Sialophorin (CD34) and the Wiskott-Aldrich syndrome. Immunodefic Rev 1990; 2:151.

473. Parkman R, Rappeport J, et al: Complete correction of the Wiskott-Aldrich syndrome by allogeneic bone-marrow transplantation. N Engl J Med 1978; 298:921.

474. Brochstein JA, Gillio AP, et al: Marrow transplantation from human leukocyte antigen-identical or haploidentical donors for correction of Wiskott-Aldrich syndrome. J Pediatr 1991; 119:907.

475. Kapoor N, Kirkpatrick D, et al: Reconstitution of normal megakaryocytopoiesis and immunologic functions in Wiskott-Aldrich syndrome by marrow transplantation following myeloablation and immunosuppression with busulfan and cyclophosphamide. Blood 1981; 57:692.

476. Mullen CA, Anderson KD, Blaese RM: Splenectomy and/or bone marrow transplantation in the management of the Wiskott-Aldrich syndrome: long-term follow-up of 62 cases. Blood 1993; 82:2961.

477. Filipovich AH, Shapiro RS, et al: Unrelated donor bone marrow transplantation for correction of lethal congenital immunodeficiencies. Blood 1992; 80:270.

478. Modell B, Berdoukas VA: The Clinical Approach to Thalassemia. New York, Grune & Stratton, Inc., 1984.

479. Brittenham GM, Griffith PM, et al: Efficacy of deferoxamine in preventing complications of iron overload in patients with thalassemia major. N Engl J Med 1994; 331:567.

480. Ehlers KH, Giardina PJ, et al: Prolonged survival in patients with beta-thalassemia major treated with deferoxamine. J Pediatr 1991; 118:540.

481. Olivieri NF, McGee A, et al: Cardiac disease-free survival in patients with thalassemia major treated with subcutaneous deferoxamine. Ann N Y Acad Sci 1990; 612:585.

482. Olivieri NF, Nathan DG, et al: Survival in medically treated patients with homozygous β-thalassemia. N Engl J Med 1994; 331:574.

483. Wolfe LC, Olivieri NF, et al: Prevention of cardiac disease with subcutaneous deferoxamine in patients with thalassemia major. N Engl J Med 1985; 312:1600.

484. Thomas ED, Buckner CD, et al: Marrow transplantation for thalassaemia. Lancet 1982; 2:227.

485. Thomas ED: Allogeneic bone marrow transplantation for blood cell disorders. Birth Defects 1978; 18:361.

486. Lucarelli G, Galimberti M, et al: Bone marrow transplantation in adult thalassemia. Blood 1992; 80:1603.

487. Lucarelli G, Galimberti M, et al: Marrow transplantation in patients with thalassemia responsive to iron chelation therapy. N Engl J Med 1993; 329:840.

488. Lucarelli G, Galimberti M, et al: Marrow transplantation in patients with advanced thalassemia. N Engl J Med 1987; 316:1050.

489. Lucarelli G, Clift RA, et al: Marrow transplantation for patients with thalassemia: results in class 3 patients. Blood 1996; 87:2082.

490. Davies SC: Bone marrow transplant for sickle cell disease—the dilemma. Blood Rev 1993; 7:4.

491. Roberts IAG, Davies SC: Sickle cell: the transplant issue. Bone Marrow Transplant 1993; 11:253.

492. Kodish E, Lantos J, et al: Bone marrow transplantation for sickle cell anemia. N Engl J Med 1991; 325:1349.

493. Ferster A, De Valck C, et al: Bone marrow transplantation for severe sickle cell anaemia. Br J Haematol 1992; 80:102.

494. Vallera DA: Immunotoxins for *ex vivo* bone marrow purging in human bone marrow transplantation. Cancer Treat Res 1988; 37:515.

495. Vermylen C, Cornu G: Bone marrow transplantation in sickle cell anemia: the European experience. Am J Pediatr Hematol Oncol 1994; 16:18.

496. Bernaudin F, Souillet G, et al: Bone marrow transplantation (BMT) in 14 children with severe sickle cell disease (SCD): the French experience. Bone Marrow Transplant 1993; 12:118.

497. Giardini C, Galimberti M, et al: Bone marrow transplantation in sickle-cell anemia in pesaro. Bone Marrow Transplant 1993; 12:122.

498. Walters MC, Sullivan KM, et al: Neurologic complications after allogeneic marrow transplantation for sickle cell anemia. Blood 1995; 85:879.

499. Walters MC, Patience M, et al: Bone marrow transplantation for sickle cell disease. N Engl J Med 1996; 335:369.

500. Ferster A, Bujan W, et al: Bone marrow transplantation corrects the splenic reticuloendothelial dysfunction in sickle cell anemia. Blood 1993; 81:1102.

501. Gluckman E, Devergie A, Dutreix J: Radiosensitivity in Fanconi anaemia: application to the conditioning regimen for bone marrow transplantation. Br J Haematol 1983; 54:431.

502. Gluckman E: Bone marrow transplantation for Fanconi's anaemia. Baillieres Clin Haematol 1989; 2:153.

503. Gluckman E: Bone marrow transplantation in Fanconi's anemia. Stem Cells 1993; 11:180.

504. Kohli-Kumar M, Morris C, et al: Bone marrow transplantation in Fanconi anemia using matched sibling donors. Blood 1994; 84:2050.

505. Hows JM, Chapple M, et al: Bone marrow transplantation for Fanconi's anaemia: the Hammersmith experience 1977–89. Bone Marrow Transplant 1989; 4:629.

506. Zanis-Neto J, Ribeiro RC, et al: Bone marrow transplantation for patients with Fanconi anemia: a study of 24 cases from a single institution. Bone Marrow Transplant 1995; 15:293.

507. Gluckman E, Auerbach AD, et al: Bone marrow transplantation for Fanconi anemia. Blood 1995; 86:2856.

508. Flowers MED, Doney KC, et al: Marrow transplantation for Fanconi anemia with or without leukemic transformation: an update of the Seattle experience. Bone Marrow Transplant 1992; 9:167.

509. Janov A, Leong T, et al: Diamond-Blackfan anemia. Natural history and sequelae of treatment. Medicine 1996; 76:1.

510. Iriondo A, Garijo J, et al: Complete recovery of hemopoiesis following bone marrow transplant in a patient with unresponsive congenital hypoplastic anemia (Blackfan-Diamond syndrome). Blood 1984; 64:348.

511. Lenarsky C, Weinber K, et al: Bone marrow transplantation for constitutional pure red cell aplasia. Blood 1988; 72:451.

512. Greinix HT, Storb R, et al: Long-term survival and cure after marrow transplantation for congenital hypoplastic anaemia (Diamond-Blackfan syndrome). Br J Haematol 1993; 84:515.

513. Mugishima H, Gale RP, et al: Bone marrow transplantation for Diamond-Blackfan anemia. Bone Marrow Transplant 1995; 15:55.

514. Wiktor-Jedrzejczak W, Szcczlik C, et al: Success of bone marrow transplantation in congenital Diamond-Blackfan anaemia: a case report. Eur J Haematol 1987; 38:204.

515. Weinberg K: White blood cell disorders. In Forman SJ, Blume KG, Thomas ED (eds): Bone Marrow Transplantation. Boston, Blackwell Scientific Publications, Inc., 1994, pp 894–901.

516. Bonilla MA: Cytokine treatment of severe chronic neutropenia. Int J Pediatr Hematol Oncol 1994; 2:117.

517. Haddad E, Le Deist F, et al: Treatment of Chédiak-Higashi syndrome by allogenic bone marrow transplantation: report of 10 cases. Blood 1995; 85:3328.

518. Gillio AP, Guinan EC: Cytokine treatment of inherited bone marrow failure syndromes. Int J Pediatr Hematol Oncol 1995; 2:125.

519. Bellucci S, Devergie A, et al: Complete correction of Glanzmann's thrombasthenia by allogeneic bone-marrow transplantation. Br J Haematol 1985; 59:635.

520. Coccia P: Bone marrow transplantation for osteopetrosis. In Forman SJ, Blume KG, Thomas ED (eds): Bone Marrow Transplantation. Boston, Blackwell Scientific Publications, Inc., 1994, pp 874–882.

521. Walker DG: Bone resorption restored in osteopetrotic mice by transplants of normal bone marrow and spleen cells. Science 1975; 190:784.

522. O'Reilly RJ, Brochstein J, et al: Marrow transplantation for congenital disorders. Semin Hematol 1984; 21:188.

523. Key LL Jr, Rodriguiz RM, et al: Cytokines and bone resorption in osteopetrosis. Int J Pediatr Hematol Oncol 1995; 2:143.

524. Barton NW, Brady RO, et al: Replacement therapy for inherited enzyme deficiency: macrophage-targeted glucocerebrosidase for Gaucher's disease. N Engl J Med 1991; 324:1464.

525. Tsai P, Lipton JM, et al: Allogeneic bone marrow transplantation in severe Gaucher disease. Pediatr Res 1992; 31:503.

526. Hopwood JJ, Vellodi A, et al: Long-term clinical progress in bone marrow transplanted mucopolysaccharidosis type I patients with a defined genotype. J Inherit Metab Dis 1993; 16:1024.

527. Krivit W, Shapiro EG: Bone marrow transplantation for storage diseases. In Forman SJ, Blume KG, Thomas ED (eds): Bone Marrow Transplantation. Boston, Blackwell Scientific Publications, Inc., 1994, pp 883–893.

528. Bergstrom SK, Quinn JJ, et al: Long-term follow-up of a patient transplanted for Hunter's disease type IIB: a case report and literature review. Bone Marrow Transplant 1994; 14:653.

529. Lenarsky C, Kohn DB, et al: Bone marrow transplant for genetic disease. Hematol Oncol Clin North Am 1990; 4:589.

530. Krivit W: Maroteaux-Lamy syndrome (mucopolysaccharidosis type VI) treatment by allogeneic BMT in 6 patients and potential for autotransplantation bone marrow gene insertion. Int Pediatr 1992; 7:47.

531. Cowan MJ: Bone marrow transplantation for the treatment of genetic diseases. Clin Biochem 1991; 24:375.

532. Krivit W, Shapiro E, et al: Treatment of late infantile metachromatic leukodystrophy by bone marrow transplantation. N Engl J Med 1990; 322:28.

533. Shapiro EG, Lipton ME, Krivit W: White matter dysfunction and its neuropsychological correlates: longitudinal study of a case of metachromatic leukodystrophy treated with bone marrow transplant. Clin Exp Neuropsychol 1992; 14:610.

IV

Disorders of Erythrocyte Production

A Diagnostic Approach to the Anemic Patient

Megaloblastic Anemia

Disorders of Iron Metabolism and
Sideroblastic Anemia

The Porphyrias

Lead Poisoning

A Diagnostic Approach to the Anemic Patient

Frank A. Oski[†] • Carlo Brugnara • David G. Nathan

Most of the chapters thus far have been devoted to descriptions of specific disorders that result in anemia. The purpose of this chapter is to provide both a more general classification of the anemias and an initial diagnostic approach to the patient with this laboratory finding. Details of the diagnostic procedures employed in the ultimate diagnosis of the various anemias are omitted because they are presented in their respective chapters.

DEFINITION OF ANEMIA

Anemia is generally defined as a reduction in red cell mass or blood hemoglobin concentration. The limit for differentiating anemic from normal states is generally set at two standard deviations below the mean for the normal population. This definition will result in 2.5% of the normal population being classified as anemic. Conversely, the values for hemoglobin-deficient individuals are distributed in such a fashion that some are placed within the normal range. These individuals, who have the potential for a hemoglobin concentration in the upper part of the normal range, may be recognized only after a response to treatment.

Because the primary function of the red cell is to deliver and release adequate quantities of oxygen to the tissues to meet their metabolic demands, it is apparent that some measures of both body oxygen metabolism and accompanying cardiovascular compensations are required to complement the current laboratory definition of anemia. The fact that hemoglobin concentration alone is insufficient to judge whether a patient is "functionally anemic" is best illustrated in a patient with cyanotic congenital heart disease or chronic respiratory insufficiency or in a patient with mutant hemoglobins that alter hemoglobin's affinity for oxygen (see Chapter 19).

With these caveats in mind, a useful statistical defi-

nition of anemia is provided in Table 9–1 that recognizes the effect of age and sex on the designation of anemia.[1]

CLASSIFICATION OF ANEMIAS

Anemias may be classified on a physiologic or a morphologic basis. A combination of both approaches is often employed in the initial differential diagnosis.

The best approach for providing an understanding of the multiple disorders capable of producing anemia is to separate the causes of anemia into two categories of functional disturbances[2]:

1. Disorders of effective red cell production, in which the net rate of red cell production is depressed. This can be due to disorders of erythrocyte maturation, in which erythropoiesis is largely ineffectual, or to an absolute failure of erythropoiesis. In the former, the marrow contains many erythroblasts that die in situ before reaching the reticulocyte stage. In the latter, there is absolute erythroblastopenia.

2. Disorders in which rapid erythrocyte destruction or red cell loss is primarily responsible for the anemia.

These two categories are not mutually exclusive. More than one mechanism may be present in some anemias, but one functional disorder is generally the major reason for the patient's anemia. Table 9–2 lists the anemias most commonly encountered in infancy and childhood and classifies them into three categories of functional disturbance.

Anemias may also be classified on the basis of red cell size and then further subdivided, according to red cell morphology. In this type of classification, anemias are subdivided into microcytic anemias, normocytic anemias, and macrocytic anemias. This classification is also arbitrary, and categories are not mutually exclu-

---

† Deceased.

Table 9–1. VALUES (NORMAL MEAN AND LOWER LIMITS OF NORMAL) FOR HEMOGLOBIN, HEMATOCRIT, AND MEAN CORPUSCULAR VOLUME (MCV) DETERMINATIONS

Age (y)	Hemoglobin (g/dL)		Hematocrit (%)		MCV (μ^3)	
	Mean	Lower Limit	Mean	Lower Limit	Mean	Lower Limit
0.5–1.9	12.5	11.0	37	33	77	70
2–4	12.5	11.0	38	34	79	73
5–7	13.0	11.5	39	35	81	75
8–11	13.5	12.0	40	36	83	76
12–14:						
Female	13.5	12.0	41	36	85	78
Male	14.0	12.5	43	37	84	77
15–17:						
Female	14.0	12.0	41	36	87	79
Male	15.0	13.0	46	38	86	78
18–49:						
Female	14.0	12.0	42	37	90	80
Male	16.0	14.0	47	40	90	80

sive. For example, macrocytic reticulocytes abound in the hemolytic anemias. Therefore, although the mature erythrocytes in the various hemolytic anemias may be normocytic, the mean corpuscular volume (MCV) of all the cells may be larger than normal, owing to the contribution of reticulocytes to the volume measurement.[3] Volume distribution curves may reveal the contribution of a subset of large cells to the MCV. Furthermore, during the course of a disease, classification of

the patient's anemia may change from one category to another as a result of other clinical or pathologic variables. In Table 9–3 the more common anemias of infancy and childhood are classified on the basis of their characteristic cell size.

EVALUATION OF THE ANEMIC PATIENT

The initial diagnostic approach to the anemic patient includes a detailed history and physical examination and a minimum of essential laboratory tests. Tables 9–4 and 9–5 list those features of the history and physical examination that are most helpful in providing clues to the etiology of anemia. The initial laboratory tests should include determination of hemoglobin and hematocrit concentration, measurement of red cell indices, platelet count, white blood cell count and differential, reticulocyte count, and examination of a peripheral blood smear. After this initial assessment, other useful and simple laboratory procedures may be employed. These include, when indicated, measurement of erythrocyte porphyrin concentration and serum ferritin concentration, supravital stains of the erythrocytes, hemoglobin electrophoresis, a screening test for the presence of unstable hemoglobins, a direct and an indirect Coombs test, a screening test for glucose-6-phosphate dehydrogenase deficiency, and an examination of the bone marrow.

Electronic Cell Counting

The most widely employed methods for determination of hemoglobin, hematocrit, and red cell indices are

Table 9–2. PHYSIOLOGIC CLASSIFICATION OF ANEMIA

A. DISORDERS OF RED CELL PRODUCTION IN WHICH THE RATE OF RED CELL PRODUCTION IS LESS THAN EXPECTED FOR THE DEGREE OF ANEMIA:
1. Marrow failure:
   a. Aplastic anemia:
      Congenital
      Acquired
   b. Pure red cell aplasia:
      Congenital:
         Diamond-Blackfan syndrome
         Aase's syndrome
      Acquired:
         Transient erythroblastopenia of childhood
      Other
   c. Marrow replacement:
      Malignancies
      Osteopetrosis
      Myelofibrosis[20]:
         Chronic renal disease[21]
         Vitamin D deficiency[22]
   d. Pancreatic insufficiency-marrow hypoplasia syndrome
2. Impaired erythropoietin production:
   a. Chronic renal disease
   b. Hypothyroidism, hypopituitarism
   c. Chronic inflammation
   d. Protein malnutrition
   e. Hemoglobin mutants with decreased affinity for oxygen

B. DISORDERS OF ERYTHROID MATURATION AND INEFFECTIVE ERYTHROPOIESIS:
1. Abnormalities of cytoplasmic maturation:
   a. Iron deficiency
   b. Thalassemia syndromes
   c. Sideroblastic anemias
   d. Lead poisoning
2. Abnormalities of nuclear maturation
   a. Vitamin B_{12} deficiency
   b. Folic acid deficiency
   c. Thiamine-responsive megaloblastic anemia
   d. Hereditary abnormalities in folate metabolism
   e. Orotic aciduria
3. Primary dyserythropoietic anemias (types I, II, III, IV)
4. Erythropoietic protoporphyria
5. Refractory sideroblastic anemia with vacuolization of marrow precursors and pancreatic dysfunction deficiency

C. HEMOLYTIC ANEMIAS:
1. Defects of hemoglobin:
   a. Structural mutants
   b. Synthetic mutants (thalassemia syndromes)
2. Defects of the red cell membrane
3. Defects of red cell metabolism
4. Antibody-mediated
5. Mechanical injury to the erythrocyte
6. Thermal injury to the erythrocyte
7. Oxidant-induced red cell injury
8. Infectious agent–induced red cell injury
9. Paroxysmal nocturnal hemoglobinuria
10. Plasma-lipid–induced abnormalities of the red cell membrane

electronic. In comparison with manual techniques, electronic methods have the advantages of greater precision and reproducibility and the capacity for completing a large number of measurements quickly.

One of two general principles is used in most of the more popular electronic counting systems. These may be simply classified as the electrical *impedance principle* and the *light scatter principle*.

The electrical impedance principle is employed in the Coulter Counter (Coulter Electronics, Hialeah, FL). With this technique, cells passing through an aperture cause changes in electrical resistance that are counted as voltage pulses, which are proportional to cell volume. The electrical pulses are amplified and are counted during the time an accurately metered volume of the suspension is drawn through the aperture. These devices can directly measure the MCV and compute the hematocrit from the MCV and red blood cell count.

The light scatter principle is used in the Technicon H*1, H*2, and H*3 Autoanalyzers (Bayer Diagnostics, Tarrytown, NY).[4-7] With this flow cytometric technique, red cells first undergo isovolumetric sphering and then MCV and mean corpuscular hemoglobin concentration (MCHC) are measured from the low-angle forward light scattering and the high-angle (refractive index) light scattering, respectively.

Readers are encouraged to consult other references[8-10] for details of operation of electronic counters and to familiarize themselves with potential sources of

Table 9–3. CLASSIFICATION OF ANEMIAS BASED ON RED CELL SIZE

A. MICROCYTIC ANEMIAS:
1. Iron deficiency (nutritional, chronic blood loss)
2. Chronic lead poisoning
3. Thalassemia syndromes
4. Sideroblastic anemias
5. Chronic inflammation
6. Some congenital hemolytic anemias with unstable hemoglobin
B. MACROCYTIC ANEMIAS:
1. With megaloblastic bone marrow:
a. Vitamin B_{12} deficiency
b. Folic acid deficiency
c. Hereditary orotic aciduria
d. Thiamine-responsive anemia[22]
2. Without megaloblastic bone marrow:
a. Aplastic anemia
b. Diamond-Blackfan syndrome
c. Hypothyroidism
d. Liver disease
e. Bone marrow infiltration
f. Dyserythropoietic anemias
C. NORMOCYTIC ANEMIAS:
1. Congenital hemolytic anemias:
a. Hemoglobin mutants
b. Red cell enzyme defects
c. Disorders of the red cell membrane
2. Acquired hemolytic anemias:
a. Antibody-mediated
b. Microangiopathic hemolytic anemias
c. Secondary to acute infections
3. Acute blood loss
4. Splenic pooling
5. Chronic renal disease (usually)

Table 9–4. HISTORICAL FACTORS OF IMPORTANCE IN EVALUATING THE PATIENT WITH ANEMIA

Age	Nutritional iron deficiency is never responsible for anemia in term infants prior to 6 months of age; rarely seen in premature infants prior to the time they have doubled their birth weight. Anemia manifesting itself in the neonatal period generally is the result of recent blood loss, isoimmunization, or initial manifestation of a congenital hemolytic anemia or congenital infection. Anemia first detected at ages 3 to 6 months suggests a congenital disorder of hemoglobin synthesis or hemoglobin structure.
Gender	Consider x-linked disorders in males (glucose-6-phosphate dehydrogenase (G6PD) deficiency, pyruvate kinase deficiency).
Race	Hemoglobins S and C more common in blacks; β-thalassemia more common in whites; α-thalassemia trait most common among black and yellow races.
Ethnicity	Thalassemia syndromes most common among patients of Mediterranean origin. G6PD deficiency is observed with increased frequency among Sephardic Jews, Filipinos, Greeks, Sardinians, and Kurds.
Neonatal	History of hyperbilirubinemia in the newborn period suggests the presence of congenital hemolytic anemia, such as hereditary spherocytosis of G6PD deficiency. Prematurity predisposes to early development of iron deficiency.
Diet	Document sources of iron, vitamin B_{12}, folic acid, or vitamin E in the diet. History of pica, geophagia, or pagophagia suggests presence of iron deficiency.
Drugs	Oxidant-induced hemolytic anemia, phenytoin (Dilantin)-induced megaloblastic anemia, drug-induced aplastic anemia.
Infection	Hepatitis-induced aplastic anemia, infection-induced red cell aplasia, or hemolytic anemia.
Inheritance	Family history of anemia, jaundice, gallstones, or splenomegaly.
Diarrhea	Suspect small bowel disease with malabsorption of folate or vitamin B_{12}. Suspect inflammatory bowel disease with blood loss. Suspect exudative enteropathy with blood loss.

error. Some of these potential errors are listed in Table 9–6. Cold agglutinins in high titer tend to cause spurious macrocytosis with low red cell counts and very high MCHCs. Warming either the blood or the diluent eliminates this problem.[11]

Electronic cell counting provides a useful means of categorizing anemias based on the MCV and MCHC. The red cell volume distribution width (RDW) is derived from the red blood cell histogram that accompanies each analysis. The RDW is an index of the variation in red cell size and thus can be used to detect anisocytosis. In the normal patient, the histogram is virtually symmetric. The RDW is calculated as a standard statis-

Table 9-5. PHYSICAL FINDINGS AS CLUES TO THE ETIOLOGY OF ANEMIA

Skin	Hyperpigmentation	Fanconi's aplastic anemia
	Petechiae, purpura	Autoimmune hemolytic anemia with thrombocytopenia, hemolytic-uremic syndrome, bone marrow aplasia, bone marrow infiltration
	Carotenemia	Suspect iron deficiency in infants
	Jaundice	Hemolytic anemia, hepatitis, and aplastic anemia
	Cavernous hemangioma	Microangiopathic hemolytic anemia
	Ulcers on lower extremities	S and C hemoglobinopathies, thalassemia
Facies	Frontal bossing, prominence of the malar and maxillary bones	Congenital hemolytic anemias, thalassemia major, severe iron deficiency
Eyes	Microcornea	Fanconi's aplastic anemia
	Tortuosity of the conjunctival and retinal vessels	S and C hemoglobinopathies
	Microaneurysms of retinal vessels	S and C hemoglobinopathies
	Cataracts	Glucose-6-phosphate dehydrogenase deficiency, galactosemia with hemolytic anemia in newborn period
	Vitreous hemorrhages	S hemoglobinopathy
	Retinal hemorrhages	Chronic, severe anemia
	Edema of the eyelids	Infectious mononucleosis, exudative enteropathy with iron deficiency, renal failure
	Blindness	Osteopetrosis
Mouth	Glossitis	Vitamin B_{12} deficiency, iron deficiency
	Angular stomatitis	Iron deficiency
Chest	Unilateral absence of the pectoral muscles	Poland's syndrome (increased incidence of leukemia)[23-25]
	Shield chest	Diamond-Blackfan syndrome
Hands	Triphalangeal thumbs	Red cell aplasia
	Hypoplasia of the thenar eminence	Fanconi's aplastic anemia
	Spoon nails	Iron deficiency
Spleen	Enlargement	Congenital hemolytic anemia, leukemia, lymphoma, acute infection, portal hypertension

tical value, the coefficient of variation of the red cell volume distribution. The formula can be expressed as:

$$RDW = SD/MCV \times 100$$

Because RDW reflects the ratio of standard deviation (SD) and MCV, a wide red cell distribution curve in a patient with a markedly increased MCV may still gen-

Table 9-6. SOURCES OF ERROR IN BLOOD CELL COUNTS SPECIFIC FOR ELECTRONIC COUNTERS

1. *Incorrect diluent or lysis agent* for particular instrument
2. *Extraneous particles in diluting fluid* (or containers, at any step)
3. *Presence of cell type that was not to be counted*
4. *Destruction of cell type that was to be counted*
5. *Error in metered delivery of cells after dilution:* pump, valves, tubing, connections, cut-off switch
6. *Partial obstruction of aperture* (impedance type instrument)
7. *Coincidence loss*
8. *Threshold setting,* sensitivity or potentiometer setting not determined by proper calibration
9. *Carry-over* from one specimen to the next
10. *Spurious pulses from sensing region* of equipment, owing to air bubbles
11. *Spurious signals* from electrical or radiofrequency interference
12. *Instability,* or intermittent failure of electronic components

erate a normal RDW number. The RDW in normal individuals ranges from 11.5% to 14.5%, but it may vary as a function of the model of the electronic cell counter employed. Normal values for infants and children appear to range from 1.5% to 15.0%.[12] The hemoglobin distribution width (HDW) is calculated in a similar manner from the histogram for MCHC. Coulter instruments do not directly measure cell hemoglobin concentration. MCHC and HDW provided by these instruments are sensitive to variations in MCV and should be used with caution in the differential diagnosis of anemias.

Bessman and associates[13] have provided a classification of anemias based on MCV and RDW. An updated version that includes MCHC and HDW appears in Table 9-7.

Visual analysis of the red cell histograms generated by automated cell counters provides essential clues for the diagnosis of anemias. Presence of either microcytes or macrocytes and of increased RDW can be readily appreciated. Histograms for MCHC are particularly useful because they allow prompt identification of dehydrated hyperchromic cells in sickle cell disease, hereditary spherocytosis, hereditary xerocytosis, and immune hemolytic anemias. Moreover, a careful study of volume and hemoglobin concentration histograms allows rapid differentiation of iron deficiency and β-

Table 9–7. THE RELATIONSHIP OF MEAN CORPUSCULAR VOLUME AND RED CELL VOLUME DISTRIBUTION WIDTH IN A VARIETY OF DISEASE STATES

RDW	MCV		
	Low	*Normal*	*High*
Normal	Heterozygous α- and β-thalassemia	Normal Lead poisoning	Aplastic anemia
High	Iron deficiency Hemoglobin H disease S β-thalassemia	Early iron deficiency Liver disease Mixed nutritional deficiencies	Newborns, prematurity Vitamin B$_{12}$ or folate deficiency
		High MCHC/HDW: Immune hemolytic anemia SS and SC disease Hereditary spherocytosis/xerocytosis	*High MCHC/HDW:* Immune hemolytic anemia

thalassemia trait and of hemoglobin H and hemoglobin H/CS disease. Figure 9–1 provides the histograms for MCV and MCHC in a normal control and in patients with β-thalassemia trait, iron deficiency, and sickle cell disease.

Automated reticulocyte counting is also available in several hematology analyzers. Automated counting has better precision and accuracy compared with manual counting.[14–16] Absolute reticulocyte counts are easily obtained with these instruments, obviating the limitations of counting reticulocytes only as a percentage or correcting for the changes in hematocrit (corrected reticulocyte count). An additional useful feature of automated reticulocyte counters is that the presence of stress reticulocytes can easily be identified based on their increased volume and RNA content. Cellular indices for reticulocytes such as volume, hemoglobin concentration, and hemoglobin content are also available in the Technicon H*3 instrument.[17]

The Blood Film

Films made on coverslips are preferable to those made on glass slides because a greater proportion of the blood on the film is technically suitable for microscopic examination. The proper processing of blood films on coverslips is fast becoming a lost art. The details of preparation and examination can be found in manuals of laboratory hematology,[18] but the lucid and succinct instructions of Wintrobe[19] deserve reproduction here:

1. Use a small drop of blood, only 2 to 3 mm in diameter, taken either from a stylet wound, as described earlier, or from a syringe or needle tip used in venipuncture immediately after the venipuncture has been performed (anticoagulants are not to be used because they will alter the morphologic appearance).

2. Hold the coverslips only by their edges, placing one crosswise over the other, and allow the blood to spread between them for about 2 seconds.

3. Quickly but gently separate the coverslips by pulling them laterally, in opposite directions to one another but in the plane of the spreading film, just before the film reaches the edges (do not squeeze or lift the coverslips from one another).

4. Quickly air-dry the films, either by placing them face up on a clean surface if the humidity is low or by moving them through the air while holding them by their edges with your fingertips.

If the procedure has been carried out successfully, the blood will be spread evenly and there will be no holes or thick areas in the preparation. A multicolored sheen will be seen on the surface of the dried, unstained film if light glances off from it at the proper angle, because the thin layer of closely fitting cells acts like a diffraction grating. Later, under the microscope, after staining, the red cells will be seen next to each other, but neither overlapping, nor in rouleau formation, and central pallor will be visible; lymphocytes will have a readily distinguished cytoplasm, rather than a minimal zone bearing closely on the nucleus as occurs in thick films or those that dry too slowly.

The examination of the peripheral blood film is the single most useful procedure in the initial evaluation of the patient with anemia. The blood film should first be examined under low power to determine the adequacy of cell distribution and staining. Signs of poor blood film preparation include loss of central pallor in red blood cells, polygonal shapes, and artifactual spherocytes. Artifactual spherocytes, in contrast to true spherocytes, show no variation in central pallor and are larger than normal red cells. One should never attempt to interpret a poorly prepared blood film.

Once the adequacy of the blood film is determined by low-power examination, the blood film should be examined under 1000× magnification. Cells should be graded as to size, staining intensity, variation in color, and abnormalities of shape. A classification of red cell hemolytic disorders based on their predominant morphology can be accomplished. An approach to such a classification is presented in Table 9–8 and is discussed in detail in Chapter 16.

The blood film should also be examined for the presence of basophilic stippling and red cell inclusions. The significance of some of these findings is described in Table 9–9.

A DIAGNOSTIC APPROACH TO THE ANEMIC PATIENT

Once the laboratory tests have been obtained, results may be employed in an initial attempt at diagnostic

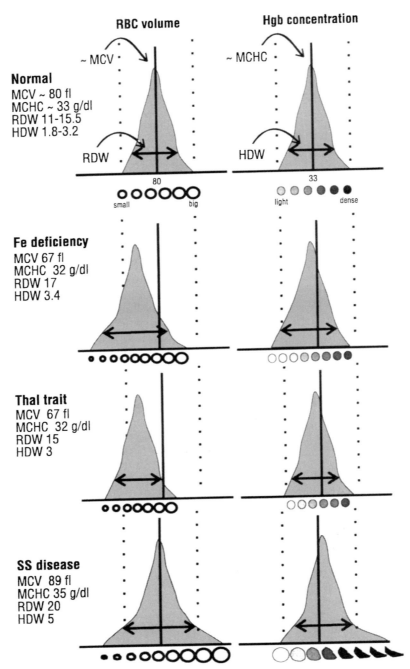

Figure 9-1. Histograms for mean value of red cell volume (MCV, *left column*) and of red cell hemoglobin concentration (MCHC, *right column*) in a normal control *(first row)*, a patient with iron deficiency *(second row)*, a subject with heterozygous β-thalassemia *(third row)*, and a patient with homozygous Hb S disease *(bottom row)*. Goal posts are placed at 60 and 120 fL for MCV and at 28 and 41 g/dL for MCHC. RDW = red cell volume distribution width; HDW = hemoglobin distribution width.

Table 9–8. CLASSIFICATION OF RED CELL HEMOLYTIC DISORDERS BY PREDOMINANT MORPHOLOGY
(Nonhemolytic Disorders of Similar Morphology Are Enclosed in Parentheses for Reference)

Spherocytes
Hereditary spherocytosis
ABO incompatibility in neonates
Immunohemolytic anemias with IgG- or C3-coated red cells*
Acute oxidant injury (hexose monophosphate shunt defects during hemolytic crisis, oxidant drugs and chemicals)
Hemolytic transfusion reactions*
Clostridium welchii septicemia
Severe burns, other red cell thermal injury
Spider, bee, and snake venoms
Severe hypophosphatemia
Hypersplenism†

Bizarre Poikilocytes
Red cell fragmentation syndromes (micro- and macroangiopathic hemolytic anemias)
Acute oxidant injury†
Hereditary elliptocytosis in neonates
Hereditary pyropoikilocytosis

Elliptocytes
Hereditary elliptocytosis
Thalassemias
(Other hypochromic-microcytic anemias)
(Megaloblastic anemias)

Stomatocytes
Hereditary stomatocytosis
Rh_null blood group
Stomatocytosis with cold hemolysis
(Liver disease, especially acute alcoholism)
(Mediterranean stomatocytosis)

Irreversibly Sickled Cells
Sickle cell anemia
Symptomatic sickle syndromes

Intraerythrocytic Parasites
Malaria
Babesiasis
Bartonellosis

Spiculated or Crenated Red Cells
Acute hepatic necrosis (spur cell anemia)
Uremia
Red cell fragmentation syndromes†
Infantile pyknocytosis
Embden-Meyerhof pathway defects†
Vitamin E deficiency†
Abetalipoproteinemia
Heat stroke†
McLeod blood group
(Postsplenectomy)
(Transiently after massive transfusion of stored blood)
(Anorexia nervosa)†

Target Cells
Hemoglobins S, C, D, and E
Hereditary xerocytosis
Thalassemias
(Other hypochromic-microcytic anemias)
(Obstructive liver disease)
(Postsplenectomy)
(Lecithin: cholesterol acyltransferase deficiency)

Prominent Basophilic Stippling
Thalassemias
Unstable hemoglobins
Lead poisoning†
Pyrimidine 5'-nucleotidase deficiency

Nonspecific or Normal Morphology
Embden-Meyerhof pathway defects
Hexose monophosphate shunt defects
Unstable hemoglobins
Paroxysmal nocturnal hemoglobinuria
Dyserythropoietic anemias
Copper toxicity (Wilson's disease)
Cation permeability defects
Erythropoietic porphyria
Vitamin E deficiency
Hemolysis with infections†
Rh hemolytic disease in neonates*
Paroxysmal cold hemoglobinuria*†
Cold hemagglutinin disease*
Hypersplenism
Immunohemolytic anemia*†

* Usually associated with positive Coombs' test.
† Disease sometimes associated with this morphology.

categorization of the patient, as illustrated by the simple algorithm in Figure 9–2. This algorithm provides for two additional diagnostic steps after the initial characterization of anemia based on the complete blood cell count, reticulocyte count, and cellular indices.

If the diagnosis of hemolytic anemia is entertained, it is useful to consider the potential pathophysiology before ordering useless and expensive screening tests. The authors have used a simple and reliable approach to pathophysiology that involves consideration of the potential assaults on the red cell from the farthest point to the inner core of the erythrocyte (Fig. 9–3).

The most common cause of rapid red cell loss with reticulocytosis is hemorrhage. In infants and children, unusual causes of hemorrhage include hemorrhage beneath the scalp and intra-abdominal, urinary tract, and pulmonary hemorrhage. In the latter two causes, hyperbilirubinemia is not present. Indeed, if the hemorrhage

is chronic, leading to iron deficiency, the plasma will be pale.

Sequestration in an abnormal spleen will usually cause spherocytosis, but if the hypersplenism is associated with liver disease, target cells are also present. In this condition, the osmotic fragility test will reveal a sensitive and a resistant population of erythrocytes.

Vascular damage to erythrocytes may be associated with thrombocytopenia and be caused by hemangiomas (the Kasabach-Merritt syndrome); intravascular coagulation, usually due to sepsis; damaged artificial heart valves; and renal vascular disease and severe hypertension. Schistocytes that resemble military helmets of various nationalities are usually present, and siderinuria and hemoglobinuria are often detected.

Abnormalities of plasma are frequent causes of hemolysis. Antibodies usually induce spherocytosis by causing splenic sequestration but sometimes merely fix

Table 9-9. DIAGNOSTIC SIGNIFICANCE OF RED CELL INCLUSIONS

Inclusion	Staining Agent	Diagnostic Significance
Basophilic stippling	Wright's stain	Represent aggregated ribosomes. May be observed in thalassemia syndromes, iron deficiency, syndromes accompanied by ineffective erythropoiesis and pyrimidine 5'-nucleotidase deficiency, particularly prominent in unstable hemoglobinopathies and lead poisoning.
Howell-Jolly bodies	Wright's stain	Represent nuclear remnants. Observed in asplenic and hyposplenic states, pernicious anemia, dyserythropoietic anemias, and severe iron deficiency anemia.
Cabot's rings	Wright's stain	Appear as basophilic rings, circular, or twisted figures-of-eight. Considered to be nuclear remnants or artifacts. Observed in lead poisoning, pernicious anemia and hemolytic anemias.
Heinz's bodies	Brilliant cresyl blue, methyl violet	Represent denatured or aggregated hemoglobin. Observed in patients with thalassemia syndromes or unstable hemoglobins, following oxidant stress in patients with enzyme deficiencies of the pentose phosphate pathway, and in patients with asplenia or chronic liver disease.
Siderocytes	Prussian blue counterstained with Safrinin	Represent nonhemoglobin iron within erythrocytes. Seen in increased numbers in peripheral circulation after splenectomy. Observed in increased numbers in patients with chronic infection, aplastic anemias, or hemolytic anemias.

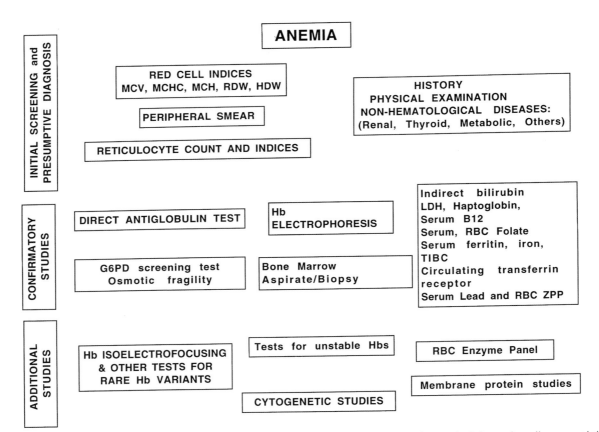

Figure 9-2. Algorithm for differential diagnosis of anemia. The initial characterization of anemia is based on the complete blood cell count, reticulocyte count, cellular indices, erythrocyte morphology, and history. This first step is followed by two additional diagnostic steps, to confirm a relatively common kind of anemia or to diagnose one of the uncommon types of anemia. G6PD = glucose-6-phosphate dehydrogenase; TIBC = total iron-binding capacity; LDH = lactate dehydrogenase; ZPP = zinc protoporphyrin.

```
┌─────────────────────────────────────────────────────────────────────┐
│ HEMORRHAGE (pale plasma, normal morphology, or microcytosis)          │
│ ┌───────────────────────────────────────────────────────────────┐    │
│ │ HYPERSPLENISM (spherocytosis, target cells)                     │    │
│ │ ┌─────────────────────────────────────────────────────────┐    │    │
│ │ │ VASCULAR DAMAGE (helmet cells, hemoglobinuria)            │    │    │
│ │ │ ┌───────────────────────────────────────────────────┐    │    │    │
│ │ │ │ PLASMA FACTORS (spherocytes, bite cells)           │    │    │    │
│ │ │ │ ┌─────────────────────────────────────────────┐    │    │    │    │
│ │ │ │ │ MEMBRANE (various shapeopathies)             │    │    │    │    │
│ │ │ │ │ ┌───────────────────────────────────────┐    │    │    │    │    │
│ │ │ │ │ │ METABOLIC (bite cells,                 │    │    │    │    │    │
│ │ │ │ │ │ contracted cells)                      │    │    │    │    │    │
│ │ │ │ │ │ ┌─────────────────────────┐            │    │    │    │    │    │
│ │ │ │ │ │ │ HBOPATHY                 │            │    │    │    │    │    │
│ │ │ │ │ │ │ (sickle, target)         │            │    │    │    │    │    │
│ │ │ │ │ │ │ SS, SC, thal             │            │    │    │    │    │    │
│ │ │ │ │ │ └─────────────────────────┘            │    │    │    │    │    │
│ │ │ │ │ │ G6PD⁻ and PK⁻                          │    │    │    │    │    │
│ │ │ │ │ └───────────────────────────────────────┘    │    │    │    │    │
│ │ │ │ │ PNH, HS, permeability defects                │    │    │    │    │
│ │ │ │ └─────────────────────────────────────────────┘    │    │    │    │
│ │ │ │ antibodies, toxins, drugs, CU⁺⁺                    │    │    │    │
│ │ │ └───────────────────────────────────────────────────┘    │    │    │
│ │ │ heart valve, hemangioma, renal vascular disease, DIC     │    │    │
│ │ └─────────────────────────────────────────────────────────┘    │    │
│ │ liver disease, portal vascular disorders, "primary" splenomegaly│    │
│ └───────────────────────────────────────────────────────────────┘    │
│ including pulmonary hemorrhage                                         │
└─────────────────────────────────────────────────────────────────────┘
```

Figure 9-3. The assaults on the red cell from the vasculature to the "center" of the cell. The site of damage is in capital letters, the laboratory findings in parentheses, and the common causes in the lower part of the square. HBOPATHY = hemoglobinopathy; SS = hemoglobin SS; SC = hemoglobin SC; thal = thalassemia; PK = pyruvate kinase; PNH = paroxysmal nocturnal hemoglobinuria; HS = hereditary spherocytosis; CU⁺⁺ = copper.

complement and cause hemoglobinuria without morphologic change. Many drugs and toxins can damage red cells either by oxidant damage with resultant schistocytosis or by direct lysis, as illustrated by bacterial lipases in septic shock. Acute hemolysis also may be caused by excessive release of hepatic copper in Wilson's disease. No morphologic change is noted.

Primary membrane abnormalities that cause hemolysis are usually congenital and associated with specific morphologic changes. An exception is paroxysmal nocturnal hemoglobinuria, which is an acquired membrane defect associated with no morphologic change. The congenital membrane defects are usually due to abnormalities of structural membrane proteins, such as in hereditary spherocytosis, but may involve cation channels (hydrocytosis and xerocytosis) and, rarely, membrane lipids (abetalipoproteinemia).

The red cell itself may contribute to its own quietus, as exemplified by glucose-6-phosphate dehydrogenase deficiency, pyruvate kinase deficiency, and deficiencies of the other enzymes involved in erythrocyte metabolic pathways. Morphologic alterations are not predictable.

Finally, the red cell may be sabotaged by its own hemoglobin, such as in sickle cell anemia, the thalassemias, and the unstable hemoglobinopathies.

If the clinician considers these options in an inclusive but systematic fashion, direct screening tests can be ordered and expert consultation avoided.

References

1. Dallman PR, Siimes MA: Percentile curves for hemoglobin and red cell volume in infancy and childhood. J Pediatr 1979; 94:26.
2. Finch CA: Red Cell Manual. Seattle, University of Washington, 1970.
3. d'Onofrio G, Chirillo R, et al: Simultaneous measurement of reticulocyte and red blood cell indices in healthy subjects and patients with microcytic and macrocytic anemia. Blood 1995; 85:818.
4. Tycko DH, Metz MH, et al: A flow-cytometric light scattering measurement of red blood cell volume and hemoglobin concentration. J Appl Opt 1985; 24:1355.
5. Fossat G, David M, et al: New parameters in erythrocyte counting. Arch Pathol Lab Med 1987; 111:1150.
6. Mohandas N, Kim YR, et al: Accurate and independent measurement of volume and hemoglobin concentration of individual red cells by laser light scattering. Blood 1986; 68:506.
7. Mohandas N, Johnson A, et al: Automated quantitation of cell density distribution and hyperdense cell fraction in RBC disorders. Blood 1989; 74:442.
8. Brittin GM, Brecher G: Instrumentation and automation in clinical hematology. In Brown E, Moore CV (eds): Progress in Hematology. Vol. VII. New York, Grune & Stratton, Inc., 1971, p 299.
9. Nelson DA, Morris MW: Basic examination of blood. In Henry JB (ed): Clinical Diagnosis & Management by Laboratory Methods. 18th ed. Philadelphia, W.B. Saunders Co., 1991, p 553.
10. Simson E: Hematology Beyond the Microscope. Tarrytown, NY, Technicon Instruments Corporation, 1984.
11. Hattersley PG, Gerard PW, et al: Erroneous values on the Model S Coulter due to high titer cold agglutinins. Am J Clin Pathol 1971; 55:442.
12. Novak RW: Red blood cell distribution width in pediatric microcytic anemias. Pediatrics 1987; 80:251.
13. Bessman JD, Gilmer PR Jr, et al: Improved classification of anemias by MCV and RDW. Am J Clin Pathol 1983; 80:322.
14. Savage RA, Skoog DP, Rabinovitch A: Analytic inaccuracy and imprecision in reticulocyte counting: a preliminary report from the College of American Pathologists reticulocyte project. Blood Cells 1985; 11:97.
15. National Committee for Clinical Laboratory Standards. Methods for Reticulocyte Counting, Proposed Standards. NCCLS document H16-P, Villanova, PA, 1985.

16. Schimenti KJ, Lacerna K, et al: Reticulocyte quantification by flow cytometry, image analysis and manual counting. Cytometry 1992; 13:853.
17. Brugnara C, Hipp MJ, et al: Automated reticulocyte counting and measurement of reticulocyte cellular indices: evaluation of the Miles H*3 blood analyzer. Am J Clin Pathol 1994; 102:623.
18. Cartwright GE: Diagnostic Laboratory Hematology. 4th ed. New York, Grune & Stratton, Inc., 1968.
19. Wintrobe MM: Clinical Hematology. 7th ed. Philadelphia, Lea & Febiger, 1974, p 24.
20. Beguin Y, Fillet G, et al: Ferrokinetic study of splenic erythropoiesis: relationships among clinical diagnosis, myelofibrosis, splenomegaly, and extramedullary erythropoiesis. Am J Hematol 1989; 32:123.
21. Geary DG, Fennel RS, et al: Hyperparathyroidism and anemia in chronic renal failure. Eur J Pediatr 1982; 139:296.
22. Abboud MR, Alexander D, et al: Diabetes mellitus, thiamine-dependent megaloblastic anemia, and sensorineural deafness associated with deficient ocketoglutarate dehydrogenase activity. J Pediatr 1985; 107:537.
23. Parikh PM, Karandikar SM, et al: Poland's syndrome with acute lymphoblastic leukemia in an adult. Med Pediatr Oncol 1988; 16:290.
24. Sackey K, Odone V, et al: Poland's syndrome associated with childhood non-Hodgkin's lymphoma. Am J Dis Child 1984; 138:600.
25. Parikh T, Karandikar SM, et al: Poland's syndrome with acute lymphoblastic leukemia in an adult. Med Pediatr Oncol 1988; 16:290.

Megaloblastic Anemia

V. Michael Whitehead • David S. Rosenblatt
Bernard A. Cooper

Before the mid-1920s, *pernicious anemia* was a disease dreaded as much as drug-resistant leukemia is today. With its characteristic megaloblastic bone marrow, pernicious anemia was a fatal illness until it was successfully treated with dietary liver in 1926.[1] It is now known that megaloblastic anemia is caused most frequently by a nutritional deficiency of folates or by a specific malabsorption of cobalamin known as pernicious anemia (Table 10–1). Precise means for diagnosing and treating these deficiencies are now available. Over the past 70 years, hematologists have gained detailed knowledge of the synthesis, biology, biochemistry, and molecular biology of both vitamin B_{12} and folate. It is extraordinary that this knowledge base is continuing to grow as new discoveries are made.

This chapter reviews aspects of this knowledge as it pertains in particular to pediatric patients. Emphasis is placed on the clinical and laboratory diagnosis of overt deficiencies of vitamin B_{12} and folates as well as on their treatment. Also, attention is focused on subclinical deficiency states as they relate to populations at increased risk, including premature newborns, the elderly, those with HIV infection, and those with elevated plasma total homocysteine levels. Consideration is given to the role of these vitamins in the prevention of neural tube defects and of cardiovascular disease and in the pathogenesis of cancer. Finally, current knowledge of inborn errors of cobalamin and folate metabolism is presented.

DEFINITIONS

Megaloblastic anemia is a macrocytic anemia that is usually accompanied by leukopenia and thrombocyto-

Table 10-1. CAUSES OF MEGALOBLASTIC ANEMIA

Vitamin B₁₂ (Cobalamin)

Defects in Absorption

Inadequate Gastric Intrinsic Factor Due to

Pernicious anemia
Gastritis
Total gastrectomy
Intrinsic factor gene mutations

Achlorhydria and Pepsin Deficiency (?)

Disease of the small intestine

Surgical resection or bypass of the terminal ileum
Regional enteritis (Crohn's disease)
Tropical and nontropical sprue
Infiltrative diseases (Whipple's syndrome, lymphoma)
Competition by parasites (fish tapeworm, blind loop
 syndrome)
Imerslund-Gräsbeck syndrome
Drugs (colchicine, PAS, neomycin)
Transcobalamin II deficiency
Secondary to megaloblastic anemia

Inadequate Nutrition

Strict vegetarians (vegans)
Maternal deficiency affecting the fetus or infant

Defects in Transport

Transcobalamin II deficiency

Defects in Metabolism

Nitrous oxide intoxication
Inherited (cblC, cblD, cblE, cblF, and cblG diseases)

Folates

Defects in Absorption

Inherited (hereditary folate malabsorption)
Tropical and nontropical sprue
Infiltrative diseases of the small bowel (Whipple's sydrome,
 lymphoma)

Inadequate Nutrition

Insufficient or poorly selected diet
Maternal deficiency affecting the fetus or infant

Increased Requirement

Alcoholism
Pregnancy
Lactation
Hemolytic anemia
Hyperthyroidism
Anticonvulsant therapy
Lesch-Nyhan syndrome
Prematurity
Homocystinuria
First trimester during neural tube development

Folate Inhibitors

Antifolates (methotrexate, pyrimethamine, trimethoprim)
Sulfones

Inherited Defects

Methylenetetrahydrofolate reductase deficiency
Methionine synthase deficiency (cblE, cblG disease)
Others

Other Causes

Defects in Purine and Pyrimidine Synthesis

Inherited
Orotic aciduria
Acquired
Myelodysplasia and leukemia
Drug-induced
HIV infection

Other

Thiamine-responsive anemia
Scurvy
Pyridoxine-responsive anemia

penia. It is characterized by a specific megaloblastic bone marrow morphology, affecting erythroid, myeloid, and platelet precursors. In this chapter, the terms *vitamin B₁₂* and *cobalamin* are used interchangeably to refer to corrins that have coenzyme activity or that can be converted to coenzymes in cells (see later). The term *folates* refers to synthetic folic acid and to the various natural folate coenzymes, which are reduced dihydrofolates (DHFs) and tetrahydrofolates (THFs) and their single-carbon substituted forms. *Natural folate coenzymes* are substrates for the enzyme folate polyglutamate synthetase and are converted by it to folate polyglutamates containing predominantly 6 or 7 γ-linked glutamate residues. Most folates in nature are present as reduced and substituted folate polyglutamates. These, too, are included under the general term *folates*.

HISTORY

Anemia associated with morphologically abnormal erythrocytes had been observed in pernicious anemia from 1876 to 1877.[2-4] By 1883, macrocytosis had been described in patients with pernicious anemia. In 1891, Ehrlich stained and described megaloblastic erythroid precursors.[5] The presence of increased numbers of nuclear segments in circulating neutrophils ("hypersegmentation") was described in 1923, and giant myeloid band forms were observed in megaloblastic bone marrow in 1920. Megaloblastic changes in the bone marrow during relapse, with the return of normal morphology during remission, were reported in 1921, 5 to 6 years before therapy for the disease was developed. In 1926, Minot and Murphy[1] described conversion of megaloblastic bone marrow to normoblastic bone marrow along with reticulocytosis and correction of the anemia following treatment with dietary liver. The sequence of these events has been summarized in several reviews.[3, 6]

Among many subsequent observations, the following are among the most important:

1. Similar clinical syndromes (*pernicious anemia of pregnancy* and *tropical anemia*) were described in 1931 and subsequently were shown to be due to deficiency in folates.[7]

2. In pernicious anemia, because of atrophy (destruction) of the gastric mucosa,[8] the stomach does not contain enough of the gastric intrinsic factor needed for absorption of vitamin B₁₂ from the gut.[9] The disease is caused by failure to absorb adequate quantities of vitamin B₁₂.[2, 10]

3. Cobalamin injections were found to correct pernicious anemia,[11] and folate administration to resolve the anemia described by Wills. Each vitamin, when given in large doses, could produce some effect on the hematologic abnormalities caused by deficiency of the other.[12, 13]

4. The cobalamin-binding protein *transcobalamin II* functions as an "intrinsic factor" within the body, permitting endocytosis-mediated utilization of cobalamin by cells.[14, 15]

5. Assays for cobalamin and folates in serum and

tissues of patients with megaloblastic anemia permitted chemical definition of the deficiency.[16-18]

6. Subacute combined degeneration of the spinal cord, a neurologic syndrome, often accompanied classic pernicious anemia but not the megaloblastic anemia caused by folate deficiency.[2, 19]

7. Pernicious anemia is probably an autoimmune disease[20] caused by lymphocyte-mediated destruction of gastric parietal cells, with the possible immunologic target being the Na⁺,K⁺ATPase on the parietal cell membrane.[21-23]

8. Inherited defects of the metabolism of cobalamin and folates may cause abnormal development in addition to megaloblastic anemia.[24-27]

9. The purification and subsequent cloning of intrinsic factor and the transcobalamins, the accumulation of information about their structure, and the study of their receptors define the function of these proteins.[28-33]

10. The complete pathway of cobalamin biosynthesis by bacteria has been elucidated.[34]

11. Elevated plasma methylmalonic acid and total homocysteine reflect tissue functional deficiency of cobalamin and of either folates or cobalamin, respectively, even in patients with vitamin levels within the normal range.[35]

12. Neural tube defects including spina bifida can be prevented by maternal folate supplementation during the periconceptual interval.[36, 37]

13. Folate supplementation can reduce the elevated plasma total homocysteine level, recognized to be a risk factor for arteriosclerotic vascular disease,[38] and it may decrease the incidence of bowel and other cancers.[39]

HEMATOLOGIC DESCRIPTION

Bone Marrow and Blood

The causes of megaloblastic anemia are classified in Table 10–1.

The megaloblastic bone marrow is hyperplastic, with erythropoiesis being stimulated by increased levels of erythropoietin acting on erythroid progenitor cells. Megaloblastic erythroid cells are more prone to undergo programmed cell death or apoptosis during maturation than when they are mature[40, 41]; this results in a predominance of young erythroid cells in the bone marrow. This "ineffective erythropoiesis" is the cause of elevated serum levels of lactate dehydrogenase, bile pigments, and iron (derived from dying erythroid precursors). Mature erythrocytes have abnormal shapes and are of various sizes, and their mean cell volume (MCV) is much greater than normal. Macrocytic and misshapen erythrocytes survive for a shorter time in the blood than do normal erythrocytes.

In megaloblastic anemia, erythroid precursors have a normal DNA content together with an elevated RNA content. For this reason, they have more cellular RNA per unit of DNA and, thus, are larger than normal cells of the same level of maturation.[42] Their nuclear

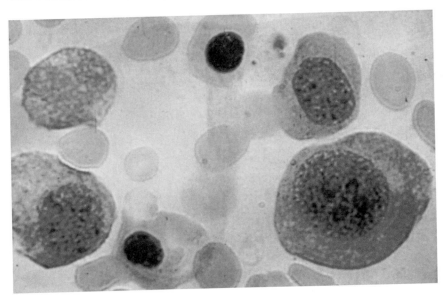

Figure 10-1. Megaloblasts in the bone marrow. (See the text for details.)

chromatin appears looser than normal on stained smears (Fig. 10–1), giving the characteristic appearance of the megaloblast. There is asynchrony of maturation of nucleus and cytoplasm, with the nucleus appearing less mature than the cytoplasm. For example, polychromatophilic erythroblasts with considerable accumulation of hemoglobin in the cytoplasm may have vesicular, open, or immature nuclei, and more mature orthochromic erythroblasts may contain nuclei that are not the dense, small, purple-staining nuclei of normal orthochromes. Experienced observers usually recognize megaloblastic erythropoiesis by noting the vesicular and open nuclear pattern in the earliest erythroblasts (proerythroblasts and basophilic erythroblasts) (see Fig. 10–1).

Myeloid precursors are larger than normal; the most striking are the giant metamyelocytes and band neutrophils in the megaloblastic bone marrow. These cells may persist in bone marrow for 10 to 14 days after the start of treatment.[43] Giant metamyelocytes and band neutrophils are not seen in the megaloblastoid bone marrow of patients with leukemia or myelodysplasia. Similar abnormalities probably affect megakaryocyte precursors, but these changes have not been well de-

scribed. Neutropenia and thrombocytopenia are more common in patients with severe than with mild anemia associated with megaloblastic bone marrow, but they may both occur in cobalamin-deficient patients who are not anemic.

Multilobar neutrophils are seen in the peripheral blood (Fig. 10–2). *Neutrophil hypersegmentation* is defined as the presence of one or more six-lobed neutrophils or of five or more neutrophils with five or more well-separated lobes among 100 segmented neutrophils. Hypersegmentation is a characteristic feature of cobalamin and folate deficiencies.

Other Tissues

Macrocytosis of buccal cells has been reported in patients with megaloblastic anemia. Similar abnormalities have been described in cells of the tongue, vaginal epithelium, urinary tract, nasal epithelium, and other lining tissues. Decreased height of gastric cells and enterocytes also has been described. These changes reverse after treatment of the megaloblastic anemia and are not found in all patients.[44, 45]

VITAMIN B₁₂ (Cobalamin)
Nutritional Sources and Requirements

Cobalamin is synthesized by bacteria and algae. The entire bacterial biosynthetic pathway for cobalamin synthesis has been elucidated and involves 20 different enzymatic steps.[34] Cobalamin is required as a vitamin by animals but is not required by higher plants. Plants neither synthesize nor accumulate cobalamin and, thus, do not contribute it to the diet. The presence of cobalamin in ground water is used as an index of fecal contamination.

Because all of the cobalamin needed by humans is provided through the diet, inadequate intake causes deficiency. Neither the dietary cobalamin needs nor the frequency of dietary cobalamin deficiency in different

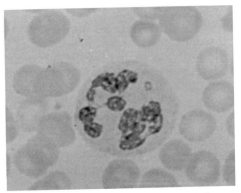

Figure 10-2. Multilobar neutrophil.

populations are well defined, but some published data do exist.[46, 47] In India, the concentration of vitamin B_{12} in serum and tissues is low[48–52]—both in vegetarians, who eat no meat but do eat dairy products, and in strict vegetarians (vegans) who consume no animal products whatever and in whom megaloblastic anemia due to inadequate cobalamin intake does occur. Neurologic disease, subacute combined degeneration of the spinal cord (SCDSC), due to cobalamin deficiency, has been described in vegans, but its frequency appears to be very low.[53, 54] It is not known why the frequency of neurologic disease in vegans with very low plasma cobalamin levels is low. Insight might be gained from studies of the frequency of neurologic disease and of biologic cobalamin deficiency as reflected by elevated plasma levels of total homocysteine and of methylmalonic acid in such vegan communities.

The World Health Organization has recommended a daily intake of cobalamin of 1 μg for normal adults; 1.3 and 1.4 μg daily for lactating and pregnant women, respectively; and 0.1 μg per day for infants, on the basis of the known physiology and turnover of cobalamin, the quantity required to treat deficiency, and a variety of other factors. The World Health Organization has calculated that mean adult cobalamin intake per day was less than 1 μg in many countries.[55]

Chemistry of Cobalamins

Cobalamins have the chemical structure shown in Figure 10–3. They belong to a class of compounds known as *corrins*, which contain a ringlike structure resembling but distinct from that of porphyrins (including hemo-

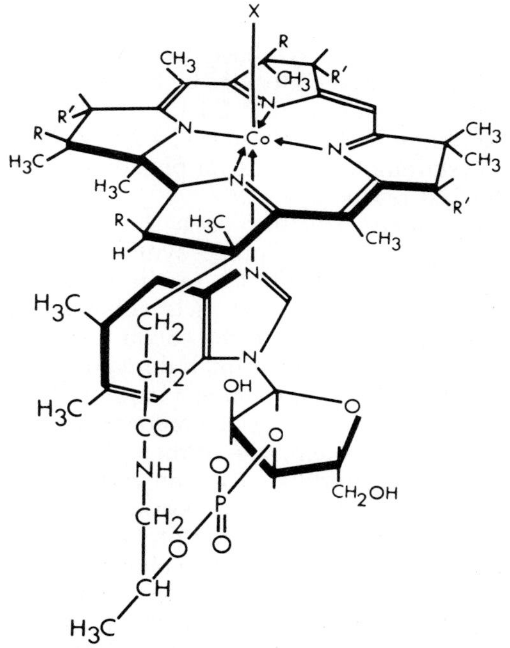

Figure 10–3. Cobalamin (vitamin B_{12}, Cbl). When X is methyl, the compound is methylcobalamin (MeCbl); when it is adenosyl, the compound is 5'-deoxyadenosylcobalamin (AdoCbl); when it is CN, the compound is cyanocobalamin (CNCbl), and so forth.

globin) and a nucleotide, 5,6-dimethylbenzimidazole, that is set almost at right angles to the corrin ring. Corrins that have coenzyme activity or can be converted to coenzymes in cells include cobalamins with CN, OH, H_2O, SH, SO_3, glutathione, methyl, or 5'-deoxyadenosyl bound to the cobalt, as well as cobalamins with the cobalt atom reduced to divalent cob(II)alamin (vitamin B_{12R}) or to monovalent cob(I)alamin (vitamin B_{12S}). When the cobalt atom is in its oxidized, trivalent state, the compounds are known as *cob(III)alamins* or are named for the group binding to the cobalt (e.g., cyanocobalamin [CNCbl], hydroxocobalamin [OHCbl], aquocobalamin [H_2OCbl]).[56–58]

Biochemistry of Vitamin B_{12}

Vitamin B_{12} functions as a coenzyme in two reactions:

1. As methylcobalamin (MeCbl) in the synthesis of methionine from homocysteine and 5-methyltetrahydrofolate (5-methyl-THF),[59] which is mediated by the cobalamin-requiring enzyme methionine synthase (5-methyl-THF–homocysteine *S*-methyltransferase, EC 2.1.1.13)[60]:

Reaction 1

Homocysteine + 5-methyl-THF → methionine + THF

2. As 5'-deoxyadenosylcobalamin (AdoCbl, Ado-B_{12}) in the conversion of methylmalonyl coenzyme A (CoA) to succinyl CoA,[2, 61] which is mediated by the cobalamin-requiring enzyme methylmalonyl-CoA mutase (MMA mutase, EC 5.4.99.2)[62–69]:

Reaction 2

Methylmalonyl CoA → succinyl CoA

In prokaryotes, a variety of other enzymes utilize cobalamin for reactions that appear not to occur in mammalian cells.

Reaction 1 is the major pathway for resynthesis of methionine in humans, and low plasma levels of methionine develop when it is impaired. Interruption of this reaction, which requires both folate and cobalamin cofactors, is considered to be the common lesion that results in megaloblastic anemia with both cobalamin and folate deficiencies (known as the "methylfolate trap" hypothesis). In addition, both cobalamin-dependent reactions reduce plasma levels of two potentially toxic materials: (1) homocysteine, which has been associated with vascular endothelial damage; and (2) methylmalonate, which can cause metabolic acidosis (limited to inborn errors of cobalamin metabolism).

Cobalamin that enters the cytoplasm does not appear to be retained in the cell unless it binds to a high-affinity binder. Methionine synthase[60] is the major such binder in the cytoplasm. Cobalamin also enters the mitochondria, in which it reacts with adenosine triphosphate (ATP)–cob(II)alamin transferase to form Ado-Cbl, which binds to MMA mutase (Fig. 10–4).[70–75] In mitochondria from rat liver, most of the cobalamin appears to be AdoCbl.[74] Cytoplasmic cobalamin is

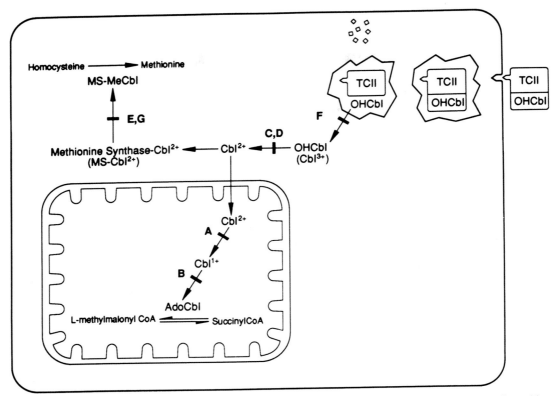

Figure 10–4. Scheme of cobalamin (vitamin B_{12}, Cbl) metabolism. The letters A through G represent the sites of known inherited defects (cblA–cblG). Cbl = cobalamin; $Cbl^{1+,2+,3+}$ = cobalamin with 1+, 2+, or 3+ oxidation states of the central cobalt; OHCbl = hydroxycobalamin; MS = methionine synthase; TC II = transcobalamin II; MeCbl = methylcobalamin; CoA = coenzyme A.

probably reduced to cob(II)alamin before binding to methionine synthase.[60] It is possible that entry into mitochondria also requires reduction or chemical modification of cobalamins because intact (unswollen) mitochondria from rat liver appear to be impermeable to cob(III)alamins.[76]

Methionine Synthesis

Methionine is consumed in the diet and is absorbed. Plasma methionine enters cells and the cerebrospinal fluid by similar membrane transport systems. Cellular methionine may be incorporated into protein or may be adenosylated to *S*-adenosylmethionine (SAMe) by the enzyme ATP-L-methionine *S*-adenosyltransferase (EC 2.5.1.6):

Reaction 3

$$Methionine + adenosine \rightarrow SAMe$$

SAMe donates methyl groups in many reactions, leaving *S*-adenosylhomocysteine (AHCy):

Reaction 4

$$SAMe + R \rightarrow AHCy + CH_3\text{-}R$$

AHCy is hydrolyzed to homocysteine and adenosine by the enzyme *S*-adenosylhomocysteine hydrolase (EC 3.3.1.1):

Reaction 5

$$AHCy \rightarrow homocysteine + adenosine$$

The homocysteine may then be remethylated to methionine by methionine synthase (see Reaction 1, presented earlier) or in hepatocytes by betaine-L-homocysteine methyltransferase (EC 2.1.1.5), or it may react with cystathionine β-synthase (EC 4.2.1.22) and serine to form cystathionine. Pyridoxal phosphate is a cofactor in this last reaction.[77–81]

The crystalline structure of a 27-kd MeCbl-containing fragment of methionine synthase from *Escherichia coli* was determined at a resolution of 0.3 nm[81a] (Fig. 10–5). This structure depicts cobalamin-protein interactions and reveals that the corrin macrocycle lies between a helical NH_2-terminal domain and an αβ carboxyl-terminal domain that is a variant of the Rossmann fold. MeCbl undergoes a conformational change on binding the protein; the dimethylbenzimidazole group, which is coordinated to the cobalt in the free cofactor, moves away from the corrin and is replaced by a histidine contributed by the protein.

Methionine synthase requires cobalamin bound to the enzyme as a prosthetic group or coenzyme. If cob(I)alamin is bound to the enzyme, it is readily methylated by 5-methyl-THF to form MeCbl. The methionine synthase then mediates transfer of this methyl from MeCbl to homocysteine to form methionine. Cob(I)alamin is readily oxidized and appears to spontaneously undergo oxidation to cob(II)alamin. Methylation

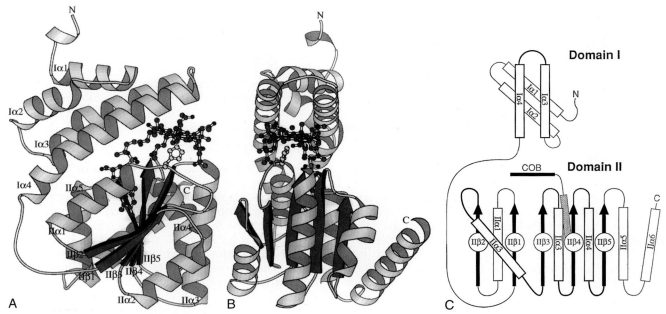

Figure 10–5. The cobalamin-binding domains of methionine synthase. *A,* A ribbon drawing with atoms of the cobalamin and His[759] in ball-and-stick mode. The drawing was generated with the use of MOLSCRIPT (see Kraulis PJ: MOLSCRIPT. A program to produce both detailed and schematic plots of protein structures. J Appl Crystallogr 1991; 24:946). The NH$_2$-terminal helical bundle domain is shown "above" the corrin. Kinks in helices in 1α3 and 1α4, evident in the drawing, occur at Pro[696] and Pro[734]. *B,* A ribbon drawing in an orientation 90 degrees from that shown in *A.* This orientation corresponds approximately to the topology diagram of *C.* In this view, a striking feature is the narrow first domain, which is similar in width to the corrin macrocycle. In the intact enzyme, substrate-binding segments are expected to adjoin this domain. *C,* Topology diagram. The helices of the first domain form a bundle according to defined criteria (see Harris NL, Presnell SR, Cohen FE: Four helix bundle diversity in globular proteins. J Molec Biol 1994; 236:1356), with the front and back pair of helices inclined at angles of 50 and 55 degrees. In domain II, a doubly wound α/β fold, helices IIα1 and IIα5 are behind the sheet and IIα2, IIα3 and IIα4 are in front. Helix IIα6 makes substantial contacts with helix IIα5 but may also pack against other domains in intact methionine synthase. The corrin (COB) is indicated above the cleft between b-sheet strands 1 and 3; the dimethylbenzimidazole tail *(shaded)* adjoins strands IIβ3 and IIβ4. (Adapted from Drennan CL, Huang S, et al: How a protein binds B$_{12}$: a 3.0 Å X-ray structure of B$_{12}$-binding domains of methionine synthase. Science 1994; 266:1669–1674.)

of cob(II)alamin requires SAMe as a methyl donor. In *E. coli,* two flavoproteins have been described that maintain cob(I)alamin in its reduced state or provide other necessary reduction in the reaction.[82] In mammalian cells, this function may be provided by an iron atom that is a part of the methionine synthase enzyme,[60] whereas a copper atom appears to serve this function in the *E. coli* enzyme.[83] Evidence for the importance of some type of reduction reaction associated with methionine synthesis is provided by patients with cblE disease (described later), in whom this activity appears to be abnormal.[84]

Methylmalonyl-CoA Mutase

For this intramitochondrial reaction to occur (see Reaction 2, presented earlier), cobalamin must undergo reduction to cob(I)alamin (either before entry or in the mitochondria), enter the mitochondria (by an unknown mechanism), and receive a 5'-deoxyadenosyl group from ATP:

Reaction 6

ATP + Cob(I)alamin → AdoCbl + Triphosphate

The resulting AdoCbl then binds to MMA mutase to produce the active enzyme.

The biochemical effects associated with impairment of this pathway due to cobalamin deficiency include (1) elevated plasma and urine methylmalonic acid levels to an extent determined by the flow of odd-chain fatty acids, valine, and threonine through the pathway; and (2) the secondary effects of MMA accumulation, which include acidosis, hyperglycinemia, the possible inhibition of other enzymes, and perhaps inhibition of proliferation of bone marrow stem cells.[85–89]

Physiology of Cobalamins

Transport

Effective transmembrane transport of cobalamins into mammalian cells at the low cobalamin levels found in nature requires mediation of a cobalamin-binding protein reacting with a receptor on the cell surface that recognizes the cobalamin-protein complex. These transporters are *intrinsic factor (IF),* which binds to the IF-Cbl receptor on the small intestinal mucosa, and *transcobalamin II (TC II),* which binds to the TC II–Cbl receptor, located on the surface of many cells.

Cobalamin-Binding Proteins

Intrinsic Factor. IF, a glycoprotein, is synthesized in gastric parietal cells in humans and guinea pigs and in chief (pepsinogen) cells in the rat stomach. It may also be secreted by pancreatic cells in dogs.[90] It is readily digested by pepsin but not by trypsin.[91] The Cbl-IF in the gut lumen is available for absorption, whereas unbound IF is not absorbed. IF binds cobalamins less tightly (K_d = 0.1 to 1.0 nmol/L)[92] than do the transcobalamins. However, its binding affinity for cobalamins is far greater than that for nonfunctional corrin analogues, such that the latter are not absorbed from the intestine. The gene for IF is located on chromosome 11.[93]

Transcobalamin II. TC II mediates the entry of cobalamin into cells. It is found in plasma, cerebrospinal fluid, seminal fluid, and transudates. It is synthesized in a variety of cells, including fibroblasts, macrophages, enterocytes, renal cells, hepatocytes, spleen, heart, gastric mucosa, and endothelium.[94] It is a nonglycosylated protein with a molecular weight of 43,000.[95] It polymerizes with itself or with another protein when it binds cobalamin. Plasma turnover of TC II is rapid.[96] It binds cobalamin tightly (K_d = 5 to 18 pmol/L) but has low affinity for corrins without vitamin B_{12} activity. A complementary DNA (cDNA) for TC II has been characterized.[28]

Haptocorrins. Haptocorrins (also variously called *TC 0, TC I, TC III, R binder,* and *cobalophilin*) are a family of proteins with similar structure but different degrees of glycosylation. They are synthesized by myeloid cells and probably by many other cells. Haptocorrins are present in many secretions, including plasma, bile, saliva, tears, breast milk, amniotic fluid, and seminal fluid, and in extracts of granulocytes, salivary gland, platelets, hepatoma cells, and breast tumors.[94, 97, 98] The fully glycosylated haptocorrin found in plasma has a low isoelectric point and a half-life of 9 days; those haptocorrins with higher pIs are cleared more rapidly from the plasma into the bile. Seventy to 90% of the cobalamin in plasma is bound to haptocorrin, with the remainder associated with TC II. Haptocorrins have the greatest affinity for cobalamins of all of the cobalamin-binding proteins (K_d = 3 to 7 pmol/L). In addition, they have considerable binding affinity for other corrins that lack vitamin B_{12} activity. It has been suggested that an important function of haptocorrins *in vivo* is the binding and excretion of such cobalamin analogues into the bile.[99] Gastric juice contains both haptocorrins, which are probably derived from saliva and perhaps gastric parietal cells,[98] and IF.

Absorption of Cobalamins

Cobalamin in meat and fish is released from intracellular enzymes and binds to haptocorrin present in saliva or the food. Haptocorrin is digested by trypsin in the stomach and duodenum, permitting binding of cobalamin to IF. The IF-Cbl complex binds to receptors on the brush border of the ileal enterocyte; after binding, the cobalamin slowly enters the portal vein bound to TC II. Whereas cobalamin fed in large quantities without IF appears in the portal vein 1 hour after feeding, cobalamin bound to IF appears about 12 hours after feeding and 8 to 12 hours after reaching the ileal lumen (Fig. 10–6).[100] Synthesis of TC II by ileal cells may be required for transport.[101, 102] The distribution of the ileal IF-Cbl receptor varies in different subjects. In some, removal of a small segment of ileum removes the majority of the absorptive surface and causes malabsorption of vitamin B_{12}; in other subjects, the absorptive mechanism extends through a considerable portion of the ileum.

The maximum quantity of IF-Cbl that can be bound to receptor in the human intestine is about 1.5 μg.[2] The IF-Cbl receptor appears to disappear from the surface of the enterocyte during IF-Cbl absorption; this limits the absorption of large doses of cobalamin bound to IF. However, receptor activity reappears rapidly, so that a second bolus can be absorbed soon after the first. When massive quantities of cobalamin (100 to 1000 μg) are fed to patients lacking IF in the gut, a small propor-

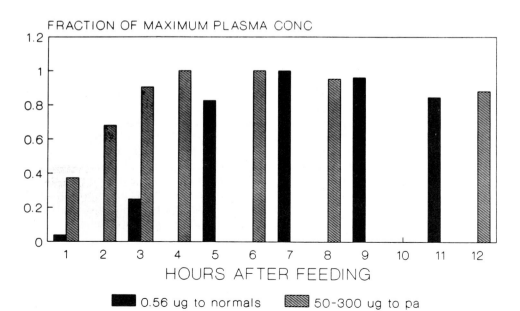

FRACTION OF MAXIMUM PLASMA CONC

HOURS AFTER FEEDING

■ 0.56 ug to normals   ▨ 50-300 ug to pa

Figure 10–6. Absorption of labeled cyanocobalamin (vitamin B_{12}) with the intrinsic factor mechanism *(black bars)* or without intrinsic factor *(shaded bars)*. (Adapted from Doscherholmen A, Hagen PS: Delay of absorption of radiolabeled cyanocobalamin in the intestinal wall in the presence of intrinsic factor. J Lab Clin Med 1959; 54:434.)

tion (0.1% to 1%) is absorbed from the jejunum, presumably by means of a nonspecific mechanism such as diffusion. The receptor for IF-Cbl has been purified.[103, 104]

Malabsorption of cobalamin caused by competition for the cobalamin in the intestinal lumen has generated some quite exotic studies. Following the demonstration that megaloblastic anemia could be corrected by removal of massive quantities of fish tapeworm (*Diphyllobothrium latum*) from some patients in Finland, the worm was studied and shown to be capable of accumulating cobalamin after releasing it from IF.[105, 106] Although this competition by 100 m of worm length was well documented, it is likely that the cobalamin deficiency caused by the worm occurred only in patients with marginal secretion of IF, and not in subjects with normal gastric secretion. The recent increase in ingestion of raw fish among some social groups may provide us with new cases for additional studies.

Cobalamin malabsorption has been observed in some patients with intestinal blind loops or with stenotic areas of the small bowel.[107] This malabsorption decreased after treatment with antibiotics (e.g., tetracyclines); this finding suggests that bacteria proliferating in stagnant intestinal areas competed with the host for cobalamin in the intestinal lumen, but the exact nature of the process remains unclear. An increased serum folate level is observed in many of these patients and is attributed to the synthesis of large amounts of folates by the intestinal bacteria.

How cobalamin is transported across the ileal cell is unknown. Indirect evidence suggests that the transport occurs by means of endocytosis,[108–112] with release of the cobalamin from IF in lysosomes. The subsequent transport of the vitamin appears to require the correct chemical configuration of the cobalamin[113] and, thus, probably involves specific binding to a transporter, possibly TC II. Chemical modification of absorbed cobalamin is not required for passage through the intestinal cell, although cobalamin may be reduced and metabolized to coenzyme forms in ileal cells, as described earlier.

Cobalamin is excreted in the bile, binds to IF in the small intestine, and is reabsorbed. Reabsorption does not occur in pernicious anemia; as a result, depletion of cobalamin stores occurs more rapidly than when absorption is unimpaired. Normal body losses have been estimated to be in the range of 2 to 4 μg cobalamin per day.

Entry of Cobalamin into Cells

Cobalamin bound to TC II enters cells by endocytosis after the complex associates with receptors on the cell surface.[14, 15, 92, 114] The TC II–Cbl receptor has been purified.[115] No chemical modification of cobalamin is required for transport. Entry into the cytoplasm is probably from lysosomes[14] and requires lysosome-mediated digestion of the TC II before the free cobalamin can enter the cell. Treatment of cells with lysosomotropic agents (e.g., chloroquine or ammonium chloride), which prevent generation of low pH in endosomes,

prevents entry of cobalamin into the cytoplasm[14, 116]; as a result, TC II–Cbl accumulates in endosomes. Penetration of free cobalamin from the lysosome into the cytoplasm appears to require a specific transport system, which is defective in children with cobalamin F disease (cblF disease; see later in this chapter).[117, 118] Excretion or loss of cobalamin from cells has not been studied.

Pernicious Anemia

Pernicious anemia is a disease that results from the destruction of IF-producing gastric parietal cells by lymphocyte-mediated immune activity. The consequent lack of IF results in vitamin B_{12} malabsorption. Patients who lack IF following gastric resection and those few in whom a presumed genetic mutation yields defective or undetectable IF are not considered to have pernicious anemia.

Age, Gender, and Race*

The frequency of pernicious anemia increases with age, with most new cases detected in the fifth to seventh decades of life. Men and women have been shown to be equally affected in most surveys. Studies in Sweden, Denmark, and the United Kingdom conducted between 1942 and 1968 found the incidence to be between 100 and 130 cases per 100,000. As American and European populations age, the frequency of pernicious anemia will probably exceed this reported incidence. In the seventh decade and later, the incidence of pernicious anemia may be as great as 250 to 500 cases per 100,000.

Pernicious anemia occurs predominantly in whites. It is less common in blacks, in whom it may appear at a younger age than in whites, and in East Indians. It is very rare in Asians. Pernicious anemia is more common among those of northern European origin than among those originating in the Mediterranean area. Such a north-south gradient of case incidence has even been reported within the United Kingdom and Holland.[2]

Genetics

The hereditary nature of pernicious anemia is unknown. Attempts to link pernicious anemia with HLA phenotypes have been inconclusive. There is an increased risk of pernicious anemia in identical twins.†

Clinical Presentations

Cobalamin deficiency is manifested clinically through its effects on rapidly proliferating tissues, principally the bone marrow and the lining of the intestinal tract, as well as on the nervous system. This can give rise to three clinical pictures in which megaloblastic anemia, gastrointestinal symptoms, or neurologic degeneration predominate.

Megaloblastic Anemia. Pernicious anemia often

---

*See reference 2, pp 316–321.
†See reference 2, p 483.

presents as severe macrocytic anemia accompanied by neutropenia and thrombocytopenia. The gradual onset of the anemia, to which the patient adjusts by gradually curtailing activity, means that the patient may be largely asymptomatic, except for some weakness. Impending or actual congestive heart failure may be present, as may postural or activity-induced shortness of breath. Usually, some neurologic or mental symptoms and signs also are present, as are glossitis and other intestinal symptoms.

Gastrointestinal Features. In some patients, the anemia and neurologic deficits are relatively mild, and the predominant symptoms are gastrointestinal. These symptoms include loss of appetite with minor weight loss (5% to 10% of body weight), nausea, constipation, occasional diarrhea, and soreness of the tongue (glossitis) or "cankers" of the tongue that are aggravated by the eating of spicy or "acid" foods. Failure to notice an accompanying mild macrocytic anemia or to elicit neurologic abnormalities may result in unwarranted intestinal visualization and imaging. Although gastrointestinal symptoms may be secondary to "megaloblastic" changes in gut cells, the relationship of such morphologic changes in buccal, esophageal, and enteric cells to glossitis, anorexia, constipation, and diarrhea is uncertain.[45]

Neurologic Disease. The neurologic syndrome of cobalamin deficiency is known as *subacute combined degeneration of the spinal cord* (SCDSC). The syndrome consists of degeneration of posterior and lateral columns of the cord and a peripheral nerve lesion,[119, 120] which is more severe in the lower than in the upper extremities. Demyelination may be secondary to axonal degeneration. Decreased vibration and position sense are usually the first objective manifestations of SCDSC, with pyramidal tract signs being observed later. The latter may be masked by a decrease in tendon reflexes secondary to the peripheral nerve lesion.[121-123] Cerebral symptoms and optic nerve degeneration also occur. SCDSC can occur with little evidence of anemia and includes some or all of the following features*:

- Degeneration of the posterior spinal columns, which results in decreased vibration sense below the iliac crests in 48%, loss of position sense in the feet in 42%, and ataxia in 64% of patients
- Degeneration of pyramidal tracts, which causes spasticity and dorsiflexion of the toes (Babinski's reflex) in 56% of patients
- Peripheral neuropathy with distal paresthesia, anesthesia, and muscular weakness in 90% of patients
- Dementia mimicking Alzheimer's disease
- Depression, with or without dementia, in 90% of patients and affecting virtually all symptomatic patients
- Optic atrophy, which is very rare in pernicious anemia

Decreased vibration sense and paresthesias in the legs probably affect most patients with symptomatic pernicious anemia, but SCDSC affects no more than 30%. In one series,* paresthesias were noted in 30% of patients, whereas SCDSC was present in only 6% to 9%.

In many of these patients with SCDSC, the MCV is elevated, and the serum cobalamin level is in the deficient range. However, patients without anemia and mainly neurologic disease may have serum cobalamin levels above the range of deficiency. The diagnosis of cobalamin deficiency in patients with neurologic problems should not be excluded only on the basis of a normal serum cobalamin level. The same applies to patients with a syndrome of senile dementia or Alzheimer's disease. In such patients, elevated levels of plasma methylmalonic acid and total homocysteine should be sought.

The pathogenesis of the neurologic lesions is not clear. A neurologic lesion similar to that in SCDSC can be produced in primates (including humans) and pigs by chronic exposure to nitrous oxide.[124] Nitrous oxide also produces megaloblastic anemia in humans. Nitrous oxide penetrates cells readily and oxidizes MeCbl bound to methionine synthase when it transfers its methyl. The cob(I)alamin remaining after the methyl group has been transferred to homocysteine is oxidized irreversibly by nitrous oxide to cobalamin catabolites, which remain bound to and inactivate methionine synthase.[125, 126] The neurologic lesion can be prevented in monkeys and pigs with methionine supplements. How this inactivation of methionine synthase causes neurologic disease and how it is prevented by methionine is unknown, but SCDSC probably is caused by the same mechanism. It should be noted that the concentration of methylmalonic acid in spinal fluid exceeds that in plasma.[127, 128]

Subclinical or Preclinical Pernicious Anemia. Many patients with pernicious anemia now come to medical attention because of erythrocyte macrocytosis detected on routine electronic blood cell analysis. Other patients are identified through screening programs in at-risk populations, such as the institutionalized and the elderly. The diagnosis is based on the detection of a low serum vitamin B_{12} level, an increased plasma holotranscobalamin II level, an elevated plasma level of methylmalonic acid, or an elevated plasma total homocysteine level.[129-134] Whether or not clinical manifestations of cobalamin deficiency are detectable, many patients who show biochemical evidence of deficiency volunteer that they "feel better" following treatment with vitamin B_{12}.

The frequency of the neurologic syndrome of SCDSC as the presenting symptoms and signs of pernicious anemia in adult patients appears to have increased over the past 30 years. In a study published in 1961,† 10% to 15% reported neurologic symptoms. Hall reported finding neurologic signs in 35% of patients with this disease.[135] In a study in California reported in 1986, neurologic or mental disorders were present in 50% of patients with cobalamin deficiency.[136] Because no data

---

*See reference 2, pp 472–473.

---

*See reference 2, pp 468–469.
†See reference 2, pp 320–322.

on change of incidence of pernicious anemia have been published during this interval, it is unclear whether the spectrum of the disease has changed or whether patients without anemia are now being recognized because of the universal availability of the red cell volume determination (MCV), as well as the availability of assays for serum cobalamin.

Maternal and Pediatric Vitamin B$_{12}$ Deficiency

In well-nourished subjects, cobalamin deficiency takes many months to develop because of the long half-life of cobalamin within the body (about 0.05% to 0.2% is lost per day)[137] and of the large hepatic stores of the vitamin. The earliest manifestations of impending deficiency are related to loss of gastric IF in pernicious anemia, with reduced capacity to absorb vitamin B$_{12}$ from the diet. At this stage, the proportion of cobalamin in plasma that is associated with TC II is decreased to below normal.[138]

During development of the deficiency, the quantities of cobalamin in the liver and in the plasma decrease progressively. In most subjects, the plasma cobalamin level falls below the normal range before other manifestations of deficiency are detected. In some, however, other manifestations of deficiency may appear before the concentration of cobalamin in the plasma reaches the levels that are usually associated with deficiency.[139, 140]

The appearance of hypersegmented neutrophils in the peripheral blood smear and the presence of increased methylmalonic acid and total homocysteine levels in the plasma may precede the development of classic megaloblastic anemia. However, bone marrow morphology, if it is examined, probably is abnormal, and oval macrocytes may be observed on blood smears. Neurologic and mental disease may develop at this stage and may not be recognized as resulting from cobalamin deficiency in the absence of anemia, elevated MCV, or decreased concentration of cobalamin in the plasma.[139, 140]

More prolonged deficiency results in anemia with a megaloblastic bone marrow accompanied by neutropenia and thrombocytopenia. These are most commonly (but not exclusively) seen in patients with the most severe anemia.[141]*

From the previous discussion, it is apparent that patients with deficiency of cobalamin without symptoms may be identified by laboratory testing, may present with unexplained neurologic signs or dementia, or may develop the full picture of megaloblastic anemia. The progression is more rapid in patients with low cobalamin stores and in those with an additional metabolic insult (exposure to nitrous oxide, simultaneous deficiency of folate, or exposure to antifols).

Maternal Vitamin B$_{12}$ Deficiency

Pernicious anemia, the most common cause of vitamin B$_{12}$ deficiency, has its greatest incidence after the child-

bearing years. However, it has been described in young women. When it is recognized, diagnosed, and treated, the infant suffers no ill effects. However, apparently asymptomatic, nonanemic cases of maternal pernicious anemia have been described.[52, 142] Such mothers have low serum and milk vitamin B$_{12}$ levels, and the infants are born with low cobalamin stores. These stores are not repleted during breast-feeding. If the mother has circulating anti-IF antibodies, these antibodies can cross the placenta and enter the fetus and impair intestinal cobalamin absorption during the first few weeks of life, particularly if the antibody titer is high.[143]

Nutritional deficiency of vitamin B$_{12}$ is seen in strict vegan mothers, whose diets contain no animal-derived components and, therefore, no source of vitamin B$_{12}$.[144] This is particularly so in immigrants to the West, where improved hygienic standards in food handling and preparation minimize the bacterial and fungal content of food, which is believed to be the source of vitamin B$_{12}$ in Asian countries.[145] Food faddists also can consume a diet deficient in vitamin B$_{12}$.

Other less common causes of maternal vitamin B$_{12}$ deficiency are secondary to gastric resection, which results in loss of IF-producing mucosa; the presence of fish tapeworms or small intestinal bacterial overgrowth; and bowel disease resulting in malabsorption of vitamin B$_{12}$ from the terminal ileum (see Table 10–1). Crohn's disease, ulcerative colitis, and surgical resection of the terminal ileum all can result in vitamin B$_{12}$ malabsorption, leading to deficiency. Because of the enterohepatic circulation of vitamin B$_{12}$, such deficiency may develop more rapidly in those with malabsorption than in those whose diet is deficient because vitamin B$_{12}$ entering the gut from the bile will not be reabsorbed.

Inhalation of the anesthetic gas nitrous oxide inactivates MeCbl, the vitamin B$_{12}$ coenzyme involved in methionine synthesis. Repeated exposure to nitrous oxide produces a full-blown clinical picture of vitamin B$_{12}$ deficiency with megaloblastic anemia and SCDSC.[124] The effect of nitrous oxide exposure on the fetus during maternal nitrous oxide inhalation is unknown.

Vitamin B$_{12}$ Deficiency in Newborns and Infants

Newborn infants born to mothers who are deficient in cobalamin may develop severe deficiency in the early weeks of life. Severely deficient mothers probably are sterile,[146] but those with marginal cobalamin stores due to diet or early pernicious anemia may produce cobalamin-deficient infants. This deficiency, if unrecognized, may cause permanent neurologic damage in the infant. The clinical manifestations in young children are predominantly those of "failure to thrive" and slow mental development.

Deficiency of vitamin B$_{12}$ is rarely recognized in newborns, presenting most often as failure to thrive, including developmental delay and mental retardation, after several months of life. The most common cause is maternal vitamin B$_{12}$ deficiency (see earlier), which

---

*See reference 2, pp 202–204.

may go unrecognized. There may be no anemia or macrocytosis in the infant, and variable degrees of pancytopenia may be present. The bone marrow may not show florid megaloblastic changes. The extent to which dietary folates or folate supplements may mask the clinical picture is unknown. The diagnosis is based on a high index of suspicion leading to demonstration of a low serum vitamin B_{12} level, other confirmatory tests, response to treatment, and investigation of the mother's diet and vitamin B_{12} status.

The other major causes of inadequate vitamin B_{12} availability in newborns, detected within the first year of life or sometimes some years later, are inborn errors of vitamin B_{12} metabolism. These are described in a later section.

Vitamin B_{12} Deficiency in Older Children and Adolescents

Deficiency in older children and adolescents has the same causes as that in adults. Pernicious anemia has been reported in children younger than 10 years of age but is very rare. Cases are also encountered in teenagers, but again, uncommonly. Diets lacking vitamin B_{12} prepared by parents or selected by teenagers[147] may be the cause. Gastric and intestinal diseases may result in vitamin B_{12} malabsorption. Vitamin B_{12} deficiency has been reported following surgery for necrotizing enterocolitis, particularly when resection has included part of the terminal ileum.[148] Low serum vitamin B_{12} levels and decreased vitamin B_{12} absorption as determined with the Schilling test have been reported in patients with HIV infection with and without AIDS.[149]

Diagnosis of Vitamin B_{12} Deficiency

Commonly, macrocytic anemia occurs and is accompanied by neutropenia and thrombocytopenia. The MCV is 120 fL or greater, unless the increase in MCV is balanced by a decrease due to a coexisting iron deficiency or a chronic inflammatory process.[150-153] The blood smear contains oval macrocytes and multilobar neutrophils. For a variety of reasons, including the use of newer automated cell counters and the varying competence of technicians analyzing blood smears, oval macrocytes and multilobar neutrophils may not be reported even if present. The bone marrow usually is megaloblastic.

Abnormal biochemical findings in the serum include increased levels of lactate dehydrogenase, bilirubin, and iron, as well as increased transferrin saturation, which reflects "ineffective erythropoiesis." Serum cholesterol, lipid, and immunoglobulin levels may be decreased. These changes are not specific to cobalamin deficiency but are corrected after cobalamin therapy.[154, 155] Equally nonspecific is the finding of increased serum gastrin levels and antibody to gastric parietal cells, which signal the presence of atrophic gastritis but do not distinguish those who lack IF from those who do not. The presence of antibody to IF in serum means that the patient has or will develop cobalamin deficiency.[20, 156]

Serum Levels of Vitamin B_{12}

The most direct evidence of cobalamin deficiency is an abnormally low serum cobalamin level. Although early studies using microbiologic assays showed that serum cobalamin level was almost always less than 100 pg/mL[141] (78 pmol/L) in patients with megaloblastic anemia due to cobalamin deficiency, megaloblastic bone marrow is found in only 20% to 30% of patients with serum cobalamin levels less than 100 pg/mL. Therefore, significant cobalamin deficiency can occur without hematologic manifestations. In some patients with deficiency of cobalamin, megaloblastic anemia and a decrease in serum cobalamin level into the deficient range occur with longer periods of deficiency. Neurologic manifestations of cobalamin deficiency may appear before macrocytic erythrocytes and classic megaloblastic anemia develop.[140]

Serum cobalamin level has been shown to reflect hepatic cobalamin in reports that describe studies of a small number of subjects,[157] but the clinical significance of isolated low levels of cobalamin in serum without other evidence of cobalamin deficiency, such as abnormal metabolism of methylmalonate or homocysteine, or a definitely abnormal deoxyuridine suppression test result, has not been determined. In many cases, these patients are treated with vitamin B_{12}, but without obvious clinical benefit.

In contrast, significant cobalamin deficiency may occur in the absence of low serum cobalamin levels in patients who do not have megaloblastic anemia. In one study, serum cobalamin level was greater than 100 pg/mL in 30% to 40% of patients demonstrated to have significant cobalamin deficiency; in 3% to 5%, the serum cobalamin level was in the normal range.[139, 140] This failure of the assay to provide a near-perfect clinical correlation[158] is due in part to technical defects in the specificity of the cobalamin binder used in some commercial ligand-binding assays. It also reflects the limits of sensitivity and specificity of the assay when used as the sole measure of cobalamin deficiency, particularly when the assay is applied to populations in which florid clinical features of cobalamin deficiency are not present. In patients with megaloblastic anemia, the finding of a normal to increased level of serum folate, together with a reduced ratio of erythrocyte to serum folate level, provides strong but indirect evidence of cobalamin deficiency.[159]

These studies suggest that evidence of functional cobalamin deficiency other than serum cobalamin levels (e.g., macrocytosis, multilobar neutrophils, and elevated levels of plasma methylmalonic acid and total homocysteine) must be sought when cobalamin sufficiency is evaluated in such populations, as well as in individuals in whom deficiency is strongly suspected.

The diagnosis of cobalamin deficiency is confirmed by the finding of increased serum levels of methylmalonic acid and total homocysteine, which is evidence of functional cobalamin deficiency, and by the demonstration of cobalamin malabsorption, which can be corrected by the administration of cobalamin with a source of IF (urinary excretion test, or Schilling test;

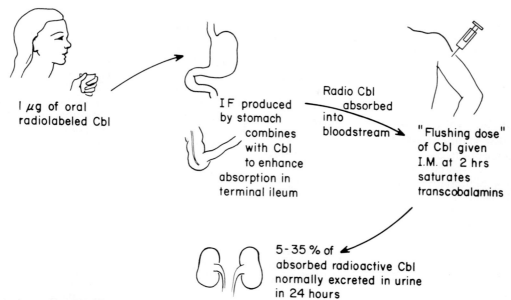

Figure 10–7. The urinary excretion (Schilling) test. Labeled cyanocobalamin is fed, and a proportion of absorbed label is flushed into the urine by subsequent injection of a large quantity (1000 μg) of unlabeled vitamin B_{12}. The oral dose must be standardized, other radioactivity must be absent from the urine, and renal function and urine collection must be adequate. If excretion is low, then the test may be repeated with the use of a source of intrinsic factor.

Fig. 10–7). Indeed, correction of the cobalamin malabsorption with the feeding of IF together with radiolabeled cobalamin confirms that a lack of IF is the cause, proving that the patient has pernicious anemia. The diagnosis can also be established on the basis of a positive therapeutic test result (described in the next section).

In patients who cannot absorb vitamin B_{12}, there is some evidence that the amount of cobalamin bound to TC II decreases before the decrease in total serum cobalamin (mostly bound to haptocorrin) occurs.[138] In such patients, the neutrophil lobe count (number of lobes per 100 cells) may increase within 6 to 8 weeks after discontinuation of cobalamin injections and will decrease again after injection of CNCbl. Plasma homocysteine and methylmalonic acid levels sometimes increase into the abnormal range in less than 6 months. Decreased TC II–Cbl might then signal a failure of vitamin B_{12} absorption, whereas increased neutrophil lobe count and homocysteine and methylmalonic acid levels would indicate tissue cobalamin functional deficiency.

A Positive Therapeutic Test Result

A positive therapeutic test result is the correction of hematologic, biochemical, and neurologic abnormalities following vitamin treatment. If cobalamin deficiency is apparent and the megaloblastic anemia is not severe, then treatment consists of the administration of one or more injections of 100 to 1000 μg of CNCbl or OHCbl (to confirm the diagnosis if megaloblastic changes in the erythroid series in the bone marrow disappear within 48 hours) and at least two of the following:

1. A decrease in serum iron by 50% over 24 hours

2. An increase in the reticulocyte count 5 to 10 days after treatment
3. The correction of thrombocytopenia over 2 weeks
4. The correction of neutropenia over 2 weeks
5. A decrease in the MCV by 5 fL or more over 2 weeks (after the reticulocytosis has subsided)
6. The correction of anemia over 2 to 4 weeks
7. A decrease in the neutrophil lobe count from the elevated to the normal range over 4 weeks
8. A decrease in elevated plasma methylmalonic acid and total homocysteine levels over 2 weeks

To establish the diagnosis of cobalamin deficiency and avoid severe metabolic disturbances, the patient should receive 10 μg CNCbl subcutaneously daily for 2 days. This therapy is sufficient for normalizing metabolic derangements such as elevated levels of serum lactate dehydrogenase and serum iron and for inducing an increase in the reticulocyte count, with a maximum level being attained at 5 to 7 days. For children, the dose of CNCbl is 0.2 μg/kg per day subcutaneously for 2 days.

The clinician can establish a diagnosis of folate deficiency by treating the patient with a low dose of folic acid (in the range of 0.5 mg/d by mouth for 2 to 3 days) and then by monitoring for metabolic normalization and reticulocytosis in the succeeding 2 weeks (see earlier). It should be noted that the administration of 2 to 5 mg of folic acid will induce reticulocytosis in almost all patients with cobalamin deficiency, whereas giving 100 to 1000 μg of cobalamin will induce reticulocytosis in some patients with folate deficiency.

Serum Cobalamin in Folate Deficiency

The serum cobalamin level is decreased in a proportion of patients with folate deficiency and megaloblastic anemia and may be in the range of deficiency. This cobalamin level increases over 7 days when folate is administered; the level does not increase in patients deficient in cobalamin.[160] The mechanism involved is unknown but may represent redistribution of cobalamin between cells and plasma.

Urinary Excretion Test (the Schilling Test)

In performing this standard test for the measurement of cobalamin absorption, the clinician feeds the fasting patient 0.5 μg of [57]Co-labeled CNCbl in water, waits 2 hours, gives a subcutaneous injection of 1000 μg of CNCbl to block tissue uptake of [57]Co-CNCbl, and measures the amount of [57]Co-CNCbl excreted in the urine in 24 hours. If malabsorption is found, the test is repeated 1 week later, with the addition of a source of IF to the 0.5 μg of oral [57]Co-CNCbl to demonstrate correction of the malabsorption by IF; such correction establishes the diagnosis of pernicious anemia (see Fig. 10–7).

Food Schilling Test

In patients with atrophic gastritis and inadequate gastric peptic activity, vitamin B_{12} may be absorbed when it is fed in water; however, cobalamin in food may not be adequately absorbed. Cobalamin in a variety of cooked foods has been demonstrated to be poorly absorbed by such patients, and this may produce decreased body stores of cobalamin and sometimes even true deficiency. In such patients, the results of the Schilling test are normal.

In the *food Schilling test*, [57]Co-CNCbl is incorporated into or added to eggs, meat, or liver and fed to the patient. Tests for this abnormality are not well standardized. Those utilizing cobalamin naturally incorporated into eggs, meat, or liver may require performance of the fecal excretion test (see the next section) because the OHCbl produced by breakdown of the natural coenzymes of cobalamin (mostly 5'-deoxyadenosyl cobalamin) binds to plasma and other proteins and may not be as well excreted into the urine as during the routine Schilling test. Absorption of 1 μg of labeled CNCbl added to eggs and fed, either cooked or uncooked, or mixed with 3 mL of chicken serum[161–163] can be tested with the standard protocol for the Schilling test; however, clinical studies remain inadequate for defining normal ranges, reliability (reproducibility, and the ability to detect abnormality, such as malabsorption), and precise procedures (with respect to types of food, food amount, and interaction of [57]Co-CNCbl with food [added or incorporated], details of feeding, B_{12} flushing, urine collection). At this time, such tests must be standardized within the institution that uses them, with development of normal ranges for each batch of cobalamin-containing food produced. If possible, the total amount of cobalamin fed in the test should not exceed 2 μg.

Single-Sample Fecal Excretion Test

The single-sample fecal excretion test of cobalamin absorption is convenient and simple, and it probably avoids the pitfalls of tests that rely on urinary excretion. The basis of this test of vitamin B_{12} absorption is the simultaneous feeding of labeled cobalamin (free or bound to food) with 2 g of a nonabsorbable dye (carmine) and 10 μCi (1 mg) of ^{51}Cr–chromic chloride. The ^{51}Cr is not absorbed. A 2- to 3-g sample of the first or second carmine (red)–stained stool is added to a counting vial, shaken with 1 to 3 mL of water, and counted for ^{51}Cr and [57]Co. The ratio of counts is compared with the ratio in the sample fed. In normal subjects, 36% to 88% of a 1- to 2-μg dose of [57]Co-labeled cobalamin is absorbed.[164]

Deoxyuridine Suppression Test

The deoxyuridine suppression test[165, 166] was developed (Fig. 10–8) on the basis of the hypothesis that the activity of thymidylate synthase is decreased in cells deficient in cobalamin or folates because of lack of the required folate coenzyme, 5,10-methylene-THF polyglutamate. Such deficient cells may have an expanded intracellular pool of deoxyuridylate, which reflects the decreased activity of thymidylate synthase. Incubation

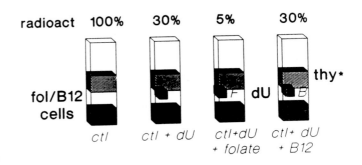

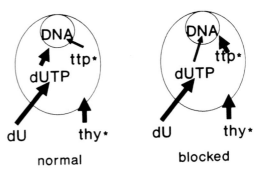

Figure 10–8. Deoxyuridine suppression test. This test, effective only with bone marrow cells, evaluates the capacity of the cells to convert deoxyuridine into thymidylate. Four test tubes containing bone marrow from a patient deficient in folate are illustrated. Labeled thymidine (*hatched area*, radioactivity) is incorporated into DNA in the presence of excess deoxyuridine (*dotted cubes*) because thymidylate synthesis from deoxyuridine is limited by the folate deficiency. Thymidylate synthesis is corrected by the addition of folate to tube No. 3 but not by the addition of cobalamin to tube No. 4. The presumed phenomenon occurring in the cells is illustrated below, with reaction rates shown as thick or thin arrows. fol = folate; dUR = deoxyuridine; thy = thymidine; ctl = control; dUTP = deoxyuridine triphosphate; ttp = thymidine triphosphate.

of deficient cells with deoxyuridine would be expected to further expand this pool. The test involves incubation of fresh washed bone marrow cells with deoxyuridine for 1 hour, followed by incubation with ^{3}H-labeled thymidine for 1 hour. The quantity of ^{3}H-thymidine incorporated into cell DNA is then determined.

In normal cells, thymidylate synthase converts the deoxyuridine to thymidylate during the initial incubation. This reduces the amount of ^{3}H-thymidine subsequently incorporated into DNA to less than 10% of that observed when the preincubation with deoxyuridine is not carried out. In bone marrow cells from a patient who is deficient in cobalamin or folates, preincubation with deoxyuridine reduces incorporation of ^{3}H-thymidine into DNA to only 30% to 40% of that observed in the absence of preincubation with deoxyuridine.

The defect in suppression of the incorporation of ^{3}H-thymidine into DNA by preincubation with deoxyuridine in cobalamin-deficient cells is corrected by the addition of either MeCbl or 5-formyl-THF (folinic acid) during the preincubation with deoxyuridine. Addition of *N*-5-methyl-THF to deoxyuridine during the preincubation corrects the defect in folate-deficient cells but not in cells deficient in cobalamin. There is uncertainty regarding the details of the actual biochemical processes being modulated during this test, but the deoxyuridine suppression test as described has proved reliable in discriminating between cobalamin and folate deficiency. The exception to this is in patients who have concomitant iron deficiency.

Methylmalonic Acid and Total Homocysteine Levels in Cobalamin Deficiency

Tissues deficient in cobalamin may not adequately metabolize substrates of cobalamin-dependent enzymes, such as methylmalonic acid. The presence of methylmalonic acid in the urine of some patients with pernicious anemia and its slow disappearance following treatment with doses of cobalamin that corrected the anemia was described in 1962.[167] It is now known that almost all subjects who are cobalamin deficient, both children and adults,[168] accumulate methylmalonic acid in the plasma.[35, 169–172] Indeed, elevated plasma levels of methylmalonic acid may be found before the appearance of macrocytosis or anemia, or of other clinical features of cobalamin deficiency. These levels return to the normal range after several days or weeks of cobalamin treatment.

Homocysteine accumulates in the plasma of patients deficient in cobalamin, as well as in that of patients who are deficient in folates.[35, 132, 139, 140, 168, 173, 174] Plasma homocysteine binds to free SH groups on proteins. Thus, it may not be detected when it is present in low concentrations unless it is released from the proteins by reducing agents to yield a measure of total plasma homocysteine. Elevated plasma total homocysteine levels are found in more than 80% of patients who are deficient in cobalamin or folates. As with elevated plasma methylmalonic acid levels, the total plasma homocysteine concentration returns to normal after

several days or weeks of therapy with the appropriate vitamin. Raised plasma total homocysteine may not decrease if the vitamin in which the patient is not deficient is given. Methylmalonic acid and total homocysteine may also accumulate in the plasma of patients with renal insufficiency. The implications of elevated levels of total homocysteine in plasma in relation to neural tube defects, cerebral and cardiovascular disease, and the incidence of cancer are discussed later in this chapter.

Treatment of Cobalamin Deficiency
General

Patients admitted to a hospital with severe anemia may have heart failure due to a combination of factors, including tachycardia, increased cardiac output, sodium retention, and inadequate oxygenation of the myocardium. The aim of emergency treatment is stabilization of the patient with the use of oxygen, diuretics, and limited slow red cell transfusion. Rapid or generous transfusion may exacerbate the cardiac failure. Immediate administration of vitamin B_{12} or folate in large doses is not required because several days must elapse before hematologic improvement can be detected. Clinical disasters sometimes occur during therapy. Treatment of severely anemic adults with pernicious anemia has been associated with immediate death in 14%[175]; however, more recent studies do not appear to confirm this.[176] Disasters include life-threatening hypokalemia and cerebral and cardiovascular accidents (usually strokes due to thrombosis or embolism).

Severe hypokalemia is most likely to occur following the administration of a large dose of cobalamin in a patient who is severely anemic. This results from a rapid recovery and retention of intracellular potassium that is accompanied by a delay in renal potassium conservation, which in turn shifts potassium from the extracellular to the intracellular compartment. Although hypokalemia may not have been the primary cause of the reported deaths, the clinician should anticipate and avoid it, if possible, by providing potassium supplements (sometimes in large doses), as needed; by initiating treatment with a low dose of cobalamin (e.g., 10 µg of CNCbl given daily subcutaneously for 2 to 3 days); and by transfusion to achieve partial correction of the anemia.

The risk of occurrence of an acute thrombotic episode may be reduced by these maneuvers, but this has not been documented. The role of potentially thrombogenic homocystinemia in causing these thrombotic episodes is not known. Also, these complications of initial therapy may affect children with severe cobalamin deficiency.

Initial Therapy

Bone marrow aspiration should be performed early to establish the presence of megaloblastic anemia because erythroid hyperplasia will decrease and cell morphology will change within a few hours following transfusion. Serum cobalamin and folate values are not significantly altered by transfusion but should be obtained before the procedure is performed. However, a whole blood sample for red cell folate determination must be collected (in citrate or ethylenediaminetetra-acetic acid [EDTA]) before transfusion. Otherwise, the red cell folate level will be that of the mixture of the patient's and donor's red cells.

A dose of 10 μg CNCbl given subcutaneously daily for 2 days is sufficient to correct metabolic abnormalities, such as the elevated serum lactate dehydrogenase and iron levels, and to induce an increase in the reticulocyte count, with a maximum count attained 5 to 7 days after the start of treatment. For children, the dose of CNCbl is 0.2 μg/kg subcutaneously daily for 2 days. Such doses given over 5 to 7 days usually do not restore elevated plasma MMA and total homocysteine levels to normal.

Complete correction of megaloblastic erythropoiesis and associated metabolic changes can occur with as little as 15 μg of CNCbl in some adults, whereas as much as 150 μg may be required in others. Dementia and depression may improve rapidly with therapy, whereas other neurologic abnormalities usually show slow improvement over 6 months and may not return to normal. However, one of the authors of this chapter (BAC) has observed complete recovery from SCDSC in a patient who was bedridden and had positive Babinski's reflexes within as short a time as 1 to 2 weeks after institution of cobalamin treatment.

Subsequently, injections of CNCbl of 1000 μg should be given daily for 1 week, followed by 100 μg of CNCbl weekly for 1 month. This therapy is required to replete body cobalamin stores.

Patients proven to be deficient in cobalamin and who cannot absorb the vitamin (i.e., those with pernicious anemia) require monthly injections of CNCbl. A prudent monthly dose is 100 μg injected subcutaneously. Failure of this regimen to maintain normal body stores is extremely rare. Similar maintenance of stores and repletion appears to follow injections of 1000 μg (1 mg) of OHCbl every 3 months[177] or of 1 mg of OHCbl daily for 1 to 2 weeks every 6 to 12 months. The binding of OHCbl to tissues permits such infrequent injection, but a small proportion of patients do develop antibodies against the TC II–Cbl complex.[178] These antibodies have not been found to affect health but do cause the accumulation of very large concentrations of TC II in plasma. It is unclear whether this rare allergy to cobalamin is more common after injections of OHCbl or of CNCbl.

In some patients with pernicious anemia, cobalamin levels in serum or plasma can be maintained in the normal range with daily ingestion of 50 to 200 μg of CNCbl, taken remote from meals. Efficacy of therapy should be monitored biochemically.

In patients with apparent deficiency of cobalamin secondary to defective peptic digestion (normal results obtained on Schilling test but abnormal absorption of cobalamin bound to food), normal cobalamin levels and stores can be maintained through feeding 10 to 25 μg/d of CNCbl; however, the efficacy of such treat-

ment should be verified periodically by the demonstration of normal levels of serum cobalamin, methylmalonic acid, and total homocysteine. In children with inherited defects of cobalamin metabolism, injections of 1000 μg OHCbl 2 to 3 times per week should be used. The effectiveness of therapy in such cases can be monitored with the measurement of serum levels of total homocysteine, methylmalonic acid, and methionine, and perhaps of additional metabolites.

Associated Diseases

Patients with pernicious anemia are at increased risk of developing carcinoma of the stomach.[179, 180] Cancer may be diagnosed before, at the same time as, or many years after the diagnosis of pernicious anemia. Currently, patients undergo follow-up that includes annual gastroscopy, with biopsy of suspicious areas. Evidence of mucosal dysplasia or the presence of chromosomal changes suggesting a premalignant state would warrant more frequent assessment. Pernicious anemia is also associated with other autoimmune diseases, particularly those involving the thyroid. Hypothyroidism is common and should be evaluated clinically and with measurement of hormone levels, as needed.[181] Pernicious anemia is associated with type I diabetes as well.[182]

Inborn Errors of Vitamin B₁₂ Transport and Metabolism

Transport Disorders

Intrinsic Factor Deficiency

A small number of children have been recognized to have megaloblastic anemia and developmental delay as a result of an absence of effective IF. Evidence of vitamin B₁₂ deficiency usually appears after the first year but before the fifth year of life, although clinical deficiency has appeared as late as age 12 years in patients with partially defective IF.[183] These patients have normal gastric acid secretion and normal findings on gastric cytologic examination. In some cases, immunologically active but nonfunctional IF is produced, whereas in others none is found at all. An IF labile to destruction by acid and pepsin and having a low affinity for vitamin B₁₂ has been reported.[184] In children with IF deficiency, absorption of cobalamin is abnormal but is normalized when the vitamin is mixed with a source of normal IF, such as human gastric juice from an unaffected individual. The gene for human IF is on chromosome 11. Southern blot analysis of DNA from patients with inherited IF deficiency has not revealed any large deletions,[93] suggesting that most mutations are the result of point mutations. As with the other disorders of cobalamin transport, inheritance appears to be autosomal recessive.

Defective Transport of Vitamin B₁₂ by Enterocytes

Defective transport of vitamin B₁₂ by enterocytes, also known as the *Imerslund-Gräsbeck syndrome*, usually presents with clinical manifestations of vitamin B_{12} deficiency in children between the ages of 1 and 15 years.[2, 185, 186] At least 150 cases have been described; they most commonly occur among Finns and Sephardic Jews. All patients who were investigated had normal IF, no evidence of antibodies to IF, and normal intestinal morphology. They had a selective defect in vitamin B_{12} absorption that was not corrected by treatment with IF. In some patients, proteinuria of the tubular type was found.

In one sibship,[187] normal quantities of IF–vitamin B_{12} receptor were found in ileal biopsy specimens. Ileal homogenates bound IF–vitamin B_{12} normally; this finding suggests that the basic defect is not an absence of receptors. In other patients,[188] an apparent absence of the ileal receptor has been observed. A canine model exists for this disorder.[189, 190]

The inheritance is autosomal recessive. Therapy with systemic vitamin B_{12} corrects the anemia but not the proteinuria.

R Binder (Haptocorrin, TC I) Deficiency

The deficiency or complete absence of R binder in the plasma, saliva, and leukocytes of six individuals has been described.[191–196] It is unclear whether R binder deficiency is the cause of disease in any of these patients. Although serum cobalamin levels are low, TC II–vitamin B_{12} levels are normal, and the patients are not clinically deficient in vitamin B_{12}.

The original report described two brothers, only one of whom had optic atrophy, ataxia, long tract signs, and dementia.[196] A more recently described patient had findings resembling those seen in SCDSC.[196] A role for R binders has been postulated in the scavenging of cobalamin analogues that may be toxic to the brain.[99]

Transcobalamin II Deficiency (see Fig. 10–4)

Clinical Findings. At least 30 patients with TC II deficiency are known.[191, 197] Although all of the TC II in fetal and cord blood is of fetal origin, infants with no detectable TC II in their plasma do not develop manifestations of cobalamin deficiency until several days after birth. TC II–deficient patients develop severe anemia much earlier than do patients with other causes of cobalamin malabsorption, usually in the first few months of life. Other symptoms include failure to thrive, weakness, and diarrhea in addition to pallor. The anemia usually is clearly megaloblastic, but some patients present with pancytopenia or even isolated erythroid hypoplasia.[198] The presence of immature white cell precursors in a marrow that is otherwise hypocellular can lead to the misdiagnosis of leukemia. Neurologic disease has appeared from 6 months to 30 months following the onset of symptoms.[199–202] Severe immunologic deficiency with defective cellular and humoral immunity has been seen, as has defective granulocyte function. Homocystinuria has been sought in at least two patients prior to their receiving vitamin B_{12} therapy. In three of five patients[191] who were tested before the initiation of therapy, methylmalonic aciduria

was found. Following discontinuation of therapy, methylmalonic aciduria may return.

In all patients except one, no TC II competent to bind cobalamin was detected. However, immunologically reactive TC II was found in three patients. In one patient, TC II was able to bind cobalamin, but the complex did not mediate vitamin uptake into cells. An abnormal Schilling test result was usually found in TC II deficiency (five of seven patients); in two patients in whom the absorption of cobalamin was normal, immunoreactive TC II was present. This suggests that the TC II molecule may have a role in the IF–vitamin B_{12}–mediated transport across the ileal cell even if it is not functional in transporting the vitamin in the circulation or in delivering it to cells.

Inheritance. On the basis of electrophoretic polymorphisms,[203, 204] the TC II gene *(TCN2)* was originally linked to the P blood group on chromosome 22.[205] The cDNA for *TCN2* has now been cloned[206] and the molecular basis of some of the variants defined.[207] The first mutant alleles in TC II deficiency have included deletions[197] and nonsense mutations.[208] Autosomal recessive inheritance for TC II deficiency has been confirmed. TC II is synthesized by cultured cells, and prenatal diagnosis is possible even when the specific mutation in a family is not yet known.

Treatment. Serum vitamin B_{12} levels must be kept very high if TC II–deficient patients are to be treated successfully. Levels ranging from 1000 to 10,000 pg/mL have been required and are achieved with doses of oral OHCbl or CNCbl twice weekly (500 to 1000 µg) or with systemic administration of CNCbl or OHCbl (1000 µg) weekly or more often. Folate in the form of folic acid or folinic acid in milligram doses has been successful in reversing the hematologic findings in most patients. Folate should not be given as the only therapy because of the danger of hematologic relapse and of neurologic damage, which has been induced in one such patient by folate supplementation without cobalamin.[191]

Disorders of Utilization

The Methylmalonic Acidurias

Those disorders causing methylmalonic aciduria[209] are characterized by severe metabolic acidosis and the accumulation of large amounts of MMA in the blood, urine, and cerebrospinal fluid. Levels are much higher than those seen in adults with cobalamin deficiency. Patients with methylmalonic acidurias have a defect in the mitochondrial matrix enzyme methylmalonyl CoA mutase, which requires AdoCbl as a cofactor and catalyses the conversion of L-methylmalonyl CoA to succinyl CoA. Classification of the methylmalonic acidurias has been made largely on the basis of studies in cultured fibroblasts. Complementation groups have been defined on the basis of whether two lines partially correct a defect in propionate incorporation following cell fusion.

Mutase Deficiency (Deficiency of Methylmalonyl CoA Mutase)

Background. Disorders of the mutase apoenzyme result in methylmalonic aciduria, which is not responsive to vitamin B_{12} therapy. Mature mutase purified from human liver is a 77,000-dalton homodimer that is coded by a nuclear gene, is found in the cytoplasm as a precursor with a leader sequence, and is processed to a mature protein in the mitochondria.[67] There are at least two separate types of mutase deficiency. The mut° cell lines have no residual mutase activity, whereas the mut⁻ cell lines show some residual mutase activity when AdoCbl is added, and the mutase in mut⁻ cell lines show decreased affinity for AdoCbl. Several of the mut° cell lines synthesize no detectable protein, whereas some synthesize unstable proteins, and at least one has a mutation that interferes with transfer of the mutase to the mitochondria.[210] Similarly, variable levels of mRNA have been demonstrated in different mut° lines. Usually, there is no complementation between mut° and mut⁻ cell lines, but intragenic (interallelic) complementation has been seen among some mut lines.[211, 212]

Clinical Syndromes. Clinically well at birth, patients with mutase deficiency rapidly become symptomatic with protein feeding. They usually come to medical attention because of lethargy, vomiting, failure to thrive, muscular hypotonia, respiratory distress, and recurrent vomiting and dehydration. In normal children, MMA level usually is less than 15 to 20 μg per gram of creatinine; in contrast, in methylmalonic aciduria, excretion is usually more than 100 mg and as much as several grams per day. In addition to methylmalonic aciduria, these patients may have ketones and glycine in both blood and urine and metabolic acidosis with elevated levels of ammonia. Many also have hypoglycemia, leukopenia, and thrombocytopenia. One study[213] has demonstrated that MMA inhibits bone marrow stem cells in a concentration-dependent manner. It is interesting that follow-up of children identified by newborn screening[214] has revealed a number of individuals who excrete MMA and have mutase deficiency as demonstrated by complementation analysis, and yet who are clinically well and have never developed acidosis. It is unclear whether these children are at risk for catastrophic acidosis later in life. The incidence of all forms of methylmalonic aciduria in Massachusetts is about 1 in 29,000.

Inheritance. The gene for the mutase is located on the short arm of chromosome 6, 6p12-21.2, spans 40 kb, and consists of 13 exons.[63, 66, 215, 216] At least 15 point mutations have been found, including a large number near the carboxyl terminus that appear to alter AdoCbl binding to the enzyme.[217, 218] A premature stop codon has been found in the mitochondrial leader sequence,[219] and a common mutation has been detected in three African-American patients who had a similar phenotype.[220] In Japan, 6 of 16 patients studied shared 1 mutation.[221] Mutase deficiency is an autosomal recessive disease, and prenatal diagnosis is possible.

Treatment. Therapy consists of protein restriction, with the goal of limiting the amino acids that use the propionate pathway. Formula deficient in valine, isoleucine, methionine, and threonine is used. Mutase-deficient patients are not responsive to vitamin B_{12}. Therapy with carnitine has been advocated in patients who are deficient.[222, 223] Lincomycin and metronidazole have been used to reduce enteric propionate production by anaerobic bacteria.[224–226] Even with therapy, prognosis is guarded, and brain infarcts and renal dysfunction have been reported as late complications.[209]

Adenosylcobalamin Deficiency (cblA and cblB Diseases)

Background. Two disorders result in vitamin B_{12}–responsive methylmalonic aciduria and an intracellular deficiency in AdoCbl. They are distinguished by complementation analysis and by the fact that cblA is capable of AdoCbl synthesis in cell extracts but not in intact cells, whereas cblB is deficient in both systems. The defect in cblA disease is in a reducing system, presumably in mitochondria, and results in the conversion of cob(III)alamin to cob(I)alamin. The defect in cblB disease lies in the adenosyltransferase, which is the final step in the synthesis of AdoCbl (see Fig. 10–4, Points A and B).

Clinical Syndromes. Most children with cblA disease become ill either in the first week of life or before the end of the first year. Similarly, most patients with cblB disease present in the first year of life. Symptoms are similar to those seen in mutase deficiency but usually are less severe and depend on the clinical response to vitamin B_{12} therapy.[227] Most cblA disease patients (90%) respond to vitamin B_{12}, with almost 70% being well by the age of 14 years. Fewer than half of cblB disease patients (40%) respond to therapy, and only 30% have long-term survival. Therapy has been with either OHCbl or CNCbl systemically. It is not clear whether AdoCbl offers any therapeutic advantage.

Inheritance. The inheritance of both cblA and cblB diseases is presumed to be autosomal recessive. Roughly equal numbers of patients of both sexes have been reported, and obligate heterozygotes of patients with cblB disease show decreased adenosyltransferase activity.[203] The mutations behave as recessive in complementation analyses.

Management. One report of prenatal therapy with vitamin B_{12} with a good therapeutic result has been published.[228] However, it is not certain whether therapy at birth would not have been equally effective.

Combined Deficiencies of Adenosylcobalamin and Methylcobalamin (cblC, cblD, and cblF Diseases)

Background. The precise defect in the cblC, cblD, and cblF disorders is not known, but all three result in failure of the cell to synthesize both cobalamin cofactors, MeCbl and adenosylcobalamin (AdoCbl).[203] Patients have a functional deficiency in both methionine synthase and MMA-CoA mutase, leading to homocystinuria and hypomethioninemia along with methylmalonic aciduria. The three defects occur subsequent to the endocytosis of TC II–vitamin B_{12} and to hydrolysis of the TC II–vitamin B_{12} complex (see Fig. 10–4, Points C, D, and F). In cblF disease, the defect appears to block the transfer of free vitamin B_{12} from the lysosome to the cytoplasm, whereas in cblC and cblD diseases, the defect is presumed to be in a cytosolic cob(III)alamin reductase or reductases, which are needed to reduce the trivalent cobalt of vitamin B_{12} before further vitamin B_{12} metabolism can occur.[229] Partial deficiencies of CNCbl β-ligand transferase and microsomal cob(III)alamin reductase in cblC and cblD fibroblasts have been described.[230, 231] When incubated with labeled CNCbl, fibroblasts from cblC and cblD accumulate very little intracellular vitamin B_{12} and virtually no AboCbl or MeCbl. In contrast, cblF fibroblasts accumulate excess vitamin B_{12}, but all of it is unmetabolized, non–protein bound, and localized to lysosomes.[117, 118]

Clinical Syndromes. There are more than 90 known cases of cblC disease[232]; 2 patients in 1 sibship with cblD disease; and 5 unrelated patients with cblF disease.

Most of the patients with cblC disease present in the first month or before the end of the first year of life with poor feeding, failure to thrive, and lethargy.[233] Most but not all have megaloblastic macrocytic anemia, and some have hypersegmented neutrophils and thrombocytopenia. Others have onset later in childhood or adolescence with spasticity, delirium, and psychosis.[234] For example, a boy presented at the age of 4 years with fatigue, delirium, and spasticity,[235] and a girl presented at the age of 14 years with mental deterioration and myelopathy.[234] In four patients, pigmentary retinopathy with perimacular degeneration was described.[191, 233, 236, 237] Other reported findings in cblC disease include hydrocephalus, cor pulmonale, and hepatic failure.[232, 238, 239] Neonatal screening for MMA was the method by which the diagnosis was made in some cases. In these patients, the MMA levels are lower than those seen in mutase deficiency but higher than those reported for the defects in vitamin B_{12} transport. Elevated serum cobalamin and folate levels have been reported in several patients.

The patients with cblD disease were more mildly affected, having come to attention because of mild mental retardation and behavioral problems.[240] Cerebrovascular disease due to thromboembolism was found at the age of 18 years in one of the brothers.[203]

The findings common to the first two patients with cblF disease include their being small for gestational age, poor feeding, growth retardation, and persistent stomatitis.[241, 242] The first patient had glossitis and an abnormal Schilling test result,[243] and the second had a persistent skin rash. Both patients had minor facial abnormalities, and the first had dextrocardia. Only the second patient had macrocytosis and homocystinemia as reflected by elevated total blood homocysteine level.[241] Both patients are female. The second patient died suddenly despite apparent clinical response to therapy with vitamin B_{12}. The third patient with cblF,

a boy, had recurrent stomatitis in infancy, arthritis at the age of 4 years, and confusion, disorientation, and a pigmentary skin abnormality at the age of 10 years. He was subsequently found to have pancytopenia, an increased MCV, low serum cobalamin levels, and abnormal cobalamin absorption.[244] The fourth patient, also a boy, had aspiration pneumonia at birth and then hypotonia, lethargy, hepatomegaly, hypoglycemia, neutropenia, and thrombocytopenia.[244] Both patients had a good response to cobalamin treatment. The fifth patient with cblF, a Native Canadian girl, was diagnosed at the age of 6 months with anemia, failure to thrive, developmental delay, and recurrent infections. Serum cobalamin levels and cobalamin absorption were both low.[245]

Inheritance. The numbers of males and females affected with cblC disease are roughly equal, and both sexes are affected with equal severity. Thus, cblC disease is probably inherited as an autosomal recessive disorder. Both of the two siblings with cblD disease are males, so the possibility of sex linkage cannot be excluded. Inheritance of cblF disease also is thought to be autosomal recessive.

Laboratory Findings. The Cbl disorders can be differentiated by the results of studies of cultured fibroblasts (Table 10–2). Uptake of labeled CNCbl can distinguish the cblC and cblD diseases from all other cobalamin mutations because its level in these two disorders is reduced. The incorporation of the substrates propionate and methyl-THF is reduced in all three disorders, as is the synthesis of the two vitamin B_{12} cofactors, AdoCbl and MeCbl. Direct measurements of total mutase and methionine synthase activity in cell extracts should be low (they are not measured in cblF disease). Complementation analysis with an unknown cell line and previously defined groups provides the specific diagnosis.[117] Prenatal diagnosis of cblC disease has been successfully accomplished with the use of amniocytes, and the diagnosis ruled out with the use of chorionic villus biopsy material and cells.[246, 247]

Management. Therapy in cblC disease can be difficult, particularly in the patient with early onset. Many patients with onset in the first month of life die.[203] Many patients have improved with OHCbl therapy, 1 mg per day by injection, by reducing MMA and homocystine excretion. Results from studies of cultured cells[248] and from clinical studies suggest that OHCbl rather than CNCbl should be used.[249] Therapy with MeCbl and AdoCbl has been employed, but it is unclear whether these agents offer a therapeutic advantage. In a detailed study of therapy,[249] the effectiveness of oral OHCbl and systemic OHCbl was compared along with the effect of carnitine, folinic acid, and betaine (250 mg/kg per day). Systemic OHCbl treatment was much more effective than oral therapy, and betaine appeared to be helpful when used in combination with OHCbl. Neither folinic acid nor carnitine had any effect. The result of therapy with daily oral betaine and biweekly injections of OHCbl was a reduction in MMA, normalization of serum methionine and homocysteine concentrations, and resolution of lethargy, irritability, and failure to thrive. However, complete rever-

Table 10–2. DIAGNOSTIC STUDIES IN cbl DISEASES: CORRELATION OF GENETIC COMPLEMENTATION GROUP WITH BIOCHEMICAL PHENOTYPE AND MAJOR CLINICAL MANIFESTATIONS

Complementation Group	cb1A	cb1B	cb1C	cb1D	cb1E	cb1G	cb1F
Major Clinical Findings							
Megaloblastic anemia	N	N	D	D	D	D	Nt
Methylmalonic aciduria	D	D	D	D	N*	N	D
Homocystinuria	N	N	D	D	D	D	Nt
Laboratory Findings							
Studies in Intact Fibroblasts							
(^{57}Co)-cyano-B$_{12}$ uptake:	N	N	D	D	N	N	I
AdoB$_{12}$ (%)	D	D	D	D	N	N	D
MeB$_{12}$ (%)	N	N	D	D	D	D	D
Propionate incorporation	D	D	D	D	N	N	D
Methyltetrahydrofolate incorporation	N	N	D	D	D	D	D
Studies in Cell Extracts							
Methylmalony-CoA mutase holoenzyme	D	D	D	D	N	N	—
Methionine synthase holonenzyme	N	N	D	D	Nt	D	D

*Transient methylmalonic aciduria reported in one patient.
tSeen in one of two cases reported.
‡Under standard reducing conditions.
N = Normal for laboratory findings, not seen for clinical findings; D = decreased for laboratory findings, detected for clinical findings; I = increased.

sal of the neurologic and retinal findings did not occur; this emphasizes the need for early diagnosis and treatment. Even with good metabolic control, surviving patients usually have moderate to severe developmental delay.[191, 203] The prognosis appears to be better in patients with a later age of onset.

The patients with cblF disease appeared to respond to systemic therapy with OHCbl, though the first patient responded to oral Cbl.[242, 244, 245, 250] A theoretic concern in cblF disease is that patients may have accumulation of vitamin B$_{12}$ in lysosomes to an extent that it in itself causes symptoms. The disease has been excluded in twins and in a single pregnancy by the results of studies on amniocytes.

Methylcobalamin Deficiency (cblE and cblG Diseases)

Background. Functional methionine synthase deficiency is characterized by homocystinuria and hypomethioninemia without methylmalonic aciduria. On the basis of complementation analysis, two distinct groups of patients have been identified: those with cblE disease, and those with cblG disease (see Fig. 10–4, Points E and G).

Clinical Syndromes. The patients usually come to medical attention in the first 2 years of life; in one case, however, the patient presented at age 21 years with symptoms that caused her to be diagnosed as having multiple sclerosis. Both males and females have been described as having cblE and cblG diseases, although there is predominance in males in cblE disease.[232] The most common findings in both cblE and cblG diseases included megaloblastic anemia and various neurologic problems, of which developmental delay and cerebral

atrophy were the most common.[251] Other findings included electroencephalographic abnormalities, nystagmus, hypotonia, hypertonia, seizures, blindness, and ataxia.

Laboratory Findings. Fibroblasts from both cblE and cblG patients show decreased intracellular levels of MeCbl and normal levels of adenosylmethionine.[252] Total CNCbl uptake and binding to the intracellular enzymes are normal in cblE fibroblasts and in fibroblasts from most cblG patients. In fibroblasts from a minority of cblG patients, binding of labeled Cbl to methionine synthase does not occur.[253] In both cblE and cblG diseases, there is decreased incorporation of methyl-THF, reflecting the functional methionine synthase deficiency. The standard assay for methionine synthase in cell extracts gives activities within the range of controls in cblE patients, but most cblG patients have low methionine synthase activity in cell extracts. In cblE cells, a relative deficiency in methionine synthase activity can be seen when the assay is performed under suboptimal reducing conditions, suggesting that the defect lies in a reducing system associated with methionine synthase.[254, 255] It has been suggested that the defect in cblG disease lies in the interaction of the enzyme with *S*-adenosylmethionine.[256]

One patient with cblE disease has had transient methylmalonic aciduria.[84] The clinical heterogeneity is evidenced by several patients who did not present for therapy until adulthood. Their disease was mainly neurologic, and the anemia was recognized only later.

Inheritance. The cblE and cblG diseases are thought to be inherited in an autosomal recessive pattern. Decreased MeCbl levels have been seen in obligate heterozygotes for cblE.[257]

Management. Generally, systemic therapy with

OHCbl, at first daily and then once or twice weekly, has been used. Usually, therapy with cobalamin results in correction of the anemia and metabolic abnormalities. The neurologic findings have been difficult to reverse, particularly in cblG disease; this stresses the importance of early diagnosis and therapy.

Prenatal diagnosis of cblE disease has been successfully performed in amniocytes, and the mother carrying the affected fetus was treated from the second trimester with systemic vitamin B$_{12}$.[257] The baby was treated from birth and, throughout the first decade of life, has done very well. It is uncertain, however, whether prenatal therapy is needed.

FOLATE

Nutritional Sources and Requirements

Sources

Folate is widespread in food.[2, 258–260] Foods with very high folate content include liver, kidney, orange juice, and spinach.[261–264] In studies of replete adult populations, about one third of the daily folate intake is provided by cereals and bread, another one third by fruits and vegetables, and the remaining one third by meats and fish.[265] Human milk provides enough folate for the infant, but heat-sterilized bovine milk may be inadequate. Goat's milk contains little folate, and children maintained on it alone develop severe folate deficiency.[266]

Requirements

Inadequate folate intake is the commonest cause of folate deficiency causing megaloblastic anemia. The reduced folates in food are labile to light and oxidation and are partly destroyed during cooking. The dietary folate requirement is a matter of dispute, but the daily intake recommended by the World Health Organization is listed in Table 10–3. It should be noted, however, that the assay of folate in diets is not standardized and that different results are obtained through the use of different techniques. Within these limits, in populations in which clinical folate deficiency is unusual, mean dietary folate intake has been about 3 μg of total folates per kg of body weight. This is about 150 μg/d for women and 200 μg/d for men. In such a population, folate levels were measured in 500 liver specimens, most of which were obtained from victims of trauma. The concentrations of hepatic folates appeared to be adequate.[267] In volunteers ingesting diets of known folate content,[268, 269] plasma and erythrocyte folate levels remained within the normal range when intakes were from 150 to 200 μg/d. Intakes of this magnitude were calculated for normal subjects by measurement of a catabolite of folate (*p*-acetamidobenzoyl glutamate) that is excreted in urine.[270, 271]

Subjects with Increased Folate Requirements

Although folate deficiency can be recognized through its hematologic effects and the lack of these combined with normal plasma methylmalonic acid and total homocysteine levels interpreted as folate sufficiency, studies linking folate status with neural tube defects and with arteriosclerotic vascular disease (see later) suggest the need to re-examine what is meant by "folate sufficiency." Intakes of folate in excess of those recommended to maintain normal red cell and serum folate levels may be necessary for maximum birth-weight gain, for prevention of neural tube defects, and for reduction of the risk of cardiovascular and cerebrovascular disease. Whether this represents a greater need for folate in the population in general or is restricted to one or more specific subpopulations with altered folate metabolism remains to be determined.

Folate requirements appear greatest per kilogram in the newborn infant and the young child,[55] in pregnant women in whom folate is shunted to the developing fetus and urinary folate loss is increased, and in lactating women who secrete 50 μg or more into each liter of milk. The folate content of milk does not correlate with the level of plasma folate,[272] folate being concentrated in milk above the level of plasma folate. Some milk folate is bound to the folate-binding protein, as described later.

Other groups with greater than normal folate requirements include patients with sprue and other diseases of the small intestine; patients chronically taking antiepileptic medication[273]; women taking the birth control pill[274]; and patients with hemolytic anemia, including those with sickle cell anemia and thalassemia.

Chemistry of Folates

Folates or pteroylglutamates are conjugates of pterin, *p*-aminobenzoate, and glutamate, and they have a molecular weight of about 450. *Folic acid* is an oxidized folate that is synthesized chemically as a stable yellow powder and sold commercially. It requires reduction to a DHF or THF to function as a coenzyme in cells. Folic acid has a low solubility in aqueous solutions and at acid pH. Reduced folates are photolabile and susceptible to destruction by oxidation. THF is very labile and readily breaks at the carbon 9–nitrogen 10 bond, producing inactive catabolites.[275]

Biochemistry of Folates

Folates bind to and act as coenzymes for enzymes that mediate single-carbon metabolism. They accept and

Table 10–3. RECOMMENDED INTAKE OF FOLATE AND COBALAMIN (WHO-FAO, 1989)

Age	Folate (μg/kg per d)	Cobalamin (μg/d)
Infants	3.6	0.1
Age 1–16	3.3	
Adults	3.1*	1.0*

*For pregnant or lactating women: folate, supplementation with 300–1000 μg/d; cobalamin, 0.3–0.4 μg/d.

donate single-carbon atoms at different states of oxidation (e.g., formaldehyde, formate, and methyl).[2, 275] Folate-dependent enzymes are inactive without their folate cofactors.[276] A scheme of folate metabolism is illustrated in Figure 10–9. The concentrations of folates found within cells are far lower than the affinity constants of most of the folate-dependent enzymes for them.[277–279] Intracellular metabolism would not occur if these affinities were not increased. This appears to depend on the enzyme *folate polyglutamate synthetase*, which converts folates to folate polyglutamates. Almost all intracellular folates in animals and humans are in the form of polyglutamates, which usually contain a total of six or seven glutamates.[279] The affinity of folate polyglutamates for most of these enzymes is much greater than that of folate monoglutamates, and this greater affinity permits intracellular folate-dependent enzyme reactions to occur.

Folate-Dependent Reactions

Folate (PteGlu) enters cells as folic acid, as 5-methyl-THF, or as 5-formyl-THF. Folic acid is successively

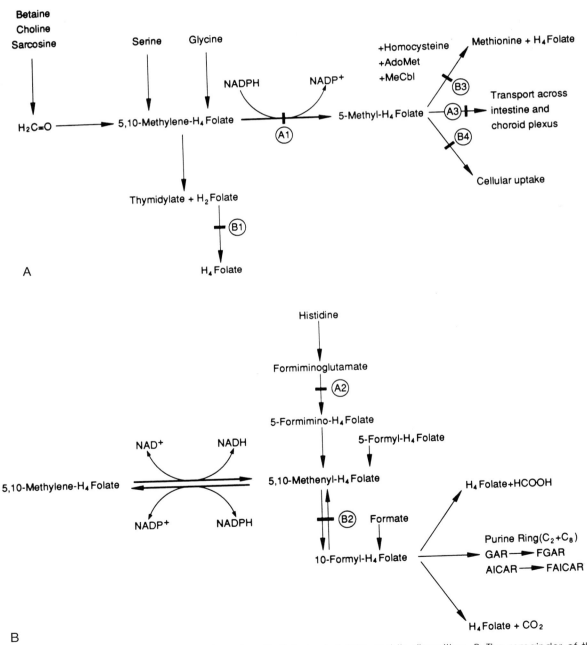

Figure 10-9. Folate metabolism. *A*, The generation of methyltetrahydrofolate and its disposition. *B*, The remainder of the folate pathway. The sites of the confirmed (A series) and suspected (B series) inborn errors of folate metabolism and transport are indicated (see text for details).

reduced to DHF and THF by the enzyme DHF reductase (EC 1.2.1.3.):

Reaction 1

$$PteGlu + H_2 \rightarrow H_2PteGlu + H_2 \rightarrow H_4PteGlu$$

5-Methyl-THF is the predominant folate in plasma and extracellular fluids. It enters cells and gives its CH_3 to homocysteine to form methionine, through the action of the cobalamin-dependent enzyme methionine synthase (see earlier). A decrease in this reaction that is related to cobalamin deficiency or a lack of folate results in increased homocysteine and decreased methionine levels:

Reaction 2

$$5\text{-}CH_3\text{—}H_4PteGlu + \text{homocysteine} \rightarrow H_4PteGlu + \text{methionine}$$

5-Formyl-THF (folinic acid, leucovorin) is a stable, reduced folate that is available commercially. It also is a natural folate and is converted to 5,10-methenyl-THF by the enzyme 5,10-methenyl-THF synthetase:

Reaction 3

$$5\text{-}CHO\text{—}H_4PteGlu \rightarrow 5,10\text{-}CH{=}H_4PteGlu$$

THF has a central role in folate metabolism, arising from 5-methyl-THF (see above) and from 10-formyl-THF during purine synthesis. It is a principal substrate for the enzyme folate polyglutamate synthetase (EC 6.3.2.17):

Reaction 4

$$H_4PteGlu + Glu \rightarrow H_4PteGlu_n$$

THF polyglutamate accepts a single carbon from serine to become 5,10-methylene-THF polyglutamate through the action of cytosolic and mitochondrial serine hydroxymethyltransferase enzymes (EC 2.1.2.1):

Reaction 5

$$H_4PteGlu_n + \text{serine} \rightarrow 5,10\text{-}CH_2\text{—}H_4PteGlu_n + \text{glycine}$$

5,10-Methylene-THF polyglutamate has a central regulatory role in folate metabolism through its reaction with thymidylate synthase (dTMP synthase) to form thymidylate and DHF polyglutamate and through the following two reactions[7, 8]:

Reaction 6

$$5,10\text{-}CH_2\text{—}H_4PteGlu_n + dUMP \rightarrow H_2PteGlu_n + dTMP$$

5,10-Methylene-THF polyglutamate is converted to 5,10-methenyl-THF polyglutamate and then to 10-formyl-THF polyglutamate, which is required for purine synthesis by a trifunctional enzyme referred to as C_1 synthase (methylene-THF dehydrogenase [EC 1.5.1.5], 5,10-methenyl-THF cyclohydrolase [EC 3.5.4.9], formyl-THF synthetase [EC 6.3.4.4]):

Reaction 7

$$5,10\text{-}CH_2\text{—}H_4PteGlu_n - H_2 \rightarrow 5,10\text{-}CH^+\text{—}H_4PteGlu_n$$
$$\rightarrow 10\text{-}CHO\text{—}H_4PteGlu_n \leftrightarrows H_4PteGlu_n + CHO$$

5,10-Methylene-THF polyglutamate is reduced to 5-methyl-THF polyglutamate by the enzyme methylene-THF reductase. Polymorphism in this gene has been linked to elevated plasma total homocysteine levels and to both arteriosclerotic vascular disease and neural tube birth defects[280, 281]:

Reaction 8

$$5,10\text{-}CH_2\text{—}H_4PteGlu_n + H_2 \rightarrow 5\text{-}CH_3\text{—}H_4PteGlu_n$$

10-Formyl-THF polyglutamate is the coenzyme for the bifunctional enzyme phosphoribosylglycinamide (GAR) transformylase (EC 2.1.2.2) and phosphoribosylaminoimidazolecarboxamide (AICAR) transformylase (EC 2.1.2.3) involved in purine synthesis:

Reaction 9

$$10\text{-}CHO\text{—}H_4PteGlu_n + GAR \text{ or } AICAR \rightarrow$$
$$H_4PteGlu_n + CHO\text{-}GAR \text{ or } CHO\text{-}AICAR$$

Histidine catabolism involves a bifunctional enzyme (formimino transferase–cyclodeaminase) that transfers a formimino (FI) group from glutamate to $H_4PteGlu_n$, with its subsequent deamination. Increased urinary excretion of formiminoglutamic acid (FIGlu) is a biochemical feature of folate deficiency. It is not measured frequently because of technical difficulties and lack of specificity.

Reaction 10

$$FIGlu + H_4PteGlu_n \rightarrow FIH_4PteGlu_n + Glu \rightarrow$$
$$5,10\text{-}CH^+\text{—}H_4PteGlu_n + NH_3$$

Folate polyglutamates are converted to monoglutamates by the enzyme γ-glutamylhydrolase (EC 3.4.22.12), which is located in lysosomes and in the intestinal brush border.[282, 283] Folate monoglutamates cross cell membranes much better than do polyglutamates, and adequate cellular nutrition is impossible without this hydrolysis.

Reaction 11

$$R\text{-}H_4PteGlu_n \rightarrow R\text{—}H_4PteGlu$$

Physiology of Folates
Absorption of Folates from the Gut

Dietary folates are principally folate polyglutamates. They are hydrolyzed within the gut lumen or brush border or in the lysosomes of enterocytes to folate monoglutamates. The monoglutamates are transported by a carrier-mediated transport system from the proximal small intestine into the portal venous plasma. In addition to this transport system, folate can diffuse across the intestine in vitro by unidentified pathways. The saturable system utilizes a folate binder on the enterocyte surface that binds most folate monoglutamates with equal affinity. Transport is affected by pH and sodium transport[284–288] and does not require metabolism of the folate.[289] Folate appears in the portal venous blood within 15 minutes of entering the stomach and reaches a maximum level in portal venous plasma about 1 hour later. Reduced folates, such as 5-formyl-

THF, are rapidly converted to 5-methyl-THF during absorption.[290]

Some folates that are presented to the liver, and some hepatic folates, are excreted into the bile and reabsorbed.[2, 291, 292] This enterohepatic circulation of folates provides a slow and more even absorption than would occur in its absence. There is evidence that the enterohepatic circulation of folates is disturbed by alcohol ingestion (i.e., it occurs more rapidly),[292, 293] and this contributes to folate deficiency.[294-296] The efficiency of utilization of folic acid, of folate polyglutamates, and of food folate is variable in different subjects. In general, folate polyglutamates are absorbed about 80% as effectively as are monoglutamates,[297] but food folate availability varies, depending on the diet. Folate absorption from a mixed diet is, on average, about 50% as efficient as absorption of synthetic folic acid—that is, about twice as much folate in food is required as is folic acid.[55, 261]

Transport of Folates in Plasma

Plasma folate consists almost entirely of 5-methyl-THF.[298] It is mostly unbound, although some of it may be bound to albumen. When absorption of food folate ceases, plasma folate decreases rapidly over days, becoming very low within 1 to 2 weeks.[299]

A small amount of plasma folate is bound to a folate-binding protein[300-303] that is homologous or identical to a folate receptor protein present on the surfaces of many cells.[303-305] Plasma folate-binding protein levels are increased in pregnancy, during folate deficiency, in renal failure, in the presence of breast and ovarian cancers, and during some types of inflammation. Its function in plasma is unclear.[306-309] In milk, it may function to improve the utilization of milk folate by the newborn animal.[307, 310, 311]

Entry of Folates into Cells

Folates enter cells principally by an anion-coupled, energy-independent, reduced folate carrier that also transports methotrexate, a widely used folate antagonist, but not folic acid. The gene for the human reduced folate carrier (RFC1) has been cloned.[311a, 311b] It is located on the long arm of chromosome 21. The reduced folate carrier also is involved in the countertransport of folates from cells.[312-315]

The folate receptor is a 38- to 39-kd glycoprotein attached to the cell membrane via a glycosylphosphatidylinositol anchor. There are three isoforms, two of which have been mapped to the human chromosomal locus 11q13. It binds 5-methyl-THF and folic acid and mediates their entry into cells by a process known as potocytosis.[316] The folate receptor increases greatly on the surface of cells grown in very low folate concentrations.[317] The extent of its contribution to total folate uptake by cells is not known. It is not expressed on hematopoietic cells.

Folate Deficiency

Folate deficiency worldwide is extremely prevalent, coexisting with poverty, malnutrition, and chronic parasitic, bacterial, and viral infections. Inadequate diet, overcooking of vegetables with loss of folates, and malabsorption secondary to tropical sprue are important contributors. Additional populations at increased risk in society are the elderly, the very young, and pregnant and lactating mothers. In Europe and North America, significant groups of the population fail to consume 200 μg of folates daily and are at increased risk of being folate deficient. Megaloblastic anemia due to folate deficiency is common worldwide, as is anemia with megaloblastosis in patients with multifactorial malnutrition and ill health. The recent findings of (1) elevated plasma total homocysteine levels in association with cerebral and cardiovascular disease, as well as their reduction with folate supplements; and (2) that a folate supplement in the periconceptual period prevents many cases of neural tube defects (even when given to mothers whose serum and red cell folate levels fall within the normal range) have raised questions about how much folate constitutes dietary sufficiency (see later).

Maternal and Pediatric Folate Deficiency

Maternal Folate Deficiency

Folate deficiency is common in mothers, particularly where poverty or malnutrition are common and dietary supplements are not provided.[318] It is usually accompanied by iron deficiency. The growing fetus imposes an increased demand for folate, which is often not met by the diet. Increased demand for folates in mothers with thalassemia minor and sickle cell disease increases further the risk of folate deficiency with full-blown megaloblastic anemia. Folate deficiency may also result from malabsorption due to disease of the small intestine. An increased need for folates in the first trimester of pregnancy has been implicated in the occurrence of neural tube defects (anencephaly, sphingomyelocele, and spina bifida) in infants (see later).

Deficiency in Newborns and Infants

The level of serum folates is higher in cord blood than maternal blood. This means that the fetus is privileged in extracting adequate folate from the mother even in the face of developing maternal folate deficiency. Therefore, clinical folate deficiency is not present at birth. The newborn has increased demands for folate for growth, which must be met by the diet. Maternal milk folate levels remain elevated during development of maternal folate deficiency, but they decrease when deficiency is present. Folate deficiency is common in premature infants unless folate supplements are given.[319] Folate must be added to hyperalimentation solutions given to newborns receiving care in intensive care units. Other factors contributing to increased folate needs are infections or other illnesses. Hemolysis due to vitamin E deficiency or due to enzyme defects, such as glucose-6-phosphate dehydrogenase deficiency, or to rarer red cell enzyme deficiencies, results in an increased demand for folates. Folate absorption is reduced in chronic diarrhea. As mentioned earlier, infants fed goat's milk develop folate deficiency because goat's milk contains almost no folate.[266]

Folate deficiency in infants may not present as classic megaloblastic anemia. Rather, the baby likely will have been transfused, and neutropenia and thrombocytopenia may be the only hematologic features. Where general malnutrition exists, features of folate deficiency may be overshadowed by the clinical picture of marasmus or protein-calorie malnutrition. The increased requirement for growth and the lack of long-term folate stores makes folate deficiency a regular component of starvation. Because folate is stored principally in the liver, hepatitis and other diseases of the liver may disturb stores and precipitate folate deficiency. Inborn errors of folate metabolism are rare but of considerable interest (discussed later).

Deficiency in Older Children and Adolescents

The most common cause of folate deficiency in older children is malnutrition. Some subgroups are particularly at risk because of increased demands, including those with sickle cell disease, thalassemia major, hepatitis, HIV infection, and malabsorption.

Certain drugs and medications predispose to folate deficiency. Alcohol abuse is associated with folate deficiency and affects a proportion of children and adolescents. Antifolate drugs such as triamterene and sulfisoxazole-trimethoprim can inhibit human DHF reductase to some degree and, in the presence of marginal folate stores, induce folate deficiency. Similarly, folate deficiency has been reported in patients taking chronic antiepileptic medication and oral contraceptives.[273, 274]

Diagnosis of Folate Deficiency

The diagnosis of folate deficiency is similar to that for cobalamin deficiency. The bone marrow is indistinguishable from that in deficiency of cobalamin, and the same abnormalities may be noted in clinical chemistry data. In most patients who are deficient in folate, serum folate and erythrocyte folate levels are low. The level of serum folate (normal range, 4 to 20 ng/mL [8.8 to 44.0 nmol/L]) decreases rapidly during folate deprivation and falls into the range of deficiency (less than 3 ng/mL [less than 6.6 nmol/L]) within 2 weeks of cessation of folate intake.[299] The erythrocyte folate level decreases slowly (normal, 200 to 800 ng/mL [440 to 1800 nmol/L]) as deficient erythrocytes replace sufficient ones (most deficient subjects have erythrocyte folate values that are less than 150 ng/mL [less than 330 nmol/L]) during the 3 to 4 months' turnover of red cells. In patients who are folate deficient because of poor intake or absorption, both values will usually be in the deficient range. In patients who develop deficiency while taking alcohol, intravenous amino acids, or possibly some antibiotics, serum folate levels are

deficient but erythrocyte folate levels may not have decreased out of the range of normal. The level of FIGlu in a 24-hour sample of urine collected in acid following a histidine load is elevated in folate deficiency. This test is infrequently performed today.

Total plasma homocysteine is increased above normal in 80% to 90% of patients with proven deficiency of folate; however, large groups of patients have not yet been studied. The level of methylmalonic acid is normal.[127, 320]

The result of the deoxyuridine suppression test with bone marrow cells is abnormal and is corrected by the addition of 5-formyl-THF, 5-methyl-THF, or other folates during the preincubation with deoxyuridine (see earlier; see also Fig. 10–8).

Erythrocyte Folate Levels in Cobalamin Deficiency

Erythroid precursors in the bone marrow accumulate 5-methyl-THF from plasma and convert it to THF by means of the cobalamin-dependent enzyme methionine synthase. THF is converted to THF polyglutamates and retained in mature red cells as 5-methyl-THF polyglutamates. This reaction is impaired in cobalamin-deficient cells, with the result that patients deficient in cobalamin have lower erythrocyte folate levels together with normal or raised serum folate levels.[159] This interpretation of the cause of erythrocyte folate changes in cobalamin deficiency is known as the "methylfolate trap hypothesis."[321]

Treatment of Folate Deficiency

In patients deficient in folate, the diet should be corrected. In those with intestinal disease, 5 mg of folic acid taken daily by mouth (or 100 µg/kg of body weight for children) is sufficient.

Folate deficiency megaloblastic anemia responds to very small doses of folic acid (200 to 500 µg/d). The response provides verification of the diagnosis, because cobalamin deficiency does not respond to such low doses of folate. Daily treatment with 1 mg is more than adequate. However, larger doses are frequently given because folic acid is manufactured in 5-mg tablets. Such treatment is without risk if cobalamin deficiency can be excluded. There is concern that large doses of folate can exacerbate neurologic damage in patients with cobalamin deficiency. Certainly, the diagnosis of megaloblastic anemia can be delayed, with the result that the duration of neurologic damage is extended and the risk of incomplete neurologic recovery increased after the correct diagnosis has been made. In some patients with inborn errors of cobalamin metabolism, neurologic degeneration has appeared during prolonged treatment with folate.[322]

The primary treatment modality for patients with nutritional folate deficiency is correction of the dietary abnormality. For patients with sprue, 5 to 15 mg/d of folate suffice and can be verified by the detection of normal or high serum and erythrocyte folate levels after therapy.

Clinical responses have been reported in a small number of patients with dementia, restless leg syndrome, and other neurologic defects following the administration of large doses of folic acid or folinic acid.[323–325] How common these responses are is unknown.

Folates and Neural Tube Defects

In North America and Europe, the population incidence of neural tube defects (anencephaly, sphingomyelocele, and spina bifida) ranges from 0.6 to 3.7 cases per 1000 live births.[326] Folate deficiency (or insufficiency) in the first trimester of pregnancy has been implicated in the occurrence of neural tube defects in infants.[327] The United Kingdom and the Hungarian studies of recurrent and occurrent neural tube defects, respectively, confirmed the findings of earlier and later studies and proved that a folate supplement taken in the periconceptual period (to include the time from initiation of pregnancy to that of closure of the neural tube at about 1 month of gestation) reduced the incidence of neural tube defects by 50% to 70%.[36, 37] Both folate and cobalamin status have been implicated in the causation of neural tube defects.[328] The incidence of neural tube defects was inversely correlated with the red cell folate level.[329] Until it is determined who is at particular risk in the population, perhaps by maternal total plasma homocysteine level or methylene-THF reductase polymorphism status,[281, 330, 331] the problem of how to provide adequate folate to mothers planning a pregnancy remains. Folate supplements are the most effective way to deliver folate, but half of all pregnancies are unplanned. Fortifying the diet (e.g., by adding folate to wheat) to increase the mean folate intake of the population has been recommended.[332] The Food and Drug Administration has recommended that folate be added to prepared foods in sufficient amounts to provide an additional intake of 150 to 200 μg/d of folate. This supplementation is likely to be more effective in improving folate nutriture in the population than would the consumption of a diet higher in natural folates.[333]

Folates and Arteriosclerotic Vascular Disease

In addition to known major risk factors for the development of atherosclerotic vascular disease involving peripheral, coronary, and cerebral arteries, such as increased serum cholesterol and low-density lipoprotein levels, the premature occurrence of arteriosclerosis in patients with severe homocystinuria has suggested that an elevated plasma homocysteine might be an atherogenic factor.[334] Subsequently, a thermolabile (at 46°C) variant of methylene-THF reductase was described and found to be associated with higher plasma homocysteine concentration and with the development of atherosclerotic vascular disease.[335] A polymorphism involving an alanine-to-valine substitution in methylene-THF reductase correlates with reduced enzyme activity and increased thermolability; individuals homozygous for

the polymorphism have significantly elevated plasma homocysteine levels[280] (Fig. 10–10). Being a heterozygosity for cystathionine β-synthase may account for a small number of cases of elevated plasma homocysteine as well.[38] Treatment of subjects with elevated total plasma homocysteine levels with either vitamin B₆ or folic acid or, occasionally, betaine normalizes the homocysteine level.[336] It appears likely that such therapy can prevent recurrent or occurrent arteriosclerotic disease.[337]

Folates and Cancer

A number of epidemiologic studies suggest an association between folate deficiency and premalignant changes in several epithelial tissues, including the cervix,[338] bronchus,[339] and colon.[39] Some of these studies have demonstrated an apparent reversal of the pathologic lesions with folate supplementation. However, difficulty in differentiating between megaloblastic and

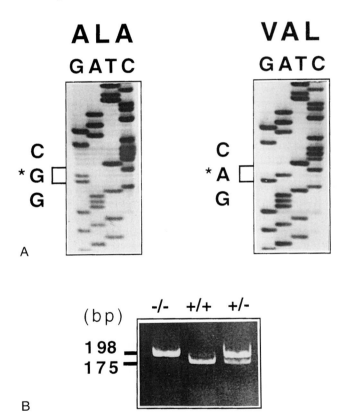

Figure 10–10. Sequence change and restriction enzyme analysis for the alanine (ALA)–to–valine (VAL) substitution in methylenetetrahydrofolate reductase. A, Sequence of two individuals, a homozygote for the alanine residue and a homozygote for the valine residue. The antisense strands are depicted. The primers for analysis of the A→V change are: 5'-TGAAGGAGAA GGTGTCTGCGGGA-3' (exonic) and 5'-AGGACGGTGC GGTGAGAGTG-3' (intronic); these primers generate a fragment of 198 bp. B, The substitution creates a Hinf1 recognition sequence, which digests the 198-bp fragment into 175- and 23-bp fragments; the latter fragment has been run off the gel. All three possible genotypes are shown. (From Frosst P, Blom HJ, et al: A candidate genetic risk factor for vascular disease: a common methylenetetrahydrofolate reductase mutation causes thermoinstability. Nat Genet 1995; 10:111.)

dysplastic changes tends to confound these results. A causal relationship between folate deficiency and the development of colon cancer has been established by comparison of folate-deficient and folate-replete rats fed the carcinogen dimethylhydrazine.[340]

Ribofolate Peptide

A thymic factor that stimulates DNA synthesis of immature thymocytes has been found to recruit G1-phase cells synchronously into the S phase, thereby functioning as a progression growth factor.[341] This thymic growth peptide consists of a formyl pteroyl group bound to the N-terminal glutamyl of a nonapeptide. The pterin part of the thymic growth peptide molecule has a ribitol substituent, in analogy with riboflavin.[342] This represents a novel folate structure with unexpected properties.

Folate Antimetabolites

Antifolates are analogues of folic acid that block folate metabolism, interrupting DNA synthesis and causing cell death. They inhibit the enzyme DHF reductase as the primary target.

Methotrexate is an effective anticancer agent widely used in combination chemotherapy of carcinomas of the breast, lung, bone, ovary, and head and neck, as well as of other cancers. It contributes to cure of choriocarcinoma and childhood acute lymphoblastic leukemia. Methotrexate is also used for its immunosuppressive and antiproliferative properties in the treatment of psoriasis, rheumatoid arthritis, and graft-versus-host disease following bone marrow transplantation.

Pyrimethamine is an antimalarial drug having greater affinity for parasitic than human DHF reductase. Trimethoprim is another antifolate with antibacterial activity and a higher affinity for bacterial than human DHF reductase. It is combined with sulfisoxazole, a sulfa drug that interferes with bacterial synthesis of folic acid, to deliver a double-dose synergistic antifolate attack on bacteria. Bactrim and Septra are such combinations widely used to treat urinary tract and other infections. They are also used to prevent *Pneumocystis carinii* pneumonia in immunocompromised patients receiving chemotherapy or in persons infected with HIV.

Newer antifolates have been synthesized and tested for the past 40 years. Currently, trimetrexate and piritrexim are two lipid-soluble antifolates that enter cells by transport routes different from those used by methotrexate. Trimetrexate appears to be useful against *P. carinii*; this is because host toxicity can be prevented with leucovorin, whereas *P. carinii* is unable to take up this folate. A series of novel antifolates that specifically inhibit thymidylate synthesis are being developed in Great Britain. The prototype, CB3717, has been proved toxic to the liver and kidneys. Newer analogues, including D-1694,[343] do not seem to be so toxic. Dideaza-THF is a new antifolate that specifically inhibits GAR transformylase, a folate-requiring enzyme involved in purine synthesis.[344]

Resistance to Methotrexate

Cancer and leukemia cells develop resistance to methotrexate in a variety of ways, including the following[345]:

1. Diminished transport of methotrexate (and of reduced folates) into the cell
2. Amplification of the DHF reductase gene, with overproduction of DHF reductase
3. Mutations of the DHF reductase gene resulting in a DHF reductase, with decreased binding affinity for methotrexate
4. Decreased folate polyglutamate synthetase activity, with diminished polyglutamylation of methotrexate
5. Increased γ-glutamyl hydrolase activity, with decreased retention of methotrexate polyglutamates

Inborn Errors of Folate Metabolism and Transport

Methylenetetrahydrofolate Reductase Deficiency

Description. Methylene-THF reductase deficiency is the most common inborn error of folate metabolism, with more than 40 cases being recognized[26, 346] (Table 10–4). It is not associated with megaloblastic anemia because the block is in the conversion of methylene-THF to methyl-THF. There is no "trapping" of folates as methyl-THF, and reduced folates are available for purine and pyrimidine metabolism. Since methyl-THF serves as a methyl donor for the conversion of homocysteine to methionine, methylene-THF reductase deficiency results in elevated homocysteine levels and decreased levels of methionine (see Fig. 10–9, Point A1).

Clinical Syndromes. This disorder may be diagnosed at any time from infancy to adulthood, and clinically asymptomatic but biochemically affected individuals have been reported.[27, 347] In general, clinical severity is related to the proportion of methyl-THF in cells. Most of the patients are brought to medical attention in infancy, with the most common clinical manifestation being developmental delay. Most of the patients have been diagnosed during the first year of life. Breathing disorders, seizures, and microcephaly are often present, and motor and gait abnormalities and psychiatric manifestations have been reported. The report of two patients with schizophrenia and methylene-THF reductase deficiency leads to speculation on the role of methylene-THF reductase deficiency in psychiatric disease.[348, 349]

Laboratory Investigation. Homocystinuria is seen in all patients, with homocystine level ranging from 15 to 667 μmol per 24 hours[350] and having a mean of 130 μmol per 24 hours. These values are much lower than those found in homocystinuria due to cystathionine synthase deficiency. If methylene-THF reductase deficiency is suspected, more than one determination of homocystine excretion should be performed to eliminate the possibility of a false-negative value. Recently, there has been interest in measurements of both pro-

Table 10-4. INHERITED DEFECTS OF FOLATE METABOLISM

	Hereditary Folate Malabsorption	Methylenetetrahydrofolate Reductase Deficiency	Glutamate Formiminotransferase Deficiency
Clinical Findings			
Prevalence	15 Cases	>25 Cases	13 Cases
Megaloblastic anemia	A	N	N*
Developmental delay	A	A	N*
Seizures	A	A	N*
Speech abnormalities	N	N	A*
Gait abnormalities*	N	A	N*
Peripheral neuropathy	N	A	N*
Apnea	N	A	N*
Biochemical Findings			
Homocystinuria(emia)	N	A	N
Hypomethioninemia	N	A	N
Formiminoglutamic aciduria	A*	N	A
Folate absorption	A	N	N
Serum folate	A	A	N*
Red cell folate	A	A*	N*
Defects Detectable in Cultured Fibroblasts			
Whole Cells			
CH$_3$-H$_4$PteGlu Uptake	N	N	N
CH$_3$-H$_4$PteGlu Content	N	A	N
Extracts			
Glutamate formiminotranferase		*Activity Undetectable in Cultured Fibroblasts*	
?Abnormal in liver and erythrocytes			
Methylene-H$_4$PteGlu reductase	N	A	N

*Exceptions described in some cases.
N = normal; A = abnormal (i.e., clinical findings or laboratory findings present).

tein-bound and total homocysteine. These measurements are performed by treating plasma or serum with reducing agents to free the homocysteine from proteins to which it is bound. These measurements have defined several patients[351] with elevated levels of homocysteine and an increased risk for cardiovascular disease.[335, 352] Measurement of methylene-THF reductase in cell extracts has revealed unusual thermolability, and the term "intermediate homocystinuria"[351] has been coined. These patients were adults without the usual manifestations of methylene-THF reductase deficiency—in particular, the absence of neurologic manifestations. An alanine-to-valine substitution in a conserved residue of the methylene-THF reductase gene on chromosome 1 has been identified as the polymorphism associated with both thermolability and susceptibility to cardiovascular disease.[280]

Plasma methionine levels have been found to be low in this deficiency. Values ranged from 0 to 18 μmol/L (mean, 12 μmol/L)[350]; normal fasting plasma methionine levels are usually in the range of 23 to 35 μmol/L. Neurotransmitter levels have been measured in the cerebrospinal fluid of only a few patients, and they usually have been low.[350] The diagnosis of methylene-THF reductase deficiency has been confirmed by direct measurement of enzyme activity in the liver, leukocytes, and cultured fibroblasts and lymphocytes. The specific activity of methylene-THF reductase in cultured fibroblasts is dependent on the stage of the culture cycle, being severalfold greater at confluence than during logarithmic growth. It is important to compare activities of unknown samples and control cell lines at confluence. A rough correlation exists between residual enzyme activity and the clinical severity.[353] In cultured fibroblasts, the proportion of total folate that is methyl-THF and the extent of labeled formate incorporated into methionine provide better correlations with clinical severity.[353, 354] Cultured fibroblasts from patients with methylene-THF reductase deficiency do not grow on tissue culture medium in which homocysteine replaces methionine.[355, 356] This methionine auxotrophy is shared by the inborn errors of vitamin B$_{12}$ metabolism that affect methionine synthase activity (cblC, cblD, cblE, cblF, and cblG diseases). The clinical heterogeneity in methylene-THF reductase deficiency is reflected at the biochemical level. Enzyme from fibroblasts of the first reported case of methylene-THF reductase deficiency had increased thermolability compared with control enzyme, especially when the assay was performed in the presence of the cofactor flavin-adenine dinucleotide.[356] As already discussed, studies have demonstrated increased thermolability in enzyme from adults who have been detected on the basis of increased total plasma homocysteine levels or of plasma protein-bound homocysteine levels. The patients were detected during screening of either patients with coronary heart disease or those with low folate and cobalamin levels. These patients had none of the other manifestations of methylene-THF reductase deficiency.

Autopsy Findings. The findings at autopsy in methylene-THF reductase deficiency[357–364] include dilation of cerebral vessels, internal hydrocephalus, and microgyria. Perivascular changes, demyelination, macrophage infiltration, gliosis, and astrocytosis have been reported. The major factor in the death of some patients was thrombosis, both of arteries and of cerebral veins.[357] The neurovascular findings in methylene-THF reductase deficiency are not dissimilar to those seen in classic homocystinuria due to cystathionine synthase deficiency. Two reports of patients with classic findings of subacute combined degeneration of the spinal cord similar to that described for vitamin B$_{12}$ deficiency have been published.[363, 364] Methionine deficiency may cause demyelination by interfering with methylation. Because methylene-THF reductase is present in the mammalian brain, and since only methyl-THF can cross the blood-brain barrier, methylene-THF reductase deficiency may result in functionally low levels of folate in the brain. Because neurologic findings in methylene-THF reductase deficiency may be present in the absence of low methionine levels, it is possible that they are due to impaired purine and pyrimidine synthesis, as opposed to methionine depletion. Also, because methylene-THF reductase has dihydropteridine reductase activity,[365] it may have a direct role in neurotransmitter synthesis. Whether most of the neuropathologic disorder arises from decreased methionine levels, elevated homocysteine levels, or the effects of low folate level other than the methylation of homocysteine to methionine has not been resolved.

Inheritance and Prenatal Diagnosis. More than one case have been reported in several families. Both affected males and females have been born to unaffected parents, and consanguinity has been reported. Methylene-THF reductase deficiency shows autosomal recessive inheritance. Phenotypic heterogeneity is associated with genotypic heterogeneity, and at least nine different mutations are known.[366, 367] Prenatal diagnosis has been reported using amniocytes,[368] and the enzyme is present in chorionic villi.

Treatment. This disease has been very difficult to treat, and the prognosis is poor once evidence of neurologic involvement has been detected. Therefore, it is important to diagnose methylene-THF reductase deficiency as early as possible. The following agents have been used for therapy:

1. Folates, to maximize any residual enzyme activity
2. Methyl-THF, to replace specifically the missing product of methylene-THF reductase
3. Methionine, to correct the deficiency of this amino acid, which requires methyl-THF for synthesis
4. Pyridoxine, because it is a cofactor for cystathionine synthase and thus may lower homocysteine levels
5. Vitamin B$_{12}$, because MeCbl is a cofactor for methionine synthase
6. Carnitine, because of its requirement for adenosylmethionine
7. Betaine, because it—along with homocysteine—is a substrate for betaine methyltransferase, an enzyme that also converts homocysteine to methionine but which is primarily active in the liver.

Betaine has the advantage of both raising methionine levels and decreasing homocysteine levels. It is to be noted, however, that because betaine methyltransferase is a liver enzyme, the effects of betaine on the brain are thought to be mediated through changes in circulating levels of metabolites. A summary of the treatment protocols for the individual patients with methylene-THF reductase deficiency has been published.[350] These protocols have been highly variable and, for the most part, unsuccessful until the introduction of betaine. Therapy either with methionine alone or with methyl-THF has not been effective. The authors[369] have suggested a regimen consisting of oral betaine, folinic acid, vitamin B$_{12}$, and vitamin B$_6$. Therapy with betaine following prenatal diagnosis has resulted in the best outcome reported to date.[370]

Glutamate Formiminotransferase Deficiency

Clinical Syndromes. It is still uncertain whether glutamate formiminotransferase deficiency (GFD) is associated with any consistent clinical findings. Only 13 patients have been described. Formiminoglutamate (FIGlu) excretion is the one constant feature of GFD. Patients with GFD range in age from 3 months to 42 years at diagnosis. Several patients had macrocytosis and hypersegmentation of neutrophils. Three patients had delayed speech, two had seizures, and two had mental retardation as their presenting signs. Two patients were studied because they were siblings of known patients. Mental retardation was described in the majority of the original patients from Japan,[371] but only three of the remaining eight patients showed mental retardation.

A mild phenotype and a severe phenotype have been described. The severe form of GFD is characterized by mental and physical retardation, abnormal electroencephalographic activity, and dilatation of the cerebral ventricles with cortical atrophy. No mental retardation occurs in the mild form, but excretion of FIGlu is greater. It has been proposed,[372] without direct enzyme measurements, that the mild form is due to a defect in the formiminotransferase enzyme, whereas the severe form results from a block in the cyclodeaminase enzyme.

Laboratory Investigation. The catabolism of histidine is associated with the transfer of a formimino group to THF, followed by the release of ammonia and the formation of 5,10-methenyl-THF (see Fig. 10–9, Point A2). Glutamate formiminotransferase and formimino-THF cyclodeaminase, two activities that share a single octameric enzyme, are involved in these reactions. These activities are found only in the liver and kidneys, and defects in these activities result in the excretion of FIGlu.

In most cases in which enzyme activity in the liver has been examined, it was higher than would be expected for an enzymatic block causing disease. This activity, measured in five patients, ranged from 14% to 54% of control values. Because the enzyme activity is expressed in the liver only, it has not been possible to confirm the diagnosis of GFD through the use of cultured cells. There has also been considerable debate as to whether the enzyme is expressed in erythrocytes.[350, 373]

Elevated FIGlu excretion as well as increased FIGlu levels in the blood following histidine load, as well as high to normal serum folate levels, have been reported in GFD. Amino acid levels, including those of histidine, were usually normal in the plasma; however, hyperhistidinemia and hyperhistidinuria have been found on occasion, as have low plasma methionine levels. The excretion of two other metabolites—hydantoin-5-propionate, the stable oxidation product of the FIGlu precursor 4-imidazolone-5-propionate; and 4-amino-5-imidazolecarboxamide, an intermediate in purine synthesis—has also been reported.

Inheritance. Offspring of both sexes with unaffected parents have been reported; however, neither enzyme levels in the livers of the parents nor reports of consanguinity have been published. Autosomal recessive inheritance is the probable means of transmission. Because GFD is not expressed in cultured cells, definitive understanding of the genetics of this disorder awaits the cloning of the gene and the localization of the molecular defect.

Treatment. Two patients in one family[374] responded with decreased FIGlu excretion to therapy with folates, whereas six other patients did not.[350] One of two patients responded to methionine supplementation.[375, 376] As the relationship between clinical expression and FIGlu excretion has not been easy to define, it is uncertain whether reducing FIGlu excretion is of any value.

Hereditary Folate Malabsorption

Clinical and Laboratory Studies. Megaloblastic anemia, diarrhea, mouth ulcers, failure to thrive, and usually progressive neurologic deterioration characterize hereditary folate malabsorption (HFM). Fifteen patients with HFM have been reported, 12 of whom were females.[322, 377] Megaloblastic anemia in the first few months of life associated with low serum folate levels is the most important diagnostic feature.

FIGlu and orotic acid excretion may be found in patients with HFM. All patients have a severe abnormality in the absorption of oral folic acid or of reduced folates. The patients with HFM provide the best evidence for a specific transport system of folates across both the intestine and the choroid plexus (see Fig 10–9, Point A3). Even when blood folate levels are raised sufficiently to correct the anemia, levels in the cerebrospinal fluid may remain low.[378] This provides evidence that the carrier system in both the intestine and the brain is coded by a single gene product. The uptake of folate into other cells is probably not defective in HFM, and uptake of folate into cultured cells is not abnormal. The hematologic findings are reversed by relatively low levels of folate.

Management. The clinical response to therapy with folates has varied among patients. Oral administration of folate in pharmacologic doses did elicit a therapeutic response in some patients through correction of the hematologic abnormality. Parenterally administered folates have been effective in reversing the anemia but have been less effective in correcting the low level of folate in the cerebrospinal fluid. Folinic acid or methyltetrahydrofolic acid may be more effective in entering the cerebrospinal fluid in HFM. In some cases, seizures were reduced in number, and in others, seizures worsened with folate therapy.[322, 379]

In treating these patients, it is essential to maintain levels of folate in the blood and in the cerebrospinal fluid in the range that is associated with folate sufficiency. Oral doses of folates may be increased to 100 mg or more daily if necessary; if oral therapy is not effective, systemic therapy must be instituted. It may be necessary to give intrathecal folate if cerebrospinal fluid levels cannot be normalized. As mentioned previously, it is thought that the reduced folates, such as folinic acid and methyl-THF, may be more effective than folic acid in treating HFM.

Inheritance. All but three of the 15 HFM patients have been female. One male had atypical clinical findings, including a lack of mental retardation and correction of cerebrospinal fluid folate levels in conjunction with correction of serum folate levels.[380] Cases of HFM may have gone unrecognized, as several of the patients had siblings who died. Consanguinity has been reported in four families, and the father of one patient has intermediate levels of folate absorption. This makes autosomal recessive inheritance probable. The need to explain the preponderance of this disorder among females remains.

Cellular Uptake Defects

A series of patients with well-characterized abnormalities of folate uptake into cells have been described (see Fig. 10–9, Point B4). It remains unclear whether any of these abnormalities represent primary defects.

In one large family,[381, 382] the prevalence of severe hematologic disease was very high, with the disorders including anemia, pancytopenia, and leukemia in 34 individuals that resulted in the death of 18. The proband had severe aplastic anemia that responded to folate therapy. The uptake of methyl-THF was markedly reduced, despite the normal uptake of folic acid in stimulated lymphocytes from the proband and from four family members. The proband and his son also had a lesser reduction of methyl-THF uptake in bone marrow cells. One son only developed the transport defect after becoming neutropenic, suggesting that the abnormality may not be the primary defect. In another family, the proband and three daughters had dyserythropoiesis without anemia.[383] An abnormality of methyl-THF uptake was detected in red cells and bone marrow cells but not in lymphocytes. There was no clear correlation in the family between the clinical findings and the disorder of cellular uptake.

Other Possible Inborn Errors of Folate Metabolism

Individual cases suggesting defects in the function of DHF reductase (see Fig. 10–9, Point B1), the synthesis of 10-formyl-THF (see Fig. 10–9, Point B2), and methionine synthase (see Fig. 10–9, Point B3) are insufficiently documented for comment at the present time.

Hums for the Humatologist

A doctor may learn to his sorrow
That his choice of disease was too narrow
For a patient's complaints
From weight loss to faints
Meant a megaloblastic bone marrow!

With many-sized red cells—oval macs, too,
Multilobed polys and platelets quite few
Diagnosis is easy—even a bore
But who ever looks at a smear anymore?!

If we from a long list of ills will select it
For protean symptoms we then must respect it
When checking our lab tests we must never neglect it
For we're certain to miss it unless we suspect it!

And if we wish to serve our patients' health interests
more proficiently
We can measure plasma MMA to find subclinical
cobalamin deficiency
And provide folate supplements periconceptually,
for elevated plasma total homocysteine and as a
dietary enhancer
To reduce neural tube defects, heart attacks and strokes
And perhaps even cancer.

References

1. Minot GR, Murphy WP: Treatment of pernicious anemia by special diet. JAMA 1926; 87:470.
2. Chanarin I: The Megaloblastic Anaemias. London, Blackwell Scientific Publications, 1979.
3. Wintrobe MM: Hematology, the Blossoming of a Science: A Story of Inspiration and Effort. Philadelphia, Lea & Febiger, 1985.
4. Castle WB: The conquest of pernicious anemia. In Wintrobe MM (ed): Blood, Pure and Eloquent. New York, McGraw-Hill Book Co., 1979, pp 283–318.
5. Ehrlich P: Untersuchungen zur Histologie und Klinik des Blutes. Berlin, Hirschwald, 1891.
6. Chanarin I: The Megaloblastic Anaemias. London, Blackwell Scientific Publications, 1979, pp 329–340.
7. Wills L: Treatment of "pernicious anaemia of pregnancy" and "tropical anaemia" with special reference to yeast extract as curative agent. BMJ 1931; 1:1059.
8. Fenwick S: On atrophy of the stomach. Lancet 1870; 2:78.
9. Castle WB: Observations on the etiologic relationship of achylia gastrica to pernicious anemia. I. The effect of administration to patients with pernicious anemia of the contents of the normal human stomach recovered after ingestion of beef muscle. Am J Med Sci 1929; 178:748.
10. Cooper BA, Castle WB: Sequential mechanisms in the enhanced absorption of vitamin B_{12} by intrinsic factor in the rat. J Clin Invest 1960; 39:199.
11. Ungley CC: Vitamin B_{12} in pernicious anaemia. Parenteral administration. BMJ 1949; 2:1370.
12. Zalusky R, Herbert V, Castle WB: Cyanocobalamin therapy effect in folic acid deficiency. Arch Intern Med 1962; 109:545.
13. Hall BE, Watkins CH: Experience with pteroylglutamate synthetic folic acid in treatment of pernicious anemia. J Lab Clin Med 1947; 32:622.
14. Youngdahl-Turner P, Rosenberg LE: Binding and uptake of transcobalamin II by human fibroblasts. J Clin Invest 1978; 61:133.
15. Cooper BA, Paranchych W: Selective uptake of specifically-bound cobalt-58 vitamin B_{12} by human and mouse tumour cells. Nature 1961; 191:393.
16. Mollin DL, Ross GIM: The vitamin B_{12} concentrations of serum and urine of normals and of patients with megaloblastic anaemias and other diseases. J Clin Pathol 1952; 5:129.
17. Gottlieb CW, Lau K-S, et al: Rapid charcoal assay for intrinsic factor (IF), gastric juice unsaturated binding capacity, antibody to IF, and serum unsaturated binding capacity. Blood 1965; 25:875.
18. Adams JF, Tankel HI, Macewan F: Estimation of the total body vitamin B_{12} in the live subject. Clin Sci 1970; 39:107.
19. Russell JSR, Batten FE, Collier J: Subacute combined degeneration of the spinal cord. Brain 1900; 23:39.
20. Jeffries GH, Hoskins DW, Sleisinger MH: Antibody to intrinsic factor in serum of patients with pernicious anemia. J Clin Invest 1962; 41:1106.
21. Dow CA, Aizpura HJ, et al: 65–70kd protein identified by immunoblotting as the presumptive gastric microsomal autoantigen in pernicious anaemia. Clin Exp Immunol 1985; 62:732.
22. Aizpura HJ, Ungar B, Toh B-H: Autoantibody to the gastric receptor in pernicious anemia. N Engl J Med 1985; 313:479.
23. Burman P, Måardh S, et al: Parietal cell antibodies in pernicious anemia inhibit H^+,K^+-adenosine triphosphatase, the proton pump of the stomach. Gastroenterology 1989; 96:1434.
24. Hakami N, Nieman PE, et al: Neonatal megaloblastic anemia due to inherited transcobalamin II deficiency in two siblings. N Engl J Med 1971; 285:1163.
25. Levy HL, Mudd SH, et al: A derangement in B_{12} metabolism associated with homocystinemia, cystathioninemia, hypomethioninemia and methylmalonic aciduria. Am J Med 1970; 48:390.
26. Erbe RW: Inborn errors of folate metabolism. In: Blakley RL, Whitehead VM (eds): Folates and Pterins: Nutritional, Pharmacological and Physiological Aspects. Vol 3. New York, John Wiley & Sons, 1986, pp 413–466.
27. Marquet J, Chadefaux B, et al: Methylenetetrahydrofolate reductase deficiency: prenatal diagnosis and family studies. Prenatal Diagn 1994; 14:29.
28. Platica O, Geneczko R, et al: Isolation of the complementary DNA for human transcobalamin II. Proc Soc Exp Biol Med 1989; 192:95.
29. Johnston J, Bollekens J, et al: Structure of the cDNA encoding transcobalamin I, a neutrophil granule protein. J Biol Chem 1989; 264:15754.
30. Hansen MR, Nexo E, et al: Human intrinsic factor. Its primary structure compared to the primary structure of rat intrinsic factor. Scand J Clin Lab Invest 1989; 49(Suppl 194):19.
31. Gueant JL, Jokinen O, et al: Purification of intrinsic factor receptor from pig ileum using as affinity medium human intrinsic factor covalently bound to Sepharose. Biochim Biophys Acta 1989; 992:281.
32. Dieckgraefe BK, Seetharam B, et al: Isolation and structural characterization of a cDNA clone encoding rat gastric intrinsic factor. Proc Natl Acad Sci U S A 1988; 85:46.
33. Gräsbeck R, Simons K, Sinkkonen I: Isolation of intrinsic factor and its probable degradation product, as their vitamin B_{12} complexes, from human gastric juice. Biochim Biophys Acta 1968; 158:292.
34. Chen P, Ailion M, et al: The end of the *cob* operon: evidence that the last gene (*cob T*) catalyses synthesis of the lower ligand of vitamin B_{12}, dimethylbenzimidazole. J Bacteriol 1995; 177:1461.
35. Savage DG, Lindenbaum J, et al: Sensitivity of serum methylmalonic acid and total homocysteine determinations for diagnosing cobalamin and folate deficiencies. Am J Med 1994; 96:239.
36. MRC Vitamin Study Research Group: Prevention of neural tube defects: results of the Medical Research Council Vitamin Study. Lancet 1991; 338:131.
37. Czeizel AE, Dudas I: Prevention of the first occurrence of neural-tube defects by periconceptional vitamin supplementation. N Engl J Med 1992; 327:1832.
38. Dudman NP, Wilcken DE, et al: Disordered methionine/homocysteine metabolism in premature vascular disease. Its occurrence, cofactor therapy, and enzymology. Arterioscler Thromb 1993; 13:1253.
39. Lashner BA, Heidenreich PA, et al: The effect of folate supplementation on the incidence of dysplasia and cancer in chronic ulcerative colitis: a case control study. Gastroenterology 1989; 97:255.

40. Finch CA, Coleman DH, et al: Erythrokinetics in pernicious anemia. Blood 1956; 11:807.
41. London IM, West R: The formation of bile pigments in pernicious anemia. J Biol Chem 1950; 184:359.
42. Glazer HS, Mueller JF, et al: Effect of vitamin B$_{12}$ and folic acid on nucleic acid composition of bone marrow of patients with megaloblastic anemia. J Lab Clin Med 1954; 43:905.
43. Nath BJ, Lindenbaum J: Persistence of neutrophil hypersegmentation during recovery from megaloblastic granulopoiesis. Ann Intern Med 1979; 90:757.
44. Chanarin I: The Megaloblastic Anaemias. London, Blackwell Scientific Publications, 1979, pp 225–226.
45. Mitchell K, Ferguson MM, et al: Epithelial dysplasia in the oral mucosa associated with pernicious anaemia. Br Dent J 1986; 161:259.
46. Levine AS, Doscherholmen A: Vitamin B$_{12}$ bioavailability from egg yolk and egg white: relationship to binding proteins. Am J Clin Nutr 1983; 38:436.
47. Doscherholmen A, McMahon J, Economon P: Vitamin B$_{12}$ absorption from fish. Proc Soc Exp Biol Med 1981; 167:480.
48. Bakker HD, van Gennip AH, et al: Methylmalonate excretion in a pregnancy at risk for methylmalonic acidaemia. Clin Chim Acta 1978; 86:349.
49. Baker SJ, Mathan VI: Evidence regarding the minimal daily requirement of dietary vitamin B$_{12}$. Am J Clin Nutr 1981; 34:2423.
50. Roberts RD, Webb JKG, et al: Vitamin B$_{12}$ deficiency in Indian infants. BMJ 1973; 3:67.
51. Banerjee DK, Chatterjea JB: Vitamin B$_{12}$ content of some articles of Indian diets and effect of cooking on it. Br J Nutr 1963; 17:385.
52. Chanarin I, Stephenson E: Vegetarian diet and cobalamin deficiency: their association with tuberculosis. J Clin Pathol 1988; 41:759.
53. Armstrong BK, Davis RE, et al: Hematological vitamin B$_{12}$ and folate studies on seventh day–adventist vegetarians. Am J Clin Nutr 1974; 27:712.
54. Abdulla M, Anderson I, et al: Nutrient uptake and health status of vegans. Chemical analyses of diets using the duplicate portion sampling technique. Am J Clin Nutr 1981; 34:2464.
55. Beaton G: Requirements of Vitamin A, Iron, Folate and Vitamin B$_{12}$: Report of a Joint FAO/WHO Expert Consultation. Rome, Food and Agriculture Organization of the United Nations, 1988.
56. Dolphin D: B$_{12}$: Chemistry. Vol. 1. New York, John Wiley & Sons, 1982.
57. Pratt JM: Inorganic Chemistry of Vitamin B$_{12}$. New York, Academic Press, 1972.
58. Hogenkamp HPC: The chemistry of cobalamins and related compounds. In Babior BM (ed): Cobalamin: Biochemistry and Pathophysiology. New York, Wiley-Interscience, 1975, pp 21–74.
59. Taylor RT: B$_{12}$-dependent methionine biosynthesis. In Dolphin D (ed): B$_{12}$: Biochemistry and Medicine. Vol 2. New York, John Wiley & Sons, 1982, pp 307–355.
60. Utley CS, Marcell PD, et al: Isolation and characterization of methionine synthetase from human placenta. J Biol Chem 1985; 260:13656.
61. Retey J: Methylmalonyl-CoA mutase. In Dolphin D (ed): B$_{12}$: Biochemistry and Medicine. Vol 2. New York, John Wiley & Sons, 1982, pp 357–380.
62. Kolhouse JF, Utley C, et al: Immunochemical studies on cultured fibroblasts from patients with inherited methylmalonic acidemia. Proc Natl Acad Sci U S A 1981; 78:7737.
63. Ledley FD, Lumetta M, et al: Molecular cloning of L-methylmalonyl-CoA mutase: gene transfer and analysis of mut cell lines. Proc Natl Acad Sci U S A 1988; 85:3518.
64. Marsh EN, McKie N, et al: Cloning and structural characterization of the genes coding for adenosylcobalamin-dependent methylmalonyl-CoA mutase from Propionibacterium shermanii. Biochem J 1989; 260:345.
65. Cameron B, Briggs K, et al: Cloning and analysis of genes involved in coenzyme-B$_{12}$ biosynthesis in Pseudomonas denitrificans. J Bacteriol 1989; 171:547.
66. Ledley FD, Lumetta MR, et al: Mapping of human methylmalonyl CoA mutase (MUT) locus on chromosome 6. Am J Hum Genet 1988; 42:839.
67. Fenton WA, Hack AM, et al: Biogenesis of the mitochondrial enzyme methylmalonyl-CoA mutase: synthesis and processing of a precursor in a cell-free system and in cultured cells. J Biol Chem 1984; 259:6616.
68. Barness LA, Morrow G 3d: Methylmalonic aciduria. A newly discovered inborn error. Ann Intern Med 1968; 69:633.
69. Morrow G 3d, Revsin B, et al: A new variant of methylmalonic acidemia: defective coenzyme-apoenzyme binding in cultured fibroblasts. Clin Chim Acta 1978; 85:67.
70. Fenton WA, Ambani LM, Rosenberg LE: Uptake of hydroxocobalamin by rat liver mitochondria. Binding to a mitochondrial protein. J Biol Chem 1976; 251:6616.
71. Fenton WA, Rosenberg LE: Genetic and biochemical analysis of human cobalamin mutants in cell culture. Ann Rev Genet 1978; 12:223.
72. Fenton WA, Rosenberg LE: The defect in the cbl B class of human methylmalonic acidemia: deficiency of cob(I)alamin adenosyltransferase activity in extracts of cultured fibroblasts. Biochem Biophys Res Commun 1981; 98:283.
73. Abe T, Gibbs B, Cooper BA: Forms of vitamin B$_{12}$ in blood and bone marrow in patients with pernicious anaemia. Br J Haematol 1975; 31:493.
74. Beck WS, Cohen R, Jorgensen J: Mitochondrial cobalamins: evidence of their noninvolvement in mitochondrial DNA synthesis. In Zagalak B, Friedrich W (eds): Vitamin B$_{12}$. Berlin, Walter de Gruyter, 1979, pp 975–977.
75. Quadros EV, Jackson B, Linnell JC: Interconversion of cobalamins in human lymphocytes in vitro and the influence of nitrous oxide on synthesis of cobalamin coenzymes. In Zagalak B, Friedrich W (eds): Vitamin B$_{12}$. Berlin, Walter de Gruyter, 1979, pp 1045–1054.
76. Fenton WA, Rosenberg LE: Mitochondrial metabolism of hydroxocobalamin: synthesis of adenosylcobalamin by intact rat liver mitochondria. Arch Biochem Biophys 1978; 189:441.
77. Finkelstein JD: Regulation of methionine metabolism in mammals. In Usdin E, Borchardt RT, Creveling CR (eds): Transmethylation. New York, Elsevier North-Holland, 1978, pp 49–68.
78. Storch KJ, Wagner DA, et al: Quantitative study in vivo of methionine cycle in humans using [methyl-^{2}H$_3$]- and [1^{13}C]methionine. Am J Physiol 1988; 255:E322.
79. Gahl WA, Finkelstein JD, et al: Hepatic methionine adenosyltransferase deficiency in a 31-year-old man. Am J Hum Genet 1987; 40:39.
80. Gahl WA, Bernardini I, et al: Transsulfuration in an adult with hepatic methionine adenosyltransferase deficiency. J Clin Invest 1988; 81:390.
81. Blom HJ, Boers GHJ, et al: Cystathionine-synthase–deficient patients do not use the transamination pathway of methionine to reduce hypermethioninemia and homocystinemia. Metabolism 1989; 38:577.
81a. Drennan CL, Huang S, et al: How a protein binds B$_{12}$: a 3.0 Å X-ray structure of B$_{12}$-binding domains of methionine synthase. Science 1994; 266:1669.
82. Fujii K, Galivan JH, Huennekens FM: Activation of methionine synthase: further characterization of the flavoprotein system. Arch Biochem Biophys 1979; 178:662.
83. Frasca V, Dunham WR, et al: Studies of cobalamin-dependent methionine synthase from Escherichia coli. In Cooper BA, Whitehead VM (eds): Chemistry and Biology of Pteridines: Pteridines and Folic Acid Derivatives. Berlin, Walter de Gruyter, 1986, pp 917–920.
84. Tuchman M, Kelly P, et al: Vitamin B$_{12}$-responsive megaloblastic anemia, homocystinuria, and transient methylmalonic aciduria in cblE disease. J Pediatr 1988; 113:1052.
85. Rosenberg LE: The inherited methylmalonic acidemias. Prog Clin Biol Res 1982; 103:187.
86. Kinnally KW, Tedeschi H: Adenosine triphosphate synthesis coupled to K$^+$ influx in mitochondria. Science 1982; 216:742.
87. Coulombe JT, Shih VE, Levy HL: Massachusetts Metabolic Disorders Screening Program. II. Methylmalonic aciduria. Pediatrics 1981; 67:26.
88. Halperin ML, Schiller CM, Fritz IB: The inhibition by methylmalonic acid of malate transport by the dicarboxylate carrier in rat liver mitochondria. A possible explanation for hypoglycemia in methylmalonic aciduria. J Clin Invest 1971; 50:2276.
89. Montgomery JA, Mamer OA, Scriver CR: Metabolism of methylmalonic acid in rats. J Clin Invest 1983; 72:1937.

90. Batt RM, Horadagoda NU: Gastric and pancreatic intrinsic factor–mediated absorption of cobalamin in the dog. Am J Physiol 1989; 257:G344.

91. Allen RH, Seetharam B, et al: Effect of proteolytic enzymes on the binding of cobalamin to R protein and intrinsic factor. J Clin Invest 1978; 61:47.

92. Sennett C, Rosenberg LE, Mellman IS: Transmembrane transport of cobalamin in prokaryotic and eukaryotic cells. Ann Rev Biochem 1981; 50:1053.

93. Hewitt JE, Gordon MM, et al: Human gastric intrinsic factor: characterization of cDNA and genomic clones and localization to human chromosome 11. Genomics 1991; 10:432.

94. Fernandez-Costa F, Metz J: Vitamin B_{12} binders (transcobalamins) in serum. CRC Crit Rev Clin Lab Sci 1982; 18:1.

95. Quadros EV, Rothenberg SP, et al: Purification and molecular characterization of human transcobalamin II. J Biol Chem 1986; 261:15455.

96. Pletsch QA, Coffey JW: Intracellular distribution of radioactive vitamin B_{12} in rat liver. J Biol Chem 1971; 246:4619.

97. Ogawa K, Kudo H, et al: Expression of vitamin B_{12} R-binder in breast tumors: an immunohistochemical study. Arch Pathol 1988; 112:1117.

98. Lee EY, Seetharam B, et al: Immunohistochemical survey of cobalamin-binding proteins. Gastroenterology 1989; 97:1171.

99. Kolhouse JF, Kondo H, et al: Cobalamin analogues are present in human plasma and can mask cobalamin deficiency because current radioisotope dilution assays are not specific for true cobalamin. N Engl J Med 1978; 299:785.

100. Doscherholmen A, Hagen PS: Delay of absorption of radiolabeled cyanocobalamin in the intestinal wall in the presence of intrinsic factor. J Lab Clin Med 1959; 54:434.

101. Rothenberg SP, Weiss JP, Cotter R: Formation of transcobalamin II–vitamin B_{12} complex by guinea-pig ileal mucosa in organ culture after *in vivo* incubation with intrinsic factor–vitamin B_{12}. Br J Haematol 1978; 40:401.

102. Chanarin I, Muir M, et al: Evidence for an intestinal origin of transcobalamin II during vitamin B_{12} absorption. BMJ 1978; 1:1453.

103. Katz M, Cooper BA: Solubilization of the receptor for intrinsic factor–B_{12} complex from guinea pig intestinal mucosa. Methods Enzymol 1980; 67:67.

104. Seetharam B, Levine JS, et al: Purification, properties, and immunochemical localization of a receptor for intrinsic factor-cobalamin complex in the rat kidney. J Biol Chem 1988; 263:4443.

105. Von Bonsdorf B: On the remission after removal of the worm in pernicious anemia in presence and absence of extrinsic factor in the food. Acta Med Scand 1943; 116:77.

106. Nyberg W, Gräsbeck R, et al: Serum vitamin B_{12} levels and incidence of tape worm anemia in a population heavily infected with *Diphyllobothrium latum*. Am J Clin Nutr 1961; 9:606.

107. Seetharam B: Gastrointestinal absorption and transport of cobalamin (vitamin B_{12}). In Johnson LR (ed): Physiology of the Gastrointestinal Tract. New York, Raven Press, 1994, pp 1997–2026.

108. Robertson JA, Gallagher ND: Intrinsic factor–cobalamin accumulates in the ilea of mice treated with chloroquine. Gastroenterology 1985; 89:1353.

109. Robertson JA, Gallagher ND: *In vivo* evidence that cobalamin is absorbed by receptor-mediated endocytosis in the mouse. Gastroenterology 1985; 88:908.

110. Kapadia CR, Serfilippi D, et al: Intrinsic factor–mediated absorption of cobalamin by guinea pig ileal cells. J Clin Invest 1983; 71:440.

111. Gueant JL, Monin GB, et al: Radioautographic localisation of iodinated human intrinsic factor in the guinea pig ileum using electron microscopy. Gut 1988; 29:1370.

112. Cooper BA: Complex of intrinsic factor and B_{12} in human ileum during vitamin B_{12} absorption. Am J Physiol 1968; 214:832.

113. Kolhouse JF, Allen RH: Absorption, plasma transport and cellular retention of cobalamin analogues. J Clin Invest 1977; 60:1381.

114. Kishimoto T, Tavassoli M, et al: Receptors for transferrin and transcobalamin II display segregated distribution on microvilli of leukemia L1210 cells. Biochem Biophys Res Commun 1987; 146:1102.

115. Seligman PA, Allen RH: Characterization of the receptor for transcobalamin II isolated from human placenta. J Biol Chem 1978; 253:1766.

116. Rosenblatt DS, Hosack A, Matiaszuk N: Expression of transcobalamin II by amniocytes. Prenat Diagn 1987; 7:35.

117. Rosenblatt DS, Cooper BA: Inherited disorders of vitamin B_{12} metabolism. Blood Rev 1987; 1:177.

118. Vassiliadis A, Rosenblatt DS, et al: Lysosomal cobalamin accumulation in fibroblasts from a patient with an inborn error of cobalamin metabolism (cblF complementation group): visualization by electron microscope radioautography. Exp Cell Res 1991; 195:295.

119. Botez MI: Neuropsychiatric illness and deficiency of vitamin B_{12} and folate. In Zittoun JA, Cooper BA (eds): Folates and Cobalamins. Berlin, Springer-Verlag, 1989, pp 145–159.

120. Ditrapani G, Barone C, et al: Dementia–peripheral neuropathy during combined deficiency of vitamin B_{12} and folate. Light microscopy and ultrastructural study of sural nerve. Ital J Neurol Sci 1986; 7:545.

121. Steiner I, Kidron D, et al: Sensory peripheral neuropathy of vitamin B_{12} deficiency: a primary demyelinating disease? J Neurol 1988; 235:163.

122. Zegers de Beyl D, Delecluse F, et al: Somatosensory conduction in vitamin B_{12} deficiency. Electrophysiol Clin Neurophysiol 1988; 69:313.

123. Perkin GD, Roche SW, et al: Delayed somatosensory evoked potentials in pernicious anaemia with intact peripheral nerves. J Neurol Neurosurg Psychiatry 1989; 52:1017.

124. Weir DG, Keating S, et al: Methylation deficiency causes vitamin B_{12}–associated neuropathy in the pig. J Neurochem 1988; 51:1949.

125. Drummond JT, Matthews RG: Nitrous oxide inactivation of cobalamin-dependent methionine synthase from *Escherichia coli*: characterization of the damage to the enzyme and prosthetic group. Biochemistry 1994; 33:3742.

126. Drummond JT, Matthews RG: Nitrous oxide degradation by cobalamin-dependent methionine synthase: characterization of the reactants and products in the inactivation reaction. Biochemistry 1994; 33:3732.

127. Stabler SP, Allen RH, et al: Marked elevation of methylmalonic acid in cerebrospinal fluid (CSF) of patients with cobalamin (Cbl) deficiency. Clin Res 1989; 37:550a.

128. Stabler SP, Allen RH, et al: Cerebrospinal fluid methylmalonic acid levels in normal subjects and patients with cobalamin deficiency. Neurology 1991; 41:1627.

129. Nilsson K, Gustafson L, et al: Plasma homocysteine in relation to serum cobalamin and blood folate in a psychogeriatric population. Eur J Clin Invest 1994; 24:600.

130. Lindenbaum J, Rosenberg IH, et al: Prevalence of cobalamin deficiency in the Framingham elderly population. Am J Clin Nutr 1994; 60:2.

131. Herbert V: Staging vitamin B_{12} (cobalamin) status in vegetarians. Am J Clin Nutr 1994; 59(5 Suppl):1213S.

132. Joosten E, Pelemans W, et al: Cobalamin absorption and serum homocysteine and methylmalonic acid in elderly subjects with low serum cobalamin. Eur J Haematol 1993; 51:25.

133. Norman EJ, Morrison JA: Screening elderly populations for cobalamin (vitamin B_{12}) deficiency using the urinary methylmalonic acid assay by gas chromatography mass spectrometry. Am J Med 1993; 94:589.

134. Pennypacker LC, Allen RH, et al: High prevalence of cobalamin deficiency in elderly outpatients. J Am Geriatr Soc 1992; 40:1197.

135. Hall CA: The nondiagnosis of pernicious anemia. Ann Intern Med 1965; 63:951.

136. Carmel R, Karnaze DS, Weiner JM: Neurologic abnormalities in cobalamin deficiency are associated with higher cobalamin "analogue" values than are hematologic abnormalities. J Lab Clin Med 1988; 111:57.

137. Reizenstein PG, Ek G, Matthews CME: Vitamin B_{12} kinetics in man: implications on total-body-B_{12}-determinations, human requirements, and normal and pathological cellular B_{12} uptake. Physics Med Biol 1966; 11:295.

138. Herzlich B, Herbert V, Drivas G: Depletion of serum homo-transcobalamin-II. An early sign of negative vitamin-B_{12} balance. Lab Invest 1988; 58:332.

139. Lindenbaum J, Healton EB, et al: Neuropsychiatric disorders caused by cobalamin deficiency in the absence of anemia or macrocytosis. N Engl J Med 1988; 318:1720.

140. Lindenbaum J, Savage DG, et al: Diagnosis of cobalamin deficiency II. Relative sensitivities of serum cobalamin, methylmalonic acid and total homocysteine concentrations. Am J Hematol 1990; 34:99.

141. Mollin DL, Anderson BB, Burman JF: The serum vitamin B_{12} level: its assay and significance. Clin Haematol 1976; 5:521.

142. Danielsson L, Enocksson E, et al: Failure to thrive due to subclinical maternal pernicious anemia. Acta Paediatr Scand 1988; 77:310.

143. Bar-Shany S, Herbert V: Transplacentally acquired antibody to intrinsic factor with vitamin B_{12} deficiency. Blood 1967; 30:777.

144. Specker BL, Miller D, et al: Increased urinary methylmalonic acid excretion in breast-fed infants of vegetarian mothers and identification of an acceptable dietary source of vitamin B_{12}. Am J Clin Nutr 1988; 47:89.

145. Herbert V: Vitamin B_{12}: plant sources, requirements, and assay. Am J Clin Nutr 1988; 48(Suppl 3):852.

146. Sanfilipo JS, Liu YK: Vitamin B_{12} deficiency and infertility: report of a case. Int J Fertility 1991; 36:36.

147. Ashkenazi S, Weitz R, et al: Vitamin B_{12} deficiency due to a strictly vegetarian diet in adolescence. Clin Pediatr 1987; 26:662.

148. Skidmore MD, Shenker N, et al: Biochemical evidence of asymptomatic vitamin B_{12} deficiency in children after ileal resection for necrotizing enterocolitis. J Pediatr 1989; 115:102.

149. Harriman GR, Smith PD, et al: Vitamin B_{12} malabsorption in patients with acquired immunodeficiency syndrome. Arch Intern Med 1989; 149:2039.

150. Saxena S, Weiner JM, Carmel R: Red blood cell distribution width in untreated pernicious anemia. Am J Clin Pathol 1988; 89:660.

151. Thong KL, Hanley SA, McBride JA: Clinical significance of a high mean corpuscular volume in nonanemic patients. Can Med Assoc J 1977; 117:908.

152. Pierce HI, Hillman RS: The value of serum vitamin B_{12} level in diagnosing B_{12} deficiency. Blood 1974; 43:915.

153. Carmel R, Karnaze DS: Physician response to low serum cobalamin levels. Arch Intern Med 1986; 146:1161.

154. Kafetz K: Immunoglobulin deficiency responding to vitamin B_{12} in two elderly patients with megaloblastic anaemia. Postgrad Med J 1985; 61:1065.

155. Wright PE, Sears DA: Hypogammaglobulinemia and pernicious anemia. South Med J 1987; 80:243.

156. Nimo R, Carmel R: Increased sensitivity of detection of the blocking (type I) anti-intrinsic factor antibody. Am J Clin Pathol 1987; 88:729.

157. Chanarin I: The Megaloblastic Anaemias. London, Blackwell Scientific Publications, 1979, pp 144–146.

158. Cooper BA, Whitehead VM: Evidence that some patients with pernicious anemia are not recognized by radiodilution assay for cobalamin in serum. N Engl J Med 1978; 299:816.

159. Cooper BA, Lowenstein L: Relative folate deficiency of erythrocytes in pernicious anemia. Blood 1964; 24:502.

160. Cooper BA, Lowenstein L: Vitamin B_{12}-folate interrelationships in megaloblastic anaemia. Br J Haematol 1966; 12:283.

161. Carmel R, Sinow RM, et al: Food cobalamin malabsorption occurs frequently in patients with unexplained low serum cobalamin levels. Arch Intern Med 1988; 148:1715.

162. Gozzard DI, Dawson DW, Lewis MJ: Experiences with dual protein-bound aqueous vitamin B_{12} absorption test in subjects with low serum vitamin B_{12} concentrations. J Clin Pathol 1987; 40:633.

163. Jones BP, Broomhead AF, et al: Incidence and clinical significance of protein-bound vitamin B_{12} malabsorption. Eur J Haematol 1987; 38:131.

164. Hippe E, Gimsing P, Hollander NH: A simplified method for quantitative determination of vitamin B_{12} absorption. In Zagalak B, Friedrich W (eds): Vitamin B_{12}. Berlin, Walter de Gruyter, 1979, pp 939–944.

165. Waxman S, Metz J, Herbert V: Defective DNA synthesis in human megaloblastic bone marrow: effects of homocysteine and methionine. J Clin Invest 1969; 48:284.

166. Wickramasinghe SN: The deoxyuridine suppression test. In Hall CA (ed): The Cobalamins. Edinburgh, Churchill Livingstone, 1983, pp 196–208.

167. Cox EV, White AM: Methylmalonic acid excretion: an index of vitamin-B_{12} deficiency. Lancet 1962; 2:853.

168. Schneede J, Dagnelie PC, et al: Methylmalonic acid and homocysteine in infants on macrobiotic diets. Pediatr Res 1994; 36:194.

169. Norman EJ: New urinary methylmalonic acid test is a sensitive indicator of cobalamin (vitamin B_{12}) deficiency: a solution for a major unrecognized medical problem. J Lab Clin Med 1987; 110:369.

170. Stabler SP, Marcell PD, et al: Assay of methylmalonic acid in the serum of patients with cobalamin deficiency using capillary gas chromatography mass spectrometry. J Clin Invest 1986; 77:1606.

171. Ho CH, Chang HC, Yeh SF: Quantitation of urinary methylmalonic acid by gas chromatography mass spectrometry and its clinical applications. Eur J Haematol 1987; 38:80.

172. Matchar DB, Feussner JR, et al: Isotope-dilution assay for urinary methylmalonic acid in the diagnosis of vitamin B_{12} deficiency. A prospective clinical evaluation. Ann Intern Med 1987; 106:707.

173. Kang S-S, Wong PWK, Norusis M: Homocystinemia due to folate deficiency. Metabolism 1987; 36:458.

174. Refsum H, Ueland PM, Svardal AM: Fully automated fluorescence assay for determining total homocysteine in plasma. Clin Chem 1989; 35:1921.

175. Lawson DH, Parker JWL: Deaths from severe megaloblastic anaemia in hospitalised patients. Scand J Haematol 1976; 17:347.

176. Carmel R: Treatment of severe pernicious anemia: no association with sudden death. Am J Clin Nutr 1988; 48:1443.

177. Skouby AP: Hydroxocobalamin for initial and long-term therapy for vitamin B_{12} deficiency. Acta Med Scand 1987; 221:399.

178. Olesen H, Hom B, Schwartz M: Antibody to transcobalamin II in patients treated with long-acting vitamin B_{12} preparations. Scand J Haematol 1968; 5:5.

179. Berendt RC, Jewell LD, et al: Multicentric gastric carcinoids complicating pernicious anemia: origin from the metaplastic endocrine cell population. Arch Pathol Lab Med 1989; 113:399.

180. Hsing AW, Hansson L-E, et al: Pernicious anemia and subsequent cancer: a population-based cohort study. Cancer 1993; 71:745.

181. Ottesen M, Feldt-Rasmussen U, et al: Thyroid function and autoimmunity in pernicious anemia before and during cyanocobalamin treatment. J Endocrinol Invest 1995; 18:91.

182. Davis RE, McCann VJ, Stanton KG: Type I diabetes and latent pernicious anemia. Med J Aust 1992; 156:160.

183. Katz M, Lee SK, Cooper BA: Vitamin B_{12} malabsorption due to a biologically inert intrinsic factor. N Engl J Med 1972; 287:425.

184. Yang Y-M, Ducos R, et al: Cobalamin malabsorption in three siblings due to abnormal intrinsic factor that is markedly susceptible to acid and proteolysis. J Clin Invest 1985; 76:2057.

185. Gräsbeck R: Familial selective vitamin B_{12} malabsorption. N Engl J Med 1972; 287:358.

186. Wulffraat NM, De Schryver J, et al: Failure to thrive is an early symptom to the Imerslund-Gräsbeck syndrome. Am J Hematol Oncol 1994; 16:177.

187. Mackenzie IL, Donaldson RM Jr, et al: Ileal mucosa in familial selective vitamin B_{12} malabsorption. N Engl J Med 1972; 286:1021.

188. Burman JF, Walker WJ, et al: Absent ileal uptake of IF-bound-vitamin B_{12} in the Imerslund-Gräsbeck syndrome (familial vitamin B_{12} malabsorption with proteinuria). Gut 1985; 26:311.

189. Fyfe JC, Ramanujam KS, et al: Defective brush-border expression of intrinsic factor–cobalamin receptor in canine inherited intestinal cobalamin malabsorption. J Biol Chem 1991; 266:4489.

190. Fyfe JC, Giger U, et al: Inherited selective intestinal cobalamin malabsorption and cobalamin deficiency in dogs. Pediatr Res 1991; 29:24.

191. Cooper BA, Rosenblatt DS: Inherited defects of vitamin B_{12} metabolism. Ann Rev Nutr 1987; 7:291.

192. Carmel R: A new case of deficiency of the R binder for cobalamin, with observations on minor cobalamin binding proteins in serum and saliva. Blood 1982; 59:152.

193. Carmel R: R-binder deficiency. A clinically benign cause of cobalamin pseudodeficiency. J Am Med Assoc 1983; 250:1886.

194. Carmel R, Herbert V: Deficiency of vitamin B_{12} α-globulin in two brothers. Blood 1969; 33:1.

195. Jenks J, Begley J, Howard L: Cobalamin–R binder deficiency in a woman with thalassemia. Nutr Rev 1983; 41:277.

196. Sigal SH, Hall CA, Antel JP: Plasma R binder deficiency and neurologic disease. N Engl J Med 1988; 317:1330.

197. Li N, Rosenblatt DS, et al: Identification of two mutant alleles of transcobalamin II in an affected family. Hum Molec Genet 1994; 3:1835.

198. Nierbrugge DJ, Benjamin DR, et al: Hereditary transcobalamin II deficiency presenting as red cell hypoplasia. J Pediatr 1982; 101:732.

199. Burman JF, Mollin DL, et al: Inherited lack of transcobalamin II in serum and megaloblastic anemia: a further patient. Br J Haematol 1979; 43:27.

200. Meyers PA, Carmel R: Hereditary transcobalamin II deficiency with subnormal serum cobalamin levels. Pediatrics 1984; 74:866.

201. Thomas PK, Hoffbrand AV, Smith IS: Neurological involvement in hereditary transcobalamin II deficiency. J Neurol Neurosurg Psychiatry 1982; 45:74.

202. Zeitlin HC, Sheppard K, et al: Homozygous transcobalamin II deficiency maintained on oral hydroxocobalamin. Blood 1985; 66:1022.

203. Fenton W, Rosenberg LE: Inherited disorders of cobalamin transport and metabolism. In Scriver CR, Beaudet AL, et al (eds): The Metabolic and Molecular Basis of Inherited Disease. New York, McGraw-Hill Book Co., 1995, pp 3129–3149.

204. Daiger SP, Labowe ML, et al: Detection of genetic variation with radioactive ligands. III. Genetic polymorphism of transcobalamin II in human plasma. Am J Hum Genet 1978; 30:202.

205. Eiberg H, Moller N, et al: Linkage of transcobalamin II (TC2) to the P blood group system and assignment to chromosome 22. Clin Genet 1986; 29:354.

206. Platica O, Janeczko R, et al: The cDNA sequence and the deduced amino acid sequence of human transcobalamin II show homology with rat intrinsic factor and human transcobalamin I. J Biol Chem 1991; 266:7860.

207. Li N, Seetharam S, et al: Isolation and sequence analysis of variant forms of human transcobalamin II. Biochim Biophys Acta 1993; 1172:21.

208. Li N, Rosenblatt DS, Seetharam B: Nonsense mutations in human transcobalamin II deficiency. Biochem Biophys Res Commun 1994; 204:1111.

209. Mahoney MJ, Bick D: Recent advances in the inherited methylmalonic acidemias. Acta Paediatr Scand 1987; 76:689.

210. Fenton WA, Hack AM, et al: Immunochemical studies of fibroblasts from patients with methylmalonyl-CoA mutase apoenzyme deficiency: detection of a mutation interfering with mitochondrial import. Proc Natl Acad Sci U S A 1987; 84:1421.

211. Raff ML, Crane AM, et al: Genetic characterization of a *mut* locus mutation discriminating heterogeneity in mut° and mut⁻ methymalonic aciduria by interallelic complementation. J Clin Invest 1991; 87:203.

212. Qureshi AA, Crane AM, et al: Cloning and expression of mutations demonstrating intragenic complementation in mut° methylmalonic aciduria. J Clin Invest 1994; 93:1812.

213. Inoue S, Krieger I, et al: Inhibition of bone marrow stem cell growth *in vitro* by methylmalonic acid: a mechanism for pancytopenia in a patient with methylmalonic acidemia. Pediatr Res 1981; 15:95.

214. Ledley FD, Levy HL, et al: Benign methylmalonic aciduria. N Engl J Med 1984; 311:1015.

215. Zoghbi HY, O'Brien WE, Ledley FD: Linkage relationships of the human methylmalonyl-CoA mutase to the *HLA* and *D6S4* loci on chromosome 6. Genomics 1988; 3:396.

216. Jansen R, Kalousek F, et al: Cloning of full-length methylmalonyl-CoA mutase from a cDNA library using the polymerase chain reaction. Genomics 1989; 4:198.

217. Crane AM, Ledley FD: Cluster of mutations in methylmalonyl CoA mutase associated with mut⁻ methylmalonic acidemia. Am J Hum Genet 1994; 55:42.

218. Crane AM, Jansen R, et al: Cloning and expression of a mutant methylmalonyl coenzyme A mutase with altered cobalamin affinity that causes mut⁻ methylmalonic aciduria. J Clin Invest 1992; 89:385.

219. Ledley FD, Jansen R, et al: Mutation eliminating mitochondrial leader sequence of methylmalonyl CoA mutase causes mut° methylmalonic aciduria. Proc Natl Acad Sci 1991; 87:3147.

220. Crane AM, Martin LS, et al: Phenotype of disease in three patients with identical mutations in methylmalonyl CoA mutase. Human Genet 1992; 89:259.

221. Ogasawara M, Matsubara Y, et al: Identification of two novel mutations in the methylmalonyl-CoA mutase gene with decreased levels of mutant mRNA in methylmalonic acidemia. Hum Mol Genet 1994; 3:867.

222. Chalmers RA, Stacey TE, et al: L-Carnitine insufficiency in disorders of organic acid metabolism: response to L-carnitine by patients with methylmalonic aciduria and 3-hydroxy-3-methylglutaric aciduria. J Inherit Metab Dis 1984; 7:109.

223. Wolff JA, Carroll JE, et al: Carnitine reduces fasting ketogenesis in patients with disorders of propionate metabolism. Lancet 1986; 1:289.

224. Bain MD, Jones M, et al: Contribution of gut bacterial metabolism to human metabolic disease. Lancet 1988; 1:1078.

225. Snyderman SE, Sansaricq C, et al: The use of neomycin in the treatment of methylmalonic aciduria. Pediatrics 1972; 50:925.

226. Koletzko B, Bachmann C, Wendel U: Antibiotic treatment for improvement of metabolic control in methylmalonic aciduria. J Pediatr 1990; 117:99.

227. Matsui SM, Mahoney MJ, Rosenberg LE: The natural history of the inherited methylmalonic acidemias. N Engl J Med 1983; 308:857.

228. Ampola MG, Mahoney MJ, et al: Prenatal therapy of a patient with vitamin B_{12} responsive methylmalonic acidemia. N Engl J Med 1975; 293:313.

229. Mellman I, Willard HF, et al: Cobalamin coenzyme synthesis in normal and mutant fibroblasts: evidence for a processing enzyme activity deficient in cblC cells. J Biol Chem 1979; 254:11847.

230. Pezacka EH: Identification and characterization of two enzymes involved in the intracellular metabolism of cobalamin. Cyanocobalamin β-ligand transferase and microsomal cob(III)alamin reductase. Biochim Biophys Acta 1993; 1157:167.

231. Pezacka EH, Rosenblatt DS: Intracellular metabolism of cobalamin. Altered activities of β-axial-ligand transferase and microsomal cob(III)alamin reductase in cblC and cblD fibroblasts. In Bhatt HR, James VHT, et al (eds): Advances in Thomas Addison's Diseases. Vol. 1. Bristol, England: Journal of Endocrinology Ltd., 1994, pp 315–323.

232. Rosenblatt DS: Inherited errors of cobalamin metabolism: an overview. In Bhatt HR, James VHT, et al (eds): Advances in Thomas Addison's Diseases. Vol. 1. Bristol, England: Journal of Endocrinology Ltd., 1994, pp 303–313.

233. Mitchell GA, Watkins D, et al: Clinical heterogeneity in cobalamin C variant of combined homocystinuria and methylmalonic aciduria. J Pediatr 1986; 108:410.

234. Shinnar S, Singer HS: Cobalamin C mutation (methylmalonic aciduria and homocystinuria) in adolescence. A treatable cause of dementia and myelopathy. N Engl J Med 1984; 311:451.

235. Mitchell GA, Watkins D, et al: Clinical heterogeneity in cobalamin C variant of combined homocystinuria and methylmalonic aciduria. J Pediatr 1986; 108:410.

236. Robb RM, Dowton SB, et al: Retinal degeneration in vitamin B_{12} disorder associated with methylmalonic aciduria and sulfur amino acid abnormalities. Am J Ophthalmol 1984; 97:691.

237. Traboulski EI, Silva JC, et al: Ocular histopathologic characteristics of cobalamin C type vitamin B_{12} defect with methylmalonic aciduria and homocystinuria. Am J Ophthalmol 1992; 113:269.

238. Weintraub L, Tardo C, et al: Hydrocephalus as a possible complication of the cblC type of methylmalonic aciduria. Am J Hum Genet 1991; 49:108. Abstract.

239. Caouette G, Rosenblatt D, Laframboise R: Hepatic dysfunction in a neonate with combined methylmalonic aciduria and homocystinuria. Clin Invest Med 1992; 15:A112. Abstract.

240. Goodman SI, Moe PG, et al: Homocystinuria with methylmalonic aciduria: two cases in a sibship. Biochem Med 1970; 4:500.

241. Shih VE, Axel SM, et al: Defective lysosomal release of vitamin B_{12} (cb1F): a hereditary cobalamin metabolic disorder associated with sudden death. Am J Med Genet 1989; 33:555.

242. Rosenblatt DS, Laframboise R, et al: New disorder of vitamin

B_{12} metabolism (cobalamin F) presenting as methylmalonic aciduria. Pediatrics 1986; 78:51.

243. Laframboise R, Cooper BA, Rosenblatt DS: Malabsorption of vitamin B_{12} from the intestine in a child with cblF disease: evidence for lysosomal-mediated absorption. Blood 1992; 80:291. Letter.

244. MacDonald MR, Wiltse HE, et al: Clinical heterogeneity in two patients with cblF disease. Am J Hum Genet 1992; 15:A353. Abstract.

245. Wong LTK, Rosenblatt DS, et al: Diagnosis and treatment of a child with cblF disease. Clin Invest Med 1992; 15:A111. Abstract.

246. Zammarchi E, Lippi A, et al: cblC disease: case report and monitoring of a pregnancy at risk by chorionic villus sampling. Clin Invest Med 1990; 13:139.

247. Chadefaux-Vekemans B, Rolland MO, et al: Prenatal diagnosis of combined methylmalonic aciduria and homocystinuria (CblC or CblD mutant). Prenat Diagn 1994; 14:417. Letter.

248. Wallis J, Clark DM, Bain BJ: The use of hydroxocobalamin in the Schilling test. Scand J Haematol 1986; 37:337.

249. Bartholomew DW, Batshaw ML, et al: Therapeutic approaches to cobalamin-C methylmalonic acidemia and homocystinuria. J Pediatr 1988; 112:32.

250. Shih VE, Axel SM, et al: Defective lysosomal release of vitamin B_{12} (cblF) a hereditary metabolic disorder associated with sudden death. Am J Hum Genet 1989; 33:555.

251. Watkins D, Rosenblatt DS: Functional methionine synthase deficiency (cblE and cblG): clinical and biochemical heterogeneity. Am J Med Genet 1989; 34:427.

252. Watkins D, Rosenblatt DS: Genetic heterogeneity among patients with methylcobalamin deficiency. J Clin Invest 1988; 81:1690.

253. Sillaots SL, Hall CA, et al: Heterogeneity in cblG: differential retention of cobalamin on methionine synthase. Biochem Med Metab Biol 1992; 47:242.

254. Rosenblatt DS, Cooper BA, et al: Altered vitamin B_{12} metabolism in fibroblasts from a patient with megaloblastic anemia and homocystinuria due to a new defect in methionine biosynthesis. J Clin Invest 1984; 74:2149.

255. Rosenblatt DS, Cooper BA: Selective deficiencies of methyl B_{12} (cblE and cblG). Clin Invest Med 1989; 12:270.

256. Hall CA, Lindenbaum RH, et al: The nature of the defect in cobalamin G mutation. Clin Invest Med 1989; 12:262.

257. Rosenblatt DS, Cooper BA, et al: Prenatal vitamin B_{12} therapy of a fetus with methylcobalamin deficiency (cobalamin E disease). Lancet 1985; 1:1127.

258. Chung ASM, Pearson WN, et al: Folic acid, vitamin B_6, pantothenic acid and vitamin B_{12} in human dietaries. Am J Clin Nutr 1961; 9:573.

259. Collins RA, Harper AE, et al: The folic acid and vitamin B_{12} content of the milk of various species. J Nutr 1951; 43:313.

260. Moscovitch LF, Cooper BA: Folate content of diets in pregnancy: comparison of diets collected at home and diets prepared from dietary records. Am J Clin Nutr 1973; 26:707.

261. Cooper BA: Reassessment of folic acid requirements. In White PL, Selvey N (eds): Nutrition in Transition: Proceedings, Western Hemisphere Nutrition Congress V. Monroe, WI, American Medical Association, 1978, pp 281–288.

262. Zittoun J: Folate and nutrition. Chemioterapia 1985; 4:388.

263. Senti FR, Pilch SM: Analysis of folate data from the second National Health and Nutrition Examination Survey (NHANES II). J Nutr 1985; 115:1398.

264. Herbert V: Making sense of laboratory tests of folate status: folate requirements to sustain normality. In Zittoun J, Cooper BA (eds): Folates and Cobalamins. Berlin, Springer-Verlag, 1989, pp 119–127.

265. Canada Department of National Health and Welfare: Food Consumption Patterns Report. A Report from Nutrition Canada by the Bureau of Nutritional Sciences, Health Protection Branch, Department of Health and Welfare. Ottawa, Ontario, Canada, Health and Welfare Canada, 1976.

266. Taitz LS, Armitage BL: Goats' milk for infants and children. BMJ [Clin Res] 1984; 288:428. Editorial.

267. Hoppner K, Lampi B: Folate levels in human liver from autopsies in Canada. Am J Clin Nutr 1980; 33:862.

268. Milne DB, Johnson L, et al: Folate status of adult males living in a metabolic unit: possible relationships with iron nutriture. Am J Clin Nutr 1983; 37:768.

269. Banerjee DK, Maitra A, et al: Minimal daily requirement of folic acid in normal Indian subjects. Ind J Med Sci 1975; 63:45.

270. McNulty H, McPartlin JM, et al: Folate catabolism in normal subjects. Hum Nutr Appl Nutr 1987; 41:338.

271. Scott JM: Catabolism of folates. In Blakley RL, Benkovic SJ (eds): Folates and Pterins: Chemistry and Biochemistry of Folates. Vol. 1. New York, John Wiley & Sons, 1984, pp 307–344.

272. Ek J: Plasma, red cell, and breast milk folacin concentration in lactating women. Am J Clin Nutr 1983; 38:929.

273. Dansky LV, Rosenblatt DS, Andermann E: Mechanisms of teratogenesis: folic acid and antiepileptic therapy. Neurology 1992; 42:32.

274. Shojania AM: Oral contraceptives: effect of folate and vitamin B_{12} metabolism. Can Med Assoc J 1982; 126:244.

275. Blakley RL, Benkovic SJ (eds): Folates and Pterins: Chemistry and Biochemistry of Folates. Vol. 1. New York, John Wiley & Sons, 1984.

276. Mackenzie RE: Biogenesis and interconversion of substituted tetrahydrofolates. In Blakley RL, Benkovic SJ (eds): Folates and Pterins: Chemistry and Biochemistry of Folates. New York, John Wiley & Sons, 1984, pp 255–306.

277. Matthews RG, Lu Y-Z, et al: The polyglutamate specificities of four folate-dependent enzymes from pig liver. In Goldman ID (ed): Proceedings of the Second Workshop on Folyl and Antifolyl Polyglutamates. New York, Praeger Publishers, 1985, pp 65–75.

278. Hilton JG, Cooper BA, Rosenblatt DS: Folate polyglutamate synthesis and turnover in cultured human fibroblasts. J Biol Chem 1979; 254:8398.

279. Foo SK, Shane B: Regulation of folylpoly-γ-glutamate synthesis in mammalian cells in vivo and in vitro synthesis of pteroylpoly-γ-glutamates by Chinese hamster ovary cells. J Biol Chem 1982; 257:13587.

280. Frosst P, Blom HJ, et al: A candidate genetic risk factor for vascular disease: a common methylenetetrahydrofolate reductase mutation causes thermoinstability. Nat Genet 1995; 10:111.

281. van der Put NMJ, Steegers-Theunissen RPM, et al: Mutated methylenetetrahydrofolate reductase as a risk factor for spina bifida. Lancet 1995; 346:1070.

282. Chandler CJ, Wang TT, Halsted CH: Pteroylpolyglutamate hydrolase from human jejunal brush borders. Purification and characterization. J Biol Chem 1986; 261:928.

283. McGuire JJ, Coward JK: Pteroylpolyglutamates: biosynthesis, degradation, and function. In Blakley RL, Benkovic SJ (eds): Folates and Pterins: Chemistry and Biochemistry of Folates. Vol. 1. New York, John Wiley & Sons, 1984, pp 135–190.

284. Rosenberg IH, Zimmerman J, Selhub J: Folate transport. Chemioterapia 1985; 4:354.

285. Selhub J, Rosenberg IH: Folate transport in isolated brush border membrane vesicles from rat intestine. J Biol Chem 1981; 256:4489.

286. Schron CM, Washington C Jr, Blitzer BL: Anion specificity of the jejunal folate carrier: effects of reduced folate analogues on folate uptake and efflux. J Membr Biol 1988; 102:175.

287. Blakeborough P, Salter DN: Folate transport in enterocytes and brush-border-membrane vesicles isolated from the small intestine of the neonatal goat. Br J Nutr 1988; 59:485.

288. Browman BB, McCormick DB, Rosenberg IH: Epithelial transport of water-soluble vitamins. Ann Rev Nutr 1989; 9:187.

289. Whitehead VM, Cooper BA: Absorption of unaltered folic acid from the gastro-intestinal tract in man. Br J Haematol 1967; 13:679.

290. Whitehead VM, Pratt R, et al: Intestinal conversion of folinic acid to 5-methyltetrahydrofolate in man. Br J Haematol 1972; 22:63.

291. Herbert V: Excretion of folic acid in the bile. Lancet 1965; 1:913.

292. Hillman RS, McGuffin R, Campbell C: Alcohol interference with the folate enterohepatic cycle. Trans Assoc Am Physicians 1977; 90:145.

293. Eisenga BH, Collins TD, McMartin KE: Differential effects of acute ethanol on urinary excretion of folate derivatives in the rat. J Pharmacol Exp Ther 1989; 248:916.

294. Blocker EB, Thenen SW: Intestinal absorption, liver uptake,

and excretion of ³H-folic acid in folic acid–deficient, alcohol-consuming nonhuman primates. Am J Clin Nutr 1987; 46:503.

295. Eichner ER, Pierce HI, Hillman RS: Folate balance in dietary-induced megaloblastic anemia. N Engl J Med 1971; 284:933.

296. Lane F, Goff P, et al: Folic acid metabolism in normal, folate deficient and alcoholic man. Br J Haematol 1976; 34:489.

297. Halsted CH: The intestinal absorption of folates. Am J Clin Nutr 1979; 32:846.

298. Herbert V, Larrabee AR, Buchanan JM: Studies on the identification of a folate compound of human serum. J Clin Invest 1962; 41:1134.

299. Herbert V: Experimental nutritional folate deficiency in man. Trans Assoc Am Physicians 1962; 75:307.

300. Waxman S, Schreiber C: Characteristics of folic acid-binding protein in folate deficient serum. Blood 1973; 42:291.

301. Wagner C: Folate-binding proteins. Nutr Rev 1985; 43:293.

302. Eichner ER, McDonald CR, Dickson VL: Elevated serum levels of unsaturated folate-binding protein: clinical correlates in a general hospital population. Am J Clin Nutr 1978; 31:1988.

303. Sadasivan E, Rothenberg SP: The complete amino acid sequence of a human folate-binding protein from KB cells determined from the cDNA. J Biol Chem 1989; 264:5806.

304. Sadasivan E, Rothenberg SP: Molecular cloning of the complementary DNA for a human folate-binding protein. Proc Soc Exp Biol Med 1988; 189:240.

305. Lacey SW, Sanders JM, et al: Complementary DNA for the folate-binding protein correctly predicts anchoring to the membrane by glycosyl-phosphatidylinositol. J Clin Invest 1989; 84:715.

306. Deutsch JC, Elwood PC, et al: Role of the membrane-associated folate-binding protein (folate receptor) in methotrexate transport by human KB cells. Arch Biochem Biophys 1989; 274:327.

307. Anonymous: Transport properties of folate bound to human milk folate-binding protein. Nutr Rev 1988; 46:230. Editorial.

308. Ratnam M, Marquardt H, et al: Homologous membrane folate-binding proteins in human placenta: cloning and sequence of a cDNA. Biochemistry 1989; 28:8249.

309. Hansen SI, Holm J, Hoier-Madsen M: A high-affinity folate-binding protein in human urine. Radioligand binding characteristics, immunological properties and molecular size. Biosci Rep 1989; 9:93.

310. Lonnerdal B: Biochemistry and physiological function of human milk proteins. Am J Clin Nutr 1985; 42:1299.

311. Said HM, Horne DW, Wagner C: Effect of human milk folate-binding protein on folate intestinal transport. Arch Biochem Biophys 1986; 251:114.

311a. Moscow JA, Gong M, et al: Isolation of a gene encoding a human reduced folate carrier (RFC1) and analysis of its expression in transport-deficient, methotrexate-resistant human breast cancer cells. Cancer Res 1995; 55:3790.

311b. Wong SC, Proefke SA, et al: Isolation of human cDNAs that restore methotrexate sensitivity and reduced folate carrier activity in methotrexate transport-defective Chinese hamster ovary cells. J Biol Chem 1995; 270:17468.

312. Henderson GB, Tsuji JM, Kumar HP: Mediated uptake of folate by a high-affinity binding protein in sublines of L1210 cells adapted to nanomolar concentrations of folate. J Membr Biol 1988; 101:247.

313. Henderson GB: Transport of folate compounds by hematopoietic cells. In Zittoun J, Cooper BA (eds): Folates and Cobalamins. Berlin, Springer-Verlag, 1989, pp 231–245.

314. Freisheim JH, Ratnam M, et al: Photoaffinity analogues of methotrexate as folate antagonist binding probes. Adv Enzyme Regul 1988; 27:15.

315. Price EM, Freisheim JH: Photoaffinity analogues of methotrexate as folate antagonist binding probes. 2. Transport studies, photoaffinity labeling, and identification of the membrane carrier protein for methotrexate from murine L1210 cells. Biochemistry 1987; 26:4757.

316. Anderson RG, Kamen BA, et al: Potocytosis: sequestration and transport of small molecules by caveolae. Science 1992; 255:410.

317. Matsue H, Rothberg KG, et al: Folate receptor allows cells to grow in low concentrations of 5-methyltetrahydrofolate. Proc Natl Acad Sci U S A 1992; 89:6006.

318. Subar AF, Block G, James LD: Folate intake and food sources in the US population. Am J Clin Nutr 1989; 50:508.

319. Worthington-White DA, Behnke M, Gross S: Premature infants require additional folate and vitamin-B₁₂ to reduce the severity of the anemia of prematurity. Am J Clin Nutr 1994; 60:930.

320. Stabler SP, Marcell PD, et al: Elevation of total homocysteine in the serum of patients with cobalamin and folate deficiency detected by capillary gas chromatography-mass spectrometry. J Clin Invest 1988; 810:4660.

321. Scott JM, Weir DG: Hypothesis: the methyl folate trap. Lancet 1981; 2:337.

322. Rosenblatt DS: Inherited disorders of folate transport and metabolism. In Scriver CR, Beaudet AL, et al (eds): The Metabolic and Molecular Basis of Inherited Disease. New York, McGraw-Hill Book Co., 1995, pp 3111–3128.

323. Reynolds EH: Neurological aspects of folate and vitamin B₁₂ metabolism. Clin Haematol 1976; 5:661.

324. Lever EG, Elwes RDC, et al: Subacute combined degeneration of the cord due to folate deficiency: response to methyl folate treatment. J Neurol Neurosurg Psychiatry 1986; 49:1203.

325. Brockner P, Lods JC: Folate deficiency in geriatric patients. In Zittoun J, Cooper BA (eds): Folates and Cobalamins. Berlin, Springer-Verlag, 1989, pp 179–189.

326. Christensen B, Rosenblatt DS: Effects of folate deficiency on embryonic development. In Wickramasinghe SN (ed): Baillière's Clinical Haematology: Megaloblastic Anemia. London, Baillière Tindall, 1995, pp 617–637.

327. Schorah CJ, Smithells RW, Scott J: Vitamin B₁₂ and anencephaly. Lancet 1980; 1: 880.

328. Kirke PN, Molloy AM, et al: Maternal plasma folate and vitamin B₁₂ are independent risk factors for neural tube defects. Q J Med 1993; 86:703.

329. Daly LE, Kirke PN, et al: Folate levels and neural tube defects. JAMA 1995; 274:1698.

330. Steegers-Theunissen RPM, Boers GHJ, et al: Maternal hyperhomocysteinemia: a risk factor for neural tube defects. Metabolism 1994; 43:1475.

331. Mills JL, McPartlin JM, et al: Homocysteine metabolism in pregnancies complicated by neural-tube defects. Lancet 1995; 345:149.

332. Oakley GP, Erickson JD, Adams MJ: Urgent need to increase folic acid supplementation. JAMA 1995; 274:1717.

333. Cuskelly GJ, McNulty H, Scott JM: Effect of increasing dietary folate on red-cell folate: implications for prevention of neural tube defects. Lancet 1996; 347:657.

334. McCully KS: Vascular pathology of homocysteinemia: implications for the pathogenesis of arteriosclerosis. Am J Pathol 1969; 56:111.

335. Kang S-S, Wong PWK, et al: Thermolabile methylenetetrahydrofolate reductase: an inherited risk factor for coronary artery disease. Am J Hum Genet 1991; 48:536.

336. Franken DG, Boers GH, et al: Treatment of mild hyperhomocysteinemia in vascular disease patients. Arterioscler Thromb 1994; 14:465.

337. Boushey CJ, Beresford SAA, et al: A quantitative assessment of plasma homocysteine as a risk factor for vascular disease: probable benefits of increasing folic acid intakes. JAMA 1995; 274:1049.

338. Butterworth CE Jr, Hatch KD, et al: Improvement in cervical dysplasia associated with folic acid therapy in users of oral contraceptives. Am J Clin Nutr 1982; 35:73.

339. Heimberger DC, Alexander CB, et al: Improvement in bronchial squamous metaplasia in smokers treated with folate and vitamin B₁₂. JAMA 1988; 259:1525.

340. Cravo ML, Mason JB, et al: Folate deficiency enhances the development of colonic neoplasia in dimethylhydrazine-treated rats. Cancer Res 1992; 52:5002.

341. Soder O, Ernstrom U: Recruitment of thymocytes from G1 into S phase by a thymic factor. Int Arch Allergy Appl Immunol 1984; 74:186.

342. Ernstrom U: Identification of a mammalian growth factor as a ribofolate peptide. Biosci Rep 1991; 11:119.

343. Jackman AL, Taylor GA, et al: ICI D1694, a quinazoline antifolate thymidylate synthase inhibitor that is a potent inhibitor of L1210 tumor cell growth in vitro and in vivo: a new agent for clinical study. Cancer Res 1991; 51:5579.

344. Beardsley GP, Moroson BA, et al: A new folate antimetabolite,

5,10-dideaza-5,6,7,8-tetrahydrofolate is a potent inhibitor of *de novo* purine synthesis. J Biol Chem 1989; 264:328.

345. Jolivet J: Methotrexate and 5-fluorouracil: cellular interactions with folates. In Zittoun J, Cooper BA (eds): Folates and Cobalamins. Berlin, Springer-Verlag, 1989, pp 247–254.

346. Marquet J, Chadefaux B, et al: Methylenetetrahydrofolate reductase deficiency: prenatal diagnosis and family studies. Prenat Diagn 1994; 14:29.

347. Haworth JC, Dilling LA, et al: Symptomatic and asymptomatic methylenetetrahydrofolate reductase deficiency in two adult brothers. Am J Med Genet 1993; 45:572.

348. Freeman JM, Finkelstein JD, et al: Homocystinuria presenting as reversible "schizophrenia": a new defect in methionine metabolism with reduced 5,10-methylenetetrahydrofolate reductase activity. Pediatr Res 1972; 6:423.

349. Pasquier F, Lebert F, et al: Methylenetetrahydrofolate reductase deficiency revealed by a neuropathy in a psychotic adult. J Neurol Neurosurg Psychiatry 1994; 57:765. Letter.

350. Erbe RW: Inborn errors of folate metabolism. In Blakley RL, Whitehead VM (eds): Folates and Pterins: Nutritional, Pharmacological and Physiological Aspects. Vol. 3. New York, John Wiley & Sons, 1986, pp 413–466.

351. Kang SS, Zhou J, et al: Intermediate homocysteinemia: a thermolabile variant of methylenetetrahydrofolate reductase. Am J Hum Genet 1988; 43:414.

352. Engbersen AMT, Franken DG, et al: Thermolabile 5,10-methylenetetrahydrofolate reductase as a cause of mild hyperhomocysteinemia. Am J Hum Genet 1995; 56:142.

353. Rosenblatt DS, Cooper BA, et al: Folate distribution in cultured human cells: studies on 5,10-CH$_2$-H$_4$PteGlu reductase deficiency. J Clin Invest 1979; 63:1019.

354. Boss GR, Erbe RW: Decreased rates of methionine synthesis by methylenetetrahydrofolate reductase–deficient fibroblasts and lymphoblasts. J Clin Invest 1981; 67:1659.

355. Mudd SH, Uhlendorf BW, et al: Homocysteinuria associated with decreased methylenetetrahydrofolate reductase activity. Biochem Biophys Res Commun 1972; 46:905.

356. Rosenblatt DS, Erbe RW: Methylenetetrahydrofolate reductase in cultured human cells. II. Studies of methylenetetrahydrofolate reductase deficiency. Pediatr Res 1977; 11:1141.

357. Kanwar YS, Manaligod JR, Wong PWK: Morphologic studies in a patient with homocystinuria due to 5,10-methylenetetrahydrofolate reductase deficiency. Pediatr Res 1976; 10:598.

358. Wong PWK, Justice P, et al: Folic acid nonresponsive homocystinuria due to methylenetetrahydrofolate reductase deficiency. Pediatrics 1977; 59:749.

359. Baumgartner ER, Schweizer K, Wick H: Different congenital forms of defective remethylation in homocystinuria. Clinical, biochemical, and morphological studies. Pediatr Res 1977; 11:1015.

360. Haan EA, Rogers JG, et al: 5,10-Methylenetetrahydrofolate reductase deficiency: clinical and biochemical features of a further case. J Inherit Metab Dis 1985; 8:53.

361. Hyland K, Smith I, et al: The determination of pterins, biogenic amine metabolites, and aromatic amino acids in cerebrospinal fluid using isocratic reverse phase liquid chromatography within series dual cell coulometric electrochemical and fluorescence determinations—use in the study of inborn errors of dihydropteridine reductase and 5,10-methylenetetrahydrofolate reductase. In Wachter H, Curtius H, Pfleiderer W (eds): Biochemical and Clinical Aspects of Pteridines. Vol. 4. Berlin, Walter de Gruyter, 1985, p 85.

362. Baumgartner ER, Stokstad ELR, et al: Comparison of folic acid coenzyme distribution patterns in patients with methylenetetrahydrofolate reductase and methionine synthetase deficiencies. Pediatr Res 1985; 19:1288.

363. Clayton, PT, Smith, et al: Subacute combined degeneration of the cord, dementia, and Parkinsonism due to an inborn error of folate metabolism. J Neurol Neurosurg Psychiatry 1986; 49:920.

364. Beckman DR, Hoganson G, et al: Pathological findings in 5,10-methylenetetrahydrofolate reductase deficiency. Birth Defects 1987; 23:47.

365. Matthews RG, Kaufman S: Characterization of dihydropteridine reductase activity of pig liver methylenetetrahydrofolate reductase. J Biol Chem 1980; 255:6014.

366. Goyette P, Frosst P, et al: Seven novel mutations in the methylenetetrahydrofolate reductase gene and genotype/phenotype correlations in severe methylenetetrahydrofolate reductase deficiency. Am J Hum Genet 1995; 56:1052.

367. Goyette P, Milos R, et al: Human methylenetetrahydrofolate reductase: isolation of cDNA, mapping and mutation identification. Nat Genet 1994; 7:195.

368. Christensen E, Brandt NJ: Prenatal diagnosis of 5,10-methylenetetrahydrofolate reductase deficiency. N Engl J Med 1985; 313:50.

369. Cooper BA: Anomalies congénitales du métabolisme des folates. In Zittoun J, Cooper BA (eds): Folates et Cobalamines. Paris, Doin, 1987, pp 193–208.

370. Brandt NJ, Christensen E, et al: Treatment of methylenetetrahydrofolate reductase deficiency from the neonatal period. The Society for the Study of Inborn Errors of Metabolism. The Netherlands, Amersfoort, 1986, p 23. Abstract.

371. Arakawa T: Congenital defects in folate utilization. Am J Med 1970; 48:594.

372. Rowe PB: Inherited disorders of folate metabolism. In Stanbury JB, Wyngaarden JB, et al (eds): The Metabolic Basis of Inherited Diseases. 5th ed. New York, McGraw-Hill Book Co., 1983, p 498.

373. Shin YS, Reiter S, et al: Orotic aciduria, homocystinuria, formiminoglutamic aciduria and megaloblastosis associated with the formimino-transferase/cyclodeaminase deficiency. In Nyhan WL, Thompson LF, Watts RWE (eds): Purine and Pyrimidine Metabolism in Man. New York, Plenum Publishing Corp., 1986, p 71.

374. Perry TL, Applegarth DA, et al: Metabolic studies of a family with massive formiminoglutamic aciduria. Pediatr Res 1975; 9:117.

375. Russel A, Statter M, Abzug S: Methionine-dependent formiminoglutamic acid transferase deficiency: human and experimental studies in its therapy. Hum Hered 1977; 27:205.

376. Duran M, Ketting D, et al: A case of formiminoglutamic aciduria. Eur J Pediatr 1981; 136:319.

377. Lankowsky P: Congenital malabsorption of folate. Am J Med 1970; 48:580.

378. Steinschneider M, Sherbany A, et al: Congenital folate malabsorption: reversible clinical and neurophysiologic abnormalities. Neurology 1990; 40:1315.

379. Buchanan JA: Fibroblast Plasma Membrane Vesicles to Study Inborn Errors of Transport. Montréal, Québec, Canada, McGill University, 1984. Doctoral thesis.

380. Urbach J, Abrahamov A, Grossowicz N: Congenital isolated folate acid malabsorption. Arch Dis Child 1987; 62:78.

381. Branda RF, Moldow CF, et al: Folate-induced remission in aplastic anemia with familial defect of cellular folate uptake. N Engl J Med 1978; 298:469.

382. Arthur DC, Danzyl TJ, Branda FR: Cytogenetic studies of a family with a hereditary defect of cellular folate uptake and high incidence of hematologic disease. In Butterworth CE, Hutchinson M (eds): Nutritional Factors in the Induction and Maintenance of Malignancy: Symposium. New York, Academic Press, 1983, pp 101–111.

383. Howe RB, Branda RF, et al: Hereditary dyserythropoiesis with abnormal membrane folate transport. Blood 1979; 54:1080.

Disorders of Iron Metabolism and Sideroblastic Anemia

Nancy C. Andrews • Kenneth R. Bridges

Cold Iron

Gold is for the mistress—silver for the maid—
Copper for the craftsman cunning at his trade.
"Good!" said the baron, sitting in his hall;
"But Iron—Cold Iron—is master of them all."
by Rudyard Kipling

Iron lacks the glitter of gold and the sparkle of silver but outshines both in biologic importance. This plebeian metal is vital to the function of a number of critical enzymes, including catalases, aconitases, ribonucleotide reductase, peroxidases, and cytochrome oxidases, that exploit the flexible redox chemistry of iron to execute a variety of chemical reactions essential for our survival. In addition, we depend on hemoglobin, another iron-containing protein, to transport inhaled oxygen from the lungs to peripheral tissues. Human existence is inextricably linked to iron, and disturbances in its metabolism may have dire consequences.

PHYSIOLOGIC CHEMISTRY OF IRON

Iron and Oxidation

The key to the biologic use of iron is its ability to exist in either of two stable oxidation states: Fe^{2+} (ferrous) or Fe^{3+} (ferric). This property permits iron to act as a redox catalyst by reversibly donating or accepting electrons. An excellent example is the electron transport chain of oxidative phosphorylation, in which adenosine triphosphate (ATP) is generated from glucose by the orderly transfer of high-energy electrons through a network of iron-containing mitochondrial cytochromes.

When dissolved in aqueous solution, ferrous iron rapidly oxidizes to its ferric form, which is insoluble at physiologic pH. The resulting ferric hydroxide salts (rust) are of no metabolic utility. To achieve solubility under physiologic conditions, iron must be complexed to iron-binding agents termed *chelators*. Chelators are synthesized by all organisms ranging from microbes (e.g., desferrioxamine produced by *Streptomyces pilosis*) to humans (e.g., transferrin in human plasma). These molecules are crucial to the acquisition of iron from the environment and to its transport and storage within the body.

Iron/Protein Complexes

Iron/protein complexes capitalize on the properties of the metal to perform metabolic functions. Stable coordination complexes form between iron and electron-donating amino acids in proteins. Iron acts as the chemical workhorse, and protein structure dictates biologic specificity.

Individual iron atoms can interact directly with amino acid side groups in proteins, as in ribonucleotide reductase. Alternatively, iron may form coordination complexes with other small molecules. Heme, the iron/protoporphyrin IX complex, is so stable that removal of the iron moiety requires the enzyme heme oxygenase. Protoporphyrin IX donates four of the six electrons needed to form a stable coordination complex with iron. The functional properties of heme are determined by the nature of the associated protein or small molecule ligands supplying the remaining two electrons. The best characterized heme protein is hemoglobin, in which a globin histidine residue donates the fifth electron and the sixth comes from molecular oxygen.[1] This configuration enables hemoglobin to transport oxygen safely throughout the body.

Iron and sulfur atoms can form stable complexes that catalyze enzymatic reactions. The Krebs cycle enzyme aconitase, for example, has an iron/sulfur cluster. Data, detailed in the discussion of iron regulatory protein later in this chapter, indicate that iron/sulfur clusters may "sense" iron concentration.

Iron Toxicity

The ability of iron to catalyze redox reactions also explains its toxicity. As an enzymatic cofactor, the element is involved in the restructuring of cellular components, including proteins, carbohydrates, and nucleic acids. Unbound iron has unbridled redox activity, however, and may wreak havoc. We live in an oxygen-rich atmosphere and require oxygen for many metabolic processes. However, oxygen is extraordinarily reactive and thus toxic. Reactive oxygen intermediates superoxide (O_2^-) and hydrogen peroxide (H_2O_2) are generated by normal cellular reactions. Oxidative stress develops when production of reactive oxygen species exceeds the body's processing capacity. Under these circumstances, reactive oxygen intermediates may be converted to injurious free radicals by the iron-catalyzed Fenton reaction[2]:

$$O_2^- + Fe^{3+} \rightarrow O_2 + Fe^{2+}$$

$$Fe^{2+} + H_2O_2 \rightarrow Fe^{3+} + HO\bullet + OH^-$$

$$O_2^- + H_2O_2 \rightarrow O_2 + HO\bullet + OH^-$$

Hydroxyl radicals (HO•) attack many biologic macromolecules, including proteins and DNA. They also promote peroxidation of membrane lipids, a problem exacerbated by iron overload and pathologic membrane binding of iron. Intracellular structures are particularly susceptible to iron-dependent peroxidation. In iron-overloaded cells, injured lysosomes become fragile and leaky.[3] Release of lysosomal proteases causes further cell injury and may ultimately lead to cell death. This process contributes to the severe tissue damage seen in liver, heart, joints, and pancreas of patients with hereditary hemochromatosis (see later).

Iron is not normally present in the membrane. However, both sickle cell disease and thalassemia promote adherence of iron, heme, ferritin, and denatured hemoglobin to the inner surface of the red cell plasma membrane.[4] The membrane complex involving denatured hemoglobin has been termed *hemichrome*.[5, 6] The red cell anion transport protein band 3 appears to nucleate the formation of these iron aggregates.[7–10] Injured cells decorated with membrane iron deposits are removed by a functioning spleen in patients with thalassemia and hemoglobin SC disease, but they circulate pathologically in patients with homozygous hemoglobin SS disease.[11] Membrane-associated iron promotes free radical formation and further membrane damage, manifested by generation of the lipid peroxidation product malonyldialdehyde and by cross-linking of membrane proteins.[4, 12] Membranes become rigid, contributing to the formation of irreversibly sickled cells, which occlude the microcirculation. Removal of these iron deposits is clearly advantageous. One report suggests that the oral iron chelator deferiprone (L1) extracts hemichrome iron, dampening lipid damage.[13]

Sometimes, reactive oxygen intermediates can be beneficial. Neutrophils contain a membrane-associated NADPH oxidase that produces superoxide to kill ingested microorganisms.[14] Superoxide and secondary reactive oxygen intermediates are potent antimicrobial agents. Congenital defects in this NADPH oxidase, collectively termed *chronic granulomatous disease* (see Chapter 22), are characterized by a serious defect in defense against bacterial pathogens.

Neutrophils and iron also injure tissues in inflammatory diseases such as rheumatoid arthritis.[15] Synovial macrophages ingest red cell hemoglobin introduced by intermittent joint hemorrhage.[16] Iron is deposited in the synovial membrane, proximate to superoxide and hydrogen peroxide generated by neutrophils and macrophages participating in the inflammatory reaction.[17] Iron catalyzes the conversion of these compounds into free radical species, which promote lipid peroxidation.[18] Iron therapy exacerbates this process. In contrast, antioxidants and iron chelators retard free radical generation, thereby affording some protection against injury in rheumatoid arthritis.[19, 20]

These deleterious properties of iron are threatening only when the element is in a "free" state or in an abnormal compartment within the cell. Protection of cell structures from iron-dependent free radical damage is crucial to survival. When bound to protein either directly or in the form of heme, iron-induced generation of free radicals is largely abrogated. Thus, tight chelation of iron is a means of controlling its reactivity. As discussed later, cytoplasmic ferritin allows iron to be stored safely within cells by sequestering it in an innocuous form. Ferritin expression is induced by oxidative stress.[22] Both prokaryotic and eukaryotic cells contain ferritin, and no mutant lacking ferritin has been discovered.[23] A cell totally lacking ferritin would likely die; the redundancy of ferritin-encoding genes may help prevent genetic loss of ferritin altogether.

ACQUISITION AND DISTRIBUTION OF IRON

Although the average adult has 4 to 5 g of iron, a meticulous balance exists between dietary uptake and loss. About 1 mg of iron is lost each day through sloughing of cells from skin and mucosal surfaces (Fig. 11–1).[24] Menstruating females average 2 mg of iron loss daily, increasing their dietary iron requirement.[25] No organ performs the physiologic role of iron excretion. Consequently, absorption is the sole means of regulating body iron stores.[26] During neonatal and childhood growth spurts, iron requirements increase in response to augmentation of body mass.[27]

Iron Absorption

Iron absorption occurs predominantly in the duodenum and upper jejunum (see Fig. 11–1).[28, 29] As discussed later, the mechanism of iron transport remains unknown despite intensive investigation. The physical state of iron entering the duodenum greatly influences its absorption, however. At physiologic pH, ferrous iron is rapidly converted to the insoluble ferric form. Acid production by the stomach serves to lower the pH in the duodenum, enhancing the solubility and uptake of ferric iron. Heme is absorbed more efficiently than inorganic iron, independently of duodenal pH (Table 11–1). Consequently, meats are excellent nutritive sources of iron. A heme oxygenase inhibitor has been shown to block heme catabolism in the intestine, resulting in an iron-deficient state.[30]

A number of dietary factors influence iron absorption. Ascorbate and citrate increase iron uptake in part by acting as weak chelators to help to solubilize the metal in the duodenum (see Table 11–1).[31] Iron is readily transferred from these compounds into the mucosal lining cells. Conversely, iron absorption is inhibited by plant phytates and tannins. These compounds also chelate iron but prevent its uptake by the absorption machinery (see later).

The mechanism of iron entry into mucosal cells lining the upper gastrointestinal tract is unknown. As detailed later, most cells are believed to acquire iron from the plasma transferrin chelate (an iron-protein chelate), by means of specific transferrin receptors and receptor-mediated endocytosis. The postulate that apotransferrin (or an equivalent molecule) secreted by intestinal cells or present in bile chelates intestinal iron[32] is unsubstantiated. The transferrin gene is not expressed in intestinal cells. Later work indicated that transferrin found in the intestinal lumen is derived from plasma.[33] Plasma transferrin entering bile is fully saturated with iron, obviating any intraluminal chelating function.[34] Furthermore, hypoxia, which greatly increases iron absorption, has no effect on intestinal transferrin levels.[35] Exogenous transferrin cannot donate iron to intestinal mucosal cells,[36] and the brush border membrane lacks transferrin receptors[37] (although they are present on the basolateral surface of intestinal epithelial cells).[38, 39] Last and perhaps most compelling, humans and mice with hypotransferrinemia paradoxically absorb more dietary iron than normal. Although the erythron is iron deficient, these individuals develop hepatic iron overload.[40, 41]

In searching for molecules involved in intestinal iron transport, Conrad and co-workers have taken the approach of characterizing proteins that bind iron.[31] They have developed a hypothesis for iron transport based on identification of iron-binding proteins at several key sites. They propose that mucins bind iron in the acid milieu of the stomach, thereby solubilizing it for uptake in the alkaline duodenum. According to their model, mucin-bound iron is then transported across the muco-

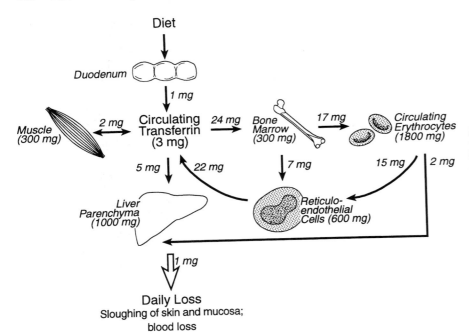

Figure 11-1. The body's iron economy. Although the average adult has 3 to 5 g of body iron, only 1 mg of dietary iron enters and leaves the iron economy on an average day. Most iron is found in the erythron and liver. Recycling through the reticuloendothelial system and circulating transferrin provide ample iron for essential functions.

sal cell membrane by associated integrins. Once inside the cell, a cytoplasmic iron-binding protein, dubbed *mobilferrin,* accepts the element and shuttles it to the basolateral surface of the cell, where it is delivered to plasma. In this model, mobilferrin could serve as a rheostat sensitive to plasma iron concentrations, with fully occupied mobilferrin down-regulating mucosal iron uptake and unsaturated mobilferrin promoting further iron uptake.[30] This model has not gained universal acceptance, however. A very different scheme has been proposed by investigators studying iron transport in yeast (Fig. 11–2). Dancis and associates[42, 43] used genetic selection to isolate *Sacchromyces cerevisiae* mutants defective in iron transport. They constructed an expression plasmid in which an enzyme necessary for histidine biosynthesis was under the control of an iron-repressible promoter. The plasmid was introduced into a yeast histidine auxotroph (i.e., a strain of yeast that requires histidine to survive). Mutants were selected in the absence of histidine, in the presence of high levels of iron. Dancis and associates discovered that membrane iron transport depends absolutely on copper transport, as shown in Figure 11–2.[44] In this model, ferric iron in yeast culture medium is reduced to its ferrous form by an externally oriented reductase (FRE1). The element is shuttled rapidly into the cell by

a ferrous transporter, which appears to be coupled to an externally oriented copper-dependent oxidase (FET3) embedded in the cell membrane.[43, 45] FET3 is strikingly homologous to the mammalian copper oxidase ceruloplasmin. The reoxidation of ferrous to ferric iron is apparently an obligatory step in the transport mechanism, although the coupling mechanism of oxidation and membrane transport is unclear.[43, 45, 46] Although the genetic evidence for this scheme is compel-

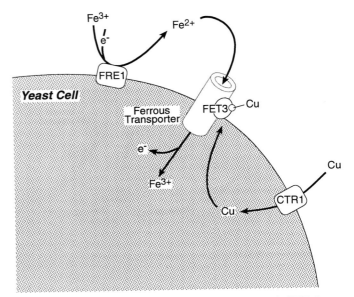

Figure 11-2. Mechanism of iron uptake in yeast. FRE1 is an externally oriented reductase embedded in the cell membrane that reduces ferric iron (Fe^{3+}) to ferrous iron (Fe^{2+}). Membrane transport involves a complex consisting of an iron permease, FTR1, and an externally oriented oxidase, FET3. FET3 requires copper, which enters the cell by means of a transmembrane copper transport protein, CTR1.

Table 11-1. FACTORS THAT MODIFY IRON ABSORPTION

Physical state (bioavailability)
   Heme >Fe^{2+} >Fe^{3+}
Inhibitors
   Phytates, tannins, soil clay, laundry starch, iron overload
Competitors
   Cobalt, lead, strontium
Facilitators
   Ascorbate, citrate, amino acids, iron deficiency

ling, the central component, the ferrous transporter itself, remains elusive. These investigators speculate that mammalian intestinal iron transport is analogous to the yeast iron uptake process.[47] This assertion is supported by studies of copper-deficient swine, which show coexisting iron deficiency unresponsive to iron therapy.[48–50]

Mouse genetics provides a different perspective on mammalian intestinal iron transport. Mouse breeders readily recognize pale animals and have developed anemic stocks with various mutations. Two mutant strains have defective intestinal mucosal iron transport. Microcytic (*mk*) mice and sex-linked anemia (*sla*) mice have severe iron deficiency due apparently to defects in iron uptake and release, respectively, from the intestinal cell.[51] Mice with the homozygous autosomal recessive *mk* mutation absorb iron poorly, have low serum iron levels, and lack stainable iron in intestinal mucosal cells. These findings are consistent with a defect in an apical iron transport molecule. Intriguingly, *mk/mk* mice are not rescued by parenteral iron treatment. Anemia develops in normal mice transplanted with *mk* bone marrow, indicating that they also have a defect in red cell iron uptake. A common component that regulates iron transport may therefore exist in intestinal cells and red cells. Mice that are homozygous or hemizygous for the *sla* mutation (*sla/sla* or *sla/y*) also have low serum iron levels. In contrast to *mk* mice, they display abnormal iron deposits within intestinal mucosal cells, suggesting that this X-linked defect impairs intracellular iron trafficking or basolateral export of iron to the plasma. The *sla* animals differ further from the *mk* mice because parenteral iron cures their anemia. Based on studies of these mutants, distinct apical and basolateral iron transport systems exist that function coordinately to transfer iron from intestinal lumen to plasma.

Whatever the mechanism of iron uptake, normally only about 10% of the elemental iron entering the duodenum is absorbed. However, this value increases markedly with iron deficiency.[52] In contrast, iron overload reduces but does not eliminate absorption, reaffirming the fact that absorption is regulated by body iron stores. In addition, both anemia and hypoxia increase iron absorption. A portion of the iron that enters the mucosal cells is retained in the form of ferritin. Intracellular intestinal iron is lost when epithelial cells are sloughed from the lining of the gastrointestinal tract. The remaining iron traverses the mucosal cells, to be coupled to transferrin for transport through the circulation.

Approximately 80% of total body iron is ultimately incorporated into hemoglobin in red blood cells. An average adult produces 2×10^{11} red cells daily, for a red cell renewal rate of 0.8% per day. Each red cell contains more than a billion atoms of iron, and each milliliter of red cells contains 1 mg of iron. To meet this daily need for 2×10^{20} atoms (or 20 mg) of elemental iron, the body has developed regulatory mechanisms whereby erythropoiesis profoundly influences iron absorption. Plasma iron turnover (PIT) represents the mass turnover of transferrin-bound iron in the circulation (expressed as milligrams per kilogram per day).[53] Accelerated erythropoiesis increases PIT, which is associated with enhanced iron uptake from the gastrointestinal tract.[54] The pathophysiologic mechanism is unknown. A circulating factor that modulates iron absorption has been hypothesized but not identified.[52, 55] Several candidate factors have been excluded, including transferrin[56] and erythropoietin.[57] Clinical manifestations of this apparent communication between the marrow and the intestine include iron overload that develops in patients with severe thalassemia without transfusion. The accelerated (but ineffective) erythropoiesis in this condition substantially boosts iron absorption. In some cases, the coupling of increased PIT and increased gastrointestinal iron absorption is beneficial. In pregnancy, PIT is accelerated by placental removal of iron. This process enhances gastrointestinal iron absorption, thereby increasing the availability of the element to meet the needs of the growing and developing fetus.

Competition studies suggest that several other heavy metals share the iron intestinal absorption pathway. These include lead, manganese, cobalt, and zinc (see Table 11–1). Increased iron absorption induced by iron deficiency also enhances the uptake of these elements. Because iron deficiency often coexists with lead intoxication, this interaction is significant and can produce particularly serious medical complications in children.[58] Interestingly, copper absorption and metabolism appear to be handled by different mechanisms, as discussed later.

Intercellular Iron Transport

As illustrated in Figure 11–1, only a small proportion of total body iron daily enters or leaves the body's stores. Consequently, intercellular iron transport is quantitatively more important than intestinal absorption. The greatest mass of iron is found in erythroid cells, making up about 80% of the total body endowment. The reticuloendothelial system recycles a substantial amount of iron from effete red cells, approximating the amount used by the erythron for new hemoglobin production.

Approximately 0.1% (3 mg) of total body iron circulates in the plasma as an exchangeable pool. In normal individuals, essentially all circulating plasma iron is bound to transferrin. This chelation serves three purposes: (1) it renders iron soluble under physiologic conditions, (2) it prevents iron-mediated free radical toxicity, and (3) it facilitates transport into cells. Transferrin is the most important physiologic supplier of iron to red cells.[59] Plasma transferrin is synthesized in the liver; it is believed to deliver iron to most tissues of the body. Transferrins are produced locally in the testes and central nervous system (CNS) because these sites are relatively inaccessible to proteins in the general circulation. Plasma transferrin is an 80-kd glycoprotein that has homologous N-terminal and C-terminal iron-binding domains.[60] The molecule is related to several other proteins, including ovotransferrin in bird and reptile eggs,[61] lactoferrin in extracellular secretions and neutrophil granules,[62, 63] and melanotransferrin (p97), a protein produced by melanoma cells.[64] The functions for these related proteins are unknown. One report indicates that lactoferrin can act as a site-specific DNA binding protein that may mediate transcriptional activation, a function at odds with its existence as an extracellular protein.[65]

X-ray crystal structures have been determined for human lactoferrin and rabbit transferrin.[66] All members of the transferrin protein superfamily have similar polypeptide folding. N-terminal and C-terminal domains are globular moieties of about 330 amino acids; each of these is divided into two subdomains, with the iron- and anion-binding sites in the intersubdomain cleft. The binding cleft opens with iron release and closes with iron binding. N-terminal and C-terminal binding sites are very similar.

The precise mechanism by which iron is loaded onto transferrin as it leaves intestinal epithelial cells or reticuloendothelial cells is unknown. The copper-dependent ferroxidase ceruloplasmin may play a role; compelling evidence indicates that the protein is involved in mobilizing tissue iron stores to produce diferric transferrin.[67–70] Transferrin binds iron avidly with a dissociation constant of approximately 10^{22} M^{-1}.[71] Ferric iron binds only in the company of an anion (usually carbonate) that serves as a bridging ligand between metal and protein, excluding water from two coordination sites.[71–73] Without the anion cofactor, iron binding is negligible; with it, ferric transferrin is resistant to all but the most potent chelators. The remaining four coordination sites are provided by the transferrin protein—a histidine nitrogen, an aspartic acid carboxylate oxygen, and two tyrosine phenolate oxygens.[74, 75] Available evidence suggests that anion binding takes place before iron binding. Iron release from transferrin involves protonation of the carbonate anion, loosening the metal-protein bond.

The sum of all iron-binding sites on transferrin constitutes the total iron-binding capacity of plasma. Under normal circumstances, about one third of transferrin iron-binding pockets are filled. Consequently, with the exception of iron overload where all the transferrin binding sites are occupied, non–transferrin-bound iron in the circulation is virtually nonexistent. Distribution of plasma and tissue iron can be traced using ^{59}Fe as a radioactive tag by reinfusing a subject with autologous transferrin loaded with radiolabeled iron. Blood samples can be analyzed at timed intervals to determine the rate of loss of the radioactive label. Such ferrokinetic studies indicate that the normal half-life of iron in the circulation is about 75 minutes.[53] The absolute amount of iron released from transferrin per unit time is the PIT (see earlier).

Such radioactive tracer studies indicate that at least 80% of the iron bound to circulating transferrin is delivered to the bone marrow and incorporated into newly formed erythrocytes (see Fig. 11–1).[76, 77] Other major sites of iron delivery include the liver, which is a primary depot for stored iron, and the spleen. Hepatic iron is found in both reticuloendothelial cells (two thirds) and hepatocytes (one third). Reticuloendothelial cells acquire iron primarily by phagocytosis and breakdown of aging red cells, extracting it from heme and returning it to the circulation bound to transferrin. Hepatocytes take up iron by at least two different pathways (see later).

Given the preeminent role of the bone marrow in the clearance of labeled iron from the circulation, ferrokinetics provide a window on erythropoietic activity. Conditions that augment erythrocyte production increase the PIT. For example, hemolytic anemias such as hereditary spherocytosis and sickle cell disease induce rapid delivery of transferrin-bound iron to the marrow. In contrast, disorders that reduce red cell production prolong the PIT. Such a picture is seen, for example, in Diamond-Blackfan anemia.

When erythrocytes are produced and released into the circulation in a normal fashion, the process of erythropoiesis is termed *effective*. In patients with certain hemolytic anemias, however, the abnormal nascent red cells are destroyed before leaving the marrow cavity. In this circumstance, the erythropoiesis is *ineffective*, meaning simply that the erythropoietic precursors have failed to accomplish their primary task: the delivery of intact erythrocytes to the circulation. The ferrokinetic profile in this case illustrates rapid removal of iron from transferrin with a delayed entry of label into the

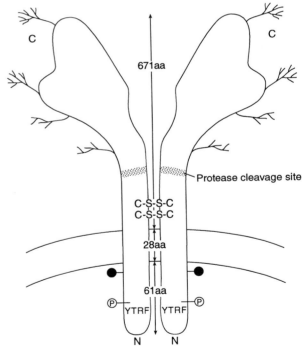

Figure 11-3. Structure of the dimeric transferrin receptor (see text for details). The N-termini of both subunits are inside the cell, and the C-termini are outside. The 61–amino acid intracellular domain has three structural features that appear to play a role in endocytosis: the YTRF amino acid motif, a phosphorylated serine residue (*encircled "P"*), and a covalently linked molecule of palmitic acid (*solid circle*). The transmembrane domain is 28 amino acids long. The extracellular domain has 671 amino acids, including disulfide linkages (C–S–S–C) as well as four glycosylation sites (*branched lines*). A potential protease cleavage site is located between amino acids 100 and 101.

pool of circulating red cell hemoglobin. β⁺-thalassemia is an important example of this pattern. In β⁺-thalassemia, ineffective erythropoiesis is coupled with a markedly enhanced PIT.

Intracellular Iron Metabolism

Although transferrin was characterized 50 years ago,[78] its receptor eluded investigators until the early 1980s. Monoclonal antibodies prepared against tumor cells targeted the transferrin receptor glycoprotein.[79] A broad body of literature now supports the concept that the iron/transferrin complex is internalized by receptor-mediated endocytosis. The general structure of the transferrin receptor is shown in Figure 11–3. This disulfide-linked homodimer has subunits containing 760 amino acids each (see Fig. 11–3).[80–82] Oligosaccharides account for about 5% of the 90-kd subunit molecular mass.[83] Four glycosylation sites (three N-linked and one O-linked) line the protein.[84] Glycosylation-defective mutants have fewer disulfide bridges, less transferrin binding, and less cell surface expression.[85, 86] The transmembrane domain, between amino acids 62 and 89, functions as an internal signal peptide, because there is none at the N-terminal end.[87] A molecule of fatty acid (usually palmitate) is also covalently linked to each subunit at the internal edge of the transmembrane domain and may play a role in membrane localization. Interestingly, nonacylated mutants mediate faster iron uptake.[88, 89] The transferrin binding regions of the protein are unidentified.[85, 86] Efforts to crystallize transferrin receptor protein are underway (Harrison S: Personal communication, 1996).

Iron is taken into cells by receptor-mediated endocytosis of monoferric and diferric transferrin (Fig. 11–4).[90–92] Receptors on the outer face of the plasma membrane bind iron-loaded transferrin with a very high affinity. The C-terminal domain of transferrin appears to mediate receptor binding.[93] Diferric transferrin binds with higher affinity than monoferric transferrin or apotransferrin.[94, 95] The dissociation constant (K_d) for bound diferric transferrin ranges from 10^{-7} M to 10^{-9} M at physiologic pH, depending on the species and tissue.[96, 97] The K_d of monoferric transferrin is approximately 10^{-6} M. The concentration of circulating transferrin is about 25 μM. Therefore, cellular transferrin receptors are ordinarily fully saturated.

After binding to its receptor on the cell surface, transferrin is rapidly internalized by invagination of clathrin-coated pits and formation of endocytic vesicles. This process requires the short, 61-amino-acid intracellular tail of the transferrin receptor molecule.[98–101] Receptors with truncated N-terminal cytoplasmic domains do not recycle properly.[98] This portion of the molecule contains a conserved tyrosine-threonine-arginine-phenylalanine (YTRF) sequence that functions as a signal for endocytosis. Genetically engineered addition of a second YTRF sequence enhances receptor endocytosis.[102] A number of stimuli reversibly phosphorylate the serine residue adjacent to the YTRF sequence at position 24 by the action of protein kinase C.[103] The role of receptor phosphorylation is unclear. Despite removal of the phosphorylation site by site-directed mutagenesis, the transferrin receptor recycles normally.[98]

An ATP-dependent proton pump lowers the pH of the endosome to about 5.5.[104–106] The acidification of the endosome weakens the association between iron and transferrin.[107] Even at pH 5.5, Fe^{3+} would not normally dissociate from transferrin in the several minutes between its endocytosis and the return of transferrin apoprotein to the cell surface.[108] A plasma membrane oxi-

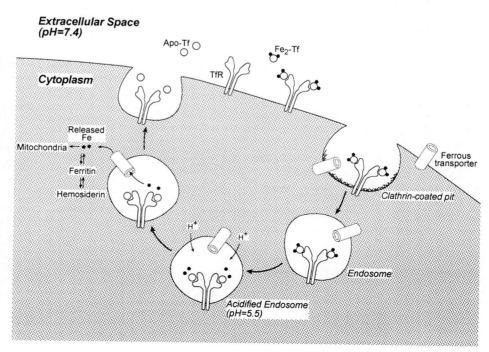

Figure 11–4. The endocytotic transferrin cycle. Apotransferrin (Apo-Tf) binds two atoms of iron per molecule to form diferric transferrin (Fe₂-Tf). Diferric transferrin binds to the transferrin receptor (TfR) on the cell surface. The complex is internalized by invagination of clathrin-coated pits to form specific endosomes. The endosomes import protons, thus lowering the pH within the organelle and transferrin's affinity for iron. Liberated iron is translocated through the endosome membrane to the cytoplasm by an unidentified transporter (dashed cylinder). Released iron is shuttled to mitochondria for heme synthesis and to ferritin for storage. The apotransferrin-transferrin receptor complex recycles to the cell surface, where the neutral pH promotes release of apotransferrin into the serum for reuse. Details are given in the text.

Extracellular Space (pH=7.4)

Apo-Tf

Fe₂-Tf

TfR

Cytoplasm

Released Fe

Mitochondria

Ferritin

Hemosiderin

Ferrous transporter

Clathrin-coated pit

H⁺

H⁺

Endosome

Acidified Endosome (pH=5.5)

doreductase reduces transferrin-bound iron from the Fe^{3+} state to Fe^{2+}, directly or indirectly facilitating the removal of iron from the protein.[109-111] Conformational changes in the transferrin receptor also play a role in iron release.[112, 113]

Rather than entering lysosomes for degradation, as do ligands in other receptor-mediated endocytosis pathways, intact receptor-bound apotransferrin recycles to the cell surface, where neutral pH promotes detachment into the circulation.[114] Thus the preservation and reuse of transferrin are accomplished by pH-dependent changes in the affinity of transferrin for its receptor.[91, 104, 105] Exported apotransferrin binds additional iron and undergoes further rounds of iron delivery to cells. The average transferrin molecule, with a half-life of 8 days, may be used up to 100 times for iron delivery.[47]

Topologically, the cell exterior and the endosome interior are equivalent compartments. The primary role of the transferrin-transferrin receptor interaction is to bring iron into the vicinity of the cell surface, thereby increasing the likelihood of iron uptake. After its release from transferrin within the endosome, iron must traverse the plasma membrane to enter the cytosol proper. The molecules effecting this transport have not been identified, but the process may be carrier mediated.[115] Two anemic, mutant animals, the Belgrade rat (b/b) and the hemoglobin deficit mouse (hbd/hbd) appear to have lesions at or near this step. Their cells take up ferrotransferrin into endosomes but fail to release iron into the cytoplasm.[116, 117] The molecular basis of the defects in these animals has not been elucidated.

The endosomal transporter may reside on the plasma membrane of the cell before endocytosis.[118] If so, it should be oriented to transport iron directly into the cell, without the assistance of transferrin (as diagrammed in Fig. 11–4). Such non–transferrin-bound iron uptake activities have been characterized in tissue culture cells (see later). This uptake system could function constitutively but inefficiently. Coupling the transferrin cycle to transport across the plasma membrane might augment iron uptake by creating an iron-rich environment for the transporter within the endosome. This same elusive transport molecule could also be involved in intestinal iron uptake. The phenotype of the mk/mk mouse (see earlier) suggests that red cell iron uptake and intestinal iron uptake share a common component that could be the "endosomal" transporter.

Once inside the cell cytoplasm, iron appears to be bound by a low-molecular-weight carrier molecule, which may assist in delivery to various intracellular locations including mitochondria (for heme biosynthesis) and ferritin (for storage). The identity of the intracellular iron carrier molecule or molecules remains unknown. The amount of iron in transit within the cell at any given time is minuscule and defies precise measurement. This minute pool of transit iron, which is believed to be in the Fe^{2+} oxidation state, is the biologically active form of the element. Metabolically inactive iron, stored in ferritin and hemosiderin, is in equilibrium with exchangeable iron bound to the low-molecular-weight carrier molecule (see Fig. 11–4).

Both prokaryotes and eukaryotes produce ferritin molecules for iron storage. Ferritins are complex 24-subunit heteropolymers of H (for heavy or heart) and L (for light or liver) protein subunits. L subunits are 19.7 kd in mass, with isoelectric points of 4.5 to 5.0; H subunits are 21 kd with isoelectric points of 5.0 to 5.7. The subunits of the ferritin molecule form a sphere with a central cavity in which up to 4500 atoms of crystalline iron is stored in the form of poly-iron-phosphate oxide.[27] Eight channels through the sphere are lined by hydrophilic amino acid residues (along the threefold axes of symmetry), and six more are lined by hydrophobic residues (along the fourfold axes).[119] Strong interspecies amino acid conservation exists in the residues that line the hydrophilic channels, whereas marked variation exists in those along the hydrophobic passages. Hydrophilic channels terminate with aspartic acid and glutamic acid residues and are lined by serine, histidine, and cysteine residues (all of which potentially bind metal ligands). The evolutionary conservation of the hydrophilic channels suggests that they provide the route for iron entry and exit from the ferritin shell, but this contention remains unproven. Little is known about how iron is released from ferritin for use.

Although the two ferritin chains are highly homologous, only H ferritin has ferroxidase activity. A mechanism involving dioxygen converts ferrous to ferric iron, promoting incorporation into ferritin.[120, 121] The composition of ferritin shells varies from H-subunit homopolymers to L-subunit homopolymers and includes all possible combinations between the two. Isoelectric focusing of ferritin from a particular tissue reveals multiple bands representing shells with different subunit compositions. These isoferritins, as they are called, show tissue-specific variation. Ferritin from liver, for instance, is rich in L subunits, as is that from the spleen. In contrast, the heart has ferritin rich in H subunits. Increased H-subunit content correlates with increased iron utilization, whereas increased L-subunit content correlates with increased iron storage.[27, 122] The H:L ratio rises with activation of heme synthesis or cell proliferation.[123, 124] Ferritin thus provides a flexible reserve of iron.

Ferritin molecules aggregate over time to form clusters, which are engulfed by lysosomes and degraded (see Fig. 11–4).[125, 126] The end product of this process, hemosiderin, is an amorphous agglomerate of denatured protein and lipid interspersed with iron oxide molecules.[127] In cells overloaded with iron, lysosomes accumulate large amounts of hemosiderin, which can be visualized by Prussian blue staining. Although the iron enmeshed in this insoluble compound constitutes an end-stage product of cellular iron storage, it remains in equilibrium with soluble ferritin. Ferritin iron, in turn, is in equilibrium with iron complexed to low-molecular-weight carrier molecules. Therefore, the introduction into the cell of an effective chelator captures iron from the low-molecular-weight "toxic iron" pool, draws iron out of ferritin, and eventually depletes iron from hemosiderin as well, though only very slowly. As might be expected, the bioavailability of hemosiderin iron is much lower than that of iron stored in ferritin.

Non–Transferrin-Bound Iron Uptake

Although compelling evidence exists that the transferrin cycle is important for iron acquisition by the erythron,[59] other tissues can import iron by alternative mechanisms. Some patients and mutant mice have little or no circulating transferrin.[128–131] Despite severe hypochromic, microcytic anemia, nonerythroid tissues are grossly normal. Whereas the red cells suffer from iron deficiency, excess iron is deposited in the liver. The iron-deprived bone marrow likely signals the gut to increase absorption, exacerbating tissue iron excess. Ponka and Schulman[59] speculate that nonerythroid cells depend less on transferrin because their modest iron needs can be met by turnover of endogenous ferritin and heme iron. Red cells are more vulnerable because of greater iron use to form hemoglobin. The transferrin cycle could serve primarily to enhance iron uptake by tissues with a great demand for the element.

Iron overload produces fully saturated transferrin and non–transferrin-bound iron circulating in a chelatable, low-molecular-weight form.[132–135] This iron is weakly complexed to albumin, citrate, amino acids, and sugars and behaves differently from iron associated with transferrin. Nonhematopoietic tissues, particularly the liver, endocrine organs, kidneys, and heart, preferentially take up this iron.

Radiolabeled iron administered to mice with and without available transferrin binding capacity has quite different patterns of distribution.[41] In normal animals, hematopoietic tissues are the prime sites of uptake. When free transferrin sites are absent, however, most iron is deposited in the liver and pancreas, indicating that these organs serve as iron reservoirs in the situation of iron overload. Notably, this pattern of distribution is similar to that seen in idiopathic hemochromatosis. These data support the idea that, while the transferrin pathway is important for meeting the needs of the erythron, it is not essential for iron uptake by all tissues.

Kaplan and coworkers have studied incorporation of iron from FeNH₄ citrate.[136, 137] Intriguingly, they find that transferrin-independent uptake increases in direct proportion to the concentration of this compound, similar to hepatic uptake of non–transferrin-bound iron in patients with saturated transferrin. They speculate that this is a protective alternative pathway that removes the toxic metal from the circulation. Other investigators have described similar uptake in HepG2 cells and have shown that it is reversible by addition of chelating compounds.[138]

A nontransferrin iron uptake mechanism with different properties has been described in K562 erythroleukemia cells.[139] In the absence of ferric transferrin, iron uptake into K562 cells is sensitive to treatment with trypsin, suggesting that it requires a protein carrier. Higher ambient iron concentrations do not increase cellular iron uptake. As discussed earlier, this transport may be accomplished by the same machinery responsible for passage of iron out of transferrin cycle endosomes into the cytoplasm.[118] These two processes accomplish essentially the same task. The putative endosomal iron transporter must be oriented to transport iron from an endocytosed extracellular compartment into the cytoplasm. This transporter may exist on the cell surface before receptor-mediated endocytosis, with the capacity to transport iron to a modest extent. This activity is not restricted to erythroid cells. Phytohemagglutinin-stimulated human peripheral lymphocytes have a similar transferrin-independent iron uptake mechanism.[140]

ROLE OF IRON IN CELL PROLIFERATION AND DIFFERENTIATION

Iron is indispensable for DNA synthesis and a host of metabolic processes.[141] Iron starvation arrests proliferation, presumably because the metal is required by ribonucleotide reductase and other enzymes.[142] Although transferrin receptors are expressed on all dividing cells in numbers that roughly reflect growth rate,[143] the erythron is the organ that relies most heavily on iron delivery by transferrin, as exemplified by atransferrinemic animals (see earlier).[40, 129, 130] But the transferrin cycle also appears to play a significant, if expendable, role in other cell types.

Studies of T lymphocytes exemplify the general relationship between transferrin receptor expression and cell proliferation. Transferrin receptors, absent from resting T cells, have long been recognized as a marker of T-cell activation. The initiation of cell division by a mitogen such as phytohemagglutinin dramatically increases both transferrin receptor surface expression and iron uptake.[144] Along the same lines, tumor cells up-regulate transferrin receptor expression to optimize iron acquisition for proliferation.

Blockade of transferrin receptor function can halt cell division. For instance, certain monoclonal antibodies against the transferrin receptor curb proliferation of tumor cells *in vitro* and *in vivo*.[145, 146] Some of these antibodies actually prevent binding of transferrin to its receptor, whereas others suppress receptor recycling but do not abrogate ligand binding.[147] Interestingly, some reports have suggested that the transferrin receptor may have an additional role in activated T cells, apart from its iron uptake function. Anti–transferrin receptor monoclonal antibodies have been described that can trigger T-cell activation and interleukin-2 secretion.[148–150] These antibodies presumably activate a signal transduction pathway beginning with the transferrin receptor but independent of iron trafficking.

The central role of iron in cell proliferation is further demonstrated by chelators that can cross the plasma membrane, bind the metal inside the cell, and limit its bioavailability. Agents such as desferrioxamine and desferrithiocin inhibit the growth of a variety of tumor cells in culture[151] and greatly reduce T-cell proliferation.[152–155] The likely inhibitory mechanism is iron deprivation, with reduced ribonucleotide reductase activity and lower levels of deoxyribonucleotides. This, in turn, leads to mitotic arrest in S phase.[156] The addition of iron to the medium reverses the growth inhibition. Chelators may also induce apoptosis or programmed cell death.[157]

Erythroid precursors need an extraordinary amount of iron to support hemoglobin synthesis and differentiation into mature red cells. The density of transferrin receptors on the cell surface changes during erythroid maturation. Transferrin receptors first appear in measurable numbers on the colony-forming unit-erythroid (CFU-E), increasing to 300,000 per cell on proerythroblasts and as many as 800,000 per cell on basophilic erythroblasts at the time of maximal iron uptake. Numbers then fall to 100,000 per cell on circulating reticulocytes and negligible levels on mature red cells.[158] A strict correlation exists between iron requirement and transferrin receptor number, indicating that the abundance of transferrin receptors on the cell surface is a major determinant of erythroid iron uptake. Because maturing red cells shed their transferrin receptors, the amount of soluble transferrin receptor in plasma reasonably reflects erythropoiesis. In culture, a monoclonal antibody to the transferrin receptor that permits ligand binding but subsequently slows receptor recycling partially blocks erythroid burst cell iron uptake. The level of iron uptake is sufficient for cell division but not hemoglobin synthesis.[159]

Beug and co-workers demonstrated that an anti–transferrin receptor monoclonal antibody to chick erythroid cells blocked erythroid differentiation at the erythroblast or early reticulocyte stage and promoted premature, pyknotic cell death.[160] The antibody apparently prevented normal cycling of transferrin receptors and inhibited efficient iron uptake. Its effects were specific for differentiation because it did not inhibit proliferation of a variety of other cell lines. Ferric salicylaldehyde-isonicotinyl-hydrazone (Fe-SIH) was added to antibody-treated cells to determine whether direct delivery of iron by this compound could rescue the normal erythroid program. Interestingly, the Fe-SIH only partially restored maturation of antibody-treated avian cells. The investigators postulated that insufficient levels of heme or hemoglobin might shut off production of proteins required for differentiation. These data are in accord with those of Ponka and Schulman,[59] who have shown that the rate of heme synthesis is influenced by the efficiency of an unknown step in iron uptake. They have localized the critical step distal to the interaction of ferric transferrin with the transferrin receptor but proximal to insertion of iron into heme by ferrochelatase.

A wealth of literature demonstrates that oxidized heme (hemin) promotes differentiation of erythroleukemia cell lines in tissue culture.[161–164] Conversely, deficient heme biosynthesis abrogates chemical induction of differentiation in an erythroleukemia cell line subclone.[162]

A hemin-inducible transcriptional regulatory element exists in the enhancer-like locus control region (LCR) upstream of the human β-globin genes.[166] Although far from the structural genes, the LCR is critical for high-level globin expression. It activates transcription, at least in part, through binding of a factor termed NF-E2 to this hemin-inducible DNA sequence element. NF-E2 DNA-binding activity has been purified from murine and human erythroleukemia cell lines.[167–169] NF-E2 activity correlates with the expression of a heterodimeric complex of a tissue-specific 45-kd polypeptide (p45 NF-E2) and a widely expressed 18-kd polypeptide (p18) that heterodimerize to form a basic-leucine zipper transcriptional regulatory protein. NF-E2 recognition elements are also found in the promoters for red cell–specific forms of the heme biosynthetic enzymes porphobilinogen deaminase and ferrochelatase.[170, 171] Interestingly, forced expression of p45 NF-E2 in nonerythroid cells stimulates iron uptake (Chang TJ, Andrews NC: Personal communication, 1996). The functional data and the fact that NF-E2 sites are found in association with this constellation of genes involved in red cell development suggest that NF-E2 coordinates hemoglobin production by regulating the expression of globin proteins, heme biosynthesis, and iron uptake.[172]

Other reports indicate that heme biosynthesis indirectly regulates the transcription of globin, transferrin receptor, and ferritin genes.[173–175] Heme also regulates globin messenger RNA (mRNA) translation. Whereas the onset of globin protein synthesis precedes that of heme in developing erythroblasts,[176] the intracellular concentration of heme directly regulates globin synthesis.[177] Although the precise mechanisms remain to be elucidated, iron uptake, heme biosynthesis, and globin protein production clearly are coordinately regulated. Interrelated regulatory networks apparently allow red cell precursors to maximize hemoglobin formation without accumulating excess globin proteins, unbound iron, or toxic protoporphyrin intermediates.

MOLECULAR GENETICS OF IRON TRANSPORT AND STORAGE PROTEINS

Ferritin and the Transferrin Receptor

Ferritin is a 24-subunit heteropolymer with a variable ratio of H and L chains. The H subunit contains 182 amino acid residues with a molecular weight of 21 kd, whereas the L subunit is composed of 174 amino acid residues with a molecular weight of 19 kd.[178] The subunits probably arose by gene duplication, although the degree of nucleotide sequence homology between the two is only about 50%.

Pinpointing the chromosomal location of ferritin genes was initially confounded by the large number of processed pseudogenes that exist for each subunit.[179–181] Functional ferritin genes have now been located on chromosomes 11 and 19 for the H and L subunits, respectively.[182, 183] Two additional H subunit–like genes have been identified on the short arm of chromosome 6.[184] These latter genes lack a defined functional status.

Ferritin formation is controlled at multiple levels—transcription, message stabilization, translation, and subunit assembly.[185, 186] In the liver and in HeLa cells, iron rapidly induces L-subunit mRNA synthesis, with no effect on H-subunit transcription.[185, 187] In contrast, induced differentiation of HL-60 promyelocytic leukemia cells and mouse erythroleukemia cells increases H-subunit mRNA production.[188, 189] Tumor necrosis factor induces H-chain transcription in human myoblasts.[190] Iron, heme, as well as reactive oxygen species and oxidative stress enhance both transcription and translation of the ferritin heavy chain.[22, 175, 186]

The murine ferritin H-chain gene has a 140-bp minimal promoter that is sufficient to direct high levels of transcription in both erythroid and liver cell lines.[191] In addition, an enhancer element located 4.5 kb upstream of the gene mediates inducible expression during erythroid differentiation in tissue culture.[191] This enhancer element contains an NF-E2 binding site whose functional role is undetermined.

Cytoplasmic ferritin mRNA forms a stable complex with several proteins. Both iron and interleukin-1β enhance translation of this messenger ribonucleoprotein (mRNP).[192–194] The influx of iron into cells shifts the message onto the ribosomes, thereby enhancing the synthesis of ferritin subunits.[194, 195] Discovery of the mechanism of this translational control revealed a previously unsuspected link between the expression of the genes encoding ferritin, the transferrin receptor, and one or more enzymes of heme biosynthesis.[196]

As mentioned earlier, levels of serum ferritin vary directly with iron status. Munro and colleagues initially showed that ferritin synthesis was regulated at the level of message translation.[194, 197, 198] Comparison of the 5′ untranslated regions of ferritin mRNAs encoding

both heavy and light chains showed striking conservation of a 28-bp sequence motif. This motif was conserved across diverse species [199–201] and correlated with the locus of ferritin translational control. Computer analysis of its predicted secondary structure shows a stable RNA stem-loop (Fig. 11–5, *inset*).

This structure, designated the iron response element (IRE), is recognized by a specific RNA-binding protein. The protein that recognizes the IRE, called IRP-1 for iron regulatory protein-1, is a 98-kd soluble polypeptide with striking homology to the mitochondrial Krebs cycle enzyme aconitase. The two have identical amino acid residues in the region corresponding to the aconitase active site.[202, 203] Under certain circumstances, IRP-1 has aconitase activity and may be one of the previously identified cytosolic aconitases. IRP-1 is an iron-regulated repressor of ferritin translation, which binds to the mRNA and blocks attachment of translation initiation factors.[204] The enzymatic active site of IRP-1 is a [4Fe-4S] cluster. When the iron concentration in the cytosol is high, the cluster is complete. This form of IRP-1 has aconitase activity but cannot bind mRNA. The ferritin message is translated efficiently. Conversely, when the iron concentration is low, aconitase activity is absent, RNA binding is avid, and message translation is blocked.[203, 205–210] IRP-1 is a dual-function protein, with ambient iron controlling the switch by its participation in the [4Fe-4S] cluster. Other molecules

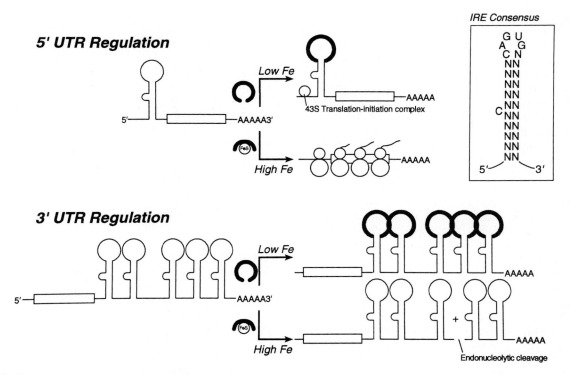

Figure 11-5. The iron regulatory protein. Two mechanisms of action of the iron regulatory protein (IRP) are shown. IRP binds to an iron response element (IRE)–stem-loop structure formed in noncoding mRNA sequences. A consensus IRE structure is shown in the *inset*. Under low iron conditions IRP binds avidly to RNA. With abundant iron, no binding occurs. IRP binding to IRE elements in the 5′ untranslated region (UTR) (e.g., ferritin and erythroid δ-aminolevulinate synthase mRNAs) blocks translation. In contrast, IRP binding to 3′ UTR IRE elements (e.g., the transferrin receptor) prevents site-specific nucleolytic cleavage, thereby stabilizing the message. A single regulator thus plays two different roles in the translational regulation of proteins involved in cellular iron metabolism.

that modulate the switch include ascorbic acid and possibly heme. Physiologic levels of ascorbic acid do not alter baseline translation of ferritin mRNA. When iron is added, however, ferritin synthesis is 50-fold more robust than is seen under ascorbate-deficient conditions. The vitamin potentiates ferritin synthesis in response to iron by activating aconitase activity of free IRP-1 in the cytosol. The molecular mechanism of the switch is unknown. The alteration in IRP-1 function by ascorbate expands further the known extensive interplay between iron and ascorbic acid.[208]

IRP-1 also modulates expression of the transferrin receptor gene. The gene encoding the transferrin receptor is located on human chromosome 3q26.2-qter, near the gene encoding transferrin at 3q21,[211, 212] and consists of 19 exons, spread over 31 kb.[213] The transferrin receptor mRNA is approximately twice the length needed to encode the receptor protein. The lengthy 3' untranslated region of the mRNA contains five potential RNA stem-loop structures that are structurally similar to those of the ferritin IRE.[214, 215] These conserved regions of the transferrin receptor mRNA bind the same protein as does the IRE of the ferritin mRNAs.[214] The attached protein increases the stability of the transferrin receptor message by obscuring a potential site of endonucleolytic cleavage. The result is a larger amount of transferrin receptor mRNA in the cell.[216] A deficit of cellular iron, then, raises transferrin receptor mRNA levels at least in part through enhanced message stability.

IRE regulation is probably not responsible for the primary increases in transferrin receptor numbers in erythroid cells, because this occurs at the transcriptional level and is unaffected by iron status.[59, 217] Relatively little is understood about the tissue-specific transcriptional regulation of the transferrin receptor, though some information has been gleaned about its regulation in nonerythroid cells.[218–220]

A second IRE-binding protein, IRP-2, also modulates post-transcriptional expression of ferritin and the transferrin receptor. Initially isolated in liver, IRP-2 has been found in all tissues examined and is more abundant than IRP-1 in some.[221, 222] Although the two proteins differ in molecular weight (90 kd for IRP-1, 118 kd for IRP-2), the key difference is that IRP-2 lacks aconitase activity.[221] Little is known about the relative roles *in vitro* of these two proteins in iron metabolism. The lack of aconitase activity in IRP-2 conceivably gives the cell wider latitude in balancing iron metabolism with intermediary energy metabolism.

The versatile regulatory functions of IREs appear also to confer iron-dependent regulation on other proteins. IREs have been detected in the 5' UTRs of the mRNAs encoding the erythroid form of the heme biosynthetic enzyme δ-aminolevulinic acid synthase and mitochondrial aconitase.[223–225] As the rate-limiting enzyme in heme biosynthesis, the IRE in the erythroid form of δ-aminolevulinic acid synthase produces a conceptually satisfying link between iron and heme production. These IREs serve the common purpose of coupling changes in the iron status of the cell with its ability to utilize and store the element (see Fig. 11–5).

When the intracellular iron concentration is low, the IRE of ferritin mRNA binds IRP, reducing ferritin synthesis, because additional iron storage capacity is not needed in this circumstance. Simultaneously, the level of transferrin receptor mRNA increases as the IRP stabilizes the message, thereby increasing transferrin receptor expression. Together these events increase the flow of iron into cells while protecting against iron toxicity. With high iron levels in the cell, the opposite scenario is operative. Although the IRPs accomplish these regulatory feats under extremes of iron status, the importance of IREs and IRPs in living animals has not yet been established. Gene targeting experiments aimed at disrupting the IRP genes in transgenic mice will help elucidate their function.

Transferrin

The liver is the major site of transferrin synthesis and secretion.[226] Other tissues can produce the protein, however, including Sertoli cells of the testes, oligodendrocytes of the CNS, lymphocytes, muscle cells, and mammary cells.[38, 227–231] Local synthesis within brain and testis apparently provides transferrin for those tissues, because serum transferrin does not penetrate the unique capillaries of these organs. The blood-testis barrier prevents the free flow of proteins from the circulation into the lumen of the seminiferous tubules. The Sertoli cells of the testis synthesize a significant quantity of transferrin that bathes developing germ cells.[227, 229] These rapidly dividing cells require substantial amounts of iron for normal growth and differentiation. Transferrin supplied by the Sertoli cells is believed to be vital to spermatocyte development.

Transferrin mRNA and protein have also been detected in oligodendrocytes.[230] Like the testis, the CNS has limited access to serum molecules because of the blood-brain barrier. Unlike the testis, however, the CNS has no cohort of rapidly proliferating cells. Iron may be needed instead to support a vast array of redox reactions that produce specialized neurotransmitter compounds such as γ-aminobutyric acid, as well as the more mundane metabolic activity required to sustain all living cells. The question of whether transferrin synthesis by oligodendrocytes is absolutely required for iron distribution to neural tissues is unanswered.

Activated T lymphocytes also synthesize and secrete transferrin.[231] At rest, the cells do not generate transferrin and do not express surface transferrin receptors. After mitogenic stimulation, however, both proteins are produced.[231, 232] The synthesis of transferrin is restricted to the CD4+ helper lymphocytes. Transferrin mRNA production and transferrin receptor synthesis by these cells precede cell division and have been postulated to be part of an autocrine regulatory loop.[231] Additional data are required to confirm this hypothesis.

Transferrin genes have been cloned from several different species. A basic similarity exists both in the protein structure of the transferrin molecule and its genomic organization.[233–236] The transferrin protein has two iron-binding pockets on either side of a central plane of symmetry, suggesting an origin by gene duplication from a primordial protein containing a single iron-binding site. No cooperativity exists in iron binding by the two sites, and the protein can be proteolytically cleaved into two halves, each of which retains iron-binding capability.[234, 235] Transferrin binds ferric iron much more avidly than ferrous iron.[71]

Human transferrin mRNA is 2.3 kb in length and encodes 679 amino acids including a 19–amino acid leader sequence. Chromosomal hybridization localized the gene to chromosome 3q, near genes for the transferrin receptor and melanotransferrin (p97).[211, 236] Both human and chicken transferrin genes have similar structures, with 17 exons. The avian gene can be expressed in transgenic mice to produce chicken transferrin, which is properly processed and secreted.[236a]

Transferrin production is regulated at multiple levels. Transcription is tissue specific and regulated by iron and hormones. Several *cis*-acting control regions exist upstream of the gene. The transferrin promoter contains binding sites for tissue-specific nuclear factors, which activate transcription differentially in liver and other tissues (e.g., Sertoli cells).[237–242] Transferrin gene expression is also modulated by iron, hormones, and inflammatory stimuli.[243–246] In the setting of iron deficiency, serum transferrin levels rise substantially, owing to enhanced transferrin mRNA synthesis by the liver.[33] In contrast, inflammation depresses levels of both serum transferrin and serum iron.

A 300-bp enhancer element approximately 3.6 kb upstream of the transferrin gene has been studied in detail.[241, 242, 247, 248] The region has two functional elements: (1) an autonomous enhancer element that binds liver-specific proteins and (2) a larger element lacking enhancer activity but able to override inhibition from a downstream negative regulatory element.

Control of transferrin gene expression contrasts to that of the transferrin receptor where iron deficiency increases message levels largely by message stabilization.[214, 215, 249] Transferrin is an abundant, secreted protein involved in iron homeostasis of the whole organism. Consequently, its expression does not have to be altered acutely to respond to external events. Primary control of transferrin expression at the level of message transcription allows modulation of systemic iron metabolism in response to a variety of factors such as inflammation or the hormonal changes of pregnancy.

Liver-derived serum transferrin levels fall in patients with hepatic iron overload due to hereditary hemochromatosis, although mRNA levels are unchanged.[250] This indicates that hepatic transferrin is also controlled at the level of translation or secretion. This regulation may involve an RNA stem-loop structure in the 5' untranslated region (5' UTR) of the transferrin messenger RNA that is functionally similar or identical to the IRE element. When reporter constructs linking this transferrin 5' untranslated sequence to a chloramphenicol acetyl transferase complementary DNA (cDNA) sequence are introduced into transgenic mice, iron regulates chloramphenicol acetyl transferase expression.[251] Translational control has been attributed to a nonconsensus IRE stem loop. The putative transferrin IRE confers a much less dramatic iron response than ferritin

IREs. Interestingly, the quantity of transferrin mRNA in nonhepatic tissues (including the testis, kidney, and spleen) is not affected by iron deficiency. The liver-derived transferrin, therefore, appears to have the unique responsibility of responding to iron status.

PLASMA FERRITIN AND TRANSFERRIN RECEPTORS

Although most ferritin is located within cells, a measurable amount of the protein exists in serum. The source of extracellular ferritin is unclear. Some apparently leaks from necrotic cells. However, the vast majority of plasma ferritin appears to be secreted. Circulating ferritin consists almost exclusively of L-chain subunits.[252] This contrasts to intracellular ferritin, which contains a mixture of H and L subunits. Also unlike intracellular ferritin, circulating ferritin is glycosylated, suggesting that it passes through the endoplasmic reticulum and Golgi apparatus as do other secreted proteins.[253–255]

Serum ferritin levels decline with iron deficiency and rise with iron loading.[256, 257] They reasonably reflect total body iron stores, in the absence of liver disease, infection, or chronic inflammation. A low serum ferritin level (less than 15 mg/L) invariably represents iron deficiency. The correlation between serum ferritin levels and body iron stores aids the evaluation of patients with possible iron deficiency or iron overload. Extreme plasma ferritin levels should be interpreted cautiously, however, because the correlation between plasma ferritin levels and body iron stores is linear in the adult only for storage pools of iron ranging between 1 and 3 g.[255] In addition, normal plasma ferritin values vary with gender and age. These considerations must be factored into any evaluation of iron stores based on plasma ferritin values, particularly with children.

Several conditions routinely modify plasma ferritin levels. Inflammation increases the plasma ferritin concentration by twofold to threefold.[258] Infections, particularly chronic conditions such as tuberculosis or osteomyelitis, increase plasma ferritin levels substantially, presumably because of the associated inflammatory response. Chronic renal disease and chronic liver disease also are associated with elevated levels. A number of tumors variably raise the level of circulating ferritin.[259, 260] Ferritin is an important prognostic factor in childhood neuroblastoma, in which serum ferritin levels correlate with disease severity.[261]

The mechanism by which inflammation or tumors increase the quantity of plasma ferritin is unknown. Interleukin-1β, a prime mediator of the inflammatory response, increases ferritin synthesis in human hepatoma cells,[192] whereas tumor necrosis factor has been shown to increase ferritin mRNA levels in murine cells in culture.[190] These cytokines may also increase ferritin synthesis in cells secreting the protein.

Soluble transferrin receptors also exist in the circulation. Small vesicles containing transferrin receptors are shed from reticulocytes during their maturation to erythrocytes.[262, 263] In addition to these vesicle-associated receptors, the extracellular portion of the transferrin receptor lacking its transmembrane anchor can be found in the circulation.[264, 265] One mechanism by which soluble transferrin receptors are generated is by a membrane-associated protease activity that clips the molecule between amino acids 100 and 101, at the base of its extracellular stem.[266, 267] The fact that this cleavage is potentiated by mutation of an O-linked glycosylation site at amino acid 104 suggests that differential glycosylation may play a regulatory role.[268] The transferrin binding domain is intact in these soluble receptors, and the receptors may be complexed with transferrin in the plasma. A second mechanism involves cleavage of soluble transferrin receptors from exocytic vesicles that are shed from erythrocytes.[269] Which mechanism is predominant in humans is unclear.

The quantity of soluble transferrin receptor in the plasma varies with the rate of erythropoiesis.[270, 271] Measurement of plasma levels of soluble transferrin receptors provides a means of estimating erythropoietic activity, which is simpler than the relatively cumbersome PIT determination. The protein exists in substantially lower amounts in patients with aplastic anemia relative to normal individuals. In contrast, the value in patients with autoimmune hemolytic anemias is markedly increased. Interestingly, patients with iron deficiency also have increased levels of circulating soluble transferrin receptors.[270–272] This may result from the increase in cellular transferrin receptor expression produced by iron starvation.

COPPER METABOLISM

Nutritional Copper Deficiency

Like iron, copper is essential for normal cell growth and metabolism but toxic in excess. Copper deficiency commonly causes hypochromic anemia among farm animals in areas of the world in which a dearth of copper exists in the soil. Nutritional copper deficiency in humans results most often from extraordinary dietary circumstances,[273, 274] such as inadvertent omission of copper from intravenous alimentation formulations for an extended time, treatment of severely malnourished patients with a copper-deficient milk diet,[275] or impaired copper absorption due to immense amounts of dietary zinc.[274] Despite their marked susceptibility to copper deficiency, the condition has been described only in preterm infants maintained on a milk diet.[276] Hypocupremia has been reported with iron deficiency and hypoproteinemia[277] and in active celiac disease[278] but must be extraordinarily uncommon.

Copper balance, in contrast to iron balance, is regulated by excretion as well as by absorption.[273, 274] The gastrointestinal tract absorbs daily about 30% of the typical 1 g of copper in an average diet. The liver promptly disposes of much of the copper in the bile, whereas a lesser amount is lost through the intestinal mucosa. Experimental animals on copper-deficient diets conserve the element by markedly decreasing biliary copper excretion.

One hundred to 150 mg of copper is present in the adult human. The liver has the highest copper content, which, together with muscle and bone, accounts for 50% to 75% of total body copper. Plasma copper, which is held much more constant than plasma iron, exists in two forms. Albumin and amino acids loosely bind 10% to 15% of circulating copper. An α_2-globulin, called ceruloplasmin or ferroxidase, tightly binds the remaining copper in the plasma. As with iron, the fetus accumulates large amounts of copper near the end of gestation, particularly in the liver, where concentrations are 5 to 10 times greater at birth than in the adult. Normally these stores do not decrease to adult levels until 5 to 15 years of age.

Copper is an essential component of cytochrome oxidase, the terminal oxidase of the electron transport chain required for the combination of hydrogen with oxygen to form water. As such, the element is essential for the oxidative production of ATP. The enzyme tyrosinase is a copper-containing protein required for melanin synthesis. Thus, copper-deficient animals have depressed cytochrome oxidase in most tissues, along with a loss of hair pigment. Another copper metalloenzyme, lysyl oxidase, plays a role in the cross-linking of collagen and elastin. Lysyl oxidase deficiency may cause the vascular defects, including aortic aneurysm, seen in copper-deficient animals.[274]

Copper deficiency and iron deficiency produce many similar abnormalities, including a low serum iron concentration and hypochromic anemia. With copper deficiency, however, iron stores are adequate or abundant.[273, 274] Copper metabolism and iron transport are intertwined, explaining the low serum iron and hypochromic anemia of copper deficiency. Ceruloplasmin catalyzes the oxidation of ferrous iron in the liver and the intestinal mucosa to the ferric transport form (transferrin) in the plasma.[67, 68] The anemia of copper deficiency reflects impaired transport of transferrin-bound iron to the bone marrow. A Japanese kindred has been reported with defective ceruloplasmin and systemic hemosiderosis,[69] consistent with the notion that ceruloplasmin is required for mobilization of tissue iron stores and loading of iron onto transferrin. Neither these patients nor those with Menkes' disease are anemic, however.

The normal copper intake is 2 to 5 mg/d in an adult and 0.04 to 0.15 mg/kg per day in the growing child. Because of its low copper content (about 0.12 mg/L), a diet consisting of milk to the exclusion of other foods risks marginal copper nutrition or deficiency during late infancy. Premature infants with low copper stores are at particular risk.

Diagnosis and Treatment

Iron deficiency or severe malnutrition can obscure the manifestations of copper deficiency. Depressed plasma copper levels are the earliest manifestations of copper deficiency. After about 6 months of age, plasma copper levels range between 70 to 140 mg/dL. The values are lower in early infancy.[279] A mild, hypochromic anemia occurs at times. Leukopenia with very marked neutropenia is particularly prevalent with copper deficiency. Osteoporosis occurs occasionally in severe cases.

Oral treatment with 0.1 to 0.3 mg/kg of copper per day (two or three times the estimated daily requirement) as 0.5% copper sulfate (containing about 2 mg of copper per milliliter) produces prompt reticulocytosis and correction of the anemia and neutropenia. Generally, the dietary imbalance that produced the deficiency can be corrected once the problem is recognized.

Inherited Disorders of Copper Metabolism

Two inherited defects of copper metabolism present as well-defined clinical syndromes. Menkes' disease, or kinky hair syndrome, is a disorder characterized by low serum copper concentration, reduced activity of copper metalloenzymes, slow growth, steely gray kinky hair, cerebral degeneration, and an X-linked pattern of inheritance.[280] Interestingly, anemia is not a prominent feature of the syndrome. Death before 3 years of age is usual. Despite a low serum copper level, the disease is characterized by copper sequestration in several tissues, particularly the kidney. Parenteral copper administration, like all other attempts at treatment, is ineffective.

Wilson's disease, in contrast, produces copper toxicity. Patients are unable to excrete copper. Systemic copper overload results, with pathology due to deposition of the metal in the liver, kidneys, and CNS.[281]

Positional cloning has led to the identification of the genes mutated in Menkes' and Wilson's diseases.[282-287] Both encode transmembrane proteins highly homologous to the P-type ATPases involved in the transport of calcium ions, sodium ions, and protons. Their N-termini have repeats of the amino acid motif Gly-Met-Thr-Cys-X-X-Cys, forming copper-binding domains. Both Menkes' and Wilson's proteins function as transmembrane copper transporters. Menkes' protein is involved in intestinal copper absorption, whereas the Wilson's protein participates in cerulosplasmin production and copper excretion. Remarkably, these human proteins share extensive homology with bacterial proteins that transport copper ions into and out of prokaryotic cells.

As noted earlier, no eukaryotic membrane iron transporters have been characterized. Because copper transport is analogous to iron transport in many respects, the identification of copper transporters and understanding copper transport mechanisms may help solve long-standing problems in understanding iron metabolism.

DISORDERED IRON METABOLISM

The journey of iron atoms from the external environment to the interior of cells is a remarkable trek. Precisely tuned machinery coordinates the element's movement across each compartment in the body. At the same time, cells must be protected from injury until the iron is stored or incorporated into proteins and enzymes. A misstep at any point along the path often produces disease.

Iron Deficiency

Etiology

Abnormal Iron Uptake from the Alimentary Tract

Poor Bioavailability. Although iron is the second most abundant metal in the earth's crust, its low solubility makes the acquisition of the element for metabolic use a major challenge. Most environmental iron exists as insoluble salts. Gastric acidity assists conversion to absorbable forms, but the efficiency of this process is limited.[288] Many plant products contain iron, but absorption frequently is limited both by low solubility and powerful chelators that bind ambient iron (see Table 11–1). The phytates (organic polyphosphates) found in wheat products, for example, bind iron with tremendous avidity.[289, 290] The challenge of acquiring sufficient iron from the environment may have been an important factor in the spread of the gene for hereditary hemochromatosis (see later).

High gastric pH reduces the solubility of inorganic iron, impeding absorption.[291] Surgical interventions, such as vagotomy or hemigastrectomy for peptic ulcer disease, formerly were the major causes of impaired gastric acidification with secondary iron deficiency. Today, the histamine-2 blockers and the more recently introduced acid pump blockers, used to treat peptic ulcer disease and acid reflux, are among the most common causes of defective iron absorption. Although the problem is infrequent, use of these medications is widespread. Peptic ulcer disease is rare in youngsters. Treatment with these drugs (and their attendant complications) is exceedingly uncommon in children.

The impaired function of the gastric parietal cells associated with pernicious anemia not only reduces the production of intrinsic factor but also lessens gastric acidity. Impaired iron absorption can result. In addition, the megaloblastic enterocytes absorb iron poorly. Frank iron deficiency can accompany the anemia produced by cobalamin deficiency.[292] The rarity of pernicious anemia in children makes this complication uncommon.

Heme is the most readily absorbed form of iron.[293] Uptake occurs independently of gastric pH. Heme absorption, like the uptake of nonheme iron, is supraphysiologic in patients with high marrow erythroid activity. The molecule is, of course, derived primarily from animal tissue. The dearth of dietary meat for much of the world's population makes iron deficiency the most common cause of anemia on the planet, affecting over 600 million persons. The fact that cultivated grasses, such as rice, are dietary staples for many persons exacerbates the problem because these plants are very poor sources of iron.[289] The consequences of iron deficiency can be quite severe (see later).

Inhibition of Iron Absorption. A number of environmental factors can produce dietary iron deficiency, including metals that share the iron absorption machinery, such as lead, cobalt, and strontium (see earlier and Table 11–1). Of these, only lead is a significant problem.[294] For children, the threat is particularly marked. Iron deficiency increases the rate of uptake both of iron and lead from the gastrointestinal tract. Iron deficiency and lead intoxication, consequently, are common companions (see Chapter 13).

Disruption of the Enteric Mucosa. Some disorders disrupt the integrity of the enteric mucosa, thereby hampering iron absorption.[295] Inflammatory bowel disease, particularly Crohn's disease, sometimes injures extensive segments of the small intestine, including the jejunum and duodenum. Invasion of the submucosa by inflammatory cells and disruption of the tissue architecture impair iron absorption and uptake of dietary nutrients.[295] Occult gastrointestinal bleeding exacerbates the problem. The result is iron deficiency anemia complicated by the anemia of chronic inflammation. Furthermore, Crohn's disease frequently involves the terminal ileum, producing concurrent cobalamin deficiency. These disorders are not diagnostic enigmas. Patients with such extensive bowel disorders are very ill. The iron deficiency is best treated by correcting the underlying inflammatory process.

Sprue, both of the tropical and nontropical variety (celiac disease), can also interfere with iron absorption.[296] Degeneration of the intestinal lining cells along with chronic inflammation causes profound malabsorption. The anemia in these patients is often complicated by a superimposed nutritional deficiency.[297] Celiac disease frequently improves dramatically with a gluten-free diet. Some patients with deranged iron absorption lack gross or even histologic changes in the structure of the bowel mucosa. A gluten-free diet improves bowel function in many such children, with secondary correction of the anemia.

Loss of Functional Bowel. Substantial segments of bowel are sometimes removed surgically, disrupting iron absorption.[298] Intractable inflammatory bowel disease is occasionally treated by surgical excision. Traumatic abdominal injury, as occurs with motor vehicle accidents, also at times requires extensive bowel resection. Structural complications, such as intestinal volvulus or intussusception, sometimes necessitate removal of significant stretches of bowel in children. Iron deficiency usually develops slowly and may not become evident for several years after the surgical procedure.

Malabsorption of iron without structurally defective intestine is exceedingly rare. Many such cases, based on negative noninvasive studies of the intestine, prove on biopsy to be celiac disease or related conditions in which the villous structure of the bowel is lost. Of the *bona fide* cases, some could be related to defects in components of the bowel absorption machinery (see earlier). The dearth of information on the normal physiology of iron absorption, unfortunately, precludes explanation of the defect in most of these rare patients.

Blood Loss

Blood loss is the world's leading cause of iron deficiency. The gastrointestinal tract is both the site of iron uptake and the most common site of blood loss. The gastrointestinal tract is unrivaled as a potential site of occult blood loss.

Gastrointestinal Blood Loss

Structural Defects. Blood loss due to gastrointestinal structural faults commonly causes iron deficiency. The most frequent congenital defect in the gastrointestinal tract is Meckel's diverticulum, a persistent omphalomesenteric duct. This flaw can produce abdominal pain and, occasionally, intestinal obstruction in young children. Occult blood loss with secondary iron deficiency is a concern in adolescents with Meckel's diverticulum.

Other structural defects of the gastrointestinal tract that produce bleeding are much less common. Arteriovenous malformations involving the superficial blood vessels along the gastrointestinal tract occur with hereditary hemorrhagic telangiectasia (the Osler-Weber-Rendu syndrome). These defective vessels frequently bleed to a degree that engenders iron deficiency. Although the disorder displays autosomal dominant transmission, the pathognomonic lesions rarely attain clinical significance before young adulthood. The condition is not a diagnostic enigma, because the mucosal lining of the oropharynx and nasal cavity exhibits characteristic telangiectasia.

Peptic ulcer disease is extremely uncommon in children. The stomach and duodenum are affected most often. Inflammation and erosion are prominent at affected sites. The discovery that many cases of peptic ulcer disease are associated with *Helicobacter pylori* infection has prompted the use of antibiotics as part of the treatment regimen.[299]

Milk-Induced Enteropathy. Whole cow's milk contains proteins that often irritate the lining of the gastrointestinal tract in infants. Low-grade hemorrhage sometimes produces iron deficiency.[300] Although cow's milk contains iron at about the same concentration as does that from humans, the bioavailability of iron in human milk is much greater.[301] In addition, the prodigious neonatal growth spurt requires a tremendous quantity of iron. The intersection of blood loss and decreased iron intake (due to the immaturity of the gastrointestinal tract; see later) with a high demand makes iron deficiency a significant problem for children nourished with whole cow's milk.[302] Although the processing that goes into the production of evaporated cow's milk apparently reduces the irritating nature of the proteins, refraining from this source of nutrition is probably the wisest course.

Parasites. The world's leading cause of gastrointestinal blood loss is parasitic infestation. Hookworm infection, caused primarily by *Necator americanus* or *Ancylostoma duodenale*, is endemic to much of the world and is often asymptomatic. Microscopic blood loss leads to significant iron deficiency, most commonly in children.[303] Over 1 billion persons, most in tropical or subtropical areas, are infested with parasites. Daily blood losses exceed 11 million liters. The larvae spawn in moist soil and penetrate the skin of unprotected feet. Hookworm infection, once prevalent in the southeastern United States, declined precipitously with better sanitation and the routine use of footwear when outside.

Trichuris trichiura, the culprit in trichuriasis or whipworm infection, is believed to infest the colon of 600 million to 700 million persons. Only 10% to 15% of these persons have worm burdens sufficiently great to produce clinical disease. Most are children between the ages of 2 and 10 years, however. Growth retardation, in addition to iron deficiency, occurs with heavy infestations. Trichuriasis is the most common helminthic infection encountered in Americans returning from visits to tropical or subtropical regions of the world.

Other Sources of Blood Loss

Urinary. Occasionally, blood loss into the urinary tract outstrips iron absorption. Urinary blood loss is usually sufficiently alarming that patients seek medical attention before substantial iron deficiency develops, however. Iron deficiency resulting from hematuria due to renal disease is relatively uncommon.

The best characterized cause of substantial renal blood loss is Berger's disease, which produces relapsing episodes of gross or microscopic hematuria. The disorder occurs most commonly in older children and young adults. Diffuse mesangial proliferation or focal and segmental glomerulonephritis are the most common renal pathologic processes. Diffuse mesangial deposits of IgA are the hallmark of the disorder. Although the disease spontaneously remits in some children, progression to end-stage renal disease occurs in a substantial minority. Occasionally, Goodpasture's syndrome produces substantial urinary blood loss. Immunofluorescent staining of biopsy specimens reveals the characteristic antibodies to basement membrane lining the glomeruli. Blood loss into the urinary bladder occurs most commonly in association with infections. Hematuria to the point of iron deficiency is extremely uncommon, however.

Pulmonary. Although pulmonary blood loss sufficiently severe to produce iron deficiency occurs, the phenomenon is distinctly rare. Chronic pulmonary hemosiderosis primarily affects children and young adolescents. The potentially deadly disorder is characterized by slow but intractable hemorrhage into the bronchioles and alveoli. The pulmonary macrophages ingest and degrade the red cells but retain the iron derived from heme. Toxic products produced by the iron that accumulates in these cells, including reactive oxygen, are probably important in the activation of the macrophages. These cells begin to damage the delicate lining of the bronchoalveolar tree, producing severe fibrosis. Oxygen exchanges poorly across the damaged alveolar surfaces, lowering the efficacy of oxygen/carbon dioxide exchange. The radiographic picture of the lungs is striking and frequently shows marked retraction and scarring.[304] The restrictive lung disease along with substantial pulmonary arterial shunting across the lung is eventually fatal.

Iron deficiency anemia is part of the clinical picture of pulmonary hemosiderosis. Because the pulmonary macrophages are distinct from the normal iron recycling circuit, iron trapped within these cells is effectively lost to body metabolism. A paradoxical situation occurs in which patients develop iron-deficiency anemia in the presence of a surfeit of total body iron.[305] Bronchoalveolar lavage reveals hemosiderin-laden macrophages that are pathognomonic of the disorder.[306] Chronic pulmonary infection with bronchiectasis, once a frequent cause of this problem, is now rare.

Most often the etiology of the disorder evades elucidation. In a number of patients, the pulmonary hemosiderosis occurs in conjunction with disorders of immune dysfunction, including celiac disease [306] and Goodpasture's syndrome.[307] Treatment of the associated disorder has been associated with remission of the pulmonary process, suggesting an immunologic mechanism to the lung injury. Chloroquine treatment has produced modest success in some patients.[308] Cyclophosphamide treatment has produced some successful responses in a number of patients.[309] A combination of prednisone and azathioprine in some patients has raised hopes about treatment.[310] Agents such as cyclosporine may be even more useful as immunologic suppressers in the treatment of this condition. The infrequency of the disorder means that a large, multicenter trial is needed to collect definitive treatment information.

Consequences of Iron Deficiency

Although anemia is most prominently linked to iron deficiency, the condition produces a wide range of abnormalities, depending on its severity. Some of these abnormalities, such as cognitive dysfunction in young children, have been recognized only recently.

Anemia

Because most iron is directed to hemoglobin synthesis, erythrocyte production is among the first casualties of iron deficiency:

1. Prelatent iron deficiency occurs when stores are depleted without a change in hematocrit or serum iron levels. This stage of iron deficiency is rarely detected.
2. Latent iron deficiency occurs when the serum iron level drops and the total iron-binding capacity increases without a change in the hematocrit. This stage is occasionally detected by a routine check of the transferrin saturation.
3. Frank iron-deficiency anemia is associated with erythrocyte microcytosis and hypochromia.

The microcytic, hypochromic anemia impairs tissue oxygen, producing weakness, fatigue, palpitations, and lightheadedness. Thalassemia trait (see Chapter 21) is sometimes confused with iron deficiency. Iron deficiency alters red cell size unevenly. Electronic blood analyzers determine the mean red cell volume as well as the range of variation in red cell size (expressed as the red cell distribution width). The red cell distribution width (determined with every electronically processed complete blood cell count) is normal in patients with thalassemia trait but is high in those with iron deficiency.[311] Other common features of thalassemia trait are basophilic stippling and target cells. These characteristics are not sufficiently distinct to be diagnostically useful, however. A simple differential approach is to examine the color of plasma. It is watery in iron deficiency and straw colored in β-thalassemia trait.

The plasma membranes of iron-deficient red cells are abnormally stiff.[312] This rigidity could contribute to poikilocytic changes, seen particularly with severe iron deficiency. These small, stiff, misshapen cells are cleared by the reticuloendothelial system, contributing to the low-grade hemolysis that often accompanies iron deficiency. The cause of this alteration in membrane fluidity is unknown.

Unexplained thrombocytosis occurs frequently with platelet counts in the range of 500,000 to 700,000 cells/fL. Megakaryocytes and normoblasts are derived from a common committed progenitor cell, the CFU-GEMM. Thrombopoietin, the molecule that stimulates the growth of megakaryocytes and the production of platelets, is structurally homologous to erythropoietin (see Chapter 6). The high levels of erythropoietin produced by iron-deficiency anemia conceivably could cross react with megakaryocyte thrombopoietin receptors, modestly raising the platelet count.

Growth and Developmental Retardation

Iron deficiency, with or without concomitant anemia, commonly impairs growth and intellectual development in children.[313] Studies of cognitive development in the setting of iron deficiency produced disparate results for a time. In some investigations, dietary iron supplementation for infants reversed cognitive dysfunction,[314] whereas others failed to show improvement.[315] Some of the disparities may have resulted from differences in the instruments used in the analyses and differences in the populations examined.

When tested using the Bayley Scale of Infant Development, abnormalities are uncovered in children as young as 9 to 12 months of age. Developmental abnormalities occur with or without anemia. In one study, iron replacement increased the Mental Development Index scores substantially in only 7 days.[316] Iron deficiency does not impair motor development even in infants with low scores on the tests of cognitive development.[317] Concomitant lead exposure can further hamper the psychological development of these children.[318]

Information on the long-term effects of iron deficiency during infancy highlights the importance of early intervention. One group of children with iron-deficiency anemia (hemoglobin less than 10 g/dL) was treated during infancy and tested for cognitive development at 5 years of age.[319] This cohort scored lower in tests of mental and motor functioning than did their counterparts, regardless of correction of the deficiency during infancy. The disparity persisted despite controls for differences in socioeconomic background. The investigators soberly concluded that children who are iron deficient in infancy are at risk of long-lasting developmental disadvantage relative to peers with better iron status. Other investigations produced concurring results.[320, 321] Correction of iron deficiency during infancy clearly improves scores in short-term tests, such as the Bayley Scale of Infant Development, without preventing longer-term, and possibly more serious, impairment in cognitive function. Health care providers, therefore, must strive to prevent iron deficiency during infancy.[322, 323]

The mechanism by which iron deficiency impairs neurologic function is unknown. Many enzymes in neural tissue require iron for normal function.[324] The cytochromes involved in energy production, for example, predominantly are heme proteins. In rats, weanlings maintained on iron-deficient diets develop severe behavioral anomalies, motor incoordination, and seizures. The abnormalities seen in iron-deficient children and adults are much less pronounced but are a source of serious concern nonetheless.[325]

The effect of iron deficiency on childhood growth is often difficult to separate from overall nutritional deficiency.[326] The high prevalence of childhood iron deficiency among less affluent persons has yoked deficiencies of iron and general nutrients. When the two factors have been separated, correction of iron deficiency improves growth independently of nutritional status.[327, 328]

Epithelial Changes

Iron deficiency produces significant gastrointestinal tract abnormalities, reflecting the enormous proliferative capacity of this organ. Some patients develop angular stomatitis and glossitis with painful swelling of the tongue. The flattened, atrophic lingual papillae make the tongue smooth and shiny. A rare complication of iron deficiency is the Plummer-Vinson syndrome with the formation of a postcricoid esophageal web. Long-standing, severe iron deficiency affects the cells that generate the fingernails, producing koilonychia, or spooning. The nail substance is soft, so that ordinary pressure on the fingertips, as occurs with writing for instance, produces a concave deformity. Most of these abnormalities are now uncommon in industrialized nations.

Miscellaneous

Pica occurs variably in patients with iron deficiency, but the precise pathophysiology of the syndrome is unknown. Patients often consume laundry starch, ice, and soil clay. Both clay and starch can bind iron in the gastrointestinal tract, exacerbating the deficiency.[329, 330] A dramatic example of the problems produced with clay consumption occurred in the 1960s with reports of iron deficiency in children along the border between Iran and Turkey.[331] These youngsters had other, peculiar abnormalities, including massive hepatosplenomegaly, poor wound healing, and a bleeding diathesis. Presumably, the children initially had simple iron deficiency associated with pica, including geophagia. The soil contained compounds that bound both iron and zinc.[332] The secondary zinc deficiency caused the hepatomegaly and other unusual features.[333]

Iron deficiency increases the gastrointestinal absorption of a number of heavy metals, including lead, that share the iron-absorption machinery. Consequently, childhood lead intoxication and iron deficiency are common bedfellows (see Chapter 13). Low-level, but persistent, exposure to environmental lead in turn exacerbates iron deficiency by competitive inhibition of the iron absorption machinery (see Table 11–1). A rare but reversible complication of severe iron deficiency is pseudotumor cerebri.[334]

Treatment of Iron Deficiency

The most important steps in the evaluation and treatment of iron deficiency are determining the cause of the deficiency and correcting the abnormality. Malignancy of the gastrointestinal tract, the haunting specter in adults with iron deficiency, is vanishingly rare in children. Growth spurts, poor dietary patterns, or benign gastrointestinal bleeding sources are much more common.[335] After these initial investigations, oral iron supplementation replaces stores most efficiently.

Oral Supplementation

Although ferrous sulfate is often recommended to treat iron deficiency, frequent problems with the drug, including gastrointestinal discomfort, bloating, and other distress, make its use unacceptable to many patients.[336] Low doses of ferrous sulfate, such as a single 325-mg tablet (containing 65 mg of elemental iron) on an empty stomach at night lessen the gastrointestinal difficulties. The absorptive capacity for iron in the duodenum is essentially saturated with about 25 mg of elemental iron in ionic form that is presented to the absorptive machinery. Ferrous gluconate, which is roughly equivalent in cost, contains about 50 mg of elemental iron per tablet. This form of replacement often produces fewer problems than ferrous sulfate and is excellent as the initial treatment of iron deficiency. Ascorbic acid supplementation enhances iron absorption. Combination tablets containing iron salts and ascorbic acid are significantly more expensive than separate tablets for each, however. Even with faithful use of oral iron, adequate replacement of body stores in patients with moderate iron deficiency anemia requires several months. With ongoing blood loss, replacement of stores with oral iron becomes a herculean task.

Polysaccharide/iron complex, a replacement form of iron that differs from the iron salts, is now available. The polar oxygen groups in the polysaccharide form coordination complexes with the iron atoms. The well-hydrated microspheres of polysaccharide iron remain in solution over a wide pH range. Most patients tolerate this form of iron better than the iron salts, even though the 150 mg of elemental iron per tablet is substantially greater than that provided by iron salts. Table 11–2 lists potential causes of a poor response to oral iron supplementation.

Parenteral Iron Replacement

Parenteral iron is available in the United States only as iron dextran. This medication is indicated when (1)

Table 11–2. POOR RESPONSE TO ORAL IRON

Noncompliance
Ongoing blood loss
Insufficient duration of therapy
High gastric pH
  Antacids
  Histamine-2 blockers
  Gastric acid pump inhibitors
Inhibitors of iron absorption/utilization
  Lead
  Aluminum intoxication (hemodialysis patients)
  Chronic inflammation
  Neoplasia
Incorrect diagnosis
  Thalassemia
  Sideroblastic anemia

oral iron is poorly tolerated, (2) rapid replacement of iron stores is needed, or (3) gastrointestinal iron absorption is compromised. Iron-dextran can be administered by intramuscular or intravenous injection.[337] Intramuscular injection of iron-dextran can be painful, and leakage into the subcutaneous tissue produces long-standing skin discoloration. A "Z-track" injection into the muscle minimizes the chance of subcutaneous leak. Suboptimal muscle mass frequently associated with nutritional deficiency further complicates this mode of replacement. Intravenous infusion of iron-dextran circumvents these problems altogether.[338] With either route of administration, a test dose of 10 mg of iron should be given and the patient observed by a physician for 30 minutes to rule out an anaphylactic reaction to the medication (such reactions are infrequent).

Ten to 15% of patients experience transient mild to moderate arthralgias the day after intramuscular or intravenous administration of iron-dextran. Acetaminophen usually effectively relieves the discomfort. Iron-dextran generally should be avoided in patients with rheumatoid arthritis, because they frequently have painful flares of their disease.[20] The symptoms may result from release of inflammatory cytokines such as interleukin-1 and tumor necrosis factor. The iron dextran is cleared from the circulation by fixed tissue macrophages, which probably are activated to release these proinflammatory peptides.

In uncomplicated cases of iron deficiency, intravenous replacement produces subjective improvement in a few days. Peak reticulocytosis occurs after about 10 days, and complete correction of the anemia can take 3 to 4 weeks.[339] The hematocrit rises sufficiently in 1 or 2 weeks to provide symptomatic relief for most patients.

Refractory bleeding that cannot be corrected, as occurs for instance with hereditary hemorrhagic telangiectasia, is a problem in management. Oral iron supplementation often fails to keep pace with losses. Blood transfusion replaces blood red cells in the short term and iron in the long term. Infection and alloimmunization alone make this an unacceptable alternative. Intermittent replacement with infusions of iron dextran is the most reasonable alternative. Replacements should occur over short intervals two or three times a year, with the aim of repleting the body stores. A simple formula can be used to determine the replacement dose:

$$\text{Dose (mL)} = 0.0442 \times (\text{desired Hb} - \text{observed Hb}) \times \text{LBW} + (0.26 \times \text{LBW})$$

where LBW = lean body weight.
The maximum adult dose is 14 mL.

Timing of Iron Replacement in Infants

Infants and children from low-income families are the most conspicuous victims of iron deficiency, despite a decline in the incidence of the condition over the past 20 years. Without iron-fortified formula, 20% of infants from inner city families develop iron deficiency, with frank iron-deficiency anemia in nearly 10% of these children.[300] The use of iron-fortified formula reduces the incidence of iron deficiency to about 1%. The aforementioned problems produced by iron deficiency prompted the Committee on Nutrition of the American Academy of Pediatrics to recommend the following[302]:

1. Breast milk should be provided for at least 5 to 6 months when possible. Iron supplementation of 1 mg/kg per day should be provided to infants who are exclusively fed breast milk beyond 6 months of age because human breast milk contains little iron.

2. Infants who are not breast fed should be nourished with an iron-supplemented formula (at least 12 mg of iron per liter) for the first year of life after 6 months of age.

3. Iron-enriched cereals should be among the first foods introduced with a solid diet.

4. Cow's milk should be avoided during the first year of life to prevent occult gastrointestinal bleeding.

5. Premature infants should receive iron supplements immediately.[340]

Iron Overload

Hereditary Hemochromatosis

Hereditary hemochromatosis reflects an alteration in the iron absorption mechanism that fractionally increases the uptake of dietary iron.[341-343] Tissue iron reaches dangerous levels after 30 or 40 years. The gene responsible for hereditary hemochromatosis is very near the A locus of the HLA class I histocompatibility antigen complex.[344, 345] Identification of the gene responsible for hereditary hemochromatosis has been hampered by extensive linkage disequilibrium in this area of the genome. Furthermore, no functional assay of iron uptake exists.

The application of yeast artificial chromosome technology to the problem led to the identification of a 4.5-Mb region immediately telomeric to HLA in which markers 700 kb apart bracketed a "critical region."[346] Additional investigation narrowed the candidate region for the hereditary hemochromatosis gene to 250 kb. Although sizable, this region was amenable to DNA sequencing, which identified 15 genes.[347] One gene has a predicted structure homologous to the HLA class I gene family and is designated *HLA-H*. A missense mutation of *HLA-H* occurs in 87% of patients with hereditary hemochromatosis who have been studied. In contrast, this mutation occurs in fewer than 5% of normal subjects. *HLA-H* is the most likely candidate for the hemochromatosis gene identified to date.[348]

The mutation of HLA-H in patients with hereditary hemochromatosis maps to the putative β_2-microglobulin–binding domain. A possible role for β_2-microglobulin in iron metabolism is suggested by studies of mice deficient for this protein who show signs of iron loading.[349-350] The mutations in HLA-H could alter the association of this protein with β_2-microglobulin and somehow enhance iron loading. Functional studies are needed to evaluate these ideas.

Hereditary hemochromatosis trait, due to the inheritance of a single gene, rarely produces clinically significant problems.[351, 352] Two genes produce the full-blown hereditary hemochromatosis syndrome. Phenotypic expression of hereditary hemochromatosis rarely occurs before early adulthood. Significant organ damage usually arises during middle age or later.[353] The most frequent question regarding hereditary hemochromatosis and children is whether the child of a person with the disorder has also inherited two genes.[354] The possibility is significant, given the 6% to 9% prevalence of the gene in persons of European ancestry.[355-358]

African Iron Overload Syndrome

During the 1960s, several groups of investigators reported that iron overload occurred unexpectedly often among sub-Saharan Africans.[359-361] Many patients had massive iron overload, approaching or exceeding that seen in those with hereditary hemochromatosis.[362] Some indigenous inhabitants of the region prepared alcoholic beverages in iron pots, raising the possibility that iron overload resulted from the extremely high iron content of these beverages. Iron loading was thought to be exacerbated by the known increase in gastrointestinal iron absorption induced by alcohol. The term *Bantu siderosis* was coined to describe the condition.[363]

Later reports cast doubt on the relationship between iron overload and iron pots.[364] Only a fraction of the persons who drank the beverage developed iron overload. In fact, more extensive study showed that similar degrees of iron overload occurred in persons who consumed little, if any, of this brew.

A study of inhabitants of Zimbabwe, where cases of massive iron overload also occurred, indicated that the disorder is an inherited defect in iron absorption.[365] The gene appears to be autosomal co-dominant, with obligate heterozygotes expressing an intermediate level of iron loading. No link to the HLA class I gene complex exists, clearly demarcating the disorder from hereditary hemochromatosis. Enhanced gastrointestinal iron absorption appears to be at fault.

The African iron overload syndrome also differs from hereditary hemochromatosis in the cellular distribution of iron. In hereditary hemochromatosis, the iron is almost entirely confined to the parenchymal cells.[366] Reticuloendothelial cells, such as the Kupffer cells of the liver, are uninvolved. In contrast, reticuloendothelial cells display massive iron deposition in the African variety of iron overload.[367]

As with hereditary hemochromatosis, our understanding of the pathophysiology of the African iron overload syndrome is hampered by incomplete information on normal iron absorption. The clinical consequences of iron overload are similar, irrespective of the cause of the accumulation (see later). The African iron overload syndrome is not confined to any ethnic group, although it appears to be restricted to the inhabitants of sub-Saharan Africa. In some areas, the incidence of heterozygosity may be as high as 10%, making it one of the most common clinically significant inherited defects in any population.

An important unanswered question is whether the gene or genes that encode this syndrome are expressed in persons of African descent elsewhere in the world. No good study exists of iron overload in blacks in the Americas, for instance. Because the gene pool of black persons in the Americas includes genes of European origin as well as those derived from Africa, any study of iron overload must account for the possible expression of the gene for hereditary hemochromatosis.

The Evolutionary Advantage of Hemochromatosis

Frequent anomalies that produce iron overload in two separate populations raises the possibility that these conditions once had a selective advantage. As previously noted, iron deficiency is the most common cause of anemia in the world. Anemia was a selective disadvantage at the dawn of human history. Today, diminished exercise tolerance is an annoyance. During much of human history, however, it would have been a fatal flaw. A change that increased the efficiency of iron absorption, therefore, would have advantages.

A person who survived into the third decade would have reproduced and passed their genes on to the next generation, including those that increase iron absorption. Survival into the fifth decade, when iron overload begins to produce problems, was uncommon. In any event, procreation had occurred by then and evolution is indifferent to events during the later stages of life. Even secondary factors, such as survival of the parent to protect young offspring, would have had diminished impact, because humans have long been a social species. Able, but young members of the community would have been protected by other adults of the clan. The fossil archive shows members of *Homo sapiens neanderthalensis* with deformities, such as congenital limb anomalies, that, if unaided, would have prohibited survival.[368] These persons doubtless survived owing to social support networks.

A problem develops with this tidy theory when the inhabitants of Asia are considered. The incidence of iron overload reportedly is quite low in this region of the world, the home to most of the Earth's popula-

tion.[369] However, medical information on Asians is not as extensive as that concerning Europeans, for instance. As more is learned about iron overload in Asia, concepts may be revised.

Neonatal Iron Overload Syndrome

The degree to which the placenta regulates access of iron to the fetus is demonstrated graphically in victims of the neonatal iron overload syndrome. Afflicted newborns have massive iron deposits in all body tissues.[370–372] Although some newborns survive for a few months, many die within days of birth of multisystemic organ failure, which includes the liver, pancreas, and heart. Patients also have an unexplained bleeding diathesis that sometimes leads to fatal internal hemorrhage. Neurologic abnormalities, including seizures, occur in some newborns.

Histologic examination shows extensive iron deposition both in parenchymal and reticuloendothelial cells.[373] At necropsy, the heavy and widespread iron deposition is accompanied by organ necrosis and fibrosis. Regenerating hepatic nodules (cirrhosis) frequently develop in newborns who survive for more than a few weeks. Many regions of the brain also display heavy iron deposits, indicating that the blood-brain barrier is effete in the face of the massive assault.

The neonatal iron overload syndrome superficially resembles hereditary hemochromatosis. The disorders are clearly distinguished on deeper examination. The most important difference is that iron is deposited *in utero* with neonatal iron overload syndrome, indicating that the defect involves iron transport across the placenta. Hereditary hemochromatosis, of course, arises from an alteration in gastrointestinal iron absorption. No clear link between gastrointestinal iron absorption and transplacental iron transport exists. The children of women with hereditary hemochromatosis are not iron loaded at birth, indicating that the placenta functions normally. Our limited understanding of the normal physiology of transplacental iron transport could obscure a functional relationship between hereditary hemochromatosis and neonatal iron overload syndrome, but the probability is low that a link exists.

The neonatal iron overload syndrome is a familial disorder whose genetics are obscure. Some mothers of affected newborns have hints of abnormal iron metabolism, such as moderately elevated saturations of plasma transferrin. Most, however, are normal. Some families have one or two offspring who were victims of the disorder, whereas others have several normal children in addition to the index case. Because the apparently defective placenta is the product of maternal and paternal genes, neonatal iron overload syndrome could result from the inheritance of two abnormal alleles of the gene or genes involved in placental iron transport. Study of this rare disorder could, therefore, provide insight into normal transplacental iron transport.

Erythroid Hyperplasia

The connection between hematopoiesis and iron absorption is most strikingly apparent in patients with ineffective erythropoiesis. Disorders such as β^+-thalassemia (thalassemia intermedia) or sideroblastic anemia increase the fractional absorption of ingested iron. Such patients can develop iron overload without transfusion.[374, 375]

The mechanism by which bone marrow activity modulates gastrointestinal iron absorption is unclear. A soluble factor appears to be released that stimulates iron uptake. In one study, reticulocytosis was induced in rats either by feeding iron-rich food to animals with severe dietary iron deficiency or by injecting phenylhydrazine, a compound that lyses circulating erythrocytes.[77] Internal iron exchange doubled, and iron absorption increased dramatically. Infusion of reticulocyte-rich blood from these animals into normal rats increased internal iron exchange and gastrointestinal iron absorption. In contrast, blood from normal animals was inert. A study involving mice produced similar results.[376] In this case, the active factor appeared to be confined solely to the red cells, with the plasma being inert. This work implies that the erythroid cells convey the iron uptake signal to the gut and that PIT influences the process little. Experiments that directly assess the activity of the iron-absorbing cells are needed to settle the issue.

In humans, robust absorption of iron from the gastrointestinal tract is associated most often with ineffective erythropoiesis, as occurs with β^+-thalassemia, for instance. Hemolytic anemias with effective erythropoiesis produce iron loading only with prodigious marrow activity. Some patients with pyruvate kinase deficiency, a condition frequently associated with reticulocyte counts as high as 70%, develop iron overload without transfusion. Without some compounding variable, such as hereditary hemochromatosis trait, iron loading without transfusion is uncommon in conditions such as sickle cell anemia or hereditary spherocytosis, where the increase in erythroid activity is less dramatic.

Consequences of Iron Overload

The effect of iron overload on some organs, such as the skin, are trivial, whereas hemosiderotic harm to others, such as the liver, can be fatal (see Chapter 21).[353] Few notable symptoms precede advanced injury. Abdominal discomfort, lethargy, and fatigue are common but nonspecific complaints. Dyspnea with exertion and peripheral edema indicate significant cardiac compromise and reflect advanced iron loading.

Liver

As the major site of iron storage, the liver is a conspicuous victim of excess iron deposition.[377] Mild to moderate hepatomegaly develops early, followed by shrinkage produced by fibrosis and cirrhosis.[353, 378] Hepatic tenderness occurs occasionally.

Hematoxylin and eosin staining reveals a brownish pigment in the hepatocytes that Perls' Prussian blue staining unmasks as iron.[379] Large amounts of iron are also deposited in Kupffer cells of patients with transfusional iron overload. Electron microscopy reveals substantial hemosiderin aggregates in addition to large quantities of ferritin.

As with many other conditions that injure the liver, hepatic damage secondary to excessive iron deposition produces fibrosis. With long-standing hemochromatosis, micronodular cirrhosis can also develop. Hemosiderotic liver damage produces very little inflammation. Consequently, significant hepatic iron deposition and even fibrosis can occur with very little increase in the serum transaminase levels. Disturbances in liver synthetic function indicate advanced disease.

Heart

Congestive cardiomyopathy is the most common defect that occurs with iron overload, but other problems have been described, including pericarditis, restrictive cardiomyopathy, and angina without coronary artery disease.[380–383] A strong correlation exists between the cumulative number of blood transfusions and functional cardiac derangements in children with thalassemia.[384, 385]

The physical examination is surprisingly benign even in patients with heavy cardiac iron deposition. Once evidence of cardiac failure appears, however, heart function rapidly deteriorates, often without response to medical intervention. Biventricular failure produces pulmonary congestion, peripheral edema, and hepatic engorgement. This potentially lethal cardiac complication has been reversed on occasion by vigorous iron extrication.[386]

Iron deposition in the bundle of His and the Purkinje system produces conduction defects.[387, 388] Sudden death is common in these patients, presumably due to arrhythmias. At one time, patients treated with the chelator desferrioxamine for transfusional iron overload received supplements of ascorbic acid in the range of 15 to 30 mg/kg per day to promote iron mobilization.[389] Reports of sudden death prompted cessation of this practice.[390] At lower doses (2 to 4 mg/kg), ascorbic acid is a safe adjunct to chelation therapy in patients with transfusional iron overload.

Cardiac dysfunction can occur with very little tissue iron deposition. The total quantity of iron is less important than the unbound, or "toxic," iron subset. The concentration of unbound iron in tissues is extremely small and virtually impossible to measure. This "toxic" iron is precisely the component bound and neutralized by iron chelators (in the case of desferrioxamine, the association constant is about 10^{32}; see later). Therefore, cardiac damage is best prevented in patients with transfusional iron overload by maintaining a constant low level of chelator in the circulation (and consequently in the tissues, where the protection is rendered). Chick cardiac myocytes in culture contract spontaneously. Iron salts added to the culture medium poison the cells and abrogate this function. Desferrioxamine chelates extracellular, and importantly, intracellular iron and restores myocyte contractility.[391]

Echocardiography in children and radionuclide ventriculography in adults are the most useful noninvasive diagnostic techniques. The echocardiographic abnormalities correlate roughly with the number of transfusions. Exercise radionuclide ventriculograms have proven to be particularly sensitive in the detection of cardiac dysfunction in patients with iron overload.[392]

Endocrine

Dysfunction of the endocrine pancreas is common in patients with iron overload.[393] Some persons develop overt diabetes mellitus requiring insulin therapy. The disturbances in carbohydrate metabolism are often more subtle, however. An oral glucose tolerance test often unmasks abnormal insulin production. Vigorous exorcism of the excess iron occasionally reverses the islet cell dysfunction.[394] Exocrine pancreatic function, in contrast, is usually well preserved.

Pituitary dysfunction produces a plethora of endocrine disturbances.[395] Reduced gonadotropin levels are common. When coupled with primary reductions in gonadal synthesis of sex steroids, this phenomenon delays sexual maturation in some children with transfusional iron overload. Secondary infertility is common.[396] Although Addison's syndrome is uncommon with iron overload, production of adrenocorticotropic hormone is occasionally deficient. A metapyrone stimulation test shows delayed or diminished pituitary secretion of this hormone.[397]

Thyroid function is usually well preserved in patients with iron overload. In contrast, parathyroid activity is frequently compromised. Functional hypoparathyroidism can be demonstrated in many patients by inducing hypocalcemia with an intravenous bolus of ethylenediaminetetraacetic acid (EDTA) while monitoring the production of parathyroid hormone.[398]

Miscellaneous Abnormalities With Iron Overload

Hyperpigmentation is a nonspecific skin response to a variety of insults, including excessive exposure to ultraviolet light (tanning), thermal injury, and drug eruptions. Cutaneous iron deposition damages the skin and enhances melanin production by melanocytes. Ultraviolet light exposure and iron are often synergistic in the induction of skin pigmentation, so that many patients tan very readily. Fair-skinned persons who routinely tan poorly often never develop hyperpigmentation despite very large body iron burdens, highlighting the genetic contribution to skin pigmentation. In contrast, patients with moderate baseline pigmentation (e.g., persons of Mediterranean descent) frequently develop a striking almond-colored hue. With particularly heavy iron overload, visible iron deposits sometimes appear in the skin as a grayish discoloration.

Arthropathy, a common feature with hereditary hemochromatosis, is rare in patients with secondary iron overload.[399] The large joints, such as the hips, are affected most commonly.[400] Decades of iron deposition in articular cartilage in hereditary hemochromatosis is the presumed cause of this condition. Chondrocalcinosis is a late but characteristic feature of the arthropathy seen in hereditary hemochromatosis. Other troubling musculoskeletal problems include severe, recurrent cramps and disabling myalgias. Muscle biopsy shows iron deposits in the myocytes, but the pathophysiologic connection to the pain and cramps is unclear.

Iron Overload and Opportunistic Infections

Withholding iron from potential pathogens is one strategy used in host defense.[401] Transferrin's extremely high affinity for iron, coupled with the fact that two thirds of the iron-binding sites of the protein normally are unoccupied, essentially eliminates free iron from plasma and extracellular tissues. Both transferrin and the structurally related protein lactoferrin are bacteriostatic *in vitro* for many bacteria.[402–404]

The very high transferrin saturations attained in patients with iron overload compromise the bacteriostatic properties of the protein. Iron sequestration is not a front-line defense against microbes. Therefore, iron overload does not produce the susceptibility to infection seen with defects in more central systems (e.g., chronic granulomatous disease). Nonetheless, a number of infections, often with unusual organisms, have been reported in patients with iron overload (Table 11–3).[405–408] Sideroblastic anemia often produces neutropenia or neutrophil dysfunction. Host defense is compromised even further in patients with sideroblastic anemia who develop secondary iron overload. Although aggressive antimicrobial therapy is often successful, some infections, such as the mucormycosis produced by *Rhizopus oryzae*, are almost uniformly fatal.

The iron chelator desferrioxamine has also been implicated in opportunistic infection with unusual organisms (e.g., *R. oryzae*) in some patients with iron overload.[409–411] *Streptomyces pilosis* synthesizes this siderophore when grown in an iron-deficient environment. Desferrioxamine is released in the vicinity of these microbes, binds iron, and returns the element to the microorganisms, where it is used for growth and replication. Some pathogenic bacteria and fungi can utilize desferrioxamine-bound iron to promote their growth, thereby enhancing the risk of severe infection.[412]

The question of when to begin chelation therapy in a patient with transfusional hemochromatosis lacks a

Table 11–3. INFECTIOUS AGENTS ASSOCIATED WITH IRON OVERLOAD

Bacterial

Listeria monocytogenes
Yersinia enterocolitica
Salmonella typhimurium
Klebsiella pneumoniae
Vibrio vulnificus
Escherichia coli

Fungal

Cunninghamella bertholeatiae
Rhizopus oryzae
Mucor sp.

simple answer.[413] The decision must be carefully individualized. Serious infection in patients treated with desferrioxamine is uncommon, and the benefits of therapy to prevent iron-induced organ damage generally outweigh the risk of infectious complications.

Treatment of Iron Overload

Phlebotomy

Phlebotomy is the most effective means of removing excess iron from patients with hereditary hemochromatosis. A single unit of blood removes about 200 mg of iron. Persons who are otherwise healthy can often tolerate phlebotomy as frequently as twice a week. Most commonly, a weekly schedule of phlebotomy is used. The process can be continued at this frequency for months in some cases. The rapid compensatory synthesis of new red cells drains iron stores. Phlebotomy is safe for adolescents or young adults. Because hereditary hemochromatosis does not cause iron overload earlier in life, phlebotomy of small children is a moot point.

The endpoint of phlebotomy is the removal of all excess iron. Iron-deficient erythropoiesis characterized by hypochromic, microcytic red cells marks the achievement of this objective. When phlebotomies are initiated, the hematocrit generally does not change from week to week. Meanwhile, the plasma ferritin level and the transferrin saturation fall. Phlebotomy therapy should not be stopped, however, because the rapid changes in iron stores greatly compromise the diagnostic value of these parameters. Transferrin saturation and plasma ferritin reasonably reflect iron status at steady state. Phlebotomy significantly shifts iron stores, which is not a steady-state condition.

After a time ranging from 1 or 2 months to as long as a year, the patient's hematocrit begins to fall several points after each phlebotomy. The transferrin saturation and plasma ferritin levels are usually in a range typical of iron deficiency at this point. The hematocrit quickly returns to baseline, however (often in 1 or 2 weeks). This rapid recovery reflects iron mobilization from the remaining stores. The timing of phlebotomy should be adjusted to compensate for the nadirs, but the therapy should not be terminated.

When the mean corpuscular volume and mean corpuscular hemoglobin concentration begin to fall, the iron stores have been exhausted. At the very least, the rate of iron egress from stores along with iron intake from food does not match the rate of utilization. At this point, the rate of phlebotomy should be reduced to two to four times per year. Erythropoiesis is the physiologic process that is most heavily dependent on iron availability. Iron-deficient erythropoiesis, then, is the best biologic indicator of depleted iron stores.

Patients with brisk hemolysis or ineffective erythropoiesis (e.g., thalassemia intermedia) sometimes develop substantial iron overload without transfusion.[414] Phlebotomy can be attempted if the patient's steady-state hematocrit is in the range of 28% to 30% and no concomitant cardiovascular disease exists. An initial regimen of unit removed every 2 weeks is reasonable. This rate of phlebotomy would remove about 450 mg of iron per month or 15 mg/d. Often this is enough to place the patient into negative iron balance, without the trouble associated with chelation therapy. The caveat to this approach is that phlebotomy can exacerbate marrow hyperplasia. Bone deformities can occur in young children. Another concern is cord compression due to compromise of the spinal canal by hyperplastic marrow (see Chapter 21). The approach to iron overload clearly demands constant vigilance.

Iron Chelation

Parenteral. Desferrioxamine (Desferal) is the only chelator available in the United States to treat chronic iron overload.[415] Several characteristics of the drug place severe constraints on its use. First, absorption from the gastrointestinal tract is limited, dictating parenteral administration. Second, the compound is excreted from the circulation with a half-life of only 10 to 15 minutes.[416] Little or no iron is bound during this time. Therefore, slow continuous parenteral administration is required. Third, desferrioxamine irritates tissues, meaning that only a small amount can be administered at a given site.

The practical translation is a drug given by continuous subcutaneous infusion using a rate-controlled pump.[417, 418] Skin irritation, manifested as raised, painful, erythematous welts, is less severe in children than adults. Nonetheless, the sites of infusion are rotated each day to minimize the problem. The infusion is given over 12 to 16 hours, allowing freedom from the pump for part of the day. Iron mobilization often falls to unacceptable levels when the infusion time is less than 12 hours. Desferrioxamine therapy is most effective when the pump is used daily. Few patients can conform to such a rigid schedule. The infusion should be conducted at least 5 days a week, however.

Subcutaneous infusion of desferrioxamine is impossible for some patients, owing, most often, to intolerable skin irritation. The skin irritation reflects the acrid character of the drug. Otovestibular toxicity occurred in one group of children treated with doses of desferrioxamine that exceeded 150 mg/kg in some instances.[419] Cessation of treatment allowed full recovery, followed by reinitiation of the drug at a level of 25 to 50 mg/kg per day. Long-term chelation therapy with desferrioxamine sometimes produces bone disease.[420] Chelation of minerals required to form hydroxyapatite in developing bone is the presumed cause of this complication. The association of desferrioxamine treatment and infection is detailed earlier.

Immunologic reactions to the drug are rare and include urticaria and anaphylaxis. Desensitization procedures, similar to those used for persons with penicillin hypersensitivity, have allowed chelation treatment of some patients with immunologic intolerance.[421] Desferrioxamine must be continued without a break in these instances, to prevent recovery of immune sensitivity.

The drug mobilizes iron more efficiently when administered as a continuous intravenous infusion (usually by way of a permanent, indwelling central venous catheter). The urine acquires an orange color, reflecting the excretion of the iron/desferrioxamine complex (ferrioxamine) by the kidneys. Desferrioxamine has been used in peritoneal dialysis fluids in some patients on chronic ambulatory peritoneal dialysis regimens, with effective removal of excess iron deposits.[422] Aggressive opportunistic infections that are sometimes fatal have occurred in some of these patients, however,[409] and other complications, described in Chapter 21, have been noted.

Oral. An orally effective iron chelator is the "Holy Grail" of chelation.[423] Many agents have been advanced, and all have failed to meet the exacting requirements. Only one drug presently occupies the field of competition, 1,2-dimethyl-3-hydroxypyrid-4-one, also called L1 or deferiprone.[424–426] After some early stumbles, L1 has emerged with clinical promise and has entered clinical trials.[427, 428] One infrequent, but serious, side effect of the drug is reversible granulocytopenia.[135, 429] The field trials will tell whether this idiosyncrasy of the drug will be its "Achilles' heel."[430] Whether the drug is actually effective in most cases has been brought into question.[430a]

Maternal-Fetal Iron Balance

Iron Delivery to the Fetus

About 1 g of iron is required for full-term fetal development, with about 300 mg incorporated into fetal tissues. Iron transport to the fetus depends completely on the placenta. This organ removes from the maternal circulation all the iron necessary for fetal development, even at the expense of maternal iron deficiency.[431, 432]

The PIT is a major determinant of gastrointestinal iron absorption. Ordinarily, the erythroid cells in the bone marrow dominate the PIT. During pregnancy, however, placental iron uptake increases the PIT, thereby boosting gastrointestinal iron absorption. This physiologic increase in iron absorption by the maternal gut raises the availability of the element to the developing fetus.

The placenta has a wealth of transferrin receptors that facilitate iron uptake, presumably by the same receptor-mediated endocytosis that occurs in other tissues.[433] The mechanics of iron transport across the placenta to the maternal circulation remain a mystery.[434] One hypothesis holds that after uptake, iron is sequestered in the abundant pool of placental ferritin, which then diffuses across the organ to the region of the fetal circulation. Although electron micrographs are consistent with this hypothesis, these static images provide no information about dynamics. The expression of transferrin receptors by the placenta increases in response to fetal iron demand, suggesting the existence of a regulatory mechanism in the placental-fetal unit.[435]

Equally mysterious is the mechanism by which iron is placed onto transferrin in the fetal circulation. Specific machinery no doubt is responsible, but information on its nature is lacking. Unlike the situation with hemoglobin, no fetal-specific transferrin exists. There-

fore the driving force for iron delivery to the fetal circulation is not an electrochemical gradient from low-affinity to high-affinity transferrin molecules.

Although iron transport across the placenta superficially resembles the uptake of the element from the gastrointestinal tract, significant differences exist between the two processes. Most important is the fact that the placenta takes up iron that is coupled to transferrin, whereas iron in the alimentary tract is liganded to inorganic molecules. The placenta is remarkably efficient at acquiring iron from the maternal circulation.

The placenta is programmed to take up iron without signals or cues from the fetus. In one study, the placentas of pregnant rats continued to remove iron efficiently from the maternal circulation for several days after excision of the fetuses.[436] Because the iron could no longer be transferred to the fetus, it accumulated abnormally in the placenta.

Effects on the Fetus of Maternal Iron Deficiency

With maternal iron deficiency, the placenta is concerned only with the welfare of the fetus. The organ will remove iron from the mother to support fetal development even at the cost of worsened maternal iron balance. For years, investigators debated the effect of maternal iron deficiency on the fetus.[257, 437, 438] The controversy was fueled by the indirect and imprecise assays of neonatal iron status, such as the cord blood ferritin level or transferrin saturation. These parameters in cord blood are subject to all the vicissitudes that buffet values in later life. Accurate determination of neonatal iron status was difficult, if not impossible. The one point on which nearly universal agreement existed was that neonatal anemia due to maternal iron deficiency is rare.

The most compelling data concerning this issue came from a study of women who had elective abortions.[439] The iron status of the mothers was determined from transferrin saturation, plasma ferritin levels, and hemoglobin values. This information was correlated with the iron status of the fetuses, which was determined by atomic absorption spectroscopy of the complete abortus. This procedure determined absolutely the fetal iron content. Fetal iron stores varied linearly with maternal hemoglobin, which ranged between 6 g/dL (severe iron deficiency) and 13 g/dL (adequate, although possibly low, iron stores). Although neonatal iron deficiency anemia is quite uncommon, maternal iron status over a wide range of values determines the iron stores of the neonate.

Consequences of Neonatal Iron Deficiency

Neonatal iron deficiency is a potentially serious problem, owing, in part, to the immaturity of the gastrointestinal tract. This organ absorbs inefficiently numerous nutrients, including iron. The placenta no longer bolsters the nutritional needs of the newborn, increasing the vulnerability of the newborn to deficiency. As detailed earlier, iron deficiency in newborns creates hazards that supersede the routine anemia and microcytosis.

Defective Plasma Iron Transport

After uptake in the duodenum and upper jejunum, iron is coupled to transferrin for its sojourn through the circulation to peripheral tissues. Disturbances in this phase of iron metabolism are unusual. When problems do occur, the consequences are often dire.

Congenital Atransferrinemia

Congenital atransferrinemia is a rare disorder in which transferrin is synthesized in such small quantities as to be virtually absent in some patients.[129] With insufficient transferrin, most dietary iron is free in the circulation or loosely bound to other plasma proteins, such as albumin. The normal pattern of iron metabolism is altered drastically. Cells that require transferrin-mediated iron uptake, such as normoblasts, develop severe iron deficiency, whereas hepatocytes (with transferrin-independent iron uptake) have a surfeit. The non–transferrin-mediated iron uptake system (see earlier) deposits much of the plasma iron in the liver and other organs. The heavy hepatic iron deposition eventually leads to cellular necrosis and fibrosis. Hepatic failure often is central to the death of these children.

Diminished delivery of iron to normoblasts reduces hemoglobin production, producing a microcytic, hypochromic anemia. Although these patients do not have systemic iron deficiency, functional deficiency of the element exists in tissues where transferrin-mediated iron uptake is crucial. Congenital atransferrinemia is very uncommon, with only a few family groups described.[440] The currently available tools of recombinant DNA technology have not been applied systematically to any of the pedigrees to elucidate the molecular mechanism. The array of possible defects that would produce the phenotype range from gene deletions or splice variants to defective glycosylation or secretion. A more thorough understanding of the disorder could also provide insight into the physiologic role of non–transferrin-mediated iron uptake.

Defective Transferrins

Defective transferrin molecules are extremely rare. These proteins disrupt the delivery of iron to the bone marrow and other tissues. In some instances, iron is weakly bound and tends to dissociate from the plasma transporter. In other instances, the protein fails to bind properly to the transferrin receptor. Affected persons have a hypochromic, microcytic anemia. Infusion of normal transferrin has not been reported but presumably would correct the defect.

Antibodies to the transferrin receptor were isolated from a patient with a lymphoproliferative disorder who acquired a refractory hypochromic, microcytic anemia.[441] The antibody blocked transferrin-mediated iron uptake. The disproportionate effect on normoblast development is consistent with the importance to these cells (as opposed to hepatocytes) of transferrin-mediated iron uptake. Siblings in another report presented with hypochromic, microcytic anemia in the presence of a high transferrin saturation.[442] Liver biopsy revealed elevated hepatic iron stores. Assessments showed that their transferrin delivered iron normally to cultured cells and *in vivo*, ruling out a problem with the protein. Impaired transferrin receptor activity of some type may have led to relative iron starvation of the normoblasts despite hepatic iron overload. The number of receptors on the cells is normal, raising the possibility of physiologically dysfunctional receptors. A second, similar kindred has been reported.[443, 444] These case reports emphasize the critical nature to normoblasts of transferrin-mediated iron uptake.

Defective Intracellular Iron Metabolism

Sideroblastic Anemia

The sideroblastic anemias are a heterogeneous group of disorders characterized by anemia, a low reticulocyte count, and ineffective erythropoiesis (Table 11–4).[445–447] Although the anemia most commonly is normochromic and normocytic, some patients have microcytosis and hypochromia. Ineffective erythropoiesis frequently produces elevated body iron stores. All patients are anemic, and thrombocytopenia and neutropenia develop commonly.[448] About 30% of patients with sideroblastic anemia have elevated levels of erythrocyte protophorins, reflecting the frequent disturbances in heme biosynthesis. The hematopoietic stem cell defect can be congenital or acquired (see Table 11–4). Either form is rare in children, although the congenital variety predominates.

The key to the diagnosis of sideroblastic anemia is Perls' Prussian blue iron staining of bone marrow samples. This procedure highlights the characteristic ring sideroblast, a normoblast with a perinuclear halo of Prussian blue–stained material (Fig. 11–6; see color section at the front of this volume). Electron microscopic examination reveals the rings to be juxtanuclear mitochondria containing large deposits of inorganic iron. In congenital sideroblastic anemia, the rings predominate in late normoblasts, whereas rings occur in early cells in the acquired form.[449]

Table 11–4. CLASSIFICATION OF SIDEROBLASTIC ANEMIAS

Congenital
  X-linked
  Autosomal

Acquired
  Idiopathic
  Alkylating agents (e.g., nitrogen mustard)
  Other drugs
  Ethanol
  Isoniazid
  Chloramphenicol

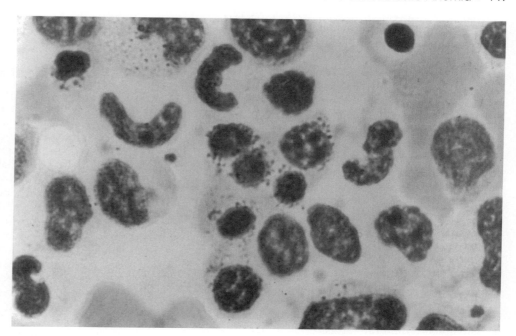

Figure 11-6. Prussian blue stain of a bone marrow aspirate from a patient with sideroblastic anemia. The greenish blue flecks that circle the nucleus of the normoblasts are iron-laden mitochondria (see color section at the front of this volume).

Bone marrow examination frequently reveals erythroid hyperplasia, despite profound anemia. This is the *sine que non* of ineffective erythropoiesis, a condition in which the normoblasts fail to supply mature erythrocytes to the circulation. The nucleus and the cytoplasm of the normoblasts commonly mature asynchronously. These megaloblastic changes (often termed *megaloblastoid*) are less pronounced than those seen with deficiencies of cobalamin or folic acid, however.

Mild to moderate hemolysis exacerbates the anemia produced by ineffective erythropoiesis.[450] The etiology of the peripheral red cell destruction is unknown. Some patients with this disorder develop an acquired form of hemoglobin H disease, which contributes to the hemolysis. Hemoglobin H (tetramers of hemoglobin β-chains) forms in a subpopulation of the developing normoblasts owing to a shutdown of α-globin production. Consequently, its distribution in the circulating erythrocytes is heterogeneous (see Chapter 21).

Chromosomal abnormalities occur frequently in sideroblastic anemia.[446, 451] Some changes, such as the loss of the long arm of chromosomes 5 or 7 (5q− and 7q−, respectively), may have pathophysiologic importance. The genes encoding a number of important growth factors are located on the long arm of chromosome 5, including granulocyte-monocyte colony-stimulating factor and the receptor for monocyte colony-stimulating factor.[452] Whether the loss of these or other genes on the chromosome is causally related to the development of sideroblastic anemia is unknown. A further complication to the conundrum is the fact that only one of the two alleles for any gene typically is lost, meaning that a dose effect of the genes in question contributes to the problem or other inconspicuous interactions occur. Most often, however, karyotype analysis reveals random loss or breaks in chromosomes. Hypodiploid karyotypic changes convey a poor prognosis.[453]

Congenital sideroblastic anemia disproportionately afflicts males. In kindreds of sufficient size to permit genetic analysis, the pattern generally is one of an X-linked recessive defect.[454, 455] Females with the disorder are usually designated simply as having congenital sideroblastic anemia, because the family trees are often too small to ascertain the pattern of inheritance.[456] As a syndrome, the sideroblastic anemia phenotype can result from any of multiple metabolic defects.

Sideroblastic anemia in children is often associated with defects in the enzymes of the heme biosynthetic pathway. The best characterized of these involves impairment of δ-aminolevulinic acid synthase (ALAS), the first and rate-limiting enzyme in heme biosynthesis.[457] Reduced ALAS activity has been reported in patients from several kindreds. A less well-characterized defect in ferrochelatase activity has been noted in a few.[458] Impaired production of heme resulting from these defects is the presumed trigger of mitochondrial iron accumulation and the formation of ring sideroblasts. Disturbed heme biosynthesis reduces hemoglobin production, leading to the microcytic, hypochromic anemia.[459]

The cloning of an erythroid-specific gene for ALAS, *eALAS* (ALAS2), opened new vistas in the understanding of sideroblastic anemia. In contrast to the autosomal gene that encodes the housekeeping form of ALAS, *eALAS* is located on the X chromosome (see earlier). Point mutations in the gene have been identified in several patients with sideroblastic anemia.[460, 461] These defects may compromise enzyme synthesis in some cases or catalytic activity in others. Possible molecular probes for the disorder open the prospect of genetic analysis even of small kindreds. Such investigations could contribute substantially to our understanding of this disorder specifically and to the coordination of heme/hemoglobin production, generally. Interestingly, the kindred described by Cooley in the initial report of familial sideroblastic anemia was analyzed using molecular techniques and found to have a defect in eALAS.[462]

A number of drugs and toxins that impair heme biosynthesis can produce sideroblastic anemia (see Table 11–4). The most important of these is lead. As noted previously, this element inhibits multiple enzymes in the heme biosynthetic pathway. Lead screening, therefore, is mandatory in any child suspected of having sideroblastic anemia, because lead poisoning can be treated. Isoniazid also produces sideroblastic anemia by inhibiting enzymes in the heme biosynthetic pathway. Prophylactic treatment with pyridoxine, which neutralizes the enzyme inhibition, is now part of the standard therapeutic regimen with this drug.

The age at clinical onset of congenital sideroblastic anemia varies greatly in the reported cases. Some children develop anemia within a few months of birth, whereas manifestations of the full-blown disorder do not appear in others before the age of 7 or 8 years.[449] Generally, the anemia is progressive, often requiring transfusions to maintain an acceptable hematocrit. Frequent transfusions can hasten the development of iron overload.

Although anemia is usually the initial manifestation of the disorder, stem cell dysfunction often produces significant thrombocytopenia and neutropenia. Polymorphonuclear leukocytes and platelets may function poorly even in patients in whom the counts are normal.[463, 464] The platelet defect produces abnormal aggregation patterns *in vitro*, including impaired responses to epinephrine, arachidonic acid, and collagen. Clinically, these changes may be manifested as a prolonged bleeding time and a predilection to frank hemorrhage. Neutrophil dysfunction, along with neutropenia, often places these children at increased risk of serious infection.

Oral pyridoxine therapy has been used in some patients with either acquired or congenital sideroblastic anemia.[465] The pyridoxine is thought to compensate partially for the defect in ALAS activity. Often, however, the correction of the anemia is incomplete. A few children who failed pyridoxine therapy have responded to the parenteral administration of pyridoxal-5-phosphate.[466] Unfortunately, most children with congenital sideroblastic anemia improve little, if at all, with either of these interventions. Because pyridoxine is inexpensive and lacks deleterious side effects, all children with sideroblastic anemia should receive a trial of vitamin therapy. Pyridoxal-5-phosphate is unavailable even for experimental therapy.

In the adult form of acquired sideroblastic anemia, conversion to acute myelogenous leukemia occurs in 15% to 20% of patients.[467–469] The rate of such conversion in children is unknown. Sometimes, patients who have received chemotherapy containing alkylating agents, such as MOPP (mechlorethamine [Mustargen], vincristine [Oncovin], procarbazine, and prednisone) for Hodgkin's disease, subsequently develop myelodysplasia, including sideroblastic anemia.[470] Conversion to a very aggressive acute leukemia that is resistant to chemotherapy occurs with dismaying frequency.

Defects in Intermediary Metabolism

Occasionally, sideroblastic anemia in children appears as a component of syndromes with disturbances in cellular metabolism. A rare cohort of children with sideroblastic anemia have an inherited defect in thiamine metabolism. These patients with Wolfram syndrome or DIDMOAD (diabetes insipidus, diabetes mellitus, optic atrophy, and deafness) sometimes develop a bizarre anemia with both megaloblastic and sideroblastic characteristics.[471] The manifestations of the syndrome frequently appear shortly after birth and progress over several years. Hematopoiesis is often markedly disturbed, with prominent sideroblastic changes in the normoblasts. Therapy with thiamine has partially reversed the anemia in some children. The disorder is believed to result from an autosomal recessive defect in thiamine phosphokinase activity. The pathophysiology of the changes that produce the clinical syndrome is unresolved.

Another metabolic defect produces Pearson's syndrome, a fatal disorder of infancy with marked disturbances in bone marrow and pancreatic function (McKusick No. 26056).[472, 473] The initial manifestation often is a severe, transfusion-dependent, macrocytic anemia plus a variable degree of neutropenia and thrombocytopenia. Striking vacuolization occurs in the erythroid and myeloid precursors, along with hemosiderosis and ringed sideroblasts. Exocrine pancreatic dysfunction occurs frequently. Necropsy reveals prominent pancreatic fibrosis. Some victims develop hepatic, renal, and neurologic dysfunction as well.

Pearson's marrow-pancreas syndrome is a mitochondrial cytopathy.[474, 475] A pair of children in one family had deletions of segments of mitochondrial DNA that encode subunits of the respiratory enzymes.[476] Defective energy production appears to be the central disturbance. The variable expression in the described patients possibly represents the inconstant inheritance of defective mitochondria, which are derived stochastically solely from the mother.[477] No treatment exists.

Systemic Defects in Iron Metabolism
Anemia of Chronic Inflammation

The anemia of chronic inflammation, sometimes called the anemia of chronic disease, is a well-recognized condition associated with a broad spectrum of maladies, the common features of which are chronicity and inflammation.[478, 479] The mild-to-moderate anemia (hemoglobin level of 10 to 11 g/dL) lacks pathognomonic features. The red cell distribution width of the normochromic, normocytic red cells is slightly elevated, reflecting a mild anisocytosis. Pappenheimer bodies (iron granules) are variably present in the erythrocytes. Together with Howell-Jolly bodies, these indicate that the underlying disorder has produced splenic dysfunction. Likewise, target cells or schistocytes, when present, are products of the primary disorder.

Inflammation is the key to the condition. Chronic disorders that lack an inflammatory component, such as congestive heart failure due to essential hypertension, for instance, do not produce the anemia of chronic inflammation. The shift in nomenclature from anemia of chronic disease emphasizes this point.

Plasma ferritin levels are almost uniformly elevated in the anemia of chronic inflammation.[258] Most often, the increase is modest (400 to 600 µg/L), but substantially greater levels sometimes occur. The transferrin saturation is usually normal or only slightly depressed (15% to 25%) and serum transferrin is usually low. A normal to low transferrin saturation in the presence of an elevated plasma ferritin distinguishes the anemia of chronic inflammation from routine iron deficiency where both values are low, as well as from iron overload where both are high.

Bone marrow examination of iron stores with Perls' Prussian blue staining reveals large deposits of iron in the reticuloendothelial cells. This characteristic feature of the anemia of chronic inflammation reflects ineffective iron reutilization. Normoblasts that fail to mature properly (a routine occurrence) and effete red cells are engulfed by marrow reticuloendothelial cells that degrade the protein and lipid and recycle the iron from hemoglobin onto transferrin for subsequent use by newly developing red cell precursors. The anemia of chronic inflammation disturbs this cycle, leaving iron stored as hemosiderin in the reticuloendothelial cells. The pattern of staining of the normoblasts is usually unremarkable. Some patients display occasional ring sideroblasts, however.

The etiology of these disturbances is unknown, although recent *in vitro* experiments have provided some clues. Proinflammatory cytokines, such as interleukin-1 and interleukin-6, activate ferritin synthesis in cultured cells in the absence of iron.[190, 193] The empty ferritin shells constitute excess iron storage capacity and could lead to the sequestration of the element due to a simple trapping process.[480] Eventually, the ferritin would be converted into hemosiderin. Antimetabolites can suppress the local inflammatory response, consistent with a role for a biologically active cell product in this condition.[481]

The fact that inflammation is a common feature to the disorders that produce this type of anemia is consistent with (but does not prove) this mechanism. Control of the chronic inflammation (e.g., patients with ulcerative colitis who undergo colectomy) usually eliminates the anemia and corrects the disturbances in iron metabolism. The anemia is recalcitrant whereas inflammation is uncontrolled. The elevated plasma ferritin level possibly relates to this process. Because plasma ferritin is a secreted protein whose site of production remains a mystery, the hypothesis cannot be directly tested.

Patients with the anemia of chronic inflammation have unusually low plasma erythropoietin levels for their degree of anemia.[482, 483] This finding is consistent with *in vitro* data in which proinflammatory cytokines suppress erythropoietin production by cells in culture (see Chapter 6).[484] The involvement of erythropoietin in the anemia of chronic inflammation reflects the multifactorial nature of the condition.

Erythropoietin and Functional Iron Deficiency

Human erythropoietin was one of the first agents of widespread clinical utility produced by recombinant DNA technology (rHepo). Used to correct the anemia of end-stage renal disease, this hormone has provided new insight into the kinetic relationship between iron and erythropoietin in red cell production. Erythropoietin treatment of anemia in patients with end-stage renal disease has also underscored the variable nature of storage iron. The shifting states of storage iron contributes to the inconsistency with which erythropoietin corrects the anemia of renal failure.

With steady-state erythropoiesis, iron and erythropoietin flow to the bone marrow at constant, low rates. In patients with end-stage renal disease, recombinant human erythropoietin (rHepo) is administered in intermittent surges, most commonly as intravenous boluses.[485] The resulting kinetics of erythropoiesis are markedly unphysiologic and strain the production process. Erythropoietin, the accelerator of erythroid proliferation, is not coordinated with the supply of iron, the fuel for erythroid proliferation. This imbalance almost never occurs naturally. The rHepo jars previously quiescent cells to proliferate and produce hemoglobin. The requirement for iron jumps dramatically and outstrips its rate of delivery by transferrin.[486]

Interplay Between Iron and Erythropoietin

Erythropoietin stimulates proliferation and differentiation of erythroid precursors, with an upsurge in heme synthesis. Iron is taken into the cells from ferrotransferrin by cell surface transferrin receptors, is transported to the mitochondria, and is inserted into the protoporphyrin IX ring by ferrochelatase. The newly synthesized heme modulates globin synthesis in part through its effect on the translational factor eIF-2. Primitive erythroid cells have relatively few transferrin receptors. The number increases with differentiation, peaking at over 10^6 per cell in the late pronormoblasts. The number subsequently declines to the point that mature erythroid cells lack transferrin receptors altogether. This variable expression of transferrin receptors means that iron delivery must be synchronized both with proliferation and stage of erythroid development.[487] Late normoblasts, for instance, cannot compensate for iron that was not delivered during the basophilic normoblast stage. These cells have fewer transferrin receptors, and those receptors are busy supplying iron for *currently* produced heme molecules.

Transferrin-bound iron is the only important source of the element for erythroid precursors. Even with normal body iron stores and transferrin saturation, robust proliferation of erythroid precursors can create a demand that outstrips the capacity of the iron-delivery system.[165, 488] Transferrin iron saturation falls as the available iron on plasma transferrin is stripped off by voracious erythroid precursors. Plasma iron turnover (PIT) rises, as does erythron iron turnover (EIT) and erythron transferrin uptake (ETU).[489, 490] The late arrival of newly mobilized storage iron fails to prevent production of hypochromic cells. This is "functional iron deficiency" or "iron-erythropoietin kinetic imbalance."

The patients with end-stage renal disease who initially received erythropoietin had substantial iron stores.[491] More importantly, supraphysiologic quantities of iron were bound to their circulating transferrin (i.e., transferrin saturations of 70% to 90%). As a result, even the bursts of heme production induced by pharmacologic levels of exogenously administered rHepo could be matched by the available transferrin-bound iron. In these patients, the rate-limiting factor in erythrocyte synthesis was the proliferative capacity of the erythroid precursors. The number of red cells produced was determined by the number of precursor cells and the quantity of erythropoietin they encountered.

When patients with "ordinary" iron stores were begun on erythropoietin, the picture was quite different. Here, the cells were jolted into accelerated proliferation while transferrin saturations ranged only between 30% and 50%. Iron was rapidly pulled into the developing erythroid cells. In some instances, transferrin-bound iron could sustain maximal synthesis of hemoglobin. In other cases, however, iron availability was suboptimal, producing mild functional iron deficiency. Even when the hemoglobin concentration increased substantially, the transferrin saturation fell, reflecting the strain on the supply system (Fig. 11–7).[165] The quantity of iron in *storage* was more than adequate to meet the demands of hemoglobin synthesis but could not be mobilized with sufficient speed to satisfy the developing normoblasts. The kinetic mismatch in *circulating* rHepo

and *circulating* ferrotransferrin is the key to functional iron deficiency.

Acknowledgment:

The authors gratefully acknowledge the expert stylistic and technical input of Ms. Marilyn Daly and Ms. Lorraine Holman. Without their help, this work would not have been completed. The chapter was prepared with the support of NIH grant R01 HL-45794.

References

1. Karlin KD: Metalloenzymes, structural motifs, and inorganic models. Science 1993; 261:701.
2. Gutteridge JMC, Rowley DA, Halliwell B: Superoxide-dependent formation of hydroxyl radicals in the presence of iron salts. Biochem J 1981; 199:263.
3. Prigerio R, Mela Q, et al: Iron overload and lysosomal stability in beta zero-thalassemia intermedia and trait: correlation between serum ferritin and serum N-acetyl-β-D-glucosaminidase levels. Scand J Haematol 1984; 33:252.
4. Hebbel RP: The sickle erythrocyte in double jeopardy: autoxidation and iron decompartmentalization. Semin Hematol 1990; 27:51.
5. Kuross SA, Rank BH, Hebbel RP: Excess heme in sickle erythrocyte inside-out membranes: possible role in thiol oxidation. Blood 1988; 71:876.
6. Kuross SA, Rank BH, Hebbel RP: Iron compartments associated with sickle cell RBC membranes: a mechanism for targeting of oxidative damage. Progr Clin Biol Res 1989; 319:601.
7. Kannan R, Labotka R, Low PS: Isolation and characterization of the hemichrome-stabilized membrane protein aggregates from sickle erythrocytes. Major site of autologous antibody binding. J Biol Chem 1988; 263:13766.
8. Schluter K, Drenckhan D: Co-clustering of denatured hemoglobin with band 3: its role in binding of autoantibodies against band 3 to abnormal and aged erythrocytes. Proc Natl Acad Sci U S A 1986; 83:6137.
9. Waugh SM, Willardson BM, et al: Heinz bodies induce clustering of band 3, glycophorin and ankyrin in sickle cell erythrocytes. J Clin Invest 1988; 78:1155.
10. Yuan J, Kannan R, et al: Isolation, characterization, and immunoprecipitation studies of immune complexes from membranes of beta-thalassemic erythrocytes. Blood 1992; 79:3007.
11. Repka T, Shalev O, et al: Nonrandom association of free iron with membranes of sickle and beta-thalassemic erythrocytes. Blood 1993; 82:3204.
12. Repka T, Hebbel RP: Hydroxyl radical formation by sickle erythrocyte membranes: role of pathologic iron deposits and cytoplasmic reducing agents. Blood 1991; 78:2753.
13. Shalev O, Repka T, et al: Deferiprone (L1) chelates pathologic iron deposits from membranes of intact thalassemic and sickle red blood cells both *in vitro* and *in vivo*. Blood 1995; 86:2008.
14. Babior BM: The respiratory burst oxidase. Trends Biochem Sci 1987; 12:241.
15. Dabbagh AJ, Trenam CW, et al: Iron in joint inflammation. Ann Rheum Dis 1993; 52:67.
16. Muirden KD: Ferritin in synovial cells in patients with rheumatoid arthritis. Ann Rheum Dis 1966; 25:387.
17. Babior BM: Oxidants from phagocytes: agents of defense and destruction. Blood 1984; 64:959.
18. Rowley D, Gutteridge JM, et al: Lipid peroxidation in rheumatoid arthritis: thiobarbituric acid-reactive material and catalytic iron salts in synovial fluid from rheumatoid patients. Clin Sci 1984; 66:691.
19. Blake DR, Hall ND, et al: Protection against superoxide and hydrogen peroxide in synovial fluid from rheumatoid patients. Clin Sci 1981; 68:483.
20. Winyard P, Blake D, et al: Mechanism of exacerbation of rheumatoid synovitis by total-dose iron-dextran infusion: *in-vivo*

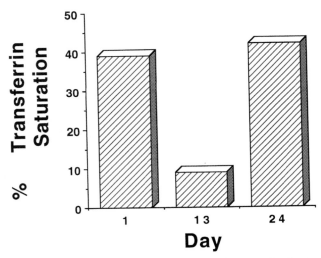

Figure 11–7. Transferrin saturation with iron in normal volunteers treated with erythropoietin. Men were treated with subcutaneous erythropoietin at a dose of 300 U/kg every 3 days for 12 days (four doses, total). During this time the patients received oral iron supplementation. The transferrin saturation was measured at the beginning of treatment (day 1), at the end (day 13), and 10 days after the completion of the study (day 24).

demonstration of iron-promoted oxidant stress. Lancet 1987; 1:69.

21. Andrews FJ, Morris CJ, et al: Effect of iron chelation on inflammatory joint disease. Ann Rheum Dis 1987; 46:327.

22. Cairo G, Tacchini L, et al: Induction of ferritin synthesis by oxidative stress. J Biol Chem 1995; 270:700.

23. Theil EC: Ferritin: structure, gene regulation and cellular function in animals, plants and microorganisms. Annu Rev Biochem 1987; 56:289.

24. Cook JD, Skikne BS, et al: Estimates of iron sufficiency in the US population. Blood 1986; 68:726.

25. Bothwell TH, Charlton RW: A general approach of the problems of iron deficiency and iron overload in the population at large. Semin Hematol 1982; 19:54.

26. McCance RA, Widdowson EM: The absorption and excretion of iron following oral and intravenous administration. J Physiol 1938; 94:148.

27. Gibson RS, MacDonald AC, Smit-Vanderkooy PD: Serum ferritin and dietary iron parameters in a sample of Canadian preschool children. J Can Diet Assoc 1988; 49:23.

28. Gitland D, Cruchard A: On the kinetics of iron absorption in mice. J Clin Invest 1962; 41:344.

29. Muir A, Hopfer U: Regional specificity of iron uptake by small intestinal brush-border membranes from normal and iron deficient mice. Gastrointest Liver Pathol 1985; 11:6376.

30. Kappas A, Drummond GS, Galbraith RA: Prolonged clinical use of a heme oxygenase inhibitor: hematological evidence for an inducible but reversible iron-deficiency state. Pediatrics 1993; 91:537.

31. Conrad ME, Umbreit JN: A concise review: iron absorption—the mucin-mobilferrin-integrin pathway. A competitive pathway for metal absorption. Am J Hematol 1993; 42:67.

32. Huebers HA, Huebers E, et al: The significance of transferrin for intestinal iron absorption. Blood 1993; 61:283.

33. Idzerda RL, Huebers H, et al: Rat transferrin gene expression: tissue-specific regulation by iron deficiency. Proc Natl Acad Sci U S A 1986; 83:3723.

34. Schumann K, Schafer SG, Forth W: Iron absorption and biliary excretion of transferrin in rats. Res Exp Med 1986; 186:215.

35. Simpson RJ, Osterloh KRS, et al: Studies on the role of transferrin and endocytosis on the uptake of Fe3+ from Fe-nitriloacetate by mouse duodenum. Biochim Biophys Acta 1986; 884:166.

36. Bezwoda WR, MacPhail AP, et al: Failure of transferrin to enhance iron absorption in achlorhydric human subjects. Br J Haematol 1986; 63:749.

37. Parmley RT, Barton JC, Conrad ME: Ultrastructural localization of transferrin, transferrin receptor and iron-binding sites on human placental and duodenal microvilli. Br J Haematol 1985; 60:81.

38. Levin MJ, Tuil D, et al: Expression of transferrin gene during development of non-hepatic tissues: high level of transferrin mRNA in fetal muscle and adult brain. Biochem Biophys Res Commun 1984; 122:212.

39. Banerjee D, Flanagan PR, et al: Transferrin receptors in the human gastrointestinal tract. Relationship to body iron stores. Gastroenterology 1986; 91:861.

40. Heilmeyer L, Keller W, et al: Congenital transferrin deficiency in a seven-year old girl. German Med Monthly 1961; 6:385.

41. Craven CM, Alexander J, et al: Tissue distribution and clearance kinetics of non-transferrin-bound iron in the hypotransferrinemic mouse: a rodent model for hemochromatosis. Proc Natl Acad Sci U S A 1987; 84:3457.

42. Dancis A, Haile D, et al: The *Saccharomyces cerevisiae* copper transport protein (Ctr1): biochemical characterization, regulation by copper, and physiologic role in copper uptake. J Biol Chem 1994; 269:25660.

43. Stearman R, Yuan DS, et al: A permease-oxidase complex involved in high-affinity iron uptake in yeast. Science 1996; 271:1552.

44. Dancis A, Yuan DS, et al: Molecular characterization of a copper transport protein in S. cerevisiae: an unexpected role for copper in iron transport. Cell 1994; 76:393.

45. De Silva DM, Askwith CC, et al: The FET3 gene product required for high affinity iron transport in yeast is a cell surface ferroxidase. J Biol Chem 1995; 270:1098.

46. Yuan DS, Stearman R, et al: The Menkes/Wilson disease gene homologue in yeast provides copper to a ceruloplasmin-like oxidase required for iron uptake. Proc Natl Acad Sci U S A 1995; 92:2632.

47. Harford JB, Rouault TA, et al: Molecular mechanisms of iron metabolism. In Stamatoyannopoulos G, Nienhuis W, et al (eds): The Molecular Basis of Blood Diseases. Philadelphia, W.B. Saunders Co., 1994.

48. Lahey ME, Gubler CJ, et al: Studies on copper metabolism: II. Hematologic manifestations of copper deficiency in swine. Blood 1952; 7:1075.

49. Gubler CJ, Lahey ME, et al: Studies on copper metabolism: III. The metabolism of iron in copper deficient swine. Blood 1952; 7:1075.

50. Cartwright GE, Gubler CJ, et al: Studies on copper metabolism: XVII. Further observations on the anemia of copper deficiency in swine. Blood 1956; 11:143.

51. Bannerman RM: Genetic defects of iron transport. Fed Proc 1976; 35:2281.

52. Finch C: Regulators of iron balance in humans. Blood 1994; 84:1697.

53. Huff RL, Hennessey TG, et al: Plasma and red cell iron turnover in normal subjects and in patients having various hematopoietic disorders. J Clin Invest 1950; 29:1041.

54. Weintraub LR, Conrad ME, Crosby WH: Regulation of the intestinal absorption of iron by the rate of erythropoiesis. Br J Hematol 1965; 2:432.

55. Beutler E, Buttenweiser E: The regulation of iron absorption: I. A search for humoral factors. J Lab Clin Med 1960; 55:274.

56. Aron J, Baynes R, et al: Does plasma transferrin regulate iron absorption? Scand J Haematol 1985; 35:451.

57. Raja KN, Pippard MJ, et al: Relationship between erythropoiesis and the enhanced intestinal uptake of ferric iron in hypoxia in the mouse. Br J Haematol 1986; 64:587.

58. Piomelli S, Seaman C, Kapoor S: Lead-induced abnormalities of porphyrin metabolism. The relationship with iron deficiency. Ann NY Acad Sci 1987; 514:278.

59. Ponka P, Schulman HM: Regulation of heme biosynthesis: distinct features in erythroid cells. Stem Cells 1993; 11(Suppl 1):24.

60. Huebers HA, Finch CA: The physiology of transferrin and transferrin receptors. Physiol Rev 1987; 67:520.

61. Williams J, Ellerman TC, et al: The primary structure of hen ovotransferrin. Eur J Biochem 1982; 122:297.

62. Mazurier J, Metz-Boutigue M, et al: Human lactotransferrin: molecular, functional and evolutionary comparisons with human serum transferrin and hen ovotransferrin. Experientia 1983; 39:135.

63. Metz-Boutigue MH, Jolies J, et al: Human lactotransferrin: amino acid sequence and structural comparison with other transferrins. Eur J Biochem 1984; 145:659.

64. Brown JP, Henwick RM, et al: Human melanoma-associated antigen p97 is structurally and functionally related to transferrin. Nature 1982; 296:171.

65. He J, Furmanski P: Sequence specificity and transcriptional activation in the binding of lactoferrin to DNA. Nature 1995; 373:721.

66. Baker EN, Lindley PF: New perspectives on the structure and function of transferrins. J Inorgan Biochem 1992; 47:147.

67. Osaki S, Johnson DA: Mobilization of liver iron by ferroxidase (ceruloplasmin). J Biol Chem 1969; 244:5757.

68. Osaki S, Johnson DA, Frieden E: The mobilization of iron from the perfused mammalian liver by a serum copper enzyme, ferroxidase I. J Biol Chem 1971; 246:3018.

69. Yoshida K, Furihata K, et al: A mutation in the ceruloplasmin gene is associated with systemic hemosiderosis in humans. Nat Genet 1995; 9:267,

70. Harris ZL, Takahashi Y, et al: Aceruloplasminemia: molecular characterization of this disorder of iron metabolism. Proc Natl Acad Sci U S A 1995; 92:2539.

71. Aisen P, Listowsky I: Iron transport and storage proteins. Annu Rev Biochem 1980; 49:357.

72. Harris DC, Aisen P: Physical biochemistry of the transferrins. In Loehr TM, Gray HB, Lever ABP (eds): Iron Carriers and Iron Proteins. Weinheim, VCH Publishers, 1989, pp 239–351.

73. Shongwe MS, Smith CA, et al: Anion binding by human lacto-

ferrin: results from crystallographic and physicochemical studies. Biochemistry 1992; 31:4451.

74. Bailey S, Evans RW, et al: Molecular structure of serum transferrin at 3.3-A resolution. Biochemistry 1988; 27:5804.

75. Anderson BF, Baker HM, et al: Structure of human lactoferrin: crystallographic structure analysis and refinement at 2.8 A resolution. J Mol Biol 1989; 209:711.

76. Jandl JH, Katz JH: The plasma-to-cell cycle of transferrin. J Clin Invest 1963; 42:314.

77. Finch C, Huebers H, et al: Effect of transfused reticulocytes on iron exchange. Blood 1982; 59:364.

78. Laurell C, Ingelman B: The iron-binding protein of swine serum. Acta Chem Scand 1947; 1:770.

79. Sutherland R, Delia D, et al: Ubiquitous cell-surface glycoprotein on tumor cells is proliferation-associated receptor for transferrin. Proc Natl Acad Sci U S A 1980; 78:4515.

80. Kuhn LC, McClelland A, Ruddle FH: Gene transfer, expression and molecular cloning of the human transferrin receptor gene. Cell 1984; 37:95.

81. Schneider C, Kurkinen M, Greaves M: Isolation of cDNA clones for the human transferrin receptor. EMBO J 1983; 2:2259.

82. Jing SQ, Trowbridge IS: Identification of the intermolecular disulfide bonds of the human transferrin receptor and its lipid-attachment site. EMBO J 1987; 6:327.

83. Reckhow CL, Enns CA: Characterization of the transferrin receptor in tunicamycin-treated A431 cells. J Biol Chem 1988; 263:7297.

84. Hayes GR, Enns CA, Lucas JJ: Identification of the O-linked glycosylation site of the human transferrin receptor. Glycobiology 1992; 2:355.

85. Williams AM, Enns CA: A mutated transferrin receptor lacking asparagine-linked glycosylation sites shows reduced functionality and an association with binding immunoglobulin protein. J Biol Chem 1993; 266:17648.

86. Williams AM, Enns CA: A region of the C-terminal portion of the human transferrin receptor contains and asparagine-linked glycosylation site critical for receptor structure and function. J Biol Chem 1993; 268:12780.

87. Zerial M, Melancon P, et al: The transmembrane segment of the human transferrin receptor functions as a signal peptide. EMBO J 1986; 5:1543.

88. Alvarez E, Girones N, Davis RJ: Inhibition of receptor-mediated endocytosis of diferric transferrin is associated with covalent modification of the transferrin receptor with palmitic acid. J Biol Chem 1990; 265:16644.

89. Jing SQ, Trowbridge IS: Nonacylated human transferrin receptors are rapidly internalized and mediate iron uptake. J Biol Chem 1990; 265: 11555.

90. Karin M, Mintz B: Receptor-mediated endocytosis of transferrin in developmentally totipotent mouse teratocarcinoma stem cells. J Biol Chem 1981; 256:3245.

91. Klausner RD, van Renswoude J, et al: Receptor-mediated endocytosis of transferrin in K562 cells. J Biol Chem 1983; 258:4715.

92. Iacopetta BJ, Morgan EH: The kinetics of transferrin endocytosis and iron uptake from transferrin in rabbit reticulocytes. J Biol Chem 1983; 258:9108.

93. Zak O, Trinder D, Aisen P: Primary receptor-recognition site of human transferrin is in the C-terminal lobe. J Biol Chem 1994; 269:7110.

94. Huebers HA, Huebers E, et al: Heterogeneity of the plasma iron pool: explanation of the Fletcher-Huehns phenomenon. Am J Physiol 1984; 247:R280.

95. Young SP, Bomford A, Williams R: The effect of the iron saturation of transferrin on its binding and uptake by rabbit reticulocytes. Biochem J 1984; 219:505.

96. Stein BS, Sussman HH: Peptide mapping of the human transferrin receptor in normal and transformed cells. J Biol Chem 1983; 58:2668.

97. Sawyer ST, Krantz SB: Transferrin receptor number, synthesis and endocytosis during erythropoietin-induced maturation of Friend virus-infected erythroid cells. J Biol Chem 1986; 261:9187.

98. Rothenberger S, Iacopetta BJ, Kuhn LC: Endocytosis of the transferrin receptor requires the cytoplasmic domain but not its phosphorylation site. Cell 1987; 49:423.

99. McGraw TE, Maxfield FR: Human transferrin receptor internalization is partly dependent upon an aromatic amino acid in the cytoplasmic domain. Cell Regulation 1990; 1:369.

100. Girones N, Alvarez E, et al: Mutational analysis of the cytoplasmic tail of the human transferrin receptor. Identification of a subdomain that is required for rapid endocytosis. J Biol Chem 1991; 266:19006.

101. Miller K, Shipman M, et al: Transferrin receptors promote the formation of clathrin lattices. Cell 1991; 65:621.

102. Collawn JF, Lai A, et al: YTRF is the conserved internalization signal of the transferrin receptor, and a second YTRF signal at position 30-34 enhances endocytosis. J Biol Chem 1993; 268:21656.

103. Davis RJ, Johnson GL, et al: Identification of serine 24 as the unique site on the transferrin receptor phosphorylated by protein kinase C. J Biol Chem 1986; 261:9034.

104. Van Renswoude J, Bridges KR, et al: Receptor-mediated endocytosis and the uptake of iron in K562 cells: identification of a non-lysosomal acidic compartment. Proc Natl Acad Sci U S A 1982; 79:6186.

105. Dautry-Varsat A, Ciechanover A, Lodish HF: pH and the recycling of transferrin during receptor-mediated endocytosis. Proc Natl Acad Sci U S A 1983; 80:2258.

106. Paterson S, Armstrong NJ, et al: Intravesicular pH and iron uptake by immature erythroid cells. J Cell Physiol 1984; 120:225.

107. Yamashiro DJ, Tycko B, et al: Segregation of transferrin to a mildly acidic (pH 6.5) para-Golgi compartment in the recycling pathway. Cell 1984; 37:789.

108. Ciechanover A, Schwartz AL, et al: Kinetics of internalization and recycling of transferrin and the transferrin receptor in a human hepatoma cell line. J Biol Chem 1983; 258:9681.

109. Low H, Grebing C, et al: Involvement of transferrin in the reduction of iron by the transplasma membrane electron transport system. J Bioenerg Biomembr 1987; 19:535.

110. Thorstensen K, Romslo I: Uptake of iron from transferrin by isolated rat hepatocytes. A redox-mediated plasma membrane process? J Biol Chem 1988; 263:8844.

111. Nunez M-T, Gaete V, et al: Mobilization of iron from endocytic vesicles. The effects of acidification and reduction. J Biol Chem 1990; 265:6688.

112. Bali PK, Zak O, Aisen P: A new role for the transferrin receptor in the release of iron from transferrin. Biochemistry 1991; 30:324.

113. Sipe DM, Murphy RF: Binding to cellular receptors results in increased iron release from transferrin at mildly acidic pH. J Biol Chem 1991; 266:8002.

114. Zak O, Aisen P: Evidence for functional differences between the two sites of rabbit transferrin: effects of serum and carbon dioxide. Biochim Biophys Acta 1990; 1052:24.

115. Egyed A: Carrier mediated iron transport through erythroid cell membrane. Br J Haematol 1988; 68:483.

116. Garrick LM, Edwards JA, et al: Diminished acquisition of iron by reticulocytes from mice with hemoglobin deficit. Exp Hematol 1987; 15:671.

117. Garrick MD, Gniecko K, et al: Transferrin and the transferrin cycle in Belgrade rat reticulocytes. J Biol Chem 1993; 20:14867.

118. Pollack S: Receptor-mediated iron uptake and intracellular iron transport. Am J Hematol 1992; 39:113. Review.

119. Harrison PM, Treffry A, Lilley TH: Ferritin as an iron storage protein: mechanisms of iron uptake. J Inorg Biochem 1986; 27:287.

120. Levi S, Luzzago A, et al: Mechanism of ferritin iron uptake: activity of the H-chain and deletion mapping of the ferro-oxidase site. A study of iron uptake and ferro-oxidase activity of human liver, recombinant H-chain ferritins, and two H-chain deletion mutants. J Biol Chem 1988; 263:18086.

121. Lawson DM, Artymiuk PJ, et al: Solving the structure of human H ferritin by genetically engineering intermolecular crystal contacts. Nature 1991; 349:541.

122. Drysdale JW: Human ferritin gene expression. Prog Nucl Acid Res 1988; 35:127. Review.

123. Pattanapanyasat K, Hoy TG, Jacobs A: The response of intracellular and surface ferritin after T-cell stimulation in vitro. Clin Sci (London) 1987; 73:605.

124. McClarty G, Chan AK, et al: Increased ferritin gene expression is associated with increased ribonucleotide reductase gene expression and the establishment of hydroxyurea resistance in mammalian cells. J Biol Chem 1990; 265:7539.

125. Iancu TC, Neustein HB, Landing BH: The liver in thalassemia major: ultrastructural observations. In Ciba Foundation Symposium. New York, Elsevier Science Publishing Co., 1977.

126. Bridges KR: Ascorbic acid inhibits lysosomal autophagy of ferritin. J Biol Chem 1987; 262:14773.

127. Wixom R, Prutkin L, Munro H: Hemosiderin: nature, formation and significance. Int Rev Exp Pathol 1980; 22:193.

128. Heilmeyer L: Atransferrinemias [German]. Acta Haematol 1966; 36:40.

129. Goya N, Miyazaki S, et al: A family of congenital atransferrinemia. Blood 1972; 40:239.

130. Bernstein SE: Hereditary hypotransferrinemia with hemosiderosis, a murine disorder resembling human atransferrinemia. J Lab Clin Med 1987; 110:690.

131. Huggenvik JI, Craven CM, et al: A splicing defect in the mouse transferrin gene leads to congenital atransferrinemia. Blood 1989; 74:482.

132. Hershko C, Graham G, et al: Non-specific serum iron in thalassemia: an abnormal serum iron fraction of potential toxicity. Br J Haematol 1978; 40:255.

133. Hershko C, Peto TE: Non-transferrin plasma iron. Br J Haematol 1987; 66:149. Editorial.

134. Grootveld M, Bell JD, et al: Non–transferrin-bound iron in plasma or serum from patients with idiopathic hemochromatosis. Characterization by high performance liquid chromatography and nuclear magnetic resonance spectroscopy. J Biol Chem 1989; 264:4417.

135. al-Refaie F, Wonke B, et al: Efficacy and possible adverse effects of the oral iron chelator 1,2-dimethyl-3-hydroxypyrid-4-one (L1) in thalassemia major. Blood 1992; 80:593.

136. Sturrock A, Alexander J, et al: Characterization of a transferrin-independent uptake system for iron in HeLa cells. J Biol Chem 1990; 265:3139.

137. Kaplan J, Jordan I, Sturrock A: Regulation of the transferrin-independent iron transport system in cultured cells. J Biol Chem 1991; 266:2997.

138. Randell EW, Parkes JG, et al: Uptake of non-transferrin bound iron by both reductive and non-reductive processes is modulated by intracellular iron. J Biol Chem 1994; 269:16046.

139. Inman RS, Wessling-Resnick M: Characterization of transferrin-independent iron transport in K562 cells. Unique properties provide evidence for multiple pathways of iron uptake. J Biol Chem 1993; 268:8521.

140. Hamazaki S, Glass J: Non-transferrin dependent ^{59}Fe uptake in phytohemagglutinin-stimulated human peripheral lymphocytes. Exp Hematol 1992; 20:436.

141. Cazzola M, Bergamaschi G, et al: Manipulations of cellular iron metabolism for modulating normal and malignant cell proliferation: achievements and prospects. Blood 1990; 75:1903.

142. Hoffbrand AV, Ganeshaguru K, et al: Effect of iron deficiency and desferrioxamine on DNA synthesis in human cells. Br J Haematol 1976; 33:517.

143. Frazier JL, Caskey JH, et al: Studies of the transferrin receptor on both human reticulocytes and nucleated human cells in culture. J Clin Invest 1982; 69:853.

144. Larrick JW, Cresswell P: Modulation of cell surface iron transferrin receptors by cellular density and state of activation. J Supramolecular Structure 1979; 11:579.

145. Lesley JF, Schulte RJ: Inhibition of cell growth by monoclonal anti-transferrin receptor antibodies. Mol Cell Biol 1985; 5:1814.

146. White S, Taetle R, et al: Combinations of anti-transferrin receptor monoclonal antibodies inhibit human tumor cell growth *in vitro* and *in vivo*: evidence for synergistic anti-proliferative effects. Cancer Res 1990; 50:6295.

147. Trowbridge IS, Lesley JF, et al: Monoclonal antibodies to transferrin receptor and assay of their biological effects. Methods Enzymol 1987; 147:265.

148. Manger B, Weiss A, et al: A transferrin receptor antibody represents one signal for the induction of IL-2 production by a human T cell line. J Immunol 1987; 136:532.

149. Cano E, Pizarro A, et al: Induction of T cell activation by monoclonal antibodies specific for the transferrin receptor. Eur J Immunol 1990; 20:765.

150. Keyna U, Platzer E, et al: Differential effects of transferrin receptor antibodies on growth and receptor expression of hu-

man lymphocytic and myelocytic cell lines. Eur J Haematol 1994; 52:169.

151. Reddel RR, Hedley DW, Sutherland RL: Cell cycle effects of iron depletion on T-47D human breast cancer cells. Exp Cell Res 1985; 161:277.

152. Chaudri G, Clark IA, et al: Effect of antioxidants on primarily alloantigen-induced T-cell activation and proliferation. J Immunol 1986; 137:2646.

153. Bierer BE, Nathan DG: The effect of desferrithiocin, an oral iron chelator, on T cell function. Blood 1990; 76:2052.

154. Polson RJ, Jenkins R, et al: Mechanisms of inhibition of mononuclear cell activation by the iron-chelating agent desferrioxamine. Immunology 1990; 71:176.

155. Pattanapanyasat K, Webster HK, et al: Effect of orally active hydroxypyridinone iron chelators on human lymphocyte function. Br J Haematol 1992; 82:13.

156. Lederman HM, Cohen A, et al: Deferoxamine: a reversible S-phase inhibitor of human lymphocyte proliferation. Blood 1984; 64:748.

157. Fukuchi K, Tomoyasu S, et al: Iron deprivation—induced apoptosis in HL-60 cells. FEBS Lett 1994; 350:139.

158. Brittenham GM: The red cell cycle. In Brock JH, Halliday JW, et al (eds): Iron Metabolism in Health and Disease. London, W.B. Saunders Co., 1994, pp 31–62.

159. Shannon KM, Larrick JW, et al: Selective inhibition of the growth of human erythroid bursts by monoclonal antibodies against transferrin or transferrin receptor. Blood 1986; 67:1631.

160. Schmidt JA, Marshall J, et al: Control of erythroid differentiation. Cell 1986; 46:41.

161. Ross J, Sautner D: Induction of globin mRNA accumulation by hemin in cultured erythroleukemic cells. Cell 1976; 8:513.

162. Rutherford TR, Clegg JB, Weatherall DJ: K562 human leukaemic cells synthesise embryonic haemoglobin in response to haemin. Nature 1979; 280:164.

163. Mager D, Bernstein A: The role of heme in the regulation of the late program of Friend cell erythroid differentiation. J Cell Physiol 1979; 100:467.

164. Bonanou-Tzedaki SA, Sohi M, Arnstein HR: Regulation of erythroid cell differentiation by haemin. Cell Differ 1981; 10:267.

165. Rutherford CJ, Schneider TJ, et al: Efficacy of different dosing regimens for recombinant human erythropoietin in a simulated perisurgical setting: the importance of iron availability in optimizing response. Am J Med 1994; 96:139.

166. Ney PA, Sorentino BP, et al: Inducibility of the HSII enhancer depends on binding of an erythroid specific nuclear protein. Nucleic Acids Res 1990; 18:6011.

167. Andrews NC, Erdjument-Bromage H, et al: Erythroid transcription factor NF-E2 is a haematopoietic-specific basic-leucine zipper protein. Nature 1993; 362:722.

168. Andrews NC, Kotkow KJ, et al: The ubiquitous subunit of erythroid transcription factor NF-E2 is a small basic-leucine zipper protein related to the v-*maf* oncogene. Proc Natl Acad Sci U S A 1993; 90:11488.

169. Ney PA, Andrews NC, et al: Purification of the human NF-E2 complex: cDNA cloning of the hematopoietic cell-specific subunit and evidence for an associated partner. Mol Cell Biol 1993; 13:5604.

170. Mignotte V, Eleouet F, et al: Cis- and transacting elements involved in the regulation of the erythroid promoter of the human porphobilinogen deaminase gene. Proc Natl Acad Sci U S A 1989; 86:6548.

171. Taketani S, Inazawa J, et al: Structure of the human ferrochelatase gene. Exon/intron gene organization and location of the gene to chromosome 18. Eur J Biochem 1992; 205:217.

172. Andrews NC: Erythroid transcription factor NF-E2 coordinates hemoglobin synthesis. Pediatr Res 1994; 36:1.

173. Battistini A, Coccia EM, et al: Intracellular heme coordinately modulates globin chain synthesis, transferrin receptor number, and ferritin content in differentiating Friend erythroleukemia cells. Blood 1991; 78:2098.

174. Battistini A, Marziali G, et al: Positive modulation of hemoglobin, heme and transferrin receptor synthesis by murine interferon-alpha and -beta in differentiating Friend cells. Pivotal role of heme synthesis. J Biol Chem 1991; 266:528.

175. Coccia E, Profita V, et al: Modulation of ferritin H-chain expres-

sion in Friend erythroleukemia cells: transcriptional and translational regulation by hemin. Mol Cell Biol 1992; 12:3015.

176. Nathan DG, Piomelli S, et al: The synthesis of heme and globin in the maturing human erythroid cell. J Clin Invest 1961; 40:940.

177. London IM, Levin DH, et al: Regulation of protein synthesis. In Boyer PD (ed): The Enzymes. New York, Academic Press, 1987.

178. Boyd D, Vecoli C, et al: Structural and functional relationships of human ferritin H and L chains deduced from cDNA clones. J Biol Chem 1985; 260:11755.

179. Cragg SJ, Drysdale J, Worwood M: Genes for the 'H' subunit of human ferritin are present on a number of human chromosomes. Hum Genet 1985; 71:108.

180. Costanzo F, Colombo M, et al: Structure of gene and pseudogenes of human apoferritin H. Nucleic Acids Res 1986; 14:721.

181. McGill JR, Naylor SL, et al: Human ferritin H and L sequences lie on ten different chromosomes. Hum Genet 1987; 76:66.

182. Santoro C, Marone M, et al: Cloning of the gene coding for human L-apoferritin. Nucleic Acids Res 1986; 14:2863.

183. Worwood M, Brook JD, et al: Assignment of human ferritin genes to chromosomes 11 and 19q13.3-19qter. Hum Genet 1985; 69:371.

184. Dugast IJ, Papadopoulos P, et al: Identification of two human ferritin H genes on the short arm of chromosome 6. Genomics 1990; 6:204.

185. White K, Munro HN: Induction of ferritin synthesis by iron is regulated at both transcriptional and translational levels. J Biol Chem 1988; 263:8938.

186. Coulson RM, Cleveland DW: Ferritin synthesis is controlled by iron-dependent translational derepression and by changes in synthesis/transport of nuclear ferritin RNAs. Proc Natl Acad Sci U S A 1993; 90:7613.

187. Cairo G, Bardella L, et al: Multiple mechanisms of iron-induced ferritin synthesis in HeLa cells. Biochem Biophys Res Commun 1985; 133:314.

188. Chou CC, Gatti RA, et al: Structure and expression of ferritin genes in a human promyelocytic cell line that differentiates in vitro. Mol Cell Biol 1986; 6:566.

189. Beaumont C, Jain SK, et al: Ferritin synthesis in differentiating Friend erythroleukemia cells. J Biol Chem 1987; 262:10619.

190. Torti SV, Kwak EL, et al: The molecular cloning and characterization of murine ferritin heavy chain, a tumor necrosis factor-inducible gene. J Biol Chem 1988; 263:12638.

191. Beaumont C, Sehan A, et al: Mouse ferritin H subunit gene: functional analysis of the promoter and identification of an upstream regulatory elements active in erythroid cells. J Biol Chem 1994; 269:20281.

192. Rogers J, Bridges KR, et al: Translational control during the acute phase response: ferritin synthesis in response to interleukin-1. J Biol Chem 1990; 265:14572.

193. Rogers J, Andriotakis J, et al: Translational enhancement of H-ferritin mRNA by interleukin-1 beta acts through 5' leader sequences distinct from the iron responsive element. Nucleic Acids Res 1994; 22:2678.

194. Rogers J, Munro H: Translation of ferritin light and heavy subunit mRNAs is regulated by intracellular chelatable iron levels in rat hepatoma cells. Proc Natl Acad Sci U S A 1987; 84:2277.

195. Aziz N, Munro HN: Both subunits of rat liver ferritin are regulated at a translational level by iron induction. Nucleic Acids Res 1986; 14:915.

196. Casey JL, Hentze MW, et al: Iron-responsive elements: regulatory RNA sequences that control mRNA levels and translation. Science 1988; 240:924.

197. Zahringer J, Baliga BS, Munro HN: Novel mechanism for translation control in regulation of ferritin synthesis by iron. Proc Natl Acad Sci U S A 1976; 73:857.

198. Munro HN, Linder MC: Ferritin: structure, biosynthesis and role in iron metabolism. Physiol Rev 1978; 58:317. Review.

199. Walden WE, Thach R: Translational control of gene expression in a normal fibroblast: characterization of a subclass of mRNAs with unusual kinetic properties. Biochemistry 1986; 25:2033.

200. Hentze MW, Rouault TA, et al: A cis-acting element is necessary and sufficient for translational regulation of human ferritin expression in response to iron. Proc Natl Acad Sci U S A 1987; 84:6730.

201. Aziz N, Munro HN: Iron regulates ferritin mRNA translation through a segment of its 5'-untranslated region. Proc Natl Acad Sci 1987; 84:8478.

202. Rouault TA, Tang CK, et al: Cloning of the cDNA encoding an RNA regulatory protein—the human iron-responsive element-binding protein. Proc Natl Acad Sci U S A 1990; 87:7958.

203. Kaptain S, Downey WE, et al: A regulated RNA binding protein also possesses aconitase activity. Proc Natl Acad Sci U S A 1991; 88:10109.

204. Gray NK, Hentze MW: Iron regulatory protein prevents binding of the 43S translation initiation complex to ferritin and eALAS mRNAs. EMBO J 1994; 13:3882.

205. Haile DJ, Rouault TA, et al: Reciprocal control of RNA-binding and aconitase activity in the regulation of the iron-responsive element binding protein: role of the iron-sulfur cluster. Proc Natl Acad Sci 1992; 89:7536.

206. Constable A, Quick S, et al: Modulation of the RNA-binding activity of a regulatory protein by iron in vitro: switching between enzymatic and genetic function? Proc Natl Acad Sci U S A 1991; 89:4554.

207. Emory-Goodman A, Hirling H, et al: Iron regulatory factor expressed from recombinant baculovirus: conversion between the RNA-binding apoprotein and Fe-S cluster containing aconitase. Nucleic Acids Res 1993; 21:1457.

208. Toth I, Bridges KR: Ascorbic acid enhances ferritin mRNA translation by an IRP/aconitase switch. J Biol Chem 1995; 270:19540.

209. Goessling LS, Daniels-McQueen S, et al: Enhanced degradation of the ferritin repressor protein during induction of ferritin messenger RNA translation. Science 1992; 256:670.

210. Lin J-J, Daniels-McQueen S, et al: Derepression of ferritin messenger RNA translation by hemin in vitro. Science 1990; 247:74.

211. Huerre C, Uzan G, et al: The structural gene for transferrin (Tf) maps to 3q21 m3qter. Ann Genet (Paris) 1984; 27:5.

212. Rabin M, McClelland A, et al: Regional localization of the human transferrin receptor gene to 3q26mqter. Am J Hum Genet 1985; 37:1112.

213. McClelland A, Kuhn LC, Ruddle FH: The human transferrin receptor gene: genomic organization, and the complete primary structure of the receptor deduced for a cDNA sequence. Cell 1984; 39:267.

214. Mullner EW, Kuhn LC: A stem-loop in the 3'-untranslated region mediates iron-dependent regulation of transferrin receptor mRNA stability in the cytoplasm. Cell 1988; 53:815.

215. Koeller DM, Casey JL, et al: A cytosolic protein binds to structural elements within the iron-responsive regulatory region of the transferrin receptor mRNA. Proc Natl Acad Sci 1989; 86:3574.

216. Binder R, Horowitz JA, et al: Evidence that the pathway of transferrin receptor mRNA degradation involves an endonucleolytic cleavage within the 3' UTR and does not involve poly(A) tail shortening. EMBO J 1994; 13:1969.

217. Chan L-NL, Gerhardt EM: Transferrin receptor gene is hyperexpressed and transcriptionally regulated in differentiating erythroid cells. J Biol Chem 1992; 267:8254.

218. Miskimins WK, McClelland A, et al: Cell proliferation and expression of the transferrin receptor gene: promoter sequence homologies and protein interactions. J Cell Biol 1986; 103:1781.

219. Miskimins WK: Interaction of multiple factors with a GC-rich element within the mitogen responsive region of the human transferrin receptor gene. J Cell Biochem 1992; 49:349.

220. Ouyang Q, Bommakanti M, Miskimins WK: A mitogen-responsive promoter region that is synergistically activated through multiple signalling pathways. Mol Cell Biol 1993; 13:1796.

221. Guo B, Brown F, et al: Characterization and expression of iron regulatory protein 2 (IRP2): presence of multiple IRP2 transcripts regulated by intracellular iron levels. J Biol Chem 1995; 270:16529.

222. Guo B, Phillips J, et al: Iron regulates the intracellular degradation of iron regulatory protein 2 by the proteasome. J Biol Chem 1995; 270:21645.

223. Dandekar T, Stripecke R, et al: Identification of a novel iron-responsive element in murine and human erythroid δ-aminolevulinic acid synthase mRNA. EMBO J 1991; 10:1903.

224. Cox TC, Bawden MJ, et al: Human erythroid 5'-aminolevulinate synthase: promoter analysis and identification of an iron-responsive element in the mRNA. EMBO J 1991; 10:1891.

225. Zheng L, Kennedy MC, et al: Binding of cytosolic aconitase to the iron responsive element of porcine mitochondrial aconitase mRNA. Arch Biochem Biophys 1992; 299:356.

226. Aisen P, Leibman A, Zweier J: Stoichiometric and site characteristics of the binding of iron to human transferrin. J Biol Chem 1978; 253:1930.

227. Skinner MK, Cosand WL, Griswold MD: Purification and characterization of testicular transferrin secreted by rat Sertoli cells. Biochem J 1984; 218:313.

228. Chen L-H, Bissel MJ: Transferrin mRNA level in the mouse mammary gland is regulated by pregnancy and extracellular matrix. J Biol Chem 1987; 262:17247.

229. Sylvester SR, Griswold MD: Localization of transferrin and transferrin receptor in rate testes. Biol Reprod 1984; 31:195.

230. Gerber MR, Connor J: Do oligodendrocytes mediate iron regulation in the human brain? Ann Neurol 1989; 26:95.

231. Lum JB, Infante AJ, et al: Transferrin synthesis by inducer T-lymphocytes. J Clin Invest 1986; 77:841.

232. Pattanapanyasat K, Hoy TG: Expression of cell surface transferrin receptor and intracellular ferritin after *in vitro* stimulation of peripheral blood T lymphocytes. Eur J Haematol 1991; 47:140.

233. Cochet M, Gannon F, et al: Organization and sequence studies of the 17-piece chicken conalbumin gene. Nature 1979; 282; 567.

234. Williams J: The formation of iron-binding fragments of hen ovotransferrin by limited proteolysis. Biochem J 1974; 141:745.

235. Zak O, Aisen P: Preparation and properties of a single-sited fragment from the C-terminal domain of human transferrin. Biochim Biophys Acta 1985; 829:348.

236. Yang F, Lum JB, et al: Human transferrin: cDNA characterization and chromosome localization. Proc Natl Acad Sci USA 1984; 81:2752.

236a. Hammer RE, Idzerda RL, et al: Estrogen regulation of the avian transferrin gene in transgenic mice. Mol Cell Biol 1986; 6:1010.

237. Brunel F, Ochoa A, et al: Interactions of DNA-binding proteins with the 5' region of the human transferrin gene. J Biol Chem 1988; 263:10180.

238. Griswold MD, Hugly S, et al: Evidence for *in vitro* transferrin synthesis and the relationship between transferrin mRNA levels and germ cells for the testes. Ann N Y Acad Sci 1988; 513:302.

239. Guillou F, Zakin MM, et al: Sertoli cell-specific expression of the human transferrin gene. Comparison with liver-specific expression. J Biol Chem 1991; 266:9876.

240. Ochoa A, Brunel F, et al: Different liver nuclear proteins bind to similar DNA sequences in the 5' flanking regions of three hepatic genes. Nucleic Acids Res 1989; 17:119.

241. Schaeffer E, Boissier F, et al: Cell type–specific expression of the human transferrin gene. J Biol Chem 1989; 264:7153.

242. Mendelzon D, Boissier F, Zakin MM: The binding site for the liver-specific transcription factor Tf-LF1 and the TATA box of the human transferrin gene promoter are the only elements necessary to direct liver-specific transcription *in vitro*. Nucleic Acids Res 1991; 18:5717.

243. Adrian GS, Korinek BW, et al: The human transferrin gene: 5' region contains conserved sequences which match the control elements regulated by heavy metals, glucocorticoids and acute phase reaction. Gene 1986; 490:167.

244. Lucerno MA, Schaeffer E, et al: The 5' region of the human transferrin gene: structure and potential regulatory sites. Nucleic Acids Res 1986; 14:8692.

245. Huggenvik JI, Idzerda RL, et al: Transferrin messenger ribonucleic acid: molecular cloning and hormonal regulation in rat Sertoli cells. Endocrinology 1987; 120:332.

246. Tsutsumi M, Skinner MK, Sanders-Bush E: Transferrin gene expression and synthesis by cultured choroid plexus epithelial cells. Regulation by serotonin and cyclic adenosine 3',5'-monophosphate. J Biol Chem 1989; 264:9226.

247. Petropoulos I, Auge-Gouillou C, Zakin MM: Characterization of the active part of the human transferrin gene enhancer and purification of two liver nuclear factors interacting with the TGTTTGC motif present in this region. J Biol Chem 1991; 266:9822.

248. Auge-Gouillou C, Petropoulos I, Zakin MM: Liver-enriched HNF-3 alpha and ubiquitous factors interact with the human transferrin gene enhancer. FEBS Lett 1993; 323:4.

249. Mullner EW, Neupert B, Kuhn LC: A specific mRNA binding factor regulates the iron-dependent stability of cytoplasmic transferrin receptor mRNA. Cell 1989; 58:373.

250. Pietrangelo A, Rocchi E, et al: Regulation of hepatic transferrin, transferrin receptor and ferritin genes in human siderosis. Hepatology 1991; 14:1083.

251. Cox LA, Adrian GS: Posttranscriptional regulation of chimeric human transferrin genes by iron. Biochemistry 1993; 32:4738.

252. Worwood M: Serum ferritin. Clin Sci 1986; 70:215.

253. Snider MD, Robbins PW: Synthesis and processing of asparagine-linked oligosaccharides of glycoproteins. Methods Cell Biol 1981; 23:89.

254. Cragg S, Wagstaff M, Worwood M: Detection of a glycosylated subunit in human serum ferritin. Biochem J 1981; 199:565.

255. Worwood M: Laboratory determination of iron status. In Brock JH, Halliday JW, et al (eds): Iron Metabolism in Health and Disease. London, W.B. Saunders Co., 1994.

256. Lipschitz DA, Cook JD, Finch CA: A clinical evaluation of serum ferritin as an index of iron stores. N Engl J Med 1974; 290:1213.

257. Rios E, Lipschitz D, et al: Relationship of maternal and infant iron stores as assessed by determination of plasma ferritin. Pediatrics 1975; 55:694.

258. Elin R, Wolff S, Finch C: Effect of induced fever on serum iron and ferritin concentrations in man. Blood 1977; 49:147.

259. Pojaznik D, de Sousa M, et al: Ferritin in neuroblastoma. Impact of tumor load and blood transfusions. Cancer Invest 1985; 3:327.

260. Zhou XD, Stahlhut MW, et al: Serum ferritin in hepatocellular carcinoma. Hepatogastroenterology 1988; 35:1.

261. Brodeur GM, Pritchard J, et al: Revisions of the international criteria for neuroblastoma diagnosis, staging and response to treatment. J Clin Oncol 1993; 11:1466. Review.

262. Pan BT, Teng K, et al: Electron microscopic evidence for externalization of the transferrin receptor in vesicular form in sheep erythrocytes. J Cell Biol 1985; 101:942.

263. Johnstone RM, Biachini A, Teng K: Reticulocyte maturation and exosome release: transferrin receptor containing exosomes show multiple plasma membrane functions. Blood 1989; 74:1844.

264. Kohgo Y, Nishisato T, et al: Circulating transferrin receptors in human serum. Br J Haematol 1986; 64:277.

265. Beguin Y, Huebers HA, et al: Transferrin receptors in rat plasma. Proc Natl Acad Sci U S A 1988; 85:637.

266. Shih YJ, Baynes RD, et al: Serum transferrin receptor is a truncated form of tissue receptor. J Biol Chem 1990; 265:19077.

267. Baynes RD, Shih YJ, Cook JD: Production of soluble transferrin receptor by K562 erythroleukemia cells. Br J Haematol 1991; 78:450.

268. Rutledge EH, Root BJ, et al: Elimination of the O-linked glycosylation site at Thr 104 results in the generation of a soluble human transferrin receptor. Blood 1994; 83:580.

269. Ahn J, Johnstone RM: Origin of a soluble truncated transferrin receptor. Blood 1993; 81:2442.

270. Kohgo Y, Niitsu Y, et al: Serum transferrin receptors as a new index of erythropoiesis. Blood 1987; 70:1955.

271. Huebers HA, Beguin Y, et al: Intact transferrin receptors in human plasma and their relation to erythropoiesis. Blood 1990; 75:102.

272. Skikne BS, Flowers CH, Cook JD: Serum transferrin receptor: a quantitative measure of tissue iron deficiency. Blood 1990; 75:1870.

273. Williams DM: Copper deficiency in humans. Semin Hematol 1983; 20:118.

274. Danks DM: Copper deficiency in humans. Ann Rev Nutr 1988; 8:235.

275. Castillo-Duran C, Uauy R: Copper deficiency impairs growth of infants recovering from malnutrition. Am J Clin Nutr 1988; 47:710.

276. Levy Y, Zeharia A, et al: Copper deficiency in infants fed cow milk. J Pediatr 1985; 106:786.

277. Celsing F, Blomstrand E, et al: Effects of iron deficiency on endurance and muscle enzyme activity in man. Med Sci Sports Exerc 1986; 18:156.

278. Goyens P, Brasseur D, et al: Copper deficiency in infants with active celiac disease. J Pediatr Gastroenterol Nutr 1985; 4:677.

279. Salmenpera L, Perheentupa J, et al: Cu nutrition in infants during prolonged exclusive breast-feeding: low intake by rising

serum concentrations of Cu and ceruloplasmin. Am J Clin Nutr 1986; 43:251.

280. Menkes JH, Alter M, et al: A sex-linked recessive disorder with retardation of growth, peculiar hair and focal cerebral and cerebellar degeneration. Pediatrics 1962; 29:764.

281. Wilson SAK: Progressive lenticular degeneration: a familial nervous disease associated with cirrhosis of the liver. Brain 1912; 34:295.

282. Vulpe C, Levinson B, et al: Isolation of a candidate gene for Menkes disease and evidence that it encodes a copper-transporting ATPase. Nat Genet 1993; 3:7.

283. Chelly J, Tumer S, et al: Isolation of a candidate gene for Menkes disease that encodes a potential heavy metal binding protein. Nat Genet 1993; 3:14.

284. Mercer JFB, Livingston J, et al: Isolation of a partial candidate gene for Menkes disease by positional cloning. Nat Genet 1993; 3:20.

285. Yamaguchi Y, Heiny ME, Gitlin JD: Isolation and characterization of a human liver cDNA as a candidate gene for Wilson's disease. Biochem Biophys Res Commun 1993; 197:271.

286. Bull PC, Thomas GR, et al: The Wilson's disease gene is a putative copper transporting P-type ATPase similar to the Menkes gene. Nat Genet 1993; 5:327.

287. Tanzi RE, Petrukhin K, et al: The Wilson's disease gene is a copper transporting ATPase with homology to the Menkes disease gene. Nat Genet 1993; 5:344.

288. Conrad M, Barton J: Factors affecting iron balance. Am J Hematol 1981; 10:199.

289. Gillooly M, Bothwell T, et al: Factors affecting the absorption of iron from cereals. Br J Nutr 1984; 51:37.

290. Ballot D, Baynes R, et al: The effects of fruit juices and fruits on the absorption of iron from a rice meal. Br J Nutr 1987; 57:331.

291. Worwood M: The clinical biochemistry of iron. Semin Hematol 1977; 14:3.

292. Stabler S, Allen R, et al: Clinical spectrum and diagnosis of cobalamin deficiency. Blood 1990; 76:871.

293. Skikne BS, Cook JD: Effect of enhanced erythropoiesis on iron absorption. J Lab Clin Res 1992; 120:746.

294. Goyer R: Lead toxicity: current concerns. Environ Health Perspect 1993; 100:177.

295. Beeken W: Absorptive defects in young people with regional enteritis. Pediatrics 1973; 52:69.

296. Anand B, Callender S, Warner G: Absorption of inorganic and haemoglobin iron in coeliac disease. Br J Haematol 1977; 37:409.

297. Sutton D, Baird I, et al: Gastrointestinal iron losses in atrophic gastritis, postgastrectomy states and adult coeliac disease. Gut 1971; 12:869.

298. Baird I, Walters R, Sutton D: Absorption of slow-release iron and effects of ascorbic acid in normal subjects and after partial gastrectomy. BMJ 1974; 4, 505.

299. Hentschel E, Brandstatter G, et al: Effect of ranitidine and amoxicillin plus metronidazole on the eradication of *Helicobacter pylori* and the recurrence of duodenal ulcer. N Engl J Med 1993; 328:308.

300. Tunnessen W Jr, Oski F: Consequences of starting whole cow's milk at 6 months of age. J Pediatr 1987; 111:813.

301. Picciano M, Deering R: The influence of feeding regiments on iron status during infancy. Am J Clin Nutr 1980; 33:746.

302. Nutrition CO: Iron supplementation for infants. Pediatrics 1976; 58:765.

303. Crompton D, Whitehead R: Hookworm infections and human iron metabolism. Parasitology 1993; 107:S137.

304. Buschman DL, Ballard R: Progressive massive fibrosis associated with idiopathic pulmonary hemosiderosis. Chest 1993; 104:293.

305. Muller N, Miller R: Diffuse pulmonary hemorrhage. Radiol Clin North Am 1991; 29:965.

306. Bouros D, Panagou P, et al: Bronchoalveolar lavage findings in a young adult with idiopathic pulmonary haemosiderosis and coeliac disease. Eur Respir J 1994; 7:1009.

307. van der Ent C, Walenkamp M, et al: Pulmonary hemosiderosis and immune complex glomerulonephritis. Clin Nephrol 1995; 43:339.

308. Bush A, Sheppard M, Warner J: Chloroquine in idiopathic pulmonary haemosiderosis. Arch Dis Child 1992; 67:625.

309. Colombo JL, Stolz SM: Treatment of life-threatening primary pulmonary hemosiderosis with cyclophosphamide. Chest 1992; 102:959.

310. Rossi GA, Balzano E, et al: Long-term prednisone and azathioprine treatment of a patient with idiopathic pulmonary hemosiderosis. Pediatr Pulmon 1992; 13:176.

311. Lin C, Lin J, et al: Comparison of hemoglobin and red blood cell distribution width in the differential diagnosis of microcytic anemia. Arch Pathol Lab Med 1992; 116:1030.

312. Tillmann W, Schroter W: Deformability of erythrocytes in iron deficiency anemia. Blut 1980; 40:179.

313. Dallman P: Iron deficiency: does it matter? J Intern Med 1989; 226:367.

314. Oski F, Honig A: The effects of therapy on the developmental scores of iron-deficient infants. J Pediatr 1978; 92:21.

315. Deinard A, List A, et al: Cognitive deficits in iron-deficient and iron-deficient anemic children. J Pediatr 1986; 108:681.

316. Oski F, Honig A, et al: Effect of iron therapy on behavior performance in nonanemic, iron-deficient infants. Pediatrics 1983; 71:877.

317. Pollitt E, Saco-Pollitt C, et al: Iron deficiency and behavioral development in infants and preschool children. Am J Clin Nutr 1986; 43:555.

318. Wasserman G, Graziano J, et al: Independent effects of lead exposure and iron deficiency anemia on developmental outcome at age 2 years. J Pediatr 1992; 121:695.

319. Lozoff B, Jimenez E, Wolf A: Long-term developmental outcome of infants with iron deficiency. N Engl J Med 1991; 325:687.

320. Walter T, De Andraca I, et al: Iron deficiency anemia: adverse effects of infant psychomotor development. Pediatrics 1991; 84:7.

321. Sheard N: Iron deficiency and infant development. Nutr Rev 1994; 52:137.

322. Lozoff B: Methodologic issues in studying behavioral effects of infant iron-deficiency anemia. Am J Clin Nutr 1989; 50:641.

323. Oski F: Iron deficiency in infancy and childhood. N Engl J Med 1993; 329:190.

324. Beard JL, Chen Q, et al: Altered monamine metabolism in caudate-putamen of iron-deficient rats. Pharmacol Biochem Behav 1994; 48:621.

325. Anezaki T, Yanagisawa K, et al: A patient with severe iron-deficiency anemia and memory disturbance. Intern Med 1992; 31:1306.

326. Grindulis H, Scott P, et al: Combined deficiency of iron and vitamin D in Asian toddlers. Arch Dis Child 1986; 61:843.

327. Aukett M, Parks Y, et al: Treatment with iron increases weight gain and psychomotor development. Arch Dis Child 1986; 61:849.

328. Angeles I, Schultink W, et al: Decreased rate of stunting among anemic Indonesian preschool children through iron supplementation. Am J Clin Nutr 1993; 58:339.

329. Roselle H: Association of laundry starch and clay ingestion with anemia in New York City. Arch Intern Med 1970; 125:57.

330. Talkington K, Gant N Jr, et al: Effect of ingestion of starch and some clays on iron absorption. Am J Obstet Gynecol 1970; 108:262.

331. Cavdar A, Arcasoy A: Hematologic and biochemical studies of Turkish children with pica. A presumptive explanation for the syndrome of geophagia, iron deficiency anemia, hepatosplenomegaly and hypogonadism. Clin Pediatr 1972; 11:215.

332. Say B, Ozsoylu S, Berkel I: Geophagia associated with iron-deficiency anemia, hepatosplenomegaly, hypogonadism and dwarfism. A syndrome probably associated with zinc deficiency. Clin Pediatr 1969; 8:661.

333. Cavdar A, Arcasoy A, et al: Zinc deficiency in geophagia in Turkish children and response to treatment with zinc sulphate. Haematologica 1980; 65:403.

334. Pless M, Lipton S: Iron deficiency in children. N Engl J Med 1993; 329:1741. Letter.

335. Kiviuori S, Anttila R, et al: Serum transferrin receptor for assessment of iron status in healthy prepubertal and early pubertal boys. Pediatr Res 1993; 34:297.

336. Milman N, Agger A, Nielsen O: Iron supplementation during pregnancy. Effect on iron status markers, serum erythropoietin and human placental lactogen. A placebo controlled study in 207 Danish women. Dan Med Bull 1991; 38:471.

337. Mays T, Mays T: Intravenous iron-dextran therapy in the treatment of anemia occurring in surgical, gynecologic and obstetric patients. Surg Gynecol Obstet 1976; 143:381.

338. Auerbach M, Witt D, et al: Clinical use of the total dose intravenous infusion of iron dextran. J Lab Clin Med 1988; 111:566.

339. Stein M, Gunston K, May R: Iron dextran in the treatment of iron-deficiency anaemia of pregnancy. Haematological response and incidence of side-effects. S Afr Med J 1991; 79:195.

340. Hall RT, Wheeler RE, et al: Feeding iron-fortified premature formula during initial hospitalization to infants less than 1800 grams birth weight. Pediatrics 1993; 92:409.

341. Cox T, Peters T: Uptake of iron by duodenal biopsy specimens from patients with iron-deficiency anaemia and primary haemochromatosis. Lancet 1978; 1:123.

342. Cox T, Peters T: *In vitro* studies of duodenal iron uptake in patients with primary and secondary iron storage disease. Q J Med 1980; 49:249.

343. Lynch S, Skikne B, Cook J: Food iron absorption in idiopathic hemochromatosis. Blood 1989; 74:2187.

344. Bassett M, Halliday J, Powell L: HLA typing in idiopathic hemochromatosis: distinction between homozygotes and heterozygotes with biochemical expression. Hepatology 1981; 1:120.

345. Edwards C, Dadone M, et al: Hereditary haemochromatosis. Clin Haematol 1982; 11:411.

346. Burt M, Smit D, et al: A 4.5 megabase YAC contig and physical map over the haemochromatosis gene region. Genomics 1996; 33:153.

347. Feder J, Gnirke A, et al: A novel MHC class I-like gene is mutated in patients with hereditary haemochromatosis. Nat Genet 1996; 13:399.

348. Cox T: Haemochromatosis: strike while the iron is hot. Nat Genet 1996; 13:386.

349. De Sousa M, et al: Iron overload in β2-microglobulin–deficient mice. Immunol Lett 1994; 39:105.

350. Rothenberg B, Voland J: β2 knockout mice develop parenchymal iron overload: a putative role for class I genes of the major histocompatibility complex in iron metabolism. Proc Natl Acad Sci U S A 1996; 93:1529.

351. McLaren G, Muir W, Kellermeyer R: Iron overload disorders: natural history, pathogenesis, diagnosis and therapy. CRC Crit Rev Clin Lab Sci. 1983; 19:205.

352. Worwood M: Iron and haemochromatosis. J Inherit Metab Dis 1983; 6:63.

353. Bassett M, Halliday J, Powell L: Value of hepatic iron measurements in early hemochromatosis and determination of the critical iron level associated with fibrosis. Hepatology 1986; 6:24.

354. Conte W, Rotter J: The use of association data to identify family members at high risk for marker-linked diseases. Am J Hum Genet 1984; 36:152.

355. Edwards C, Griffen L, et al: Prevalence of hemochromatosis among 11,065 presumably healthy blood donors. N Engl J Med 1988; 318:1355.

356. Olsson K, Ritter B, et al: Prevalence of iron overload in central Sweden. Acta Med Scand 1983; 213:145.

357. Meyer T, Ballot D, et al: The HLA linked iron loading gene in an Afrikaner population. J Med Genet 1987; 24:348.

358. McLaren C, Gordeuk V, et al: Prevalence of heterozygotes for hemochromatosis in the white population of the United States. Blood 1995; 86:2021.

359. Bothwell T, Bradlow B: Siderosis in the Bantu. A combined histopathological and chemical study. Arch Pathol 1960; 70:279.

360. Bothwell T, Charlton R, Seftel H: Oral iron overload. S Afr Med J 1965; 39:892.

361. Brink B, Disler P, et al: Patterns of iron storage in dietary iron overload and idiopathic hemochromatosis. J Lab Clin Med 1976; 88:725.

362. Isaacson C, Bothwell T: Synovial iron deposits in black subjects with iron overload. Arch Pathol Lab Med 1981; 105:487.

363. Seftel H, Malkin C, et al: Osteoporosis, scurvy, and siderosis in Johannesburg Bantu. BMJ 1966; 1:642.

364. MacPhail A, Simon M, et al: Changing patterns of dietary iron overload in black South Africans. Am J Clin Nutr 1979; 32:1272.

365. Gordeuk V, Boyd R, Brittenham G: Dietary iron overload persists in rural sub-Saharan Africa. Lancet 1986; 1:1310.

366. Bacon B, Britton R: The pathology of hepatic iron overload: a free radical-mediated process? Hepatology 1990; 11:127.

367. Friedman B, Baynes R, et al: Dietary iron overload in southern African rural blacks. S Afr Med J 1990; 78:301.

368. Wright D: Syphilis and Neanderthal man. Nature 1971; 229:409.

369. Oliver M, Scully L, et al: Non-HLA-linked hemochromatosis in a Chinese woman. Dig Dis Sci 1995; 40:1589.

370. Goldfischer S, Grotsky H, et al: Idiopathic neonatal iron storage involving the liver, pancreas, heart, and endocrine and exocrine glands. Hepatology 1981; 1:58.

371. Knisely A, Magid M, et al: Neonatal hemochromatosis. Birth Defects 1987; 23:75.

372. Knisely A, Harford J, et al: Neonatal hemochromatosis: the regulation of transferrin-receptor and ferritin synthesis by iron in cultured fibroblastic-line cells. Am J Pathol 1989; 134:439.

373. Silver M, Beverley D, et al: Perinatal hemochromatosis: clinical, morphological, and quantitative iron studies. Am J Pathol 1987; 128:538.

374. Pippard M, Callender S, et al: Iron absorption and loading in β-thalassemia intermedia. Lancet 1979; 2:819.

375. Celada A: Iron overload in a non-transfused patient with thalassaemia intermedia. Scand J Haematol 1982; 28:169.

376. Raja K, Simpson R, Peters T: Effect of exchange transfusion of reticulocytes on *in vitro* and *in vivo* intestinal iron (Fe3+) absorption in mice. Br J Haematol 1989; 73:254.

377. Bonkovsky H: Iron and the liver. Am J Med Sci 1991; 301:32.

378. Conte D, Piperno A, et al: Clinical, biochemical and histological features of primary haemochromatosis: a report of 67 cases. Liver 1986; 6:310.

379. Hultcrantz R, Glaumann H: Studies on the rat liver following iron overload. Biochemical analysis following iron mobilization. Lab Invest 1982; 46:383.

380. Schellhammer P, Engle M, Hagstrom J: Histochemical studies of the myocardium and conduction system in acquired iron-storage disease. Circulation 1967; 35:631.

381. Fitchett D, Coltart D, et al: Cardiac involvement in secondary hemochromatosis. Cardiovasc Res 1980; 14:7199.

382. Sanyal S, Johnson W, et al: Fatal "iron heart" in an adolescent: biochemical and ultrastructural aspects of the heart. Pediatrics 1975; 55:336.

383. Liu P, Olivieri N: Iron overload cardiomyopathies: new insights into an old disease. Cardiovasc Drugs Ther 1994; 8:101.

384. Wolfe L, Olivieri N, et al: Prevention of cardiac disease by subcutaneous deferoxamine in patients with thalassemia major. N Engl J Med 1985; 312:1600.

385. Koren A, Garty I, et al: Right ventricular cardiac dysfunction in β-thalassemia major. Am J Dis Child 1987; 141:93.

386. Rahko P, Salerni R, Uretsky B: Successful reversal by chelation therapy of congestive cardiomyopathy due to iron overload. J Am Coll Cardiol 1986; 8:436.

387. Buja L, Roberts W: Iron in the heart. Am J Med 1971; 51:209.

388. Olson L, Edwards W, et al: Cardiac iron deposition in idiopathic hemochromatosis: histologic and analytic assessment of 14 hearts from autopsy. J Am Coll Cardiol 1987; 10:1239.

389. O'Brien R: Iron overload: clinical and pathologic aspects in pediatrics. Semin Haematol 1977; 14:115.

390. Nienhuis A: Vitamin C and iron. N Engl J Med 1981; 304:170.

391. Link G, Pinson A, Hershko C: Heart cells in culture: a model of myocardial iron overload and chelation. J Lab Clin Med 1985; 106:147.

392. Leon M, Borer J, et al: Detection of early cardiac dysfunction in patients with severe beta-thalassemia and chronic iron overload. N Engl J Med 1979; 301:1143.

393. Flynn D, Fairney A, et al: Hormonal changes in thalassemia major. Arch Dis Child 1976; 51:828.

394. Bomford A, Williams R: Long term results of venesection therapy in idiopathic haemochromatosis. Q J Med 1976; 45:611.

395. Costin G, Kogut M, et al: Endocrine abnormalities in thalassemia major. Am J Dis Child 1979; 133:497.

396. Schafer A, Cheron R, et al: Clinical consequences of acquired transfusional iron overload in adults. N Engl J Med 1981; 304:319.

397. Schafer A, Rabinowe S, et al: Long-term efficacy of deferoxamine iron chelation therapy in adults with acquired transfusional iron overload. Arch Intern Med 1985; 45:1217.

398. Gertner J, Broadus A, et al: Impaired parathyroid response to induced hypocalcemia in thalassemia major. J Pediatr 1979; 95:210.

399. Mathews J, Williams H: Arthritis in hereditary hemochromatosis. Arthritis Rheum 1987; 30:1137.

400. Axford J, Bomford A, et al: Hip arthropathy in genetic hemochromatosis. Radiographic and histologic features. Arthritis Rheum 1991; 34:357.

401. Weinberg E: Iron and infection. Microb Rev 1978; 42:46.

402. Bullen J, Rogers H, Lewin J: The bacteriostatic effect of serum on *Pasteurella septica* and its abolition by iron compounds. Immunology 1971; 20:391.

403. Reiter B, Brock J, Steel E: Inhibition of *Escherichia coli* by bovine colostrum and post-colostral milk: II. The bacteriostatic effect of lactoferrin on a serum susceptible and serum resistant strain of *E. coli*. Immunology 1975; 28:83.

404. Lawrence T III, Biggers C, Simonton P: Bacteriostatic inhibition of *Klebsiella pneumoniae* by three human transferrins. Ann Hum Biol 1977; 4:281.

405. Abbott M, Galloway A, Cunningham J: Haemochromatosis presenting with a double *Yersinia* infection. J Infect 1986; 13:143.

406. Brennan R, Crain B, et al: *Cunninghamella*: a newly recognized cause of rhinocerebral mucormycosis. Am J Clin Pathol 1983; 80:98.

407. Bullen JJ, Spaulding PB, et al: Hemochromatosis, iron and septicemia caused by *Vibrio vulnificus*. Arch Intern Med 1991; 151:1606.

408. Capron J, Capron-Chivrac D, et al: Spontaneous *Yersinia enterocolitica* peritonitis in idiopathic hemochromatosis. Gastroenterology 1984; 87:1372.

409. Boelaert J, van Roost G, et al: The role of desferrioxamine in dialysis-associated mucormycosis: report of three cases and review of the literature. Clin Nephrol 1988; 29:261.

410. Rex J, Ginsberg A, et al: *Cunninghamella bertholetiae* infection associated with deferoxamine therapy. Rev Infect Dis 1988; 10:1187.

411. Daly A, Velazquez L, et al: Mucormycosis: association with deferoxamine therapy. Am J Med 1989; 87:468.

412. Robins-Browne R, Prpic J: Effects of iron and desferrioxamine on infections with *Yersinia enterocolitica*. Infect Immun 1985; 47:774.

413. Fargion S, Taddei M, et al: Early iron overload in beta-thalassaemia major: when to start chelation therapy? Arch Dis Child 1982; 57:929.

414. Zanella A, Berzuini A, et al: Iron status in red cell pyruvate kinase deficiency: study of Italian cases. Br J Haematol 1993; 83:485.

415. Modell B, Letsky E, et al: Survival and desferrioxamine in thalassaemia major. BMJ 1982; 284:1081.

416. Keberle H: The biochemistry of desferrioxamine and its relation to iron metabolism. Ann N Y Acad Sci 1964; 119:758.

417. Propper R, Cooper B, et al: Continuous subcutaneous administration of deferoxamine in patients with iron overload. N Engl J Med 1977; 297:418.

418. Cooper B, Bunn H, et al: Treatment of iron overload in adults with continuous parenteral desferrioxamine. Am J Med 1977; 63:958.

419. Olivieri N, Buncic J, et al: Visual and auditory neurotoxicity in patients receiving subcutaneous deferoxamine infusions. N Engl J Med 1986; 314:869.

420. Orizincolo L, Scatellari P, Castaldi G: Growth plate abnormalities in the long bones in treated β-thalassemia. Skeletal Radiol 1992; 21:39.

421. Bousquet J, Navarro M, et al: Rapid desensitisation for desferrioxamine anaphylactoid reaction. Lancet 1983; 2:859. Letter.

422. Falk R, Mattern W, et al: Iron removal during continuous ambulatory peritoneal dialysis using deferoxamine. Kidney Int 1983; 24:110.

423. Nathan D, Piomelli S: Oral iron chelators. Semin Hematol 1990; 27:83.

424. Kontoghiorghes GJ, Aldouri MA, et al: Effective chelation of iron in β-thalassemia with the oral chelator 1,2-dimethyl-3-hydroxypyrid-4-one. BMJ 1987; 295:1509.

425. Kontoghiorghes GJ, Bartlet TAN, et al: Continuous efficacy and no toxic side effects in eight months trials with the oral iron chelator 1,2-dimethyl-3-hydroxypyrid-4-one in iron overloaded thalassaemia and myelodysplastic patients. Blood 1988; 72:64a.

426. Bartlett A, Hoffbrand A, Kontoghiorghes G: Long-term trial with the oral iron chelator 1,2-dimethyl-3-hydroxypyrid-4-one (L1): II. Clinical observations. Br J Haematol 1990; 76:301.

427. Collins A, Fassos F, et al: Iron-balance and dose-response studies of the oral iron chelator 1,2-dimethyl-3-hydroxypyrid-4-one (L1) in iron-loaded patients with sickle cell disease. Blood 1994; 83; 2329.

428. Olivieri N, Brittenham G, et al: Iron-chelation therapy with oral deferiprone in patients with thalassemia major. N Engl J Med 1995; 332:918.

429. al-Refaie F, Wonke B, Hoffbrand A: Deferiprone-associated myelotoxicity. Eur J Haematol 1994; 535:298.

430. Nathan D: An orally effective iron chelator. N Engl J Med 1995; 322:1315. Editorial.

430a. Olivieri N, et al: Long-term followup of body iron in patients with thalassemia major during therapy with the orally active iron chelator deferiprone (L1). Blood. 1996; 88(Suppl 1):310a.

431. MacPhail A, Charlton R, et al: The relationship between maternal and infant iron status. Scand J Haematol 1980; 25:141.

432. Murray M, Murray A, Murray N, Murray M: The effect of iron status of Nigerian mothers on that of their infants at birth and 6 months, and on the concentration of Fe in breast milk. Br J Nutr 1978; 39:627.

433. Seligman P, Schleicher R, Allen R: Isolation and characterization of the transferrin receptor from human placenta. J Biol Chem 1979; 254:9943.

434. Okuyama T, Tawada T, et al: The role of transferrin and ferritin in the fetal-maternal-placental unit. Am J Obstet Gynecol 1985; 152:344.

435. Petry C, Wobken J, et al: Placental transferrin receptor in diabetic pregnancies with increased fetal iron demand. Am J Physiol 1994; 267:E507.

436. McArdle H, Morgan E: Transferrin and iron movements in the rat conceptus during gestation. J Reprod Fertil 1982; 66:529.

437. Hussain M, Gaafar T, et al: Relation of maternal and cord blood serum ferritin. Arch Dis Child 1977; 52:782.

438. Mau G: Hemoglobin changes during pregnancy and growth disturbances in the neonate. J Perinatal Med 1977; 5:172.

439. Ahamad S, Amir M, et al: Influence of maternal iron deficiency anemia on the fetal total body iron. Indian Pediatr 1983; 20:643.

440. Hamill R, Woods J, Cook B: Congenital atransferrinemia. A case report and review of the literature. Am J Clin Pathol 1991; 96:215.

441. Larrick J, Hyman E: Acquired iron-deficiency anemia caused by an antibody against the transferrin receptor. N Engl J Med 1984; 311:214.

442. Shahidi N, Nathan D, Diamond L: Iron deficiency anemia associated with an error of iron metabolism in two siblings. J Clin Invest 1964; 43:510.

443. Staven P, Saltvedt E, et al: Congenital hypochromic microcytic anaemia with iron overload of the liver and hyperferraemia. Scand J Haematol 1973; 10:153.

444. Staven P, Romslo I, et al: Ferrochelatase deficiency of the bone marrow in a syndrome of congenital microcytic anaemia with iron overload of the liver and hyperferraemia. Scand J Haematol 1985; 34:204.

445. Romslo I, Brun A, et al: Sideroblastic anemia with markedly increased free erythrocyte protoporphyrin without dermal photosensitivity. Blood 1982; 59:628.

446. Kardon N, Schulman P, et al: Cytogenetic findings in the dysmyelopoietic syndrome. Cancer 1982; 50:2834.

447. Gattermann N, Aul C, Schneider W: Two types of acquired idiopathic sideroblastic anaemia (AISA). Br J Haematol 1990; 74:45.

448. Bottomley SS: Sideroblastic anemia. Clin Haematol 1982; 11:389.

449. Hamel B, Schretlen E: Sideroblastic anaemia: a review of seven paediatric cases. Eur J Pediatr 1982; 138:130.

450. Barosi G, Cazzola M, et al: Estimation of ferrokinetic parameters by a mathematical model in patients with primary acquired sideroblastic anaemia. Br J Haematol 1978; 39:409.

451. Parlier V, Tiainen M, et al: Trisomy 8 detection in granulomonocytic, erythrocytic and megakaryocytic lineages by chromosomal *in situ* suppression hybridization in a case of refractory

anaemia with ringed sideroblasts complicating the course of paroxysmal nocturnal haemoglobinuria. Br J Haematol 1992; 81:296.

452. Nienhuis A, Bunn H, et al: Expression of the human c-*fms* proto-oncogene in hematopoietic cells and its deletion in the 5q − syndrome. Cell 1985; 42:421.

453. Clark R, Peters S, et al: Prognostic importance of hypodiploid hematopoietic precursors in myelodysplastic syndromes. N Engl J Med 1986; 314:1472.

454. Raskind W, Wijsman E, et al: X-linked sideroblastic anemia and ataxia: linkage to phosphoglycerate kinase at Xq13. Am J Hum Genet 1991; 48:335.

455. Harris JW: X-linked, pyridoxine-responsive sideroblastic anemia. N Engl J Med 1994; 330:709.

456. Dolan G, Reid M: Congenital sideroblastic anaemia in two girls. J Clin Pathol 1991; 44:464.

457. Buchanan G, Bottomley S, Nitchke R: Bone marrow δ-aminolevulinic acid synthetase deficiency in a female with congenital sideroblastic anemia. Blood 1980; 55:109.

458. Verhoef N, Noodeloos P, Leijnse H: Heme synthetase activity in normal human and rat erythroid cells and in sideroblastic anemia. Clin Chim Acta 1978; 82:45.

459. Ibraham N, Lutton J, et al: Regulation of heme metabolism in normal and sideroblastic bone marrow cells in culture. J Lab Clin Med 1985; 105:593.

460. Cox T, Bottomley S, et al: X-linked pyridoxine-responsive sideroblastic anemia due to a Thr(388)-to-Ser substitution in erythroid 5-aminolevulinate synthase. N Engl J Med 1994; 330:675.

461. Bottomley S, May B, et al: Molecular defects of erythroid 5-aminolevulinate synthase in X-linked sideroblastic anemia. J Bioenerg Biomembr 1995; 27:161.

462. Cotter P, Rucknagel D, Bishop D: X-linked sideroblastic anemia: identification of the mutation in the erythroid-specific delta-aminolevulinate synthase gene (*ALAS2*) in the original family described by Cooley. Blood 1994; 84:3915.

463. Ruutu P, Ruutu T, et al: A function of neutrophils in preleukemia. Scand J Haematol 1977; 18:317.

464. Sultan Y, Caen JP: Platelet dysfunction in preleukemic states and various types of leukemia. Ann N Y Acad Sci 1972; 201:300.

465. Hines J: Effect of pyridoxine plus chronic phlebotomy on the function and morphology of bone marrow and liver in pyridoxine-responsive sideroblastic anemia. Semin Hematol 1976; 13:133.

466. Mason D, Emerson P: Primary acquired sideroblastic anemia: response to treatment with pyridoxal-5-phosphate. BMJ 1973; 1:389.

467. Lewy R, Kansu E, Gabuzda T: Leukemia in patients with acquired idiopathic sideroblastic anemia: an evaluation of prognostic indicators. Am J Hematol 1979; 6:323.

468. Bolwell B, Cassileth P, Gale R: Low dose cytosine arabinoside in myelodysplasia and acute myelogenous leukemia: a review. Leukemia 1986; 1:575.

469. Estey EH, Keating MJ, et al: Karyotype is prognostically more important than the FAB system's distinction between myelodysplastic syndrome and acute myelogenous leukemia. Hematol Pathol 1987; 1:203.

470. Kitahara M, Cosgriff T, Eyre H: Sideroblastic anemia as a preleukemic event in patients treated for Hodgkin's disease. Ann Intern Med 1980; 92:625.

471. Borgna-Pignatti C, Marradi P, et al: Thiamine-responsive anemia in DIDMOAD syndrome. J Pediatr 1989; 114:405.

472. Pearson H, Lobel J, et al: A new syndrome of refractory sideroblastic anemia with vacuolization of marrow precursors and exocrine pancreatic dysfunction. J Pediatr 1979; 95:976.

473. Stoddard R, McCurnin D, et al: Syndrome of refractory sideroblastic anemia with vacuolization of marrow precursors and exocrine pancreatic dysfunction presenting in the neonate. J Pediatr 1981; 99:259.

474. McShane M, Hammans S, et al: Pearson syndrome and mitochondrial encephalomyopathy in a patient with a deletion of mtDNA. Am J Hum Genet 1991; 48:39.

475. Rotig A, Cormier V, et al: Pearson's marrow-pancreas syndrome: a multisystem mitochondrial disorder in infancy. J Clin Invest 1990; 86:1601.

476. Sano T, Ban K, et al: Molecular and genetic analyses of two patients with Pearson's marrow-pancreas syndrome. Pediatr Res 1993; 34:105.

477. Gurgey A, Rotig A, et al: Pearson's marrow-pancreas syndrome in 2 Turkish children. Acta Haematol 1992; 87:206.

478. Vreugdene G, Lowenberer B, et al: Anemia of chronic disease in rheumatoid arthritis-raised serum interleukin-6 (IL-6) levels and effects of Il-6 and anti-IL-6 on *in vitro* erythropoiesis. Rheumatol Int 1990; 10:127.

479. Sears D: Anemia of chronic disease. Med Clin North Am 1992; 76:567.

480. Konijn A, Hershko C: Ferritin synthesis in inflammation: I. Pathogenesis of impaired iron release. Br J Haematol 1977; 37:7.

481. Hersh EM, Wong VG, Freireich EJ: Inhibition of the local inflammatory response in man by antimetabolites. Blood 1966; 27:38.

482. Gasche C, Reinisch W, et al: Anemia in Crohn's disease. Importance of inadequate erythropoietin production and iron deficiency. Dig Dis Sci 1994; 39:1930.

483. Means R Jr: Clinical application of recombinant erythropoietin in the anemia of chronic disease. Hematol Oncol Clin North Am 1994; 8:933.

484. Faquin W, Schneider T, Goldberg M: Effect of inflammatory cytokines on hypoxia-induced erythropoietin production. Blood 1992; 79:1987.

485. Eschbach J, Haley N, et al: A comparison of the responses to recombinant human erythropoietin in normal and uremic subjects. Kidney Int 1992; 42:407.

486. Adamson J: The relationship of erythropoietin and iron metabolism to red blood cell production in humans. Semin Oncol 1994; 21:9.

487. Chan R, Seiser C, et al: Regulation of transferrin receptor mRNA expression. Distinct regulatory features in erythroid cells. Eur J Biochem 1994; 220:683.

488. Brugnara C, Colella G, et al: Effects of subcutaneous recombinant human erythropoietin in normal subjects: development of decreased reticulocyte hemoglobin content and iron-deficient erythropoiesis. J Lab Clin Med 1994; 123:660.

489. Hotta T, Ogawa H, et al: Iron balance following recombinant human erythropoietin therapy for anemia associated with chronic renal failure. Int J Hematol 1991; 54:195.

490. Kooistra M, van Es A, et al: Iron metabolism in patients with the anaemia of end-stage renal disease during treatment with recombinant human erythropoietin. Br J Haematol 1991; 79:634.

491. Hughes R, Smith T, et al: Regulation of iron absorption in iron loaded subjects with end stage renal disease: effects of treatment with recombinant human erythropoietin and reduction of iron stores. Br J Haematol 1992; 82:445.

The Porphyrias

Shigeru Sassa • Attallah Kappas

The porphyrias are a group of disorders caused by deficiencies in the activities of the enzymes of the heme biosynthetic pathway. The enzyme deficiencies can be either partial or nearly complete. As a result, porphyrins and/or their precursors, such as δ-aminolevulinic acid (ALA) and porphobilinogen (PBG), are abnormally produced in excess, accumulate in tissues, and are excreted in urine and stool. Two cardinal symptoms of the porphyrias are cutaneous photosensitivity and neurologic disturbances.

ENZYMES AND INTERMEDIATES IN THE HEME BIOSYNTHETIC PATHWAY

Outline of the Pathway

The enzymatic and intermediate steps in the heme biosynthetic pathway are illustrated in Figure 12–1. In animal cells, the first step and the last three steps occur in mitochondria; the intermediate steps take place in the cytosol. The two major organs that are active in heme synthesis are the liver and the erythroid bone marrow, and inherited enzymatic defects in the porphyrias are mainly expressed in these tissues.

Delta-Aminolevulinate Synthase (ALAS). ALAS is the first enzyme of the heme biosynthetic pathway and catalyzes the condensation of glycine and succinyl coenzyme A to form ALA (see Fig. 12–1). The enzyme is localized in the inner membrane of mitochondria and requires pyridoxal 5′-phosphate as a cofactor.[1] ALAS activity is very low and is rate limiting for heme formation.[2] Hepatic (or nonspecific) and erythroid ALASs are isozymes that are encoded by two distinct nuclear genes,[3, 4] *ALAS1* and *ALAS2* genes, respectively. The two human ALAS genes appear to have evolved by

duplication of a common ancestral gene that encoded a primitive catalytic site, with subsequent addition of DNA sequences encoding variable functions.[5] The locus for human gene *ALAS1* is at chromosome 3p21.1, and that for *ALAS2* is at Xp11.21.[4] Inherited deficiency of ALAS2 is associated with X-linked sideroblastic anemia.[6]

Delta-Aminolevulinate Dehydratase (ALAD). Two molecules of ALA are converted by a cytosolic enzyme, ALAD, to a monopyrrole, PBG, with the removal of two molecules of water (see Fig. 12–1). ALAD deficiency porphyria (ADP) is due to an almost complete lack of enzyme activity. The human *ALAD* gene is localized at chromosome 9q34.[7] The enzyme is a homo-octamer with a subunit size of 36,274 daltons[8] and requires an intact sulfhydryl group and a zinc atom per subunit for full activity.[9] Lead inhibits ALAD by displacing zinc from the enzyme. Zinc is the essential metal for enzyme activity, thus this results in neurologic disturbances, some of which resemble those of ADP.[10] The most potent inhibitor of the enzyme is succinylacetone,[11] a structural analogue of ALA, which is found in urine and blood of patients with hereditary tyrosinemia who frequently develop a syndrome similar to ADP.[12]

Porphobilinogen Deaminase (PBGD). PBGD catalyzes the condensation of four molecules of PBG to yield a linear tetrapyrrole, hydroxymethylbilane. In the absence of the subsequent enzyme, uroporphyrinogen III cosynthase, hydroxymethylbilane is spontaneously converted into a ring-form tetrapyrrole, uroporphyrinogen I. In contrast, in the presence of the cosynthase, uroporphyrinogen III that has an inverted D-ring pyrrole is formed (see Fig. 12–1).

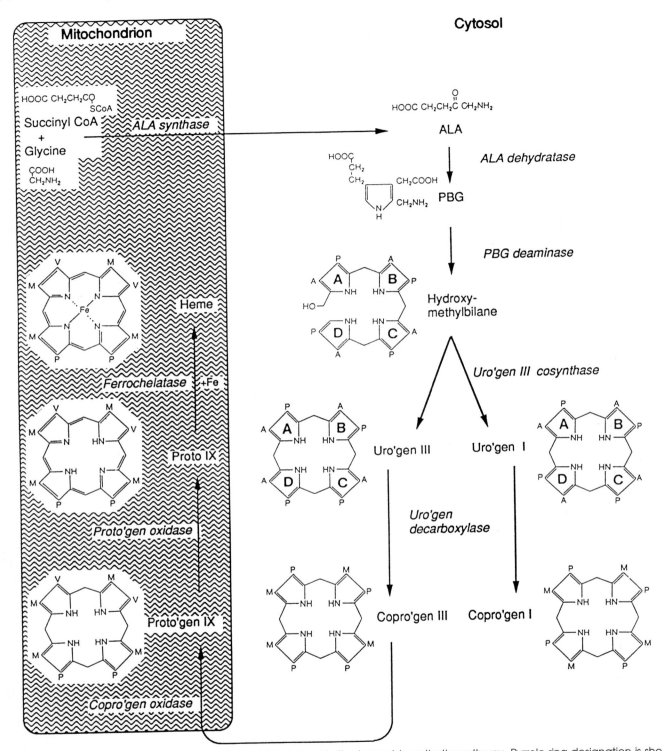

Figure 12–1. Enzymes *(italics)* and intermediates *(plain letters)* in the heme biosynthetic pathway. Pyrrole ring designation is shown in the structures of hydroxymethylbilane and uroporphyrinogen (uro'gen) I and III. In uro'gen III, substituent groups in the D ring have undergone "flipping," that is, the pyrrole ring is reversed. A = —CH₂COOH; ALA = δ-aminolevulinic acid; copro'gen = coproporphyrinogen; M = —CH₃; P = —CH₂CH₂COOH; PBG = porphobilinogen; proto = protoporphyrin; proto'gen = protoporphyrinogen; uro'gen = uroporphyrinogen; V = —CHCH₂.

The gene locus for human PBGD is at chromosome 11q23→11qter.[13] The human *PBGD* gene is split into 15 exons, spread over 10 kb of DNA.[14] There are two isozymes of PBGD: erythroid specific and nonspecific.[15]

The two isoforms of PBGD are produced by distinct messenger RNAs (mRNAs), which are transcribed from a single gene by alternate transcription and splicing of its mRNA. A partial (or heterozygous) deficiency of PBGD is associated with acute intermittent porphyria (AIP).

Uroporphyrinogen III Cosynthase (UCS). UCS catalyzes the formation of uroporphyrinogen III from hydroxymethylbilane. This involves an intramolecular rearrangement that affects only the D-ring of the uroporphyrinogen (see Fig. 12–1). Human UCS predicted from its complementary DNA (cDNA) consists of 263 amino acid residues, with a molecular mass of 28,607 daltons.[16] Homozygous deficiency of UCS is associated with congenital erythropoietic porphyria (CEP).

Uroporphyrinogen Decarboxylase (UROD). UROD is a cytosolic enzyme and catalyzes the sequential removal of the four carboxylic groups of the carboxymethyl side chains in uroporphyrinogen to yield coproporphyrinogen (see Fig. 12–1). Human UROD cDNA consists of 10 exons that are spread over 3 kb.[17] The gene for UROD has been localized to chromosome 1pter→p21.[18] Porphyria cutanea tarda (PCT) is due to a partial (or heterozygous) deficiency of UROD, whereas hepatoerythropoietic porphyria (HEP) is due to a homozygous deficiency of the enzyme.

Coproporphyrinogen Oxidase (CPO). CPO is a mitochondrial enzyme that catalyzes the removal of the carboxyl group and two hydrogens from the propionic groups of pyrrole rings A and B of coproporphyrinogen to form vinyl groups at these positions (see Fig. 12–1). The gene for human CPO is localized to chromosome 9.[19] Human CPO predicted from its cDNA is a protein of 354 amino acid residues.[20] Hereditary coproporphyria (HCP) is due to a partial (or heterozygous) deficiency of CPO.

Protoporphyrinogen Oxidase (PPOX). The oxidation of protoporphyrinogen to protoporphyrin is mediated by a mitochondrial enzyme, PPOX, which catalyzes the removal of six hydrogen atoms from the porphyrinogen nucleus (see Fig. 12–1). Variegate porphyria (VP) is due to a partial (or heterozygous) deficiency of PPOX. This is the only enzyme in the heme pathway for which no cDNA cloning has been reported.

Ferrochelatase (FECH). The final step of heme biosynthesis is the insertion of iron into protoporphyrin (see Fig. 12–1). This reaction is catalyzed by a mitochondrial enzyme, FECH. Unlike other steps in the heme biosynthetic pathway, this enzyme utilizes protoporphyrin IX as substrate, rather than its reduced form. However, the enzyme specifically requires ferrous, but not ferric, iron. The gene for human FECH has been assigned to chromosome 18q21.3.[21] The human *FECH* gene contains 11 exons and has a minimum size of about 45 kb.[21] Erythropoietic protoporphyria (EPP) is due to a partial (or heterozygous) FECH deficiency.

CONTROL OF HEME SYNTHESIS IN THE LIVER AND ERYTHROID CELLS

Biosynthesis of heme in the liver is controlled largely by the rate of formation of ALAS,[2] that is, ALAS1 (Fig. 12–2). The enzyme activity in normal liver cells is very low, whereas its level increases dramatically when the liver needs to make more heme in response to various chemical treatments.[22] The synthesis of the enzyme is also regulated in a feedback fashion by heme, which is the end product of the biosynthetic pathway.[23] At higher heme concentrations than those that repress the synthesis of ALAS1, heme induces microsomal heme oxygenase, resulting in an enhancement of its own catabolism.[23] Conceptually, therefore, the hepatic heme concentration is maintained by a balance between the synthesis of ALAS1 and heme oxygenase, both of which are under the regulatory influence of heme. In contrast, ALAS2 synthesis in erythroid cells is either refractory to or stimulated by heme treatment or is developmentally increased when heme content increases in the cell. Thus, regulation of heme synthesis in erythroid cells is different from that in the liver.[24]

PATHOPHYSIOLOGY OF PORPHYRINS AND THEIR PRECURSORS

Photosensitivity

Photosensitivity in cutaneous forms of porphyria is due to the accumulation of free porphyrins in the skin. Free porphyrins occur only in small amounts in normal tissues, but their levels may become markedly elevated in the porphyrias. On illumination at wavelengths of about 400 nm (Soret band) and in the presence of oxygen, porphyrins cause photodynamic damage to tissues, cells, subcellular elements, and biomolecules through the formation of singlet oxygen.[25]

Neurologic Disturbances

Acute hepatic porphyrias (ADP, AIP, HCP, and VP) are characterized by neurologic disturbances. The most common symptoms are abdominal pain, disturbances in intestinal motility (e.g., diarrhea and constipation), dysesthesias, muscular paralysis, and respiratory failure, which can be fatal. Despite the fact that a few theories have been put forth, the exact nature of the neurologic disturbances in the porphyrias remains obscure.[26]

CLASSIFICATION OF PORPHYRIAS

Porphyrias were traditionally classified as either hepatic or erythropoietic, depending on the principal site of expression of the specific enzymatic defect. They can also be classified as acute hepatic or cutaneous porphyrias. *Acute hepatic porphyrias* are characterized clinically by neurologic disturbances and biochemically by an overproduction of porphyrin precursors (e.g., ALA or PBG), whereas *cutaneous porphyrias* are characterized clinically by cutaneous photosensitivity and biochemically by an excessive production of porphyrins. These classifications are not necessarily absolute, because some porphyrias (e.g., HEP) show a major biochemical expression in both the liver and the bone marrow or are associated with both cutaneous and neurologic disturbances, as are HCP and VP. Eight enzymes are involved in the synthesis of heme and,

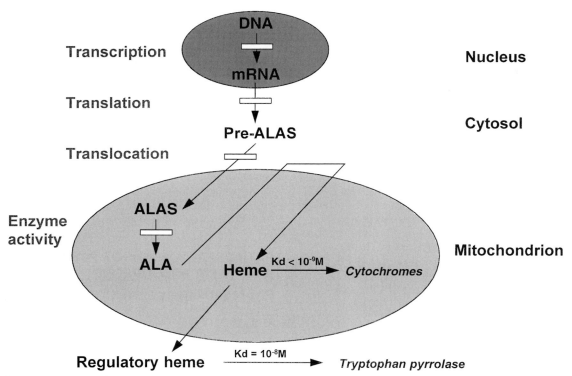

Figure 12-2. Regulation of heme synthesis in the liver. The rate of heme synthesis in the liver is determined largely by the level of ALA synthase (ALAS). The regulatory function of heme can be exerted by the regulatory heme, which is in equilibrium with the heme moiety of tryptophan pyrrolase. Excess heme may be degraded by microsomal heme oxygenase; heme also may induce heme oxygenase *(not shown)*. All these changes ultimately result in the normalization of the concentration of regulatory heme when all pools that require heme (e.g., cytochromes) have been filled. mRNA = messenger RNA.

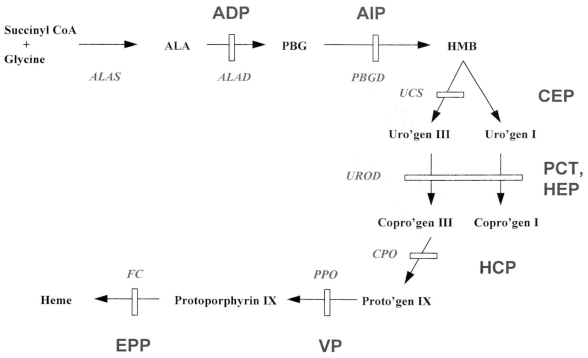

Figure 12-3. Enzymatic defects in the porphyrias. Porphyrias and their enzymatic defects *(open bars)* are shown. ALA = δ-aminolevulinic acid; ADP = ALAD deficiency porphyria; AIP = acute intermittent porphyria; ALAD = ALA dehydratase; CEP = congenital erythropoietic porphyria; copro'gen = coproporphyrinogen; CPO = copro'gen oxidase; EPP = erythropoietic protoporphyria; FC = ferrochelatase; HCP = hereditary coproporphyria; HEP = hepatoerythropoietic porphyria; HMB = hydroxy-methylbilane; PBG = porphobilinogen; PBGD = PBG deaminase; proto'gen = protoporphyrinogen; PCT = porphyria cutanea tarda; PPO = proto'gen oxidase; uro'gen = uroporphyrinogen; UCS = uro'gen III cosynthase; UROD = uro'gen decarboxylase; VP = variegate porphyria.

Table 12-1. THE PORPHYRIAS AND THEIR ENZYMATIC DEFECTS

Enzyme Deficiency	Porphyria	Principal Site of Expression	Mode of Transmission	Remarks
ALAD	ADP	Liver	Recessive	
PBGD	AIP	Liver	Dominant	
	Type I			CRIM (−)
	Type II			Normal erythrocyte PBGD
	Type III			CRIM (+)
UCS	CEP	Bone marrow	Recessive	
UROD	PCT	Liver		Acquired
	Type I			UROD decreased in all tissues
	Type II		Dominant	UROD decreased in the liver, but
	Type III		Dominant	not in erythrocytes
	HEP	Liver and bone marrow	Recessive	
CPO	HCP	Liver	Dominant	
PPOX	VP	Liver	Dominant	
FECH	EPP	Bone marrow	Dominant	

ALAD = δ-aminolevulinate dehydratase; ADP = δ-aminolevulinate dehydratase deficiency porphyria; PBGD = porphobilinogen deaminase; AIP = acute intermittent porphyria; UCS = uroporphyrinogen III cosynthase; CEP = congenital erythropoietic porphyria; UROD = uroporphyrinogen decarboxylase; PCT = porphyria cutanea tarda; HEP = hepatoerythropoietic porphyria; CPO = coproporphyrinogen oxidase; HCP = hereditary coproporphyria; PPOX = protoporphyrinogen oxidase; VP = variegate porphyria; FECH = ferrochelatase; EPP = erythropoietic protoporphyria; CRIM = cross-reactive immunologic material.
Data from Sassa S, Kappas A: The porphyrias. In Nathan DG, Oski FA (eds): Hematology of Infancy and Childhood. Philadelphia, W.B. Saunders Co., 1993, p 451.

with the exception of the first enzyme (i.e., ALAS), an enzymatic defect at each step of heme synthesis is associated with each form of porphyria (Fig. 12–3 and Table 12–1). In this chapter, each porphyria is described according to the order of the enzymes in the heme biosynthetic sequence (see Fig. 12–3). Cardinal symptoms and laboratory findings of each porphyria are summarized in Table 12–2.

ALAD Deficiency Porphyria

ADP is an autosomal recessive disorder resulting from a homozygous ALAD deficiency (see Fig. 12–3 and

Table 12-2. CLINICAL AND LABORATORY FEATURES OF THE PORPHYRIAS

Porphyria	Clinical Features	Laboratory Features			
		Erythrocytes	Plasma	Urine	Stool
ADP	Neurologic (as in AIP)	ZnPP	—	ALA	—
AIP	Neurologic: nausea, vomiting, abdominal pain, diarrhea, constipation, ileus, dysuria, muscle hypotonia, respiratory failure, sensory neuropathy, seizures	—	—	ALA, PBG	—
CEP	Photosensitivity: bullae, crusts, scar formation, sclerodermoid change, hyperpigmentation and hypopigmentation, hypertrichosis, erythrodontia, hemolytic anemia, splenomegaly	Uro I, copro I	Uro I, copro I	Uro, 7-carboxyl	—
PCT	Photosensitivity: skin fragility, bullae, crusts, scar formation, sclerodermoid change, hyperpigmentation and hypopigmentation, hypertrichosis	—	Uro, 7-carboxyl	Uro, 7-carboxyl	Uro, 7-carboxyl, isocopro
HEP	Photosensitivity (as in CEP)	ZnPP	Uro, 7-carboxyl	Uro, 7-carboxyl	Uro, 7-carboxyl, isocopro
HCP	Neurologic (as in ADP, AIP, and VP) and photosensitive (as in VP)	—	Copro	Copro, ALA, PBG	Copro
VP	Neurologic (as in ADP, AIP, and HCP) and photosensitive (as in HCP)	—	Proto	ALA, PBG	Proto
EPP	Photosensitivity: burning sensation, edema, erythema, itching, scarring, vesicles	Proto	Proto	—	Proto

7-carboxyl = 7-carboxylporphyrin; copro = coproporphyrin; isocopro = isocoproporphyrin; uro = uroporphyrin; ZnPP = zinc protoporphyrin.
Data from Sassa S, Kappas A: The porphyrias. In Nathan DG, Oski FA (eds): Hematology of Infancy and Childhood. Philadelphia, W. B. Saunders Co., 1993, p 451.

Table 12–1). This is the rarest form of the porphyrias; only four cases have been reported. The symptomatology is similar to that seen in AIP, but ADP can be differentiated from AIP by the lack of PBG overproduction.

Clinical Findings. Signs and symptoms of ADP include vomiting, pain in the arms and legs, and neuropathy, which are exacerbated after stress, alcohol use, or decreased food intake[27] (see Table 12–2). One infant with ADP has been described who, unusually, had a clinical course from birth onward that included general muscle hypotonia and respiratory insufficiency.[28]

Biochemical Findings. Urinary ALA excretion is very elevated, whereas urinary PBG excretion is within the normal range (see Table 12–2). Urinary and erythrocyte porphyrin levels are also markedly elevated (about 100-fold), but PBG excretion is normal; no satisfactory explanation has been advanced to account for these observations. A primary block in a distal enzyme is unlikely. Fecal porphyrin excretion is normal or marginally elevated. Furthermore, patients with ADP display markedly decreased activity of ALAD in erythrocytes, as well as in nonerythroid cells (less than or equal to 2% of normal), and their parents show approximately 50% decreases in enzyme activities.

Molecular Biology. In a patient with an adult onset of the disease, separate point mutations were identified, one occurring in each ALAD allele.[29] One was a base transition, $G^{820} \rightarrow A$, resulting in an amino acid change, $Ala^{274} \rightarrow Thr$, whereas the other was a base transition, $C^{718} \rightarrow T$, which resulted in an amino acid change, $Arg^{240} \rightarrow Trp$. The former mutation accompanied markedly reduced enzyme activity, whereas the latter accompanied instability of the enzyme.[30] These findings indicated that the proband was a compound heterozygote for two separate point mutations and accounted for the almost complete lack of enzymatic activity in the proband's cells and the half-normal activity in cells from his family members. Another compound heterozygosity with point mutations distinct from the previously discussed proband was also demonstrated in a child with ADP.[31] The four distinct point mutations in two pedigrees suggest a marked heterogeneity in the mutations in this disorder.

Diagnosis. Definitive diagnosis depends on the demonstration of impaired ALAD activity and deficiency of enzyme protein in erythrocytes. Supporting evidence for the diagnosis includes massive elevations of urinary ALA (but not of PBG) and substantial elevations of porphyrins in urine and erythrocytes. Clinical symptoms of ADP occur only in homozygous patients, whereas heterozygous subjects (i.e., parents and certain siblings of the proband) remain clinically unaffected.

Treatment. The clinical management of ADP should be carried out as described for AIP.

Acute Intermittent Porphyria

AIP, which is also known as *Swedish porphyria, pyrroloporphyria,* or *intermittent acute porphyria,* is an autosomal dominant disorder resulting from a partial PBGD deficiency (see Fig. 12–3 and Table 12–1). The deficient enzyme activity (about 50% of normal) is found in all tissues, including erythrocytes, in the majority of patients (85% or more). However, a subset of patients (15% or less) shows deficient enzyme activity only in nonerythroid cells. The majority (about 90%) of individuals with this genetic enzyme deficiency remain clinically normal throughout life. Clinical expression of the disease is usually linked to environmental or acquired factors (e.g., nutritional status, drugs, corticosteroids, and other chemicals of endogenous or exogenous origin). The cardinal pathobiologic defect of the disease is a neurologic dysfunction that may affect the peripheral, autonomic, and central nervous systems (see Table 12–2).

Prevalence. AIP is probably the most common of the genetic porphyrias. The highest incidence of AIP occurs in Lapland, Scandinavia, and the United Kingdom, although it has been reported in many population groups. The prevalence of AIP was estimated to be 1 to 2 per 100,000 in Europe[32] and 2.4 per 100,000 in Finland.[33] The frequency of low PBGD activity, which includes both patients with clinically manifest AIP and latent gene carriers, is, however, as high as 1 per 500 in the general population of Finland.[34] The disorder is expressed clinically almost invariably after puberty and more often in women than in men.

Clinical Findings. Like ADP, AIP is a severely debilitating form of acute hepatic porphyria. Abdominal pain, which may be generalized or localized, is the most common symptom and is often the initial sign of an acute attack. Other gastroenterologic features may include nausea, vomiting, constipation or diarrhea, abdominal distention, and ileus. Urinary retention, incontinence, and dysuria may frequently be observed. Tachycardia and hypertension, and less often fever, sweating, restlessness, and tremor, also are observed. In up to 40% of patients, hypertension may become sustained between acute attacks.

Peripheral neuropathy is a common feature of AIP. Muscle weakness often begins proximally in the legs but may involve the arms or the distal extremities. Motor neuropathy also may involve the cranial nerves or lead to bulbar paralysis, respiratory impairment, and death. Sensory, patchy neuropathy also may occur. Acute attacks of AIP may be accompanied by seizures, especially in patients with hyponatremia due to vomiting, inappropriate fluid therapy, or the syndrome of inappropriate antidiuretic hormone release. The course of an acute attack of AIP is highly variable both in individuals and among patients, with attacks lasting from a few days to several months. No cutaneous manifestations are associated with this enzyme deficiency.

Precipitating Factors. Asymptomatic heterozygotes (about 90% of subjects with documented PBGD deficiency) may display neither abnormalities in concentrations of porphyrin precursors nor clinical symptoms. Individuals with both latent or previously clinically expressed AIP may be precipitated into an acute attack by endogenous or exogenous environmental factors. There are at least five different classes of precipitating factors in this disease.[26]

ALAS1 Inducers. Most precipitating factors can be related to an associated increase in the activity of ALAS1 in the liver.[26] Overproduction of ALA then makes the partially deficient PBGD activity rate-limiting.

Endocrine Factors. The clinical disease is more common in women especially at the time of menses. A subset of female patients experiences cyclical premenstrual exacerbations of the disease.[35]

Calorie Intake. Loss of appetite or reduced calorie intake often leads to exacerbations of AIP.[36] Caloric supplementation may reduce PBG excretion and suppress clinical symptoms.[37]

Drugs and Foreign Chemicals. Many chemicals (e.g., barbiturates, certain steroids, and other foreign substances) that exacerbate porphyria have the potential to induce cytochrome P-450.[26] The resultant enhanced demand for heme synthesis may lead to induction of hepatic ALAS1.

Stress. Various forms of stress, including intercurrent illnesses, infections, alcoholic excess, and surgery, are known to upregulate the heme oxygenase gene, leading to excessive heme catabolism and derepression of ALAS1, with clinical expression of AIP.

Biochemical Findings. Patients with clinically expressed AIP, and a few individuals with latent AIP, excrete variably increased amounts of ALA and PBG in the urine between attacks. In the majority of cases, the onset of an acute attack is accompanied by further marked increases in excretion of these precursors. In severe cases, the urine develops a port-wine color from a high content of porphobilin, an auto-oxidation product of PBG. Acute attacks may also be associated with elevations in the serum concentrations of ALA, PBG, and porphyrins, which are normally undetectable. Stool porphyrin levels are usually normal or only slightly elevated. The Watson-Schwartz test is widely used as a screening test for urinary PBG. This test is, however, neither specific nor quantitative, and its results need to be confirmed and quantified by the column method of Mauzerall and Granick.[38] Hemoglobin levels and bilirubin production are normal in AIP.

Molecular Biology. Patients with AIP can be classified into three subsets (Table 12–3):

1. Patients with type I mutations are characterized by cross-reactive immunologic material (CRIM)-negative PBGD mutations; they exhibit both reduced enzyme activity and reduced PBGD protein content (about 50% of normal).

2. Type II mutations are observed in fewer than 15% of all AIP patients and are characterized by decreased PBGD activity in nonerythroid cells, such as liver (about 50% of normal), but with normal erythroid PBGD activity.

3. Patients with type III mutations are characterized by CRIM-positive mutations, that is, decreased enzyme activity (about 50% of normal) with the presence of structurally abnormal enzyme protein.[39]

Various mutations of the human *PBGD* gene have been described in patients with AIP (Table 12–4). Mutations found in type I AIP are single-base substitutions or deletions that lead to a single amino acid change or to truncated proteins, which result in the loss of expression of the enzyme protein. The mutations found in type II AIP are single-base substitutions that occur in the exon/intron boundary of exon 1, resulting in a splicing defect that affects only the nonspecific form of PBGD, but not the erythroid-specific PBGD, because the transcription of the gene in erythroid cells starts downstream of the site of mutation. Mutations characterizing type III AIP, mostly occurring in exons 10 and 12, are observed in the region that is thought to be essential for catalytic activity. In addition to these mutations or deletions (see Table 12–4), a few intragenic restriction fragment length polymorphisms that are unique to certain AIP families have been reported, but their mutations have not yet been identified.[40–47]

Diagnosis. The diagnosis of type I and III AIP can be made by demonstrating decreased PBGD activity in erythrocytes in the majority of patients (85% or more), whereas the distinction between carrier or latent status and clinically expressed AIP requires demonstration of elevated urinary excretion of PBG and ALA. Elevated urinary levels of both ALA and PBG also may be seen in HCP and VP; measurement of urinary and stool porphyrins usually differentiates these conditions from AIP. The diagnosis of type II AIP requires either the demonstration of PBGD deficiency in nonerythroid cells (e.g., lymphocytes or fibroblasts) or DNA hybridization with allele-specific oligonucleotides specific for the mutation.

Treatment. The treatment of AIP as well as that of ADP, HCP, and VP is essentially identical. Treatment between attacks comprises adequate nutritional intake, avoidance of drugs and chemicals known to exacerbate porphyria, and prompt treatment of other intercurrent diseases or infections. Unresponsive severe cases should be treated with intravenous administration of carbohydrate initiated with dextrose to provide a minimum of 300 g of carbohydrate per day. Intravenous hematin (4 mg/kg every 12 hours) is probably most effective in reducing ALA and PBG excretion as well as in curtailing acute attacks.[48] Nasal or subcutaneous administration of long-acting agonistic analogues of luteinizing hormone–releasing hormone have been shown to inhibit ovulation and greatly reduce the incidence of perimenstrual attacks of AIP in some women with cyclic exacerbations of the disease.[49] Synthetic heme analogues (e.g., tin mesoporphyrin, which inhibits heme catabolism) have also been shown to diminish the output of ALA, PBG, or porphyrins in patients with AIP and VP.[50]

Table 12-3. SUBSETS OF ACUTE INTERMITTENT PORPHYRIA

| | Erythrocyte PBGD | | | |
Type	Activity (% of Control)	Mass (% of Control)	Mass/Activity	CRIM
I	50	50	1	(−)
II	100	100	1	(−)
III	50	>50	>1	(+)

Table 12-4. MUTATIONS OF THE *PBGD* GENE IN ACUTE INTERMITTENT PORPHYRIA

Mutation in Genomic DNA	Location in cDNA and Protein	Amino Acid Substitution or Protein Abnormality	Subset Type	Reference
G→T	Exon 1 IVS1−1	Splicing defect on cDNA	II	104
G→A	Exon 1 M1I	Splicing defect on cDNA	II	105
G→A	Intron 1 IVS1+1	Splicing defect on cDNA	II	106
G→A	Exon 3 R26H	Arg→His (cofactor binding)	III	107
G→A	Exon 4 A31T	Ala→Thr	III	108
C→A	Exon 4 Q34K	Gln→Lys		109
G→A	Exon 4 S45S	Ser→Ser (silent mutation)		109
G→T	Exon 5 A55S	Ala→Ser	III	108
	Exon 7 V93F	Val→Phe (minimal activity)		105
G→A	Intron 5 IVS5+1	Splicing defect on cDNA		108
G→A	Exon 7 G111R	Gly→Arg		110
G→A	Intron 7 Last position	Splicing defect on cDNA		111
C→T	Exon 8 R116W*	Arg→Try (minimal activity)	I	105, 112
G→T	Exon 9 Q137x	Gln→stop (truncated protein)	I	113
G→A	Exon 9 R149Q	Arg→Gln (cofactor binding)	I	114
G→T	Exon 9 R149L	Arg→Leu (cofactor binding)	I	108
G→A	Intron 9 Last position	Splicing defect on cDNA		115
G→A	Exon 10 R167Q	Arg→Gln	III	109, 116
G→A	Exon 10 R167W	Arg→Try	III	117, 118
C→T	Exon 10 R173Q	Arg→Gln	III	116, 118
G→A	Exon 10 L177R	Leu→Arg		109
T→G	Exon 10 W198X†	Try→stop (truncated protein)	I	105, 119
G→A	Exon 10 R201W	Arg→Try (unstable protein)		105
	Exon 10 V202V	Val→Val (silent mutation)		109
G→T	Exon 10 E223K	Glu→Lys		108
G→A	Exon 10 Deletion	9 bp (truncated protein)	I	114
G→T	Exon 12 L245R	Leu→Arg	I	114
T→G	Exon 12 C247R	Cys→Arg		120
T→C	Exon 12 C247F	Cys→Phe (unstable protein)		105
	Exon 12 E250K	Glu→Lys (structural abnormality)	I	108
G→A	Exon 12 A252T	Ala→Thr		120
G→A	Exon 12 A252V	Ala→Val		120
C→T	Exon 12 H256N	His→Asn		109
C→A	Exon 12 Skipping exon 12	Truncated protein	III	39
G→A	Exon 12 Skipping exon 12	Truncated protein	III	121
G→C	Exon 12 Silent mutation			120
G→A	Exon 12 Premature stop codon	Truncated protein		120
CT deletion	Exon 12 Frameshift	Truncated protein	I	114
T deletion	Exon 14 Frameshift	Truncated protein	I	114
G→A	Exon 14 W283X	Try→stop (truncated protein)		105
G→A	Exon 14 IVS14+1	Exon 14 skipping		110

*Prevalent among Dutch families.
†Prevalent among Swedish families.

Congenital Erythropoietic Porphyria

CEP, which is also referred to as Günther's disease, is an autosomal recessive disorder (see Fig. 12–3 and Table 12–1). The primary abnormality is a decreased activity of UCS that results in accumulation and hyperexcretion of predominantly type I porphyrins (see Table 12–2). A fetus with this enzymatic defect shows brownish amniotic fluid from excessive amounts of porphyrins, and after birth the homozygous gene carriers manifest cutaneous photosensitivity, hemolysis, and a decreased life expectancy.

Prevalence. Fewer than 200 cases have been reported, and some of these cases may really have been PCT or HEP. No clear racial or sexual predilection is apparent.

Clinical Findings. The first clue suggesting the diagnosis of CEP at birth is pink to dark-brown staining of diapers, which is caused by large amounts of porphyrins in the urine. Early onset of cutaneous photosensitivity is characteristic and is exacerbated by exposure to sunlight. Subepidermal bullous lesions progress to crusted ero-sions that heal with scarring and either hyperpigmentation or, less commonly, hypopigmentation. Hypertrichosis and alopecia are frequent, and erythrodontia (with red fluorescence under ultraviolet light) is virtually pathognomonic of CEP (Fig. 12–4; see color section at front of this volume). Patients may display symptoms and signs of hemolytic anemia with splenomegaly and porphyrin-rich gallstones. Occasionally, anemia may be severe and require transfusion. Bone marrow shows erythroid hyperplasia, which may result in pathologic fractures or vertebral compression-collapse and shortness of stature. Although the onset of symptoms of CEP is most often observed in early infancy, a few patients may first present with the syndrome as adults.

Pathogenesis. The primary site of expression of the enzymatic defect is the bone marrow, wherein fluorescence secondary to porphyrin accumulation is variably distributed but invariably present. Many marrow normoblasts (30% to 70%) display fluorescence, principally localized in the nuclei of the cells.[51] Massive accumula-

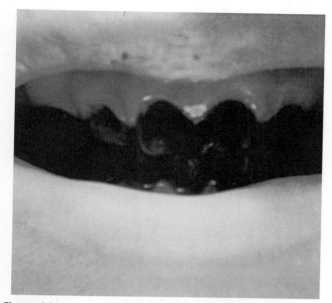

Figure 12-4. Erythrodontia of a patient with CEP. Dark reddish brown discoloration of teeth is noted. When the teeth are exposed to ultraviolet light they emit the intense red fluorescence of porphyrins. Discoloration is usually more pronounced in decidual teeth than in permanent teeth (see color section at front of this volume). (Courtesy of H. M. Nitowsky, MD.)

found in CEP, indicating that the nature of the enzymatic defect in CEP is heterogeneous, as is the case in other porphyrias.

Diagnosis. Pink urine or the onset of severe cutaneous photosensitivity in infancy (or rarely in adults) suggests the diagnosis of CEP. Demonstration of elevated levels of urinary, fecal, and erythrocyte porphyrins, with elevated type I isomers of uroporphyrin and coproporphyrin establishes the diagnosis of CEP. Demonstration of a deficiency of UCS activity constitutes the definitive diagnosis.

Treatment. The avoidance of sunlight, trauma to the skin, and infections is the most important preventive measure. Topical sunscreens may be of some help, as may oral treatment with β-carotene.[54] Transfusions with packed erythrocytes transiently decrease hemolysis and its attendant drive to increased erythropoiesis and also decrease porphyrin excretion.[55] Splenectomy has been used fairly frequently and has produced short-term reductions in hemolysis, porphyrin excretion, and skin manifestations, but not all patients respond.[56] Treatment with charcoal in a man with CEP was reported to have lowered porphyrin excretion levels and induced complete clinical remission during therapy.[57]

tions of porphyrins systemically in CEP are derived from porphyrin-laden erythrocytes, which accounts for the multiple lesions of the integument.

Biochemical Findings. Urinary levels of uroporphyrins and coproporphyrins are always elevated (20- to 60-fold), with predominant elevations of type I isomers. Erythrocyte uroporphyrins and coproporphyrins also are elevated.

Molecular Biology. A heterogeneity of mutations in the UCS gene exists in patients with CEP (Table 12–5). The first molecular analysis in a patient with CEP revealed the compound heterozygosity: →C transition resulting in an amino acid change of Cys[73]→Arg, and a C→T transition resulting in Pro[53]→Leu.[52] The second case was, however, homozygous for the mutation Cys[73]→Arg.[52] This point mutation (Cys[73]→Arg) appears to occur frequently because it was found in 8 of 21 unrelated patients with CEP (about 21% of CEP alleles).[53] Subsequently, however, other mutations have been

Porphyria Cutanea Tarda

PCT refers to a heterogeneous group of cutaneous porphyric diseases due to UROD deficiency, which may be either inherited or, more commonly, acquired.[58] Both forms of the disease display reductions in hepatic UROD activity, but erythrocyte UROD activity may or may not be decreased, depending on their types (Table 12–6).

Type I PCT is an acquired disease that typically presents in adults as decreased hepatic, but not erythrocyte, UROD activity. The disease may occur spontaneously but more commonly occurs in conjunction with precipitating environmental factors, such as alcohol, estrogen, or drug use, or in association with other disorders.[58]

Type II PCT is, in contrast, inherited in an autosomal dominant fashion and is associated with decreased UROD activity in all tissues.

Type III PCT is also inherited, but the defect is con-

Table 12-5. MUTATIONS IN THE *UCS* GENE IN CONGENITAL ERYTHROPOIETIC PORPHYRIA

Mutation in Genomic DNA	Location in cDNA or Protein		Amino Acid Substitution or Protein Abnormality	Frequency	Reference
C→T	10	L04F	Leu→Phe	1/14	122
G→A	27	A9A	Ala→Ala*		53
C→T	158	P53L	Leu→Leu	1/14	52, 53, 122, 123
A→G	184	T62A	Thr→Ala		53
C→T	197	A66V	Ala→Val		53, 124
T→C	217	C73R	Vys→Arg	7/36	52, 53, 122–124
C→T	683	T228M	Thr→Met	1/14	53, 122
98-bp deletion			55 Amino acids deletion	2/14	122
80-bp insertion	C-extremity		45 Amino acids insertion	1/14	122

*Silent substitution.

Table 12-6. SUBSETS OF PORPHYRIA CUTANEA TARDA

| Type | Familial Occurrence | UROD Activity | |
		Liver	Erythrocytes
I	(−)	Decreased	Normal
II	(+)	Decreased	Decreased
III	(+)	Decreased	Normal

fined to the liver,[59–61] and erythrocyte UROD activity and concentrations are normal.[60, 61]

Prevalence. PCT is probably the most common of all forms of the porphyrias, but its exact incidence is not clear. The disease is recognized worldwide, and there is no racial predilection except among the Bantus in South Africa, secondary to their high incidence of hemosiderosis. Type I PCT is generally more common than type II PCT in Europe, South Africa, and South America, although the trend may be less obvious in North America. Previously, PCT was thought to be more common in men, perhaps because their alcohol intake is greater than that of women; the incidence in females has recently increased to the level seen in males, perhaps from increased use of contraceptive steroids, postmenopausal estrogens, and alcohol.

Clinical Findings. The pathognomonic clinical feature of PCT is the formation of vesicles on sun-exposed areas of the skin, particularly the dorsum of the hands (Fig. 12–5; see color section at front of this volume). The vesicles are superseded by crusting, superficial scarring, or milia formation and by residual pigmentation. Facial hypertrichosis may be present (Fig. 12–6;

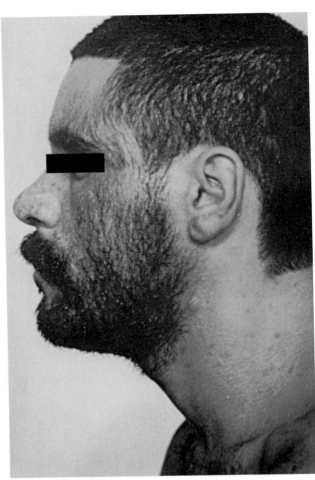

Figure 12-6. Hypertrichosis of the face of a patient with PCT. Note the erosions and pigmentations over the nose and cheeks (see color section at front of this volume). (From Poh-Fitzpatrick MB: Porphyrin-sensitized cutaneous photosensitivity. Pathogenesis and treatment. Clin Dermatol 1985; 3:41.)

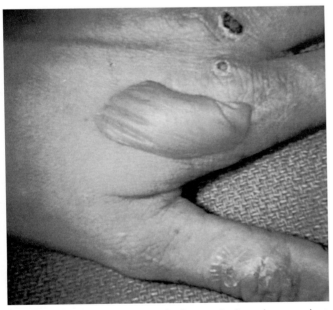

Figure 12-5. A large fluid-like bulla, crusted erosions, and unsightly scarring are typical findings in patients with PCT. These changes may also be seen in other forms of cutaneous porphyrias, but adult onset of lesions suggests either PCT, HEP, HCP, or VP (see color section at front of this volume). (From Poh-Fitzpatrick MB: Porphyrin-sensitized cutaneous photosensitivity. Pathogenesis and treatment. Clin Dermatol 1985; 3:41.)

see color section at front of this volume) and is conspicuous in women. Hypopigmented indurated plaques of skin may develop and resemble those seen in scleroderma. Photo-onycholysis is occasionally present. In contrast to the acute hepatic porphyrias, neurologic dysfunction does not occur in PCT.

Pathogenesis. Phototoxic porphyrins in the skin may be largely derived from the liver and, to some extent, formed locally in the skin. Activation of the complement system after light irradiation has been demonstrated in patients with PCT both *in vivo*,[62, 63] and *in vitro* in sera[64, 65] and is presumed to result from the generation of reactive oxygen species, most likely singlet oxygen. Bullous fluid is known to contain prostaglandin E_2, and photoactivation of uroporphyrin damages lysosomes.[66] Liver from patients with PCT almost invariably displays siderosis with fatty changes, necrosis, chronic inflammatory changes, and granuloma formation.[66] Iron, estrogens, alcohol, and chlorinated hydrocarbons, which are all potential hepatotoxins, may also aggravate PCT. The incidence of hepatitis B and C infection may also be higher than normal in patients with PCT.[67] The incidence of hepatocellular carcinoma in PCT is known to be greater than in the general population.[68] Several patients with PCT who were infected with the human immunodeficiency virus have been reported.[69–71]

Biochemical Findings. Increased concentrations of uroporphyrin (mainly isomer I) and 7-carboxylic porphyrins (isomer III) are found in the urine in PCT, with lesser increases of coproporphyrin and 5-carboxylic and 6-carboxylic porphyrins. Small quantities of isocoproporphyrin may be detected in serum or in urine, but in feces this is often the dominant porphyrin and represents the most important diagnostic criterion for PCT (Fig. 12–7).[72] Total daily fecal porphyrin excretion exceeds total urinary porphyrin excretion. Skin porphyrins are increased especially in areas that are protected from photoactivation. Serum iron and ferritin concentrations are frequently elevated.

Diagnosis. The clinical picture in PCT is fairly specific but can be confused with other porphyric (e.g., VP) and nonporphyric (e.g., systemic lupus erythematosus, scleroderma) diseases. Urinary fluorescence under ultraviolet light illumination and quantification of porphyrins and separation and identification of porphyrins by thin-layer chromatography and high-performance liquid chromatography assist the diagnosis. Plasma porphyrin levels are elevated in PCT and in other photosensitizing porphyrias. Fecal porphyrin levels are often elevated; isocoproporphyrin (or an isocoproporphyrin:coproporphyrin ratio greater than or equal to 0.1) is diagnostic of PCT.

Treatment. In type I PCT, the identification and avoidance of precipitating factors is the first line of treatment.[73] The clinical response to cessation of alcohol ingestion is highly variable; nonetheless, abstinence should be recommended. Phlebotomy is usually effective in reducing urinary porphyrin concentrations and in induction of clinical remissions.[74] Strong evidence exists that the beneficial effects of phlebotomy result from a diminution in the stores of body iron.[75] If phlebotomy is ineffective or contraindicated owing to the presence of other diseases such as anemia, low-dose chloroquine therapy may be effective.[76] Efficacy of chloroquine therapy and phlebotomy is probably similar, and a combined approach may diminish the incidence of side effects. The mechanism of action of chloroquine therapy is thought to be related to its ability to chelate porphyrins in a water-soluble, and hence more easily excretable, form.

Hepatoerythropoietic Porphyria

HEP is a rare form of porphyria probably resulting from a homozygous defect of UROD.[77] Clinically, HEP is characterized by the childhood onset of severe photosensitivity and skin fragility and is indistinguishable from CEP. Some 20 cases have been reported worldwide.[78]

Clinical Findings. Clinical findings of HEP are very similar to those seen in CEP. Pink urine, severe photosensitivity leading to scarring and mutilation of sun-exposed areas of skin, sclerodermoid changes, hypertrichosis, erythrodontia, anemia (often hemolytic), and hepatosplenomegaly are characteristic. Onset is usually

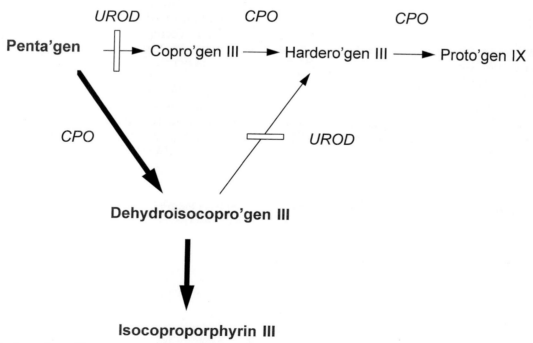

Figure 12-7. The formation of isocoproporphyrin in PCT and HEP. The normal route in heme biosynthesis is shown in the top line. In patients with PCT and HEP, the conversion of 5-carboxylate porphyrinogen (penta'gen) III to coproporphyrinogen (copro'gen) III is impaired because of a deficiency of UROD. Increased penta'gen is metabolized by CPO, yielding dehydroisocoproporphyrinogen (dehydroisocopro'gen). The latter accumulates and autoxidizes to isocoproporphyrin, because its further metabolism to harderoporphyrinogen is impaired owing to the decarboxylase defect. The enzymatic block is shown by an *open bar*, and abnormally elevated intermediates are shown in *bold*.

in early infancy or childhood, but adult onset has also been described. In contrast to PCT, serum iron concentrations are usually normal, and phlebotomy has no beneficial effects in patients with HEP.

Biochemical Findings. Elevations in the levels of urinary porphyrins—predominantly uroporphyrin of isomer type I with lesser quantities of 7-carboxylic porphyrins, mainly type III—are commonly found. Isocoproporphyrin concentrations equal to or greater than coproporphyrin are also found in urine and feces. An elevated erythrocyte zinc protoporphyrin concentration is commonly observed (see Table 12–2). Anemia and biochemical evidence of impaired hepatic function are highly variable.

Molecular Biology. Cloning and sequencing of a cDNA of the mutated gene in a patient with HEP revealed that the enzymatic defect was due to a base transition of $G^{860} \rightarrow A$, resulting in an amino acid change of $Gly^{281} \rightarrow Glu$.[79] This point mutation resulted in an unstable protein. Several other mutations were also reported. None of the mutations found in HEP have been found in familial PCT, suggesting that HEP may not be a homozygous form of PCT[80] (Table 12–7). Various mutations of the human *UROD* gene described in patients with PCT and HEP are summarized in Table 12–7.

Diagnosis. The diagnosis must be suspected in patients with severe photosensitivity and especially considered in the differential diagnosis of CEP. Diagnostic criteria include elevated levels of fecal or urinary isocoproporphyrin and erythrocyte zinc protoporphyrin. Differential diagnosis of HEP includes EPP, in which the erythrocyte protoporphyrin concentration also is elevated but in which, in contrast to HEP, urinary porphyrin levels are normal. EPP is clinically milder than HEP. Measurement of erythrocyte or fibroblast UROD activity typically shows reductions to 2% to 10% of normal control values with intermediate reductions of UROD activities in family members.[80]

Treatment. Avoidance of the sun and the use of topical sunscreens are essentially all that can be recommended to these patients. Unlike in patients with PCT, phlebotomy provides no beneficial response.

Hereditary Coproporphyria

HCP is a disease caused by a heterozygous deficiency of CPO activity that is inherited in an autosomal dominant manner (see Fig. 12–3 and Table 12–1). Clinically, the disease is similar to ADP, or AIP, although it is often milder; additionally, HCP may be associated with photosensitivity. Expression of the disease is variable and influenced by the same precipitating factors responsible for the exacerbation of AIP. Very rarely, homozygous deficiency of this enzyme may occur and is associated with a more severe form of the disease.[81]

Prevalence. Clinically expressed HCP is much less common than is clinically expressed AIP, but as in the latter disease, latent HCP or HCP gene carriers are being recognized with greater frequency since the advent of improved laboratory techniques for their detection.

Clinical Findings. Neurovisceral symptoms are predominant and are essentially indistinguishable from that of ADP, AIP, or VP. Abdominal pain, vomiting, constipation, neuropathies, and psychiatric manifestations are common. Cutaneous photosensitivity is a feature in about 30% of cases. Attacks can be precipitated by pregnancy, the menstrual cycle, and contraceptive steroids, but the most common precipitating factor is drug administration, most notably of barbiturates.

Biochemical Findings. The biochemical hallmark of HCP is hyperexcretion of coproporphyrin (predominantly type III) into the urine and feces. Fecal coproporphyrin may be chelated with copper, and the fecal protoporphyrin level may be modestly elevated. Hyperexcretion of ALA, PBG, and uroporphyrin into the urine may accompany exacerbations of the disease, but in contrast to AIP these findings generally return to normal between attacks. CPO activity is typically reduced by about 50% in heterozygotes and by 90% to 98% in rare homozygotes.[81]

Molecular Biology. A molecular analysis in HCP has been made in two patients. In the first patient who was homozygous for the CPO deficiency,[82] a $C^{691} \rightarrow T$ transition in CPO cDNA that resulted in an $Arg^{231} \rightarrow Trp$

Table 12–7. MUTATIONS/DELETIONS IN THE *UROD* GENE IN PORPHYRIA CUTANEA TARDA AND HEPATOERYTHROPOIETIC PORPHYRIA

Disease	Mutation / Deletion	Allelic Status	UROD Activity in Lymphocytes	Character of Mutations*		References
				Stability	*Activity*	
HEP	G281E	Homo	≈ 5%	Decreased	Unknown	125, 126
HEP	E167L	Homo	≈ 10%	Decreased	Unknown	79
	R292G	Hetero		Normal	Unknown	
HEP	Large deletion	Hetero	6.3–8.3%†	No product		127‡
	V134Q	Hetero		Normal	≈ 80%	
HEP	H220P	Hetero	≈ 4%	Normal	≈ 40%	80‡
f-PCT	G281V	Hetero	≈ 50%	Decreased	Unknown	128
f-PCT	Exon 6 deletion	Hetero	≈ 50%	Decreased	≈ 0%	129, 130

*Examined in vitro.
†UROD activity in hemolysate.
‡A compound heterozygote.

substitution was found. In the second patient with a heterozygous CPO defect, a single-base substitution of $G^{265} \rightarrow A$ resulting in an amino acid substitution of $Gly^{89} \rightarrow Ser$ was detected.[83]

Diagnosis. A diagnosis of HCP should be suspected in patients with the signs, symptoms, and clinical course characteristic of the acute hepatic porphyrias but in whom PBGD activity is normal. Urinary excretion of heme precursors is similar in HCP and VP, but the predominant or exclusive presence of fecal coproporphyrin is highly suggestive of HCP. Fecal or urinary predominance of harderoporphyrin, with greatly reduced CPO activity, was reported in a case of harderoporphyria,[84] a variant form of HCP.

Treatment. The identification and avoidance of precipitating factors is essential. Treatment of acute attacks is similar to the treatment of AIP.

Variegate Porphyria

VP, which is also known as *porphyria variegata, proto-coproporphyria, South African genetic porphyria,* or *royal malady* (referring to George III and the House of Hanover), is caused by a heterozygous deficiency in PPOX activity and is inherited in an autosomal dominant manner (see Fig. 12–3 and Table 12–1). Patients with this disorder may show neurovisceral symptoms or photosensitivity, or both (see Table 12–2). Very rare forms of VP are seen with homozygous deficiencies in PPOX activity.[85-87]

Prevalence. The incidence of VP of 3 per 1000 in South Africa is substantially higher than elsewhere.[88] In 1980, it was estimated that there were 10,000 affected individuals in South Africa, and there is good evidence to suggest that they are all descendants of a single union between two Dutch settlers in 1680.[89] However, the disease is recognized worldwide, and with the exception of South Africa, there is probably no racial or geographic predilection. The incidence in Finland is reported at 1.3 per 100,000. Elsewhere than South Africa, VP is probably less common than AIP.

Clinical Findings. The neurovisceral symptomatology is identical to that observed in ADP, AIP, and HCP, which has been described previously. Photosensitivity is more common, and the resulting lesions tend to be more chronic in VP than in HCP. Cutaneous manifestations include vesicles, bullae, hyperpigmentation, milia, hypertrichosis, and increased skin fragility. Lesions are clinically and histologically indistinguishable from PCT. Skin manifestations are less frequently observed in cold climates than in hot climates. The same spectrum of factors that leads to activation of ADP, AIP, and HCP may also exacerbate VP. Thus, barbiturates, dapsone, lead from "moonshine" whiskey, contraceptive steroids, pregnancy, and decreased carbohydrate intake have all been reported to induce or exacerbate VP.

Pathogenesis. PPOX activity in most patients with VP is decreased about 50%. In very rare cases of homozygous VP, however, a virtual absence of PPOX activity has been documented,[85] and symptoms in homozygous VP patients were severe photosensitivity, growth and mental retardation, and marked neurologic abnormalities; onset of the homozygous disease was in childhood in all cases.

Biochemical Findings. The biochemical hallmark of VP is elevated fecal porphyrin levels, with levels of protoporphyrin usually exceeding those of coproporphyrin (mostly isomer III). Fecal X-porphyrins (ether-acetic acid–insoluble, extracted with urea-Triton), a heterogeneous group of porphyrin-peptide conjugates, are elevated in VP more than in any other type of porphyria. Urinary coproporphyrin (type III), ALA, and PBG values are often normal between attacks but may become markedly elevated during acute exacerbations of the disease. Plasma invariably shows a fluorescence emission that probably represents a protoporphyrin-peptide conjugate.[90]

Diagnosis. VP should be considered in the differential diagnosis of acute porphyria, especially if PBGD activity is normal. Characteristic plasma porphyrin fluorescence, having a different emission maximum from PCT, is seen in VP.[79] The differentiation of VP from HCP is usually possible after fecal porphyrin analysis and in patients with only cutaneous manifestations. The demonstration of urinary 8- and 7-carboxylic porphyrins and isocoproporphyrin in PCT is usually sufficient for differentiation from VP. PPOX deficiency can be demonstrated in fibroblasts or lymphocytes.

Treatment. Identification and avoidance of precipitating factors is essential. Photosensitivity can be minimized by the wearing of protective clothing, and the use of canthaxanthrin (a β-carotene analogue) may be of some help. The treatment of neurovisceral symptoms is identical to that described for AIP.

Erythropoietic Protoporphyria

EPP, which is also referred to as *protoporphyria* or *erythrohepatic protoporphyria,* is associated with a partial deficiency of FECH and is inherited in an autosomal dominant fashion (see Fig. 12–3 and Table 12–1). Biochemically, this defect results in massive accumulations of protoporphyrin in erythrocytes, plasma, and feces. Clinically, the disease is characterized by the childhood onset of cutaneous photosensitivity in light-exposed areas, but skin lesions are milder and less disfiguring than those seen in CEP.

Prevalence. EPP is the most common form of erythropoietic porphyria. Three hundred case reports were reported as of 1976. There is no racial or sexual predilection, and onset is typically in childhood.

Clinical Findings. Cutaneous photosensitivity of EPP is quite different from that seen in CEP or PCT. Stinging or painful burning sensations in the skin occur within 1 hour of exposure to the sun and are followed several hours later by erythema and edema. Some patients experience only burning sensations in the absence of such objective signs of cutaneous phototoxicity, resulting in the erroneous diagnosis of a psychiatric illness. Petechiae or, more rarely, purpura, vesicles, and crusting may develop and persist for several days after sun exposure. Artificial lights also may cause photosensitivity, especially operating theater lights. Symptoms

Table 12–8. MUTATIONS OF THE *FECH* GENE IN ERYTHROPOIETIC PROTOPORPHYRIA

| Genomic DNA | | Effect on cDNA and / or Protein | References |
Mutation	Location		
C→T	−23 to the 1st of exon 2	Exon 2 skipping	95, 131
T→G	+2 of the donor site	Exon 3 skipping	132
99-bp deletion	706–804 from N-terminus	Exon 7 skipping	96
G→A	+1 of the donor site	Exon 9 skipping	97
A→T	−3 of the donor site	Exon 10 skipping	98, 131
A→G	+3 at the donor site	Exon 10 skipping	133
G deletion	40 in exon 1	Truncated protein	134
D→T	175 from N-terminus	Gln→a stop condon	135
G→T	163 from N-terminus	G55C	100*
G→A	801 from N-terminus	M2671	100*
2-bp deletion	899–900 from N-terminus	Frameshift	135
T→G	1088 from N-terminus	G363V	133
T→C		F417S	99

*Compound heterozygosity.

are usually worse during spring and summer and occur in light-exposed areas, especially on the face and hands. Intense and repeated exposure to the sun may result in onycholysis, leathery hyperkeratotic skin over the dorsum of the hands, and mild scarring. Gallstones, sometimes presenting at an unusually early age, are fairly common; and hepatic disease, although unusual, may be severe and associated with significant morbidity. Anemia is uncommon. There are no known precipitating factors and no neurovisceral manifestations.

Pathogenesis. The peak light absorption range for porphyrins corresponds well to the wavelength of light (about 400 nm) known to trigger photosensitivity reactions in the skin of patients with EPP. Light-excited porphyrins generate free radicals and singlet oxygen.[91] Such radicals, notably singlet oxygen, may lead to peroxidation of lipids and cross-linking of membrane proteins, which, in erythrocytes, may result in reduced deformability and thus hemolysis. Protoporphyrin, but not zinc protoporphyrin, can be released from erythrocytes after irradiation.[92] This finding may explain why patients with EPP with elevated levels of free protoporphyrin manifest photosensitivity whereas patients with lead intoxication and iron deficiency, which are predominantly associated with elevated zinc protoporphyrin levels, do not.[92] Forearm irradiation in patients with EPP leads to complement activation and polymorphonuclear chemotaxis. Similar results have been obtained *in vitro,* and these events may also contribute to the pathogenesis of skin lesions in EPP.[62]

Biochemical Findings. The biochemical hallmark of EPP is excessive concentrations of protoporphyrin in erythrocytes, plasma, bile, and feces but, because of its poor solubility in water, not in urine. The bone marrow and the newly released erythrocytes appear to be the major source of elevated protoporphyrin concentrations,[93] although the liver may contribute in certain cases.

Molecular Biology. The first molecular analysis of the FECH defect in EPP was made in a patient who had about 50% FECH activity, its enzyme protein, and its mRNA.[94] The patient's cells contained an unstable transcript encoding an abnormally short protein that completely lacked exon 2.[94, 95] Subsequently, several other mutations were found in other families. Thus far, skipping of exon 2,[95] exon 7,[96] exon 9,[97] and exon 10[98] and three point mutations[99, 100] have been reported. One patient had a heteroallelic mutation, whereas five others had a single point mutation in one allele.[95–99] Various mutations of the human *FECH* gene found in patients with EPP are summarized in Table 12–8.

Diagnosis. Photosensitivity should suggest the diagnosis, which can be confirmed by the demonstration of elevated concentrations of free protoporphyrin in erythrocytes, plasma, and stools with normal urinary porphyrins. The presence of protoporphyrin in both plasma and erythrocytes is a finding specific for EPP. Fluorescent reticulocytes on examination of peripheral blood smear may also suggest the diagnosis.

Treatment. Avoidance of the sun and use of topical sunscreen agents may be helpful. Oral administration of β-carotene may afford systemic photoprotection, resulting in improved, although highly variable, tolerance to the sun. The recommended serum β-carotene level of 600 to 800 μg/dL is usually achieved with oral doses of 120 to 180 mg daily, and beneficial effects are typically seen 1 to 3 months after the onset of therapy.[101] The mechanism of this beneficial effect of β-carotene probably involves quenching of activated oxygen radicals.[102]

References

1. McKay R, Druyan R, et al: Intramitochondrial localization of δ-aminolevulinate synthase and ferrochelatase in rat liver. Biochem J 1969; 114:455.
2. Granick S, Urata G: Increase in activity of δ-aminolevulinic acid synthetase in liver mitochondria induced by feeding of 3,5-dicarbethoxy-1,4-dihydrocollidine. J Biol Chem 1963; 238:821.
3. Riddle RD, Yamamoto M, Engel JD: Expression of δ-aminolevulinate synthase in avian cells: Separate genes encode erythroid-specific and nonspecific isozymes. Proc Natl Acad Sci U S A 1989; 86:792.
4. Bishop DF, Astrin KH, Ioannou YA: Human δ-aminolevulinate synthase: Isolation, characterization, and mapping of housekeeping and erythroid-specific genes. Am J Hum Genet 1989; 45:A176.
5. Cox TC, Bawden MJ, et al: Human erythroid 5-aminolevulinate

synthase: promoter analysis and identification of an iron-responsive element in the mRNA. EMBO J 1991; 10:1891.

6. Cotter PD, Baumann M, Bishop DF: Enzymatic defect in "X-linked" sideroblastic anemia: Molecular evidence for erythroid δ-aminolevulinate synthase deficiency. Proc Natl Acad Sci U S A 1992; 89:4028.

7. Potluri VR, Astrin KH, et al: Human 5-aminolevulinate dehydratase: Chromosomal localization to 9q34 by *in situ* hybridization. Hum Genet 1987; 76:236.

8. Wetmur JG, Bishop DF, et al: Molecular cloning of a cDNA for human δ-aminolevulinate dehydratase. Gene 1986; 43:123.

9. Sassa S: δ-Aminolevulinic acid dehydratase assay. Enzyme 1982; 28:133.

10. Granick JL, Sassa S, Kappas A: Some biochemical and clinical aspects of lead intoxication. In Bodansky O, Latner AL (eds): Advances in Clinical Chemistry. New York, Academic Press, Inc., 1978, p 287.

11. Sassa S, Kappas A: Hereditary tyrosinemia and the heme biosynthetic pathway. Profound inhibition of δ-aminolevulinic acid dehydratase activity by succinylacetone. J Clin Invest 1983; 71:625.

12. Lindblad B, Lindstedt S, Steen G: On the genetic defects in hereditary tyrosinemia. Proc Natl Acad Sci U S A 1977; 74:4641.

13. Meisler M, Wanner L, et al: The UPS locus encoding uroporphyrinogen I synthase is located on human chromosome 11. Biochem Biophys Res Commun 1980; 95:170.

14. Chretien S, Dubart A, et al: Alternative transcription and splicing of the human porphobilinogen deaminase gene result either in tissue-specific or in housekeeping expression. Proc Natl Acad Sci U S A 1988; 85:6.

15. Grandchamp B, Beaumont C, et al: Genetic expression of porphobilinogen deaminase and uroporphyrinogen decarboxylase during the erythroid differentiation of mouse erythroleukemic cells. In Nordmann Y (ed): Porphyrins and Porphyrias. London, John Libbey & Co., 1986, p 35.

16. Tsai SF, Bishop DF, Desnick RJ: Human uroporphyrinogen III synthase: molecular cloning, nucleotide sequence, and expression of a full-length cDNA. Proc Natl Acad Sci U S A 1988; 85:7049.

17. Romana M, Dubart A, et al: Structure of the gene for human uroporphyrinogen decarboxylase. Nucleic Acids Res 1987; 15:7343.

18. McLellan T, Pryor MA, et al: Assignment of uroporphyrinogen decarboxylase (UROD) to the pter-p21 region of human chromosome 1. Cytogenet Cell Genet 1985; 39:224.

19. Grandchamp B, Weil D, et al: Assignment of the human coproporphyrinogen oxidase to chromosome 9. Hum Genet 1983; 64:180.

20. Taketani S, Kohno H, et al: Molecular cloning, sequencing and expression of cDNA encoding human coproporphyrinogen oxidase. Biochim Biophys Acta 1994; 1183:547.

21. Taketani S, Inazawa J, et al: Structure of the human ferrochelatase gene. Exon/intron gene organization and location of the gene to chromosome 18. Eur J Biochem 1992; 205:217.

22. Sassa S, Granick S: Induction of δ-aminolevulinic acid synthetase in chick embryo liver cells in culture. Proc Natl Acad Sci U S A 1970; 67:517.

23. Granick S, Sinclair P, et al: Effects by heme, insulin, and serum albumin on heme and protein synthesis in chick embryo liver cells cultured in a chemically defined medium, and a spectrofluorometric assay for porphyrin composition. J Biol Chem 1975; 250:9215.

24. Sassa S: Heme biosynthesis in erythroid cells. The distinctive aspects of the regulatory mechanism. In Goldwasser E (ed): Regulation of Hemoglobin Biosynthesis. Boston, Elsevier North-Holland, 1983, p 359.

25. Lim HW, Sassa S: The porphyrias. In Lim HW, Soter NA (eds): Photomedicine for Clinical Dermatologists. New York, Marcel Dekker, Inc., 1993, p 241.

26. Kappas A, Sassa S, et al: The porphyrias. In Scriver CR, Beaudet AL, et al (eds): The Metabolic Basis of Inherited Disease. New York, McGraw-Hill Book Co., 1989, p 1305.

27. Doss M, von Tiepermann R, et al: New type of hepatic porphyria with porphobilinogen synthase defect and intermittent acute clinical manifestation. Klin Wochenschr 1979; 57:1123.

28. Thunell S, Holmberg L, Lundgreen J: Aminolevulinate dehydratase porphyria in infancy. A clinical and biochemical study. J Clin Chem Clin Biochem 1987; 25:5.

29. Ishida N, Fujita H, et al: Message amplification phenotyping of an inherited δ-aminolevulinate dehydratase deficiency in a family with acute hepatic porphyria. Biochem Biophys Res Commun 1990; 172:237.

30. Ishida N, Fujita H, et al: Cloning and expression of the defective genes from a patient with δ-aminolevulinate dehydratase porphyria. J Clin Invest 1992; 89:1431.

31. Plewinska M, Thunell S, et al: δ-Aminolevulinate dehydratase deficient porphyria: Identification of the molecular lesions in a severely affected homozygote. Am J Hum Genet 1991; 49:167.

32. Goldberg A, Moore MR, et al: Porphyrin metabolism and the porphyrias. In Ledingham JGG, Warrell DA, Weatherall DJ (eds): Oxford Textbook of Medicine. Oxford, Oxford University Press, Inc., 1987, p 9136.

33. Mustajoki P, Koskelo P: Hereditary hepatic porphyrias in Finland. Acta Med Scand 1976; 200:171.

34. Mustajoki P, Kauppinen R, et al: Frequency of low porphobilinogen deaminase activity in Finland. J Intern Med 1992; 231:389.

35. McColl KEL, Wallace AM, et al: Alterations in haem biosynthesis during the human menstrual cycle: Studies in normal subjects and patients with latent and active acute intermittent porphyria. Clin Sci 1982; 62:183.

36. Felsher BF, Redeker AG: Acute intermittent porphyria: Effect of diet and griseofulvin. Medicine 1967; 46:217.

37. Welland FH, Hellman ES, et al: Factors affecting the excretion of porphyrin precursors by patients with acute intermittent porphyria. I. The effects of diet. Metabolism 1964; 13:232.

38. Mauzerall D, Granick S: The occurrence and determination of δ-aminolevulinic acid and porphobilinogen in urine. J Biol Chem 1956; 219:435.

39. Grandchamp B, Picat C, et al: A point mutation G→A in exon 12 of the porphobilinogen deaminase gene results in exon skipping and is responsible for acute intermittent porphyria. Nucleic Acids Res 1989; 17:6637.

40. Llewellyn DH, Kalsheker NA, et al: A MspI polymorphism for the human porphobilinogen deaminase gene. Nucleic Acids Res 1987; 15:1349.

41. Lee JS, Anvret M: A PstI polymorphism for the human porphobilinogen deaminase gene (PBG). Nucleic Acids Res 1987; 15:6307.

42. Picat C, Bourgeois F, Grandchamp B: PCR detection of a C/T polymorphism in exon 1 of the porphobilinogen deaminase gene (PBGD). Nucleic Acids Res 1988; 19:5099.

43. Gu X-F, Lee JS, et al: PCR detection of a G/T polymorphism at exon 10 of the porphobilinogen deaminase gene (PBG-D). Nucleic Acids Res 1991; 19:1966.

44. Lee JS, Anvret M, et al: DNA polymorphisms within the porphobilinogen deaminase gene in two Swedish families with acute intermittent porphyria. Hum Genet 1988; 79:379.

45. Daimon M, Morita Y, et al: Two new polymorphisms in introns 2 and 3 of the human porphobilinogen deaminase gene. Hum Genet 1993; 92:115.

46. Schreiber WE, Jamani A, Ritchie B: Detection of a T/C polymorphism in the porphobilinogen deaminase gene by polymerase chain reaction amplification of specific alleles. Clin Chem 1992; 38:2153.

47. Sagen E, Laegreid A, et al: Genetic carrier detection in Norwegian families with acute intermittent porphyria. Scand J Clin Lab Invest 1993; 53:687.

48. Mustajoki P, Tenhunen R, et al: Heme in the treatment of porphyrias and hematological disorders. Semin Hematol 1989; 26:1.

49. Anderson KE, Spitz IM, et al: Prevention of cyclical attacks of acute intermittent porphyria with a long-acting agonist of luteinizing hormone–releasing hormone. N Engl J Med 1984; 311:643.

50. Galbraith RA, Kappas A: Pharmacokinetics of tin-mesoporphyrin in man and the effects of tin-chelated porphyrins on hyperexcretion of heme pathway precursors in patients with acute inducible porphyria. Hepatology 1989; 9:882.

51. Schmid R, Schwartz S, Sundberg RD: Erythropoietic (congenital) porphyria: a rare abnormality of normoblasts. Blood 1955; 10:416.

52. Deybach J-C, de Verneuil H, et al: Point mutations in the uroporphyrinogen III synthase gene in congenital erythropoietic porphyria (Gunther's disease). Blood 1990; 75:1763.

53. Warner CA, Yoo HW, et al: Congenital erythropoietic porphyria: Identification of exonic mutations in the uroporphyrinogen III synthase gene. J Clin Invest 1992; 89:693.

54. Seip M, Thune PO, Eriksen L: Treatment of photosensitivity in congenital erythropoietic porphyria (CEP) with beta-carotene. Acta Derm Venereol 1974; 54:239.

55. Haining RG, Cowger ML, et al: Congenital erythropoietic porphyria. II. The effects of induced polycythemia. Blood 1970; 36:297.

56. Varadi S: Haematological aspects in a case of erythropoietic porphyria. Br J Haematol 1958; 4:270.

57. Pimstone NR, Gandhi SN, Mukerji SK: Therapeutic efficacy of oral charcoal in congenital erythropoietic porphyria. N Engl J Med 1987; 316:390.

58. de Verneuil H, Aitken G, Nordmann Y: Familial and sporadic porphyria cutanea: Two different diseases. Hum Genet 1978; 44:145.

59. Elder GH, Lee GB, Tovey JA: Decreased activity of hepatic uroporphyrinogen decarboxylase in sporadic porphyria cutanea tarda. N Engl J Med 1978; 299:274.

60. Elder GH: Human uroporphyrinogen decarboxylase defects. In Orfanos CS, Stadler R, Gollnick H (eds): Dermatology in Five Continents. Berlin, Springer-Verlag, 1988, p 857.

61. Held JL, Sassa S, et al: Erythrocyte uroporphyrinogen decarboxylase activity in porphyria cutanea tarda: a study of 40 consecutive patients. J Invest Dermatol 1989; 93:332.

62. Lim HW, Poh-Fitzpatrick MB, Gigli I: Activation of the complement system in patients with porphyrias after irradiation *in vivo*. J Clin Invest 1984; 74:1961.

63. Meurer M, Schulte C, et al: Photodynamic action of uroporphyrin on the complement system in porphyria cutanea tarda. Arch Dermatol Res 1985; 277:293.

64. Torinuki W, Miura T, Tagami H: Activation of complement by 405-nm light in serum from porphyria cutanea tarda. Arch Dermatol Res 1985; 277:174.

65. Pigatto PD, Polenghi MM, et al: Complement cleavage products in the phototoxic reaction of porphyria cutanea tarda. Br J Dermatol 1986; 114:567.

66. Sandberg S, Romslo I, et al: Porphyrin-induced photodamage as related to the subcellular localization of the porphyrins. Acta Derm Venereol Suppl (Stockh) 1982; 100:75.

67. Herrero C, Vicente A, et al: Is hepatitis C virus infection a trigger of porphyria cutanea tarda? Lancet 1993; 341:788.

68. Pierach C: Porphyria and hepatocellular carcinoma. Br J Cancer 1987; 55:111.

69. Wissel PS, Sordillo P, et al: Porphyria cutanea tarda associated with the acquired immune deficiency syndrome. Am J Hematol 1987; 25:107.

70. Lobato MN, Berger TG: Porphyria cutanea tarda associated with the acquired immunodeficiency syndrome. Arch Dermatol 1988; 124:1009.

71. Blauvelt A, Harris HR, et al: Porphyria cutanea tarda and human immunodeficiency virus infection. Int J Dermatol 1992; 31:474.

72. Lockwood WH, Poulos V, et al: Rapid procedure for fecal porphyrin assay. Clin Chem 1985; 31:1163.

73. Topi GC, Amantea A, Griso D: Recovery from porphyria cutanea tarda with no specific therapy other than avoidance of hepatic toxins. Br J Dermatol 1984; 111:75.

74. Ippen H: Allgemeine Symptome. Der späten Hautporphyrie (Porphyria Cutanea Tarda) als Hinweise für deren Behandlung. Dtsch Med Wochenschr 1961; 86:127.

75. Ippen H: Treatment of porphyria cutanea tarda by phlebotomy. Semin Hematol 1977; 14:253.

76. Felsher BF, Redeker AG: Effect of chloroquine on hepatic uroporphyrin metabolism in patients with porphyria cutanea tarda. Medicine 1966; 45:575.

77. Elder GH, Smith SG, et al: Hepatoerythropoietic porphyria: A new uroporphyrinogen decarboxylase defect or homozygous porphyria cutanea tarda? Lancet 1981; 1:916.

78. Toback AC, Sassa S, et al: Hepatoerythropoietic porphyria: clinical, biochemical, and enzymatic studies in a three-generation family lineage. N Engl J Med 1987; 316:645.

79. Romana M, Grandchamp B, et al: Identification of a new mutation responsible for hepatoerythropoietic porphyria. Eur J Clin Invest 1991; 21:225.

80. Meguro K, Fujita H, et al: Molecular defects of uroporphyrinogen decarboxylase in a patient with mild hepatoerythropoietic porphyria. J Invest Dermatol 1994; 102:681.

81. Grandchamp B, Phung N, Nordmann Y: Homozygous case of hereditary coproporphyria. Lancet 1977; 2:1348. Letter.

82. Martasek P, Nordmann Y, Grandchamp B: Homozygous hereditary coproporphyria caused by an arginine to tryptophan substitution in coproporphyrinogen oxidase and common intragenic polymorphisms. Hum Mol Genet 1994; 3:477.

83. Fujita H, Kondo M, et al: Characterization of cDNA encoding coproporphyrinogen oxidase from a patient with hereditary coproporphyria. Hum Mol Genet 1994; 3:1807.

84. Nordmann Y, Grandchamp B, et al: Harderoporphyria: a variant hereditary coproporphyria. J Clin Invest 1983; 72:1139.

85. Kordac V, Deybach JC, et al: Homozygous variegate porphyria. Lancet 1984; 1:851.

86. Murphy GM, Hawk JL, et al: Homozygous variegate porphyria: two similar cases in unrelated families. J R Soc Med 1986; 79:361.

87. Mustajoki P, Tenhunen R, et al: Homozygous variegate porphyria. A severe skin disease of infancy. Clin Genet 1987; 32:300.

88. Eales L, Day RS, Blekkenhorst GH: The clinical and biochemical features of variegate porphyria: An analysis of 300 cases studied at Groote Schuur Hospital, Cape Town. Int J Biochem 1980; 12:837.

89. Dean G: The porphyrias. A study of inheritance and environment. London, Pitman Medical, 1971.

90. Rimington C, Lockwood WH, Belcher RV: The excretion of porphyrin-peptide conjugates in porphyria variegata. Clin Sci 1968; 35:211.

91. Spikes JD: Porphyrins and related compounds as photodynamic sensitizers. Ann N Y Acad Sci 1975; 244:496.

92. Sandberg S, Talstad I, et al: Light-induced release of protoporphyrin, but not of zinc protoporphyrin, from erythrocytes in a patient with greatly elevated erythropoietic protoporphyria. Blood 1983; 62:846.

93. Bottomley SS, Tanaka M, Everett MA: Diminished erythroid ferrochelatase activity in protoporphyria. J Lab Clin Med 1975; 86:126.

94. Nakahashi Y, Fujita H, et al: The molecular defect of ferrochelatase in a patient with erythropoietic protoporphyria. Presented before the Fourth Congress of the European Society for Photobiology, Amsterdam, 1991, p 197.

95. Nakahashi Y, Fujita H, et al: The molecular defect of ferrochelatase in a patient with erythropoietic protoporphyria. Proc Natl Acad Sci U S A 1992; 89:281.

96. Nakahashi Y, Miyazaki H, et al: Human erythropoietic protoporphyria: Identification of a mutation at the splice donor site of intron 7 causing exon 7 skipping of the ferrochelatase gene. Hum Mol Genet 1993; 2:1069.

97. Nakahashi Y, Miyazaki H, et al: Molecular defect in human erythropoietic protoporphyria with fatal liver failure. Hum Genet 1993; 91:303.

98. Wang X, Poh-Fitzpatrick M, et al: A novel mutation in erythropoietic protoporphyria: an aberrant ferrochelatase mRNA caused by exon skipping during RNA splicing. Biochim Biophys Acta 1993; 1181:198.

99. Brenner DA, Didier JM, et al: A molecular defect in human protoporphyria. Am J Hum Genet 1992; 50:1203.

100. Lamoril J, Boulechfar S, et al: Human erythropoietic protoporphyria: two point mutations in the ferrochelatase gene. Biochem Biophys Res Commun 1991; 181:594.

101. Mathews-Roth MM: Systemic photoprotection. Dermatol Clin 1986; 4:335.

102. Mathews-Roth MM, Pathak MA, et al: Beta carotene therapy for erythropoietic protoporphyria and other photosensitivity diseases. Arch Dermatol 1977; 113:1229.

103. Sassa S, Kappas A: The porphyrias. In Nathan DG, Oski FA (eds): Hematology of Infancy and Childhood. Philadelphia, W. B. Saunders Co., 1993, p 451.

104. Grandchamp B, Picat C, et al: Molecular analysis of acute intermittent porphyria in a Finnish family with normal erythrocyte porphobilinogen deaminase. Eur J Clin Invest 1989; 19:415.

105. Chen C-H, Astrin KH, et al: Acute intermittent porphyria. Identification and expression of exonic mutations in the hydroxymethylbilane synthase gene. J Clin Invest 1994; 94:1927.

106. Grandchamp B, Picat C, et al: Tissue-specific splicing mutation in acute intermittent porphyria. Proc Natl Acad Sci U S A 1989; 86:661.

107. Llewellyn DH, Whatley S, Elder GH: Acute intermittent porphyria caused by an arginine to histidine substitution (R26H) in the cofactor-binding cleft of porphobilinogen deaminase. Hum Mol Genet 1993; 2:1315.

108. Gu X-F, de Rooij F, et al: Detection of eleven mutations causing acute intermittent porphyria using denaturing gradient gel electrophoresis. Hum Genet 1993; 93:47.

109. Mgone CS, Lanyon WG, et al: Detection of seven point mutations in the porphobilinogen deaminase gene in patients with acute intermittent porphyria, by direct sequencing of *in vitro* amplified cDNA. Hum Genet 1992; 90:12.

110. Gu X-F, de Rooij F, et al: Two novel mutations of the porphobilinogen deaminase gene in acute intermittent porphyria. Hum Mol Genet 1993; 2:1735.

111. Schreiber WE, Fong F, Jamani A: Molecular diagnosis of acute intermittent porphyria by analysis of DNA extracted from hair roots. Clin Chem 1994; 40:1744.

112. Gu X-F, de Rooij F, et al: High prevalence of a point mutation in the porphobilinogen deaminase gene in Dutch patients with acute intermittent porphyria. Hum Genet 1993; 91:128.

113. Scobie GA, Llewellyn DH, et al: Acute intermittent porphyria caused by a C→T mutation that produces a stop codon in the porphobilinogen deaminase gene. Hum Genet 1990; 85:631.

114. Delfau MH, Picat C, et al: Molecular heterogeneity of acute intermittent porphyria: identification of four additional mutations resulting in the CRIM-negative subtype of the disease. Am J Hum Genet 1991; 49:421.

115. Lundin G, Wedell A, et al: Two new mutations in the porphobilinogen deaminase gene and a screening method using PCR amplification of specific alleles. Hum Genet 1994; 93:59.

116. Delfau MH, Picat C, et al: Two different point G to A mutations in exon 10 of the porphobilinogen deaminase gene are responsible for acute intermittent porphyria. J Clin Invest 1990; 86:1511.

117. Gu X-F, de Rooij F, et al: High frequency of mutations in exon 10 of the porphobilinogen deaminase gene in patients with a CRIM-positive subtype of acute intermittent porphyria. Am J Hum Genet 1992; 51:660.

118. Kauppinen R, Peltonen L, et al: CRIM-positive mutations of acute intermittent porphyria in Finland. Hum Mutat 1992; 1:392.

119. Lee JS, Anvret M: Identification of the most common mutation within the porphobilinogen deaminase gene in Swedish patients with acute intermittent porphyria. Proc Natl Acad Sci U S A 1991; 88:10912.

120. Mgone CS, Lanyon WG, et al: Detection of a high mutation frequency in exon 12 of the porphobilinogen deaminase gene in patients with acute intermittent porphyria. Hum Genet 1993; 92:619.

121. Daimon M, Yamatani K, et al: Acute intermittent porphyria caused by a G to C mutation in exon 12 of the porphobilinogen deaminase gene that results in exon skipping. Hum Genet 1993; 92:549.

122. Boulechfar S, Da Silva V, et al: Heterogeneity of mutations in the uroporphyrinogen III synthase gene in congenital erythropoietic porphyria. Hum Genet 1992; 88:320.

123. de Verneuil H, Deybach JC, et al: Coexistence of two point mutations in the uroporphyrinogen III synthase gene in one case of CEP. Blood 1989; 74:105A.

124. Warner CA, Poh-Fitzpatrick MB, et al: Congenital erythropoietic porphyria. A mild variant with low uroporphyrin I levels due to a missense mutation (A66V) encoding residual uroporphyrinogen III synthase activity. Arch Dermatol 1992; 128:1243.

125. de Verneuil H, Grandchamp B, et al: Uroporphyrinogen decarboxylase structural mutant (Gly281 Glu) in a case of porphyria. Science 1986; 234:732.

126. de Verneuil H, Grandchamp B, et al: Molecular analysis of uroporphyrinogen decarboxylase deficiency in a family with two cases of hepatoerythropoietic porphyria. J Clin Invest 1986; 77:431.

127. de Verneuil H, Bourgeois F, et al: Characterization of a new mutation (R292G) and a detection at the human uroporphyrinogen decarboxylase locus in two patients with hepatoerythropoietic porphyria. Hum Genet 1992; 89:548.

128. Garey JR, Hansen JL, et al: A point mutation in the coding region of uroporphyrinogen decarboxylase associated with familial porphyria cutanea tarda. Blood 1989; 73:892.

129. Garey JR, Harrison LM, et al: Uroporphyrinogen decarboxylase: a splice site mutation causes the deletion of exon 6 in multiple families with porphyria cutanea tarda. J Clin Invest 1990; 86:1416.

130. Hansen JL, Pryor MA, et al: Steady-state levels of uroporphyrinogen decarboxylase mRNA in lymphoblastoid cell lines from patients with familial porphyria cutanea tarda and their relatives. Am J Hum Genet 1988; 42:847.

131. Wang X, Poh-Fitzpatrick M, et al: Screening for ferrochelatase mutations: Molecular heterogeneity of erythropoietic protoporphyria. Biochem Biophys Acta 1994; 1225:187.

132. Sarkany RPE, Whitcombe DM, Cox TM: Molecular characterization of a ferrochelatase gene defect causing anomalous RNA splicing in erythropoietic protoporphyria. J Invest Dermatol 1994; 102:481.

133. Sarkany RPE, Alexander GJMA, Cox TM: Recessive inheritance of erythropoietic protoporphyria with liver failure. Lancet 1994; 343:1394.

134. Todd DJ, Hughes AE, et al: Identification of a single base pair deletion (40 del G) in exon 1 of the ferrochelatase gene in patients with erythropoietic protoporphyria. Hum Mol Genet 1993; 2:1495.

135. Schneider-Yin X, Schäfer BW, et al: Molecular defects in erythropoietic protoporphyria with terminal liver failure. Hum Genet 1994; 93:711.

CHAPTER

13

Lead Poisoning

Sergio Piomelli

SOURCES OF LEAD

Lead (Pb) is a toxic metal without any function in the human body. Because of its affinity for sulfhydryl groups, it damages a multitude of enzymes and essential cellular structures, such as mitochondria.[1] This useful metal has been mined for several centuries: as a result, progressively larger amounts have been removed from the depths of the earth and introduced into the biosphere. Enough lead has found its way into humans that nowadays it is practically impossible, at least in the industrialized parts of the world, to find a human being who does not have some lead in the body and hence in the blood.[2] It has thus become customary to refer to the blood lead values found in apparently healthy populations as "normal" blood lead levels. This term is an obvious misnomer, because it implies some kind of minimum physiologic requirement for lead. Yet, when a truly "unacculturated" population, such as the Yanomamo (who live in remote areas at the sources of the Orinoco River in Venezuela), was examined, the average blood lead level was found to be extremely low (less than 1 μg/dL)[3] and was of the same minuscule order of magnitude predicted by Patterson in 1976 for the "natural" blood lead level on

the basis of pure geophysical considerations.[4] In a remote Himalayan population, the blood lead level was approximately 3 μg/dL, with no difference between children and adults.[5] Even this small amount of lead in the blood could be explained by the practice, in this area at high elevation, of burning wood and organic materials indoors without ventilation. Hence, even in the Himalayas, whereas the outdoor air is essentially free of lead, the indoor air contains a concentration of lead that is very small (0.0009 μg/m³) but yet yields a perceptible concentration of lead in the blood.[6]

Air. Airborne lead enters the human body through the process of respiration; about 35% is absorbed and 15% to 18% is retained.[7] In small children, the intake of airborne lead by inhalation is greater than in adults, because children breathe at a lower height, where lead concentration is greater, and have a greater respiratory rate per unit of body weight.[8, 9] The progressive increase of lead in the biosphere can be followed by studies of lead concentrations in materials that can be accurately dated. Murozumi and associates[10] measured the concentration of lead at various depths of the glaciers of Greenland. Only a slight increase of lead content was found from 800 BC to AD 1740, the beginning of the industrialized era, when a gradual increase occurred. In 1930, with the use of lead as a gasoline additive, the increase abruptly became much faster. There is a clear correlation between air lead concentrations and blood lead levels; Goldsmith and Hexter, in 1957, demonstrated a logarithmic-logarithmic relationship.[11] An essentially identical relationship was found in a well-controlled study by Azar and associates, who used personal respirators to monitor air exposure.[12] The nature of this relationship implies that blood lead levels are minimal at minimal air lead concentrations, as predicted by Patterson[4] and observed in the Yanomamo.[3] As soon as the concentration of air lead increases, there is an initial rapid rise of blood lead levels, followed by a progressively slower increase (Fig. 13–1). The source of air lead was primarily the emission of lead by combustion engines. Locally, there may be emission by stationary sources, such as primary and secondary (recycling) lead smelters.[13] The concentration of lead in the air in the proximity of smelters may be extremely high; in several instances, this has resulted in local epidemics of lead poisoning.[14]

Food and Water. Additional sources of lead for humans are contained in food, water, and beverages. As much as 80% of the lead content of food is of direct or indirect atmospheric origin.[8] The high content of lead in canned foods was due to the can solder. This has been largely removed, at least in cans manufactured in the United States, by the introduction of solderless extruded cans. A 2-year-old child ingests almost as much lead as an adult because of the great caloric requirements of growing children. The average retention of ingested lead is only 10% for adults but is almost 50% for children.[15, 16] Hence, in terms of body weight, a 2-year-old child ingests at least three times as much lead as the adult receiving the same diet but absorbs five times as much lead. Lead absorption is increased by dietary deficiencies, such as iron and calcium,[17] common among children of the low socioeconomic group.

Paint: the Dust Route. Children living in old houses are exposed to the additional risk of lead in paint.[1] Although lead in air, food, and beverages can be considered *"low-dose"* sources, lead in paint is by far the most concentrated source. As much as 40% lead by weight can be present in dried paint used before World War II. Since then, lead in paint has been progressively reduced to 0.006% by weight of the dried product, a value already found in the majority of samples of paint recently tested.[1] In 1971, the maximum tolerable intake of lead suggested for children was 300 mg/d to prevent the blood lead level from exceeding 40 μg/dL. In view of the evidence that adverse health effects of lead can be seen at blood lead levels below 40 μg/dL[18] and that the absorption of lead by small children is now known to be 50% of the amount ingested (or five times higher than it was thought to be in 1971),[15] it is clear that the maximum tolerable intake of lead should be reduced by at least 10 to 20 times to 10 to 15 mg/d. For many years, it has been believed that lead poisoning in children occurs primarily as a result of "pica" (an urge to ingest nonfood material), with consequent ingestion of paint chips.[19] Although this is not an uncommon occurrence, it is certainly neither the only nor even the prevailing mechanism of ingestion of lead paint. Small children, through their ordinary hand-to-mouth activities (such as thumb sucking) directly ingest dust and thus take in large amounts of lead. Elevated blood lead levels were found in children of lead factory workers, for whom the only source of exposure was the lead dust brought home on their parents' clothing.[20] In inner-city homes, large amounts of lead are present in household dust obtained from the hands of children residing in these houses. The dust was measured and was found to contain 2.5 mg of lead per gram; the mean weight of dust per hand was 11 mg. Another study showed that old inner-city housing contained up to 0.5 mg of lead per square foot of floor surface.[21-23] These findings indicate clearly that in the highly contaminated environment of an old house, the ordinary

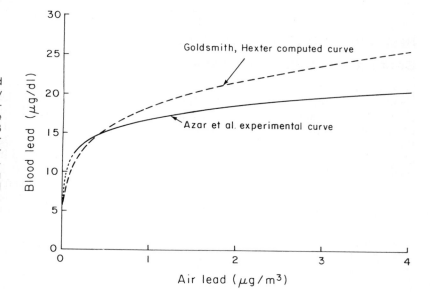

Figure 13–1. Relationship between air lead and blood lead. *Dashed line,* Curve computed by Goldsmith and Hexter[11] on the basis of epidemiologic and experimental studies published before 1967 (log blood lead (μg/dL) = 1.265 + 0.2433 log air lead (μg/m³)). *Solid line,* Essentially similar relationship determined experimentally by Azar and co-workers in 1975,[12] who used personal respirators to quantify individuals' air lead exposure (log blood lead (μg/dL) = 1.2257 + 0.153 log air lead (μg/m³)). No measurements at air lead below 0.14 μg/m³ were obtained; the *dotted part* of the line is the extrapolation to air lead = 0.01 μg/m³.

hand-to-mouth activity is sufficient to account for the intake of excessive quantities of lead by preschool children even in the absence of pathologic ingestion of nonfood objects. When pica is a factor, together with the additional ingestion of paint chips, the problem may reach catastrophic proportions with extreme rapidity. Despite legislative efforts and scientific advances in the United States, 15 to 20 million dwellings still contain leaded paint. These dwellings present an obvious risk, particularly to the children of the poor, who tend to live in the oldest houses. The state of repair of the dwelling is almost as important as the lead content of the paint; peeling or flaking paint is obviously more accessible to small children.[8]

Other Sources. Less common sources of lead include fumes from old battery casings; illegally distilled whiskey; printed paper, particularly colored magazines; and lead-painted toys.[8] An uncommon source of lead that may result in severe poisoning is improperly glazed earthenware vessels used to store acidic beverages (such as fruit juices or cider). More recent problems have been identified in gasoline sniffing by teenagers and the use of herbal medications.[24]

Additive Lead Intake. Several factors contribute simultaneously to increased intake as well as retention of lead by small children. Dietary intake of lead is additive to the ingestion of lead in dust; this is peculiar to children and is aggravated by their greater intestinal absorption of lead. It is not surprising that children, particularly preschoolers, have higher blood lead values than adults living in the same environment. The small child, between 18 months and 4 years of age (the age of greatest hand-to-mouth activity), is at the greatest risk of lead poisoning. Because lead from all sources is additive, the urban child is at a greater risk because of the higher environmental pollution. The children of the poor, who live in the oldest houses with lead-laden walls in the worst state of repair and who tend to have additional nutritional deficiency, are at the greatest risk of all. In fact, the incidence of lead poisoning is highest among the urban children of the lowest socioeconomic class.[25]

HEMATOLOGIC EFFECTS OF LEAD
General Biochemical Effects of Lead

Lead has a strong affinity for the sulfhydryl groups of cysteine, the amino group of lysine, the carboxyl group of the glutamic and aspartic acids, and the hydroxyl group of tyrosine. Lead binds to proteins, modifies their tertiary structure, and inactivates enzymatic properties.[8] Enzymes that are rich in sulfhydryl groups appear to be most sensitive to the smallest concentrations. The mitochondria are among the cellular structures that are particularly sensitive to lead.[8] Studies using ^{210}Pb and ^{203}Pb have shown the tendency of lead to accumulate in the mitochondria.[26, 27] Lead granules were shown on the membrane of isolated rat liver mitochondria incubated with lead at concentrations in the same range as observed in childhood lead poisoning.[28] Effects of lead on mitochondrial function have

been shown by depression of respiration[29, 30] and by a marked inhibition of the pyruvate-nicotinamide adenine dinucleotide system.[31] Many prominent effects of lead on heme synthesis are mediated through the alterations of the mitochondrial membrane.

Effects of Lead on Heme Synthesis

The effects of lead on heme synthesis observed in the peripheral blood represent only the visible "tip of the iceberg." Heme is the respiratory pigment of hemoglobin in erythrocytes but also the respiratory pigment in all cells of the ubiquitous cytochrome system. Heme synthesis proceeds from small building blocks, glycine and succinyl coenzyme A, to the complex molecule of protoporphyrin IX; the pathway culminates in the insertion of iron into the protoporphyrin ring (see Chapter 12). Heme synthesis starts and ends inside the mitochondria; intermediate steps take place in the cytoplasm. The first enzyme of the pathway, δ-aminolevulinic (δ-ALA) synthetase, and the last one, ferrochelatase, are located in the mitochondrial cristae. Because heme, the final product, regulates its own synthesis by feedback repression, this close anatomic arrangement is particularly convenient. In all cells, the heme formed becomes an integral part of the cytochrome system, also located inside the mitochondria. In erythropoietic precursors, additionally, very large amounts of heme are formed to make hemoglobin. Lead interferes at several points in the heme synthetic pathway in all cells. The two most important steps affected are those catalyzed by δ-ALA dehydratase (a cytoplasmic enzyme rich in sulfhydryl groups) and ferrochelatase (an intramitochondrial enzyme).

Effects of Lead on δ-Aminolevulinic Acid Dehydratase

Delta-aminolevulinic acid dehydratase (δ-ALAD) is a cytosol enzyme that contains essential sulfhydryl groups. Direct binding of lead to these sulfhydryl groups results in its inhibition: this may be completely reversed by mercaptoethanol or dithioerythritol.[32] In 1970, Hernberg and Nikkanen demonstrated in humans a negative correlation between the logarithm of the enzyme activity in the erythrocytes and the blood lead level, starting at values as low as 5 μg/dL.[33] The inhibition is very pronounced, with 50% inactivation at blood lead levels of 16 μg/dL and 90% inactivation at levels of 55 μg/dL. The effect of lead on δ-ALA is evident at extremely low levels of exposure and is already significant in the range of blood lead levels observed in most American populations. The inhibition observed in the erythrocytes reflects that in other tissues, such as liver and brain.[34, 35] The enzyme is present in great excess, and its partial inhibition may be relatively unnoticed in the overall process of heme synthesis. The metabolic effect of its inhibition is the accumulation of δ-ALA in the plasma and its excess excretion in the urine. An excess of δ-ALA has toxic systemic effects by itself[36]; hence, inhibition of δ-ALAD, resulting in the accumulation of this substrate, cannot be considered innocuous. There is a correlation between blood lead level and the logarithm of urinary δ-ALA.[37] This exponential relation leads to a curvilinear increase in δ-ALA excretion; the rise is slow at the lowest blood lead level, but it increases rapidly above 40 μg/dL. The activity of δ-ALAD is influenced also by the presence of zinc, present in the purified enzyme in the ratio of 1 mol of zinc for 1 mol of enzyme.[38] Zinc may reverse δ-ALAD inhibition, but large concentrations are required. Lead and zinc compete for the same binding site, in a location close to the active sulfhydryl groups.[39]

Accumulation of Erythrocyte Protoporphyrin

The last step of heme synthesis is catalyzed by the enzyme ferrochelatase, located in the inner matrix of the mitochondria. In humans, the concentration of lead is severalfold higher in the bone marrow mitochondria than in the peripheral blood. Ferrochelatase contains sulfhydryl groups sensitive to lead. The inhibition by lead of the step catalyzed by this enzyme, the insertion of iron into the protoporphyrin ring, results in the accumulation of the latter compound in the maturing erythrocyte. *In vitro*, sulfhydryl compounds protect the ferrochelatase activity, an effect probably mediated by the need to maintain iron in the reduced form.[40] The effect of lead on ferrochelatase *in vivo* is more likely to reflect the interference of lead with the transmitochondrial transport of iron than a direct effect on the enzyme itself. *In vitro*, ferrochelatase is inhibited directly only by rather high (10^{-3} mol/L) concentration of lead, whereas *in vivo* its inhibition has been observed at much lower concentrations, as demonstrated both by direct measurements in bone marrow reticulocytes and indirectly by the observation of increased levels of erythrocyte protoporphyrin.[41] In the presence of lead, iron uptake by the reticulocyte is diminished but heme synthesis is completely suppressed. Iron transport through the mitochondrial membrane requires energy-dependent mechanisms, inhibited by lead.[42] Ultimately, despite the presence of a normal or an increased intracellular content of iron, the mitochondria remain starved for iron. Metalloporphyrins inhibit several mitochondrial enzymes; the increased concentration of zinc protoporphyrin resulting from lead toxicity, in turn, further impairs mitochondrial function.[40] There is a relation between the concentration of lead that inhibits ferrochelatase in mitochondria *in vitro* and the concentration of iron in the medium. At any concentration of lead, ferrochelatase inhibition is most marked when the iron concentration is the lowest.[43] This biochemical mechanism explains the greater elevation of erythrocyte protoporphyrin observed, at equal lead exposure, in children with concomitant iron deficiency.[44]

Accumulation of protoporphyrin in the erythrocytes of individuals with lead poisoning has been known for almost 50 years.[45] Its clinical use was limited, however, by the need for multiple partitions through solvents to separate protoporphyrin from heme and by the poor sensitivity of spectrophotometric techniques. In 1972, the development of a simplified extraction method combined with fluorometry made the measurement of erythrocyte protoporphyrin a widely accessible test.[41] The term *free* erythrocyte protoporphyrin had been used to indicate the lack of iron at the center of the tetrapyrrole ring. In lead intoxication, protoporphyrin is bound firmly to hemoglobin, in the heme pockets made available by the decreased heme synthesis (Fig. 13–2).[46] The protoporphyrin found in the erythrocytes of patients with both iron deficiency and lead intoxication is the zinc chelate, zinc protoporphyrin.[47] Sequential studies of lead-poisoned rabbits and children[48] indicate that the compound initially formed is the free protoporphyrin base; this binds at the heme pocket and in the circulation it progressively chelates zinc nonenzymatically. In lead intoxication, protoporphyrin remains within the erythrocyte throughout the cell's life span.[49] No diffusion into the plasma takes place, and, hence, no protoporphyrin is released into the skin. Thus, photosensitivity is prominently lacking, even in the presence of high levels of erythrocyte protoporphyrin. The hemoglobin-bound protoporphyrin in children with lead poisoning has explained the nature of the fast hemoglobin component observed in their hemolysates.[50] This consists of molecules in which one or more of the hemes are replaced by protoporphyrin, with a resulting altered charge. Most of the protoporphyrin in lead-intoxicated children appears, in fact, in the fastest moving hemoglobin band. In erythropoietic protoporphyria, the protoporphyrin instead diffuses into the skin from the plasma and its photosensitizing effect results in severe clinical symptoms (see Chapter 12).

The pathogenesis of the accumulation of protoporphyrin is profoundly different in lead poisoning than in erythropoietic protoporphyria. In lead intoxication, the overall production of protoporphyrin (free base plus heme protoporphyrin) is decreased,[51] whereas in erythropoietic protoporphyria it is markedly increased. In lead poisoning, despite the large increase in protoporphyrin concentration observed, the number of protoporphyrin molecules remains a very small fraction (1 in 300 at the most) of the large number present in heme. In erythropoietic protoporphyria, instead, accumulation of protoporphyrin occurs in the late stage of erythrocyte maturation and takes place almost exclusively in the reticulocytes, when most of the hemoglobin synthesis has been completed.[52] The protoporphyrin produced is thus in absolute excess, because all heme sites are already occupied by heme. The excess protoporphyrin binds to the surface of the hemoglobin molecule at a site that bridges the α and the β chains. This is a loose bond, and protoporphyrin rapidly diffuses through the plasma into the skin, where it induces photosensitivity.[49] The amount of protoporphyrin free base formed in the erythroid tissue in erythropoietic protoporphyria is a much greater proportion (1:20) of the total protoporphyrin formed. In erythropoietic protoporphyria, the amount of protoporphyrin formed in the erythropoietic tissue is great enough to account for nearly all the excess fecal excretion, without need to invoke a large hepatic component. The *in vivo* life span of the protoporphyrin within the erythrocyte is extremely short (less than 1 or 2 days).[49] The free proto-

MITOCHONDRIA IN THE BONE MARROW

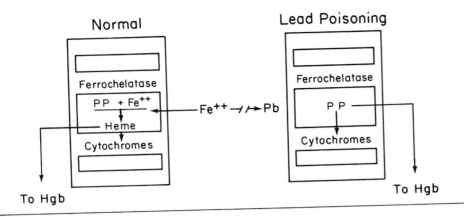

Figure 13-2. Mechanism of the accumulation of erythrocyte protoporphyrin in lead intoxication. *Top,* In the bone marrow, lead inhibits the transport of iron across the mitochondrial membrane in the maturing normoblasts; thus, protoporphyrin accumulates. *Bottom,* In the circulation erythrocytes, some of the heme pockets of hemoglobin are occupied by protoporphyrin free base instead of heme. Protoporphyrin nonenzymatically chelates zinc. Finally, the predominant protoporphyrin species found in circulating erythrocytes is Zn-protoporphyrin.

PROTOPORPHYRIN SPECIES IN THE ERYTHROCYTES IN LEAD INTOXICATION

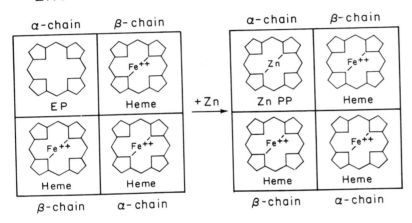

porphyrin base does not persist long enough in the circulation to bind zinc significantly. Hence, there is a preponderance of free protoporphyrin base; only small amounts of zinc protoporphyrin are found in the oldest erythrocytes. The spectrofluorometric characteristics of free protoporphyrin base in the plasma permit a clear differential diagnosis from other porphyrias.[53]

Correlation Between Protoporphyrin Level and Lead Intoxication

A progressive exponential increase in erythrocyte protoporphyrin concentration is observed at blood lead levels from 5 to 90 μg/dL.[41] In every child with blood lead levels above 55 μg/dL, the concentration of protoporphyrin is elevated, and a majority of children with blood lead levels between 40 and 60 μg/dL also have values above this range. The correlation between the logarithm of the erythrocyte protoporphyrin level and the blood lead level fits the concept of a dose-effect response, because blood lead concentration is, in turn, exponentially correlated to overall body burden of lead. The increase in protoporphyrin reflects a progressive impairment of the last step of heme synthesis in the bone marrow normoblasts with exponential accu-

mulation of substrate. In a large study of children with lower blood lead levels, the dose-effect relationship has been further confirmed by the technique of probit analysis. The blood lead level at which the erythrocyte protoporphyrin level is abnormal in 50% of the cases is 32 μg/dL.[44] The rate of exponential rise of erythrocyte protoporphyrin levels is steeper in children and women than it is in men.[37] Erythrocyte protoporphyrin level is an indicator of adverse metabolic effects. It is very effective as a screening test for severe lead poisoning, but it cannot be used to screen for blood lead levels below 40 to 50 μg/dL.

Erythrocyte Protoporphyrin Levels in Iron Deficiency

In lead intoxication the incorporation of iron into protoporphyrin is blocked despite the availability of both substrates. On the other hand, in iron deficiency an accumulation of erythrocyte protoporphyrin is a direct result of the specific lack of iron. In iron deficiency, as in lead poisoning, protoporphyrin is bound to hemoglobin at the available heme site[46, 49]; there, it binds zinc as the erythrocytes circulate. Ultimately, the prevalent protoporphyrin species becomes the zinc chelate.[47] An elevation of erythrocyte protoporphyrin levels in iron deficiency has been known since the 1940s.[54] In 1966, Dagg and co-workers concluded that protoporphyrin levels rise in iron depletion before frank anemia develops.[55] Langer and associates, on the other hand, in 1972, concluded that the elevation of protoporphyrin levels reflects the degree of anemia.[56] Studies have shown that the elevation of erythrocyte protoporphyrin levels is inversely correlated with both transferrin saturation and hemoglobin level.[57, 58] Every child with iron deficiency and anemia has elevated erythrocyte protoporphyrin levels. Most children with iron deficiency and no or minimal anemia also have an elevation of erythrocyte protoporphyrin. Early in the development of iron deficiency the depletion of iron stores is reflected by decreased transferrin saturation. This is followed next by an elevation of protoporphyrin levels, which in turn precedes the occurrence of anemia. In children younger than 2 years of age, when iron stores have not yet accumulated, elevated erythrocyte protoporphyrin levels provide an indication of impending anemia and a rational indication for iron therapy. The sensitivity of measurement of erythrocyte protoporphyrin in iron deficiency is greatly improved if the results are expressed as micrograms of erythrocyte protoporphyrin per gram of hemoglobin, rather than per deciliter of blood, the units commonly used for the diagnosis of lead poisoning.[57]

Erythrocyte Protoporphyrin Levels Distinguish Iron Deficiency from Thalassemia

Stockman and co-workers first noticed that an elevation of free erythrocyte protoporphyrin is invariably present when iron deficiency is severe enough to induce microcytosis.[59] They suggested that this could be advantageously used for discriminating between the microcytosis of iron deficiency and that of the β-thalassemia trait. Similar observations in α-thalassemia trait were shortly thereafter reported by Koenig.[60] Microcytosis without elevated protoporphyrin levels rules out iron deficiency, and it is thus diagnostic of the thalassemia trait. Occasional elevation of erythrocyte protoporphyrin levels has been observed in patients with sickle cell anemia. This may reflect the concomitant presence of iron deficiency.[61] When the erythrocyte protoporphyrin level is measured with the hematofluorometer, falsely elevated values are always observed in sickle cell anemia, owing to the interference of the moderate elevation of serum bilirubin levels usually present in this condition. However, no such artifact occurs when the extraction procedure is used. Modest elevations of erythrocyte protoporphyrin levels have been observed in chronic inflammatory disease.[62]

Anemia of Lead Poisoning

The bulk of lead in blood (greater than 90%) is in the erythrocytes, bound to a protein of approximately 240,000 daltons, a molecular weight quite close to that of δ-ALAD.[40] Lead is rapidly transferred from plasma to the erythrocytes; the plasma lead levels remain constant at 2 to 3 μg/dL, while the lead levels in whole blood may range between 10 and 150 μg/dL.[63] Kochen and Greener have shown that the erythrocytes serve as the primary carrier for lead in the blood and that their binding capacity for lead is well above the levels associated with even very heavy exposure.[64] The blood lead content is therefore independent of the hematocrit. Corrections for hematocrit are not warranted, and their use may result in spurious associations.[65] The presence of basophilic stippling in the erythrocytes of patients with lead intoxication has been shown by electron microscopy to result from deposition of ribosomal DNA and mitochondrial fragments.[30] Paglia and co-workers have provided a biochemical explanation for this microscopic finding with the demonstration that lead inhibits the enzyme pyrimidine-5′-nucleotidase, which under normal conditions plays a prominent role in the cleavage of residual nucleotides after nuclear extrusion.[66] The activity of this enzyme is decreased in lead poisoning, even in the absence of detectable basophilic stippling. The defect in pyrimidine-5′-nucleotidase probably contributes to the shortening of erythrocyte survival. Individuals genetically defective in this enzyme in fact exhibit marked chronic hemolysis. The osmotic fragility of the erythrocytes is modestly decreased in severe lead poisoning.[67] This effect is exerted directly on the red cell membrane, as it may also be produced *in vitro* by incubation of normal erythrocytes with lead. A large efflux of potassium, due to lowering of the activity of the Na^+/K^+-dependent membrane adenosine triphosphatase, is observed in lead poisoning[68] as well as an increase in the mechanical fragility of the erythrocytes. Lead intoxication also leads to ineffective erythropoiesis. Because of these multiple alterations of erythrocyte functions, the red cell survival is considerably shortened, when studied by either ^{3}H-DFP[33] or ^{14}C-glycine.[69] However, Leikin and Eng observed a decreased erythrocyte survival in only three of seven children with lead poisoning and anemia.[70] These findings suggest that hemolysis is only one of the component mechanisms of anemia and that erythrocyte underproduction also plays a role. There are so many mechanisms of interference by lead on heme and hemoglobin synthesis as well as on erythrocyte function and survival that it is almost surprising that anemia is a rather late sign of lead intoxication, particularly in children. A moderate decline in hemoglobin concentration starts in adults at blood lead levels of 50 μg/dL.[8] In newly hired adult lead workers a noticeable decrease in hemoglobin level (13.4 vs. 14 g/dL) was noted after approximately 3 months of exposure.[8] A negative correlation between hemoglobin level and blood lead level was observed by Pueschel and co-workers in 40 children with blood lead levels ranging between 30 and 120 μg/dL.[8] However, because it is known that in normal children between the ages of 1 and 6 years there is a physiologic increase in hemoglobin level, the observed correlation may have only reflected the greater frequency of lead poisoning in the youngest children. In the author's clinic, anemia has been observed in children with lead poisoning only in severe cases or in the presence of concomitant iron deficiency.[62] This is not an unexpected finding, as the defect in heme synthesis affects only a very small fraction of the total protoporphyrin production, and clinically significant anemia usually develops in the late stages. It is not uncommon to observe severe neurologic toxicity in the absence of anemia in children. On the other hand, lead intoxication and iron deficiency anemia tend to occur in the same lower socioeconomic population, and both are aggravated by each other. Iron deficiency increases lead retention and toxicity; uptake by erythrocytes and intestinal absorption of lead are decreased in the presence of iron.[71, 72] The impairment of heme synthesis in all body tissues may be one of the mechanisms of actual lead toxicity; this is synergistically aggravated by concomitant lead poisoning and iron deficiency.[43] The iron-deficient child is in increased jeopardy because the defect increases lead absorption, enhances the defect in heme synthesis, and increases the toxicity of lead.[58]

Additional Effects on Heme Synthesis

The primary effects of lead on heme synthesis are exerted on the cytosol enzyme δ-ALAD and the mitochondrial step mediated by ferrochelatase. Additional effects occur at other steps; however, it is not clear to what extent these are a direct consequence of lead inhibition or merely secondary to the alterations in the two previous steps. A modest increase in δ-ALA synthetase can be induced by lead in experimental animals and *in vitro*.[73] This appears to be due to *de novo* synthesis of the enzyme, because it can be completely blocked by cycloheximide.[74] The induction of δ-ALA synthetase is most likely mediated by the depression of feedback inhibition by heme, when heme synthesis is decreased. Both δ-ALA synthetase and ferrochelatase are mitochondrial enzymes in a close anatomic relationship, which facilitates the regulation of the synthetic pathway by heme, its end product. *In vivo*, very little increase in δ-ALA synthetase occurs; instead, there is a progressive decline with increasing lead concentration.[40] Uroporphyrinogen synthetase activity is inhibited only by rather high (10^{-4} mol/L) lead concentration.[40] Very little inhibition occurs *in vivo*, except probably in extreme lead intoxication, when the urinary excretion of both porphobilinogen and uroporphyrin is increased. Coproporphyrinogen decarboxylase, another mitochondrial enzyme, also is inhibited by lead.[40] It is well known that in lead intoxication there is a marked increase in urinary coproporphyrin level. Measurement of urinary coproporphyrin has been widely used for the diagnosis of childhood lead poisoning, particularly in emergency departments. Although this test has been superseded by the easier measurement of erythrocyte protoporphyrin, it is important to recognize its usefulness in discriminating between recent and past lead exposure. In view of the long persistence of protoporphyrin within the erythrocyte, significant elevations may last as long as 2 to 3 months after exposure to lead.[49] On the other hand, increased coproporphyrin production, because of its high solubility, is immediately reflected in excess urinary excretion. Hence, when exposure to lead is current, both erythrocyte protoporphyrin level and urinary coproporphyrin level are increased; when exposure to lead is no longer present, there is a discrepancy between the elevated erythrocyte protoporphyrin level and the normal urinary coproporphyrin excretion. The effects of lead on hemoglobin synthesis are not only limited to an overall decrease in heme production but also are seen in the synthesis of globin. A more marked decrease occurs in the synthesis of α chains than of β chains; an effect of lead on globin synthesis in human reticulocytes *in vitro* was found at concentrations as low as 10^{-5} mol/L, equivalent to a blood lead level of 20 μg/dL.[75]

Nonerythropoietic Effects of Lead on Heme Synthesis: Mechanisms of Toxicity

The process of heme synthesis is not exclusive to the erythropoietic tissue. All cells contain essential heme proteins, at least in the form of the respiratory cytochrome system, also located in the mitochondria. The most visible effects of lead on heme synthesis are those detectable in the peripheral blood, because this is the easiest tissue to sample. However, the ubiquitous presence of active heme synthesis in the mitochondria of all body cells and the affinity of lead for mitochondria result in widespread impairment of cellular function. This effect has been shown in several other tissues. Lead intoxication inhibits the synthesis of cytochrome P-450, the key enzyme in the mixed oxidase system. Its inhibition has been shown in experimental animals and, indirectly, through the measurement of antipyrine clearance, in children and workers with severe lead poisoning.[76, 77] The inhibition of the enzymatic system involved with ethanol metabolism represents the biochemical basis for the "Monday morning colic" observed in lead workers after weekend alcohol consumption.[78] Studies by Rosen and co-workers have shown that lead intoxication interferes profoundly, even at low level of exposure, with vitamin D metabolism, particularly through the reduction of the biosynthesis of 1,25-dihydroxyvitamin D.[79]

Damage by Lead of the Heme Synthetic Pathway, As a Mediator of Neurotoxicity

Of greater relevance to the pathogenesis of childhood lead encephalopathy is the demonstration that lead induces accumulation of protoporphyrin in chick dorsal root ganglions in tissue culture.[80] This effect was most obvious in the glial elements, which are known to be involved directly in the development of childhood lead encephalopathy. Exposure of neural tissue in culture to lead results in demyelination, which is reversible by the addition of heme.[80] Increased plasma levels of δ-ALA have been shown to be associated with pharmacologic, biochemical, and behavioral effects: δ-ALA inhibits ion transport across membranes and affects neuromuscular functions. Also δ-ALA is known to concentrate in the hypothalamus.[81, 82] These extra-erythropoietic effects provide an interesting model of the mechanism of clinical lead toxicity. It appears likely that toxic effects of lead, particularly in the nervous system, reflect the derangement of heme synthesis in this tissue. It is well known that there is a parallel between the clinical symptoms of lead poisoning and those of some porphyrias.[83] Silbergeld has shown that exposure to lead interacts with the neurotransmitter γ-aminobutyric acid, a compound very similar to δ-ALA, by preventing its synaptosomal release. She also demonstrated the comparative effects of lead and succinyl-acetone (a potent inhibitor of heme synthesis).[84] Exposure to lead reduces the free hepatic heme pool, with inhibition of tryptophan pyrrolase. This results in elevated brain levels of tryptophan, serotonin, and 5-hydroxyindoleacetic acid. All these effects are reversible by heme infusion.[36] Angle and McIntire pointed out how many features of lead poisoning are consistent with altered hematopoiesis.[65] The effects of lead on the heme synthetic pathway, through involvement of several organ systems, contribute, both directly and indirectly, to the neurologic toxicity.

CLINICAL ASPECTS OF LEAD POISONING

Severe Lead Poisoning

In children, the clinical effects of excessive exposure to lead are apparent primarily in the central nervous system; alterations of renal function and anemia occur only in the most severe cases. In adults, peripheral neuropathy, abdominal colic, and anemia are the most common initial signs. Acute encephalopathy can be the first presentation of severe childhood lead poisoning. The onset is usually marked by seizures, often intractable, followed by coma and cardiorespiratory arrest. The syndrome may be fatal within 24 to 48 hours. Survivors often remain with permanent neurologic damage.[85] Acute encephalopathy is often accompanied by Fanconi's syndrome with aminoaciduria, glycosuria, and hyperphosphaturia.[86] Anemia is often present and is most severe when there is associated iron deficiency. When severe, the anemia should be treated with transfusions, since iron administration may be a powerful emetic, when given in concomitance with dimercaprol. The sequelae of lead encephalopathy are particularly serious, with behavior abnormalities and seizure disorders throughout childhood and ultimately permanent mental incompetence. These sequelae are more frequent in children who had the most severe initial symptoms and especially in those children who, by returning to the original contaminated environment, have repeated exposure. It is essential to prolong therapy well after the initial, and usually transient, chelation effect and to be assured that symptomatic children do not return to the same source of lead, unless the appropriate measures have been taken to modify the environment.[87]

Chronic Lead Intoxication

The chronic phase of lead toxicity is extremely vague: abdominal pain, vomiting, general malaise, and changes in behavior may occur. These symptoms are often nonspecific and of little diagnostic help, particularly in the youngest children, aged 1 to 3 years, who are the most frequently affected.[18] The extremely rapid transition from a state of good health to a rapidly progressing encephalopathy is the main reason to screen for lead poisoning at once, whenever a child presents with any of the vague prodromic symptoms. A peripheral neuropathy of the type seen in adults appears to be uniquely frequent in children with sickle cell anemia.[88] The threshold blood lead level at which encephalopathy occurs in children is difficult to define. *Acute lead poisoning* with clinical signs other than encephalopathy has been observed at blood lead levels ranging between 60 and 450 μg/dL.[8] On the other hand, it is possible to observe children with blood lead levels as high as 200 μg/dL without overt neurologic symptoms. The probability of overt neurologic problems increases with the blood lead level and becomes significant when the blood lead level rises above 70 μg/dL. For these reasons, and because of the impending risk of an unpredictable clinical deterioration, children found to have blood lead levels of 70 μg/dL or more should be treated as medical emergencies, even in the absence of symptoms.[18]

In adults, the symptomatology of lead poisoning is primarily one of peripheral neuropathy, with peripheral extensor weakness, pain and weakness in the trunk and extremities, and uricopathic features. Progressive renal failure (lead nephropathy) is frequent. Gout (saturnine gout) results from inhibition of guanine deaminase.[89] The long persistence of alcohol-induced symptoms in adults with lead poisoning is mediated by the lead-induced depression of the cytochrome P-450 system.[78]

HEALTH EFFECTS OF LOW-LEVEL EXPOSURE TO LEAD

As a result of the greater awareness of childhood lead poisoning by physicians, extensive screening programs in several large cities, and the reduction of air lead subsequent to the wider use of lead-free gasoline,[25, 90] severe lead poisoning is extremely rare. On the other hand, there is a greater awareness of the subclinical effects of lead and of its deleterious health effects at low concentrations. As with any other toxic agent, the effects of lead are dose related, and it cannot be expected that they be limited to the acute overwhelming effect at the highest dose, without any effect at lower exposure. In recent years, evidence has accumulated to show that the gradual effects of progressively increasing doses of lead in children start at very low levels of exposure and culminate in acute lead encephalopathy at the highest levels of exposure. Much emphasis has been placed on the concept of threshold effect. Because it is known that lead can specifically affect proteins and other macromolecules in the body, it is clear that even a single atom of lead can induce biochemical damage. Therefore, the threshold of lead toxicity can theoretically be infinitesimally small; it thus appears more important to establish at what lead concentration the effect becomes more than trivial.[91] Subclinical effects of lead have been clearly demonstrated in the nervous and the hematopoietic systems of adult lead workers and in children. De la Burdé and Choate observed dysfunction of the central nervous system, motor defects, and altered behavioral profiles in preschool children having lead levels above 30 μg/dL and elevated levels of urinary coproporphyrin.[92] These persisted in a follow-up study of the same children at ages 7 to 8 years, despite the fact that the blood lead level had significantly decreased. Needleman and associates observed a significant neuropsychological impairment in children in the second grade whose previous moderate exposure to lead was documented by the deposition of lead in the dentine of deciduous teeth.[93] In this study, the children were compared with a control group matched for a variety of independent factors. This study was the first to clearly demonstrate an effect of relatively low exposure to lead on childhood neuropsychological development. This study has been confirmed by several others in various countries. Although the adverse effects of lead have been confirmed by all these studies, their extent varied in different reports. In two meta-analyses researchers have tried to summarize the results of several studies and to provide an estimate of the effects of low level lead exposure on children's intelligence and behavior.[94, 95] Although these two meta-analyses were different in methodology, in the studies enclosed, and in opposing hypothesis, the final estimates were ultimately very similar. For an increase of blood lead level from 10 to 20 μg/dL, one meta-analysis estimated the loss in intelligence quotient (IQ) to be between 1 and 2 points, and the other estimated it at 2.6 points. These values apply to a population of children and not to any specific individuals. Because the increase in loss of IQ appears to be progressive, it is clear that, as the blood level increases above 20 μg/dL, the loss of IQ points becomes more relevant and the neuropsychological damage becomes progressively severe.

Childhood Lead Poisoning in the United States

The magnitude of the problem of lead exposure in the United States has been assessed in detail by the two consecutive National Health and Nutrition Surveys (NHANES-II[25] and NHANES-III[96]). These studies surveyed a carefully selected cross section of the U.S. population and measured blood lead levels in over 10,000 individuals. The NHANES-II was done between 1976 and 1980, and the NHANES-III studies took place from 1988 to 1991.[96] The estimated average national blood lead level was found to have declined dramatically from 12.8 μg/dL in 1980 to 3.2 μg/dL in 1991. There was a continuous trend to a decrease from 1976 (the beginning of NHANES II) to 1990 (the end of NHANES-III).[90, 97] This was clearly correlated to the

Table 13–1. CHANGES IN THE BLOOD LEAD LEVELS OF U.S. CHILDREN, WITH THE PROGRESSIVE REMOVAL OF LEAD IN GASOLINE 1976–1991

Blood Lead Level	NHANES II 1976–1980 No. of Children (Age, 5 Mo to 5 Y)*	NHANES III 1988–1991 No. of Children (Age, 1 to 6 Y)*
≥30 μg/dL	540,000	42,000
≥25 μg/dL	940,000	93,000
≥20 μg/dL	3,335,000	206,000
≥15 μg/dL	8,200,000	300,000
≥10 μg/dL	12,000,000	1,700,000
Total	13,500,000	18,640,000

NHANES = National Health and Nutrition Survey.
*Cumulative number (each category includes all the previous ones).

total lead used in gasoline production throughout the active period of study. By 1990, in fact, 98% of the lead in gasoline had been removed. These results are not surprising, because most of the lead present in human blood originates directly from lead released by gasoline combustion.[98]

The reduction in atmospheric lead has had a tremendous impact on the frequency of childhood lead poisoning (Table 13–1). The number of U.S. children estimated by the two consecutive surveys to have markedly elevated blood lead levels has decreased more than 10-fold. The NHANES-II estimated 940,000 children had blood lead levels of 25 μg/dL or more; the NHANES-III estimate decreased this to 89,000. For children with blood lead levels of 30 μg/dL or more, the estimate decreased from 540,000 to 40,000. The downward trend was present for each subgroup tested (defined by race, urbanization, sex, and age).

Both NHANES studies clearly indicated that the blood lead levels were inversely correlated to income, with the highest blood lead levels being those of the poorest urban children. For instance, in NHANES-II, 10% of black children were estimated to have blood lead levels of 30 μg/dL or more, but for those from low income families the percentage was as high as 18.5%.

In fact, of the 89,000 U.S. children that the NHANES-III study estimated to have blood lead levels of 25 μg/dL or more, 49,500 are non-Latino black; 7,500 are Latino, and the remaining 32,000 are non-Latino white. Therefore, 2 of 3 children with blood lead levels of 25 μg/dL or more belong to a minority group, although these groups represent only 27% of the total population of children.

These findings clearly indicate that the magnitude of the problem of lead poisoning in the United States has been changed drastically by the removal of lead from gasoline. Although other sources of lead remain, the background created by atmospheric lead has been removed. This is a great success of preventive medicine. The severe lead intoxication common in the 1970s is a disease of the past. Although attention is now focused on the effects of low level exposure, among the poorest children, mostly in the urban areas, pockets of significant lead poisoning remain.

DEFINITION OF LEAD POISONING AND SCREENING

In view of the evidence of adverse effects of exposure to lead, even at low levels, the Centers for Disease Control and Prevention (CDC) has convened periodic meetings of a committee of "experts" to determine the blood lead level at which asymptomatic children detected by screening programs should come to medical attention. As the evidence of effects of low level lead exposure continued accumulating, there has been a progressive lowering of the "acceptable" blood lead level. (However, this definition never implied that there were no adverse effects below it.)

A *case* of lead poisoning was defined in the 1960s as a blood lead level of 80 μg/dL or more; in the 1970s it was reduced first to a blood lead level of 60 μg/dL or more and then to 40 μg/dL or more.[99–102]

In the 1980s, the definition used a combination of evidence of increased absorption (blood lead) with evidence of biologic damage. A *case* of lead poisoning was thus defined as a child with a blood lead level of 30 μg/dL or more and an associated erythrocyte protoporphyrin level of 50 μg/dL or more. This definition was then lowered to a blood lead level of 25 μg/dL or more, with an associated erythrocyte protoporphyrin level of 35 μg/dL or more.[101, 102]

In recent years, it has become obvious that adverse effects of lead occur at blood lead levels well below 25 μg/dL. These effects are not demonstrable in the individual child but are, however, seen at an epidemiologic level. At the 1991 meeting of the CDC committee, the concept of screening was changed and an additional task was included: the detection of communities with a large percentage of children with blood lead levels higher than average. *Lead poisoning* was defined as a blood lead level greater than or equal to 10 μg/dL[18] (Table 13–2). This definition has led to extensive

Table 13–2. 1991 CENTERS FOR DISEASE CONTROL CLASSIFICATION FOR ASYMPTOMATIC CHILDREN EXPOSED TO LEAD

Blood Lead Level (μg/dL)	Action Recommended
0–9	No immediate concern
	"Lead poisoning"
	Level of concern:
10–14	Community/environmental survey
15–19	Educational intervention, monitor periodically
	Level of intervention:
20–24	Medical attention, house visit
25–54	Remove lead source, medical attention, CaNaEDTA test
55–69	Remove lead source, treat with CaNaEDTA alone
≥70	Emergency hospitalization, treat with dimercaprol and CaNaEDTA
	ALWAYS RETURN TO A "CLEAN" HOME

EDTA = ethylenediaminetetraacetic acid; CaNaEDTA = calcium disodium edetate.

controversy,[103–106] and it has been said that it has created "an epidemic by edict."[107, 108] A report of the NHANES III study affirmed that as many as 1.7 million children in the United States have blood lead "above the level of concern" (10 μg/dL or more).[96] This alarmist assessment could however be moderated by reflection that two thirds of these children (or 1.3 million) have blood lead levels between only 10 and 14 μg/dL. This may result (as shown by the previously mentioned meta-analyses)[94, 95] in the loss in IQ of between 0.5 and 1.25 points, an effect so trivial as to be unmeasurable. The same study demonstrated that the greatest incidence of markedly elevated blood lead levels (25 μg/dL or more), although decreased over 10-fold from the previous 1980 study, still persists among the children of the most unprivileged segments of the population (mostly blacks and Latinos living in the inner cities). At any age, the blood lead level was shown to be inversely proportional to income.[97]

As discussed earlier, the "natural" blood lead level is below 1 μg/dL and even minuscule amounts of lead produce detectable biochemical effects. It is important not to confuse "intervention levels" (decided on pragmatic considerations) with "safe" levels. The insidious nature of lead toxicity mandates the detection of excessive exposure in apparently asymptomatic children before irreparable damage occurs. Screening for lead poisoning is made particularly difficult by the fact that the most commonly affected children are those of preschool age who are also the least accessible, as a group, to mass testing. Screening in this age group is most often performed at child health stations. It would be most desirable, instead, that screening programs reach out to the community, in search of the most economically deprived children, who are at the same time the least accessible to medical care as well as at the highest risk.

The new CDC guidelines require that the screening by blood lead measurement should be universal for all children below the age of 6.[18] Measurements of blood lead require exacting atomic absorption spectrophotometric techniques. The need for large venous samples has in the past few years been obviated by the development of microtechniques that can analyze samples as small as a few microliters. These techniques are capable of precise measurements of small amounts of lead, in the minute quantity that is present in human blood. When performed with exacting technique, measurements of blood lead on capillary samples can be reliable.[109] However, because the absolute lead content of "normal" blood is of the order of magnitude of 1 to 2 ng/mL, contamination with as little as subnanogram amounts of ubiquitous lead at the time of collection may yield falsely elevated values. The results of blood lead measurements from capillary blood obtained by finger puncture can only be considered valid when low: when these measurements are elevated, they always require confirmation by venous sampling. Under no circumstance should an asymptomatic child be treated on the basis of a capillary blood lead result.[87] Measurements of erythrocyte protoporphyrin levels that can be obtained from capillary blood with an excellent degree of precision and are not subjected to environmental contamination can be useful in emergencies, when blood lead measurements are not rapidly available. Measurements of blood lead levels or erythrocyte protoporphyrin detect different aspects of excessive exposure to lead. The blood lead levels reflect absorption of excess lead from the environment, whereas erythrocyte protoporphyrin levels indicate adverse metabolic effects of lead.

Nationwide programs for screening children must be primarily directed at identifying those in need of medical attention. The definition of *lead poisoning* by the CDC now includes the category of children with blood lead levels of 10 to 19 μg/dL.[18] Yet it has been shown that, at this level, the potential loss of IQ is so low that most people would agree it is trivial.[94, 95]

It is not suggested, in fact, by the CDC that children with blood lead levels in this range be referred to medical attention, because they do not need it. These children are used only as "living detectors" of excessive exposure to lead in their community. Yet, their parents will be advised that their child has "lead poisoning" but will be offered no recourse. For children with blood lead levels of 15 to 19 μg/dL, educational and dietary advice are recommended.[18] This advice, however, is indicated for all children, regardless of blood lead level.

If screening is designed to detect those children in need of medical attention, an appropriate definition of "lead poisoning" should have been set at a blood lead level of 20 μg/dL or more. At this level, the loss of IQ starts becoming relevant[94, 95,] and it becomes more likely that a source of lead exposure may be identified and remedied.

For children with blood lead levels of 20 to 25 μg/dL, environmental analysis, including home visits, is recommended to ascertain the source of lead.

At blood lead levels of greater than or equal to 25 μg/dL, the recommended management of asymptomatic children is as follows:

- *For all children with blood lead levels of 25 μg/dL or more:* institute environmental scrutiny and remove the source of lead.
- *For children with blood lead levels of 25 to 44 μg/dL:* treat with chelation based on the ethylenediaminetetraacetic acid (EDTA) provocation test.
- *For children with blood lead levels of 45 to 69 μg/dL:* treat with calcium-disodium EDTA (CaNaEDTA), or succimer (dimercaptosuccinic acid [DMSA]) (only if the environment is lead free).
- *For children with blood lead levels of 70 μg/dL or more:* treat with emergency hospitalization and begin therapy with dimercaprol or CaNaEDTA.

These guidelines are meant to set priorities for environmental and medical intervention and do not represent a diagnostic schema. They should not be used as a rigid set of slots but must be tempered by appropriate medical judgment. For instance, a 13-month-old child with a blood lead level of 26 μg/dL is at much greater risk than an 8-year-old child with a blood lead level of 29 μg/dL; yet both cases would fit into the same category by rigid criteria.

The impact of the new screening regulations is going to be profound. Universal screening of all American children is going to be a formidable task.[103, 106] On the other hand, the results of the NHANES-III study indicate that screening is most urgent for poor urban children, the largest "at risk" group.[96] These observations cast a serious shadow of doubt about the wisdom of universal screening, as suggested by the CDC statement.[103, 106] A major additional problem is the fact that the current technology is not adequate to the task of accurately measuring low blood lead levels. Measurements of blood lead in the 5 to 10 μg/dL range by present techniques carry an inherent error of ± 3 μg/dL (in the best of laboratories) and, moreover, significant day-by-day fluctuations are an additional source of imprecision.[106, 110]

Such a massive effort to achieve universal screening, already set in motion, without funding for education and cleanup, will be costly but not be very effective. It would be most important to remove the residual sources of lead, primarily lead-containing paint in old housing.[106, 111] Complete removal of lead from the environment remains a formidable task for modern society, but this, and not universal screening, is the only viable solution to complete the elimination of lead toxicity to children.

The removal of automobile-generated lead from the air already has had a profound impact on the problem of urban lead poisoning. In New York City, the number of children at the upper end of the distribution, with blood lead levels of 60 μg/dL or more, decreased from over 3000 per year in the 1970s to less than 12 per year in the 1990s, despite an increase in the number of children tested each year. These data indicate that a significant reduction in airborne lead causes a decrease in the background body burden of lead. Because all sources of lead are additive, this also causes a reduction in the number of children who may develop extreme blood lead levels and clinical toxicity when they are additionally exposed to lead-containing paint. Yet, a significant number of children remain at risk in dwellings with lead-containing paint. The cost of removing lead-containing paint from the homes is not irrelevant. There are approximately 50 million dwellings in the United States: children younger than the age of 6 live in at least 10 million of these. Of these dwellings, at least one third have serious lead problems.[111] Cleaning 1 million homes per year would cost no less than 5 to 7 billion dollars each year. A program of universal screening of children, without support for the environmental clean-up necessary, will not lead to the total eradication of lead intoxication in the United States.

TREATMENT OF LEAD POISONING

The first and most essential part of treatment of childhood poisoning is the identification and removal of the source of lead. Without correction of the exposure, any treatment is futile.[87]

There is no doubt that children who are symptomatic

require urgent treatment.[87] However, because the symptoms of lead poisoning may be elusive, treatment is indicated even in their absence, when there is clear evidence of excessive body burden of lead. No absolute criterion exists for treatment in the absence of symptoms, and all guidelines are arbitrary. The goal of treatment is prevention of subclinical damage without inducing damage with therapy itself; it is necessary to exercise judicious compromise.[87]

Drugs That Enhance Lead Excretion

The available chelating agents are shown in Figure 13–3. Two of them are used in severe lead poisoning: dimercaprol (formerly called BAL for British Anti-Lewisite and originally developed by the British to counteract German arsenical war gases) and CaNaEDTA. Both of these agents chelate lead and induce its excretion.

Dimercaprol is a smelly, oily compound, particularly unpleasant to patients. It forms an emetic compound with iron: iron therapy should not be given to a patient receiving dimercaprol.[87] It is dissolved in peanut oil and thus is contraindicated in children allergic to peanuts.

CaNaEDTA is water soluble. It is best administered by continuous intravenous infusion; when administered intramuscularly (a less preferable and much more painful option), 2% procaine should be added to avoid severe local pain. CaNaEDTA may itself be toxic, particularly to the renal system; overdosage may induce tubular necrosis directly or renal toxicity because of hypercalcemia. The maximum safe dose in humans is 2500 mg/m^2 per day. Only in the most severe cases should a dose of 1500 mg/m^2 be given daily. In other situations, a total dose of 1000 mg/m^2 provides a greater margin of safety. An additional risk of CaNaEDTA results from its ability to chelate zinc as well.

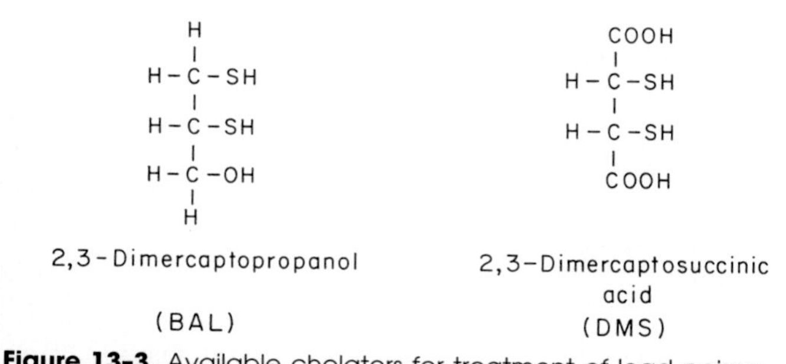

Because δ-ALAD, a zinc-dependent enzyme is already damaged by lead, the additional removal of zinc leads to its complete paralysis. This leads to a burst of neurotoxic δ-ALA into the plasma, which may aggravate (and even induce) convulsions. For these reasons, CaNaEDTA should never be given alone to symptomatic children or to asymptomatic children with blood lead levels of 70 μg/dL or more; instead, it should be given after administration of dimercaprol to prevent these acute effects.[87] An additional note of caution is necessary with regard to the use of EDTA. Besides CaNaEDTA, a commercial preparation of disodium EDTA is also available and occasionally used for hyperparathyroidism. Disodium EDTA should never be used for treatment of lead poisoning, because it may induce acute hypocalcemia, which may be fatal. Only CaNaEDTA should be used for the treatment of lead poisoning. Hospital pharmacies should exercise maximum caution in dispensing disodium EDTA, which could be fatal if erroneously given to a child with lead poisoning but without hypercalcemia.

Succimer, an oral chelating agent for lead, has completed successfully the testing stage in animals and humans. It is a derivative of dimercaprol, in which the methyl groups are replaced by carboxylic groups; this results in excellent water solubility, which allows it to be used orally. Succimer was developed by Fredheim in Geneva as a vehicle to bind arsenic to treat trypanosomiasis. In 1978, he noticed that this compound was an excellent lead chelator. He came to the United States, where, together with Graziano, developed succimer as an effective lead chelator.[112] Whereas the advantages of an oral chelator are obvious, it is crucial to be cautious in its use, because, owing to its great water solubility and affinity for lead, it may result in increased absorption if used in a lead-laden environment. For this reason, succimer should only be used when it is absolutely certain that the child has been removed from the lead-containing environment and is in a safe home. The suggested dose is 10 mg/kg, given every 8 hours for 5 days, then every 12 hours for 14 additional days, for a total cycle of 19 days. This regimen is the one with which there is the most experience. At this dose, side effects appear minimal. Large-scale clinical trials are underway to refine the dosage and to assess potential rare side effects. Succimer is licensed by the Food and Drug Administration for treatment of children with blood lead levels of 45 μg/dL or more. Experience with this drug in treating children with blood lead levels of 70 μg/dL or more is very limited. In these cases, as well as in symptomatic children, in the author's clinic, treatment is still based on a combination of dimercaprol and CaNaEDTA.

Penicillamine can be administered orally; however, it is much less effective than CaNaEDTA.[113] It is not approved by the Food and Drug Administration for treatment of lead poisoning (only for the treatment of Wilson's disease), and its use is considered experimental.[18] In addition, it may induce allergic rashes and impairment of renal function. It is not recommended for general use.[18]

Figure 13-3. Available chelators for treatment of lead poisoning. Notice that penicillamine is not approved by the Food and Drug Administration for this use.

Treatment of Symptomatic Children

The criteria for treatment are different if a child is symptomatic[87] (Table 13–3). In this case the treatment is urgent, and it should not be withheld when there is a clear index of suspicion. It is preferable, whenever possible, to obtain a firm diagnosis before treatment is initiated. However, in the presence of symptoms compatible with lead poisoning, even in doubt, it may be better to draw the appropriate blood samples and to initiate therapy at once, without awaiting the results. Measurements of blood lead levels are seldom immediately accessible to many hospitals and often are available only after hours or days of delay. Measurements of erythrocyte protoporphyrin are much more accessible and can be conveniently used for emergency diagnosis: a negative value (less than 35 µg/dL) rules out lead poisoning as the cause of the symptoms. Another useful emergency diagnostic tool is the radiologic examination of the abdomen and the long bones. If there is evidence of radiopaque material in the abdomen, the suspicion of lead poisoning is reinforced; if there are opacities of the long bones (lead lines), these also reinforce the suspicion. However, it must be remembered that the absence of radiologic evidence does not rule out lead poisoning: on the other hand, when present it reinforces the clinical suspicion. The principles for treatment of symptomatic children with lead poisoning are based on (1) control of convulsions, if present; (2) maintenance of diuresis without inducing overhydration; and (3) chelation therapy to remove lead. When symptoms are present it is unnecessary to waste time giving cathartics or enemas to evacuate the intestine. Spinal puncture can be dangerous because of the possi-

bility of increased intracranial pressure, and it should be avoided. A spinal puncture should be performed only if it is absolutely necessary to rule out meningitis. Even in this case it is important to avoid removing too much fluid. Once convulsions are controlled and diuresis is well established, chelation therapy is started.

Because of their different pharmacologic properties, dimercaprol and CaNaEDTA are advantageously used in combination to treat children with symptomatic lead poisoning, with or without concomitant encephalopathy, as well as asymptomatic children with blood lead levels greater than 70 µg/dL. The combined use of dimercaprol and CaNaEDTA is both safer and more effective than the use of CaNaEDTA alone. Treatment should always start first with dimercaprol.[87] Shortly after treatment is started, a rapid fall occurs in the blood lead level; it is therefore possible to discontinue the uncomfortable dimercaprol and to continue with CaNaEDTA alone. This decision is reached by observing the blood lead level; only when this goes below 50 µg/dL can dimercaprol be discontinued. The initial decrease in the blood lead level after therapy is rapid, as a result of its removal from the blood and the exchangeable lead pool; however, as soon as therapy is interrupted, re-equilibration occurs and the blood lead level rises again. The blood lead concentration should be remeasured at the end of the 5-day course of treatment; if by then it remains 40 µg/dL or more, additional courses of therapy of 5 days each should be given, after 2 days of interruption. If the blood lead level at the end of treatment is less than 40 µg/dL, treatment may be interrupted. However, the blood lead value should be remeasured 6 to 7 days after the end of therapy, when a significant rise (rebound phenome-

Table 13–3. TREATMENT OF SYMPTOMATIC LEAD POISONING IN CHILDREN

Presentation	Treatment	Details
Encephalopathy	Control convulsions.	Use diazepam, 0.15 mg/kg, given slowly; repeat, if needed in 20–30 minutes (keep assisted respiration equipment at hand). Maintain control with paraldehyde, 0.15 mg/kg. Reserve barbiturates for the recovery phase. Do not perform spinal puncture; if unavoidable, take less than 1 mL of fluid.
	Maintain diuresis.	Use 10% dextrose in water; maintain urine flow of 350–500 mL/m² per d.
	Treat with dimercaprol and CaNaEDTA.	Start dimercaprol, 75 mg/m² IM every 4 hours (450 mg/d). At 4 hours, start infusion of CaNaEDTA, 1000 mg/m² per d. Continue both dimercaprol and CaNaEDTA for 5 days. Interrupt therapy for 2 days. Treat for 5 additional days with both dimercaprol and CaNaEDTA; when blood lead level is ≤ 50 µg/dL, use CaNaEDTA only.
No encephalopathy	Maintain diuresis.	Use 10% dextrose in water; maintain flow of 350–500 mL/m² per d.
	Treat with dimercaprol and CaNaEDTA.	Start dimercaprol, 75 mg/m² IM every 4 hours (450 mg/d) At 4 hours, start infusion of CaNaEDTA, 1000 mg/m² Discontinue dimercaprol after 3 days, if blood lead level is ≤ 50 µg/dL. Continue therapy with CaNaEDTA for 5 days. Interrupt therapy for 2 days. Treat for 5 additional days: including dimercaprol if blood lead level is > 50 µg/dL; otherwise treat with CaNaEDTA alone. Other cycles may be needed, depending on rebound.

non) is often observed, and weekly thereafter. It is extremely unwise to consider that the lead poisoning is resolved just because the blood lead concentration has been rapidly reduced by chelation therapy. Children discharged after a single cycle of therapy are often readmitted within a few days when both the blood lead and the symptomatology return to the pretreatment level. Children with a large body burden of lead, as in those with clinical symptomatology or blood lead levels in excess of 70 μg/dL, invariably require several cycles of chelation therapy before substantial reduction of the body burden of lead is obtained.[87]

The need for additional cycles of therapy can be established by the measurement of urinary lead excretion during the first days of treatment. The lead excreted should be related to the amount of EDTA given (see EDTA provocation test). Those children who excrete lead in larger proportions are in greater need of additional cycles of therapy. It is not uncommon that a child may require several months of chelation therapy, initially with both dimercaprol and CaNaEDTA, and later with CaNaEDTA alone, before the urinary lead excretion declines and the blood lead level stabilizes below 30 μg/dL. Only at that point can chelation therapy be stopped.[87]

Treatment of Asymptomatic Children

In the case of asymptomatic children, there is no emergency; thus it is absolutely necessary to have a firm diagnosis based on an elevated blood lead level before treatment is initiated (Table 13–4). Measurements of blood lead on capillary blood samples are often falsely high because of contamination. Under no circumstances should treatment be administered to an asymptomatic child without a confirmatory measurement on venous blood.[87]

If the venous blood lead level is 70 μg/dL or more, the treatment should be the same as for symptomatic children without encephalopathy.

If the venous blood lead is 45 to 69 μg/dL, treatment should be limited to CaNaEDTA, which is easily administered in the outpatient area. Only if the child can be completely and safely removed from the source of lead should ambulatory treatment with the more pleasant oral succimer be considered.

In children with blood lead levels between 25 μg/dL and 44 μg/dL, the most logical guideline to start chelation therapy is the evaluation of the effectiveness of treatment after a test dose. There is no value in giving chelation therapy to those children in whom this does not induce an adequate excretion of lead. The EDTA provocative test is used extensively in the author's clinic, as well as in other clinics where large numbers of children are treated.[114, 115] A statement by the Committee on Drugs of the American Academy of Pediatrics that this test is "obsolete" is, in this author's opinion, unfounded and arbitrary.[116] The CaNaEDTA mobilization test is administered by giving an injection of 500 mg/m² of CaNaEDTA (not to exceed a total of 1 g) and collecting the urine for 8 hours to measure lead content. The amount of lead excreted is then related to the amount of CaNaEDTA given. If more than 1.0 μg of lead is excreted for each milligram of CaNaEDTA given, the test is strongly positive; if the lead excreted is between 0.7 and 1 μg/mg of CaNaEDTA given, the test is moderately positive; if the amount of lead excreted is between 0.7 and 0.5 μg/mg of CaNaEDTA given, the test is barely positive; below this value, the test is considered negative. The EDTA provocative test, as described, has the advantage that it can be performed in the clinic without need for hospitalization of an asymptomatic child. Several variations of the EDTA provocative test have been suggested.

Table 13–4. TREATMENT OF ASYMPTOMATIC LEAD POISONING IN CHILDREN

Blood Lead Level	Drug Treatment	Details
≥ 70 μg/dL	Dimercaprol and CaNaEDTA	Start with dimercaprol, 50 mg/m² IM every 4 hours (300 mg/d). After 4 hours, start CaNaEDTA, 1000 mg/m² per d, preferably by continuous IV infusion, or in divided doses through a heparin lock. Discontinue dimercaprol on day 3, if blood lead level is ≤ 50 μg/dL. Continue therapy with CaNaEDTA for 5 days. Interrupt therapy for 2 days. Measure blood lead level, and repeat cycle, if needed. If blood lead level is ≤ 50 μg/dL, use CaNaEDTA only.

45–69 μg/dL	CaNaEDTA alone	CaNaEDTA, 1000 mg/m² per d for 5 days IV in clinic.
		Interrupt therapy for 10 days, then measure blood lead level.
		Only if lead exposure is completely controlled:
		  Oral succimer, 10 mg/kg q8h for 5 days, then
		  Oral succimer, 10 mg/kg q12h for 14 days,
		  Interrupt therapy for 10 days, then measure blood lead level.
		Several cycles may be needed, until blood lead level remains steadily ≤ 30 μg/dL.

29–45 μg/dL	EDTA provocation test If lead/EDTA ratio is ≥ 0.7 0.6–0.7 and age <3 y 0.6–0.7 and age >3 y < 0.6	CaNaEDTA, 1000 mg/m² per d for 5 days, in clinic. CaNaEDTA, 1000 mg/m² per d for 3 days, in clinic. Repeat blood lead measurement every 2 weeks. No treatment.
≤ 30 μg/dL	No treatment	Removal of lead source; education.

By using the ratio of milligrams of lead excreted per milligrams of CaNaEDTA given, the results are essentially the same, regardless of the technique used.[87]

Once the effectiveness of chelation therapy has been evaluated for the individual child, a rational decision can be made concerning the future treatment.

Children with a strongly positive CaNaEDTA provocation test will benefit from chelation therapy; children with a less positive test will obviously be poor responders.

In children with a moderately positive test, a course of EDTA or succimer is indicated.[87]

In children with a barely positive EDTA response, the preferable course of action is to remove the source of lead (if identified) and await the slow, natural decline of the excessive body burden of lead. Under these circumstances no treatment is best.[87]

References

1. Committee on Biological Effects of Atmospheric Pollutants: Lead: Airborne Lead in Perspective. Washington, DC, National Academy of Sciences, 1972.
2. Lin-Fu JS: Vulnerability of children to lead exposure and toxicity. N Engl J Med 1973; 289:1229.
3. Hecker L, Allen HE, et al: Heavy metal levels in acculturated and unacculturated populations. Arch Environ Health 1974; 29:181.
4. Patterson CC: Contaminated and natural lead environments of man. Arch Environ Health 1965; 11:344.
5. Piomelli S, Corash L, et al: Blood lead concentrations in a remote Himalayan population. Science 1980; 210:1135.
6. Davidson CI, Grimm TC, et al: Airborne lead and other elements derived from local fires in the Himalayas. Science 1961; 214:1344.
7. Chamberlain AC, Clough WS, et al: Uptake of lead by inhalation of motor exhausts. Proc R Soc Lond B Biol Sci 1975; 192:77.
8. Environmental Protection Agency: Air Quality Criteria for Lead. Publication No. 600/80770017. Washington, DC, Environmental Protection Agency, 1977.
9. Knelson JHE: Problem of estimating respiratory lead dose in children. Health Perspect 1974; 7:53.
10. Murozumi M, Chow TJ, et al: Chemical concentrations of pollutant lead aerosols, terrestrial dusts, and sea salts in Greenland and Antarctic snow strata. Geochim Cosmochim Acta 1969; 33:1247.
11. Goldsmith JR, Hexter AC: Respiratory exposure to lead: Epidemiological experimental dose-response relationships. Science 1967; 158:132.
12. Azar A, Snee RD, et al: An epidemiologic approach to community air lead exposure using personal air samples. Environ Qual Safety Suppl 1976; 11:254.
13. Landrigan PJ, Baker EL, et al: Increased lead absorption with anemia and slowed nerve conduction in children near a lead smelter. J Pediatr 1976; 89:904.
14. Yankel AI, vonLindern J, et al: The Silver Valley lead study. The relationship between childhood blood lead levels and environmental exposure. J Air Pollut Cont Assoc 1977; 27:736.
15. Alexander FW, Delves HT, et al: The uptake and excretion by children of lead and other contaminants. In Barth D, Berlin A, et al (eds): Environmental Health Aspects of Lead: Proceedings, International Symposium. Amsterdam, Luxembourg, Commission of the European Communities, October 1972, pp 319–331.
16. Ziegler EE, Edwards BB, et al: Absorption and retention of lead by infants. Pediatr Res 1978; 12:29.
17. Mahaffey KR: Exposure to lead in childhood. The importance of prevention. N Engl J Med 1992; 327:1308. Editorial; comment.
18. Centers for Disease Control: Preventing Lead Poisoning in Young Children. Atlanta, U.S. Department of Health and Human Services, 1991.
19. Chisolm JJ, Jr, Harrison HE: The exposure of children to lead. Pediatrics 1956; 18:943.
20. Baker EL, Holland DS, et al: Lead poisoning in children of lead workers; house contamination with industrial dust. N Engl J Med 1977; 296:260.
21. Sayre W, Charney E, et al: House and hand dust as a potential source of childhood lead exposure. Am J Dis Child 1974; 127:167.
22. Vostal JJ, Taves E, et al: Lead analysis of house dust: A method for the detection of another source of lead exposure in inner city children. Environ Health Perspect 1974; 7:91.
23. Lepow ML, Bruckman L, et al: Role of airborne lead in increased body burden of lead in Hartford children. Environ Health Perspect 1974; 7:99.
24. Goodheart RS, Dunne JW: Petrol sniffer's encephalopathy. A study of 25 patients. Med J Aust 1994; 160:178.
25. Annest JS, Mahaffey KR, et al: Blood lead levels for persons 6 months—74 years of age: United States, 1976–80. Hyattsville, MD, U. S. Department of Health, 1981.
26. Castellino N, Aloj S: Intracellular distribution of lead in the liver and kidney of the rat. Br J Industr Med 1969; 26:139.
27. Barltrop D, Barrett A, et al: Subcellular distribution of lead in the rat. J Lab Clin Med 1974; 77:705.
28. Walton JR: Granules containing lead in isolated mitochondria. Nature 1973; 243:100.
29. Holtzman D, Shenshu J: Early effects of inorganic lead on immature rat brain mitochondrial respiration. Pediatr Res 1976; 10:70.
30. Bessis MC, Breton-Gorius J: Ferritin and ferruginous micelles in normal erythroblasts and hypochromic hypersideremic anemias. Blood 1959; 14:423.
31. Goyer RA, Krull R: Further observations on the morphology and biochemistry of mitochondria from kidneys of normal and lead-intoxicated rats. Fed Proc 1969; 26:619A.
32. Granick JL, Sassa S, et al: Studies in lead poisoning. II. Correlation between the ratio of activated to inactivated δ-aminolevulinic acid dehydratase of whole blood and the blood lead level. Biochem Med 1973; 8:149.
33. Hernberg S, Nikkanen G: Enzyme inhibition by lead under normal urban conditions. Lancet 1970; 1:63.
34. Millar JA, Cummings RLC, et al: Lead and δ-aminolevulinic acid dehydratase levels in mentally retarded children and lead-poisoned suckling rats. Lancet 1970; 2:695.
35. Secchi GC, Erba I, et al: δ-Amino levulinic acid dehydratase activity of erythrocytes and liver tissue in man. Relationship to lead exposure. Arch Environ Health 1974; 28:130.
36. Litman DA, Correia MA: L-Tryptophan: a common denominator of biochemical and neurological events of acute hepatic porphyrins? Science 1983; 222:1031.
37. Roels H, Bruaux I, et al: Impact of air pollution by lead on the heme biosynthetic pathway in school-age children. Arch Environ Health 1976; 31:1976.
38. Gurba PE, Sennet RE, et al: Studies on the mechanism of action of δ-aminolevulinate dehydratase from bovine and rat liver. Arch Biochem 1972; 150:130.
39. Abdulla M, Haeger-Aronsen B: ALA dehydratase activation by zinc. Enzyme 1971; 12:708.
40. Sassa S: Toxic effects of Icad, with particular reference to porphyrin and heme metabolism. In DeMatteis F, Aldridge W (eds): Handbook of Experimental Pharmacology, New Series, Vol. 44, Heme & Hemoprotein. Berlin, Springer-Verlag, 1973, p 333.
41. Piomelli S: A micromethod for free erythrocyte porphyrins: the FEP test. J Lab Clin Med 1973; 81:932.
42. Flatmark R, Romslo I: Energy-dependent accumulation of iron by isolated rat liver mitochondria. J Biol Chem 1975; 250:6433.
43. Piomelli S, Seaman C, et al: Lead-induced abnormalities of porphyrin metabolism. The relationship with iron deficiency. Ann N Y Acad Sci 1987; 514:278. Review.
44. Piomelli S, Seaman C, et al: Threshold for lead damage to heme synthesis in urban children. Proc Natl Acad Sci U S A 1982; 79:3335.
45. Van Den Bergh AAH, Grotepass W: Porphyrinamie ohne Porphyrinurie. Klin Wochenschr 1933; 22:586.
46. Lamola AA, Piomelli S, et al: Erythropoietic protoporphyria and lead intoxication: the molecular basis for difference in cutaneous photosensitivity. II. Different binding of erythrocyte protoporphyrin to hemoglobin. J Clin Invest 1975; 56:1528.

47. Lamola AA, Yamane T: Zinc protoporphyrin in the erythrocytes of patients with lead intoxication and iron deficiency anemia. Science 1974; 186:936.

48. Hart D, Graziano J, Piomelli S: Red blood cell protoporphyrin accumulation in experimental lead poisoning. Biochem Med 1980; 23:167.

49. Piomelli S, Lamola AA, et al: Erythropoietic protoporphyria and lead intoxication: the molecular basis for difference in cutaneous photosensitivity. I. Different rates of disappearance of protoporphyrin from the erythrocytes, both *in vivo* and *in vitro*. J Clin Invest 1975; 56:1519.

50. Charache S, Weatherall J: Fast hemoglobin in lead poisoning. Blood 1966; 28:377.

51. Licktman HC, Feldman F: *In vitro* pyrrol and porphyrin synthesis in lead poisoning and iron deficiency. J Clin Invest 1963; 42:380.

52. Clark KGA, Nicholson DC: Erythrocyte protoporphyrin and iron uptake in erythropoietic protoporphyria. Clin Sci 1971; 42:363.

53. Poh-Fitzpatrick MB, Lamola AA: Direct spectrofluorometry of diluted erythrocytes and plasma: A rapid diagnostic method in primary and secondary porphyrinemias. J Lab Clin Med 1976; 87:362.

54. Cartwright GQ, Huguley CM, Jr, et al: Studies on free erythrocyte protoporphyrin, plasma iron and plasma copper in normal and anemic subjects. Blood 1948; 3:501.

55. Dagg LH, Goldberg A, et al: Value of erythrocyte protoporphyrin in the diagnosis of latent iron deficiency (sideropenia). Br J Haematol 1966; 12:326.

56. Langer EE, Haining RG, et al: Erythrocyte protoporphyrin. Blood 1972; 40:112.

57. Piomelli S, Brickman A, et al: Rapid diagnosis of iron deficiency by measurement of free erythrocyte porphyrins and hemoglobin: the FEP/hemoglobin ratio. Pediatrics 1976; 57:136.

58. Yip R, Schwartz S, et al: Screening for iron deficiency with the erythrocyte protoporphyrin test. Pediatrics 1988; 72:214.

59. Stockman JA, III, Weiner LR, et al: The measurement of free erythrocyte porphyrin (FEP) as a simple means of distinguishing iron deficiency from β-thalassemia trait in subjects with microcytosis. J Lab Clin Med 1975; 85:113.

60. Koenig HM, Lightsey AL, Schanberger JE: The micromeasurement of free erythrocyte protoporphyrin as a means of differentiating α-thalassemia trait from iron deficiency anemia. J Pediatr 1975; 86:539.

61. Vichinsky E, Kleman K, et al: The diagnosis of iron deficiency anemia in sickle cell disease. Blood 1981; 58:963.

62. Piomelli S: The diagnostic utility of measurements of erythrocyte porphyrins. Hematol Oncol Clin North Am 1987; 1:419. Review.

63. Rosen IF, Zarate-Salvador C, et al: Plasma lead levels in normal and lead intoxicated children. J Pediatr 1974; 84:45.

64. Kochen JA, Greener Y: Levels of lead in blood and hematocrit: Implications for the evaluation of newborn and anemic patients. Pediatr Res 1973; 7:937.

65. Angle CR, McIntire MS: Children, the barometer of environmental lead. Adv Pediatr 1982; 27:3.

66. Paglia DE, Valentine WN, et al: Effects of low-level lead exposure on pyrimidine-5′-nucleodase and other erythrocyte enzymes. Possible role of pyrimidine-5′-nucleotidase in the pathogenesis of lead-induced anemia. J Clin Invest 1975; 56:1164.

67. Qazi QH, Madahar DP: A simple rapid test for lead poisoning. J Pediatr 1971; 79:805.

68. Waldron HA: The effect of lead on the fragility of the red cell incubated *in vitro*. J Clin Pathol 1964; 17:405.

69. Berk PD, Tschudy DP, et al: Hematologic and biochemical studio in a case of lead poisoning. Am J Med 1970; 48:137.

70. Leikin S, Eng G: Erythrokinetic studies of the anemia of lead poisoning. Pediatrics 1963; 31:916.

71. Barton C, Conrad ME, et al: Effects of calcium on the absorption and retention of lead. J Lab Clin Med 1978; 91:366.

72. Kaplan ML, Jones AG, et al: Inhibitory effect of iron on the uptake of lead by erythrocytes. Life Sci 1975; 16:1975.

73. Maines MD, Kappas A: Studies on the mechanism of induction of heme oxygenase by cobalt and other metal ions. Biochem J 1976; 154:125.

74. Strand LJ, Manning J, et al: The induction of δ-aminolevulinic acid synthetase in cultured liver cells: The effect on end product and inhibitors of heme biosynthesis. J Biol Chem 1972; 2047:2828.

75. Ali MAM, Quinlan A: Effect of lead on globin synthesis *in vitro*. Am J Clin Pathol 1977; 67:77.

76. Alvares AP, Kapelner S, et al: Drug metabolism in normal children, lead poisoned children, and normal adults. Clin Pharmacol 1975; 17:179.

77. Meredith IA, Campbell BC, et al: The effects of industrial lead poisoning on cytochrome P450 mediated phenazone (anti-pyrine) hydroxylation. Eur J Clin Pharmcol 1977; 12:235.

78. Kappas A, Alvarez PA: How the liver metabolizes foreign substances. Sci Am 1976; 22:233.

79. Rosen IF, Chesney RW, et al: Reduction in 1,25-dihydroxyvitamin D in children with increased lead absorption. N Engl J Med 1980; 302:1128.

80. Whetsell WOJ, Sassa S, et al: Porphyrin-heme biosynthesis in organotypic cultures of mouse dorsal root ganglia. J Clin Invest 1984; 74:600.

81. Becker D, Viljoen JD, et al: The inhibition of red cell and brain ATPase by δ-aminolaevulinic acid. Biochim Biophys Acta 1971; 225:26.

82. Moore MR, Meredith PA: The association of δ-aminolaevulinic acid with the neurological and behavioural effects of lead exposure. In Hemphill DD (ed): Trace Metals in Environmental Health. Columbia, MO, University of Missouri Press, 1976, p 363.

83. Dagg JH, Goldberg A, et al: The relationship of lead poisoning to acute intermittent porphyria. Q J Med 1965; 34:163.

84. Silbergeld EK: Mechanisms of lead neurotoxicity, or looking beyond the lamppost. FASEB J 1992; 6:3201. Review.

85. Byers RK, Lord EE: Late effects of lead poisoning on mental development. Am J Dis Child 1943; 6:471.

86. Chisolm JJ Jr: Aminoaciduria as a manifestation of renal tubular injury in lead intoxication and a comparison with patterns of aminoaciduria seen in other disease. J Pediatr 1962; 60:1.

87. Piomelli S, Rosen JF, et al: Management of childhood lead poisoning. J Pediatr 1984; 105:523.

88. Seto DSU, Freeman JM: Lead neuropathy in childhood. Am J Dis Child 1964; 107:337.

89. Farkas WR, Stanawitz R, et al: Saturnine gout: Lead induced formation of guanine crystals. Science 1978; 199:786.

90. Annest JL, Pirkle JL, et al: Chronological trend in blood lead levels between 1976 and 1980. N Engl J Med 1983; 308:1373.

91. Dinman BI: The non-concept of no threshold. Science 1972; 175:495.

92. De la Burdé B, Choate MS Jr: Does asymptomatic lead exposure in children have latent sequelae? J Pediatr 1972; 81:1088.

93. Needleman HL, Gunroe C, et al: Deficits in psychologic and classroom performance of children with elevated dentine lead levels. N Engl J Med 1979; 300:689.

94. Pocock SJ, Smith M, et al: Environmental lead and children's intelligence: a systematic review of the epidemiological evidence. BMJ 1994; 309:1189.

95. Schwartz J: Low-level lead exposure and children's IQ: a meta-analysis and search for a threshold. Environ Res 1994; 65:42.

96. Brody DJ, Pirkle JL, et al: Blood lead levels in the US population. Phase 1 of the Third National Health and Nutrition Examination Survey (NHANES III, 1988 to 1991). JAMA 1994; 272:277. See Comments.

97. Pirkle JL, Brody DJ, et al: The decline in blood lead levels in the United States. The National Health and Nutrition Examination Surveys (NHANES). JAMA 1994; 272:284. See Comments.

98. Facchetti S, Geiss R: Isotopic lead experiment: Status report. Publication No. EUR 8352 EN. Luxembourg, Commission of the European Communities, 1982.

99. Steinfeld L: Medical aspects of childhood lead poisoning. Pediatrics 1971; 48:464.

100. Anonymous: Increased lead absorption and lead poisoning in young children: A statement by the Centers for Disease Control. J Pediatr 1975; 87:824.

101. Centers for Disease Control: Prevention of Lead Poisoning in Children. Atlanta, U.S. Department of Health, Education and Welfare, 1978.

102. Centers for Disease Control: Prevention of Lead Poisoning in Children. Atlanta, U.S. Department of Health, Education and Welfare, 1985.

103. Harvey B: Should blood lead screening recommendations be revised? Pediatrics 1994; 93:201.

104. Hoekelman RA: A pediatrician's view. A lead balloon. Pediatr Ann 1992; 21:335. Editorial.

105. Hoekelman RA: Can we ever get the lead out of our environment? Pediatr Ann 1994; 23:589. Editorial.

106. Piomelli S: Childhood lead poisoning in the '90s. Pediatrics 1994; 93:508.

107. Schoen EJ: Exaggerated threat of childhood lead poisoning in California—epidemic by edict. West J Med 1992; 157:470. Letter.

108. Schoen EJ: Blood lead screening: the argument against it. Am Fam Physician 1993; 48:1371. Editorial.

109. Schonfeld DJ, Rainey PM, et al: Screening for lead poisoning by fingerstick in suburban pediatric practices. Arch Pediatr Adolesc Med 1995; 149:447.

110. Schonfeld DJ, Cullen MR, et al: Screening for lead poisoning in an urban pediatric clinic using samples obtained by fingerstick. Pediatrics 1994; 94:174.

111. Centers for Disease Control: Strategic Plan for Eradicating Childhood Lead Poisoning in the 1990s. Atlanta, U.S. Department of Health, Education and Welfare, 1991.

112. Friedheim E, Graziano JH, et al: Treatment of lead poisoning by 2,3-dimercaptosuccinic acid. Lancet 1978; 2:1234.

113. Shannon M, Graef J, Lovejoy FH Jr: Efficacy and toxicity of D-penicillamine in low-level lead poisoning. J Pediatr 1988; 112:799.

114. Markowitz ME, Rosen JF: Need for the lead mobilization test in children with lead poisoning. J Pediatr 1991; 119:305.

115. Markowitz ME, Bijur PE, et al: Effects of calcium disodium versenate (CaNa2EDTA) chelation in moderate childhood lead poisoning. Pediatrics 1993; 92:265.

116. American Academy of Pediatrics: Treatment guidelines for lead exposure in children. Pediatrics 1995; 96:155.

V

Hemolytic Anemias

Autoimmune Hemolytic Anemia

Destruction of Red Cells by the Vasculature and
Reticuloendothelial System

Disorders of the Erythrocyte Membrane

Pyruvate Kinase Deficiency and Disorders of
Glycolysis

Glucose-6-Phosphate Dehydrogenase
Deficiency and Hemolytic Anemia

Autoimmune Hemolytic Anemia

Russell E. Ware • Wendell F. Rosse

The vast majority of erythrocyte disorders that occur in the pediatric age group result from abnormalities within the red blood cell, that is, they are intracorpuscular defects. These intrinsic red cell defects include a wide variety of inherited genetic mutations as well as acquired nutritional deficiencies and lead to defects in globin chain and heme synthesis, abnormal membrane structural proteins, or defective intracellular enzymes. Particularly in the congenital conditions, intracorpuscular defects often lead to a shortened erythrocyte life span, hemolysis, and anemia.

A less common category of erythrocyte disorders includes conditions characterized by abnormalities external to the red cells, known as extracorpuscular defects. Examples include environmental stress (oxidative, heat, mechanical injury), microangiopathic erythrocyte damage (hemolytic-uremic syndrome, thrombotic thrombocytopenic purpura), or immune-mediated red blood cell destruction. Like many of the intrinsic conditions, extrinsic erythrocyte disorders are typically associated with hemolysis and anemia.

Those conditions that result from abnormal interactions between erythrocytes and the immune system are collectively referred to as *autoimmune hemolytic anemia (AIHA)*. AIHA is characterized by the presence of autoantibodies that bind to the erythrocyte surface membrane and lead to premature red cell destruction. Specific characteristics of the autoantibodies, particularly the isotype, thermal reactivity, and ability to fix complement, help shape the resulting clinical picture. In all cases of AIHA, however, the autoantibody leads to a shortened red blood cell survival, hemolysis, and anemia.

In this chapter, three important clinical forms of AIHA are described: (1) *warm-reactive AIHA*, characterized by an autoantibody (usually IgG) that binds preferentially to erythrocyte antigens at 37°C, fixes complement in some cases, and leads to extravascular hemolysis; (2) *paroxysmal cold hemoglobinuria (PCH)*, in which an IgG erythrocyte autoantibody binds optimally at 4°C, fixes complement efficiently, and causes intravascular hemolysis, and (3) *cold agglutinin disease*, characterized by an autoantibody (typically IgM), which binds optimally to erythrocytes below 37°C, fixes complement efficiently, and also leads to intravascular hemolysis. These three disorders are discussed together because of their many similarities, although differences in pathophysiology and therapy are emphasized. A fourth related condition, *paroxysmal nocturnal hemoglobinuria (PNH)*, is a rare and fascinating acquired hematologic disorder that features hemolysis due to abnormal interactions between erythrocytes and the complement system. Unlike true AIHA, the defect in PNH is intracorpuscular, but the presentation and clinical manifestations may be similar. Research advances in the understanding of PNH are described, including the identification of specific mutations in the phosphatidylinositol glycan class A *(PIGA)* gene in affected patients.

HISTORICAL PERSPECTIVE

Erythrocyte hemolysis, characterized by anemia, shortened red blood cell survival, jaundice, and occasionally hemoglobinuria, has been recognized as a clinical entity for almost a century.[1, 2] In the early 1900s, it was noted that the serum from some patients with hemolytic anemia had the ability to agglutinate or hemolyze erythrocytes *in vitro*; such patients had "agglutinins" or "hemolysins," respectively, which suggested an immune basis for the hemolysis.[3] The majority of patients, however, did not have these laboratory findings, and the mechanism by which their erythrocytes were destroyed was unknown. In fact, it was often impossible to distinguish acquired immune hemolytic anemia (an extracorpuscular defect) from the intracorpuscular defect known as congenital hemolytic jaundice (now called hereditary spherocytosis).

A major advance occurred in 1945, when Coombs and co-workers reported the use of a rabbit antihuman globulin serum to detect Rh agglutinins.[4] This so-called Coombs' reagent amplified the weak agglutinins present on sensitized red cells and allowed serologic identification of previously undetectable autoantibodies on the erythrocyte surface. The authors noted that their reagent "promises to be of practical use" but likely did not foresee that it would completely revolutionize the field of immunohematology. The demonstration that the sensitizing agent on the erythrocytes was γ-globulin strengthened the idea of an autoimmune process,[5] and it was later documented that IgG warm-reactive antibodies were the most common form of AIHA.[6] For the first time, it was possible to distinguish accurately between intrinsic erythrocyte defects and extrinsic erythrocyte destruction.[7]

Over the next few years, several investigators reported the presence of complement components as well as γ-globulins on the red cell surface; and by the late 1960s, the role of complement in immune-mediated destruction of erythrocytes was appreciated.[8–12] Interactions between IgG-sensitized red cells and monocytes were investigated,[13–15] including differences related to IgG subtypes[16, 17] or red cell antigens.[18] These early studies helped to elucidate the immune mechanisms of erythrocyte clearance by the reticuloendothelial system.

The development of an animal model, using guinea pigs deficient in complement components C3 or C4, represented an experimental breakthrough that led to a greater understanding of both the pathophysiology[19–21] and therapy[22, 23] of AIHA. With this model, the important contributions of antibody, complement, and the reticuloendothelial system to the pathophysiology of erythrocyte hemolysis could be studied. Taken together, these laboratory investigations led to models of the immune-mediated clearance of erythrocytes by the reticuloendothelial system that are still accepted today.

Over the next 15 years there were relatively fewer advances in the field, chiefly ones involving increased precision of serologic diagnosis,[24, 25] newer therapeutic options,[26–28] or large clinical reviews of patient outcome.[29–31] Within the past 5 years, however, there has been a rapid increase in our knowledge of the basic immunologic abnormalities that may be important in the generation and expansion of erythrocyte autoantibodies in AIHA. The stage is therefore set for focused research on the T and B lymphocytes in patients with AIHA, with the goal of understanding the pathogenesis of AIHA at the molecular level. Specific questions remain unanswered regarding the loss of self-tolerance, the formation of autoreactive antibodies, and the lack of regulation and suppression of these autoantibodies by the immune system.

CLASSIFICATION

Classification of AIHA can be done by a variety of different ways, such as by the thermal sensitivity or isotype of the autoantibodies, but a simple and convenient classification scheme separates the disorders into a primary versus a secondary process (Table 14–1). In primary AIHA, hemolytic anemia is the only clinical finding and there is no identifiable systemic illness to explain the presence of erythrocyte autoantibodies. Many children with this form of AIHA will, however, have had a recent viral-like illness. The most common form of primary AIHA in children involves warm-reactive autoantibodies, usually IgG, which sensitize erythrocytes and lead to extravascular immune clearance and hemolysis. A second category of primary AIHA, particularly common in children after a viral-like illness, is PCH. PCH is a particularly interesting form of AIHA characterized by an IgG autoantibody that binds at cold temperatures, fixes complement efficiently, and causes intravascular hemolysis. The third major form of primary AIHA, cold agglutinin disease, is more frequently observed in adults, but commonly follows *Mycoplasma* infections in children. In this disorder, an IgM autoantibody binds to erythrocytes optimally below 37°C and fixes complement; erythrocytes either undergo intravascular hemolysis or immune clearance from surface-bound complement components.

Table 14–1. CLASSIFICATION OF AUTOIMMUNE HEMOLYTIC ANEMIA (AIHA) IN CHILDREN

Primary AIHA*

Warm-reactive autoantibodies, usually IgG
Paroxysmal cold hemoglobinuria, usually IgG
Cold-agglutinin disease, usually IgM

Secondary AIHA†

Systemic autoimmune disease (e.g., lupus)
Malignancy (Hodgkin's and non-Hodgkin's lymphoma)
Immunodeficiency
Infection (*Mycoplasma*, viruses)
Drug-induced

*Occurs in majority of affected children and often follows a nonspecific viral-like syndrome but in the absence of another systemic illness.
†Occurs in association with another systemic process.

Secondary AIHA occurs in the context of another clinical diagnosis, with hemolytic anemia being only one manifestation of a systemic illness. Secondary AIHA can occur in patients with generalized autoimmune disease, such as systemic lupus erythematosus or other autoimmune inflammatory disorders.

AIHA also occurs in patients with malignancy, immunodeficiency states, drug therapy, or specific infections. Because the AIHA may be the initial presenting manifestation, however, it is imperative to evaluate each patient with AIHA for the presence of an underlying illness.

As is discussed later, Evans' syndrome is a unique entity that features autoimmune pancytopenia, although the erythrocytes and platelets are more frequently involved.

PRIMARY AUTOIMMUNE HEMOLYTIC ANEMIA

Incidence

Primary AIHA is not a rare disorder. The disease has been estimated to occur at an annual incidence of 1 in 80,000 persons in the general population,[32] making it more common than acquired aplastic anemia[33, 34] but less common than immune thrombocytopenic purpura.[35] In children, AIHA may occur even in infants and toddlers, especially after an infection[29, 31, 36]; teenagers with AIHA are more likely to have an associated underlying systemic illness and therefore have secondary disease.[37–39] Cold agglutinin disease occurs in the pediatric age group but is particularly common in the elderly.[40–43] In summary, it is fair to say that AIHA can affect persons of any age, race, or nationality. The issue of gender preference is somewhat more controversial; in children, males may be affected more frequently, whereas affected teenagers are more commonly female.[29, 36, 44]

Natural History

The prognosis for the majority of children with primary AIHA is good.[30, 38, 45–47] Overall, young patients with cold-reactive autoantibodies appear to have a better clinical outcome than those with warm-reactive antibodies. The former patients tend to have an acute self-limited illness but may require aggressive supportive care. In contrast, children with warm-reactive AIHA often have a chronic clinical course characterized by intermittent remissions and relapses.

Older series reported a high mortality rate in AIHA, but these studies included many adults with AIHA secondary to malignancy.[6, 48] More recent series, including several that focused exclusively on children, have demonstrated a much better prognosis. Buchanan and colleagues reported that 77% of children with AIHA had an acute self-limited disease and that the majority of children responded well to short-term therapy[45]; these results were later confirmed in a review of 42 children.[31] In the modern era, mortality in children with primary AIHA appears to be no more than 10%, occurring primarily in teenagers with chronic unrelenting disease.[29, 31, 36]

Heisel and Ortega attempted to define prognostic factors for AIHA in childhood.[37] They concluded that children between 2 and 12 years of age had the best prognosis; these patients tended to have an abrupt onset of symptoms with low numbers of reticulocytes but otherwise normal blood cell counts. The children who fared worse were either infants younger than 2 years of age or teenagers; these patients had a more prolonged onset of symptoms, had an increased reticulocyte count with nucleated erythrocyte precursors in the peripheral blood, and often had decreased platelet counts.[37] Other studies have confirmed the observation that younger children with an abrupt onset of symptoms have a better prognosis than older patients.[29, 36, 44]

Clinical Presentation

The proper evaluation of a patient with AIHA begins with a careful history and physical examination. Many patients with AIHA present with signs and symptoms referable to anemia, such as pallor, weakness, exercise intolerance, or dizziness. The anemia is usually well compensated from a cardiovascular standpoint, so that symptoms of congestive heart failure or circulatory collapse are rare. Occasionally, a patient presents with jaundice, typically noted in the sclerae, owing to accelerated erythrocyte destruction and bilirubin turnover. The symptom of dark urine reflects intravascular hemolysis rather than bilirubin and has been described by patients using a variety of flavorful terms, including cola, iced tea, mahogany, or motor oil. Less commonly, the patient will describe abdominal pain or fever.

The patient often has a benign previous medical history, although questions should be asked regarding prior similar episodes. The review of systems should include questions regarding concurrent medications and the possibility of an underlying systemic illness. The family history is frequently negative in AIHA; rare cases of apparent familial AIHA[29, 49, 50] likely reflect a tendency toward a systemic autoimmune disorder such as systemic lupus erythematosus.

On physical examination, the patient with AIHA is often pale and jaundiced, with pallor and icterus especially apparent in the conjunctivae and palms. The patient should have no physical stigmata of congenital disorders such as Blackfan-Diamond anemia, Fanconi's anemia, or constitutional aplastic anemia. Jaundice may be apparent, especially if hemolysis is brisk, reflecting the breakdown and recycling of unconjugated bilirubin from the destroyed erythrocytes. Depending on the skill of the examiner, scleral icterus can be detected at a bilirubin concentration of 3 to 4 mg/dL. Examination of the heart typically reveals tachycardia and a systolic flow murmur that results from the high-output anemic state. The liver and spleen may be palpable, owing in the latter case to an increase in red pulp.[51] However, the presence of massive splenomegaly, hepatomegaly, or enlarged lymph nodes should suggest an underlying infection or malignant process.

Laboratory Evaluation

Similar to other forms of anemia found in young patients, such as aplastic anemia or transient erythroblastopenia of childhood, the degree of anemia in AIHA may be surprisingly marked at presentation. A child with AIHA frequently has a hemoglobin concentration of 4 to 7 g/dL with no apparent cardiovascular compromise. Red blood cell indices are not generally helpful in establishing the diagnosis, because a normal mean corpuscular volume may reflect the weighted average of small microspherocytes and large reticulocytes. Erythrocyte agglutination within the sample tube may give an artificially large mean corpuscular volume on an automated counter.[52] An elevated mean corpuscular hemoglobin concentration (greater than 36 g/dL) is more suggestive of hereditary spherocytosis, because the spherical erythrocyte volume in hereditary spherocytosis is below normal but contains a normal amount of hemoglobin (see Chapter 16). The leukocyte count and platelet count should be normal. Concurrent thrombocytopenia may indicate a bone marrow failure syndrome (e.g., aplastic anemia) or microangiopathic hemolytic anemia (e.g., hemolytic-uremic syndrome, thrombotic thrombocytopenic purpura). Combined AIHA and thrombocytopenia is referred to as Evans'

syndrome and is characterized by a broader immune dysregulation.[53] Granulocytopenia also may be present in Evans' syndrome.

Evaluation of the peripheral blood smear is very useful in establishing the diagnosis of AIHA. Numerous small spherocytes are usually present in warm-reactive AIHA; splenic ingestion of a portion of the erythrocyte allows the cell to re-form into the entropically favored spherical shape,[13] and surface complement also may induce spherocytosis.[54] Occasionally, teardrop shapes or even schistocytes may be observed[55]; the presence of target cells are more consistent with a hemoglobinopathy or primary hepatic disease. Polychromasia is a common finding, because the bone marrow releases large numbers of reticulocytes and even nucleated red blood cells to compensate for the accelerated erythrocyte destruction. Figure 14–1A shows the peripheral blood smear from a patient with warm-reactive AIHA and demonstrates numerous small microspherocytes and large reticulocytes (see color section at the front of this volume). Numerous Howell-Jolly bodies are present, because this patient had previously undergone splenectomy. In contrast, Figure 14–1B shows the blood smear of a patient with hereditary spherocytosis and illustrates the morphologic similarities between these two conditions. Sphero-

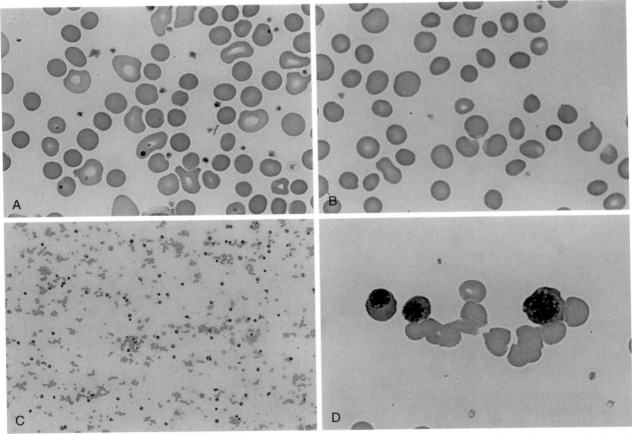

Figure 14–1. Examination of the peripheral blood in autoimmune hemolytic anemia (AIHA). *A,* Blood from a patient with IgG (warm-reactive) AIHA illustrates many small microspherocytes and larger reticulocytes (×1000). *B,* Blood from a patient with hereditary spherocytosis illustrates the morphologic similarities between spherocytosis and AIHA. *C,* Agglutinated erythrocytes from a patient with IgM (cold-reactive) AIHA are clearly visible at low power (×100). *D,* At higher power in this patient (×1000), the nucleated cells in the peripheral blood are identified as erythroid progenitor cells prematurely released from the bone marrow (see color section at the front of this volume).

cytes are less commonly seen in cold-reactive AIHA, but erythrocyte agglutination can be observed on the blood film if the binding affinity of the antibody reaches room temperature. Figure 14–1C illustrates agglutinated red cells in a case of cold-reactive (IgM) AIHA; at higher power (see Fig. 14–1D) the nucleated cells are seen to be immature erythroid cells prematurely released from the bone marrow.

Reticulocytosis is often present in AIHA, owing to the bone marrow's compensation for the shortened red cell survival in the peripheral blood.[56] Absolute reticulocyte counts are typically 300 to 600 $\times$ 10³/μL, representing 10% to 20% of circulating erythrocytes. However, reticulocytopenia is well described in AIHA.[57–59] Several explanations have been offered to explain a low reticulocyte count in the presence of accelerated erythrocyte clearance. The autoantibody may react with antigens on the reticulocytes and lead to immune-mediated clearance within the marrow. Alternatively, the AIHA may be well compensated and subclinical until infection with parvovirus B19 temporarily shuts off erythropoiesis and leads to worse and symptomatic anemia.[60, 61] Aspiration of the bone marrow is not mandatory but may be helpful to exclude a malignant process, myelodysplasia, or a bone marrow failure syndrome. In AIHA, the marrow aspirate usually reveals erythroid hyperplasia, with a myeloid/erythroid ratio below unity.

Examination of the urine may be unremarkable. In cases of AIHA with intravascular hemolysis, however, free plasma hemoglobin is cleared through the renal filtration system and leads to darkened urine. When hemoglobinuria is present, urine dipstick analysis will indicate the presence of blood, but microscopic examination will reveal few red blood cells. Chronic hemoglobinuria will lead to hemosiderin accumulation in uroepithelial cells, which can be detected in the urinary sediment.

The results of a variety of serum chemistries may be abnormal owing to erythrocyte hemolysis, but their routine measurement should not be essential to establishing the diagnosis of AIHA. Elevations in lactate dehydrogenase and aspartate aminotransferase levels reflect the release of intraerythrocyte enzymes; in contrast, the serum alanine aminotransferase level or levels of other hepatic enzymes should not be elevated in AIHA. The serum haptoglobin level is typically low, because it acts as a scavenger for free plasma hemoglobin. However, haptoglobin is not synthesized well in young infants and is an acute phase reactant[62]; for these reasons, quantitation of the haptoglobin level may not be helpful in the evaluation of a patient with AIHA (or for that matter, in any patient). The serum total bilirubin concentration is elevated in most patients with AIHA, although levels above 5 mg/dL are unusual and suggest abnormal hepatic function. Because the elevated bilirubin value in AIHA reflects accelerated erythrocyte destruction rather than hepatic disease, virtually all of the bilirubin is unconjugated. The direct (conjugated) fraction should not exceed 10% to 20% of the total bilirubin concentration.

The most important and useful laboratory test to establish the diagnosis of AIHA is the direct antiglobulin test (DAT or Coombs' test), which identifies antibodies and complement components on the surface of circulating erythrocytes. Therefore, a thorough understanding of the individual laboratory steps that constitute the DAT is essential for the accurate interpretation of the test results.

Anticoagulated patient erythrocytes are washed several times to remove all plasma proteins and then mixed with rabbit polyclonal antiserum that binds to human γ-globulin and human complement (usually C3). First described 50 years ago,[4] this Coombs' reagent is clearly the most important diagnostic laboratory tool for the patient with AIHA. IgM autoantibodies are pentameric and can act as a bridge between adjacent erythrocytes (Fig. 14–2A). In contrast, IgG autoantibodies are smaller and are unable to bridge the surface repulsion between adjacent erythrocytes known as the zeta potential (see Fig. 14–2B), unless the distance imposed by the zeta potential is reduced (see Fig. 14–2C). The broad-spectrum Coombs' reagent, however, can bridge the zeta potential and cause agglutination (see Fig. 14–2D). A positive result at this point, therefore, leads to testing with more specific antisera, to discriminate between IgG and complement on the red blood cell surface. The presence of IgG on the erythrocyte is sufficient evidence for an IgG autoantibody; simultaneous detection of complement indicates that the antibody can fix complement as well. In contrast, the presence of complement alone (with no IgG detected) suggests a cold-reactive autoantibody that fixes complement at lower temperatures but binds poorly to the erythrocyte at 37°C; in this setting, the serum should be analyzed for the presence of either an IgM autoantibody or the unique IgG Donath-Landsteiner autoantibody (see later).

The DAT report on a patient with AIHA should describe the agglutination results of the polyspecific Coombs' reagent and, if positive, the results of the specific IgG and C3 reagents. The DAT can be performed at lower temperatures, such as 4°C and 10°C, and at room temperature, 23°C, to assist with the detection of cold-reactive autoantibodies and characterization of their thermal reactivity and amplitude. The DAT results are scored based on the amount of agglutination, historically on a scale of 1 to 4. At many institutions, including Duke University Medical Center, DAT results are reported using a scale ranging from 1 to 12, with a value of 5 or above reflecting macroscopic agglutination.

On occasion, the DAT is negative despite good clinical evidence for autoimmune hemolysis. One explanation for this apparent paradox is that the amount of IgG present on the erythrocyte may be below the threshold for detection by standard Coombs testing. In this setting, a more sensitive assay for surface-bound IgG such as a radioimmunoassay,[63] enzyme-linked immunosorbent assay,[64, 65] or rosette formation[66] is helpful in identifying IgG on the cell surface. Alternatively, the lack of surface IgG may indicate the presence of a surface antibody other than an IgG molecule, such as an IgA autoantibody[25, 67–69] or even a warm-reactive IgM autoantibody.[70, 71]

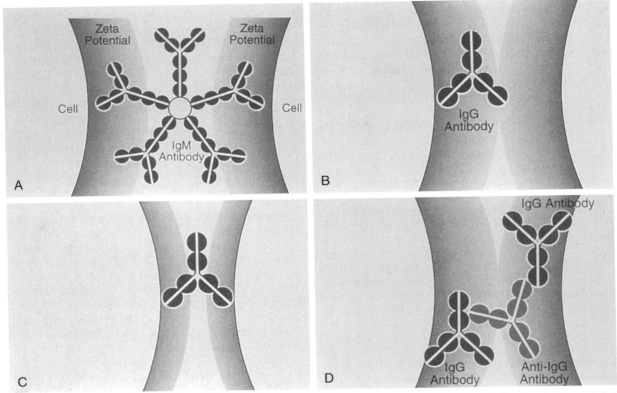

Figure 14-2. Interactions between immunoglobulin molecules and the erythrocyte during agglutination tests and the direct antiglobulin test (DAT). *A,* An IgM autoantibody can simultaneously bind two erythrocytes owing to its multiple antigen binding sites. The large size of the IgM molecule allows it to bridge the zeta potential between erythrocytes and cause agglutination. *B,* An IgG autoantibody is too small to bridge the zeta potential. *C,* Hence, there is no agglutination of erythrocytes unless the zeta potential is reduced. *D,* On the addition of the Coombs' reagent, which is a rabbit antiglobulin that recognizes human IgG, the zeta potential is successfully bridged and red cells agglutinate.

Also of interest is the observation that the DAT may be positive in an otherwise normal person. This result is apparently a biologically false-positive result, because these individuals develop no evidence of AIHA even with long follow-up.[72, 73] Analysis of the immune system of such persons revealed normal T-cell subsets, although the number of B cells was significantly increased.[74]

Differential Diagnosis

The typical patient with AIHA presents with clear evidence of hemolytic anemia, including jaundice and splenomegaly on physical examination and spherocytes and reticulocytes on the peripheral blood smear. In this setting, the differential diagnosis includes certain forms of nonimmune hemolytic anemia, including intrinsic red cell membrane or enzyme defects as well as extrinsic causes of hemolysis. Hereditary spherocytosis, described more fully in Chapter 16, can be confused with AIHA. The osmotic fragility test, often erroneously considered to be a pathognomonic test for hereditary spherocytosis, is positive in both hereditary spherocytosis and AIHA. It also can be positive in patients with congestive splenomegaly. Patients with other rare disorders, such as clostridial sepsis, early stages of Wilson's disease,[75] or hyperlipoproteinemic

liver disease,[76] can also present with numerous spherocytes and hemolytic anemia. Patients with microangiopathic hemolytic anemia, such as hemolytic-uremic syndrome and thrombotic thrombocytopenic purpura, typically have schistocytes rather than spherocytes and usually have severe thrombocytopenia as well. Furthermore, the diagnosis of AIHA is most easily and accurately made on the basis of the positive DAT.

If the patient presents with anemia and reticulocytopenia, the differential diagnosis should include acquired forms of hypoplastic anemia, such as transient erythroblastopenia of childhood or acquired aplastic anemia. In addition, patients with nonimmune hemolytic anemia who develop transient hypoplastic anemia from parvovirus B19 infection may present with this clinical picture.[77] In these patients, the underlying hemolytic anemia may not have been clinically recognizable until the parvovirus infection.

Characteristics of Erythrocyte Autoantibodies

The *sine qua non* of both primary and secondary AIHA is the presence of antibodies that bind to erythrocytes. As a direct consequence of the binding of this erythrocyte autoantibody, circulating erythrocytes have a shortened life span with hemolysis or accelerated clear-

Table 14-2. COMMON CHARACTERISTICS OF ERYTHROCYTE AUTOANTIBODIES IN AUTOIMMUNE HEMOLYTIC ANEMIA

Characteristic*	Warm-Reactive	Paroxysmal Cold Hemoglobinuria	Cold Agglutinin
Immunoglobulin isotype	IgG	IgG	IgM
Thermal reactivity	37°C	4°C	4°C
Fixes complement	Variable	Yes	Yes
Direct antiglobulin test			
4°C	Not performed	IgG, C3	C3
37°C	IgG, ± C3	C3	C3
Plasma titer	Low/absent	Moderate	High
Hemolysin	No	Yes	Variable
Antigenic specificity	Rh and others	P	I/i
Site of red blood cell destruction	Spleen	Intravascular	Liver, intravascular
Common therapy	Corticosteroids	Avoidance of cold	Avoidance of cold
	Splenectomy	Corticosteroids	Plasmapheresis

*Many characteristics of the autoantibodies differ between warm-reactive AIHA, paroxysmal cold hemoglobinuria, and cold agglutinin disease. See text for additional descriptions and details.

ance by the reticuloendothelial system. However, the clinical complexity and variability of AIHA depends in large part on immunologic characteristics of the autoantibody, including its isotype, thermal reactivity, ability to fix complement, binding affinity, and antigenic specificity. Elucidation of each of these characteristics is important to understanding the pathophysiology and clinical course of AIHA in a given patient.[43, 78-83] Table 14-2 is a summary of the important characteristics of erythrocyte autoantibodies in AIHA, emphasizing the differences among the three major clinical conditions: warm-reactive AIHA, PCH, and cold agglutinin disease.

Antibody Isotype

One of the most important tasks for the immunohematology laboratory in the evaluation of a new patient with AIHA is determination of the isotype of the erythrocyte autoantibody. In most cases, the pathogenic antibody is identified as an IgG molecule.[31, 46, 84, 85] In general, IgG autoantibodies bind to red cell antigens optimally at 37°C, hence the descriptive term *warm-reactive* autoantibodies. All IgG molecules are heterodimers, with two heavy chains noncovalently linked to two light chains. The heavy and light chains together form two variable antigen-binding sites known as the Fab portions, and the heavy chains also contain a constant structural domain (the Fc portion), which includes the binding site for complement and the binding site for the Fc receptor.

There are four subtypes of IgG antibodies, which are designated IgG1, IgG2, IgG3, and IgG4. These different subtypes have important implications for the fixation of complement, hemolysis, and clearance by the reticuloendothelial system. IgG1 and IgG3 antibodies fix complement better than do IgG2 and IgG4 antibodies.[86, 87] A patient who had only IgG4 autoantibody on his erythrocytes was reported to have little hemolysis, presumably due to weak interactions with the Fc receptor on macrophages.[88] Adapted from the review of several thousand patients with AIHA by Engelfriet and colleagues,[85] Table 14-3 lists the relative frequency of each IgG subclass identified in patients with warm IgG

autoantibody AIHA. IgG1 autoantibodies were by far the predominant subclass identified, followed by multiple subclasses that typically included IgG1.

Less commonly, IgG antibodies are cold reactive; these autoantibodies are characteristic of childhood PCH but also have been reported rarely in cold hemagglutinin disease.[89] In the unusual setting of a pregnant woman with AIHA, certain IgG autoantibodies can cross the placenta and cause acquired neonatal AIHA.[90-92]

In other cases of AIHA, IgM autoantibodies are identified, particularly after a defined infection such as from *Mycoplasma pneumoniae*.[93] In one series, IgM autoantibodies represented a significant proportion of AIHA in early childhood.[94] The IgM molecule is a pentameric structure that contains five covalently linked domains, each of which is structurally similar to a single IgG molecule. The large size of IgM autoantibodies can span the zeta potential between adjacent erythrocytes. Erythrocytes that are connected by a bridging IgM molecule become too dense to remain in suspension and agglutinate.

Although IgG and IgM autoantibodies represent the vast majority of cases of AIHA, rarely an IgA autoantibody is identified.[25, 68, 69, 95] IgA antibodies are not reactive with the standard Coombs' reagent, and therefore specific research reagents must be used for their identification. Finally, a combination of different isotypes,

Table 14-3. FREQUENCY OF IgG SUBCLASSES IDENTIFIED IN WARM-REACTIVE (IgG AUTOANTIBODY) AUTOIMMUNE HEMOLYTIC ANEMIA

IgG Subclass	Percentage of Total Cases
IgG1	74.0
IgG2	0.7
IgG3	2.1
IgG4	0.9
Multiple, including IgG1	20.1
Multiple, not including IgG1	0.3
None detectable	1.9

Adapted from Engelfriet CP, Overbeeke MAM, von dem Borne AE: Autoimmune hemolytic anemia. Semin Hematol 1992; 29:3.

especially simultaneous IgG and IgM autoantibodies, has been reported on several occasions.[96-102]

Thermal Reactivity

The thermal reactivity (sometimes called the thermal amplitude) of an erythrocyte autoantibody is another important parameter to determine; although the core temperature of humans is 37°C, temperatures in superficial vessels (particularly in the digits) may fall below 30°C. Binding of antibody to erythrocytes may therefore be considered a process of dynamic equilibrium, depending on the location of a given erythrocyte within the circulation. The thermal reactivity of most IgG autoantibodies is 37°C, meaning that binding to erythrocytes occurs best at the normal body temperature. These antibodies are therefore referred to as warm-reactive autoantibodies. Occasionally, warm-reactive IgM autoantibodies are identified, although these are rare.[70, 71, 94]

Cold-reactive (Donath-Landsteiner) IgG autoantibodies have an optimal binding at 4°C and are clinically important as the cause of PCH. Because of their unusual characteristics, the DAT is negative or demonstrates the presence of complement only, because the cold-reacting antibodies are removed during the washing of the erythrocytes. A special procedure must therefore be followed to detect the Donath-Landsteiner antibody characteristic of PCH.

This autoantibody is a biphasic hemolysin, meaning it binds to erythrocytes and fixes complement at 4°C, but on warming to 37°C the complement cascade is amplified and leads to hemolysis. Two samples of blood should be drawn simultaneously from the patient and kept at 37°C until the serum is separated. The serum samples are then incubated with normal erythrocytes and a source of complement, either in a melting ice bath or at 37°C. Both reactions are then warmed to 37°C and examined for the presence of hemolysis. In the first sample, the cold incubation allows the IgG autoantibody to bind and fix complement, after which the warming step allows complement amplification to occur with resultant red cell lysis. In contrast, the sample maintained at 37°C shows no lysis, because no significant IgG autoantibody binding or complement fixation occurs at the warmer temperature.

In contrast to many IgG autoantibodies, IgM autoantibodies typically have optimal binding to erythrocytes at 0°C to 4°C, and hence are called cold-reactive antibodies. The thermal range over which the autoantibody is active is crucial and determines the amount of hemolysis observed (Fig. 14–3). The IgM autoantibody binds optimally in the cold, but complement activation proceeds optimally at warmer temperatures. The overlap between the range of antibody activity and complement activation is the so-called zone of hemolysis.[103]

Complement Fixation

The ability of an erythrocyte autoantibody to fix complement plays a critical role in the pathophysiology of

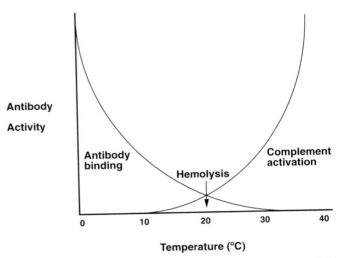

Figure 14-3. Thermal reactivity curve of a cold-reactive IgM autoantibody. The antibody is optimally reactive at 0°C to 4°C, whereas complement is amplified most efficiently at 37°C. The overlap area is the so-called zone of hemolysis and determines the amount of hemolysis observed. (Adapted from Issitt PD: Applied Blood Group Serology, 3rd ed. Miami, Montgomery Scientific Publication, 1985, p 545.)

immune clearance and the clinical manifestations of hemolysis, because complement augments the destructive effects of the autoantibody. The process of complement deposition, amplification, and pore formation involves a complex series of intravascular enzymatic events.

In the classical complement activation pathway, the Fc portion of the bound immunoglobulin molecule interacts with C1q, the first component of the complement cascade. Two IgG molecules in close proximity are required to bind C1q to the erythrocyte (Fig. 14–4A), whereas a single IgM molecule is sufficient to bind C1q (see Fig. 14–4B). Components C1r and C1s then bind to C1q to form a multiunit protein complex on the red cell surface. This active complex binds and enzymatically cleaves C4, followed by additional enzymatic events that lead to the deposition of component C3b on the surface of the erythrocyte. At this point, the erythrocyte may be cleared by the spleen, liver, or other parts of the reticuloendothelial system that recognize C3b by means of specific surface receptors. Alternatively, amplification of the complement cascade may continue, leading to the formation of the C5b-7 membrane attack complex, followed by fixation of C8 and C9, and the polymerization of C9 to form pores within the cell membrane (Fig. 14–5). These pores breach the erythrocyte membrane integrity and cause hemolysis of the cell.

IgM autoantibodies fix complement very efficiently, because distinct binding sites within the IgM pentamer are close enough to bind C1q (see Fig. 14–4B). In fact, the "hemolysins" that were identified at the turn of the century were actually IgM autoantibodies that fixed complement efficiently and completely, resulting in membrane pore formation and erythrocyte lysis. Rarely, IgM antibodies that do not fix complement have

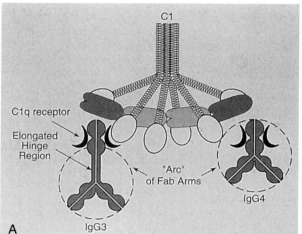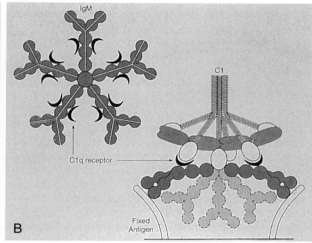

Figure 14-4. The binding of C1, the first component of complement, to antibodies. *A,* Binding of C1 to IgG molecules occurs through the Fc portion of the immunoglobulin molecule. Binding is inhibited by interference from the Fab arms, which is minimized when the hinge region is elongated, as in an IgG3 molecule; hence, IgG3 fixes complement more efficiently than IgG4. *B,* The complement binding sites of IgM molecules are not available when the antibody is in its fluid-phase planar form. When two of the monomers are affixed, however, the IgM molecule assumes an arched form and the C1 binding sites become available for reaction.

been reported.[94, 104] In contrast, IgG autoantibodies do not fix complement as efficiently as their IgM counterparts, owing in part to the necessity of two distinct IgG molecules being in close proximity to allow the initial binding of C1q.[11] If the target autoantigens on the erythrocyte membrane are not mobile or are spaced too far apart, complement cannot be fixed. Moreover, not all IgG molecules are equivalent in their ability to fix complement; the IgG1 and IgG3 subclasses are able to fix complement far better than the IgG2 and IgG4 subtypes.[86, 87] The Donath-Landsteiner antibodies, although IgG autoantibodies, fix complement very efficiently and lead to intravascular lysis.

Antibody Binding Affinity

The binding affinity of an erythrocyte autoantibody for its antigen also has implications both for the likelihood

Figure 14-5. Electron micrograph of the lesions that appear in the cell membrane after completion of the complement membrane attack complex. The dark lesions are hydrophilic complexes of protein about 10 nm in diameter.

of *in vitro* detection and for the pathophysiology of erythrocyte clearance.[79, 83] An IgG autoantibody typically has a high affinity for its antigen on the erythrocyte surface and therefore can be identified readily by the DAT. For this same reason, the indirect antiglobulin test may be negative with an IgG autoantibody, because there may be very little unbound antibody circulating in the plasma. In contrast, most IgM autoantibodies have little binding affinity at 37°C and therefore are more easily detected as high-titer unbound antibody within the plasma.

When testing the serologic specificity of most cases of warm-reactive AIHA, the blood bank frequently identifies reactivity with all cells tested. This "nonspecific" or "panreactive" pattern of reactivity suggests that the autoantibody is binding to a surface antigenic structure that is common to all human red cells. Interestingly, the autoantibody may not react with cells that lack the entire Rh protein complex; experiments with these rare Rh_null erythrocytes provide evidence that the Rh protein cluster is the main antigenic determinant for some warm-reactive autoantibodies[10, 103] (see Chapter 49). More recent studies have confirmed that autoantibodies bind to Rh in about 50% of patients with warm-reactive AIHA,[81, 82, 105] although other candidate autoantigens have been identified.[106] Reactivity with the ABO blood group antigens[107] or other major systems such as Lewis or Kell are extremely rare.[85, 103, 108] Autoantibodies with defined specificity against unusual protein antigens have also been described, including protein 4.1,[109] Ge,[110] Wr^b,[24] Sc1,[111] and many others. Occasionally, reactivity against a particular Rh antigen such as c or e is identified,[42, 112] although this is not common. In contrast, IgM autoantibodies frequently have reactivity against polysaccharides on the red cell rather than surface proteins. The I/i surface structure is a prototypic polysaccharide autoantigen on the red cell surface and is the target of many IgM antibodies that develop in response to infections.[93] In addition to the important I/i surface antigens, other autoantigens have also been reported in IgM AIHA,[42, 43, 113–115] including the polysaccharide P autoantigen in PCH.[116]

Antigenic Specificity

Elucidation of the antigenic specificity of autoreactive erythrocyte antibodies provides information that is useful for several reasons. One is the likelihood of finding compatible blood for transfusion. If an autoantibody is a "panreactive" antibody that binds to all cells with no apparent specificity, then compatible blood will not likely become available. Identification of the antigenic specificity may also help predict intravascular lysis due to complement activation. If the antigen is within the Rh complex, then the antigenic density on the erythrocytes makes complement activation remote, and therefore complement-mediated intravascular hemolysis unlikely. The P antigen system, in contrast, is densely populated on the erythrocyte surface and capable of binding sufficient IgG antibody to allow Donath-Landsteiner antibodies to fix complement completely and allow intravascular lysis.[11]

Immune Clearance of Sensitized Erythrocytes

Much of our understanding about the pathophysiology of immune-mediated erythrocyte clearance derives from experiments performed over 20 years ago. An elegant series of *in vitro* and *in vivo* studies by Jandl[7, 13, 14, 16] and by Rosse[11, 12, 18] clarified the role of antibody, complement, and the reticuloendothelial system in the pathophysiology of autoimmune erythrocyte clearance. In the early 1970s, Frank and colleagues developed a guinea pig model for AIHA that permitted the dissection of the steps involved in the clearance of erythrocytes coated with antibody or complement. Using ^{51}Cr-labeled cells that were sensitized *in vitro* using rabbit IgG or IgM anti-guinea pig erythrocyte antibodies, these investigators analyzed the rate and pattern of clearance, as well as the sites of sequestration. IgG-coated erythrocytes were removed predominantly by the spleen, regardless of concurrent complement activation, and the amount of surface IgG was correlated with the rate of splenic clearance. The liver was the predominant clearance site when very large amounts of IgG were present. Fc receptors on macrophages were responsible for the binding and phagocytosis of IgG-coated erythrocytes.[19, 20] In contrast to these findings for IgG-mediated hemolysis, IgM-coated erythrocytes were cleared rapidly within the liver and the amount of bound IgM was correlated with the rate of erythrocyte clearance. However, there was an absolute dependence on complement for the clearance of IgM-coated cells, with macrophage receptors for the C3b molecule responsible for binding and phagocytosis of erythrocytes.[19, 21] More recently, several investigators have attempted to mimic erythrocyte-monocyte interactions and correlate *in vitro* results with *in vivo* hemolysis.[117–120]

These and other laboratory experiments, coupled with careful clinical observations, have led to the development of a general understanding regarding immune-mediated clearance of erythrocytes in AIHA (Fig. 14–6). In warm-reactive AIHA, the IgG autoantibodies coat autologous erythrocytes and may fix complement. The sensitized cells pass through the spleen and other parts of the reticuloendothelial system, where they interact with complement and Fc receptors on the macrophages. The macrophage has three distinct classes of receptor for the Fc portion of the IgG molecule, designated FcγRI, FcγRII, and FcγRIII. Whereas each form of Fc receptor binds IgG with similar specificity, the binding affinity varies for individual subclasses of IgG autoantibodies.[121] The erythrocytes may be fully ingested by macrophages; however, if only a portion of the surface membrane is removed, the erythrocyte reforms into a spherocyte that is identifiable on the peripheral blood smear. For IgG-coated erythrocytes, the majority of immune clearance occurs within the cords of the spleen[122]; hence the hemolysis is extravascular. If the IgG antibody fixes complement, the erythrocyte will also be cleared by macrophages bearing receptors for complement receptors.[19, 23, 123]

In cold agglutinin disease or PCH, the autoreactive antibody binds preferentially at 4°C and fixes complement very well. At normal body temperature, there is virtually no antibody identifiable on the cell surface, but complement components, particularly C3b, can be identified using the Coombs reagent. If complement is activated to completion on the cell surface *in vivo*, the erythrocytes will hemolyze intravascularly and cause hemoglobinuria. When C3b is present on the red cell surface, however, then macrophages within the reticuloendothelial system can bind the erythrocytes by means of specific complement receptors and engulf

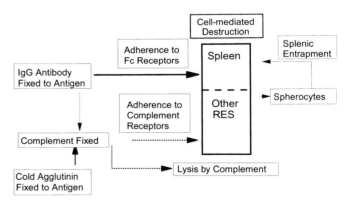

Figure 14-6. Immune-mediated clearance of erythrocytes in AIHA. In warm-reactive disease, the IgG autoantibodies are bound to erythrocytes but typically do not fix complement efficiently. The coated cells enter the spleen and other parts of the reticuloendothelial system (RES), where they interact with Fc receptors on macrophages. Erythrocytes may be completely engulfed and destroyed by this interaction or may have only a portion of their membrane removed. In this case, the red cells will reshape into spherocytes, which are then doomed on their next passage through the spleen. In cold-reactive disease, complement is typically fixed very efficiently and intravascular lysis by the complement cascade can occur. Alternatively, the presence of surface-bound complement (C3) can lead to extravascular red cell destruction by the spleen and RES.

them in a manner similar to warm-reactive AIHA.[124, 125] Complement-coated erythrocytes are cleared by macrophages primarily within the liver rather than the spleen.

Therapy

The need for treatment of a patient with AIHA depends on the severity and rapidity with which the anemia develops. A child with relatively mild anemia (9 to 12 g/dL), especially one who has a recent viral infection, will benefit from observation. If the patient has a more severe level of anemia (6 to 9 g/dL), or if the hemoglobin concentration is observed to fall precipitously, then therapy should be instituted. Optimal therapy depends on the clinical picture as well as on the form of AIHA. If the autoantibodies are cold reactive, for example, then the patient should be kept warm with avoidance of all cold stimuli. Strict adherence to this recommendation is difficult but is often the best therapy for a cold-reactive autoantibody. In the setting of severe intravascular hemolysis, it is imperative to maintain good renal blood flow and urine output.[47]

In the acute setting, therapy for AIHA in children should begin with close observation, the judicious use of erythrocyte transfusions, and corticosteroid therapy. Second-line therapy includes intravenous immunoglobulin therapy and plasma (exchange) transfusion. Other therapeutic modalities such as cyclosporin A, vinblastine, danazol, azathioprine, cyclophosphamide, and other agents are not yet widely accepted in the pediatric age group and therefore have no therapeutic role in the acute setting of childhood AIHA. Table 14–4 lists these various treatment modalities; and in the following sections, clinical responses and mechanisms of action are described.

When the anemia is severe enough to cause cardiovascular compromise, usually at a level below 5 g/dL, strong consideration must be given to transfusing the patient with erythrocytes in an attempt to provide additional oxygen-carrying capacity. Although the transfusion process for a patient with AIHA is complicated and somewhat intimidating, an erythrocyte transfusion may be lifesaving and should not be withheld from a patient who may die as a result of complications related to anemia.[126]

The first problem related to the transfusion of a patient with AIHA is the identification of compatible erythrocytes. It is important to provide the blood bank with a relatively large amount of serum and cells for testing, well in advance of an anticipated erythrocyte transfusion. Particularly if the antigenic specificity is panreactive, the crossmatch will likely identify no units of blood that are compatible. In this case, the blood bank will designate certain units that are "least incompatible" with the patient's serum. Of great importance is the ability to identify alloantibodies that may be masked by the stronger autoantibody.[127, 128] Adsorption techniques are designed to remove autoantibodies and allow the identification of clinically important alloantibodies.[129, 130]

The second difficulty regarding transfusion of a patient with AIHA is the actual transfusion itself. Fortunately, acute symptomatic transfusion reactions are infrequent, even when transfusing units of blood that indicate strong *in vitro* reactivity with the patient's serum.[127, 131] The transfused cells have an *in vivo* survival that is approximately equivalent to endogenous erythrocytes, and so are often beneficial even if only for a short time. On occasion, however, the transfusion results in severe hemolysis with hemoglobinemia, hemoglobinuria, and renal failure. For this reason, it is prudent to begin the transfusion at a slow rate, checking both plasma and urine samples periodically for free hemoglobin. For patients with cold-reactive antibodies, it is useful to warm the patient and the entire room; a blood warmer should be used to raise the temperature of the transfused blood.

The use of corticosteroids is widely accepted therapy

Table 14–4. TREATMENT MODALITIES FOR AUTOIMMUNE HEMOLYTIC ANEMIA

Treatment*	Dose	Comments
Red blood cell transfusions	Sufficient to reach 6–8 g/dL	Incompatibility may cause hemolysis
		Alloantibodies may be present
Corticosteroids	1–2 mg/kg IV q6h acutely	Useful for IgG more than IgM
	5–30 mg PO qod chronically	High doses for short-term use only
Intravenous immunoglobulin	1.0 g/kg per d for 1–5 d	Expensive, inconvenient to administer
		Effective in one third of patients
Exchange transfusion or plasmapheresis	Daily until stable	Useful for IgM more than IgG
		Requires large-caliber intravenous access
Splenectomy	—	Curative in 60–80% of patients
		Risk of postsplenectomy sepsis
Danazol	50–800 mg/d PO	Hepatic dysfunction
		Androgenic side effects
Vincristine	1 mg/m² IV every wk	Neurotoxicity
Cyclophosphamide	50–100 mg/d PO	Carcinogenesis
Azathioprine	25–200 mg/d PO	Immunosuppression
Cyclosporin A	2–10 mg/kg per d PO	Nephrotoxicity, hypertension
		Immunosuppression

IV = intravenously; PO = perorally.
*See text for further description and discussion of each therapeutic agent.

for AIHA, particularly for IgG antibodies. From the initial report almost 50 years ago,[132] glucocorticoids have been used to interfere with the basic pathophysiology and immune destruction observed in AIHA. The guinea pig model of AIHA demonstrated that steroids increased the survival of both IgG- and IgM-sensitized erythrocytes by decreasing sequestration within the spleen and liver, respectively.[20, 21] Corticosteroids are believed to inhibit the Fc receptor–mediated clearance of sensitized erythrocytes,[23, 133] which likely accounts for their effect within 24 to 48 hours of institution. Corticosteroids may also inhibit autoantibody synthesis, although this effect may require several weeks to occur.

For the patient with warm-reactive AIHA or PCH, a typical dosing regimen of corticosteroids is 1 to 2 mg/kg of methylprednisolone given intravenously every 6 hours for the first 24 to 72 hours, usually while the patient is the sickest. Oral prednisone at 2 mg/kg per day may then be used when the patient is clinically stable. Typically, these high doses of therapy are used for 2 to 4 weeks, followed by a taper that may take 1 to 3 months. The tapering of the steroid dose should be based on the patient's hemoglobin concentration, reticulocyte count, and DAT result. In general, the tapering should be slower when active disease is evident. An overall response rate of approximately 80% has been reported.[134] On occasion, corticosteroids may be beneficial in cold-agglutinin disease.[135]

Intravenous immunoglobulin (IVIG) became popular as a therapy for immune thrombocytopenic purpura in the 1980s.[136] Able to induce a potent blockade of the reticuloendothelial system,[137] IVIG was therefore an attractive option for the treatment of AIHA as well. Unfortunately, many early patients appeared to be refractory to IVIG therapy.[138, 139] Bussel and colleagues then reported that very high doses of IVIG (5.0 g/kg over 5 days) were necessary to derive a therapeutic benefit, perhaps because the size of the reticuloendothelial system was enlarged in AIHA patients.[28] Even at this high dose, however, only approximately one third of patients with warm-reactive AIHA responded to IVIG therapy.[28, 140] Prognostic factors that predicted IVIG response included a lower pretreatment hemoglobin concentration and the presence of hepatomegaly.[141] Based on these results, as well as on a variety of safety and cost issues,[142] IVIG should not be considered standard treatment of AIHA in children. However, continued investigation of its potential role in modulation of the immune response may shed light on important mechanisms of autoantibody production and immune-mediated clearance.[143]

Exchange transfusion is a reasonable therapeutic option for AIHA, because soluble plasma autoantibodies, soluble activated complement components, and sensitized erythrocytes can all be removed from the patient simultaneously.[144] More commonly, however, plasmapheresis or plasma exchange has been employed,[145–148] even in very small infants.[149, 150] It is generally accepted that patients with IgM autoantibodies respond better to plasmapheresis than those with IgG autoantibodies,[147, 151] presumably due to differences in the size and binding characteristics of the two molecules. The larger size of the IgM molecules keeps them within the intravascular space and amenable to removal by plasmapheresis. In contrast, IgG autoantibodies can diffuse into the extravascular space; plasmapheresis removes therefore only a fraction of the total IgG autoantibodies. In addition, IgM autoantibodies are less tightly affixed than IgG autoantibodies to erythrocytes at warm temperatures and are therefore more likely to be removed by plasmapheresis. For this reason, the extracorporeal circuit should be warmed during exchange transfusion of a patient with cold-reactive autoantibodies.[152]

For the child with chronic or refractory AIHA, more aggressive therapy is often required to alleviate the symptoms of anemia and to help the child achieve a more normal lifestyle. The long-term use of corticosteroids or immunoglobulin is generally unacceptable, because of side effects, costs, and inconvenience. A variety of additional therapeutic agents are available, however, as well as surgical intervention. No simple algorithm can be proposed that is correct for all patients. The clinician should individualize therapy for each patient, depending on the hematologic response and side effects.

Splenectomy is the time-honored therapy for the patient with chronic AIHA.[134, 153] The rationale for splenectomy is based in part on the animal model of AIHA, which demonstrated that IgG-sensitized erythrocytes were cleared almost exclusively within the spleen, regardless of whether complement was activated as well.[22] In keeping with this model, patients with IgG autoantibodies respond better to splenectomy than those patients with IgM autoantibodies.[154] However, prediction of the clinical response to splenectomy, based on the observation of splenic uptake of radiolabeled red cells,[155] has been described as having a variable reliability.[29, 48] In 12 patients with AIHA, Parker and colleagues found a poor correlation between ^{51}Cr-labeled red cell survival and eventual response to splenectomy.[156] Only 3 of 5 patients with a highly elevated spleen:liver uptake ratio had a clinical remission, whereas 3 of 5 with a very low ratio did have a remission after splenectomy. The authors concluded that radiolabeled red cell survival studies were not reliable indicators of the clinical response to splenectomy.[156] Splenectomy also may benefit the patient with AIHA by removing a major site of autoantibody production, similar to the pathophysiology of antiplatelet autoantibody production in immune thrombocytopenic purpura.[35]

In 52 patients with AIHA who underwent splenectomy with absent surgical mortality and low morbidity, Coon reported an excellent response in 64% and an improved status in another 21% of patients.[157] However, splenectomy is to be avoided in young children if possible, because of the possibility of postsplenectomy sepsis due to encapsulated bacterial organisms. Before splenectomy, or certainly shortly thereafter, children should receive immunization with a polyvalent vaccine against *Streptococcus pneumoniae* to enhance their humoral immune response. Children who undergo splenectomy also should be prescribed twice-daily penicillin for at least 2 years after surgery; some clinicians prefer life-long penicillin prophylaxis after splenectomy. Erythromycin should be used if the patient is allergic to penicillin. After splenectomy, children with fever over 38.5°C (101.5°F) should seek prompt medical attention for the possibility of bacterial sepsis.

Additional therapeutic agents have been used less frequently in children with AIHA. Danazol, a semisynthetic androgen, has been reported to have efficacy in patients with AIHA,[27, 158, 159] although no young children were included in these reports. One report suggested that danazol was more effective when used as first-line therapy in conjunction with corticosteroids,[159] whereas another demonstrated excellent responses even in refractory patients who had received previous therapy including splenectomy.[27] The mechanisms of action of danazol are not known, but decreases in titers of cell-bound IgG and complement were noted in most responders.[27] Danazol has been shown to decrease IgG production,[160] suggesting that this therapy may have multiple mechanisms of action that could be beneficial for the patient with AIHA. The primary side effects of danazol are elevations in the hepatic transaminases and mild masculinizing effects.

Cytotoxic agents also have been used in the treatment of AIHA, with the intent of reducing autoantibody formation. Vincristine and vinblastine have limited use in the pediatric age group but should be considered for the refractory patient.[26, 161, 162] *In vitro* incubation of platelets with *Vinca* alkaloids followed by transfusion of these "loaded" platelets has been used to poison the reticuloendothelial macrophages directly.[161] Other cytotoxic agents, including cyclophosphamide, chlorambucil, 6-mercaptopurine, and 6-thioguanine, have had limited success in adults, and no trials in children with AIHA have been reported. A typical daily dose of cyclophosphamide for an adult is 50 to 100 mg orally. These agents are generally myelosuppressive and potentially mutagenic[163] and therefore should be used with great caution in children. Similarly, combination chemotherapy for autoimmune disease has significant side effects related to granulocytopenia and thrombocytopenia.

Azathioprine is an immunosuppressive agent that affects both the humoral and cellular arms of the immune response, but its greatest effects are on the T lymphocytes.[134] By affecting T-cell helper function, azathioprine can interfere with autoantibody synthesis. Azathioprine is unlikely to induce a clinical remission as a single agent but could be used as a corticosteroid-sparing agent. A starting dose of azathioprine would be 25 to 50 mg/d, and side effects include leukopenia and thrombocytopenia. Because the goal of azathioprine is a reduction in autoantibody synthesis, responses may not be noted until after 2 to 3 months of therapy.[134]

Cyclosporin A, another immunosuppressive agent that focuses primarily on T lymphocytes, has been reported to be successful in a few patients with AIHA.[164] Because of significant side effects associated with long-term use of cyclosporin A, including nephro-

toxicity, hypertension, and the risk of second malignancy, it should not be used in children with AIHA except as a last resort.

Finally, several agents have been reported anecdotally as having beneficial effects in the treatment of AIHA. Alpha-interferon therapy has led to a response in a case of cold agglutinin disease[165] and therefore merits additional investigation. The effects of soluble growth factors on erythrocyte phagocytosis by macrophages in AIHA have been reported, suggesting a potential role for cytokine therapy.[166] As with many other autoimmune diseases, therapy specific for autoreactive T or B lymphocytes is clearly needed and would allow clinical benefit without hazardous side effects.

Pathogenesis of Autoantibody Formation

The autoantibodies produced in AIHA are clearly pathogenic, and the amount of antibody bound to the cell surface is proportional to the rate of erythrocyte removal by the reticuloendothelial system. Much less is known about the origin of autoantibody formation and why certain individuals have *in vivo* expansion of cells that should normally be suppressed or eliminated by the immune system.

Case reports have suggested an association between AIHA and certain immune response genes, especially the HLA-B locus.[167] Patients with HLA-B8 may have an increased risk for AIHA,[168] although a linkage with HLA-B27 has also been reported.[169] One large investigation of familial autoimmune cytopenias concluded that genetic factors were present, but they were not linked to the HLA complex.[170] In cold agglutinin disease, trisomy 3 has been identified as a frequent chromosomal abnormality and the autoantibodies are produced by defined abnormal clones of B lymphocytes.[171, 172]

The antierythrocyte antibodies that develop in most patients with AIHA represent a polyclonal B-lymphocyte response. The mechanisms by which these autoreactive B cells proliferate without proper immune surveillance are still poorly understood at this time, although new data are beginning to shed light on these processes. Expansion of autoreactive B cells could result from *in vivo* stimulation of normal B lymphocytes[173]; two reports support this idea.[174, 175] However, a considerable amount of data suggest that autoreactive antibodies develop after a specific immune stimulation, rather than a consequence of polyclonal antibody formation.[176, 177] Sequence analysis of the immunoglobulin gene rearrangements used by autoreactive autoantibodies has demonstrated a restricted repertoire of variable gene usage and evidence of somatic mutation.[178–181] These results suggest that autoreactive B cells undergo *in vivo* antigen-driven selection and mutation. The ability to clone individual autoreactive B cells, either by Epstein-Barr virus transformation[181, 182] or hybridoma formation,[183] should facilitate additional molecular analysis of the immunoglobulin response.

Although the pathogenic autoantibodies are produced by B lymphocytes, it is quite possible that the underlying immune defect in many patients with AIHA lies with the T lymphocytes.[184] T cells help to orchestrate the immune response by interacting with antigen-presenting mononuclear cells and helping B cells produce specific antibody. Previous reports have documented a variety of T-lymphocyte abnormalities in patients with AIHA, including an increase in activated T lymphocytes,[185] an imbalance in T-cell subsets,[186] a deficiency in the autologous mixed lymphocyte reaction,[187] and a deficiency of suppressor T-cell function.[188, 189] Experimental results from a murine model of AIHA also have implicated T lymphocytes in the pathogenesis of the disorder.[190, 191] Finally, several cases of AIHA have been reported in the clinical setting of T-lymphocyte immunosuppression from cyclosporin A treatment[192, 193]; these may result from dysregulation of transplanted donor lymphocytes.[194, 195] AIHA is also a well-recognized clinical manifestation of infection with the human immunodeficiency virus.[196, 197] Taken together, these data support the hypothesis that autoreactive B lymphocytes are present in the immune repertoire of normal individuals but expand and proliferate only in certain clinical settings, such as genetically susceptible individuals or T-lymphocyte dysregulation.

SECONDARY AUTOIMMUNE HEMOLYTIC ANEMIA

The classification scheme described in Table 14–1 indicates that AIHA can be a primary disorder or can occur in association with another systemic illness. These latter cases are known as secondary AIHA, because they occur in the setting of a much broader immune dysregulation. In one large series, secondary cases of AIHA represented over half of the total cases of warm-reactive AIHA.[85] It is therefore important to evaluate all patients with AIHA for the presence of another illness.

A common form of secondary AIHA is that which occurs in the presence of another autoimmune disease such as systemic lupus erythematosus.[198] Other generalized autoimmune and inflammatory disorders, including Sjögren's syndrome,[199, 200] scleroderma,[201] dermatomyositis,[202] ulcerative colitis,[203, 204] rheumatoid arthritis, autoimmune thyroiditis, and others,[85] are also associated with AIHA. It is believed that patients with these disorders have a genetic susceptibility and immune dysregulation that leads to the expansion and proliferation of autoreactive B lymphocytes. A special association exists between AIHA and other autoimmune cytopenias, especially thrombocytopenia.[205, 206] First noted by Evans and colleagues,[53] the combination of autoimmune anemia and thrombocytopenia is usually referred to as Evans' syndrome. In a large review of childhood Evans' syndrome, it was reported that the typical clinical course is chronic and relapsing and the therapy is generally unsatisfactory.[207] A variety of immunoregulatory abnormalities have been suggested in this disorder,[206, 208] although no single underlying specific immune defect has been identified. The autoantibodies are apparently directed against specific antigens on each of the various blood cell types; that is,

the antibodies against erythrocytes, platelets, and occasionally granulocytes are not cross reactive.[209]

AIHA can also occur in the setting of malignancy, in some cases as a clinical presentation before the diagnosis. In adults, the erythrocyte autoantibody may reflect an abnormal B-lymphocyte clone found in chronic lymphocytic leukemia,[210, 211] lymphoma,[210, 212] or multiple myeloma.[213] AIHA may also occur in young patients with Hodgkin's disease,[214-217] leukemia,[218] or myelodysplasia.[219] Although the etiology of AIHA in cancer patients is not known, it is possible that an underlying immune deficiency is the origin of both the autoimmune phenomena and the malignancy.

Children with congenital immunodeficiency can also develop AIHA, probably due to the lack of proper immune regulation.[220-222] Similarly, patients with acquired immunosuppression can develop AIHA.[193, 223] Patients infected with the human immunodeficiency virus are particularly susceptible to the development of erythrocyte autoantibodies,[196, 197] probably due to both the polyclonal B-lymphocyte activation and lack of immune regulation by T lymphocytes.

The majority of young children who present with PCH have had a recent viral-like illness,[36, 44, 47] although a pathogen is rarely identified. Historically, PCH developed in patients with syphilis, although this is rarely observed today. On occasion, however, a well-defined infection triggers an episode of AIHA. Multiple infectious agents have been reported, including *Mycoplasma pneumoniae*,[224] as well as Epstein-Barr virus,[225, 226] measles, varicella, mumps, rubella,[227] and other viruses.[228] Most of these autoantibodies are IgM with a specificity for the I/i polysaccharide antigen system on the red blood cells,[93] although occasionally specificity against the P polysaccharide antigen has been reported.[229] Reactivity of anti-I antibodies with mycoplasmal antigens suggests that autoantibodies may result from immunologic cross-reactivity.[230]

Acute bacterial infections also can cause hemolytic anemia, but from a different mechanism. The T antigen on the erythrocyte surface is known as a "cryptic" antigen, because it is not normally available for binding. In the presence of bacteria with neuraminidase activity, such as clostridial or pneumococcal species, however, sialic acid removal leads to exposure of the T antigen. Because many people have naturally occurring cold-reactive IgM plasma antibodies with anti-T specificity, hemolysis can result.[231] Although the practice is somewhat controversial, transfusions of erythrocytes are often washed in this clinical setting, to avoid transfusing additional anti-T antibodies.[232]

Although they are not common in childhood, drug-induced autoantibodies should be mentioned as a final category of secondary AIHA. Classically described after therapy with methyldopa,[233] red cell antibodies have been reported in association with literally dozens of different pharmaceutical agents.[234] Medications of particular importance in the pediatric age range that can cause AIHA include a variety of antibiotics: penicillins,[235, 236] cephalosporins,[237, 238] tetracycline,[239] erythromycin,[240] and probenecid.[241] Common agents such as acetaminophen[242] and ibuprofen[243] have also been implicated in hemolysis. The mechanism of drug-induced hemolytic anemia typically results from generation of autoantibodies, although the drug may be required to form a hapten or even a ternary complex with the erythrocyte.[234, 244, 245]

PAROXYSMAL NOCTURNAL HEMOGLOBINURIA

A rare condition, PNH has fascinated hematologists for over a century. In its classic presentation, patients with PNH have intermittent episodes of dark urine, most commonly on awakening in the morning. The hemolysis of PNH is due to an abnormal interaction between the erythrocytes and the complement system and, as such, is appropriate for this chapter on AIHA. However, the hemolysis results from an increased sensitivity of the patient's erythrocytes to complement-mediated lysis, and thus PNH (unlike AIHA) is an intracorpuscular defect. In addition, PNH is a very complex disease with protean clinical manifestations, only one of which is the hemolytic anemia. The secrets of this enigmatic disorder have only recently yielded to the efforts of modern molecular biology, culminating with the identification of *PIGA*, which is mutated in patients with PNH.

Historical Perspective

Clinicians first described PNH in the latter part of the 19th century,[246, 247] although it took many years to recognize several important facts: (1) the dark pigment in the urine was actually hemoglobin; (2) the serum of patients with PNH did not induce hemolysis of normal erythrocytes, thus distinguishing PNH from PCH; (3) the hemolysis was due to an intrinsic defect in the patient's own erythrocytes; and (4) the hemolysis was due to the lytic action of serum complement. Many of the initial insights into the pathophysiology of the hemolysis were due to the efforts of Dr. Thomas Ham, who first clearly demonstrated that acidified serum enhanced the hemolysis of PNH erythrocytes[248–250]; this test that bears his name has until recently been the simplest definitive laboratory method to establish the diagnosis of PNH. It is now recognized that the complement lysis sensitivity is not all or none; patients often have a population of erythrocytes that have a 15- to 25-fold increased complement sensitivity (type III cells), another population with a 3- to 5-fold increased sensitivity (type II cells), and a population of normal type I erythrocytes.[251–253]

Clinical Manifestations

The passing of dark urine is the classic symptom for which the disorder is named. As noted earlier, patients with PNH have hemoglobinuria rather than hematuria, resulting from chronic intravascular hemolysis from complement. Although the original descriptions accurately indicated that dark urine occurs more frequently on awakening, the cause for this temporal variation is not clear. Moreover, many patients have dark urine throughout the day whereas some never develop it. The typical patient with PNH reports an episode every few weeks, although some have chronic unrelenting hemolysis. Patients will describe massive hemoglobinuria with a variety of colorful descriptions, ranging from iced tea to cola to motor oil, and may describe the urine as various combinations of red, orange, brown, and black. Infections tend to trigger hemolysis, although frequently there is no identifiable reason. Therapy with oral corticosteroids (1 to 2 mg/kg of prednisone) ameliorates the hemolysis and is often required for only 24 to 72 hours around the time of a hemolytic episode.

The clinical manifestations of PNH include much more than simply hemolytic anemia, however.[254] Table 14–5 lists the more common signs and symptoms observed in patients with PNH. In addition to hemolysis, patients with PNH tend to have an increased number of infections, particularly those that are sinopulmonary and bloodborne. Another severe clinical complication is venous thrombosis, which often occurs in unusual locations such as the hepatic veins (Budd-Chiari syndrome), mesenteric veins, and sagittal veins. The complications of venous thrombosis are often fatal, because the hypercoagulability observed in PNH is very difficult to treat even with thrombolytic agents. Defective hematopoiesis is present in the majority of patients with PNH, either at presentation or during the course of the disease. Most patients have peripheral macrocytic anemia and erythroid hyperplasia in the bone marrow, but some develop severe aplastic anemia and suffer the clinical consequences of pancytopenia. Treatment with antithymocyte globulin seems to help in a portion of cases. Finally, PNH can evolve into acute nonlymphoblastic leukemia, which typically occurs within the first 5 years of disease.[255] The incidence of leukemic transformation is only 1% to 3%; however, this rate far exceeds that of the general population.

Although primarily a disease of adults, PNH definitely occurs in children and adolescents. The authors reported a cohort of 26 young patients with PNH and noted several important differences as compared with the clinical descriptions of adults.[256] Many children

Table 14–5. SIGNS AND SYMPTOMS COMMONLY OBSERVED IN PAROXYSMAL NOCTURNAL HEMOGLOBINURIA

Intravascular hemolysis
  Dark urine
  Iron deficiency
  Acute renal failure
Infections
  Sinopulmonary
  Bloodborne
Venous thrombosis
  Occurs in one third of patients
  Unusual locations
Defective hematopoiesis
  Macrocytosis, pancytopenia
  Association with aplastic anemia
Transition to malignancy
  Nonlymphoblastic leukemia

were initially misdiagnosed, with an average of almost 2 years from initial symptoms to the correct diagnosis. Very few children had dark urine as a presenting symptom, and only 65% of children ever developed clinically evident hemoglobinuria. Thrombosis occurred in approximately one third of patients, and some died of this dreaded complication. All patients had laboratory evidence of defective or ineffective hematopoiesis, either at diagnosis or over the course of their disease. The survival curve for these patients indicated that the 10-year survival was only 60%, although several deaths were due to complications of aplastic anemia in an era before modern antibiotic and transfusion therapy. Because bone marrow transplantation can be curative therapy for PNH,[257, 258, 258a] it should be considered in select patients with this disorder.

Biochemical Basis

Important clues to the etiology of PNH emerged with the identification of two complement regulatory proteins, CD55 (decay accelerating factor)[259] and CD59 (membrane inhibitor of reactive lysis)[260] in the 1980s. The abnormal peripheral blood cells in patients with PNH were noted to be lacking both CD55 and CD59.

As a result of these deficiencies, randomly deposited complement factors and C3 convertase complexes cannot be cleared from the erythrocyte membrane and lead to the formation of the membrane attack complex, pore formation, and cell lysis.[251]

The commonality of these two complement regulatory proteins goes beyond function, however, because both use a novel motif for anchoring into the plasma membrane (Fig. 14–7). Unlike the majority of surface proteins that contain a highly hydrophobic domain that serves as a transmembrane region between the intracellular domain and the extracellular domain of the polypeptide, certain proteins use a glycosylphosphatidyl-inositol (GPI) anchor for membrane attachment.[261, 262] By definition, GPI-linked proteins are covalently attached at their C-terminus to a variable glycan moiety, which is itself attached to a phosphatidyl-inositol molecule in the outer leaflet of the cell membrane lipid bilayer. This glycolipid structure is presumably assembled within the endoplasmic reticulum and coupled to the protein precursor as a preformed unit.[262, 263] Initially described for the alkaline phosphatase enzyme,[264] GPI linkage is now known to be used by a diverse set of surface proteins (Table 14–6), including acetylcholinesterase,[265] Thy-1,[266] lymphocyte function-

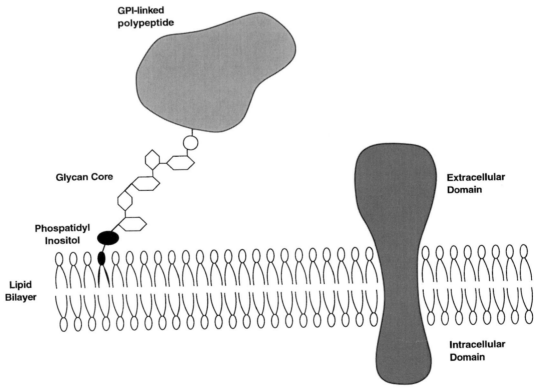

Figure 14-7. The glycosylphosphatidylinositol (GPI) anchor for attachment of surface proteins to the cell membrane. The structure of a GPI-linked protein is shown on the left. The GPI anchor consists of a phosphatidylinositol molecule in the outer leaflet of the lipid bilayer, which is connected to a glycan core consisting of multiple sugars and side chains. The polypeptide is then linked to the anchor at its C-terminus by an amide bond. The result is a surface protein with a fluid and mobile attachment to the cell surface. The entire polypeptide is present in the extracellular milieu. In contrast, a transmembrane protein is shown on the right, with an extracellular domain, a short transmembrane domain, and an intracellular domain.

Table 14-6. SURFACE PROTEINS ABSENT FROM
AFFECTED HEMATOPOIETIC CELLS IN PAROXYSMAL
NOCTURNAL HEMOGLOBINURIA

Complement regulatory proteins
    Decay accelerating factor (CD55)
    Membrane inhibitor of reactive lysis (CD59)
Immunologically important proteins
    Lymphocyte function antigen-3 (LFA-3, CD58)
    Fc receptor gamma III (FcγRIII, CD16)
    Endotoxin binding protein receptor (CD14)
Receptors
    Urokinase receptor (UPAR)
    Folate receptor
Enzymes
    Alkaline phosphatase
    Acetylcholinesterase
    5'-*ecto*nucleotidase
Proteins with unknown functions
    CD24
    CD48
    CD52 (Campath-1)
    CD66
    CD67
    JMH-bearing protein

Adapted from Rosse WF, Ware RE: The molecular basis of paroxysmal nocturnal hemoglobinuria. Blood 1995; 86:3277.

associated antigen 3,[267] Fcγ receptor type III,[268] the complement regulatory proteins CD55 and CD59,[259, 260] and others.[269, 270] The functional advantages of GPI-linkage for surface proteins are speculative but include increased lateral diffusional mobility,[271, 272] second messenger generation,[273] signal transduction,[274, 275] and the ability to be cleaved from the cell surface into the extracellular milieu.[276]

The primary defect in PNH resides in the incomplete bioassembly of GPI anchors, because all GPI-linked surface proteins are absent on the surface of the abnormal PNH cells.[277–283] Biochemical analysis of GPI-deficient cells localized the defect in PNH to an early step in GPI anchor biosynthesis.[284–287] Mammalian mutant cell lines deficient in GPI-linked surface proteins have been established and can be classified into different complementation classes.[288, 289] Class A, C, and H mutants cannot transfer the initial *N*-acetylglucosamine to the phosphatidyl-inositol acceptor, suggesting that at least three genes control this step. Fusion experiments of PNH cells with murine GPI-deficient cell lines further identified the defect as a class A mutation in all patients tested.[286, 290, 291] Therefore, despite the possibility of various enzymatic defects along the GPI anchor biosynthetic pathway, all patients with PNH who have been tested have a class A defect.[292]

The absence of GPI-linked surface proteins on the abnormal cells in PNH has led to a simpler and more accurate diagnostic test than older methods of complement-mediated lysis. Peripheral blood erythrocytes and granulocytes can be analyzed by flow cytometry for surface expression of GPI-linked proteins such as CD16, CD48, CD55, or CD59.[293, 294] Erythrocytes that are completely deficient in GPI-linked surface proteins are present in most patients and correspond to the PNH type III cells. Partially deficient cells can be detected in approximately 50% of patients and correspond to type II cells.[294, 295] Examples of these cell populations are shown in Figure 14–8; the surface CD59 expression on circulating erythrocytes from a patient with type I and type III cells is shown in Figure 14–8*A*; that for a patient with type I, II, and III cells is shown in Figure 14–8*B*; and that for a patient with predominantly type III cells but a few type II cells is shown in Figure 14–8*C*. A blood sample from a normal control is shown in Figure 14–8*D*.

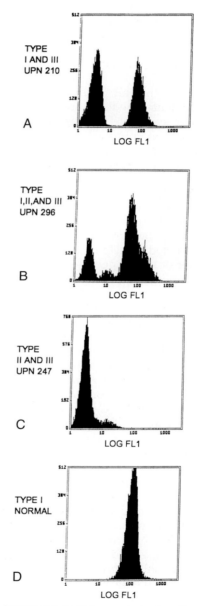

Figure 14-8. Immunophenotype analysis of erythrocytes in paroxysmal nocturnal hemoglobinuria (PNH) by flow cytometry. Examples of surface CD59 expression are shown for three patients and a control. *A*, Data for unique patient number (UPN) 210, who had both type I and type III erythrocytes. *B*, Data for UPN 296 with type I, II, and III cells. *C*, Data for UPN 247 with predominantly type III erythrocytes and a few type II cells. *D*, Normal expression from a control. (Data from Ware RE, Rosse WF, Hall SE: Immunophenotypic analysis of reticulocytes in paroxysmal nocturnal hemoglobinuria. Blood 1995; 86:1586.)

Molecular Basis

Analysis of glucose-6-phosphate dehydrogenase allozymes[296] and a monoclonal pattern of X chromosome inactivation[297, 298] have suggested that PNH is a clonal abnormality. The abnormal clone is believed to originate at the level of a primitive multipotent bone marrow progenitor cell, in that all cells of the myeloerythroid lineage, including erythrocytes, granulocytes, platelets, and monocytes, are affected.[283] Lymphocytes[290, 299] and natural killer cells[300] also have been reported to be deficient in GPI to varying degrees, suggesting that in some cases a totipotent lymphohematopoietic stem cell may be affected. The abnormal PNH clone is usually dominant, with some patients having over 95% GPI-deficient circulating erythrocytes and granulocytes.

The recognition that all patients with PNH have a class A complementation defect suggested that a single gene might be responsible for this disorder. Using the strategy of a human complementary DNA expression library, Miyata and associates identified a gene that repaired the defect in a class A GPI-deficient cell line.[301] Designated PIGA because it repaired the phosphoinositol glycan defect in a class A mutant, this complementary DNA encodes a novel polypeptide with homology to other known glycosyltransferases. The cloned complementary DNA was 3589 nucleotides in length and encoded a predicted protein of 484 amino acids. No N-terminal leader or signal peptide sequence was apparent, but a highly hydrophobic region near the C-terminus might form a transmembrane domain for insertion through the endoplasmic reticulum membrane. Northern blot analysis indicated a single transcript of approximately 4.2 kb.[301]

PIGA was quickly considered to be a candidate gene for PNH, so several groups analyzed their patients for genetic mutations. PIGA abnormalities in PNH have now been reported from laboratories around the world, confirming that PIGA is the gene defective in PNH.[302–309] Interestingly, the majority of mutations are short (1 to 2 nucleotides) insertions or deletions that occur throughout the coding region of the PIGA gene. These nucleotide changes cause frameshift mutations, as the triplet nucleotide coding sequence is altered; frequently, a premature termination codon is present after the frameshift mutation. Missense mutations that substitute a single amino acid residue account for only 25% of the PIGA abnormalities reported and seem to be clustered in the 5' end of the coding region.[310]

The chromosomal assignment of PIGA to the X chromosome,[302, 311] and the recent assignment of other genes involved in GPI anchor biosynthesis (PIGF and PIGH) to autosomes,[311] helps to explain the predominant class A defect in PNH. Whereas a single gene mutation in PIGA could result in abnormal GPI anchor biosynthesis, mutations in both alleles of other genes involved in GPI anchor biosynthesis would likely be required to produce clinically overt disease. It is therefore possible that a patient with PNH will yet be identified with a complementation other than class A.

How *PIGA* Mutations Cause Paroxysmal Nocturnal Hemoglobinuria

With the biochemical and molecular basis of PNH in hand, it is perhaps surprising that the pathophysiology of many clinical manifestations of PNH remains unclear. The hemoglobinuria is readily explainable by the absence of surface CD55 and CD59, which allows chronic complement-mediated intravascular hemolysis. In contrast, the etiology of the hypercoagulable state in PNH is not well understood. PNH platelets lack the GPI-linked complement regulatory proteins CD55 and CD59 and respond to the deposition of terminal complement components by vesiculation of portions of their plasma membrane. These resultant platelet microparticles have increased procoagulant properties.[312] PNH cells also lack the receptor for the GPI-linked urokinase plasminogen activator, which may result in impaired fibrinolysis.[313] However, PNH patients have normal plasma levels of natural anticoagulants, including protein C and S, thrombomodulin, and antithrombin III.[314]

The defective hematopoiesis that affects so many patients with PNH is also not well understood. An unusual association occurs between PNH and aplastic anemia, in that one frequently evolves clinically into the other.[315, 316] For example, some patients with near-normal blood cell counts and a hypercellular bone marrow slowly develop hypoplasia. In contrast, others have severe aplastic anemia and eventually develop PNH, often after immunosuppressive therapy such as with antithymocyte globulin or cyclosporin A.[317] Several possible explanations for the defective hematopoiesis include (1) the PNH clone suppresses normal marrow progenitors; (2) the marrow has been injured by an extrinsic agent, and the PNH clone is relatively resistant to the damage; and (3) the PNH clone has an intrinsic growth and proliferative advantage compared with normal stem cells. It is impossible to distinguish among these possibilities, but circumstantial evidence supports the last possibility. A proliferative advantage would help explain the increased rate of leukemic transformation that occurs in patients with PNH. In addition, the identification of more than one mutant clone in several PNH patients suggests a selection pressure for the PIGA mutation.[308, 309, 318] In the setting of marrow hypoplasia, the emergence of any proliferative clone would presumably be advantageous. To paraphrase Bessler and co-workers,[318] "acquired PIGA mutations may be nature's gene therapy for aplastic anemia, and the price to pay is PNH."

References

1. Hayem G: Sur une variété particulière d'ictère chronique. Ictère infectieux chronique splenomégalique. Presse Med 1898; 6:121.
2. Donath J, Landsteiner K: Über paroxysmale Hämoglobinurie. Munchen Med Wochenschr 1904; 51:1590.
3. Landsteiner K: Über Beziehungen zwischen dem Blutserum und den Körperzellen. Munchen Med Wochenschr 1903; 50:1812.
4. Coombs RRA, Mourant AE, Race RR: A new test for the detec-

tion of weak and "incomplete" Rh agglutinins. Br J Exp Pathol 1945; 26:255.

5. Coombs RRA, Mourant AE: On certain properties of antisera prepared against human serum and its various protein fractions: Their use in the detection of sensitization of human red cells with "incomplete" Rh antibody, and on the nature of this antibody. J Pathol Bacteriol 1947; 59:105.

6. Dausset J, Colombani J: The serology and the prognosis of 128 cases of autoimmune hemolytic anemia. Blood 1959; 14:1280.

7. Jandl JH, Jones AR, Castle WB: The destruction of red cells by antibodies in man. I. Observations on the sequestration and lysis of red cells altered by immune mechanisms. J Clin Invest 1957; 30:1428.

8. Borsos T, Rapp HJ: Complement fixation on cell surfaces by 19S and 7S antibodies. Science 1965; 150:505.

9. Eyster ME, Jenkins DE Jr: Erythrocyte coating substances in patients with positive direct antiglobulin reactions. Correlation of γ-G globulin and complement coating with underlying diseases, overt hemolysis and response to therapy. Am J Med 1969; 46:360.

10. Eyster ME, Jenkins DE Jr: Gamma G erythrocyte autoantibodies: Comparison of *in vivo* complement coating and *in vitro* "Rh" specificity. J Immunol 1970; 105:221.

11. Rosse WF: Fixation of the first component of complement (C'1a) by human antibodies. J Clin Invest 1968; 47:2430.

12. Rosse WF: Quantitative immunology of immune hemolytic anemia. I. The fixation of C1 by autoimmune antibody and heterologous anti-IgG antibody. J Clin Invest 1971; 50:727.

13. LoBuglio AF, Cotran RS, Jandl JH: Red cells coated with immunoglobulin G: Binding and sphering by mononuclear cells in man. Science 1967; 158:1582.

14. Abramson N, LoBuglio AF, et al: The interaction between human monocytes and red cells. Binding characteristics. J Exp Med 1970; 132:1191.

15. Kay NE, Douglas SD: Monocyte-erythrocyte interaction *in vitro* in immune hemolytic anemias. Blood 1977; 50:889.

16. Abramson N, Gelfand EW, et al: The interaction between human monocytes and red cells. Specificity for IgG subclasses and IgG fragments. J Exp Med 1970; 132:1207.

17. Huber H, Douglas SD, et al: IgG subclass specificity of human monocyte receptor sites. Nature 1971; 229:419.

18. Kurlander RJ, Rosse WF, Logue GL: Quantitative influence of antibody and complement coating of red cells on monocyte-mediated cell lysis. J Clin Invest 1978; 61:1309.

19. Schreiber AD, Frank MM: Role of antibody and complement in the immune clearance and destruction of erythrocytes. I. *In vivo* effects of IgG and IgM complement-fixing sites. J Clin Invest 1972; 51:575.

20. Atkinson JP, Frank MM: Complement-independent clearance of IgG-sensitized erythrocytes: Inhibition by cortisone. Blood 1974; 44:629.

21. Atkinson JP, Frank MM: Studies on *in vivo* effects of antibody: Interaction of IgM antibody and complement in the immune clearance and destruction of erythrocytes in man. J Clin Invest 1974; 54:339.

22. Atkinson JP, Schreiber AD, Frank MM: Effects of corticosteroids and splenectomy on the immune clearance and destruction of erythrocytes. J Clin Invest 1973; 52:1509.

23. Schreiber AD, Parsons J, et al: Effect of corticosteroids on the human monocyte IgG and complement receptors. J Clin Invest 1975; 56:1189.

24. Issitt PD, Pavone BG, et al: Anti-Wr^b, and other autoantibodies responsible for positive direct antiglobulin tests in 150 individuals. Br J Haematol 1976; 34:5.

25. Reusser P, Osterwalder B, et al: Autoimmune hemolytic anemia associated with IgA—Diagnostic and therapeutic aspects in a case with long-term follow-up. Acta Haematol 1987; 77:53.

26. Ahn YS, Harrington WJ, et al: Treatment of autoimmune hemolytic anemia with *Vinca*-loaded platelets. JAMA 1983; 249:2189.

27. Ahn YS, Harrington WJ, et al: Danazol therapy for autoimmune hemolytic anemia. Ann Intern Med 1985; 102:298.

28. Bussel JB, Cunningham-Rundles C, Abraham C: Intravenous treatment of autoimmune hemolytic anemia with very high dose gammaglobulin. Vox Sang 1986; 51:264.

29. Habibi B, Homberg J-C, et al: Autoimmune hemolytic anemia in children. A review of 80 cases. Am J Med 1974; 56:61.

30. Carapella de Luca E, Casadei AM, et al: Auto-immune haemolytic anaemia in childhood. Follow-up in 29 cases. Vox Sang 1979; 36:13.

31. Sokol RJ, Hewitt S, et al: Autoimmune haemolysis in childhood and adolesence. Acta Haematol 1984; 72:245.

32. Schreiber AD, Rosse WF, Frank MM: Autoimmune hemolytic anemia. In Frank MM, Austen KF, et al (eds): Samter's Immunologic Diseases. 5th ed. Vol. II. Boston, Little, Brown & Co., 1995, p 903.

33. Clausen N: A population study of severe aplastic anemia in children. Acta Paediatr Scand 1986; 75:58.

34. Szklo M, Sensenbrenner L, et al: Incidence of aplastic anemia in metropolitan Baltimore: a population-based study. Blood 1985; 66:115.

35. Ware R, Kinney TR: Immunopathology of childhood idiopathic thrombocytopenia. Crit Rev Oncol Hematol 1987; 7:169.

36. Sokol RJ, Hewitt S, Stamps BK: Autoimmune haemolysis associated with Donath-Landsteiner antibodies. Acta Haematol 1982; 68:268.

37. Heisel MA, Ortega JA: Factors influencing prognosis in childhood autoimmune hemolytic anemia. Am J Pediatr Hematol Oncol 1983; 5:147.

38. Zupanska B, Lawkowicz W, et al: Autoimmune haemolytic anaemia in children. Br J Hematol 1976; 34:511.

39. Wolach B, Heddle N, et al: Transient Donath-Landsteiner hemolytic anemia. Br J Haematol 1981; 48:425.

40. Schubothe H: The cold hemagglutinin disease. Semin Hematol 1966; 3:27.

41. Schreiber AD, Herskovitz BS, Goldwein M: Low-titer cold-hemagglutinin disease. N Engl J Med 1977; 296:1490.

42. Sokol RJ, Hewitt S, Stamps BK: Autoimmune haemolysis: an 18-year study of 865 cases referred to a regional transfusion centre. BMJ 1981; 282:2023.

43. Nydegger UE, Kazatchkine MD, Miescher PA: Immunopathologic and clinical features of hemolytic anemia due to cold agglutinins. Semin Hematol 1991; 28:66.

44. Gottsche B, Salama A, Mueller-Eckhardt C: Donath-Landsteiner autoimmune hemolytic anemia in children. A study of 22 cases. Vox Sang 1990; 58:281.

45. Buchanan GR, Boxer LA, Nathan DG: The acute and transient nature of idiopathic immune hemolytic anemia in childhood. J Pediatr 1976; 88:780.

46. Nordhagen R, Stensvold K, et al: Paroxysmal cold hemoglobinuria. The most frequent autoimmune hemolytic anemia in children? Acta Paediatr Scand 1984; 73:258.

47. Warren RW, Collins ML: Immune hemolytic anemia in children. Crit Rev Oncol Hematol 1988; 8:65.

48. Allgood JW, Chaplin H Jr: Idiopathic acquired autoimmune hemolytic anemia. A review of forty-seven cases treated from 1955 through 1965. Am J Med 1967; 43:254.

49. Dobbs CE: Familial auto-immune hemolytic anemia. Arch Intern Med 1965; 116:273.

50. Toolis F, Parker AC, et al: Familial autoimmune haemolytic anaemia. BMJ 1977; 1:1392.

51. Jensen OM, Kristensen J: Red pulp of the spleen in autoimmune haemolytic anaemia and hereditary spherocytosis: Morphometric light and electron microscopy studies. Scand J Haematol 1986; 36:263.

52. Weiss GB, Bessman JD: Spurious automated red cell values in warm autoimmune hemolytic anemia. Am J Hematol 1984; 17:433.

53. Evans RS, Takahashi K, et al: Primary thrombocytopenic purpura and acquired hemolytic anemia. Evidence for a common etiology. Arch Intern Med 1951; 87:48.

54. Brown DL, Nelson DA: Surface microfragmentation of red cells as a mechanism for complement-mediated immune spherocytosis. Br J Haematol 1973; 24:301.

55. Farolino DL, Rustagi PK, et al: Teardrop-shaped red cells in autoimmune hemolytic anemia. Am J Hematol 1986; 21:415.

56. Stefanelli M, Barosi G, et al: Quantitative assessment of erythropoiesis in haemolytic disease. Br J Haematol 1980; 45:297.

57. Greenberg J, Curtis-Cohen M, et al: Prolonged reticulocytopenia in autoimmune hemolytic anemia of childhood. J Pediatr 1980; 97:784.

58. Hauke G, Fauser AA, et al: Reticulocytopenia in severe autoim-

mune hemolytic anemia (AIHA) of the warm antibody type. Blut 1983; 46:321.

59. Liesveld JL, Rowe JM, Lichtman MA: Variability of the erythropoietic response in autoimmune hemolytic anemia: Analysis of 109 cases. Blood 1987; 69:820.

60. Bertrand Y, Lefrere JJ, et al: Autoimmune haemolytic anaemia revealed by human parvovirus linked erythroblastopenia. Lancet 1985; 2:382. Letter.

61. Smith MA, Shah NS, Lobel JS: Parvovirus B19 infection associated with reticulocytopenia and chronic autoimmune hemolytic anemia. Am J Pediatr Hematol Oncol 1989; 11:167.

62. Javid J: Human serum haptoglobins. Semin Hematol 1967; 4:35.

63. Yam P, Petz LD, Spath P: Detection of IgG sensitization of red cells with ^{125}I staphylococcal Protein A. Am J Hematol 1982; 12:337.

64. Bodensteiner D, Brown P, et al: The enzyme-linked immunosorbent assay: Accurate detection of red blood cell antibodies in autoimmune hemolytic anemia. Am J Clin Pathol 1983; 79:182.

65. Sokol RJ, Hewitt S, et al: Small quantities of erythrocyte bound immunoglobulins and autoimmune haemolysis. J Clin Pathol 1987; 40:254.

66. Galili U, Manny N, Izak G: EA rosette formation: A simple means to increase sensitivity of the antiglobulin test in patients with anti red cell antibodies. Br J Haematol 1981; 47:227.

67. Angevine CD, Anderson BR, Barnett EV: A cold agglutinin of the IgA class. J Immunol 1966; 96:578.

68. Suzuki S, Amano T, et al: Autoimmune hemolytic anemia associated with IgA autoantibody. Clin Immunol Immunopathol 1981; 21:247.

69. Kowal-Vern A, Jacobson P, et al: Negative direct antiglobulin test in autoimmune hemolytic anemia. Am J Pediatr Hematol Oncol 1986; 8:349.

70. Freedman J, Wright J, et al: Hemolytic warm IgM autoagglutinins in autoimmune hemolytic anemia. Transfusion 1987; 27:464.

71. Shirey RS, Kickler TS, et al: Fatal immune hemolytic anemia and hepatic failure associated with a warm-reacting IgM autoantibody. Vox Sang 1987; 52:219.

72. Worlledge SM: The interpretation of a positive direct antiglobulin test. Br J Haematol 1978; 39:157.

73. Gorst DW, Rawlinson VI, et al: Positive direct antiglobulin test in normal individuals. Vox Sang 1980; 38:99.

74. Bareford D, Longster G, et al: Follow-up of normal individuals with a positive antiglobulin test. Scand J Haematol 1985; 35:348.

75. Forman SJ, Kumar KS, et al: Hemolytic anemia in Wilson disease: Clinical findings and biochemical mechanisms. Am J Hematol 1980; 9:269.

76. Zieve L: Jaundice, hyperlipemia and hemolytic anemia: A heretofore unrecognized syndrome associated with alcoholic fatty liver and cirrhosis. Ann Intern Med 1958; 48:471.

77. Ware R: Human parvovirus infection. J Pediatr 1989; 114:343.

78. Rubin H: Autoimmune hemolytic anemias. Warm and cold antibody types. Am J Clin Pathol 1977; 68:638.

79. Joshi SR, Iyer YS, Bhatia HM: Serological and immunoglobulin studies in autoimmune haemolytic anaemia with emphasis on the nature of biphasic antibodies. Acta Haematol 1980; 64:31.

80. Garratty G: Mechanisms of immune red cell destruction, and red cell compatibility testing. Hum Pathol 1983; 14:204.

81. Wolf MW, Roelcke D: Incomplete warm hemolysins. I. Case reports, serology, and immunoglobulin classes. Clin Immunol Immunopathol 1989; 51:55.

82. Wolf MW, Roelcke D: Incomplete warm hemolysins. II. Corresponding antigens and pathogenetic mechanisms in autoimmune hemolytic anemias induced by incomplete warm hemolysins. Clin Immunol Immunopathol 1989; 51:68.

83. Andrzejewski C Jr, Young PJ, et al: Heterogeneity of human red cell autoantibodies assessed by isoelectric focusing. Transfusion 1991; 31:236.

84. Bell CA, Zwicker H, Sacks HJ: Autoimmune hemolytic anemia: Routine serologic evaluation in a general hospital population. Am J Clin Pathol 1973; 60:903.

85. Engelfriet CP, Overbeeke MAM, von dem Borne AE: Autoimmune hemolytic anemia. Semin Hematol 1992; 29:3.

86. Ishizaka T, Ishizaka K, et al: Biologic activities of aggregated γ-globulin. VIII. Aggregated immunoglobulins of different classes. J Immunol 1967; 99:82.

87. Augener W, Grey HM, et al: The reaction of monomeric and aggregated immunoglobulins with C1. Immunochemistry 1971; 8:1011.

88. von dem Borne AE, Beckers D, et al: IgG₄ autoantibodies against erythrocytes, without increased haemolysis: a case report. Br J Haematol 1977; 37:137.

89. Silberstein LE, Berkman EM, Schreiber AD: Cold hemagglutinin disease associated with IgG cold-reactive antibody. Ann Intern Med 1987; 106:238.

90. Chaplin H Jr, Cohen R, et al: Pregnancy and idiopathic autoimmune haemolytic anaemia: A prospective study during 6 months' gestation and 3 months' post partum. Br J Haematol 1973; 24:219.

91. Sacks DA, Platt LD, Johnson CS: Autoimmune hemolytic disease during pregnancy. Am J Obstet Gynecol 1981; 140:942.

92. Sokol RJ, Hewitt S, Stamps BK: Erythrocyte autoantibodies, autoimmune haemolysis and pregnancy. Vox Sang 1982; 43:169.

93. Bell CA, Zwicker H, Rosenbaum DL: Paroxysmal cold hemoglobinuria (P.C.H.) following mycoplasma infection: Anti-I specificity of the biphasic hemolysin. Transfusion 1973; 13:138.

94. Salama A, Mueller-Eckhardt C: Autoimmune haemolytic anaemia in childhood associated with non-complement binding IgM autoantibodies. Br J Haematol 1987; 65:67.

95. Gottsche B, Salama A, Mueller-Eckhardt C: Autoimmune haemolytic anemia associated with an IgA autoanti-Gerbich. Vox Sang 1990; 58:211.

96. Sokol RJ, Hewitt S, Stamps BK: Autoimmune hemolysis: Mixed warm and cold antibody type. Acta Haematol 1983; 69:266.

97. Silberstein LE, Shoenfeld Y, et al: Combination of IgG and IgM autoantibodies in chronic cold agglutinin disease: Immunologic studies and response to splenectomy. Vox Sang 1985; 48:105.

98. Shulman IA, Branch DR, et al: Autoimmune hemolytic anemia with both cold and warm autoantibodies. JAMA 1985; 253:1746.

99. Nusbaum NJ, Khosla S: Autoimmune hemolytic anemia with both cold and warm autoantibodies. JAMA 1985; 254:1175.

100. Freedman J, Lim FC, et al: Autoimmune hemolytic anemia with concurrence of warm and cold red cell autoantibodies and a warm hemolysin. Transfusion 1985; 25:368.

101. Szymanski IO, Teno R, Rybak ME: Hemolytic anemia due to a mixture of low-titer IgG lambda and IgM lambda agglutinins reacting optimally at 22°C. Vox Sang 1986; 51:112.

102. McCann EL, Shirey RS, et al: IgM autoagglutinins in warm autoimmune hemolytic anemia: A poor prognostic feature. Acta Haematol 1992; 88:120.

103. Issitt PD: Applied Blood Group Serology. 3rd ed. Miami, Montgomery Scientific Publication, 1985, p 545.

104. Szymanski IO, Huff SR, et al: Erythrocyte sensitization with monomeric IgM in a patient with hemolytic anemia. Am J Hematol 1984; 17:71.

105. Barker RN, Casswell KM, et al: Identification of autoantigens in autoimmune haemolytic anaemia by a non-radioisotope immunoprecipitation method. Br J Haematol 1992; 82:126.

106. Leddy JP, Falany JL, et al: Erythrocyte membrane proteins reactive with human (warm-reacting) anti-red cell autoantibodies. J Clin Invest 1993; 91:1672.

107. Szymanski IO, Roberts PL, Rosenfield RE: Anti-A autoantibody with severe intravascular hemolysis. N Engl J Med 1976; 294:995.

108. Marsh WL, Oyen R, et al: Autoimmune hemolytic anemia and the Kell blood groups. Am J Hematol 1979; 7:155.

109. Wakui H, Imai H, et al: Autoantibody against erythrocyte protein 4.1 in a patient with autoimmune hemolytic anemia. Blood 1988; 72:408.

110. Shulman IA, Vengelen-Tyler V, et al: Autoanti-Ge associated with severe autoimmune hemolytic anemia. Vox Sang 1990; 59:232.

111. Owen I, Chowdhury V, et al: Autoimmune hemolytic anemia associated with anti-Sc1. Transfusion 1992; 32:173.

112. van't Veer MB, van Wieringen PMV, et al: A negative direct antiglobulin test with strong IgG red cell autoantibodies present in the serum of a patient with autoimmune haemolytic anaemia. Br J Haematol 1981; 49:383.

113. von dem Borne AE, Mol JJ, et al: Autoimmune haemolytic anemia with monoclonal IgM (K) anti-P cold autohaemolysins. Br J Haematol 1982; 50:345.

114. Longster GH, Johnson E: IgM anti-D as autoantibody in a case of "cold" autoimmune haemolytic anaemia. Vox Sang 1988; 54:174.

115. Rousey SR, Smith RE: A fatal case of low titer anti-Pr cold agglutinin disease. Am J Hematol 1990; 35:286.

116. Levine P, Celano MJ, Falkowski F: The specificity of the antibody in paroxysmal cold hemoglobinuria (P.C.H.). Transfusion 1963; 3:278.

117. Gallagher MT, Branch DR, et al: Evaluation of reticuloendothelial function in autoimmune hemolytic anemia using an *in vitro* assay of monocyte-macrophage interaction with erythrocytes. Exp Hematol 1983; 11:82.

118. Zupanska B, Brojer E, et al: Monocyte-erythrocyte interaction in autoimmune haemolytic anaemia in relation to the number of erythrocyte-bound IgG molecules and subclass specificity of autoantibodies. Vox Sang 1987; 52:212.

119. Garratty G, Nance SJ: Correlation between *in vivo* hemolysis and the amount of red cell-bound IgG measured by flow cytometry. Transfusion 1990; 30:617.

120. Zupanska B, Sokol RJ, et al: Erythrocyte autoantibodies, the monocyte monolayer assay and *in vivo* haemolysis. Br J Haematol 1993; 84:144.

121. Anderson CL, Looney RJ: Human leukocyte IgG Fc receptors. Immunol Today 1986; 7:264.

122. Ferreira JA, Feliu E, et al: Morphologic and morphometric light and electron microscopic studies of the spleen in patients with hereditary spherocytosis and autoimmune haemolytic anaemia. Br J Haematol 1989; 72:246.

123. Fischer JT, Petz LD, et al: Correlations between quantitative assay of red cell-bound C3, serologic reactions, and hemolytic anemia. Blood 1974; 44:359.

124. Logue GL, Rosse WF, Gockerman JP: Measurement of the third component of complement bound to red blood cells in patients with the cold agglutinin syndrome. J Clin Invest 1973; 52:493.

125. Jaffe CH, Atkinson JP, Frank MM: The role of complement in the clearance of cold agglutinin-sensitized erythrocytes in man. J Clin Invest 1976; 58:942.

126. Garratty G, Petz LD: Transfusing patients with autoimmune haemolytic anaemia. Lancet 1993; 341:1220.

127. Sokol RJ, Hewitt S, et al: Patients with red cell autoantibodies: selection of blood for transfusion. Clin Lab Haematol 1988; 10:257.

128. James P, Rowe GP, Tozzo GG: Elucidation of alloantibodies in autoimmune haemolytic anaemia. Vox Sang 1988; 54:167.

129. Petz LD: Transfusing the patient with autoimmune hemolytic anemia. Clin Lab Med 1982; 2:193.

130. Wallhermfechtel MA, Pohl BA, Chaplin H: Alloimmunization in patients with warm autoantibodies. A retrospective study employing three donor alloabsorptions to aid in antibody detection. Transfusion 1984; 24:482.

131. Salama A, Berghofer H, Mueller-Eckhardt C: Red blood cell transfusion in warm-type autoimmune haemolytic anaemia. Lancet 1992; 340:1515.

132. Dameshek W, Rosenthal MC, Schwartz LI: The treatment of acquired hemolytic anemia with adrenocorticotrophic hormone (ACTH). N Engl J Med 1951; 244:117.

133. Fries LF, Brickman CM, Frank MM: Monocyte receptors for the Fc portion of IgG increase in number in autoimmune hemolytic anemia and other hemolytic states and are decreased by glucocorticoid therapy. J Immunol 1983; 131:1240.

134. Collins PW, Newland AC: Treatment modalities of autoimmune blood disorders. Semin Hematol 1992; 29:64.

135. Meytes D, Adler M, et al: High dose methylprednisolone in acute immune cold hemolysis. N Engl J Med 1985; 312:318.

136. Ware R, Kinney TR: Therapeutic considerations in childhood idiopathic thrombocytopenic purpura. Crit Rev Oncol Hematol 1987; 7:169.

137. Fehr J, Hofmann V, Kappeler U: Transient reversal of thrombocytopenia in idiopathic thrombocytopenic purpura by high-dose intravenous gamma globulin. N Engl J Med 1982; 306:1254.

138. Salama A, Mueller-Eckhardt C, Kiefel V: Effect of intravenous immunoglobulin in immune thrombocytopenia: Competitive inhibition of reticuloendothelial system function by sequestration of autologous red blood cells? Lancet 1983; 2:193.

139. Mueller-Eckhardt C, Salama A, et al: Lack of efficacy of high-dose intravenous immunoglobulin in autoimmune hemolytic anemia: A clue to its mechanism. Scand J Hematol 1985; 34:394.

140. Hilgartner MW, Bussel J: Use of intravenous gamma globulin for the treatment of autoimmune neutropenia of childhood and autoimmune hemolytic anemia. Am J Med 1987; 83:25.

141. Flores G, Cunningham-Rundles C, et al: Efficacy of intravenous immunoglobulin in the treatment of autoimmune hemolytic anemia: Results in 73 patients. Am J Hematol 1993; 44:237.

142. Ware RE: The use of intravenous immunoglobulin in hematologic disorders. Semin Pediatr Infect Dis 1992; 3:179.

143. Klaesson S, Ringden O, et al: Immune modulatory effects of immunoglobulins on cell-mediated immune responses *in vitro*. Scand J Immunol 1993; 38:477.

144. Heidemann SM, Sarnaik SA, Sarnaik AP: Exchange transfusion for severe autoimmune hemolytic anemia. Am J Pediatr Hematol Oncol 1987; 9:302.

145. Bernstein ML, Schneider BK, Naiman JL: Plasma exchange in refractory acute autoimmune hemolytic anemia. J Pediatr 1981; 98:774.

146. Brooks BD, Steane EA, et al: Therapeutic plasma exchange in the immune hemolytic anemias and immunologic thrombocytopenic purpura. Prog Clin Biol Res 1982; 106:317.

147. Silberstein LE, Berkman EM: Plasma exchange in autoimmune hemolytic anemia (AIHA). J Clin Apheresis 1983; 1:238.

148. McConnell ME, Atchison JA, et al: Successful use of plasma exchange in a child with refractory immune hemolytic anemia. Am J Pediatr Hematol Oncol 1987; 9:158.

149. Fosburg M, Dolan M, et al: Intensive plasma exchange in small and critically ill pediatric patients: Techniques and clinical outcome. J Clin Apheresis 1983; 1:215.

150. Greuth M, Wagner HP, et al: Plasma exchange: An important part of the therapeutic procedure of a small child with autoimmune hemolytic anemia. Acta Pediatr Scand 1986; 75:1037.

151. Council on Scientific Affairs: Current status of therapeutic plasmapheresis and related techniques. Report of the AMA panel on therapeutic plasmapheresis. JAMA 1985; 253:819.

152. Andrzejewski C Jr, Gault E, et al: Benefit of a 37°C extracorporeal circuit in plasma exchange therapy for selected cases with cold agglutinin disease. J Clin Apheresis 1988; 4:13.

153. Chertkow G, Davie JV: Results of splenectomy in auto-immune haemolytic anaemia. Br J Haematol 1956; 2:237.

154. Dacie JV: Autoimmune hemolytic anaemia. Arch Intern Med 1975; 135:1293.

155. Mollison PL: Survival curves of incompatible red cells. An analytical review. Transfusion 1986; 26:43.

156. Parker AC, Macpherson AIS, Richmond J: Value of radiochromium investigation in autoimmune haemolytic anaemia. BMJ 1977; 1:208.

157. Coon WW: Splenectomy in the treatment of hemolytic anemia. Arch Surg 1985; 120:625.

158. Chan AC, Sack K: Danazol therapy in autoimmune hemolytic anemia associated with systemic lupus erythematosus. J Rheumatol 1991; 18:280.

159. Pignon J-M, Poirson E, Rochant H: Danazol in autoimmune haemolytic anaemia. Br J Haematol 1993; 83:343.

160. Agnello V, Pariser K, et al: Preliminary observations on danazol therapy of systemic lupus erythematosus: Effects on DNA antibodies, thrombocytopenia and complement. Rheumatol 1983; 10:682.

161. Gertz MA, Petitt RM, et al: Vinblastine-loaded platelets for autoimmune hemolytic anemia. Ann Intern Med 1981; 95:325.

162. Medellin PL, Patten E, Weiss GB: Vinblastine for autoimmune hemolytic anemia. Ann Intern Med 1982; 96:123.

163. Seiber SM, Adamson RH: Toxicity of antineoplastic agents in man: Chromosomal aberrations, antifertility effects, congenital malformations, and carcinogenic potential. Adv Cancer Res 1975; 22:57.

164. Dundar S, Ozdemir O, Ozcebe O: Cyclosporin in steroid-resistant autoimmune haemolytic anaemia. Acta Haematol 1991; 86:200.

165. O'Connor BM, Clifford JS, et al: Alpha-interferon for severe cold agglutinin disease. Ann Intern Med 1989; 111:255.

166. Berney T, Shibata T, et al: Murine autoimmune hemolytic anemia resulting from Fcγ receptor-mediated erythrophagocytosis: Protection by erythropoietin but not by interleukin-3, and ag-

gravation by granulocyte-macrophage colony-stimulating factor. Blood 1992; 79:2960.

167. Abdel-Khalik A, Paton L, et al: Human leucocyte antigens A, B, C, and DRW in idiopathic "warm" autoimmune haemolytic anaemia. BMJ 1980; 280:760.

168. Kleiner-Baumgarten A, Schlaeffer F, Keynan A: Multiple autoimmune manifestations in a splenectomized subject with HLA-B8. Arch Intern Med 1983; 143:1987.

169. Lortholary O, Valeyre D, et al: Autoimmune haemolytic anaemia and idiopathic pulmonary fibrosis associated with HLA-B27 antigen. Eur J Haematol 1990; 45:112.

170. Lippman SM, Arnett FC, et al: Genetic factors predisposing to autoimmune diseases. Autoimmune hemolytic anemia, chronic thrombocytopenic purpura, and systemic lupus erythematosus. Am J Med 1982; 73:827.

171. Silberstein LE, Robertson GA, et al: Etiologic aspects of cold agglutinin disease: Evidence for cytogenetically defined clones of lymphoid cells and the demonstration that an anti-Pr cold autoantibody is derived from a chromosomally aberrant B cell clone. Blood 1986; 67:1705.

172. Gordon J, Silberstein L, et al: Trisomy 3 in cold agglutinin disease. Cancer Genet Cytogenet 1990; 46:89.

173. Haneberg B, Matre R, et al: Acute hemolytic anemia related to diphtheria-pertussis-tetanus vaccination. Acta Paediatr Scand 1978; 67:345.

174. Stevenson FK, Smith GJ, et al: Identification of normal B-cell counterparts of neoplastic cells which secrete cold agglutinins of anti-I and anti-i specificity. Br J Haematol 1989; 72:9.

175. Stellrecht KA, Vella AT: Evidence for polyclonal B cell activation as the mechanism for LCMB-induced autoimmune hemolytic anemia. Immunol Lett 1992; 31:273.

176. Reininger L, Shibata T, et al: Spontaneous production of anti-mouse red blood cell autoantibodies is independent of the polyclonal activation in NZB mice. Eur J Immunol 1990; 20:2405.

177. Scott BB, Sadigh S, et al: Molecular mechanisms resulting in pathogenic anti-mouse erythrocyte antibodies in New Zealand black mice. Clin Exp Immunol 1993; 93:26.

178. Sanz I, Casali P, et al: Nucleotide sequences of eight human natural autoantibody V_H regions reveals apparent restricted use of V_H families. J Immunol 1989; 142:4054.

179. Silverman GJ, Carson DA: Structural characterization of human monoclonal cold agglutinins: Evidence for a distinct primary sequence-defined V_H4 idiotype. Eur J Immunol 1990; 20:351.

180. Friedman DF, Cho EA, et al: The role of clonal selection in the pathogenesis of an autoreactive human B cell lymphoma. J Exp Med 1991; 174:525.

181. Silberstein LE, Jefferies LC, et al: Variable region gene analysis of pathologic human autoantibodies to the related i and I red blood cell antigens. Blood 1991; 78:2372.

182. Andrzejewski C, Young PJ, et al: Production of human warm-reacting red cell monoclonal autoantibodies by Epstein-Barr virus transformation. Transfusion 1989; 29:196.

183. Shoenfeld Y, Hsu-Lin SC, et al: Production of autoantibodies by human-human hybridomas. J Clin Invest 1982; 70:205.

184. Parkman R: Cellular basis of autoimmune hemolytic anemia. Am J Pediatr Hematol Oncol 1981; 3:105.

185. Parker AC, Stuart AE, Dewar AE: Activated T-cells in autoimmune haemolytic anaemia. Br J Haematol 1977; 36:337.

186. Phan-Dinh-Tuy F, Habibi R, et al: T cell subpopulations defined by monoclonal antibodies in autoimmune hemolytic anemia. Biomed Pharmacother 1983; 37:75.

187. Conte R, Tazzari PL, Finelli C: Deficiency of autologous mixed lymphocyte reaction in patients with idiopathic autoimmune hemolytic anemia. Vox Sang 1985; 49:285.

188. Soyano A, Romano E, Linares J: Abnormal generation of concanavalin A—induced suppressor cell function in human autoimmune hemolytic anemia. Clin Immunol Immunopathol 1982; 23:70.

189. Horowitz SD, Borcherding W, Hong R: Autoimmune hemolytic anemia as a manifestation of T-suppressor-cell deficiency. Clin Immunol Immunopathol 1984; 33:313.

190. Calkins CE, Cochran SA, et al: Evidence for regulation of the autoimmune antierythrocyte response by idiotype-specific suppressor T cells in NZB mice. Int Immunol 1990; 2:127.

191. Young JL, Hooper DC: Characterization of autoreactive helper T cells in a murine model of autoimmune haemolytic disease. Immunology 1993; 80:13.

192. Albrechtsen D, Solheim BG, et al: Autoimmune haemolytic anemia in cyclosporine-treated organ allograft recipients. Transplant Proc 1988; 20:959.

193. Sniecinski IJ, Oien L, et al: Immunohematologic consequences of major ABO-mismatched bone marrow transplantation. Transplantation 1988; 45:530.

194. Solheim BG, Albrechtsen D, et al: Auto-antibodies against erythrocytes in transplant patients produced by donor lymphocytes. Transplant Proc 1987; 19:4520.

195. Tamura T, Kanamori H, et al: Cold agglutinin disease following allogeneic bone marrow transplantation. Bone Marrow Transplant 1994; 13:321.

196. Puppo F, Torresin A, et al: Autoimmune hemolytic anemia and human immunodeficiency virus (HIV) infection. Ann Intern Med 1988; 1:249.

197. Scadden DT, Zon LI, Groopman JE: Pathophysiology and management of HIV-associated hematologic disorders. Blood 1988; 74:1455.

198. Fong KY, Loisou S, et al: Anticardiolipin antibodies, haemolytic anaemia and thrombocytopenia in systemic lupus erythematosus. Br J Rheumatol 1992; 31:453.

199. Boling EP, Wen J, et al: Primary Sjögren's syndrome and autoimmune hemolytic anemia in sisters. Am J Med 1983; 74:1066.

200. Kondo H, Sakai S, Sakai Y: Autoimmune haemolytic anaemia, Sjögren's syndrome and idiopathic thrombocytopenic purpura in a patient with sarcoidosis. Acta Haematol 1993; 89:209.

201. Jones E, Jones JV, et al: Scleroderma and hemolytic anemia in a patient with deficiency of IgA and C4: A hitherto undescribed association. J Rheumatol 1987; 14:609.

202. Kay EM, Makris M, et al: Evans' syndrome associated with dermatomyositis. Ann Rheum Dis 1990; 49:793.

203. Veloso T, Fraga J, et al: Autoimmune hemolytic anemia in ulcerative colitis. A case report with review of the literature. J Clin Gastroenterol 1991; 13:445.

204. Yates P, Macht LM, et al: Red cell autoantibody production by colonic mononuclear cells from a patient with ulcerative colitis and autoimmune haemolytic anaemia. Br J Haematol 1992; 82:753.

205. Fagiolo E: Platelet and leukocyte antibodies in autoimmune hemolytic anemia. Acta Haematol 1976; 56:97.

206. Miller BA, Beardsley DS: Autoimmune pancytopenia of childhood associated with multisystem disease manifestations. J Pediatr 1983; 103:877.

207. Pui C-H, Wilimas J, Wang W: Evans syndrome in childhood. J Pediatr 1980; 97:754.

208. Wang W, Herrod H, et al: Immunoregulatory abnormalities in Evans Syndrome. Am J Hematol 1983; 15:381.

209. Pegels JG, Helmerhorst FM, et al: The Evans syndrome: Characterization of the responsible autoantibodies. Br J Haematol 1982; 51:445.

210. Kuipers EJ, van Imhoff GW, et al: Anti-H IgM (kappa) autoantibody mediated severe intravascular haemolysis associated with malignant lymphoma. Br J Haematol 1991; 78:283.

211. Sthoeger ZM, Sthoeger D, et al: Mechanism of autoimmune hemolytic anemia in chronic lymphocytic leukemia. Am J Hematol 1993; 43:259.

212. Crisp D, Pruzanski W: B-cell neoplasms with homogeneous cold-reacting antibodies (cold agglutinins). Am J Med 1982; 72:915.

213. Pereira A, Mazzara R, et al: Anti-Sa cold agglutinin of IgA class requiring plasma-exchange therapy as early manifestation of multiple myeloma. Ann Hematol 1993; 66:315.

214. Kedar A, Khan AB, et al: Autoimmune disorders complicating adolescent Hodgkin's disease. Cancer 1979; 44:112.

215. Chu J-Y: Autoimmune hemolytic anemia in childhood Hodgkin's disease. Am J Pediatr Hematol Oncol 1982; 4:125.

216. Xiros N, Binder T, et al: Idiopathic thrombocytopenic purpura and autoimmune hemolytic anemia in Hodgkin's disease. Eur J Haematol 1988; 40:437.

217. Strickland DK, Ware RE: Urticarial vasculitis: An autoimmune disorder following therapy for Hodgkin's disease. Med Pediatr Oncol 1995; 25:208.

218. Arbaje YM, Beltran G: Chronic myelogenous leukemia complicated by autoimmune hemolytic anemia. Am J Med 1990; 88:197.

219. Sokol RJ, Hewitt S, Booker DJ: Erythrocyte autoantibodies, autoimmune haemolysis, and myelodysplastic syndromes. J Clin Pathol 1989; 42:1088.

220. Blanchette VS, Hallett JJ, et al: Abnormalities of the peripheral blood as a presenting feature of immunodeficiency. Am J Hematol 1978; 4:87.

221. Rich KC, Arnold WJ, et al: Cellular immune deficiency with autoimmune hemolytic anemia in purine nucleoside phosphorylase deficiency. Am J Med 1979; 67:172.

222. Leickly FE, Buckley RH: Successful treatment of autoimmune hemolytic anemia in common variable immunodeficiency with high-dose intravenous gamma globulin. Am J Med 1987; 82:159.

223. Bapat AR, Schuster SJ, et al: Thrombocytopenia and autoimmune hemolytic anemia following renal transplantation. Transplantation 1987; 44:157.

224. Murray HW, Masur H, et al: The protean manifestations of *Mycoplasma pneumoniae* infection in adults. Am J Med 1975; 58:229.

225. Rosenfield RE, Schmidt PJ, et al: Anti-i, a frequent cold agglutinin in infectious mononucleosis. Vox Sang 1965; 10:631.

226. Rollof J, Eklund PO: Infectious mononucleosis complicated by severe immune hemolysis. Eur J Haematol 1989; 43:81.

227. Miyazaki S, Ohtsuka M, et al: Coombs positive hemolytic anemia in congenital rubella. J Pediatr 1979; 94:759.

228. Burstein Y, Berns L: Acquired immune hemolytic anemia in children. Pediatr Ann 1982; 11:301.

229. Boccardi V, D'Annibali S, et al: *Mycoplasma pneumoniae* infection complicated by paroxysmal cold hemoglobinuria with anti-P specificity of biphasic hemolysin. Blut 1977; 34:211.

230. Costea N, Yakulis VJ, Heller P: Inhibition of cold agglutinins (anti-I) by *M. pneumoniae* antigens. Proc Soc Exp Biol Med 1972; 139:476.

231. Richard KA, Robinson RJ, et al: Acute acquired haemolytic anaemia associated with polyagglutination. Arch Dis Child 1969; 44:102.

232. Williams RA, Brown EF, et al: Transfusion of infants with activation of T antigen. J Pediatr 1989; 115:949.

233. Murphy WG, Kelton JG: Methyldopa-induced autoantibodies against red blood cells. Blood Rev 1988; 2:36.

234. Petz LD: Drug-induced immune haemolytic anaemia. Clin Haematol 1980; 9:455.

235. Petz LD, Fudenberg HH: Coombs-positive hemolytic anemia caused by penicillin administration. N Engl J Med 1966; 274:171.

236. Seldon MR, Bain B, et al: Ticarcillin-induced immune haemolytic anaemia. Scand J Haematol 1982; 28:459.

237. Molthan L, Reidenberg MM, Eichman MF: Positive direct Coombs tests due to cephalothin. N Engl J Med 1967; 277:123.

238. Branch DR, Berkowitz LR, et al: Extravascular hemolysis following the administration of cefamandole. Am J Hematol 1985; 18:213.

239. Simpson MB, Pryzbylik J, et al: Hemolytic anemia after tetracycline therapy. N Engl J Med 1985; 312:840.

240. Wong KY, Boose GM, Issitt CH: Erythromycin-induced hemolytic anemia. J Pediatr 1981; 98:647.

241. Sosler SD, Behzad O, et al: Immune hemolytic anemia associated with probenecid. Am J Clin Pathol 1985; 84:391.

242. Manor E, Marmor A, et al: Massive hemolysis caused by acetaminophen. JAMA 1976; 236:2777.

243. Korsager S, Sorensen H, et al: Antiglobulin-tests for detection of auto-immunohaemolytic anaemia during long-term treatment with ibuprofen. Scand J Rheumatol 1981; 10:174.

244. Salama A, Mueller-Eckhardt C: On the mechanisms of sensitization and attachment of antibodies to RBC in drug-induced immune hemolytic anemia. Blood 1987; 69:1006.

245. Packman CH, Leddy JP: Drug-related immunologic injury of erythrocytes. In Williams WJ, Beutler E, et al (eds): Hematology. 4th ed. New York, McGraw-Hill Book Co., 1990, p 681.

246. Gull WW: A case of intermittent haematinuria, with remarks. Guy's Hosp Rep 1866; 12:381.

247. Strubing P: Paroxysmale Haemoglobinurie. Dtsch Med Wochenschr 1882; 8:1.

248. Ham TH: Chronic hemolytic anemia with paroxysmal nocturnal hemoglobinuria. A study of the mechanism of hemolysis in relation to acid-base equilibrium. N Engl J Med 1937; 217:915.

249. Ham TH: Studies on the destruction of red blood cells. I. Chronic hemolytic anemia with paroxysmal nocturnal hemoglobinuria: An investigation of the mechanism of hemolysis with observations on five cases. Arch Intern Med 1939; 64:127

250. Ham TH, Dingle JH: Studies on destruction of red blood cells. II. Chronic hemolytic anemia with paroxysmal nocturnal hemoglobinuria: Certain immunological aspects of the hemolytic mechanism with special reference to serum complement. J Clin Invest 1939; 18:657.

251. Rosse WF, Dacie JV: Immune lysis of normal human and paroxysmal nocturnal hemoglobinuria red blood cells. I. The sensitivity of PNH red cells to lysis by complement and specific antibody. J Clin Invest 1966; 45:736.

252. Rosse WF: Variations in the red cells in paroxysmal nocturnal hemoglobinuria. Br J Haematol 1973; 24:327.

253. Rosse WF, Adams JP, Thorpe AM: The population of cells in paroxysmal nocturnal hemoglobinuria of intermediate sensitivity to complement lysis–significance and mechanism of increased immune lysis. Br J Haematol 1974; 28:181.

254. Rosse WF: Evolution of clinical understanding: Paroxysmal nocturnal hemoglobinuria as a paradigm. Am J Hematol 1993; 42:122.

255. Devine DV, Gluck WL, et al: Acute myeloblastic leukemia in paroxysmal nocturnal hemoglobinuria: Evidence of evolution for the abnormal paroxysmal nocturnal hemoglobinuria clone. J Clin Invest 1987; 79:314.

256. Ware RE, Hall SG, Rosse WF: Paroxysmal nocturnal hemoglobinuria with onset in childhood and adolescence. N Engl J Med 1991; 325:991.

257. Antin JH, Ginsburg D, et al: Bone marrow transplantation for paroxysmal nocturnal hemoglobinuria: Eradication of the PNH clone and documentation of complete lymphohematopoietic engraftment. Blood 1985; 66:1247.

258. Kawahara K, Witherspoon RP, Storb R: Marrow transplantation for paroxysmal nocturnal hemoglobinuria. Am J Hematol 1992; 39:283.

258a. Hillman P, Lewis SM, et al: Natural history of paroxysmal nocturnal hemoglobinuria. N Engl J Med 1995; 333:1253.

259. Medof ME, Walter EI, et al: Decay accelerating factor of complement is anchored to cells by a C-terminal glycolipid. Biochemistry 1986; 25:6740.

260. Stefanova I, Hilgert I, et al: Characterization of a broadly expressed human leucocyte surface antigen MEM43 anchored in membrane through phosphatidylinositol. Mol Immunol 1989; 26:153.

261. Low MG: Biochemistry of the glycosylphosphatidyl-inositol membrane protein anchors. Biochem J 1987; 244:1.

262. Low MG, Saltiel AR: Structural and functional roles of glycosylphosphatidylinositol in membranes. Science 1988; 239:268.

263. Bangs JD, Hereld D, et al: Rapid processing of the carboxyl terminus of a trypanosome variant surface glycoprotein. Biochemistry 1985; 82:3207.

264. Low MG, Zilversmit DB: Role of phosphatidylinositol in attachment of alkaline phosphatase to membranes. Biochemistry 1980; 19:3913.

265. Haas R, Brandt PT, et al: Identification of amine components in a glycolipid membrane-binding domain at the C-terminus of human erythrocyte acetylcholinesterase. Biochemistry 1986; 25:3098.

266. Fatemi SH, Haas R, et al: The glyco-phospholipid anchor of Thy-1. J Biol Chem 1987; 262:4728.

267. Dustin ML, Selvaraj P, et al: Anchoring mechanisms for LFA-3 cell adhesion glycoprotein at membrane surface. Nature 1987; 329:846.

268. Selvaraj P, Rosse WF, et al: The major Fc receptor in blood has a phosphatidylinositol anchor and is deficient in paroxysmal nocturnal hemoglobinuria. Nature 1988; 333:565.

269. Reiser H, Oettgen H, et al: Structural characterization of the TAP molecule: A phosphatidylinositol-linked glycoprotein distinct from the T cell receptor T3 complex and Thy-1. Cell 1986; 47:365.

270. Stiernberg J, Low MG, et al: Removal of lymphocyte surface molecules with phosphatidylinositol-specific phospholipase C: Effects on mitogen responses and evidence that ThB and certain Qa antigens are membrane-anchored via phosphatidylinositol. J Immunol 1987; 38:3877.

271. Ishihara A, Hou Y, Jacobson K: The Thy-1 antigen exhibits rapid

lateral diffusion in the plasma membrane of rodent lymphoid cells and fibroblasts. Proc Natl Acad Sci U S A 1987; 84:1290.

272. Noda M, Yoon K, et al: High lateral mobility of endogenous and transfected alkaline phosphatase: A phosphatidylinositol-anchored membrane protein. J Cell Biol 1987; 105:1671.

273. Romero G, Luttrell L, et al: Phosphatidyl-inositol-glycan anchors of membrane proteins: Potential precursors of insulin mediators. Science 1988; 240:509.

274. Yeh ETH, Reiser H, et al: TAP transcription and phosphatidyl-inositol linkage mutants are defective in activation through the T cell receptor. Cell 1988; 52:665.

275. Presky DH, Low MG, Shevach EM: Role of phosphatidylinositol-anchored proteins in T cell activation. J Immunol 1990; 144:860.

276. Roy-Choudhury S, Mishra VS, et al: A phospholipid is the membrane-anchoring domain of a protein growth factor of molecular mass 34 kDa in placental trophoblasts. Proc Natl Acad Sci U S A 1988; 85:2014.

277. Auditore JV, Hartmann RC, et al: The erythrocyte acetylcholinesterase enzyme in paroxysmal nocturnal hemoglobinuria. Arch Pathol 1960; 69:534.

278. Tanaka KR, Valentine WN, Fredricks RE: Diseases or clinical conditions associated with low leukocyte alkaline phosphatase. N Engl J Med 1960; 262:912.

279. Nicholson-Weller A, March JP, et al: Affected erythrocytes of patients with paroxysmal nocturnal hemoglobinuria are deficient in the complement regulatory protein, decay accelerating factor. Proc Natl Acad Sci U S A 1983; 80:5066.

280. Selvaraj P, Dustin ML, et al: Deficiency of lymphocyte function-associated antigen 3 (LFA-3) in paroxysmal nocturnal hemoglobinuria. J Exp Med 1987; 166:1011.

281. Holguin MH, Fredrick LR, et al: Isolation and characterization of a membrane protein from normal human erythrocytes that inhibits reactive lysis of the erythrocytes of paroxysmal nocturnal hemoglobinuria. J Clin Invest 1989; 84:7.

282. Simmons DL, Tan S, et al: Monocyte antigen CD14 is a phospholipid anchored membrane protein. Blood 1989; 73:284.

283. Rosse, WF: Phosphatidylinositol-linked proteins and paroxysmal nocturnal hemoglobinuria. Blood 1990; 75:1595.

284. Hirose S, Ravi L, et al: Synthesis of mannosylglucosaminylinositol phospholipids in normal but not paroxysmal nocturnal hemoglobinuria cells. Proc Natl Acad Sci U S A 1992; 89:6025.

285. Mahoney JF, Urakaze M, et al: Defective glycosylphosphatidylinositol anchor synthesis in paroxysmal nocturnal hemoglobinuria granulocytes. Blood 1992; 79:1400.

286. Takahashi M, Takeda J, et al: Deficient biosynthesis of N-acetylglucosaminyl-phosphatidylinositol, the first intermediate of glycosyl phosphatidylinositol anchor biosynthesis, in cell lines established from patients with paroxysmal nocturnal hemoglobinuria. J Exp Med 1993; 177:517.

287. Hillmen P, Bessler M, et al: Specific defect in N-acetylglucosamine incorporation in the biosynthesis of the glycosylphosphatidylinositol anchor in cloned cell lines from patients with paroxysmal nocturnal hemoglobinuria. Proc Natl Acad Sci U S A 1993; 90:5272.

288. Hyman R: Somatic genetic analysis of the expression of cell surface molecules. Trends Genet 1988; 4:5.

289. Sugiyama E, DeGasperi R, et al: Identification of defects in glycosylphosphatidylinositol anchor biosynthesis in the Thy-1 expression mutants. J Biol Chem 1991; 266:12119.

290. Armstrong C, Schubert J, et al: Affected paroxysmal nocturnal hemoglobinuria T lymphocytes harbor a common defect in assembly of N-acetyl-D-glucosamine inositol phospholipid corresponding to that in Class A Thy-1⁻ murine lymphoma mutants. J Biol Chem 1992; 267:25347.

291. Norris J, Hoffman S, et al: Glycosyl-phosphatidylinositol anchor synthesis in paroxysmal nocturnal hemoglobinuria: Partial or complete defect in an early step. Blood 1994; 83:816.

292. Yeh ETH, Rosse WF: Paroxysmal nocturnal hemoglobinuria and the glycosylphosphatidylinositol anchor. J Clin Invest 1994; 93:2305.

293. Schubert J, Alvarado M, et al: Diagnosis of paroxysmal nocturnal hemoglobinuria using immunophenotyping of peripheral blood cells. Br J Haematol 1991; 79:487.

294. Hall SE, Rosse WF: The use of monoclonal antibodies and flow cytometry in the diagnosis of paroxysmal nocturnal hemoglobinuria. Blood 1996; 87:5332.

295. Ware RE, Rosse WF, Hall SE: Immunophenotypic analysis of reticulocytes in paroxysmal nocturnal hemoglobinuria. Blood 1995; 86:1586.

296. Oni SB, Osunkoya BO, Luzzato L: Paroxysmal nocturnal hemoglobinuria: Evidence for monoclonal origin of abnormal red cells. Blood 1970; 36:145.

297. Josten KM, Tooze JA, et al: Acquired aplastic anemia and paroxysmal nocturnal hemoglobinuria: Studies on clonality. Blood 1991; 78:3162.

298. Ohashi H, Hotta T, et al: Peripheral blood cells are predominantly chimeric of affected and normal cells in patients with paroxysmal nocturnal hemoglobinuria: Simultaneous investigation on clonality and expression of glycophosphatidylinositol-anchored proteins. Blood 1994; 83:853.

299. Tseng JE, Hall SE, et al: Phenotypic and functional analysis of lymphocytes in paroxysmal nocturnal hemoglobinuria. Am J Hematol 1995; 50:244.

300. Nicholson-Weller A, Russian DA, Austen KF: Natural killer cells are deficient in the surface expression of the complement regulatory protein, decay accelerating factor (DAF). J Immunol 1986; 137:1275.

301. Miyata T, Takeda J, et al: The cloning of PIG-A, a component in the early step of GPI-anchor biosynthesis. Science 1993; 259:1318.

302. Takeda J, Miyata T, Kawagoe K: Deficiency of the GPI anchor caused by a somatic mutation of the PIG-A gene in paroxysmal nocturnal hemoglobinuria. Cell 1993; 73:703.

303. Bessler M, Mason PJ, et al: Paroxysmal nocturnal haemoglobinuria (PNH) is caused by somatic mutations in the PIG-A gene. EMBO J 1994; 13:110.

304. Miyata T, Yamada N, et al: Abnormalities of PIG-A transcripts in granulocytes from patients with paroxysmal nocturnal hemoglobinuria. N Engl J Med 1994; 330:249.

305. Schwartz RS: PIG-A: the target gene in paroxysmal nocturnal hemoglobinuria. N Engl J Med 1994; 330:283.

306. Ware RE, Rosse WF, Howard TA: Mutations within the Piga gene in patients with paroxysmal nocturnal hemoglobinuria. Blood 1994; 83:2418.

307. Bessler M, Mason PJ, et al: Mutations in the PIG-A gene causing partial deficiency of GPI-linked surface proteins (PNH II) in patients with paroxysmal nocturnal hemoglobinuria. Br J Haematol 1994; 87:863.

308. Yamada N, Miyata T, et al: Somatic mutations of the PIG-A gene found in Japanese patients with paroxysmal nocturnal hemoglobinuria. Blood 1995; 85:885.

309. Ostendorf T, Nischan C, et al: Heterogeneous PIG-A mutations in different cell lineages in paroxysmal nocturnal hemoglobinuria. Blood 1995; 85:1640.

310. Rosse WF, Ware RE: The molecular basis of paroxysmal nocturnal hemoglobinuria. Blood 1995; 86:3277.

311. Ware RE, Howard TA, et al: Chromosomal assignment of genes involved in glycosylphosphatidylinositol anchor biosynthesis: Implications for the pathogenesis of paroxysmal nocturnal hemoglobinuria. Blood 1994; 83:3753.

312. Wiedmer T, Hall SE, et al: Complement-induced vesiculation and exposure of membrane prothrombinase sites in platelets of paroxysmal nocturnal hemoglobinuria. Blood 1993; 82:1192.

313. Ploug M, Plesner T, et al: The receptor for urokinase-type plasminogen activator is deficient on peripheral blood leukocytes in patients with paroxysmal nocturnal hemoglobinuria. Blood 1992; 79:1447.

314. Griscelli-Bennaceur A, Gluckman E, et al: Aplastic anemia and paroxysmal nocturnal hemoglobinuria: Search for a pathogenetic link. Blood 1995; 85:1354.

315. Rosse WF: Paroxysmal nocturnal hemoglobinuria in aplastic anemia. Clin Haematol 1985; 14:105.

316. Lewis SM, Dacie JV: The aplastic anaemia-paroxysmal nocturnal haemoglobinuria syndrome. Br J Haematol 1967; 13:236.

317. Schubert J, Vogt HG, et al: Development of the glycosylphosphatidylinositol-anchoring defect characteristic for paroxysmal nocturnal hemoglobinuria in patients with aplastic anemia. Blood 1994; 83:2323.

318. Bessler M, Mason P, et al: Somatic mutations and cellular selection in paroxysmal nocturnal haemoglobinuria. Lancet 1994; 343:951.

Destruction of Red Cells by the Vasculature and Reticuloendothelial System

Lisa G. Payne • Catherine P. M. Hayward
John G. Kelton

Red blood cells enter the circulation from the bone marrow as reticulocytes. Because their surface properties differ from mature red cells, their first 1 to 2 days are spent in the pulp of the spleen. Once the reticulocytes have remaining cytoplasmic organelles removed by the cells of the reticuloendothelial (RE) system, they exit the spleen as mature red blood cells with a life span of about 120 days.[1] "Senescent" red blood cells are removed from the circulation by the phagocytic cells of the RE system. To survive in the circulation, the red blood cells must withstand the physical stresses produced by the rapid blood flow in the heart and arteries and the repetitive deformation they undergo to pass through the capillaries of the microcirculation. *Hemolytic anemia* is defined as a shortened red blood cell survival and can be due to either intrinsic defects in the red blood cells (usually hereditary) or external factors. The red blood cells can be destroyed either within the circulation (intravascular hemolysis) or by

RE cells that are outside the circulation (extravascular hemolysis).

The focus of this chapter is a discussion of the destruction of red blood cells by the vasculature and RE system.

OVERVIEW OF THE STRUCTURE AND FUNCTION OF THE RETICULOENDOTHELIAL SYSTEM

The term *reticuloendothelial system* was introduced by Aschoff in 1924 to describe specialized cells found throughout the body. These cells are characterized by their ability to phagocytose particulate material in blood.[2] The name is a misnomer because the cells of this system, the monocytes and monocyte-derived tissue macrophages, neither form reticulum nor are derived from endothelium.[3] Nevertheless, the term is used in this chapter because it has led to an understanding of the cellular origin and function of these cells.[4-6]

RE cells are mesenchyme-derived cells distributed throughout the body, with the highest concentrations found in the spleen. Lower concentrations are present in the lungs, liver, and bone marrow. RE cells include monocytes, macrophages, histiocytes, Kupffer's cells, and osteoclasts. The RE system has a number of important functions, including antigen processing and the generation of an early immune response, iron clearance, removal of antibody and complement-sensitized cells, and removal of senescent cells. The RE system performs a number of important physiologic functions in the regulation of hematopoiesis. Perhaps its most important job is scavenging. RE cells remove abnormal red blood cells from the bone marrow in disorders accompanied by ineffective erythropoiesis.[7-9] After phagocytosis by the RE cells, the red blood cells are lysed and digested to yield amino acids, iron, and bilirubin. The amino acids and iron enter their respective metabolic pools for reutilization. The bilirubin is returned to the circulation for transport to the liver, where it is conjugated and excreted in the bile.

The survival of red blood cells in the circulation is markedly reduced in all hemolytic anemias, with a corresponding increase in the ability of the RE system to remove and, in most situations, to destroy the abnormal red blood cells. A compensatory proliferative response by the phagocytic cells in the spleen results in splenic hypertrophy.[10, 11] Certain diseases associated with splenic enlargement result in increased sequestration, phagocytosis, and destruction of normal red blood cells, which can result in both anemia and shortened red blood cell survival. In other diseases, altered splenic filtration is secondary to microcirculatory changes, which results in increased splenic clearance of red blood cells in the absence of detectable splenic hypertrophy.[12] The association of splenomegaly with some of these situations and functional "hypersplenism" is discussed in greater detail in Chapter 26.

RETICULOENDOTHELIAL CELL-MEDIATED RED CELL CLEARANCE

The RE cell plays a major role in both physiologic and pathologic red cell clearance.

Physiologic Clearance: Senescent Red Blood Cells

The interactions between red blood cells and RE cells depend in part on the size, shape, and deformability of the red blood cells, as well as on the "occupants" of the cell membrane receptors (e.g., complement and immunoglobulins). As red cells age they progressively lose volume, leading to increased density, reduced deformability, and increased osmotic fragility. These changes are a consequence of electrolyte loss and microvesiculation.[13] In addition, enzymatic activities decrease and lipid peroxidation products accumulate.

Phosphatidylserine, which is usually found on the internal red blood cell membrane, is externalized on senescent red blood cells, possibly due to age-dependent rearrangements in the membrane lipid transport mechanisms.[14] Cells that express phosphatidylserine in their outer membrane surface are cleared by the spleen through endocytosis by macrophages and monocytes.[14]

Other signals have been suggested to trigger the removal of senescent red blood cells from the circulation. Kay and co-workers[15] proposed that senescent red cells are cleared from the circulation because of the exposure of a "senescent antigen" on the cell membrane that reacts with naturally occurring IgG. In support of the hypothesis, the IgG eluted from senescent red blood cells has been shown to preferentially rebind to senescent red cells.[16] This senescent antigen has now been identified as band 3, an integral protein of the red cell membrane.[17-21] The phagocytosis of senescent red blood cells can be enhanced by naturally occurring anti–band 3 antibodies (IgG) through increased binding of complement to the red blood cell surface,[21, 22] and the complement-activating properties of the IgG.[23] The change in band 3 that produces the age-dependent antigenic changes is unknown. It has been postulated that proteolytic cleavage of band 3 may produce the senescent antigen[24] or that the antigen may be formed by the oligomerization of band 3.[16] Based on these studies, it appears that several mechanisms may be involved in the clearance of senescent red blood cells. Because the red blood cells expressing phosphatidylserine on their outer membrane are cleared in antibody-deficient mice with severe combined immunodeficiency, antibody-independent mechanisms must exist.[14]

Similar mechanisms involving senescent antigens may be involved in the clearance of other circulating cells. Small, low-density platelets from healthy individuals (the oldest platelets) have been shown to have large amounts of IgG on their surfaces.[25] In patients with sickle cell anemia, increased red blood cell IgG has been observed.[26, 27] Thus, increased IgG binding and RE phagocytosis may represent a ubiquitous clearance mechanism, with respect to both cells and disease states.

Pathologic Clearance: Autoimmune Hemolytic Anemia

IgG-sensitized red blood cells are cleared by RE cells throughout the body. The spleen is important but not the only determinant, as shown by the normal life span of red cells after splenectomy. Complement-fixing antibodies cause destruction of the red blood cells in three ways: (1) many complement components are potent opsonins; (2) partial phagocytosis initiated by complement can alter the red cell membrane leading to red cell clearance; and (3) complement can lead to cell lysis, a dramatic, but uncommon endpoint.[28]

Complement-coated red blood cells are cleared by C3b receptors on liver monocytes and macrophages,[29] whereas cells coated with IgG are primarily sequestered within the spleen.[30] Red cells coated with both

IgG and C3b are phagocytosed more efficiently than those coated by either IgG or C3b alone. Red cells sensitized by IgG are often cleared, whereas complement sensitized red cells are initially sequestered (within the liver) but most eventually return to the circulation.[30] This release is postulated to be due to degradation of the cell-associated C3b to C3d; this change causes the cells to "break free" because there are C3b but no C3d receptors on macrophages. Although C3d levels increase with the age of the cell, no evidence exists that this contributes to increased rigidity of the red cell membrane or to accelerated clearance.

THE SPLEEN AND RETICULOENDOTHELIAL CELL FUNCTION

The greatest concentration of RE cells is within the spleen, and in the following section a very brief overview of splenic RE activity is presented. A more detailed discussion is found in Chapter 26.

Anatomy of the Spleen

The spleen is rich in lymphatic and RE tissue, which reflects its function both as a clearance organ and as an organ important in immune response. Consistent with its importance, the spleen receives a disproportionately large share of the total cardiac output (about 6%). The arterial blood enters the spleen through the splenic artery. The splenic artery branches into the trabecular arteries. The trabecular arteries supply the central arteries, which are surrounded by the white pulp, so named because it is rich in lymphoid tissue (see Fig. 26–1). The central arteries flowing into the white pulp take off from their supply vessels at near right angles. The anatomic arrangement of these arteries produces a unique flow pattern: the plasma and soluble antigens are skimmed from the column of blood as they enter the white pulp (Fig. 15–1). As the arteries become progressively smaller they become surrounded by a sheath of lymphocytes (predominantly T cells) with adjacent nodules that are rich in B cells. Because of plasma skimming, the cellular elements of the blood are progressively more hemoconcentrated as they flow into the red pulp. The white pulp is important for the immune response, whereas the red pulp has an important role in immune-mediated clearance.[31–33]

The spleen contains approximately 50% of all of the T lymphocytes and about 10% of all B lymphocytes.[34] The splenic lymphocyte population is not static because there is continuous trafficking of these cells in and out of the spleen. The spleen is especially important for generating a primary IgM response to antigens,[35–37] which may explain the fall in serum IgM levels observed after splenectomy.[38, 39] Soluble antigens, such as foreign proteins in the plasma, are directed into the white pulp, where they are captured by specialized RE cells termed *follicular dendritic cells*. These cells partially digest the protein for presentation to splenic T and B cells to initiate the immune response.

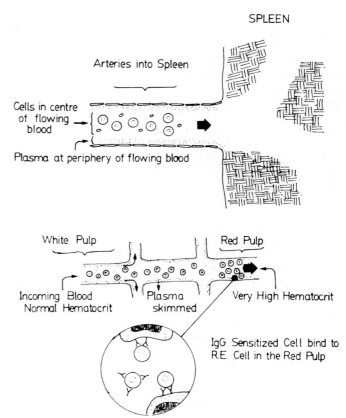

Figure 15–1. Schematic representation of the way in which the spleen separates the plasma from the cellular elements. Within the arterial circulation of the spleen, the cellular elements are in the middle of the column of flowing blood and the plasma is at the periphery. Plasma is skimmed from the cellular elements by arteries that come off perpendicular to the perfusing arteries. In the red pulp of the spleen, monocytes and macrophages are able to phagocytose the IgG and complement-sensitized cells with minimal inhibition by monomeric IgG. (Reprinted from Pochedly C (ed): Disorders of the Spleen. Pathophysiology and Management. New York, Marcel Dekker, 1989, p 188, by courtesy of Marcel Dekker, Inc.)

The spleen helps regulate the immune response by producing regulating factors, such as anti-idiotypic antibodies, that limit the production of specific antibodies.[40, 41] This may explain why impaired or altered splenic function occasionally leads to the unregulated production of autoantibodies and why splenic dysfunction is associated with certain autoimmune diseases.[42] However, owing to the overlap in the immunologic functions of the spleen with lymphocytes and RE cells in other parts of the body, abnormal immune responses, such as an overwhelming infection, occur only in a minority of individuals with impaired or absent splenic function.

The red pulp occupies the majority of the spleen (about 75%) and includes those areas not taken up by the connective tissue support system and the white pulp. Blood flows through the white pulp to enter the red pulp, where it collects in the venous sinuses. Blood can enter the venous sinuses through several routes. There are direct connections between the arterial capillaries and the venous sinuses, but most capillaries end in splenic cords. The blood cells must traverse the endothelial cells lining the cords to enter the splenic sinuses (Fig. 15–2; see also Fig. 26–2). The cords and sinus are separated by a fenestrated basement membrane that contains openings 3 to 4 μm in diameter.

Clearance Function of the Spleen

Every circulating cell in the body passes through the spleen numerous times each day.[43–51]

The spleen sequesters red blood cells with abnormalities caused by increased cytoplasmic viscosity (sickled hemoglobin, cellular dehydration); intracellular particles (Heinz bodies, parasites); decreased surface-to-volume ratio (spherocytes); and cells sensitized by antibodies or complement. The splenic environment of high hematocrit, low glucose, and low pH also conditions susceptible cells (e.g., those with primary membrane defects) and renders them even more prone to sequestration. The immune and filtration roles of the spleen are discussed separately.

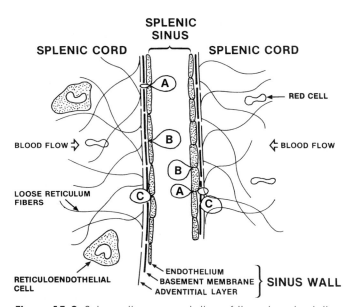

Figure 15–2. Schematic representation of the microcirculation of the red pulp. Blood flows from the splenic cords to the sinuses. The sinus endothelium is incompletely covered by a basement membrane and the adventitial cell lining. Red cells must undergo dramatic changes in shape to pass through the interendothelial cell slits. Alterations in red cell deformability may slow or prevent the passage of the cells. In the diagram the red cells labeled A contain inclusion bodies. Although the greater part of the cell may pass through the sinus endothelium, the inclusions are pinched off and remain in the splenic cord. Removal of pathologic inclusions by the spleen results in the loss of small amounts of the red cell membrane. The loss of membrane further reduces the red cell deformability and increases the likelihood of subsequent splenic retention. The red cells labeled B are normal red cells, which are able to pass through the sinus endothelium unhindered. The red cells labeled C are spherocytes that, because of their reduced deformability, are unable to pass through the interendothelial slits. Red cells and inclusions unable to penetrate the sinus endothelium will be removed by the RE cells. (Reprinted with permission from Bowdler AJ (ed): The Spleen. Structure, Function and Clinical Significance. London, Chapman & Hall Medical, 1990, p 296.)

Immune Clearance Function of the Spleen

The spleen is especially important for immune clearance because it contains a high concentration of monocytes and macrophages capable of recognizing, binding, and ultimately phagocytosing any cell with antibody (IgG) or complement (usually in the presence of IgG) on its surface.[33, 52–54] The RE system possesses no receptors for IgM. As noted previously, the cellular elements of the blood are directed into the red pulp, where the blood flows through splenic cords. The blood flow in the red pulp is slow, allowing the cellular elements to come into close contact with the monocytes and macrophages. There are few direct connections between the cords and the sinuses; and to enter the splenic sinuses, the cells must squeeze through the spaces between the endothelial cells (see Figs. 15–2 and 26–2). The entire red pulp is rich in monocytes and macrophages that carry receptors for opsonins, especially IgG. IgG-mediated phagocytosis requires that the Fc receptors on the monocytes and macrophages bind the Fc portion of the IgG molecule. IgG that is bound to a cell is no more likely to interact with the Fc receptors of the RE cells than uncomplexed (monomeric) IgG in the plasma. However, the multiple antigenic determinants (epitopes) on most antigens have the net effect of concentrating the IgG on a target cell. As a result, the monomeric IgG is displaced from the Fc receptors on the RE cells and the complexed IgG binds (Fig. 15–3). Because the red pulp is relatively poor in plasma, less monomeric IgG is present to compete with Fc receptors on the RE cells. As a result, most cells with IgG on their surface will bind to the RE cells and be phagocytosed (see Fig. 15–3). When IgG and complement are bound to red blood cells, the rate and amount of *in vivo* red cell clearance is often greater than when IgG alone is present.[55] Binding of complement alone to the red cells does not initiate phagocytosis, and a second signal, usually IgG binding to the macrophage Fc receptors, is needed.[56]

High concentrations of IgG in the plasma raise the concentration of IgG in the red pulp of the spleen and compete for Fc receptors. This explains why patients with hypergammaglobulinemia have impaired Fc-dependent RE function. This observation has been exploited in the treatment of patients with immune cytopenias through the administration of large doses of intravenous IgG. Treatment with high doses of intravenous IgG to produce RE blockade (sometimes called a medical splenectomy) is effective but of short duration for IgG-mediated cytopenias such as acute immune thrombocytopenia of children (see Fig. 15–3).

Filtering Capacity of the Spleen

The spleen has the capacity to clear bacteria and abnormal cells from the circulation. Red blood cells with congenital abnormalities (e.g., sickle cell anemia) or acquired abnormalities (e.g., autoimmune hemolytic anemia) are removed.[57–64] Inclusions within red blood cells such as Howell-Jolly bodies, siderotic granules,

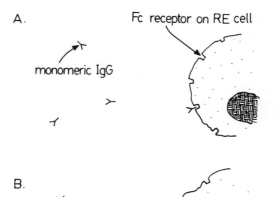

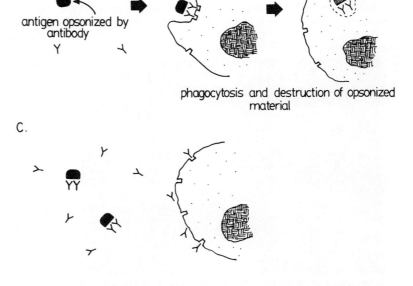

Figure 15–3. Schematic representation of the interaction of IgG with Fc receptors on reticuloendothelial cells. *A,* Monomeric IgG in the plasma is in equilibrium with monomeric IgG bound to the Fc receptors on the RE cells. *B,* The binding of the IgG to an antigen alters the equilibrium so that the antigen-bound IgG displaces monomeric IgG from the Fc receptors, binds to the Fc receptors, and ultimately triggers phagocytosis and destruction of the opsonized material. *C,* The dynamics of this equilibrium indicate an increased concentration of monomeric IgG, which can be secondary to the basic disease process or can be iatrogenic and prevent the IgG opsonized material from interacting with the Fc receptors.

Heinz bodies,[65–66a] and malarial parasites are trapped in the tail of the red blood cell and removed during the passage of red blood cells through the interendothelial slits (see Figs. 15–2 and 15–4).[44–51]

Red blood cells with reduced deformability are also removed by the spleen. An important cause of reduced red blood cell deformity is the spherocytic change caused by the loss of a portion of the membrane. Typically, this occurs in patients with autoimmune hemolytic anemia; however, certain inherited abnormalities of spectrin or spectrin-binding proteins can also lead to spherocyte formation. Because spherical red blood cells have reduced deformability, they are unable to pass through the interendothelial slits in the spleen. Consequently, spherocytes become physically trapped and are phagocytosed by the RE cells. The slow transit of red blood cells through the spleen may also contribute to damage to the red blood cell membrane, through depletion of the energy stores.[67–70] This, in turn, produces diminished deformability (Table 15–1). Thus, a cycle of red blood cell damage and splenic sequestration can be established when primarily defective red blood cells are further injured during passage through the spleen. Under such circumstances, splenectomy can be palliative or even curative treatment for the anemia[69–71] (Table 15–2).

Hazards of Splenectomy and Hyposplenism

The absence of the spleen is associated with an increased susceptibility to bacterial infections secondary to impairment of the immune response. Splenectomy may result in overwhelming septicemia, which occasionally is fatal, especially in infants and young children.[72–80] The risk of sepsis and mortality from septicemia is greatest with an underlying condition that is in itself associated with an increased susceptibility to

Table 15–1. DISORDERS ASSOCIATED WITH DIMINISHED RED CELL DEFORMABILITY

Abnormalities of Hemoglobin Structure or Stability

Sickle cell anemia (Hb SS)
Sickle cell trait (Hb SA)
Hemoglobin C disease (Hb CC)
Heinz body formation

Abnormalities of Red Cell Membrane or Metabolism

Hereditary spherocytosis
Hereditary pyropoikilocytosis
Antibody-induced spherocytosis
Acanthocytosis (abetalipoproteinemia)
Heinz body formation

infection, such as sickle cell disease, thalassemia major, or Hodgkin's disease. In children who undergo splenectomy for traumatic splenic rupture, or as treatment for an underlying red cell membrane disorder (such as hereditary spherocytosis), the risk of infection is lower (for details see Chapter 26).[76]

Immunologic alterations after splenectomy include a reduction of total serum IgM concentration.[80–82] In addition, the antibody response to lipopolysaccharides is also impaired,[83] and the total T-lymphocyte (CD2, CD3) counts and helper-inducer subpopulation (CD4CD29) are significantly lower in splenectomized children compared with normal children.[84] The deficiency of the CD4CD29 cell subset, which is thought to mediate bacterial surveillance, may explain the influence of age at splenectomy on the incidence of subsequent bacterial

Table 15–2. INDICATIONS FOR SPLENECTOMY IN HEMOLYTIC ANEMIA

Probable or Predictable Improvement in Anemia
Hereditary spherocytosis
Hereditary elliptocytosis
Pyruvate kinase deficiency
Hexokinase deficiency
Glucose phosphate isomerase deficiency
Possible But Not Always Unpredictable Benefit
Acquired idiopathic autoimmune hemolytic anemia

infections. This subset of T cells is virtually absent in cord blood,[85] increases with age, and is significantly lower in normal children compared with adults.[84–87]

The postsplenectomy alterations are not limited to the immunologic effector cells. Functional neutrophil defects have been described, involving defects in oxidative metabolism and Fc receptor–dependent phagocytosis.[88] One postulated mechanism is that defective polymorphonuclear leukocytes accumulate because of loss of the filtering capacity of the spleen. In at least two studies these changes have been associated with an increased frequency of infections after splenectomy.[88, 89]

Overwhelming postsplenectomy infection by encapsulated organisms is an important complication of splenectomy. Patients suffer an acute onset of nausea, vomiting, and confusion that can lead to death within hours.[90–95] The case-fatality rate is about 50%, and many patients have evidence of disseminated intravascular coagulation, hypoglycemia, electrolyte imbalance, and shock. Although splenectomized individuals can produce antibodies in response to immunization or infection, the levels achieved are less than those in normal controls,[96–103] and postsplenectomy patients undergoing chemotherapy may have poor responses to vaccinations against encapsulated organisms.[104] All individuals who have had a splenectomy should receive 23 valent pneumococcal vaccination and probably also vaccines against *Neisseria meningitidis* and *Haemophilus influenzae* group B, irrespective of when they had the splenectomy.[105] With an elective splenectomy, immunization with 23 valent pneumococcal vaccine, meningococcal vaccine, and a vaccine for *H. influenzae* group B should be offered to all patients at least 2 weeks before surgery. Pneumococcal vaccination should be repeated at 5 to 10 years as antibody titers fall with time.[106, 107] The use of long-term prophylactic antibiotics (e.g., penicillin, 250 mg twice daily) combined with vaccination has been recommended for asplenic children,[81,108–110] but there are reports of pneumococcal sepsis, some of which resulted in death, despite penicillin prophylaxis and vaccination.[108,111–113] Patient and parent education is an important factor in managing potential health problems after splenectomy, including the early recognition, prevention, and treatment of infection.[114] In one survey, only 16% of postsplenectomy patients were aware of any special health precautions to be taken after splenectomy.[115]

SCHISTOCYTIC HEMOLYTIC ANEMIA

Hemolytic anemia characterized by red blood cell fragments, spherocytes (Fig. 15–5), and evidence of intra-

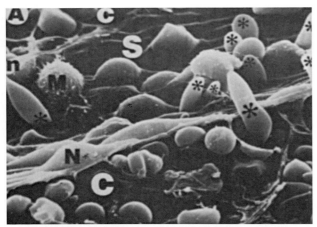
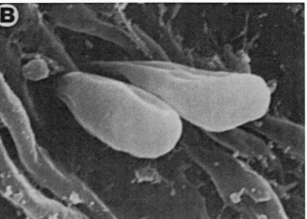

Figure 15–4. Erythrocytes entering sinus *(S)* from splenic cord *(C)*. Endothelial cells arrayed longitudinally in the direction of flowing blood occasionally present nuclear *(N)* bulges. *A,* Red pulp from patient with hereditary spherocytosis. Note spherocytes in cord. Several red blood cells (*) enter the sinus as spindle-shaped forms. A splenic macrophage *(M)* bearing many tiny villous projections is anchored to the sinus wall (×3500). n = endothelial cell. *B,* Erythrocyte caught astraddle an endothelial cell while trying to enter the sinus through two windows at the same time. Breakage of such a straplike connection between the two bulging ends could produce two schizocytes. Note the short, minute filamentous processes that partially bind two endothelial cells together (×10,600). (From Barnhart MI, Lusher MI: The human spleen as revealed by scanning electron microscopy. Am J Hematol 1976; 1:252.)

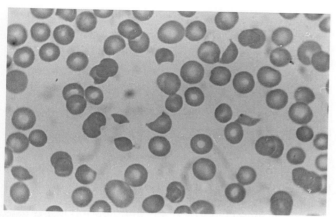

Figure 15-5. Peripheral blood smear of a patient with acute thrombotic thrombocytopenic purpura. Note the fragmented cells.

vascular hemolysis is called schistocytic hemolytic anemia. Such fragmentation is common in newborns, particularly in preterm infants, and may have no clinical significance in that setting. Schistocytic hemolysis can complicate valvular heart disease, the surgical repair of intracardiac defects, and the insertion of prosthetic heart valves. Schistocytic hemolytic anemia is also associated with a variety of disorders of the microcirculation (Table 15–3). In some patients, the mechanism of hemolysis can be explained by the interaction of the circulating red blood cells with an abnormal hemodynamic or physical environment within the heart or blood vessels. In a large group of disorders, including hemolytic-uremic syndrome, thrombotic thrombocytopenia purpura, and preeclampsia, the cause of the schistocytic hemolytic anemia remains obscure.

The original description of microangiopathic hemolytic anemia suggested that the red blood cell damage was caused by red blood cells passing through partially obstructed blood vessels.[116, 117] Studies in experimental

Table 15-3. CAUSES OF SCHISTOCYTIC HEMOLYTIC ANEMIA

Mechanical Hemolysis Secondary to Macrovascular Abnormalities

Hemolysis with Microvascular Abnormalities

Congenital
Kasabach-Merritt syndrome
Familial hemolytic-uremic syndrome
Acquired
Immunologic vasculitides: acute glomerulonephritis, polyarteritis, scleroderma, Wegener's granulomatosis
Acute renal allograft rejection
Allergic vasculitides
Microangiopathy with hypertension
Malignant hypertension
Preeclampsia and eclampsia
Microangiopathy with malignancy
Hemolytic-uremic syndrome
Thrombotic thrombocytopenic purpura

Hemolysis with Disseminated Intravascular Coagulation

animals indicated that the blockage of small blood vessels by platelet and fibrin thrombi due to intravascular coagulation[118] and by alterations in the blood vessel wall due to malignant hypertension[119] could induce intravascular hemolysis and red blood cell fragmentation. The mechanism of red blood cell fragmentation complicating disseminated intravascular coagulation has been clarified: red blood cells in the flowing blood must navigate a series of fibrin strands crossing the vessel wall. Some of the red blood cells are physically cut in half by the strands, like pancakes thrown across clotheslines. The size and shape of the red blood cell fragments are related to how the red blood cell hits the fibrin strand, the proportion of the membrane lost, and the amount of hemoglobin retained within the red blood cell.[120, 121]

The mechanism of the red blood cell fragmentation in other schistocytic hemolytic anemias that are not characterized by disseminated intravascular coagulation is less certain. It has been suggested that the red blood cell damage is sustained by partial entrapment of red blood cells by damaged vessel walls in malignant hypertension. This interaction would mechanically damage the red blood cells. Other possible causes of red blood cell fragmentation include the action of proteolytic enzymes on the red blood cell membrane. It is probable that more than one mechanism can cause red blood cell fragmentation.

The hallmark of all schistocytic hemolytic anemias is laboratory evidence of intravascular hemolysis, in particular elevations in the level of the red blood cell enzyme lactate dehydrogenase. Intravascular hemolysis results in reduced or absent levels of haptoglobin, the formation of heme-albumin, and the presence of free hemoglobin. The morphologic picture is characteristic, with red blood cell fragmentation predominating, but occasionally other red blood cell morphologic abnormalities are noted, including spherocytosis and teardrop-shaped changes. For purposes of this discussion, schistocytic hemolytic anemia is divided into two general groups of disorders: those in which thrombocytopenia is mild or absent and those in which thrombocytopenia is usually severe. In general, thrombocytopenia is a more common accompaniment of schistocytic hemolytic anemia secondary to disorders of the microcirculation.

Schistocytic Hemolytic Anemia with a Normal Platelet Count or Mild Thrombocytopenia

Mild hemolytic anemia has been associated with both congenital and acquired disease of the heart valves and aorta.[122–126] The most severe episodes of cardiac hemolytic anemia follow the repair of intracardiac defects and the insertion of prosthetic heart valves.[127] Open heart surgery for the repair of congenital cardiac defects and the replacement of malfunctioning and diseased heart valves can be followed by postoperative hemolytic anemia and is characterized by the presence of fragmented, distorted, and spherocytic red blood cells and hemoglobinemia, hemoglobinuria, and hemosiderinuria. The insertion of a prosthetic heart valve is often followed by a mild, compensated hemolytic anemia with shortened red blood cell survival and a lowering of serum haptoglobin levels; however, with improvement in surgical techniques and the design of prosthetic heart valves, especially xenografts, the incidence of severe hemolytic anemia has been reduced.[128]

Cardiac hemolytic anemia is often associated with a new hemodynamic abnormality or with the persistence of a preoperative abnormality. For example, schistocytic hemolytic anemia has been reported to complicate the incomplete repair of an intracardiac defect, abnormal function of the prosthetic valve, and, more frequently, defective attachment of the base of the prosthetic valve to the adjacent cardiac tissue. In the last situation, a regurgitant jet of blood flows past the valve and hits a nonendothelialized prosthetic surface. The hemodynamic abnormality is usually readily detected, but sometimes severe hemolytic anemia occurs in the absence of cardiac signs. The successful repair of the cardiac defect or replacement of a malfunctioning prosthetic valve can dramatically relieve the hemolysis.

Pathogenesis

Cardiac schistocytic hemolytic anemia almost always involves the high pressures and flow rates of the left side of the heart. Presumably, the red blood cells are mechanically damaged by the high shear forces produced by the abnormal blood flow. Studies of red cells in cone-plate viscometers demonstrate that red blood cells will be hemolyzed when shear forces exceed 3000 dynes/cm^2, especially if the surface of the plate has irregularities.[129, 130] Sheer forces of this magnitude can be generated within the heart by the pressure gradient between the aorta and left ventricle or between the left ventricle and the left atrium. Yet, red blood cells can withstand shear forces up to 15,000 dynes/cm^2 without hemolysis, provided these forces are generated at a fluid-fluid interface.[131] Sheer forces of this magnitude far exceed those encountered within the heart or circulation. Therefore, the red blood cell damage and hemolysis observed in cardiac hemolytic anemia require both high shear forces and the interaction of red blood cells with abnormal surfaces within the heart or vessels. This conclusion is supported by reports that hemolysis resolves when an abnormal intracardiac prosthetic surface is covered with endothelium.[127]

The importance of hemodynamic factors in the pathogenesis of cardiac hemolytic anemia is also borne out by the increase in the rate of hemolysis that accompanies a rise in cardiac output with exercise or with anemia.[132] The loss of hemoglobin in the urine is diurnal, being greatest during the day in the ambulatory patient and least during the night.[132] Hemoglobinuria also lessens as the cardiac output falls when the anemia is corrected by blood transfusion.

Diagnosis and Treatment

Postoperative cardiac hemolytic anemia should be suspected in any patient who develops hemolytic anemia after cardiac surgery. Its onset is usually immediately after surgery. The development of hemolysis some time after surgery may indicate failure or infection of the prosthetic heart valve.

The diagnosis of cardiac hemolysis is supported by the finding of fragmented and spherocytic red blood cells in the peripheral blood, evidence of intravascular hemolysis with free hemoglobin, and the demonstration of hemosiderin in the urinary deposits. The intravascular hemolysis is accompanied by the release of the red blood cell enzyme lactate dehydrogenase into the plasma. The level of serum lactate dehydrogenase has been found to correlate with the shortened ^{51}Cr-labeled red blood cell survival in patients with cardiac hemolytic anemia.[133] The direct antiglobulin test is usually negative, but occasionally, and for uncertain reasons, the test result may be positive.[127]

In some patients the hemolysis lessens in the first few weeks after surgery, but in most it persists and can become more severe as the patient ambulates and the cardiac output rises. The anemia may be so severe that blood transfusions are necessary, and the loss of hemoglobin and hemosiderin in the urine can result in iron deficiency.[133, 134] Iron and folic acid should be prescribed to achieve a maximal erythropoietic response, but this may be insufficient to compensate for the hemolysis. Blood transfusions may be useful because they raise the hemoglobin level and reduce hemolysis by lowering cardiac output.

The definitive treatment is surgical correction of the underlying hemodynamic abnormality. The decision to reoperate can be delayed for weeks or months, depending on the severity of the hemolysis and the hemodynamic status of the patient, in the hope that hemolysis may lessen. In mild cases of postoperative cardiac hemolytic anemia, the risks of operation usually outweigh the problems of a compensated hemolytic anemia.

Malignant Hypertension

Microangiopathic hemolytic anemia and mild to moderate thrombocytopenia can be the hematologic manifestation of malignant hypertension. The lowering of blood pressure with antihypertensive drugs results in improvement in the hemolysis and thrombocytopenia. These patients seldom have evidence of activation of the coagulation cascade, and anticoagulants are not indicated. When the hypertension is resistant to drug therapy, nephrectomy and hemodialysis have been reported to lower blood pressure and stop hemolysis in adults.[135, 136]

March Hemoglobinuria

Although hemoglobinuria in association with severe exercise was first reported in the late 1800s, it was not until 1964 that Davidson[137] demonstrated that the hemoglobinuria that followed strenuous physical exertion when running on hard surfaces was brought about by the physical injuries sustained by the red blood cells within the blood vessels in the feet. This observation was subsequently confirmed.[138] Hemoglobinuria has also been observed after repeated blows to the hands from karate exercises[139] and in conga-drum players.[140]

Burns

Extensive body burns may induce spherocytosis and intravascular hemolysis because of thermal damage to the red blood cell membrane.[141]

Schistocytic Hemolytic Anemia with Severe Thrombocytopenia

Hemolytic-Uremic Syndrome

The term *hemolytic-uremic syndrome* (HUS) was first used by Gasser and co-workers to describe the association of acute hemolytic anemia, thrombocytopenia, and renal failure in infants and young children. It has subsequently been shown that HUS encompasses a group of pathologically similar disorders that have different initiating events or disease association. All patients with HUS have a variable degree of renal failure, thrombocytopenia, and schistocytic hemolytic anemia. Less frequently, platelet-mediated thrombi cause other manifestations, including strokes. Many cases of idiopathic HUS have now been associated with verocytotoxin-producing infecting organisms. The incidence of HUS appears to be increasing.[142]

Clinical Features

Hemolytic-uremic syndrome affects healthy young children. About 90% of cases occur in early childhood (after the age of 6 months and before 5 years) and are preceded by watery diarrhea, which can evolve to hemorrhagic colitis.[143] Typically, the diarrhea precedes the hemolytic anemia and thrombocytopenia by 5 to 7 days. The severity of the colitis is predictive of other complications and long-term renal sequelae.[144] Several days later, oliguria can develop. The oliguria and azoturia contribute to the hypertension that is often seen in these patients.[145] Some children have gastrointestinal symptoms with abdominal pain, nausea, vomiting, and diarrhea. Rarely, an abdominal mass may be noted, reflecting intussusception or gangrenous bowel.[146] Pancreatic insufficiency (diabetes mellitus) has been reported in 4% to 15% of patients; this may be transient or permanent. Pancreatic exocrine dysfunction may also rarely be noted.[146] Fever may or may not occur.[147] Despite the frequent occurrence of thrombocytopenia, bleeding is uncommon. Neurologic involvement occurs in 20% to 30% of children with HUS. Seizures are the most frequent neurologic manifestation, with drowsiness, personality changes, coma, and hemiparesis occurring less commonly.[148–150] Cranial nerve involvement may be present, and pale or hemorrhagic cerebral infarcts are present in 3% to 5% of children.

Renal involvement may be of variable severity, ranging from mild oliguria to complete anuria. HUS is the most frequent cause of childhood acute renal failure; and although most patients have a return of renal function to normal, some have persisting renal failure. In those countries with a high frequency of HUS, such as Argentina, HUS represents the single most important cause of end-stage renal disease in children.[151]

Laboratory abnormalities in HUS include anemia with evidence of red blood cell fragmentation and elevated levels of lactate dehydrogenase, reticulocytes, and unconjugated bilirubin reflecting intravascular hemolysis. The degree of anemia is not related to acute renal failure. Haptoglobin is decreased, the direct antiglobulin test is negative, and osmotic fragility is normal. Thrombocytopenia is usually observed, with median platelet counts around $50 \times 10^9/L$, although they can fall as low as $5 \times 10^9/L$. At presentation, 50% of patients will have counts greater than $100 \times 10^9/L$. Red cell fragments may artificially raise the platelet count on automated cell counters. Thrombocytopenia lasts 7 to 20 days; however, platelet abnormalities (low concentrations of serotonin and adenosine diphosphate) can persist for several weeks after normalization of the platelet count. Neither the severity nor the duration of thrombocytopenia correlates with the overall severity of the disorder. In most instances, leukocytosis is present, with one study demonstrating more severe disease and a poorer prognosis with white blood cell counts greater than $20 \times 10^9/L$.[152] The prothrombin and partial thromboplastin times are usually normal; and if they are abnormal, then septicemia should be suspected. Elevated levels of fibrin degradation products and slight reductions in fibrinogen levels may be observed; but despite the often fulminant microangiopathy, coagulation and fibrinolysis are only mildly disturbed. One study demonstrated elevated plasma levels of tissue plasminogen activator antigen and plasminogen activator inhibitor type I activity in patients with HUS, which presumably reflected endothelial cell activation or injury[153]; these values normalized during remission. The urinalysis reveals proteinuria (typically 1 to 2 g/24 h) with microscopic hematuria and cellular casts. Because of endothelial damage and "capillary leakiness," crystalloid and colloid can escape to the extracellular space, causing a low plasma albumin level. Rhabdomyolysis has occurred very rarely in association with HUS.

Pathologic Findings

Pathologic findings are not limited to the kidneys. They range from endothelial cell swelling to thrombotic ischemia. The thrombi can be found in many organs, lending support to the concept that HUS is caused by a systemic "toxin."[154]

Two different histologic patterns are seen. With diarrhea-associated HUS, glomerular capillary thrombosis is present, with some arteriolar thrombosis and necrosis.[155, 156] In idiopathic forms of HUS (usually the adult form), small arteries exhibit intimal proliferation and narrowing of the capillary lumen.

HUS can produce ischemic damage throughout the entire gut, but the colon is typically affected the most severely. Pathologic findings in the gut include microangiopathy with endothelial cell injury and thrombosis with submucosal edema and hemorrhage.[154]

The central nervous system can also suffer ischemic damage caused by microthrombi. Patients may demonstrate irritability, restlessness, drowsiness, cerebellar ataxia, seizures (generalized or focal) or coma.[143] Possible factors for central nervous system involvement include female sex, a raised packed cell volume, and prolonged use of antimotility drugs.[148]

Role of Infectious Agents. For many years, an infectious etiology causing or initiating HUS has been postulated. The basis for this hypothesis is a strong association of prodromal diarrhea or respiratory illness in patients who subsequently developed HUS. Many case reports have described the sporadic association of cases of HUS with certain infecting agents. At other times, an infection is associated with a cluster of cases of HUS within a family. In some countries, viral infections have been associated with epidemics of HUS, but bacterial infections, especially *Escherichia coli, Shigella,* and *Salmonella,* have been the infectious agents most commonly associated. However, it was not until an epidemic of HUS was traced to *E. coli*–contaminated apple juice that a causal association between infection and HUS was confirmed. In Ontario, Canada, apple juice sold at fall fairs was responsible for 14 cases of HUS.[157] This clustering of infections was described by Steele and colleagues,[156] and subsequent work by this group of investigators demonstrated that the common factor was a toxin-producing strain of *E. coli.*[158] It is now recognized that certain strains of *E. coli,* especially 0157:H7, are strongly associated with HUS.[147, 158, 159] Presumably, this is related to the ability of the *E. coli* to produce a verocytotoxin. Other infectious organisms, including *Shigella dysenteriae* types 1 and 234 and other subtypes of *E. coli* (026:H11), also can produce verocytotoxin and are capable of causing HUS.[147, 159] After ingesting contaminated food products, approximately 40% of persons will develop bloody diarrhea 1 day later, and of these patients, 2% to 4% will develop HUS.[147]

Epidemiologic studies of endemic and epidemic outbreaks of these infections have now produced a clearer picture of the disorder. Verocytotoxin-producing organisms can be spread by contaminated food and by person-to-person contact. Poorly cooked ground beef, unpasteurized milk, and contaminated apple juice all have been implicated as sources of the infection. Often, the origin of the infection is not known but it is assumed to be a fecal-oral transmission because of the frequent occurrence of epidemics in daycare centers and nursing homes.[147, 159] The most recent large scale outbreak of hemorrhagic colitis was in the Seattle-Tacoma, Washington, area[160] and was associated with the ingestion of undercooked hamburgers from a chain of fast-food restaurants. Between December 1, 1992, and February 28, 1993, the Centers for Disease Control and Prevention reported 501 cases of culture-confirmed *E. coli* 0157:H7 gastroenteritis. Six per cent of these patients developed HUS, and 371 of these cases occurred in children. One study, examining pediatric outcomes, reported a mortality rate of 8% (similar to other published accounts) and a similar incidence of extrarenal manifestations, with the exception of a higher incidence of bowel gangrene requiring colectomy.[161] A case-control study during an *E. coli* 0157:H7 infection epidemic in a remote Inuit community in northern Canada demonstrated also that the main risk factor for childhood infection with *E. coli* 0157:H7 and the subsequent development of HUS was exposure to a family member with diarrhea.[162] The diarrhea with *E. coli* 0157:H7 infection typically lasts 1 week, and HUS develops in fewer than 10% of children with symptomatic infections.[147, 159] Infections caused by *E. coli* produce a spectrum of illnesses ranging from an asymptomatic infection, to diarrhea that may be watery or bloody, to mild hemolysis and thrombocytopenia alone, to HUS that ranges in severity from mild to fatal. In some patients, neurologic events predominate and the patient has a syndrome identical to thrombotic thrombocytopenic purpura (TTP) (discussed subsequently).

The annual incidence of HUS in Washington, DC, and Baltimore has been estimated at 1.08 per 100,000 children younger than 5 years of age.[163] In Canada, the United States, and Argentina, the majority of cases of HUS are now associated with evidence of verocytotoxin-producing organisms.[164] Epidemiologic studies may explain the high frequency of HUS in certain countries, such as Argentina, compared with North America. It has been estimated that verocytotoxin-producing *E. coli* accounts for approximately 3% of the diarrheal illness in North America, compared with up to 30% in Argentina.[160] The other significant diarrhea-producing organism that is associated with HUS is *Shigella dysenteriae* serotype I, which is a major cause of acute renal failure and HUS in India.[143]

Role of Verocytotoxin. After being ingested in contaminated food that is insufficiently cooked, the verocytotoxin producing microbes that produce either one or more of the Shiga-like toxins (VT-1, VT-2, VT-2c), bind to colonic mucosal epithelial cells and subsequently invade and destroy these cells.[165, 166] The factors that predispose certain individuals to the development of HUS are unclear. Damage to the underlying vasculature and tissues follows, producing bloody diarrhea.[166] The verocytotoxins then enter the systemic circulation and attach to globotriaosylceramide (Gb3) molecules, the predominant membrane glycosphingolipid receptor for verocytotoxins, in glomerular capillary endothelial cells. This receptor has also been found on cultured endothelial cells. In response to these toxins, endothelial cells swell and release von Willebrand factor (vWf) along with other substances. The A-subunit of the verocytotoxin is endocytosed, and after proteolysis and disulfide bond reduction, a 27-kd intracellular enzyme is generated from the toxin. This enzyme then cleaves ribosomal RNA in the affected cell, leading to a suppression in overall protein synthesis (Fig. 15–6).[166] Despite the very strong association of verocytotoxin-producing infectious organisms with HUS, a causal link remains to be established. Animals infected with enterohemorrhagic *E. coli* that produces verocytotoxins develop diarrhea that can be bloody; however, HUS has not been observed.[159] A variety of hypothetical

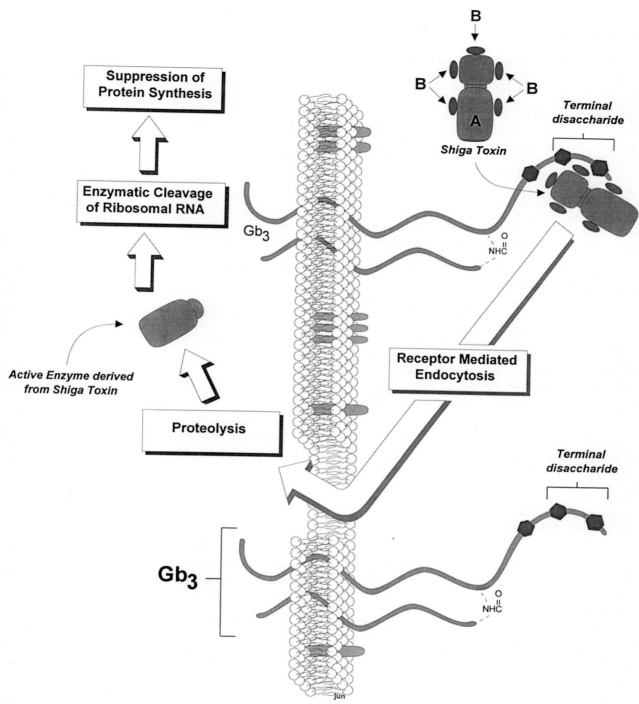

Figure 15-6. The binding, internalization, and processing of Shiga toxin in endothelial cells. Shiga toxin binds to the terminal component of Gb3 molecules on endothelial cell surfaces. The toxin is then internalized and proteolyzed; this process generates an active enzyme that suppresses the cellular protein synthesis. (Modified from Moake JL: Haemolytic-uraemic syndrome: basic science. Lancet 1994; 343:395. © by The Lancet Ltd., 1994.)

mechanisms have been postulated, including a direct toxic effect of the cytotoxin on endothelial cells. Three different types of verocytotoxins (also known as Shiga-like toxins, [SLT]) have been identified: verocytotoxin-1 (VT-1 or SLT-I), verocytotoxin-2 (VT-2 or SLT-II), and verocytotoxin-2 variant (VT-2C). The genes for these toxins have been cloned.[167] Both VT-1 and VT-2 are composed of A and B subunits.[144] Verocytotoxin 1 differs in only one amino acid from the A subunit of Shiga toxin.[168] Verocytotoxins 1 and 2 exhibit 58% homology in their nucleotide base sequence[169] and are serologically distinct, demonstrating no cross-neutralization by homologous antisera, whereas VT-2 is completely neutralized by antisera to VT-2c.[170] Although there are structural differences in the two types of verocytotoxins, both forms share an identical mechanism of toxicity. The virulence of verocytotoxin-producing organisms has been postulated to be related to the production of verocytotoxin and is dependent on microfilament-mediated invasion of intestinal cells.[171] E. coli serotypes that are associated with HUS may produce VT-1 alone, VT-2 alone, VT-2c alone, or two in combination. In patients infected with enterohemorrhagic E. coli 0157:H7 strains that produce VT-1, or VT-1 and VT-2 together, an incidence of 3% to 6% of HUS is reported, as compared with 39% for strains producing only VT-2 verocytotoxin.[172] One mice model supports this observation, because VT-2 was found to be 400 times more toxic than VT-1 alone or the combination.[173] Of interest, in the outbreak in Washington state, the E. coli strain produced both VT-1 and VT-2.

Verocytotoxin binds specifically to globotriaosylceramide on cell surfaces.[174] Cells that are resistant to the toxin fail to express the surface receptor.[175] The receptor has been demonstrated in human renal tissue, and its distribution correlates with the regions of the kidney that are clinically affected in HUS.[176] Several other factors have been postulated to participate in the pathogenesis of HUS, and these are briefly reviewed.

A Platelet-Aggregating Factor. Patients with HUS have disseminated platelet thrombi that can cause ischemic damage to kidneys, brain, and other organs. Consequently, it is possible that platelets participate in the process either directly or indirectly by being the target of an aggregating factor. A platelet-aggregating factor has been postulated to cause episodes of TTP (described subsequently).

Patients with HUS have been shown to have a platelet function defect that can range from impaired or absent platelet aggregation to standard aggregating agents such as adenosine diphosphate and collagen.[177, 178] Platelets from patients with HUS also have reduced levels of the platelet granular substance β-thromboglobulin. However, the role of the platelet in HUS remains uncertain.

Participation of von Willebrand Factor. The coagulation protein vWf is often abnormal in character and amount in some patients with TTP. Some investigators believe that abnormalities of vWf are causally related to TTP. Similar abnormalities have been observed in patients with both sporadic (presumably infectious) and familial HUS.

A large multimeric protein, vWf is important in platelet adhesion, linking platelets to the vessel wall through platelet glycoprotein Ib.[179] It also binds to platelet glycoprotein IIb/IIIa after platelet activation.[180] Several groups of investigators have demonstrated that some patients with HUS have abnormal vWf,[181, 182] in the form of ultra-large multimers (ULvWf). One group of investigators noted high levels of plasma vWf without a marked increase in the plasma concentration of β-thromboglobulin, suggesting that the elevated vWf level was caused by endothelial cell release and not platelet granular release. However, the pathophysiologic role of vWf in HUS remains uncertain, and indeed it is even possible that some of the alterations of vWf in patients with HUS could be related to in vitro proteolysis[182] or damage to endothelial cells.[182a]

Endothelial Cell Injury. In most patients, the kidney is the main site of endothelial cell damage. Endothelial cell injury induced by cytotoxic antiendothelial cell antibodies has also been proposed as a possible mechanism that induces the microangiopathy of HUS. One group of investigators described the presence of cytotoxic antiendothelial cell antibodies in sera from a group of children with HUS.[183] They postulated that HUS is a disorder of immune regulation leading to an autoantibody-mediated endothelial injury. Because most episodes of childhood HUS are associated with verocytotoxin-producing E. coli, the relationship between the infection and the autoantibodies is not clear. Although HUS has been reported in patients with immune abnormalities, including thymic lymphoplasia[184] and Wiskott-Aldrich syndrome,[185] and in patients treated with immunosuppressive agents,[186, 187] most children who develop HUS are healthy and have no predisposing immunologic abnormalities. Inflammatory mediators, such as tumor necrosis factor-α and interleukin-1, may also regulate endothelial cell sensitivity to verocytotoxins. In one study researchers demonstrated that tumor necrosis factor-α and, to a lesser extent, interleukin-1 potentiated the toxic effects of VT-1 by increasing the synthesis of the VT-1 receptor (globotriaosylceramide).[188]

A Deficiency of Prostaglandin I_2. A deficiency of prostaglandin I_2 (PGI_2) has been postulated to play a role in the microangiopathy of HUS. PGI_2 is produced by the vessel wall and is both a potent vasodilator and an inhibitor of platelet aggregation. Thus, it is conceivable that a deficiency of PGI_2 could result in increased platelet aggregation and vessel thrombosis. Plasma from patients with HUS reduces PGI_2 release from cultured endothelial cells,[189] and its metabolite, 6-keto-$PGF_1\alpha$, is reduced in HUS.[190] However, the lack of therapeutic response to infusions of PGI_2 in patients with HUS[189] suggests that this deficiency is not of major pathogenic significance, and it may merely reflect a secondary disturbance in vessel function.

Other Proposed Causes. The first proposed cause of schistocytic hemolytic anemia and thrombocytopenia was disseminated intravascular coagulation. However, there is little evidence implicating disseminated intravascular coagulation in the pathophysiology of HUS. The fibrinogen turnover and the level of fibrinopeptide A are normal in patients with HUS.[191] Mild elevations of fibrin degradation products have been reported, but their relevance remains uncertain.[192] Furthermore, anticoagulants and fibrolytic therapy have been tried, without benefit.

Leukocytosis is commonly observed during acute episodes of HUS. This has led one group of investigators[193] to question whether elevations in serum leukocyte enzymes (elastase and α_1-antitrypsin) might participate in the disease.

A number of investigators have also demonstrated abnormalities of the red blood cell membrane or content. Abnormalities include reductions in red blood cell arachidonic acid,[194] alterations in the ratio of membrane phosphatidylethanolamine to lysolecithin,[195] and variably abnormal levels of vitamin E.[196, 197] The implications of all these observations remain uncertain. With respect to the fragmentation, young erythrocytes may possess receptors for endothelial-cell derived ULvWf multimers and may attach to endothelial cells, fragmenting because of heightened shear stresses in narrowed vessel lumina. These receptors may be part of the P₁ antigen system. In certain disease states, reticulocytes have been demonstrated to bind thrombospondin, a protein involved in cell adhesion and platelet aggregation, via its receptor, glycoprotein IV (GPIV, also known as CD36).[198] As microvascular endothelial cells also express CD36, this may explain another mechanism of red cell adherence and fragmentation. Which of these potential pathogenic mechanisms is important for pathogenesis is not clear.

Diagnosis

Patients with the complete syndrome of renal failure, thrombocytopenia, and microangiopathy almost certainly have HUS, although other causes of thrombotic microangiopathy, including disseminated intravascular coagulation, cavernous sinus hemangioma, and vasculitis, should be excluded.

Verocytotoxin-producing *E. coli* is associated with diarrhea, hemorrhagic colitis, and HUS. The detection of this organism in the stools is definitive evidence of this infection; however, it is present in the stool for a short time only after the onset of diarrhea, and symptoms of HUS usually appear a week later. It is imperative to demonstrate the presence of the verocytotoxin to distinguish the organism associated with HUS from non–toxin-producing strains of *E. coli* 0157 LPS (lipopolysaccharide). The combination of stool culture and an enzyme-linked immunosorbent assay for antibodies (IgG and IgM) to *E. coli* 0157:H7 confirmed infection by verotoxin-producing *E. coli* in 82% of patients (mainly children) with HUS in one study.[199] Other laboratory investigations such as DNA hybridization, toxin detection by cytotoxicity assays, and polymerase chain reaction techniques are occasionally used as adjunctive techniques.[144, 158, 159, 200, 201] However, despite these technologies, HUS remains a diagnosis of exclusion.

Treatment

Improvements in the management of acute renal failure and hypertension have reduced the mortality of HUS to 5% to 10% in most centers.[149, 151] However, about 25% of the survivors suffer lasting renal impairment. To reduce the morbidity and mortality of HUS, a number of treatment modalities have been tried, but acceptable randomized clinical trials addressing treatment issues have been impeded by the rarity of the disorder. Consequently, the optimal treatment remains unknown. Because most patients do well, any randomized trial of long-term efficacy will require large numbers of patients to demonstrate statistically any therapeutic benefit.

Supportive Therapy. The general management of renal failure and hypertension is the mainstay of treatment. Dialysis may be required to manage uremia, volume, and electrolyte problems in many patients.[149] Hypertension is present in 50% of children with HUS and should be treated.[149, 150] Angiotensin-converting enzyme inhibitors are often used because the hypertension is usually renal mediated. Anemia should be corrected with red blood cell transfusions. Thrombocytopenia is rarely of severe magnitude, and severe hemorrhage is extremely uncommon. Platelet transfusions may potentially worsen the thrombotic process and should be given only for life-threatening bleeding. Seizures are the most common neurologic complication in HUS and should be managed with anticonvulsant therapy.[149, 150]

Interventional Therapies

Plasma Infusion or Exchange. Although the use of plasma therapy has dramatically reduced the mortality of acute TTP, the role of plasma therapy in HUS is unclear. Plasma infusion could replace a deficient factor and has a major role in the treatment of familial HUS. Plasma exchange could potentially remove causative factors in the plasma. Because of the problems of maintaining euvolemia with plasma infusion, plasma exchange may be more feasible but has the disadvantage of requiring vascular access. Results of a prospective, randomized trial of plasma infusion (17 patients) compared with supportive therapy (15 patients) in patients who required dialysis for HUS demonstrated no benefit of the intervention in reducing short- or long-term sequelae.[202] However, the small numbers of patients in this trial make it of little general value. The role of plasma therapy remains uncertain, and a large clinical trial would be useful. Plasma therapy should be used when a congenital or familial form of the disorder is suspected, because dramatic responses to plasma infusion are the norm.[203]

Antiplatelet Agents. Because the microthrombi in HUS are rich in platelets, antiplatelet therapy has been used. In one study, therapy was associated with a faster rise in platelet count in the treated group.[204] Benefit in terms of renal function has not been demonstrated. A prospective, randomized trial combining dipyridamole and heparin in HUS showed no benefit.[205] Because aspirin and dipyridamole are unlikely to be associated with serious adverse effects, the authors favor their use, although clinical benefit probably is small.

Intravenous IgG. There have been anecdotal reports of benefit from intravenous IgG in TTP. In one study, patients with HUS treated with intravenous IgG were compared with historical controls. Intravenous IgG treatment was associated with a significantly faster recovery from thrombocytopenia and oliguria, with a reduction in neurologic sequelae in the treatment group.[206] Although intravenous IgG appeared useful in this study, it has not been shown to be effective in familial HUS and TTP or in classic adult TTP.

Other Therapies. Although anticoagulants, corticosteroids, and prostacyclin infusions all have been tried in this disorder, no evidence of beneficial therapeutic effect from any of these treatments has been reported.

Fibrinolytic therapy has been associated with increased bleeding and is not recommended.[207-209] Vitamin E has been reported to be of benefit in one uncontrolled study, but this finding was not confirmed in another.[210, 211]

Prognosis

Sixty-four to 85% of children with HUS recover completely, with a mortality of 5% to 10% during the acute illness.[149-151] Some patients fail to recover renal function, and in some patients a slow progression to end-stage renal disease is seen.[150] Low serum calcium levels and severe oliguria or anuria are associated with a poor outcome.[212] After recovery from HUS, patients should be monitored for the development of arterial hypertension and proteinuria. Recurrence of the disorder is very uncommon and suggests a genetic predisposition. Recurrent HUS after renal transplantation has been reported.[213, 214]

Thrombotic Thrombocytopenic Purpura

Thrombotic thrombocytopenic purpura shares many features with HUS, including consumptive thrombocytopenia, microangiopathic hemolytic anemia, and renal dysfunction. Most of the data on treatment and pathogenesis of TTP is based on studies of adults; much less is known about this disorder in children. Whereas a prodromal diarrheal illness is the most common presenting feature in childhood HUS, it is uncommon in TTP. The other classic features of TTP are neurologic dysfunction and fever. However, only 40% of patients present with the classic pentad (thrombocytopenia, fragmentation hemolysis, fever, neurologic dysfunction, and renal impairment) of symptoms.

The pathogenesis of TTP is not known. The development of TTP has been linked to exposure to chemotherapeutic agents,[215-219] oral contraceptives[220, 221] and pregnancy (89% of patients develop it during the antepartum period),[221-224] collagen vascular diseases,[225-229] and cyclosporin A immunosuppression after solid organ or bone marrow transplantation.[214] Infections, including that of human immunodeficiency virus, have also been implicated in up to 40% of patients.[223, 230-232] The incidence of TTP is approximately 1 per million, with a female-to-male ratio of 2:1 and a median age at diagnosis of 35 years.

The microangiopathy of TTP can affect any organ but primarily targets the central nervous system, kidneys, pancreas, heart, and adrenal glands. Pathologically, capillaries and precapillary arterioles have occlusive intraluminal hyaline thrombi, which may also form subendothelial deposits.[233] Gingival biopsy samples demonstrate these abnormalities in 50% of cases,[244] and a bone marrow sample may show these findings in 10% to 20% of cases.[255] Some features of the pathogenesis of TTP are shared with HUS. Evidence exists for endothelial cell damage or activation (PGI$_2$ deficiency,[189, 236, 237] decreased levels of tissue factor pathway inhibitor,[238] and elevated levels of plasma P-selectin).[239] Additionally, similar abnormalities in vWf occur in both

diseases.[240-244] Calpain, a platelet-associated calcium-dependent cysteine protease,[245] is present during acute episodes of TTP.[246] This enzyme has been shown to "modify" the structure and binding characteristics of vWf, so that it will bind to the platelet membrane glycoprotein IIbIIIa, enhancing platelet aggregation.[247] Calpain-induced proteolysis may explain both the loss of the large multimers of vWf from the plasma of patients with acute episodes of TTP and the increased platelet aggregation, which may contribute to microvascular thrombi and end-organ dysfunction.

If untreated, TTP has a 90% mortality. The clinical course of TTP is variable, ranging from a single episode to relapsing or chronic TTP. Plasma infusion was first suggested to be beneficial as a treatment modality in 1963, and this was confirmed in 1977.[248] With plasma therapy, most patients recover from acute TTP; however, 10% to 61% of patients will experience relapse.[220, 221] Plasma exchange has been shown to be superior to plasma infusion in a randomized clinical trial.[249, 250] Initial therapy can be started using infusion if plasma exchange is not available. Patients with TTP can also be treated with the cryosupernatant fraction of plasma.[251, 252] This may be beneficial because the largest plasma vWf multimers are missing from this fraction and because the aggregation induced by TTP plasma is enhanced (*in vitro*) by the addition of the cryoprecipitate.[240, 253] The role of other therapies, including corticosteroids and platelet inhibitor drugs, is controversial.[254] Platelet transfusions should be avoided, because they may accelerate clinical deterioration.[255, 256] The role of splenectomy is uncertain,[257] but it may be of benefit in patients with relapsing TTP.[255, 256, 258]

Familial Hemolytic-Uremic Syndrome

A familial HUS, known in the past by the eponyms Upshaw's syndrome and Shulman's syndrome, is an uncommon, but not rare, disorder.[203, 246, 260] Indeed, most large medical centers have at least one family with this disorder. Some patients have intermittent episodes of classic HUS with azotemia, abdominal pain, thrombocytopenia, and schistocytic hemolytic anemia. Other patients have only schistocytic hemolytic anemia and thrombocytopenia. Less commonly, they have a syndrome that appears identical to TTP. The pathophysiology remains unknown, and there is no diagnostic test for this disorder. The authors and other investigators have demonstrated abnormalities of vWF both at the time of acute illness and after recovery. The authors also observed that a platelet-aggregating factor (the enzyme calpain) is present in the serum of a patient with familial HUS.[260, 261] The enzyme had similar reactivity to the platelet-aggregating factor found in patients with TTP.

Recognition of familial HUS is important because the natural history is of recurring episodes of thrombotic microangiopathy that primarily affects the kidneys. Some patients ultimately progress to end-stage renal failure. Patients with familial HUS respond to plasma infusion. They respond best if the plasma is administered before the disorder becomes severe. The approach the authors use is to treat patients who have recurring episodes with intermittent plasma infusion of 10 to 20 mL/kg. The plasma is given when the patient's platelet count begins to drop. In this way, the majority of acute episodes can be prevented. Over time, many patients fail this therapy and must be managed with more plasma delivered by plasma exchanges.

Kasabach-Merritt Syndrome

The association of congenital capillary hemangiomas with thrombocytopenia was first described in 1940 by Kasabach and Merritt.[262] This lesion typically presents in infancy, although thrombocytopenia and schistocytic hemolytic anemia also can be seen with hemangiomas that present late in life.[263] Most hemangiomas in children regress by 8 years of age. These lesions are more common on the extremities, and removal or regression of the tumor is associated with amelioration of the hematologic abnormalities. Studies suggest that both local and splenic platelet clearance contribute to the thrombocytopenia.[264] Present treatment options include the use of corticosteroids, embolization, radiation therapy, or chemotherapy. A consumptive coagulopathy may also complicate the hemostatic defect in this disorder and may improve with antifibrinolytic therapy.[266] Treatment with interferon alfa may be effective in this disorder and has been used in children with life-threatening complications.[267, 268]

Preeclampsia and Eclampsia

Preeclampsia and eclampsia are microangiopathic disorders of uncertain pathogenesis that occur with pregnancy. These disorders share certain features with both HUS or TTP; however, HUS and TTP are less common causes of schistocytic anemia in pregnancy. Clinical and pathologic findings in these disorders can overlap considerably.[269, 270] Preeclampsia and eclampsia resolve spontaneously after delivery. Because the treatment of TTP and HUS differs considerably from the treatment of preeclampsia and eclampsia, a correct diagnosis is important.[224] Patients who present with an acute microangiopathy early in pregnancy should be managed as if they had acute TTP. Failure of microangiopathy to resolve after delivery should alert the physician to the possibility of TTP or HUS.

Microangiopathy with Malignancy

Schistocytic hemolytic anemia with thrombocytopenia may be seen in association with a number of malignancies, most typically with adenocarcinoma of the stomach or breast.[271] Almost always, the patient has evidence of activation of the coagulation cascade with clinical or subclinical disseminated intravascular coagulation. The hemolytic anemia may resolve with response to therapy. The prognosis for patients with this disorder and an unresponsive tumor is extremely poor. Additionally, patients treated with a number of chemotherapeutic agents, especially mitomycin C, are at risk of developing a microangiopathic hemolytic anemia.[216, 217]

The risk of developing microangiopathy after therapy with mitomycin C is estimated between 4% and 15%.[218] Other chemotherapeutic agents, including cisplatin and bleomycin, have also been implicated.[216] The patient may be in complete remission from his or her tumor at the time he or she presents with anemia and thrombocytopenia. Noncardiogenic pulmonary edema is often noted in patients with this disorder.[271] Poor response to plasma therapy is common, and the mortality is high. Plasma therapy is seldom of benefit, and other treatments must be considered as experimental.[216] Elevation in plasma vWf antigen levels after administration of chemotherapy has been reported.[218, 219] In contrast to HUS, the vWf multimeric profile distribution was not altered in spite of the elevation in antigen levels.

Acquired Microangiopathy with Immunologic Vasculitides

A wide variety of immunologic disorders have been associated with fragmentation hemolysis thrombocytopenia and microangiopathy.[225] These disorders are diseases in which immune complex–mediated endothelial damage is postulated to occur. Immunologic vasculitides with microangiopathy have been reported with systemic lupus erythematosus,[226, 227] polyarteritis nodosa,[228] scleroderma,[228] Goodpasture's syndrome, and glomerulonephritis[272, 273] and after transplantation.[274–276] Because of the considerable overlap in pathologic findings between these disorders and TTP and HUS, the clinical presentation is important in establishing a correct diagnosis.

TTP can occur in patients with pre-existing collagen vascular disorders; however, TTP is an uncommon manifestation or complication of systemic lupus.[226] Distinction between the disorders may be difficult because of the multisystemic involvement seen in both diseases. Additionally, the vasculitides within the central nervous system of patients with systemic lupus erythematosus are identical to the microangiopathic lesions of TTP.[226] Response to plasma exchange therapy in patients with acute, severe microangiopathy has been reported.[226] The authors favor this approach for patients presenting with an episode clinically indistinguishable from TTP.

HUS may occur in patients who have undergone allogeneic kidney transplantation.[275] Sometimes it recurs, destroying the graft. Additionally, HUS may occur in association with other glomerular diseases.[273] Thrombotic microangiopathy can arise as a complication of solid organ transplantation and can be difficult to distinguish from allograft rejection and cyclosporin A toxicity.[273–277] Immunologic injury to the vessel is thought to be the cause of the microangiopathy of organ rejection. Because the management of recurrent HUS and allograft rejection is different, the presence of a cellular infiltrate on a biopsy specimen may help exclude HUS.

Patients who develop microangiopathy after allogeneic bone marrow transplantation have an extremely poor prognosis.[278] Unlike patients with TTP and HUS, most of these patients have laboratory evidence of disseminated intravascular coagulation. The disorder is often associated with the use of cyclosporin A prophylaxis. Plasma levels of vWf are elevated, reflecting endothelial injury.[278] The precise mechanism of endothelial injury is not known, but the correlation with severe acute graft-versus-host disease in many patients suggests that the microangiopathy is secondary to an immunologic injury. Responses to therapy are uncommon.

References

1. Berendes M: The proportion of reticulocytes in the erythrocytes of the spleen as compared with those of circulating blood, with special reference to hemolytic states. Blood 1959; 14:558.
2. Aschoff L: Das Reticulo-endotheliale System. Ergeb Inn Med Kinderheilkd 1924; 26:1.
3. Van Furth R, Cohn ZA, et al: The mononuclear phagocytic system: a new classification of macrophages, monocytes and their precursor cells. Bull World Health Organ 1972; 46:845.
4. Groopman JE, Golde DW: Biochemistry and function of monocytes and macrophages. In Williams WJ, Beutler E, et al (eds): Hematology. New York, McGraw-Hill Book Co., 1983, p 848.
5. Golde DW, Groopman JE: Cellular kinetics of monocytes and macrophages. In Williams WJ, Beutler E, et al (eds): Hematology. New York, McGraw-Hill Book Co., 1983, p 854.
6. Bainton DF, Golde DW: Differentiation of macrophages from normal human bone marrow in liquid culture. J Clin Invest 1978; 61:1555.
7. Goodman JR, Wallerstein AO, et al: The ultrastructure of bone marrow histiocytes in megaloblastic anaemia and the anaemia of infection. Br J Haematol 1968; 14:471.
8. Wickramasinghe SM, Bush V: Observations on the ultrastructure of erythropoietic cells and reticulum cells in the bone marrow of patients with homozygous beta-thalassemia. Br J Haematol 1975; 30:395.
9. Wickramasinghe SN, Hughes M: Some features of bone marrow macrophages in patients with homozygous beta-thalassemia. Br J Haematol 1978; 38:23.
10. Jacob HS, MacDonald RA, et al: Regulation of spleen growth and sequestering function. J Clin Invest 1963; 42:1476.
11. Jandl JH, Files NM, et al: Proliferative response of the spleen and liver to hemolysis. J Exp Med 1965; 122:299.
12. Louareesuwan S, Ho M, et al: Dynamic alteration in splenic function during acute falciparum malaria. N Engl J Med 1987; 317:675.
13. Clark MR, Mohandas M, et al: Osmotic gradient ektacytometry: Comprehensive characterization of red cell volume and surface maintenance. Blood 1983; 61:899.
14. Connor J, Pak CC, et al: Exposure of phosphatidylserine in the outer leaflet of human red blood cells. J Biol Chem 1994; 269:2399.
15. Kay MMB: Mechanism of removal of senescent cells by human macrophages in situ. Proc Natl Acad Sci U S A 1975; 72:3521.
16. Kay MMB: Localization of senescent cell antigen on band 3. Proc Natl Acad Sci U S A 1984; 81:5753.
17. Lutz H, Fasler S, et al: Naturally occurring anti-band 3 antibodies and complement in phagocytosis of oxidatively-stressed land in clearance of senescent red cells. Blood Cells 1988; 14:175.
18. Low PS, Waugh SM, et al: The role of hemoglobin denaturation and band 3 clustering in red blood cell aging. Science 1985; 227:531.
19. Lutz HU, Wipf G: Naturally occurring autoantibodies to skeletal proteins from human red blood cells. J Immunol 1982; 128:1695.
20. Kay MMB, Sorensen K, et al: Antigenicity, storage, and aging: Physiologic autoantibodies to cell membrane and serum proteins and the senescent cell antigen. Mol Cell Biochem 1982; 49:65.
21. Szymanski I, Odgren PR: Studies on the preservation of red blood cells. Attachment of the third component of human complement to erythrocytes during storage at 4°C. Vox Sang 1979; 36:213.
22. Khansari N, Fudenberg HH: Phagocytosis of senescent erythrocytes by autologous monocytes: Requirement of membrane-specific autologous IgG for immune eliminations of aging red blood cells. Cell Immunol 1983; 78:114.
23. Freedman J: Membrane-bound immunoglobulins and complement components on young and old red blood cells. Transfusion 1984; 21:477.
24. Lutz HU, Flepp R, Strgaro-Wipf G: Naturally occurring autoantibodies to exoplasmic and cryptic regions of band 3 protein, the major integral membrane protein of human red blood cells. J Immunol 1984; 133:2610.
25. Kelton JG, Denomme G: The quantitation of platelet-associated IgG on cohorts of platelets separated from healthy individuals by buoyant density centrifugation. Blood 1982; 60:136.
26. Green GA, Rehn MM, Kalra VK: Cell-bound autologous immunoglobulin in erythrocyte subpopulations from patients with sickle cell disease. Blood 1985; 65:1127.
27. Galili U, Clark MR, Shohet SB: Excessive binding of natural anti-alpha-galactosyl immunoglobulin G to sickle erythrocytes may contribute to extravascular cell destruction. J Clin Invest 1986; 77:27.
28. Müller-Eberhard HJ: Complement. Springer Semin Immunopathol 1983; 6:2.
29. Bokisch VA, Dririch MP, et al: Third component of complement (C3): Structural properties in relation to functions. Proc Natl Acad Sci U S A 1975; 72:1989.
30. Jaffe C, Atkinson JP, et al: The role of complement in the clearance of cold agglutinin-sensitized erythrocytes in man. J Clin Invest 1976; 58:942.
31. Schreiber AD, Frank MM: Role of antibody and complement in the immune clearance and destruction of erythrocytes. J Clin Invest 1972; 51:575.
32. King HK, Schumaker HB: Splenic studies. I. Susceptibility to infection after splenectomy in infancy. Ann Surg 1952; 136:239.
33. Lockwood CM: Immunological functions of the spleen. Clin Haematol 1983; 12:449.
34. Christensen BE, Jonsson V, et al: Traffic of T and B lymphocytes in the normal spleen. Scand J Haematol 1978; 20:246.
35. Rowley DA: The formation of circulating antibody in the splenectomized human being following intravenous injection of heterologous erythrocytes. J Immunol 1950; 65:515.
36. Rowley DA: The effect of splenectomy on the formation of circulating antibody in the adult male albino rat. J Immunol 1959; 64:289.
37. Sullivan JL, Ochs HD, et al: Immune response after splenectomy. Lancet 1978; 1:178.
38. Schumacher MJ: Serum immunoglobulin and transferrin levels after childhood splenectomy. Arch Dis Child 1970; 45:114.
39. Claret I, Morals L, et al: Immunological studies in the postsplenectomy syndrome. J Pediatr Surg 1975; 10:59.
40. Romball CG, Weigle WO: Splenic role in the regulation of immune responses. Cell Immunol 1977; 34:376.
41. Klaus GGB: Antigen-antibody complexes elicit antiidiopathic antibodies to self idiotypes. Nature 1978; 272:265.
42. Spirer Z, Hauser GJ, et al: Autoimmune antibodies after splenectomy. Acta Haematol 1980; 63:230.
43. Toghill PJ: Red cell pooling in enlarged spleens. Br J Haematol 1964; 10:347.
44. Jandl JH, Aster RH: Increased splenic pooling and the pathogenesis of hypersplenism. Am J Med 1967; 253:383.
45. Song SH, Groom AC: The distribution of red cells in the spleen. Can J Physiol Pharmacol 1971; 49:734.
46. Wennberg E, Weiss L: The structure of the spleen and hemolysis. Annu Rev Med 1969; 20:29.
47. Burke JS, Simon GT: Electron microscopy of the spleen. I. Anatomy and microcirculation. Am J Pathol 1970; 58:127.
48. Hirasawa Y, Tokuhiro H: Electron microscopic studies on the normal spleen: especially on the red pulp and the reticuloendothelial cells. Blood 1970; 35:201.
49. Weiss L, Tavassoli M: Anatomical hazards to the passage of erythrocytes through the spleen. Semin Hematol 1970; 7:372.
50. Chen IT, Weiss I: Electron microscopy of the red pulp of the human spleen. Am J Anat 1972; 134:425.
51. Barnhart MI, Lusher JM: The human spleen as revealed by scanning electron microscopy. Am J Hematol 1976; 1:243.

52. Bowdler AJ: Splenomegaly and hypersplenism. Clin Haematol 1983; 12:467.

53. Bishop MB, Lansing LS: The spleen: a correlative overview of normal and pathologic anatomy. Hum Pathol 1982; 13:334.

54. Coetzee T: Clinical anatomy and physiology of the spleen. S Afr Med J 1982; 61:737.

55. Schreiber AD, Frank MM: Role of antibody and complement in the immune clearance and destruction of erythrocytes. J Clin Invest 1972; 51:575.

56. Unkeless JC, Wright SD: Phagocytic cells: Fly and complement receptors. In Gallin JI, Synderman R (eds): Inflammation: Basic Principles and Chemical Correlates. New York: Raven Press, 1988, p 343.

57. Crosby WH: Normal functions of the spleen relative to red blood cells: a review. Blood 1959; 14:399.

58. Jacob HS, Jandl HH: Effects of sulfhydryl inhibition on red blood cells. II. Studies *in vivo.* J Clin Invest 1962; 41:1514.

59. Rifkind RA: Destruction of injured red cells *in vivo.* Am J Med 1966; 41:721.

60. Weed RI, Weiss L: The relationship of red cell fragmentation occurring within the spleen to cell destruction. Trans Assoc Am Physicians 1966; 179:426.

61. Seeler RA, Shwiaki MZ: Acute splenic sequestration crises in young children with sickle-cell anemia. Clin Pediatr 1972; 1:701.

62. Bowdler AJ: The role of the spleen and splenectomy in autoimmune hemolytic anemia. Semin Hematol 1976; 13:335.

63. Lewis SM, Szur L, et al: The pattern of erythrocyte destruction in haemolytic anaemia, as studied with radioactive chromium. Br J Haematol 1960; 6:122.

64. Mollison PL, Crome P, et al: Rate of removal from the circulation of red cells sensitized with different amounts of antibody. Br J Haematol 1969; 11:461.

65. Wennberg E, Weiss L: Splenic erythroclasia: An electron microscopic study of hemoglobin H disease. Blood 1968; 31:778.

66. Nathan DG, Gunn RB: Thalassemia: consequences of unbalanced hemoglobin synthesis. Am J Med 1966; 41:815.

66a. Nathan DG: Rubbish in the red cell. N Engl J Med 1969; 281:558. Editorial.

67. Weed RI, Lacelle PL, et al: Metabolic dependence of red cell deformability. J Clin Invest 1969; 45:1137.

68. Nathan DG, Shohet SB: Erythrocyte ion transport defects and hemolytic anemia. Semin Hematol 1970; 7:381.

69. Mentzer WC Jr, Baehner RL, et al: Selective reticulocyte destruction in erythrocyte pyruvate kinase deficiency. J Clin Invest 1971; 50:688.

70. Murphy JR: The influence of pH and temperature on some physical properties of normal erythrocytes and erythrocytes from patients with hereditary spherocytosis. J Lab Clin Med 1967; 69:756.

71. Smith CH, Erlandson ME, et al: The role of splenectomy in the management of thalassemia. Blood 1960; 15:197.

72. Smith CH, Erlandson ME, et al: Postsplenectomy infection in Cooley's anemia. An appraisal of the problem in this and other blood disorders. N Engl J Med 1962; 266:737.

73. Eraklis AJ, Kevy SV, et al: Hazard of overwhelming infection after splenectomy in childhood. N Engl J Med 1967; 276:1225.

74. Eraklis AJ, Filler RM: Splenectomy in childhood. A review of 1413 cases. J Pediatr Surg 1972; 7:382.

75. Edwards LD: Infections in splenectomized patients. A study of 131 patients. Scand J Infect Dis 1976; 8:255.

76. Krivey N, Tatarski I: Infections after splenectomy. N Engl J Med 1978; 298:165.

77. Chilcote RR, Baehner RL, et al: Septicemia and meningitis in children splenectomized for Hodgkin's disease. N Engl J Med 1976; 295:789.

78. Singer DB: Postsplenectomy sepsis. Perspect Pediatr Pathol 1973; 1:285.

79. Gwaltney JM Jr, Sande MA, et al: Spread of *Streptococcus pneumoniae* in families. II. Relation of transfer of *S. pneumoniae* to incidence of colds and serum antibody. J Infect Dis 1975; 132:62.

80. Claret J, Morales L, et al: Immunological studies in the postsplenectomy syndrome. J Pediatr Surg 1975; 10:59.

81. Golematis B, Tzarchis P, et al: Overwhelming postsplenectomy infection in patients with thalassemia major. Mt Sinai J Med 1989; 56:97.

82. Gavrillis P, Rothenberg SP, et al: Correlation of low serum IgM levels with absence of functional splenic tissue in sickle cell disease syndromes. Am J Med 1974; 57:542.

83. Ciebink GS, Foker JE, et al: Serum antibody and opsonic responses to vaccination with pneumococcal capsular polysaccharide in normal and splenectomized children. J Infect Dis 1980; 141:404.

84. Kreuzfelder E, Obertacke MD, et al: Alterations of the immune system following splenectomy in childhood. J Trauma 1991; 31:358.

85. Kingsley G, Pitzalis C, et al: Correlation of immunoregulatory function with cell phenotype in cord blood lymphocytes. Clin Exp Immunol 1988; 73:40.

86. Bottomly K: A functional dichotomy in CD4+ T lymphocytes. Immunol Today 1988; 9:268.

87. DePaoli P, Battistin S, et al: Age-related changes in human lymphocyte subsets: Progressive reduction of CD4CD45R (suppressor inducer) population. Clin Immunol Immunopathol 1988; 48:290.

88. Dahl M, Håakansson A, et al: Polymorphonuclear neutrophil function and infections following splenectomy in childhood. Scand J Haematol 1986; 37:137.

89. Håakansson L, Foucard T, et al: Neutrophil function in infection-prone children. Arch Dis Child 1980; 55:776.

90. Posey DL, Marks C: Overwhelming postsplenectomy sepsis in childhood. Am J Surg 1983; 145:318.

91. Hague AU, Min KW: Postsplenectomy pneumococcemia in adults. Arch Pathol Lab Med 1980; 104:258.

92. Krivit W: Overwhelming postsplenectomy infection. Surg Clin North Am 1979; 59:223.

93. Schwartz PE, Sterioff S, et al: Postsplenectomy sepsis and mortality in adults. JAMA 1982; 248:2279.

94. Kingston ME, MacKenzie CR: The syndrome of pneumococcemia, disseminated intravascular coagulation and asplenia. Can Med Assoc J 1979; 121:57.

95. Whittaker AN: Infection and the spleen: Association between hyposplenism, pneumococcal sepsis and disseminated intravascular coagulation. Med J Aust 1969; 1:1213.

96. Sullivan JL, Ochs HD, et al: Immune response after splenectomy. Lancet 1978; 1:178.

97. Siber GR, Weitzman SA: Antibody response of patients with Hodgkin's disease to protein and polysaccharide antigens. Rev Infect Dis 1981; 3:S144.

98. Lawrence EM, Edwards KM: Pneumococcal vaccine in normal children. Am J Dis Child 1983; 137:846.

99. Pedersen FK, Henrichsen J, et al: Antibody response to vaccination with pneumococcal capsular polysaccharides in splenectomized children. Acta Paediatr Scand 1982; 71:451.

100. Austrian R: Pneumococcal infection and pneumococcal vaccine. N Engl J Med 1977; 297:938.

101. Ammann AJ, Addiego J, et al: Polyvalent pneumococcal-polysaccharide immunization of patients with sickle-cell anemia and patients with splenectomy. N Engl J Med 1977; 297:897.

102. Austrian R: A reassessment of pneumococcal vaccine. N Engl J Med 1984; 310:651.

103. Siber GR, Gorham C, et al: Antibody response to pretreatment immunization and posttreatment boosting with bacterial polysaccharide vaccines in patients with Hodgkin's disease. Ann Intern Med 1986; 104:467.

104. Obaro S, Henderson DC, et al: Long-term management after splenectomy. Monitor antibody levels after vaccination. BMJ 1994; 308:339.

105. Lanzkowsky P, Karayalcain G, et al: Complications of laparotomy and splenectomy in stages of Hodgkin's disease in children. Am J Hematol 1976; 1:393.

106. Advisory Committee on Immunization Practices: Recommendations of the Advisory Committee on Immunization Practices (ACIP): Use of vaccines and immune globulins in persons with altered immunocompetence. MMWR 1993; 42:1.

107. McMullin M, Johnstone G: Long-term management of patients after splenectomy. BMJ 1993; 307:1372.

108. Gonzaga RAF: Fatal post-splenectomy pneumococcal sepsis despite prophylaxis. Lancet 1984; 2:694.

109. John AB, Ramlal A, et al: Prevention of pneumococcal infection in children with homozygous sickle cell disease. BMJ 1984; 288:1567.

110. Hays DM, Lernberg JL, et al: Postsplenectomy sepsis and other complications following staging laparotomy for Hodgkin's disease in childhood. J Pediatr 1986; 21:628.

111. Broome CV, Facklam RR, et al: Pneumococcal disease after pneumococcal vaccination. An alternative method to estimate the efficacy of pneumococcal vaccine. N Engl J Med 1980; 303:549.

112. Ahonkhai VI, Landesman SH, et al: Failure of pneumococcal vaccine in children with sickle-cell disease. N Engl J Med 1979; 301:26.

113. Overturf GD, Field R: Death from type 6 pneumococcal septicemia in a vaccinated child with sickle-cell disease. N Engl J Med 1979; 300:143.

114. Krivit W: Overwhelming post-splenectomy infection. Am J Hematol 1977; 2:193.

115. White KS, Covington D, et al: Patients awareness of health precautions after splenectomy. Am J Infect Control 1991; 19:36.

116. Brain MC, Dacie JV, et al: Microangiopathic haemolytic anaemia: The possible role of vascular lesions in pathogenesis. Br J Haematol 1962; 8:358.

117. Monroe WM, Strauss AF: Intravascular hemolysis: A morphologic study of schistocytes in thrombotic purpura and other disease. South Med J 1953; 46:837.

118. Rubenberg ML, Regoeczi E, et al: Microangiopathic haemolytic anaemia: the experimental production of haemolysis and red-cell fragmentation by defibrination in vivo. Br J Haematol 1967; 14:627.

119. Venkatachalam MA, Jones DB, et al: Microangiopathic haemolytic anemia in rats with malignant hypertension. Blood 1968; 32:278.

120. Bull BS, Rubenberg ML, et al: Microangiopathic haemolytic anaemia: mechanisms of red-cell fragmentation: In vitro studies. Br J Haematol 1968; 14:643.

121. Bull BS, Kuhn IN: The production of schistocytes by fibrin strands (a scanning electron microscope study). Blood 1970; 35:104.

122. Brodeur MTH, Sutherland DW, et al: Red cell survival in patients with aortic valvular disease and ball valve prosthesis. Circulation 1965; 32:570.

123. Westring DW: Aortic valve disease and hemolytic anemia. Ann Intern Med 1966; 65:203.

124. Ravenel SD, Johnson JD, et al: Intravascular hemolysis associated with coarctation of the aorta. J Pediatr 1969; 75:67.

125. Westphal RG, Azem EA: Macroangiopathic hemolytic anemia due to congenital cardiac anomalies. JAMA 1971; 216:1477.

126. Moisey CU, Manohitharajah SM, et al: Hemolytic anemia in a child in association with congenital mitral valve disease. J Thorac Cardiovasc Surg 1972; 63:765.

127. Marsh GW, Lewis SM: Cardiac haemolytic anaemia. Semin Hematol 1969; 6:133.

128. Thompson ME, Lewis JH, et al: Indexes of intravascular hemolysis, quantification of coagulation factors and platelet survival in patients with porcine heterograft valves. Am J Cardiol 1983; 51:489.

129. Nevaril CG, Lynch EC, et al: Erythrocyte destruction and damage induced by shearing stress. J Lab Clin Med 1968; 71:784.

130. Monroe JM, True DE, et al: Surface roughness and edge geometrics in hemolysis with rotating disc flow. J Biomed Mater Res 1981; 15:923.

131. Blackshear PL Jr, Dorman FD, et al: Shear wall interaction and hemolysis. Trans Am Soc Artif Intern Organs 1966; 12:113.

132. Sears DA, Crosby WH: Intravascular hemolysis due to intracardiac prosthetic devices. Diurnal variations related to activity. Am J Med 1965; 39:341.

133. Myhre E, Rasmussen K, et al: Serum lactic dehydrogenase activity in patients with prosthetic heart valves: A parameter of intravascular hemolysis. Am Heart J 1970; 80:463.

134. Eysters E, Mayer K, et al: Traumatic hemolysis with iron deficiency anemia in patients with aortic valve lesions. Ann Intern Med 1968; 68:995.

135. Giromini M, Laperbonza C: Prolonged survival after bilateral nephrectomy in an adult with haemolytic uraemic syndrome. Lancet 1969; 2:169.

136. Gavras H, Brown WCB, et al: Microangiopathic hemolytic anemia and the development of malignant phase of hypertension. Circ Res 1971; 28:127.

137. Davidson RJL: Exertional haemoglobinuria: A report on three cases with studies on the hemolytic mechanism. J Clin Pathol 1964; 17:536.

138. Buckle RM: Exertional (march) hemoglobinuria. Reduction of hemolytic episodes by use of sorbo-rubber insoles in shoes. Lancet 1965; 1:1136.

139. Streeton JA: Traumatic haemoglobinuria caused by karate exercises. Lancet 1967; 2:191.

140. Kaden WS: Traumatic hemoglobinuria in conga drum players. Lancet 1970; 1:1341.

141. Shen SC, Ham TH, et al: Studies in the destruction of red blood cells. III. Mechanisms and complications of hemoglobinuria in patients with thermal burns: spherocytosis and increased osmotic fragility of red blood cells. N Engl J Med 1943; 229:701.

142. Tarr PI, Neill MA, et al: Increasing incidence of the hemolytic-uremic syndrome in King County, Washington: Lack of evidence for ascertainment bias. Am J Epidemiol 1989; 129:582.

143. Neild GH: Hemolytic-uraemic syndrome in practice. Lancet 1994; 343:398.

144. Smith HR, Scotland SM: Vero cytotoxin-producing strains of Escherichia coli. J Med Microbiol 1988; 26:77.

145. Brasher C, Siegler RL: The hemolytic-uremic syndrome. West J Med 1981; 134:193.

146. Siegler RL: Spectrum of extrarenal involvement in postdiarrheal hemolytic-uremic syndrome. J Pediatr 1994; 125:511.

147. Griffin PM, Ostroff SM, et al: Illnesses associated with Escherichia coli 0157-H7 infections. Ann Intern Med 1988; 109:705.

148. Cimolai N, Morrison BJ, et al: Risk factors for the central nervous system manifestations of gastroenteritis-associated hemolytic-uremic syndrome. Paediatrics 1992; 90:616.

149. Rasoulpour M, Leichtner A, et al: Cerebral vascular accident during the recovery phase of hemolytic-uremic syndrome. Int J Pediatr Nephrol 1985; 6:287.

150. Siegler RL: Central nervous system involvement in hemolytic-uremic syndrome. J Pediatr 1989; 114:901.

151. Van Dyck M, Proesmans W, et al: Hemolytic uremic syndrome in childhood: Renal function ten years later. Clin Nephrol 1988; 19:109.

152. Milford DV, Staten I, et al: Prognostic markers in diarrhoea-associated haemolytic-uremic syndrome: Initial neutrophil count, human neutrophil elastase and von Willebrand factor antigen. Nephrol Dial Transplant 1991; 6:232.

153. Bergstein JM, Riley M, et al: Role of plasminogen-activator inhibitor type 1 in the pathogenesis and outcome of the hemolytic uremic syndrome. N Engl J Med 1992; 327:755.

154. Richardson SE, Karmali MA, et al: This histopathology of the hemolytic uremic syndrome associated with verocytotoxin-producing Escherichia coli infections. Hum Pathol 1988; 19:1102.

155. Levy M, Gagnadous MF, et al: Pathology of hemolytic-uremic syndrome in children. In Remuzzi G, Mecca G, et al (eds): Hemostasis, Prostaglandins, and Renal Disease. New York, Raven Press, 1980, p 383.

156. Fong JSC, de Chadarevian JP, et al: Hemolytic-uremic syndrome. Current concepts and management. Pediatr Clin North Am 1982; 29:835.

157. Steele BT, Murphy N, Rance CP: An outbreak of hemolytic uremic syndrome associated with ingestion of fresh apple juice. J Pediatr 1982; 101:963.

158. Karmali MA, Petric M, et al: The association between idiopathic hemolytic uremic syndrome and infection by verotoxin-producing Escherichia coli. J Infect Dis 1985; 151:775.

159. Cleary TG: Cytotoxin-producing Escherichia coli and the hemolytic uremic syndrome. Pediatr Clin North Am 1988; 35:485.

160. O'Brien A, Melton AR, et al: Profile of Escherichia coli 0157:H7 pathogen responsible for hamburger-bovine outbreak of hemorrhagic colitis and hemolytic uremic syndrome in Washington. J Clin Microbiol 1993; 31:2799.

161. Brandt JR, Fouser LS, et al: Escherichia coli 0157:H7–associated hemolytic uremic syndrome after ingestion of contaminated hamburgers. J Pediatr 1994; 125:519.

162. Rowe PC, Orrkine E, et al: Epidemic Escherichia coli 0157:H7 gastroenteritis and hemolytic-uremic syndrome in a Canadian Inuit community: intestinal illness in family members as a risk factor. J Pediatr 1994; 124:21.

163. Kinney JS, Gross TP, et al: Hemolytic-uremic syndrome: A pop-

ulation-based study in Washington, DC, and Baltimore, Maryland. Am J Public Health 1988; 78:64.

164. Cleary TG, Lopez EL: The Shiga-like toxin-producing *Escherichia coli* and the hemolytic uremic syndrome. Pediatr Infect Dis J 1989; 8:720.

165. Obrig TG: Pathogenesis of Shiga toxin (verotoxin)-induced endothelial cell injury. In Kaplan BS, Trompeter RS, Moake JL (eds): Hemolytic-uraemic syndrome and thrombotic thrombocytopenic purpura. New York, Marcel Dekker, 1992, p 405.

166. Ashkenazi S: Role of bacterial cytokine in hemolytic uremic syndrome and thrombotic thrombocytopenic purpura. Ann Rev Med 1993; 44:11.

167. Jackson MP, Newland JW, et al: Nucleotide sequence analysis of the structural gene for Shiga-like toxin I by bacteriophage 933J from E. coli. Microb Pathog 1987; 2:147.

168. Jackson MP, Strockbine NA, et al: DNA sequence comparisons of Shiga toxin, Shiga-like toxin I and Shiga-like toxin II. Presented before the International Symposium and Workshop on Verocytotoxin-Producing *E. coli* Infections. Toronto, Canada, July 1987.

169. Igarashi K, Ogasawara T, et al: Mode of action of verotoxins. Presented before the International Symposium and Workshop on Verocytotoxin-Producing *E. coli* Infections. Toronto, Canada, July 1987.

170. Head SC, Karmali MA, et al: Serological differences between verocytotoxin 2 and Shiga-like toxin II. Lancet 1988; 2:751.

171. Karch H, Hessemann J, et al: A plasmid of enterohemorrhagic *Escherichia coli* 0157-H7 is required for expression of a new fimbrial antigen and for adhesion to epithelial cell. Infect Immunol 1986; 55:455.

172. Ostroff SM, Tam PI, et al: Toxin genotypes and plasmid profiles as determinants of systemic sequelae in *Escherichia coli* 0157:H7 infections. J Infect Dis 1989; 160:994.

173. Tesh VL, Burris JA, et al: Comparison of the relative toxicities of Shiga-like toxins type I and type II for mice. Infect Immun 61:3392, 1993.

174. Lingwood CA, Law H, et al: Glycolipid binding of purified and recombinant *Escherichia coli* produced verotoxin *in vitro*. J Biol Chem 1987; 262:8834.

175. Cohen A, Hannigan GE, et al: Role of globotriosyl- and galabiosylceramide in verotoxin binding and high-affinity interferon receptor. J Biol Chem 1987; 262:17088.

176. Boyd B, Lingwood C: Verotoxin receptor glycolipid in human renal tissue. Nephron 1989; 51:207.

177. Fong JSC, Kaplan BS: Impairment of platelet aggregation in hemolytic uremic syndrome: Evidence for platelet "exhaustion." Blood 1982; 60:564.

178. Kaplan BS, Fong JSC: Reduced platelet aggregation in hemolytic-uremic syndrome. Thromb Haemost 1980; 43:154.

179. Bockenstedt P, Greenberg JM, Handin RI: Structural basis of von Willebrand factor binding to platelet glycoprotein Ib and collagen. J Clin Invest 1986; 17:743.

180. Ruggeri ZM, Demarco L, et al: Platelets have more than one binding site for von Willebrand factor. J Clin Invest 1983; 72:1.

181. Moake JL, Byrnes JJ, et al: Abnormal VIII: von Willebrand factor patterns in the plasma of patients with the hemolytic-uremic syndrome. Blood 1984; 64:59.

182. Mannucci PM, Lombardi R, et al: Enhanced proteolysis of plasma von Willebrand factor in thrombotic thrombocytopenic purpura and the hemolytic uremic syndrome. Blood 1989; 74:978.

182a. Forsyth KD, Simpson AC, et al: Neutrophil-mediated endothelial injury in haemolytic uraemic syndrome. Lancet 1989; 2:411.

183. Leung DYM, Moake JL, et al: Lytic anti-endothelial cell antibodies in haemolytic-uraemic syndrome. Lancet 1988; 2:183.

184. Dubilier LD, Chadwick JA, et al: Thymic lymphoplasia associated with the hemolytic uremic syndrome. J Pediatr 1968; 73:714.

185. Krivit W, Good RA: Aldrich's syndrome (thrombocytopenia, eczema and infection in infants). Studies of the defense mechanisms. Am J Dis Child 1959; 97:137.

186. Fluge G, Moe PJ: Hemolytic uremic (nephropathic) syndrome. Acta Pediatr Scand 1967; 56:665.

187. Mathieu H, Lederc F, et al: Étude clinique et biologique de 38 obsérvations de syndrome hémolytique et urémique. Arch Fr Pediatr 1969; 26:369.

188. van de Kar N, Kooistra T, et al: Tumor necrosis factor α induces endothelial galactosyl transferase activity and verocytotoxin receptors. Role of specific tumor necrosis factor receptors and protein kinase C. Blood 1995; 85:734.

189. Defreyn G, Proesmans W, et al: Abnormal prostacyclin metabolism in the hemolytic uremic syndrome: equivocal effect of prostacyclin infusions. Clin Nephrol 1982; 18:43.

190. Webster J, Rees AJ, et al: Prostacyclin deficiency in haemolytic-uraemic syndrome. BMJ 1980; 281:271.

191. George CR, Slichter SJ, et al: A kinetic evaluation of hemostasis in renal disease. N Engl J Med 1974; 291:1111.

192. Badami KG, Srivastava RN, et al: Disseminated intravascular coagulation in post-dysenteric haemolytic uraemic syndrome. Acta Pediatr Scand 1987; 76:919.

193. Kaplan BS, Mills M: Elevated serum elastase and alpha-1-antitrypsin levels in hemolytic uremic syndrome. Clin Nephrol 1988; 30:193.

194. Powell HR, Groves V, et al: Arachidonic acid in haemolytic uraemic syndrome. Pediatr Nephrol 1987; 1:C52.

195. O'Regan S, Chesney RW, et al: Red cell membrane phospholipid abnormalities in the hemolytic uremic syndrome. Clin Nephrol 1980; 15:14.

196. Taylor CM, Situnayake RD, et al: A marker of lipid peroxidation in haemolytic uraemic syndrome (HUS). Pediatr Nephrol 1987; 1:C52.

197. Siegler RL, Smith JB, et al: Prostacyclin production and vitamin E in the haemolytic uremic syndrome. Pediatr Res 1984; 18:370A.

198. Sugihara K, Sugihara T, et al: Thrombospondin mediates adherence of CD36+ sickle reticulocytes to endothelial cells. Blood 1992; 80:2634.

199. Greatorex J, Thorne CM: Humoral immune responses to Shiga-like toxins and *Escherichia coli* 0157 lipopolysaccharide in hemolytic-uremic syndrome patients and healthy subjects. J Clin Microbiol 1994; 32:1172.

200. Chart H, Scotland SM, et al: Serum antibodies to *Escherichia coli* serotype 0157:H7 in patients with hemolytic uremic syndrome. J Clin Microbiol 1989; 27:285.

201. Scotland SM, Rowe B, et al: Vero cytotoxin-producing strains of *Escherichia coli* from children with haemolytic uraemic syndrome and their detection by specific DNA probes. J Med Microbiol 1988; 25:237.

202. Rizzoni G, Claris-Appiani A, et al: Plasma infusion for hemolytic uremic syndrome in children: Results of a multi-center controlled trial. J Pediatr 1988; 112:284.

203. Upshaw JD Jr: Congenital deficiency of a factor in normal plasma that reverses microangiopathic hemolysis and thrombocytopenia. N Engl J Med 1978; 298:1350.

204. O'Regan S, Chesney RW, et al: Aspirin and dipyridamole therapy in the hemolytic uremic syndrome. J Pediatr 1980; 97:473.

205. Van Damme-Lombaerts R, Proesmans W, et al: Heparin plus dipyridamole in childhood hemolytic uremic syndrome: A prospective, randomized study. J Pediatr 1988; 113:913.

206. Sheth KJ, Gill JC, et al: High-dose intravenous gamma globulin infusions in hemolytic-uremic syndrome: A preliminary report. Am J Dis Child 1990; 144:268.

207. Powell HR, Ekert H: Streptokinase and antithrombotic therapy in the hemolytic uremic syndrome. J Pediatr 1974; 845:345.

208. Stewart J, Winterborn MH, et al: Thrombolytic therapy in haemolytic uraemic syndrome. BMJ 1974; 3:217.

209. Stuart J, White RHR: Thrombolytic therapy in haemolytic uraemic syndrome. BMJ 1975; 1:152.

210. Powell HR, McCredie DA, et al: Vitamin E treatment of haemolytic uraemic syndrome. Arch Dis Child 1984; 59:401.

211. Thomson PD, Milner LS: A randomized selected trial of vitamin E in the haemolytic uraemic syndrome (HUS). Presented before the Tenth International Congress on Nephrology, London, 1987, p 98A.

212. Havens PL, O'Rourke RP, et al: Laboratory and clinical variables to predict outcome in hemolytic-uremic syndrome. Am J Dis Child 1988; 142:961.

213. Van den Berg-Wolf MG, Koote AMM, et al: Recurrent hemolytic uremic syndrome in a renal transplant recipient and review of the Leiden experience. Transplantation 1988; 45:248.

214. Springate J, Fildes R, et al: Recurrent hemolytic syndrome after renal transplantation. Transplant Proc 1988; 20:559.

215. Jackson AM, Rose BD, et al: Thrombotic microangiopathy and renal failure associated with antiplastic chemotherapy. Ann Intern Med 1984; 101:41.

216. Murgo AJ: Thrombotic microangiopathy in the cancer patient including those induced by chemotherapeutic agents. Semin Hematol 1987; 24:161.

217. Doll DC, Ringenberg QA, et al: Vascular toxicity associated with antineoplastic agents. J Clin Oncol 1986; 4:1405.

218. Cantrell JE, Phillips TM, Schein PS: Carcinoma-associated hemolytic-uremic syndrome: A complication of mitomycin C chemotherapy. J Clin Oncol 1985; 3:723.

219. Licciardello JT, Moake JL, et al: Elevated plasma von Willebrand factor levels and arterial occlusive complications associated with cisplatin-based chemotherapy. Oncology 1985; 42:296.

220. Cuttner J: Thrombotic thrombocytopenic purpura: A ten year experience. Blood 1980; 56:30.

221. Holdrinet RSG, Namdar Z, et al: Thrombotic thrombocytopenic purpura: Clinical course and response to therapy in twelve patients. Neth J Med 1988; 33:113.

222. Neame PD: Immunologic and other factors in TTP. Semin Thromb Hemost 1980; 6:416.

223. Wurzel JM: TTP lesions in placenta but not fetus. N Engl J Med 1979; 301:503.

224. Weiner CP: Thrombotic microangiopathy in pregnancy and the postpartum period. Semin Hematol 1987; 24:119.

225. Kwaan HC: Miscellaneous secondary thrombotic microangiopathy. Semin Hematol 1987; 24:141.

226. Gelfran J, Truong L, et al: Thrombotic thrombocytopenic purpura syndrome in systemic lupus erythematosus: Treatment with plasma infusion. Am J Kidney Dis 1985; 6:154.

227. Devinsky O, Petito CK, et al: Clinical and neuropathological finding in systemic lupus erythematosus: The role of vasculitis, heart emboli and thrombotic thrombocytopenic purpura. Ann Neurol 1988; 23:380.

228. Benitez L, Mathews M, et al: Platelet thrombosis with polyarteritis nodosa. Arch Pathol 1964; 77:116.

229. Frayha RA, Shulman LE, et al: Hematological abnormalities in scleroderma. A study of 180 cases. Acta Haematol 1980; 64:25.

230. Leaf AN, Laubenstein LJ, et al: TTP associated with immunodeficiency virus type I (HIV-1) infection. Ann Intern Med 1988; 109:209.

231. Platanias LC, Paiusco D, et al: Thrombotic thrombocytopenic purpura as the first manifestation of human immunodeficiency virus infection. Am J Med 1989; 87:699.

232. Ucar A, Fernandez HF, et al: Thrombotic microangiopathy and retroviral infections: A 13-year experience. Am J Hematol 1994; 45:304.

233. Berkowitz LR, Dalldorf FG, et al. TTP: A pathology review. JAMA 1979; 241:1709.

234. Goodman A, Ramos R, et al: Gingival biopsy in TTP. Ann Intern Med 1978; 89:501.

235. Ridolfi RL, Bell WR: Thrombotic thrombocytopenic purpura: Report of 25 cases and review of the literature. Medicine 1981; 60:413.

236. Remuzzi G, Zoja C, et al: Prostacyclin in thrombotic microangiopathy. Semin Thromb Hemost 1987; 6:391.

237. Chen YC, McLeod B, et al: Accelerated prostacyclin degradation in thrombotic thrombocytopenic purpura. Lancet 1981; 2:267.

238. Kobayashi M, Wada H, et al: Decreased plasma tissue factor pathway inhibitor levels in patients with thrombotic thrombocytopenic purpura. Thromb Hemost 1995; 73:10.

239. Katayama M, Handa M, et al: Soluble P-selection is present in normal circulation and its plasma level is elevated in patients with thrombotic thrombocytopenic purpura and haemolytic uremic syndrome. Br J Haematol 1993; 84:702.

240. Kelton JG, Moore J, et al: Studies investigating platelet aggregation and release initiated by sera from patients with thrombotic thrombocytopenic purpura. Blood 1987; 69:924.

241. Miura M, Koezumi S, et al: Efficacy of several plasma components in a young boy with chronic thrombocytopenic and hemolytic anemia who responds repeatedly to normal plasma infusion. Am J Hematol 1984; 17:307.

242. Moake JL, Rudy CK, et al: Therapy of chronic relapsing thrombotic thrombocytopenic purpura with prednisone and azathioprine. Am J Hematol 1985; 20:73.

243. Moake JL, Rudy CK, et al: Unusually large plasma factor VIII: von Willebrand factor multimers in chronic relapsing thrombotic thrombocytopenic purpura. N Engl J Med 1982; 307:1432.

244. Moake JL, McPherson PD: Abnormalities of von Willebrand factor multimers in thrombotic thrombocytopenic purpura and the hemolytic-uremic syndrome. Am J Med 1989; 87:3-9N.

245. Suzuki K: Calcium-activated neutral protease: Domain structure and activity regulation. Trends Biochem Sci 1987; 12:103.

246. Murphy WG, Moore JC, et al: Relationship between platelet-aggregating factor and von Willebrand factor in thrombotic thrombocytopenic purpura. Br J Haematol 1987; 66:509.

247. Moore JC, Murphy WG, Kelton JG: Calpain proteolysis of von Willebrand factor enhances its binding to platelet membrane glycoprotein IIb/IIIa: An explanation for platelet aggregation in thrombotic thrombocytopenic purpura. Br J Hematol 1990; 74:457.

248. Byrnes JJ, Khurana M: Treatment of TTP with plasma. N Engl J Med 1977; 297:1386.

249. Rock GA, Shumak KH, et al: Comparison of plasma exchange with plasma infusion in the treatment of thrombotic thrombocytopenic purpura. N Engl J Med 1991; 325:393.

250. Shepard KV, Bukowski RM: The treatment of TTP with exchange transfusions, plasma infusions, and plasma exchange. Semin Hematol 1987; 24:178.

251. Byrnes JJ, Moake JL, et al: Effectiveness of the cryosupernatant fraction of plasma in the treatment of refractory thrombotic thrombocytopenic purpura. Am J Hematol 1990; 34:169.

252. Naumovski L, Pillsbury HE: Treatment of thrombotic thrombocytopenic purpura with cryosupernatant. Am J Hematol 1991; 38:250. Letter.

253. Kelton JG, Moore J, et al: The detection of a platelet-agglutinating factor in thrombotic thrombocytopenic purpura. Ann Intern Med 1984; 101:589.

254. DePasquale A, Venturoni L, et al: Possible usefulness of ticlopidine in combined treatment of thrombotic thrombocytopenic purpura. Report of one case. Haematologica 1986; 71:53.

255. Gordon LI, Kwaan HC, Rossi EC: Deleterious effects of platelet transfusions and recovery thrombocytosis in patients with thrombotic microangiopathy. Semin Hematol 1987; 24:194.

256. Rose M, Eldor A: High incidence of relapses in thrombotic thrombocytopenic purpura. Clinical study of 38 patients. Am J Med 1987; 83:437.

257. Hayward CPM, Sutton DMC, et al: Treatment outcomes in patients with adult thrombotic thrombocytopenic purpura–hemolytic uremic syndrome. Arch Intern Med 1994; 154.

258. Onundarson PT, Rowe JM, et al: Response to plasma exchange and splenectomy in thrombotic thrombocytopenic purpura. A 10-year experience of a single institution. Arch Intern Med 1992; 152:791.

259. Wells AD, Majumdar G, et al: Role of splenectomy as a salvage procedure in thrombotic thrombocytopenic purpura. Br J Surg 1991; 78:1389.

260. Schulman I, Pierce M, et al: Studies on thrombopoiesis. I. A factor in normal plasma required for platelet production; chronic thrombocytopenia due to its deficiency. Blood 1960; 16:943.

261. Murphy WG, Moore JC, Kelton JG: Calcium-dependent cysteine protease activity in the sera of patients with thrombotic thrombocytopenic purpura. Blood 1987; 70:1683.

262. Kasabach HH, Merritt KK: Capillary hemangioma with extensive purpura. Am J Dis Child 1940; 59:1063.

263. Shim WKT: Hemangiomas of infancy complicated by thrombocytopenia. Am J Surg 1968; 116:896.

264. Brizel HE, Raccuglia G: Giant hemangioma with thrombocytopenia: Radioisotopic demonstration of platelet sequestration. Blood 1965; 26:751.

265. Warrell RP, Kempin SJ: Treatment of severe coagulopathy in the Kasabach-Merritt syndrome with aminocaproic acid and cryoprecipitate. N Engl J Med 1985; 314:309.

266. Blix S, Aas K: Giant hemangioma, thrombocytopenia, fibrinogenopenia and fibrinolytic activity. Acta Med Scand 1961; 169:63.

267. Hatley RM, Sabio H, et al: Successful management of an infant with a giant hemangioma of the retroperitoneum and Kasabach-Merritt syndrome with alpha-interferon. J Pediatr Surg 1993; 28:1356.

268. Chui HH, Chen RL, et al: Recombinant alpha-interferon treatment of intracranial hemangioma and Kasabach-Merritt syndrome in an infant with cytomegalovirus. J Formos Med Assoc 1995; 94:261.

269. Gibson B, Hunter D, et al: Thrombocytopenia in pre-eclampsia and eclampsia. Semin Thromb Hemost 1982; 8:234.

270. Kelton J, Hunter DJ, Neame PB: A platelet function defect of pre-eclampsia. Obstet Gynecol 1985; 65:107.

271. Bancroft Lesesne J, Rothschild N, et al: Cancer-associated hemolytic-uremic syndrome: Analysis of 85 cases from a national registry. J Clin Oncol 1989; 7:781.

272. Stave GM, Croker BP: Thrombotic microangiopathy in anti-glomerular basement membrane glomerulonephritis. Arch Pathol Lab Med 1984; 108:747.

273. Siegler RL, Brewer ED, et al: Hemolytic uremic syndrome associated with glomerular disease. Am J Kidney Dis 1989; 13:144.

274. Lichtman MA, Hoyer LW, et al: Erythrocyte deformation and hemolytic anemia coincident with the microvascular disease of rejecting renal homotransplants. Am J Med Sci 1968; 256:239.

275. Grino JM, Caralps A, et al: Apparent recurrence of hemolytic uremic syndrome in azathioprine-treated allograft recipients. Nephron 1988; 49:301.

276. Springate J, Fildes R, et al: Recurrent hemolytic syndrome after renal transplantation. Transplant Proc 1988; 20:559.

277. Sommer BG, Innes JT, et al: Cyclosporine-associated renal arteriopathy resulting in loss of allograft function. Am J Surg 1985; 149:756.

278. Holler E, Kolb HJ, et al: Microangiopathy in patients on cyclosporine prophylaxis who develop acute graft-versus-host disease after HLA-identical bone marrow transplantation. Blood 1989; 73:2018.

CHAPTER

16

Disorders of the Erythrocyte Membrane

Patrick G. Gallagher • Bernard G. Forget • Samuel E. Lux

The erythrocyte membrane is the most thoroughly studied biologic membrane. Its easy accessibility has enabled researchers to characterize both its primary structure and a number of its important functions. Although it constitutes only about 1% of the total weight of the red cell, the membrane plays a pivotal role in the maintenance of erythrocyte integrity in a number of ways. It responds to erythropoietin during erythropoiesis and imports the iron required by the cell for hemoglobin synthesis. It retains vital compounds such as organic phosphates and removes metabolic waste. The erythrocyte membrane sequesters the reductants required to prevent corrosion by oxygen. It helps regulate erythrocyte metabolism by selectively and reversibly binding and inactivating glycolytic enzymes. It exchanges chloride and bicarbonate ions and helps the body maintain an adequate pH. The membrane maintains a slippery exterior so that erythrocytes do not adhere to endothelial cells or aggregate and occlude the microcirculation, and it provides strength and flexibility to the red cell to allow it to maintain its integrity while enduring circulatory stresses during its 4-month life span.

The red cell membrane is an excellent illustration of the fluid mosaic model proposed by Singer and Nicholson.[1] The erythrocyte membrane is composed of mobile, asymmetrically distributed proteins and lipids

that interact in a variety of ways.[2] In this chapter, the normal erythrocyte membrane is discussed, with particular emphasis placed on aspects that are critical in the genesis of membrane abnormalities. The focus then shifts to the defects that lead to abnormalities of red cell shape, particularly hereditary spherocytosis and elliptocytosis. These are two of the most common and best understood disorders of the erythrocyte membrane.

COMPOSITION OF THE ERYTHROCYTE MEMBRANE

Membrane Lipids

Lipid Composition

Lipids compose about 50% by weight of the red cell membrane (Table 16–1). Phospholipids and unesterified (free) cholesterol predominate and are present in nearly equal proportions (cholesterol:phospholipid molar ratio = 0.80).[3–5] Small amounts of glycolipids, principally globoside, are also present (Fig. 16–1).[3] The average red cell contains about 250 million phospholipid molecules, 195 million cholesterol molecules, 10 million glycolipid molecules, and 4 million protein molecules in a membrane whose total surface area is about 140 mm^2.[6, 7] Phosphatidylcholine (PC), phospha-

Table 16-1. COMPOSITION OF NORMAL HUMAN RED CELL MEMBRANES

Component	Weight (%)	Grams per Membrane (×10⁻¹³)	Approximate Number of Molecules per Membrane (×10⁶)	Percentage in Outer Half of Bilayer	Percentage in Inner Half of Bilayer
Proteins and glycoproteins	55	5.7	6		
Lipids	45	4.7	475		
Phospholipids	28	3.0	250		
Sphingomyelin	6.8	0.73	60	80	20
Phosphatidylcholine	7.0	0.75	65	75	25
Phosphatidylethanolamine	7.4	0.79	65	20	80
Phosphatidylserine	4.3	0.46	40	0	100
Phosphatidylinositol (PI)	1.0	0.10	8	0	100
PI	0.34	0.036	3		
PI-4-P	0.22	0.024	2		
PI-4,5-PP	0.39	0.042	3		
Phosphatidic acid	1.0	0.10	8	Unknown	Unknown
Lysophosphatidylcholine	0.3	0.03	3	Unknown	Unknown
Lysophosphatidylethanolamine	0.3	0.03	3	Unknown	Unknown
Cholesterol	13	1.3	195	50	50
Glycolipids	3	0.3	10	100	0
Free fatty acids	1	0.1	20	Unknown	Unknown
	100	10.4	481		

From Lux SE, Palek J: Disorders of the red cell membrane. In Handin RI, Lux SE, Stossel TP (eds): Blood: Principles and Practice of Hematology. Philadelphia, J.B. Lippincott Co., 1995, pp 1701–1818.

tidylethanolamine (PE), sphingomyelin (SM), and phosphatidylserine (PS) are the predominant phospholipids. Their structures are shown in Figure 16–1. Small amounts of phosphatidic acid (PA), phosphatidylinositol (PI), and lysophosphatidylcholine (lyso-PC) are also present. It is notable that at physiologic pH, PS, PA,

and PI have a net negative charge whereas the other phospholipids are electrically neutral. With the exception of SM and lyso-PC, these lipids have two fatty acids attached to a glycerol backbone. These are usually in ester linkage, although sometimes, particularly in PE, one of the fatty acids is a vinyl ether (plasmalo-

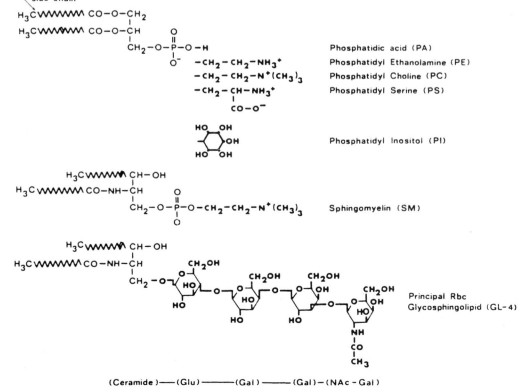

Figure 16-1. Chemical structures of the major phospholipids and the principal glycosphingolipid (GL-4) of the red cell membrane. Note that phosphatidylcholine (PC) and sphingomyelin (SM) share the same polar moiety (choline) and that SM and GL-4 share the same nonpolar moiety (ceramide).

gen).[8] The lysophospholipids have only one fatty acid and are named for the hemolysis induced because of their detergent-like properties.

Lipid Organization

The majority of the phospholipids in the red cell membrane are in a planar bilayer with their polar head groups exposed at each surface and their hydrophobic fatty acyl side chains buried in the bilayer core. It is possible, but unproved, that small foci of nonbilayer phospholipids may also exist in localized regions of the membrane, presumably for specific functional reasons. For example, some theories require the interaction of nonbilayer regions of micellar-like phospholipid as the initiating event in membrane fusion.[9] Glycolipids and cholesterol are intercalated between the phospholipids in the bilayer with their long axes perpendicular to the bilayer plane. Red cell glycolipids are located entirely in the external half of the bilayer with their carbohydrate moieties extending into the aqueous phase. They carry several important red cell antigens, including A, B, H, Le[a], Le[b], and P[10–15] and may serve other important functions. The location of membrane cholesterol molecules is less certain. It is likely that cholesterol is present in about equal proportions on both sides of the bilayer,[16] although some data suggest that it is somewhat more prevalent in the outer half.[17, 18] However, because all of the membrane cholesterol is available for exchange within 24 hours,[19] inner and outer membrane cholesterol must also be exchangeable. Measurements indicate that this transfer occurs rapidly, with a half-time of only seconds.[20] Cholesterol molecules are relatively buried, because the 3-OH group, the part of the molecule that is closest to the aqueous interface, lies approximately at the level of the carbonyl group of the phospholipid fatty acids.[21]

Phospholipid Asymmetry

There is now convincing evidence that red cell membrane lipids, like membrane proteins (to be discussed), are asymmetrically distributed across the bilayer plane (*trans* asymmetry).[22–24] The asymmetric distribution of phospholipids reflects a steady state involving a constant exchange (flip/flop) of phospholipids between the two bilayer hemileaflets. In pure phospholipid bilayers, this transmembrane diffusion is slow, lasting several hours to days. In contrast, the transmembrane shuttle of phospholipids in biologic membranes is very fast. In addition to enzymatic phospholipid translocation, described in the next paragraph, phospholipid flip/flop is accelerated by transmembrane proteins, which produce localized discontinuities in the bilayer, or, in the case of neutral phospholipids, by transmembrane pH gradients.[25]

***Trans* Asymmetry.** *Trans* asymmetry of phospholipids is produced and maintained by an adenosine triphosphate (ATP)-dependent transport system, called the aminophospholipid translocase or "flippase."[26, 27] This enzyme translocates PS, and to a lesser extent PE, from the outer to the inner bilayer.[28–32] The half-times

for PS and PE are about 5 and 60 minutes, respectively, at 37°C.[33] A similar activity exists in all mammalian red cells[34] and in at least some nonerythroid cells and cell organelles.[35] The aminophospholipid translocase requires Mg^{2+}-ATP at the inner membrane surface[30] and may contain an active site cysteine, because it is inhibited by sulfhydryl modifying reagents.[36] It is also inhibited by vanadate (50 μM) and free calcium (Ca^{2+}) (>0.2 μM).[32]

The enzyme has been cloned.[37] It is a 130-kDa integral membrane protein and a member of a previously unrecognized subfamily of Mg^{2+}-dependent, P-glycoprotein ATPases. Closely related enzymes exist in yeast, the malaria parasite *Plasmodium falciparum*, and the worm *Caenorhabditis elegans*. A yeast strain that lacks the homologous enzyme cannot transport PS from the outer to the inner membrane surface,[37] which confirms the function of this family of proteins. More distantly related P-glycoprotein ATPases include the multidrug resistance proteins—MRP1, MRP2, and MRP3—which also appear to be lipid translocases.[38–40] Mdr1 has broad specificity,[38] which explains why it is able to excrete many different amphipathic drugs. Perhaps its normal function is to organize a variety of lipids in membranes—both long chain and short chain. Mdr2 is required for biliary phospholipid secretion[40] and probably functions as a PC-specific translocase[41] in hepatocyte canalicular membranes. Mdr3 can substitute for mdr2 in mice and is known to be specific for PC.[38, 42] Presumably, other P-glycoprotein–related ATPases, such as the chloride transporter that is defective in cystic fibrosis, may also be lipid translocases.

There may also be a "floppase." PC and SM are not transported inward by the flippase enzyme[30, 32, 37]; however, there is some evidence that red cells are able to transport PC, along with PS and PE, from the inner to the outer bilayer.[43] It is not clear whether this floppase activity is a second function of the flippase or whether it is generated by a separate enzyme.[43]

For a while it appeared that the Rh protein might be the aminophospholipid translocase. A photoactivatable PS analogue that was transported to the inner bilayer by the translocase, selectively labeled a 31-kDa protein[44] that was precipitated by monoclonal anti-Rh antibodies.[45] The 31-kDa protein, which is the same size as Rh proteins,[46] was also labeled by an inhibitor of the translocase.[35] However, the Rh proteins[46] differ from the recently cloned flippase[37] and Rh null erythrocytes, which lack all Rh antigens, have normal translocase activity.[45] Most likely the Rh proteins are associated with the translocase, perhaps as part of a complex,[47] and are labeled by an "innocent bystander" mechanism.

Early experiments suggested that membrane skeletal proteins such as spectrin might help stabilize phospholipid asymmetry through interactions with inner membrane lipids. Spectrin interacts weakly with anionic phospholipids *in vitro*,[48–51] and phospholipid asymmetry is lost when spectrin is oxidized and cross-linked.[52–55] However, it is now known that the translocase is also sensitive to oxidation[27, 31, 35] and would have been damaged by the treatments used to oxidize spectrin.[52–55] In addition, heat-treated ghosts, heat-induced vesicles that are spectrin depleted, and spectrin-deficient hereditary spherocytes are capable of translocating aminophospholipids with the same efficiency as normal ghosts.[56, 57] It appears the aminophospholipid translocase can maintain phospholipid asymmetry without help from the membrane skeleton, at least under normal conditions.

Increase in intracellular Ca^{2+} leads to activation of a poorly defined lipid translocation pathway in which both PS and PE flip to the outer bilayer leaflet while PC flops inside.[43, 58–60] In addition to the inhibitory effect of Ca^{2+} on the aminophospholipid translocase, this rapid phospholipid scrambling may represent yet another mechanism underlying altered phospholipid asymmetry. The molecular basis of the phenomenon is unknown. Hypothetical possibilities include phospholipase activation leading to formation of diacylglycerol, which may destabilize the lipid bilayer by forming nonbilayer structures, or disruption of lipid bilayer integrity during the plasma membrane fusion that follows Ca^{2+}-induced shedding of membrane microvesicles.[43, 60]

Phospholipid asymmetry results from the balance of the active translocation of PS and PE and the passive, slow bidirectional flip/flop of phospholipids. Changes in the equilibrium distribution of phospholipids could occur by inhibition of the translocase, acceleration of basal flip/flop rates to a degree that overwhelms the translocase, or both. Phospholipid flip/flop is increased and phospholipid asymmetry is lost in sickle cells,[61–63] in which several forms of skeletal protein damage have been documented,[64] including decreased phospholipid translocase activity[61] and uncoupling of the lipid bilayer from the underlying skeleton in the sickle cell spicules.[65] Phospholipid asymmetry is also altered in diabetic red cells,[66] which, like sickle cells, tend to adhere to endothelial cells.[66–69]

It is generally believed that red cells, and perhaps other cells,[24] sequester aminophospholipids on the cytoplasmic side of the membrane because the exposed lipids trigger the conversion of prothrombin to thrombin and promote intravascular clotting.[70–72] In addition, macrophages bind and ingest red cells, or even liposomes, that have PS exposed on their outer surfaces.[73–78] Little is known of the receptor involved, whether it is a unique PS receptor or a receptor of known function that also binds PS. It is also unclear whether the PS receptor actually participates in the removal of sickle cells or other damaged cells from the circulation or whether it has other functions, such as the scavenging of dead or dying cells that have lost the ability to internalize PS.

Down-regulation of the aminophospholipid translocase is an early step in apoptosis (programmed cell death) in lymphocytes[79] and is followed by the appearance of PS on the cell surface and phagocytosis. Involvement of the translocase in a fundamental process like apoptosis could explain the wide cellular distribution and evolutionary preservation of the enzyme. Finally, there is some speculation that the aminophospholipid translocase might also power another fundamental process, endocytosis, by "pumping" PS and PE into the inner bilayer.[26] Even a small excess of inner bilayer phospholipids would tend to make the membrane invaginate.

Cis Asymmetry. Red cell lipids exist in different domains within each of the bilayer planes (cis asymmetry).

Macroscopic Domains. Fluorescent phospholipids partition into doughnut-shaped lipid domains up to several microns in diameter within the membrane of red cells or ghosts.[80] These lipid-rich domains are intrinsic structural features of the membrane, not just "gel-phase" or "fluid-phase" domains.[80] They increase in size when membrane proteins aggregate, and they are lacking in large liposomes made solely of membrane lipids, which suggests that proteins play a role in their formation. How and why this occurs is a mystery.

Microscopic Domains: Protein-Bound Lipids. Lipids may also partition on a more microscopic scale within the membrane. Early experiments[81] detected a layer of tightly associated "boundary lipids" attached to membrane proteins that intruded into the bilayer core, but subsequent work[82] suggested that such lipids were bound only transiently ($<10^{-7}$ second) and probably were not distinguishable from other lipids in the bilayer on the time scale of enzyme reactions and other cellular events. However, there are probably exceptions to this generalization, because specific lipids are required for the enzymatic functions of some transport proteins, such as the sodium (Na^+) and Ca^{2+} pumps, and because some membrane proteins, such as glycophorin A (to be discussed), bind anionic (PS, PI) but not choline (PC, SM) phospholipids. Positively charged amino acids are concentrated on the cytoplasmic side of the bilayer-spanning domains of glycophorins and other membrane proteins, in part because their position determines the orientation of the protein.[83–85] Although it is not well documented, anionic phospholipids probably cluster near these regions of positive charge. Surface-bound membrane proteins such as spectrin and protein 4.1, which bind preferentially to anionic phospholipids,[48–51] may also contribute to the nonrandom topography of inner membrane phospholipids.

Bilayer Couple Hypothesis. The shape of the lipid bilayer is responsive to very slight variations ($<0.4\%$) in the surface area of its inner and outer halves.[86, 87] This is termed the *bilayer couple effect*.[88] It reflects the tight packing of membrane lipids, the independent motion of lipids in each half of the bilayer, and the extreme thinness of the membrane ($<0.1\%$ of the diameter of the cell). Processes that expand the outer bilayer (or contract the inner) will produce uniform membrane spiculation, called *echinocytosis*. Conversely, relative expansion of the inner bilayer will lead to membrane invagination and cup-shaped red cells, *stomatocytosis*. Strongly charged amphipathic compounds, such as phospholipids, cause echinocytosis.[87, 89] They are trapped in the outer bilayer by their fixed charge. Permeable amphipaths (e.g., weak acids and bases that can cross the membrane in their uncharged form) will cause the membrane to extend toward the side of greater accumulation.[90, 91] In general, cationic compounds accumulate in the negatively charged inner bilayer and anionic compounds partition to the neutral outer bilayer. Even subtle effects, such as differences in the cross-sectional area of lipid head groups or fatty acyl tails, can lead to changes in membrane curvature.[89]

The bilayer couple hypothesis predicts that shape changes resulting from expansion of one lipid leaflet can be reversed by a commensurate alteration in the other. For example, the intensely spiculated red cells of patients with abetalipoproteinemia can be almost completely converted to biconcave disks by the addition of small amounts (0.1 mM) of chlorpromazine, a cationic amphipath.[92] Unfortunately, this simple test has not been widely applied to pathologic red cells, so it is difficult to estimate how often bilayer couple effects dictate cell shape *in vivo*.

Glycolipids and Cholesterol. Glycolipids and cholesterol are intercalated between the phospholipids in the bilayer with their long axes perpendicular to the bilayer plane. Red cell glycolipids are located entirely in the external half of the bilayer with their carbohydrate moieties extending into the aqueous phase. They carry several important red cell antigens, including A, B, H, Le[a], Le[b], and P, and may serve other important functions. The P glycolipid, for example, serves as the receptor for parvovirus B19,[93] the agent responsible for most aplastic crises.

Cholesterol is present in about equal proportions on both sides of the bilayer[16] (see Table 16–1) and equilibrates between them in seconds or less. This facilitates membrane bending, because the movement of cholesterol can offset the difference in surface pressure caused by bending and compressing one of the bilayers relative to the other. Cholesterol depletion promotes inward curvature of the membrane, whereas cholesterol enrichment favors outward deflection.[94] Cholesterol molecules are relatively buried, because the 3-OH group (the part of the molecule that is closest to the aqueous interface) lies approximately at the level of the carbonyl group of the phospholipid fatty acids.[95]

Membrane Phosphoinositides. The polar head group of this interesting class of phospholipids contains phosphatidylinositol (PI),[43] or its phosphorylated forms, PI-4-monophosphate and PI-4,5-bisphosphate (PIP and PIP$_2$, respectively). In nucleated cells, phosphoinositides are precursors of important intracellular second messengers such as inositol-1,4,5-trisphosphate (IP$_3$) and diacylglycerol.[96] In mature erythrocytes, phosphoinositides represent 2% to 5% of the total phospholipids. They reside largely at the inner membrane surface and undergo rapid phosphorylation and dephosphorylation.[96] They help regulate Ca^{2+} transport, interact with membrane proteins such as glycophorin C and protein 4.1 (see later), and may influence discocyte-echinocyte shape transformation.

Lipid Mobility

Purified phospholipids exhibit discrete, liquid crystalline to gel phase transitions that are dependent on the length and degree of unsaturation of their acyl side chains. Above the temperature of this transition, the acyl side chains waggle very rapidly (10^8 to 10^9 times per second) from side to side, with progressively greater excursions as one proceeds from the glycerol ester linkage to the terminal methyl group.[97, 98] The presence of a double bond in the acyl chain increases the disorder and flexibility all along the hydrocarbon chain,[99, 100] especially toward the terminal methyl end.[99] Below the temperature of the liquid crystalline to gel transition, acyl chains of purified lipids are extended in stiff, parallel, hexagonally packed arrays that are more nearly solid than liquid.

Cholesterol as an Intermediate. Cholesterol buffers the extremes of the gel and liquid crystalline states. At temperatures above the gel/liquid phase transition, cholesterol partially immobilizes the acyl chains of phospholipids, particularly the proximal 8 to 10 carbons that are adjacent to the bulky steroid nucleus.[98] Below this transition, cholesterol disrupts the ordering of the acyl chains, in effect preserving membrane fluidity.[101] The net result is that cholesterol tends to abolish the gel to liquid crystalline transition and create a condition of intermediate fluidity in which the proximal ends of the hydrocarbon chains are extended and relatively rigid and the distal ends are disordered and fluid. The red cell membrane contains relatively large amounts of cholesterol (cholesterol/phospholipid = 0.8 mol/mol) and is relatively less fluid than other plasma membranes.[102] The inner bilayer is somewhat more fluid than the outer,[29] probably because it contains more unsaturated fatty acids.[8] The significance of this difference is unknown.

Spectroscopic techniques are available for assessing the motion of various lipid-soluble probes and are widely used to measure lipid "fluidity." Decreased red cell lipid fluidity due to membrane cholesterol accumulation has been implicated in the pathogenesis of acanthocytosis associated with abetalipoproteinemia[103] or liver disease (spur cell anemia)[104, 105] and with a number of other conditions; however, it remains to be determined whether these changes are due to true alterations in lipid fluidity or to changes in lipid organization that alter the location and spectroscopic properties of the probe.

Lateral Diffusion. Phospholipids move about rapidly within each plane of model lipid bilayers.[102, 106, 107] From the measured lateral diffusion constants (2 to 5 $\times$ 10^{-8} cm^2/s), one can calculate that phospholipids exchange places with each other about 10^7 times per second. This rate is somewhat damped in the red cell membrane (estimated diffusion constant of 1.4×10^{-8} cm^2/s),[108] but the difference is about what would be expected, considering the effects of cholesterol on the lateral mobility of phospholipids.[107]

Lipid Renewal Pathways

Mature erythrocytes are unable to synthesize fatty acids, phospholipids, or cholesterol *de novo* and depend on lipid exchange and fatty acid acylation as mechanisms for phospholipid repair and renewal (Fig. 16–2). Outer bilayer phospholipids (PC, SM) exchange slowly (approximate turnover time of 5 days)[109] with the phos-

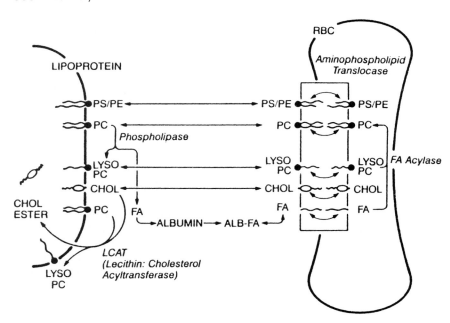

Figure 16–2. Fatty acid renewal and lipid exchange pathways in the human erythrocyte.

pholipids of plasma lipoproteins.[110, 111] Inner bilayer phospholipids (PS, PE) are unable to participate in this process and are virtually unexchangeable.[109]

Fatty acids and lysophosphatides exchange more rapidly. Red cell membrane cholesterol (unesterified) also exchanges readily with the unesterified cholesterol in plasma lipoproteins (half-life = 7 hours), where it is partially converted to esterified cholesterol by the action of lecithin:cholesterol acyltransferase (LCAT). Because the newly formed cholesteryl ester cannot return to the red cell membrane (there is virtually no esterified cholesterol in the membrane), LCAT catalyzes a unidirectional pathway that depletes the membrane of cholesterol and decreases its surface area. Conversely, if LCAT is absent or inhibited, excess membrane cholesterol accumulates, expanding the membrane surface area.[112]

The fatty acid acylation pathway is an active metabolic pathway and requires ATP energy. This system combines fatty acids with lysophosphatides (principally lyso-PC) to remake the native phospholipid.[113–115] The acylase enzyme and its phospholipid products are located in the inner bilayer.[116] In theory, this enzyme should facilitate the renewal of lost or damaged fatty acid side chains and should prevent the accumulation of deleterious lysophosphatides within the membrane; however, it is not certain that the phospholipases necessary to remove damaged fatty acids operate in the red cell.

These renewal pathways, although limited, permit a slow replacement of membrane lipid components. Approximately 30 days are required before erythrocyte lipids reach equilibrium after a change in dietary fatty acids. Theoretically, this could be pathologically significant in persons on unusual diets (e.g., infants receiving a high intake of medium-chain triglycerides); however, no pathologic consequences have been reported.

Membrane Proteins

The red cell membrane contains at least a dozen major proteins[117] and hundreds of minor ones.[118] The major proteins of the red cell membrane (Fig. 16–3) and their disorders have been intensively studied,[119–169] and, in most cases, their genes have been cloned. It is important to realize that the enumeration and characterization of all the proteins of the red cell membrane may never be achieved because the membrane is not a separate, discontinuous structure but one that extends into both the cytoplasm and the extracellular space. Isolation of many of these minor proteins may be technically challenging because some of these proteins may be sensitive to even minor variations in isolation conditions, as are some of the proteins already characterized.

Traditionally, components of the erythrocyte membrane have been analyzed after hypotonic hemolysis[117, 170] and separation by sodium dodecyl sulfate (SDS) polyacrylamide gel electrophoresis (Fig. 16–4).[117, 171, 172] Various classifications for proteins of the erythrocyte membrane exist based on electrophoretic mobility, protein function, location, and so on (Table 16–2). For example, the network of proteins on the inner surface of the red cell that is responsible for maintaining the shape and deformability of the erythrocyte is called the erythrocyte membrane skeleton. The principal proteins of the membrane skeleton include spectrin, actin, and protein 4.1. In another classification that uses location for classification, membrane proteins of the red cell may be classified as either integral or peripheral. Integral membrane proteins penetrate or traverse the lipid bilayer and interact with the hydrophobic lipid core. They include glycophorins A, B, C, and D, which possess membrane receptors and antigens, and transport proteins such as band 3, the erythrocyte anion exchanger. Peripheral proteins interact with integral proteins or lipids at the membrane surface but do not penetrate into the bilayer core. In the red cell, the

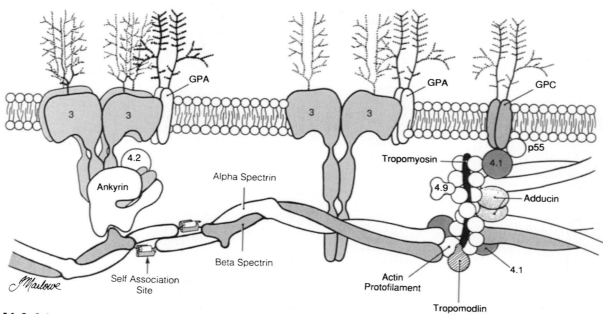

Figure 16-3. Schematic model of the red cell membrane. The relative position of the various proteins is correct, but the proteins and lipids are not drawn to scale. (From Lux SE, Palek J: Disorders of the red cell membrane. In Handin RJ, Lux SE, Stossel TP (eds): Blood: Principles and Practice of Hematology. Philadelphia, Lippincott-Raven, 1995, pp 1701–1818.)

Figure 16-4. Protein composition of the red blood cell membrane skeleton. The major components of the erythrocyte membrane are separated by sodium dodecyl sulfate–polyacrylamide gel electrophoresis (SDS-PAGE) and revealed by Coomassie blue staining. (Adapted from Gallagher PG, Tse WT, Forget BG: Clinical and molecular aspects of disorders of the erythrocyte membrane skeleton. Semin Perinatol 1990; 14:352.)

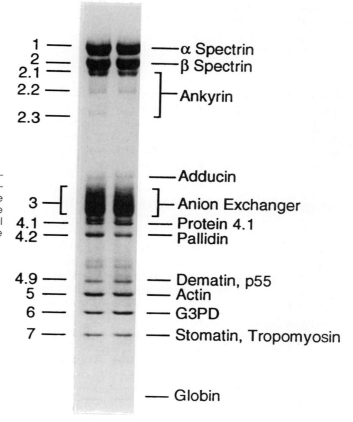

Table 16-2. MAJOR HUMAN

SDS Gel Band‡	Protein	Peripheral or Integral	Molecular Wt. $\times 10^3$ (Gel/Calculated)	Approx. Proportion (Wt%)	Monomer Copies per Cell ($\times 10^{-3}$)†	Oligomeric State	Chromosome Location
1	α spectrin	P	240/281	14	242 ± 20	Heterodimer/tetramer	1q22 q23
2	β spectrin	P	220/246	13	242 ± 20		14q23 p24.2
2.1¶	Ankyrin	P	210/206	6¶	124 ± 11¶	Monomer	8p11.2
2.9	α adducin	P	103/81	<1	≈30	Heterodimer/tetramer	4p16.3
	β adducin	P	97/80	<1	≈30		2p13 p14
3#	AE1‖	I	90–100**/102††	29	≈1200	Dimer or tetramer	17q12 p21
4.1	Protein 4.1	P	80 + 78††/66§§	5	≈200	Monomer	1p33 p34.2
4.2	Protein 4.2	P	72/77	5	≈250	Dimer or trimer	15q15 q21
4.9#	Dematin	P	48 + 52/43 + 46	1	≈140	Trimer¶¶	8p21.1
	p55	P	55/53		≈80	Dimer	Xq28
5#	β actin	P	43/42	6	≈500	Oligomer (≈14)	7pter q22
	Tropomodulin	P	43/41		≈30	Monomer	9q22
6	G3PD‖	P	35/36	5##	≈500	Tetramer	12p13
7#	Stomatin	I	31/32	4	—	Heterodimer***	9q33 q34
	Tropomyosin	P	27 + 29/28***		≈70		1q31
8	Protein 8	P	23/	1–2	≈200	Dimer	—
PAS-1	Glycophorin A†††	I	36†††/14††	1.6	≈1000		4q31
PAS-2	Glycophorin C†††	I	32†††/14††	0.1	≈200(C + D)§§	Dimer	2q14 q21
PAS-3	Glycophorin B†††	I	20†††/8††	0.2	≈200		4q31
	Glycophorin D†††	I	23†††/11††	0.02	≈200(C + D)§§		2q14 q21
	Glycophorin E†††	I	—‖[21]/6††	—‖ ‖	—‖ ‖	—‖ ‖	4q31

*Calculated from amino acid sequences.

†Based on an estimate of 5.7 × 10⁻¹³ g protein/ghost[117] and on the approximate proportions of each protein, estimated from densitometry of SDS gels. The data for spectrin and ankyrin were measured directly by radioimmunoassay.

‡Proteins 1 to 8 were estimated from the data in Fairbanks et al,[117] Palek and Jarolim,[159] and from unpublished data.

§Numbering system of Fairbanks et al[117] and Steck.[172] Bands 1 to 8 refer to Coomassie blue-stained gels. PAS-1 to PAS-3 refer to periodic acid–Schiff-stained gels.

‖HE, hereditary elliptocytosis; HS, hereditary spherocytosis; HPP, hereditary pyropoikilocytosis; HAc, hereditary acanthocytosis; HSt, hereditary stomatocytosis; SAO, Southeast Asian ovalocytosis; AE1, anion exchange protein 1 (erythroid anion exchange protein); G3PD, glyceraldehyde-3-phosphate dehydrogenase.

¶Protein 2.1 is full-length ankyrin. Other isoforms are evident on SDS gels including band 2.2, 195 kd; band 2.3, 175 kd; and band 2.6, 145 kd. Band 2.2 is produced by alternate splicing. The origin of the other bands is unknown. The data shown are for ankyrin 2.1 except for the number of copies/cell and approximate proportion (wt%), which include all isoforms.

#The α and β adducins lie in the upper part of SDS gel band 3. Band 4.9 contains both dematin and p55; band 5 contains β actin and tropomodulin; band 7 contains stomatin and tropomyosin.

**The protein runs as a broad band on SDS gels due to heterogeneous glycosylation.

major peripheral membrane proteins are located on the cytoplasmic membrane face and include enzymes such as glyceraldehyde-3-phosphate dehydrogenase and structural proteins such as spectrin. With this classification as a guide, significant features of the major erythrocyte membrane proteins are delineated.

Integral Membrane Proteins

Glycophorins

Study of red cell antigens has led to our knowledge of the glycophorin proteins. Glycophorins A, B, and E[132, 137] are associated with the MNSs antigens, and glycophorins C and D are associated with the Gerbich (Ge) blood groups.[131, 168]

Glycophorin A. Glycophorin A (GPA), the major sialoglycoprotein of the red cell, is present in approximately 1 million copies per cell. Three GPA complementary DNA (cDNA) transcripts are expressed from the gene (transcripts of 2.8, 1.7, and 1.0 kb) that vary only by usage of alternate polyadenylation sites. GPA is synthesized with a cleavable leader sequence that produces a mature protein of 181 amino acids (Fig. 16–5). The 36-kDa protein has an extracellular NH₂-terminus, a single transmembrane region, and a cytoplasmic COOH-terminus.[173–175] The extracellular domain (residues 1 to 61) contains 15 tetrasaccharides that are O-glycosidically linked to serine or threonine residues and one complex oligosaccharide attached to asparagine 26.[176] Overall, the carbohydrate accounts for about 60% of the mass of the molecule. This includes much of the sialic acid on the red cell membrane as well as the M and N blood group antigens. The M and N antigens on GPA are determined by polymorphic amino acids at residues 1 and 5 of the mature protein.[173] The M antigen is defined by a serine at residue 1 and a glycine at residue 5, whereas the N antigen is defined by a leucine at position 1 and a glutamine at position 5 (Table 16–3). M and N antibodies usually recognize these peptide determinants exclusively, but some may exhibit carbohydrate-dependent recognition characteristics.

Little is known about the membrane domain (amino acids 62 to 95), except that it binds negatively charged phospholipids,[213–216] such as PS and PI, and is probably the site of GPA dimerization.[132, 213–216] The dimeric interaction is strong and difficult to dissociate, even in detergents. Conventional SDS gels contain monomers, dimers, and heterodimers of GPA and similar oligomers of some of the other glycophorins. All of these species run anomalously on SDS gels because the large

ERYTHROCYTE MEMBRANE PROTEINS

Gene Size (kb)	Number of Exons	Amino Acids	Gene Symbol	Associated Diseases‖
80	52	2429	*SPTA1*	HE, HPP, HS
>100	≈32	2137	*SPTB*	HE, HPP, HS, HAc
>120	42	1880	*ANK1*	HS
—	—	737	*ADDA*	—
—	—	726	*ADDB*	—
17	20	911	*EPB3*	HS, SAO, HAc
>250	23	588	*EL1*	HE
20	13	691	*ELB42*	HS‖ ‖
—	—	383¶¶	—	—
>4	6	466	*MPP1*	—
—	—	375	*ACTB*	—
5	9	359	*TMOD*	—
12	7	335	*GAPD*	—
—	—	288	*EPB72*	HSt
—	—	239***	*TPM3*	—
>40	7	131	*GYPA*	—
14	4	128	*GYPC*	HE
>30	5	72	*GYPB*	None
14	4	107	*GYPD*	HE
>30	4	59	*GYPE*	—

††The calculated molecular weight does not include the contribution of the carbohydrate chains.
‡‡¹¹Protein 4.1 is a doublet (4.1a and 4.1b) on SDS gels. Protein 4.1a is derived from 4.1b by slow deamidation. Its proportion is a measure of RBC age.
§§Protein 4.1 exists in a very large number of isoforms. The major erythroid isoform is listed here. It is not known why its calculated molecular weight deviates so much from the apparent molecular weight on SDS gels.
‖ ‖Deficiency of protein 4.2 is associated with a variety of morphologies (see text), but spherocytes predominate.
¶¶Although dematin is present as a trimer in solution, the 48- and 52-kd subunits have an apparent stoichiometry of 3:1 on SDS gels.
##The amount of G3PD (band 6) associated with the membrane varies from person to person (≈3 to 6 wt%).
***Tropomyosin is a heterodimer of the 27-kd and 29-kd subunits. There are about 70,000 copies of each chain per RBC. Data for the calculated molecular weight and the number of amino acids are for fibroblast tropomyosin.
†††The glycophorins (GPA to GPD) are visible only on PAS-stained gels.
‡‡‡Molecular weights, including carbohydrate, estimated from mobilities on SDS gels.
§§§Glycophorins C and D are probably synthesized from the same mRNA using different translational start sites. The total number of GPC and GPD molecules is about 200,000.
‖ ‖ ‖Glycophorin E mRNA has been identified but it is not certain that the mRNA is translated.
From Lux SE, Palek J: Disorders of the red cell membrane. In Handin RI, Lux SE, Stossel TP (eds): Blood: Principles and Practice of Hematology. Philadelphia, J.B. Lippincott Co., 1995, pp 1701–1818.

amount of carbohydrate interferes with SDS binding.[217] The carbohydrate also interferes with Coomassie blue staining to the extent that the glycophorins are invisible unless special stains (e.g., periodic acid–Schiff) are used. The function of the cytoplasmic domain (residues 96 to 131) is also largely unknown. The protein is first detectable in proerythroblasts and is a specific marker for erythroid cells.[218]

Glycophorin B. Glycophorin B (GPB) is structurally similar to GPA but is present at a much lower level than GPA, with only about 150,000 copies per cell. A single 0.6-kb cDNA transcript gives rise to a protein with a cleavable leader sequence yielding a mature protein 72 amino acids in length (see Fig. 16–5). The protein is almost identical to the N blood group form of GPA for the first 26-amino acid residues except that it lacks the complex oligosaccharide at position 21.[173, 177] Subsequently, it lacks a piece of the extracellular domain of GPA corresponding to exon 3 and almost all of the cytoplasmic domain. Thus, there are no asparagine-linked carbohydrate chains on GPB but there are about 11 serine/threonine-linked oligosaccharide chains. Besides the peptide sequence that carries the N antigen reactivity, which is also found on GPA, GPB carries the

S, s, and U antigens. The S and s antigens differ by an amino acid polymorphism at residue 29; S is a methionine, s is a threonine.[177] There is evidence that GPB forms a macromolecular complex with the Rh glycoproteins, which form the Rh antigens, the Rh50 glycoprotein, CD47, and proteins bearing the Duffy and LW antigens.[169, 219]

Glycophorin E. Glycophorin E (GPE) is a glycophorin identified by molecular cloning.[220, 221] It resides on chromosome 4 just beyond GPB, which it resembles in structure, except that it lacks amino acid residues 27 to 39 of GPB, and it contains an in-frame insertion of 8 amino acids in the region corresponding to the transmembrane domain of GPA. The function of GPE is unknown. In fact it is not even known if the GPE messenger RNA (mRNA) is translated. The GPA, GPB, and GPE genes are oriented in tandem on chromosome 4. They apparently arose by gene duplication during primate evolution.

Glycophorins C and D. Glycophorins C (GPC) and D (GPD) have a general domain structure similar to GPA, GPB, and GPE, but they are located on a different chromosome and their amino acid sequences are unique.[222] GPC contains one N-linked and about 12 O-

Gene

Protein

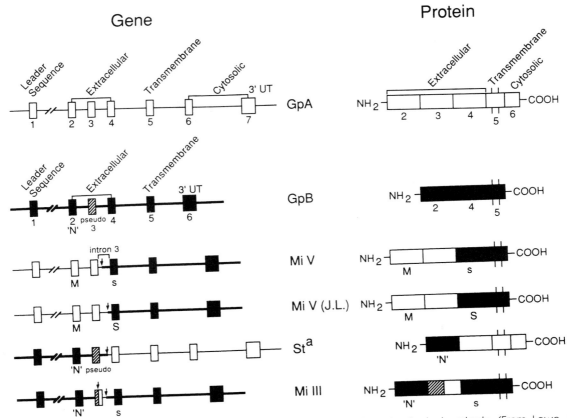

Figure 16–5. Genomic structures and polypeptides of glycophorins A and B and selected variants. (From Lowe JB: Red cell membrane antigens. In Stamatoyannopoulos G, Nienhuis AW, et al (eds): The Molecular Basis of Blood Diseases, 2nd ed. Philadelphia, W.B. Saunders Co., 1994, pp 293–319.)

linked oligosaccharides as well as the Gerbich (Ge:3) blood group antigens (amino acids 41 to 50). The GPC cDNA predicts a protein of about 14 kDa (Fig. 16–6), a size substantially smaller than the observed size of 32 kDa on SDS polyacrylamide gels. This discrepancy is thought to be due to extensive glycosylation at sites within a 57-amino acid stretch at the NH₂-terminus predicted to be at the surface of the erythrocyte mem-

Table 16–3. VARIANTS OF GLYCOPHORINS A, B, AND E

Variant	Defect	References
Amino terminal	Amino terminal sequence	173, 177
M	Ser-Ser*-Thr*-Thr*-Gly-Val...	173, 177
N	Leu-Ser*-Thr*-Thr*-Glu-Val...	178, 179
Mᶜ	Ser-Ser*-Thr*-Thr*-Glu-Val...	178, 179
Mᵍ	Leu-Ser-Thr-Asn-Glu-Val...	180
Hᵉ (Henshaw)	Trp-Ser*-Thr*-Ser*-Gly-Val...	
Other	Structural defects	
En(a−)	Absence of glycophorin A†	137, 173, 181–184
S-s-U−	Absence of glycophorin B†	137, 185–187
Mᵏ	Absence of glycophorin A & B†	137, 188
MiI (Miltenberger I). MiII, MiVII, MiVIII	Variants of glycophorin A that differ by one or two amino acids.	189–193
MiIII, MiJ.L., MiV, MiVI, MiIX, MiX, Ph, Pj, Dantu, Stᵃ (types A, B, & C)	Variants due to formation of Lepore-like and anti–Lepore-like hybrids of glycophorins A, B, and E	137, 189, 194–209
Cad	Carbohydrate variant with an abnormal O-linked oligosaccharide containing an extra β(1 → 4)–linked galactosamine on the penultimate galactose residue of both glycophorins A and B	210–212

*O-glycosylation site.
†Due to homologous recombination and unequal crossover → partial gene deletions.

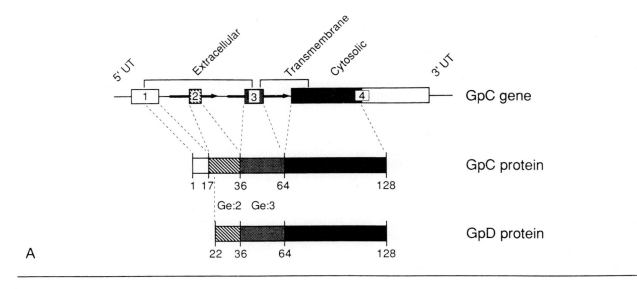

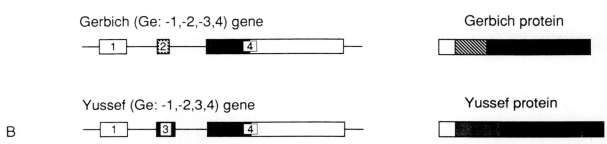

Figure 16–6. Genomic structures and polypeptides of glycophorins C and D and representative variants. *(A)* Wild-type glycophorin C (GPC) gene and derived protein products. The GPC gene comprises four exons. The extracellular domain of GPC is encoded by exons 1 and 2. Its transmembrane segment is encoded by exons 3 and 4, and the cytosolic portion is encoded by exon 4. Arrows encompassing exons 2 and 3 represent repeat sequences believed to be involved in recombination events that have deleted exon 2 or 3 in some GPC variants (see *B*). Glycophorin D (GPD) is believed to be derived from the same transcript that yields GPC, by means of translation initiation at an internal methionine residue corresponding to residue 22 of GPC. Positions of amino acid residues corresponding to exon boundaries are indicated below the GPC and GPD proteins. The Ge:2 and Ge:3 antigenic determinants have been localized to positions corresponding to exons 2 and 3, respectively. *(B)* Variant GPC proteins. The Gerbich-type variant GPC gene lacks sequences corresponding to exon 3, by means of a postulated recombination event occurring between repeated sequences depicted in *A*. This variant gene encodes a shortened GPC molecule deficient in amino acid residues corresponding to exon 3. The Yussef-type variant GPC gene lacks sequences corresponding to exon 2, by means of a similar mechanism, and is predicted to express a shortened protein deficient in amino acid residues corresponding to exon 2. (From Lowe JB: In Stamatoyannopoulos G, Nienhuis AW, et al (eds): The Molecular Basis of Blood Diseases, 2nd ed. Philadelphia, W.B. Saunders Co., 1994, pp 293–319.)

brane. Unlike GPA, GPC is not erythroid specific. Monoclonal antibodies to GPC stain neural tissue in a distinctive fibrillar pattern.[223] In red cells a desialylated form of GPC is exposed on the surface of very early progenitors (erythrocyte burst-forming unit [E-BFU]) and can be a useful marker of early normal or leukemic erythroid differentiation.[224] Normally glycosylated GPC first appears in the erythrocyte colony-forming unit (E-CFU).[132] GPD is a shortened form of GPC, lacking its NH₂-terminal 21 amino acids. It arises from the same mRNA as GPC by use of an alternate initiation codon.[131, 225] There are 143,000 copies of GPC and 82,000 copies of GPD per red cell.[226]

Association of Glycophorin A with Band 3. GPA and band 3 are associated in the membrane. The Wr^b antigen is caused by interaction of a site on band 3 (Glu[658]) with a site or sites located near the end of the extracellular domain of GPA or in the adjacent transmembrane domain.[227, 228] A monoclonal antibody to the Wr^b blood group antigen immunoprecipitates both GPA and band 3.[229, 230] Antibodies to glycophorin, including monovalent Fab fragments, decrease the lateral[231] and rotational[232] mobility of band 3. The coexpression of GPA in *Xenopus* oocytes enhances expression of band 3, by facilitating transport of band 3 from the endoplasmic reticulum to the cell surface.[233]

Glycophorin Functions. The functions of the glycophorins are uncertain, except for the observation that they provide most of the negative surface charge red cells require to avoid sticking to each other and to the vascular wall. GPC binds to protein 4.1 and p55 and may help anchor the skeleton to the membrane.

The glycophorins have been considered as possible conduits for transmembrane signaling and carry receptors for *P. falciparum* and for a number of viruses and bacteria. When wheat germ agglutinin or specific antibodies are attached to the external domain of GPA, the protein binds to the underlying membrane skeleton,[225, 234] probably through its interactions with band 3.[231, 235] The effect seems to involve transmembrane communication rather than antibody or lectin cross-linking, because it is also observed with monovalent Fab fragments but is not observed in red cells bearing variant glycophorins that lack a cytoplasmic domain (e.g., Miltenberger V).[236] The increased cross-links dramatically rigidify the membrane and cause it to acquire irreversible, plastic-like properties on deformation. The reason why red cells have this interesting property is a mystery. Chasis and Mohandas[132] note that a number of pathogens adhere to red cells and suggest the consequently stiffened erythrocytes may hasten reticuloendothelial removal of the invaders.

Recent work indicates that GPA bears receptors for *P. falciparum*. This was first discovered by Perkins[237] and has now been confirmed in many other laboratories either by direct competition, using the purified sialoglycoproteins, or by the inability of *P. falciparum* to infect red cells with various glycophorin abnormalities.[238–240] The principal ligand appears to be sialic acid attached through an $\alpha 2$–3 linkage to galactose,[241] but recognition also requires the peptide backbone of GPA.[242] GPA binds to EBA-175, a 175-kDa erythrocyte-binding antigen located on the surface of *P. falciparum* merozoites.[242]

Glycophorin Variants. The realization that the MNSs blood group antigens are carried by the glycophorins led to the discovery of a large number of glycophorin defects in persons with variants of this blood group system, some of which are listed in Table 16–3.

Glycophorin A-B-E Variants. Variants of the GPA-GPB-GPE locus have been classified according to the mechanism that brought about the alteration, including deletions of the GPA or GPB genes, or both, recombination due to genetic crossover or gene replacement (either double crossover events or gene conversion), and variants with altered antigenic properties due to alterations in the glycans attached to otherwise normal GPA or GPB proteins. Variants derived from complete or partial deletion of the GPA or GPB genes lead to the most dramatic phenotypes. Red cells with little or no detectable MN antigens, En(a−) cells, have been described with the underlying genetic defect being homozygous GPA gene deletion or the creation of chimeric molecule with the 5′ end of the GPA gene linked to the 3′ end of the GPB gene. En(a−) red cells have very weak MN blood group antigens and, as expected from the gene defect, lack GPA.[181–184] Surprisingly, the red cell compensates for this loss of surface charge by increasing the glycosylation of band 3.[181, 183, 188] As a result the surface charge is only about 20% less than expected.

Erythrocytes lacking the Ss and U determinants are found in individuals from some regions of Africa[243] but are rarely seen in North Americans. These cells are deficient in GPB or express a defective, nonglycosylated form of GPB.[185, 186] In most instances, Southern

blot analysis of DNA from GPB-deficient S-s-U− individuals has identified large GPB gene deletions.[187, 244] Rarely, S-s-U− individuals have been identified without detectable GPB gene deletions on Southern blotting. In these individuals, point mutations or microdeletions have been hypothesized to be causative.

Recombination events leading to hybrid glycophorin molecules are relatively common among the glycophorin A-B-E variants, as would be expected for a cluster of recently duplicated genes.[137, 189, 195–209] They are believed to result from chromosomal misalignment during meiosis and subsequent nonhomologous crossing over of the chromosomes in the region of GPA and GPB. A similar process is known to be responsible for the Lepore hemoglobins. Both Lepore-like and anti–Lepore-like unequal crossover of the glycophorins occur. In the former, illustrated by the Miltenberger V (MiV) variants,[199, 208, 209] the normal GPA gene is replaced by a fusion gene containing the NH$_2$-terminal end of GPA (first three exons) and the COOH-terminal end of GPB (last three exons). These two phenotypes vary in the particular Ss allele derived from the GPB gene. In the St^a variant,[198, 200, 203, 209] the hybrid protein is reversed and is derived from the NH$_2$-terminal end of GPB (first two exons) and the COOH-terminal of GPA (last three exons). Variants produced by sequence replacements include the MiIII, MiX, and MiVI types.

Individuals with homozygous deletions of both GPA and GPB genes have been described. Red cells from these individuals lack GPA and GPB proteins, as well as the MN, Ss, and En^a antigens and the Wr^b determinants. It is important to note that none of the GPA or GPB variants produce any detectable change in erythropoiesis or in the shape, function, or life span of the affected red cells. This is true even in these rare individuals with complete absence of both GPA and GPB. This observation indicates either that GPA, GPB, and GPE have no essential function or that such functions are redundant or can be performed by another protein such as band 3 or GPC.

Glycophorin C-D Variants. Antigens of the Gerbich blood group correspond to determinants on GPC and GPD. The four most common variants are

1. The Melanesian type. This variant lacks the Ge:1 determinant (Ge: -1, 2, 3, 4). Its molecular basis is not known.
2. The Yussef type (Ge: -1, -2, 3, 4) lacks exon 2 due to a 3.4-kb DNA deletion.
3. The Gerbich type (-1, -2, -3, 4) which lacks exon 3 also due to a 3.4-kb DNA deletion
4. The Leach variant (see later).

Other less common variants include the Webb type, a trypsin-sensitive antigen created by a single nucleotide substitution that changes an asparagine to a serine, removing the single asparagine-linked glycosylation site on GPC.[245] This, in turn, is responsible for the smaller size of W$_b$ GPC. Red cells of the Yussef, Gerbich, and Webb phenotypes have mutations in the extracellular domain of GPC, and in all three cases the mutant GPC protein is present, though its antigenicity is altered. In the rare Ls^a phenotype, erythrocytes display elongated GPC and GPD, owing to a duplication of exon 3.

In the Leach phenotype, GPC protein is absent, owing either to deletion of both exons 3 and 4[246–248] or to a frameshift mutation.[248] The Leach phenotype does not result in significant anemia, but it does cause elliptocytosis, as well as a decrease in membrane deformability and mechanical stability.[249–252] In contrast, red cells with the extracellular Ge- mutants and red cells that lack GPA or GPB have normal mechanical properties.[132, 253] Studies suggest that the deficiency of GPC is not directly responsible for the altered mechanical properties observed in Leach erythrocytes. Instead, the mechanical instability appears to be due to a concomitant partial deficiency of protein 4.1.[254] The instability is fully corrected by introducing protein 4.1 or its spectrin-binding domain (which facilitates spectrin/actin interactions) into GPC-deficient red cells. Why protein 4.1 and another recently described protein, p55, are deficient is not completely clear. However, the cytoplasmic domain of GPC interacts with both proteins[255] and presumably helps bind them to the membrane.

Band 3 (Anion Exchanger-1)

Band 3 (or AE1), the erythroid anion exchange protein, is the major integral protein of the red cell, comprising 25% to 30% of the membrane protein (see Fig. 16–3). It is expressed in great abundance, about 1.2 million copies per cell. The human band 3 cDNA is about 4.7 kb in length and encodes a 911-amino acid polypeptide (Fig. 16–7).[256, 257] Band 3 migrates as a diffuse band on SDS gels due to heterogeneous glycosylation (see Fig. 16–4). In addition to its critical role as the conduit for chloride-bicarbonate exchange,[258–262] there is some evidence that band 3 may be a flippase,[263, 264] and considerable evidence that it influences red cell deformability, intermediary metabolism, senescence, and possibly even shape.[265] Band 3 is also a major binding site for a variety of enzymes and cytoplasmic membrane components. Two of these functions, transport and binding, are relegated to two structurally separate domains of the protein.[266–268]

Structure and Functions of Band 3

The NH$_2$-Terminal Domain (Cytoplasmic Domain) of Band 3. The NH$_2$-terminal domain of band 3, consisting of the first 403 amino acids, binds glycolytic enzymes, hemoglobin, and skeletal proteins. The majority of this domain can be released from the membrane by treatment with chymotrypsin or trypsin as a 43-kDa fragment. The domain is an elongated, water-soluble, 403-amino acid segment, with a pliant, proline-rich hinge near the center. This hinge is thought to be located between amino acids 175 and 190 of the NH$_2$-terminal domain. The first 45 amino acids are highly acidic (20 are acidic and none are basic) and are thought to extend into the cytoplasm. The remainder of the domain is quite mobile, extending at high pH and contracting at low pH, presumably flexing about the hinge region.[267]

The acidic NH$_2$-terminal sequence contains the binding sites for the glycolytic enzymes glyceraldehyde-3-phosphate dehydrogenase (G3PD),[269–271] phosphoglycerate kinase (PGK),[272] and aldolase.[273–276] About 65% of G3PD, 50% of PGK, and 40% of aldolase are bound in the intact red cell.[269, 273] Membrane attachment inhibits enzyme activity[270, 275, 276] and is regulated by substrates, cofactors, and inhibitors of the three enzymes and by phosphorylation of tyrosine 8.[277] The phosphorus is added by the kinase p72syk[278] and may be removed by a phosphotyrosine phosphatase that is bound to band 3.[279] These observations suggest that band 3 may be an important regulator of red cell glycolysis. In fact, mild oxidants, which stimulate tyrosine phosphorylation in intact red cells, elevate glycolytic rates.[280]

The NH$_2$-terminus also weakly ($K_d < 10^{-4}$ M) binds hemoglobin,[281, 282] deoxyhemoglobin binds better than the oxyhemoglobin, but 2,3-diphosphoglycerate (2,3-DPG) inhibits deoxyhemoglobin binding.[281] This is understandable from x-ray diffraction studies, which show that the first five to seven amino acids of band 3 insert deeply into the 2,3-DPG–binding cleft of hemoglobin.[282] However, owing to high hemoglobin concentrations, approximately half the band 3 molecules have hemoglobin attached under physiologic conditions. Hemichromes, a partially denatured form of hemoglobin, bind much better and copolymerize with band 3, forming an aggregate.[283–286] These aggregates may play a role in red cell senescence.

Band 3 Cytoplasmic Domain—Peripheral Membrane Protein Interactions. Three peripheral membrane proteins, ankyrin,[268, 287–291] protein 4.1,[292, 293] and protein 4.2[271, 294–296] also bind to the cytoplasmic domain of band 3. The ankyrin-binding site has been partially characterized and includes sequences from the proximal, middle, and distal portions of the cytoplasmic domain.[288, 290, 297] This and other evidence suggests that the cytoplasmic domain has a complex folded structure. Ankyrin binds to the flexed conformations of band 3, most likely to band 3 tetramers.[291] Proteins 4.1 and 4.2 may also have more than one site of attachment. Protein 4.1 competes with antibodies specific for the NH$_2$-terminus, protects NH$_2$-terminal sites from proteolysis, and inhibits ankyrin binding, which occurs partly at the NH$_2$-terminus.[293] However, it also binds to peptides containing clustered basic residues (LRRRY and IRRRY) that are located at the COOH-terminal of the domain.[298] The protein 4.2 sites are less well defined, but mutations that inhibit binding occur at both the NH$_2$-[296] and COOH-terminal[299] ends of the domain.

The COOH-Terminal Domain of Band 3. The 52-kDa COOH-terminal domain of band 3 (amino acids 404–911) contains the anion exchange channel. The 1.2 million channels in each red cell can exchange 10^{10} to 10^{11} bicarbonate and chloride anions per second. This allows most of the bicarbonate produced in red cells by carbonic anhydrase to be carried in the plasma and increases CO_2 transport from the tissues to the lungs by about 60%.[300] The hydrogen (H^+) byproduct of the carbonic anhydrase reaction binds to hemoglobin and facilitates O_2 release to the tissues (Bohr effect). All of these reactions are reversed in the lungs.

The relationship of band 3 structure and the ion

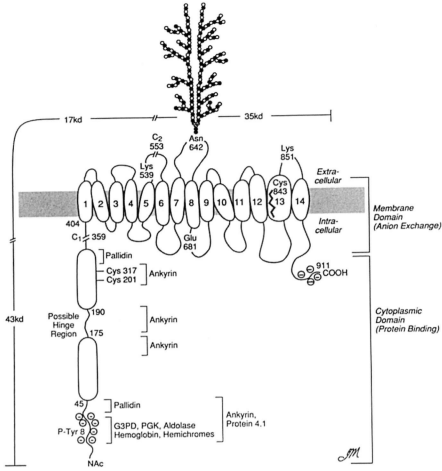

Figure 16–7. Organizational model of band 3, or AE1, the human erythrocyte anion exchange protein. The protein is divided into two structurally and functionally distinct domains: an approximately 43-kd cytoplasmic domain (amino acids 1 to 359), which contains binding sites for several cellular proteins, and an approximately 52-kd (17 + 35 kd) transmembrane domain (amino acids 360 to 911), which forms the anion exchange channel. The two regions can be separated by chymotrypsin cleavage at the inner membrane (C1). A second chymotryptic site (C2) is accessible at the external surface. *Cytoplasmic Domain.* The highly acidic NH_2 terminal region (amino acids 1 to 45) binds hemoglobin, hemichromes, protein 4.1, and the glycolytic enzymes phosphoglycerate kinase (PGK), aldolase, and glyceraldehyde-3-phosphate dehydrogenase (G3PD). Enzyme attachment is blocked by phosphorylation of tyrosine 8. Ankyrin and probably protein 4.2 binding involves several noncontiguous regions scattered throughout the cytoplasmic domain, which suggests that these binding sites are formed by protein folding. A functional hinge exists in the middle of the domain. *Transmembrane Domain.* Band 3 may contain as many as 14 transmembrane segments. Their orientation with respect to the inside and outside of the membrane has been extensively studied, but almost nothing is known about how they are positioned, relative to each other, to form the anion channel. Lys^{539} and Lys^{851} are probably the sites where H_2-DIDS, a covalent inhibitor of anion transport, attaches to band 3. Glu^{681} is probably one of the specific sites involved in anion exchange. A fatty acid, indicated by the *zig-zag symbol*, is esterified to Cys^{843}, and a complex carbohydrate structure is attached to Asn^{642}. Within the carbohydrate structure, *solid circles* represent *N*-acetylglucosamine; *hatched circles*, mannose; and *open circles*, galactose. (From Lux SE, Palek J: Disorders of the red cell membrane. In Handin RJ, Lux SE, Stossel TP (eds): Blood: Principles and Practice of Hematology. Philadelphia, Lippincott-Raven, 1995, pp 1701–1818.)

transport mechanism is under investigation. The COOH-terminal membrane domain is composed of 12 or 14 transmembrane helices connected by hydrophilic segments.[147, 256] The location and orientation of these structures (i.e., which are cytoplasmic and which are extracellular) has been studied in great detail.[142, 147, 256, 301, 302] The helices form the transport channel, but how they do so is unknown. Low-resolution structure image analysis of negatively stained two-dimensional crystals of the membrane domain revealed that two different conformations exist, represented by two crystal structures.[303] Perhaps these are the inward- and outward-facing transporters. The basic structural unit in both is an oblong band 3 dimer (~40 × 11 Angstrom). At the center of the dimer, the two monomers abut and appear to form a channel, presumably the transport channel.[303] There is also a flexible subdomain on the far side of each monomer, which might be formed by one or more of the large cytoplasmic loops between transmembrane helices.

It is unknown whether the apparent morphologic channel is actually one or two functional channels. A variety of studies suggest that each monomer contains a functional anion channel.[304, 305] If two channels exist, their location, at the interface of band 3 monomers, raises the possibility that two anions may be translocated simultaneously in opposite directions or that allosteric interactions between the subunits may regulate transport.[306, 307]

Anion exchange probably occurs by a ping-pong mechanism in which an intracellular anion enters the transport channel and is translocated outward and released, with the channel remaining in the outward conformation until an extracellular anion enters and triggers the reverse cycle.[142, 147, 308, 309] Whatever the mechanism, it probably involves a fairly large conformational change, because anion transport has a high energy and volume of activation.[310, 311] The specific residues involved in transport have not been identified, although there is evidence that a glutamic acid, four histidines, and one or more arginines are involved.[312–316] Anion exchange is extremely rapid (half-life = 50 milliseconds) for chloride and bicarbonate, the physiologic anions. The specificity of the channel is quite broad, and larger anions such as sulfate, phosphate, pyruvate, and superoxide are also transported, though at much slower rates.[142]

Finally, a large number of potent and useful anion transport inhibitors are known, especially various stilbene disulfonates such as DIDS (4,4'-diisothiocyanostilbene-2,2'-disulfonate). These bind to two lysine residues, probably Lys^{539} and Lys^{851}, on externally exposed portions of the protein in or near the entrance of the channel.[142, 259] These inhibitors have been of great benefit in the study of normal and mutant band 3 states.

Band 3-Related Antigens and Polymorphisms. Four to 20%[317] are heterozygous for a polymorphic, but functionally normal band 3 called band 3 Memphis (Lys^{56} →Glu).[318] Band 3 also carries the Diego (Dia) blood group (Pro^{854}→Leu plus Lys^{56}→Glu)[318] and the Wright a (Wr^a)/Wright b (Wr^b) blood groups (Lys^{658}/Glu^{658}, respectively).[228]

Self-Association of Band 3. Band 3 is extracted from the membrane by the nonionic detergent octaethylene glycol n-dodecyl monoether as stable dimers, tetramers, and higher-order oligomers. Quantitation of these species after separation on sizing columns shows that 70% of band 3 is in the dimer form and 30% is tetramers and oligomers. Almost all of the latter is associated with the membrane skeleton. This correlates with studies that show ankyrin binds preferentially to band 3 tetramers.[289, 291, 319] Isolated membrane domains only form dimers[320]; thus, tetramers are probably assembled by cross-linking neighboring dimers through the cytoplasmic domain, either with ankyrin (the physiologic cross-linker) or by oxidation (disulfide cross-linking),[297] hemichromes,[284–286] or other means.

Association of Band 3 with Glycophorin A. As noted earlier, GPA and band 3 are associated in the membrane. GPA facilitates migration of band 3 from its site of synthesis in the endoplasmic reticulum to the plasma membrane under experimental conditions[233] but probably is not critical *in vivo* because M^kM^k red cells, which lack GPA and GPB, contain normal amounts of band 3.[321] Band 3, on the other hand, does seem to be critical for GPA synthesis or stability because red cells that lack band 3 (described later in the

section on band 3 defects in hereditary spherocytosis) also lack GPA.[322]

Intramembranous Particles. Freeze-cleave electron microscopy of erythrocyte membranes reveals randomly distributed intramembranous particles (IMP) of 80 to 100 Angstrom on both the inner (P, protoplasmic) and outer (E, external) bilayer faces. Some studies suggest the more numerous IMP_P are primarily band 3 dimers and tetramers and that IMP_E are mostly glycophorins or the glucose transport protein.[323, 324]

Defects of Band 3 and Human Disease. Defects of band 3 have been identified in four disorders: (1) hereditary spherocytosis, owing to decreased synthesis, membrane insertion, or stability of band 3, or to mutations in the protein 4.2–binding sites[121, 156, 159]; (2) Southeast Asian ovalocytosis, owing to deletion of amino acids 400 to 408[159]; (3) rare forms of inherited acanthocytosis in which band 3 variants exhibit increased anion transport[325–328]; and (4) congenital dyserythropoietic anemia, type II, in which the lactosaminoglycan side chain is improperly constructed due to lack of the relevant glycosyl transferases.

Anion Exchangers in Nonerythroid Tissues. Erythroid band 3 (AE1) is a member of a multigene family of ion transporters. Two other genes encoding band 3–related anion exchange proteins have been identified: AE2 and AE3.[119, 329–331] AE2 is widely distributed and is probably the general tissue anion antiporter. AE3 expression is restricted to the heart and the brain. Both proteins are larger than AE1, owing to addition of about 300 amino acids at the NH_2-terminus. There is distinct homology between the three transporters, particularly in the membrane domain.[332–334] AE1 itself is expressed outside the red cell, in the acid-secreting, type A–intercalated cells in the collecting ducts of the kidney,[335–336] and possibly in cardiac myocytes.[337] The kidney transcript lacks the first 66 amino acids and is unable to bind glycolytic enzymes, protein 4.1, or ankyrin.[338, 339]

Other Integral Membrane Proteins

The red cell membrane contains over 100 other integral proteins. These include the Rh protein(s); the Kell antigen; the Duffy antigen; transporters for glucose, urea and amino acids; ATPases including Na^+,K^+-ATPase, Ca^{2+}-ATPase, and Mg^{2+}-ATPase; various kinases and phosphatases; acetylcholinesterase; decay accelerating factor; complement proteins (C3b and C4b); receptors for transferrin, insulin, insulin-like growth factors, thyroid hormone, parathyroid hormone, β-adrenergic agonists, cholinergic agents, diphtheria toxin, ceruloplasmin, and opiates; and many more.

Peripheral Membrane Proteins

The erythrocyte membrane skeleton (see Fig. 16–3) comprises 55% to 60% of the membrane protein mass and includes spectrin, actin, tropomyosin, tropomodulin, adducin, ankyrin, protein 4.1, dematin (protein 4.9), a portion of band 3, protein 4.2, and the proteins in the band 7 region of the SDS gel. Spectrin, actin, protein 4.1, and dematin (and perhaps tropomodulin and adducin) form the core of the structure because the skeleton retains its shape when other components are eluted with hypertonic KCl but disintegrates if spectrin or actin are removed. Operationally, the red cell membrane skeleton is the insoluble proteinaceous residue that remains after extraction of red cells[340] or their ghosts[341] with the nonionic detergent Triton X-100.

Spectrin

Structure and Function of Erythrocyte Spectrin. Spectrin is composed of two subunits, α and β, that, despite some similarities, are structurally distinct (Fig. 16–8) and are encoded by separate genes.[342, 343] On SDS polyacrylamide gels,[117] α-spectrin (~280 kDa) and β-spectrin (~246 kDa) (see Fig. 16–4) are the most abundant proteins of the red cell membrane skeleton, comprising 25% to 30% of total membrane protein and are present in approximately 200,000 copies per cell. The α- and β-spectrin chains intertwine in an antiparallel manner to form 100-nm long heterodimers, which in turn self-associate head to head to form tetramers and some larger oligomers.[344–347] Spectrin is highly flexible[346, 347] and is able to assume a variety of configurations, a property that may be critical for normal membrane function.

Spectrin tetramers, which have a contour length of 200 nm,[346, 347] are tightly coiled *in vivo*, with an end to end distance of only about 76 nm.[348] Spectrin molecules condense by twisting their α and β subunits around a common axis and regulate the degree of condensation by varying the pitch and diameter of the twisted double strand.[349] The native molecule has about 10 turns with a pitch of 7 nm and a diameter of 5.9 nm. The coiled spectrin tetramers can extend reversibly when the membrane is stretched but cannot exceed their contour length without rupturing.

Alpha-spectrin migrates on SDS polyacrylamide gels as a 240-kDa polypeptide. It begins with an isolated, unpaired helix (helix C) followed by nine typical 106-amino acid repeats (conformational segments 1 to 9), a short central segment that lacks homology to the repeats, but is related to SH3 domains (segment 10), followed by 12 more repeats (segments 11 to 22) and ends in a longer COOH-terminal segment that potentially encodes Ca²⁺-binding EF hand structures.[342, 350] The function of the spectrin SH3 domain is unknown. In other structural proteins, SH3 domains function as sites for the attachment of various molecules to membranes.[351] The ligand or ligands for α-spectrin have not yet been identified. The COOH-terminus of α-spectrin contains two EF hands, structures that participate in Ca²⁺ binding and regulate Ca²⁺ action in other proteins, including α-actinin[352, 353] and probably fodrin.[354, 355] Whereas one of the EF hands can bind Ca²⁺ at high concentrations (millimoles),[356–358] there is no evidence that spectrin binds Ca²⁺ *in vivo* or that its interactions with actin and protein 4.1 are regulated by Ca²⁺.

Beta-spectrin migrates on SDS polyacrylamide gels as a 220-kDa polypeptide. It consists of 17 homologous 106-amino acid repeat segments,[343, 359] a nonhomologous NH₂-terminal segment that contains an actin-binding domain,[360–363] the putative protein 4.1–binding site,[361, 364] and a short nonhomologous COOH-terminal segment that contains a consensus sequence for at least four casein kinase I phosphorylation sites.[365, 366] Evidence shows that membrane mechanical stability is sensitive to the state of phosphorylation.[367] Increased phosphorylation decreases and decreased phosphorylation increases membrane stability. Repeat 15 and part of repeat 16 are arranged in a β sheet structure and form the binding site for ankyrin.[359]

Seminal studies utilizing limited tryptic digestion of spectrin showed that the α- and β-spectrin chains are

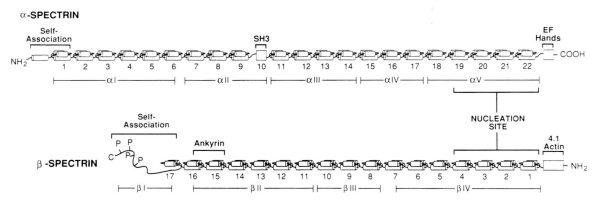

Figure 16–8. Spectrin structure. The α and β chains are aligned antiparallel with respect to their NH₂- and COOH-terminal ends. The approximately 106 amino acid "spectrin repeats" are numbered from the NH₂-terminus of each chain. In this model, each repeat is composed of three α helices (A, B, and C). The spectrin self-association site is formed by joining parts of two repeats that are left over at the "head" ends of the two chains. The α chain contributes helix C, the β chain, helices A and B. Some repeats are specialized, such as β15 and part of β16, which form the ankyrin-binding site, and the first four repeats at the "tail" of each chain, which nucleate interchain interactions. *Rectangles* denote peptide segments that differ from the repeats. They include the actin/protein 4.1 binding sites, a potential Ca²⁺ binding region (EF hands), and an SH3 domain. Each chain can be further divided into large structural domains by gentle proteolysis with trypsin. These domains are marked below each chain. In patients with hereditary elliptocytosis or pyropoikilocytosis due to defects in spectrin, the defects lie in the α I, α II, or β I domains. (From Lux SE, Palek J: Disorders of the red cell membrane. In Handin RJ, Lux SE, Stossel TP (eds): Blood: Principles and Practice of Hematology. Philadelphia, Lippincott-Raven, 1995, pp 1701–1818.)

divided into five and four domains, respectively, designated α I to α V and β I to β IV (Fig. 16–9).[344, 368] This technique allowed the isolation and characterization of functional domains of normal spectrin and the identification of mutant spectrins from patients with hereditary elliptocytosis and pyropoikilocytosis (see later).

Spectrin is Composed of Homologous Triple-Helical Repeats. The homologous 106-amino acid repeats in α- and β-spectrin fold into α-helical segments containing three antiparallel helices connected by short nonhelical segments (Fig. 16–10).[342, 343, 350, 369, 370] Each repeat forms a triple-helical structure that is about 5 nm long, is 2 nm wide, and is rotated 60° (right-handed) relative to the neighboring repeats.[350] Evidence for this model comes from circular dichroism measurements of spectrin length, biochemical analyses, comparison of spectrin flexibility in solution with other coiled-coil α-helical proteins, expression studies, and x-ray crystallography.

Each repeat begins with a straight, 28-amino acid α helix (helix A) (see Fig. 16–10). The polypeptide chain then reverses itself and forms a second, 34-amino acid long α helix (helix B). This is followed by another reverse turn and the 31-amino acid C helix, which bends in the middle. The helices are in a triangular array and are held together by both hydrophobic and electrostatic interactions.[350] One face of each helix is lined with mostly hydrophobic amino acids. Because an α helix makes one turn every 3.6 residues, the hydrophobic amino acids are spaced every third or fourth residue, at the positions designated "a" and "d" in Figure 16–10. Additional salt bonds occur between the mostly polar amino acids at positions "e" and "g" of the helices, particularly between helices A and C and B and C.[350] The three helices are tilted away from each other by 10° to 20° so that the COOH-terminal end of each repeat is wider than the NH₂-terminal end. This allows for the attachment of the following repeat without any adjustment of the structure. The repeats connect to each other through the A and C helices, forming one long α helix.[350] Because of the tight connection, the B helix of the proximal repeat overlaps the A helix of the distal repeat. Interactions between the two helices appear to restrict the mobility of the repeats at the repeat junction, at least in *Drosophila* tissue spectrin (also called fodrin), which was used for the structural studies. It is not clear whether this inter-repeat interaction is present in the more flexible erythrocyte spectrin molecule.

Speicher and Marchesi[370] note that several residues appeared to be highly conserved in the repeat segments, particularly at position 45, where there is an invariant tryptophan, and position 26, where there is almost always a leucine. Other conserved residues in-

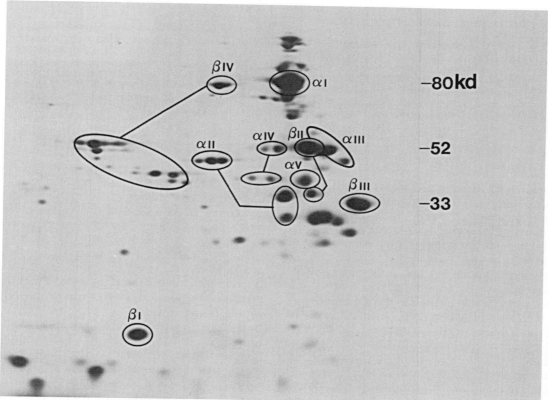

Figure 16–9. Mild (partial) tryptic digestion of spectrin. The resulting tryptic peptide domains are separated by two-dimensional gel electrophoresis. Isoelectric focusing is performed in the first dimension *(left to right)* and SDS-PAGE *(top to bottom)* in the second dimension. The major tryptic peptides of the α- and β-spectrin chains are circled and labeled. *Connected circles* indicate peptides that are related to each other. The smaller peptides in each connected pair result from additional tryptic cleavages. The numbers on the right indicate apparent molecular weights. (From Marchesi SL, Letsinger JT, et al: Mutant forms of spectrin α-subunits in hereditary elliptocytosis. J Clin Invest 1987; 80:191.)

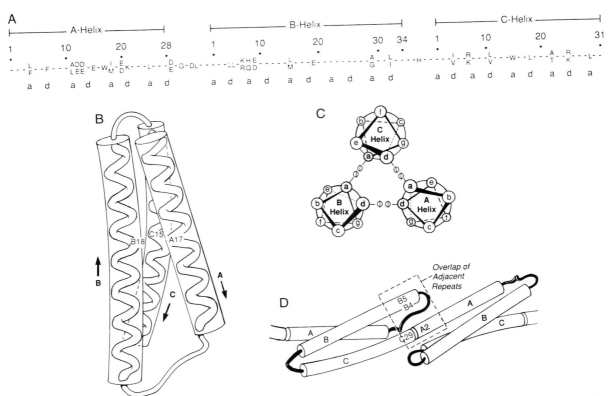

Figure 16-10. Structure of spectrin repeats. *A*, Consensus sequence of human erythrocyte spectrin phased according to crystallographic data, which defines three α helices that encompass the amino acids shown. Less conserved residues are marked with a dash. Residues a and d are the major contact points between helices. They tend to be hydrophobic and are conserved in most spectrins. *B*, Model of a single repeat based on the crystal structure of *Drosophila* α-fodrin. The positions of the nearly invariant tryptophans at A17 and C15 are shown. They interact with surrounding residues, including B18, at the central junction where the A helix crosses over from B to C. *C*, Cross section of a typical repeat. The A, B, and C helices are in a triangular array, and the a and d residues lie on one face of each helix. The side chains of these amino acids are usually hydrophobic (Φ) and interact with each other to stabilize the triple helical configuration. Salt bonds between the typically polar amino acids at positions e and g also help attach the B and C and A and C helices to each other. *D*, Interconnection of two adjacent repeats. The A and C helices are directly connected, forming one long helix. The distal repeat of each pair is rotated 60 degrees (right-handed). The B helix of the proximal repeat (*black and white*) overlaps the A helix of the following repeat (*shaded*). Interactions in the overlap region among conserved hydrophobic residues such as C29, B4, and B5 and the mostly hydrophobic residues at A2 probably stabilize the connection and limit mobility at the repeat junction. (From Lux SE, Palek J: Disorders of the red cell membrane. In Handin RJ, Lux SE, Stossel TP (eds): Blood: Principles and Practice of Hematology. Philadelphia, W.B. Saunders Co., 1995, pp 1701–1818.)

clude positions 1, 12, 15, 26, 35, 46, 68 (hydrophobic amino acids), 22 (arginine), 38 (aspartate), 41 (aspartate or glutamate), 71 (lysine), 72, and 101 (histidine). Studies of spectrin mutations in hereditary elliptocytosis and pyropoikilocytosis highlight the importance of these conserved residues.

The presence of homologous 106-amino acid repeats suggests that spectrin evolved from duplication of a single ancestral minigene. However, the genomic organization of both human α- and β-spectrin genes reveals that, with only a few exceptions, the size and position of exons does not correspond with the structural or conformational unit of spectrin repeats.[371, 372] This lack of correlation suggests that if an ancestral minigene did exist very early in evolution, the original distribution of introns within the minigene has been lost owing to the subsequent loss or acquisition of various introns.

Spectrin Functions. The functions of erythrocyte spectrin are to maintain cellular shape, regulate the lateral mobility of integral membrane proteins, and provide structural support for the lipid bilayer. In non-erythroid cells, spectrin may establish or maintain local concentrations of proteins of the plasma membrane, participate in the early stages of cell junction formation, and regulate access of secretory vesicles to the plasma membrane. Many of these important functions are mediated through spectrin/protein interactions.

Spectrin Self-Association. Self-association of spectrin dimers into tetramers (Fig. 16–11) and higher-order oligomers is perhaps the best characterized interaction of the spectrin proteins, allowing the erythrocyte membrane to acquire its mechanical properties. Disruption of spectrin self-association has been shown to lead to abnormally shaped erythrocytes and, in a number of cases, hemolytic anemia. Study of spectrin mutants reveals that defects of either the NH_2-terminal end of the α chain or the COOH-terminal end of the β chain (the "head" end of the molecule) may lead to impaired spectrin self-association.

Spectrin heterodimers (αβ) associate at the head end to form heterotetramers ($\alpha_2\beta_2$) and higher oligomers.[346, 347, 373, 374] Both tetramers and oligomers exist on the

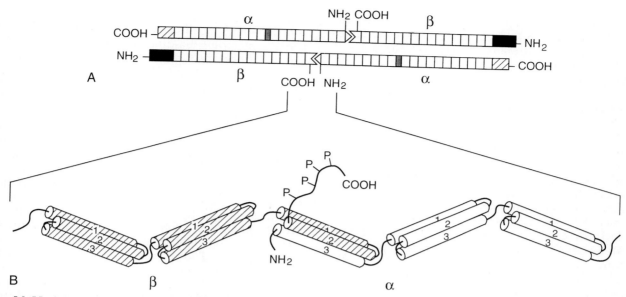

Figure 16-11. A model of spectrin heterodimer self-association. The NH₂-terminus of the α subunit and the COOH-terminus of the β subunit interact in an antiparallel fashion to form the spectrin heterodimer. Two spectrin dimers interact in a head-to-head fashion to form a spectrin tetramer, the basic building block of the erythrocyte membrane skeleton network. (From Tse WT, Lecomte MC, Costa FF, et al: A point mutation in the β spectrin gene associated with αI/74 hereditary elliptocytosis: implications for the mechanism of spectrin dimer self-association. J Clin Invest 1990; 86:909.)

membrane, but tetramers predominate, probably because the association constant for formation of tetramers is substantially higher than for the larger species. At low ionic strength and physiologic temperature (37°C), spectrin dissociates into dimers, whereas physiologic ionic strength and lower temperatures (25°C) favor the tetramer and oligomer species.[373–376] At 0°C the equilibrium is kinetically frozen.[374] It is possible to extract spectrin from the membrane at such temperatures and examine its association state directly or manipulate it, *in vitro* or on the membrane, to produce any desired oligomeric species.[347, 374, 375, 377] Measurements of spectrin eluted from normal ghosts indicate that about 5% of the spectrin is in the dimer form and about 50% is tetramers. The remainder is divided between higher-order spectrin oligomers and very high-molecular-weight complexes of spectrin, actin, protein 4.1, and dematin.[347, 378] Studies of this type have contributed to our fundamental understanding of abnormalities in many cases of hereditary elliptocytosis and pyropoikilocytosis.

The interconversion of spectrin dimers to tetramers involves a reversible opening of the dimer bond and formation of two new αβ attachments. The αβ contact closely resembles the triple-helical structure of native spectrin repeats except that in the contact site two of the helices are contributed by the COOH-terminus of the β chain (helices A and B) and one (helix C) comes from the NH₂-terminus of the α chain.[345] Spectrin dimers exist in "open" and "closed" forms, depending on whether the ends of the α and β chains are free (open) or bound to each other (closed). The open and closed states are distinguished by their reactivity and susceptibility to proteases.[345, 379, 380] Newly assembled spectrin heterodimers open and close by interaction

with each other, forming heterotetramers, or by forming an internal αβ bond. In the latter case, the longer α chain probably folds back in a hairpin structure to engage the β subunit. Opening the αβ contact (either the internal bond in closed dimers or the first αβ bond in tetramers) is the rate-limiting step in dimer-tetramer interconversion.[380]

The Nucleation Site of Spectrin. The side-to-side assembly of the α- and β-spectrin chains occurs in a zipper-like fashion, beginning with a defined nucleation site composed of four repeats from each chain, α19 to α22 and β1 to β4, respectively (see Fig. 16–5).[381] These are located at the tail end of the molecule, where actin binds. Two of the α repeats and one of the β repeats have 8-residue insertions that participate in the interchain interaction.[382, 383] These are located between conformational segments α20/α21, and β2/β3. The model suggests that after the initial tight association of the complementary nucleation sites, a conformational change is initiated that promotes the pairing of the remaining length of the two chains.[381] Interestingly, in support of this hypothesis is the finding of a common polymorphism, a low expression allele called αᴸᴱᴸʸ or αⱽ/⁴¹, which interferes with nucleation and effectively decreases synthesis of functionally competent α-spectrin (see later).

Ankyrin-Dependent and Ankyrin-Independent Binding of Spectrin to Membranes. The primary linkage of spectrin to the erythrocyte membrane is mediated by the binding of β-spectrin to ankyrin, which in turn binds to band 3. By functional analyses of truncated recombinant β-spectrin peptides, Kennedy and colleagues[359] showed that ankyrin binding requires almost the entire 15th repeat segment of β-spectrin and a small portion of the 16th. A similar ankyrin-binding site exists in nonerythroid β-spectrin (β-fodrin). Abnormalities of the spectrin/ankyrin-binding site would be expected to lead to abnormally shaped erythrocytes with unstable membranes.

Beta-spectrin and β-fodrin also contain an ankyrin-*independent* site in the NH₂-terminal half (tail half) of each molecule, which binds to brain membranes that have been stripped of peripheral membrane proteins,[384, 385] and possibly to stripped erythrocyte membranes. Binding is inhibited by Ca^{2+}/calmodulin.[384] This site is called membrane association domain 1 (MAD1). Beta-fodrin and the muscle/brain isoform of erythrocyte β-spectrin (see later) have a second, Ca^{2+}/calmodulin-independent site, MAD2, near the COOH-terminus.[384, 385] MAD2 contains a sequence motif called the pleckstrin homology domain,[386, 387] which binds to "WD40 repeats" within the $G_β$ subunit of G proteins[388] and similar repeats in other proteins, to the phospholipid phosphatidylinositol-4,5-bisphosphate, and to the intracellular messenger IP_3.[389–391] It is assumed but not proven that this motif mediates membrane binding.

The Junctional Complex of the Erythrocyte Membrane Skeleton. A second linkage of spectrin to the plasma membrane is mediated by its association with the junctional complex that includes spectrin, actin, and protein 4.1.[127, 128, 139] Spectrin, protein 4.1, and actin form a ternary or higher-order complex that links spectrin tetramers to one another in a tail-to-tail fashion. The spectrin/actin-binding site has been mapped to a region near the NH₂-terminus of β spectrin[362] that contains a 27-amino acid sequence that is highly conserved between a number of actin-binding proteins, including α actinin, dystrophin, filamin, fimbrin, and ABP-120.[363] This site was identified as the actin-binding site in ABP-120 and is presumed to be the actin-binding site of these proteins, including β-spectrin. Protein 4.1 is also thought to bind β-spectrin near its NH₂-terminus, as demonstrated by electron microscopy; however, the precise site of this interaction is unknown. A mutation in this region of β-spectrin has been described in a spherocytosis kindred whose erythrocyte membranes demonstrated impaired spectrin/protein 4.1 binding (see later). Intact spectrin dimers appear to be required for formation of the spectrin/protein 4.1 complex.

Nonerythroid Spectrins (Fodrins). Spectrin-related proteins exist in a wide variety of tissues and species.[127, 128, 148] There are two closely related, yet distinct mammalian α subunits of spectrin. One, α-spectrin, is expressed in mature erythroid cells; the other, α-fodrin, is expressed in all other tissues.[138] Birds have a single α-spectrin subunit that is expressed in all tissues, including erythrocytes. Similarly there are two β subunits in mammals: β-spectrin and β-fodrin. *Drosophila* also have a third subunit called β-heavy spectrin (M_r = 430 kDa). Beta-spectrin, in turn, exists in both erythroid and muscle/brain isoforms (see later). With a few exceptions, nonerythroid spectrins are composed of two nonidentical, high-molecular-weight subunits, α and β, which, like spectrin, are composed primarily of homologous repeat units of 106 amino acids.

Fodrin (also called tissue spectrin, brain spectrin, spectrin II or spectrin G) is a heterodimer of α- and β-fodrin chains. It shares a number of common biologic functions with erythrocyte spectrin (spectrin I or spectrin R), including binding to actin, ankyrin, and adducin.[148] Other features differ. For example, the α-fodrin contains a calmodulin-binding site that is lacking in α-spectrin, and β-fodrin contains a pleckstrin homology domain (see earlier) that is not present in erythrocyte spectrin.

There is great variability in subcellular localization or subunit composition of erythroid and nonerythroid spectrins. Although typically thought to be localized in the membrane skeleton of the mammalian erythrocyte, spectrin exhibits developmentally regulated patterns of expression and differences in cellular distribution between various tissues.[128, 134, 148] This is observed in diverse processes, such as neural development, *Drosophila* oogenesis, epithelial cell polarity, and sea urchin embryogenesis. Fodrins have been shown to redistribute with some types of cellular activation such as the binding of ligands or IgG to cell surface receptors, dimethyl sulfoxide–induced differentiation, cell polarization, and viral transformation. Proteolysis of fodrin is an early event in apoptosis and may contribute to the membrane blebbing in apoptotic cells. A β-fodrin homologue has even been identified in tomatoes.

Winkelmann and co-workers showed that tissue-specific differential processing of the 3' end of β-spectrin pre-mRNA generates a β-spectrin cDNA isoform in human skeletal muscle and brain encoding a COOH-terminus different from that present in erythrocyte β-spectrin.[392] The encoded isoform replaces the last 22 amino acids of erythrocyte β-spectrin, a region that contains a casein kinase I consensus sequence, with a new sequence of 213 amino acids that includes the pleckstrin homology domain. The identification of frameshift mutations in the region of the β-spectrin gene 5' to this tissue-specific splice site in the DNA of patients with membrane-related hemolytic anemias raises interesting questions regarding the expression and function of this β-spectrin isoform in muscle and brain.

The Spectrin Superfamily of Proteins. The spectrin superfamily of proteins includes the erythroid and nonerythroid spectrins, dystrophin, a dystrophin homologue, and α-actinin. These proteins share a number of structural properties including flexible, rodlike shapes of side-to-side subunits arranged in an antiparallel manner. Members of the spectrin superfamily are composed of homologous amino acid repeats of 106, 109, and 120 residues for spectrin, dystrophin, and α-actinin, respectively, that are thought to be folded into triple α-helical segments.[138, 148, 166] Members of this family are actin-binding proteins. Sequence comparison reveals a number of similarities between members of the spectrin superfamily of proteins.[138] There is homology in the sequence of the triple-helical repeats of spectrin, dystrophin, and actinin across species, with conservation of the invariant tryptophan at position 45 or 46. The repeats of dystrophin and spectrin are most homologous, whereas the actinin repeat is more distantly related. The COOH-terminal regions of α-spectrin, α-actinin, and dystrophin are homologous, containing potential Ca^{2+}-binding, EF hand structures. The NH_2-termini of β-spectrin, dystrophin, and α-actinin are also homologous, encoding a potential actin-binding site. The similarities in both structure and function suggest a common ancestral origin for the genes of this group of proteins.

Ankyrin (Bands 2.1, 2.2, 2.3, and 2.6)

Ankyrin is a large, 206-kDa, 8.3×10-nm protein (see Fig. 16–3)[393] that provides the primary linkage between the spectrin/actin-based erythrocyte membrane skeleton and the plasma membrane.[122, 146] Ankyrin is composed of an NH_2-terminal 89-kDa membrane (band 3)-binding domain, a 62-kDa spectrin-binding domain, and a COOH-terminal 55-kDa regulatory region (Fig. 16–12).[394–403] In the red cell, ankyrin makes up approximately 5% of total membrane protein.[128, 130] It provides the connection between spectrin and band 3 through a high affinity linkage ($K_d \sim 10^{-7}$ M) with β spectrin[394] and a high-affinity linkage ($K_d \sim 10^{-7}$ to 10^{-8} M) with the cytoplasmic domain of band 3.[268, 287, 289] Selective disruption of the ankyrin/band 3 interaction in *intact* red cells, at slightly alkaline pH,[404] markedly decreases membrane stability, emphasizing the importance of the interaction.

Ankyrin appears to be involved in the local segregation of integral membrane proteins within functional domains on the plasma membrane. This important polarization of membrane proteins may be generated by the relative affinities of the different isoforms of ankyrins for target proteins.[130] The composition and specialized functions of membrane skeletons differ in erythroid and nonerythroid cells. This specialization appears to have evolved through the tissue-specific, developmentally regulated expression of multiple protein isoforms.

Ankyrin Structure and Functions

The Membrane Domain (or Repeat Domain) of Ankyrin. The 89-kDa NH_2-terminal domain is almost entirely composed of 24 consecutive 33-amino acid repeats called cdc10/ankyrin repeats, or just ankyrin repeats,[146] which are subdivided into 6-repeat folding units.[402, 403] The repeats are quite similar to each other and must have formed by repeated duplications of a primordial minigene. Binding sites for band 3[395, 397–400] and at least six other families of integral membrane proteins are located in this domain. Repeats 7 through 12 (folding unit 2) and repeats 13 through 24 (folding units 3 and 4) form two distinct but cooperative binding sites for band 3.[405] Because band 3 exists as a dimer on the membrane, the presence of two binding sites potentially allows ankyrin to interact with four band 3 molecules simultaneously, which is the normal stoichiometry of ankyrin/band 3 complexes.[406–409] Whether ankyrin actually binds to different band 3 molecules in the tetrameric complex is unknown. Alternatively, ankyrin may bind to two different sites on one band 3 molecule but prefer the conformation these sites assume in the band 3 tetramer. Selective disruption of the ankyrin/band 3 interaction, at slightly alkaline pH, markedly decreases membrane stability, emphasizing the importance of the interaction.[410]

The NH_2-terminal domain of ankyrin also binds tubulin *in vitro*, especially unpolymerized tubulin,[411, 412] but this may be a spurious interaction because there is no persuasive evidence that the two proteins interact *in vivo*.

The ankyrin repeats consist of 33 amino acids, 15 of which are conserved. Very similar repeats are found in an enormous variety of proteins in all phyla, including bacteria and viruses.[146] These proteins have little in common except, perhaps, the ability to interact with other proteins or DNA. The cdc10/ankyrin repeats must have been propagated throughout evolution because of their ability to generate versatile modules that could be tailored to interact with specific ligands.

The Spectrin-Binding Domain. The spectrin-binding site is located within a 62-kDa globular, central domain of ankyrin (also called the 72-kDa domain[411–413]) and

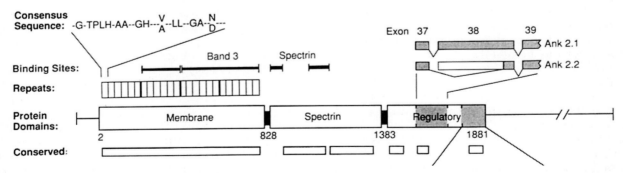

Figure 16–12. Structure of erythrocyte ankyrin, ANK1. The membrane domain (89 kDa) contains 24 repeats (33 amino acids each), grouped in folding units of six. Their consensus sequence is shown at the top left in single-letter amino acid code. Dashes indicate less conserved residues. Repeats 7–12 (folding unit 2) and repeats 13–24 (folding units 3 and 4) form two distinct but cooperative binding sites for band 3. The spectrin domain (62 kDa) contains the binding site or sites for spectrin. These two domains are the most conserved. The regulatory domain (55 kDa) is thought to modulate the binding functions of the other two domains. In the middle of the domain, a highly acidic inhibitory region in exon 38 is spliced out of full-length ankyrin (ANK2.1) to make ANK2.2. At least eight isoforms of the last three exons exist. The last three isoforms contain a basic sequence (*open area*) that is common in brain ANK1 but rare in the red cell protein. In addition, isoforms lacking exons 38 and 39, 36 through 39, and 36 through 41 have been detected. The *asterisk* indicates the location of the translation terminator codon. (From Lux SE, Palek J: Disorders of the red cell membrane. In Handin RJ, Lux SE, Stossel TP (eds): Blood: Principles and Practice of Hematology. Philadelphia, Lippincott-Raven, 1995, pp 1701–1818.)

appears to involve regions at both the beginning[398] and middle[401] of the domain. The complementary binding site for ankyrin on spectrin is formed by spectrin repeats 15 and 16 near the end of the molecule involved in dimer-tetramer self-association.[359] Each spectrin tetramer apparently binds only one ankyrin molecule, even though two binding sites are available. This is probably because ankyrin binds about 10 times more avidly to spectrin tetramer than to spectrin dimer.[395, 404]

The Regulatory Domain. The 55-kDa, proteolytically sensitive, COOH-terminal domain contains regulatory sequences that enhance and diminish the binding of ankyrin to spectrin and the anion exchange protein.[402, 413–415] Some of these are alternatively spliced, creating ankyrin isoforms of different sizes and functions. For example, ankyrin 2.2 (band 2.2) lacks an acidic 162-amino acid sequence from exon 38 that is found in full-sized ankyrin (band 2.1).[402] The smaller isoform functions like an activated ankyrin, with enhanced binding to band 3 and spectrin and the ability to bind to new sites on some other plasma membranes. The 162-amino acid "repressor sequence," expressed as a separate protein, binds to ankyrin 2.2 and inhibits its interaction with band 3.[413] Eight alternatively spliced isoforms of the three COOH-terminal exons have been identified. In addition, isoforms lacking (1) exons 38 and 39, (2) exons 36 through 39, and (3) exons 36 through 41 have been detected.[416, 417] Some of these shortened RNAs probably form the smallest ankyrin isoforms (e.g., bands 2.3, 2.6). The COOH-terminal exons are highly conserved,[418] unlike most of the 55-kDa domain, which suggests they also encode regulatory sequences. These may be activating sequences because proteolytic removal of the last 196 amino acids partially deactivates ankyrin, muting its affinity for band 3.[415]

Curiously, the regulatory domain also contains a "death domain" near its NH$_2$-terminal end.[419] Other proteins that carry this lethal motif are part of a pathway or pathways that trigger NF-κB activation and apoptosis.[420–431] Examples include the tumor necrosis factor receptor and the proteins Fas/APO1, TRADD, RIP, FADD/MORT1, WSL-1, and *Drosophila* reaper. There is no evidence that ankyrin is involved in apoptosis, but this possibility should be investigated, especially because fodrin (tissue spectrin) is cleaved at a specific site in the α chain by a protease generated during apoptosis,[432, 433] a process that is thought to be related to the characteristic membrane blebbing observed in apoptotic cells.

The function of ankyrin is also regulated by phosphorylation.[414, 434, 435] *In vitro*, up to seven phosphates are added to ankyrin by the red cell membrane casein kinase I.[434] Unphosphorylated ankyrin binds preferentially to spectrin tetramers and oligomers rather than to spectrin dimers.[395, 414, 434] This preference is abolished by phosphorylation, which also reduces the capacity of ankyrin to bind band 3.[435] Ankyrin is also phosphorylated by protein kinase A, but the functional effect of the modification has not been studied.

The Ankyrin Gene Family. Ankyrins, like spectrins, are members of a family of proteins.[146] Ankyrin-like molecules have a wide distribution, with immunoreactive forms found in almost all tissues. Nonerythroid ankyrins bind a variety of integral membrane proteins other than band 3, including Na$^+$,K$^+$-ATPase, the voltage-dependent axonal Na$^+$ channel, the amiloride-sensitive epithelial Na$^+$ channel, the cardiac Na$^+$/Ca^{2+} exchanger, H$^+$,K$^+$-ATPase, the IP$_3$ receptor, CD44, and a group of neurofascin-related brain adhesive proteins. The available data suggest that ankyrins localize these proteins to particular membrane domains, presumably by local interactions with cytoskeletal proteins. ANK1, erythrocyte ankyrin, is also found in myocytes[436, 437] and brain, particularly in the Purkinje cells of the cerebellum.[438, 439] ANK2 is an exclusively neural form that is localized to neuronal cell bodies and dendrites.[440–442] ANK3 is the most widely distributed, particularly in epithelia and axons.[443–445] It is also expressed in megakaryocytes, macrophages, myocytes, melanocytes, hepatocytes, and testicular Leydig cells.

Protein 4.1

Protein 4.1 is a member of the erythrocyte membrane skeleton that interacts with spectrin and actin, as well as proteins in the overlying lipid bilayer (see Fig. 16–3).[135, 136] The cloned protein is globular (5.7 nm diameter) and has a molecular weight of 66 kDa but migrates as a 78- to 80-kDa protein on SDS polyacrylamide gels. The reason for this difference is unknown. There are approximately 2 × 10^5 copies of protein 4.1 per cell. Chymotryptic digestion and limited sequencing have divided protein 4.1 into four domains (Fig. 16–13).[446] Beginning at the NH$_2$-terminal end they are a 30-kDa domain (residues 1 to ~300), a 16-kDa domain (residues ~300–404), a 10-kDa domain (residues 405–471), and a 22- to 24-kDa domain (residues 472–622). Two forms of the intact protein, designated 4.1a (80 kDa) and 4.1b (78 kDa), are separated on high-resolution SDS gels. Protein 4.1a is derived from protein 4.1b by gradual deamidation of Asn^{502} within the 22- to 24-kDa domain,[447] leading to a predominance of protein 4.1a in older erythrocytes.[448]

Proteins that Interact with Protein 4.1. Protein 4.1 binds tightly (K$_d$ ~10^{-7} M) to β-spectrin,[361, 364, 449] very near the actin-binding site,[360, 393] and greatly amplifies the otherwise weak spectrin/actin interaction.[450–452] This activity can be traced to the 10-kDa domain[453, 454] and, at least partly, to a 21-amino acid peptide within the domain.[455–458] Protein 4.1 also binds directly to F-actin (K$_d$ ~10^{-7} M).[459] This suggests it works by bridging spectrin and actin, although other mechanisms have not been excluded. The interaction of protein 4.1 with spectrin and actin is blocked by protein kinase A phosphorylation, which labels residues in the 16-kDa (Ser^{331}) and 10-kd (Ser^{467}) domains,[460, 461] and by tyrosine kinase phosphorylation, which labels a site (Tyr^{418}) in the 10-kDa domain.[462] The ternary complex also appears to be regulated by Ca^{2+} and calmodulin.[463–465] Calmodulin binds to protein 4.1 in a Ca^{2+}-independent manner (K$_d$ ~5 × 10^{-7} M) but, once bound, the calmodulin/protein 4.1 complex confers Ca^{2+} sensitivity on the viscosity increase produced by spectrin/actin/pro-

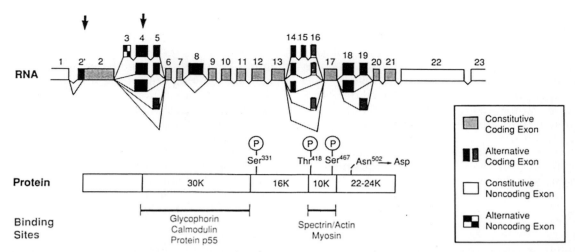

Figure 16-13. Protein 4.1. *Top,* Alternative splicing map of protein 4.1 mRNA. Reticulocyte 4.1 is translated from the downstream AUG (*arrow* over exon 4) and includes a 63-bp (21-amino acid) erythroid-specific sequence within exon 16 that is critical for spectrin/actin interactions. Many combinations of exons are expressed, although some are observed only in nonerythroid tissues. *Middle and Bottom,* Domain map of the 80-kd (erythroid) form of protein 4.1, indicating binding sites, phosphorylation sites, and the location of a COOH-terminal asparagine that is deamidated in aged red cells. (From Conboy JG: Structure, function, and molecular genetics of erythroid membrane skeletal protein 4.1 in normal and abnormal red blood cells. Semin Hematol 1993; 30:138.)

tein 4.1 binding.[465] The calmodulin-binding site is located within the 30-kDa domain.[465]

Protein 4.1 also binds to the membrane and serves as a secondary attachment site for spectrin. The binding involves the 30-kDa domain of protein 4.1[466, 467] and is blocked by Ca^{2+} and calmodulin[468] or by phosphorylation of protein 4.1 with protein kinase C (but not protein kinase A).[469] The identity of the membrane attachment site is controversial. GPA, GPC, and band 3 are the major candidates. The putative interaction with GPA depends on the presence of phosphatidyl inositol-4,5-bisphosphate (PI-PP),[470] and therefore could be regulated metabolically or through various signaling pathways. The interaction with band 3 has a high capacity but relatively low affinity.[292, 466] Protein 4.1 binds directly to GPC, to a site near amino acids 82 through 98 in the GPC tail.[466] It also binds indirectly, by means of protein p55 (see later), to a more distal site, near residues 112 through 128.[466]

The major question is whether one or all of these protein/protein interactions occurs *in vivo*. Although there is evidence that all three *can* occur, the interaction with GPC is the only one that has been shown to have functional consequences in intact red cells[251, 471]: (1) protein 4.1-deficient red cells are also deficient in GPC but not GPA or band 3[471–473]; (2) the residual GPC is only loosely bound to the skeleton but becomes tightly bound if the deficient cells are reconstituted with protein 4.1[472]; and (3) GPC-deficient red cells are structurally unstable, whereas GPA-deficient cells are mechanically normal.[132, 251] In addition, both protein 4.1 and GPC bind p55, which may augment or regulate their interaction.[466, 467, 474–476] There is preliminary evidence that these effects are due to protein 4.1 deficiency rather than protein 4.1/GPC or protein 4.1/protein p55 interactions, because the mechanical weakness of GPC-deficient membranes is fully restored by reconstitution with protein 4.1 or its spectrin/actin-binding domain.

In one study it was concluded that, *in vivo*, approximately 40% of protein 4.1 is bound directly to GPC, 40% is bound indirectly through protein p55, and 20% is bound to band 3.[466]

Protein 4.1 also interacts with myosin,[477] tubulin,[478] and phosphatidyl serine.[479, 480] The interaction with myosin (K_d 1.4×10^{-7} M) is particularly interesting because the myosin-binding site lies within the 10-kDa domain that regulates spectrin/actin/protein 4.1 complex formation and because protein 4.1 inhibits the actin-activated Mg^{2+}-ATPase activity of myosin.[477] Finally, protein 4.1 is modified by the addition of the O-linked monosaccharide N-acetylglucosamine to a site in the 22- to 24-kDa domain.[481] The function of this unusual alteration is unknown.

Alternatively Spliced Isoforms of Protein 4.1. Protein 4.1 is expressed as many alternatively spliced forms. The protein 4.1 gene is over 90 kb in length and encodes at least 23 exons, including 10 alternatively spliced exons or "motifs" (see Fig. 16–13).[482] This leads to a remarkably diverse collection of protein 4.1 isoforms in both erythroid and nonerythroid cells.[482–487] Both tissue- and stage-specific isoforms have been observed. Protein 4.1 utilizes two different initiation codons, termed *upstream* and *downstream initiation codons*, which translate to isoforms of 135 and 80 kDa, respectively. The 80-kDa isoform is created by the splicing out of a 17-nt motif that contains the upstream translation initiator. In most tissues this sequence is spliced in and a downstream 80-bp motif is spliced out. This gives rise to the elongated, 135-kDa isoform that contains an additional 209 amino acids attached to the NH_2-terminus of erythroid protein 4.1. Another important protein 4.1 isoform is created by the splicing in/out of a 63-bp motif within the 10-kDa domain. This motif is expressed primarily in erythroid cells and muscle and contains the 21-amino acid spectrin/actin-binding site. Expression of this motif is linked to terminal erythroid differentiation.[486]

Protein 4.1 is expressed in most tissues. It appears as a variety of isoforms that are related to the 80- and 135-kDa species. Protein 4.1 is not limited to the plasma membrane in nonerythroid cells. It is also located in the nucleus[488] and decorating actin/stress fibers.[489] It is part of a superfamily of proteins that includes talin, ezrin, moesin, radixin, merlin/schwannomin, and the human protein tyrosine phosphatases PTP H1 and PTP-MEG. These proteins, which share homology to the NH$_2$-terminal (30 kDa) domain of protein 4.1, appear to be involved in the linkage of actin filaments to the plasma membrane.

Protein 4.2

Protein 4.2 is a 78-kDa peripheral membrane protein that helps link the skeleton to the lipid bilayer.[133, 490] It binds to band 3 (AE1) and probably binds to ankyrin, possibly promoting their interaction. Protein 4.2 binds to ankyrin in solution,[295] but it has been difficult to prove that it binds ankyrin when ankyrin is attached to band 3. It is possible that protein 4.2 and ankyrin can only bind to different band 3 molecules. However, in nb/nb mice, which lack ankyrin, and in a child with hereditary spherocytosis and deletion of one ankyrin gene, a considerable reduction in protein 4.2 is observed in erythrocyte membranes.[491, 492] In addition, ankyrin elutes more easily from the red cell membranes of some humans with protein 4.2 deficiency.[493, 494] These observations strongly suggest that the two proteins sometimes interact in vivo. Protein 4.2 is myristylated[495] and palmitoylated,[496] but the function of these modifications is unknown. It also binds ATP,[497] conceivably supplying a membrane pool of ATP for transporters, kinases, flippases, and other local needs.

Protein 4.2 is homologous to transglutaminases,[498, 499] although it possesses no transglutaminase activity. A critical residue in the active site of transglutaminases is not conserved in protein 4.2. Perhaps some other common property, as yet unknown, of these proteins maintains their structural homology. The protein 4.2 gene resembles transglutaminases in its intron-exon organization.[500] Four isoforms exist owing to alternative splicing of 90-bp and 234-bp exons in the region corresponding to the NH$_2$-terminal end of the protein.[501] The respective proteins are 80 kDa (both exons present), 78 kDa (small exon absent), 71 kDa (large exon absent), and 69 kDa (both exons absent). The 78-kDa protein is the predominant species (97%) in normal red cells[490]; isoforms lacking the 234-bp exon are rare.

Protein 4.2 has been linked to the mouse pallid mutation (pa/pa).[502] However, recombinants between the two loci have been identified, indicating they are genetically separate (Peters LL: Personal communication, 1996).

Protein p55

Protein p55 is the human homolog of dlg, a Drosophila tumor suppressor gene.[503] It contains three domains: an NH$_2$-terminal domain of unknown function that is also present in dlg, a central SH3 domain that may be a binding site for other proteins, and a COOH-terminal guanylate kinase domain.[476, 504] There are 80,000 copies of p55 per red cell, probably assembled into dimers. The protein is extensively palmitoylated[504] and is tightly bound to the membrane. The p55 gene is located on the long arm of the X chromosome, at Xq28, just beyond the factor VIII gene.[505] It is expressed throughout erythroid differentiation and is widely expressed in nonerythroid tissues. p55 interacts with protein 4.1 and GPC, linking them together.[466, 467, 474] Patients who lack either protein 4.1 or GPC also lack p55,[475] and direct binding studies show that p55 binds to the 30-kDa domain of protein 4.1 (K_d ~2 × 10^{-9} M) and to the cytoplasmic domain of GPC (K_d ~7 × 10^{-9} M).[466, 467, 475, 476] Considering the wide tissue distribution of all three proteins, it is likely this interaction, or interactions of p55 with other members of the protein 4.1 superfamily, will have a variety of important functions.

Actin

Red cell actin is structurally and functionally similar to other actins.[506–508] It is the β subtype, which is found in a variety of other nonmuscle cells.[508] However, unlike other nonmuscle actins, red cell actin is organized as short, double-helical F-actin "protofilaments" 12 to 13 monomers long.[509, 510] These short filaments appear to be stabilized by their interactions with spectrin, adducin, protein 4.1, and tropomyosin and by capping of the slow growing or "pointed" end of the actin filament by tropomodulin.[511] It is not clear what caps the rapidly growing, "barbed" end—perhaps adducin (see later).

Evidence exists that the state of actin polymerization is functionally important to the red cell because compounds that inhibit actin polymerization increase membrane flexibility, whereas compounds that promote its polymerization make the membrane rigid.[512] Spectrin dimers bind to the side of actin filaments at a site near the tail end of the spectrin molecule.[360, 362, 450, 509, 510] Spectrin tetramers are therefore bivalent and can crosslink actin filaments; however, binding is weak (K_d ~10^{-3} M) and ineffectual in the absence of protein 4.1.[513]

Adducin

Adducin is a heteromer of structurally related proteins,[514, 515] α-adducin (81 kDa) and β-adducin (80 kDa), encoded by separate genes. A third, nonerythroid adducin (γ-adducin) has also been described.[516] The α and β subunits each have three domains: an NH$_2$-terminal 39-kDa, globular "head"; a 9-kDa, connecting "neck"; and a 33-kDa, protease-sensitive, extended, COOH-terminal "tail."[515] The last domain contains mostly hydrophilic residues and 22-amino acid segments with homology to the MARCKS proteins. In solution, adducin is a mixture of heterodimers and heterotetramers.[517] Models suggest the four head domains cluster in a globular core whereas the tail domains extend to interact with spectrin and actin.[517] Alternatively, spliced isoforms of both adducin subunits have been described[518–520]; the function or functions of these isoforms are unknown. It has been estimated that there are ~30,000 copies of adducin per cell or one adducin per actin protofilament. Adducin is present at the erythroblast stage but is not incorporated into the red cell membrane until late in erythroid development.[521]

Adducin is believed to play a role in the early assembly of the spectrin/actin complex by promoting the interaction of spectrin and actin.[514] This interaction is regulated by phosphorylation of the COOH-terminal domain of adducin by protein kinase C. Because of its role in spectrin/actin interactions, adducin is frequently compared with protein 4.1. However, unlike protein 4.1, adducin does not bind directly to spectrin in the absence of actin. *In vitro*, the actin-binding domain of β-spectrin plus the first two spectrin repeats are sufficient for assembly of a spectrin/actin/adducin ternary complex. The complex promotes binding of additional spectrin, an interaction that is blocked by calmodulin.[514] The COOH-terminal tail of adducin contains the spectrin-, actin-, and calmodulin-binding sites and the sites of phosphorylation. It has the same ability to promote spectrin/actin interactions as the intact molecule. Evidence suggests that adducin also acts as a barbed-end capping protein for actin filaments.[522]

Adducin is present in a number of nonerythroid cells and is concentrated at sites of cell-to-cell contact.[523] The protein assembles at these sites in response to extracellular Ca^{2+} and dissociates after treatment of the cells with phorbol esters, which stimulate phosphorylation of the protein by protein kinase C.[523, 524] The protein is also phosphorylated by protein kinase A, but the effect of this phosphorylation is unknown. Thus, adducin may locally regulate the membrane skeleton through Ca^{2+} and protein kinase C and promote attachment of the membrane skeleton to certain parts of the membrane, such as sites of cell contact that require reinforcement. Defects of adducin have not been identified, although there is evidence that a polymorphism within α-adducin may be associated with some cases of essential hypertension.[525, 526]

Dematin (Protein 4.9)

Human erythrocyte dematin consists of two chains of 48 kDa and 52 kDa, present in a ratio of 3:1 (48 kDa:52 kDa).[527–529] The native protein is a trimer. It binds to F-actin (two sites per molecule) and bundles actin filaments into cables.[529, 530] This action is abolished by protein kinase A phosphorylation[527] but is not affected by protein kinase C. The COOH-terminal half of the 48-kDa subunit is similar to villin,[531] an actin-binding protein that induces growth of microvilli and reorganizes actin filaments in brush borders. In contrast to villin, dematin is widely distributed, which raises the possibility that it may substitute for villin and regulate actin organization, under phosphorylation control, in tissues that lack villin. The 52-kDa subunit differs from the 48-kDa subunit by insertion of a 22-amino acid sequence in the C-terminal domain that resembles a sequence in protein 4.2[530] and contains an ATP-binding site.[496] The

function of this site is unknown. Dematin must also attach to a lipid or integral membrane protein, because it remains associated with the membrane when the other skeletal proteins are extracted; however, this site has not been identified.

Tropomyosin

Erythrocyte tropomyosin is a heterodimer of 27- and 29-kDa subunits that run on SDS gels in the region of band 7.[532] The red cell analogue is similar to other nonmuscle tropomyosins by many criteria, except that it polymerizes poorly.[532, 533] This makes sense in the red cell where the double-helical actin filaments are short (two chains, each containing six to seven monomers). There is one copy of tropomyosin for each six to eight actin monomers, which is just enough to line both grooves of the actin protofilament. The binding of tropomyosin to actin is not affected by spectrin, but spectrin/actin interactions are inhibited by saturating concentrations of tropomyosin.[533] Possible functions of tropomyosin include stabilizing the short erythroid actin filaments and helping determine the sites of spectrin/actin interactions.

Tropomodulin

Tropomodulin is a 41-kDa protein that binds to tropomyosin in a 2:1 molar ratio with a K_d of 5×10^{-7} M.[534, 535] Each protein binds to the NH_2-terminal region of the other.[536, 537] Tropomodulin also binds to actin.[538] It associates with the slowly growing, pointed end of actin filaments, after tropomyosin binds,[539] and blocks growth at that end.[511, 540] This is consistent with the fact that there are 30,000 copies of tropomodulin per red cell, or one per actin protofilament. Capping is enhanced if the grooves of the actin filament are lined with tropomyosin.[541] Tropomodulin remains attached to the membrane when spectrin, actin, and tropomyosin are removed. Its binding site has not yet been identified.

Myosin

Red cells contain a nonmuscle myosin composed of two light chains of 19 and 25 kDa associated with a 200-kDa heavy chain.[542, 543] The protein forms bipolar filaments and has typical ATPase activities. There are about 4300 copies of myosin in adult red cells and 2.5 times as many in neonatal erythrocytes,[544] or about one myosin per 50 to 100 actin monomers. This may explain the greater motility of neonatal reticulocytes.

Caldesmon

Erythrocytes contain caldesmon, a 71-kDa, calmodulin-binding protein that regulates myosin ATPase.[545] The amount of caldesmon corresponds precisely to the amount of tropomyosin (1 caldesmon:1 tropomyosin:seven to nine actin monomers), suggesting that caldesmon may also be part of the junctional complex. Its function in the mature erythrocyte is a mystery.

Membrane Physiology

Studies of the evolution of the red cell suggest that the sequestration of hemoglobin inside a cell membrane was necessary to protect hemoglobin from oxidative threats and to permit its concentrations to rise to levels that would support mammalian metabolism. Metabolism, in turn, places certain constraints on the red cell membrane. In humans, the red cell must be flexible enough to negotiate splenic and capillary channels and still be durable enough to survive the turbulent journey through the circulatory system approximately half a million times during its 120-day life span. In addition, for blood to flow at reasonable rates, the red cell membrane must behave as a fluid in its interactions with other cells and plasma. In this section, some of the characteristics of the red cell membrane that allow the red cell to achieve these goals are described.

Red Cell Deformability

The material properties of the membrane reflect the properties of both the lipid bilayer and the skeleton. During deformation of the red cell membrane, bending is restricted by the incompressibility of the lipid bilayer and is facilitated by rapid translocation of cholesterol from the inner to the outer half of the bilayer.[20] The lipid bilayer cannot expand its surface area more than 3% to 4%. Consequently, when red cells are suspended in hypotonic solutions, such as during osmotic fragility testing, they swell to a spherical shape and then rupture, discharging their hemoglobin into the supernatant.[546]

The membrane skeleton determines both the solid and semisolid properties of the membrane.[145] The solid properties are exemplified by the elastic extension of red cells, which completely restore their normal shape after the applied force has been removed. An example is red cells that have been deformed when passing through fenestrations of the splenic sinus wall. This elastic recovery of the biconcave shape is facilitated by the unique molecular anatomy of the skeletal lattice. In normal red cells, individual spectrin molecules are arranged in a hexagonal array and are folded in a compact configuration. The junctional complexes are close to each other and are linked by shortened spectrin tetramers, thus allowing large unidirectional extensions without disruption of the lattice. The skeletal connections are unperturbed during such deformations. On the other hand, application of large or prolonged forces allows the skeletal elements to reorganize and make new connections. This produces a permanent "plastic" deformation. When the force is excessive, membrane fragmentation ensues. An example is the poikilocytosis produced in microangiopathic blood vessels where red cells may adhere to damaged endothelium and be stretched by the vascular torrent or may be clotheslined by fibrin strands.[547] After release, many of the cells are either permanently deformed or fragmented.

The need to undergo large deformations is best exemplified in the wall of the splenic sinus where red cells have to squeeze through narrow slits between the endothelial cells that line the splenic sinus wall. This "whole cell deformability" is determined by three factors: (1) cell geometry, that is, a large cell surface/volume ratio, which allows cells to undergo large deformations at a constant volume; (2) viscosity of the cell contents, which is principally determined by the properties and the concentration of hemoglobin in the cells; and (3) intrinsic viscoelastic properties of the red cell membrane.[145] Among these factors, the contribution of the surface/volume ratio and the viscosity of the cell contents are the most important, as exemplified by the cellular lesion of hereditary spherocytosis and other red cell disorders, discussed later in this chapter. On the other hand, the intrinsic deformability of the red cell membrane has a relatively small effect on red cell survival. This is best illustrated by the red cell membrane properties of Southeast Asian ovalocytes (SAO), which carry a mutant band 3 protein. Both the intact SAO red cells and their membranes are extremely rigid, yet the SAO red cells have a nearly normal survival *in vivo*.[145, 159]

Structural Integrity of the Membrane

The skeleton is the principal determinant of membrane stability. As noted earlier, it is possible to manipulate the proportion of spectrin dimers and tetramers *in situ* by exposing ghosts to temperatures and salt concentrations that favor or discourage self-association. Ghosts enriched in spectrin dimers are strikingly fragile.[377] Similarly, hereditary elliptocytosis and pyropoikilocytosis are often due to α- or β-spectrin mutations that weaken spectrin self-association (see later). In such cells the hexagonal skeletal lattice is disrupted,[548] usually in association with red cell fragmentation and poikilocytosis.

The fluid lipid bilayer is stabilized both by the underlying membrane skeleton and the transmembrane proteins. *In vitro*, the bilayer can be uncoupled from the skeleton at the tips of spiculated red cells by various treatments.[549] The lipids are released in the form of microvesicles, which contain integral proteins but lack skeletal components.[143] Such loss of membrane material may underlie the surface area deficiency of red cells subjected to prolonged storage[550, 551] or of ATP-depleted red cells.[552] Aggregation of the band 3–containing intramembrane particles in the membrane also destabilizes the lipid bilayer.[553] In ghosts, such aggregation can be induced by treatment with Ca^{2+}, magnesium, polylysine, or basic proteins.[553] The particle-free regions bleb and release lipid microvesicles. As discussed later, all these pathways may contribute to the surface deficiency of hereditary spherocytes.

The role of the membrane skeleton in red cell shape is best illustrated by irreversibly sickled cells or hereditary elliptocytes, in which the abnormal shape is retained in the ghosts and membrane skeletons.[554, 555] This process is probably an example of "plastic deformation," the result of prolonged exposure of red cells to deforming forces, when the proteins of the deformed skeleton undergo active rearrangement that permanently stabilize the cells in the deformed shape.[145] Existing protein/protein contacts disconnect, and new associations form. In hereditary elliptocytosis, shape transformations may be facilitated by the weakened skeletal protein interactions.

In addition, both normal and abnormal red cell shapes can be stabilized by intermolecular cross-linking of membrane proteins, either due to formation of intermolecular disulfide bridges induced by oxidants or by transamidative protein cross-linking catalyzed by a Ca^{2+}-activated cytosolic transglutaminase.[556, 557] These protein modifications are like endogenous fixatives and permanently stabilize cell shape *in vitro*.

The Red Cell Surface

The red cell surface is rich in sialic acid residues, accounting for the negative surface charge. The majority of these residues reside on glycophorin A; the remainder are shared by other glycophorins, the anion exchange protein, and glycolipids.[131, 132, 137, 147] Alterations in surface charge distribution are deleterious. For example, surface charge clustering may contribute to adhesion of sickle red cells to the surface of endothelial cells.[558] Several proteins are removed from the surface of reticulocytes that participate in cell/cell and cell/matrix interactions during erythroid differentiation.[559–561] One example, $\alpha_4\beta_1$ integrin, interacts with VCAM-1, an endothelial cell adhesion molecule, and may contribute to attachment of sickle cells to the endothelium[560] (see Chapter 20).

The structure and the genetic origins of red cell surface antigens, residing either on glycolipids, on externally exposed portions of transmembrane proteins or their carbohydrate side chains, or on the proteins linked by a glycosylphosphatidylinositol anchor, are discussed in Chapter 49. Furthermore, several surface receptors are involved in attachment of malarial parasites to the cells, including glycophorins, band 3 protein, and the Duffy blood group antigen.[155, 562]

Glycosylphosphatidylinositol-Anchored Membrane Proteins

A hydrophobic glycosylphosphatidylinositol (GPI) anchor is embedded in the outer leaflet of the bilayer to connect externally exposed hydrophilic proteins with the hydrophobic lipid bilayer. Among the large number of GPI-linked surface proteins, a group of complement-regulatory proteins are clinically the most important.[162] Defective biosynthesis of the GPI anchor precludes attachment of these proteins to the membrane, causing increased susceptibility to hemolysis by complement, as clinically manifest by paroxysmal nocturnal hemoglobinuria (see Chapter 14). Because this glycolipid anchor is embedded only in the outer leaflet of the bilayer, anchored surface proteins are not restricted by the membrane skeleton, in contrast to most transmembrane proteins, and are much more laterally mobile.[162] This high mobility may be important in recruiting complement regulatory proteins to sites of complement activation. These regulatory proteins are preferentially enriched in the lipid vesicles that are released from abnormal red cells,[562] such as vesicles derived from spicules of deoxygenated sickle cells. Consequently, GPI-linked proteins are diminished in the densest fraction of sickle cells, rendering them more susceptible to complement-mediated injury.[563]

Lateral Mobility of Transmembrane and Surface Proteins

The mobilities of membrane surface molecules influence the interaction of red cells with the outside environment. For example, cell agglutination requires rapid lateral movements of surface antigens. Their immobilization (e.g., by glutaraldehyde) inhibits agglutination.[564] The lateral mobility of proteins that are anchored exclusively in the outer leaflet of the bilayer (e.g., GPI-linked proteins) is very fast. Conversely, transmembrane proteins, such as band 3, are much less mobile. In the case of band 3, this occurs because of specific binding to ankyrin and the skeleton, steric hindrance by spectrin strands, which entangle the internal portions of band 3, self-association of band 3 into tetramers and higher oligomers, and interaction of band 3 with other transmembrane proteins, such as the glycophorins.

Organization of the Membrane Skeleton

Nodes and individual filaments of the membrane skeleton are visible when stretched but not when collapsed. Stretched skeletons reveal complexes of F-actin (the nodes) cross-linked by molecular filaments of spectrin when viewed by high-resolution, negative-stain electron microscopy.[143, 509, 510] Dematin, adducin, and protein 4.1 co-localize with these complexes on immunoelectron microscopy.[143] Most of the complexes are connected by spectrin tetramers (85%) and three-armed hexamers (10%).[510] Ankyrin and band 3–containing globular complexes attach to spectrin near the site of self-association. The average thickness of the skeletal protein layer has been estimated to be 3 to 6 nm from x-ray diffraction data[565] and 7 to 10 nm from electron micrographs.[566] These dimensions suggest the skeleton is only one or two molecules thick on average, which means it must cover 25% to 50% of the inner membrane surface area. This corresponds reasonably to micrographs of unspread skeletons, where the contracted, collapsed spectrin filaments appear to cover much but not all of the inner membrane surface.

A model of the membrane skeleton based on this is shown in Figure 16–3. Spectrin dimers are depicted as twisted, flexible polymers joined head to head to form tetramers and higher-order oligomers. Self-association occurs between the NH_2-terminal end of the spectrin α chain and the COOH-terminal end of the β chain, as described in detail in the earlier section on spectrin. Spectrin molecules are linked into a two-dimensional network by interactions with a complex of actin protofilaments, protein 4.1, dematin, adducin, and tropomyosin.[139] These associations occur at the tail ends of the bifunctional spectrin tetramer. The predicted complexes are morphologically similar to isolated spectrin/actin/protein 4.1 complexes and to structures observed *in situ* in normal ghosts. They serve as branch points in skeletal construction. On average, six spectrin molecules emanate from each complex, although there is some variation. This leads to a hexagonal arrangement of spectrin in spread skeletons. In unperturbed skeletons, most spectrin molecules probably fold up to about one third their length and do not extensively overlap or intertwine.[349]

Individual spectrin tetramers and oligomers are attached to the overlying lipid bilayer through high-affinity interactions with ankyrin and band 3, probably with the assistance of protein 4.2. Current evidence suggests that band 3 is a mixture of dimers and tetramers in the membrane[320] and that the tetramer probably binds only one molecule of ankyrin.[289, 291, 319] If so, about 40% of the band 3 molecules are involved in anchoring the membrane skeleton. Although the spectrin tetramer contains two ankyrin-binding sites, there is only enough ankyrin to fill one, and, on average, only one is filled *in situ*. Interactions between protein 4.1, protein p55, and GPC or between protein 4.1 and band 3 provide secondary sites of attachment.

Modulation of Membrane Skeletal Structure

Red cell membrane proteins are subject to a large number of post-translational modifications or other regulatory effects, including phosphorylation, fatty acid acylation, methylation, glycosylation, deamidation, calpain cleavage, polyphosphoinositide and calmodulin regulation, oxidation, and modification by polyanions.[2, 567]

Phosphorylation

Almost all of the membrane skeletal proteins are phosphorylated by one or more protein kinases. These include casein kinases (spectrin, ankyrin, band 3, protein 4.1, and dematin); protein kinase A (ankyrin, adducin, protein 4.1, and dematin); protein kinase C (adducin, protein 4.1, and dematin); and tyrosine kinases (band 3 and protein 4.1).[567] In all cases studied so far, phosphorylation inhibits membrane protein interactions. Ankyrin phosphorylation (casein kinase) abolishes the preference of ankyrin for spectrin tetramer[410, 434] and decreases binding to band 3.[435] Phosphorylation of protein 4.1 (several kinases) diminishes its binding to spectrin and its ability to promote spectrin/actin binding[461, 462, 568] and decreases its attachment to the membrane.[569] Phosphorylation by protein kinase C also inhibits binding of protein 4.1 to band 3.[469] Phosphorylation of protein 4.9 by protein kinase A prevents actin bundling.[527] Phosphorylation of Tyr[8] at the NH_2-terminus of band 3 blocks the binding of glycolytic enzymes,[277] and presumably hemoglobin, and results in increased glycolysis.[570] Many studies[374, 375, 434, 571, 572] failed to identify a functional effect of spectrin phosphorylation; however, evidence shows that membrane mechanical stability is very sensitive to the state of phosphorylation.[367] Increased phosphorylation decreases and decreased phosphorylation increases membrane stability.

Polyanions

Physiologic concentrations of organic polyanions such as 2,3-DPG and ATP weaken and dissociate the membrane skeleton[573] and increase the lateral mobility of band 3 in ghosts.[574] *In vitro* these compounds dramatically inhibit spectrin/actin interactions, even in the presence of protein 4.1.[575] However, it is still not clear whether these or other polyanions (e.g., polyphosphorylated phosphoinositides) are "physiologic" mediators *in vivo*. Some studies suggest that even supraphysiologic concentrations of 2,3-DPG have little or no effect on intact erythrocytes.[576, 577]

Calcium and Calmodulin

There is good evidence that calmodulin modifies the membrane properties of the red cell.[464] Physiologic concentrations of calmodulin, sealed in red cell ghosts, destabilize membranes in the presence of micromolar concentrations of Ca^{2+}. Studies suggest the effect may result from interactions of calmodulin with protein 4.1.[465] Submicromolar concentrations of calmodulin, even lower than those that exist in the red cell (approximately 3 to 6 μM), block protein 4.1–induced gelation of actin in the presence of spectrin.[465] The effect is Ca^{2+} dependent. It begins at a Ca^{2+} concentration of 10^{-6} to 10^{-7} M, which is relatively low but still higher than the free Ca^{2+} concentration in the erythrocyte (20 to 40 nM). Surprisingly, Ca^{2+}-calmodulin does not block spectrin/actin/protein 4.1 complex formation under these conditions,[465] only the extensive cross-linking needed to cause gelation. Calmodulin also binds to the spectrin β chain in a Ca^{2+}-dependent manner[463]; however, the affinity of spectrin for calmodulin is not great and it is unclear whether this effect occurs at the concentrations of calmodulin that exist in erythrocytes. Beta-adducin also binds calmodulin ($K_d = 2.3 \times 10^{-7}$ M).[578] Adducin that is bound to spectrin and actin fosters the attachment of a second, neighboring spectrin. This reaction is blocked by calmodulin in the presence of Ca^{2+} ($>10^{-7}$ M).[514, 579] The physiologic consequences of this effect are unclear.

Several other Ca^{2+}-dependent events do not require the presence of calmodulin. One of them is membrane protein cross-linking, catalyzed by Ca^{2+}-dependent transglutaminase.[556] This cross-linking acts as an endogenous fixative, stabilizing red cell shape.[579] However, the Ca^{2+} concentration required by this reaction is more than 100-fold greater than the normal red cell Ca^{2+} concentration, making it unlikely that transglutaminase permanently stabilizes red cell shape *in vivo*.[579] A second calmodulin-independent effect of Ca^{2+} is the so-called Gárdos phenomenon,[580] a unidirectional K^+ and water loss, producing cellular dehydration. In contrast to transamidative cross-linking, the Ca^{2+} concentration required to trigger the Gárdos channel is low (in the micromolar range) and thus physiologically significant. This pathway contributes to

Table 16–4. PROPERTIES AND CAPACITIES OF MAJOR CATION TRANSPORTERS IDENTIFIED IN THE NORMAL HUMAN RED CELL MEMBRANE

System	Inhibitor	Capacity (mmol/L cells per h)	Potential Maximum Capacity (mmol/Liter cells per h)	Activator*	Role
$Na^+ K^+$ pump	Oubain	1–2	No further activation possible		Long-term volume regulation, with passive leak
Passive leak	No specific	1–2	Unknown	Various	
$Na^+ K^+ 2Cl^-$ cotransport	Loop diuretics Cl^- dependent‡	0.1–1.2†	No further activation possible	Cyclic AMP, cell shrinkage in other cell types	Volume-regulatory increase in other cell types
$K^+ Cl^-$ cotransport	DHIOA, others Cl^- dependent	0–0.2†§	0.5 10	Cell swelling N-Ethyl-malemide	Small role in short-term volume regulation
$Na^+ Na^+$ exchange		~0.5†	No further activation possible		
Ca^{2+}-activated K^+ channel	Charybdotoxin quinidine	0	50	Internal Ca^{2+}	Role in human RBC unknown; related to Ca^{2+}-activated channel in nerve
Band 3 (anion exchanger-1)	SITS, DIDS	Cations: zero, in HCO_3^- free media Anions: >1000	No further activation possible		Anion exchange services carbonic anhydrase
Na^+-linked amino acid transporters		Zero in the absence of amino acids	No further activation possible		Amino acid supply to (e.g., glutathione synthesis)

DHIOA = (dihydroinenyloxy) alkanoic acid; DIDS = 4,4'-diisothiocyanostilbene-2,2-disulfonic acid; SITS = 4-acetamido-4'-isothiocyanostilbene-2,2'-disulfonic acid.
Activator implies physical or pharmacologic maneuver aside from manipulation of substrate concentration.
†Shows major interindividual variation within normal population.
‡*Cl⁻ dependent* implies that the cation flux is inhibited by the replacement of Cl⁻ by an "inert" cation such as nitrate.
§Enhanced in capacity in reticulocytes.
From Stewart GW, Argent AC, Dash BCJ: Stomatin: A putative cation transport regulator in the red cell membrane. Biochim Biophys Acta 1993; 1225:15–25. Copyright 1993 with permission of Elsevier Science, NL, Amsterdam, The Netherlands.

cellular dehydration of sickle red cells. A third calmodulin-independent Ca^{2+} effect involves calpain, one of a family of Ca^{2+}-stimulated neutral proteases, which are present in a variety of tissues, including red cells.[567] Susceptible membrane substrates include band 3, ankyrin, protein 4.1, and, to a lesser extent, spectrin. Finally, Ca^{2+} also induces phospholipid scrambling, as discussed earlier in the chapter.

Thus, increases in intracellular Ca^{2+} produce a wide range of deleterious effects. Although these phenomena are well studied *in vitro,* their role in erythrocyte pathology, particularly in acquired disorders associated with abnormal red cell shape, is not well understood.

Membrane Permeability

Normally the red cell membrane is nearly impermeable to monovalent and divalent cations, thereby maintaining a high K^+, low Na^+, and very low Ca^{2+} content. In contrast, the red cell is highly permeable to water and anions, which are readily exchanged by the water channel and the anion transport protein, respectively. Glucose is taken up by the glucose transporter,[581, 582] whereas larger charged molecules, such as ATP and related compounds, do not cross the normal red cell membrane.

The transport pathways for cations and anions in the human red cell membrane (Table 16–4) can be divided into five categories: (1) exchangers, such as the Na^+/H^+ exchanger and anion exchanger discussed earlier; (2) cotransporters, in which the transmembrane movements of more than one solute are coupled in the same direction (e.g., the K^+/Cl^- cotransporter and the $Na^+/K^+/Cl^-$ cotransporter); (3) the Ca^{2+}-activated K^+ channel (Gárdos channel), discussed later; (4) the cation "leak" pathways, which allow Na^+ and K^+ to move in the direction of their concentration gradients; and (5) membrane pumps, such as the ouabain-inhibitable Na^+/K^+ pump and the Ca^{2+} pump, respectively. Detailed reviews of these pathways are available.[583–587]

An important feature of the normal red cell is its ability to maintain a constant volume. One of the very intriguing, yet unanswered, questions is how cells "sense" changes in cell volume and activate appropriate volume regulatory pathways. One possibility is that they sense mechanical events, such as membrane stretching.[588] Such a mechanism is unlikely to operate in red cells that, by virtue of their large surface area, can undergo a substantial volume increase without stretching. Another possibility is that cell volume is controlled by the crowding of cytoplasmic macromolecules.[588] According to this theory, cell shrinkage stimulates and swelling inhibits a putative protein kinase, which, in turn, changes the activity of a volume regulatory cation transporter, such as the K^+/Cl^- cotransporter.

Water Permeability

Water permeability in most cells is similar to the permeability of pure lipid bilayer membranes, in which water is postulated to enter through small holes in the bilayer.[589] When phospholipids are in the liquid crystalline state, these cavities are thought to be caused by a noncooperative rotation and kinking around the C—C bonds. In addition, water permeability may be facilitated by lipids with large polar head groups, such as gangliosides and lysophospholipids, which, when dispersed in water, prefer a micellar rather than bilayer configuration. Additionally, integral proteins are likely to enhance water diffusion by producing localized discontinuities in the lipid bilayer.[589] Membranes of red cells and some kidney tubules differ from membranes of most other cells in that they have a high water permeability, being endowed by a molecular water channel protein.[590, 591] This protein, designated "CHIP 28" (channel-like integral protein of 28 kDa) or "aquaporin," has been cloned.[592] The hydropathy analysis indicates six highly hydrophobic membrane segments. Both the NH_2-terminus and COOH-terminus are exposed in the cytoplasm, and there are two external potential glycosylation sites. There are about 200,000 copies of the channel per cell. The suggested function of CHIP 28 is to facilitate rehydration of red cells after their shrinkage in the hypertonic environment of the renal medulla.[593]

Transport Pathways

Two pathways exert a critical volume regulatory effect (Fig. 16–14). One is the K^+/Cl^- cotransporter, a typical carrier-mediated cotransport pathway, which is particularly active in reticulocytes. It is activated by cell swelling, acidification, depletion of intracellular magnesium, and thiol oxidation. It is increased in sickle red cells and hemoglobin C erythrocytes, accounting, in part, for cellular dehydration of these cells.[584–586]

The second transporter is the Gárdos channel, which causes selective loss of K^+ in response to an increase in intracellular ionized Ca^{2+}. This channel appears to be regulated by a cytoplasmic protein called calpromotin and by cyclic adenosine monophosphate (AMP). The channel is inhibited by insect toxins, such as charybdotoxin, and by the calcium channel blockers nitrendipine and nifedipine.[584, 585] In sickle cells, the combination of the Gárdos pathway and the K^+/Cl^- cotransporter account for the net loss of K^+ and water, leading to cellular dehydration.

Disruption of the Permeability Barrier in Abnormal Erythrocytes. The effects of breaching the red cell permeability barrier are well illustrated by complement hemolysis. Complement activation on the red cell surface leads to formation of the membrane attack complex, composed of the terminal complement components embedded in the lipid bilayer. This multimolecular complex acts as a cation channel, allowing passive movements of Na^+, K^+, and Ca^{2+} across the membrane according to their concentration gradients. Attracted by fixed anions, such as hemoglobin, ATP, and 2,3-DPG, Na^+ accumulates in the cells in excess of K^+ loss and in excess of the compensatory efforts of the Na^+/K^+ pump. The resulting increase in intracellular monovalent cations and water is followed by cell swelling and, ultimately, colloid osmotic hemolysis.

An alternate leak pathway in sickle cells involves an influx of Na^+ and Ca^{2+} and an efflux of K^+ during deoxygenation and sickling.[584, 585] Although the molecular basis of this diffusional pathway is unknown, the magnitude of the Na^+ and K^+ leaks correlates with the degree of morphologic sickling and with lipid bilayer/skeleton uncoupling, suggesting it is caused by mechanical events.[585–597] This conclusion is further supported by the observation that Ca^{2+} permeability is increased by mechanical stress.[594] Such permeability pathways may be related to stretch-activated channels, described in various tissues, including endothelial, epithelial, and muscle cells.[595] The mechanism of activation of these channels is unknown, but one of the possibilities involves deformation of the submembrane skeleton.[596, 597]

Membrane Pumps

To maintain low intracellular concentrations of Na^+ and Ca^{2+} and a high K^+ concentration, the membrane is endowed with two cation pumps, both utilizing intracellular ATP as an energy source. The ouabain-inhibitable Na^+/K^+ pump, extrudes Na^+ and takes up K^+, with a stoichiometry of three Na^+ ions pumped outward for two K^+ ions pumped inward. This exactly balances the normal passive leaks (Na^+ = 1.0–2.0 mEq/LRBC per hour; K^+ efflux = 0.8–1.5 mEq/LRBC per hour). The enzyme is activated by intracellular Na^+ (K_M = 25 mM) and extracellular K^+ (K_M = 2.5 mM).[598] Because plasma K^+ is high enough to saturate the extracellular K^+ site, Na^+ and K^+ transport is primarily regulated by increases in red cell Na^+ concentration, and cell K^+ losses are rectified only if there is a concomitant Na^+ gain to stimulate active transport. Even then the ratio between the inward Na^+ leak and outward K^+ leak must not be less than the physiologic ratio of 3:2. At lower ratios, the Na^+/K^+ pump, driven by the Na^+ leak and internal Na^+ concentration will not balance the leaks and will actually exacerbate K^+ loss.[599, 600] Consequently, conditions in which K^+ loss approaches or exceeds Na^+ gain lead to irreversible K^+ depletion and cell dehydration such as hereditary spherocytosis and sickle cell anemia.

The calmodulin-activated, Mg^{2+}-dependent Ca^{2+} pump extrudes Ca^{2+} and maintains a very low intracellular free Ca^{2+} concentration ($\sim$20–40 nM). It protects red cells from the multiple deleterious effects of Ca^{2+} (echinocytosis, membrane vesiculation, calpain activation, membrane proteolysis, and cell dehydration) described earlier in the chapter. The structure and function of the Na^+/K^+ and Ca^{2+} pumps has been reviewed.[587]

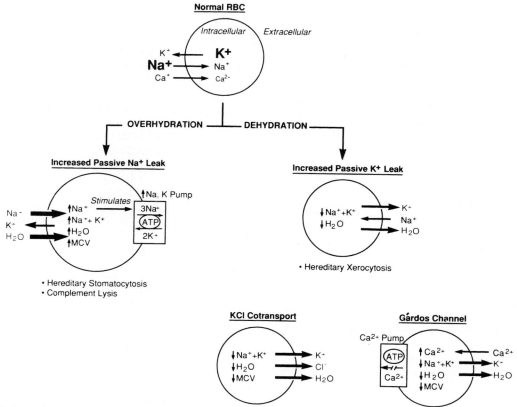

Figure 16–14. Cation changes leading to dehydration or overhydration of red cells. *Left,* Overhydration is caused by a massive unbalanced influx of Na+, which overwhelms the Na+/K+ pump and leads to an increase in total monovalent cations (Na+ + K+) and cell water. *Right,* Dehydration is caused by excess, unbalanced K+ leakage, or activation of K+-losing channels such as the K+/Cl- cotransport channel or the Ca2+-activated Gárdos pathway. Dehydration is associated with a decline in total monovalent cations (Na+ + K+) and cell water. (From Lux SE, Palek J: Disorders of the red cell membrane. In Handin RJ, Lux SE, Stossel TP (eds): Blood: Principles and Practice of Hematology. Philadelphia, Lippincott-Raven, 1995, pp 1701–1818.)

Membrane Development and Aging

Assembly of a Stable Membrane Skeleton

Spectrin and ankyrin synthesis is detectable at very early stages of erythroid development in avian and mammalian erythroid cells.[141, 601, 602] However, these proteins turn over rapidly and do not assemble into a permanent network. Synthesis of band 3 and protein 4.1 begins at the proerythroblast stage and increases throughout terminal erythroid maturation, up to the late erythroblast stage. During the same time, the mRNA levels and synthesis of spectrin and ankyrin decline. Even so, the proportion of newly assembled spectrin and ankyrin on the membrane progressively increase, and these proteins become more stable, as indicated by their slower turnover. This increased recruitment and stabilization of spectrin and ankyrin, in spite of declining synthesis, is thought to be related to the progressive increase in the synthesis of band 3 and protein 4.1, because these proteins are the principal sites for attachment of the skeleton to the membrane.[141] However, mice that lack band 3, owing to a targeted gene disruption, have a normal or near-normal membrane skeleton,[603] indicating that band 3 is not required or can be adequately compensated.

Skeletal Proteins Synthesized in Excess. The synthesis of membrane skeletal proteins is wasteful. Only fractions of newly synthesized spectrin, ankyrin, band 3, and protein 4.1 are assembled into the permanent skeletal network. The excess proteins are rapidly catabolized.[601, 604, 605] Furthermore, skeletal protein synthesis is highly asymmetric. This is most striking in the case of spectrin, where twofold to threefold more α-spectrin is produced than β-spectrin. Yet, the two chains are assembled into the membrane skeleton in equimolar amounts as mixed heterodimers. Because of this high α-spectrin to β-spectrin synthetic ratio, heterozygotes for a deleted or synthetically inactive α-spectrin allele should be asymptomatic, because sufficient α-spectrin should still be made to pair with all the β-spectrin.

Rate-Limiting Steps of Membrane Skeletal Assembly. The principal rate-limiting step in membrane skeletal assembly is the synthesis of band 3, which contains a high-affinity ankyrin-binding site that recruits and stabilizes spectrin and ankyrin on the membrane.[606, 607] This view, however, has to be reconciled with recent observations that some patients with dominantly inherited hereditary spherocytosis and partial band 3 deficiency,[409, 608] and in mice lacking band 3,[603] do not have a proportional decrease in the amounts of spectrin and ankyrin in their membranes.

The second rate-limiting step is the availability of ankyrin, which provides the high-affinity binding sites for β-spectrin. This is best illustrated by studies of membrane skeletal synthesis in *nb/nb* spherocytic mice[380] and in a severe form of human hereditary spherocytosis associated with combined deficiency of spectrin and ankyrin.[381] In both disorders, ankyrin synthesis is markedly reduced, which leads to decreased assembly of spectrin and ankyrin on the membrane, in spite of normal spectrin synthesis.[381]

The third rate-limiting step involves synthesis of β-spectrin. Because α- and β-spectrin polypeptides are assembled on the membrane in equimolar amounts, and because β-spectrin binds to ankyrin with high affinity, the availability of β-spectrin seems to regulate the amounts of membrane-assembled αβ-spectrin heterodimers. This regulatory role of β-spectrin is illustrated by the effects of erythropoietin on membrane protein assembly. Erythropoietin stimulates the synthesis of β-spectrin and increases assembly of αβ-spectrin heterodimers on the membrane.[609] In contrast, α-spectrin, which is made in excess, does not seem to have a limiting role in the skeletal assembly. Alpha-spectrin becomes rate limiting only when its synthesis is markedly reduced, as it is in some patients with nondominant hereditary spherocytosis or hereditary pyropoikilocytosis.

Membrane Remodeling During Enucleation and Reticulocyte Maturation

At the orthochromic erythroblast stage, when membrane biogenesis is nearly complete, the cell membrane undergoes a series of critical remodeling steps. The cell nucleus is surrounded by an actin ring, which likely participates in the expulsion of the nucleus from the erythroblast. At the same time, the spectrin skeleton segregates into the incipient reticulocyte, whereas some surface receptors cluster in the membrane surrounding the soon to be extruded nucleus.[377] Further membrane remodeling takes place as the young multilobular reticulocyte attains the biconcave shape.[561, 610, 611] This involves a loss of lipids and certain surface proteins, including receptors for transferrin and fibronectin.

Fetal Red Cells

Fetal erythrocytes possess a myriad of differences from adult erythrocytes. There are differences in carbohydrate metabolism, activity of both glycolytic and nonglycolytic enzymes, altered ATP and phosphate metabolism, differences in methemoglobin content and oxygen affinity, and altered storage characteristics.[612–617] There are also differences in the membranes of fetal and adult erythrocytes. ABO and I antigens and the receptors for the adsorbed serum antigens of the Lewis system are incompletely expressed.[618]

Band 3 and the Ii Blood Group. A single *N*-glycan chain is attached at Asn in the COOH-terminal membrane domain of band 3.[619] This chain is composed of a number of *N*-acetyllactosamine units of variable length arranged in an unbranched, linear fashion (i antigen) in fetal erythrocytes and has i reactivity.[620–622] In adult erythrocytes, it exists in a branched fashion (I antigen) and has I reactivity.[621, 622] Removal of the carbohydrate does not affect anion exchange. The rare absence of the I antigen in adult cells apparently results from the lack of the branching enzyme.[622]

Fetal membranes are more permeable to monovalent cations[623] and contain less of the Na$^+$,K$^+$-ATPase activity required for monovalent cation removal.[624] They contain more phospholipid and cholesterol per cell[625] and, as a consequence, have a larger surface/volume ratio and are slightly more osmotically resistant than adult cells.[626] The ratio of sphingomyelin to phosphatidylcholine is increased in fetal membranes and differences in fatty acid composition exist, but these changes evidently tend to balance each other, because membrane fluidity is normal.[625, 627] The protein composition of fetal red cell membrane is quantitatively normal[628]; however, most of the major membrane proteins of fetal cells have not been purified and characterized, so it is uncertain whether they are all genetically and functionally identical to their counterparts in adult red cells. The fact that hereditary spherocytosis and elliptocytosis are expressed in the neonatal period indicates that the fetal and adult forms of the involved proteins—spectrin, ankyrin, band 3, protein 4.1, and protein 4.2—probably arise from the same gene. There is some evidence that band 3 may be functionally different from its adult counterpart[629] and that fetal red cells may contain more myosin[630]; however neither of these differences is well proved.

Nothing is known about the arrangement of membrane proteins in fetal red cells, as compared with adult red cells, but there are indications that subtle differences may exist. For example, clustering and endocytosis of con-A receptors can be induced in fetal but not adult human erythrocytes.[631] This endocytosis occurs through spectrin-free regions of fetal membranes.[632] Similar regions exist on adult rabbit reticulocytes, and probably on adult human reticulocytes, but are eliminated on maturation of these cells.[632, 633] This suggests that fetal and adult membrane skeletons differ in organization, at least in certain membrane domains. If so, this might help to explain the increased rigidity,[634] increased mechanical fragility,[626] and decreased life span (average 45 to 70 days)[635] of fetal red cells. It also offers a potential explanation for the observation that fetal red cells contain numerous surface pits and vacuoles not found in adult cells[636, 637]—a fact that has generally been used as evidence for immaturity of the fetal and neonatal spleen. It is possible, however, that apparent cause and effect are reversed and that splenic immaturity is responsible for persistence of the spectrin-free domains, particularly because adult red cells of splenectomized persons are excessively vacuolated[636] and because it is known that the spleen normally pares lipids and some proteins from reticulocytes.[638–640]

Membrane Alterations in Senescent Red Cells

The removal of senescent red cells from the circulation is a subject of long-standing interest. The concept of red cell senescence is based on results of radioactive labeling of a cohort of reticulocytes and bone marrow erythroblasts.[641] In many species, including humans, the fraction of labeled cells remains constant for a defined time period, followed by a rapid decline of radioactivity, suggesting that the red cells are removed from the circulation in an age-dependent manner. Many techniques have been employed to isolate senescent red cells, including methods based on differences in cell density, osmotic fragility, and cell size.[641, 642] Density separation is most widely used, but the results obtained by this technique must be interpreted with caution. Although red cells exhibit a progressive increase in density as they age *in vivo*, not all dense red cells are senescent.[641, 643, 644]

In addition to *in vitro* separation techniques, various *in vivo* animal models have been employed to study red cell aging.[641] Red cells can be labeled with biotin and then removed at defined times with avidin, which complexes tightly to biotin.[645] The senescent cells defined by these techniques exhibit numerous membrane abnormalities.[641, 643, 646, 647] Of particular note is the loss of K^+ and water, leading to cell dehydration and increased cell density, and the loss of surface area, presumably due to gradual release of membrane microvesicles.[641, 642, 647, 648] The latter phenomenon is probably caused by constant exposure of red cells to the shearing forces of the microcirculation. In addition, red cell membrane proteins and lipids experience oxidative damage, as evidenced by high-molecular-weight aggregates containing hemoglobin, spectrin, and band 3,[649, 650] and by adducts of proteins and malonylaldehyde, a product of lipid peroxidation.[651]

Early results suggested that loss of red cell surface charge,[652] due to *in vivo* loss of sialic acid residues, and exposure of the penultimate β-galactose residues[653] of the carbohydrate side chains were important factors in the recognition and removal of aged erythrocytes. More recent studies reveal that the mild surface charge loss can be entirely explained by the loss of cell surface area[654] and that the surface charge density and the number of sialic acid residues per sialoglycoprotein in senescent red cells is normal.[655, 656]

In addition to red cell membrane abnormalities, red cell aging is associated with a decline of many red cell enzyme activities.[657] However, red cell ATP concentration is normal.[641] Likewise no major abnormalities have been detected in Ca^{2+} transport and there is no compelling evidence that Ca^{2+} accumulates in senescent cells.[641]

Targeting Senescent Red Cells for Destruction. Although some of the above alterations may compromise red cell microcirculatory flow, none is likely to destroy old cells. In a series of studies, senescent red cells were shown to have small amounts (a few hundred molecules per cell) of autologous IgG on their surface that target the cells for destruction by macrophages.[658] The nature of the "senescent antigen" has been a source of some dispute. Possibilities include band 3 molecules[659-661] and exposed α-galactosyl residues on membrane glycoproteins.[662, 663] The contribution of the latter modification is probably minimal, because the removal

of α-galactosyl residues by extensive washing does not affect phagocytosis of senescent erythrocytes.[664] On the other hand, there is considerable evidence that antibodies are bound to band 3 in aged and pathologic red cells.[285, 327, 328, 659-661, 665-668] One explanation for this phenomenon is that antibodies to senescent antigen bind to aggregated or oligomerized band 3.[649, 660, 666] Band 3 clusters have been visualized by immunofluorescence microscopy and detected by biochemical methods in aged red cells. Aggregation probably results from cumulative oxidative damage because similar damage, including the binding of autologous IgG, takes place on oxidized red cells or red cells containing Heinz bodies, a product of oxidative denaturation of hemoglobin.[285, 665, 667-669] The senescent antigen is also exposed on red cells infected with the knobby variant of *P. falciparum*.[670]

In addition to targeting senescent red cells for macrophage destruction, band 3 antibodies also trigger complement deposition on senescent cells.[668] As noted earlier, this process may be facilitated by loss of GPI-linked complement regulatory proteins from old cells through microvesiculation. Although the role of autologous IgG in the destruction of senescent erythrocytes is widely accepted, two observations suggest that other mechanisms must be considered. First, blockade of the Fc portion of autologous "senescent" IgG with protein G fails to inhibit red cell phagocytosis.[646] Second, red cell survival is the same in agammaglobulinemic mice as in controls.[646] However, this may not be applicable to humans, because the removal of mouse red cells from the circulation is random.[641]

Altered phospholipid asymmetry might also contribute to removal of senescent erythrocytes. This could occur from damage to the aminophospholipid translocase by products of lipid peroxidation.[671] Disordered phospholipid asymmetry reportedly activates the alternate complement pathway[672] and targets red cells for destruction by macrophages.[673]

Other alterations of possible pathologic significance include postsynthetic modification of red cell proteins by nonenzymatic glycosylation[674] or carboxymethylation.[675, 676] Glycosylation of proteins, like hemoglobin (to form hemoglobin A_{1c}), occurs gradually over the life of the cell and is proportional to the glucose concentration. Methylation of membrane proteins occurs primarily in older red cells. Ankyrin and protein 4.1 are the principal substrates.

Surface/Volume Ratio

From both a diagnostic and pathophysiologic point of view, it is useful to consider red cell morphology and membrane disorders in terms of changes in membrane surface area or cell volume. These parameters reflect two of the membrane's major functions discussed earlier: maintenance of structural integrity and control of cation permeability. Surface loss occurs by membrane fragmentation due either to inherent skeletal weakness or to acquired membrane damage and leads eventually to microspherocytosis. Some microspherocytes are usually present in patients with "surface loss disorders"

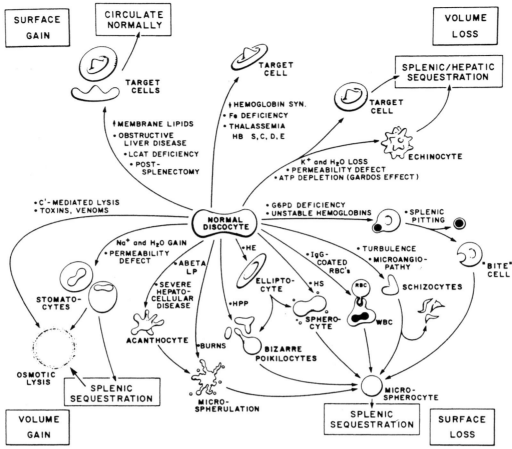

Figure 16–15. Summary of the major abnormalities of red cell shape and major red cell membrane disorders in relation to their effects on red cell surface area and volume. (Adapted from Lux SE, Glader BE: Hemolytic anemias III. Membrane and metabolic disorders. In Beck WS (ed): Hematology. Cambridge, MA, MIT Press, 1977, pp 269–298.)

who are hemolyzing; often, however, other morphologic forms predominate (e.g., bizarre poikilocytes, spiculated red cells, "bite cells," or elliptocytes), which may be viewed as intermediates in the surface loss pathway. Volume gain occurs because of changes in membrane permeability that permit cations and water to accumulate and lead to the formation of stomatocytes. Surface gain is caused by the accretion of membrane lipid; volume loss results from failure of hemoglobin synthesis or from the loss of cations and water. Both result in the formation of target cells.

These processes are all related by the surface/volume ratio. This ratio is indirectly measured by the unincubated osmotic fragility test, which assesses the ability of red cells to swell in increasingly hypotonic salt solutions. Cells with a decreased surface/volume ratio (spherocytes, stomatocytes) can tolerate less swelling than normal cells before they burst and are termed *osmotically fragile*. Target cells, with their increased surface/volume ratio, are relatively osmotically resistant.

In general, a decrease in surface/volume ratio is deleterious to the red cell, because the cell's ability to negotiate the narrow passageways separating the splenic cords and sinuses is seriously compromised as its surface/volume ratio approaches the limiting spherical form. In contrast, an increase in surface/volume ratio is usually innocuous, except in those cells that lose cations and water and become dehydrated. A summary of the major abnormalities of red cell surface area, volume, and shape is presented diagrammatically in Figure 16–15. This diagram attempts to correlate pathophysiologic processes with morphologic characteristics. Some of these processes are due to alterations in membrane structure and are discussed in the remainder of this chapter. Others are discussed more fully in other chapters in this text.

INHERITED ABNORMALITIES OF THE ERYTHROCYTE MEMBRANE

Hereditary Spherocytosis

Hereditary spherocytosis (HS) (Table 16–5) is a common, inherited hemolytic anemia in which defects of spectrin or proteins that participate in the attachment of spectrin to the membrane, ankyrin, protein 4.2, or band 3, lead to spheroidal, osmotically fragile cells that are selectively trapped in the spleen, resulting in a shortened red cell life span.

Table 16-5. CLASSIFICATION OF RED CELL HEMOLYTIC DISORDERS BY PREDOMINANT MORPHOLOGY*

Spherocytes

Hereditary spherocytosis
ABO incompatibility in neonates
Immunohemolytic anemias with IgG- or C3-coated red cells†
Acute oxidant injury (hexose monophosphate shunt defects during hemolytic crisis, oxidant drugs, and chemicals)
Hemolytic transfusion reactions†
Clostridial sepsis
Severe burns, other red cell thermal injuries
Spider, bee, and snake venoms
Severe hypophosphatemia
Hypersplenism‡

Bizarre Poikilocytes

Red cell fragmentation syndromes (microangiopathic and macroangiopathic hemolytic anemias)
Acute oxidant injury‡
Hereditary elliptocytosis in neonates
Hereditary pyropoikilocytosis
Homozygous hereditary elliptocytosis

Elliptocytes

Hereditary elliptocytosis
Thalassemias
(Other hypochromic-microcytic anemias)
(Megaloblastic anemias)

Stomatocytes

Hereditary stomatocytosis
Rh$_{null}$ or Rh$_{mod}$ blood group
Cryohydrocytosis
Adenosine deaminase hyperactivity with low red cell ATP‡
(Liver diseases, especially acute alcoholism)
(Mediterranean stomatocytosis)
(Duchenne muscular dystrophy)‡
(Marathon runners)‡
(Various medications)

Irreversibly Sickled Cells

Sickle cell anemia
Symptomatic sickle syndromes

Intraerythrocytic Parasites

Malaria
Bartonellosis
Babesiosis

Prominent Basophilic Stippling

Thalassemias
Unstable hemoglobinopathies
Lead poisoning‡
Pyridine-5′-nucleotidase deficiency

Spiculated or Crenated Red Cells

Acute hepatic necrosis (spur cell anemia)
Uremia
Red cell fragmentation syndromes‡
Infantile pyknocytosis
Embden-Meyerhof pathway defects‡
Vitamin E deficiency‡
Abetalipoproteinemia
Heat stroke‡
McLeod blood group
(Postsplenectomy)
(Transiently after massive transfusion of stored blood)
(Anorexia nervosa)‡
(Decompression from hyperbaric exposure)‡
(Woronet's trait)

Target Cells

Hemoglobins S, C, D, and E
Hereditary xerocytosis
Thalassemias
(Lecithin:cholesterol acyltransferase deficiency)
(Other hypochromic-microcytic anemias)
(Obstructive liver disease)
(Postsplenectomy)

Nonspecific or Normal Morphology

Embden-Meyerhof pathway defects‡
Hexose monophosphate shunt defects‡
Adenosine deaminase hyperactivity with low red cell ATP‡
Unstable hemoglobinopathies‡
Paroxysmal nocturnal hemoglobinuria
Dyserythropoietic anemias‡
Copper toxicity (Wilson's disease)
Cation permeability defects‡
Erythropoietic porphyria
Vitamin E deficiency
Hemolysis with infections†
Hemolysis with infections
Rh hemolytic disease in neonates†
Paroxysmal cold hemoglobinuria†
Cold hemagglutinin disease†
Hypersplenism
Immunohemolytic anemia†‡

*Nonhemolytic disorders of similar morphology are enclosed in parentheses for reference.
†Usually associated with positive Coombs' test.
‡Disease or condition sometimes associated with this morphology.

History

Hereditary spherocytosis was first recognized more than 100 years ago by two Belgian physicians, Vanlair and Masius, who gave a remarkably thorough account of the disease.[677] They described a woman who suffered from anemia, jaundice, splenomegaly, and recurrent abdominal pain. The authors noted that most of the woman's red cells were spherical and hypothesized that a combination of splenic enlargement and liver atrophy led to their rapid destruction and their patient's anemia. They also noted that the patient's sister had suffered from an identical illness and that her mother was also subject to jaundice. In the 1890s, the British physicians Wilson and Stanley recognized the hereditary nature of the disease and were the first to recognize the characteristic pathology of the spleen engorged with red cells.[678, 679] However, a report by Minkowski in 1900, in the German literature, received wide attention,[680] and many additional papers soon appeared, including Chauffard's classic description of osmotic fragility[681] and reticulocytosis[682] as hallmarks of the disease. The use of splenectomy was advocated and its success led to rapid acceptance of the procedure. The first successful splenectomy for HS was unintentionally performed by Wells in England 20 years before,[683] 3 years before Wilson's description of HS. While operating on a jaundiced woman for a supposed uterine fibroid, he encountered and removed an enormous spleen. The patient recovered and her jaundice disappeared. The events were reconstructed 40 years later by Dawson,[683] who found the abnormal erythrocyte osmotic fragility during an examination of the woman and her son. Thus, the major clinical features of HS were defined by the 1920s, although nothing was known about the pathophysiology of the disease. Readers interested in more details about these and other aspects of the history of HS should consult the chapters by Dacie, Crosby, and Wintrobe in *Blood, Pure and Eloquent*.[684]

Prevalence and Genetics

Hereditary spherocytosis occurs in all racial and ethnic groups. It is particularly common in Northern European peoples, where it affects about 1 person in 5000.[685] In fact, this is probably an underestimate of the prevalence. Surveys of red cell osmotic fragility, using sensitive assays, suggest that very mild forms of the disease may be four or five times as common.[686, 687] There are no good estimates of the prevalence in other populations, but clinical experience suggests it is less common in African-Americans and Southeast Asians.

The disorder exhibits both dominant and recessive phenotypes. About 75% of families have the autosomal dominant disease.[685, 688, 689] No definite homozygotes for typical dominant HS have ever been identified, which suggests that homozygosity may be incompatible with life. A report of near-lethal HS (severe intrauterine hydrops fetalis, marked spherocytosis, and extreme spectrin deficiency) in a family where one parent has moderate dominant HS and the other has clinically silent disease, with only a slightly abnormal osmotic fragility test, supports this supposition.[690] The single exception may be a Portuguese family where both parents have very mild HS and the affected children have moderately severe hemolysis and anemia (Hb: 7 to 8 g/dL; reticulocytes: 7% to 20%).[691] Two other reports of less severe "homozygous" HS have appeared, but in neither case was homozygosity proved.[692, 693]

In 20% to 25% of HS cases both parents are clinically normal but have subtle laboratory abnormalities that suggest a carrier state.[688, 694] These patients probably have an autosomal recessive form of the disease, although it is not always possible to exclude dominant HS with reduced penetrance or dominant HS due to a new mutation. However, for simplicity the term *recessive HS* is used to identify patients who do not have typical dominant HS. By definition, patients whose parents are completely normal (5% to 10%) are considered to have new mutations. This may occur more commonly than is recognized.[688]

Etiology

The primary molecular defects in HS reside in membrane skeletal proteins, particularly the proteins whose vertical interactions connect the membrane skeleton to the lipid bilayer: spectrin, ankyrin, protein 4.2, and band 3 (Tables 16–6 and 16–7). Red cells from the majority of European and American HS patients are spectrin and ankyrin deficient, including both the dominant and recessive forms.[608, 694, 713, 714] The degree of spectrin deficiency (and by deduction ankyrin defi-

ciency) correlates well with the spheroidicity of HS erythrocytes, the severity of hemolysis, and the response of patients to splenectomy (Fig. 16–16).[688, 694, 715] The mechanical properties of the cells, particularly their ability to withstand shear stress, also correlate with their spectrin content.[715, 716] Microscopically, HS red cells show fewer spectrin filaments interconnecting spectrin/actin/protein 4.1 junctional complexes, but overall skeletal architecture is preserved,[548] except in the most severe forms of HS.

A minority of European and American HS patients are deficient in band 3 and protein 4.2 (dominant HS) or protein 4.2 alone (recessive HS).[490, 493, 608, 707] In contrast, these are the most common forms of HS in Japan.[120]

Alpha-Spectrin Defects

The mechanisms of spectrin deficiency are unknown in most HS patients. Initially it seemed probable that recessive and dominant HS would be due to defects in α-spectrin and β-spectrin, respectively. In humans, α-spectrin exceeds β-spectrin synthesis by 3 or 4 to 1.[381] Heterozygotes for α-spectrin synthetic defects should still produce enough normal α-spectrin chains to pair with all or nearly all of the β chains that are made, so spectrin deficiency would only be evident in the homozygous state. In fact, this fits with what is observed. Even in the most severe forms of recessive HS, obligate heterozygotes show little or no spectrin deficiency.[694, 713, 717]

Approximately one half of patients with severe recessive HS and marked spectrin deficiency (20% to 40% of normal) have a mutation in the ninth 106-amino acid repeat of α-spectrin, Ala^{969}→Asp, termed the *spectrin α IIa variant*.[718, 719] This mutation is not the cause of HS because it is present in 2% to 15% of normal individuals[718–720] and, in many HS families, it is located on a different chromosome and inherited independently from the HS gene.[719, 720] These findings, combined with work by Jarolim and associates[721] suggest that the α IIa variant is a polymorphism in linkage disequilibrium with a second variant called α spectrin^{LEPRA} (*Low Expression PRAgue*). This variant, a C to T substitution 99 nt upstream of the acceptor splice site of intron 30, produces an aberrantly spliced α-spectrin mRNA. The variant allele produces approximately six times less of the correctly spliced α-spectrin transcript than the normal allele. In the heterozygous state, α-spectrin^{LEPRA}, as would be expected, is asymptomatic. The combination of α-spectrin^{LEPRA} with other defects of α-spectrin in *trans*, leads to significant α-spectrin deficiency and severe spherocytic anemia.[721]

Beta-Spectrin Defects

Deficiency of the scarce β-spectrin chains, on the other hand, should limit formation of αβ-spectrin heterodimers and be expressed as a dominant defect. So should a deficiency of ankyrin, because spectrin heterodimers are only stable when bound to the membrane[722] and ankyrin, the high-affinity binding site, is normally pres-

Table 16-6. ANKYRIN MUTATIONS ASSOCIATED WITH HEREDITARY SPHEROCYTOSIS

| Variant | Inheritance | Mutations | | | | Exon | Ankyrin Domain | Comment | Reference |
		Type	Codon	Gene	Protein				
Unnamed	AD	Substitution	—	C → G −204	—	—	—	5'UTR	695
Unnamed	AR	Substitution	—	T → C −108	—	—	—	5' UTR, recurrent: 4/7 families	695
Bugey	—	Deletion, frameshift	146	−C	PCT	6	Membrane	De novo	696
Osterholz	—	Deletion, frameshift	173	20 nt deletion	PCT	6	Membrane	De novo	695
Stuttgart	AD	Deletion, frameshift	329	−GC	PCT	10	Membrane		695
Walsrode	AR	Substitution	463	GTC → ATC	Val → Ile	13	Membrane		695
Florianopolis	AD	Insertion, frameshift	506	+C	PCT	14	Membrane	Recurrent	702
Unnamed	AD	Deletion, frameshift	535	−A	PCT	15	Membrane		702
Napoli	—	Deletion, frameshift	573	−T	PCT	16	Membrane	De novo	697
Einbeck	AD	Insertion, frameshift	573	+C	PCT	16	Membrane		695
Duisburg	AD	Substitution, splicing	ivs 16*	C → A	PCT	16/17	Membrane		695
Unnamed	AD	Nonsense	631	GAG → TAG	PCT	17	Membrane		701
Unnamed	AD	Nonsense	765	TCG → TAG	PCT	20	Membrane		701
Marburg	AD	Deletion, frameshift	797–798	−TAGT	PCT	22	Membrane		695
Unnamed	AD	Deletion, frameshift	907	−G	PCT	25	Spectrin		701
Unnamed	AD	Nonsense	1053	CGA → TGA	PCT	28	Spectrin		701
Unnamed	AD	Missense	1075	ATC → ACC	Ile → Thr	28	Spectrin		702
Porta Westfalica	—	Deletion, frameshift	1127	−C	PCT	29	Spectrin	De novo	695
Bovenden	AD	Nonsense	1436	CGA → TGA	PCT	36	Regulatory		695
Unnamed	AD	Nonsense	1488	CGA → TGA	PCT	37	Regulatory		701
Prague	AD	Insertion	1512–1513†	201 nt insertion	67 aa insertion	37/38	Regulatory		698, 699
Dusseldorf	AR	Substitution	1592	GAC → AAC	Asp → Asn	38	Regulatory		696
Rakovnik	AD	Nonsense	1669‡	GAA → TAA	PCT	38	Regulatory		700
Unnamed	AD	Substitution	ivs 38§	C → T	?PCT	38/39	Regulatory		695
Bocholt	AR	? splicing Substitution	1879	CGG → TGG	Arg → Trp	41	Regulatory		695

PCT, premature chain termination due to a frameshift or nonsense mutation; AD, autosomal dominant; AR, autosomal recessive; UTR, untranslated region.

*18 nt before start of exon 17.
†Insertion between exons 37 and 38.
‡Decreased ankyrin 2.1 isoform.
§34 nt before start of exon 39.

Table 16-7. BAND 3 MUTATIONS ASSOCIATED WITH HEREDITARY SPHEROCYTOSIS

Variant	Inheritance	Type	Mutations Codon	Mutations Gene	Mutations Protein	Exon	Band 3 Domain	Comment	Reference
Coimbra	AD	Substitution	488	CTG → ATG	Val → Met	4	Cyto	? Hydrops	705
Tuscaloosa	?AD	Substitution	40	CCG → CGC	Pro → Arg	4	Cyto	Decreased binding of protein 4.2	299
Foggia	AD	Deletion, frameshift	54–55	−C	PCT	4	Cyto		711
Hodonin	AD	Nonsense	81	TGG → TGA	PCT	5	Cyto		709
Napoli	AD	Insertion, frameshift	99–100	+T	PCT	5	Cyto		711
Lyon, Osnabruck I*	AD	Nonsense	150	CGA → TGA	PCT	6	Cyto, two unrelated families		156, 695
Nachod	AD	Splicing	117–121	−3, C → A (splicing)	GTVLL deleted	6	Cyto	?Decreased ankyrin binding	709
Wilson	AD	Deletion, frameshift	171	−G	PCT	7	Cyto		703
Worcester	AD	Insertion, frameshift	170–172	+G	PCT	7	Cyto		709
Campinas	AD	Splicing, frameshift		+1, G → T (splicing)†	PCT	8	Cyto	RTA	712
Noirterre	AD	Nonsense	330	CAG → TAG	PCT	10	Cyto		704
Montefiore	?AR	Substitution	327	GAG → AAG	Glu → Lys	10	Cyto	Decreased binding of protein 4.2	296
Bruggen	AD	Deletion, frameshift	419	−C	PCT	11	TM		695
Benesov	AD	Duplication	455	GGG → GAG	Gly → Glu	12	TM		709
Pribram	AD	Splicing, frameshift	477	−1, G → A (splicing)‡	PCT	12	TM	RTA‡	709, 710
Milano	AD	In-frame duplication		69 bp duplication	23 aa insertion	13	TM		706
Dresden	AD	Substitution	518	CGC → TGC	Arg → Cys	13	TM		695
Smichov	AD	Deletion, frameshift	616	−C	PCT	15	TM		709
Truthov	AD	Nonsense	628	TAC → TAA	PCT	15	TM		709
Osnabruck I	AD	Inframe deletion	663 or 664	− ATG	?	16	TM		695
Hobart	AD	Deletion, frameshift	646–647	−G	PCT	16	TM		709
Hradec Kralove	AD	Substitution	760	CGG → TGG	Arg → Trp	17	TM		707
Prague II	AD	Substitution	760	CGG → CAG	Arg → Gln	17	TM		409
Most	AD	Substitution	707	CTG → CCG	Leu → Pro	17	TM		709
Jablonec	AD	Substitution	808	CGC → TGC	Arg → Cys	18	TM		707
Prague	AD	Insertion, frameshift	819–822	+CAC CCAGATC	PCT	18	TM		707
Chur	AD	Substitution	771	GGC → GAC	Gly → Asp	18	TM		708
Prague III	AD	Substitution	870	CGG → TGG	Arg → Trp	19	TM		707
Birmingham	AD	Substitution	834	CAC → CCC	His → Pro	19	TM		709
Philadelphia	AD	Substitution	837	ACG → ATG	Thr → Met	19	TM		709

PCT, premature chain termination due to a frameshift or nonsense mutation; AD, autosomal dominant; AR, autosomal recessive; Cyto, cytoplasmic; TM, transmembrane; RTA, renal tubular acidosis.
*Two mutations were described independently but refer to the same defect.
†Skipping of exon 8.
‡Intron 12 inserted into coding sequence.

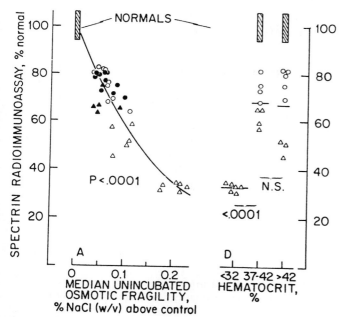

Figure 16-16. Correlation between red cell spectrin deficiency and unincubated osmotic fragility (a measure of spheroidicity) in hereditary spherocytosis. Spectrin content, as measured by radioimmunoassay, is shown on the vertical axis; and osmotic fragility, as measured by NaCl concentration producing 50% hemolysis of erythrocytes, is shown on the horizontal axis. *Circles* represent patients with typical autosomal dominant hereditary spherocytosis, and *triangles* represent patients with atypical, nondominant spherocytosis. *Open symbols* represent patients who have undergone splenectomy. The *right panel* shows the hematocrit of each patient at least 4 months after splenectomy. Note that very spectrin deficient patients have more spherical red cells and an incomplete response to splenectomy. (With permission from Agre P, Asimos A, Casella JF, et al: Inheritance pattern and clinical response to splenectomy as a reflection of erythrocyte spectrin deficiency in hereditary spherocytosis. The New England Journal of Medicine 1986; 315:1579. Copyright 1986, Massachusetts Medical Society.)

ent in limiting amounts. By the same reasoning band 3 should also be a culprit, because ankyrin and spectrin bind to band 3 and only a fraction of the band 3 molecules are available to bind ankyrin.[289]

Initially, cytogenetic studies supported the hypothesis that some patients with dominant HS have defects in β-spectrin. Kimberling and colleagues[723] detected a loose linkage between polymorphisms of the immunoglobulin heavy chains (IgH) and an HS locus (now called SPH1) by combining observations on 70 patients in 11 informative families. IgH was subsequently localized to chromosome 14q32.3, reasonably close to β-spectrin (14q23–q24.2).[724] Defects in β-spectrin, a large gene spanning over 200 kb, are now being discovered.

Mutations have been identified in a number of unrelated dominant HS families, all of whom are heterozygotes for a β-spectrin defect. Spectrin[Kissimmee] is an unstable β-spectrin that lacks the ability to bind protein 4.1 and as a consequence, binds poorly to actin.[364, 725-727] This variant is due to a point mutation, $Trp^{202} \rightarrow Arg^{364}$, in a conserved region near the NH_2-terminus of β-spectrin, which probably forms part of the protein 4.1–binding site.[393, 728] Truncated β-spectrin mutations due

to (1) a large genomic deletion that leads to exon skipping of exons 22 and 23, β-spectrin[Durham] and to (2) a splicing mutation, β-spectrin[Winston-Salem], have been described.[729, 730] A screen of the β-spectrin gene of 40 HS patients with spectrin deficiency identified several nonsense and frameshift mutations.[731] One of these, spectrin[Houston], a frameshift mutation due to a single nucleotide deletion, was found in patients from several unrelated kindreds[731] and may be a common β-spectrin mutation associated with dominant HS. The spectrum of HS-causing β-spectrin mutations is just now beginning to be revealed. Interestingly, in the few cases in which peripheral blood morphology has been described, patients with β-spectrin mutations have had acanthocytes as well as spherocytes. This may prove to be a characteristic finding.

Ankyrin Defects

Evidence implicating defects of ankyrin in many cases of HS comes from a variety of sources, including biochemical analyses, genetic studies, and study of a murine model of HS. Biochemical studies suggested a defect of ankyrin in two patients with an atypical, unusually severe form of HS characterized by bizarre-shaped microspherocytes.[732] Red cell spectrin and ankyrin levels were approximately half normal, apparently owing to failure of ankyrin synthesis or to synthesis of an unstable molecule.[733] Ankyrin mRNA concentrations were also half normal, and pulse chase studies showed that newly synthesized ankyrin did not accumulate in the cytoplasm and only reached half-normal levels on the membrane. In contrast, spectrin mRNA concentrations were normal, though only half of the synthesized spectrin attached to the membrane, presumably owing to the lack of ankyrin sites. Spectrin synthesis was either normal or increased; however, spectrin incorporation into the membrane skeleton was diminished owing to a marked deficiency of membrane-associated ankyrin. These studies support the hypothesis that ankyrin deficiency or dysfunction may lead to spectrin deficiency in HS.

Evidence of ankyrin deficiency has been found in many cases of typical HS. Savvides and colleagues[608] measured red cell spectrin and ankyrin levels by radioimmunoassay in the erythrocyte membranes of 39 patients from 20 typical dominant HS kindreds. The values ranged from 40% to 100% of the normal cellular levels of 242,000 ± 20,500 spectrin heterodimers and 124,500 ± 11,000 ankyrins. Both spectrin and ankyrin levels were less than the normal range in 75% to 80% of kindreds. The degree of spectrin and ankyrin deficiency was very similar in 19 of the 20 kindreds studied. Similar data have been observed in other studies.[714, 734-738] Concomitant spectrin and ankyrin deficiency is not unexpected. Decreased ankyrin synthesis or accumulation on the erythrocyte membrane could lead to decreased assembly of spectrin on the membrane because spectrin-binding sites in ankyrin may be absent or defective.

Two abnormally migrating ankyrins associated with dominantly inherited HS have been described.[698-700] In ankyrin[Prague], normal ankyrin (206 kDa) is replaced by a 174-kDa variant, presumably due to abnormal splicing.[698, 699] The variant contains 67 new amino acids inserted at the splice junction between exons 37 and 38 (Asn[1512]/Gly[1513]). In ankyrin[Rakovnik], a nonsense mutation in the regulatory region leads to a selective deficiency of the 2.1 ankyrin isoform.[700]

Additional genetic studies also support the initial hypothesis that a defect of the ankyrin gene can be associated with HS. Studies of atypical HS patients with karyotypic abnormalities including translocations and interstitial deletions have defined a locus for HS at chromosomal segments 8p11.2-21.1.[491, 739–743] In situ hybridization analysis has located the ankyrin gene at chromosomal segment 8p11.2.[491] Karyotype analysis of an HS patient with mental retardation revealed an interstitial deletion of chromosome 8, band p11.1-p21.1.[491] Fluorescence-based in situ hybridization of lymphocyte metaphase spreads from this patient with an ankyrin genomic probe provided direct evidence that one copy of the erythrocyte ankyrin gene was deleted (Fig. 16–17). There was also a 50% reduction in ankyrin content of the patient's red blood cell membranes. These results demonstrated that a deficiency of ankyrin due to a gene deletion may be a cause of HS.

A similar phenotype has been reported in a patient with an 8p11.1-p21.3 deletion.[742]

Linkage of HS and the ankyrin gene has been proved, using restriction enzyme polymorphisms, in a large family with typical dominant HS.[744] In other studies, using an ankyrin intragenic microsatellite polymorphism, one third of spectrin/ankyrin-deficient dominant HS patients were found to carry only one of their two alleles in reticulocyte RNA, demonstrating reduced ankyrin expression from one allele.[745] These combined observations suggest that ankyrin deficiency is the primary defect in the majority of patients with dominant HS and that spectrin deficiency is secondary to the loss of ankyrin attachment sites.

The precise genetic defects in ankyrin that cause HS are beginning to be described (see Tables 16–6 and 16–7). These have been detected primarily by mutation screening using PCR-based single-stranded conformational polymorphism (SSCP) techniques.[695–697, 701, 702] Analysis of the initial mutations detected suggests that (1) ankyrin mutations are common, affecting patients with both dominant and recessive HS; (2) mutations that abolish the normal ankyrin product are prevalent in dominant HS (e.g., frameshift mutations or mutations that introduce a stop codon in the coding sequence);

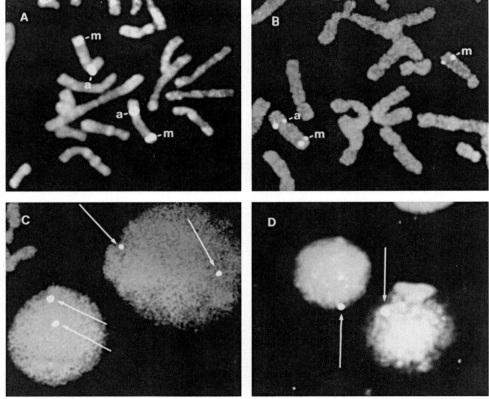

Figure 16–17. Demonstration of absence of one copy of the *ANK1* gene in a patient with hereditary spherocytosis (HS) using fluorescence *in situ* hybridization (FISH). The patient is heterozygous for a deletion of part of the short arm of chromosome 8. Metaphase spreads prepared with cells from a normal control subject (*A*) or the patient (*B*) were labeled with both *MYC* (m) and ankyrin (a) genomic probes. Note that the ankyrin probe hybridized to only one of the HS chromosomes 8, each of which is marked by the control *MYC* probe. Interphase nuclei from a normal control subject (*C*) or the patient (*D*) hybridized to the ankyrin probe (*arrows*). Note that there is only one hybridization signal per cell for the HS cells. (Reprinted with permission from Tse WT, Menninger JC, et al: Demonstration of the deletion of a copy of the ankyrin gene in a patient with hereditary spherocytosis by *in situ* hybridization. Trans Assoc Am Phys 1990; 103:242.)

and (3) defects upstream of the coding region are frequent in recessive HS, particularly a T→C nucleotide substitution in the ankyrin gene promoter (CCTGG→CCCGG), −108 bp from the translation start site, which is present on one chromosome in 4 of 13 recessive HS families. This defect lies next to one of the several transcriptional start sites of ankyrin. Because this defect is silent in obligate heterozygotes, recessive HS patients must have a second mutation. This has been discovered in two patients: a man with mild HS who carries the −108 mutation and a silent defect in *trans*, ankyrin[Walsrode] (Val[463]→Ile), and a man with moderate HS, the −108 mutation, and ankyrin[Bocholt], an Arg→Trp mutation in an alternatively spliced region near the COOH-terminus. Additionally, variations in the clinical severity and red cell ankyrin content of similar mutations indicate that other factors modify the expression of the primary ankyrin defects. For example, ankyrin[Marburg] and ankyrin[Einbeck] are frameshift mutations that occur in the NH$_2$-terminal (membrane) domain and do not produce a detectable product in mature red cells. They would be expected to have a similar phenotype but patients with ankyrin[Marburg] have moderate to severe HS and moderate ankyrin deficiency (64% of normal), whereas patients with ankyrin[Einbeck] have very mild disease and normal ankyrin levels. Understanding this and similar variations will be one of the critical problems in HS research in the next few years.

The majority of ankyrin mutations are private, that is, each individual kindred has a unique mutation. One frameshift mutation associated with severe dominant HS, ankyrin[Florianopolis], has been identified in HS patients from three different kindreds from different genetic backgrounds.[702] Analysis of an ankyrin gene polymorphism in these individuals demonstrated that this mutation is on different ankyrin alleles, suggesting that the ankyrin[Florianopolis] mutation has occurred more than once.

Band 3 Defects

In about one third of patients with dominant HS, the primary protein defect resides in band 3, as evidenced by band 3 deficiency.[707] In fact, these patients probably always have a combined deficiency of band 3 and protein 4.2.[120] Mice and cows that lack band 3 also lack protein 4.2,[603, 746] and, when tested, human patients are also deficient in both proteins.[120] Genetic linkage of HS to the band 3 gene has been described, and mutations of the band 3 gene have been identified in several HS kindreds.[409, 695, 704–712] Affected patients have mild to moderate HS and a 20% to 40% deficiency of band 3 and protein 4.2, which is usually detected as an increase in the spectrin/band 3 ratio on SDS gels. Red cell spectrin content is normal. Most band 3–deficient patients also have a small number of mushroom-shaped or "pincered" erythrocytes on peripheral blood smears. This morphology is not observed in the other protein defects.

A variety of band 3 mutations have been described in cases of HS (see Table 16–7). One of the initial band 3 mutants associated with HS was band 3[Prague].[409] This mutant is due to a 10-nucleotide duplication in the band 3 gene that leads to a shift in the reading frame and results in premature chain termination. The mutation occurs in a region encoding the COOH-terminus of the protein, leading to an altered COOH-terminus after amino acid 821 (70 new amino acids). The mutation affects the last transmembrane helix and probably alters insertion of band 3 into the membrane because the mutant protein is not detectable in mature red cells. Interestingly, the decrease in band 3 content occurs principally in the mobile, dimeric fraction of band 3. Immobilized band 3, which probably includes band 3 bound to ankyrin, was not greatly affected.

A group of band 3 mutations that cluster near the COOH-terminus and replace a conserved arginine with another amino acid have been described.[707] These arginines are all located at the cytoplasmic end of a predicted transmembrane helix. Arginine residues are located in the same position in most transmembrane proteins and are thought to help orient the membrane-spanning segments. This suggests the mutant band 3 proteins may be absent from the mature red cell because they do not fold and insert into the endoplasmic reticulum and ultimately into the erythrocyte membrane correctly after synthesis. In addition, some arginines in band 3 appear to be involved in anion transport.

Other band 3 mutations have been described.[156, 695, 704–706, 708–712] In two French families with dominant HS, nonsense mutations (band 3 Noirterre and band 3 Lyon) led to markedly decreased mRNA accumulation, presumably due to mRNA instability[156, 704]; a similar mechanism is hypothesized in band 3[Osnabruck I,695] which appears to be the same mutation as band 3[Lyon] (see Table 16–7). The band 3[Lyon] phenotype was reported to be aggravated by a modifying allele in *trans*, band 3[Genas], which is characterized by a G→A substitution at a position 89 nt from the cap site in the 5′-untranslated region of the band 3 cDNA.[156] Frameshift mutations other than band 3[Prague] have been described, such as band 3[Wilson,747] which occurred in the first patient described with band 3 deficiency,[703] and band 3[Bruggen.695] Band 3[Milano] is a 23-amino acid, in-frame duplication in transmembrane domain 4 that is probably not incorporated into the erythrocyte membrane.[706] This duplication is present in the genomic DNA and is thought to have arisen from an unequal recombination of the anti-Lepore type. Band 3[Chur], Gly[771]→Asp,[708] and band 3[Coimbra], Val[488]→Met,[705] are missense mutations in the band 3 gene associated with dominant HS. Other missense mutations in band 3 have been associated with protein 4.2 deficiency and HS or with acanthocytosis alone (see later). In HS patients with band 3[Pribram] or band 3[Campinas], which are defects in band 3 mRNA processing, renal tubular acidosis has also been observed.[709, 710, 712] The precise pathogenesis of the renal tubular acidosis, attributed in part to the defective band 3 protein expressed in the kidney, is unknown.

In cows, homozygosity for a nonsense mutation in the band 3 gene leads to absence of band 3 and protein 4.2.[746] Red cell membranes are unstable and show surface area loss, as evidenced by invagination, vesiculation, and extrusion of microvesicles. There is defective anion transport and a mild acidosis. In mice, targeted disruption of the band 3 gene causes a severe spherocytic hemolytic anemia, with exuberant loss of the membrane surface as vesicles, tubules, and myelin forms.[603] Red cell membranes also lack protein 4.2. Surprisingly, the content of membrane skeletal proteins and the architecture of negative-stained, spread skeletons is normal or nearly normal.[603]

Together, these studies suggest that (1) homozygosity for a band 3 defect causes a severe, nonlethal hemolytic anemia, (2) band 3 is not critical for assembly of the membrane skeleton, and (3) band 3 provides the sole membrane attachment for protein 4.2.

Protein 4.2 Defects

Several investigators have described families with clinically typical recessive HS in which affected patients lack red cell protein 4.2.[296, 297, 490, 493, 747-753] In the most common variant, 4.2^{Nippon}, the red cells contain only a small quantity of a 74/72-kDa doublet of protein 4.2 instead of the usual 72-kDa species, because of a Ala^{142}→Thr mutation that affects the processing of the protein 4.2 mRNA.[501] Protein 4.2^{Nippon}–deficient membranes lose 70% of their ankyrin with low ionic strength extraction, and the ankyrin loss is blocked by preincubation of the membranes with purified 4.2, which suggests protein 4.2 stabilizes ankyrin on the membrane.[493, 494] This hypothesis is supported by the observations that the amount of protein 4.2 is low in the red cell membranes of ankyrin-deficient nb/nb mice and in HS patients who lack one ankyrin gene. In addition, red cells from patients homozygous for 4.2^{Nippon} are fragile and have heat-sensitive skeletons, clumped intramembranous particles (probably band 3 molecules), and increased lateral mobility of band 3.[494] However, ankyrin lability is not evident in other patients with protein 4.2 deficiency,[748, 753] some of whom have normal morphology, acanthopoikilocytosis,[753] or ovalostomatocytosis instead of spherocytosis. Presumably, these differences are examples of allelic variation.

Finally, erythrocyte protein 4.2 deficiency has been associated with mutations in the cytoplasmic domain of band 3 in two patients. One of the mutations (band 3^{Montefiore}) lies near the NH$_2$-terminus of band 3 (Glu^{40}→Lys).[296] The other (band 3^{Tuscaloosa}) is near the end of the cytoplasmic domain (Pro^{327}→Thr).[299] Presumably the protein 4.2–binding site involves both regions.

Other Membrane Protein Defects

Inextractable spectrin was first observed some years ago in 2 of 12 HS patients in whom spectrin failed to elute from the membrane after exposure to low ionic strength for 72 hours.[754] These are conditions that generally produce greater than 90% spectrin extraction. A second patient was discovered more recently.[755] The molecular basis of this phenomenon has not subsequently been investigated, although the possibility that

it might be secondary to a defect in ankyrin or β-spectrin seems obvious. In addition, some tightly bound spectrin is palmitoylated and this fraction might be increased.[756] HS membranes contain increased amounts of hemoglobin and catalase.[757] This is a relatively nonspecific finding that is observed in a number of hemolytic anemias, particularly if red cell dehydration occurs. Its molecular basis is not understood. Two reports of apparent HS combined with partial enolase deficiency (~50%) have appeared.[758, 759] In the first patient, a French woman, red cell osmotic fragility and autohemolysis tests were typical of HS, although spherocytes were not apparent on the blood smear. Dominant inheritance was suggested by history but could not be established because the affected father was deceased. However, dominant inheritance of both HS and partial enolase deficiency was clearly evident in the second family when both diseases could be traced through four generations. In this kindred, the enolase-deficient spherocytes resisted lysis in the acidified glycerol lysis test, another characteristic of typical HS (see later). The similarity of these two cases suggests that they may represent a unique subgroup of HS. In particular, the combination of dominant inheritance and half-normal levels of enolase raises the possibility that the primary defect could lie in an enolase-binding membrane protein, assuming such a protein exists.

The discovery that red cell membrane proteins are phosphorylated was followed by numerous reports that phosphorylation was defective in HS. These reports are summarized and analyzed in previous reviews.[760, 761] In short, the effects were variable and generally were only demonstrable in ghosts incubated in low ionic strength buffers for relatively long periods. Initial rates of phosphorylation in HS ghosts were normal[762-764] as was membrane protein phosphorylation of intact spherocytes from splenectomized individuals.[764] It now appears that the phosphorylation defects were probably secondary effects.

Homogenized suspensions of membrane skeletons from hereditary spherocytes gel poorly or not at all when treated with spectrin kinase, whereas normal skeletons gel firmly under the same conditions.[765, 766] The phenomenon is not understood on a molecular level, but it is specific and reproducibly abnormal in HS.

Secondary Membrane Effects

A large number of secondary abnormalities have been identified over the years. These are catalogued and discussed in detail in earlier reviews[760, 761] and are briefly summarized below.

Membrane Lipids. The principal lipid abnormality of hereditary spherocytes is a symmetric loss of membrane lipids as part of the overall loss of membrane surface, the hallmark of HS pathobiology. The relative proportions of cholesterol and the various phospholipids are normal,[767] and the phospholipids show the usual transmembrane asymmetry, even in severe cases,[57, 768] It has been reported that very long chain fatty acids are missing from certain classes of phospholipids,[769] but this has not been confirmed.[770] It is unclear whether this difference is due to technical factors or to genetic heterogeneity of the disease. Even if real, however, it seems likely that the changes in fatty acid composition will be secondary to underlying membrane protein defects.

Cations and Transport. It has been known for many years that HS red cells are intrinsically more leaky to Na^+ and K^+ ions than normal cells.[771-774] Interestingly, a similar defect exists in spectrin-deficient mice.[775] The excessive Na^+ influx activates Na^+,K^+-ATPase and the monovalent cation pump, and the accelerated pumping, in turn, increases ATP turnover and glycolysis. At one time, it was believed that this modest Na^+ leak was responsible for the hemolysis of hereditary spherocytes,[773] particularly those cells trapped in the unfavorable metabolic environment of the spleen, but it now is clear that this is incorrect, because the magnitude of the Na^+ flux does not correlate with the extent of hemolysis in HS.[776] In addition, patients with hereditary stomatocytosis (to be discussed) and a much greater defect in Na^+ permeability do not develop microspherocytes, and sometimes have very little hemolysis.[777] The leak of Na^+ into red cells in hereditary stomatocytosis is accompanied by the entry of water and cell swelling, a finding that contrasts to the well-established dehydration of hereditary spherocytes.

The dehydration of HS red cells is likely to be inflicted, at least in part, by the adverse environment of the spleen, because spherocytes from surgically removed spleens are the most dehydrated.[778] The pathways causing HS red cell dehydration have not been clearly defined. One likely candidate is increased K^+/Cl^- cotransport, which is activated by acid pH.[586] HS red cells, particularly from unsplenectomized subjects, have a low intracellular pH,[779] reflecting the low pH of the splenic environment (see later). The K^+/Cl^--cotransport pathway is also activated by oxidation,[780] which is likely to be inflicted by splenic macrophages (see later). Lastly, hyperactivity of the Na^+/K^+ pump, triggered by increased intracellular Na^+, can dehydrate red cells directly, because three Na^+ ions are extruded in exchange for only two K^+ ions.[639, 640] The loss of monovalent cations is accompanied by water.

Glycolysis. In general, glycolysis is mildly accelerated in HS red cells,[773, 781, 782] mostly to support increased cation pumping,[773] and 2,3-DPG concentrations are slightly depressed,[779, 783, 784] probably due to activation of 2,3-DPG phosphatase by the acidic intracellular pH of the cell.[784] The latter abnormalities are at least partly due to splenic detention, because the acidosis and DPG deficiency both improve after splenectomy.[779, 783]

An apparently specific decrease in carrier-mediated transport of phosphoenolpyruvate has been noted in red cells of some patients with HS.[785] Unfortunately, only nonsplenectomized patients were studied, so it is possible that the defect is secondary to the metabolic derangements these cells acquire during their detention in the spleen. More likely it is caused by diminished anion exchange. Band 3 transports pyruvate and probably phosphoenolpyruvate. If so, reduced phosphoenolpyruvate transport would be expected in HS patients with band 3 deficiency. Surprisingly, anion transport is also suppressed (30% to 35%) in patients with known ankyrin defects.[786] The molecular explanation is unknown. It should be noted that diminished phosphoenolpyruvate transport has only been reported in Japanese patients with HS, a population in whom combined band 3 and protein 4.2 deficiency is particularly common.[120]

Murine Models

Six types of autosomal recessive, spherocytic hereditary hemolytic anemias have been described in the common house mouse, *Mus musculus*.[380, 438, 787-793] These are designated *ja/ja* (jaundiced), *sph/sph* (spherocytosis), *sph^ha/sph^ha* (hemolytic anemia), *sph^2BC/sph^2BC*, *sph^2J/sph^2J*, and *nb/nb* (normoblastosis). The nomenclature indicates that the six mutants represent three alleles: *ja*, *sph*, and *nb*. The *sph^ha*, *sph^2BC*, and *sph^2J* mutations are allelic variants at the *sph* locus.[788, 792] All of the mutants have severe hemolysis with marked spherocytosis, bilirubin gallstones, massive hepatosplenomegaly, and reticulocyte counts that approach 100%.[787] Anemia is observed only in the homozygous state and is associated with decreased viability.

All of the mouse mutants are spectrin or spectrin/ankyrin deficient and have extremely fragile red cells. Red cells spontaneously vesiculate and ghosts disintegrate during preparation. The *ja/ja* mutant has a defect in the spectrin β chain ($Arg^{1160} \rightarrow Stop$) and no detectable spectrin.[791] The *sph/sph* variants have α spectrin mutations[380] They lack α chains, either due to decreased synthesis (*sph*, *sph^2BC*, *sph^2J*) or to synthesis of an unstable chain (*sph^ha*) but have small amounts of β-spectrin. Disruption of the α-spectrin gene by accidental insertion of a transgene has also been reported.[794] Homozygous animals have a severe spherocytic anemia that is lethal in the first few days of life.

Mice with the *nb* mutation have a primary defect in ankyrin-1 (erythrocyte ankyrin). The mutation maps to the *Ank-1* locus on mouse chromosome 8.[793] *nb/nb* red cells have only a trace of ankyrin-1 mRNA and protein[438, 787] but only a partial deficiency of spectrin (50% to 70% of normal). This is different than ankyrin defects in human HS, in which ankyrin and spectrin levels are comparably depressed.[608, 714] *nb/nb* mice also lack ankyrin-1 in cerebellar Purkinje cells.[438, 439] This leads to an age-related loss of Purkinje cells during the first 5 to 7 months of life and the emergence of cerebellar ataxia.[438] Spinocerebellar degeneration and related syndromes have also been reported in a few adult humans with HS,[795-803] although it is not yet known whether ankyrin-1 is affected. Fetal *nb/nb* mice have no anemia and normal reticulocyte counts at birth,[804] apparently owing to expression of ankyrin-related proteins *in utero*.[805] Humans may also be protected *in utero*, at least partially, because hydrops fetalis has not been reported in patients with probable ankyrin defects (i.e., combined spectrin/ankyrin deficiency), even in patients who become transfusion dependent after birth.

Another recessive spherocytic hemolytic anemia has been described in the deer mouse, *Peromyscus maniculatus*.[806] This disorder is less severe and closely resembles the autosomal dominant form of human HS. The spectrin content of deer mouse erythrocytes is reduced about 20%.[807]

Pathophysiology

Mechanisms of Membrane Surface Loss

Vesiculation. The primary membrane lesions described earlier, all involving vertical interactions between the skeleton and the bilayer, fit the prevailing theory that HS is caused by local disconnection of the skeleton and bilayer, followed by vesiculation of the unsupported surface components. This, in turn, leads to progressive reduction in membrane surface area and to a shape called a spherocyte, although it usually ranges between a thickened discocyte and a spherostomatocyte.[808] The phospholipid and cholesterol contents of isolated spherocytes are decreased by 15% to 20%, consistent with the loss of surface area.[809–812] Despite its popularity, the evidence supporting the vesiculation theory is surprisingly scant. On the plus side, careful biomechanical measurements show that HS membranes are fragile. The force required to fragment the membrane is diminished and is proportional to the density of spectrin on the membrane.[715, 716] Membrane elasticity and bending stiffness are also reduced and proportional to spectrin density.[716, 813] In addition, HS red cells lose membrane more readily than normal when metabolically deprived[812, 814–816] or when their ghosts are subjected to conditions facilitating vesiculation.[817] However, this has not been shown to occur in metabolically healthy spherocytes, perhaps because it occurs slowly (1% to 2% per day) under such conditions. Because budding red cells are rarely observed in typical HS blood smears, the postulated vesiculation must either involve microscopic vesicles or occur in bywaters of the circulation such as the reticuloendothelial system. Probably both explanations are true. When membrane vesicles are induced in normal red cells, they originate at the tips of spicules, where the lipid bilayer uncouples from the underlying skeleton.[549] The vesicles are small (about 100 nm) and devoid of hemoglobin and skeletal proteins, so that they are invisible during a conventional examination of stained blood films. Tiny (50 to 80 nm) bumps have been detected in preliminary studies with an atomic force microscope, on the surface of HS red cells obtained from patients who are actively hemolyzing.[818] The bumps could be microvesicles, although this needs to be proven using more conventional microscopic techniques. They are less than the length of a spectrin molecule (100 nm) and are not present on red cells from splenectomized patients.

Models Relating Membrane Defects and Surface Loss. The observation that spectrin or spectrin/ankyrin deficiencies are common in HS has led to the suggestion that they are the primary cause of spherocytosis. According to this hypothesis, interactions of spectrin with bilayer lipids or proteins are required to stabilize the membrane. Spectrin-deficient areas would tend to bud off, leading to spherocytosis. However, this conjecture does not explain how spherocytes develop in patients whose red cells are deficient in band 3 or protein 4.2 but have normal amounts of spectrin.[493, 608, 819] An alternate hypothesis argues that the bilayer is stabilized by interactions between lipids and the abundant band 3 molecules (Fig. 16–18). Each band 3 contains about 14 hydrophobic transmembrane helices, many of which must interact with lipids. Such interactions presumably spread beyond the first layer of lipids and influence the mobility of lipids in successive layers. In deficient red cells the area between band 3 molecules would increase, on average, and the stabilizing effect would diminish. Transient fluctuations in the local density of band 3 could aggravate this situation and allow unsupported lipids to be lost, resulting in spherocytosis. Such an hypothesis is supported by band 3 gene "knock-out" mice that lose massive amounts of membrane surface despite a normal membrane skeleton.[603] This concept is also consistent with early studies of intramembrane particle aggregation, which leads to particle-free domains, as discussed earlier in the chapter. These domains are unstable, giving rise to surface blebs that are subsequently released from the cells as vesicles.[553] Additionally, in a subset of patients with band 3 deficiency, the protein appears to be lost from the cells during their residence in the circulation. The concomitant loss of the "boundary" lipids may contribute to the deficiency of surface area. Spectrin- and ankyrin-deficient red cells could become spherocytic by a similar mechanism. Because spectrin filaments corral band 3 molecules and limit their lateral movement,[820] a decrease in spectrin would allow band 3 molecules to diffuse and transiently cluster, fostering vesiculation.

Loss of Cellular Deformability. Hereditary spherocytes hemolyze because of the rheologic consequences of their decreased surface/volume ratio. The red cell membrane is very flexible, but it can only expand its surface area about 3% before rupturing.[821] Hence the cell becomes less and less deformable as surface area is lost. For HS red cells, poor deformability is only a hindrance in the spleen, because the cells have a nearly normal life span after splenectomy.[822, 823]

Splenic Sequestration and Conditioning

Spherocytes are detained at the cord/sinus junction. In the spleen most of the arterial blood empties directly into the splenic cords, a tortuous maze of interconnecting narrow passages formed by reticular cells and lined with phagocytes.[824–829] Histologically, this is an "open" circulation, but apparently most of the blood that enters the cords normally travels by fairly direct (i.e., functionally closed) pathways.[828, 829] If passage through these channels is impeded, red cells are diverted deeper into the labyrinthine portions of the cords where blood flow is slow and the cells may be detained for minutes to hours. Whichever route is taken, to re-enter the circulation red cells must squeeze through

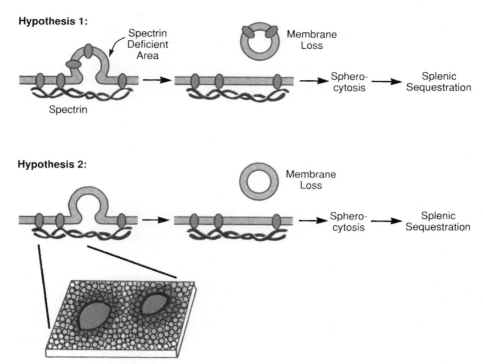

Figure 16–18. Two hypotheses concerning the mechanism of membrane loss in hereditary spherocytosis. *Hypothesis 1* assumes that the "membrane" (i.e., the lipid bilayer and integral membrane proteins) is directly stabilized by interactions with spectrin or other elements of the membrane skeleton. Spectrin-deficient areas, lacking support, bud off, leading to spherocytosis. *Hypothesis 2* assumes the membrane is stabilized by interactions of band 3 with neighboring lipids. The influence of band 3 extends into the lipid milieu because the first layer of immobilized lipids slows the lipids in the next layer and so on. In band 3–deficient cells the area between lipid molecules increases and unsupported lipids are lost. Spectrin/ankyrin deficiency allows band 3 molecules to diffuse and transiently cluster, with the same consequences. This hypothesis is supported by the fact that mice that lack band 3, owing to a targeted gene disruption, have marked membrane vesiculation and spherocytosis despite a nearly intact membrane skeleton.[603] (From Lux SE, Palek J: Disorders of the red cell membrane. In Handin RJ, Lux SE, Stossel TP (eds): Blood: Principles and Practice of Hematology. Philadelphia, Lippincott-Raven, 1995, pp 1701–1818.)

spaces between the endothelial cells that form the walls of the venous sinuses. Even when maximally distended, these narrow slits are always much smaller than red cells, which are greatly distorted during their passage.[826, 827] Numerous experiments show that spherocytes are selectively sequestered at this juncture.[830–832] As a consequence, spleens from patients with HS have massively congested cords and relatively empty sinuses.[824, 833–835] In electron micrographs, few spherocytes are seen in transit through the sinus wall,[824, 834, 836] which contrasts to the situation in normal spleens where cells in transit are readily found.[828]

Evidence is also abundant that HS red cells suffer during detention in the spleen. In unsplenectomized HS patients two populations of spherocytes are detectable: a minor population of hyperchromic "microspherocytes" that form the "tail" of very fragile cells in the unincubated osmotic fragility test and a major population that may be only slightly more spheroidal than normal. It was known by 1913 that red cells obtained from the splenic vein were more osmotically fragile than those in the peripheral circulation,[837] and this fact was confirmed by other hematologists of the time[683, 838]; however, its significance was not clear until the classic studies of Emerson and Young in the 1950s.[832, 839] These investigators showed that osmotically fragile microspherocytes are concentrated in and

emanate from the splenic pulp. After splenectomy, spherocytosis persists, but the tail of hyperfragile red cells is no longer evident. These and other data led to the conclusion that the spleen detains and "conditions" circulating HS red cells in a way that increases their spheroidicity and hastens their demise.[832, 840–842] The kinetics of this process were beautifully illustrated *in vivo* by Griggs, who found that a cohort of ^{59}Fe-labeled HS red cells gradually shifted from the major, less fragile population to the more fragile, conditioned population 7 to 11 days after their release into the circulation.[842] Although most conditioned HS red cells that escape the spleen are probably recaptured and destroyed, the damage incurred is sufficient to permit extrasplenic recognition and removal, because conditioned spherocytes, isolated from the spleen and reinfused postoperatively, are rapidly eliminated.[842, 843]

The mechanism of splenic conditioning is less certain. It is difficult to obtain accurate information about the cordal environment, but the existing data suggest it is metabolically inhospitable,[831, 840, 844, 845] though perhaps less so than originally believed.[829] Crowded red cells must compete for limited supplies of glucose[844] in acidic surroundings (pH $\sim$6.6–7.2)[829, 831, 840, 845] where glycolysis is inhibited.[846, 847] The acidic environment also induces Cl$^-$ and water entry and cell swelling[848] but, as discussed earlier, it also stimulates the K$^+$/Cl$^-$

cotransporter, which produces a net loss of K$^+$ and water from the cells. The adverse effects of the cordal environment are further compounded by the oxidant-producing macrophages. Hence, the spherocyte, detained in the splenic cords because of its surface deficiency, is stressed by erythrostasis in a metabolically threatening environment.

Erythrostasis. The hereditary spherocyte is particularly vulnerable to erythrostasis. This is the basis of the well known autohemolysis test.[849] During prolonged sterile incubation in the absence of supplemental glucose, red cells undergo a series of changes that culminate in hemolysis.[149] The sequence of the changes is the same for HS and normal erythrocytes; however, because HS cells are abnormally leaky and bear unstable membranes, their degeneration is accelerated. HS red cells are initially jeopardized because their membrane permeability to Na$^+$ is mildly increased.[772, 773] Their propensity to accumulate Na$^+$ and water is normally balanced by increased Na$^+$ pumping; however, the increased dependence on glycolysis is detrimental in erythrostasis where substrate is limited.[773] HS red cells exhaust serum glucose and become ATP depleted more rapidly than normal red cells. As ATP levels fall, ATP-dependent Na$^+$/K$^+$ and Ca^{2+} pumps fail, and the cells gain Na$^+$ and water and swell. Later, when the Ca^{2+}-dependent K$^+$ (Gárdos) pathway is activated, K$^+$ loss predominates and the cells lose water and shrink. The Na$^+$ gain is accelerated in HS red cells but is insufficient by itself to induce hemolysis. However, HS red cells are doubly jeopardized. As noted earlier, they are inherently unstable and fragment excessively during metabolic depletion.[812–816] Membrane lipids (and probably integral membrane proteins) are lost at more than twice the normal rate.[814] At first this surface loss is balanced by cell dehydration, but eventually (30 to 48 hours) membrane loss predominates, the cells exceed their critical hemolytic volume, and autohemolysis ensues.[149]

Splenic Trapping. Calculations indicate the average normal red cell passes through the splenic cords about 14,000 times during its lifetime[149] and has an average transit time of 30 to 40 seconds, surprisingly close to measured transient times in normal human spleens *in vivo*.[850] The calculated residence time of the average HS red cell in the splenic cords is much longer, perhaps as long as 15 to 150 minutes, but still far short of the time required for metabolic depletion to occur. This conclusion is supported by direct analysis of splenic red cells. HS red cells obtained from the splenic pulp and containing 80% to 100% conditioned cells are moderately cation depleted and show changes in adenosine diphosphate and 2,3-DPG concentrations consistent with metabolism in an acidic environment, but their ATP levels are normal.[778] Others have reported similar results.[851, 852]

The data suggest that splenic conditioning is caused by mechanisms other than ATP depletion. For example, K$^+$ loss and membrane instability may be exacerbated by the high concentrations of acids and oxidants that must exist in a spleen filled with activated macrophages lunching on trapped HS red cells. *In vitro*, oxi-

dants from activated phagocytes can diffuse across the membranes of bystander red cells and damage intracellular proteins within minutes. Red cells moving through the rapid transit pathways in the spleen might escape damage, but those caught in cordal traffic would be vulnerable. Oxidants, even in relatively low concentrations, cause selective K$^+$ loss by a variety of mechanisms[853–857] and also damage membrane skeletal proteins.[650, 667, 668, 858–861] Finally, there is preliminary evidence that HS red cells may be abnormally sensitive to oxidants.[862] When exposed to peroxides they undergo remarkable blebbing and, presumably, vesiculation.[862] If a similar process occurs in the spleen, it could be responsible for the excessive surface loss observed in conditioned cells.

Residence in the spleen may also activate proteolytic enzymes in the red cell membrane. Membrane proteins of HS red cells from patients with splenomegaly are excessively digested during *in vitro* incubations, and the degree of proteolysis correlates with splenic size.[863] Whether this occurs *in vivo* is uncertain, but if so it could contribute to skeletal weakness and membrane loss. The possibility that macrophages may directly condition HS red cells must also be considered. It is well known that spherocytosis often results from the interaction of IgG-coated red cells with macrophages, but HS red cells do not have abnormal levels of surface IgG.[864] Macrophages also bear receptors for oxidized lipids (scavenger receptor) and phosphatidyl serine, but there is no evidence at present that HS red cells expose the relevant ligands. The involvement of macrophages is supported by the old observations of Coleman and Finch,[865] recently confirmed,[866] that large doses of corticosteroids markedly ameliorate HS in nonsplenectomized patients. The effects are similar to those produced by splenectomy. Coleman and Finch observed that hemoglobin production, reticulocytosis, and fecal urobilinogen level declined; red cell life span doubled; and hyperspheroidal, conditioned red cells disappeared from the circulation. It is well known that similar doses of corticosteroids inhibit splenic processing and destruction of IgG- or C3b-coated red cells in patients with immunohemolytic anemias, probably by suppressing macrophage-induced red cell sphering and phagocytosis.[867, 868] Electron microscopy shows that splenic erythrophagocytosis is common in HS, particularly in the splenic cords.[834, 836, 869] In addition, phagocytes expressed from the cords of HS patients contain bits of ghostlike "debris,"[870] presumably resulting from membrane fragmentation.

In summary, it is clear that HS red cells are selectively detained by the spleen and that this custody is detrimental, leading to a loss of membrane surface that fosters further splenic trapping and eventual destruction. It appears that the primary membrane defects involve deficiencies or defects of spectrin, ankyrin, protein 4.2, or band 3, but much remains to be learned about why these proteins are defective and how this causes surface loss. Obvious membrane budding and fragmentation are rare in HS patients. The current speculation is that the HS skeleton (including band 3) may not adequately support all regions of the lipid bilayer,

Table 16-8. CHARACTERISTICS OF HEREDITARY SPHEROCYTOSIS

Clinical Manifestations

Anemia
Splenomegaly
Intermittent jaundice
  From hemolysis
  From biliary obstruction
Aplastic crises
Inheritance
  Dominant ~75%
  Nondominant ~25% *de novo* or recessive
Rare manifestations
  Leg ulcers
  Extramedullary hematopoietic tumors
  Myopathy or myocardiopathy
  Spinocerebellar ataxia
Excellent response to splenectomy

Laboratory Characteristics

Reticulocytosis
Spherocytosis
Elevated mean corpuscular hemoglobin concentration
Increased osmotic fragility and acidified glycerol lysis tests
Normal direct antiglobulin test

leading to loss of small areas of untethered lipids and integral membrane proteins (see Fig. 16–18). As discussed earlier, it is not clear whether this is due directly to deficiency of spectrin and ankyrin or whether spectrin/ankyrin deficiency operates indirectly by increasing the lateral mobility of band 3 molecules and decreasing their stabilization of the lipid bilayer. The mechanisms of splenic conditioning and red cell destruction are also uncertain. Kinetic considerations make it unlikely that HS red cells are continuously trapped in the cords for the long periods required to induce passive sphering and autohemolysis by metabolic depletion; however, repetitive accrual of metabolic damage remains a possibility. A special suscepti-

bility of the HS red cell to the acidic, oxidant-rich environment of the spleen and active intervention of macrophages in the processing of erythrostatically damaged spherocytes must also be considered.

Clinical and Laboratory Characteristics

Clinical Characteristics

Classification

Typical HS. The typical clinical picture of HS combines evidence of hemolysis (anemia, jaundice, reticulocytosis, gallstones, and splenomegaly) with spherocytosis (spherocytes on peripheral blood smear, positive osmotic fragility or acidified glycerol lysis tests), and a positive family history (Table 16–8). Mild, moderate, and severe forms of HS have been defined according to differences in the hemoglobin and bilirubin concentrations and the reticulocyte count (Table 16–9).[688, 714] Typical HS is associated with both dominant and recessive inheritance. In most cases, the recessive disease is more severe. There is, however, considerable overlap.[688, 694] Clinical severity and the response to splenectomy roughly parallel the degree of spectrin (or ankyrin) deficiency in patients with defects in either protein.[688, 694, 714, 717, 733] It is unknown if analogous correlations are true for patients with other HS-related mutations.

HS typically presents in infancy or childhood but may present at any age.[871] In children, anemia is the most frequent presenting complaint (50%), followed by splenomegaly, jaundice, or a positive family history.[872] No comparable data exist for adults. Two thirds to three fourths of HS patients have incompletely compensated hemolysis and mild to moderate anemia. The anemia is often asymptomatic except for fatigue and mild pallor or, in children, nonspecific parental complaints such as irritability. Jaundice is seen at some time in about half of patients, usually in association

Table 16-9. CLINICAL CLASSIFICATION OF HEREDITARY SPHEROCYTOSIS

Trait	Trait	Mild Spherocytosis	Moderate Spherocytosis	Moderately Severe Spherocytosis*	Severe Spherocytosis†
Hemoglobin (g/dL)	Normal	11–15	8–12	6–8	<6
Reticulocytes (%)	1–3	3–8	≥8	≥10	≥10
Bilirubin (mg/dL)	0–1	1–2	≥2	2–3	≥3
Spectrin content (% of normal)‡	100	80–100	50–80	40–80§	20–50
Peripheral smear	Normal	Mild spherocytosis	Spherocytosis	Spherocytosis	Spherocytosis and poikilocytosis
Osmotic fragility Fresh blood	Normal	Normal or slightly increased	Distinctly increased	Distinctly increased	Distinctly increased
Incubated blood	Slightly increased	Distinctly increased	Distinctly increased	Distinctly increased	Markedly increased

*Values in untransfused patients.
†By definition, patients with severe spherocytosis are transfusion dependent.
‡Normal (±SD) = 245 ± 27 × 10[5] spectrin dimers per erythrocyte. In most patients ankyrin content is decreased to a comparable degree. A minority of HS patients lack band 3 or protein 4.2 and may have mild to moderate spherocytosis with normal amounts of spectrin and ankyrin.
§The spectrin content is variable in this group of patients, presumably reflecting heterogeneity of the underlying pathophysiology.
Adapted from Eber SW, Armbrust R, Schröter W: Variable clinical severity of hereditary spherocytosis: relation to erythrocytic spectrin concentration, osmotic fragility and autohemolysis. J Pediatr 1990; 177: 409; Pekrun A, Eber SW, et al: Combined ankyrin and spectrin deficiency in hereditary spherocytosis. Ann Hematol 1993; 67: 89; and Lux SE, J Palek: Disorders of the red cell membrane. In Handin RI, Lux SE, Stossel TP (eds): Blood: Principles and Practice of Hematology. Philadelphia, J.B. Lippincott Co., 1995, pp 1701–1818.

with viral infections. When jaundice is present it is acholuric (i.e., unconjugated [indirect] hyperbilirubinemia without detectable direct bilirubinuria). Palpable splenomegaly is detectable in about half of infants and most (75% to 95%) older children and adults.[872–874] Typically, the spleen is modestly enlarged (2 to 6 cm), but it may be massive.[875, 876] There is no proven correlation between the size of the spleen and the severity of HS, although, given the pathophysiology and the response of the disease to splenectomy, such a correlation probably exists.

Silent Carrier State. The parents of patients with "nondominant" HS are clinically asymptomatic and do not have anemia, splenomegaly, hyperbilirubinemia, or spherocytosis on peripheral blood smears.[610, 694] But most do have subtle laboratory signs of HS, including slight reticulocytosis (average $2.1 \pm 0.8\%$), diminished haptoglobin levels, slightly elevated osmotic fragility, shortened acidified glycerol lysis time, or elevated autohemolysis. The incubated osmotic fragility test is probably the most sensitive measure of this condition, particularly the 100% lysis point, which is significantly elevated in carriers (0.43 ± 0.05 g NaCl/dL) compared with normal subjects (0.23 ± 0.07).[688] However, no single test is sufficient. Carriers can only be detected reliably by considering the results of a battery of tests. From the prevalence of recessive HS (1 in 20,000; that is, 25% of all HS, which is 1 in 5000 in the United States)[685] one can estimate that roughly 1.4% of the population should be silent carriers. Interestingly, screens of normal Norwegian[686] or German[687] blood donors with osmotic fragility or acidified glycerol lysis tests show a 0.9% to 1.1% incidence of previously unsuspected "very mild" HS. Presumably, many of these individuals are silent carriers.

Mild HS. Red cell production and destruction are balanced or nearly balanced in 20% to 30% of HS patients.[873, 877] These persons are considered to have "compensated hemolysis." Such patients are not anemic and are usually asymptomatic. In some cases, diagnosis may be difficult because hemolysis, splenomegaly, and spherocytosis are unusually mild. For example, in this group of patients, reticulocyte counts are generally less than 6% and only 60% have significant spherocytosis on peripheral blood smears[688]; red cell spectrin and ankyrin levels are typically more than 80% of normal.[688] Hemolysis may become severe with illnesses that cause splenomegaly, such as infectious mononucleosis.[878] Hemolysis may also be exacerbated by pregnancy[879, 880] or exercise,[881] to the point where it may impair athletic performance in endurance sports, even in patients with mild disease. Many of these patients are diagnosed during family studies or discovered as adults when splenomegaly or gallstones appear. Although mild HS is usually familial, it develops sporadically in families with more severe disease.[882] Presumably this is due to the co-inheritance of modifying genes, such as those affecting spectrin or ankyrin synthesis or splenic function.

One of the interesting mysteries about HS is why patients with compensated hemolysis continue to have erythroid hyperplasia when their hemoglobin levels are normal. It is difficult to reconcile this phenomenon with the generally accepted theory that erythropoiesis is regulated by tissue hypoxia. One possibility is the concentration of 2,3-DPG, which reportedly is low in hereditary spherocytes before splenectomy (although the P_{50} of HS blood is normal).[779, 783] Another possibility is that the dehydrated HS red cells are rheologically impaired[783] and do not perfuse the juxtaglomerular renal vessels, the site or erythropoietin production, normally, even when the hematocrit is normal. In fact, recent measurements show that erythropoietin is overproduced and serum erythropoietin is inappropriately elevated (up to eight times normal) in HS,[883] which is compatible with either possibility.

Moderate and Severe HS. A small fraction of HS patients (5% to 10%) have moderately severe to severe anemia.* Patients with "moderately severe" disease typically have a hemoglobin value of 6 to 8 g/dL, reticulocyte count of about 10%, a bilirubin level of 2 to 3 mg/dL, and 40% to 80% of the normal red cell spectrin content. This category includes patients with both dominant and recessive HS and a variety of molecular defects. Patients with "severe" disease, by definition, have life-threatening anemia and are transfusion dependent. They almost always have recessive HS. Most probably have isolated, severe spectrin deficiency (<40% of normal), which is thought to be due to a defect in α-spectrin.[718, 719] Some may have ankyrin defects.[732] Patients with severe HS are also distinguished by red cell morphology. They often have some irregularly contoured or budding spherocytes or bizarre poikilocytes in addition to typical spherocytes.[713, 732] Such cells are rare before splenectomy in patients with moderately severe disease, though some may be seen after splenectomy. In addition to the risks of recurrent transfusions, these patients often suffer from an aplastic crisis and those with severe HS may develop growth retardation, delayed sexual maturation, or aspects of thalassemic facies.[713, 875, 876]

HS in Pregnancy. In general, unsplenectomized patients with HS have no significant complications during pregnancy except for anemia, which worsens due to plasma volume expansion[886] and sometimes due to increased hemolysis.[879, 880] Hemolytic crises during pregnancy requiring transfusion have been reported.[880] Folic acid deficiency is also a risk.[887, 888] One group reported that 20% of HS patients were transfused during pregnancy,[880] but in the authors' experience, pregnant HS patients rarely need transfusion.

HS in the Neonate. HS frequently presents as jaundice in the first few days of life.[889–891] Perhaps as many as half of all HS patients have a history of neonatal jaundice[892] and 91% of infants discovered to have HS in the first week of life are jaundiced (bilirubin >10 mg/dL).[890] Hyperbilirubinemia usually appears in the first 2 days of life and may rise rapidly,[889, 891, 892] driven by the combination of hemolysis and the reduced capacity of the neonatal liver to conjugate bilirubin. Kernicterus is a risk,[889] so exchange transfusions

---

*See references 688, 690, 713, 717, 732, 882, 884, and 885.

are sometimes necessary, but in most cases the jaundice is controlled with phototherapy. Only 43% of neonates with HS are anemic (hemoglobin less than 15 g/dL), and severe anemia is rare.[890] Possibly, human infants with ankyrin defects, such as ankyrin-deficient *nb/nb* mice,[804, 805] are partially protected *in utero* by the expression of ankyrin-related proteins in embryonic and fetal erythroblasts. Hydrops fetalis has been reported in an infant with an apparent defect in α-spectrin.[690] Such infants may require intrauterine transfusions.

The diagnosis of HS is often more difficult in the neonatal period than later in life. Splenomegaly is uncommon; at most the spleen tip is palpable and reticulocytosis is variable and usually not severe.[891, 892] Only 35% of affected neonates have a reticulocyte count greater than 10%.[890] In addition, the haptoglobin level is not a reliable indicator of hemolysis during the first few months of life.[893] An even greater problem is that 33% of neonates with HS do not have significant numbers of spherocytes on their peripheral blood smears.[890] Moreover, because fetal red cells are more osmotically resistant than adult cells when fresh, and more osmotically sensitive after incubation at 37°C for 24 hours,[890, 894] the osmotic fragility test may give false-positive (incubated) or false-negative (unincubated) results unless fetal controls are used. Fortunately, these have been published[890] and they appear to reliably discriminate neonates with HS, particularly when the incubated osmotic fragility test is used.[890–892]

No evidence exists that patients with HS who are symptomatic as neonates have a more severe form of the disease. In fact, most become asymptomatic within the first few weeks of life. However, some infants become progressively more anemic and require transfusion. In the authors' experience this usually happens because the marrow response to anemia is more sluggish than normal. The reticulocyte count is relatively low for the degree of anemia. Fortunately, the problem is transient, except in rare patients with severe HS, and

usually remits after one or two transfusions. If the child is otherwise well, the authors allow the hemoglobin level to fall to 5.5 to 6.5 g/dL before transfusing to try and stimulate the marrow, and they only raise the hemoglobin to 9 to 11 g/dL after transfusion to avoid suppressing the desired marrow response. Once the bone marrow responds, the course of the disease depends on the equilibrium between the rates of red cell production and destruction.

Laboratory Features

Peripheral Blood Smear. Spherocytes (Fig. 16–19) are the hallmark of HS. They are dense, round, and hyperchromic, lack central pallor, and have a decreased mean cell diameter. They are almost uniformly present (up to 97%) on blood smears from patients with moderate or moderately severe HS[688] but are present in only 25% to 35% of patients with mild HS.[688, 872, 873] Hereditary spherocytes are technically misnamed; they range in shape from thickened discocytes to spherostomatocytes.[808]

In most HS patients, spherocytes and microspherocytes are the only abnormal cells on the peripheral smear (other than polychromatophils). Rarely, a few stomatospherocytes may be seen. In severe HS, dense, irregular, contracted, or budding spherocytes may appear; and in the most severe cases, these abnormal forms may dominate the blood smear.

Specific morphologic abnormalities have been described in association with some membrane defects in HS. Before splenectomy, patients with band 3–deficient HS may have a small number of mushroom-shaped red cells or "pincered" cells on peripheral blood films.[158] Acanthocytes or hyperchromic echinocytes are present in many patients with β-spectrin defects[725] before splenectomy and increase after the operation. Other patients with β-spectrin defects, especially truncated β chains, have spherocytic elliptocytosis (to be dis-

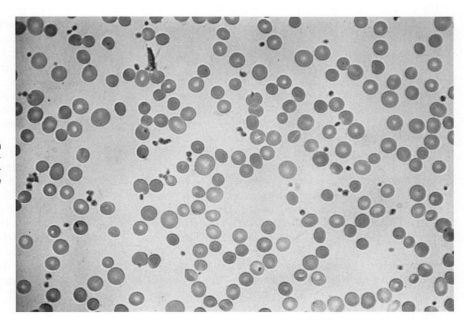

Figure 16–19. Peripheral blood smear from a patient with typical hereditary spherocytosis. Small, dense, round, conditioned microspherocytes are visible throughout the smear.

cussed). Acanthopoikilocytes[753] and ovalostomatocytes[751] have been observed in some patients with protein 4.2 deficiency. Other patients have typical spherocytosis.[493] No specific morphologic abnormality other than spherocytosis has been identified in patients with ankyrin defects—probably the most common subgroup.[695] Bone marrow erythroblasts are morphologically normal[895] and reticulocytes are only slightly spheroidal[896] in typical HS, because erythrocytes gradually acquire the spherocytic shape in the circulation. Nucleated red cells are uncommon in blood smears[872] except in the most severe forms of HS.[713] Howell-Jolly bodies are also uncommon before splenectomy (4% of patients)[872] and suggest reticuloendothelial blockade.[885] When examining a smear in a case of suspected spherocytosis, it is important that it be a high-quality smear with the erythrocytes well separated and some cells with central pallor in the field of examination, because spherocytes are a common artifact on peripheral blood smears.

Red Cell Indices. Most patients have mild to moderate HS with mild anemia (hemoglobin = 9 to 12 g/dL) or no anemia at all (so-called compensated hemolysis). In moderate to severe HS, the hemoglobin concentration ranges from 6 to 9 g/dL. In the most severe cases, the hemoglobin may drop to levels as low as 4 to 5 g/dL. The mean corpuscular hemoglobin concentration (MCHC) of HS red cells is increased, owing to relative cellular dehydration.[873] Spherocyte Na^+ concentrations are normal or slightly increased, but K^+ concentration and water content are low, particularly in cells harvested from the splenic pulp.[778, 897–898] The average MCHC exceeds the upper limit of normal (36%) in about half of HS patients, but all patients have some dehydrated cells.[873] The Technicon H1 blood counter and its successors (Technicon Corp., Tarrytown, NY), which measure mean corpuscular volume (MCV) by light scattering, provide a histogram of MCHCs that has been claimed to be accurate enough to identify nearly all HS patients.[899–901] This may be one of the easiest and most accurate ways to diagnose HS, particularly when one member of a family is already known to have HS and an inexpensive method of screening other family members is desired. The MCH and MCV fall within the normal range in HS,[873] except in severe HS in which the MCV may be slightly low.[713] However, the MCV is relatively low for the age of the cells (reticulocytes have a high MCV) in all HS patients, reflecting the dehydrated state of HS red cells.

Osmotic Fragility Test. In the normal erythrocyte, a redundancy of cell membrane gives the cell its characteristic discoid shape and provides it with abundant surface area relative to cell volume. In spherocytes, there is a decrease in surface area relative to cell volume, resulting in the characteristic osmotic fragility. Osmotic fragility testing (Fig. 16–20) is performed by suspending red cells in increasingly hypotonic buffered NaCl.[840, 902, 903] In hypotonic solutions, normal erythrocytes are able to increase their volume by swelling until they become spherical and burst, releasing hemoglobin into the supernatant. Cells that begin with a decreased surface/volume ratio, like spherocytes or stomatocytes,

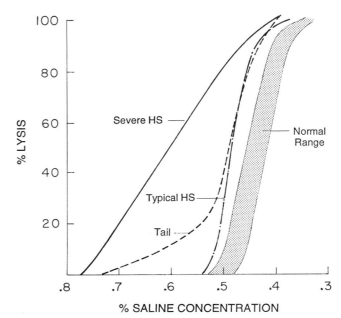

Figure 16–20. Osmotic fragility curves in hereditary spherocytosis. The *shaded area* is the normal range. Results representative of both typical and severe spherocytosis are shown. A "tail," representing very fragile erythrocytes that have been conditioned by the spleen, is common in many patients with hereditary spherocytosis before splenectomy.

reach the spherical limit at a higher NaCl concentration than normal cells, and are termed *osmotically fragile.* Approximately one fourth of individuals with HS will have a normal osmotic fragility on freshly drawn red cells, with the osmotic fragility curve approximating the number of spherocytes seen on peripheral smear.[874, 904] However, after incubation at 37°C for 24 hours, HS red cells lose membrane surface area more readily than normal because their membranes are leaky and unstable. This incubation accentuates the defect in HS erythrocytes and brings out the defect on osmotic fragility, making osmotic fragility testing the most sensitive test routinely available for diagnosing HS.[904] This is surprising because osmotic fragility reflects a secondary property of HS red cells, the loss of surface area, instead of the primary molecular defect. When the spleen is present, a subpopulation of very fragile erythrocytes that have been conditioned by the spleen form the "tail" of the osmotic fragility curve. This tail disappears after splenectomy.

Modifications of the osmotic fragility test have been proposed. Some have suggested that addition of 3 μM of ouabain during the 24-hour preincubation increases the sensitivity of the incubated osmotic fragility test, particularly for mildly affected subjects.[905, 906] Unfortunately, this was not confirmed in a separate study.[907] Another group has employed logarithmic transforms of the osmotic fragility curve to simplify calculation of the 50% hemolysis point[908]; however, this de-emphasizes the beginning and endpoints of hemolysis, which can be diagnostically useful in some patients and in silent carriers.[688] The state-of-the-art method for demonstrating the low surface/volume ratio of hereditary spherocytes is osmotic gradient ektacytometry.[909] However, only a few clinical laboratories are equipped with this instrumentation.

Additional Diagnostic Tests

Acidified Glycerol Lysis Test and Pink Test. The glycerol lysis test, in which glycerol is employed to retard the osmotic swelling of red cells, was developed as an alternative to the osmotic fragility test. It is based on the rate rather than the extent of hemolysis. The original glycerol lysis test[910] lacked sensitivity and specificity.[911] An acidified version, the acidified glycerol lysis test (AGLT), was more sensitive in some hands[912] but was not completely specific.[913] For unknown reasons, the accuracy of the standard AGLT is greatly improved if the samples are preincubated at room temperature for 24 hours (incubated AGLT).[914-916] Under these conditions, in some investigators hands, the sensitivity and specificity of the test approach 100%, similar to the incubated osmotic fragility test. Eber found that changing the concentration of the sodium phosphate buffer from 5.3 to 9.3 mM gives 100% sensitivity and specificity without the need for preincubation.[687] The modified test is easy to perform and requires very little blood. Ethylenediaminetetraacetic acid (EDTA)-anticoagulated blood (20 μL) is diluted into a solution of 9.3 mM sodium phosphate and buffered 2 M glycerol-saline (pH 6.90), and the fall in absorbance at 625 nm (largely turbidity) is measured as the red cells hemolyze. The half-time for AGLT lysis is more than 30 minutes for normal samples and less than 5 minutes for HS samples. Another adaptation of the original glycerol lysis test, called the Pink test, is more reproducible and accurate than the original[917] but requires a 1-day preincubation.[918] Modifications of the test have made it adaptable to micro size samples (e.g., use fingerstick blood samples).[918, 919] However, direct comparisons suggest it is less specific than the osmotic fragility or incubated AGLT tests.[914] Because the modified AGLT test has also been adapted to micro samples,[687] it would appear to be the test of choice if osmotic fragility testing is not available.

Hypertonic Cryohemolysis Test. This method is based on the fact that HS red cells are particularly sensitive to cooling at 0°C in hypertonic solutions.[920] It has been claimed that this test is 100% sensitive for HS, but the specificity is only 94% for normal individuals and 86% for patients with autoimmune hemolytic anemia. The test is independent of the surface/volume ratio of the cells, which is an advantage compared with other diagnostic tests. The use of this test awaits independent verification of its sensitivity and specificity.

Autohemolysis Test. The autohemolysis of erythrocytes after 48 hours at 37°C is normally less than 5% in the absence of glucose or less than 1% in the presence of glucose. Autohemolysis of spherocytes is increased to 15% to 45% in the absence of glucose.[849, 874, 921] In HS, the degree of autohemolysis is reduced by the addition of glucose,[874, 898, 921] whereas in acquired disorders such as immune-mediated anemias, the degree of autohemolysis is not reduced. Thus, if positive, the autohemolysis test suggests an intrinsic red cell abnormality whereas a negative test is noncontributory. Although this differentiation may be helpful, the autohemolysis test is time consuming, cumbersome, variable, and only rarely performed.

Membrane Protein Analysis. Specialized testing is available for studying difficult cases or cases in which additional information is desired. Useful tests for these purposes include structural and functional studies of erythrocyte membrane proteins such as protein quantitation (see later), limited tryptic digestion of spectrin, membrane protein synthesis and assembly, or ion transport studies. Membrane rigidity and fragility may be examined using an ektacytometer.

Membrane Protein Quantitation. Membrane protein concentrations are usually assessed using SDS gels. Individual stained bands are quantified by densitometry or by eluting the dye from an excised band and measuring its concentration spectrophotometrically. This technique is satisfactory for detecting spectrin deficiency (expressed as a spectrin/band 3 ratio),[922] although it is not as accurate as a radioimmunoassay[608, 713] or enzyme-linked immunoassay.[714] Densitometry may underestimate spectrin and ankyrin deficiencies because it normalizes them to band 3, which is partially lost along with membrane lipids as spherocytes circulate. As a result, the spectrin/band 3 ratio is lower after splenectomy. This is even more true for ankyrin, which is present in smaller amounts and migrates close to β-spectrin on gels. SDS gels do not routinely give reliable results even with a gel system that optimizes the spectrin/ankyrin separation.[713] The popular Laemmli gels are completely unsatisfactory because ankyrin migrates between the spectrin bands in this system. Immunoassays, on the other hand, work well.[714, 733] SDS gels are satisfactory for detecting band 3 deficiency (elevated spectrin/band 3 ratio) or protein 4.2 deficiency and are useful in combination with antibody staining (Western blots) for detecting mutant proteins of altered size. However, in the authors' experience direct quantitation of membrane proteins rarely detects patients missed by the incubated osmotic fragility test[2] and is a lot more difficult and expensive to perform.

Determination of the Molecular Defect. In cases in which molecular diagnosis is desired, studies of membrane proteins, as described earlier, may implicate a specific membrane protein. In other cases there is no clue to the underlying molecular defect. In these cases, linkage analysis has been performed to include or exclude the candidate genes. Various mutation detection screening techniques have been employed, the most popular of which is single-stranded conformation polymorphism (SSCP) analysis. Mutation detection can be performed using direct nucleotide sequence analysis of polymerase chain reaction (PCR)-amplified cDNA or genomic DNA.

Other Laboratory Findings. Other laboratory features in HS are manifestations of ongoing hemolysis and reflect increased erythrocyte destruction and production. These include reticulocytosis, erythroid hyperplasia of the bone marrow, indirect hyperbilirubinemia, and increased fecal urobilinogens.[872, 873, 923] The plasma hemoglobin level is frequently normal,[924] and the haptoglobin value is only variably reduced,[925] because most of the hemoglobin that is released when hereditary spherocytes are destroyed is catabolized at the site of destruction, so-called extravascular hemolysis. Haptoglobin may be decreased or absent in neonates, and thus is an unreliable marker of hemolysis in the newborn.

Complications

Most patients with HS have a well-compensated hemolysis and are rarely symptomatic. It is only when complications occur that these patients are brought to medical attention. Complications are generally related to chronic hemolysis and anemia.

Gallstones. The formation of bilirubinate gallstones is one of the most common complications of HS and is a major impetus for splenectomy in many patients. Cases of gallstones occurring in infancy[926] have been reported, but most appear in adolescents and young adults. In a retrospective study of 152 consecutive cases of HS, conducted before the development of ultrasonography, approximately half of HS patients developed detectable gallstones between 10 and 30 years of age.[927] Gallstones were detected in only 5% of children younger than 10 years old who were adequately examined. The rise in the incidence of gallstones after age 30 paralleled the incidence in the general population,[927] which suggests that cholelithiasis owing to HS is primarily manifest in the second and third decades.

Unfortunately, longitudinal studies using modern techniques (i.e., liver and biliary tree ultrasonography) are not available, making the true incidence and natural history of gallstones in this population unknown. Indeed, many patients with gallstones are asymptomatic, and it is unclear how many will develop symptomatic gallbladder disease or biliary obstruction. Anecdotal reports in the old HS literature suggested that 40% to 50% of HS patients with cholelithiasis had symptoms and that a high proportion of stone-containing gallbladders had histologic evidence of cholecystitis.[928] However, studies that include large numbers of patients with mild HS show a much lower incidence of symptomatic gallbladder disease.[929] Clearly, more accurate data about the long-term complications of pigment stone disease are needed to assess the risk-benefit ratio of splenectomy in HS and the need for cholecystectomy in the asymptomatic patient with cholelithiasis. Because the pigment stones typical of HS are easily detected by ultrasonography, all HS patients should have ultrasound examinations about every 5 years and before splenectomy.

Crises

Hemolytic Crises. Patients with HS, like patients with other hemolytic diseases such as sickle cell disease, face a number of potential "crises." Hemolytic crises are probably the most frequent of these, particularly mild hemolytic crises, which usually occur with viral syndromes, particularly in children younger than age 6. They are characterized by a mild transient increase in jaundice, splenomegaly, anemia, and reticulocytosis. No medical intervention is required. Some of these patients may actually be in the recovery phase of an aplastic crisis. Severe hemolytic crises occur, but they are rare. Characteristic features include jaundice, anemia, vomiting, abdominal pain, and tender splenomegaly. Hospitalization, erythrocyte transfusion, and careful monitoring may be required.

Aplastic Crises, Parvovirus B19. Aplastic crises are less frequent than hemolytic crises but are more serious and may lead to severe anemia, resulting in congestive heart failure or even death.[683, 875] They are usually caused by parvovirus B19, the etiologic of erythema infectiosum (fifth disease).[930] Parvovirus B19 infection may present as fever, chills, lethargy, vomiting, diarrhea, myalgias, and a maculopapular rash on the face (slapped cheek syndrome), trunk, and extremities. In addition, the HS patient with an aplastic crisis may experience anemia, jaundice, pallor, and weakness.[931, 932] Parvovirus B19 selectively infects erythropoietic precursors and inhibits their growth.[933, 934] Parvovirus infections are often associated with mild neutropenia or thrombocytopenia, and a few cases of transient pancytopenia have been reported.[935, 936] Infection with parvovirus B19 is a particular danger to susceptible pregnant women, because it can infect the fetus, leading to fetal anemia, nonimmune hydrops fetalis, and fetal demise.[937–939] The risk of nonimmune hydrops fetalis to the fetus of women who become infected with B19 during pregnancy is low.[938] Nevertheless, because the virus is highly contagious and is easily transmitted to patients and staff,[940, 941] and because only about half of the pregnant population have acquired protective antibodies, it has been suggested that patients who have or are suspected of having an aplastic crisis should be placed on precautions while hospitalized and IgG-negative contacts who are pregnant should be tested for evidence of seroconversion. Nonimmune hydrops fetalis can be detected by ultrasonography and has been successfully treated with intrauterine transfusions.[942] Parvovirus may infect multiple members of a family simultaneously.[943]

The sequence of events in an aplastic crisis is well described in the classic article of Owren[931] and is illustrated in Figure 16–21. During the aplastic phase, the hematocrit level and reticulocyte count fall, marrow erythroblasts disappear, and unused iron accumulates in the serum. Giant pronormoblasts often appear and are a hallmark of the cytopathic effects of parvovirus B19.[944] As production of new red cells declines, the cells that remain age and microspherocytosis and osmotic fragility increase. Bilirubin levels may decrease as the number of abnormal red cells that can be destroyed declines. The return of marrow function is heralded by a fall in the serum iron concentration and the emergence of granulocytes, platelets, and, finally, reticulocytes. The lack of reticulocytes early in the recovery phase should not eliminate hemolytic anemias from diagnostic consideration.

It is during an aplastic crisis that many asymptomatic HS patients with normally compensated hemolysis come to medical attention.[945, 946] As would be expected, multiple family members with undiagnosed HS who

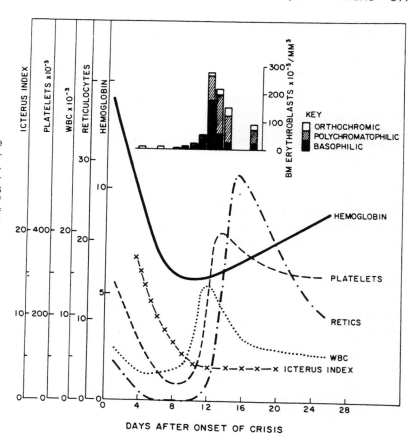

Figure 16–21. The temporal sequence of a severe aplastic crisis in a patient with hereditary spherocytosis who previously had well-compensated hemolysis. Note the profound reticulocytopenia and mild leukopenia and thrombocytopenia in the early phases of the reaction. Note also that the re-emergence of reticulocytes is heralded by the sequential return of peripheral blood granulocytes and platelets and bone marrow normoblasts. As in this patient, jaundice frequently declines during an aplastic crisis because of a decrease in the total number of abnormal red cells that have to be destroyed. (Data replotted from Owren PA: Congenital hemolytic jaundice. The pathogenesis of the "hemolytic crisis." Blood 1948; 3:231.)

are infected with parvovirus B19 have developed aplastic crises at the same time.[943] This phenomenon has led to reports of "epidemics" or "outbreaks" of HS. Diagnostic confusion may arise during re-emergence of marrow function, when the physician may mistake an aplastic crisis for a hemolytic one. Because aplastic crises usually last 10 to 14 days[931] (about half the life span of HS red cells),[850, 947] the hemoglobin value typically falls to about half its usual level before recovery occurs. Thus, aplastic crises are a serious threat to young children with HS, particularly children with more severe forms of the disease. Intensive medical management is required in these cases. The alert clinician will recognize the signs and symptoms of an aplastic crisis and be prepared for expectant management. A phase I vaccine trial with recombinant parvovirus B19–like particles is underway.

Megaloblastic Crises. Rarely, patients may present with megaloblastic crises due to folate deficiency. This typically occurs in HS patients recovering from an aplastic crisis or in the pregnant HS patient.[887, 888] In these cases, the dietary intake of folic acid is inadequate for the increased needs of the erythroid HS bone marrow. Megaloblastic crisis in pregnancy has been reported as the first manifestation of HS. All patients with hemolytic anemias, including HS, should routinely receive folic acid supplements (~1 mg/d) to prevent this complication.

Other Complications

Gout, Leg Ulcers. Rarely, adults with HS develop gout,[948, 949] indolent leg ulcers,[950, 951] or a chronic erythematous dermatitis on the legs.[952] All three problems are corrected by splenectomy.

Extramedullary Hematopoiesis. Adults with HS may also develop extramedullary masses of hematopoietic tissue, particularly alongside the posterior thoracic or lumbar spine[683, 949, 953–957] or in the hila of the kidneys.[683] Surprisingly, these tumors often arise in patients with mild HS, perhaps because they frequently escape splenectomy, and are the first manifestations of HS. The masses gradually enlarge and may be mistaken for neoplasms.[949] Biopsy may lead to extensive bleeding.[949] If necessary, an open biopsy should be performed. These bone marrow tumors can be diagnosed by magnetic resonance imaging,[957] which may make biopsies unnecessary. The masses stop growing and undergo fatty metamorphosis after splenectomy, but they do not shrink in size.[953, 955]

Multiple Myeloma. Untreated HS may predispose patients to multiple myeloma. Four patients with HS and myeloma have been reported.[958–960] None was splenectomized, two had gallbladder disease, and one had silicosis. It has been suggested that the association may be due to chronic reticuloendothelial stimulation because splenic clearance of abnormal red cells induces proliferation of lymphocytes and plasma cells as well as macrophages.[961] HS patients have a mild, polyclonal hypergammaglobulinemia,[958, 962] and there is a small amount of evidence favoring the association of myeloma and chronic gallbladder disease.[958, 963] Untreated HS may also exacerbate hemochromatosis in patients who are heterozygous for the hereditary disease.[964–967]

Several HS patients subsequently died of liver failure or hepatoma.

Heart Disease. Untreated HS may aggravate underlying heart disease and precipitate heart failure.[968] Gradually worsening congestive heart failure may rarely be the presenting complaint in an elderly HS patient who has developed progressively worsening anemia as marrow senescence evolves.

Angioid Streaks. These brownish or gray streaks resembling veins in the optic fundus have been described in adult members of several HS kindreds.[969, 970] The frequency of this association is unknown. Angioid streaks are relatively common in some other hematologic disorders, notably sickle cell disease and thalassemia,[969, 971] and may be complicated by retinal vascular proliferation requiring treatment.[972]

Diagnostic Problems

In general, HS is easily diagnosed and differentiated from other causes of spherocytosis, but there are several situations in which diagnosis can be difficult. In the neonatal period it may be hard to differentiate HS from ABO incompatibility. Anemia, hyperbilirubinemia, circulating microspherocytes, and altered osmotic fragility are found in both conditions and the direct antiglobulin test is sometimes negative in ABO incompatibility. However, in most affected infants with ABO incompatibility, anti-A (or -B) antibodies can be eluted from the red cells, and free anti-A (or -B) IgG antibodies can be detected in the infant's serum. Occasionally, older patients with immunohemolytic anemias and spherocytosis also have so few antibody molecules attached to their red cells that the direct antiglobulin test is negative and differentiation of the disease from HS is possible only with the use of radioactive antiglobulin reagents.[973]

Spherocytosis is also seen in Heinz body hemolytic anemias during an acute hemolytic crisis and occasionally in the steady state. The diagnosis of Heinz body anemia is suggested by the presence of bite cells and blister cells on peripheral blood films and by detecting Heinz bodies in red cells stained with methyl violet.

As noted earlier, diagnostic difficulties also arise in patients who present during an aplastic crisis. Early in the crisis, the acute nature of the symptoms may suggest an acquired process and the absence of reticulocytes may divert the physician from a diagnosis of hemolytic anemia. Later, as marrow function returns, physicians may occasionally be misled by the properties of the emerging young HS red cells, which are less spherocytic and osmotically fragile than usual.[896]

HS may be camouflaged by disorders that increase the surface/volume ratio of the red cells, such as obstructive jaundice,[809] iron deficiency,[974] β-thalassemia,[975] vitamin B_{12} or folate deficiency,[976] or hemoglobin SC disease.[977] Spherocytosis is transiently improved and both the osmotic fragility test and hemolysis normalize when obstructive jaundice develops.[809] This is due to the expansion of red cell membrane surface area that follows the increased uptake of cholesterol and phospholipids from the abnormal plasma lipoproteins. In normal cells, this increase in surface area leads to the formation of target cells (see later), but, in spherocytes, it leads to the appearance of discocytes. For example, we have seen a young girl who developed jaundice and symptoms of biliary obstruction at 6 years of age. She had a palpable spleen tip, evidence of mild compensated hemolysis (hemoglobin = 14 g/dL; reticulocytes = 3.3%), and a normal peripheral blood smear and osmotic fragility test (fresh and incubated). Abdominal radiographic studies showed calcified stones in the gallbladder and common bile duct. After cholecystectomy and relief of the partial biliary obstruction, the child's hemolysis worsened (reticulocytes = 10.8%) and she developed anemia (hemoglobin = 10.2 g/dL), spherocytosis, and a definitely abnormal incubated osmotic fragility test. She subsequently responded to splenectomy.

In a similar manner, iron deficiency corrects the abnormal shape, fragility, and high MCHC of hereditary spherocytes but does not improve their life span.[974] Megaloblastic anemia can also mask HS, at least the morphologic characteristics of the disease.[976] Osmotic fragility is also improved. The masking effect is observed in both vitamin B_{12} and folate deficiencies and is rapidly reversed after correction of the nutritional deficit.

The coexistence of HS and β-thalassemia trait has been described in a few case reports. It has been reported to worsen,[978, 979] ameliorate,[975, 980] or have no effect on the clinical status of the patient. In a large French family with independently segregating HS and β-thalassemia trait, patients with both traits had signs of both diseases: small, hemoglobin A_2-rich, osmotically fragile cells and some spherocytes on peripheral blood smears. However, the HS phenotype in these patients was less severe than that of HS family members without β-thalassemia trait.[975]

Co-inheritance of HS and hemoglobin SC disease may exacerbate the hemoglobinopathy.[977] A 14-year-old boy with both diseases was much more anemic than his SC siblings and had experienced five splenic sequestration crises. However, the two diseases may also disguise each other, at least partially. Only a few spherocytes or target cells were evident on the boy's blood smear and the surface/volume ratio of his red cells (and probably their osmotic fragility) was normal. Presumably this is due to the balancing effects of HS (loss of surface area) and hemoglobin SC (loss of cell volume) on red cells. Even sickle trait may be worsened by HS. Yang and colleagues[981] reported two patients with the combination who suffered multiple splenic sequestration crises. On the other hand, spontaneous regression of HS, presumably due to development of a hyposplenic state, has been observed in two family members who had HS and sickle cell trait.[982]

Nonerythroid Manifestations

Kindreds with HS and neurologic or muscular manifestations have been described. Patients with interstitial gene deletions (chromosome 8p11.1–8p21.1) that include ankyrin and many neighboring genes have psychomotor retardation and hypogonadism.[491, 739–742] Coetzer and co-workers[732] described a patient with an-kyrin-deficient atypical HS and various neurologic manifestations. Two patients with HS and slowly pro-gressive spinocerebellar degenerative disease were re-ported by McCann and Jacob.[796] Two brothers with HS, a movement disorder, and myopathy have also been described.[803] A three-generation Russian family with co-segregating HS and hypertrophic cardiomyopathy has been reported.[983] Additional case reports in the older literature describe patients with HS and various neurologic abnormalities such as Friedreich's disease, cerebellar disturbances, muscle atrophy, and a tabes-like syndrome.[795–799]

The observation that erythrocyte ankyrin and eryth-rocyte β-spectrin are also expressed in muscle,[148, 436, 437] brain, and the spinal cord[148, 438, 443] raises the possibility that these HS patients may suffer from defects of one of these proteins. This hypothesis is further supported by studies of ankyrin-deficient *nb/nb* mice. These mice have almost no detectable ankyrin-1 and suffer from a severe, spherocytic hemolytic anemia and a late-onset cerebellar ataxia that parallels a gradual loss of Purkinje cells.[438]

Treatment and Outcome

Splenectomy

Splenectomy cures almost all patients with typical HS, eliminating anemia and hyperbilirubinemia, and re-ducing the reticulocyte count to near-normal levels (1% to 3%). In most patients, red cell survival becomes normal or remains only slightly shortened. Spherocyto-sis and altered osmotic fragility persist, but the "tail" of the osmotic fragility curve, created by conditioning of a subpopulation of spherocytes by the spleen, disap-pears. After splenectomy, patients with the most severe forms of HS still suffer from shortened erythrocyte survival and hemolysis but their clinical improvement is striking.[694, 713]

Early complications of splenectomy include local in-fection or bleeding and pancreatitis, presumably due to injury to the tail of the pancreas incurred during removal of the spleen.[984] In general, the morbidity of splenectomy for HS is lower than that of other hemato-logic disorders. However, the indications for splenec-tomy should be weighed carefully, because a small fraction of patients will die of overwhelming postsple-nectomy infections.[985–993] Because the risk of postsple-nectomy sepsis is very high in infancy and early child-hood, splenectomy should be delayed until the age of 5 to 9 years if possible, and to at least 3 years in all cases, even if chronic transfusions are required in the interim. There is no evidence that further delay is useful, and it may be harmful, because the risk of cholelithiasis increases dramatically in children after the age of 10 years.[927]

Risks

Postsplenectomy Sepsis. It is difficult to estimate the risk of postsplenectomy infections after infancy (see also Chapter 26). The surveys of Schwartz and col-leagues[991] and Green and co-workers[987] are limited to adults and largely predate immunization for *Streptococ-cus pneumoniae* and other bacteria. They show an incidence of fulminant sepsis of 0.2 to 0.5/100 person-years of follow-up and a death rate of 0.1/100 person-years. In addition, other serious bacterial infections (e.g., pneumonia, meningitis, peritonitis, bacteremia) were much more common (4.5/100 person-years) than normal, particularly in the first few years after the operation. More recently, Schilling[993] reported a post-splenectomy mortality rate of 0.073/100 person-years, which is substantially better than the risk reported in the earlier studies.[987, 991] There was no significant difference in the risk of fatal sepsis for splenectomies performed before or after the age of 6 in the Schilling study, and three of the four deaths occurred 18 years or more after the operation. None of the patients who died had received pneumococcal vaccine, and none were taking prophylactic penicillin. The risk of infec-tion would presumably be lower today, when pneumo-coccal immunization is routine (see later), because 50% to 70% of postsplenectomy sepsis is due to *S. pneumon-iae* and about 80% of pneumococcal disease is due to strains contained in the vaccine. Further risk reduction would be anticipated from the chronic use of prophy-lactic penicillin. In fact, Danish researchers have shown that the incidence of pneumococcal infection after sple-nectomy is dramatically lower since the introduction of pneumococcal vaccine and the promotion of early antibiotic therapy for febrile children who have had a splenectomy.[994] Nevertheless, the risk cannot be re-duced to zero. Postsplenectomy infections occur occa-sionally in successfully immunized patients,[995–998] and compliance regarding prophylactic medications is a problem, particularly in teenagers.[999]

Penicillin-Resistant Pneumococci. Penicillin-resis-tant pneumococci are increasing very rapidly all over the world.[1000–1002] In some countries, more than half of all isolates are resistant.[1003] In the United States, the prevalence is 5% to 10% but is much higher in some localities and is rising.[1000, 1004] Risk factors for the devel-opment of resistant strains include previous antibiotic use, repeat hospitalizations, and day care attendance. Although most of the strains show some sensitivity to penicillin, some are highly resistant and others are multiply resistant.[1005–1007] The emergence of these strains will greatly complicate the use of antibiotics for pneu-mococcal prophylaxis during the next decade. Already, multidrug resistant strains have been isolated from pediatric patients in the United States with sickle cell anemia.[1006] For patients in selected parts of the world, consideration must also be given to the greater risk of red cell parasitic diseases, such as falciparum malaria and babesiosis, in splenectomized hosts.[1008–1011]

Ischemic Heart Disease. The risk of ischemic heart disease may also increase after splenectomy. In one study, Robinette and Fraumeni[1012] observed that death from ischemic heart disease occurred 1.86 times as often in splenectomized young men as in matched controls during a 28-year period of follow-up, a sig-nificant difference. The reason for this observation is unknown, but it has been attributed to the chronically higher platelet count observed after splenectomy.

Indications

Considering the risks and benefits, the following approach is recommended:

1. All patients with severe spherocytosis, including those with growth failure or skeletal changes, should be splenectomized.

2. Splenectomy is usually recommended for patients with moderate HS if they suffer from reduced vitality or physical stamina due to anemia, if, later in life, anemia compromises vascular perfusion of vital organs, or if leg ulcers or extramedullary hematopoietic tumors develop.

3. Whether patients with moderate HS and asymptomatic anemia should have a splenectomy remains controversial.

4. Splenectomy can be deferred, probably indefinitely, in patients with mild HS and compensated hemolysis.

5. The treatment of patients with mild to moderate HS and gallstones is also debatable, particularly because new treatments for gallstones such as laparoscopic cholecystectomy, endoscopic sphincterotomy, and extracorporal choletripsy, lower the risk of this complication.[1013–1015] If such patients have symptomatic gallstones, the authors and others favor a combined cholecystectomy and splenectomy,[1016] particularly if acute cholecystitis or biliary obstruction has occurred. There is no evidence that staging cholecystectomy and splenectomy, as was done in the past, is of any benefit.

Laparoscopic Splenectomy. When splenectomy is warranted, laparoscopic splenectomy is becoming the method of choice in many centers.[1017–1026] The procedure can be combined with laparoscopic cholecystectomy if desired.[1018, 1019, 1025] Although laparoscopic splenectomy requires a longer operative time than open splenectomy,[1017, 1025] it results in less postoperative discomfort, a quicker return to preoperative diet and activities, shorter hospitalization, decreased costs, and smaller scars.[1022, 1024, 1025] However, there is an increased risk of bleeding during the operation and 10% to 15% of the laparoscopic operations (for all causes) have to be converted to standard splenectomies.[1018, 1019, 1026] It is also not clear whether accessory spleens are more easily missed during laparoscopic splenectomies. Even enormous spleens (>600 g) can be removed laparoscopically,[1021, 1023] because the spleen is placed in a large nylon bag, diced, and eliminated by suction catheters. However, some surgeons believe the risk of blood loss is greater when large spleens are removed and recommend the technique be limited to small spleens.[1023, 1026] The longer operative times required for the procedure undoubtedly decrease with experience.

Partial (Subtotal) Splenectomy. The emergence of antibiotic-resistant pneumococci has led to re-examination of the role of alternate treatment modalities. Partial splenectomy has been suggested for selected HS patients, especially patients with mild to moderate disease. The goal of this operation is to decrease the hemolysis while maintaining some residual splenic phagocytic function. In practice, at least 90% of the enlarged organ is removed (Fig. 16–22). In a study by Tchernia and colleagues,[1027] complications of partial splenectomy were low and regrowth of the splenic remnant was not observed during a 4-year follow-up period. However, splenic tissue has tremendous regeneration potential, as attested to by reports of previously splenectomized HS individuals who developed enlarged accessory spleens or ectopic splenic tissue, together with recurrent hemolysis, later in life.[1028, 1029] More experience and longer follow-up are needed before partial splenectomy can be routinely recommended.

Embolization. A case report detailing partial splenic arterial embolization in a child with HS has been published.[1030] The technique has also been used to decrease operative blood loss in patients with very large spleens before laparoscopic splenectomy.[1021] There are no additional data on this treatment in pediatric patients with HS.

Prophylaxis. All splenectomized patients must receive polyvalent pneumococcal vaccine, preferably given several weeks preoperatively. The Centers for Disease Control and Prevention recommends pneumo-

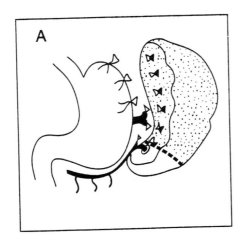
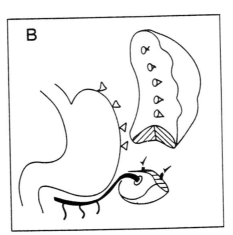

Figure 16-22. Surgical technique used for partial (about 80%) splenectomy. *A,* All vascular pedicles supplying the spleen are divided except those arising from the left gastroepiploic vessels. *B,* The upper pole of the spleen is removed at the boundary between the well-perfused and poorly perfused tissue. (From Tchernia G, Gauthier F, et al: Initial assessment of the beneficial effect of partial splenectomy in hereditary spherocytosis. Blood 1993; 81:2014.)

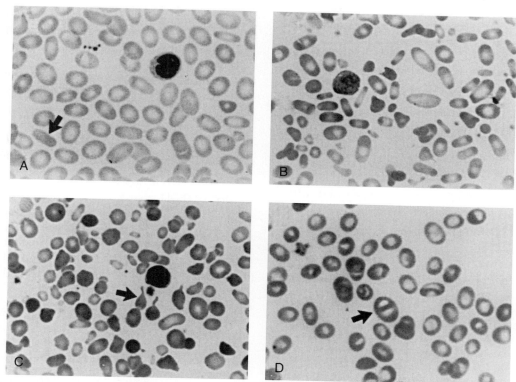

Figure 16–23. Peripheral blood smears from subjects with various forms of hereditary elliptocytosis (HE). *A,* Simple heterozygote with mild common HE associated with an elliptogenic spectrin mutation. Note predominant elliptocytosis with occasional rod-shaped cells *(arrow)* and virtual absence of poikilocytes. *B,* ``Homozygous'' common HE due to compound heterozygosity for two α-spectrin mutations. Both parents have mild HE. There are many elliptocytes as well as numerous fragments and poikilocytes. *C,* Hereditary pyropoikilocytosis (HPP). The patient is a compound heterozygote for a mutant α-spectrin and a defect characterized by reduced synthesis of the normal α-spectrin allele. Note prominent microspherocytosis, micropoikilocytosis, and fragmentation. Only a few elliptocytes are present. Some poikilocytes are in the process of budding *(arrow)*. *D,* Southeast Asian ovalocytosis (SAO). The majority of cells are oval, some of them containing either a longitudinal slit or a transverse ridge *(arrow)*. (From Palek J, Jarolim P: Clinical expression and laboratory detection of red blood cell membrane protein mutations. Semin Hematol 1993; 30:266.)

coccal vaccine for all children 2 years of age and older with splenic absence or dysfunction.[1031] Immunization with *H. influenzae* and, in some countries, meningococcal vaccines is also recommended, particularly in children. We advocate prophylactic antibiotics after splenectomy, with emphasis on protection against pneumococcal sepsis (i.e., penicillin V or equivalent, 125 mg orally twice daily in young children (<7 years) and 250 mg twice daily in older children and adults), at least for the first 5 years after surgery and preferably for life. Before splenectomy, HS patients, like patients with other hemolytic disorders, should take folic acid (1 mg/d orally), to prevent folate deficiency.

Postsplenectomy Changes. After splenectomy, spherocytosis persists but conditioned microspherocytes disappear; and changes typical of the postsplenectomy state, including Howell-Jolly bodies, target cells, siderocytes, and acanthocytes, become evident in the peripheral blood smear. On average, the MCV and mean red cell surface area increase and the MCHC and osmotic fragility decrease, but the effects are modest (5% to 10%).[1032] In typical dominant HS, reticulocyte counts fall to normal or near-normal levels,[733] although red cell life span, if carefully measured, remains slightly shortened (96 ± 13 days).[823] In all but the most severe cases, anemia and jaundice remit and do not recur.

Splenectomy Failure. The rare splenectomy failure (i.e., recurrence of hemolysis) is usually caused by an accessory spleen that was missed during surgery[1028, 1029] or by another red cell disorder, such as pyruvate kinase deficiency.[1033, 1034] Accessory spleens occur in 15% to 40% of patients and must always be sought.[928, 984, 1035] Recurrence of hemolytic anemia years[1029] or even decades[1028] after splenectomy should raise suspicion of an accessory spleen, particularly if Howell-Jolly bodies are no longer evident on peripheral blood smears. The absence of "pitted" red cells with crater-like surface indentations, readily seen by interference contrast microscopy, is also a sensitive measure of recrudescent splenic function.[1036, 1037] The ectopic splenic tissue can be confirmed by a radiocolloid liver/spleen scan or a scan using ^{51}Cr-labeled, heat-damaged red cells.[1028, 1038]

Hereditary Elliptocytosis, Hereditary Pyropoikilocytosis, and Related Disorders

Hereditary elliptocytosis (HE) is characterized by the presence of elliptical or oval erythrocytes on peripheral blood smears (Fig. 16–23). Although oval or elliptical erythrocytes are normally found in camels, llamas, birds, and reptiles, in humans the presence of elliptocytes indicates a defect in the erythrocyte membrane skeleton. HE and the related disorder hereditary pyropoikilocytosis (HPP) are characterized by clinical, biochemical, and genetic heterogeneity. Clinically, these disorders range from the asymptomatic carrier to severe hemolysis and even death *in utero* due to hydrops fetalis. Erythrocyte biochemical defects range from none to severe. Four different genetic loci have been implicated in the pathogenesis of these disorders.

In the past, hereditary elliptocytic disorders have simply been considered variants of HS and worthy of little further attention. However, the membrane defects and their pathophysiologic consequences in HE differ fundamentally from those of HS, leading to the difference in erythrocyte shape.

History

Hereditary elliptocytosis was first reported in 1904 by Dresbach, a physiologist at Ohio State University in Columbus, who discovered the condition in one of his histology students during a laboratory exercise in which the students were examining their own blood.[1039] This report elicited some controversy, because the student died soon thereafter, leading to speculation that the student actually suffered from incipient pernicious anemia.[1040] A number of famous pathologists supported Dresbach's view that the elliptocytosis was a primary disorder,[1041] and this was substantiated during the next two decades by the reports of Bishop[1042] and Huck and Bigalow.[1043] The demonstration of the disease in three generations of one family clearly established the hereditary nature of this disorder.[1044, 1045]

In the 1930s and 1940s there was some debate as to whether HE was a disease or simply a morphologic curiosity.[1044–1049] Early on, some confusion also existed in differentiating HE from sickle cell anemia, from hypochromic elliptocytosis (probably thalassemia), and later, from HS.[1047] These reports emphasize an important fact: HE and its hemolytic variants can sometimes be morphologically deceptive. Additional historical and clinical features of the disease are found in the reports of Wyandt and associates,[1048] Wolman and Ozge,[1049] and Dacie.[1050]

HE is common in people of African and Mediterranean ancestry.[1051–1059] In the United States, HE has been estimated to occur in 1 in 2000 to 4000 of the population.[1048, 1051] The true incidence of HE is unknown because its clinical severity is heterogeneous and many patients are asymptomatic and without anemia. In a study of HE in Benin, an incidence of 1.6% was observed.[1052] One common elliptocytic mutation of α-spectrin, $\alpha^{1/65-68}$, has an incidence that approaches 1% in Central Africa. It has a worldwide distribution in people of African ancestry. Genetic haplotyping studies suggest that this mutation may have a "founder affect" with origins of this mutation in central Africa similar to that attributed to hemoglobin S Benin-type.[1052]

HE variants are inherited predominantly in an autosomal dominant manner. Typically, individuals whom are heterozygous for an elliptocytic variant have asymptomatic elliptocytosis without anemia. Individuals who are homozygotes or compound heterozygotes for HE variants may suffer from mild to severe hemolysis with moderate to marked anemia. Spontaneous elliptocytogenic mutations have been reported. Presumably, they will also be inherited in an autosomal dominant fashion.

Clinical and Laboratory Characteristics of Hereditary Elliptocytosis and Related Disorders

Classification

Most of the reported cases of HE can be classified into one of three clinical categories: common HE, spherocytic HE, and Southeast Asian ovalocytosis (SAO). With the exception of SAO, which is homogeneous in molecular genetic terms (see later), these classifications denote clinical phenotypes and not specific molecular etiologies, although correlations between the two exist. Numerous molecular defects in the membrane proteins of HE have been identified, and HE can also be classified based on these defects (see later).

Heterozygous Common HE. Common HE is, by far, the most prevalent form of HE, particularly in African populations.[1052, 1053] It is frequently classified into several subtypes. The clinical characteristics of common HE trait vary enormously, defining several clinical subtypes. It is important to note that different members of the same family may exhibit different clinical patterns, and even single individuals may exhibit variability in their clinical presentation over time. Thus the clinical patterns defined below are probably more useful for illustrating the spectrum of common HE than for classifying the disease.

Silent Carrier State. This condition was identified by analyzing asymptomatic members of kindreds with HE or HPP. The affected persons have normal red cell morphology and no evidence of hemolysis, but detailed investigations show a subtle defect in their membrane skeletons, with decreased red cell thermal stability, decreased mechanical stability of isolated skeletons, an increased fraction of spectrin dimers in 0°C spectrin extracts, abnormal tryptic peptide maps of spectrin, or various combinations of these defects.[1055–1061] It is notable that some patients classified as "silent carriers" have the same molecular defect as patients with mild common HE,[1058–1061] emphasizing the variability of clinical expression.

Mild HE. This is the most common clinical form of HE.[250, 1062–1077] Patients are asymptomatic and are often diagnosed incidentally when undergoing screening for an unrelated condition. They are not anemic and only very rarely exhibit splenomegaly. Red cell survival may be normal,[1076] but more often there is very mild, compensated hemolysis with a slight reticulocytosis and a decreased haptoglobin level.[1066, 1069, 1074, 1075, 1078] In these patients HE is hardly more than a morphologic curiosity. The peripheral blood smear shows prominent elliptocytosis with little red cell budding or fragmentation and no spherocytosis. Elliptocytes (by definition) usually exceed 30% of the red cells and in some cases approach 100%.[1048, 1060, 1061, 1074, 1078] Very elongated elliptocytes are common (>10%). These patients are easily separated from normal individuals, who have less than 2% to 5% elliptocytes.[1061, 1072, 1078] Somewhat higher proportions of elliptocytes are seen in patients with anemia, particularly megaloblastic anemias, hypochromic-microcytic anemias, myelodysplastic syndromes, and myelofibrosis[1079]; but even in these individuals elliptocytes do not exceed 35%.[1072] Thus the diagnosis of common HE is rarely difficult.

Common HE with Chronic Hemolysis. More severe variants of common HE occur frequently, even within members of the same kindred.[1066, 1080–1083] In general, the hemolysis is accompanied by evidence of membrane instability on the peripheral blood smear: budding red cells, fragments, and other bizarre poikilocytes. In patients with α-spectrin mutations, significant hemolysis is frequently due to co-inheritance of a spectrin allele that leads to decreased α-spectrin expression, such as the α^{LELY} allele, and one of the more deleterious HE alleles affecting α-spectrin (see later).[1067, 1084–1089] Of the common mutations, $\alpha^{I/74}$-spectrin is more severe than $\alpha^{I/46-50a}$-spectrin and much more severe than $\alpha^{I/65-68}$-spectrin. Patients with α^{LELY} in *trans* to $\alpha^{I/74}$ have marked hemolysis and elliptopoikilocytosis compared with their siblings with wild type α-spectrin and $\alpha^{I/74}$ ($+/\alpha^{I/74}$), whereas patients with $\alpha^{LELY}/\alpha^{I/65-68}$ have more elliptocytes than their $+/\alpha^{I/65-68}$ siblings but no significant hemolysis.[1087] Less often hemolysis is caused by inheritance of a mutant spectrin that is grossly dysfunctional.[1080] This is indicated by dominant transmission of the hemolytic syndrome and by an unusually high fraction of spectrin dimers in 0°C spectrin extracts.

Common HE with Sporadic Hemolysis. Patients with common HE may also develop uncompensated hemolysis in response to stimuli that cause hyperplasia of the reticuloendothelial system, particularly if the spleen is involved. Examples include viral hepatitis, cirrhosis, infectious mononucleosis, bacterial infections, and malaria.[1075, 1090–1092] Hemolysis has also been observed with thrombotic thrombocytopenic purpura and during renal transplant rejection complicated by disseminated intravascular coagulation, which suggests that elliptocytes may be especially susceptible to microangiopathic damage.[1093] For unknown reasons pregnancy and cobalamin (vitamin B$_{12}$) deficiency may also transiently aggravate the disease.[880, 1094]

HE with Infantile Poikilocytosis. Infants with mild common HE often begin life with moderately severe hemolytic anemia, characterized by marked red cell budding, fragmentation, and poikilocytosis and by neonatal jaundice, which may require an exchange transfusion.[1056, 1068, 1078, 1095–1100] In most cases, enough elliptocytes are present to suggest the diagnosis, but sometimes this is not so and the disorder is mistaken for sepsis, infantile pyknocytosis, or a microangiopathic or oxidant-induced hemolytic anemia.[1097, 1098] Neonatal HE can easily be distinguished from these conditions if the parents' smears are examined, because one will have common HE. However, it is more diffi-

cult to distinguish HE with neonatal poikilocytosis from HPP (see later). Most α-spectrin variants have been associated with the neonatal poikilocytosis syndrome. The factors that determine susceptibility are unknown. With time, fragmentation and hemolysis decline, and the clinical picture of mild common HE emerges.[1101] This transition requires 4 months to 2 years. Subsequently, the disease is clinically indistinguishable from typical mild common HE. The prevalence is unknown, but in the authors' experience it is not rare.

The fragmenting neonatal red cells are very sensitive to heat, like hereditary pyropoikilocytes (see later), but unlike pyropoikilocytes, this sensitivity lessens over time.[1100] During the conversion, the poikilocytic red cells are dense and rich in hemoglobin F whereas the smooth elliptocytes are light and enriched in hemoglobin A. This suggests the change in the disease corresponds to the change from fetal to adult erythropoiesis. No variations in the primary α-spectrin defect or its functional effects on spectrin self-association occur during the conversion, so other skeletal interactions must differ in fetal and adult red cells. Mentzer[573] has made the interesting suggestion that 2,3-DPG is the critical agent. Because it is not bound by hemoglobin F, 2,3-DPG is elevated in fetal red cells. The free anion is known to weaken spectrin/actin/protein 4.1 interactions[367, 574, 575] and to increase the fragility of isolated ghosts at physiologic concentrations *in vitro*.[1094] It is unclear if this occurs in intact red cells.[576, 577] If so, this would certainly aggravate the underlying defect in spectrin self-association.

HE with Dyserythropoiesis. In a small number of families with otherwise typical common HE, the sporadic occurrence of hemolysis and anemia is at least partially due to the development of dysplastic and ineffective erythropoiesis. All the reported patients with this rare syndrome are from Italy, have somewhat less elongated red cells than is typical for common HE, and show the characteristic findings of ineffective erythropoiesis, relatively low reticulocyte counts, indirect hyperbilirubinemia, high serum iron and ferritin, and rapid clearance of ^{59}Fe combined with poor incorporation of ^{59}Fe into new erythrocytes.[1102, 1103] Erythrocytes from some patients exhibit macrocytic changes. Other patients have a few spherocytes, but these are probably an artifact because osmotic fragility test results are normal.[1102] The patient's bone marrow is hyperplastic, with decreased late erythroblasts and dysplastic features (asynchrony of nuclear-cytoplasmic maturation, binuclearity, internuclear bridges, and small numbers of ringed sideroblasts). Anemia and, presumably, erythroid dysplasia usually commence during adolescence or early adult life and advance gradually over years. Because dysplasia persists after splenectomy, response to the operation is incomplete. The available data suggest that dysplasia and elliptocytosis co-segregate because no individuals with dysplasia have been observed who did not have elliptocytosis.[1102, 1103] If so, these families must represent a unique subtype of mild common HE. This is supported by the fact that none of the typical HE protein defects were observed in one well-studied family. Spectrin self-association, spectrin peptide maps, and the concentration of protein 4.1 and other major membrane proteins were normal.

Homozygous Common HE. A number of patients who are homozygotes or compound heterozygotes for common HE have been reported.[1062, 1078, 1104–1116] Some have had very severe, even fatal, transfusion-dependent hemolytic anemia (Hb 2 to 6 g/dL) with marked fragmentation, poikilocytosis, spherocytosis, and elliptocytosis. Others experience hemolysis to a lesser degree (Hb 7 to 11 g/dL). It appears these differences reflect variations in the severity of the many α-spectrin mutations that produce HE.[1078, 1117] Clinically, the disease resembles HPP,[1078, 1117] except for the mildest forms. Patients have an excellent response to splenectomy.

Hereditary Pyropoikilocytosis. This uncommon disorder presents in infancy or early childhood as a severe hemolytic anemia (hemoglobin 4 to 8 g/dL)[1078] characterized by extreme poikilocytosis with budding red cells, fragments, spherocytes, triangulocytes, and other bizarre-shaped cells and, in some cases, with few or no elliptocytes (Fig. 16–24).[1058, 1118–1121] This morphology is similar to that seen in patients who have severe thermal burns. It is also similar to that observed in homozygous common HE and common HE with neonatal poikilocytosis. Most of the cases have occurred in individuals of African origin. Patients typically present with hyperbilirubinemia in the neonatal period or with marked anemia in the first few months of life.[1122] There is red cell fragmentation, erythroblastosis, and splenomegaly.[1122, 1123] Complications of severe anemia including growth retardation, frontal bossing, and early gallbladder disease have been reported.[1120, 1121] Osmotic fragility tests are very abnormal, particularly after incubation,[1105, 1119–1121] and autohemolysis is greatly elevated.[1119–1121] A significant characteristic, microcytosis is reflected by very low MCVs (25 to 75 fL) because of the large number of fragmented red cells.[1059–1061, 1078, 1119, 1120] Another characteristic feature of these cells is their remarkable thermal sensitivity. Hereditary pyropoikilocytes fragment at 45° to 46°C (normal = 49°C) after short periods of heating (10 to 15 minutes).[1121] After splenectomy, hemolysis is markedly decreased, but not eliminated.[1120, 1121] After splenectomy, the hemoglobin typically ranges from 10 to 14 g/dL with 3% to 10% reticulocytes.[1078]

Although HPP was initially considered as a separate disease, there is convincing evidence that it is related to HE. As noted earlier, HPP is clinically and morphologically similar to the more severe forms of hemolytic elliptocytosis. In addition, in many cases, one of the parents or siblings has typical mild common HE and in some of these kindreds an identical molecular defect is observed in siblings with phenotypically different diseases (i.e., HPP and common HE). In other families, all the first-degree relatives are phenotypically normal. A number of biochemical and molecular defects are shared between HE and HPP. However, HPP red cells, but not hereditary elliptocytes, are usually markedly deficient in spectrin.[606, 1078, 1123] Typically, one parent of the HPP offspring carries an α-spectrin mutation whereas the other parent is fully asymptomatic and has no detectable biochemical abnormality.[606] Studies of spectrin synthesis and mRNA levels reveal that such asymptomatic parents carry a silent "thalassemia-like" defect of spectrin synthesis. When co-inherited with the elliptocytogenic spectrin mutation in the HPP offspring, this thalassemia-like defect enhances the expression of the mutant spectrin in the cells and leads to a superimposed spectrin deficiency. The spectrin deficiency is thought to be responsible for the large number of spherocytes and relative paucity of elliptocytes in some patients. Other HPP patients are homozygotes or compound heterozygotes for structural defects of spectrin.

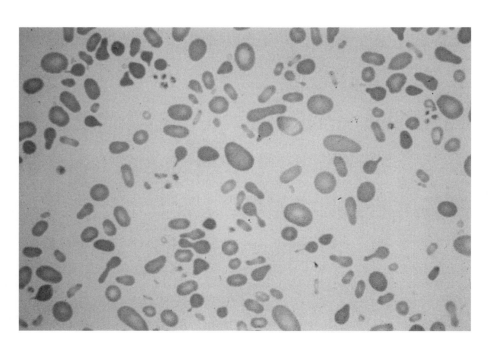

Figure 16–24. Peripheral blood smear from a patient with hereditary pyropoikilocytosis. Poikilocytes, budding and fragmented erythrocytes, spherocytes, and a few elliptocytes are seen.

Spherocytic HE. This dominant disorder is a phenotypic hybrid of common HE and HS. It has been reported only in white families of European descent, is not linked to the Rh gene, and appears to be a unique subtype.[1046, 1075, 1124–1127] Its prevalence is unknown, but, judging from the number of published reports, it is relatively rare, probably accounting for no more than 5% of HE in patients of European ancestry. Unlike mild common HE, almost all the affected patients have some hemolysis. This is usually mild to moderate and is often incompletely compensated. The elliptocytes are fewer and plumper than in mild common HE, and some spherocytes, microspherocytes, and microelliptocytes are usually present. Poikilocytes and red cell fragments are uncommon, which distinguishes this disorder from common HE with hemolysis. Red cell morphology may vary, even within the same family. Some family members may have relatively prominent spherocytes and as few as 10% to 20% elliptocytes, whereas in others elliptocytes predominate and spherocytes are rare.[1046, 1124] This may cause diagnostic confusion initially, particularly if the propositus has few elliptocytes. Family studies almost always reveal some members with obvious elliptocytosis.

Spherocytic elliptocytes are osmotically fragile,[1046, 1124, 1126, 1127] particularly after incubation. Excessive mechanical fragility and increased autohemolysis that responds to glucose are also characteristic. Gallbladder disease is common, and aplastic crises are a risk.[1124, 1126] The splenic pathology of spherocytic HE mimics HS.[1128, 1129] Splenic sequestration is evident, red cells are conditioned during splenic passage, and hemolysis abates after splenectomy.[1124, 1126, 1129]

The molecular pathology of classic spherocytic HE is unknown. However, patients with COOH-terminal truncations of β-spectrin (see later) have many of the clinical features of spherocytic HE and probably are an example of the disorder.[1130–1139] A number of such truncations have been identified. The affected patients typically have moderate hemolysis and anemia, punctuated by recurrent, severe hemolytic crises.[1131, 1132, 1135] Blood smears show plump and usually smooth elliptocytes; although in two cases, poikilocytosis was prominent.[1131, 1132, 1134, 1139] In all but one instance the HE red cells were mildly heat sensitive.[1131] All patients have a positive osmotic fragility test or an osmotic gradient ektacytometry pattern that resembles the pattern in HS. Like HS, the spleen is enlarged and selectively destroys labeled elliptocytes (half-life = 11 days; normal, 24 to 34 days),[1137] and splenectomy is effective.

Patients who lack GPC (see later) also have positive osmotic fragility tests and rounded, smooth elliptocytes.[369, 1140, 1141] They should probably also be classified as having a recessive (and unusually mild) variant of spherocytic HE. Patients who lack protein 4.2 (another recessive condition) sometimes display features of spherocytic HE, such as ovalostomatocytosis[490, 751]; however, protein 4.2 deficiency more often resembles HS, morphologically and pathophysiologically, and is better classified as a variant of that disorder.

Rare patients appear to be compound heterozygotes for HS and HE. One Turkish girl is a particularly good candidate.[1142] Her mother and father had mild HS and very mild common HE (probably), respectively, whereas she suffered from a moderately severe hemolytic anemia (hemoglobin, 8.4; reticulocytes, 24%; bilirubin, 1.6 mg/dL) with frontal bossing, osteoporosis, splenomegaly (10 cm), and a mixture of microspherocytes and rounded elliptocytes.

Southeast Asian Ovalocytosis. This condition, which has a unique phenotype, a unique molecular defect, and a unique geographic distribution, is discussed separately, later in the chapter.

Analysis of Membrane Structure and Function

Thermal Sensitivity of Red Cells and Spectrin. Red cells heated to temperatures approaching 50°C for short periods of time become unstable and fragment spontaneously (Fig. 16–25),[1143–1145] probably owing to denaturation of spectrin.[1146] Normal spectrin denatures at 49°C (10-minute exposure),[555, 1146] and normal red cells fragment at the same temperature.[444, 1121, 1147] As noted earlier, almost all patients with HPP and some patients with other forms of HE have thermally sensitive red cells. Hereditary pyropoikilocytes and red cells from infants with common HE and neonatal poikilocytosis fragment after 10 minutes at 44° to 46°C.[1100, 1121] Red cells from some but not all patients with common HE

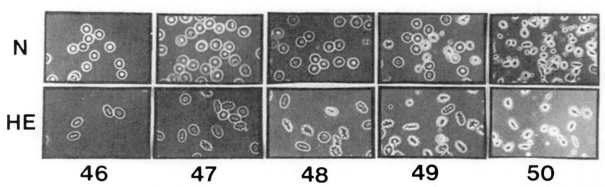

Figure 16–25. Effects of heat on the morphology of normal and hereditary elliptocytosis red cells. Note that crenation and membrane budding are first evident in hereditary elliptocytosis red cells at 47°C to 48°C but do not appear in normal cells until they are heated to 49°C.

fragment at 47° to 48°C.[555, 1121] As expected, purified spectrin from these red cells is also heat sensitive.[555, 1146] This test is limited because we do not understand, in molecular terms, why specific mutations are thermally sensitive. However, it remains one of the simplest tests available for assessing HPP in laboratories that do not specialize in membrane protein analysis.

Abnormal Spectrin Oligomerization. Many patients with HE and all patients with HPP are unable to properly convert spectrin dimers to tetramers and higher oligomers *in vitro* or on the membrane. This important functional property is easily assessed in low temperature spectrin extracts (Fig. 16–26). At 0°C the equilibrium between spectrin dimer and tetramer is greatly slowed.[562] If spectrin is extracted from the membrane at 0°C and carefully protected from warming during separation of dimers, tetramers, and oligomers (usually on nondenaturing polyacrylamide gels), the proportion of each spectrin species reflects its relative proportion on the membrane.[347] Patients with defects in spectrin self-association have abnormally high proportions of spectrin dimer in 0°C spectrin extracts (i.e., more than 10% of total spectrin dimers and tetramers).[1082, 1147, 1148] The fraction of spectrin dimers is an important functional assessment in patients with α-spectrin defects. It correlates well with clinical severity[1088] and accurately predicts unusually severe mutations.[1080] Conversely, discordance between the degree of hemolysis and fraction of spectrin dimers may alert the physician to an underlying, secondary complication (see earlier section on common HE with hemolysis).

Ektacytometry. The ektacytometer can be used to assess red cell membrane deformability and stability in patients with hemolytic disorders.[1149–1151] Isolated red cell ghosts are subjected to a high shear stress in a laser diffraction viscometer, and the "deformability index" (a measure of the average elongation of the sheared ghosts) is recorded as a function of time. Fragile ghosts fragment more quickly than normal, causing their "deformability" to fall. The technique is a useful screening test because membrane stability is reduced in almost all membrane skeletal diseases. In addition, the ektacytometer can be modified to measure cellular deformability at different osmolalities, a technique termed *osmotic gradient ektacytometry.*[909] The resulting curves depend on both membrane surface area and cell volume and are a sensitive measure of the surface loss that characterizes many skeletal defects.

Tryptic Maps of Spectrin. Limited tryptic digestion of spectrin extracted from erythrocytes, performed at 0°C, followed by SDS polyacrylamide gel electrophoresis (SDS-PAGE) or isoelectric focusing combined with SDS-PAGE (two-dimensional gels) separates the resulting trypsin-resistant domains of α- and β-spectrin.[346, 368] The gels are stained with Coomassie blue, and characteristic, reproducible maps are obtained. A two-dimensional separation of normal spectrin domains is shown in Figure 16–9. Among these peptides, the 80-kDa α I domain peptide, which contains the self-association site of normal α-spectrin, is the most prominent. Many of the known elliptocytogenic α-spectrin mutations affect the 80-kDa domain and yield

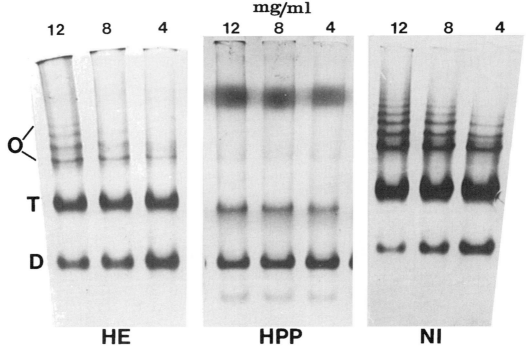

Figure 16–26. Nondenaturing gel electrophoresis of spectrin dimers and oligomers from erythrocytes of normal (NI) individuals and patients with hereditary elliptocytosis (HE) and hereditary pyropoikilocytosis (HPP). Low ionic strength spectrin extracts were concentrated to 12.5, 8, and 4 mg/mL and equilibrated at 30°C for 3 hours. Note the markedly reduced amounts of tetramer (T) and oligomer (O) at each concentration of HPP spectrin (the diffuse band at the top of the HPP gels is hemoglobin). HE spectrin shows intermediate behavior. (From Knowles WJ, Morrow JS, et al: Molecular and functional changes in spectrin from patients with hereditary pyropoikilocytosis. J Clin Invest 1983; 71:1867. By copyright permission of The American Society for Clinical Investigation.)

peptide maps containing one or more fragments of the domain. One-dimensional maps of spectrin domains from patients with some of these HE defects are shown in Figure 16–27. In most of the defects, tryptic cleavage occurs in the third helix of the triple-helical spectrin repeats.[154] The reported mutations reside in the vicinity of these cleavage sites either in the same helix or, less commonly, at neighboring sites in the first and second helices. Interestingly, HE mutations near the COOH-terminus of β-spectrin may also alter tryptic cleavage of the neighboring 80-kDa α-spectrin domain (to be discussed). Thus, tryptic peptide mapping is a powerful tool to map the approximate sites of the underlying spectrin mutations; the mutations can subsequently be defined by examination of the corresponding region at the cDNA or genomic DNA level.

Genetic Analyses. Genomic DNA isolated from peripheral blood leukocytes or reverse-transcribed reticulocyte or bone marrow mRNA can be amplified by PCR utilizing specific DNA oligonucleotide primers flanking the region suspected to contain a mutation. The amplification product is then subjected to nucleic acid sequencing or other forms of analysis. There are many individual variations of this technique that have been used to identify the mutations described in the following sections. Screening techniques can be used when there are no biochemical clues to the location of the mutation. These techniques are particularly advantageous when analyzing the genes of large proteins, such as spectrin or ankyrin. Genomic DNA is tested in most cases because the mutant mRNA species may not accumulate in significant amounts. The SSCP method is a simple, sensitive, and appropriately popular example of such a screening test. Labeled, PCR-amplified DNA fragments (100 to 400 bp) are denatured and the single strands are refolded before running on a nondenaturing gel.[1152, 1153] Surprisingly, even a single nucleotide change usually alters the folding pattern enough to allow mutant and normal fragments to separate on the gel (70% to 90% of mutations). Abnormal fragments are subcloned and sequenced. In some regions where common elliptocytogenic mutations have been identified, multiplex PCR techniques or simple restriction endonuclease digestion of amplified DNA can be used to screen rapidly for these mutations.

Etiology of Common Hereditary Elliptocytosis and Related Disorders

Spectrin Defects

Abnormalities of either α- or β-spectrin are associated with many cases of HE and HPP. The majority are due to mutations in the spectrin heterodimer self-association site (Figs. 16–28 and 16–29) with defective ability of spectrin dimers to form tetramers, resulting in destabilization of the erythrocyte membrane skeleton.

Alpha-Spectrin Defects. Most of the HE defects lie in the 80-kDa α I domain at the NH$_2$-terminus of the α-spectrin chain. Nine tryptic cleavage defects of the normal 80-kDa α I domain peptide have been identified by tryptic mapping, characterized by loss of the normal 80-kDa peptide and the appearance of one of the following: a new 78-kDa peptide ($\alpha^{I/74}$), a new 74-kDa peptide ($\alpha^{I/74}$), a new 65- or 68-kDa peptide ($\alpha^{I/65-68}$), a new 61-kDa peptide ($\alpha^{I/61}$), a new 46-kDa peptide

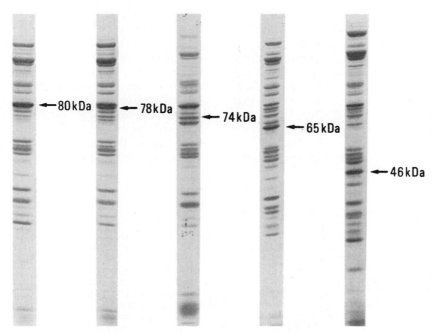

Figure 16–27. One-dimensional peptide maps after partial trypsin digestion of spectrin variants. In normal individuals, most of the α I domain appears as an 80-kd fragment. In spectrin mutants with various alterations of the α chain, the main fragment representing the α I domain is shorter, because of abnormal cleavages that reflect, in turn, local conformational changes. The $\alpha^{I/78}$, $\alpha^{I/74}$, $\alpha^{I/65-68}$, and $\alpha^{I/46-50a}$ phenotypes are shown. (From Delaunay J, Dhermy D: Mutations involving the spectrin heterodimer contact site: clinical expression and alterations in specific function. Semin Hematol 1993; 30:21.)

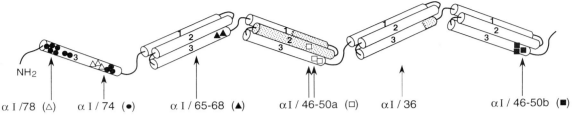

Figure 16–28. Triple helical model of spectrin depicting currently known mutations of the α I domain (also described in Table 16–9). The abnormal tryptic cleavage sites in the different forms of HE/HPP are indicated by the *arrows*. The open and filled symbols mark the positions of various missense mutations or in-frame amino acid insertions that are associated with the abnormal cleavages. Note that in most cases the mutation is adjacent to the abnormal cleavage site, either in the same helical coil or in neighboring helices in the triple helical model. The *shaded areas* represent deletions in the second or third triple helical repeats, respectively, that are associated with the α$^{I/46-50a}$ phenotype (Sp Dayton) or the α$^{I/36}$ phenotype (Sp Sfax). (From Gallagher PG, Tse WT, Forget BG: Clinical and molecular aspects of disorders of the erythrocyte membrane skeleton. Semin Perinatol 1990; 14:351.)

(α$^{I/46}$), a new 50- or 46-kDa peptide (α$^{I/46-50a}$), a new 50-kDa peptide with a more basic isoelectric point than α$^{I/46-50a}$ (α$^{I/50b}$), two new peptides of 43 and 42 kDa (α$^{I/43}$), or two new peptides of 36 and 33 kDa (α$^{I/36-33}$). In general, these defects produce decreased spectrin self-association, reflected in an increased proportion of spectrin dimers in 0°C low ionic strength extracts of spectrin and decreased conversion of spectrin dimers to tetramers in solution, in ghosts, and on inside-out vesicles. The fragile spectrin/spectrin links weaken the membrane skeleton and diminish the resistance of the isolated membrane or skeleton to shear stress.[573, 909, 1096, 1150] Surprisingly, this results in a stiff membrane[1154] (elevated elastic shear modulus) rather than a lax one. The dependence of the pathophysiology on spectrin/spectrin attachments fits with the observation that the severity of an α-spectrin mutation is inversely proportional to its distance from the contact site of self-association. There are two exceptions to this observation: α$^{I/65-68}$ is unusually mild given its relative proximity to the contact site, and α$^{I/50a}$ and α$^{I/50b}$ are unusually severe relative to their positions. Most α-spectrin defects occur in helix C of the proposed model of triple-helical repeats. The precise mutations responsible for HE/HPP have been identified in most of these tryptic variants (see Fig. 16–28; Tables 16–10 and 16–11).

Spectrin Alpha$^{I/74}$. This is a heterogeneous collection of defects that result in enhanced tryptic cleavage following Arg^{45} or Lys^{48} in an extrahelical segment (helix C in the crystallographic structure of the repeat) that juts out from the NH$_2$-terminal end of the α-spectrin chain. This is the end that participates in the formation of the spectrin self-association contact site. The corresponding (COOH-terminal) end of the β chain also contains extra helices (helices A and B) in repeat 17, followed by a phosphorylated segment. Tse and Speicher and their colleagues[345, 1055] proposed that these three helices pair up, as they do all along the spectrin chain, and that this is the bond responsible for spectrin self-association. Increasing evidence indicates that this hypothesis is true.

Spectrin α$^{I/74}$ mutations disrupt one of the three interacting terminal helices of the contact site and markedly disrupt spectrin self-association. As a result, they are generally the most severe of the common α-spectrin mutations that cause HE/HPP. Patients who are homozygous for α$^{I/74}$ defects usually have life-threatening hemolysis and an HPP-like syndrome.[1078, 1088] Patients who are compound heterozygotes for an α$^{I/74}$ mutation and an α$^{I/46-50a}$ or α$^{I/61}$ defect also have severe hemolysis. Both groups of patients have partial (about 30%) spectrin deficiency,[1123] similar to HS. Spectrin deficiency and the appearance of spherocytes along with elliptocytes and poikilocytes is a common feature of the most severe forms of HE and HPP. Sometimes α$^{I/74}$ patients have so many microspherocytes and so few elliptocytes on their blood smears that the diagnosis of HE is not considered until smears from family members are examined.

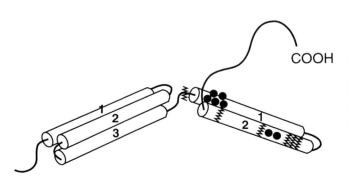

Figure 16–29. Triple helical mode of spectrin demonstrating currently known mutations of the COOH-terminal end of β-spectrin (also described in Table 16–9). The *filled circles* mark positions of various missense mutations associated with the HE or HPP phenotype. The *jagged lines* indicate truncations of the β-spectrin chain due to insertions, deletions, and exon skipping. Note that all of the mutations affect the two unpaired helical coils that participate in the spectrin self-association interaction. (From Gallagher PG, Tse WT, Forget BG: Clinical and molecular aspects of disorders of the erythrocyte membrane skeleton. Semin Perinatol 1990; 14:351.)

Table 16-10. ALPHA-SPECTRIN MUTATIONS ASSOCIATED WITH HEREDITARY ELLIPTOCYTOSIS AND HEREDITARY PYROPOIKILOCYTOSIS*

Variant	Tryptic Phenotype	Mutation			Exon	Repeat Segment	α Helix	Reference
		Codon	**Gene**	**Protein**				
Lograno	$\alpha^{I/74}$	24	ATC → AGC	Ile → Ser	2	α1	3	1155
Corbeil	$\alpha^{I/74}$	28	CGT → CAT	Arg → His	2	α1	3	1081
Unnamed	$\alpha^{I/74}$	28	CGT → CTT	Arg → Leu	2	α1	3	1080, 1118
Unnamed	$\alpha^{I/74}$	28	CGT → AGT	Arg → Ser	2	α1	3	1080, 1118
Unnamed	$\alpha^{I/74}$	28	CGT → TGT	Arg → Cys	2	α1	3	1080
Marseille	$\alpha^{I/74}$	31	GTG → GCG	Val → Ala	2	α1	3	1156
Genova	$\alpha^{I/74}$	34	CGG → TGG	Arg → Trp	2	α1	3	1157
Tunis	$\alpha^{I/78}$	41	CGG → TGG	Arg → Trp	2	α1	3	1063, 1064
Clichy	$\alpha^{I/78}$	45	AGG → AGT	Arg → Ser	2	α1	3	1095
Anastasia	$\alpha^{I/78}$	45	AGG → ACG	Arg → Thr	2	α1	3	1158
Culoz	$\alpha^{I/74}$	46	GGT → GTT	Gly → Val	2	α1	3	1159
Unnamed	$\alpha^{I/74}$	48	AAG → AGG	Lys → Arg	2	α1	3	1118
Lyon	$\alpha^{I/74}$	49	CTT → TTT	Leu → Phe	2	α1	3	1159
Ponte de Sôr	$\alpha^{I/65}$	151	GGT → GAT	Gly → Asp	4	α2	3	1160
Unnamed	$\alpha^{I/65}$	154	+TTG	+Leu	4	α2	3	1161
Dayton	$\alpha^{I/46-50a}$	178–226	insertion in intron 4†	−48 residues	5	α2		1162
Saint-Louis	$\alpha^{I/46-50a}$	207	CTG → CCG	Leu → Pro	5	α2	2	1163
Nigerian	$\alpha^{I/46-50a}$	260	CTG → CCG	Leu → Pro	6	α3	3	1164
Unnamed	$\alpha^{I/46-50a}$	261	TCC → CCC	Ser → Pro	6	α3	3	1164
Sfax	$\alpha^{I/36}$	362–371	AGAT → AG/gt‡	−9 residues	8	α4	3	1085
Alexandria	$\alpha^{I/46-50b}$	469	CAT → Del	His → Del	11	α5	3	1181
Barcelona	$\alpha^{I/46-50b}$	469	CAT → CCT	His → Pro	11	α5	3	1086
Unnamed	$\alpha^{I/46-50b}$	471	CAG → CCG	Gln → Pro	11	α5	3	1164
Jendouba	$\alpha^{II/31}$	791	GAC → GAA	Asp → Glu	17	α7	3	1166
Oran	$\alpha^{II/21}$	822–863	ivs 17 − 1 g → a§	−41 residues		α8		1107

*References are limited to the first description of the genomic mutation. In some cases, the names of the variants have been coined subsequently. The protein phenotype is based on an initial terminology after mild trypsin digestion and peptide mapping.
†Skipping of exon 5.
‡Creation of cryptic splice site, partial inframe skipping of exon 8.
§Skipping of exon 18.

Table 16-11. BETA-SPECTRIN MUTATIONS ASSOCIATED WITH HEREDITARY ELLIPTOCYTOSIS AND HEREDITARY PYROPOIKILOCYTOSIS

Variant	Tryptic Phenotype	Mutation			Exon	Repeat Segment	β Helix	Reference
		Codon	**Gene**	**Protein**				
Cagliari	$\alpha^{I/74}$	2018	GCC → GGC	Ala → Gly	30	β17	1	1167
Providence	$\alpha^{I/74}$	2019	TCT → CCT	Ser → Pro	30	β17	1	1168
Paris	$\alpha^{I/74}$	2023	GCG → GTG	Ala → Val	30	β17	1	1155
Linguere	$\alpha^{I/74}$	2024	TGG → AGG	Trp → Arg	30	β17	1	1155
Buffalo	$\alpha^{I/74}$	2025	CTG → CGG	Leu → Arg	30	β17	1	1169
Tandil*	$\alpha^{I/74}$	2041	−7nt; GGACAGTGT → GT	PCT‡	30	β17	2	1134
Nice*	$\alpha^{I/74}$	2046	+2nt; GAAG → GAGAAG	PCT	30	β17	2	1132, 1133
Kayes	$\alpha^{I/74}$	2053	GCT → CCT	Ala → Pro	30	β17	2	1055
Napoli*	$\alpha^{I/74}$	2053	−8nt; TTTTGAGAAG → TG	PCT	30	β17	2	1170
Tokyo*	$\alpha^{I/74}$	2059	−1nt; GCCAGC → GCAGC	PCT	30	β17	2	1165
Cotonou	$\alpha^{I/74}$	2061	TGG → AGG	Trp → Arg	30	β17	2	1052
Nagoya*	$\alpha^{I/74}$	2069	GAG → TAG	PCT	30	β17	2	1171
Göttingen*	$\alpha^{I/74}$	Intron 30	ivs 30 − 2 t → a§	PCT	30	β17	2	1135, 1136
Le Puy*	$\alpha^{I/74}$	Intron 30	ivs 30 − 4 a → g§	PCT	30	β17	2	1137, 1138
Rouen*	$\alpha^{I/74}$	Intron 31	ivs 31 − 3 g → t‖	PCT	31	β17	2	1130, 1131

*Truncated β-chain detectable on gel.
†PCT: premature chain termination due to a frameshift or nonsense mutation.
§Skipping of exon 30.
‖Skipping of exon 31.

In most cases, the primary defect in spectrin $\alpha^{1/74}$ variants is an amino acid substitution near the site of enhanced tryptic cleavage in the α chain.[1080, 1081, 1084, 1118, 1157, 1159, 1172] Codon 28, a CpG dinucleotide, is a "hot spot" for mutation and has been associated with four different sequence variations. In addition, in an increasing number of $\alpha^{1/74}$ HE/HPP kindreds, the primary defect occurs in helices A or B of repeat 17 of β-spectrin (see later). These two helices are adjacent to the $\alpha^{1/74}$ cleavage site in helix C at the NH_2-terminus of the α chain. These mutations support the self-association model of Tse, Speicher and colleagues.[345, 1055]

Spectrin Alpha$^{1/46-50a}$. This disorder is also heterogeneous and variable in severity. Generally it is less severe than spectrin $\alpha^{1/74}$ and more severe than spectrin $\alpha^{1/65-68}$.* It is particularly common in black populations. Mutations cluster around the site of abnormal tryptic cleavage in helix C of α-spectrin repeat 2, with one informative exception,[1163] which occurs at an adjacent site in helix B of repeat 2.

Spectrin Alpha$^{1/65-68}$. This common α-spectrin mutation is widely distributed in blacks in West Africa (where the prevalence of HE is 0.67%),[1168] in blacks in Central Africa,[157] and in their descendants in the West Indies and North America.[1160, 1161, 1175-1179] It is also seen in Arab populations and is the most common cause of HE in North Africa. The disorder is quite mild. It causes mild common HE in blacks and is even milder in North Africans, who sometimes have little or no elliptocytosis (i.e., are silent carriers). Even homozygotes have only mild to moderate hemolysis. Studies indicate that, with one exception,[1160] all patients have an extra leucine inserted between codons 154 and 155, probably due to duplication of codon 154.[1160, 1161, 1164, 1173] The high frequency of $\alpha^{1/65-68}$ and its homogeneous expression strongly suggest that it has experienced genetic selection.[1052] This has led to the hypothesis that it may provide some protection from malaria or other tropical blood-borne parasites. This has not yet been systematically tested, although there is preliminary evidence that growth of *P. falciparum* is inhibited in $\alpha^{1/65-68}$ erythrocytes.[1180]

Spectrin Alpha$^{1/78}$. This defect has been observed mostly in North Africans.[1063, 1064, 1095] Symptoms are quite variable, ranging from asymptomatic to moderately severe hemolysis, perhaps related to co-inheritance of spectrin α^{LELY} (see later). The primary mutations are located amid those that cause spectrin $\alpha^{1/74}$ defects,[1064, 1095] but, for unknown reasons, they cause tryptic cleavage at a more proximal site (Lys^{16}).

Spectrin Alpha$^{1/50b}$. This defect has been observed primarily in patients of African ancestry. The clinical phenotype ranges from asymptomatic elliptocytosis to poikilocytic elliptocytosis with hemolysis.[1086, 1164, 1165, 1181] Two point mutations and a single amino acid substitution have been associated with this disorder.

Spectrin Alpha$^{1/36}$. A truncated α-spectrin with the protein phenotype of $\alpha^{1/36}$ is spectrin^{Sfax}. This mutant spectrin is shortened by 9 amino acids owing to a point mutation that creates an alternate splice junction.[1085]

*See references 1068, 1078, 1082, 1117, 1163, 1164, 1173, and 1174.

Beta-Spectrin Defects. Beta chain abnormalities have been identified in patients with HE, defective spectrin self-association, and $\alpha^{1/74}$-spectrin on tryptic digests. All mutants described occur in repeat 17, the region involved in spectrin self-association (see Fig. 16–29). A variety of mutations have been described that are either associated with a structurally abnormal β-spectrin chain or a β chain with a truncated COOH-terminus. Truncated β chains have been reported in a number of kindreds with HE and chronic hemolysis.[1130-1134, 1170, 1171] SDS gels show two spectrin β bands: β and β'. The β component comigrates with the normal spectrin β chain (220 kDa), whereas β' moves faster, consistent with loss of a portion of the peptide chain. The size of the β' band varies from 210 to 218 kDa. This end of β-spectrin contains at least four phosphorylation sites within 10 kDa of the COOH-terminus.[572] In most patients the β' component is not phosphorylated, which localizes the deletion to the COOH-terminal end of the β chain. Spectrin^{Rouen} (218 kDa) is an exception; it has the shortest deletion and retains at least one phosphorylation site.[1130, 1131] Low temperature extracts of truncated β-spectrin variants contain increased spectrin dimer (approximately 50% of the spectrin dimer plus tetramer pool), and nearly all of the mutant β'-spectrin is found in the dimer fraction, proving that it is responsible for the functional defect.

The primary genetic defect in the β-spectrin gene has been identified in several HE kindreds. In cases associated with truncated β-spectrin chains, the coding sequence terminates because of a frameshift. In three instances a splice site mutation causes the adjacent exon to be skipped.[1130, 1131, 1136, 1138] In the other cases, insertions or deletions in the coding region alter the reading frame[1132-1134, 1165, 1170] or there is a nonsense mutation[1171] that leads to a shortened β-spectrin chain. The other variants probably induce conformational changes that alter the ability of spectrin to self-associate.

Spectrin Defects Outside the Heterodimer Self-Association Site. A few cases of mutant spectrins outside the heterodimer self-association site have been described in patients with HE and HPP. Some of these variants have an effect on spectrin dimer self-association, the basis of which is largely unknown. Lane and colleagues reported a truncated α-spectrin chain variant associated with HE in three generations of a family.[1096] The affected red cells had decreased stability and impaired spectrin self-association. Truncated α-spectrin varied from 10% to 45% of total α-spectrin. Two-dimensional tryptic peptide maps were qualitatively normal but showed a decrease in the quantity of one of the α IV domain peptides. The genetic defect underlying this variant α-spectrin chain remains unknown.

A severe neonatal poikilocytic anemia associated with impaired spectrin dimer self-association was observed in an infant whose parents were clinically and biochemically normal.[1108] There was increased tryptic cleavage at the junction of the α II and α III domains and a slight modification of the molecular weights of the two major peptides of the α II domain. The proband is homozygous for a splice junction mutation that leads to two variant mRNA species: One species encodes a truncated α-spectrin chain that is not assembled on the membrane. The other species encodes a protein that lacks exon 20 but is attached to the membrane.[1182] Because α-spectrin is produced in excess, the heterozygous parents are clinically and biochemically asymptomatic.

Spectrin^{Oran} is a variant of the α II domain that is expressed at low levels. It is asymptomatic in the heterozygous state but causes severe HE in the homozygous state. Tryptic peptide mapping and amino acid sequencing of a variant peptide reveals an abnormal cleavage after Arg^{890},[1107] owing to a mutation of the acceptor splice site upstream of exon 18 (-1, a→g) that causes exon 18 to be skipped. A minor mRNA species utilizes an alternative acceptor site one base downstream from the mutated intron/exon boundary. The skipping of exon 18 probably changes the conformation of the α II domain of spectrin, leading to its abnormal pattern of tryptic digestion.

Spectrin^{Jendouba} ($\alpha^{II/31}$) is a variant associated with asymptomatic HE, a mild defect in spectrin self-association,[1166] and abnormal tryptic cleavage after Lys^{788} due to an Asp→Glu mutation at codon 791. This mutation apparently has a long-range effect on the self-association of spectrin dimers.

A large β-spectrin chain variant, spectrin^{Detroit}, with an estimated molecular weight of 330 kDa, was isolated from a child with HE.[1183] Further study of this patient and his family members demonstrated that HE was caused by co-inheritance of an α-spectrin chain variant (the $\alpha^{I/65-68}$ abnormality) rather than by the elongated β-spectrin chain. Family members with normal α-spectrin and heterozygous for the elongated β chain variant had normal red cell morphology and no clinical abnormalities, but their erythrocyte membranes were more rigid and fragile than normal. The fragility is probably a consequence of both weaker spectrin dimer association and spectrin deficiency (total spectrin was about 80% of normal). The underlying molecular defect of this elongated β-spectrin chain is unknown.

Low Expression Alpha-Spectrin Allele: Alpha^{LELY}. In some cases, HE/HPP patients are *heterozygous* for a structural variant of spectrin involving the self-association site but have a more severe phenotype than expected, including marked hemolysis and anemia requiring blood transfusions or splenectomy. These patients also have spectrin deficiency. They are usually categorized as having hemolytic HE, poikilocytic HE, or HPP. It has been postulated that they possess a second defect of α-spectrin that affects spectrin production or accumulation. The parents who transmit the postulated defect are clinically and biochemically normal. Studies of patients have focused on associated α-spectrin polymorphisms, studies of α-spectrin chain synthesis *in vitro*, and PCR-based analyses.

The best-characterized low expression allele of α-spectrin is the α^{LELY} allele. In initial studies, a polymorphism of the α V domain, referred to as $\alpha^{V/41}$ and associated with increased proteolytic susceptibility of the junction between the α IV and α V domains, was identified in tryptic digests of spectrin.[1087] HE patients who were heterozygous for various mutant α spectrins

and who possessed the $\alpha^{V/41}$ polymorphism in *trans* were more severe than expected.[154] However, the polymorphism itself was asymptomatic in either the heterozygous or homozygous state. Molecular studies identified two linked abnormalities: (1) a C→T substitution at position -12 of intron 45, immediately upstream of exon 46, which is thought to cause the six amino acids encoded by exon 46 to be skipped, and (2) an amino acid substitution, Leu→Val at codon 1857 in exon 40, owing to a C→G substitution.[1184] Together, these changes identify the α^{LELY} allele, which has a wide ethnic distribution and is *very common* (gene frequencies of 31% in whites, 21% in African blacks, 20% in Japanese, and 22% in Chinese).[1185] In patients who are heterozygous for α^{LELY} and an α-spectrin mutation causing HE, the limited synthesis of α^{LELY} protein decreases the amount of spectrin containing α^{LELY} that is incorporated into the membrane by around 50% and increases the relative incorporation of spectrin containing the HE α chain. It is postulated that α^{LELY} is poorly expressed owing to defective spectrin nucleation because the six deleted amino acids lie within the nucleation site that joins the α- and β-spectrin chains[372] (see earlier discussion). Alpha chains that lack exon 46 fail to assemble into stable spectrin dimers and are degraded.

The α^{LELY} allele is clinically silent by itself, even when homozygous, probably because α-spectrin is normally synthesized in a threefold or fourfold excess.[604] As explained earlier, when spectrin α^{LELY} is inherited in *trans* to an α-spectrin mutation, it has the effect of increasing the concentration of the mutant spectrin and the severity of the associated disease. The effect can be quite dramatic. For example, in one family a patient who was heterozygous for the $\alpha^{I/74}$ mutation ($+/\alpha^{I/74}$) had very mild disease and almost no morphologic abnormality, whereas a relative who had also inherited the α^{LELY} allele ($\alpha^{I/74}\alpha^{LELY}$) had severe elliptocytosis.[1087] Similarly, in another family the α^{LELY} allele increased the proportion of spectrin $\alpha^{I/65-68}$ in heterozygotes from 45% to 65% of the total spectrin.[1087] This was associated with an increase in the proportion of elliptocytes from none or only a few to nearly 100%. All α-spectrin mutations seem to be similarly affected (Fig. 16–30). Conversely, when the α^{LELY} allele is on the same chromosome as an α-spectrin mutation it mutes the elliptocytic phenotype.

Although the synthesis of α^{LELY} subunits is decreased, owing to poor incorporation of the peptide lacking exon 46, the production of α^{LELY} mRNA is normal. In particular, spectrin α^{LELY} should be distinguished from thalassemia-like defects of α-spectrin synthesis that, when co-inherited with some of the α-spectrin mutations, also produce a phenotype of HPP. The latter defects are characterized by reduced α-spectrin mRNA levels and diminished α-spectrin synthesis. None is well characterized. Preliminary studies in an HPP patient heterozygous for the $\alpha^{I/50a}$-spectrin variant and an asymptomatic parent show that α-spectrin protein synthesis is decreased, as measured by pulse-labeling of late erythroblasts.[606] Competitive PCR studies in the same patient show that α-spectrin mRNA is decreased

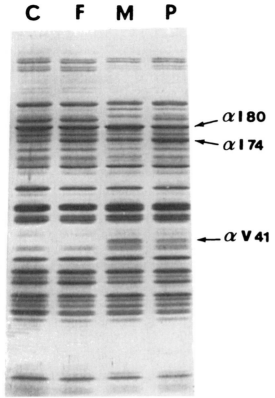

C F M P

αI80
αI74

αV41

Figure 16-30. One-dimensional gel electrophoresis of partial tryptic digests of spectrin. Lane C contains spectrin of a normal control subject. Lane P contains spectrin from a hereditary elliptocytosis proband who is a compound heterozygote for the $\alpha^{I/74}$ variant and the $\alpha^{V/41}$ polymorphism that marks the presence of spectrin α^{LELY}. Lane F contains spectrin of the proband's father, who is heterozygous for the $\alpha^{I/74}$ variant and lacks the $\alpha^{V/41}/\alpha^{LEVY}$ polymorphism. Lane M contains spectrin of the proband's mother, who lacks the $\alpha^{I/74}$ variant and is homozygous for the $\alpha^{V/41}/\alpha^{LELY}$ polymorphism. (From Baklouti F, Maréchal J, et al: Occurrence of the αI 22 Arg→His (CGT→CAT) spectrin mutation in Tunisia: potential association with severe elliptocytosis. Br J Haematol 1991; 78:108.)

compared with controls. In another example, three patients who are heterozygous for distinct mutations of the α I domain of spectrin, have markedly decreased amounts of α spectrin mRNA derived from the companion allele, leading to a phenotype of HPP.[1186] In these cases, the structural mutation either created or abolished a restriction enzyme site, creating a marker for the production-defective allele.

Molecular Determinants of the Clinical Severity of HE/HPP Spectrin Mutations. The two principal determinants of severity are the spectrin content of the cells and the percentage of dimeric spectrin in crude spectrin extracts.[157, 1088] The fraction of dimeric spectrin, in turn, depends principally on two factors. The first is the dysfunction of the mutant spectrin. Mutations within or near the site of self-association produce a more profound defect of spectrin function and a more severe clinical phenotype than point mutations in more distant triple-helical repeats.[154] The second factor is the fraction of the mutant spectrin in the cells. This is determined by the gene dose (i.e., simple heterozygote

versus homozygote or double heterozygote) and by other genetic defects such as the presence of α^{LELY}-spectrin or another defect leading to reduced synthesis of α-spectrin.[1087, 1184]

Polymorphisms of Spectrin. Spectrin polymorphisms are useful markers in genetic studies of erythrocyte membrane defects. A number of protein polymorphisms have been identified by tryptic mapping of spectrin. Variant peptides have been identified in the α II and α III domains.[1052, 1187–1189] Four polymorphisms of the α II domain occur primarily in people of African origin and have been characterized at the levels of protein and DNA sequence.[1187, 1188] All four polymorphisms involve various combinations of amino acids at residues 701, 809, and 853: type 1—normal, Arg/Ile/Thr; type 2—apparent increase in molecular weight and basic shift in isoelectric point, His/Val/Arg; type 3—apparent increase in molecular weight, His/Ile/Thr; and type 4—basic shift in isoelectric point, Arg/Val/Arg. All of the amino acid variations are due to single base substitutions. These polymorphisms occur in distinct haplotypes and have been correlated with specific HE/HPP α-spectrin mutations.[1189] The α III domain protein polymorphism is also a point mutation.[1052]

Protein 4.1 Defects

The link between protein 4.1 deficiency and elliptocytosis was first described in a consanguineous Algerian family.[1062, 1109] Partial absence of the protein is found in the 4.1(−) trait, which appears to be a common cause of elliptocytosis, accounting for 30% to 40% of cases in some Arab and European populations.[1069–1071, 1117, 1190] It is not observed in individuals of African ancestry.[1053]

Heterozygous Protein 4.1 Deficiency. Protein 4.1(−) heterozygotes have clinically mild HE with little or no hemolysis, prominent elliptocytosis, often approaching 100%, and minimal red cell fragmentation.[1191]

Homozygous Protein 4.1 Deficiency. Erythrocytes from patients homozygous for the protein 4.1(−) trait (i.e., complete protein 4.1 deficiency) are elliptical, fragmented, and poikilocytic.[1062, 1109, 1192] They are very osmotically fragile and possess normal thermal stability. Membranes from homozygous protein 4.1(−) red cells fragment much more rapidly than normal at moderate sheer stresses, an indication of their intrinsic instability.[1150] Membrane mechanical stability can be completely restored by reconstituting the deficient red cells with normal protein 4.1 or the protein 4.1/spectrin/actin-binding site.[1193, 1194] In addition to complete deficiency of protein 4.1, erythrocytes from protein 4.1(−) homozygotes lack protein p55[475, 1195] and have only 30% of the normal content of GPC and GPD.[473, 477, 1109, 1195, 1196] This adds evidence to the hypothesis that GPC is one of the membrane attachment sites for protein 4.1.[283, 472] In addition, protein 4.9 is absent from isolated membrane skeletons but not intact red cell membranes, and membrane phospholipid asymmetry is perturbed.[479, 1062] Homozygous patients have a severe hemolytic anemia, requiring transfusions and splenectomy.[1062, 1109, 1192] There appears to be a good response to splenectomy.

In the original Algerian kindred,[1062] protein 4.1(−) mRNA is not translated,[1197] owing to a 318-bp deletion, which includes the downstream translation initiation site that is utilized in reticulocytes (Fig. 16–31).[136] In other patients, point mutations of the downstream initiator codon (AUG→AGG[1109] and AUG→ACG[1198]) have been identified. Interestingly (and probably fortunately), expression of protein 4.1 is relatively unimpaired in nonerythroid tissues and early erythroblasts[484–486, 1199] because most of the protein 4.1 isoforms in these tissues initiate translation at the alternatively spliced, upstream translation initiation site.

Protein 4.1 Structural Defects. Variants with abnormal molecular weights have also been described in association with HE.[1071, 1200, 1201] A shortened protein 4.1 was discovered in an Italian family with very mild common HE and mechanically unstable red cells. The patients are heterozygous for a protein 4.1 variant that has lost the two exons encoding the spectrin/actin-binding domain. The mutant protein runs as a doublet of 65 and 68 kDa on SDS gels and seems to be present in nearly normal amounts. It is presumed, but not proven, to be functionally inept. A high-molecular-weight variant, protein 4.1[95] or protein 4.1[Hurdle-Mills, 1071] was discovered in a family of Scottish-Irish ancestry with very mild common HE. The patients are heterozygous for a duplication of three exons that include the spectrin/actin-binding domain.[1200, 1201] Membrane function appears to be preserved because red cell membranes have normal mechanical stability.[136] It is not clear how this variant causes HE.

Glycophorin C Defects

Elliptocytes are noted on peripheral blood smears of patients whose erythrocytes carry the Leach phenotype (i.e., lacking the Gerbich antigens, Ge: −1, −2, −3, −4).[248–250, 1140, 1141, 1202, 1203] These erythrocytes are devoid of GPC and GPD and, presumably secondarily, lack protein p55 and are deficient in protein 4.1. It has been speculated that the protein 4.1 deficiency in Leach erythrocytes is the cause of their elliptocytic shape. Interestingly, the relative deficiency of protein 4.1 in Leach erythrocytes is less than the degree of GPC deficiency in homozygous protein 4.1(−) erythrocytes. These findings add supportive evidence to the hypothesis that GPC and protein p55 provide a binding site for protein 4.1 in the red cell.[475]

The Leach phenotype is usually due to a deletion of 7 kb of genomic DNA that removes exons 3 and 4 from the *GPC/GPD* locus.[1203, 1204] One individual has a single nucleotide deletion preceded by a missense mutation,[1205] TGGCCG→TTGCG, leading to a frameshift with premature chain termination. Patients carrying the Leach phenotype suffer from a mild spherocytic HE with increased erythrocyte osmotic fragility.[246, 249, 250, 1140] In some individuals, no elliptocytes are detected on peripheral smear.[473] In one patient, transient elliptocytosis and GPC deficiency were associated with development of an autoantibody to GPC.[1143]

Individuals whose erythrocytes lack several of the Gerbich antigens, that is, the Yusef type (−1, −2, 3, 4) and Gerbich type (−1, −2, −3, 4), owing to large deletions of genomic DNA, lack GPC and GPD. Instead, these erythrocytes possess a single structurally related functional protein of molecular weight intermediate between that of GPC and GPD.[1206] These erythrocytes are not elliptocytic and have normal amounts of protein 4.1 and protein p55, suggesting that the hybrid protein is functionally active and fully capable of interacting with the two skeletal proteins. Individuals whose erythrocytes lack GPA, GPB, or both, are asymptomatic and have erythrocytes of normal shape and mechanical stability.

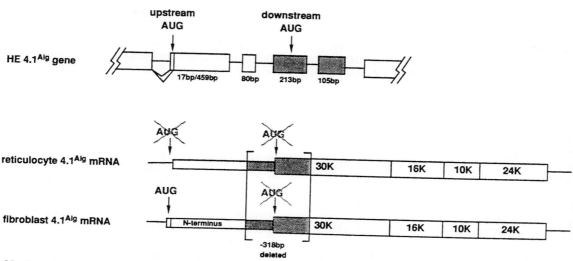

Figure 16–31. Genetic model of the defect causing protein 4.1(−) HE in a well-described Algerian family. The *upper panel* shows the 5′ portion of the 4.1 gene, including the exons encoding the upstream and downstream AUGs. In the mutant gene, the shaded exons are not spliced into 4.1 mRNAs. Reticulocyte 4.1 mRNA thus lacks any functional translation initiation site and cannot make any protein 4.1. Fibroblast 4.1 mRNA retains the upstream AUG and can synthesize high-molecular-weight 4.1 isoforms with an NH₂-terminal extension. (From Conboy JG: Structure, function, and molecular genetics of erythroid membrane skeletal protein 4.1 in normal and abnormal red blood cells. Semin Hematol 1993; 30:138.)

Pathophysiology of HE/HPP
Spectrin Mutations

The principal functional consequence of the elliptocytogenic spectrin mutations is a weakening or even disruption of the spectrin dimer-tetramer contact, and, consequently, the two-dimensional integrity of the membrane skeleton. These horizontal defects are readily detected by ultrastructural examination of membrane skeletons, which reveals disruption of the normally uniform hexagonal lattice. Consequently, membrane skeletons, cell membranes, and the red cells are mechanically unstable. In patients carrying severely dysfunctional spectrin mutations, or in subjects who are homozygous or compound heterozygous for such mutant proteins, this membrane instability is sufficient to cause hemolytic anemia with red cell fragmentation.

How elliptocytes are formed is less clear. In common HE, red cell precursors are round and the cells become progressively more elliptical as they age *in vivo*.[1048, 1072, 1207] Red cells distorted by shear stress *in vitro* or flowing through the microcirculation *in vivo* have elliptical or parachute-like shapes, respectively.[145, 1208] Perhaps elliptocytes and poikilocytes are permanently stabilized in their abnormal shape because the weakened skeletal interactions facilitate skeletal reorganization after prolonged or repetitive cellular deformation. Skeletal reorganization is likely to involve breakage of the unidirectionally stretched protein connections and formation of new contacts that reduce stress on the skeleton and stabilize the deformed shape.[145] This process, first proposed in 1978, has been shown to account for permanent deformation of irreversibly sickled cells.[1209, 1210]

HPP red cells have two abnormalities: they contain a mutant spectrin that disrupts spectrin self-association and they are partially deficient in spectrin.[606, 1123] This is either due to an elliptocytogenic α-spectrin mutation and a defect involving reduced α-spectrin synthesis or to two elliptocytogenic spectrin alleles. In the latter situation, spectrin deficiency might be a consequence of spectrin instability, which would reduce the amount of spectrin available for membrane assembly. In red cells carrying a lot of unassembled spectrin dimers, the fact that one ankyrin is bound per one spectrin tetramer (i.e., two spectrin heterodimers) may also contribute to spectrin deficiency. At best only about one half of the spectrin dimers could succeed in attaching to the available ankyrin binding sites. Probably it would be less because unphosphorylated ankyrin binds spectrin dimers about 10 times less avidly than spectrin tetramers.[395, 414, 434]

The phenotype of HPP, characterized by the presence of fragments and elliptocytes, together with evidence of red cell surface area deficiency (i.e., microspherocytes), suggests that the membrane dysfunction involves both vertical interactions (a consequence of the spectrin deficiency) and horizontal interactions (a consequence of the elliptocytogenic spectrin mutations).

Protein 4.1 Variants

Hereditary elliptocytes that are deficient in protein 4.1 are similar in shape and membrane instability to elliptocytes that result from spectrin mutations.[145] This suggests that protein 4.1 deficiency principally affects the spectrin/actin contact (i.e., a horizontal interaction) rather than the skeletal attachment to GPC (a vertical interaction).

Permeability of HE Red Cells

Red cells of HE consume more ATP and 2,3-DPG than normal erythrocytes,[1211] probably owing to increased transmembrane Na^+ movements.[1212] As a result of the underlying skeletal defect, HE and HPP red cells are abnormally permeable to Na^+, K^+, and Ca^{2+} ions.[1120, 1212] The excessive Ca^{2+} leak was originally thought to be the primary molecular lesion in a patient with a severe microcytic hemolytic anemia and red cell thermal instability,[1120] who was subsequently shown to have a spectrin mutation and probably HPP.[1174]

Common HE and Malaria

Epidemiologic studies of the elliptocytogenic mutations of spectrin in Central Western Africa suggest that their prevalence is considerably greater than would be expected for sporadic mutations. For example, the prevalence of the spectrin $\alpha^{I/65-68}$ mutation approaches 1%[1053] and the mutation is always associated with the same α-spectrin haplotype.[1188] Similar findings were reported for two α-spectrin mutations producing the spectrin $\alpha^{I/46-50a}$ phenotype (Leu[207]→Pro and Leu[260]→Pro). These data are of considerable interest in light of recent *in vitro* studies, demonstrating diminished malarial parasite entry or growth in red cells that contain some of the elliptocytogenic spectrin mutants or are deficient in protein 4.1.[1180, 1213, 1214]

Treatment

In typical HE, the condition is mild and splenectomy is rarely required. Splenectomy to decrease hemolysis, ameliorate anemia, and avoid the formation of bilirubinate gallstones has been the cornerstone of therapy for cases of severe hemolytic HE and HPP. Most practitioners believe that the same indications for splenectomy in HS should be applied to patients with symptomatic HE and HPP. Patients with HE/HPP who have been splenectomized have experienced increased hematocrits, decreased reticulocytosis, and improvement in clinical symptoms. If hemolysis is still active after splenectomy, folate should be administered daily. Recommendations for antibiotic prophylaxis, immunization, and monitoring during intercurrent illnesses are similar to those noted for HS patients before and after splenectomy. Serial interval ultrasound examinations, beginning around age 6 years, to detect gallstones should be performed in patients with brisk hemolysis.

Neonates should be managed as any patient with hemolytic anemia. Phototherapy and exchange transfusions are warranted in cases of severe anemia and pathologic hyperbilirubinemia. Splenectomy is rarely necessary in the neonatal period.

Southeast Asian Ovalocytosis

This condition, also known as Melanesian elliptocytosis or stomatocytic elliptocytosis, is inherited in an autosomal dominant pattern.[1215–1220] It is observed in the aboriginal populations of Melanesia and Malaysia and in portions of Indonesia and the Philippines.[1215–1218, 1221–1223] The abnormality is very common in Melanesia, particularly in lowland tribes where malaria is endemic.[1216, 1220, 1223, 1224] In these tribes, 5% to 25% of the natives are affected. *In vivo*, there is evidence that SAO provides some protection against all forms of malaria, particularly against heavy infections and cerebral malaria.[1216, 1217, 1220, 1224–1226] The prevalence of SAO increases with age in populations challenged by malaria, suggesting that individuals with SAO have a selective advantage.[1225] *In vitro*, SAO red cells are resistant to invasion by malarial parasites,[1227–1229] apparently because the membrane is 10 to 20 times more rigid than normal.[1147, 1230–1233] Other membrane characteristics reflect this property,[1147] including unusually high heat resistance, lack of endocytosis in response to drugs that produce dramatic endocytosis in normal cells, and strong resistance to crenation, even after several days' storage in plasma or buffered salt solutions. The latter property, combined with the distinctive red cell morphology (see later), provides a simple means of diagnosing the disease.

Most of the cells are rounded elliptocytes, but a few are traversed by one or two transverse bars that divide the central clear space (see Fig. 16–23D).[1215, 1219, 1221–1223] These "elliptical knizocytes" or "stomatocytic elliptocytes" are not seen in any other condition. Hemolysis is apparently mild or absent, although extensive hematologic data are not available.[1215, 1217, 1221, 1222] One patient had compensated hemolysis (no anemia), with mild splenomegaly, an absolute reticulocyte count of 150 to 300×10^{-3} (normal 10 to 100×10^{-3}), mild hyperbilirubinemia, and gallstones.[1234] This indicates that membrane rigidity is not a major determinant of red cell survival. In another well-studied patient,[1222] red cell Na^+ and K^+ permeability was increased, glucose consumption was elevated to compensate for increased cation pumping, autohemolysis was increased, and the cells were osmotically resistant. Curiously, many blood group antigens are poorly expressed on the surface of SAO red cells,[1223] possibly because the rigid membrane inhibits their clustering and impedes agglutination.

Etiology

The finding of tight linkage between an abnormal proteolytic digest of band 3 protein and the SAO phenotype led to detection of the underlying molecular defect.[1219] All carriers of the SAO phenotype are heterozygotes. One band 3 allele is normal, and the other contains two mutations in *cis*: a deletion of nine codons encoding amino acids 400 through 408, located at the boundary of the cytoplasmic and membrane domains and the replacement of Lys^{56} by Glu.[1232, 1233, 1235–1238] The $Lys^{56} \rightarrow Glu$ substitution is an asymptomatic polymorphism known as band 3 Memphis. The mutant

SAO band 3 exhibits tight binding to ankyrin,[1219] increased tyrosine phosphorylation,[1239–1241] inability to transport anions,[1242, 1243] and markedly restricted lateral and rotational mobility in the membrane.[1219, 1232] Because SAO is caused by deletion of 27 bases from the band 3 gene, amplification of the deleted region in genomic DNA or reticulocyte cDNA is the most specific diagnostic test. This produces a single band in control red cells and a doublet with the second band shorter by 27 bp in SAO cells.[1232, 1235, 1244] No SAO homozygotes have been identified; it has been hypothesized that this would lead to embryonic or fetal lethality.

Molecular Basis of Membrane Rigidity and Malaria Resistance

SAO red cells are unique among elliptocytes in that they are rigid and hyperstable rather than unstable.[1231] The SAO band 3 mutation is the first example of a defect of an integral membrane protein leading to red cell membrane rigidity, a property that had previously been attributed to the membrane skeleton.[1245] The explanation of the rigidity is presently not clear. One hypothesis proposes that conformational changes of the cytoplasmic domain of SAO band 3 preclude lateral movement (extension) of the skeletal network during deformation.[1147, 1233] A second possibility is that SAO band 3 binds abnormally tightly to ankyrin and thus to the underlying skeleton.[1219] The increased propensity of SAO band 3 to aggregate into higher oligomers may be important as the oligomers can strengthen band 3 attachment to ankyrin.[1246] The tendency of SAO band 3 to form linear arrays would also decrease its mobility within the bilayer.[1247] Finally, SAO band 3 may adhere to the skeleton in a nonspecific manner, possibly due to denaturation of the membrane spanning domain.[1248]

The resistance of SAO red cells to malaria is presumably related to the altered properties of SAO band 3. Band 3 serves as one of the malaria receptors, because invasion by the parasite *in vitro* is inhibited by band 3–containing liposomes.[1249] In normal red cells, parasite invasion is associated with marked membrane remodeling and redistribution of band 3–containing intramembrane particles.[1250] Intramembrane particles cluster at the site of parasite invasion, forming a ring around the orifice through which the parasite enters the cell. The invaginated red cell membrane, which surrounds the invading parasite, is free from intramembrane particles. The reduced lateral mobility of band 3 protein in SAO red cells may preclude band 3 receptor clustering and thus prevent attachment or entry of the parasites.[1219, 1232] Resistance to malaria has also been attributed to diminished anion exchange, owing to the inability of SAO band 3 to transport anions.[1242, 1243] In addition, SAO red cells consume ATP at a higher rate than normal cells; the ensuing partial depletion of ATP levels in ovalocytes has been proposed to account, at least in part, for the resistance of these cells to malaria invasion *in vitro*.[1230] However, diminished anion transport and ATP depletion do not appear to play a critical role in malaria resistance of SAO erythrocytes *in vivo*. This is evidenced by the fact that band 3–deficient

HS red cells are considerably less resistant to malaria invasion than SAO red cells, although both cell types have a similar decrease of anion transport, and by the fact that malaria resistance of SAO red cells is detected *in vitro* even when red cell ATP levels are maintained.

Hydrops Fetalis Syndromes and Disorders of the Erythrocyte Membrane

Defects of the erythrocyte membrane have been well characterized in cases of severe neonatal hemolytic anemia due to recessive HS and homozygous HE/pyro-poikilocytosis (HE/HPP). Three well-documented kindreds with fatal or near-fatal anemia and hydrops fetalis associated with erythrocyte membrane defects have been described. In all three cases, defects were identified in spectrin, the principal structural protein of the erythrocyte membrane. Based on the authors' experience, membrane defects have been suspected, but not proven, in numerous other cases of nonimmune hydrops fetalis with severe hemolytic anemia.

An infant has been described who had hydrops fetalis, severe spherocytic anemia, extremely abnormal red blood cell osmotic fragility, and transfusion-dependent anemia that failed to respond to splenectomy.[690] The patient's mother had typical autosomal dominant HS and her father, although clinically and hematologically normal, had red cells with slightly abnormal osmotic fragility. Cultured progenitor-derived erythroblasts from this patient showed a decrease in total cell spectrin content to 26% of normal. Metabolic labeling studies of cultured erythroblasts using ^{35}S-methionine revealed markedly decreased α-spectrin synthesis and absence of α-spectrin chain degradation products. It was thought that two different genetic defects caused the severe reduction of α-spectrin synthesis in the affected child's erythroid cells and that the profound spectrin deficiency resulted in cell destruction during egress of reticulocytes from the marrow or during enucleation of normoblasts. The precise genetic defect or defects in this family have not been characterized.

In a second kindred,[1168] four third-trimester fetal losses occurred associated with hemolytic anemia and hydrops fetalis. Studies of erythrocytes and erythrocyte membranes from the parents showed abnormal membrane stability as well as structural and functional abnormalities of spectrin. A point mutation in the β-spectrin gene, Ser[2019]→Pro, spectrin[Providence], was identified in the heterozygous state in the parents and two living children and in the homozygous state in the three deceased infants studied.

A Laotian infant was born with severe Coombs-negative hemolytic anemia (Hb 2.7 g/dL) and gross hydrops fetalis at birth.[1169] His neonatal course was marked by ongoing hemolytic anemia requiring erythrocyte transfusions. He has remained transfusion dependent for 2 years; his blood smears reveal only normal erythrocytes, which represent transfused cells and nucleated erythrocytes. Family history is remarkable for a previous sibling born with hemolytic anemia and hydrops fetalis who died on the second day of life. At autopsy it was revealed that she had diffuse tissue anoxia and marked extramedullary erythropoiesis. The parents had very rare elliptocytes and fragile erythrocyte membranes. Their spectrin exhibited weak self-association *in vitro* and displayed the mutant α[1/74] peptide on two-dimensional peptide maps. The proband and his deceased sister were homozygous for a point mutation of β-spectrin, Leu[2025]→Arg, spectrin[Buffalo], in the region of spectrin that participates in spectrin self-association. The parents were heterozygous for this mutation.

Stomatocytosis and Xerocytosis

Red cell hydration is largely determined by the intracellular concentration of monovalent cations. A net increase in Na$^+$ and K$^+$ ions causes water to enter, forming "stomatocytes" or "hydrocytes," whereas a net loss of monovalent cations produces dehydrated red cells or "xerocytes" (see Fig. 16–14).[1251, 1252] In the past 35 years, numerous descriptions of congenital or familial hemolytic anemias associated with abnormal cation permeability and, in some cases, disturbed red cell hydration have been reported.[1251–1286] These span the range from severe stomatocytosis to severe xerocytosis. They can be divided into six provisional categories based on differences of severity, morphology, cation content, lipid and protein composition, genetics, and response to splenectomy (Table 16–12). It is unknown if these categories are unique entities. Indeed, none of these apparent disorders is precisely defined in either clinical or molecular terms.

Hereditary Stomatocytosis

Hereditary stomatocytosis, the name given by Lock and co-workers to the first reported case,[1253] is characterized by erythrocytes with a mouth-shaped (stoma) area of central pallor on peripheral blood smears (Fig. 16–32). The clinical severity of hereditary stomatocytosis is variable; some patients experience hemolysis and anemia whereas others are asymptomatic.[777, 1251–1253] At least 10 families have been described.*

Stomatocyte membranes are remarkably permeable to Na$^+$ and K$^+$ ions, particularly Na$^+$ ions. Intracellular Na$^+$ is increased and K$^+$ is decreased, but the total monovalent cation content (Na$^+$ + K$^+$) is high, which leads to an increase in cell water and cell volume. As a consequence, the "edematous cells" are sometimes called "hydrocytes" or "overhydrated stomatocytes."[1288]

Pathophysiology

The major detectable defect in hereditary stomatocytosis is a marked asymmetric increase in passive Na$^+$ and K$^+$ permeability (Na$^+$ in > K$^+$ out). Permeabilities as great as 15 to 40 times normal are observed.[1254, 1280, 1287] Because the influx of Na$^+$ exceeds the loss of K$^+$, stomatocytic red cells progressively gain cations

---

*See references 777, 1251, 1253–1256, 1263, 1264, 1267, 1268, 1271, 1272, 1274, and 1287.

Table 16-12. CLINICAL HETEROGENEITY OF HEREDITARY HYDROCYTOSIS-XEROCYTOSIS SYNDROMES

| | Stomatocytosis (Hydrocytosis) | | Intermediate Syndromes | | | |
	Severe Hemolysis	Mild Hemolysis	Cryohydrocytosis	Stomatocytic Xerocytosis	Xerocytosis with High PC	Xerocytosis
Hemolysis	Severe	Mild-moderate	Moderate	Mild	Moderate	Moderate
Anemia	Severe	Mild-moderate	Mild-moderate	None	Mild	Moderate
Blood smear	Stomatocytes	Stomatocytes	Stomatocytes*	Stomatocytes	Targets	Targets, echinocytes
MCV (80–100 fL³)†	110–150	95–130	90–105	91–98	84–92	100–110
MCHC (32%–36%)	24–30	26–29	34–40	33–39	34–38	100–110
Unincubated osmotic fragility	Very increased	Increased	Normal	Decreased	Very decreased	34–38 Very decreased
RBC Na⁺ (5–12 mEq/LRBC)	60–100	30–60	40–50	10–20	10–15	10–20
RBC K⁺ (90–103 mEq/LRBC)	20–55	40–85	55–65	75–85	75–90	60–80
RBC Na⁺ + K⁺ (95–110 mEq/LRBC)	110–140	115–145	100–105	87–103	93–99	75–90
Phosphatidylcholine content	Normal	±Increased	Normal	Normal	Increased	Normal
Cold autohemolysis	No	No	Yes	No	No	?
Effect of splenectomy	Good	Good	Fair	?	?	?Poor
Genetics	AD, ?AR	AD	AD	AD	AD	AD

PC, phosphatidylcholine; MCV, mean corpuscular volume; MCHC, mean corpuscular hemoglobin concentration; AR, autosomal recessive; AD, autosomal dominant; LRBC, liter of red blood cells.
*In the few reported patients the stomatocytes have had a unique *curved* slit of central pallor.
†Values in parentheses are the normal range.

and water and swell. As a result, their average density is less than normal and the swollen stomatocytes are osmotically fragile. Unlike normal cells, aged stomatocytes are less dense and more stomatocytic than stomatocytic reticulocytes.[777, 1251]

The transporters of the red cell are similar to those of other cells in many respects.[1288, 1289] However, the rate of cation transport is less in the erythrocyte than any other cell. In addition, the erythrocyte is relatively sluggish in responding to pharmacologic or other stimuli with changes in Na⁺ or K⁺ transport. Finally, the red cell is equipped with a high-capacity anion exchanger to service carbonic anhydrase, an intracellular respiratory enzyme, making red cell chloride transport much faster than in other cells. The different transporters identified in the red cell are described in Table 16–4.

In stomatocytosis, monovalent cation transporters are stimulated by the influx of Na⁺, particularly the Na⁺/K⁺-pump and K⁺/Cl⁻ cotransporter,[1271] but are unable to keep up with the exaggerated cation leaks. There is no convincing evidence that Na⁺/K⁺ pumping is defective. Pump kinetics are normal,[777] and the number of pumps is increased severalfold,[1251, 1282] even after correcting for red cell age.[1290] Some authors have observed that Na⁺ and K⁺ are not transported in the usual ratio, 3 Na⁺:2 K⁺,[777, 1265, 1272] and have argued that the Na⁺/K⁺ pump is "decoupled."[1272] Other work suggests that this is, at least partly, an artifact of the methods used to measure cation permeability.[1291]

Bifunctional imidoesters, which cross-link proteins, reverse the abnormal shape and permeability of hereditary stomatocytes and normalize their survival in the circulation.[1287, 1292, 1293] The critical proteins involved have not been identified using these agents because many red cell membrane proteins are cross-linked at the concentrations required to achieve this effect. Stomatocytes are relatively rigid[1268] and expend extraordinary amounts of ATP pumping Na⁺ and K⁺, attempting to maintain homeostasis. They are vulnerable to splenic sequestration and, predictably, splenectomy has been beneficial in some patients with severe hemolysis,[1251, 1267, 1271, 1272, 1274] but not, without risk (see later).[1294]

Stomatin

The red cell membranes of all or almost all patients with the classic overhydrated form of stomatocytosis, described earlier, lack a 31-kDa protein called stomatin or band 7.2b (Fig. 16–33).[1256, 1259, 1260, 1271, 1287, 1295] Stomatin is an integral membrane phosphoprotein whose function is not completely understood[1287, 1288, 1295–1297]. Its importance, however, is underscored by its wide tissue and species distribution. In humans, stomatin mRNA has been detected in every tissue and cell tested, except for brain and neutrophils.[1287, 1288, 1296–1298] Protein immunoblotting using a polyclonal anti–human stomatin antibody showed reactivity in human liver and kidney tissue but none in brain, cardiac tissue, or ileum.[1295] Reactivity to a monoclonal antibody directed against human erythrocyte stomatin has been observed in the erythrocyte membranes of a wide variety of species, including frog, rat, chicken, rabbit, pig, cow, and sheep.[1297] It has been hypothesized that stomatin may support, activate, or regulate an unidentified ion channel.[1287, 1288] Evidence showing a potential interaction between stomatin and the membrane skeleton protein adducin[1299] suggests that stomatin may also be a part of the junctional complex of the membrane skeleton.[139] In this capacity, it may participate in a variety of spe-

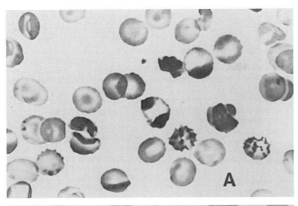

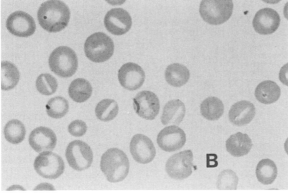

Figure 16–32. Peripheral blood morphology in hereditary xero-cytosis and hereditary stomatocytosis. *A,* Hereditary xerocytosis: note the presence of target cells, echinocytes and some dense cells in which the hemoglobin is puddled at the periphery. Red cell morphology is usually much less dramatic in this disease, especially before splenectomy. Often, modest targeting is the only detectable abnormality. *B,* Hereditary stomatocytosis: many stomatocytes and occasional target cells are seen. (From Lande WM, Mentzer WC: Haemolytic anaemia associated with increased cation permeability. Clin Haematol 1985; 14:89.)

cialized cellular functions. A homologue of stomatin, *mec2,* a protein involved in mechanosensation that is linked to a Na$^+$ channel, has been cloned from *Caeno-rhabditis elegans.*[1300] Compared with the human protein, it has extended NH$_2$- and COOH-terminal extensions. However, the proteins are very homologous, particularly in a region encoding glutamate and alanine residues. It is this region that has been suggested as an adducin-binding site.

Although hereditary stomatocytosis appears to be a dominantly inherited condition and affected individuals are presumably heterozygotes, stomatin protein is completely absent (mRNA levels are normal).[1288] This suggests a dominant-negative effect, where a mutant stomatin interacts with the wild-type protein, forming an unstable oligomeric protein complex.[1287] Stomatin protein does appear to form oligomers; however, four groups have cloned and sequenced cDNAs from stomatocytosis patients with stomatin deficiency,[1289, 1301–1303] including the most severely affected patient that has been reported,[1251, 1303] and all four find the coding sequence is *normal.* This makes it much more likely that the defect resides in a protein that interacts with stomatin and causes its destruction secondarily. For exam-

ple, the defect could activate a protein that modifies stomatin (e.g., a kinase, phosphatase, or ubiquitinating enzyme) so that it is recognized and destroyed, that destroys stomatin directly (e.g., a protease), or that directs it to be lost along with other proteins and organelles during reticulocyte maturation.

Finally, stomatin-deficient patients apparently do not suffer any nonhematologic symptoms,[1289] which suggests that either the deficiency is confined to erythrocytes or stomatin is not essential for the function of other tissues.

Clinical Features

Typical Stomatin-Deficient Stomatocytosis. The diagnostic features of the classic type of hereditary stomatocytosis include the unique red cell morphology (5% to 50% stomatocytes), severe hemolysis, macrocytosis (110–150 fL), elevated erythrocyte Na$^+$ concentration of 60–100 mEq/L (normal range, 5–12 mEq/L), reduced K$^+$ concentration of 20–55 mEq/L (normal range, 90–103 mEq/L), and increased total Na$^+$ + K$^+$ content of 110–140 mEq/L (normal range, 95–110 mEq/L). The excess cations elevate cell water, producing large, osmotically fragile cells with a low MCHC (24%–30%). In many patients, hereditary stomatocytes are also moderately deficient in 2,3-DPG.[1251, 1268, 1282] Perhaps a portion of the 1,3-DPG normally used for 2,3-DPG synthesis is diverted through phosphoglycerate kinase to provide extra ATP for cation transport.[1282] The 2,3-DPG deficiency mildly enhances oxygen affinity and causes additional water entry and cell swelling. Some patients[1264, 1270] and dogs[1304, 1305] with hereditary stomatocytosis have an unexplained decrease in red cell glutathione; however, it is unlikely that this is pathophysiologically significant.

Hereditary Stomatocytosis Variants. Hereditary stomatocytosis is probably more heterogeneous than suggested earlier. Some patients with severe permeability defects have little or no hemolysis.[777] In addition, studies of 44 Japanese patients with stomatocytosis show that the proportion of stomatocytes and the degree of Na$^+$ influx do not correlate with each other, and neither correlates with the amount of hemolysis or anemia.[1259] Furthermore, stomatin deficiency was not observed in Japanese patients with the most severe permeability defects and was only present, to a mild degree, in 5 of 9 patients with more moderate Na$^+$ leaks. This suggests that hereditary stomatocytosis is a complex mixture of diseases or that factors other than Na$^+$ leak and stomatin content are critical to the demise of the stomatocyte.

Treatment

Splenectomy reduces the hemolytic rate in patients with severe hereditary stomatocytosis[1251, 1255, 1268, 1271, 1272, 1274] and can be beneficial; however, a high proportion of patients have experienced thrombotic complications, in some cases with disastrous results.[1294] *In vitro,* stomatocytic erythrocytes from a hypercoagulable, splenectomized xerocytotic individual demonstrated

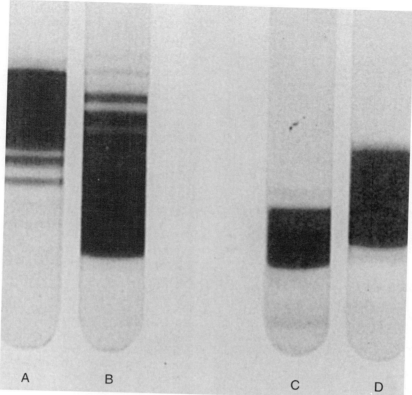

Figure 16–33. Separation of stomatocytes (hydrocytes) and xerocytes by density on Stractan density gradients. *Left,* Normal *(A)* and hereditary xerocytosis *(B)* samples. The xerocytes extend to higher densities than the normal red cells. *Right,* Normal *(C)* and hereditary stomatocytosis *(D)* samples. Many of the stomatocytes are less dense than the normal erythrocytes. (From Lande WM, Mentzer WC: Haemolytic anaemia associated with increased cation permeability. Clin Haematol 1985; 14:89.)

increased endothelial adherence compared with stomatocytic erythrocytes from unsplenectomized family members without hypercoagulability.[1306] *In vivo,* venous thromboemboli predominate, sometimes with complicating pulmonary or portal hypertension.[1294] Thrombotic episodes have not occurred before splenectomy.

Hereditary Xerocytosis (High Phosphatidylcholine Hemolytic Anemia)

Several families have been described with a hemolytic anemia in which the red cells are markedly dehydrated, as manifested by an elevated MCHC.[815, 1263, 1273, 1276, 1279–1286, 1307] Physiologically, the major red cell abnormality is a change in the relative membrane permeability to K^+. Efflux of K^+ is increased twofold to fourfold and approximates Na^+ influx. There is no metabolic or hemoglobin abnormality to account for this permeability lesion, and red cell Ca^{2+} content is not increased. The nature of the permeability defect is unknown. Monovalent cation pump activity is increased appropriately for the slightly elevated Na^+ content, but the Na^+/K^+ pump cannot compensate for K^+ losses in excess of Na^+ gain. In fact, the action of the pump significantly exacerbates the rate of K^+ loss

because three Na^+ ions are pumped out for every two K^+ ions returned.[639, 640] As a consequence, xerocytes gradually become cation depleted and lose water in response to decreased intracellular osmolality. This is easily detected by centrifugation on Stractan gradients (Fig. 16–34). Little is known about the molecular pathology of this rare disease. Where measured, the proportion of red cell membrane phosphatidylcholine is increased (12–20 fmol/cell; normal range, 10–12 fmol/cell).[1276] The combination of hereditary xerocytosis and high phosphatidylcholine is sometimes given the name high phosphatidylcholine hemolytic anemia (HPCHA),[1262, 1276, 1277, 1280, 1282, 1308] but there appears to be little reason to distinguish HPCHA from hereditary xerocytosis.[1276] Early studies suggested the excess phosphatidylcholine was due to diminished transfer of phosphatidylcholine fatty acids to phosphatidylethanolamine,[1277] a pathway that is normally stimulated by cellular dehydration.[1309] It is not clear why this pathway is inhibited in hereditary xerocytosis or how it relates to the underlying membrane leakiness and hemolysis.

Xerocytic red cells are also shear sensitive[1281] and are exceptionally prone to membrane fragmentation in response to metabolic stress.[815] This suggests a membrane skeletal defect, but no systematic studies of xerocytic skeletons have been conducted. Results of con-

Normal

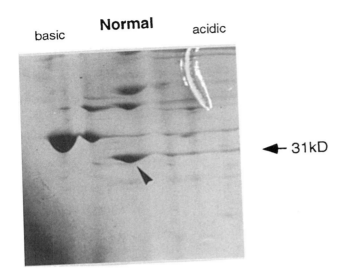

basic　　　　　　　　　acidic

←— 31kD

Stomatocytic

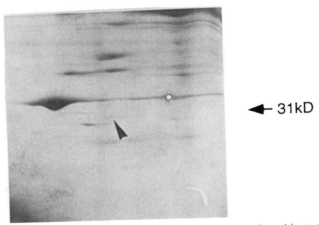

←— 31kD

Figure 16–34. Two-dimensional analysis of normal and hereditary stomatocytosis red cell membranes. Membranes were prepared by hypotonic lysis, stripped of peripheral proteins, and subjected to nonequilibrium pH gradient electrophoresis (NEPHGE) in the horizontal dimension followed by SDS-PAGE in the vertical dimension and Coomassie blue staining. The *arrowheads* mark the location of the basic 31-kd protein (band 7.2b or stomatin) that is deficient in the stomatocytic red cells. (From Stewart GW, Argent AC, Dash BCJ: Stomatin: a putative cation transport regulator in the red cell membrane. Biochim Biophys Acta 1993; 1225:15. Copyright 1993 with permission of Elsevier Science, NL, Amsterdam, The Netherlands.)

bin to methemoglobin, and cross-linking of hemoglobin to spectrin.[1314, 1315] Similar sensitivity occurs in dehydrated normal red cells. Conversely, rehydrated xerocytes exhibit a normal reaction to H_2O_2. Native xerocytes contain the abnormal spectrin/globin complex, and the amount correlates with the extent of dehydration in various cellular fractions and with membrane rigidity.[1316] Oxidation of normal erythrocytes with peroxide generates the spectrin/globin complex and rigid membranes.[650] Complex formation is blocked by carbon monoxide, which prevents hemoglobin oxidation, but is not blocked by lipid antioxidants.[650] This implies a direct role for hemoglobin in cross-linking spectrin.

Clinical Features

In all families with hereditary xerocytosis studied, inheritance appears to be autosomal dominant. Diagnostic red cell features include an increased MCHC and decreased osmotic fragility (i.e., resistance to osmotic lysis). In the most severely affected patients,[1257] blood smears display contracted and spiculated red cells in which the hemoglobin appears to be aggregated in one portion of the cell. Most patients, however, have nearly normal erythrocyte morphology, with only a few target cells and an occasional echinocyte or stomatocyte. The characteristic biochemical abnormality is a reduced K^+ concentration and total monovalent cation content. In older erythrocytes, K^+ levels approach half normal.[1276] Red cell 2,3-DPG concentrations are moderately decreased in hereditary xerocytosis,[815, 1257, 1265, 1273, 1317] as well as in hereditary stomatocytosis. The reasons are unknown. Because loss of the polyvalent DPG is compensated by an influx of monovalent chloride ions and water, patients with xerocytosis and unusually low DPG levels have fewer dehydrated red cells than expected for the degree of cation loss and in rare cases have no dehydration at all.[1317] Patients with low DPG also have increased whole blood oxygen affinity and, consequently, may have little apparent anemia.[1307, 1317] Autohemolysis is increased and responds to glucose, similar to the pattern in HS.[815, 1265, 1279, 1282]

Hereditary xerocytes appear to be macrocytic, despite their dehydration. This, however, is partially, an artifact of cellular stiffness. In Coulter-type electronic counters, the conversion of pulse height (from the resistance of a cell passing through an electric field) to a cellular volume is dependent on cell shape. Xerocytes do not deform to the same degree as normal cells, which causes the electronically measured MCV to be about 10% too high.[1311] This also affects the hematocrit, which is calculated from the MCV.

Splenectomy is probably not beneficial in hereditary xerocytosis. The limited experience available suggests that removing the spleen does not significantly reduce hemolysis.[1257, 1262] Presumably, xerocytes are so functionally compromised that they are easily detected and eliminated in other areas of the reticuloendothelial system. Splenectomy may even be contraindicated. One 46-year-old xerocytosis patient had fatal pulmonary emboli after splenectomy.[1262] Fortunately, most patients

ventional analyses of red cell membrane proteins have been normal,[815] except for an increase in the proportion of membrane-associated G3PD in one family.[1310] Quantitatively, all membrane components are increased, because, for unknown reasons, xerocytes have 15% to 25% more surface area than normal.[1311] Xerocytes are relatively rigid cells[1261] and probably develop a dehydration-induced membrane injury.[1281] This poorly defined lesion is also found in irreversibly sickled cells[1312] and presumably is important in the pathophysiology of hemolysis. Hereditary xerocytes are unusually sensitive to oxidants.[1313–1315] Exposure of xerocytes to concentrations of H_2O_2 that do not affect normal cells causes a rapid loss of intracellular K^+, conversion of hemoglo-

are able to maintain a hemoglobin level of at least 9 g/dL, so that splenectomy is not required.

Intermediate Syndromes

Hydrocytosis and xerocytosis represent the extremes of a spectrum of red cell permeability defects. A number of families with features of both conditions have been reported. The reported cases seem to fall into three groups whose red cells differ principally in morphology, osmotic fragility, and sensitivity to cold.

Cryohydrocytosis

Patients with this disorder have a mild congenital hemolytic anemia characterized by marked autohemolysis that is greater at 4°C than at 37°C.[1266, 1269, 1285] The mode of inheritance of this disorder is unknown, but one of the authors (S.E.L.)[1318] has seen a family with 12 affected members in four generations, suggesting autosomal dominant transmission. The cold autohemolysis is sensitive to the method of anticoagulation. It is increased in the cold in heparin, EDTA, and defibrinated plasma but not in acid citrate dextrose.[1266, 1269] This may reflect unusual pH sensitivity of the abnormal red cells, because cold hemolysis is accentuated at pH 8 (the pH of blood in the first three anticoagulants at 4°C) compared with pH 7.6 (the pH of acid citrate dextrose plasma at 4°C).[1266, 1269, 1283–1285] Blood smears show stomatocytes, some of which have an eccentric or curvilinear slit or a transverse bar bisecting the area of central pallor. Fresh erythrocytes are Na^+ loaded and K^+ depleted, but the total concentration of Na^+ and K^+ is normal.[1266] In the cold, Na^+ and K^+ permeabilities are markedly increased; however, because Na^+ entry greatly predominates, the red cells rapidly swell and lyse. The primary molecular lesion of these erythrocytes is unknown. Membrane lipids are quantitatively normal, and with the exception of a mild decrease in red cell glutathione, no defects in metabolism have been detected.[1266, 1269] In one patient, stomatin was missing when red cell membrane proteins were analyzed,[1260] but this defect was not observed in the authors' patients.[1318]

Pseudohyperkalemia

Stewart and co-workers[1283, 1284] have reported a family with a dominantly inherited disorder characterized by erythrocyte K^+ loss that is exaggerated in the cold. Electrolyte analyses of plasma obtained from blood samples stored for just a few hours at room temperature or below may falsely suggest that affected individuals are hyperkalemic. The disorder resembles cryohydrocytosis except that K^+ loss and dehydration predominate (?cryoxerocytosis) instead of Na^+ gain and cryohemolysis. Fortunately, there is little K^+ loss at physiologic temperatures, so patients have only mildly dehydrated red cells and little or no hemolysis and anemia.

Stomatocytic Xerocytosis

In 1971, Miller and colleagues reported 54 patients with dominantly inherited stomatocytosis in a large Swiss-German family.[1270] Apparent heterozygotes (51 of 54 patients) had mild hemolysis, 1% to 25% stomatocytes on their peripheral blood smears, and no anemia. Intracellular K^+ and total monovalent cations were mildly decreased, and fresh red cells were osmotically resistant. Three probable homozygotes from a consanguineous mating had mild anemia, moderately severe hemolysis, marked stomatocytosis (20% to 35%), and greater cation permeability[1270, 1291]; however, because net Na^+ and K^+ levels were relatively balanced, cell hydration was not seriously deranged. The molecular defect in this kindred is unknown.

Other Disorders Characterized By Stomatocytosis

Acquired Stomatocytosis

In normal individuals, 3% or less of the red cells on peripheral blood smears are stomatocytic,[1319, 1320] although more stomatocytic forms are evident (up to 10%) if sensitive techniques such as scanning electron microscopy are used.[1321] Because stomatocytes may occasionally occur as a drying artifact in limited areas of the smear, care must be taken to examine multiple areas on several smears before diagnosing stomatocytosis. In wet preparations, stomatocytes are bowl shaped (uniconcave). Such preparations are useful in excluding artifactual stomatocytes, but the presence of bowl-shaped cells cannot be used as proof of stomatocytes because target cells are also bowl shaped in solution.[1322]

Drugs. In a prospective study of 4291 peripheral blood smears, Davidson and co-workers[1323] found increased numbers of stomatocytes in 2.3% of the preparations. Fifty-nine per cent of these smears had 5% to 20% stomatocytes, 35% had 20% to 50% stomatocytes, and 6% had more than 50% stomatocytes. In this and other studies, a wide variety of drugs and diagnoses were associated with stomatocytosis.[1261, 1270, 1323–1325] Further studies are needed to determine which associations are specific and reproducible. As discussed early in the chapter, in the section on the bilayer couple hypothesis,[86–91] amphophilic, lipid-soluble drugs can cause red cells to assume a stomatocytic shape if the drug partitions preferentially into the inner half of the lipid bilayer. The affected red cells are misshapen but are not cation loaded or hydrocytic and do not usually hemolyze.

Alcoholism. Acquired stomatocytosis is common in alcoholics, particularly in those with acute alcoholism (Fig. 16–35), and may be associated with moderate hemolysis.[1319, 1320] Red cell cation measurements have not been reported; however, severe hydrocytosis is unlikely, because osmotic fragility tests have been normal.[1319]

***Vinca* Alkaloids.** *Vinca* alkaloids (e.g., vincristine, vinblastine) frequently induce hemolysis, sometimes with increased membrane Na^+ permeability and sto-

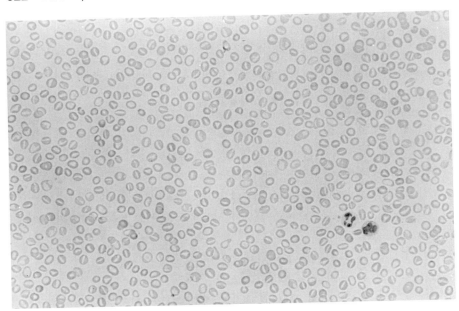

Figure 16–35. Peripheral blood smear from a patient with acute alcoholism. Acquired stomatocytic morphology is seen in almost all erythrocytes.

matocytosis, in the doses used for chemotherapy of leukemias and lymphomas.[1325] This is a particular problem in the rare instances where these drugs must be given to patients with cancer who also have HS. We have seen two such patients and in both cases very severe hemolysis occurred. Presumably the explanation is that spherocytes and stomatocytes both have a decreased surface/volume ratio. Imposing a stomatocytic stress on HS red cells will make them even more spheroidal and hasten their demise.

Marathon Runners, March Hemoglobinuria. Stomatocytes have also been observed, transiently, on wet preparations of blood from marathon runners immediately after a race.[1326] Because some marathon runners develop transient intravascular hemolysis after running (march hemoglobinuria),[1327] there is a possibility that the two phenomena are related. Interestingly, some years ago, Banga and colleagues[1328] reported that three patients with march hemoglobinuria lacked a 29-kDa protein (presumably stomatin) in the band 7.2 region of red cell membranes. The defect was very similar and probably identical to the defect observed in hereditary stomatocytosis. Patients with march hemoglobinuria do not have any significant hemolysis or abnormal red cell morphology under basal conditions.

Rh Null Disease

The Rh(D) antigen and the other antigens of the Rh group (cCeE) are part of two minor red cell membrane proteins whose structure has been identified.[160, 169] Patients who lack all Rh antigens (Rh_{null})[1329] have a moderately severe hemolytic anemia (^{51}Cr-labeled red cell half-life of 10 to 14 days)[1330–1333] characterized by stomatocytosis and spherocytosis. Osmotic fragility is only mildly increased,[1330, 1333] but ektacytometry shows a significant loss of membrane surface, particularly in denser (and presumably older) cells.[1330] Red cell membrane K^+ or Rb^+ (a K^+ analogue) permeability is about twice normal, which is compatible with a mild xerocytosis syndrome.[1330, 1334] Indeed, in one patient, a majority of the Rh_{null} cells were dense and K^+ depleted.[1330] In another, cation and water concentrations were normal.[1334] Stomatocytosis and hemolysis are also features of Rh_{mod} disease, a related anomaly, in which the expression of Rh antigens is suppressed but not absent, owing to the influence of a suppressor gene.[1335, 1336]

Tangier Disease

Tangier disease is an autosomal recessive condition characterized by splenomegaly, absence of high-density lipoproteins (HDLs), hypertriglyceridemia, mild corneal clouding, peripheral neuropathy, bone marrow foam cells (70% of patients), and characteristic orange-colored, cholesterol ester–laden tonsils.[1337, 1338] Cholesterol esters are greatly elevated in tissue macrophages in Tangier disease owing to the lack of HDLs, which normally returns cholesterol esters to the liver. The HDL deficiency is caused by hypercatabolism of the lipoprotein.[1337] Normally, HDLs bind to specific receptors on macrophages, are internalized (presumably to load up on cholesterol esters), and then recycle to the membrane surface. In Tangier disease, for unknown reasons, HDLs are misrouted to macrophage lysosomes and destroyed. Hematologic examination of one patient with Tangier disease disclosed stomatocytosis, hemolysis (hemoglobin 8.5 g/dL; reticulocytes 6% to 9%), and osmotically sensitive red cells.[1339] Membrane cholesterol was low, the cholesterol:phospholipid ratio was decreased, and phospholipid analysis showed high phosphatidylcholine and low sphingomyelin.[1339] Red cell cation concentrations and permeabilities were not investigated. Because hematologic data have rarely been reported in Tangier disease, it is difficult to be certain that this patient is not exceptional. However, previous reports of unexplained hemolysis in three patients suggest that he is not.[1340–1342]

Mediterranean Stomatocytosis

About 25 years ago several groups observed that stomatocytosis was remarkably common among Mediterranean immigrants to Australia.[1324, 1343–1345] The typical stomatocytic morphology was associated with mild-to-moderate hemolytic anemia, normal red cell cations, and normal osmotic fragility.[1324, 1344] Many patients also had macrothrombocytopenia (40,000 to 150,000 platelets, 3 to 120 μm^3) and slight splenomegaly. A study of healthy Mediterranean immigrants confirmed the increased incidence of stomatocytosis (36% of patients with more than 5% stomatocytes); however, affected individuals were not anemic.[1346] Splenomegaly and macrothrombocytopenia were also common, but they segregated independently of the red cell defect. The cause of this phenomenon remains a mystery. Indeed, it is not even clear if it still exists, because no further reports have appeared in recent years. There is a general impression that stomatocytosis is not unusually prevalent in Mediterranean countries or in Mediterranean immigrants in other parts of the world, which suggests an environmental influence. Accurate data concerning the prevalence of stomatocytosis are lacking.

Other Disorders

Stomatocytosis is also observed in at least some patients with the hemolytic anemia that results from adenosine deaminase overproduction.[1347] A preliminary report of mild stomatocytosis and uncompensated hemolysis in a Japanese woman with polyagglutinable red cells and an apparent defect in sialylation of band 3 and glycophorin has also appeared.[1348]

Other Disorders Characterized By Xerocytosis

ATP Depletion

When red cell ATP concentrations fall below 5% to 15% of normal, the cells leak cations and become rigid and echinocytic.[1349] In plasma or other Ca^{2+}-containing media, a specific K^+ permeability lesion (the Gárdos phenomenon) is superimposed on the unchecked normal leak of Na^+ and K^+ and leads to cation depletion and dehydration. Coincidentally, poorly defined changes occur in membrane skeletal structure.[1350, 1351]

Presumably these phenomena are involved in the hemolysis that occurs in inherited defects of glycolysis such as pyruvate kinase (PK) deficiency. Studies by Nathan, Mentzer, and Glader and their co-workers[1352–1354] showed that PK-deficient red cells rapidly lose ATP and K^+ and become dehydrated, spiculated, and viscous when incubated *in vitro*, particularly under conditions in which residual mitochondrial production of ATP is curtailed. Contracted, crenated red cells are observed in PK deficiency[1355, 1356] and other disorders of red cell glycolysis. These "deflated echinocytes"[1356] are more rigid than normal[1357] and are relatively scarce in unsplenectomized patients,[1355, 1356] which implies they are premorbid cells given temporary reprieve by removal of the spleen.

Little is known about the status of membrane proteins in red cells with compromised ATP production. Small amounts of disulfide-linked spectrin complexes and marked diminution of spectrin extractability were detected in a patient with glucose phosphate isomerase deficiency,[1358] which suggests that membrane protein damage may be pathologically relevant in these disorders.

Irreversibly Sickled Cells

Irreversibly sickled cells are circulating erythrocytes from patients with sickle cell anemia that retain a sickled shape when oxygenated because of an acquired defect in the membrane skeleton.[554] Biochemically, irreversibly sickled cells are deficient in total monovalent cations and water.[1359, 1360] The mechanism of their formation and the nature of the acquired membrane defects responsible for their abnormal shape, cation content, and surface topography are detailed in Chapter 20.

MISCELLANEOUS DISORDERS AFFECTING THE ERYTHROCYTE MEMBRANE

Other Causes of Decreased Erythrocyte Membrane Surface

Excluding HS, only a few conditions cause decreased membrane surface area, leading to spherocytosis on the peripheral blood smear.

Immune Adherence

Other than HS, immunohemolytic anemias are the most common cause of spherocytosis in infants and children: AB(H)-related hemolysis in neonates and warm antibody–type autoimmune (or drug-related) hemolytic anemias in older children and adults. (For unknown reasons Rh-related hemolysis in neonates rarely causes spherocytosis, whereas it does so readily later in life.) Patients who suffer from severe transfusion reactions with immunohemolysis may also have spherocytes on their peripheral blood smears. The pathophysiology of these disorders is discussed in Chapter 14.

Thermal Injury

More than 130 years ago Schultze observed that red cells heated to temperatures approaching 50°C for short periods developed membrane budding, fragmentation, and microspherocytosis.[1361] This phenomenon was further defined by the careful studies of Ham and co-workers and others[1143–1145] and is now believed to be due to heat denaturation of spectrin or other membrane proteins.[1146] Similar changes are observed acutely in patients with major cutaneous burns, presumably due to heat exposure of red cells in the skin and subcutaneous tissues. During the first 24 to 48 hours after the burn, intravascular hemolysis develops, which is associated with red cell fragmentation and spherocytosis.[1362, 1363] The severity of the reaction is related to the extent and degree of the burn. Generally, hemolysis is evident in patients with third-degree burns involving 15% to 20% or more of the body surface area.[1362, 1364] In severely burned patients, up to 30% of the red cell mass may be destroyed. This acute hemolytic process is usually complete by the third day after the burn and is followed by a chronic anemia resembling that seen in various chronic disorders.[1365, 1366] An unusual variant of this disorder has been reported after infusion of red cells that were inadvertently overheated in a blood warmer.[1367, 1368]

Mechanical Injury

Hemolysis can be caused by direct physical trauma to the red cell membrane. This occurs in a variety of disorders, which are grouped under the terms *microangiopathic* and *macroangiopathic hemolytic anemias*. Membrane damage leading to intravascular hemolysis is apparently inflicted by the interaction of red cells (flowing at arterial speeds) with prosthetic materials, damaged endothelial surfaces, or intravascular fibrin strands.[547, 1369, 1370] Dense microspherocytes are almost always produced by this process, but usually bizarre-shaped schizocytes and red cell fragments dominate the morphology. How such cells form is still not completely clear, because simple fragmentation of red cells generates spherocytes but not schizocytes. Perhaps red cells draped over fibrin strands or attached to abnormal surfaces not only are distorted by shear but also are held in the distorted position for some time, permitting rearrangement of the stressed membrane skeleton and assumption of a new, irreversibly misshapen form. This concept is strengthened by the observation that fragmentation is worsened by the presence of underlying skeletal weakness.[1093]

Hypophosphatemia

Red cell glucose metabolism is compromised in patients with severe hypophosphatemia (serum phosphorus level less than 0.1 to 0.3 mg/dL).[1371, 1372] ATP and DPG levels decline and hemoglobin-oxygen affinity increases. If red cell ATP concentration falls to very low levels (10% to 20% of normal), a severe hemolytic anemia characterized by marked microspherocytosis, spheroacanthocytosis, and red cell rigidity results.[1371] Hemolysis is reversible after phosphate repletion and ATP regeneration.

Toxins and Venoms

Clostridial Sepsis. *Clostridium welchii* and *C. perfringens* septicemias are seen in a variety of clinical situations but must particularly be considered in patients with penetrating wounds, septic abortions, peritonitis after a perforated viscus, or cholecystitis or cholangitis and in immunosuppressed patients with gastrointestinal or hematologic malignancies or neonates with necrotizing enterocolitis.[1373–1384] In patients with clostridial sepsis, severe, rapidly progressive intravascular hemolysis and microspherocytosis may occur.[1374, 1381] Hemolysis of the entire red cell mass has been reported.[1373, 1380, 1385, 1386] Complications include shock, acute renal failure, and death. Transfusion therapy may be ineffective. Antibiotics and hyperbaric oxygen have occasionally been successful in treating clostridial infections.[1377, 1382, 1383]

The mechanism of red cell damage is uncertain and may vary between patients. The bacteria produce several hemolytic toxins including α toxin, a 43-kDa protein that contains an NH_2-terminal phospholipase domain and a COOH-terminal domain required for hemolysis,[1382, 1387, 1388] and θ toxin, a 54-kDa cholesterol-binding protein[1389–1391] that aggregates and forms membrane pores[1390, 1392] leading to colloid osmotic hemolysis. *C. perfringens* contains a neuraminidase that cleaves terminal sialic acids from red cell glycoproteins in some patients.[1393] The underlying galactose residues form the Thomsen-Friedenreich cryptoantigen (or T antigen). The antigen is easily detected because affected erythrocytes are agglutinated by peanut lectin.[1376] Anti-T antibodies are present in almost all adult plasma, thus T-antigen activation can lead to significant hemolysis.[1381, 1382, 1384] In infected infants and children who lack T antibodies, transfusion may lead to massive hemolysis. Rarely, T-antigen activation may precede the intravascular hemolysis, leading to early detection of clostridial sepsis and life-saving therapeutic intervention.[1376]

In one patient with severe hemolysis, red cells showed profound proteolytic damage to membrane proteins, particularly spectrin, and no significant lipid alterations.[1394] This suggests that proteolytic rather than lipolytic bacterial toxins are primarily responsible for red cell destruction.

Venoms. The venoms of cobras and certain vipers and rattlesnakes may produce severe hemolysis and spherocytosis.[1395–1397] Spherocytic hemolytic anemia may also be seen in patients bitten by the common brown spiders (*Loxosceles reclusus* and *L. lata*) of South America and the central and southern sections of the United States[1398, 1399] and in individuals with massive numbers of honeybee, wasp, or yellow jacket stings.[1400–1403] Hemolysis in a child stung by a Portuguese man-of-war jellyfish has also been reported.[1404]

A full description of the numerous toxins in these venoms and their mechanisms of action is beyond the scope of this chapter. In general, the mechanisms of hemolysis after envenomation are not fully understood. The venoms of snakes and insects often contain phospholipases (particularly phospholipase A_2) and protein toxins that enhance their action. Examples of toxins include the mastoparans of wasp and hornet venoms[1405–1407] and melittin, a polypeptide contained in honeybee (*Apis mellifera*) venom[1408–1411] that immobilizes and clusters erythrocyte protein 3, producing protein-free areas of the lipid bilayer that are susceptible to phospholipase action.[1410]

Hemolysis after brown spider bites is characteristically delayed from 1 to 5 days and is caused by a different mechanism.[1399] Affected patients develop a transient, spherocytic, Coombs-positive hemolytic anemia[1412-1414] with erythrophagocytosis and IgG[1413] and C3[1412] deposition on the red cell surface. *In vitro*, venom components bind to the red cell membrane[1415] and induce IgG attachment and activation of complement by the alternative pathway.[1416] The hemolysis usually subsides within a week, but it may be fatal.[1399, 1417, 1418] Complement appears to play a critical role because complement-deficient guinea pigs are resistant to the venom.[1419] The venom also contains a phospholipase D that may contribute to the hemolysis.[1420]

Excepting spider bites, which may be clinically deceptive initially, the potential for a hemolytic catastrophe should be obvious in patients who have been bitten or stung.[1399] An early sign of impending hemolysis may be a rapid rise in the serum K^+ level caused by the prelytic leak of this ion from the red cells. Once hemolysis is established, therapy other than transfusions is usually of little use. In snake bites, localization or drainage of the venom and prompt administration of antivenom can be lifesaving.

Hypersplenism

Occasionally, patients with infections associated with splenomegaly develop transient hemolysis associated with spherocytosis and splenic sequestration of red cells.[1421-1423] In some instances, this may be attributed to latent red cell defects such as HS; but in others, no red cell abnormalities can be identified. Typically, the latter patients have subacute infections with persistent fever, splenomegaly, and numerous cells of lymphocytic or reticuloendothelial derivation (atypical lymphocytes, monocytes, histiocytes, or plasma cells) in the peripheral blood. Only a minor population of the red cells (10% to 50%) are spherical on peripheral blood smears or unincubated osmotic fragility tests. Presumably the combination of delayed splenic passage caused by splenomegaly and pyrogenic stimulation of the reticuloendothelial system is sufficient to permit detention and conditioning of even normal red cells—a form of hypersplenism.

Disorders Associated with Increased Membrane Surface

Target Cells

Red cells increase their surface area by an increase in membrane lipids. In dried smears the excess surface accumulates and bulges outward in the red cell's central clearing, producing the characteristic target cell morphology. Target cells are also seen when red cell volume is diminished, owing to decreased hemoglobin synthesis (e.g., thalassemia, iron deficiency), abnormal hemoglobin charge or aggregation (e.g., hemoglobins S, C, D, and E), or decreased cell cations and water. In these cases there is a relative increase in the surface/volume ratio. With the exception of dehydrated red cells, an increase in membrane surface, whether relative or absolute, has little effect on red cell deformability or life span and hence is usually innocuous.

Liver Disease. Target cells are particularly characteristic of biliary obstruction[1322, 1424] but also occur in other forms of liver disease. Like spur cells (see later), they form when red cells accumulate excess lipids from abnormal lipoproteins. However, unlike spur cells, target cells are characterized by a balanced increase in both free cholesterol and phospholipids.[1425-1427] The phospholipid increase is confined to phosphatidylcholine.[1425]

The pathogenesis of lipid accumulation in target cells is relatively clear. The process is extracorpuscular, reversible, and due to an abnormal serum component. Normal cells acquire target cell surface area, morphologic characteristics, and osmotic resistance when transfused into patients with obstructive jaundice or incubated in their serum, whereas target cells from such patients lose their excess lipids and revert to biconcave discs in normal persons or their sera.[1424] Cooper and co-workers[1425] find a close relation between the cholesterol/phospholipid ratios of target cells and serum lipoproteins, particularly low-density lipoproteins (LDLs). It is known that in obstructive jaundice a unique, abnormal lipoprotein called LP-X accumulates in the LDL density class,[1428, 1429] possibly caused, at least in part, by an acquired deficiency of the hepatic enzyme lecithin:cholesterol acyltransferase (LCAT). LP-X contains approximately equal amounts of free cholesterol and phosphatidylcholine, plus a small amount of protein, cholesterol esters, triglycerides, and lithocholic acid.[1428] Normal red cells rapidly acquire excess cholesterol, phosphatidylcholine, and surface area when incubated with LP-X *in vitro*,[1427] and it seems likely that this may be the source of lipids for membrane expansion and targeting *in vivo*.

Membrane proteins may also be abnormal in these cells. Iida and co-workers[1430] found that protein 4.2 was diminished or absent in 11 Japanese patients with obstructive jaundice and typical lipid-laden target cells. Red cell morphology, membrane lipids, and protein 4.2 content returned to normal in 1 patient after surgical relief of the biliary obstruction. This curious observation has been neither confirmed nor denied, and its relevance, if any, to the pathophysiology of targeting remains obscure.

Familial Lecithin:Cholesterol Acyltransferase Deficiency. Familial LCAT deficiency is a rare autosomal recessive disorder characterized by anemia, corneal opacities, hyperlipemia, proteinuria, chronic nephritis, and premature atherosclerosis.[112, 1431] LCAT deficiency is relatively asymptomatic during childhood. Proteinuria and corneal opacities are among the earliest manifestations. The latter consist of minute grayish dots that concentrate near the edge of the cornea, resembling arcus senilis. Almost all of the reported patients have had a moderate normochromic anemia (hemoglobin = 8 to 11 g/dL) characterized by prominent target cell formation and decreased osmotic fragility.[1432-1434] Hematologic studies suggest that the anemia is due to a combination of moderate hemolysis and decreased erythropoietic compensation, but interpretation of the evidence is complicated by the coexisting renal disease. Other studies have shown that the red cells are abnormally susceptible to peroxidative threat and have mechanically fragile membranes.[1433] There is no obvious explanation for these changes, but it is possible that they contribute to the shortened red cell life span.

LCAT deficiency is caused by a variety of mutations in the LCAT gene; affected individuals are either homozygotes or compound heterozygotes for these mutations.[1435-1439] As expected from the absence of LCAT activity, there is a pronounced decrease in cholesteryl esters and an increase in free cholesterol and phosphatidylcholine in plasma lipoproteins. Because LCAT is required for normal lipoprotein formation and catabolism, nascent lipoproteins and abnormal lipoprotein remnants accumulate in the plasma. One of the latter is LP-X.[1440] As discussed in the previous section, this lipoprotein is believed to be responsible for target cell formation in patients with the acquired LCAT deficiency of obstructive liver disease.[1427] Free cholesterol and phosphatidylcholine levels are markedly elevated in the red cell membranes of LCAT-deficient patients[112]; however, total red cell phospholipid levels are normal because the increase in phosphatidylcholine is balanced by a decrease in phosphatidylethanolamine and sphingomyelin. As in liver disease, red cell targeting and lipid abnormalities can be induced by incubation of normal red cells in LCAT-deficient lipoproteins and reversed by incubation in normal serum.[1441] Other plasma membranes are also probably affected by the abnormal LCAT-deficient lipoproteins. For example, accumulations of lipid in endothelial membranes may underlie the atherosclerotic and nephritic complications seen in some patients. Phagocytosis of abnormal lipoproteins by reticuloendothelial cells leads to the appearance of foam cells and sea-blue histiocytes in the bone marrow, spleen, and other organs.[1432, 1442] Serum and red cell lipids are improved *in vivo* when LCAT is supplied by infusions of normal plasma; however, the short half-life of this protein, 4 to 5 days, and the large amounts of plasma required make chronic replacement therapy impractical.

Fish-Eye Disease. Fish-eye disease is caused by partial deficiency of LCAT and is also associated with mutations in the LCAT gene.[112] It is characterized by corneal opacities (which give the disease its name), hypertriglyceridemia, and very low levels of HDLs. One report notes increased target cells and decreased osmotic fragility.[1443]

Post Splenectomy. In the first several weeks after splenectomy, target cells gradually increase in number,[1322, 1444-1446] eventually (in otherwise normal persons) reaching levels of 2% to 10%. This change is associated with an increase in osmotic resistance, membrane lipid content, and mean surface area relative to volume, indicating expansion of the red cell membrane surface. By deduction, the spleen must normally remove surplus membrane from such cells, a process referred to as "surface remodeling."[638, 1447] Experimental studies have clearly documented that the stress reticulocytes induced by acute blood loss or hemolysis undergo extensive surface remodeling and suggest that normal reticulocytes are remodeled to a lesser degree. In addition to membrane lipids, transferrin receptors, fibronectin receptors, and a high-molecular-weight membrane protein complex[639] are also removed during the remodeling process. Postsplenectomy blood smears also show increased numbers of acanthocytes, poikilocytes, and red cells burdened with useless or potentially harmful inclusions (e.g., Heinz bodies, Howell-Jolly bodies, siderotic granules, and endocytic vesicles).[1036, 1037, 1448, 1449] The presence of these inclusions attest to the "culling" and "pitting" functions of the spleen.[1449]

Spiculated Red Cells: Echinocytes and Acanthocytes

There are two basic types of spiculated red cells—echinocytes and acanthocytes. Echinocytes typically have a serrated outline with small, uniform projections more or less evenly spread over the circumference of the cell, whereas acanthocytes have a few spicules of varying size that project irregularly from the red cell surface. These differences are easily appreciated in scanning electron micrographs and can usually be discerned in wet preparations, but it is often quite difficult to make the distinction in dried smears. In general, echinocytes appear crenated in smears, that is, as cells with relatively uniform scalloped edges, whereas acanthocytes appear contracted, dense, and irregular.

Echinocytes are readily produced *in vitro* by washing red cells in saline,[1450] by the interaction of red cells with glass surfaces,[1450, 1451] and by amphipathic molecules that partition into and expand the outer half of the lipid bilayer. High pH values, ATP depletion, and Ca^{2+} accumulation also cause echinocytosis.[1452, 1453] *In vivo*, echinocytes are most often found in patients with advanced uremia,[1454, 1455] with defects of glycolytic metabolism,[1355] after splenectomy[1450] and in some patients with microangiopathic hemolytic anemias. Echinocytes are also common in neonates, especially those who are premature,[1456, 1457] and in divers after decompression from pressures of more than 3 to 4 bar.[1458] They are seen transiently after transfusions with large amounts of stored blood, because red cells become echinocytic after a few days of storage. Acanthocytes and echinocytes may be found in patients with severe hepatocellular damage,[1459] abetalipoproteinemia,[1460] infantile pyknocytosis,[1461] anorexia nervosa,[1462, 1463] McLeod[1464] and In(Lu)[1465] blood groups, and hypothyroidism.[1466] Occasionally, they are the predominant morphologic feature in patients with myelodysplasia.[1467, 1468]

Abetalipoproteinemia

Abetalipoproteinemia (Bassen-Kornzweig syndrome) is the paradigm of the disorders associated with acanthocytosis.[1460, 1469] Progressive ataxic neurologic disease, retinitis pigmentosa, celiac syndrome, and acanthocytosis are the primary manifestations of this disorder.[1470] Intestinal absorption of lipids is defective, serum cholesterol level is extremely low, and serum β-lipoprotein is absent. The disease is caused by failure to synthesize or secrete lipoproteins containing products of the apolipoprotein B gene. In some patients, this is due to lack of microsomal triglyceride transfer protein (MTP), which catalyzes the transport of triglyceride, cholesterol ester, and phospholipid from phospholipid surfaces.[1471, 1472] MTP is a heterodimer of protein disulfide isomerase and a unique large subunit with apparent molecular weight of 88 kDa. It is located in the lumen of hepatic microsomes and intestinal epithelia, the sites of lipoprotein synthesis,[1473, 1474] and is the only tissue-specific component, other than apolipoprotein B, required for secretion of apolipoprotein B–containing lipoproteins.[1475] Mutations in the MTP subunits have been described.[1471, 1472, 1476, 1477]

Related entities (hypobetalipoproteinemia, normotriglyceridemic abetalipoproteinemia, and chylomicron retention disease) exist that are associated with partial production of apolipoprotein B–containing lipoproteins or with secretion of lipoproteins containing truncated forms of apolipoprotein B.[1470, 1478] Patients with these diseases may also manifest acanthocytosis and neurologic disease, depending on the severity of the lipoprotein defect.[1471] Even patients with heterozygous hypobetalipoproteinemia may have acanthocytosis, although often they do not.

Characteristically, 50% to 90% of the red cells are acanthocytes.[1470, 1479] The shape defect is not evident in nucleated red cells or reticulocytes and worsens as the erythrocytes age. Membrane protein composition is normal, but membrane lipid composition is not. Phosphatidylcholine concentration is decreased by about 20%, and the amount of sphingomyelin is correspondingly increased. The cholesterol/phospholipid ratio is normal to mildly elevated.[1480–1482] These changes reflect abnormalities in the distribution of plasma phospholipids and a decrease in LCAT activity.[1483] The relative increases in cholesterol and sphingomyelin concentration both decrease lipid fluidity,[1481] particularly in the outer half of the bilayer,[1484] and presumably contribute to the acanthocytic shape. They probably do so by expanding the outer bilayer relative to the inner bilayer, because drugs that selectively intercalate into the inner bilayer convert acanthocytes to biconcave disks.[92] However, this is almost impossible to prove, because the difference in the surface areas of the outer bilayers of an acanthocyte and a discocyte is less than 0.4%.

Because of fat malabsorption and the absence of LDLs, which transport vitamin E,[1485] the red cells of these patients are markedly deficient in vitamin E.[1486] Exposure to lipid-soluble oxidants such as H_2O_2 leads to an increase in lipid peroxides, a decrease in phospholipids rich in unsaturated fatty acids such as phosphatidylethanolamine and phosphatidylserine, damage to membrane proteins, and hemolysis. Oxidant sensitivity can be prevented by treatment with a water-soluble form of vitamin E (e.g., D-α-tocopherol polyethylene glycol succinate).[1486] The role of vitamin E deficiency in the pathophysiology of the disease is uncertain. It is widely believed that such deficiency may be the primary stimulus for secondary manifestations of the disease, such as neuropathy,[1470] because a similar neuropathy is observed in rare patients with chronic cholestasis[1487–1489] or selective malabsorption of vitamin E.[1490] In these latter defects[1491] and probably in abetalipoproteinemia,[1470, 1492] the neurologic disease can be delayed or prevented by chronic vitamin E administration.

Despite increased lipid viscosity and vitamin E deficiency, the hemolysis experienced by these patients is mild.[1470, 1480] This is in striking contrast to spur cell anemia (see later), in which hemolysis of similarly shaped cells is often quite severe. It has been suggested that the difference is explained by the fact that the spleen is normal in abetalipoproteinemia, whereas it is enlarged and congested by portal hypertension in spur cell anemia. Whether this is a sufficient explanation is unknown.

Acanthocytosis with Neurologic Disease and Normal Lipoproteins (Amyotrophic Chorea-Acanthocytosis)

This syndrome was first described by Estes and coworkers.[1493, 1494] Since then, additional reports have appeared, particularly from Japan.[1495–1507] The disorder is characterized by acanthocytosis, normolipoproteinemia, and progressive neurologic disease beginning in adolescence or adult life (8 to 62 years), including orofacial dyskinesia, lip and tongue biting, limb chorea, axonal sensorimotor polyneuropathy, decreased or absent tendon reflexes, muscle hypotonia, distal muscle wasting, and increased creatine phosphokinase. Mental deterioration is variable.[1502] Magnetic resonance imaging and pathologic examinations show atrophy of the basal ganglia, particularly the caudate and putamen. In some patients, little or no hemolysis occurs; in others, acanthocytosis precedes the onset of neurologic symptoms.[1502]

It is likely that more than one disorder is represented by these reports, because both dominant and recessive inheritance is recorded. In addition, variant syndromes with chorea-acanthocytosis and myopathy[1508] and with chorea-acanthocytosis, spherocytosis, and hemolysis[803] have been observed. Acanthocytosis is also associated with other unusual hereditary neurologic syndromes. One of these appears to be recessively inherited and features acanthocytosis, tics, and parkinsonism and is sometimes associated with motor neuron disease or diurnal dystonia.[1509, 1510] A second syndrome combines acanthocytosis, mitochondrial myopathy, encephalopathy, lactic acidosis, and strokelike symptoms.[1509] A third is characterized by acanthocytosis and Hallervorden-Spatz disease (progressive dementia, dystonia, spasticity, pallidal degeneration with iron deposition, and frequently retinal degeneration).[1511–1513] A fourth syndrome combines acanthocytosis with abnormal lipoproteins and a Hallervorden-Spatz–like disorder (HARP syndrome—hypoprebetalipoproteinemia, acanthocytosis, retinitis pigmentosa, and pallidal degeneration with iron deposition).[1514, 1515]

The cause or causes of these disorders are unknown, but there is evidence that the red cell membrane is defective. The red cells from patients with chorea-acanthocytosis are dense, owing to excessive K$^+$ loss,[1498] and may or may not have an increased proportion of sphingomyelin.[1498, 1506] Ankyrin, band 3, and protein 4.2 self digest more rapidly than normal in the red cells of these patients, suggesting a defect in the vertical connections between the membrane skeleton and the lipid bilayer.[1507] Intramembranous particles are more clustered in the chorea-acanthocytosis red cells, which is compatible with this type of defect. A defect near the COOH-terminal end of band 3, Pro^{868}→Leu, has been identified in one family with chorea-acanthocytosis.[325] Hematologically, affected individuals of the latter kindred have 20% to 25% acanthocytes and mild anemia with reticulocytosis. Finally, abnormal cyclic AMP phosphorylation of red cell dematin has been observed in a kindred with mild spheroacanthocytosis and a choreiform movement disorder or dementia.[1516]

Anorexia Nervosa

Acanthocytosis is common in many patients with severe anorexia nervosa.[1462, 1463] The cause of the acanthocytosis is unknown. Plasma lipid and LDL levels are normal or slightly decreased; however, even in those patients with low levels of LDLs,[1517] acanthocytosis may not be due solely to the lipoprotein deficiency, because patients with much lower concentrations of LDLs (e.g., those with hypobetalipoproteinemia) usually have normal red cell morphology.[1470] Severe starvation or malnutrition due to causes other than anorexia nervosa can also produce acanthocytosis[1518–1520] or target cells and hypobetalipoproteinemia.[1521]

Despite the acanthocytosis, only a small fraction of these patients experience significant anemia. Red cell life span is normal or only slightly shortened. Leukopenia and neutropenia are common, and mild thrombocytopenia is not rare.[1462, 1463, 1522] Based on morphology, these cytopenias are due to a hypoproliferative bone marrow[1463] and their severity correlates with weight.[1523] The hypoplastic marrow is also deficient in fat, which is replaced by an amorphous ground substance, perhaps acid mucopolysaccharide.[1463]

Hepatocellular Damage (Spur Cell Anemia)

The anemia seen in patients with liver disease is of complex etiology. Common causes include blood loss, hypersplenism, iron deficiency, folic acid deficiency, and marrow suppression from alcohol ingestion, hepatitis virus, and other poorly understood factors.[1524, 1525] In addition, in some patients, acquired abnormalities of the red cell membrane may contribute to anemia. Two morphologic syndromes are recognized. In one, target cells predominate. In the other, a syndrome of brisk hemolysis develops in association with acanthocytes or "spur" cells, so-called spur cell anemia.[1459, 1525–1535]

Typically, target cells are associated with obstructive liver disease and acanthocytes are associated with hepatocellular disease. In practice, the situation is more complex. It is not uncommon for both morphologies to coexist, and some experimental data suggest they are different stages of the same process. For example, when the bile duct is ligated in a rat, acanthocytes appear within 8 hours, but they convert to target cells if the obstruction persists for 7 days or more.[1536] Nevertheless, acanthocytes (spur cells) and target cells differ in many important respects, and they are considered separately in this chapter.

Spur cell anemia has most often been described in patients with alcoholic cirrhosis.[1459, 1527–1529, 1533, 1534] However, it is also reported in those with cardiac cirrhosis,[1529] metastatic liver disease,[1532] hemochromatosis,[1531] neonatal hepatitis,[1537] cholestasis,[1525, 1526, 1535] Wilson's disease,[2] and severe acute hepatitis.[2] This suggests that it may occur in any disease in which damage to hepatocytes is severe.

Typically, patients have moderately severe hemolysis (hematocrit of 20% to 30%), marked indirect hyperbilirubinemia, splenomegaly, and clinical and laboratory evidence of severe hepatic dysfunction. By definition, more than 20% acanthocytes are evident in multiple areas on several peripheral blood smears. Because crenated and spiculated cells are a frequent artifact of improperly dried smears, the authors believe it is useful to demonstrate that such cells are also present in wet preparations. (The freshly drawn cells should either be fixed or be examined immediately after dilution in their own plasma.) Morphologically, the acanthocytes of spur cell anemia are indistinguishable from those seen in patients with abetalipoproteinemia. In some patients significant numbers of echinocytes and target cells may be present, and spherocytes may develop, presumably as a result of microspherulation. Occasionally, this may cause some diagnostic confusion. In our experience, however, many of these "spherocytes" have fine spicules, evident on close examination, which distinguish them from true microspherocytes.

The red cell life span of spur cells is markedly shortened because of splenic sequestration,[1459, 1528, 1533, 1538] and, as expected, hemolysis abates after splenectomy.[1538] Unfortunately, splenectomy is a dangerous and often fatal procedure in these very sick patients and is not generally recommended.[1538] In addition, spur cell anemia has been reported in a splenectomized patient.[1530] Some success has been reported in treating the anemia of these patients with either phospholipid infusions[1539] or flunarizine[1540]; however, these approaches are still experimental.

The clinical syndrome of spur cell anemia can be produced by at least two different pathogenic mechanisms. In one group, typically consisting of patients with alcoholic cirrhosis,[1459, 1529, 1534] the disorder is due to an acquired abnormality of red cell lipids. The pathophysiology of spurring in these patients has been defined and reviewed by Cooper and associates[1425, 1459, 1538, 1541, 1542] and is illustrated in Figure 16–36. It occurs in two stages: cholesterol loading and splenic remodeling. In the first stage, abnormal, cholesterol-laden, apolipoprotein A-II–deficient lipoproteins, produced by the spur cell patient's diseased liver, transfer their excess cholesterol to circulating erythrocytes and increase the membrane cholesterol concentration, the

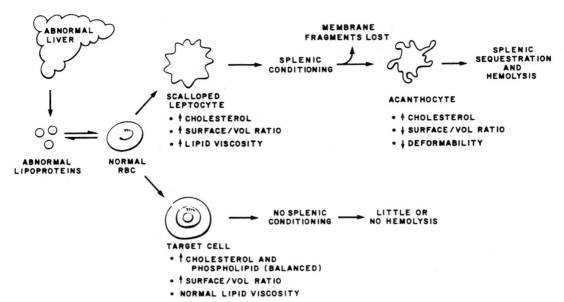

Figure 16-36. Schematic illustration of the pathophysiology of acanthocyte (''spur cell'') and target cell formation in liver disease.

cholesterol/phospholipid ratio, and the membrane surface area (Fig. 16–37).[1425, 1543] This is an acquired process and can be mimicked *in vitro* by incubating normal red cells in spur cell plasma[1459, 1538] or in artificial media containing cholesterol-phospholipid dispersions with a cholesterol:phospholipid ratio greater than 1.0.[1541] It can be reproduced *in vivo* in dogs fed a high cholesterol diet.[1542] In scanning electron micrographs, these cholesterol-laden cells are flattened and often folded, with an undulating periphery.[1542] They appear scalloped or crenated on dried smears.[1459, 1538] *In vivo*, scalloped cells are converted into spur cells by a process of splenic conditioning. Over a period of 1 to 7 days, membrane

lipids and surface area are lost, cellular rigidity increases, presumably because of the decline in surface/volume ratio, and the cell assumes a typical acanthocytic form.[1459, 1538]

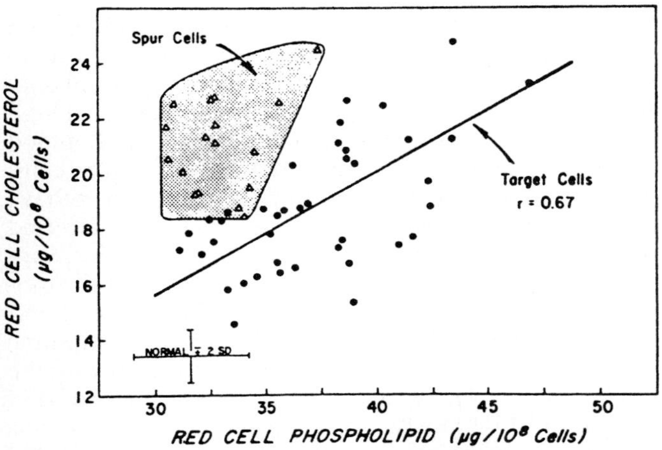

Splenectomy prevents both the formation of spur cells and their premature destruction; but as noted earlier, it is a high-risk procedure and is seldom indicated.

The cholesterol-laden, incipient spur cell is presumably detained and conditioned by the spleen because it is less deformable than normal. The molecular explanation for this change in deformability is unknown. There is evidence that cholesterol affects the function of band 3.[1544] Perhaps it also influences band 3 oligomerization or its interaction with other membrane proteins. A slight increase in the cholesterol/phospholipid ratio above normal markedly alters cholesterol organization in the membrane[1545] and increases the helical content of one or more of the major membrane proteins.[1546, 1547] There is also evidence that membrane proteolytic activity is increased in spur cells and that spur cell plasma can stimulate membrane degradation in normal erythrocytes.

Other studies have identified a defect in phospholipid repair.[1548, 1549] Spur cells and cholesterol-laden normal red cells readily incorporate arachidonic acid, a polyunsaturated fatty acid, into acylcarnitine, a fatty acid membrane repair intermediate, but further incorporation of arachidonate into phospholipids is slowed, and activity of the involved enzyme, lysophosphocholine acyl transferase (or arachidonoyl-CoA:1-palmitoyl-sn-glycero-3-phosphocholine acyl transferase), is decreased. Inhibition of this pathway impairs the red cell's ability to replace peroxidized fatty acyl side chains of phospholipids. The role of this defect in the pathophysiology of spur cell anemia is not yet clear.

The second group of patients with liver disease and spur cell anemia differs in that red cell membrane lipids are normal and incubation of normal red cells in

Figure 16-37. The cholesterol and phospholipid content of target *(filled symbols)* and spur *(open symbols)* cells. Note that target cells tend to have a balanced increase in cholesterol and phospholipid whereas spur cells are usually selectively enriched in cholesterol. (From Cooper RA, Diloy-Puray M, et al: An analysis of lipoproteins, bile acids, and red cell membranes associated with target cells and spur cells in patients with liver disease. J Clin Invest 1972; 51:3182. By copyright permission of the American Society for Clinical Investigation.)

the patients' plasma does not induce spurring.[1528, 1532, 1533] The pathophysiology of this condition is unknown and largely unstudied. It has been reported in patients with alcoholic cirrhosis[1528, 1533] and metastatic liver disease,[1532] and this is the form of the disease most often seen in children with spur cells and severe hepatocellular dysfunction.[2]

Both of these disorders appear to differ from Zieve's syndrome, a poorly defined syndrome of hyperlipoproteinemia, jaundice, and spherocytic hemolytic anemia that occurs in occasional patients with alcoholic liver disease.[1550]

Vitamin E Deficiency

Premature infants (less than 36 weeks' gestation or weighing less than 2000 g) and children or adults with steatorrhea are susceptible to vitamin E deficiency because of decreased absorption of the vitamin.[1551–1553] Discussion of this disorder in preterm infants is now primarily of historical interest.[1554] Infants described with this syndrome were being fed formulas that were very low in vitamin E and very high in polyunsaturated fatty acids. As the interactions among dietary iron, polyunsaturated fatty acids, and vitamin E were elucidated, infant formulas were altered so that this condition has virtually disappeared in most nurseries. However, vitamin E deficiency may cause a hemolytic anemia in infancy in patients with fat malabsorption such as cystic fibrosis or abetalipoproteinemia.[1470, 1555, 1556]

The features of severe vitamin E deficiency in infants are hemolysis, thrombocytosis, and a generalized edema.[1557–1559] Peripheral blood smears are often normal but sometimes show variable numbers of irregularly contracted, spiculated cells (acanthocytes or pyknocytes) and small numbers of spherocytes and fragmented red cells.[1556, 1558] The mechanism of hemolysis is uncertain. Vitamin E is a lipid-soluble antioxidant, and in its absence lipid peroxidation occurs, with damage to the double bonds of unsaturated fatty acids. Phospholipids rich in unsaturated acyl chains, such as phosphatidyl ethanolamine, are particularly susceptible.[1482, 1486, 1560] However, there is some evidence that damage to the sulfhydryl groups of membrane proteins may also contribute to hemolysis.[1561]

Kay and co-workers found that vitamin E–deficient rat erythrocytes have many of the characteristics of aged normal red cells, especially exposure of the so-called senescent antigen.[1562] This "neoantigen," described in detail earlier in the chapter, apparently results from proteolysis, clustering, or oxidation of protein 3. It is recognized by an IgG, anti–band 3 autoantibody that initiates removal of the cells by macrophages. Autoantibody attachment is blocked by vitamin E and reversed by thiol-reducing agents in experimental situations, which suggest that membrane lipid oxidation occurs first and leads to the oxidation of band 3 thiols. Presumably, similar processes accelerate red cell destruction *in vivo* in vitamin E deficiency.

Infantile Pyknocytosis

In 1959, Tuffy and colleagues described a syndrome of neonatal jaundice and hemolysis associated with variable numbers of distorted, irregularly contracted, spiculated cells, which they called pyknocytes.[1461] Morphologically, these cells are very similar (and possibly identical) to acanthocytes. Normal full-term infants have 0.3% to 1.9% pyknocytes/acanthocytes on peripheral blood smears. In premature infants the normal range is 0.3% to 5.6%. The affected infants typically present with jaundice and slight hepatosplenomegaly in the first few days of life. Pyknocytosis and hemolytic anemia peak at 3 to 4 weeks of age and then decline spontaneously. Clinical severity is variable; however, some infants are severely affected (hemoglobin = 4.6 g/dL; 15% to 20% reticulocytes; 25% to 50% pyknocytes), and some require exchange transfusions. Transfused erythrocytes become pyknocytic and survive poorly,[1461, 1563, 1564] indicating an extracorpuscular defect. The syndrome is seen in both premature and term infants. The only consistent chemical abnormality is a mild elevation in serum aspartate transaminase (50 to 250 IU). Parents and siblings are normal.

The cause of this syndrome has not been clearly defined, and, for unknown reasons, the diagnosis is seldom made today. Infants with severe G6PD deficiency,[1565] neonatal Heinz body hemolytic anemias,[1461, 1566] vitamin E deficiency,[1556, 1558] glycolytic enzyme deficiencies,[1355] neonatal hepatitis,[1537] HE,[1197, 1198] and microangiopathic hemolytic anemias may present with hemolysis and pyknocytes and are sometimes misdiagnosed as having infantile pyknocytosis. However, in most of the original case reports, evidence is sufficient to exclude those disorders, which suggests that infantile pyknocytosis may be a valid entity. The transient nature, mild transaminase elevation, morphology, and extracorpuscular etiology suggest a metabolic defect, possibly involving a circulating oxidant; however, other hypotheses are equally tenable.

McLeod's Syndrome

McLeod's syndrome is a multisystemic disorder with acanthocytosis and, in some patients, late-onset myopathy or chorea.[1567, 1568] The McLeod blood group phenotype, first discovered in a blood donor named Hugh McLeod, is an X-linked anomaly of the Kell blood group system in which either red cells or white cells, or both, react poorly with Kell antisera but behave normally in other blood group reactions. The affected cells lack Kx, the product of the *XK* gene, which appears to be a membrane precursor of the Kell antigens.[1567, 1569, 1570] The relevant gene has been cloned and encodes a novel 444-amino acid integral membrane protein that has some of the features of a membrane transporter.[1571] As expected, Kx is defective in McLeod patients.[1571, 1572] Male hemizygotes who lack Kx on their red cells have variable acanthocytosis (8% to 85%) and mild, compensated hemolysis (3% to 7% reticulocytes).[1464, 1573, 1574] Some teardrop erythrocytes and bizarre poikilocytes are also present. Female heterozygotes have occasional acanthocytes (as expected by the Lyon hypothesis) and very mild hemolysis,[1464, 1573] although lyonized women with more severe symptoms are described.[1572]

Some McLeod patients also develop a neuropathy or myopathy. This is first manifest as areflexia or an elevated creatine phosphokinase.[1575] Later in adult life, a cardiomyopathy or slowly progressive neuropathy may appear.[1576–1581] The neuropathy is characterized by various combinations of dystonic or choreiform movements, orofacial dyskinesia, dysarthria, tongue biting, and caudate atrophy on cerebral imaging. Psychiatric symptoms, seizures, and peripheral neuropathy with muscle denervation are also reported. These features, combined with acanthocytosis, can mimic the chorea-acanthocytosis syndromes described in a previous section.

The *XK* gene is less than 500 kb beyond the chronic granulomatous disease locus on the short arm of the X chromosome (p21.1).[1582] Consequently, males with deletions encompassing both loci have both chronic granulomatous disease and McLeod's syndrome.[1583] It is important to recognize patients with McLeod's syndrome because, if they receive transfusions, they may develop antibodies that are only compatible with McLeod's syndrome red cells.[1584, 1585]

Uremia

Red cell survival is reduced in patients with advanced renal failure.[1586–1588] An extracorporeal factor is involved, because red cells from uremic patients survive normally when infused into normal persons, whereas normal red cells survive poorly in uremic patients.[1587] The factor is nondialyzable, and some studies suggest that it is parathyroid hormone (PTH).[1589–1591] PTH levels are elevated in renal failure, owing to hyperphosphatemia and secondary hyperparathyroidism. PTH levels correlate closely with red cell survival in chronic renal failure patients on dialysis,[1591] and parathyroidectomy abolishes hemolysis in dogs with uremia.[1589] *In vitro*, relevant levels of PTH or its bioactive NH_2-terminal peptide augment Ca^{2+} entry into red cells through a cyclic AMP–independent pathway and cause the cells to develop filamentous extensions and lose membrane surface, presumably by vesiculation.[1590] These effects are largely blocked by the Ca^{2+} channel blocker verapamil. It is possible that they are responsible for the increased numbers of echinocytes observed in some uremic patients, because increased intracellular Ca^{2+} is markedly echinocytogenic.[1592]

In(Lu) Gene

The major antigens of the Lutheran blood group system are Lu^a and Lu^b. They are located on two low abundance glycoproteins of 80 and 85 kDa.[1593] About 1 person in 5000 inherits a dominantly acting inhibitor, called In(Lu),[1465, 1594] which partially suppresses expression of Lu^a and Lu^b such that they are undetectable by standard agglutination tests. This inhibition is the most common cause of the null Lutheran phenotype, Lu(a−b−). The In(Lu) gene product inhibits expression of CD44, an adhesive protein; MER2, a common red cell antigen; CR1, the C3b/C4b complement receptor; AnWj, the erythroid *Haemophilus influenzae* receptor; and the glycolipid antigens P1 and i, as well as the Lu antigens.[1595] Although several of these proteins are widely expressed, the action of In(Lu) is limited only to red cells.[1596] Patients with the In(Lu) Lu(a−b−) phenotype have abnormally shaped red cells but no hemolysis.[1465] The morphology varies from normal or mild poikilocytosis to acanthocytosis. Osmotic fragility of fresh In(Lu) Lu(a−b−) red cells is normal[1465] but during *in vitro* incubation the cells lose K^+ and become osmotically resistant.

Woronet's Trait

Beutler and associates have reported a benign, dominantly inherited abnormality of red cell shape in a single family, characterized by the presence of 5% to 10% irregularly spiculated red cells bearing 1 to 10 spicules (acanthocytes or keratocytes).[1597] A larger proportion of the cells showed slight echinocytosis. The abnormal cells were equally prevalent in young and old red cell fractions. Red cell life span, cations, enzymes, and Kell antigens were normal.

Hypothyroidism

Patients with hypothyroidism frequently (20% to 65%) have a small number (0.5% to 2%) of acanthocytes on peripheral blood smears.[1450, 1466, 1598, 1599] Given the high incidence of hypothyroidism relative to other disorders that cause acanthocytosis, it has been suggested that the presence of acanthocytes should prompt physicians to consider thyroid testing, especially in adults. This approach has led to the diagnosis of hypothyroidism in previously unsuspected cases.[1600]

Other Membrane Disorders

Oxidant Hemolysis

Oxidant damage is incurred by the red cell membrane in a variety of inherited disorders involving abnormal hemoglobins of defects in the cells' endogenous system for detoxification of oxidants. These include sickle cell disease, thalassemias, unstable hemoglobinopathies, G6PD deficiency, and disorders of glutathione metabolism. Membrane oxidant damage may also result from encounters with exogenous oxidants, one of the most important of these being copper.

Copper Toxicity

Acute copper-induced hemolysis has been reported in humans after accidental or suicidal ingestion of copper or copper-containing compounds, copper sulfate therapy for burns, copper contamination of hemodialysis units, and Wilson's disease.[1601–1605] In the first three instances, acute intoxication is characterized by flushing, chills, nausea and vomiting, diarrhea, abdominal pain, a metallic taste in the mouth, excessive salivation, headache, weakness, and acute intravascular hemolysis.[1601–1606]

Wilson's Disease (Hepatolenticular Degeneration)

Wilson's disease is an autosomal recessive disorder of copper metabolism characterized by defective biliary excretion of copper, low plasma ceruloplasmin, and toxic accumulation of copper in liver, erythrocytes, kidneys, cornea, and brain.[1607, 1608] Consequences include cirrhosis, hemolysis, corneal Kayser-Fleischer rings, and a progressive neurologic syndrome.[1609–1622] The Wilson disease gene, *ATP7B*, encodes an integral membrane protein that has the features of a copper-transporting ATPase.[1623–1627] A wide variety of mutations have been described in this gene in Wilson's disease patients.[1628, 1629]

Hemolysis is an early feature of Wilson's disease; it is seen in 20% of patients who present with liver disease[1609] and may be the presenting manifestation of the disorder.[1610–1616] Because the disease is treatable and because hemolysis may presage fulminant liver disease by days to years,[1607, 1613, 1615, 1616] the clinician must always consider Wilson's disease in children and young adults with Coombs'-negative hemolytic anemia. Typically, these previously well children have chemical evidence of liver disease, mild hepatosplenomegaly, low ceruloplasmin concentration, increased erythrocyte and hepatic copper levels, and increased urinary copper excretion.[1607] Jaundice is frequent and may be extreme. The hemolysis observed in Wilson's disease is also acute, but the clinical features, although similar to acute copper poisoning, are usually more subtle. Hemoglobin may be detected on urinalysis, but gross hemoglobinuria is unusual. Peripheral blood smears are usually uncharacteristic, although we have seen one child in whom spur cells and target cells were prominent.

It is believed that in Wilson's disease copper initially accumulates in the liver, where it eventually reaches a toxic level and is released into the blood stream by hepatocellular necrosis.[1615] Plasma copper is rapidly taken up by red cells.[1630] Intravascular hemolysis occurs as a consequence of oxidative damage. The oxidative effects of copper are manifold. *In vitro*, copper inactivates numerous red cell glycolytic and hexose monophosphate shunt enzymes; directly oxidizes NADPH and glutathione; oxidizes and denatures hemoglobin; damages membrane ATPases, fatty acid acylase, and probably other membrane enzymes; generates lipid peroxides; and cross-links membrane skeletal proteins into disulfide-bonded high-molecular-weight complexes, increasing membrane permeability and rigidity.[1606, 1631] However, many of these effects have not been demonstrated at concentrations of copper observed in hemolyzing erythrocytes (150 to 400 mg/dL red cells = 2.4×10^{-5} to 6.3×10^{-5} M).[1617, 1621] It is likely that oxidation results from the reaction of copper with protein thiols to yield superoxide and its subsequent conversion to peroxide and other forms of activated oxygen. So far it has not been possible to determine the exact cause of the red cells' demise.

References

1. Singer SJ, Nicolson GL: The fluid-mosaic model of the structure of cell membranes. Science 1972; 175:720.
2. Lux SE, Palek J: Disorders of the red cell membrane. In Handin RI, Lux SE, Stossel TP (eds): Blood: Principles and Practice of Hematology. Philadelphia, J.B. Lippincott Co., 1995, p 1701.
3. Sweeley CC, Dawson G: Lipids of the erythrocyte. In Jamieson GA, Greenwalt TJ (eds): Red Cell Membrane Structure and Function. Philadelphia, J.B. Lippincott Co., 1969, p 172.
4. Turner JD, Rouser G: Precise quantitative determination of human blood lipids by thin layer and triethylaminoethyl cellulose column chromatography. Ann Biochem 1970; 38:437.
5. Ways P, Hanahan DJ: Characterization and quantification of red cell lipids in normal man. J Lipid Res 1964; 5:318.
6. Marchesi VT, Tillack TW, et al: Chemical characterization and surface orientation of the major glycoprotein of the human erythrocyte membrane. Proc Natl Acad Sci U S A 1972; 69:1445.
7. Weinstein RS: The morphology of adult red cells. In Surgenor DM (ed): The Red Blood Cell. 2nd ed. Vol. I. New York, Academic Press, 1974, p 214.
8. Van Deenen LLM, De Gier J: Lipids of the red blood cell membrane. In Surgenor DM (ed): The Red Blood Cell. 2nd ed. New York, Academic Press, 1974, p 148.
9. Cullis PR, Hope MJ: Effects of fusogenic agents on membrane structure of erythrocyte ghosts and the mechanism of membrane fusion. Nature 1978; 271:672.
10. Spitalnik SL: Human blood group antigens and antibodies: I. Carbohydrate determinants. In Hoffman R, Benz EJ Jr, et al (eds): Hematology. 2nd ed. New York, Churchill Livingstone, Inc., 1995, p 1948.
11. Telen MJ: Human blood group antigens and antibodies: I. Protein determinants. In Hoffman R, Benz EJ Jr, et al (eds): Hematology. 2nd ed. New York, Churchill Livingstone, Inc., 1995, p 1954.
12. King MJ: Blood group antigens on human erythrocytes: distribution, structure and possible functions. Biochim Biophys Acta 1994; 1197:15.
13. Watkins WM: Blood-group substances: Their nature and genetics. In Surgenor DM (ed): The Red Blood Cell. 2nd ed. Vol. I. New York, Academic Press, 1974, p 293.
14. Naiki M, Marcus DM: Human erythrocyte P and Pk blood group antigens: Identification as glycosphingolipids. Biochem Biophys Res Commun 1974; 60:1105.
15. Dejter-Juszynski M, Harpaz N, et al: Blood-group ABH-specific macroglycolipids of human erythrocytes: Isolation in high yield from a crude membrane glycoprotein fraction. Eur J Biochem 1978; 83:363.
16. Blau L, Bittman R: Cholesterol distribution between the two halves of the lipid bilayer of human erythrocyte ghost membranes. J Biol Chem 1978; 253:8366.
17. Hale JE, Schroeder F: Asymmetric transbilayer distribution of sterol across plasma membranes determined by fluorescence quenching of dehydroergosterol. Eur J Biochem 1982; 122:649.
18. Fisher KA: Analysis of membrane halves: Cholesterol. Proc Natl Acad Sci U S A 1976; 73:173.
19. Hubbell WL, McConnell HM: Orientation and motion of amphiphilic spin labels in membranes. Proc Natl Acad Sci U S A 1969; 64:20.
20. Lange Y, Dolde J, Steck TL: The rate of transmembrane movement of cholesterol in the human erythrocyte. J Biol Chem 1981; 256:5321.
21. Huang CH: A structural model for the cholesterol-phosphatidylcholine complexes in bilayer membranes. Lipids 1977; 12:348.
22. Bergelson LD, Barsukov LI: Topological asymmetry of phospholipids in membranes. Science 1977; 197:224.
23. Etemadi AH: Membrane asymmetry: A survey and critical appraisal of the methodology. Methods for assessing the unequal distribution of lipids. Biochim Biophys Acta 1980; 604:423.
24. Op den Kamp JAF: Lipid asymmetry in membranes. Annu Rev Biochem 1979; 48:47.
25. Devaux PF: Protein involvement in transmembrane lipid asymmetry. Annu Rev Biophys Biomol Struct 1992; 21:417.
26. Devaux PF: Lipid transmembrane asymmetry and flip-flip in biological membranes and in lipid bilayers. Curr Opin Struct Biol 1993; 3:489.
27. Devaux PF: Static and dynamic lipid asymmetry in cell membranes. Biochemistry 1991; 30:1163.

28. Connor J, Schroit AJ: Determination of lipid asymmetry in human red cells by resonance energy transfer. Biochemistry 1987; 26:5099.

29. Daleke DL, Huestis WH: Incorporation and translocation of aminophospholipids in human erythrocytes. Biochemistry 1985; 24:5406.

30. Seigneuret M, Devaux PF: ATP-dependent asymmetric distribution of spin-labeled phospholipids in the erythrocyte membrane: Relation to shape changes. Proc Natl Acad Sci U S A 1984; 81:3751.

31. Tilley L, Cribier S, et al: ATP-dependent translocation of amino phospholipids across the human erythrocyte membrane. FEBS Lett 1986; 194:21.

32. Zachowski A, Favre E, et al: Outside-inside translocation of aminophospholipids in the human erythrocyte membrane is mediated by a specific enzyme. Biochemistry 1986; 25:2585.

33. Morrot G, Hervé P, et al: Aminophospholipid translocase of human erythrocytes: Phospholipid substrate specificity and effect of cholesterol. Biochemistry 1989; 28:3456.

34. Connor J, Schroit AJ: Transbilayer movement of phosphatidyl-serine in nonhuman erythrocytes: Evidence that the amino-phospholipid transporter is a ubiquitous membrane protein. Biochemistry 1989; 28:9680.

35. Zachowski A, Henry J-P, Devaux PF: Control of transmembrane lipid asymmetry in chromaffin granules by an ATP-dependent protein. Nature 1989; 340:75.

36. Connor J, Schroit AJ: Transbilayer movement of phosphatidyl-serine in erythrocytes: Inhibition of transport and preferential labeling of a 31,000-dalton protein by sulfhydryl reactive reagents. Biochemistry 1988; 27:848.

37. Tang X, Halleck MS, et al: A subfamily of P-type ATPases with aminophospholipid transporting activity. Science 1996; 272:1495.

38. van Helvoort A, Smith AJ, et al: MDR1 P-glycoprotein is a lipid translocase of broad specificity, while MDR3 P-glycoprotein specifically translocates phosphatidylcholine. Cell 1996; 87:507.

39. Higgins CF, Gottesman MM: Is the multidrug transporter a flippase? Trends Biochem Sci 1992; 17:18.

40. Smit JJ, Schinkel AH, et al: Homozygous disruption of the murine mdr2 P-glycoprotein gene leads to a complete absence of phospholipid from bile and to liver disease. Cell 1993; 75:451.

41. Ruetz S, Gros P: Phosphatidylcholine translocase: a physiological role for the mdr2 gene. Cell 1994; 77:1071.

42. Smith AJ, Timmermans-Hereijgers JL, et al: The human MDR3 P-glycoprotein promotes translocation of phosphatidylcholine through the plasma membrane of fibroblasts from transgenic mice. FEBS Lett 1994; 354:263.

43. Connor J, Pak CH, et al: Bidirectional transbilayer movement of phospholipid analogs in human red blood cells: Evidence for an ATP-dependent and protein-mediated process. J Biol Chem 1992; 267:19412.

44. Schroit AJ, Madsen J, Ruoho AE: Radioiodinated, photoactivatable phosphatidylcholine and phosphatidylserine transfer properties and differential photoreactive interaction with human erythrocyte membrane proteins. Biochemistry 1987; 26:1812.

45. Schroit AJ, Bloy C, et al: Involvement of Rh blood group polypeptides in the maintenance of aminophospholipid asymmetry. Biochemistry 1990; 29:10303.

46. Chérif-Zahar B, Bloy C, et al: Molecular cloning and protein structure of a human blood group Rh polypeptide. Proc Natl Acad Sci U S A 1990; 87:6243.

47. Bruckheimer EM, Gillum KD, Schroit AJ: Colocalization of Rh polypeptides and the aminophospholipid transporter in dilauroylphosphatidylcholine-induced erythrocyte vesicles. Biochem Biophys Acta 1995; 1235:147.

48. Bonnet D, Begard E: Interaction of anilinonapthyl labeled spectrin with fatty acids and phospholipids: Fluorescence study. Biochem Biophys Res Comm 1984; 120:344.

49. Cohen AM, Liu S-C, et al: Ultrastructural studies of the interaction of spectrin with phosphatidylserine liposomes. Blood 1986; 68:920.

50. Maksymiw R, Sui S-F, et al: Electrostatic coupling of spectrin dimers to phosphatidylserine containing lipid lamellae. Biochemistry 1987; 26:2983.

51. Mombers C, De Gier J, et al: Spectrin-phospholipid interaction. A monolayer study. Biochim Biophys Acta 1980; 603:52.

52. Bergmann WL, Dressler V, et al: Crosslinking of SH groups in the erythrocyte membrane enhances transbilayer orientation of phospholipids: Evidence for a limited access of phospholipids to the reorientation sites. Biochim Biophys Acta 1984; 769:390.

53. Dressler V, Haest CWM, et al: Stabilizing factors of phospho-lipid asymmetry in the erythrocyte membrane. Biochim Biophys Acta 1984; 775:189.

54. Franck PFH, Roelofsen B, Op den Kamp JA: Complete exchange of phosphatidylcholine from intact erythrocytes after protein crosslinking. Biochim Biophys Acta 1982; 687:105.

55. Haest CWM, Plasa G, et al: Spectrin as a stabilizer of the phospholipid asymmetry in the human erythrocyte membrane. Biochim Biophys Acta 1978; 509:21.

56. Calvez J-Y, Zachowski A, et al: Asymmetric distribution of phospholipids in spectrin-poor erythrocyte vesicles. Biochemistry 1988; 27:5666.

57. Kuypers FA, Lubin BH, et al: The distribution of erythrocyte phospholipids in hereditary spherocytosis demonstrates a minimal role for erythrocyte spectrin on phospholipid diffusion and asymmetry. Blood 1993; 81:1051.

58. Verhoven B, Schlegel RA, Williamson P: Rapid loss and restoration of lipid asymmetry by different pathways in resealed erythrocyte ghosts. Biochim Biophys Acta 1992; 1104:15.

59. Williamson P, Kulick A, et al: Ca^{2+} induces transbilayer redistribution of all major phospholipids in human erythrocytes. Biochemistry 1992; 31:6355.

60. Zwaal RFA, Comfurius P, Bevers EM: Mechanism and function of changes in membrane phospholipid asymmetry in platelets and erythrocytes. Biochem Soc Trans 1993; 21:248.

61. Blumenfeld N, Zachowski A, et al: Transmembrane mobility of phospholipids in sickle erythrocytes: Effect of deoxygenation on diffusion and asymmetry. Blood 1991; 77:849.

62. Franck PFH, Chiu DT-Y, et al: Accelerated transbilayer movement of phosphatidylcholine in sickled erythrocytes: A reversible process. J Biol Chem 1983; 258:8436.

63. Lubin B, Chiu D, et al: Abnormalities in membrane phospholipid organization in sickled erythrocytes. J Clin Invest 1981; 67:1643.

64. Platt OS, Falcone JF, Lux SE: Molecular defect in the sickle erythrocyte skeleton. Abnormal spectrin binding to sickle inside-out vesicles. J Clin Invest 1985; 75:266.

65. Liu S-C, Derick LH, et al: Uncoupling of the spectrin-based skeleton from the lipid bilayer in sickled red cells. Science 1991; 252:574.

66. Wautier JL, Paton RC, et al: Increased adhesion of erythrocytes to endothelial cells in diabetes mellitus and its relationship to vascular complications. N Engl J Med 1981; 305:237.

67. Hebbel RP, Yamada O, et al: Abnormal adherence of sickle erythrocytes to cultured vascular endothelium: Possible mechanism for microvascular occlusion in sickle cell disease. J Clin Invest 1980; 65:154.

68. Hebbel RP, Boogaerts MA, et al: Erythrocyte adherence to endothelium in sickle-cell anemia: A possible determinant of disease severity. N Engl J Med 1980; 302:992.

69. Mohandas N, Evans E: Adherence of sickle erythrocytes to vascular endothelial cells: Requirement for both cell membrane changes and plasma factors. Blood 1984; 64:282.

70. Bevers EM, Comfurius P, et al: Generation of prothrombin-converting activity and the exposure of phosphatidyl serine at the outer surface of platelets. Eur J Biochem 1982; 122:429.

71. Chiu D, Lubin B, et al: Sickled erythrocytes accelerate clotting *in vitro*: An effect of abnormal membrane lipid asymmetry. Blood 1981; 58:398.

72. Zwaal RF, Comfurius P, van Deenen LL: Membrane asymmetry and blood coagulation. Nature 1977; 268:358.

73. Allen TM, Williamson P, Schlegel RA: Phosphatidylserine as a determinant of reticuloendothelial recognition of liposome models of the erythrocyte surface. Proc Natl Acad Sci U S A 1988; 85:8067.

74. McEvoy L, Williamson P, Schlegel RA: Membrane phospholipid asymmetry as a determinant of erythrocyte recognition by macrophages. Proc Natl Acad Sci U S A 1986; 83:3311.

75. Pradhan D, Williamson PL, Schlegel RA: Phosphatidylserine

as a signal for recognition and phagocytosis of erythrocytes by macrophages. Mol Biol Cell 1993; 4(Suppl):84a. Abstract.

76. Schwartz RS, Chiu DT, Lubin B: Plasma membrane phospholipid organization in human erythrocytes. Curr Topics Hematol 1985; 5:63.

77. Tanaka Y, Schroit AJ: Insertion of fluorescent phosphatidylserine into the plasma membrane of red blood cells: Recognition by autologous macrophages. J Biol Chem 1983; 258:11335.

78. Pradhan D, Williamson P, Schlegel RA: Phosphatidylserine vesicles inhibit phagocytosis of erythrocytes with a symmetric transbilayer distribution of phospholipids. Mol Membr Biol 1994; 11:181.

79. Verhoven B, Schlegel RA, Williamson P: Mechanisms of phosphatidylserine exposure, a phagocyte recognition signal, on apoptotic T lymphocytes. J Exp Med 1995; 182:1597.

80. Rodgers W, Glaser M: Characterization of lipid domains in erythrocyte membranes. Proc Natl Acad Sci U S A 1991; 88:1364.

81. Jost PC, Nadakavukaren KK, Griffith OH: Phosphatidyl choline exchange between the boundary lipid and bilayer domains in cytochrome oxidase containing membranes. Biochemistry 1977; 16:3110.

82. Smith RL, Oldfield E: Dynamic structure of membranes by deuterium NMR. Science 1984; 225:280.

83. Boyd D, Beckwith J: The role of charged amino acids in the localization of secreted and membrane proteins. Cell 1990; 62:1031.

84. Parks GD, Lamb RA: Topology of eukaryotic type II membrane proteins: Importance of N-terminal positively charged residues flanking the hydrophobic domain. Cell 1991; 64:777.

85. Yamane K, Akiyama Y, et al: A positively charged region is a determinant of the orientation of cytoplasmic membrane proteins in *Escherichia coli*. J Biol Chem 1990; 265:21166.

86. Beck JS: Relations between membrane monolayers in some red cell shape transformations. J Theor Biol 1978; 75:487.

87. Ferrell JE Jr, Lee KJ, Huestis WH: Membrane bilayer balance and erythrocyte shape: A quantitative assessment. Biochemistry 1985; 24:2849.

88. Sheetz MP, Singer SJ: Biological membranes as bilayer couples: A molecular mechanism of drug-erythrocyte interactions. Proc Natl Acad Sci U S A 1974; 71:4457.

89. Christiansson A, Kuypers FA, et al: Lipid molecular shape effects erythrocyte morphology: A study involving replacement of native phosphatidylcholine with different species followed by treatment of cells with sphingomyelinase C or phospholipase A. J Cell Biol 1985; 101:1455.

90. Isomaa B, Hagerstrand H, Paatero G: Shape transformation induced by amphiphiles in erythrocytes. Biochim Biophys Acta 1987; 899:93.

91. Sheetz MP, Painter RG, Singer SJ: Biological membranes as bilayer couples: III. Compensatory shape changes induced in membranes. J Cell Biol 1976; 70:193.

92. Lange Y, Steck TL: Mechanism of red blood cell acanthocytosis and echinocytosis *in vivo*. J Membr Biol 1984; 77:153.

93. Brown KE, Anderson SM, Young NS: Erythrocyte P antigen: Cellular receptor for B19 parvovirus. Science 1993; 262:114.

94. Lange Y, Slayton JM: Interaction of cholesterol and lysophosphatidylcholine in determining red cell shape. J Lipid Res 1982; 23:1121.

95. Huang C-H: A structural model for the cholesterol-phosphatidyl choline complexes in bilayer membranes. Lipids 1977; 12:348.

96. Berridge MJ: Inositol trisphosphate and calcium signalling. Nature 1993; 361:315.

97. Levine YK, Birdsall NJM, et al: ¹³C nuclear magnetic resonance relaxation measurements of synthetic lecithins and the effect of spin-labeled lipids. Biochemistry 1972; 11:1416.

98. McConnell HM, McFarland BG: The flexibility gradient in biological membranes. Ann NY Acad Sci 1972; 195:207.

99. Barton PG, Gunstone FD: Hydrocarbon chain packing and molecular motion in phospholipid bilayers formed from unsaturated lecithins. J Biol Chem 1975; 250:4470.

100. Seelig A, Seelig J: Effect of a single *cis* double bond on the structure of a phospholipid bilayer. Biochemistry 1977; 16:45.

101. Oldfield E, Chapman D: Effects of cholesterol and cholesterol derivatives on hydrocarbon chain mobility in lipids. Biochem Biophys Res Commun 1971; 43:610.

102. Lee AG, Birdsall NJM, Metcalfe JC: Measurement of fast lateral diffusion of lipids in vesicles and in biological membranes by ³H nuclear magnetic resonance. Biochemistry 1973; 12:1650.

103. Cooper RA, Durocher JR, Leslie MH: Decreased fluidity of red cell membrane lipid in abetalipoproteinemia. J Clin Invest 1977; 60:115.

104. Cooper RA: Abnormalities of cell membrane fluidity in the pathogenesis of disease. N Engl J Med 1977; 297:371.

105. Vanderkooi J, Fischkoff S, Chance B: Fluorescent probe analysis of the lipid architecture of natural and experimental cholesterol-rich membranes. Biochemistry 1974; 13:1589.

106. Devaux P, McConnell HM: Lateral diffusion in spin-labeled phosphatidyl choline multilayers. J Am Chem Soc 1972; 94:4475.

107. Wu E-S, Jacobson K, Papahadjopoulos D: Lateral diffusion in phospholipid multilayers measured by fluorescence recovery after photobleaching. Biochemistry 1977; 16:3936.

108. Koppel DE, Sheetz MP, Schindler M: Matrix control of protein diffusion in biological membranes. Proc Natl Acad Sci U S A 1981; 78:3576.

109. Reed CF: Incorporation of orthophosphate-³²P into erythrocyte phospholipids in normal subjects and in patients with hereditary spherocytosis. J Clin Invest 1968; 47:2630.

110. Renooij W, Van Golde LMG: The transposition of molecular classes of phosphatidyl choline across the rat erythrocyte membrane and their exchange between the red cell membrane and plasma lipoproteins. Biochim Biophys Acta 1977; 470:465.

111. Shohet SB: Release of phospholipid fatty acid from human erythrocytes. J Clin Invest 1970; 49:1668.

112. Glomset JA, Assmann G, et al: Lecithin:cholesterol acyltransferase deficiency and fish eye disease. In Scriver CS, Beaudet AL, et al (eds): The Metabolic and Molecular Bases of Inherited Disease. 7th ed. New York, McGraw-Hill Book Co., 1995, p 1933.

113. Mulder E, Van Deenen LLM: Metabolism of red cell lipids: I. Incorporation *in vitro* of fatty acids into phospholipids from mature erythrocytes. Biochim Biophys Acta 1965; 106:106.

114. Oliveria MM, Vaughan M: Incorporation of fatty acids into phospholipids of erythrocyte membranes. J Lipid Res 1964; 5:156.

115. Shohet SB, Nathan DG, Karnovsky ML: Stages in the incorporation of fatty acids into red blood cells. J Clin Invest 1968; 47:1096.

116. Renooij W, Van Golde LMG, et al: Preferential incorporation of fatty acids at the inside of human erythrocyte membranes. Biochim Biophys Acta 1974; 363:287.

117. Fairbanks G, Steck TL, Wallach DFH: Electrophoretic analysis of the major polypeptides of the human erythrocyte membrane. Biochemistry 1971; 10:2606.

118. Rubin RW, Milikowski C: Over two hundred polypeptides resolved from the human erythrocyte membrane. Biochim Biophys Acta 1978; 509:100.

119. Alper SL: The band 3-related anion exchanger (AE) gene family. Annu Rev Physiol 1991; 53:549.

120. Inoue T, Kanzaki A, et al: Uniquely higher incidence of isolated or combined deficiency of band 3 and/or band 4.2 as the pathogenesis of autosomal dominantly inherited hereditary spherocytosis in the Japanese population. Int J Hematol 1994; 60:227.

121. Bennett V, Stenbuck PJ: Identification and partial purification of ankyrin, the high affinity membrane attachment site for human erythrocyte spectrin. J Biol Chem 1979; 254:2533.

122. Bennett V, Stenbuck PJ: Human erythrocyte ankyrin. Purification and properties. J Biol Chem 1980; 255:2540.

123. Calvert R, Ungewickell E, Gratzer W: A conformational study of human spectrin. Eur J Biochem 1980; 107:363.

124. Cartron JP, Rahuel C: Human erythrocyte glycophorins: Protein and gene structure analysis. Transfusion Med Rev 1992; 6:63.

125. Colin Y, Le Van Kim C, et al: Human erythrocyte glycophorin C: Gene structure and rearrangement in genetic variants. J Biol Chem 1989; 264:3773.

126. Colin Y, Rahuel C, et al: Isolation of cDNA clones and complete

amino acid sequence of human erythrocyte glycophorin C. J Biol Chem 1986; 261:229.

127. Bennett V: The spectrin-actin junction of erythrocyte membrane skeletons. Biochim Biophys Acta 1989; 988:107.

128. Bennett V: Spectrin-based membrane skeleton: A multipotential adaptor between plasma membrane and cytoskeleton. Physiol Rev 1990; 70:1029.

129. Bennett V, Lambert S: The spectrin skeleton from red cells to brain. J Clin Invest 1991; 87:1483.

130. Bennett V: Ankyrins: Adaptors between diverse plasma membrane proteins and the cytoplasm. J Biol Chem 1992; 267:8703.

131. Cartron JP, Le Van Kim C, Colin Y: Glycophorin C and related glycoproteins: Structure, function, and regulation. Semin Hematol 1993; 30:152.

132. Chasis JA, Mohandas M: Red blood cell glycophorins. Blood 1992; 8:1869.

133. Cohen CM, Dotimas E, Korsgren C: Human erythrocyte membrane protein band 4.2 (pallidin). Semin Hematol 1993; 30:119.

134. Coleman TR, Fishkind DJ, et al: Contributions of the beta-subunit to spectrin structure and function. Cell Motil Cytoskeleton 1989; 12:248.

135. Conboy JG, Mohandas N: Characterization of the gene coding human erythrocyte protein 4.1: Implications for understanding hereditary elliptocytosis. In Agre P, Parker JC (eds): Red Blood Cell Membranes: Structure, Function, Clinical Implications. New York, Marcel Dekker, Inc., 1989, p 167.

136. Conboy JG: Structure, function, and molecular genetics of erythroid membrane skeletal protein 4.1 in normal and abnormal red blood cells. Semin Hematol 1993; 30:58.

137. Fukuda M: Molecular genetics of the glycophorin A gene cluster. Semin Hematol 1993; 30:138.

138. Gallagher PG, Forget BG: Spectrin genes in health and disease. Semin Hematol 1993; 30:4.

139. Gilligan DM, Bennett V: The junctional complex of the membrane skeleton. Semin Hematol 1993; 30:74.

140. Goodman SR, Krebs KE, et al: Spectrin and related molecules. CRC Crit Rev Biochem 1988; 23:171.

141. Hanspal M, Palek J: Biogenesis of normal and abnormal red blood cell membrane skeletons. Semin Hematol 1992; 29:305.

142. Jennings ML: Structure and function of the red blood cell anion transport protein. Annu Rev Biophys Chem 1989; 18:397.

143. Liu S-C, Derick LH: Molecular anatomy of the red blood cell membrane skeleton: Structure-function relationships. Semin Hematol 1992; 29:231.

144. Low PS, Willardson BM, et al: The other functions of erythrocyte membrane band 3. In Hamasaki N, Jennings ML (eds): Anion Transport Protein of the Red Blood Cell Membrane. New York, Elsevier Science Publishing Co., 1989, p 103.

145. Mohandas N, Chasis JA: Red cell deformability, membrane material properties, and shape: Regulation by transmembrane, skeletal, and cytosolic proteins and lipids. Semin Hematol 1993; 30:171.

146. Peters LL, Lux SE: Ankyrins: Structure and function in normal cells and hereditary spherocytes. Semin Hematol 1993; 30:85.

147. Tanner MJA: Molecular and cellular biology of the erythrocyte anion exchanger (AE1). Semin Hematol 1993; 30:34.

148. Winkelmann JC, Forget BG: Erythroid and nonerythroid spectrins. Blood 1993; 81:3173.

149. Becker PS, Lux SE: Disorders of the red cell membrane. In Nathan DG, Oski FA (eds): Hematology of Infancy and Childhood. 4th ed. Philadelphia, W.B. Saunders Co., 1993, p 529.

150. Becker PS, Lux SE: Disorders of the red cell membrane skeleton: Hereditary spherocytosis and hereditary elliptocytosis. In Scriver CS, Beaudet AL, et al (eds): The Metabolic and Molecular Bases of Inherited Disease. 7th ed. New York, McGraw-Hill Book Co., 1995, p 3513.

151. Boivin P, Lecomte MC, et al: Clinical expression of spectrin alpha I variants. In Cohen CM, Palek J (eds): Cellular and Molecular Biology of Normal and Abnormal Erythroid Membranes. New York, Wiley-Liss, 1990, p 235.

152. Davies KA, Lux SE: Hereditary disorders of the red cell membrane skeleton. Trends Genet 1989; 5:222.

153. Delaunay J, Alloisio N, et al: The red cell skeleton and its genetic disorders. Mol Aspects Med 1990; 11:161.

154. Delaunay J, Dhermy D: Mutations involving the spectrin heter-

155. Gratzer WB, Dluzewski AR: The red blood cell and malaria parasite invasion. Semin Hematol 1993; 30:232.

156. Alloisio N, Maillet P, et al: Hereditary spherocytosis with band 3 deficiency. Association with a nonsense mutation of the band 3 gene (allele Lyon) and aggravation by a low-expression allele occurring in *trans* (allele Genas). Blood 1996; 88:1062.

157. Palek J, Lambert S: Genetics of the red cell membrane skeleton. Semin Hematol 1990; 27:290.

158. Palek J, Sahr KE: Mutations of the red blood cell membrane proteins: From clinical evaluation to detection of the underlying genetic defect. Blood 1992; 80:308.

159. Palek J, Jarolim P: Clinical expression and laboratory detection of red cell membrane protein mutations. Semin Hematol 1993; 30:249.

160. Cartron JP, Agre P: Rh blood group antigens: Protein and gene structure. Semin Hematol 1993; 30:193.

161. Redman CM, Marsh WL: The Kell blood group system and the McLeod phenotype. Semin Hematol 1993; 30:209.

162. Rosse WF: The glycolipid anchor of membrane surface proteins. Semin Hematol 1993; 30:219.

163. Telen MJ: Erythrocyte blood group antigens: Not so simple after all. Blood 1995; 85:299.

164. Delaunay J: Genetic disorders of the red cell membrane. Crit Rev Oncol Hematol 1994; 19:79.

165. Hitt AL, Luna EJ: Membrane interactions with the actin cytoskeleton. Curr Opin Cell Biol 1994; 6:120.

166. Dhermy D: The spectrin super-family. Biol Cell 1991; 71:249.

167. Anstee DJ, Hemming NJ, Tanner MJA: Functional factors in the red cell membrane: Interactions between the membrane and its underlying skeleton. Immun Invest 1995; 24:187.

168. Colin Y: Gerbich blood groups and minor glycophorins of human erythrocytes. Transfus Clin Biol 1995; 2:259.

169. Cartron JP: Defining the Rh blood group antigens: Biochemistry and molecular genetics. Blood 1994; 8:199.

170. Dodge JT, Mitchell C, et al: The preparation and chemical characteristics of hemoglobin-free ghosts of human erythrocytes. Arch Biochem Biophys 1963; 100:119.

171. Laemmli UK: Cleavage of structural proteins during the assembly of the head of bacteriophage T4. Nature 1970; 227:680.

172. Steck TL: Cross-linking the major proteins of the isolated erythrocyte membrane. J Mol Biol 1972; 66:295.

173. Furthmayr H: Structural comparison of glycophorins and immunochemical analysis of genetic variants. Nature 1978; 271:519.

174. Siebert PD, Fukuda M: Isolation and characterization of human glycophorin A cDNA clones by a synthetic oligonucleotide approach: Nucleotide sequence and mRNA structure. Proc Natl Acad Sci U S A 1986; 83:1665.

175. Rahuel C, London J, et al: Characterization of cDNA clones for human glycophorin A: Use for gene localization and for analysis of normal glycophorin-A–deficient (Finnish type) genomic DNA. Eur J Biochem 1988; 172:147.

176. Irimura T, Tsuji T, et al: Structure of a complex-type sugar chain of human glycophorin A. Biochemistry 1981; 20:560.

177. Dahr W, Gielen W, et al: Structure of the Ss blood group antigens: I. Isolation of Ss-active glycopeptides and differentiation of the antigens by modification of methionine. Hoppe Seylers Z Physiol Chem 1980; 361:145.

178. Dahr W, Kordowicz M, et al: The amino acid sequence of the M^c-specific major red cell membrane sialoglycoprotein—an intermediate of the blood group M- and N-active molecules. Hoppe Seylers Z Physiol Chem 1981; 362:363.

179. Dahr W, Beyreuther K, et al: Amino acid sequence of the blood group M^c-specific major human erythrocyte membrane sialoglycoprotein. Hoppe Seylers Z Physiol Chem 1981; 362:81.

180. Dahr W, Kordowicz M, et al: Structural analysis of the Ss sialoglycoprotein specific for Henshaw blood group from human erythrocyte membranes. Eur J Biochem 1984; 141:51.

181. Tanner MJA, Anstee DJ: The membrane change in En(a−) human erythrocytes. Biochem J 1976; 153:271.

182. Tanner MJA, Jenkins RE, Anstee DJ: Abnormal carbohydrate composition of the major penetrating membrane protein of En(a−) human erythrocytes. Biochem J 1976; 155:701.

183. Gahmberg CG, Myllyla G, Leikola J: Absence of the major sialoglycoprotein in the membrane of human En(a−) erythrocytes and increased glycosylation of band 3. J Biol Chem 1976; 251:6108.

184. Dahr W, Uhlenbruck G, Leikola J: Studies on the membrane glycoprotein defect of En(a−) erythrocytes. I. Biochemical aspects. J Immunogenet 1976; 3:329.

185. Tanner MJ, Anstee DJ, Judson PA: A carbohydrate-deficient membrane glycoprotein in human erythrocytes of phenotype S−s−. Biochem J 1977; 165:151.

186. Dahr W, Uhlenbruck G, et al: SDS-polyacrylamide gel electrophoretic analysis of the membrane glycoproteins from S−s−U− erythrocytes. J Immunogenet 1975; 2:249.

187. Huang C-H, Johe K, et al: δ Glycophorin (glycophorin B) gene deletion in two individuals homozygous for the S−s−U− blood group phenotype. Blood 1987; 70:1830.

188. Tokunaga E, Sasakawa S, Tamaka K: Two apparently healthy Japanese individuals of type MᵏMᵏ have erythrocytes which lack both blood group MN and Ss-active sialoglycoproteins. J Immunogenet 1979; 6:383.

189. Anstee DJ: The blood group MNSs-active sialoglycoproteins. Semin Hematol 1981; 15:13.

190. Blanchard D, Asseraf A, Prigent MJ: Miltenberger class I and II erythrocytes carry a variant of glycophorin A. Biochem J 1983; 213:399.

191. Dahr W, Newman RA, et al: Structures of Miltenberger class I and II specific major human erythrocyte membrane sialoglycoproteins. Eur J Biochem 1984; 138:259.

192. Dahr W, Beyreuther K, Moulds JJ: Structural analysis of the major human erythrocyte membrane sialoglycoproteins from Miltenberger class VII cells. Eur J Biochem 1987; 166:27.

193. Dahr W, Vengelen-Tyler V, et al: Structural analysis of glycophorin A from Miltenberger class VIII erythrocytes. Biol Chem Hoppe Seyler 1989; 370:855.

194. Johe KK, Smith AJ, Blumenfeld OO: Amino acid sequence of MiIII glycophorin: Demonstration of δ-α and α-δ junction regions and expression of δ pseudoexon by direct protein sequencing. J Biol Chem 1991; 266:7256.

195. Johe KK, Vengelen-Tyler V, et al: Synthetic peptides homologous to human glycophorins of the Miltenberger complex of variants of MNSs blood group system specify the epitopes for Hil, Sᴶᴸ, Hop, and Mur antisera. Blood 1991; 78:2456.

196. Mawby WJ, Anstee DJ, Tanner MJ: Immunochemical evidence for hybrid sialoglycoproteins of human erythrocytes. Nature 1981; 291:161.

197. Tanner MJ, Anstee DJ, Mawby WJ: A new human erythrocyte variant (Ph) containing an abnormal membrane sialoglycoprotein. Biochem J 1980; 187:493.

198. Johe KK, Smith AJ, et al: Amino acid sequence of an α-δ glycophorin hybrid: A structure reciprocal to Stᵃ δ-α glycophorin hybrid. J Biol Chem 1989; 264:17486.

199. Anstee DJ, Mawby WJ, Tanner MJ: Abnormal blood group Ss-active sialoglycoproteins in the membrane of Miltenberger class III, IV, and V erythrocytes. Biochem J 1979; 183:193.

200. Huang C-H, Guizzo ML, et al: Molecular genetic analysis of a hybrid gene encoding Stᵃ glycophorin of the human erythrocyte membrane. Blood 1989; 74:836.

201. Blumenfeld OO, Smith AJ, Moulds JJ: Membrane glycophorins of Dantu blood group erythrocytes. J Biol Chem 1987; 262:11864.

202. Blanchard D, Cartron JP, et al: Pj variant, a new, hybrid MNSs glycoprotein of the human red cell membrane. Biochem J 1982; 203:419.

203. Huang C-H, Blumenfeld OO: Identification of recombination events resulting in three hybrid genes encoding human MiV, MiV(J.L.), and Stᵃ glycophorins. Blood 1991; 77:1813.

204. Huang C-H, Blumenfeld OO: Molecular genetics of human erythrocyte MiIII and MiVI glycophorins. Use of a pseudoexon in construction of two δ-α-δ hybrid genes resulting in antigenic diversification. J Biol Chem 1991; 266:7248.

205. Huang C-H, Blumenfeld OO: Multiple origins of the human glycophorin Stᵃ gene. Identification of hot spots for independent unequal homologous recombinations. J Biol Chem 1991; 266:23306.

206. Huang C-H, Kikuchi M, et al: Gene conversion confined to a direct repeat of the acceptor splice site generates allelic diversity at human glycophorin (GYP) locus. J Biol Chem 1992; 267:3336.

207. Huang C-H, Skov F, et al: Molecular analysis of human glycophorin MiIX gene shows a silent segment transfer and untemplated mutation resulting from gene conversion via sequence repeats. Blood 1992; 80:2379.

208. Huang C-H, Blumenfeld OO: Characterization of a genomic hybrid specifying the human erythrocyte antigen Dantu: Dantu gene is duplicated and linked to a δ glycophorin gene deletion. Proc Natl Acad Sci U S A 1988; 85:9640.

209. Kudo S, Fukuda M: Structural organization of glycophorin A and B genes: Glycophorin B gene evolved by homologous recombination at Alu repeat sequences. Proc Natl Acad Sci U S A 1989; 86:4619.

210. Cartron JP, Blanchard D: Association of human erythrocyte membrane glycoproteins with blood group Cad specificity. Biochem J 1982; 207:497.

211. Blanchard D, Cartron JP, et al: Primary structure of the oligosaccharide determinant of blood group Cad specificity. J Biol Chem 1983; 258:7691.

212. Herkt F, Parente JP, et al: Structure determination of oligosaccharides isolated from Cad erythrocyte membranes by permethylation analysis and 500 MHz ¹H-NMR spectroscopy. Eur J Biochem 1985; 146:125.

213. Armitage IM, Shapiro DL, et al: ³¹P nuclear magnetic resonance evidence for polyphosphoinositide associated with the hydrophobic segment of glycophorin A. Biochemistry 1977; 16:1317.

214. Mendelsohn R, Dluhy RA, et al: Interaction of glycophorin with phosphatidylserine: A Fourier transform infrared investigation. Biochemistry 1984; 23:1498.

215. Ong RL: ³¹P and ¹⁹F NMR studies of glycophorin-reconstituted membranes: Preferential interaction of glycophorin with phosphatidylserine. J Membr Biol 1984; 78:1.

216. Yeagle PL, Kelsey D: Phosphorus nuclear magnetic resonance studies of lipid-protein interactions: Human erythrocyte glycophorin and phospholipids. Biochemistry 1989; 28:2210.

217. Segrest JP, Jackson RL, et al: Human erythrocyte membrane glycoprotein: A reevaluation of the molecular weight as determined by SDS polyacrylamide gel electrophoresis. Biochem Biophys Res Commun 1971; 44:390.

218. Gahmberg CG, Jokinen M, et al: Expression of the major sialoglycoprotein (glycophorin) on erythroid cells in human bone marrow. Blood 1978; 52:379.

219. Ridgwell K, Eyers SA, et al: Studies on the glycoprotein associated with Rh (rhesus) blood group antigen expression in the human red blood cell membrane. J Biol Chem 1994; 269:6410.

220. Kudo S, Fukuda M: Identification of a novel human glycophorin, glycophorin E, by isolation of genomic clones and complementary DNA clones utilizing polymerase chain reaction. J Biol Chem 1990; 65:1102.

221. Vignal A, London J, et al: Promoter sequence and chromosomal organization of the genes encoding glycophorins A, B, and E. Gene 1990; 95:289.

222. Anstee DJ: The nature and abundance of human red cell surface glycoproteins. J Immunogenet 1990; 17:219.

223. King MJ, Holmes CH, et al: Reactivity with erythroid and non-erythroid tissues of a murine monoclonal antibody to a synthetic peptide having amino acid sequence common to cytoplasmic domain of human glycophorins C and D. Br J Haematol 1995; 89:440.

224. Villeval JL, LeVan Kim C, et al: Early expression of glycophorin-C during normal and leukemic erythroid differentiation. Cancer Res 1989; 49:2626.

225. Chasis JA, Mohandas N, Shohet SB: Erythrocyte membrane rigidity induced by glycophorin A-ligand interaction. Evidence for a ligand-induced association between glycophorin A and skeletal proteins. J Clin Invest 1985; 75:1919.

226. Smythe J, Gardner B, Anstee DJ: Quantitation of the number of molecules of glycophorins C and D on normal red blood cells using radioiodinated Fab fragments of monoclonal antibodies. Blood 1994; 83:1668.

227. Huang C-H, Reid ME, et al: Human red blood cell Wright antigens: A genetic and evolutionary perspective on glycophorin A-band 3 interaction. Blood 1996; 87:3942.

228. Bruce LJ, Ring SM, et al: Changes in the blood group Wright antigens are associated with a mutation at amino acid 658 in human erythrocyte band 3: A site of interaction between band 3 and glycophorin A under certain conditions. Blood 1995; 85:541.

229. Leddy JP, WIlkinson SL, et al: Erythrocyte membrane proteins reactive with IgG (warm-reacting) anti-red blood cell autoantibodies: II. Antibodies coprecipitating band 3 and glycophorin A. Blood 1994; 84:650.

230. Telen MJ, Chasis JA: Relationship of the human erythrocyte Wr^b antigen to an interaction between glycophorin A and band 3. Blood 1990; 76:842.

231. Knowles DW, Chasis JA, et al: Cooperative action between band 3 and glycophorin A in human erythrocytes: Immobilization of band 3 induced by antibodies to glycophorin A. Biophys J 1994; 66:1726.

232. Che A, Cherry RJ: Loss of rotational mobility of band 3 proteins in human erythrocyte membranes induced by antibodies to glycophorin A. Biophys J 1995; 68:1881.

233. Groves JD, Tanner MJ: Glycophorin A facilitates the expression of human band 3-mediated anion transport in *Xenopus* oocytes. J Biol Chem 1992; 267:22163.

234. Chasis JA, Reid ME, et al: Signal transduction by glycophorin A: Role of extracellular and cytoplasmic domains in a modulatable process. J Cell Biol 1988; 107:1351.

235. Paulitschke M, Nash GB, et al: Perturbation of red blood cell membrane rigidity by extracellular ligands. Blood 1995; 86:342.

236. Chasis JA, Knowles D, et al: Conformational changes in cytoplasmic domains of band 3 and glycophorin-A affect red cell membrane properties. Blood 1991; 78(Suppl 1):252a. Abstract.

237. Perkins M: Inhibitory effects of erythrocyte membrane proteins on the *in vitro* invasion of the human malarial parasite *(Plasmodium falciparum)* into its host cell. J Cell Biol 1981; 90:563.

238. Pasvol G, Wainscoat JS, Weatherall DJ: Erythrocytes deficient in glycophorin resist invasion by the malarial parasite *Plasmodium falciparum*. Nature 1982; 297:64.

239. Cartron JP, Prou O, et al: Susceptibility to invasion by *Plasmodium falciparum* of some human erythrocytes carrying rare blood groups. Br J Haematol 1983; 55:639.

240. Hadley TJ, Klotz FW, et al: Falciparum malaria parasites invade erythrocytes that lack glycophorin A and B (M^{k}M^k). Strain differences indicate heterogeneity and two pathways for invasion. J Clin Invest 1988; 80:1190.

241. Orlandi PA, Klotz FW, Haynes JD: A malaria invasion receptor, the 175-kilodalton erythrocyte binding antigen of *Plasmodium falciparum* recognizes the terminal Neu5Ac(α2-3)Gal- sequences of glycophorin A. J Cell Biol 1992; 116:901.

242. Sim BK, Chitnis CE, et al: Receptor and ligand domains for invasion of erythrocytes by *Plasmodium falciparum*. Science 1994; 264:1941.

243. Lowe RF, Moores PP: Red cell factor in Africans of Rhodesia, Malawi, Mozambique and Natal. Hum Hered 1972; 22:344.

244. Rahuel C, London J, et al: Erythrocyte glycophorin B deficiency may occur by two distinct gene alterations. Am J Hematol 1991; 37:57.

245. Chang S, Reid ME, et al: Molecular characterization of erythrocyte glycophorin-C variants. Blood 1991; 77:644.

246. Anstee DJ, Ridgewell K, et al: Individuals lacking the Gerbich blood-group antigens have alterations in the human erythrocyte membrane sialoglycoproteins β and α. Biochem J 1984; 221:97.

247. High S, Tanner MJA, et al: Rearrangements of the red cell membrane glycophorin C (sialoglycoprotein β) gene: A further study of alterations in the glycophorin C gene. Biochem J 1989; 262:47.

248. Telen MJ, Le Van Kim C, et al: Molecular basis for elliptocytosis associated with glycophorin C and glycophorin D deficiency in the Leach phenotype. Blood 1991; 78:1603.

249. Anstee DJ, Parsons SF, et al: Two individuals with elliptocytic red cells apparently lack three minor sialoglycoproteins. Biochem J 1984; 218:615.

250. Daniels GL, Shaw M-A, et al: A family demonstrating inheritance of the Leach phenotype, a Gerbich-negative phenotype associated with elliptocytosis. Vox Sang 1986; 50:117.

251. Reid ME, Chasis JA, Mohandas N: Identification of a functional role for human erythrocyte sialoglycoproteins beta and gamma. Blood 1987; 69:1068.

252. Nash GB, Parmar J, Reid ME: Effects of deficiencies of glycophorins C and D on the physical properties of the red cell. Br J Haematol 1990; 76:282.

253. Reid ME, Anstee DJ, et al: Normal membrane function of abnormal β-related erythrocyte sialoglycoproteins. Br J Haematol 1987; 67:467.

254. Discher D, Knowles D, et al: Mechanical linkage between red cell skeleton and plasma membrane is *not* a demonstrated function of protein 4.1. Blood 1993; 82(Suppl 1):309a. Abstract.

255. Marfatia SM, Lue RA, et al: *In vitro* binding studies suggests a membrane-associated complex between erythroid p55, protein 4.1, and glycophorin C. J Biol Chem 1994; 269:8631.

256. Lux SE, John KM, et al: Cloning and characterization of band 3, the human erythrocyte anion exchange protein (AE1). Proc Natl Acad Sci U S A 1989; 86:9089.

257. Tanner MJ, Martin PG, et al: The complete amino acid sequence of the human erythrocyte membrane anion-transport protein deduced from the cDNA sequence. Biochem J 1988; 256:703.

258. Bar-Noy S, Cabantchik I: Transport domain of the erythrocyte anion exchange protein. J Membr Biol 1990; 115:217.

259. Bartel D, Hans H, Passow H: Identification by site-directed mutagenesis of Lys-558 as the covalent attachment site of H$_2$DIDS in the mouse erythroid band 3 protein. Biochim Biophys Acta 1989; 985:355.

260. Cabantchik ZI, Rothstein A: Membrane proteins related to anion permeability of human red blood cells: I. Localization of disulfonic stilbene binding sites in proteins involved in permeation. J Membr Biol 1974; 15:207.

261. Ho MK, Guidotti G: A membrane protein from human erythrocytes involved in anion exchange. J Biol Chem 1975; 250:675.

262. Jennings ML: Topography of membrane proteins. Annu Rev Biochem 1989; 58:999.

263. Ortwein R, Oslender-Kohnen A, Deuticke B: Band 3, the anion exchanger of the erythrocyte membrane, is also a flippase. Biochim Biophys Acta 1994; 1191:317.

264. Vondenhof A, Oslender A, et al: Band 3, an accidental flippase for anionic phospholipids? Biochemistry 1994; 33:4517.

265. Gimsa J, Ried C: Do band 3 protein conformational changes mediate shape changes of human erythrocytes? Mol Membr Biol 1995; 12:247.

266. Low PS, Westfall MA, et al: Characterization of the reversible conformational equilibrium of the cytoplasmic domain of erythrocyte membrane band 3. J Biol Chem 1984; 259:13070.

267. Low PS: Structure and function of the cytoplasmic domain of band 3: Center of erythrocyte membrane-peripheral protein interactions. Biochim Biophys Acta 1986; 864:145.

268. Bennett V, Stenbuck PJ: Association between ankyrin and the cytoplasmic domain of band 3 isolated from human erythrocyte membrane. J Biol Chem 1980; 255:6424.

269. Kliman HJ, Steck TL: Association of glyceraldehyde-3-phosphate dehydrogenase with the human red cell membrane. A kinetic analysis. J Biol Chem 1980; 255:6314.

270. Tsai I-H, Prasanna-Murthy SN, Steck TL: Effect of red cell membrane binding on the catalytic activity of glyceraldehyde-3-phosphate dehydrogenase. J Biol Chem 1982; 257:1438.

271. Yu J, Steck TL: Isolation and characterization of band 3, the predominant polypeptide of the human erythrocyte membrane. J Biol Chem 1975; 250:9170.

272. De BK, Kirtley ME: Interaction of phosphoglycerate kinase with human erythrocyte membranes. J Biol Chem 1977; 252:6715.

273. Jenkins JD, Madden DP, Steck TL: Association of phosphofructokinase and aldolase with the membrane of the intact erythrocyte. J Biol Chem 1984; 259:9374.

274. Higashi T, Richards CS, Uyeda K: The interaction of phosphofructokinase with erythrocyte membranes. J Biol Chem 1979; 254:9542.

275. Murthy SNP, Liu T, et al: The aldolase binding site of the human erythrocyte membrane is at the NH$_2$ terminus of band 3. J Biol Chem 1981; 256:11203.

276. Strapazon E, Steck TL: Interaction of the aldolase and the membrane of human erythrocytes. Biochemistry 1977; 16:2966.

277. Low PS, Allen DP, et al: Tyrosine phosphorylation of band 3 inhibits peripheral protein binding. J Biol Chem 1987; 262:4592.

278. Harrison ML, Isaacson CC, et al: Phosphorylation of human erythrocyte band 3 by endogenous p72^{syk}. J Biol Chem 1994; 269:955.

279. Zipser Y, Kosower NS: Phosphotyrosine phosphatase associated with band 3 protein in the human erythrocyte membrane. Biochem J 1996; 314:881.

280. Harrison ML, Rathinavelu P, et al: Role of band 3 tyrosine phosphorylation in the regulation of erythrocyte glycolysis. J Biol Chem 1991; 266:4106.

281. Chétrite G, Cassoly R: Affinity of hemoglobin for the cytoplasmic fragment of human erythrocyte membrane band 3. Equilibrium measurements at physiological pH using matrix-bound proteins: The effects of ionic strength, deoxygenation and of 2,3-diphosphoglycerate. J Mol Biol 1985; 185:639.

282. Walder JA, Chatterjee R, et al: The interaction of hemoglobin with the cytoplasmic domain of band 3 of the human erythrocyte membrane. J Biol Chem 1984; 259:10238.

283. Waugh SM, Low PS: Hemichrome binding to band 3: Nucleation of Heinz bodies on the erythrocyte membrane. Biochemistry 1985; 24:34.

284. Waugh SM, Walder JA, Low PS: Partial characterization of the copolymerization reaction of erythrocyte membrane band 3 with hemichromes. Biochemistry 1987; 26:1777.

285. Kannan R, Labotka R, Low PS: Isolation and characterization of the hemichrome-stabilized membrane protein aggregates from sickle erythrocytes. Major site of autologous antibody binding. J Biol Chem 1988; 263:13766.

286. McPherson RA, Sawyer WH, Tilley L: Rotational diffusion of the erythrocyte integral membrane protein band 3: Effect of hemichrome binding. Biochemistry 1992; 31:512.

287. Bennett V, Stenbuck, PJ: The membrane attachment protein for spectrin is associated with band 3 in human erythrocyte membranes. Nature 1979; 280:468.

288. Davis L, Lux SE, Bennett V: Mapping the ankyrin-binding site of the human erythrocyte anion exchanger. J Biol Chem 1989; 264:9665.

289. Hargreaves WR, Giedd KN, et al: Reassociation of ankyrin with band 3 in erythrocyte membranes and in lipid vesicles. J Biol Chem 1980; 255:11965.

290. Willardson BM, Thevenin BJ-M, et al: Localization of the ankyrin binding site on erythrocyte membrane protein, band 3. J Biol Chem 1989; 264:15893.

291. Thevenin BJ, Low PS: Kinetics and regulation of the ankyrin-band 3 interaction of the human red blood cell membrane. J Biol Chem 1990; 265:16166.

292. Pasternack GR, Anderson RA, et al: Interactions between protein 4.1 and band 3: An alternative binding site for an element of the membrane skeleton. J Biol Chem 1985; 260:3676.

293. Lombardo CR, Willardson BM, Low PS: Localization of the protein 4.1-binding site on the cytoplasmic domain of erythrocyte membrane band 3. J Biol Chem 1992; 267:9540.

294. Korsgren C, Cohen CM: Purification and properties of human erythrocyte band 4.2. Association with the cytoplasmic domain of band 3. J Biol Chem 1986; 261:5536.

295. Korsgren C, Cohen CM: Associations of human erythrocyte protein 4.2. Binding to ankyrin and to the cytoplasmic domain of band 3. J Biol Chem 1988; 263:10212.

296. Rybicki AC, Qiu JJH, Musto S, et al: Human erythrocyte protein 4.2 deficiency associated with hemolytic anemia and a homozygous ^{40}glutamic acid-lysine substitution in the cytoplasmic domain of band 3 (band 3^{Montefiore}). Blood 1993; 81:2155.

297. Thevenin BJ, Willardson BM, Low PS: The redox state of cysteines 201 and 317 of the erythrocyte anion exchanger is critical for ankyrin binding. J Biol Chem 1989; 264:15886.

298. Jöns T, Drenckhahn D: Identification of the binding interface involved in linkage of cytoskeletal protein 4.1 to the erythrocyte anion exchanger. EMBO J 1992; 11:2863.

299. Jarolim P, Palek J, et al: Band 3 Tuscaloosa: Pro^{327}-Arg^{327} substitution in the cytoplasmic domain of erythrocyte band 3 protein associated with spherocytic hemolytic anemia and partial deficiency of protein 4.2. Blood 1992; 80:523.

300. Wieth JO, Andersen OS, et al: Chloride-bicarbonate exchange in red blood cells: Physiology of transport and chemical modification of the binding sites. Phil Trans R Soc Lond [Biol] 1982; 299:383.

301. Cabantchik ZI: The anion transport system of red blood cell membranes. In Harris JR (ed): Blood Cell Biochemistry. Vol. I. New York, Plenum Press, 1990, p 337.

302. Reithmeier RAF: The erythrocyte anion transporter (band 3). Curr Opin Struct Biol 1993; 3:515.

303. Wang DN, Kühlbrandt W, et al: Two-dimensional structure of the membrane domain of human band 3, the anion transport protein of the erythrocyte membrane. EMBO J 1993; 12:2233.

304. Jennings ML: Topical review: Oligomeric structure and the anion transport function of human erythrocyte band 3 protein. J Membr Biol 1984; 80:105.

305. Lindenthal S, Schubert D: Monomeric erythrocyte band 3 protein transports anions. Proc Natl Acad Sci U S A 1991; 88:6540.

306. Salhany JM, Sloan RL, Cordes KA: In situ cross-linking of human erythrocyte band 3 by bis(sulfosuccinimidyl)suberate: Evidence for ligand modulation of two alternate quaternary forms: Covalent band 3 dimers and noncovalent tetramers formed by the association of two covalent dimers. J Biol Chem 1990; 265:17688.

307. Salhany JM, Sloan RL, Cordes KA: Evidence for the development of an intermonomeric asymmetry in the covalent binding of 4,4'-diisothiocyanato-2,2'-disulphonate to human erythrocyte band 3. Biochemistry 1991; 30:4097.

308. Falke JJ, Pace RJ, Chan SI: Direct observation of the transmembrane recruitment of band 3 transport sites by competitive inhibitors: A ^{35}Cl NMR study. J Biol Chem 1984; 259:6481.

309. Gunn RB, Fröhlich O: Asymmetry in the mechanism for anion exchange in human red blood cell membranes: Evidence for reciprocating sites that react with one transported anion at a time. J Gen Physiol 1979; 74:351.

310. Canfield VA, Macey RI: Anion exchange in human erythrocytes has a large activation volume. Biochim Biophys Acta 1984; 778:379.

311. Dalmark M, Wieth JO: Temperature dependence of chloride, bromide, iodide, thiocyanate and salicylate transport in human red cells. J Physiol 1972; 224:583.

312. Sekler I, Lo RS, Kopito RR: A conserved glutamate is responsible for ion selectivity and pH dependence of mammalian anion exchangers AE1 and AE2. J Biol Chem 1995; 270:28751.

313. Jennings ML: Rapid electrogenic sulfate-chloride exchange mediated by chemically modified band 3 in human erythrocytes. J Gen Physiol 1995; 105:21.

314. Muller-Berger S, Karbach D, et al: Inhibition of mouse erythroid band 3-mediated chloride transport by site-directed mutagenesis of histidine residues and its reversal by second site mutation of Lys 558, the locus of covalent H$_2$DIDS binding. Biochemistry 1995; 34:9315.

315. Muller-Berger S, Karbach D, et al: Roles of histidine 752 and glutamate 699 in the pH dependence of mouse band 3 protein-mediated anion transport. Biochemistry 1995; 34:9352.

316. Bohm R, Zaki L: Towards the localization of the essential arginine residues in the band 3 protein of human red blood cell membranes. Biochim Biophys Acta 1996; 1280:238.

317. Ranney HM, Rosenberg GH, et al: Frequencies of band 3 variants of human red cell membranes in some different populations. Br J Haematol 1990; 76:262.

318. Bruce LJ, Anstee DM, et al: Band 3 Memphis variant II. Altered stilbene disulfonate binding and the Diego (Dia) blood group antigen are associated with the human erythrocyte band 3 mutation Pro^{854}→Leu. J Biol Chem 1994; 269:16155.

319. Mulzer K, Kampmann L, et al: Complex associations between membrane proteins analyzed by analytical ultracentrifugation: Studies on the erythrocyte membrane proteins band 3 and ankyrin. Colloid Polym Sci 1990; 268:60.

320. Casey JR, Reithmeier RAF: Analysis of the oligomeric state of band 3, the anion transport protein of the human erythrocyte membrane, by size exclusion high performance liquid chromatography. J Biol Chem 1991; 266:15726.

321. Bruce LJ, Groves JD, et al: Altered band 3 structure and function in glycophorin A- and B-deficient (M^{k}M^k) red blood cells. Blood 1994; 84:916.

322. Chishti AH: Personal communication, 1996.

323. Edwards HH, Mueller TJ, Morrison M: Distribution of transmembrane polypeptides in freeze fracture. Science 1979; 203:1343.

324. Pinto da Silva P, Torrisi MR: Freeze-fracture cytochemistry: Partition of glycophorin in freeze-fractured human erythrocyte membranes. J Cell Biol 1982; 93:463.

325. Bruce LJ, Kay MM, et al: Band 3 HT, a human red-cell variant associated with acanthocytosis and increased anion transport, carries the mutation Pro[868]→Leu in the membrane domain of band 3. Biochem J 1993; 293:317.

326. Kay MM, Bosman GM, et al: Functional topography of band 3: Specific structural alteration linked to functional aberrations in human erythrocytes. Proc Natl Acad Sci U S A 1988; 85:492.

327. Kay MM: Band 3 in aging and neurological disease. Ann NY Acad Sci 1991; 621:179.

328. Kay MM, Marchalonis JJ, et al: Human erythrocyte aging: Cellular and molecular biology. Transfusion Med Rev 1991; 5:173.

329. Alper SL, Kopito RR, et al: Cloning and characterization of a murine band 3-related cDNA from kidney and from a lymphoid cell line. J Biol Chem 1988; 263:17092.

330. Demuth DR, Showe LC, et al: Cloning and structural characterization of a human non-erythroid band 3-like protein. EMBO J 1986; 5:1205.

331. Kopito RR, Lee BS, et al: Regulation of intracellular pH by a neuronal homologue of the erythrocyte anion exchanger. Cell 1989; 59:927.

332. Brosius FC III, Alper SL, et al: The major kidney band 3 transcript predicts an aminoterminal truncated band 3 polypeptide. J Biol Chem 1989; 264:7784.

333. Kudrycki KE, Schull GE: Primary structure of the rat kidney band 3 anion exchange protein deduced from a cDNA. J Biol Chem 1989; 264:8185.

334. Kudrycki KE, Newman PR, Schull GE: cDNA cloning and tissue distribution of mRNAs for two proteins that are related to the band 3 chloride-bicarbonate exchanger. J Biol Chem 1990; 265:462.

335. Drenckhahn D, Schluter K, et al: Colocalization of band 3 with ankyrin and spectrin at the basal membrane of intercalated cells in the rat kidney. Science 1985; 230:1287.

336. Alper SL, Natale J, et al: Subtypes of intercalated cells in rat kidney collecting duct defined by antibodies against erythroid band 3 and renal vacuolar H[+]-ATPase. Proc Natl Acad Sci U S A 1989; 86:5429.

337. Puceat M, Korichneva I, et al: Identification of band 3-like proteins and Cl[−]/HCO$_3^-$ exchange in isolated cardiomyocytes. J Biol Chem 1995; 270:1315.

338. Ding Y, Casey JR, Kopito RR: The major kidney AE1 isoform does not bind ankyrin (Ank1) *in vitro*. An essential role for the 79 NH$_2$-terminal amino acid residues of band 3. J Biol Chem 1994; 269:32201.

339. Wang CC, Moriyama R, et al: Partial characterization of the cytoplasmic domain of human kidney band 3. J Biol Chem 1995; 270:17892.

340. Sheetz MP: Integral membrane protein interaction with Triton cytoskeletons of erythrocytes. Biochim Biophys Acta 1979; 557:122.

341. Yu J, Fischman DA, Steck TL: Selective solubilization of proteins and phospholipids of red blood cell membranes by nonionic detergents. J Supramol Struct 1973; 1:233.

342. Sahr KE, Laurila P, et al: The complete cDNA and polypeptide sequences of human erythroid alpha-spectrin. J Biol Chem 1990; 265:4434.

343. Winkelmann JC, Chang J-G, et al: Full length sequence of the cDNA for human erythroid beta-spectrin. J Biol Chem 1990; 265:11827.

344. Speicher DW, Morrow JS, et al: A structural model of human erythrocyte spectrin: Alignment of chemical and functional domains. J Biol Chem 1982; 257:9093.

345. Speicher DW, DeSilva TM, et al: Location of the human red cell spectrin tetramer binding site and detection of a related "closed" hairpin loop dimer using proteolytic footprinting. J Biol Chem 1993; 268:4227.

346. Shotton DM, Burke BE, Branton D: The molecular structure of human erythrocyte spectrin. Biophysical and electron microscopic studies. J Mol Biol 1979; 131:303.

347. Liu S-C, Windisch P, et al: Oligomeric states of spectrin in normal erythrocyte membranes. Biochemical and electron microscopic studies. Cell 1984; 37:587.

348. Vertessy BG, Steck TL: Elasticity of the human red cell membrane skeleton. Effects of temperature and denaturants. Biophys J 1989; 55:255.

349. McGough AM, Josephs R: On the structure of erythrocyte spectrin in partially expanded membrane skeletons. Proc Natl Acad Sci U S A 1990; 87:5208.

350. Yan Y, Winograd E, et al: Crystal structure of the repetitive segments of spectrin. Science 1993; 262:2027.

351. Koch CA, Anderson D, et al: SH2 and SH3 domains: Elements that control interactions of cytoplasmic signaling proteins. Science 1991; 252:668.

352. Noegel A, Witke W, Schleicher M: Calcium-sensitive non-muscle α-actinin contains EF-hand structures and highly conserved regions. FEBS Lett 1987; 221:391.

353. Waites GT, Graham IR, et al: Mutually exclusive splicing of calcium-binding domain exons in chick α-actinin. J Biol Chem 1992; 267:6263.

354. Fishkind DJ, Bonder EM, Begg DA: Isolation and characterization of sea urchin egg spectrin: Calcium modulation of the spectrin-actin interaction. Cell Motil Cytoskeleton 1987; 7:304.

355. Wallis CJ, Wenegieme EF, Babitch JA: Characterization of calcium binding to brain spectrin. J Biol Chem 1992; 267:4333.

356. Trave G, Lacombe PJ, et al: Molecular mechanism of the calcium-induced conformational change in the spectrin EF-hands. EMBO J 1995; 14:4922.

357. Lundberg S, Bjork J, et al: Cloning, expression and characterization of two putative calcium-binding sites in human non-erythroid alpha-spectrin. Eur J Biochem 1995; 230:658.

358. Trave G, Pastore A, et al: The C-terminal domain of alpha-spectrin is structurally related to calmodulin. Eur J Biochem 1995; 227:35.

359. Kennedy SP, Warren SL, et al: Ankyrin binds to the 15th repetitive unit of erythroid and nonerythroid β-spectrin. J Cell Biol 1991; 115:267.

360. Cohen CM, Tyler JM, Branton D: Spectrin-actin associations studied by electron microscopy of shadowed preparations. Cell 1980; 21:875.

361. Becker PS, Schwartz MA, et al: Radiolabel-transfer crosslinking demonstrates that protein 4.1 binds to the N-terminal region of beta spectrin and to actin in binary interactions. Eur J Biol Chem 1990; 193:827.

362. Karinch AM, Zimmer WE, Goodman SR: The identification and sequence of the actin-binding domain of human red blood cell β-spectrin. J Biol Chem 1990; 265:11833.

363. Bresnick AR, Janmey PA, Condeelis J: Evidence that a 27-residue sequence is the actin-binding site of ABP-120. J Biol Chem 1991; 266:12989.

364. Becker PS, Tse WT, et al: β Spectrin Kissimmee: A spectrin variant associated with autosomal dominant hereditary spherocytosis and defective binding to protein 4.1. J Clin Invest 1993; 92:612.

365. Harris HW Jr, Lux SE: Structural characterization of the phosphorylation sites of human erythrocyte spectrin. J Biol Chem 1980; 255:11512.

366. Tao M, Conway R, Cheta S: Purification and characterization of a membrane-bound protein kinase from human erythrocytes. J Biol Chem 1980; 255:2563.

367. Manno S, Takakuwa Y, et al: Modulation of erythrocyte membrane mechanical function by beta-spectrin phosphorylation and dephosphorylation. J Biol Chem 1995; 270:5659.

368. Speicher DW, Morrow JS, et al: Identification of proteolytically resistant domains of human erythrocyte spectrin. Proc Natl Acad Sci U S A 1980; 77:5673.

369. Winograd E, Hume D, Branton D: Phasing the conformational unit of spectrin. Proc Natl Acad Sci U S A 1991; 88:10788.

370. Speicher DW, Marchesi VT: Erythrocyte spectrin is comprised of many homologous triple helical segments. Nature 1984; 311:177.

371. Kotula L, Laury-Kleintop LD, et al: The exon-intron organization of the human erythrocyte α-spectrin gene. Genomics 1991; 9:131.

372. Amin KM, Scarpa AL, et al: The exon-intron organization of the human erythroid beta-spectrin gene. Genomics 1993; 18:118.

373. Morrow JS, Marchesi VT: Self-assembly of spectrin oligomers

in vitro: A basis for a dynamic cytoskeleton. J Cell Biol 1981; 88:463.

374. Ungewickell E, Gratzer W: Self-association of human spectrin: A thermodynamic and kinetic study. Eur J Biochem 1978; 88:379.

375. Shahbakhti F, Gratzer WB: Analysis of the self-association of human red cell spectrin. Biochemistry 1986; 25:5969.

376. Ralston G, Dunbar J, White M: The temperature-dependent dissociation of spectrin. Biochim Biophys Acta 1977; 491:345.

377. Liu S-C, Palek J: Spectrin tetramer-dimer equilibrium and the stability of erythrocyte membrane skeletons. Nature 1980; 285:586.

378. Beaven GH, Jean-Baptiste L, et al: An examination of the soluble oligomeric complexes extracted from the red cell membrane and their relation to the membrane cytoskeleton. Eur J Cell Biol 1985; 36:299.

379. Morris SA, Eber SW, Gratzer WB: Structural basis for the high activation energy of spectrin self-association. FEBS Lett 1989; 244:68.

380. DeSilva TM, Peng K, et al: Analysis of human red cell spectrin tetramer (head-to-head) assembly using complementary univalent peptides. Biochemistry 1992; 31:10872.

381. Speicher DW, Weglarz L, DeSilva TM: Properties of human red cell spectrin heterodimer (side-to-side) assembly and identification of an essential nucleation site. J Biol Chem 1992; 267:14775.

382. Viel A, Branton D: Interchain binding at the tail end of the spectrin *D. melanogaster* molecule. Proc Natl Acad Sci U S A 1994; 91:10839.

383. Ursitti JA, Kotula L, et al: Mapping the human erythrocyte beta-spectrin dimer initiation site using recombinant peptides and correlation of its phasing with the alpha-actinin dimer site. J Biol Chem 1996; 271:6636.

384. Davis LH, Bennett V: Identification of two regions of beta$_G$ spectrin that bind to distinct sites in brain membranes. J Biol Chem 1994; 269:4409.

385. Lombardo CR, Weed SA, et al: βII-spectrin (fodrin) and βIΣ2-spectrin (muscle) contain NH$_2$- and COOH-terminal membrane association domains (MAD1 and MAD2). J Biol Chem 1994; 269:29212.

386. Macias MJ, Musacchio A, et al: Structure of the pleckstrin homology domain from beta-spectrin. Nature 1994; 369:675.

387. Shaw G: The pleckstrin homology domain: An intriguing multifunctional protein module. Bioessays 1996; 18:35.

388. Wang DS, Shaw R, et al: Binding of pleckstrin homology domains to WD40/beta-transducin repeat containing segments of the protein product of the *Lis-1* gene. Biochem Biophys Res Commun 1995; 209:622.

389. Hyvonen M, Macias MJ, et al: Structure of the binding site for inositol phosphates in a PH domain. EMBO J 1995; 14:4676.

390. Wang DS, Shaw G: The association of the C-terminal region of βIΣII spectrin to brain membranes is mediated by a PH domain, does not require membrane proteins, and coincides with an inositol-1,4,5 triphosphate binding site. Biochem Biophys Res Commun 1995; 217:608.

391. Ferguson KM, Lemmon MA, et al: Structure of the high affinity complex of inositol trisphosphate with a phospholipase C pleckstrin homology domain. Cell 1995; 83:1037.

392. Winkelmann JC, Costa FF, et al: Beta spectrin in human skeletal muscle: Tissue-specific differential processing of 3′ beta spectrin pre-mRNA generates a beta spectrin isoform with a unique carboxyl terminus. J Biol Chem 1990; 265:20449.

393. Tyler JM, Reinhardt BN, Branton D: Associations of erythrocyte membrane proteins: Binding of purified bands 2.1 and 4.1 to spectrin. J Biol Chem 1980; 255:7034.

394. Yu J, Goodman SR: Syndeins: The spectrin-binding protein(s) of the human erythrocyte membrane. Proc Natl Acad Sci U S A 1979; 76:2340.

395. Weaver DC, Pasternack GR, Marchesi VT: The structural basis of ankyrin function: II. Identification of two functional domains. J Biol Chem 1984; 259:6170.

396. Weaver DC, Marchesi VT: The structural basis of ankyrin function: I. Identification of two structural domains. J Biol Chem 1984; 259:6165.

397. Wallin R, Culp EN, et al: A structural model of human erythrocyte band 2.1: Alignment of chemical and functional domains. Proc Natl Acad Sci U S A 1984; 81:4095.

398. Davis LH, Bennett V: Mapping the binding sites of human erythrocyte ankyrin for the anion exchanger and spectrin. J Biol Chem 1990; 265:10589.

399. Davis LH, Otto E, Bennett V: Specific 33-residue repeat(s) of erythrocyte ankyrin associate with the anion exchanger. J Biol Chem 1991; 266:11163.

400. Michaely P, Bennett V: The membrane-binding domain of ankyrin contains four independently folded subdomains, each comprised of six ankyrin repeats. J Biol Chem 1993; 268:22703.

401. Platt OS, Lux SE, Falcone JF: A highly conserved region of human erythrocyte ankyrin contains the capacity to bind spectrin. J Biol Chem 1993; 268:24421.

402. Lux SE, John KM, Bennett V: Analysis of cDNA for human erythrocyte ankyrin indicates a repeated structure with homology to tissue-differentiation and cell-cycle control proteins. Nature 1990; 344:36.

403. Lambert S, Yu H, et al: cDNA sequence for human erythrocyte ankyrin. Proc Natl Acad Sci U S A 1990; 87:1730.

404. Low PS, Willardson BM, et al: Contribution of the band 3-ankyrin interaction to erythrocyte membrane mechanical stability. Blood 1991; 77:1581.

405. Michaely P, Bennett V: The ANK repeats of erythrocyte ankyrin form two distinct but cooperative binding sites for the erythrocyte anion exchanger. J Biol Chem 1995; 270:22050.

406. Hargreaves WR, Giedd KN, et al: Reassociation of ankyrin with band 3 in erythrocyte membranes and in lipid vesicles. J Biol Chem 1980; 255:11965.

407. Thevenin BJM, Low PS: Kinetics and regulation of the ankyrin-band 3 interaction of the human red blood cell membrane. J Biol Chem 1990; 265:16166.

408. Mulzer K, Kampmann L, et al: Complex associations between membrane proteins analyzed by analytical ultracentrifugation: Studies on the erythrocyte membrane proteins band 3 and ankyrin. Colloid Polym Sci 1990; 268:60.

409. Jarolim P, Rubin HL, et al: Duplication of 10 nucleotides in the erythroid band 3 (AE1) gene is a kindred with hereditary spherocytosis and band 3 protein deficiency (Band 3^{PRAGUE}). J Clin Invest 1994; 93:121.

410. Low PS, Willardson BM, et al: Contribution of the band 3-ankyrin interaction to erythrocyte membrane mechanical stability. Blood 1991; 77:1581.

411. Bennett V, Davis J: Erythrocyte ankyrin: Immunoreactive analogues are associated with mitotic structures in cultured cells and with microtubules in brain. Proc Natl Acad Sci U S A 1981; 78:7550.

412. Davis JQ, Bennett V: Brain ankyrin. A membrane-associated protein with binding sites for spectrin, tubulin, and the cytoplasmic domain of the erythrocyte anion channel. J Biol Chem 1984; 259:13550.

413. Davis LH, Davis JQ, Bennett V: Ankyrin regulation: An alternatively spliced segment of the regulatory domain functions as an intramolecular modulator. J Biol Chem 1992; 267:18966.

414. Cianci CD, Giorgi M, Morrow JS: Phosphorylation of ankyrin down-regulates its cooperative interaction with spectrin and protein 3. J Cell Biochem 1988; 37:301.

415. Hall TG, Bennett V: Regulatory domains of erythrocyte ankyrin. J Biol Chem 1987; 262:10537.

416. Gallagher PG, Tse WT, et al: Large number of alternatively spliced isoforms of the regulatory region of human erythrocyte ankyrin. Trans Assoc Am Phys 1992; 105:268.

417. Jarolim P, Rubin H, Palek J: Multiple alternate splices are detected in reticulocyte mRNA coding for the regulatory domain of human erythroid ankyrin. Blood 1992; 80(Suppl 1):144a. Abstract.

418. White RA, Birkenmeier CS, et al: Murine erythrocyte ankyrin cDNA: Highly conserved regions of the regulatory domain. Mamm Genome 1992; 3:281.

419. Cleveland JL, Ihle JN: Contenders in FasL/TNF death signaling. Cell 1995; 81:479.

420. Tartaglia LA, Ayres TM, et al: A novel domain within the 55 kd TNF receptor signals cell death. Cell 1993; 74:845.

421. Chinnaiyan AM, O'Rourke K, et al: FADD, a novel death domain-containing protein, interacts with the death domain of Fas and initiates apoptosis. Cell 1995; 81:505.

422. Boldin MP, Varfolomeev EE, et al: A novel protein that interacts with the death domain of Fas/APO1 contains a sequence motif related to the death domain. J Biol Chem 1995; 270:7795.

423. Hsu H, Xiong J, Goeddel DV: The TNF receptor 1-associated protein TRADD signals cell death and NF-κB activation. Cell 1995; 81:495.

424. Stanger BZ, Leder P, et al: RIP: A novel protein containing a death domain that interacts with Fas/APO1 (CD95) in yeast and causes cell death. Cell 1995; 81:513.

425. Kitson J, Raven T, et al: A death domain-containing receptor that mediates apoptosis. Nature 1996; 384:372.

426. Boldin MP, Mett IL, et al: Self-association of the "death domains" of the p55 tumor necrosis factor (TNF) receptor and Fas/APO1 prompts signaling for TNF and Fas/APO1 effects. J Biol Chem 1995; 270:387.

427. Adam D, Wiegmann K, et al: A novel cytoplasmic domain of the p55 tumor necrosis factor receptor initiates the neutral sphingomyelinase pathway. J Biol Chem 1996; 271:14617.

428. Hsu H, Huang J, et al: TNF-dependent recruitment of the protein kinase RIP to the TNF receptor-1 signaling complex. Immunity 1996; 4:387.

429. Hsu H, Shu H-B, et al: TRADD-TRAF2 and TRADD-FADD interactions define two distinct TNF receptor 1 signal transduction pathways. Cell 1996; 84:299.

430. Varfolomeev EE, Boldin MP, et al: A potent mechanism of "cross-talk" between the p55 tumor necrosis factor receptor and Fas/APO1: Proteins binding to the death domains of the two receptors also bind to each other. J Exp Med 1996; 183:1271.

431. Machleidt T, Kramer B, et al: Function of the p55 tumor necrosis factor receptor "death domain" mediated by phosphatidylcholine-specific phospholipase C. J Exp Med 1996; 184:725.

432. Martin SJ, O'Brien GA, et al: Proteolysis of fodrin (non-erythroid spectrin) during apoptosis. J Biol Chem 1995; 270:6425.

433. Cryns VL, Bergeron L, et al: Specific cleavage of α-fodrin during Fas- and tumor necrosis factor-induced apoptosis is mediated by an interleukin-1β-converting enzyme/Ced-3 protease distinct from the poly(ADP-ribose) polymerase protease. J Biol Chem 1996; 271:31277.

434. Lu P-W, Soong C-J, Tao M: Phosphorylation of ankyrin decreases its affinity for spectrin tetramer. J Biol Chem 1985; 260:14958.

435. Soong CJ, Lu PW, Tao M: Analysis of band 3 cytoplasmic domain phosphorylation and association with ankyrin. Arch Biochem Biophys 1987; 254:509.

436. Moon RT, Ngai J, et al: Tissue-specific expression of distinct spectrin and ankyrin transcripts in erythroid and nonerythroid cells. J Cell Biol 1985; 100:152.

437. Nelson WJ, Lazarides E: Goblin (ankyrin) in striated muscle: Identification of the potential membrane receptor for erythroid spectrin in muscle cells. Proc Natl Acad Sci U S A 1984; 81:3292.

438. Peters LL, Birkenmeier CS, et al: Purkinje cell degeneration associated with erythroid ankyrin deficiency in *nb/nb* mice. J Cell Biol 1991; 114:1233.

439. Kordeli E, Bennett V: Distinct ankyrin isoforms at neuron cell bodies and nodes of Ranvier resolved using erythrocyte ankyrin-deficient mice. J Cell Biol 1991; 114:1243.

440. Otto E, Kunimoto M, et al: Isolation and characterization of cDNAs encoding human brain ankyrins reveal a family of alternatively spliced genes. J Cell Biol 1991; 114:241.

441. Chan W, Kordeli E, Bennett V: 440-kD ankyrin_B: Structure of the major developmentally regulated domain and selective localization in unmyelinated axons. J Cell Biol 1993; 123:1463.

442. Kunimoto M, Otto E, Bennett V: A new 440-kD isoform is the major ankyrin in neonatal rat brain. J Cell Biol 1991; 115:1319.

443. Kordeli E, Lambert S, Bennett V: Ankyrin_G: A new ankyrin gene with neural-specific isoforms localized at the axonal initial segment and node of Ranvier. J Biol Chem 1995; 270:2352.

444. Peters LL, John KM, et al: Ank3 (epithelial ankyrin), a widely distributed new member of the ankyrin gene family and the major ankyrin in kidney, is expressed in alternatively spliced forms, including forms that lack the repeat domain. J Cell Biol 1995; 130:313.

445. Devarajan P, Stabach PR, et al: Identification of a small cyto-plasmic ankyrin (Ank_G119) in kidney and muscle that binds βIε spectrin and associated with the Golgi apparatus. J Cell Biol 1996; 133:819.

446. Leto TL, Marchesi VT: A structural model of human erythrocyte protein 4.1. J Biol Chem 1984; 259:4603.

447. Inaba M, Gupta KC, et al: Deamidation of human erythrocyte membrane protein 4.1: Possible role in aging. Blood 1992; 79:3355.

448. Mueller TJ, Jackson CW, et al: Membrane skeletal alterations during *in vivo* mouse red cell aging: Increase in the band 4.1a:4.1b ratio. J Clin Invest 1987; 79:492.

449. Coleman TR, Harris AS, et al: Beta spectrin bestows protein 4.1 sensitivity on spectrin-actin interactions. J Cell Biol 1987; 104:519.

450. Ungewickell E, Bennett PM, et al: *In vitro* formation of a complex between cytoskeletal proteins of the human erythrocyte. Nature 1979; 280:811.

451. Cohen CM, Foley SF: The role of band 4.1 in the association of actin with erythrocyte membranes. Biochim Biophys Acta 1982; 688:691.

452. Ohanian V, Wolfe LC, et al: Analysis of the ternary interaction of the red cell membrane skeletal proteins spectrin, actin, and 4.1. Biochemistry 1984; 23:4416.

453. Correas I, Leto TL, et al: Identification of the functional site of erythrocyte protein 4.1 involved in spectrin-actin associations. J Biol Chem 1986; 261:3310.

454. Correas I, Speicher DW, Marchesi VT: Structure of the spectrin-actin binding site of erythrocyte protein 4.1. J Biol Chem 1986; 261:13362.

455. Conboy JG, Shitamoto R, et al: Hereditary elliptocytosis due to both qualitative and quantitative defects in membrane skeletal protein 4.1. Blood 1991; 78:2438.

456. Discher D, Parra M, et al: Mechanochemistry of the alternatively spliced spectrin-actin binding domain in membrane skeletal protein 4.1. J Biol Chem 1993; 268:7186.

457. Discher DE, Winardi R, et al: Mechanochemistry of protein 4.1's spectrin-actin-binding domain: Ternary complex interactions, membrane binding, network integration, structural strengthening. J Cell Biol 1995; 130:897.

458. Schischmanoff P, Winardi R, et al: Defining the minimal domain of protein 4.1 involved in spectrin-actin binding. J Biol Chem 1995; 270:21243.

459. Morris MB, Lux SE: Characterization of the binary interaction between human erythrocyte protein 4.1 and actin. Eur J Biochem 1995; 231:644.

460. Horne WC, Prinz WC, Tang EK-Y: Identification of two cAMP-dependent phosphorylation sites on erythrocyte protein 4.1. Biochim Biophys Acta 1990; 1055:87.

461. Ling E, Danilov YN, Cohen CM: Modulation of red cell band 4.1 function by cAMP-dependent kinase and protein kinase C phosphorylation. J Biol Chem 1988; 263:2209.

462. Subrahmanyam G, Bertics PJ, Anderson RA: Phosphorylation of protein 4.1 on tyrosine-418 modulates its function *in vitro*. Proc Natl Acad Sci U S A 1991; 88:5222.

463. Anderson JP, Morrow JS: The interaction of calmodulin with erythrocyte spectrin. Inhibition of protein 4.1-stimulated actin binding. J Biol Chem 1987; 262:6365

464. Takakuwa Y, Mohandas N: Modulation of erythrocyte membrane material properties by Ca^{2+} and calmodulin. Implications for their role in regulation of skeletal protein interactions. J Clin Invest 1988; 78:80.

465. Tanaka T, Kadowaki K, et al: Ca^{2+}-dependent regulation of the spectrin/actin interaction by calmodulin and protein 4.1. J Biol Chem 1991; 266:1134.

466. Hemming NJ, Anstee DJ, et al: Identification of the membrane attachment sites for protein 4.1 in the human erythrocyte. J Biol Chem 1995; 270:5360.

467. Marfatia SM, Leu RA, et al: Identification of the protein 4.1 binding interface on glycophorin C and p55, a homologue of the *Drosophila* discs-large tumor suppressor protein. J Biol Chem 1995; 270:715.

468. Lombardo CR, Low PS: Calmodulin modulates protein 4.1 binding to human erythrocyte membranes. Biochim Biophys Acta 1994; 1196:139.

469. Danilov YN, Fennell R, et al: Selective modulation of band 4.1

binding to erythrocyte membranes by protein kinase C. J Biol Chem 1990; 265:2556.

470. Anderson RA, Marchesi VT: Regulation of the association of membrane skeletal protein 4.1 with glycophorin by polyphosphoinositide. Nature 1985; 318:295.

471. Mueller T, Manson M: Glycoconnectin (PAS2) a membrane attachment site for the human erythrocyte cytoskeleton. In Kruckeberg W, Eaton J, Greuner G (eds): Erythrocyte Membranes 2: Recent Clinical and Experimental Advances. New York, Alan R. Liss, Inc., 1981, p 95.

472. Reid ME, Takakuwa Y, et al: Glycophorin C content of human erythrocyte membrane is regulated by protein 4.1. Blood 1990; 75:2229.

473. Sondag D, Alloisio N, et al: Gerbich reactivity in 4.1 (−) hereditary elliptocytosis and protein 4.1 level in blood group Gerbich deficiency. Br J Haematol 1987; 65:43.

474. Marfatia SM, Lue RA, et al: In vitro binding studies suggests a membrane-associated complex between erythroid p55, protein 4.1, and glycophorin C. J Biol Chem 1994; 269:8631.

475. Alloisio N, Dalla Venezia N, et al: Evidence that red blood cell protein p55 may participate in the skeleton-membrane linkage that involves protein 4.1 and glycophorin C. Blood 1993; 82:1323.

476. Lue RA, Marfatia SM, et al: Cloning and characterization of hdlg: The human homologue of the Drosophila discs large tumor suppressor binds to protein 4.1. Proc Natl Acad Sci U S A 1994; 91:9818.

477. Pasternack GR, Racusen RH: Erythrocyte protein 4.1 binds and regulates myosin. Proc Natl Acad Sci U S A 1989; 86:9712.

478. Correas I, Avila J: Erythrocyte protein 4.1 associates with tubulin. Biochem J 1988; 255:217.

479. Rybicki AC, Heath R, et al: Human erythrocyte protein 4.1 is a phosphatidylserine binding protein. J Clin Invest 1988; 81:255.

480. Sato SB, Ohnishi S: Interaction of a peripheral protein of the erythrocyte membrane, band 4.1, with phosphatidylserine-containing liposomes and erythrocyte inside-out vesicles. Eur J Biochem 1983; 130:19.

481. Holt GD, Haltiwanger RS, et al: Erythrocytes contain cytoplasmic glycoproteins. O-linked GlcNAc on band 4.1. J Biol Chem 1987; 262:14847.

482. Huang J-P, Tang C-JC, et al: Genomic structure of the locus encoding protein 4.1. Structural basis for complex combinational patterns of tissue-specific alternative RNA splicing. J Biol Chem 1993; 268:3758.

483. Conboy JG, Chan J, et al: Multiple protein 4.1 isoforms produced by alternative splicing in human erythroid cells. Proc Natl Acad Sci U S A 1988; 85:9062.

484. Conboy JG, Chan JY, et al: Tissue- and development-specific alternative RNA splicing regulates expression of multiple isoforms of erythroid membrane protein 4.1. J Biol Chem 1991; 266:8273.

485. Tang TK, Qin Z, et al: Heterogeneity of mRNA and protein products arising from the protein 4.1 gene in erythroid and non-erythroid tissues. J Cell Biol 1990; 110:617.

486. Chasis JA, Coulombel L, et al: Differentiation-associated switches in protein 4.1 expression: Synthesis of multiple structural isoforms during normal human erythropoiesis. J Clin Invest 1993; 91:329.

487. Winardi R, Discher D, et al: Evolutionarily conserved alternative pre-mRNA splicing regulates structure and function of the spectrin-actin binding domain of erythroid protein 4.1. Blood 1995; 86:4315.

488. De Carcer G, Lallena MJ, Correas I: Protein 4.1 is a component of the nuclear matrix of mammalian cells. Biochem J 1995; 312:871.

489. Cohen CM, Foley SF, Korsgren C: A protein immunologically related to erythrocyte band 4.1 is found on stress fibers of nonerythroid cells. Nature 1982; 299:648.

490. Yawata Y: Red cell membrane protein band 4.2: Phenotypic, genetic and electron microscopic aspects. Biochim Biophys Acta 1994; 1204:131.

491. Lux SE, Tse WT, et al: Hereditary spherocytosis associated with deletion of the human erythrocyte ankyrin gene on chromosome 8. Nature 1990; 345:736.

492. Rybicki AC, Musto S, Schwartz RS: Decreased content of pro-

tein 4.2 in ankyrin-deficient normoblastosis (nb/nb) mouse red blood cells: Evidence for ankyrin enhancement of protein 4.2 membrane binding. Blood 1995; 86:3583.

493. Rybicki AC, Heath R, et al: Deficiency of protein 4.2 in erythrocytes from a patient with a Coombs negative hemolytic anemia: Evidence for a role of protein 4.2 in stabilizing ankyrin on the membrane. J Clin Invest 1988; 81:893.

494. Inoue T, Kanzaki A, et al: Electron microscopic and physico-chemical studies on disorganization of the cytoskeletal network and integral protein (band 3) in red cells of band 4.2 deficiency with a mutation (codon 142:GCT→ACT). Int J Hematol 1994; 59:157.

495. Risinger M, Dotimas E, Cohen CM: Human erythrocyte protein 4.2, a high copy number membrane protein, is N-myristylated. J Biol Chem 1992; 267:5680.

496. Das AK, Bhattacharya R, et al: Human erythrocyte membrane protein 4.2 is palmitoylated. Eur J Biochem 1994; 224:575.

497. Azim AC, Marfatia SM, et al: Human erythrocyte dematin and protein 4.2 (pallidin) are ATP binding proteins. Biochemistry 1996; 35:3001.

498. Korsgren C, Lawler J, et al: Complete amino acid sequence and homologies of human erythrocyte membrane protein band 4.2. Proc Natl Acad Sci U S A 1990; 87:613.

499. Sung LA, Chien S, et al: Molecular cloning of human protein 4.2: A major component of the erythrocyte membrane. Proc Natl Acad Sci U S A 1990; 87:955.

500. Korsgren C, Cohen CM: Organization of the gene for human erythrocyte membrane protein 4.2: Structural similarities with the gene for the a subunit of factor XIII. Proc Natl Acad Sci U S A 1991; 88:4840.

501. Bouhassira EE, Schwartz RS, et al: An alanine to threonine substitution in protein 4.2 cDNA is associated with a Japanese form of hereditary hemolytic anemia (protein 4.2^Nippon). Blood 1992; 79:1846.

502. White RA, Peters LL, et al: The murine pallid mutation is a platelet storage pool disease associated with the protein 4.2 (pallidin) gene. Nat Genet 1992; 2:80.

503. Bryant PJ, Woods DF: A major palmitoylated membrane protein of human erythrocytes shows homology to yeast guanylate kinase and to the product of a Drosophila tumor suppressor gene. Cell 1992; 68:621. Letter.

504. Ruff P, Speicher DW, Husain-Chishti A: Molecular identification of a major palmitoylated erythrocyte membrane protein containing the src homology 3 motif. Proc Natl Acad Sci U S A 1991; 88:6595.

505. Metzenberg AB, Gitschier J: The gene encoding the palmitoylated erythrocyte membrane protein, p55, originates at the CpG island 3′ to the factor VIII gene. Hum Mol Genet 1992; 1:97.

506. Tilney LG, Detmers P: Actin in erythrocyte ghosts in its association with spectrin: Evidence for a nonfilamentous form of these two molecules in situ. J Cell Biol 1975; 66:508.

507. Pinder JC, Sleep JA, et al: Concentrated Tris solutions for the preparation, depolymerization, and assay of actin: application to erythroid actin. Anal Biochem 1995; 225:291.

508. Pinder JC, Gratzer WB: Structural and dynamic states of actin in the erythrocyte. J Cell Biol 1983; 96:768.

509. Byers T, Branton D: Visualization of the protein associations in the erythrocyte membrane skeleton. Proc Natl Acad Sci U S A 1985; 82:6153.

510. Liu S-C, Derick LH, Palek J: Visualization of the hexagonal lattice in the erythrocyte membrane skeleton. J Cell Biol 1987; 104:527.

511. Fowler VM, Sussmann MA, et al: Tropomodulin is associated with the free (pointed) ends of the thin filaments in rat skeletal muscle. J Cell Biol 1993; 120:411.

512. Nakashima K, Beutler E: Comparison of structure and function of human erythrocyte and human muscle actin. Proc Natl Acad Sci U S A 1979; 76:935.

513. Ohanian V, Wolfe LC, et al: Analysis of the ternary interaction of the red cell membrane skeletal proteins spectrin, actin, and 4.1. Biochemistry 1984; 23:4416.

514. Gardner K, Bennett V: Modulation of spectrin-actin assembly by erythrocyte adducin. Nature 1987; 328:359.

515. Joshi R, Gilligan DM, et al: Primary structure and domain

organization of human alpha and beta adducin. J Cell Biol 1991; 115:665.

516. Dong L, Chapline C, et al: 35H, a sequence isolated as a protein kinase C binding protein, is a novel member of the adducin family. J Biol Chem 1995; 270:25534.

517. Hughes CA, Bennett V: Adducin: A physical model with implications for function in assembly of spectrin-actin complexes. J Biol Chem 1995; 270:18990.

518. Lin B, Nasir J, et al: Genomic organization of the human alpha-adducin gene and its alternately spliced isoforms. Genomics 1995; 25:93.

519. Tisminetzky S, Devescovi G, et al: Genomic organization and chromosomal localization of the gene encoding human beta adducin. Gene 1995; 167:313.

520. Sinard JH, Stewart GW, et al: A novel isoform of beta adducin utilizes an alternatively spliced exon near the C-terminus. Mol Biol Cell 1995; 6:269a. Abstract.

521. Nehls V, Drenckhahn D, et al: Adducin in erythrocyte precursor cells of rats and humans: Expression and compartmentalization. Blood 1991; 78:1692.

522. Kuhlman PA, Hughes CA, et al: A new function for adducin. Calcium/calmodulin-regulated capping of the barbed ends of actin filaments. J Biol Chem 1996; 271:7986.

523. Kaiser HW, O'Keefe E, Bennett V: Adducin: Ca^{++}-dependent association with sites of cell-cell contact. J Cell Biol 1989; 109:557.

524. Ling E, Gardner K, Bennett V: Protein kinase C phosphorylates a recently identified membrane skeleton-associated calmodulin-binding protein in human erythrocytes. J Biol Chem 1986; 261:13875.

525. Bianchi G, Tripodi G, et al: Two point mutations within the adducin genes are involved in blood pressure variation. Proc Natl Acad Sci U S A 1994; 91:3999.

526. Casari G, Barlassina C, et al: Association of the alpha-adducin locus with essential hypertension. Hypertension 1995; 25:320.

527. Husain-Chishti A, Levin A, Branton D: Abolition of actin-bundling by phosphorylation of human erythrocyte protein 4.9. Nature 1988; 334:718.

528. Husain-Chishti A, Faquin W, et al: Purification of erythrocyte dematin (protein 4.9) reveals an endogenous protein kinase that modulates actin-bundling activity. J Biol Chem 1989; 264:8985.

529. Siegel DL, Branton D: Partial purification and characterization of an actin-binding protein, band 4.9, from human erythrocytes. J Cell Biol 1985; 100:775.

530. Azim AC, Knoll JH, et al: Isoform cloning, actin binding, and chromosomal localization of human erythroid dematin, a member of the villin superfamily. J Biol Chem 1995; 270:17407.

531. Rana AP, Ruff P, et al: Cloning of human erythroid dematin reveals another member of the villin family. Proc Natl Acad Sci U S A 1993; 90:6651.

532. Fowler VM, Bennett V: Erythrocyte membrane tropomyosin: Purification and properties. J Biol Chem 1984; 259:5978.

533. Mak AS, Roseborough G, Baker H: Tropomyosin from human erythrocyte membrane polymerizes poorly but binds F-actin effectively in the presence and absence of spectrin. Biochim Biophys Acta 1987; 912:157.

534. Fowler VM: Identification and purification of a novel M_r 43,000 tropomyosin-binding protein from human erythrocyte membranes. J Biol Chem 1987; 262:12792.

535. Fowler VM: Tropomodulin: A cytoskeletal protein that binds to the end of erythrocyte tropomyosin and inhibits tropomyosin binding to actin. J Cell Biol 1990; 111:471.

536. Babcock GG, Fowler VM: Isoform-specific interaction of tropomodulin with skeletal muscle and erythrocyte tropomyosins. J Biol Chem 1994; 269:27510.

537. Sung LA, Lin JJ: Erythrocyte tropomodulin binds to the N-terminus of hTM5, a tropomyosin isoform encoded by the gamma-tropomyosin gene. Biochem Biophys Res Commun 1994; 201:627.

538. Ursitti JA, Fowler VM: Immunolocalization of tropomodulin, tropomyosin and actin in spread human erythrocyte skeletons. J Cell Sci 1994; 107:1633.

539. Gregorio CC, Fowler VM: Mechanisms of thin filament assembly in embryonic chick cardiac myocytes: Tropomodulin requires tropomyosin for assembly. J Cell Biol 1995; 129:683.

540. Gregorio CC, Weber A, et al: Requirement of pointed-end capping by tropomodulin to maintain actin filament length in embryonic chick cardiac myocytes. Nature 1995; 376:83.

541. Weber A, Pennise CR, et al: Tropomodulin caps the pointed ends of actin filaments. J Cell Biol 1994; 127:1627.

542. Fowler VM, Davis JP, Bennett V: Human erythrocyte myosin. Identification and purification. J Cell Biol 1985; 100:47.

543. Wong AJ, Kiehart DP, Pollard TD: Myosin from human erythrocytes. J Biol Chem 1984; 260:46.

544. Colin FC, Schrier SL: Myosin content and distribution in human neonatal erythrocytes are different from adult erythrocytes. Blood 1991; 78:3052.

545. der Terrossian E, Deprette C, et al: Purification and characterization of erythrocyte caldesmon. Hypothesis for an actin-linked regulation of a contractile activity in the red blood cell membrane. Eur J Biochem 1994; 219:503.

546. Rand RP, Burton AC: Area and volume changes in hemolysis of single erythrocytes. J Cell Comp Physiol 1963; 61:245.

547. Bull BS, Kuhn IN: The production of schistocytes by fibrin strands (a scanning electron microscope study). Blood 1970; 35:104.

548. Liu S-C, Derick LH, et al: Alteration of the erythrocyte membrane skeletal ultrastructure in hereditary spherocytosis, hereditary elliptocytosis, and pyropoikilocytosis. Blood 1990; 76:198.

549. Liu S-C, Derick LH, et al: Separation of the lipid bilayer from the membrane skeleton during discocyte-echinocyte transformation of human erythrocyte ghosts. Eur J Cell Biol 1989; 49:358.

550. Wagner GM, Chiu DT-Y, et al: Spectrin oxidation correlates with membrane vesiculation in stored RBC's. Blood 1987; 69:1777.

551. Wolfe LC: The membrane and the lesions of storage in preserved red cells. Transfusion 1985; 25:185.

552. Lutz HU, Liu S-C, Palek J: Release of spectrin-free vesicles from human erythrocytes during ATP depletion. Characterization of spectrin-free vesicles. J Cell Biol 1977; 73:548.

553. Elgsaeter A, Shotton DM, Branton D: Intramembrane particle aggregation in erythrocyte ghosts: II. The influence of spectrin aggregation. Biochim Biophys Acta 1976; 426:101.

554. Lux SE, John KM, Karnovsky MJ: Irreversible deformation of the spectrin-actin lattice in irreversibly sickled cells. J Clin Invest 1976; 58:955.

555. Tomaselli MB, John KM, Lux SE: Elliptical erythrocyte membrane skeletons and heat-sensitive spectrin in hereditary elliptocytosis. Proc Natl Acad Sci U S A 1981; 78:1911.

556. Lorand L, Siefring GE Jr, Lowe-Krentz L: Enzymatic basis of membrane stiffening in human erythrocytes. Semin Hematol 1979; 16:65.

557. Haest CWM, Fischer TM, et al: Stabilization of erythrocyte shape by a chemical increase in membrane shear stiffness. Blood Cells 1980; 6:539.

558. Hebbel RP: Beyond hemoglobin polymerization: The red blood cell membrane and sickle cell disease pathophysiology. Blood 1991; 77:214.

559. Patel VP, Lodish HF: A fibronectin matrix is required for differentiation of murine erythroleukemia cells into reticulocytes. J Cell Biol 1987; 105:3105.

560. Swerlick RA, Eckman JR, et al: $\alpha_4\beta_1$ integrin expression on sickle reticulocytes: Vascular cell adhesion molecule 1-dependent binding to endothelium. Blood 1993; 82:1891.

561. Patel VP, Lodish HF: The fibronectin receptor on mammalian erythroid precursor cells: Characterization and developmental regulation. J Cell Biol 1986; 102:449.

562. Pasvol G, Carlsson J, Clough B: The red cell membrane and invasion by malarial parasites. Bailliéres Clin Haematol 1993; 6:513.

563. Test ST, Butikofer P, et al: Characterization of the complement sensitivity of calcium-loaded human erythrocytes. Blood 1991; 78:3056.

564. Victoria EJ, Muchmore EA, et al: The role of antigen mobility in anti-Rh(D)-induced agglutination. J Clin Invest 1975; 56:292.

565. McCaughan L, Krimm S: X-ray and neutron scattering density profiles of the intact human red blood cell membrane. Science 1980; 207:1481.

566. Tsukita S, Tsukita S, Ishikawa H: Cytoskeletal network underlying the human erythrocyte membrane. Thin-section electron microscopy. J Cell Biol 1980; 85:567.

567. Cohen CM, Gascard P: Regulation and post-translational modification of the erythrocyte membrane and membrane-skeletal proteins. Semin Hematol 1992; 29:244.

568. Eder PS, Soong CJ, Tao M: Phosphorylation reduces the affinity of protein 4.1 for spectrin. Biochemistry 1986; 25:1764.

569. Chao T-S, Tao M: Modulation of protein 4.1 binding to inside-out membrane vesicles by phosphorylation. Biochemistry 1991; 30:10529.

570. Harrison ML, Rathinavelu P, et al: Role of band 3 tyrosine phosphorylation in the regulation of erythrocyte glycolysis. J Biol Chem 1991; 266:4106.

571. Anderson JM, Tyler JM: State of spectrin phosphorylation does not affect erythrocyte shape or spectrin binding to erythrocyte membranes. J Biol Chem 1980; 255:1259.

572. Harris HW Jr, Levin N, Lux SE: Comparison of the phosphorylation of human erythrocyte spectrin in the intact red cell and in various cell-free systems. J Biol Chem 1980; 255:11521.

573. Mentzer WC Jr, Iarocci TA, et al: Modulation of erythrocyte membrane mechanical fragility by 2,3-diphosphoglycerate in the neonatal poikilocytosis/elliptocytosis syndrome. J Clin Invest 1987; 79:943.

574. Schindler M, Koppel D, Sheetz MP: Modulation of membrane protein lateral mobility by polyphosphates and polyamines. Proc Natl Acad Sci U S A 1980; 77:1457.

575. Wolfe LC, Lux SE, Ohanian V: Spectrin-actin binding in vitro; effect of protein 4.1 and polyphosphates. J Supramol Struct Cell Biochem 1981; 5 (Suppl 5):123. Abstract.

576. Suzuki Y, Nakajima T, et al: Influence of 2,3-diphosphoglycerate on the deformability of human erythrocytes. Biochim Biophys Acta 1990; 1029:85.

577. Waugh RE: Effects of 2,3-diphosphoglycerate on the mechanical properties of erythrocyte membrane. Blood 1986; 68:231.

578. Gardner K, Bennett V: A new erythrocyte membrane-associated protein with calmodulin binding activity. Identification and purification. J Biol Chem 1986; 261:1339.

579. Palek J, Liu PA, Liu SC: Polymerization of red cell membrane protein contributes to spheroechinocyte shape irreversibility. Nature 1978; 274:505.

580. Flynn TP, Allen DW, et al: Oxidant damage of the lipids and proteins of the erythrocyte membranes in unstable hemoglobin disease. Evidence for the role of lipid peroxidation. J Clin Invest 1983; 71:1215.

581. Chin JJ, Jung EKY, Yung CY: Structural basis of human erythrocyte glucose transporter function in reconstituted vesicles. J Biol Chem 1986; 261:7101.

582. Mueckler MM, Caruso C, et al: Sequence and structure of a human glucose transporter. Science 1985; 229:941.

583. Agre P, Parker JC: Red Blood Cell Membranes: Structure, Function, Clinical Implications. New York, Marcel Dekker, Inc., 1989.

584. Brugnara C: Membrane transport of Na and K and cell dehydration in sickle erythrocytes. Experientia 1993; 49:100.

585. Joiner CH: Cation transport and volume regulation in sickle red blood cells. Am J Physiol 1993; 264:C251.

586. Lauf PK, Bauer J, et al: Erythrocyte K-Cl cotransport: Properties and regulation. Am J Physiol 1992 263:C917.

587. Raess BU, Tunnicliff G: The Red Cell Membrane: A Model for Solute Transport. Clifton, NJ, Humana Press, 1989.

588. Parker JC: In defense of cell volume? Am J Physiol 1993; 265:1191.

589. De Gier J: Permeability barriers formed by membrane lipids. Bioelectrochem Bioenerg 1992; 27:1.

590. Nielsen S, Smith BL, et al: CHIP28 water channels are localized in constitutively water-permeable segments of the nephron. J Cell Biol 1993; 120:371.

591. Zeidel ML, Ambudkar SV, et al: Reconstitution of functional water channels in liposomes containing purified red cell CHIP28 protein. Biochemistry 1992; 31:7436.

592. Preston GM, Agre P: Isolation of the cDNA for erythrocyte integral membrane protein of 28 kilodaltons: Member of an ancient channel family. Proc Natl Acad Sci U S A 1991; 88:11110.

593. Smith BL, Baumgarten R, et al: Concurrent expression of erythroid and renal aquaporin CHIP and appearance of water channel activity in perinatal rats. J Clin Invest 1993; 92:2035.

594. Johnson RM, Gannon SA: Erythrocyte cation permeability induced by mechanical stress: A model for sickle cell cation loss. Am J Physiol 1990; 259:C746.

595. Kim Y-K, Dirksen ER, Sanderson MJ: Stretch-activated channels in airway epithelial cells. Am J Physiol 1993; 265:1306.

596. Sachs F: Ion channels as mechanical transducers. In Stein WD, Bronner F (eds): Cell Shape: Determinants, Regulation, and Regulatory Role. New York, Academic Press, 1989, p 63.

597. Sachs F: Stretch-sensitive ion channels: An update. In Corey DP, Roper SD (eds): Sensory Transduction. New York, Rockefeller University Press, 1992, p 242.

598. Garrahan PJ, Glynn IM: Factors affecting the relative magnitude of the sodium:potassium and sodium:sodium exchanges catalyzed by the sodium pump. J Physiol 1967; 192:189.

599. Clark MR, Guatelli JC, et al: Study of dehydrating effect of the red cell Na$^+$/K$^+$ pump in nystatin-treated cells with varying Na$^+$ and water content. Biochim Biophys Acta 1981; 646:422.

600. Joiner CH, Platt OS, Lux SE: Cation depletion by the sodium pump in red cells with pathologic cation leaks. J Clin Invest 1986; 78:1487.

601. Lazarides E: From genes to structural morphogenesis: The genesis and epigenesis of a red blood cell. Cell 1987; 51:345.

602. Lazarides E, Woods C: Biogenesis of the red blood cell membrane-skeleton and the control of erythroid morphogenesis. Annu Rev Cell Biol 1989; 5:427.

603. Peters LL, Shivdasani RA, et al: Anion exchanger 1 (band 3) is required to prevent erythrocyte membrane surface loss but not to form the membrane skeleton. Cell 1996; 86:917.

604. Hanspal M, Palek J: Synthesis and assembly of membrane skeletal proteins in mammalian red cell precursors. J Cell Biol 1987; 105:1417.

605. Hanspal M, Hanspal J, Kalraiya R: Asynchronous synthesis of membrane skeletal proteins during terminal maturation of murine erythroblasts. Blood 1992; 80:530.

606. Hanspal M, Hanspal JS, et al: Molecular basis of spectrin deficiency in hereditary pyropoikilocytosis. Blood 1993; 82:1652.

607. Woods CM, Boyer B, et al: Control of erythroid differentiation: Asynchronous expression of the anion transporter and the peripheral components of the membrane skeleton in AEV- and S13-transformed cells. J Cell Biol 1986; 103:1789.

608. Savvides P, Shalev O, et al: Combined spectrin and ankyrin deficiency is common in autosomal dominant hereditary spherocytosis. Blood 1993; 82:2953.

609. Hanspal M, Kalraiya R, et al: Erythropoietin enhances the assembly of β spectrin heterodimers on the murine erythroblast membranes by increasing spectrin synthesis. J Biol Chem 1991; 266:15626.

610. Chasis JA, Prenant M, et al: Membrane assembly and remodeling during reticulocyte maturation. Blood 1989; 74:1112.

611. Johnstone RM: The transferrin receptor. In Agre P, Parker JC (eds): Red Blood Cell Membranes: Structure, Function, and Clinical Implications. New York, Marcel Dekker, Inc., 1989, p 325.

612. Oski FA, Naiman JL: Red cell metabolism in the premature infant: I. Adenosine triphosphate levels, adenosine triphosphate stability, and glucose consumption. Pediatrics 1965; 36:104.

613. Ng WG, Donnell GN, Bergren WR: Galactokinase activity in human erythrocytes of individuals at different ages. J Lab Clin Med 1965; 66:115.

614. Travis SF, Kumar SP, et al: Red cell metabolic alterations and postnatal life in term infants: Glycolytic enzymes and glucose-6-phosphate dehydrogenase. Pediatr Res 1980; 14:1349.

615. Wimberley PD: A review of oxygen delivery in the neonate. Scand J Clin Lab Invest 1982; 160(Suppl):1.

616. Stockman JA, deAlarcon PA: Hematopoiesis and granulopoiesis. In Polin RA, Fox WW (eds): Fetal and Neonatal Physiology. Vol. II. Philadelphia, W.B. Saunders Co., 1992, p 1327.

617. Oski FA, Naiman JL (eds): Hematologic Problems in the Newborn. 3rd ed. Vol. IV. Philadelphia, W.B. Saunders Co., 1982.

618. Mollison PL: Blood Transfusion in Clinical Medicine. Oxford, Blackwell Scientific Publications, Inc., 1967, p 275.

619. Jay DG: Glycosylation site of band 3, the human erythrocyte anion-exchange protein. Biochemistry 1986; 25:554.

620. Fukuda M, Dell A, Fukuda MN: Structure of fetal lactosaminoglycan: The carbohydrate moiety of band 3 isolated from human umbilical cord erythrocytes. J Biol Chem 1984; 259:4782.

621. Fukuda M, Dell A, et al: Structure of branched lactosaminoglycan, the carbohydrate moiety of band 3 isolated from adult erythrocytes. J Biol Chem 1984; 259:8260.

622. Fukuda M, Fukuda MN, Hakomori S: Developmental change and genetic defect in the carbohydrate structure of band 3 glycoprotein of human erythrocyte membrane. J Biol Chem 1979; 254:3700.

623. Zipursky A, LaRue T, Israels LG: The *in vitro* metabolism of erythrocytes from newborn infants. Can J Biochem 1960; 38:727.

624. Whaun JM, Oski FA: Red cell stromal adenosine triphosphatase (ATPase) of newborn infants. Pediatr Res 1969; 3:105.

625. Neerhout RC: Erythrocyte lipids in the neonate. Pediatr Res 1968; 2:172.

626. Sjolin S: The resistance of red cell *in vitro*: A study of the osmotic properties, the mechanical resistance and the storage behavior of red cells of fetuses, children and adults. Acta Paediatr 1954; 43:1.

627. Kehry M, Yguerabide J, Singer SJ: Fluidity in the membranes of adult and neonatal human erythrocytes. Science 1977; 195:486.

628. Shapiro DL, Pasqualini P: Erythrocyte membrane proteins of premature and full-term newborn infants. Pediatr Res 1978; 12:176.

629. Chow EI, Chen D: Kinetic characteristics of bicarbonate-chloride exchange across the neonatal human red cell membrane. Biochim Biophys Acta 1982; 685:196.

630. Matovick LM, Groschel-Stewart U, et al: Myosin is a component of the erythrocyte membrane. J Cell Biol 1984; 99:2a. Abstract.

631. Schekman R, Singer SJ: Clustering and endocytosis of membrane receptors can be induced in mature erythrocytes of neonatal but not adult humans. Proc Natl Acad Sci U S A 1976; 73:4075.

632. Tokuyasu KT, Schekman R, Singer SJ: Domains of receptor mobility and endocytosis in the membranes of neonatal human erythrocytes and reticulocytes are deficient in spectrin. J Cell Biol 1979; 80:481.

633. Zweig S, Singer SJ: Concanavalin A–induced endocytosis in rabbit reticulocytes, and its decrease with reticulocyte maturation. J Cell Biol 1979; 80:487.

634. Gross GP, Hathaway WE: Fetal erythrocyte deformability. Pediatr Res 1972; 6:593.

635. Bratteby LE, Garby L, et al: Studies on erythrokinetics in infancy: 13. The mean life span and the life span frequency function of red blood cells formed during foetal life. Acta Paediatr Scand 1968; 57:311.

636. Holroyde CP, Oski FA, Gardner FH: The "pocked" erythrocyte: Red-cell surface alterations in reticuloendothelial immaturity of the neonate. N Engl J Med 1969; 281:516.

637. Tsukada M, Hanamura K, et al: Scanning electron microscopic study on red blood cells in several diseases of newborns and infants. Acta Paediatr Jpn 1976; 18:4.

638. Shattil SJ, Cooper RA: Maturation of macroreticulocyte membranes *in vivo*. J Lab Clin Med 1972; 79:215.

639. Lux SE, John KM: Isolation and partial characterization of a high molecular weight red cell membrane protein complex normally removed by the spleen. Blood 1977; 50:625.

640. Patel VP, Ciechanover A, et al: Mammalian reticulocytes lose adhesion to fibronectin during maturation to erythrocytes. Proc Natl Acad Sci U S A 1985; 82:440.

641. Clark MR: Senescence of red blood cells: Progress and problems. Physiol Rev 1988; 68:503.

642. Clark MR, Shohet SB: Red cell senescence. Clin Haematol 1985; 14:223.

643. Beutler E: Isolation of the aged. Blood Cells 1988; 14:1.

644. Dale GL, Norenberg SL: Density fractionation of erythrocytes by Percoll/hypaque results in only a slight enrichment for aged cells. Biochim Biophys Acta 1990; 1036:183.

645. Suzuki T, Dale GL: Senescent erythrocytes: Isolation of *in vivo* aged cells and their biochemical characteristics. Proc Natl Acad Sci U S A 1988; 85:1647.

646. Gershon H: Is the sequestration of aged erythrocytes mediated by natural autoantibodies? Isr J Med Sci 1992; 28:818.

647. Lutz HU: Erythrocyte Clearance. In Harris JR (ed): Blood Cell Biochemistry, Erythroid Cells. Vol. I. New York, Plenum Press, 1990, p 81.

648. Waugh RE, Mohandas N, et al: Rheologic properties of senescent erythrocytes: Loss of surface area and volume with red blood cell age. Blood 1992; 79:1351.

649. Jain SK, Hochstein P: Polymerization of membrane components in aging red blood cells. Biochem Biophys Res Commun 1980; 92:247.

650. Snyder LM, Fortier NL, et al: Effect of hydrogen peroxide exposure on normal human erythrocyte deformability, morphology, surface characteristics and spectrin hemoglobin cross-linking. J Clin Invest 1985; 76:1971.

651. Jain SK: Evidence for membrane lipid peroxidation during the *in vivo* aging of human erythrocytes. Biochim Biophys Acta 1988; 937:205.

652. Danon D, Marikovsky Y: The aging of the red blood cell: A multifactor process. Blood Cells 1988; 14:7.

653. Aminoff D, Ghalambor MA, Henrich CJ: GOST, galactose oxidase and sialyl transferase: substrate and receptor sites in erythrocyte senescence. In Eaton JW (ed): Erythrocyte Membranes: 2. Recent Clinical and Experimental Advances. New York, Alan R. Liss, Inc., 1981, p 269.

654. Gattegno L, Bladier D, Garnier M: Changes in carbohydrate content of surface membranes of human erythrocytes during aging. Carbohyd Res 1976; 52:197.

655. Lutz HU, Fehr J: Total sialic acid content of glycophorins during senescence of human red blood cells. J Biol Chem 1979; 254:11177.

656. Seaman GV, Knox RJ, Nordt FJ: Red cell aging: I. Surface charge density and sialic acid content of density-fractionated human erythrocytes. Blood 1977; 50:1001.

657. Beutler E: Biphasic loss of red cell enzyme activity during *in vivo* aging. Prog Clin Biol Res 1985; 95:317.

658. Kay MM: Mechanism of removal of senescent cells by human macrophages *in situ*. Proc Natl Acad Sci U S A 1975; 72:3521.

659. Kay MM: Localization of senescent cell antigen on band 3. Proc Natl Acad Sci U S A 1984; 81:5753.

660. Schlüter K, Drenckhahn D: Co-clustering of denatured hemoglobin with band 3: Its role in binding of autoantibodies against band 3 to abnormal and aged erythrocytes. Proc Natl Acad Sci U S A 1986; 83:6137.

661. Lutz HU, Stringaro-Wipf G: Senescent red cell bound IgG is attached to band 3 protein. Biomed Biochim Acta 1983; 42:117.

662. Galili U, Macher BA, et al: Human natural anti-α-galactosyl IgG: II. The specific recognition of α(113)-linked galactose residues. J Exp Med 1985; 162:573.

663. Galili U, Flechner I, et al: The natural anti-α-galactosyl IgG on human normal senescent red blood cells. Br J Haematol 1986; 62:317.

664. Kay MM, Bosman GJ: Naturally occurring human "anti-galactosyl" IgG antibodies are heterophile antibodies recognizing blood-group-related substances. Exp Hematol 1985; 13:1103.

665. Kay MM, Marchalonis JJ, et al: Definition of a physiologic aging autoantigen by using synthetic peptides of membrane protein band 3: Localization of the active antigenic sites. Proc Natl Acad Sci U S A 1990; 87:5734.

666. Turrini F, Arese P, et al: Clustering of integral membrane proteins of the human erythrocyte membrane stimulates autologous IgG binding, complement deposition, and phagocytosis. J Biol Chem 1991; 266:23611.

667. Beppu M, Mizukami A, et al: Binding of anti-band 3 autoantibody to oxidatively damaged erythrocytes: Formation of senescent antigen on erythrocyte surface by an oxidative mechanism. J Biol Chem 1990; 265:3226.

668. Lutz HU, Bussolino F, et al: Naturally occurring anti-band-3 antibodies and complement together mediate phagocytosis of oxidatively stressed human erythrocytes. Proc Natl Acad Sci U S A 1987; 84:7368.

669. Waugh SM, Willardson BM, et al: Heinz bodies induce clustering of band 3, glycophorin, and ankyrin in sickle cell erythrocytes. J Clin Invest 1986; 78:1155.

670. Winograd E, Greenan JR, Sherman IW: Expression of senescent antigen on erythrocytes infected with a knobby variant of the human malaria parasite *Plasmodium falciparum*. Proc Natl Acad Sci U S A 1987; 84:1931.

671. Herrmann A, Devaux PF: Alteration of the aminophospholipid translocase activity during *in vivo* and artificial aging of human erythrocytes. Biochim Biophys Acta 1990; 1027:41.

672. Wang RH, Phillips G Jr, et al: Activation of the alternative complement pathway by exposure of phosphatidylethanolamine and phosphatidylserine on erythrocytes from sickle cell disease patients. J Clin Invest 1993; 92:1326.

673. Schroit AJ, Madsen JW, Tanaka Y: *In vivo* recognition and clearance of red blood cells containing phosphatidylserine in their plasma membranes. J Biol Chem 1985; 260:5131.

674. Vlassara H, Valinsky J, et al: Advanced glycosylation end products on erythrocyte cell surface induce receptor-mediated phagocytosis by macrophages. A model for turnover of aging cells. J Exp Med 1987; 166:539.

675. Barber JR, Clarke S: Membrane protein carboxyl methylation increases with human erythrocyte age. J Biol Chem 1983; 258:1189.

676. Galletti P, Ingrosso D, et al: Increased methyl esterification of membrane proteins in aged red-blood cells: Preferential esterification of ankyrin and band-4.1 cytoskeletal proteins. Eur J Biochem 1983; 135:25.

677. Vanlair CF, Masius JB: De la microcythémie. Bull R Acad Med Belg 1871; 5:515.

678. Wilson C: Some cases showing hereditary enlargement of the spleen. Trans Clin Soc (London) 1890; 23:162.

679. Wilson C, Stanley D: A sequel to some cases showing hereditary enlargement of the spleen. Trans Clin Soc (London) 1893; 26:163.

680. Minkowski O: Über eine hereditäre, unter dem Bilde eines chronischen Ikterus mit Urobilinurie, Splenomegalie und Nierensiderosis verlaufende Affektion. Verh Dtsch Kongr Med 1900; 18:316.

681. Chauffard MA: Pathogénie de l'ictère congénital de l'adulte. Semaine Méd (Paris) 1907; 27:25.

682. Chauffard MA: Les ictères hémolytiques. Semaine Méd (Paris) 1908; 28:49.

683. Dawson of Penn. The Hume Lectures on haemolytic icterus. BMJ 1931; 1:921, 963.

684. Wintrobe MM: Blood, Pure and Eloquent. New York, McGraw-Hill Book Co., 1980.

685. Morton NE, MacKinney AA, et al: Genetics of spherocytosis. Am J Hum Genet 1962; 14:170.

686. Godal HC, Heist H: High prevalence of increased osmotic fragility of red blood cells among Norwegian donors. Scand J Haematol 1981; 27:30.

687. Eber SW, Pekrun A, et al: Prevalence of increased osmotic fragility of erythrocytes in German blood donors: Screening using a modified glycerol lysis test. Ann Hematol 1992; 64:88.

688. Eber SW, Armbrust R, Schröter W: Variable clinical severity of hereditary spherocytosis: Relation to erythrocytic spectrin concentration, osmotic fragility and autohemolysis. J Pediatr 1990; 177:409.

689. Race RR: On the inheritance and linkage relations of acholuric jaundice. Ann Eugenics 1942; 11:365.

690. Whitfield CF, Follweiler JB, et al: Deficiency of α-spectrin synthesis in burst-forming units-erythroid in lethal hereditary spherocytosis. Blood 1991; 78:3043.

691. Olim G, Marques S, et al: Red cell abnormalities in a kindred with an uncommon form of hereditary spherocytosis. Acta Méd Portug 1984; 6:137.

692. Bernard J, Boiron M, Estager J: Une grand famille hémolytique: Trieze cas de maladie de Minkowski-Chauffard observés dans la même fratrie. Semaine Hôp Paris 1952; 28:3741.

693. Duru F, Gürgey A, et al: Homozygosity for dominant form of hereditary spherocytosis. Br J Haematol 1992; 82:596.

694. Agre P, Asimos A, et al: Inheritance pattern and clinical response to splenectomy as a reflection of erythrocyte spectrin deficiency in hereditary spherocytosis. N Engl J Med 1986; 315:1579.

695. Eber SW, Gonzalez JM, et al: Ankyrin-1 mutations are a major cause of dominant and recessive hereditary spherocytosis. Nature Genet 1996; 13:214.

696. Morlé L, Bozon M, et al: Allele Bugey: a *de novo* deletional frameshift variant in exon 6 of the ankyrin gene associated with spherocytosis. Am J Hematol 1997; 54:242.

697. Miraglia del Giudice E, Hayette S, et al: Ankyrin Napoli: A *de novo* deletional frameshift mutation in exon 16 of ankyrin gene (ANK1) associated with spherocytosis. Br J Haematol 1996; 93:828.

698. Jarolim P, Brabec V, et al: Ankyrin Prague: A dominantly inherited mutation of the regulatory domain of ankyrin associated with hereditary spherocytosis. Blood 1990; 76(Suppl 1):37a. Abstract.

699. Jarolim P, Rubin HL, et al: Abnormal alternative splicing of erythroid ankyrin mRNA in two kindred with hereditary spherocytosis (Ankyrin^Prague and Ankyrin^Rakovnik). Blood 1993; 82(Suppl 1):5a. Abstract.

700. Jarolim P, Rubin HL, et al: A nonsense mutation 1669Glu→Ter within the regulatory domain of human erythroid ankyrin leads to a selective deficiency of the major ankyrin isoform (band 2.1) and a phenotype of autosomal dominant hereditary spherocytosis. J Clin Invest 1995; 95:941.

701. Özcan R, Jarolim P, et al: High frequency of frameshift/nonsense mutations of ankyrin-1 in Czech patients with dominant hereditary spherocytosis. Blood 1996; 88(Suppl 1):10a. Abstract.

702. Gallagher PG, Ferreira JDS, et al: A recurring frameshift mutation of the ankyrin-1 gene associated with severe hereditary spherocytosis in Brazil. Blood 1996; 88(Suppl 1):11a. Abstract.

703. Lux S, Bedrosian C, et al: Deficiency of band 3 in dominant hereditary spherocytosis with normal spectrin content. Clin Res 1990; 38:300a. Abstract.

704. Jenkins PB, Abou-Alfa GK, et al: A nonsense mutation in the erythrocyte band 3 gene associated with decreased mRNA accumulation in a kindred with dominant hereditary spherocytosis. J Clin Invest 1996; 97:373.

705. Alloisio N, Inoue T, et al: Modulation of clinical expression and band 3 deficiency in hereditary spherocytosis. Blood 1997 (in press).

706. Bianchi P, Zanella A, et al: Band 3 Milano: A large duplication (69 bp) of the erythrocyte band 3 gene associated with dominant hereditary spherocytosis. Blood 1995; 86(Suppl 1):468a. Abstract.

707. Jarolim P, Rubin HL, et al: Mutations of conserved arginines in the membrane domain of erythroid band 3 lead to a decrease in membrane-associated band 3 and to the phenotype of hereditary spherocytosis. Blood 1995; 85:634.

708. Maillet P, Vallier A, et al: Band 3 Chur: A variant associated with band 3-deficient hereditary spherocytosis and substitution in a highly conserved position of transmembrane segment 11. Br J Haematol 1995; 91:804.

709. Jarolim P, Murray JL, et al: Characterization of 13 novel band 3 gene defects in hereditary spherocytosis with band 3 deficiency. Blood 1996; 88:4366.

710. Jarolim P, Brabec V, et al: Association of a band 3 gene mutation with renal tubular acidosis. Blood 1996; 88(Suppl 1):3a. Abstract.

711. Miraglia del Giudice E, Vallier A, et al: Novel band 3 variants (bands 3 Foggia, Napoli I and Napoli II) associated with hereditary spherocytosis and band 3 deficiency: status of the D38A polymorphism within the EPB3 locus. Br J Haematol 1997; 96:70.

712. Lima PRM, Gontijo JAR, et al: Band 3 Campinas: A novel splicing mutation in the band 3 gene (AE1) associated with hereditary spherocytosis, hyperactivity of Na+/Li+ countertransport and an abnormal renal bicarbonate handling. Blood 1996; 88(Suppl 1):462a. Abstract.

713. Agre P, Orringer EP, Bennett V: Deficient red-cell spectrin in severe, recessively inherited spherocytosis. N Engl J Med 1982; 306:1155.

714. Pekrun A, Eber SW, et al: Combined ankyrin and spectrin deficiency in hereditary spherocytosis. Ann Hematol 1993; 67:89.

715. Chasis JA, Agre PA, Mohandas N: Decreased membrane mechanical stability and *in vivo* loss of surface area reflect spectrin deficiencies in hereditary spherocytosis. J Clin Invest 1988; 82:617.

716. Waugh RE, Agre P: Reductions of erythrocyte membrane viscoelastic coefficients reflect spectrin deficiencies in hereditary spherocytosis. J Clin Invest 1988; 81:133.

717. Agre P, Casella JF, et al: Partial deficiency of erythrocyte spectrin in hereditary spherocytosis. Nature 1985; 314:380.

718. Marchesi SL, Agre PL, et al: Mutant spectrin α^{II} domain in recessively inherited spherocytosis. Blood 1989; 74(Suppl 1):182a. Abstract.

719. Tse WT, Gallagher PG, et al: Amino acid substitution in α-spectrin commonly co-inherited with nondominant hereditary spherocytosis. Am J Hematol 1997; 54:233.

720. Boivin P, Galand C, et al: Spectrin alpha IIa variant in dominant and non-dominant spherocytosis. Hum Genet 1993; 92:153.

721. Wichterle H, Hanspal M, et al: Combination of two mutant alpha spectrin alleles underlies a severe spherocytic hemolytic anemia. J Clin Invest 1996; 98:2300.

722. Woods CM, Lazarides E: Spectrin assembly in avian erythroid development is determined by competing reactions of subunit homo- and hetero-oligomerization. Nature 1986; 321:85.

723. Kimberling WJ, Taylor RA, et al: Linkage and gene localization of hereditary spherocytosis (HS). Blood 1978; 52:859.

724. Fukushima Y, Byers MG, et al: Assignment of the gene for β-spectrin (SPTB) to chromosome 14q23→q24.2 by *in situ* hybridization. Cytogenet Cell Genet 1990; 53:232.

725. Goodman SR, Shiffer KA, et al: Identification of the molecular defect in the erythrocyte membrane skeleton of some kindreds with hereditary spherocytosis. Blood 1982; 60:772.

726. Wolfe LC, John KM, et al: A genetic defect in the binding of protein 4.1 to spectrin in a kindred with hereditary spherocytosis. N Engl J Med 1982; 307:1367.

727. Becker PS, Morrow JS, Lux SE: Abnormal oxidant sensitivity and beta-chain structure of spectrin in hereditary spherocytosis associated with defective spectrin-protein 4.1 binding. J Clin Invest 1987; 80:557.

728. Tyler JM, Hargreaves WR, Branton D: Purification of two spectrin-binding proteins: Biochemical and electron microscopical evidence for site specific reassociation between spectrin bands 2.1 and 4.1. Proc Natl Acad Sci U S A 1979; 76:5192.

729. Hassoun H, Vassiliadis JN, et al: Molecular basis of spectrin deficiency in beta spectrin Durham. A deletion within beta spectrin adjacent to the ankyrin-binding site precludes spectrin attachment to the membrane in hereditary spherocytosis. J Clin Invest 1995; 96:2623.

730. Hassoun H, Vassiliadis JN, et al: Hereditary spherocytosis with spectrin deficiency due to an unstable truncated beta spectrin. Blood 1996; 87:2538.

731. Hassoun H, Vassiliadis JN, et al: Characterization of the underlying molecular defect in hereditary spherocytosis associated with spectrin deficiency. Blood 1995; 86(Suppl 1):467a. Abstract.

732. Coetzer TL, Lawler J, et al: Partial ankyrin and spectrin deficiency in severe, atypical hereditary spherocytosis. N Engl J Med 1988; 318:230.

733. Hanspal M, Yoon SH, et al: Molecular basis of spectrin and ankyrin deficiencies in severe hereditary spherocytosis: Evidence implicating a primary defect of ankyrin. Blood 1991; 77:165.

734. Iolascon A, Miraglia del Giudice E, et al: Ankyrin deficiency in dominant hereditary spherocytosis: Report of three cases. Br J Haematol 1991; 78:551.

735. Miraglia del Giudice E, Iolascon A, et al: Erythrocyte membrane protein alterations underlying clinical heterogeneity in hereditary spherocytosis. Br J Haematol 1994; 88:52.

736. Yawata Y, Kanzaki A, et al: Red cell membrane disorders in the Japanese population: Clinical, biochemical, electron microscopic, and genetic studies. Int J Hematol 1994; 60:23.

737. Saad ST, Costa FF, et al: Red cell membrane protein abnormalities in hereditary spherocytosis in Brazil. Br J Haematol 1994; 88:295.

738. Rizk SH, Ibrahim AM, et al: Red cell membrane defects and inheritance in 20 Egyptian families with hereditary spherocytosis: Correlation with clinical severity. Cell Vision 1996; 3:137.

739. Chilcote RR, Le Beau MM, et al: Association of red cell spherocytosis with deletion of the short arm of chromosome 8. Blood 1987; 69:156.

740. Cohen H, Walker H, et al: Congenital spherocytosis, B19 parvovirus infection and inherited deletion of the short arm of chromosome 8. Br J Haematol 1991; 78:251.

741. Kitatani M, Chiyo H, et al: Localization of the spherocytosis gene to chromosome segment 8p11.22–8p21.1. Hum Genet 1988; 78:94.

742. Okamoto N, Wada Y, et al: Hereditary spherocytic anemia with deletion of the short arm of chromosome 8. Am J Med Genet 1995; 58:225.

743. Kimberling WJ, Fulbeck T, et al: Localization of spherocytosis to chromosome 8 or 12 and report of a family with spherocytosis and a reciprocal translocation. Am J Hum Genet 1975; 27:586.

744. Costa FF, Agre P, et al: Linkage of dominant hereditary spherocytosis to the gene for the erythrocyte membrane-skeleton protein ankyrin. N Engl J Med 1990; 323:1046.

745. Jarolim P, Rubin HL, et al: Comparison of the ankyrin (AC)$_n$ microsatellites in genomic DNA and mRNA reveals absence of one ankyrin mRNA allele in 20% of patients with hereditary spherocytosis. Blood 1995; 85:3278.

746. Inaba M, Yawata A, et al: Defective anion transport and marked spherocytosis with membrane instability caused by hereditary total deficiency of red cell band 3 in cattle due to a nonsense mutation. J Clin Invest 1996; 97:1804.

747. Takaoka Y, Ideguchi H, et al: A novel mutation in the erythrocyte protein 4.2 gene of Japanese patients with hereditary spherocytosis (protein 4.2 Fukuoda). Br J Haematol 1994; 88:527.

748. Ideguchi H, Nishimura J, et al: A genetic defect of erythrocyte band 4.2 protein associated with hereditary spherocytosis. Br J Haematol 1990; 74:347.

749. Hayashi S, Koomoto R, et al: Abnormality in a specific protein of the erythrocyte membrane in hereditary spherocytosis. Biochem Biophys Res Commun 1974; 57:1038.

750. Hayette S, Dhermy D, et al: A deletional frameshift mutation in protein 4.2 gene (allele 4.2 Lisboa) associated with hereditary hemolytic anemia. Blood 1995; 85:250.

751. Hayette S, Morle L, et al: A point mutation in the protein 4.2 gene (allele 4.2 Tozeur) associated with hereditary haemolytic anaemia. Br J Haematol 1995; 89:762.

751a. Matsuda M, Hatano N, et al: A novel mutation causing an aberrant splicing in the protein 4.2 gene associated with hereditary spherocytosis (protein 4.2 Notame). Hum Mol Genet 1995; 4:1187.

751b. Kanzaki A, Yasunaga M, et al: Band 4.2 Shiga: 317CGC→TGC in compound heterozygotes with 142 GCT→ACT results in band 4.2 deficiency and microspherocytosis. Br J Haematol 1995; 91:333.

752. Kanzaki A, Yawata Y, et al: Band 4.2 Komatsu: 526 GAT→TAT (175 Asp→Tyr) in exon 4 of the band 4.2 gene associated with total deficiency of band 4.2, hemolytic anemia with ovalostomatocytosis and marked disruption of the cytoskeletal network. Int J Hematol 1995; 61:165.

753. Ghanem A, Pothier B, et al: A haemolytic syndrome associated with the complete absence of red cell membrane protein 4.2 in two Tunisian siblings. Br J Haematol 1990; 75:414.

754. Sheehy R, Ralston GB: Abnormal binding of spectrin to the membrane of erythrocytes in some cases of hereditary spherocytosis. Blut 1978; 36:145.

755. Price Evans DA, Mackie MJ, Anand R: Diminished extractable spectrin in the erythrocytes of a patient with 'sporadic' hereditary spherocytosis. Acta Haematol 1986; 76:136.

756. Mariani M, Maretzki D, Lutz HU: A tightly membrane-associated subpopulation of spectrin is ^{3}H palmitoylated. J Biol Chem 1993; 268:12996.

757. Allen DW, Cadman S, et al: Increased membrane binding of erythrocyte catalase in hereditary spherocytosis and in metabolically stressed normal cells. Blood 1977; 49:113.

758. Boulard-Heitzmann P, Boulard M, et al: Decreased red cell enolase activity in a 40-year-old woman with compensated hemolysis. Scand J Haematol 1984; 33:401.

759. Lachant NA, Jennings MA, Tanaka KR: Partial erythrocyte enolase deficiency: A hereditary disorder with variable clinical expression. Blood 1986; 68(Suppl 1):55a. Abstract.

760. Lux SE, Glader BE: Disorders of the red cell membrane. In

Nathan DG, Oski FA (eds): Hematology of Infancy and Childhood. 2nd ed. Philadelphia, W.B. Saunders Co., 1981, p 456.

761. Lux SE: Disorders of the red cell membrane. In Nathan DG, Oski FA (eds): Hematology of Infancy and Childhood. 3rd ed. Philadelphia, W.B. Saunders Co., 1987, p 444.

762. Beutler E, Guinto E, Johnson C: Human red cell protein kinase in normal subjects and patients with hereditary spherocytosis, sickle cell disease, and autoimmune hemolytic anemia. Blood 1976; 48:887.

763. Boivin P, Delaunay J, Galand C: Altered erythrocyte membrane protein phosphorylation in an unusual case of hereditary spherocytosis. Scand J Haematol 1979; 23:251.

764. Wolfe LC, Lux SE: Membrane protein phosphorylation of intact normal and hereditary spherocytic erythrocytes. J Biol Chem 1978; 253:3336.

765. Pinder JC, Dhermy D, et al: A phenomenological difference between membrane skeletal protein complexes isolated from normal and hereditary spherocytosis erythrocytes. Br J Haematol 1983; 55:455.

766. Armbrust R, Eber SW, Schröter W: Absence of phosphorylation-induced gelation of erythrocyte membrane skeletons: A diagnostic tool for hereditary spherocytosis. Ann Hematol 1992; 64:93.

767. De Gier J, Van Deenen LLM: Phospholipid and fatty acid characteristics of erythrocytes in some cases of anaemia. Br J Haematol 1964; 10:246.

768. Vermeulen WP, Briede JJ, et al: Enhanced Mg^{2+}-ATPase activity in ghosts from HS erythrocytes and in normal ghosts stripped of membrane skeletal proteins may reflect enhanced aminophospholipid translocase activity. Br J Haematol 1995; 90:56.

769. Kuiper PJ, Livne A: Differences in fatty acid composition between normal erythrocytes and hereditary spherocytosis affected cells. Biochim Biophys Acta 1972; 260:755.

770. Zail SS, Pickering A: Fatty acid composition of erythrocytes in hereditary spherocytosis. Br J Haematol 1979; 42:399.

771. Kanzake A, Ikeda A, Yawata Y: Membrane studies on rod-shaped red cells in hereditary elliptocytosis: Least hemolysis and normal sodium influx with decreased membrane lipids. Br J Haematol 1988; 70:105.

772. Bertles JE: Sodium transport across the surface of red blood cells in hereditary spherocytosis. J Clin Invest 1957; 36:816.

773. Jacob HS, Jandl JH: Cell membrane permeability in the pathogenesis of hereditary spherocytosis (HS). J Clin Invest 1964; 43:1704.

774. Zipursky A, Israels LG: Significance of erythrocyte sodium flux in the pathophysiology and genetic expression of hereditary spherocytosis. Pediatr Res 1971; 5:614.

775. Joiner CH, Franco RS, et al: Increased cation permeability in mutant mouse red cells with defective membrane skeletons. Blood 1994; 86:4307.

776. Wiley JS: Red cell survival in hereditary spherocytosis. J Clin Invest 1970; 49:666.

777. Oski FA, Naiman JL, Blum SF: Congenital hemolytic anemia with high-sodium, low-potassium red cells: Studies of three generations of a family with a new variant. N Engl J Med 1969; 280:909.

778. Mayman D, Zipursky A: Hereditary spherocytosis: The metabolism of erythrocytes in the peripheral blood and in the splenic pulp. Br J Haematol 1974; 27:201.

779. Palek J, Mirevova L, Brabcu V: 2,3-Diphosphoglycerate metabolism in hereditary spherocytosis. Br J Haematol 1969; 17:59.

780. Olivieri O, Bonollo M, et al: Activation of K^+/Cl^- cotransport in human erythrocytes exposed to oxidative agents. Biochim Biophys Acta 1993; 1176:37.

781. Loder PB, Babarczy G, de Gruchy GC: Red cell metabolism in hereditary spherocytosis. Br J Haematol 1967; 13:95.

782. Mohler DN: Adenosine triphosphate metabolism in hereditary spherocytosis. J Clin Invest 1965; 44:1417.

783. Fernandez LA, Erslev AJ: Oxygen affinity and compensated hemolysis in hereditary spherocytosis. J Lab Clin Med 1972; 80:780.

784. Kagimoto T, Hayashi F, et al: Phosphorus ^{31}NMR study on nucleotides and intracellular pH of hereditary spherocytes. Experientia 1978; 34:1092.

785. Ideguchi H, Hamasaki N, Ikehara Y: Abnormal phosphoenol-

786. pyruvate transport in erythrocytes of hereditary spherocytosis. Blood 1981; 58:426.

786. Eber SW, Cho M, et al: Increased band 3 mobility and decreased anion transport in ankyrin deficient hereditary spherocytes. Blood 1993; 82(Suppl 1):175a. Abstract.

787. Bodine DM, Birkenmeier CS, Barker JE: Spectrin deficient inherited hemolytic anemias in the mouse: Characterization by spectrin synthesis and mRNA activity in reticulocytes. Cell 1984; 37:721.

788. Bernstein SE: Hereditary disorders of the rodent erythron. In: Genetics in Laboratory Medicine. Publication No. 1679. Washington, DC, National Academy of Sciences, 1969, p 9.

789. Birkenmeier CS, McFarland-Starr EC, Barker JE: Chromosomal location of three spectrin genes: Relationship to the inherited hemolytic anemias of mouse and man. Proc Natl Acad Sci U S A 1988; 85:8121.

790. Greenquist AC, Shohet SB, Bernstein SE: Marked reduction of spectrin in hereditary spherocytosis in the common house mouse. Blood 1978; 51:1149.

791. Bloom ML, Kaysser TM, et al: The murine mutation jaundiced is caused by replacement of an arginine with a stop codon in the mRNA encoding the ninth repeat of beta-spectrin. Proc Natl Acad Sci U S A 1994; 91:10099.

792. Unger AE, Harris MJ, et al: Hemolytic anemia in the mouse: Report of a new mutation and clarification of its genetics. J Hered 1983; 74:88.

793. White RA, Birkenmeier CS, et al: Ankyrin and the hemolytic anemia mutation, nb, map to mouse chromosome 8: Presence of the nb allele is associated with a truncated erythrocyte ankyrin. Proc Natl Acad Sci U S A 1990; 87:3117.

794. Grimber G, Galand C, et al: Inherited haemolytic anaemia created by insertional inactivation of the alpha-spectrin gene. Transgenic Res 1992; 1:268.

795. d'Ermao N, Levi M: Neurological symptoms in anemia. In: Neurological Symptoms in Blood Diseases. Baltimore, University Park Press, 1972, p 1.

796. McCann SR, Jacob HS: Spinal cord disease in hereditary spherocytosis: Report of two cases with a hypothesized common mechanism for neurologic and red cell abnormalities. Blood 1976; 48:259.

797. Curshmann H: Über funikuläre Myelose bei hämolytischem Ikterus. Dtsch A Nervenheilkd 1931; 122:119.

798. Dumolard C, Sarrovy C, Portier A: Ataxie cerebelleuse assoc iée à un syndrome de splenomegalie chronique avec anemie. Bull Soc Med Hop (Paris) 1938; 54:71.

799. Lemaire A, Dumolard A, Portici A: Deux cas familiaux de maladie de Friedreich avec maladie hemolytique chez des indigenes Algeriens. Bull Soc Med Hop (Paris) 1937; 53:1084.

800. Michelazzi AM: Anemia emolitica familiare con sinomatoligia nervosa. Rass Fisiopat Clin Ter 1940; 12:145.

801. Percorella F: Sindrome neuroanemica in soggetto con ittero imolitico familiare. Riv Clin Pediatr 1946; 44:690.

802. Salmon H: Hämolytischer Ikterus und Degeneration der Hinterstränge. Med Klin 1914; 10:312c.

803. Spencer SE, Walker FO, Moore SA: Chorea-amyotrophy with chronic hemolytic anemia: A variant of chorea-amyotrophy with acanthocytosis. Neurology 1987; 37:645.

804. Peters LL, White RA, et al: Changes in cytoskeletal mRNA expression and protein synthesis during murine erythropoiesis in vivo. Proc Natl Acad Sci U S A 1992; 89:5749.

805. Peters LL, Turtzo C, et al: Distinct fetal Ank-1 and Ank-2 related proteins and mRNAs in normal and nb/nb mice. Blood 1993; 81:2144.

806. Anderson R, Huestis RR, Motulsky AG: Hereditary spherocytosis in the deer mouse. Its similarity to the human disease. Blood 1960; 15:491.

807. Falcone J, Lux SE: Unpublished observations, 1996.

808. LeBlond PF, De Boisfleury A, Bessis M: La forme des érythrocytes dans la sphérocytose héréditaire. Étude au microscope à balayage. Rélation avec déformabilité. Nouv Rev Fr Hématol 1973; 13:873.

809. Cooper RA, Jandl JH: The role of membrane lipids in the survival of red cells in hereditary spherocytosis. J Clin Invest 1969; 48:736.

810. Johnsson R: Red cell membrane proteins and lipids in spherocytosis. Scand J Haematol 1978; 20:341.

811. Langley GR, Feldherhof CH: Atypical autohemolysis in hereditary spherocytosis as a reflection of two cell populations: Relationship of cell lipids to conditioning by the spleen. Blood 1968; 32:569.

812. Reed CF, Swisher SN: Erythrocyte lipid loss in hereditary spherocytosis. J Clin Invest 1966; 45:777.

813. Waugh RE: Effects of inherited membrane abnormalities on the viscoelastic properties of erythrocyte membranes. Biophys J 1987; 51:363.

814. Cooper RA, Jandl JH: The selective and conjoint loss of red cell lipids. J Clin Invest 1969; 48:906.

815. Snyder LM, Lutz HU, et al: Fragmentation and myelin formation in hereditary xerocytosis and other hemolytic anemias. Blood 1978; 52:750.

816. Weed RI, Bowdler AJ: Metabolic dependence of the critical hemolytic volume of human erythrocytes: Relationship to osmotic fragility and autohemolysis in hereditary spherocytosis and normal red cells. J Clin Invest 1966; 45:1137.

817. Liu S-C, Derick LH, Duquette MA: Surface area density of membrane skeleton (MS) in normal red cells and severe hereditary spherocytosis (HS): Role in lipid bilayer destabilization. Blood 1988; 72(Suppl 1):31a. Abstract.

818. Zachée P, Boogaerts MA, et al: Adverse role of the spleen in hereditary spherocytosis: Evidence by the use of the atomic force microscope. Br J Haematol 1992; 80:264.

819. Miraglia del Giudice E, Perrotta S, et al: Hereditary spherocytosis characterized by increased spectrin/band 3 ratio. Br J Haematol 1990; 80:133. Letter.

820. Golan DE, Palek J, Agre PA: Red cell membrane spectrin content regulates band 3 and glycophorin lateral diffusion. Blood 1990; 76(Suppl 1):8a. Abstract.

821. Evans EA, Waugh R, Melnik C: Elastic area compressibility modulus of red cell membranes. Biophys J 1976; 16:585.

822. Baird R, McPherson AI, Richmond J: Red blood cell survival after splenectomy in congenital spherocytosis. Lancet 1971; 2:1060.

823. Chapman RG: Red cell life span after splenectomy in hereditary spherocytosis. J Clin Invest 1968; 47:2263.

824. Barnhart MI, Lusher JM: The human spleen as revealed by scanning electron microscopy. Am J Hematol 1976; 1:243.

825. Chen L-T, Weiss L: Electron microscopy of red pulp of human spleen. Am J Anat 1972; 134:425.

826. Chen L-T, Weiss L: The role of the sinus wall in the passage of erythrocytes through the spleen. Blood 1973; 41:529.

827. Weiss L, Tavassoli M: Anatomical hazards to the passage of erythrocytes through the spleen. Semin Hematol 1970; 7:372.

828. Weiss L: A scanning electron microscopic study of the spleen. Blood 1974; 43:665.

829. Groom AC: Microcirculation of the spleen: New concepts, new challenges. Microvasc Res 1987; 34:269.

830. Johnsson R, Vuopio P: Studies on red cell flexibility in spherocytosis using a polycarbonate membrane filtration method. Acta Haematol 1978; 60:329.

831. Murphy JR: The influence of pH and temperature on some physical properties of normal erythrocytes and erythrocytes from patients with hereditary spherocytosis. J Lab Clin Med 1967; 69:758.

832. Young LE, Platzer RF, et al: Hereditary spherocytosis: II. Observations on the role of the spleen. Blood 1951; 6:1099.

833. Ferreira JA, Feliu E, et al: Morphologic and morphometric light and electron microscopic studies of the spleen in patients with hereditary spherocytosis and autoimmune haemolytic anaemia. Br J Haematol 1989; 72:246.

834. Molnar Z, Rappaport H: Fine structure of the red pulp of the spleen in hereditary spherocytosis. Blood 1972; 39:81.

835. Wiland OK, Smith EB: The morphology of the spleen in congenital hemolytic anemia (hereditary spherocytosis). Am J Clin Pathol 1956; 26:619.

836. Fujita T, Kashimura M, Adachi K: Scanning electron microscopy (SEM) studies of the spleen-normal and pathological. Scand Electron Microsc 1982; 1:435.

837. Banti G: Splenomegalie hemolytique au hemopoietique: Le role de la rate dans l'hemolyse. Sémaine Méd 1913; 33:313.

838. MacAdam W, Shiskin C: The cholesterol content of the blood in anaemia and its relation to splenic function. Q J Med 1922; 16:193.

839. Emerson CP Jr, Shen SC, et al: Studies on the destruction of red blood cells: IX. Quantitative methods for determining the osmotic and mechanical fragility of red cells in the peripheral blood and splenic pulp; the mechanism of increased hemolysis in hereditary spherocytosis (congenital hemolytic jaundice) as related to the function of the spleen. Arch Intern Med 1956; 97:1.

840. Dacie JV: Familial haemolytic anaemia (acholuric jaundice), with particular reference to changes in fragility produced by splenectomy. Q J Med (New Series) 1943; 12:101.

841. Iolascon A, Miraglia del Giudice E, et al: Hereditary spherocytosis (HS) due to loss of anion exchange transporter. Haematologica 1992; 77:450.

842. Griggs RC, Weisman R Jr, Harris JW: Alterations in osmotic and mechanical fragility related to *in vivo* erythrocyte aging and splenic sequestration in hereditary spherocytosis. J Clin Invest 1960; 39:89.

843. MacPherson AIS, Richmond J, et al: The role of the spleen in congenital spherocytosis. Am J Med 1971; 50:35.

844. Jandl JH, Aster RH: Increased splenic pooling and the pathogenesis of hypersplenism. Am J Med Sci 1967; 253:383.

845. LaCelle PL: pH in the mouse spleen and its effect on erythrocyte flow properties. Blood 1974; 44(Suppl 1):910. Abstract.

846. Minakami S, Yoshikawa HL: Studies on erythrocyte glycolysis: III. The effects of active cation transport, pH and inorganic phosphate concentration on erythrocyte glycolysis. J Biochem (Tokyo) 1966; 59:145.

847. Rakitzis ET, Mills GC: Relation of red cell hexokinase activity to extracellular pH. Biochim Biophys Acta 1967; 141:439.

848. Parker JC: Ouabain-insensitive effects of metabolism on ion and water content in red blood cells. Am J Physiol 1971; 221:338.

849. Dacie JV: Observations on autohemolysis in familial acholuric jaundice. J Pathol Bacteriol 1941; 52:331.

850. Ferrant A, Leners N, et al: The spleen and haemolysis: Evaluation of the intrasplenic transit time. Br J Haematol 1987; 65:331.

851. Motulsky AG, Casserd F, et al: Anemia and the spleen. N Engl J Med 1958; 259:1164, 1212.

852. Prankerd TAJ: Studies on the pathogenesis of haemolysis in hereditary spherocytosis. Q J Med 1960; 24:199.

853. Maridonneau I, Braquet P, Garay RP: Na+ and K+ transport damage induced by oxygen free radicals in human red cell membranes. J Biol Chem 1983; 258:3107.

854. Orringer EP, Parker JC: Selective increase of potassium permeability in red blood cells exposed to acetylphenylhydrazine. Blood 1977; 50:1013.

855. Orringer EP: A further characterization of the selective K movements observed in human red blood cells following acetylphenylhydrazine exposure. Am J Hematol 1984; 16:355.

856. Sugihara T, Evans EA, Hebbel RP: Lipid hydroperoxides promote deformation-dependent leak of monovalent cation from erythrocytes. Blood 1990; 76(Suppl 1):18a. Abstract.

857. Wiater LA, Dunham PB: Passive transport of K+ and Na+ in human red blood cells: Sulfhydryl binding agents and furosemide. Am J Physiol 1983; 245:C348.

858. Becker PS, Cohen CM, Lux SE: The effect of mild diamide oxidation on the structure and function of human erythrocyte spectrin. J Biol Chem 1986; 261:4620.

859. Caprari P, Bozzi A, et al: Oxidative erythrocyte membrane damage in hereditary spherocytosis. Biochem Int 1992; 26:265.

860. Platt OS, Falcone JF: Membrane protein lesions in erythrocytes with Heinz bodies. J Clin Invest 1988; 82:1051.

861. Schwartz RS, Rybicki AC, et al: Protein 4.1 in sickle erythrocytes. Evidence for oxidative damage. J Biol Chem 1987; 62:15666.

862. Malorni W, Iosi F, et al: A new, striking morphologic feature for the human erythrocyte in hereditary spherocytosis: The blebbing pattern. Blood 1993; 81:2821. Letter.

863. De Matteis MC, De Angelis V, et al: Role of spleen in hereditary spherocytosis: Evidence for increased *in vitro* proteolysis of red cell membrane. Br J Haematol 1991; 79:108.

864. Szymanski IO, Odgren PR, et al: Red blood cell associated IgG in normal and pathologic states. Blood 1980; 55:48.

865. Coleman DH, Finch CA: Effect of adrenal steroids in hereditary spherocytic anemia. J Lab Clin Med 1956; 47:602.

866. Duru F, Gürgey A: Effect of corticosteriods in hereditary sphe-rocytosis. Acta Paediatr Jpn 1994; 36:666.

867. Atkinson JP, Schreiber AS, Frank MM: Effects of corticosteroids and splenectomy on the immune clearance and destruction of erythrocytes. J Clin Invest 1973; 52:1509.

868. Schreiber AD, Parsons J, et al: Effect of corticosteroids on the human monocyte IgG and complement receptors. J Clin Invest 1975; 56:1189.

869. Matsumoto N, Ishihara T, et al: Electron microscopic studies of the spleen and liver in hereditary spherocytosis. Acta Pathol Jpn 1973; 23:507.

870. Bowman HS, Oski FA: Splenic macrophage interaction with red cells in pyruvate kinase deficiency and hereditary sphero-cytosis. Vox Sang 1970; 19:168.

871. Friedman EW, Williams JC, Van Hook L: Hereditary spherocy-tosis in the elderly. Am J Med 1988; 84:513.

872. Krueger HC, Burgert EO Jr: Hereditary spherocytosis in 100 children. Mayo Clin Proc 1966; 41:821.

873. MacKinney AA Jr, Morton NE, et al: Ascertaining genetic carriers of hereditary spherocytosis by statistical analysis of multiple laboratory tests. J Clin Invest 1962; 41:554.

874. Young LE, Izzo MJ, Platzer RF: Hereditary spherocytosis: I. Clinical, hematologic and genetic features in 28 cases, with particular reference to the osmotic and mechanical fragility of incubated erythrocytes. Blood 1951; 6:1073.

875. Debre R, Lamy M, et al: Congenital and familial hemolytic disease in children. Am J Dis Child 1938; 56:1189.

876. Diamond LK: Indications for splenectomy in childhood: Re-sults in fifty-two operated cases. Am J Surg 1938; 39:400.

877. Jensson O, Jonasson JL, et al: Studies on hereditary spherocyto-sis in Iceland. Acta Med Scand 1977; 201:187.

878. Gehlbach SH, Cooper BA: Haemolytic anaemia in infectious mononucleosis due to inapparent congenital spherocytosis. Scand J Haematol 1970; 7:141.

879. Ho-Yen DO: Hereditary spherocytosis presenting in pregnancy. Acta Haematol (Basel) 1984; 72:29.

880. Pajor A, Lehoczky D, Szakacs Z: Pregnancy and hereditary spherocytosis: Report of 8 patients and a review. Arch Gynecol Obstet 1993; 253:37.

881. Godal HC, Refsum HE: Haemolysis in athletes due to heredi-tary spherocytosis. Scand J Haematol 1979; 22:83.

882. Garwicz S: Atypical spherocytosis, a disease of spleen as well as of red blood cells. Lancet 1975; 1:956.

883. Guarnone R, Centenara E, et al: Erythropoietin production and erythropoiesis in compensated and anaemic states of heredi-tary spherocytosis. Br J Haematol 1996; 92:150.

884. Eber SW, Pekrun A, et al: Decreased and increased membrane protein densities in severe recessive spherocytosis. Blood 1991; 78(Suppl 1):84. Abstract.

885. Wiley JS, Firkin BG: An unusual variant of hereditary sphero-cytosis. Am J Med 1970; 48:63.

886. Maberry MC, Mason RA, et al: Pregnancy complicated by hereditary spherocytosis. Obstet Gynecol 1992; 79:735.

887. Delamore IW, Richmond J, Davies SH: Megaloblastic anaemia in congenital spherocytosis. BMJ 1961; 1:543.

888. Kohler HG, Meynell MJ, Cooke WT: Spherocytic anaemia, complicated by megaloblastic anaemia of pregnancy. BMJ 1960; 1:779.

889. Burman D: Congenital spherocytosis in infancy. Arch Dis Child 1958; 33:335.

890. Schröter W, Kahsnitz E: Diagnosis of hereditary spherocytosis in newborn infants. J Pediatr 1983; 103:460.

891. Trucco JI, Brown AK: Neonatal manifestations of hereditary spherocytosis. Am J Dis Child 1967; 113:263.

892. Stamey CC, Diamond LK: Congenital hemolytic anemia in the newborn. Am J Dis Child 1957; 94:616.

893. Bergstrand CG, Czar B: Serum haptoglobin in infancy. J Clin Lab Invest 1961; 13:576.

894. Erlandson ME, Hilgartner M: Hemolytic disease in the neona-tal period and early infancy. J Pediatr 1959; 54:566.

895. LeBlond PF, LaCelle PL, Weed RI: Rhéologie des érythroblastes et des érythrocytes dans la sphérocytose congénital. Nouv Rev Fr Hématol 1971; 11:537.

896. Bell CM, Parker AC, Maddy AH: Abnormal pattern of erythro-cyte ageing in hereditary spherocytosis as shown by Percoll density gradient centrifugation. Clin Chim Acta 1984; 142:91.

897. Maizels M: The anion and cation content of normal and anae-mic bloods. Biochem J 1936; 30:821.

898. Selwyn JG, Dacie JV: Autohemolysis and other changes re-sulting from the incubation in vitro of red cells from patients with congenital hemolytic anemia. Blood 1954; 9:414.

899. Mohandas N, Kim YR, et al: Accurate and independent mea-surement of volume and hemoglobin concentration of individ-ual red cells by laser light scattering. Blood 1986; 68:506.

900. Gilsanz F, Ricard MP, Millan I: Diagnosis of hereditary sphero-cytosis with dual-angle differential light scattering. Am J Clin Pathol 1993; 100:119.

901. Pati AR, Patton WN, Harris RI: The use of the Technicon H1 in the diagnosis of hereditary spherocytosis. Clin Lab Haemat 1989; 11:27.

902. Parpart AK, Lorenz PB, et al: The osmotic resistance (fragility) of human red cells. J Clin Invest 1947; 26:636.

903. Godal HC, Nyvold N, Russtad A: The osmotic fragility of red blood cells: A re-evaluation of technical conditions. Scand J Haematol 1979; 23:55.

904. Young LE: Observations on inheritance and heterogeneity of chronic spherocytosis. Trans Assoc Am Phys 1955; 68:141.

905. Jacob HS: Hereditary spherocytosis: A disease of the red cell membrane. Semin Hematol 1965; 2:139.

906. Johnsson R, Salminen S: Effect of ouabain on osmotic resistance and monovalent cation transport of red cells in hereditary spherocytosis. Scand J Haematol 1980; 29:323.

907. Godal HC, Gjonnes G, Ruyter R: Does preincubation of the red blood cells contribute to the capacity of the osmotic fragil-ity test to detect very mild forms of hereditary spherocytosis? Scand J Haematol 1982; 29:89.

908. Judkiewicz L, Bartosz G, et al: Modified osmotic fragility test for the laboratory diagnosis of hereditary spherocytosis. Am J Hematol 1989; 31:136.

909. Clark MR, Mohandas N, Shohet SB: Osmotic gradient ektacy-tometry: Comprehensive characterization of red cell volume and surface maintenance. Blood 1983; 61:899.

910. Gottfried EL, Robertson NA: Glycerol lysis time of incubated erythrocytes in the diagnosis of hereditary spherocytosis. J Lab Clin Med 1974; 84:746.

911. Zanella A, Milani S, et al: Diagnostic value of the glycerol lysis test. J Lab Clin Med 1983; 102:743.

912. Zanella A, Izzo C, et al: Acidified glycerol lysis test: A screen-ing test for spherocytosis. Br J Haematol 1980; 45:481.

913. Rutherford CJ, Postlewaight BF, Hallowes M: An evaluation of the acidified glycerol lysis test. Br J Haematol 1986; 63:119.

914. Bucx MJ, Breed WP, Hoffman JJ: Comparison of acidified glyc-erol lysis test, Pink test and osmotic fragility test in hereditary spherocytosis: Effect of incubation. Eur J Haematol 1988; 40:227.

915. Hoffmann JJ, Swaak-Lammers N, et al: Diagnostic utility of the pre-incubated acidified glycerol lysis test in haemolytic and non-haemolytic anaemias. Eur J Haematol 1991; 47:367.

916. Marik T, Brabec V: Acidified glycerol lysis test in various haemolytic anaemias. Folia Haematol Int Mag Klin Morphol Blutforsch 1990; 117:259.

917. Vettore L, Zanella A, et al: A new test for the laboratory diagnosis of spherocytosis. Acta Haematol (Basel) 1984; 72:258.

918. Sureda-Balari A, Villarrvoia-Espinosa J, Fernandez-Fuertes I: A new modification of the 'Pink test' for the diagnosis of hereditary spherocytosis. Acta Haematol 1989; 82:213.

919. Pinto L, Iolascon A, et al: A modification of the 'Pink test' may improve the diagnosis of hereditary spherocytosis. Acta Haematol 1989; 82:53.

920. Streichman S, Gesheidt Y, Tatarsky I: Hypertonic cryohemo-lysis: A diagnostic test for hereditary spherocytosis. Am J Hematol 1990; 35:104.

921. Young LE, Izzo MJ, et al: Studies on spontaneous in vitro autohemolysis in hemolytic disorders. Blood 1956; 11:977.

922. Cutillo S, Pinto L, et al: Spectrin/band 3 ratio as diagnostic tool in hereditary spherocytosis. Eur J Pediatr 1992; 151:35.

923. Watson CJ: Studies of urobilinogen. III. The per diem excretion of urobilinogen in the common forms of jaundice and disease of the liver. Arch Intern Med 1937; 59:206.

924. Sears DA, Anderson RP, et al: Urinary iron excretion and renal metabolism of hemoglobin in hemolytic disease. Blood 1966; 28:708.

925. Muller-Eberhard U, Javid J, et al: Plasma concentrations of hemopexin, haptoglobin and heme in patients with various hemolytic diseases. Blood 1968; 32:811.

926. Gairdner D: The association of gall-stones with acholuric jaundice in children. Arch Dis Child 1939; 14:109.

927. Bates GC, Brown CH: Incidence of gallbladder disease in chronic hemolytic anemia (spherocytosis). Gastroenterology 1952; 21:104.

928. Lawrie GM, Ham JM: The surgical treatment of hereditary spherocytosis. Surg Gynecol Obstet 1974; 139:208.

929. MacKinney AA Jr: Hereditary spherocytosis. Clinical family studies. Arch Intern Med 1965; 116:257.

930. Young N: Hematologic and hematopoietic consequences of B19 parvovirus infection. Semin Hematol 1988; 25:159.

931. Owren PA: Congenital hemolytic jaundice. The pathogenesis of the hemolytic crisis. Blood 1948; 3:231.

932. Lefrére JJ, Courouce AM, et al: Human parvovirus and aplastic crisis in chronic hemolytic anemias: A study of 24 observations. Am J Hematol 1986; 23:271.

933. Mortimer PP, Humphries RK, et al: A human parvovirus-like virus inhibits haematopoietic colony formation *in vitro*. Nature 1983; 302:426.

934. Ozawa K, Kurtzman G, Young N: Replication of the B19 parvovirus in human bone marrow cell cultures. Science 1986; 233:883.

935. Hanada T, Koike K, et al: Human parvovirus B19-induced transient pancytopenia in a child with hereditary spherocytosis. Br J Haematol 1988; 70:113.

936. Saunders PW, Reid MM, Cohen BJ: Human parvovirus induced cytopenias: A report of five cases. Br J Haematol 1986; 53:407. Letter.

937. Anand A, Gray ES, et al: Human parvovirus infection in pregnancy and hydrops fetalis. N Engl J Med 1987; 316:183.

938. Anderson LJ, Hurwitz ES: Human parvovirus B19 and pregnancy. Clin Perinatol 1988; 15:273.

939. Leads from the MMWR. Risks associated with human parvovirus B19 infection. JAMA 1989; 261:1406.

940. Bell LM, Nasides SJ, et al: Human parvovirus B19 infection among hospital staff members after contact with infected patients. N Engl J Med 1989; 321:485.

941. Shneerson JM, Mortimer PP, Vandervelde EM: Febrile illness due to a parvovirus. BMJ 1980; 280:1580.

942. Schwarz TF, Roggendorf M, et al: Human parvovirus B19 infection in pregnancy. Lancet 1988; 2:566. Letter.

943. Robins MM: Familial crisis in hereditary spherocytosis: Report of six affected siblings. Clin Pediatr 1965; 4:210.

944. Ozawa K, Kurtzman G, Young N: Productive infection by B19 parvovirus of human erythroid bone marrow cells *in vitro*. Blood 1987; 70:384.

945. Lefrére JJ, Courouce A-M, et al: Six cases of hereditary spherocytosis revealed by human parvovirus infection. Br J Haematol 1986; 62:653.

946. McLellan NJ, Rutter N: Hereditary spherocytosis in sisters unmasked by parvovirus infection. Postgrad Med J 1987; 63:49.

947. Stefanelli M, Barosi G, et al: Quantitative assessment of erythropoiesis in haemolytic disease. Br J Haematol 1980; 45:297.

948. Tileston W: Hemolytic jaundice. Medicine 1922; 1:355.

949. Hanford RB, Schneider GF, MacCarthy JD: Massive thoracic extramedullary hemopoiesis. N Engl J Med 1960; 263:120.

950. Lawrence P, Aronson I, et al: Leg ulcers in hereditary spherocytosis. Clin Exp Dermatol 1991; 16:28.

951. Vanscheidt W, Leder O, et al: Leg ulcers in a patient with spherocytosis: A clinicopathological report. Dermatologica 1990; 181:56.

952. Beinhauer LG, Gruhn JG: Dermatologic aspects of congenital spherocytic anemia. Arch Dermatol 1957; 75:642.

953. Abe T, Yachi A, et al: Thoracic extramedullary hematopoiesis associated with hereditary spherocytosis. Intern Med 1992; 31:1151.

954. Bastion Y, Coiffier B, et al: Massive mediastinal extramedullary hematopoiesis in hereditary spherocytosis: A case report. Am J Hematol 1990; 35:263.

955. Martin J, Palacio A, et al: Fatty transformation of thoracic extramedullary hematopoiesis following splenectomy: CT features. J Comput Assist Tomogr 1990; 14:477.

956. Pulsoni A, Ferrazza G, et al: Mediastinal extramedullary hematopoiesis as first manifestation of hereditary spherocytosis [clinical conference]. Ann Hematol 1992; 65:196.

957. Pietsch B, Sigmund G, Wurtemberger G: Kernspintomographische Befunde der kompensierten chronischen Hamolyse. Fallbericht uber eine hereditare Spharozytose. Aktuelle Radiol 1993; 3:266.

958. Schafer AI, Miller JB, et al: Monoclonal gammopathy in hereditary spherocytosis: A possible pathogenic relation. Ann Intern Med 1978; 88:45.

959. Fukata S, Tamai H, et al: A patient with hereditary spherocytosis and silicosis who developed an IgA (lambda) monoclonal gammopathy. Jpn J Med 1987; 26:81.

960. Lempert KD: Gammopathy and spherocytosis. Ann Intern Med 1978; 89:145.

961. Jandl JH, Files NM, et al: Proliferative response of the spleen and liver to hemolysis. J Exp Med 1965; 122:299.

962. Schilling RF: Hereditary spherocytosis; a study of splenectomized persons. Semin Hematol 1976; 13:169.

963. Isobe T, Osserman EF: Pathologic conditions associated with plasma cell dyscrasias: A study of 806 cases. Ann NY Acad Sci 1971; 190:507.

964. Blacklock HA, Meerkin M: Serum ferritin in patients with hereditary spherocytosis. Br J Haematol 1981; 49:117.

965. Edwards CQ, Skolnick MH, et al: Iron overload in hereditary spherocytosis: Association with HLA-linked hemochromatosis. Am J Hematol 1982; 13:101.

966. Fargion S, Cappellini MD, et al: Association of hereditary spherocytosis and idiopathic hemochromatosis: A synergistic effect in determining iron overload. Am J Clin Pathol 1986; 86:645.

967. Mohler DN, Wheby MS: Hemochromatosis heterozygotes may have significant iron overload when they also have hereditary spherocytosis. Am J Med Sci 1986; 292:320.

968. Morita M, Hashizume M, et al: Hereditary spherocytosis with congestive heart failure: Report of a case. Surg Today 1993; 23:458.

969. Clarkson JG, Altman RD: Angioid streaks. Surv Ophthalmol 1982; 26:235.

970. McLane NJ, Grizzard WS, et al: Angioid streaks associated with hereditary spherocytosis. Am J Ophthalmol 1984; 97:444.

971. Gibson JM, Chaudhuri PR, Rosenthal AR: Angioid streaks in a case of beta thalassemia major. Br J Ophthalmol 1983; 67:29.

972. Deutman AF, Kovacs B: Argon laser treatment in complications of angioid streaks. Am J Ophthalmol 1979; 88:12.

973. Gilliland BC, Baxter E, Evans RS: Red cell antibodies in acquired hemolytic anemia with negative antiglobulin serum tests. N Engl J Med 1971; 85:252.

974. Crosby WH, Conrad ME: Hereditary spherocytosis: Observations on hemolytic mechanisms and iron metabolism. Blood 1960; 15:662.

975. Pautard B, Féo C, et al: Occurrence of hereditary spherocytosis and β thalassemia in the same family: Globin chain synthesis and viscodiffractometric studies. Br J Haematol 1988; 70:239.

976. Blecher TE: What happens to the microspherocytosis of hereditary spherocytosis in folate deficiency? Clin Lab Haemat 1988; 10:403.

977. Warkentin TE, Barr RD, et al: Recurrent acute splenic sequestration crisis due to interacting genetic defects: Hemoglobin SC disease and hereditary spherocytosis. Blood 1990; 75:266.

978. Aksoy M, Erdem S: The combination of hereditary spherocytosis and heterozygous beta-thalassaemia: A family study. Acta Haematol 1968; 39:183.

979. White BP, Farver M: Coexistence of hereditary spherocytosis and beta-thalassemia: Case report of severe hemolytic anemia in an American black. S D J Med 1991; 44:257.

980. Miraglia del Giudice E, Perrotta S, et al: Coexistence of hereditary spherocytosis (HS) due to band 3 deficiency and beta-thalassaemia trait: Partial correction of HS phenotype. Br J Haematol 1993; 85:553.

981. Yang YM, Donnell C, et al: Splenic sequestration associated with sickle cell trait and hereditary spherocytosis. Am J Hematol 1992; 40:110.

982. Babiker MA, El Seed FA: A family with sickle cell trait and hereditary spherocytosis. Scand J Haematol 1984; 33:54.

983. Moiseyev VS, Korovina EA, et al: Hypertrophic cardiomyopathy associated with hereditary spherocytosis in three generations of one family. Lancet 1987; 2:853. Letter.

984. Eraklis AJ, Filler RM: Splenectomy in childhood: A review of 1413 cases. J Pediatr Surg 1972; 7:382.

985. Heier HE: Splenectomy and serious infection. Scand J Haematol 1980; 24:5.

986. Eraklis AJ, Kevy SV, et al: Hazard of overwhelming infection after splenectomy in childhood. N Engl J Med 1967; 276:1225.

987. Green JB, Shackford SR, et al: Late septic complications in adults following splenectomy for trauma: A prospective analysis in 144 patients. J Trauma 1986; 26:999.

988. Evans DI: Postsplenectomy sepsis 10 years or more after operation. J Clin Pathol 1985; 38:309.

989. Holdsworth RJ, Irving AD, Cuschieri A: Postsplenectomy sepsis and its mortality rate: Actual versus perceived risks. Br J Surg 1991; 78:1031.

990. Krivit W: Overwhelming post-splenectomy infection. Am J Hematol 1977; 2:193.

991. Schwartz PE, Sterioff S, et al: Postsplenectomy sepsis and mortality in adults. JAMA 1982; 248:2279.

992. Singer DB: Postsplenectomy sepsis. In Rosenberg HS, Bolande RP (eds): Perspectives in Pediatric Pathology. Vol. I. Chicago, Year Book Medical Publishers, 1973, p 285.

993. Schilling RF: Estimating the risk for sepsis after splenectomy in hereditary spherocytosis. Ann Intern Med 1995; 122:187.

994. Konradsen HB, Henrichsen J: Pneumococcal infections in splenectomized children are preventable. Acta Pediatr Scand 1991; 80:423.

995. Brivet F, Herer B, et al: Fatal postsplenectomy pneumococcal sepsis despite pneumococcal vaccine and penicillin prophylaxis. Lancet 1984; 1:356. Letter.

996. Buchanan GR, Smith SJ: Pneumococcal septicemia despite pneumococcal vaccine and prescription of penicillin prophylaxis in patients with sickle cell anemia. Am J Dis Child 1986; 140:428.

997. Gonzaga RA: Fatal post-splenectomy pneumococcal sepsis despite prophylaxis. Lancet 1984; 2:694.

998. Wong WY, Overturf GD, Powers DR: Infection caused by *Streptococcus pneumoniae* in children with sickle cell disease: Epidemiology, immunologic mechanisms, prophylaxis and vaccination. Clin Infect Dis 1992; 14:1124.

999. Buchanan GR, Siegel JD, et al: Oral penicillin prophylaxis in children with impaired splenic function: A study of compliance. Pediatrics 1982; 70:926.

1000. Caputo GM, Appelbaum PC, Liu HH: Infections due to penicillin-resistant pneumococci. Clinical, epidemiologic, and microbiologic features. Arch Intern Med 1993; 153:1301.

1001. Musher DM: Pneumococcal pneumonia including diagnosis and therapy of infection caused by penicillin resistant strains. Infect Dis Clin North Am 1991; 5:509.

1002. Chesney PJ: The escalating problem of antimicrobial resistance in *Streptococcus pneumoniae*. Am J Dis Child 1992; 146:912.

1003. Marton A, Gulyas M, et al: Extremely high incidence of antibiotic resistance in clinical isolates of *Streptococcus pneumoniae* in Hungary. J Infect Dis 1991; 163:542.

1004. Spika JS, Facklam RR, et al: Antimicrobial resistance of *Streptococcus pneumoniae* in the United States, 1979–1987. The Pneumococcal Surveillance Working Group. J Infect Dis 1991; 163:1273.

1005. Friedland IR, McCracken GH Jr: Management of infections caused by antibiotic-resistant *Streptococcus pneumoniae*. N Engl J Med 1994; 331:377.

1006. Wong WY, Powars DR, Hiti AL: Multi-drug resistance to *Streptococcus pneumoniae* in sickle cell anemia. Am J Hematol 1995; 48:278.

1007. Steele RW, Warrier R, et al: Colonization with antibiotic-resistant *Streptococcus pneumoniae* in children with sickle cell disease. J Pediatr 1996; 128:531.

1008. Golightly LM, Hirschhorn LR, Weller PF: Infectious disease rounds: Fever and headache in a splenectomized woman. Rev Infect Dis 1989; 11:629.

1009. Mathewson HO: Self-limited babesiosis in a splenectomized child. Pediatr Infect Dis 1984; 3:148.

1010. Rosner F, Zarrabi MH, et al: Babesiosis in splenectomized adults: Review of 22 reported cases. Am J Med 1984; 76:696.

1011. Teutsch S, Etkind P, et al: Babesiosis in post-splenectomy hosts. Am J Trop Med Hyg 1980; 29:738.

1012. Robinette CD, Fraumeni JF Jr: Splenectomy and subsequent mortality in veterans of the 1939–45 war. Lancet 1977; 2:127.

1013. Gokcora IH, Ormeci N, et al: Treatment of biliary fistulas and cholelithiasis: Is endoscopic sphincterotomy acceptable in the paediatric age group? Int Surg 1989; 74:51.

1014. Holcomb GW III, Olsen DO, Sharp KW: Laparoscopic cholecystectomy in the pediatric patient. J Pediatr Surg 1991; 26:1186.

1015. Sackmann M, Delius M, et al: Shock wave lithotripsy of gallbladder stones. The first 175 patients. N Engl J Med 1988; 318:393.

1016. Pappis CH, Galanakis S, et al: Experience of splenectomy and cholecystectomy in children with chronic haemolytic anaemia. J Pediatr Surg 1989; 24:543.

1017. Lobe TE, Presbury GJ, et al: Laparascopic splenectomy. Pediatr Ann 1993; 22:671.

1018. Trias M, Taragarona EM, et al: Laparoscopic splenectomy: Technical aspects and preliminary results. Endosc Surg Allied Technol 1994; 2:288.

1019. Smith BM, Schropp KP, et al: Laparoscopic splenectomy in childhood. J Pediatr Surg 1994; 29:975.

1020. Yee JC, Akpata MO: Laparoscopic splenectomy for congenital spherocytosis with splenomegaly: A case report. Can J Surg 1995; 38:73.

1021. Poulin EC, Thibault C: Laparoscopic splenectomy for massive splenomegaly: Operative technique and case report. Can J Surg 1995; 38:69.

1022. Farah RA, Rogers ZR, et al: Laparoscopic splenectomy in children with hematologic disorders. Blood 1995; 86(Suppl 1):135a. Abstract.

1023. Liew SC, Storey DW: Laparoscopic splenectomy. Aust N Z J Surg 1995; 65:743.

1024. Silvestri F, Russo D, et al: Laparoscopic splenectomy in the management of hematological diseases. Haematologica 1995; 80:47.

1025. Yoshida K, Yamazaki Y, et al: Laparoscopic splenectomy in children. Preliminary results and comparison with the open technique. Surg Endosc 1995; 9:1279.

1026. Gigot JF, de Ville de Goyet J, et al: Laparoscopic splenectomy in adults and children: Experience with 31 patients. Surgery 1996; 119:384.

1027. Tchernia G, Gauthier F, et al: Initial assessment of the beneficial effect of partial splenectomy in hereditary spherocytosis. Blood 1993; 81:2014.

1028. Bart JB, Appel MF: Recurrent hemolytic anemia secondary to accessory spleens. South Med J 1978; 71:608.

1029. MacKenzie FA, Elliot DH, et al: Relapse in hereditary spherocytosis with proven splenunculus. Lancet 1962; 1:1102.

1030. Jimenez M, Azcona C, et al: Partial splenic embolization in a child with hereditary spherocytosis. Eur J Pediatr 1995; 154:501. Letter.

1031. Atkinson W, Furphy L, et al (eds): Pneumococcal disease. In: Epidemiology and Prevention of Vaccine-Preventable Diseases. 3rd ed. Atlanta, Centers for Disease Control and Prevention, 1996, p 175.

1032. De Haan LD, Werre JM, et al: Alterations in size, shape and osmotic behaviour of red cells after splenectomy: A study of their age dependence. Br J Haematol 1988; 69:71.

1033. Brook J, Tanaka KR: Combination of pyruvate kinase (PK) deficiency and hereditary spherocytosis (HS). Clin Res 1970; 18:176A. Abstract.

1034. Valentine WN: Hereditary spherocytosis revisited. West J Med 1978; 128:35.

1035. Rutkow IM: Twenty years of splenectomy for hereditary spherocytosis. Arch Surg 1981; 116:306.

1036. Buchanan GR, Holtkamp CA: Pocked erythrocyte counts in patients with hereditary spherocytosis before and after splenectomy. Am J Hematol 1987; 25:253.

1037. Kvindesdal BB, Jensen MK: Pitted erythrocytes in splenectomized subjects with congenital spherocytosis and in subjects splenectomized for other reasons. Scand J Haematol 1986; 37:41.

1038. Satou S, Yokota E, et al: Relapse of hereditary spherocytosis following splenectomy. Acta Haematol Jpn 1985; 48:1337.

1039. Dresbach M: Elliptical human red corpuscles. Science 1904; 19:469.
1040. Flint A: Elliptical human erythrocytes. Science 1904; 19:796.
1041. Dresbach M: Elliptical human erythrocytes. Science 1905; 21:473.
1042. Bishop FW: Elliptical human erythrocytes. Arch Intern Med 1914; 14:388.
1043. Huck JG, Bigelow RM: Poikilocytes in otherwise normal blood (elliptical human erythrocytes). Bull Johns Hopkins Hosp 1923; 34:390.
1044. Hunter WC, Adams RB: Hematologic study of three generations of a white family showing elliptical erythrocytes. Ann Intern Med 1929; 2:1162.
1045. Hunter WC: Further study of a white family showing elliptical erythrocytes. Ann Intern Med 1932; 6:775.
1046. Giffin HZ, Watkins CH: Ovalocytosis with features of hemolytic icterus. Trans Assoc Am Physicians 1939; 54:355.
1047. Penfold J, Lipscomb JM: Elliptocytosis in man, associated with hereditary haemorrhagic telangiectasis. Q J Med 1943; 12:157.
1048. Wyandt H, Bancroft PM, Winship TO: Elliptic erythrocytes in man. Arch Intern Med 1941; 68:1043.
1049. Wolman IJ, Ozge A: Studies on elliptocytosis. I. Hereditary elliptocytosis in the pediatric age period: A review of recent literature. Am J Med Sci 1957; 234:702.
1050. Dacie JV: The lifespan of the red blood cell and circumstances of its premature death. In Wintrobe MM (ed): Blood, Pure and Eloquent. New York, McGraw-Hill Book Co., 1980, p 210.
1051. McCarty SH: Elliptical red blood cells in man. A report of eleven cases. J Lab Clin Med 1934; 19:612.
1052. Glele-Kakai C, Garbarz M, et al: Epidemiological studies of spectrin mutations related to hereditary elliptocytosis and spectrin polymorphisms in Benin. Br J Haematol 1996; 95:57.
1053. Lecomte MC, Dhermy D, et al: L'elliptocytose hereditaire en Afrique de l'Ouest: Frequence et repartition des variants de la spectrine. C R Acad Sci Paris 1988; 306:43.
1054. Ganesan J, George R, Lie-Injo LE: Abnormal haemoglobins and hereditary ovalocytosis in the Ulu Jempul district of Kuala Pilah, West Malaysia. Southeast Asian J Trop Med Public Health 1976; 7:430.
1055. Tse WT, Lecomte MC, et al: Point mutation in the β-spectrin gene associated with $\alpha^{1/74}$ hereditary elliptocytosis. Implications for the mechanism of spectrin dimer self-association. J Clin Invest 1990; 86:909.
1056. Lawler J, Liu S-C, et al: Molecular defect of spectrin in hereditary pyropoikilocytosis: Alterations in the trypsin resistant domain involved in spectrin self-association. J Clin Invest 1982; 70:1019.
1057. Dalla Venezia N, Wilmotte R, et al: An α-spectrin mutation responsible for hereditary elliptocytosis associated in *cis* with the $\alpha^{V/41}$ polymorphism. Hum Genet 1993; 90:641.
1058. Mentzer WC, Turetsky T, et al: Identification of the hereditary pyropoikilocytosis carrier state. Blood 1984; 63:1439.
1059. Palek J, Lux SE: Red cell membrane skeletal defects in hereditary and acquired hemolytic anemias. Semin Hematol 1983; 20:189.
1060. Palek J: Hereditary elliptocytosis and related disorders. Clin Haematol 1985; 14:45.
1061. Palek J: Hereditary elliptocytosis, spherocytosis and related disorders: Consequences of a deficiency or a mutation of membrane skeletal proteins. Blood Rev 1987; 1:147.
1062. Tchernia G, Mohandas N, Shohet SB: Deficiency of cytoskeletal membrane protein band 4.1 in homozygous hereditary elliptocytosis: Implications for erythrocyte membrane stability. J Clin Invest 1981; 68:454.
1063. Morlé L, Alloisio N, et al: Spectrin Tunis ($\alpha^{1/78}$), a new α^I variant that causes asymptomatic hereditary elliptocytosis in the heterozygous state. Blood 1988; 71:508.
1064. Morlé L, Morlé F, et al: Spectrin Tunis (Sp $\alpha^{1/78}$), an elliptocytogenic variant, is due to the CGG→TGG codon change (Arg→Trp) at position 35 of the α^I domain. Blood 1989; 75:828.
1065. Lecomte MC, Dhermy D, et al: Hereditary elliptocytosis with spectrin molecular defect in a white patient. Acta Haematol (Basel) 1984; 71:235.
1066. Alloisio N, Guetorni D, et al: Sp $\alpha^{1/65}$ hereditary elliptocytosis in North Africa. Am J Hematol 1986; 23:113.
1067. Guetarni D, Roux A-F, et al: Evidence that expression of Sp $\alpha^{1/65}$ hereditary elliptocytosis is compounded by a genetic factor that is linked to the homologous α-spectrin allele. Hum Genet 1990; 85:627.
1068. Marchesi SL, Knowles WT, et al: Abnormal spectrin in hereditary elliptocytosis. Blood 1986; 67:141.
1069. Feddal S, Brunet G, et al: Molecular analysis of hereditary elliptocytosis with reduced protein 4.1 in the French Northern Alps. Blood 1991; 78:2113.
1070. Lambert S, Zail S: Partial deficiency of protein 4.1 in hereditary elliptocytosis. Am J Hematol 1987; 26:263.
1071. McGuire M, Smith BL, Agre P: Distinct variants of erythrocyte protein 4.1 inherited in linkage with elliptocytosis and Rh type in three white families. Blood 1988; 72:287.
1072. Florman AL, Wintrobe MM: Human elliptical red corpuscles. Bull Johns Hopkins Hosp 1938; 63:209.
1073. Garrdo-Lacca G, Merino C, Luna G: Hereditary elliptocytosis in a Peruvian family. N Engl J Med 1957; 256:311.
1074. Geerdink RA, Helleman PW, Verloop MC: Hereditary elliptocytosis and hyperhaemolysis: A comparative study of 6 families with 145 patients. Acta Med Scand 1966; 179:715.
1075. Jensson O, Jonasson TH, Olafsson O: Hereditary elliptocytosis in Iceland. Br J Haematol 1967; 13:844.
1076. Motulsky AG, Singer K, et al: The life span of the elliptocyte: Hereditary elliptocytosis and its relationship to other familial hemolytic diseases. Blood 1954; 9:57.
1077. Pothier B, Alloisio N, et al: Assignment of spectrin alpha$^{1/74}$ hereditary elliptocytosis to the alpha or beta chain of spectrin through *in vitro* dimer reconstitution. Blood 1990; 75:2001.
1078. Coetzer T, Lawler J, et al: Molecular determinants of clinical expression of hereditary elliptocytosis and pyropoikilocytosis. Blood 1987; 70:766.
1079. Rummens JL, Verfaillie C, et al: Elliptocytosis and schistocytosis in myelodysplasia: Report of two cases. Acta Haematol 1986; 75:174.
1080. Coetzer T, Sahr K, et al: Four different mutations in codon 28 of α spectrin are associated with structurally and functionally abnormal spectrin $\alpha^{1/74}$ in hereditary elliptocytosis. J Clin Invest 1991; 88:743.
1081. Garbarz M, Lecomte MC, et al: Hereditary pyropoikilocytosis and elliptocytosis in a white French family with the spectrin $\alpha^{1/74}$ variant related to a CGT→CAT codon change (Arg→His) at position 22 of the spectrin α I domain. Blood 1990; 75:1691.
1082. Lawler J, Liu S-C, et al: Molecular defect of spectrin in a subgroup of patients with hereditary elliptocytosis: Alteration in the alpha subunit involved in spectrin self association. J Clin Invest 1984; 73:1688.
1083. Lecomte MC, Féo C, et al: Severe hereditary elliptocytosis in two related Caucasian children with a decreased amount of spectrin (Sp) α chain. J Cell Biochem 1989; 13B:230. Abstract.
1084. Baklouti F, Maréchal J, et al: Occurrence of the αI 22 Arg→His (CGT→CAT) spectrin mutation in Tunisia: Potential association with severe elliptocytosis. Br J Haematol 1991; 78:108.
1085. Baklouti F, Maréchal J, et al: Elliptocytogenic $\alpha^{1/36}$ spectrin Sfax lacks nine amino acids in helix 3 of repeat 4. Evidence for the activation of a cryptic 5'-splice site in exon 8 of spectrin α-gene. Blood 1992; 79:2464.
1086. Dalla Venezia N, Alloisio N, et al: Elliptopoikilocytosis associated with the α69 His→Pro mutation in Spectrin Barcelona ($\alpha^{1/50-46b}$). Blood 1993; 82:1661.
1087. Alloisio N, Morlé L, et al: Sp $\alpha^{V/41}$: A common spectrin polymorphism at the α^{IV}-α^V domain junction. Relevance to the expression level of hereditary elliptocytosis due to α-spectrin variants located in *trans*. J Clin Invest 1991; 87:2169.
1088. Coetzer T, Palek J, et al: Structural and functional heterogeneity of α spectrin mutations involving the spectrin heterodimer self-association site: Relationships to hematologic expression of homozygous hereditary elliptocytosis and hereditary pyropoikilocytosis. Blood 1990; 75:2235.
1089. Randon J, Boulanger L, et al: A variant of spectrin low expression allele alpha^{LELY} carrying a hereditary elliptocytosis mutation in codon 28. Br J Haematol 1994; 88:534.
1090. Ozer L, Mills GC: Elliptocytosis with haemolytic anaemia. Br J Haematol 1964; 10:468.
1091. Kruetrachuo M, Asawapokee N: Hereditary elliptocytosis and

Plasmodium falciparum malaria. Ann Trop Med Parasitol 1972; 66:161.

1092. Nkrumah FK: Hereditary elliptocytosis associated with severe haemolytic anaemia and malaria. Afr J Med Sci 1972; 3:131.

1093. Jarolim P, Palek J, et al: Severe hemolysis and red cell fragmentation due to a combination of a spectrin mutation with a thrombotic microangiopathy. Am J Hematol 1989; 32:50.

1094. Schoomaker EB, Butler WM, Diehl LF: Increased heat sensitivity of red blood cells in hereditary elliptocytosis with acquired cobalamin (vitamin B_{12}) deficiency. Blood 1982; 59:1213.

1095. Lecomte MC, Garbarz M, et al: Sp $\alpha^{I/78}$: A mutation of the α I spectrin domain in a white kindred with HE and HPP phenotypes. Blood 1989; 74:1126.

1096. Lane PA, Shew RL, et al: Unique α-spectrin mutant in a kindred with common hereditary elliptocytosis. J Clin Invest 1987; 79:989.

1097. Austin RF, Desforges JF: Hereditary elliptocytosis: An unusual presentation of hemolysis in the newborn associated with transient morphologic abnormalities. Pediatrics 1969; 44:196.

1098. Carpentieri U, Gustavson LP, Haggard ME: Pyknocytosis in a neonate: An unusual presentation of hereditary elliptocytosis. Clin Pediatr 1977; 16:76.

1099. Josephs HW, Avery ME: Hereditary elliptocytosis associated with increased hemolysis. Pediatrics 1965; 16:741.

1100. Zarkowsky HS: Heat-induced erythrocyte fragmentation in neonatal elliptocytosis. Br J Haematol 1979; 41:515.

1101. Prchal JT, Castleberry RP, et al: Hereditary pyropoikilocytosis and elliptocytosis: Clinical, laboratory, and ultrastructural features in infants and children. Pediatr Res 1982; 16:484.

1102. Torlontano G, Fioritoni G, Salvati AM: Hereditary haemolytic ovalocytosis with defective erythropoiesis. Br J Haematol 1979; 43:435.

1103. Jankovic M, Sansone G, et al: Atypical hereditary ovalocytosis associated with defective dyserythropoietic anemia. Acta Haematol 1993; 89:35.

1104. Dhermy D, Lecomte MC, et al: Molecular defect of spectrin in the family of a child with congenital hemolytic poikilocytic anemia. Pediatr Res 1984; 18:1005.

1105. Garbarz M, Lecomte MC, et al: Double inheritance of an $\alpha^{I/65}$ spectrin variant in a child with homozygous elliptocytosis. Blood 1986; 67:1661.

1106. Lawler J, Coetzer TL, et al: Spectrin $\alpha^{I/61}$: A new structural variant of α spectrin in a double heterozygous form of hereditary pyropoikilocytosis. Blood 1988; 72:1412.

1107. Alloisio N, Morlé L, et al: Spectrin Oran ($\alpha^{II/21}$), a new spectrin variant concerning the α^{II} domain and causing severe elliptocytosis in the homozygous state. Blood 1988; 71:1039.

1108. Lecomte MC, Féo C, et al: Severe recessive poikilocytic anemia with a new spectrin α chain variant. Br J Haematol 1990; 74:497.

1109. Dalla Venezia N, Gilsanz F, et al: Homozygous 4.1 ($-$) hereditary elliptocytosis associated with a point mutation in the downstream initiation codon of protein 4.1 gene. J Clin Invest 1992; 90:1713.

1110. Alloisio N, Wilmotte R, et al: A splice site mutation of alpha-spectrin gene causing skipping of exon 18 in hereditary elliptocytosis. Blood 1993; 81:2791.

1111. Grech JL, Cachia EA, et al: Hereditary elliptocytosis in two Maltese families. J Clin Pathol 1961; 14:365.

1112. Haddy TB, Rana SR: Homozygous hereditary elliptocytosis with hemolytic anemia. South Med J 1984; 77:631.

1113. Iarocci TA, Wagner GM, et al: Hereditary poikilocytic anemia associated with the coinheritance of two α spectrin abnormalities. Blood 1988; 71:1390.

1114. Lipton EL: Elliptocytosis with hemolytic anemia: the effects of splenectomy. Pediatrics 1955; 15:67.

1115. Nielsen JA, Strunk KW: Homozygous hereditary elliptocytosis as a cause of haemolytic anaemia in infancy. Scand J Haematol 1968; 5:486.

1116. Pryor DS, Pitney WR: Hereditary elliptocytosis: A report of two families from New Guinea. Br J Haematol 1967; 13:126.

1117. Dhermy D, Garbarz M, et al: Hereditary elliptocytosis: Clinical, morphological, and biochemical studies of 38 cases. Nouv Rev Fr Hématol 1986; 28:129.

1118. Floyd PB, Gallagher PG, et al: Heterogeneity in the molecular basis of hereditary pyropoikilocytosis and hereditary elliptocytosis associated with increased levels of the spectrin $\alpha^{I/74}$-kilodalton tryptic peptide. Blood 1991; 78:1364.

1119. Dacie JV, Mollison PL, et al: Atypical congenital haemolytic anaemia. Q J Med 1953; 22:79.

1120. Wiley JS, Gill FM: Red cell calcium leak in congenital hemolytic anemia with extreme microcytosis. Blood 1976; 47:197.

1121. Zarkowsky HS, Mohandas N, et al: A congenital haemolytic anaemia with thermal sensitivity of the erythrocyte membrane. Br J Haematol 1975; 29:537.

1122. DePalma L, Luban NL: Hereditary pyropoikilocytosis: Clinical and laboratory analysis in eight infants and young children. Am J Dis Child 1993; 147:93.

1123. Coetzer T, Palek J: Partial spectrin deficiency in hereditary pyropoikilocytosis. Blood 1986; 59:919.

1124. Cutting HO, McHugh WJ, et al: Autosomal dominant hemolytic anemia characterized by ovalocytosis: A family study of seven involved members. Am J Med 1965; 39:21.

1125. Dacie JV: Hereditary elliptocytosis (HE). In: The Haemolytic Anaemias. 3rd ed. Vol. I. Edinburgh, Churchill Livingstone, 1985, p 216.

1126. Greenberg LH, Tanaka KR: Hereditary elliptocytosis with hemolytic anemia—a family study of five affected members. Calif Med 1969; 110:389.

1127. Weiss HJ: Hereditary elliptocytosis with hemolytic anemia. Am J Med 1963; 35:455.

1128. Matsumoto N, Ishihara T, et al: Fine structure of the spleen in hereditary elliptocytosis. Acta Pathol Jpn 1976; 26:533.

1129. Wilson HE, Long MJ: Hereditary ovalocytosis (elliptocytosis) with hypersplenism. Arch Intern Med 1955, 95:438.

1130. Garbarz M, Tse WT, et al: Spectrin Rouen (β220-218), a novel shortened β-chain variant in a kindred with hereditary elliptocytosis. Characterization of the molecular defect as exon skipping due to a splice site mutation. J Clin Invest 1991; 88:76.

1131. Lecomte MC, Gautero H, et al: Elliptocytosis-associated spectrin Rouen ($\beta^{220/218}$) has a truncated but still phosphorylatable beta-chain. Br J Haematol 1992; 80:242.

1132. Pothier B, Morlé L, et al: Spectrin Nice ($\beta^{220/216}$): A shortened β chain variant associated with an increase of the $\alpha^{I/74}$ fragment in a case of elliptocytosis. Blood 1987; 69:1759.

1133. Tse WT, Gallagher PG, et al: An insertional frameshift mutation of the beta-spectrin gene associated with elliptocytosis in spectrin Nice ($\beta^{220/216}$). Blood 1991; 78:517.

1134. Garbarz M, Boulanger L, et al: Spectrin β^{Tandil}, a novel shortened β-chain variant associated with hereditary elliptocytosis is due to a deletional frameshift mutation in the β-spectrin gene. Blood 1992; 80:1066.

1135. Eber SW, Morris SA, et al: Interactions of spectrin in hereditary elliptocytes containing truncated spectrin β-chains. J Clin Invest 1988; 81:523.

1136. Yoon SH, Yu H, et al: Molecular defect of truncated β-spectrin associated with hereditary elliptocytosis. β-spectrin Göttingen. J Biol Chem 1991; 266:8490.

1137. Dhermy D, Lecomte MC, et al: Spectrin beta-chain variant associated with hereditary elliptocytosis. J Clin Invest 1982; 70:707.

1138. Gallagher PG, Tse WT, et al: A splice site mutation of the β-spectrin gene causing exon skipping in hereditary elliptocytosis associated with a truncated β-spectrin chain. J Biol Chem 1991; 266:15154.

1139. Ohanian V, Evans JP, Gratzer WB: A case of elliptocytosis associated with a truncated spectrin chain. Br J Haematol 1985; 61:31.

1140. Dahr W, Moulds J, et al: Altered membrane sialoglycoproteins in human erythrocytes lacking the Gerbich blood group antigen. Biol Chem Hoppe Seyler 1985; 366:201.

1141. Daniels GL, Reid ME, et al: Transient reduction in erythrocyte membrane sialoglycoprotein β associated with the presence of elliptocytes. Br J Haematol 1988; 70:477.

1142. Aksoy M, Erdem S, et al: Combination of hereditary elliptocytosis and hereditary spherocytosis. Clin Genet 1974; 6:46.

1143. Ham TH, Shen SC, et al: Studies on the destruction of red blood cells: IV. Thermal injury: Action of heat in causing increased spheroidicity, osmotic and mechanical fragilities and hemolysis of erythrocytes: observations on the mechanisms of destruction in such erythrocytes in dogs and in a patient with a fatal thermal burn. Blood 1948; 3:373.

1144. Ham TH, Sayre RW, et al: Physical properties of red cells as related to effects *in vivo*: II. Effect of thermal treatment on rigidity of red cells, stroma and the sickle cell. Blood 1968; 32:862.

1145. Kimber RJ, Lander H: The effect of heat on human red cell morphology, fragility and subsequent survival *in vivo*. J Lab Clin Med 1964; 64:922.

1146. Chang K, Williamson JR, Zarkowsky HS: Effect of heat on the circular dichroism of spectrin in hereditary pyropoikilocytosis. J Clin Invest 1979; 64:326.

1147. Liu S-C, Palek J, et al: Altered spectrin dimer-dimer association and instability of erythrocyte membrane skeletons in hereditary pyropoikilocytosis. J Clin Invest 1981; 68:597.

1148. Liu S-C, Palek J, Prchal J: Defective spectrin dimer-dimer association in hereditary elliptocytosis. Proc Natl Acad Sci U S A 1982; 79:2072.

1149. Chasis JA, Mohandas N: Erythrocyte membrane deformability and stability: Two distinct membrane properties that are independently regulated by skeletal protein interactions. J Cell Biol 1986; 103:343.

1150. Mohandas N, Clark MR, et al: A technique to detect reduced mechanical stability of red cell membranes: Relevance to elliptocytic disorders. Blood 1982; 59:768.

1151. Mohandas N, Clark MR, et al: Analysis of factors regulating erythrocyte deformability. J Clin Invest 1980; 66:563.

1152. Orita M, Iwahana H, et al: Detection of polymorphisms of human DNA by gel electrophoresis as single-strand conformation polymorphisms. Proc Natl Acad Sci U S A 1989; 86:2766.

1153. Sarkar G, Yoon H-S, Sommer SS: Screening for mutations by RNA single-strand conformation polymorphism (rSSCP): Comparison with DNA-SSCP. Nucleic Acids Res 1992; 20:871.

1154. Chabanel A, Sung K-LP, et al: Viscoelastic properties of red cell membranes in hereditary elliptocytosis. Blood 1989; 73:592.

1155. Parquet N, Devaux I, et al: Identification of three novel spectrin $\alpha^{1/74}$ mutations in hereditary elliptocytosis: Further support for a triple-stranded folding unit model of the spectrin heterodimer contact site. Blood 1994; 84:303.

1156. Lecomte MC, Garbarz M, et al: Molecular basis of clinical and morphological heterogeneity in hereditary elliptocytosis (HE) with spectrin αI variants. Br J Haematol 1993; 85:584.

1157. Perrotta S, Miraglia del Giudice E, et al: Mild elliptocytosis associated with the α34 Arg→Trp mutation in spectrin Genova (α1/74). Blood 1994; 83:3346.

1158. Perrotta S, Iolascon A, et al: Spectrin Anastasia (alpha I/78): A new spectrin variant (alpha 45 Arg→Thr) with moderate elliptocytogenic potential. Br J Haematol 1995; 89:933.

1159. Morlé L, Roux AF, et al: Two elliptocytogenic $\alpha^{1/74}$ variants of the spectrin α^1 domain. Spectrin Culoz (GGT→GTT; αI 40 Gly→Val) and spectrin Lyon, (CTT→TTT; αI 43 Leu→Phe). J Clin Invest 1990; 86:548.

1160. Boulanger L, Dhermy D, et al: A second allele of spectrin α-gene associated with the αI/65 phenotype (allele alpha Ponte de Sor). Blood 1994; 84:2056. Letter.

1161. Roux AF, Morlé F, et al: Molecular basis of Sp $\alpha^{1/65}$ hereditary elliptocytosis in North Africa: Insertion of a TTG triplet between codons 147 and 149 in the α-spectrin gene from five unrelated families. Blood 1989; 73:2196.

1162. Hassoun H, Coetzer TL, et al: A novel mobile element inserted in the α spectrin gene: spectrin Dayton. A truncated α spectrin associated with hereditary elliptocytosis. J Clin Invest 1994; 94:643.

1163. Gallagher PG, Tse WT, et al: A common type of the spectrin αI 46-50a-kD peptide abnormality in hereditary elliptocytosis and hereditary pyropoikilocytosis is associated with a mutation distant from the proteolytic cleavage site: Evidence for the functional importance of the triple helical model of spectrin. J Clin Invest 1992; 89:892.

1164. Sahr KE, Tobe T, et al: Sequence and exon-intron organization of the DNA encoding the alpha I domain of human spectrin: Application to the study of mutations causing hereditary elliptocytosis. J Clin Invest 1989; 84:1243.

1165. Kanzaki A, Rabodonirina M, et al: A deletion frameshift mutation of the β-spectrin gene associated with elliptocytosis in spectrin Tokyo ($\beta^{220/216}$). Blood 1992; 80:2115.

1166. Alloisio N, Wilmotte R, et al: Spectrin Jendouba: An $\alpha^{II/31}$ spectrin variant that is associated with elliptocytosis and carries a mutation distant from the dimer self-association site. Blood 1992; 80:809.

1167. Sahr KE, Coetzer TL, et al: Spectrin Cagliari: An Ala→Gly substitution in helix 1 of β spectrin repeat 17 that severely disrupts the structure and self-association of the erythrocyte spectrin heterodimer. J Biol Chem 1993; 268:22656.

1168. Gallagher PG, Weed SA, et al: Recurrent fatal hydrops fetalis associated with a nucleotide substitution in the erythrocyte beta-spectrin gene. J Clin Invest 1995; 95:1174.

1169. Gallagher PG, Petruzzi MJ, et al: Mutation of a highly conserved residue of βI-spectrin associated with fatal and near-fatal neonatal hemolytic anemia. J Clin Invest 1997; 99:267.

1170. Wilmotte R, Miraglia del Guidice E, et al: A deletional frameshift mutation in the β-spectrin gene associated with hereditary elliptocytosis in spectrin Napoli. Br J Haematol 1994; 88:437.

1171. Maillet P, Inoue T, et al: A stop codon in exon 30 of β-spectrin gene associated with hereditary elliptocytosis in spectrin Nagoya. Hum Mutation 1996; 8:366.

1172. Lorenzo F, Miraglia del Giudice E, et al: Severe poikilocytosis associated with a *de novo* alpha 28 Arg→Cys mutation in spectrin. Br J Haematol 1993; 83:152.

1173. Marchesi SL, Letsinger JT, et al: Mutant forms of spectrin alpha-subunits in hereditary elliptocytosis. J Clin Invest 1987; 80:191.

1174. Lawler J, Palek J, et al: Molecular heterogeneity of a hereditary pyropoikilocytosis: Identification of a second variant of the spectrin alpha-subunit. Blood 1983; 62:1182.

1175. Dhermy D, Garbarz M, et al: Abnormal electrophoretic mobility of spectrin tetramers in hereditary elliptocytosis. Hum Genet 1986; 74:363.

1176. Lawler J, Coetzer TL, et al: Sp $\alpha^{1/65}$: A new variant of the alpha subunit of spectrin in hereditary elliptocytosis. Blood 1985; 66:706.

1177. Lecomte MC, Dhermy D, et al: Pathologic and non-pathologic variants of the spectrin molecule in two black families with hereditary elliptocytosis. Hum Genet 1985; 71:351.

1178. Lecomte MC, Dhermy D, et al: A new abnormal variant of spectrin in black patients with hereditary elliptocytosis. Blood 1985; 65:1208.

1179. Miraglia del Giudice E, Ducluzeau MT, et al: $\alpha^{1/65}$ hereditary elliptocytosis in Southern Italy: Evidence for an African origin. Hum Genet 1992; 89:553.

1180. Schulman S, Roth EF Jr, et al: Growth of *Plasmodium falciparum* in human erythrocytes containing abnormal membrane proteins. Proc Natl Acad Sci U S A 1990; 87:7339.

1181. Gallagher PG, Roberts WE, et al: Poikilocytic hereditary elliptocytosis associated with Spectrin Alexandria: An α I/50b kD variant that is caused by a single amino acid deletion. Blood 1993; 82:2210.

1182. Fournier CM, Nicolas G, et al: Spectrin St Claude, a splicing mutation of the human alpha spectrin gene associated with severe poikilocytic anemia. Blood 1997 (in press).

1183. Johnson RM, Ravindranath Y, et al: A large erythroid spectrin β-chain variant. Br J Haematol 1992; 80:6.

1184. Wilmotte R, Maréchal J, et al: Low expression allele α^{LELY} of red cell spectrin is associated with mutations in exon 40 ($\alpha^{V/41}$ polymorphism) and intron 45 and with partial skipping of exon 46. J Clin Invest 1993; 91:2091.

1185. Maréchal J, Wilmotte R, et al: Ethnic distribution of allele alpha^{LELY}, a low-expression allele of red-cell spectrin alpha-gene. Br J Haematol 1995; 90:553.

1186. Gallagher PG, Tse WT, et al: A defect in alpha-spectrin mRNA accumulation in hereditary pyropoikilocytosis. Trans Assoc Am Phys 1991; 104:32.

1187. Knowles WJ, Bologna ML, Chasis JA: Common structural polymorphisms in human erythrocyte spectrin. J Clin Invest 1984; 73:973.

1188. DiPaolo BR, Speicher KD, Speicher DW: Identification of the amino acid mutations associated with human erythrocyte spectrin αII domain polymorphisms. Blood 1993; 82:284.

1189. Gallagher PG, Kotula L, et al: Molecular basis and haplotyping of the alpha II domain polymorphisms of spectrin: Application to the study of hereditary elliptocytosis and pyropoikilocytosis. Am J Hum Genet 1996; 59:351.

1190. Féo CJ, Fischer S, et al: Première observation de l'absence d'une protéine de la membrane érythrocytaire (band-4₁) dans un cas d'anémie elliptocytaire familiale. Nouv Rev Fr Hématol 1981; 22:315.

1191. Alloisio N, Mark L, et al: The heterozygous form of 4.1(−) hereditary elliptocytosis [the 4.1(−) trait]. Blood 1985; 65:46.

1192. Alloisio N, Dorléac E, et al: Analysis of the red cell membrane in a family with hereditary elliptocytosis—total or partial absence of protein 4.1. Hum Genet 1981; 59:68.

1193. Takakuwa Y, Tchernia G, et al: Restoration of normal membrane stability to unstable protein 4.1-deficient erythrocyte membranes by incorporation of purified protein 4.1. J Clin Invest 1986; 78:80.

1194. Discher D, Parra M, et al: Identification of the minimal domain of protein 4.1 involved in skeletal interactions. Blood 1993; 82(Suppl 1):4a. Abstract.

1195. Alloisio N, Morlé L, et al: Red cell membrane sialoglycoprotein beta in homozygous and heterozygous 4.1(−) hereditary elliptocytosis. Biochim Biophys Acta 1985; 816:57.

1196. Lambert S, Conboy J, Zail S: A molecular study of heterozygous protein 4.1 deficiency in hereditary elliptocytosis. Blood 1988; 72:1926.

1197. Conboy J, Mohandas N, et al: Molecular basis of hereditary elliptocytosis due to protein 4.1 deficiency. N Engl J Med 1986; 315:680.

1198. Garbarz M, Devaux I, et al: Protein 4.1 Lille, a novel mutation in the downstream initiation codon of protein 4.1 gene associated with heterozygous 4.1(−) hereditary elliptocytosis. Hum Mutat 1995; 5:339.

1199. Conboy JG, Chasis JA, et al: An isoform-specific mutation in the protein 4.1 gene results in hereditary elliptocytosis and complete deficiency of protein 4.1 in erythrocytes but not in nonerythroid cells. J Clin Invest 1993; 91:77.

1200. Conboy J, Marchesi S, et al: Molecular analysis of insertion/deletion mutations in protein 4.1 in elliptocytosis: II. Determination of molecular genetic origins of rearrangements. J Clin Invest 1990; 86:524.

1201. Marchesi S, Conboy J, et al: Molecular analysis of insertion/deletion mutations in protein 4.1 in elliptocytosis: I. Biochemical identification of rearrangements in the spectrin/actin binding domain and functional characterizations. J Clin Invest 1990; 86:515.

1202. Reid ME, Matynewycz MA, et al: Leach type Ge− red cells and elliptocytosis. Transfusion 1987; 27:213.

1203. Tanner MJ, High S, et al: Genetic variants of human red cell membrane sialoglycoprotein β: Study of the alterations occurring in the sialoglycoprotein β gene. Biochem J 1988; 250:407.

1204. Winardi R, Reid M, et al: Molecular analysis of glycophorin C deficiency human erythrocytes. Blood 1993; 81:2799.

1205. Lowe JB: Red cell membrane antigens. In Stamatoyannopoulos G, Nienhuis AW, et al (eds): The Molecular Basis of Blood Diseases. 2nd ed. Philadelphia, W.B. Saunders Co., 1994, p 293.

1206. Le Van Kim C, Colin Y, et al: Gerbich blood group of the Ge: -1, -2, -3 types: Immunochemical study and genomic analysis with cDNA probes. Eur J Biochem 1987; 165:571.

1207. Rebuck JW, van Slyck EJ: An unsuspected ultrastructural fault in human elliptocytes. Am J Clin Pathol 1968; 49:19.

1208. Bessis M: Living Blood Cells and Their Ultrastructure. New York, Springer-Verlag, 1973, p 140.

1209. Lux SE, John KM: The role of spectrin and actin in irreversibly sickled cells: Unsickling of "irreversibly" sickled ghosts by conditions which interfere with spectrin-actin polymerization. In Caughey WS (ed): Biochemical and Clinical Aspects of Hemoglobin Abnormalities. New York, Academic Press, 1978, p 335.

1210. Liu S-C, Derick LH, Palek J: Dependence of the permanent deformation of red blood cell membranes on spectrin dimer-tetramer equilibrium: Implication for permanent membrane deformation of irreversibly sickled cells. Blood 1993; 81:522.

1211. De Gruchy GC, Loder PB, Hennessy IV: Haemolysis and glycolytic metabolism in hereditary elliptocytosis. Br J Haematol 1962; 8:168.

1212. Peters JC, Rowland M, et al: Erythrocyte sodium transport in hereditary elliptocytosis. Can J Physiol Pharmacol 1966; 44:817.

1213. Facer CA: Malaria, hereditary elliptocytosis, and pyropoikilocytosis. Lancet 1989; 1:897. Letter.

1214. Chishti AH, Palek J, et al: Reduced invasion and growth of Plasmodium falciparum into elliptocytic red blood cells with a combined deficiency of protein 4.1, glycophorin C, and p55. Blood 1996; 87:3462.

1215. Amato D, Booth PB: Hereditary ovalocytosis in Melanesians. Papua New Guinea Med J 1977; 20:26.

1216. Castelino D, Saul A, et al: Ovalocytosis in Papua New Guinea—dominantly inherited resistance to malaria. Southeast Asian J Trop Med Public Health 1981; 12:549.

1217. Cattani JA, Gibson FD, et al: Hereditary ovalocytosis and reduced susceptibility to malaria in Papua New Guinea. Trans R Soc Trop Med Hyg 1987; 81:705.

1218. Fix AG, Baer AS, Lie-Injo LE: The mode of inheritance of ovalocytosis/elliptocytosis in Malaysian Orang Asli families. Hum Genet 1982; 61:250.

1219. Liu S-C, Zhai S, et al: Molecular defect of the band 3 protein in Southeast Asian ovalocytosis. N Engl J Med 1990; 323:1530.

1220. Baer A, Lie-Injo LE, et al: Genetic factors and malaria in the Temuan. Am J Hum Genet 1976; 28:179.

1221. Harrison KL, Collins KA, McKenna HW: Hereditary elliptical stomatocytosis; a case report. Pathology 1976; 8:307.

1222. Honig GR, Lacson PS, Maurer HS: A new familial disorder with abnormal erythrocyte morphology and increased permeability of the erythrocytes to sodium and potassium. Pediatr Res 1971; 5:159.

1223. Booth PB, Serjeantson S, et al: Selective depression of blood group antigens associated with hereditary ovalocytosis among Melanesians. Vox Sang 1977; 32:99.

1224. Serjeantson S, Bryson K, et al: Malaria and hereditary ovalocytosis. Hum Genet 1977; 37:161.

1225. Foo LC, Rekhra J-V, et al: Ovalocytosis protects against severe malaria parasitemia in the Malayan aborigines. Am J Trop Med Hyg 1992; 47:271.

1226. Genton B, al-Yaman F, et al: Ovalocytosis and cerebral malaria. Nature 1995; 378:564.

1227. Hadley T, Saul A, et al: Resistance of Melanesian elliptocytes (ovalocytes) to invasion by Plasmodium knowlesi and Plasmodium falciparum malaria parasites in vitro. J Clin Invest 1983; 71:780.

1228. Dluzewski AR, Nash GB, et al: Invasion of hereditary ovalocytes by Plasmodium falciparum in vitro and its relation to intracellular ATP concentration. Mol Biochem Parasitol 1992; 55:1.

1229. Kidson C, Lamont G, et al: Ovalocytic erythrocytes from Melanesians are resistant to invasion by malaria parasites in culture. Proc Natl Acad Sci U S A 1981; 78:5829.

1230. Saul A, Lamont G, et al: Decreased membrane deformability in Melanesian ovalocytes from Papua New Guinea. J Cell Biol 1984; 98:1348.

1231. Mohandas N, Lie-Injo LE, et al: Rigid membranes of Malayan ovalocytes: A likely genetic barrier against malaria. Blood 1984; 63:1385.

1232. Mohandas N, Winardi R, et al: Molecular basis for membrane rigidity of hereditary ovalocytosis: A novel mechanism involving the cytoplasmic domain of band 3. J Clin Invest 1992: 89:686.

1233. Schofield AE, Tanner MJ, et al: Basis of unique red cell membrane properties in hereditary ovalocytosis. J Mol Biol 1992; 223:949.

1234. Reardon DM, Seymour CA, et al: Hereditary ovalocytosis with compensated haemolysis. Br J Haematol 1993; 85:197.

1235. Jarolim P, Palek J, et al: Deletion in the band 3 gene in malaria resistant Southeast Asian ovalocytosis. Proc Natl Acad Sci U S A 1991; 88:11022.

1236. Mueller TJ, Morrison M: Detection of a variant of protein 3, the major transmembrane protein of the human erythrocyte. J Biol Chem 1977; 252:6573.

1237. Jarolim P, Rubin HL, et al: Band 3 Memphis: A widespread polymorphism with abnormal electrophoretic mobility of erythrocyte band 3 protein caused by the substitution AAG→GAG (Lys→Glu) in codon 56. Blood 1992; 80:1592.

1238. Yannoukakos D, Vasseur C, et al: Human erythrocyte band

3 polymorphism (band 3 Memphis): Characterization of the structural modification (Lys[56]→Glu) by protein chemistry methods. Blood 1991; 78:1117.

1239. Jones GL: Red cell membrane proteins in Melanesian ovalocytosis autophosphorylation and proteolysis. Proc Australian Biochem Soc 1984; 16:34. Abstract

1240. Jones GL, McLemore-Edmundson H, et al: Human erythrocyte band 3 has an altered N-terminus in malaria-resistant Melanesian ovalocytosis. Biochem Biophys Acta 1991; 1096:33.

1241. Husain-Chishti A, Andrabi K, et al: Altered tyrosine phosphorylation of the red cell band 3 protein in malaria resistant Southeast Asian ovalocytosis (SAO). Blood 1991; 78(Suppl 1):80a. Abstract.

1242. Schofield AE, Rearden DM, Tanner MJA: Defective anion transport activity of the abnormal band 3 in hereditary ovalocytic red cells. Nature 1992; 335:836.

1243. Tanner MJ, Bruce L, et al: The defective red cell anion transporter (band 3) in hereditary Southeast Asian ovalocytosis and the role of glycophorin A in the expression of band 3 anion transport activity in *Xenopus* oocytes. Biochem Soc Trans 1992; 20:542.

1244. Tanner MJ, Bruce L, et al: Melanesian hereditary ovalocytes have a deletion in red cell band 3. Blood 1991; 78:2785.

1245. Mohandas N, Chasis JA, Shohet SB: The influence of membrane skeleton on red cell deformability, membrane material properties, and shape. Semin Hematol 1983; 20:225.

1246. Liu S-C, Palek J, et al: Molecular basis of altered red blood cell membrane properties in Southeast Asian ovalocytosis: Role of the mutant band 3 protein in band 3 oligomerization and retention by the membrane skeleton. Blood 1995; 86:349.

1247. Che A, Cherry RJ, et al: Aggregation of band 3 in hereditary ovalocytic red blood cell membranes. Electron microscopy and protein rotational diffusion studies. J Cell Sci 1993; 105:655.

1248. Moriyama R, Ideguchi H, et al: Structural and functional characterization of band 3 from Southeast Asian ovalocytes. J Biol Chem 1992; 267:25792.

1249. Okoye VC, Bennett V: *Plasmodium falciparum* malaria. Band 3 as a possible receptor during invasion of human erythrocytes. Science 1985; 227:169.

1250. Dluzewski AR, Fryer PR, et al: Red cell membrane protein distribution during malarial invasion. J Cell Sci 1989; 92:691.

1251. Zarkowsky HS, Oski FA, Sha'afi R: Congenital hemolytic anemia with high-sodium, low-potassium red cells: I. Studies of membrane permeability. N Engl J Med 1968; 278:573.

1252. Lande WM, Mentzer WC: Haemolytic anaemia associated with increased cation permeability. Clin Haematol 1985; 14:89.

1253. Lock SP, Smith RS, et al: Stomatocytosis: A hereditary red cell anomaly associated with haemolytic anaemia. Br J Haematol 1961; 7:303.

1254. Rix M, Bjerrum PJ, et al: Medfodt stomatocytose med haemolytisk anaemi—med abnorm kationpermeabilitet og defekte membranproteiner. (Congenital stomatocytosis with hemolytic anemia—with abnormal cation permeability and defective membrane proteins.) Ugeskr Laeger 1991; 153:724.

1255. Bienzle U, Niethammer D, et al.: Congenital stomatocytosis and chronic haemolytic anaemia. Scand J Haematol 1975; 15:339.

1256. Eber SW, Lande WM, et al: Hereditary stomatocytosis: Consistent association with an integral membrane protein deficiency. Br J Haematol 1989; 72:452.

1257. Glader BE, Fortier N, et al: Congenital hemolytic anemia associated with dehydrated erythrocytes and increased potassium loss. N Engl J Med 1974; 291:491.

1258. Huppi PS, Ott P, et al: Congenital haemolytic anaemia in a low birth weight infant due to congenital stomatocytosis. Eur J Haematol 1991; 47:1.

1259. Kanzaki A, Yawata Y: Hereditary stomatocytosis: Phenotypical expression of sodium transport and band 7 peptides in 44 cases. Br J Haematol 1992; 82:133.

1260. Lande WM, Thiemann PV, Mentzer WC Jr: Missing band 7 membrane protein in two patients with high Na, low K erythrocytes. J Clin Invest 1982; 70:1273.

1261. Clark MR, Mohandas N, et al: Effects of abnormal cation transport on deformability of desicytes. J Supramol Struct 1978; 8:521.

1262. Lane PA, Kuypers FA, et al: Excess of red cell membrane proteins in hereditary high-phosphatidylcholine hemolytic anemia. Am J Hematol 1990; 34:186.

1263. Lo SS, Hitzig WH, Marti HR: Stomatozytose. Schweiz Med Wochenschr 1970; 100:1977.

1264. Lo SS, Marti HR, Hitzig WH: Haemolytic anaemia associated with decreased concentration of reduced glutathione in red cells. Acta Haematol 1971; 46:14.

1265. McGrath KM: Dehydrated hereditary stomatocytosis—a report of two families and a review of the literature. Pathology 1984; 16:146.

1266. Lande W, Cerrone K, et al: Congenital anemia with abnormal cation permeability and cold hemolysis *in vitro*. Blood 1979; 54(Suppl 1):29a. Abstract.

1267. Meadow SR: Stomatocytosis. Proc R Soc Med 1967; 60:13.

1268. Mentzer WC Jr, Smith WB, et al: Hereditary stomatocytosis membranes and metabolism studies. Blood 1975; 46:659.

1269. Miller G, Townes PL, et al: A new congenital hemolytic anemia with deformed erythrocytes (?"stomatocytes") and remarkable susceptibility of erythrocytes to cold hemolysis *in vitro*. I. Clinical and hematologic studies. Pediatrics 1965; 35:906.

1270. Miller DR, Rickles FR, et al: A new variant of hereditary hemolytic anemia with stomatocytosis and erythrocyte cation abnormality. Blood 1971; 38:184.

1271. Morlé L, Pothier B, et al: Reduction of membrane band 7 and activation of volume stimulated (K+, Cl−)-cotransport in a case of congenital stomatocytosis. Br J Haematol 1989; 71:141.

1272. Mutoh S, Sasaki R, et al: A family of hereditary stomatocytosis associated with normal level of Na-K-ATPase activity of red blood cells. Am J Hematol 1983; 14:113.

1273. Nolan GR: Hereditary xerocytosis: A case history and review of the literature. Pathology 1984; 16:151.

1274. Schröter W, Ungefehr K, Tillmann W: Role of the spleen in congenital stomatocytosis associated with high sodium-low potassium erythrocytes. Klin Wochenschr 1981; 59:173.

1275. Shohet SB, Nathan DG, Livermore BM: Hereditary hemolytic anemia associated with abnormal membrane lipids. II. Ion permeability and transport abnormalities. Blood 1973; 42:1.

1276. Clark MR, Shohet SB, Gottfried EL: Hereditary hemolytic disease with increased red blood cell phosphatidylcholine and dehydration: One, two, or many disorders? Am J Hematol 1993; 42:25.

1277. Shohet SB, Livermore BM, et al: Hereditary hemolytic anemia associated with abnormal membrane lipids: Mechanism of accumulation of phosphatidyl choline. Blood 1971; 38:445.

1278. Turpin F, Lortholary P, et al: Un cas d'anémie hémolytique avec stomatocytose. Nouv Rev Fr Hématol 1971; 11:585.

1279. Wiley JS, Ellory JC, et al: Characteristics of the membrane defect in the hereditary stomatocytosis syndrome. Blood 1975; 46:337.

1280. Yawata Y, Takemoto Y, et al: The Japanese family of congenital hemolytic anemia with high red cell phosphatidyl choline and increased sodium transport. Acta Haematol Jpn 1982; 45:672.

1281. Platt OS, Lux SE, Nathan DG: Exercise-induced hemolysis in xerocytosis: Erythrocyte dehydration and shear sensitivity. J Clin Invest 1981; 68:631.

1282. Wiley JS, Cooper RA, et al: Hereditary stomatocytosis: Association of low 2,3-diphosphoglycerate with increased cation pumping by the red cell. Br J Haematol 1979; 41:133.

1283. Stewart GW, Corrall RJ, et al: Familial pseudohyperkalemia. Lancet 1979; 2:175.

1284. Stewart GW, Ellory JC: A family with mild hereditary xerocytosis showing high membrane cation permeability at low temperatures. Clin Sci 1985; 69:309.

1285. Lande WM, Andrews DL, et al: Temperature dependence of RBC passive K efflux in primary permeability disorders: Unique finding in a patient with cryohydrocytosis. Blood 1985; 66(Suppl 1):34a. Abstract.

1286. McCormack MK, Geller GR, et al: Hemolytic anemia associated with a cation abnormality. J Cell Biol 1975; 67:271a. Abstract.

1287. Stewart GW, Hepworth-Jones BE, et al: Isolation of cDNA coding for an ubiquitous membrane protein deficient in high Na+, low K+ stomatocytic erythrocytes. Blood 1992; 79:1593.

1288. Stewart GW, Argent AC, Dash BC: Stomatin: A putative cation transport regulator in the red cell membrane. Biochim Biophys Acta 1993; 1225:15.

1289. Stewart GW, Argent AC: Integral band 7 protein of the human erythrocyte membrane. Biochem Soc Trans 1992; 20:785.

1290. Wiley JS, Shaller CC: Selective loss of calcium permeability on maturation of reticulocytes. J Clin Invest 1977; 59:1113.

1291. Dutcher PO, Segel GB, et al: Cation transport and its altered regulation in human stomatocytic erythrocytes. Pediatr Res 1975; 9:924.

1292. Mentzer WC, Lubin BH, Emmons S: Correction of the permeability defect in hereditary stomatocytosis by dimethyl adipimidate. N Engl J Med 1976; 294:1200.

1293. Mentzer WC, Lam G, et al: Membrane effects of imidoesters in hereditary stomatocytosis. In Lux SE, Marchesi VT, et al (eds): Normal and Abnormal Red Cell Membranes. New York, Alan R. Liss, Inc., 1979, p 265.

1294. Stewart GW, Amess JA, et al: Thrombo-embolic disease after splenectomy for hereditary stomatocytosis. Br J Haematol 1996; 93:303.

1295. Wang D, Mentzer WC, et al: Purification of band 7.2b, a 31-kd integral membrane phosphoprotein absent in hereditary stomatocytosis. J Biol Chem 1991; 266:17826.

1296. Hiebl-Dirschmied CM, Adolf GR, Prohaska R: Isolation and partial characterization of the human erythrocyte band 7 integral membrane protein. Biochim Biophys Acta 1991; 1065:195.

1297. Hiebl-Dirschmied C, Entler B, et al: Cloning and nucleotide sequence of cDNA encoding human erythrocyte band 7 integral membrane protein. Biochim Biophys Acta 1991; 1090:123.

1298. Gallagher PG, Forget BG: Structure, organization, and expression of the human band 7.2b gene, a candidate gene for hereditary hydrocytosis. J Biol Chem 1995; 270:26358.

1299. Sinard JH, Stewart GW, et al: Stomatin binding to adducin: A novel link between transmembrane transport and the cytoskeleton. Mol Cell Biol 1994; 5:421a. Abstract.

1300. Huang M, Gu G, et al: A stomatin-like protein necessary for mechanosensation in C. elegans. Nature 1995; 378:292.

1301. Gallagher PG, Segel G, et al: The gene for erythrocyte band 7.2b in hereditary stomatocytosis. Blood 1992; 80(Suppl 1):276a. Abstract.

1302. Wang D, Turetsky T, et al: Further studies on RBC membrane protein 7.2b deficiency in hereditary stomatocytosis. Blood 1992; 80(Suppl 1):275a. Abstract.

1303. Lux SE, John KM: Unpublished observations, 1996.

1304. Pinkerton PH, Fletch SM, et al: Hereditary stomatocytosis with hemolytic anemia in the dog. Blood 1974; 44:557.

1305. Smith JE, Moore K, et al: Glutathione metabolism in canine hereditary stomatocytosis with mild erythrocyte glutathione deficiency. J Lab Clin Med 1983; 101:611.

1306. Smith BD, Segel GB: Abnormal erythrocyte adherence in hereditary stomatocytosis. Blood 1997 (in press).

1307. Vives-Corrons JL, Besson I, et al: Hereditary xerocytosis: A report of six unrelated Spanish families with leaky red cell syndrome and increased heat stability of the erythrocyte membrane. Br J Haematol 1995; 90:817.

1308. Jaffe ER, Gottfried EL: Hereditary nonspherocytic hemolytic disease associated with an altered phospholipid composition of the erythrocytes. J Clin Invest 1968; 47:1375.

1309. Dise CA, Goodman DBP, Rasmussen H: Selective stimulation of erythrocyte membrane phospholipid fatty acid turnover associated with decreased volume. J Biol Chem 1980; 255:5201.

1310. Fairbanks G, Dino JE, et al: Membrane alterations in hereditary xerocytosis: Elevated levels of glyceraldehyde-3-phosphate dehydrogenase. In Kruckeberg WC, Eaton JW, et al (eds): Erythrocyte Membranes: Recent Clinical and Experimental Advances. New York, Alan R. Liss, Inc., 1978, p 173.

1311. Sauberman N, Fairbanks G, et al: Altered red blood cell surface area in hereditary xerocytosis. Clin Chim Med 1981; 114:149.

1312. Platt OS: Exercise-induced hemolysis in sickle cell anemia: Shear-sensitivity and erythrocyte dehydration. Blood 1982; 59:1055.

1313. Harm W, Fortier NL, et al: Increased erythrocyte lipid peroxidation in hereditary xerocytosis. Clin Chim Acta 1979; 99:121.

1314. Sauberman N, Fortier NL, et al: Spectrin-hemoglobin cross-linkages associated with in vitro oxidant hypersensitivity in pathologic and artificially dehydrated red cells. Br J Haematol 1983; 54:15.

1315. Snyder LM, Sauberman N, et al: Red cell membrane response

1316. Fortier N, Snyder LM, et al: The relationship between in vivo generated hemoglobin skeletal protein complex and increased red cell membrane rigidity. Blood 1988; 71:1427.

1317. Albala MM, Fortier NL, Glader BE: Physiologic features of hemolysis associated with altered cation and 2,3-diphosphoglycerate content. Blood 1978; 52:135.

1318. Lux SE, John KM, Landrigan P: Unpublished observations, 1996.

1319. Douglass CC, Twomey JJ: Transient stomatocytosis with hemolysis: A previously unrecognized complication of alcoholism. Ann Intern Med 1970; 72:159.

1320. Wislöff F, Boman D: Acquired stomatocytosis in alcoholic liver disease. Scand J Haematol 1979; 23:43.

1321. Simpson LO: Blood from healthy animals and humans contains nondiscocytic erythrocytes. Br J Haematol 1989; 73:561.

1322. Barrett AM: A special form of erythrocyte possessing increased resistance to hypotonic saline. J Pathol Bacteriol 1938; 46:603.

1323. Davidson RJ, How J, Lessels S: Acquired stomatocytosis: Its prevalence and significance in routine haematology. Scand J Haematol 1977; 19:47.

1324. Ducrou W, Kimber RJ: Stomatocytes, haemolytic anaemia and abdominal pain in Mediterranean migrants. Some examples of a new syndrome? Med J Aust 1969; 2:1087.

1325. Ohsaka A, Kano Y, et al: A transient hemolytic reaction and stomatocytosis following Vinca alkaloid administration. Acta Haematol Jpn 1989; 52:7.

1326. Reinhart WH, Chien S: Stomatocytic transformation of red blood cells after marathon running. Am J Hematol 1985; 19:201.

1327. Davidson RJ: March or exertional hemoglobinuria. Semin Hematol 1969; 6:150.

1328. Banga JP, Pinder JC, et al: An erythrocyte membrane protein anomaly in march haemoglobinuria. Lancet 1979; 2:1048.

1329. Vos GH, Vos D, et al: A sample of blood with no detectable Rh antigens. Lancet 1961; 1:14.

1330. Ballas SK, Clark MR, et al: Red cell membrane and cation deficiency in Rh$_{null}$ syndrome. Blood 1984; 63:1046.

1331. Seidl S, Spielmann W, Martin H: Two siblings with Rh$_{null}$ disease. Vox Sang 1972; 23:182.

1332. Senhauser DA, Mitchell MW, et al: Another example of phenotype Rh$_{null}$. Transfusion 1970; 10:89.

1333. Sturgeon P: Hematological observations on the anemia associated with blood type Rh$_{null}$. Blood 1970; 36:310.

1334. Lauf PK, Joiner CH: Increased potassium transport and ouabain binding in human Rh$_{null}$ red blood cells. Blood 1976; 48:457.

1335. McGuire DM, Rosenfield RE, et al: Rh$_{mod}$. A second kindred (Craig). Vox Sang 1976; 30:430.

1336. Saji H, Hosoi T: A Japanese Rh$_{mod}$ family: Serological and haematological observations. Vox Sang 1979; 37:296.

1337. Assmann G, von Eckardstein A, Brewer HB Jr: Familial high density lipoprotein deficiency: Tangier disease. In: Scriver CS, Beaudet AL, et al (eds): The Metabolic and Molecular Bases of Inherited Disease. 7th ed. New York, McGraw-Hill Book Co., 1995, p 2053.

1338. Schmitz G, Assmann G, et al: Tangier disease: A disorder of intracellular membrane traffic. Proc Natl Acad Sci U S A 1985; 82:6305.

1339. Reinhart WH, Gössi U, et al: Haemolytic anaemia in alpha-lipoproteinaemia (Tangier disease): Morphological, biochemical, and biophysical properties of the red blood cell. Br J Haematol 1989; 72:272.

1340. Hoffman HN, Fredrickson DS: Tangier disease (familial high density lipoprotein deficiency): Clinical and genetic features in two adults. Am J Med 1965; 39:582.

1341. Kummer H, Laissue J, et al: Familiäre analphalipoproteinämie (Tangier-Krankheit). Schweiz Med Wochenschr 1968; 98(11):406.

1342. Shaklady MM, Djardjouras EM, Lloyd JK: Red-cell lipids in familial alphalipoprotein deficiency (Tangier disease). Lancet 1968; 2:151.

1343. Norman JG: Stomatocytosis in migrants in Mediterranean origin. Med J Aust 1969; 1:315. Letter.

1344. Jackson JM, Knight D: Stomatocytosis in migrants of Mediterranean origin. Med J Aust 1969; 1:939. Letter.

1345. Lander H: More maladies in Mediterranean migrants. Stomatocytosis and macrothrombocytopenia. Med J Aust 1971; 1:438.

1346. von Behrens WE: Splenomegaly, macrothrombocytopenia and stomatocytosis in healthy Mediterranean subjects (splenomegaly in Mediterranean macrothrombocytopenia). Scand J Haematol 1975; 14:258.

1347. Miwa S, Fujii H, et al: A case of red-cell adenosine deaminase overproduction associated with hereditary hemolytic anemia found in Japan. Am J Hematol 1978; 5:107.

1348. Wada H, Kanzaki A, et al: A new band 3 variant with increased hemolysis, decreased anion transport, glycophorin A anomaly and abnormal rheology. Blood 1990; 76(Suppl 1):20a. Abstract.

1349. Weed RI, LaCelle PL, Merrill EW: Metabolic dependence of red cell deformability. J Clin Invest 1969; 48:795.

1350. Lux SE, John KM, Ukena TE: Diminished spectrin extraction from ATP-depleted human erythrocytes. Evidence relating spectrin to changes in erythrocyte shape and deformability. J Clin Invest 1978; 61:815.

1351. Palek J, Liu SC, Snyder LM: Metabolic dependence of protein arrangement in human erythrocyte membranes. I. Analysis of spectrin-rich complexes in ATP-depleted red cells. Blood 1978; 51:385.

1352. Nathan DG, Oski FA, et al: Extreme hemolysis and red cell distortion in erythrocyte pyruvate kinase deficiency. II. Measurements of erythrocyte glucose consumption, potassium flux and adenosine triphosphate stability. N Engl J Med 1965; 272:118.

1353. Mentzer WC Jr, Baehner RL, et al: Selective reticulocyte destruction in erythrocyte pyruvate kinase deficiency. J Clin Invest 1971; 50:688.

1354. Glader BE: Salicylate-induced injury of pyruvate kinase deficient erythrocytes. N Engl J Med 1976; 294:916.

1355. Oski FA, Nathan DG, et al: Extreme hemolysis and red cell distortion in erythrocyte pyruvate kinase deficiency. I. Morphology, erythrokinetics and family enzyme studies. N Engl J Med 1964; 270:1023.

1356. Leblond PF, Lyonnais J, Delage JM: Erythrocyte populations in pyruvate kinase deficiency anaemia following splenectomy. I. Cell morphology. Br J Haematol 1978; 39:55.

1357. Leblond PF, Coulombe L, Lyonnais J: Erythrocyte populations in pyruvate kinase deficiency anaemia following splenectomy: II. Cell deformability. Br J Haematol 1978; 31:63.

1358. Coetzer T, Zail SS: Erythrocyte membrane proteins in hereditary glucose phosphate isomerase deficiency. J Clin Invest 1979; 63:552.

1359. Clark MR, Unger RC, Shohet SB: Monovalent cation composition and ATP and lipid content of irreversibly sickled cells. Blood 1978; 51:1169.

1360. Glader BE, Lux SE, Muller-Soyano A: Energy-reserve and cation composition of irreversibly sickled cells (ISCs) *in vivo*. Br J Haematol 1978; 40:527.

1361. Schultze M: Ein Heizbarer objectisch und seine Verwendung bei Untersuchungen des Blutes. Arch Mikrok Anat 1865; 1:1.

1362. Shen SC, Ham TH, Fleming AB: Studies on the destruction of red blood cells: III. Mechanism and complication of hemoglobinuria in patients with thermal burns: Spherocytosis and increased osmotic fragility of red blood cells. N Engl J Med 1943; 229:701.

1363. Topley E: The usefulness of counting "heat-affected" red cells as a guide to the risk of the later disappearance of red cells after burns. J Clin Pathol 1961; 14:295.

1364. James GW III, Purnell OJ, et al: The anemia of thermal injury: I. Studies of pigment excretion. J Clin Invest 1951; 30:181.

1365. James GW III, Abbott LD, et al: The anemia of thermal injury: III. Erythropoiesis and hemoglobin metabolism studied with N[15]-glycine in dog and man. J Clin Invest 1954; 33:150.

1366. Moore FD, Peacock WC, et al: The anemia of thermal burns. Ann Surg 1946; 124:811.

1367. McCollough J, Polesky HF, et al: Iatrogenic hemolysis: A complication of blood warmed by a microwave device. Anesth Analg 1972; 51:102.

1368. Staples PJ, Griner PF: Extracorporeal hemolysis of blood in a microwave blood warmer. N Engl J Med 1971; 285:317.

1369. Brain MC, Dacie JV: Microangiopathic haemolytic anaemia: The possible role of vascular lesions in pathogenesis. Br J Haematol 1962; 8:358.

1370. Nevaril CG, Lynch EC: Erythrocyte damage and destruction induced by shearing stress. J Lab Clin Med 1968; 71:784.

1371. Jacob HS, Amsden T: Acute hemolytic anemia with rigid red cells in hypophosphatemia. N Engl J Med 1971; 285:1446.

1372. Lichtman MA, Miller DR, et al: Reduced red cell glycolysis, 2,3-diphosphoglycerate and adenosine triphosphate concentration, and increased hemoglobin-oxygen affinity caused by hypophosphatemia. Ann Intern Med 1971; 74:562.

1373. Dean HM, Decker CL, Baker LD: Temporary survival in clostridial hemolysis with absence of circulating red cells. N Engl J Med 1967; 277:700.

1374. Myers G, Ngoi SS, et al: Clostridial septicemia in an urban hospital. Surg Gynecol Obstet 1992; 174:291.

1375. Ifthikaruddin JJ, Holmes JA: *Clostridium perfringens* septicaemia and massive intravascular haemolysis as a terminal complication of autologous bone marrow transplant. Clin Lab Haematol 1992; 14:159.

1376. Batge B, Filejski W, et al: Clostridial sepsis with massive intravascular hemolysis: Rapid diagnosis and successful treatment. Intensive Care Med 1992; 18:488.

1377. Tsai IK, Yen MY, et al: *Clostridium perfringens* septicemia with massive hemolysis. Scand J Infect Dis 1989; 21:467.

1378. Becker RC, Giuliani M, et al: Massive hemolysis in *Clostridium perfringens* infections. J Surg Oncol 1987; 35:13.

1379. Bennett JM, Healey PJM: Spherocytic hemolytic anemia and acute cholecystitis caused by *Clostridium welchii*. N Engl J Med 1963; 268:1070.

1380. Mera CL, Freedman MH: *Clostridium* liver abscess and massive hemolysis: Unique demise in Fanconi's aplastic anemia. Clin Pediatr 1984; 23:126.

1381. Mupanemunda RH, Kenyon CF, et al: Bacterial-induced activation of erythrocyte T-antigen complicating necrotizing enterocolitis: A case report. Eur J Pediatr 1993; 152:325.

1382. Placzek MM, Gorst DW: T activation haemolysis and death after blood transfusion. Arch Dis Child 1987; 62:743.

1383. Warren S, Schreiber JR, Epstein MF: Necrotizing enterocolitis and hemolysis associated with *Clostridium perfringens*. Am J Dis Child 1984; 138:686.

1384. Williams RA, Brown EF, et al: Transfusion of infants with activation of erythrocyte T antigen. J Pediatr 1989; 115:949.

1385. Abdominal pain, total intravascular hemolysis, and death in a 53 year old woman (clinical conference). Am J Med 1990; 88:667.

1386. Terebelo HR, McCue RL, Lenneville MS: Implication of plasma free hemoglobin in massive clostridial hemolysis. JAMA 1982; 248:2028.

1387. Titball RW, Leslie DL, et al: Hemolytic and sphingomyelinase activities of *Clostridium perfringens* alpha toxin are dependent on a domain homologous to that of an enzyme from the human arachidonic acid pathway. Infect Immun 1991; 59:1872.

1388. Leslie D, Fairweather N, et al: Phospholipase C and haemolytic activities of *Clostridium perfringens* alpha toxin cloned in *Escherichia coli*: Sequence and homology with a *Bacillus cereus* phospholipase C. Mol Microbiol 1989; 3:383.

1389. Iwamoto M, Ohno-Iwashita Y, Ando S: Role of the essential thiol group in the thiol-activated cytolysin from *Clostridium perfringens*. Eur J Biochem 1987; 194:25.

1390. Iwamoto M, Ohno-Iwashita Y, Ando S: Effect of isolated C-terminal fragment of theta toxin (perfringolysin O) on toxin assembly and membrane lysis. Eur J Biochem 1990; 194:25.

1391. Tweten RK: Cloning and expression in *Escherichia coli* of the perfringolysin O (theta toxin) from *Clostridium perfringens* and characterization of the gene product. Infect Immun 1988; 56:3228.

1392. Harris RW, Sims PJ, Tweten RK: Kinetic aspects of the aggregation of *Clostridium perfringens* theta-toxin on erythrocyte membranes. A fluorescence energy transfer study. J Biol Chem 1991; 266:6936.

1393. Hubl W, Mostbeck B, et al: Investigation of the pathogenesis of massive hemolysis in a case of *Clostridium perfringens* septicemia. Ann Hematol 1993; 67:145.

1394. Simpkins H, Kahlenberg A: Structural and compositional changes in the red cell membrane during *Clostridium welchii* infection. Br J Haematol 1971; 21:173.

1395. Iyaniwura TT: Snake venom constituents: Biochemistry and toxicology (Part 1). Vet Hum Toxicol 1991; 33:468.

1396. Perkash A, Sarup BM: Red cell abnormalities after snake bite. J Trop Med Hyg 1972; 75:85.

1397. Reid HA: Cobra-bites. BMJ 1964; 2:540.

1398. Foil LD, Norment BR: Envenomation by *Loxosceles reclusa.* J Med Entomol 1979; 16:18. Review.

1399. Nance WE: Hemolytic anemia of necrotic anachnoidism. Am J Med 1961; 31:801.

1400. Dacie JV: Haemolytic anemias due to drugs, chemicals and venoms: Glucose-6-phosphate dehydrogenase deficiency and favism. In The Haemolytic Anaemias, Congenital and Acquired. 2nd ed. New York, Grune & Stratton, 1967, part IV, p 993.

1401. Monzon C, Miles J: Hemolytic anemia following a wasp sting. J Pediatr 1980; 96:1039.

1402. Schulte KL, Kochen MM: Haemolytic anemia in an adult after a wasp sting. Lancet 1981; 2:478. Letter.

1403. Bousquet J, Huchard G, Michel FB: Toxic reactions induced by hymenoptera venom. Ann Allergy 1984; 52:371.

1404. Guess HA, Saviteer PL, Morris CR: Hemolysis and acute renal failure following a Portuguese man-of-war sting. Pediatrics 1982; 70:979.

1405. Argiolas A, Pisano JJ: Facilitation of phospholipase A2 activity by mastoparans, a new class of mast cell degranulation peptides from wasp venom. J Biol Chem 1983; 25:13697.

1406. Ho CL, Hwang LL: Structure and biological activities of a new mastoparan isolated from the venom of the hornet *Vespa basalis.* Biochem J 1991; 274: 453.

1407. Katsu T, Kuroko M, et al: Interaction of wasp venom mastoparan with biomembranes. Biochim Biophys Acta 1990; 1027:85.

1408. Claque MJ, Cherry RJ: A comparative study of band 3 aggregation in erythrocyte membranes by melittin and other cationic agents. Biochim Biophys Acta 1989; 980:93.

1409. Dempsey CE: The actions of melittin on membranes. Biochim Biophys Acta 1990; 1031:143.

1410. Dufton MJ, Hider RC, Cherry RJ: The influence of melittin on the rotation of band 3 protein in the human erythrocyte membrane. Eur Biophys J 1984; 11:17.

1411. Hui SW, Stewart CM, Cherry RJ: Electron microscopic observation of the aggregation of membrane proteins in human erythrocyte by melittin. Biochim Biophys Acta 1990; 1023:335.

1412. Eichner ER: Spider bite hemolytic anemia: Positive Coombs' test, erythrophagocytosis, and leukoerythroblastic smear. Am J Clin Pathol 1984; 81:683.

1413. Hardman JT, Beck ML, et al: Incompatibility associated with the bite of a brown recluse spider *(Loxosceles reclusa).* Transfusion 1983; 23:233.

1414. Madrigal GC, Ercolani RL, Wenzl JE: Toxicity from a bite of the brown spider *(Loxosceles reclusus):* Skin necrosis, hemolytic anemia, and hemoglobinuria in a nine-year-old child. Clin Pediatr 1972; 11:641.

1415. Futrell JM, Morgan PN, et al: Location of brown recluse venom attachment sites on human erythrocytes by the ferritin-labeled antibody technique. Am J Pathol 1979; 95:675.

1416. Kurpiewski G, Campbell BJ, et al: Alternate complement pathway activation by recluse spider venom. Int J Tissue React 1981; 3:39.

1417. Taylor EH, Denny WF: Hemolysis, renal failure and death, presumed secondary to bite of brown recluse spider. South Med J 1966, 59:1209.

1418. Vorse H, Seccareccio P, et al: Disseminated intravascular coagulopathy following fatal brown spider bite (necrotic arachnidism). J Pediatr 1972; 80:1035.

1419. Gebel HM, Finke JH, et al: Inactivation of complement by *Loxosceles reclusa* spider venom. Am J Trop Med Hyg 1979; 28:756.

1420. Bernheimer AW, Campbell BJ, Forrester LJ: Comparative toxicology of *Loxosceles reclusa* and *Corynebacterium pseudotuberculosis.* Science 1985; 228:590.

1421. Jandl JH, Jacob HS: Hypersplenism due to infection: A study of five cases manifesting hemolytic anemia. N Engl J Med 1961; 264:1063.

1422. Harris IM, McAlister J, et al: Splenomegaly and the circulating red cell. Br J Haematol 1958; 4:97.

1423. Crane GG: The anemia of hyperreactive malarious splenomegaly. Rev Soc Bras Med Trop 1992; 25:1.

1424. Cooper RA, Jandl JH: Bile salts and cholesterol in the pathogenesis of target cells in obstructive jaundice. J Clin Invest 1968; 47:809.

1425. Cooper RA, Diloy-Puray M, et al: An analysis of lipoproteins, bile acids, and red cell membranes associated with target cells and spur cells in patients with liver disease. J Clin Invest 1972; 31:3182.

1426. Neerhout RC: Abnormalities of erythrocyte stromal lipids in hepatic disease: Erythrocyte stromal lipids in hyperlipemic states. J Lab Clin Med 1968; 71:438.

1427. Verkleij AJ, Nanta ICD, et al: The fusion of abnormal plasma lipoprotein (LP-X) and the erythrocyte membrane in patients with cholestasis studied by electron microscopy. Biochim Biophys Acta 1976; 436:366.

1428. Narayanan S: Biochemistry and clinical relevance of lipoprotein X. Am Clin Lab Sci 1984; 14:371. Review.

1429. Seidel D, Alaupovic P, Furman RH: A lipoprotein characterizing obstructive jaundice: I. Method for quantitative separation and identification of lipoproteins in jaundice subjects. J Clin Invest 1969; 48:1211.

1430. Iida H, Hasegawa I, Nozawa Y: Biochemical studies on abnormal membranes: Protein abnormality of erythrocyte membrane in biliary obstruction. Biochem Biophys Acta 1976; 443:394.

1431. Norum KR, Gjone E: Familial serum-cholesterol esterification failure: A new inborn error of metabolism. Biochim Biophys Acta 1967; 144:698.

1432. Gjone E, Torsvik H, Norum KR: Familial plasma cholesterol ester deficiency: A study of the erythrocytes. Scand J Clin Lab Invest 1968; 21:327.

1433. Jain SK, Mohandas N, Sensabaugh GF: Hereditary plasma lecithin-cholesterol acyl transferase deficiency: A heterozygous variant with erythrocyte membrane abnormalities. J Lab Clin Med 1982; 99:816.

1434. Murayama N, Asano Y, Hosoda S: Decreased sodium influx and abnormal red cell membrane lipids in a patient with familial plasma lecithin:cholesterol acyltransferase deficiency. Am J Hematol 1984; 16:129.

1435. Bujo H, Kusunoki J, et al: Molecular defect in familial lecithin:cholesterol acyltransferase (LCAT) deficiency: A single nucleotide insertion in LCAT gene causes a complete deficient type of the disease. Biochem Biophys Res Commun 1991; 181:933.

1436. Funke H, von Eckardstein A, et al: Genetic and phenotypic heterogeneity in familial lecithin:cholesterol acyltransferase (LCAT) deficiency: Six newly identified defective alleles further contribute to the structural heterogeneity in this disease. J Clin Invest 1993; 91:677.

1437. Klein HG, Lohse P, et al: Two different allelic mutations in the lecithin:cholesterol acyltransferase (LCAT) gene resulting in classic LCAT deficiency: LCAT (Tyr 83 Stop) and LCAT (Tyr 156 Asn). J Lipid Res 1993; 34:49.

1438. Maeda E, Naka Y, et al: Lecithin-cholesterol acyltransferase (LCAT) deficiency with a missense mutation in exon 6 of the LCAT gene. Biochem Biophys Res Commun 1991; 178:460.

1439. Skretting G, Blomhoff JP, et al: The genetic defect in the original Norwegian lecithin:cholesterol acyltransferase deficiency families. FEBS Lett 1992; 309:307.

1440. Gjone E, Javitt NB, et al: Studies of lipoprotein-X (LP-X) and bile acids in familial lecithin:cholesterol acyltransferase deficiency. Acta Med Scand 1973; 194:377.

1441. Norum KR, Gjone E: The influence of plasma from patients with familial lecithin:cholesterol acyltransferase deficiency on the lipid pattern of erythrocytes. Scand J Clin Lab Invest 1968; 22:94.

1442. Jacobsen CD, Gjone E, Hovig T: Sea-blue histiocytes in familial lecithin:cholesterol acyltransferase deficiency. Scand J Haematol 1972; 9:106.

1443. Frohlich J, Hoag G, et al: Hypoalphalipoproteinemia resembling fish eye disease. Acta Med Scand 1987; 221:291.

1444. Singer K, Miller EB, et al: Hematologic changes following splenectomy in man, with particular reference to target cells, hemolytic index and lysolecithin. Am J Med Sci 1941; 202:171.

1445. Singer K, Weisz L: The life cycle of the erythrocyte after splenectomy and the problems of splenic hemolysis and target cell formation. Am J Med Sci 1945; 210:301.

1446. DeHaan LD, Werre JM, et al: Alterations in size, shape and osmotic behaviour of red cells after splenectomy: A study of their age dependence. Br J Haematol 1988; 69:71.
1447. Come SE, Shohet SB, Robinson SH: Surface remodeling vs whole-cell hemolysis of reticulocytes produced with erythroid stimulation or iron-deficiency anemia. Blood 1974; 44:817.
1448. Smith CH, Khakoo Y: Burr cells: Classification and effect of splenectomy. J Pediatr 1970; 76:99.
1449. Crosby WH.: Normal function of the spleen relative to red blood cells: A review. Blood 1959; 14:399.
1450. Brecher G, Haley JE, Wallerstein RO: Spiculated erythrocytes after splenectomy: Acanthocytes or non-specific poikilocytes? Nouv Rev Fr Hématol 1972; 12:751.
1451. Furchgott RF: Disk-sphere transformation in mammalian red cells. J Exp Biol 1940; 17:30.
1452. Nakao M, Nakao T, Yamazoe S: Adenosine triphosphate and shape of erythrocytes. J Biochem 1961; 45:487.
1453. Palek J, Stewart G, Lionetti FJ: The dependence of shape of human erythrocyte ghosts on calcium, magnesium, and adenosine triphosphate. Blood 1974; 44:583.
1454. Aherne WA: The "burr" red cell and azotaemia. J Clin Pathol 1957; 10:252.
1455. Schwartz SO, Motto SA: The diagnostic significance of "burr" red blood cells. Am J Med Sci 1949; 218:513.
1456. Féo CJ, Tchernia G, et al: Observation of echinocytosis in eight patients: A phase contrast and SEM study. Br J Haematol 1978; 40:519.
1457. Zipursky A, Brown E, et al: The erythrocyte differential count in newborn infants. Am J Pediatr Hematol 1983; 5:45.
1458. Carlyle RF, Nichols G, Rowles PM: Abnormal red cells in blood of men subjected to simulated dives. Lancet 1979; 1:1114.
1459. Cooper RA: Anemia with spur cells: A red cell defect acquired in serum and modified in the circulation. J Clin Invest 1969; 48:1820.
1460. Bassen FA, Kornzweig AL: Malformation of the erythrocytes in a case of atypical retinitis pigmentosa. Blood 1950; 5:381.
1461. Tuffy P, Brown AK, et al: Infantile pyknocytosis: A common erythrocyte abnormality of the first trimester. Am J Dis Child 1959; 98:227.
1462. Kay J, Stricker RB: Hematologic and immunologic abnormalities in anorexia nervosa. South Med J 1983 76:1008.
1463. Mant MJ, Faragher BS: The haematology of anorexia nervosa. Br J Haematol 1972; 23:737.
1464. Symmans WA, Shepard CS, et al: Hereditary acanthocytosis associated with the McLeod phenotype of the Kell blood group system. Br J Haematol 1979; 42:575.
1465. Udden MM, Umeda M, et al: New abnormalities in the morphology, cell surface receptors, and electrolyte metabolism of In(Lu) erythrocytes. Blood 1987; 69:52.
1466. Wardrop C, Hutchison HE: Red-cell shape in hypothyroidism. Lancet 1969; 1:1243.
1467. Doll DC, List AF, et al: Acanthocytosis associated with myelodysplasia. J Clin Oncol 1989; 7:1569.
1468. Ohsaka A, Yawata Y, et al: Abnormal calcium transport of acanthocytes in acute myelodysplasia with myelofibrosis. Br J Haematol 1989; 73:568.
1469. Salt HB, Wolff OH, et al: On having no beta-lipoprotein. A syndrome comprising a-beta-lipoproteinaemia, acanthocytosis, and steatorrhoea. Lancet 1960; 2:326.
1470. Kane JP, Havel RJ: Disorders of the biogenesis and secretion of lipoproteins containing the B apolipoproteins. In: Scriver CS, Beaudet AL, et al (eds): The Metabolic and Molecular Bases of Inherited Disease. 7th ed. New York, McGraw-Hill Book Co., 1995, p 1853.
1471. Sharp D, Blinderman L, et al: Cloning and gene defects in microsomal triglyceride transfer protein associated with abetalipoproteinaemia. Nature 1993; 365:65.
1472. Wetterau JR, Aggerbeck LP, et al: Absence of microsomal triglyceride transfer protein in individuals with abetalipoproteinemia. Science 1992; 258:999.
1473. Black DD, Hay RV, et al: Intestinal and hepatic apolipoprotein B gene expression in abetalipoproteinemia. Gastroenterology 1991; 101:520.
1474. Glickman RM, Glickman JN, et al: Apolipoprotein synthesis in normal and abetalipoproteinemic intestinal mucosa. Gastroenterology 1991; 101:749.
1475. Lieper JM, Bayliss JD, et al: Microsomal triglyceride transfer protein, the abetalipoproteinemia gene product, mediates the secretion of apolipoprotein B–containing lipoproteins from heterologous cells. J Biol Chem 1994; 269:21951.
1476. Ricci B, Sharp D, et al: A 30-amino acid truncation of the microsomal triglyceride transfer protein large protein subunit disrupts its interaction with protein disulfide-isomerase and causes abetalipoproteinemia. J Biol Chem 1995; 270:14281.
1477. Narcisi TM, Shoulders CC, et al: Mutations of the microsomal-triglyceride-transfer-protein gene in abetalipoproteinemia. Am J Hum Genet 1995; 57:1298.
1478. Hardman DA, Pullinger CR, et al: Molecular and metabolic basis for the metabolic disorder normotriglyceridemic abetalipoproteinemia. J Clin Invest 1991; 88:1722.
1479. Gheeraert P, DeBuyzere M, et al: Plasma and erythrocyte lipids in two families with heterozygous hypobetalipoproteinemia. Clin Biochem 1988; 21:371.
1480. Simon ER, Ways P: Incubation hemolysis and red cell metabolism in acanthocytosis. J Clin Invest 1964; 43:1311.
1481. Barenholz Y, Yechiel E, et al: Importance of cholesterol-phospholipid interaction in determining dynamics of normal and abetalipoproteinemia red blood cell membrane. Cell Biophys 1981; 3:115.
1482. Iida H, Takashima Y, et al: Alterations in erythrocyte membrane lipids in abetalipoproteinemia: Phospholipid and fatty acyl composition. Biochem Med 1984; 32:79.
1483. Cooper RA, Gulbrandsen CL: The relationship between serum lipoproteins and red cell membranes in abetalipoproteinemia: Deficiency of lecithin:cholesterol acyltransferase. J Lab Clin Med 1971; 78:323.
1484. Flamm M, Schachter D: Acanthocytosis and cholesterol enrichment decrease lipid fluidity of only the outer human erythrocyte membrane leaflet. Nature 1982; 298:290.
1485. McCormick EC, Cornwell DG, et al: Studies on the distribution of tocopherol in human serum lipoproteins. J Lipid Res 1969; 1:211.
1486. Dodge JT, Cohen G, et al: Peroxidative hemolysis of red blood cells from patients with abetalipoproteinemia (acanthocytosis). J Clin Invest 1967; 46:357.
1487. Elias E, Muller DP, Scott J: Association of spinocerebellar disorders with cystic fibrosis or chronic childhood cholestasis and very low serum vitamin E. Lancet 1981; 2:1319.
1488. Alvarez F, Landrieu P, et al: Vitamin E deficiency is responsible for neurologic abnormalities in cholestatic children. J Pediatr 1985; 107:422.
1489. Sokol RJ, Guggenheim MA, et al: Frequency and clinical progression of the vitamin E deficiency neurologic disorder in children with prolonged neonatal cholestasis. Am J Dis Child 1985; 139:1211.
1490. Harding AE, Matthews S, et al: Spinocerebellar degeneration associated with a selective defect of vitamin E absorption. N Engl J Med 1985; 313:32.
1491. Sokol RJ, Guggenheim M, et al: Improved neurologic function after long-term correction of vitamin E deficiency in children with chronic cholestasis. N Engl J Med 1985; 313:1580.
1492. Muller DPR, Lloyd JK, Bird AC: Long-term management of abetalipoproteinaemia. Arch Dis Child 1977; 52:209.
1493. Estes JW, Morléy JT, et al: A new hereditary acanthocytosis syndrome. Am J Med 1967; 42:868.
1494. Levine IM, Estes JW, Looney JM: Hereditary neurological disease with acanthocytosis. Arch Neurol 1968; 19:403.
1495. Hardie RJ: Acanthocytosis and neurological impairment—a review. Q J Med 1989; 71:291.
1496. Alonso ME, Teixeira F, et al: Chorea-acanthocytosis: A report of a family and neuropathological study of two cases. Can J Neurol Sci 1989; 16:426.
1497. Asano K, Osawa Y, et al: Erythrocyte membrane abnormalities in patients with amyotrophic chorea with acanthocytosis: II. Abnormal degradation of membrane proteins. J Neurol Sci 1985; 68:161.
1498. Clark MR, Aminoff MJ, et al: Red cell deformability and lipid composition in two forms of acanthocytosis: Enrichment of acanthocytic populations by density gradient centrifugation. J Lab Clin Med 1989; 113:469.
1499. Critchley EM, Clark DB, Wikler A: Acanthocytosis and neuro-

logical disorder without abetalipoproteinemia. Arch Neurol 1968; 18:134.

1500. Faillace RT, Kingston WJ, et al: Cardiomyopathy associated with the syndrome of amyotrophic chorea and acanthocytosis. Ann Intern Med 1982; 96:616.

1501. Gross KB, Skrivanek JA, et al: Familial amyotrophic chorea with acanthocytosis: New clinical and laboratory investigations. Arch Neurol 1985; 42:753.

1502. Hardie RJ, Pullon HW, et al: Neuroacanthocytosis: A clinical, haematological and pathological study of 19 cases. Brain 1991; 114:13.

1503. Sotaniemi KA: Chorea-acanthocytosis: Neurological disease with acanthocytosis. Acta Neurol Scand 1983; 68:53.

1504. Ueno E, Oguchi K, et al: Morphological abnormalities of erythrocyte membrane in the hereditary neurological disease with chorea, areflexia and acanthocytosis. J Neurol Sci 1982; 56:89.

1505. Vance JM, Pericak-Vance MA, et al: Chorea-acanthocytosis: A report of three new families and implications for genetic counseling. Am J Med Genet 1987; 28:403.

1506. Villegas A, Moscat J, et al: A new family with choreo-acanthocytosis. Acta Haematol (Basel) 1987; 77:215.

1507. Vita G, Serra S, et al: Peripheral neuropathy in amyotrophic chorea-acanthocytosis. Ann Neurol 1989; 26:583.

1508. Lupo I, Aragona F, et al: Choreo-acanthocytosis with myopathy: Report of a case. Acta Neurol (Napoli) 1987; 9:334.

1509. Spitz MC, Jankovic J, Killian JM: Familial tic disorder, parkinsonism, motor neuron disease, and acanthocytosis: A new syndrome. Neurology 1985; 35:366.

1510. Peppard RF, Lu CS, et al: Parkinsonism with neuroacanthocytosis. Can J Neurol Sci 1990; 17:298.

1511. Roth AM, Hepler RS, et al: Pigmentary retinal dystrophy in Hallervorden-Spatz disease: Clinicopathological report of a case. Surv Ophthalmol 1971; 16:24.

1512. Swisher CN, Menkes JH, et al: Coexistence of Hallervorden-Spatz disease with acanthocytosis. Trans Am Neurol Assoc 1972; 97:212.

1513. Luckenbach MW, Green WR, et al: Ocular clinicopathologic correlation of Hallervorden-Spatz syndrome with acanthocytosis and pigmentary retinopathy. Am J Ophthalmol 1983; 95:369.

1514. Higgins JJ, Patterson MC, et al: Hypoprebetalipoproteinemia, acanthocytosis, retinitis pigmentosa, and pallidal degeneration (HARP syndrome). Neurology 1992; 42:194.

1515. Orrell RW, Amrolia PJ, et al: Acanthocytosis, retinitis pigmentosa, and pallidal degeneration: A report of three patients with hypoprebetalipoproteinemia (HARP syndrome). Neurology 1995; 45:487.

1516. Cianci CD, Mische SM, Morrow JS: Impaired cAMP dependent phosphorylation of erythrocyte protein 4.9 in patients with hereditary spheroechinocytosis and neurodegenerative disease. J Cell Biol 1989; 107:469a. Abstract.

1517. Amrein PC, Friedman R, et al: Hematologic changes in anorexia nervosa. JAMA 1979; 241:2190.

1518. Eto Y, Kitagawa T: Wolman's disease with hypobetalipoproteinemia and acanthocytosis: Clinical and biochemical observations. J Pediatr 1970; 77:862.

1519. Gracey M, Hilton HB: Acanthocytes and hypobetalipoproteinemia. Lancet 1973; 1:679.

1520. Paramathypathy K, Aw SE: Acanthocytosis with beta-lipoprotein deficiency in an Indian girl. Med J Aust 1970; 2:1081.

1521. Fondu P, Mozes N, et al: The erythrocyte membrane disturbances in protein-energy malnutrition: Nature and mechanisms. Br J Haematol 1980; 44:605.

1522. Warren MP, Vande Wiele RL: Clinical and metabolic features of anorexia nervosa. Am J Obstet Gynecol 1973; 117:435.

1523. Herpertz-Dahlmann B, Remschmidt H: Blutbildveränderungen bei Anorexia nervosa in Abhängigkeit vom Gewicht. Monatsschr Kinderheilkd 1988; 136:739.

1524. Kimber CD, Deller J, et al: The mechanism of anaemia in chronic liver disease. Q J Med 1965; 34:33.

1525. Balistreri WF, Leslie MH, Cooper RA: Increased cholesterol and decreased fluidity of red cell membranes (spur cell anemia) in progressive intrahepatic cholestasis. Pediatrics 1981; 67:461.

1526. Cynamon HA, Isenberg JN, et al: Erythrocyte lipid alterations in pediatric cholestatic liver disease: Spur cell anemia of infancy. J Pediatr Gastroenterol Nutr 1985; 4:542.

1527. Doll DC, Doll NJ: Spur cell anemia. South Med J 1982; 75:1205.

1528. Douglass CC, McCall MS, Frenel EP: The acanthocyte in cirrhosis with hemolytic anemia. Ann Intern Med 1968; 68:390.

1529. Grahn EP, Dietz AA, et al: Burr cells, hemolytic anemia and cirrhosis. Am J Med 1968; 45:78.

1530. Greenberg MS, Choi ES: Post-splenectomy spur cell hemolytic anemia. Am J Med Sci 1975; 269:277.

1531. Hitchins R, Naughton L, et al: Spur cell anemia (acanthocytosis) complicating idiopathic hemochromatosis. Pathology 1988; 20:59.

1532. Keller JW, Majerus PW, Finke EH: An unusual type of spiculated erythrocyte in metastatic liver disease and hemolytic anemia: Report of a case. Ann Intern Med 1971; 74:732.

1533. Silber R, Amorosi E, et al: Spur-shaped erythrocytes in Laennec's cirrhosis. N Engl J Med 1966; 275:639.

1534. Smith JA, Lonergan ET, et al: Spur cell anemia: Hemolytic anemia with red cells resembling acanthocytes in alcoholic cirrhosis. N Engl J Med 1964; 276:396.

1535. Stillman AE, Giordano GF: Spur cell anemia associated with extrahepatic biliary tract obstruction. Am J Gastroenterol 1983; 78:589.

1536. Taniguchi M, Tanabe F, et al: Experimental biliary obstruction of rat: Initial changes in the structure and lipid content of erythrocytes. Biochim Biophys Acta 1983; 753:22.

1537. Tchernia G, Navarro J, et al: Anemie hemolytique avec acanthocytose et dyslipidemie au cours de deux hepatites neonatales. Arch Fr Pediatr 1968; 25:729.

1538. Cooper RA, Kimball DB, Dorocher JR: Role of the spleen in membrane conditioning and hemolysis of spur cells in liver disease. N Engl J Med 1974; 290:1279.

1539. Salvioli G, Rioli G, et al: Membrane lipid composition of red blood cells in liver disease: Regression of spur cell anaemia after infusion of polyunsaturated phosphatidylcholine. Gut 1978; 19:844.

1540. Fossaluzza V, Rossi P: Flunarizine treatment for spur cell anaemia. Br J Haematol 1983; 55:715.

1541. Cooper RA, Leslie MH, et al: Factors influencing the lipid composition and fluidity of red cell membranes in vitro: Production of red cells possessing more than two cholesterols per phospholipid. Biochemistry 1978; 17:327.

1542. Cooper RA, Leslie MH, et al: Red cell cholesterol enrichment and spur cell anemia in dogs fed a cholesterolenriched atherogenic diet. J Lipid Res 1980; 21:1082.

1543. Duhamel G, Forgez P, et al: Spur cells in patients with alcoholic liver cirrhosis are associated with reduced plasma levels of apo A-II, HDL, and LDL. J Lipid Res 1983; 24:1612.

1544. Schubert D, Boss K: Band 3 protein-cholesterol interactions in erythrocyte membranes: Possible role in anion transport and dependency on membrane phospholipid. FEBS Lett 1982; 150:4.

1545. Lange Y, Cutler HB, Steck TL: The effect of cholesterol and other interrelated amphipaths on the contour and stability of the isolated red cell membrane. J Biol Chem 1980; 255:9331.

1546. Seigneuret M, Favre E, et al: Strong interactions between a spin-labeled cholesterol analog and erythrocyte proteins in the human erythrocyte membrane. Biochim Biophys Acta 1985; 813:174.

1547. Rooney MW, Lange Y, Kauffman JW: Acyl chain organization and protein secondary structure in cholesterol-modified erythrocyte membranes. J Biol Chem 1984; 259:8281.

1548. Allen DW, Manning N: Abnormal phospholipid metabolism in spur cell anemia: Decreased fatty acid incorporation into phosphatidylethanolamine and increased incorporation into acylcarnitine in spur cell anemia erythrocytes. Blood 1994; 84:1283.

1549. Allen DW, Manning N: Cholesterol-loading of membranes of normal erythrocytes inhibits phospholipid repair and arachadonoyl-CoA:1-palmitoyl-sn-glycero-3-phosphocholine acyl transferase: A model of spur cell anemia. Blood 1996; 87:3489.

1550. Zieve L: Jaundice, hyperlipemia and hemolytic anemia: A heretofore unrecognized syndrome associated with alcoholic fatty liver and cirrhosis. Ann Intern Med 1958; 48:471.

1551. Melhorn DK, Gross S: Vitamin E–dependent anemia in the premature infant: II. Relationships between gestational age and absorption of vitamin E. J Pediatr 1971; 79:581.

1552. Ehrenkranz RA: Vitamin E and the neonate. Am J Dis Child 1980; 134:1157.

1553. Zipursky A: Vitamin E deficiency anemia in newborn infants. Clin Perinatol 1984; 11:393.

1554. Gallagher PG, Ehrenkranz RA: Nutritional anemias in infancy. Perinatal Hematol 1995; 22:671.

1555. Dolan TF Jr: Hemolytic anemia and edema as the initial signs in infants with cystic fibrosis. Clin Pediatr 1976; 15:597.

1556. Monzon CM, Woodruff CW: Anemia and edema as presenting signs in cystic fibrosis: A case report. J Med 1986; 17:135.

1557. Melhorn DK, Gross S: Vitamin E–dependent anemia in the premature infant: I. Effects of large doses of medicinal iron. J Pediatr 1971; 79:569.

1558. Oski FA, Barness LA: Vitamin E deficiency: A previously unrecognized cause of hemolytic anemia in the premature infant. J Pediatr 1967; 70:211.

1559. Ritchie JH, Fish MB, et al: Edema and hemolytic anemia in premature infants: A vitamin E deficiency syndrome. N Engl J Med 1968; 279:1185.

1560. Jacob HS, Lux SE: Degradation of membrane phospholipids and thiols in peroxide hemolysis: Studies in vitamin E deficiency. Blood 1968; 32:549.

1561. Brownlee NR, Huttner JJ, et al: Role of vitamin E in glutathione-induced oxidant stress: Methemoglobin, lipid peroxidation, and hemolysis. J Lipid Res 1977; 18:635.

1562. Kay MM, Bosman GJ, et al: Oxidation as a possible mechanism of cellular aging: Vitamin E deficiency causes premature aging and IgG binding to erythrocytes. Proc Natl Acad Sci U S A 1986; 83:2463.

1563. Ackerman BD: Infantile pyknocytosis in Mexican-American infants. Am J Dis Child 1969; 117:417.

1564. Keimowitz R, Desforges JF: Infantile pyknocytosis. N Engl J Med 1965; 273:1152.

1565. Zannos-Mariola L, Kattamis C, et al: Infantile pyknocytosis and glucose-6-phosphate dehydrogenase deficiency. Br J Haematol 1962; 8:258.

1566. Allison AC: Acute haemolytic anaemia with distortion and fragmentation of erythrocytes in children. Br J Haematol 1957; 3:1.

1567. Redman CM, Marsh WL: The Kell antigens and McLeod red cells. In Agre PC, Cartron JP (eds): Protein Blood Group Antigens of the Human Red Cell: Structure, Function and Clinical Significance. Baltimore, Johns Hopkins University Press, 1992, p 53.

1568. Redman CM, Marsh WL: The Kell blood group system and the McLeod phenotype. Semin Hematol 1993; 30:209.

1569. Redman CM, Marsh WL, et al: Biochemical studies on McLeod phenotype red cells and isolation of Kx antigen. Br J Haematol 1988; 68:131.

1570. Khamlichi S, Bailly P, et al: Purification and partial characterization of the erythrocyte Kx protein deficient in McLeod patients. Eur J Biochem 1995; 228:931.

1571. Ho M, Chelly J, Carter N: Isolation of the gene for McLeod syndrome that encodes a novel membrane transport protein. Cell 1994; 77:869.

1572. Ho MF, Chalmers RM, et al: A novel point mutation in the McLeod syndrome gene in neuroacanthocytosis. Ann Neurol 1996; 39:672.

1573. Taswell HF, Lewis JC, et al: Erythrocyte morphology in genetic defects of the Rh and Kell blood group systems. Mayo Clin Proc 1977; 52:157.

1574. Wimmer BM, Marsh WL, et al: Haematological changes associated with the McLeod phenotype of the Kell blood group system. Br J Haematol 1977; 36:219.

1575. Marsh WL, Marsh NJ, et al: Elevated serum creatine phosphokinase in subjects with McLeod syndrome. Vox Sang 1981; 40:403.

1576. Hardie RJ: Acanthocytosis and neurological impairment—a review. Q J Med 1989; 71:291.

1577. Swash M, Schwartz MS, et al: Benign X-linked myopathy with acanthocytosis (McLeod syndrome): Its relationship to X-linked muscular dystrophy. Brain 1983; 106:717.

1578. Witt TN, Danek A, et al: McLeod syndrome: A distinct form

of neuroacanthocytosis: Report of two cases and literature review with emphasis on neuromuscular manifestations. J Neurol 1992; 239:302.

1579. Danek A, Uttner I, et al: Cerebral involvement in McLeod syndrome. Neurology 1994; 44:117.

1580. Takashima H, Sakai T, et al: A family of McLeod syndrome, masquerading as chorea-acanthocytosis. J Neurol Sci 1994; 124:56.

1581. Malandrini A, Fabrizi GM, et al: Atypical McLeod syndrome manifested as X-linked chorea-acanthocytosis, neuromyopathy and dilated cardiomyopathy: Report of a family. J Neurol Sci 1994; 124:89.

1582. Bertelson CJ, Pogo AO, et al: Localization of the McLeod locus (XK) within Xp21 by deletion analysis. Am J Hum Genet 1988; 42:703.

1583. Francke U, Ochs HD, et al: Minor Xp21 chromosome deletion in a male associated with expression of Duchenne muscular dystrophy, chronic granulomatous disease, retinitis pigmentosa, and McLeod's syndrome. Am J Hum Genet 1985; 37:250.

1584. Giblett ER, Klebanoff SJ, et al: Kell phenotypes in chronic granulomatous disease: A potential transfusion hazard. Lancet 1971; 1:1235.

1585. Hart MVD, Szaloky A, van Loghem JJ: A "new" antibody associated with the Kell blood group system. Vox Sang 1968; 15:456.

1586. Joske RA, McAlister JM, et al: Isotope investigations of red cell production and destruction in chronic renal disease. Clin Sci (Oxford) 1956; 15:511.

1587. Loge JP, Lange RD, et al: Characterization of the anemia associated with chronic renal insufficiency. Am J Med 1958; 24:4.

1588. Nathan DG, Schupak E, et al: Erythropoiesis in anephric man. J Clin Invest 1964; 43:2158.

1589. Akmal M, Telfer N, et al: Erythrocyte survival in chronic renal failure: Role of secondary hyperparathyroidism. J Clin Invest 1985; 76:1695.

1590. Bogin E, Massry SG, et al: Effect of parathyroid hormone on osmotic fragility of human erythrocytes. J Clin Invest 1982; 69:1017.

1591. Saltissi D, Carter GD: Association of secondary hyperparathyroidism with red cell survival in chronic haemodialysis patients. Clin Sci 1985; 68:29.

1592. White JG: Effects of an ionophore A23187 on the surface morphology of normal erythrocytes. Am J Pathol 1974; 77:507.

1593. Parsons SF, Mallinson G, et al: Evidence that the Lu^b blood group antigen is located on red cell membrane glycoproteins of 85 and 78 kd. Transfusion 1987; 27:61.

1594. Shaw MA, Leak MR, et al: The rare Lutheran blood group phenotype Lu(a−b−): A genetic study. Ann Hum Genet 1984; 48:229.

1595. Telen MJ: The Lutheran antigens and proteins affected by Lutheran regulatory genes. In Agre PC, Cartron JP (eds): Protein Blood Group Antigens of the Human Red Cell: Structure, Function and Clinical Significance. Baltimore, Johns Hopkins University Press, 1992, p 70.

1596. Telen MJ, Eisenbarth GS, Haynes BF: Human erythrocyte antigens: Regulation of a novel red cell surface antigen by the inhibitor Lutheran In(Lu) gene. J Clin Invest 1983; 71:1878.

1597. Beutler E, West C: The Woronet's trait: A new familial erythrocyte anomaly. Blood Cells 1980; 6:281.

1598. Horton L, Coburn RJ, et al: The haematology of hypothyroidism. Q J Med 1976; 45:101.

1599. Perillie PE, Tembrevilla C: Red-cell changes in hypothyroidism. Lancet 1975; 2:1151.

1600. Betticher DC, Pugin P: Hypothyroidie et acanthocytes: Importance diagnostique du frottis sanguin. Schweiz Med Wochenschr 1991; 121:1127.

1601. Chuttani HK, Gupta PS, et al: Acute copper sulfate poisoning. Am J Med 1965; 39:849.

1602. Fairbanks VF: Copper sulfate induced hemolytic anemia: Inhibition of glucose-6-phosphate dehydrogenase and other possible etiologic mechanisms. Arch Intern Med 1967; 120:428.

1603. Holtzman NA, Elliott DA, Heller RH: Copper intoxication. N Engl J Med 1966; 275:347.

1604. Manzler AD, Schreiner AW: Copper-induced acute hemolytic anemia: A new complication of hemodialysis. Ann Intern Med 1970; 73:409.

1605. Roberts RH: Hemolytic anemia associated with copper sulfate poisoning. Mississippi Doctor 1956; 33:292.

1606. Oski FA: Chickee, the copper. Ann Intern Med 1970; 73:485. Editorial.

1607. Cartwright GE: Diagnosis of treatable Wilson's disease. N Engl J Med 1978; 298:1347.

1608. Danks DM: Disorders of copper transport. In: Scriver CS, Beaudet AL, et al (eds): The Metabolic and Molecular Bases of Inherited Disease. 7th ed. New York, McGraw-Hill Book Co., 1995, p 2211.

1609. Walshe JM: Wilson's disease: The presenting symptoms. Arch Dis Child 1962; 37:253.

1610. Buchanan GR: Acute hemolytic anemia as a presenting manifestation of Wilson's disease. J Pediatr 1975; 86:245.

1611. Forman SJ, Kumar KS, et al: Hemolytic anemia in Wilson disease: Clinical findings and biochemical mechanisms. Am J Hematol 1980; 9:269.

1612. Grüter W: Hämolytische Krisen als Frühmanifestation der Wilson'schen Krankheit. Dtsch Z Nervenheilkd 1959; 179:401.

1613. Lehr H, Pauschinger M, et al: Haemolytic anaemia as initial manifestation of Wilson's disease. Blut 1988; 56:45.

1614. Robitaille GA, Piscatelli RL, et al: Hemolytic anemia in Wilson's disease. JAMA 1977; 237:2402.

1615. Roche-Sicot J, Benhamou J-P: Acute intravascular hemolysis and acute liver failure associated as a first manifestation of Wilson's disease. Ann Intern Med 1977; 86:301.

1616. Willms KG, Blume KG, Löhr GW: Hämolytische Anämie bei Morbus Wilson (Hepatolentikuläre Degeneration). Klin Wochenschr 1972; 50:995.

1617. Deiss A, Lee GR, Cartwright GE: Hemolytic anemia in Wilson's disease. Ann Intern Med 1970; 73:413.

1618. Dobyns WB, Goldstein NP, Gordon H: Clinical spectrum of Wilson's disease (hepatolenticular degeneration). Mayo Clin Proc 1979; 54:35.

1619. Hoagland HC, Goldstein NP: Hematologic (cytopenic) manifestations of Wilson's disease. Mayo Clin Proc 1978; 53:498.

1620. Iser JH, Stevens BJ, et al: Hemolytic anemia of Wilson's disease. Gastroenterology 1974; 67:290.

1621. McIntyre N, Clink HM, Levi AJ: Hemolytic anemia in Wilson's disease. N Engl J Med 1967; 276:439.

1622. Meyer RJ, Zalusky R: The mechanisms of hemolysis in Wilson's disease: Study of a case and review of the literature. Mt Sinai J Med 1977; 44:530.

1623. Petrukhin K, Fischer SG, et al: Mapping, cloning and genetic characterization of the region containing the Wilson disease gene. Nature Genet 1993; 5:338.

1624. Bull PC, Thomas GR, et al: The Wilson disease gene is a putative copper transporting P-type ATPase similar to the Menkes gene. Nature Genet 1993; 5:327.

1625. Tanzi RE, Petrukhin K, et al: The Wilson disease gene is a copper transporting ATPase with homology to the Menkes disease gene. Nature Genet 1993; 5:344.

1626. Yamaguchi Y, Heiny ME, Gitlin JD: Isolation and characterization of a human liver cDNA as a candidate gene for Wilson disease. Biochem Biophys Res Commun 1993; 197:271.

1627. Chelly J, Monaco AP: Cloning the Wilson disease gene. Nature Genet 1993; 5:317.

1628. Thomas GR, Forbes JR, et al: The Wilson disease gene: Spectrum of mutations and their consequences. Nature Genet 1995; 9:210.

1629. Figus A, Angius A, et al: Molecular pathology and haplotype analysis of Wilson disease in Mediterranean populations. Am J Hum Genet 1995; 57:1318.

1630. Gubler CJ, Labey ME, et al: Studies on copper metabolism. IX. Transportation of copper in blood. J Clin Invest 1953; 32:405.

1631. Hochstein P, Kumar KS, Forman SJ: Mechanisms of copper toxicity in red cells. In Brewer GJ (ed): The Red Cell. New York, Alan R. Liss, Inc., 1978.

Pyruvate Kinase Deficiency and Disorders of Glycolysis

William C. Mentzer

The erythrocyte, devoid of nucleus, mitochondria, ribosomes, and other organelles, has no capacity for cell replication, protein synthesis, or oxidative phosphorylation. The glycolytic production of adenosine triphosphate (ATP), the sole known energy source of such erythrocytes, is sufficient to meet their limited metabolic requirements. The discovery that hemolytic anemia may result from any of several glycolytic enzymopathies has underscored the dependence of erythrocytes on glycolysis. Acquired abnormalities of the chemical milieu within the erythrocyte may also influence glycolysis, alter hemoglobin function, and sometimes shorten red cell life span. Acquired deficiencies of erythrocyte glycolytic enzymes have also been found in malignancies of the hematopoietic system, but, in general, they have not resulted in hemolytic anemia.

In the following paragraphs, the clinical, biochemical and genetic features associated with abnormalities of erythrocyte glycolysis are described in detail. Because they have been more thoroughly studied, the congenital hemolytic anemias are discussed at length, whereas the various acquired disorders are dealt with more briefly.

Hereditary anemias resulting from altered erythrocyte metabolism are distinguished from hereditary spherocytosis by the absence of spherocytes on the peripheral blood smear, by normal osmotic fragility of fresh erythrocytes, by a partial therapeutic response to splenectomy, and by a recessive mode of inheritance. Hemoglobin structure and synthesis are normal. Because no specific morphologic abnormality is associated with these disorders, they have become known as congenital nonspherocytic hemolytic anemias (CNSHAs).[1] Although these anemias are usually transmitted in an autosomal recessive fashion, phosphoglycerate kinase (PGK) deficiency is an X-linked abnormality and adenosine deaminase (ADA) excess is an autosomal dominant disorder. Symptoms and signs may be limited to the manifestations of hemolysis or, if the enzymopathy is present in other tissues, may involve other organ systems. In the latter instance, the specific pattern of involvement of nonerythroid tissues may be of real assistance in diagnosis.[2]

Initial attempts at classification were based on the autohemolysis test, in which saline-washed erythrocytes were incubated *in vitro* at 37°C under sterile conditions and the percentage of hemolysis determined after 48 hours.[3] Autohemolysis was greater than normal in almost all cases of CNSHA. If glucose was added before incubation, hemolysis was reduced in control subjects and in some patients with CNSHA (type I), but was unchanged, or actually increased, in others (type II). Robinson and associates[4] found that type II erythrocytes contained subnormal amounts of ATP but markedly increased amounts of 2,3-diphosphoglycerate (2,3-DPG). These observations, coupled with the inability of such cells to metabolize glucose,[3] led Robinson and co-workers to suggest the existence of a specific glycolytic enzyme defect below the site of 2,3-DPG synthesis. In 1961, Valentine and associates provided dramatic confirmation of the suggested glycolytic defect by reporting a deficiency of erythrocyte pyruvate kinase (PK) in three patients with CNSHA.[5] Subsequently, abnormalities of other glycolytic enzymes have been associated with CNSHA, as indicated in Figure 17–1.

During the past two decades, specific alterations in protein structure have been found to underlie many of the enzyme deficiency states, and the tools of molecular biology are beginning to identify the genetic basis for these defects.[6, 7]

The presence of a glycolytic enzymopathy should be suspected when chronic hemolysis occurs in the absence of marked abnormalities of erythrocyte morphology or osmotic fragility. An exception to the usually unremarkable red cell morphology in CNSHA is the pronounced basophilic stippling found in pyrimidine-5'-nucleotidase (P-5'-N) deficiency.[8] Hemoglobin elec-

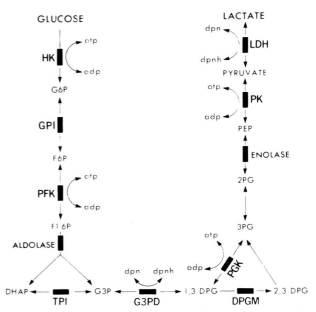

Figure 17-1. The Embden-Meyerhof pathway. Recognized enzyme defects are indicated by solid bars. HK = hexokinase; GPI = glucose phosphate isomerase; PFK = phosphofructokinase; TPI = triose phosphate isomerase, G3PD = glucose-3-phosphate dehydrogenase; PGK = phosphoglycerate kinase; DPGM = 2,3-diphosphoglycerate mutase; PK = pyruvate kinase; LDH = lactate dehydrogenase.

trophoresis, stains for inclusion bodies, hemoglobin heat stability, acid hemolysis, and appropriate studies for immune hemolysis are normal. Despite its initial usefulness in directing the attention of investigators to the glycolytic pathway, further experience with the autohemolysis test has shown that it lacks specificity and is, at best, of limited value in the evaluation of CNSHA.[9] Unfortunately, no other simple, convenient laboratory screening test has been developed that unequivocally reveals the presence of a glycolytic enzymopathy. Therefore, the appropriate diagnostic strategy for the evaluation of a suspected enzymopathy is first to eliminate easily identified causes of hemolysis, such as hemoglobinopathies or spherocytosis, before proceeding to tests for enzyme disorders.[10] Definitive diagnosis depends on quantitative assay of the activity of the suspected enzyme or identification of a specific mutation by DNA analysis. The availability of such assays is limited, but screening tests for deficiencies of PK, triose phosphate isomerase (TPI), and phosphoglucose isomerase can be carried out in any well-equipped clinical laboratory.[11] Mutant enzyme proteins vary in their *in vitro* properties (Table 17–1), and characterization of such properties has improved understanding of the genetics and pathogenesis of anemias associated with defective glycolytic enzymes. Measurement of glycolytic intermediates extracted from freshly obtained erythrocytes has provided confirmation of the *in vivo* significance of *in vitro* abnormalities of enzyme function. The usual finding is an accumulation of proximal and a depletion of distal intermediates, giving rise to a characteristic transition or crossover pattern at the locus of an abnormal enzyme. Secondary crossovers

1. Vmax	Maximal enzyme velocity obtainable with saturating substrate concentrations
2. K_m	The substrate concentration yielding half maximal activity; an index of catalytic efficiency
3. pH optimum	That pH at which maximal enzyme activity is present
4. Heat stability	Resistance of enzyme protein to heat denaturation
5. Electrophoretic mobility	Migration of enzyme protein in an electric field
6. Specific activity	Enzyme activity per defined amount of enzyme protein (e.g., mg); enzyme protein is measured immunologically with antienzyme antibodies

are sometimes observed, reflecting the influence of altered concentrations of metabolites on key regulatory enzymes such as hexokinase (HK), phosphofructokinase (PFK), and PK. As a result of secondary crossovers, the pattern of glycolytic intermediates may become so complex as to be of only limited usefulness in the identification of an enzymopathy. On the other hand, measurement of intracellular metabolites are the most convenient way to screen for abnormalities of nucleotide metabolism. Red cell ATP levels are below normal in ADA excess, whereas pyrimidine-5'-nucleotidase deficiency is associated with increased concentrations of red cell ATP and reduced levels of glutathione. The apparent increase in ATP is, in fact, due to the presence of large amounts of cytidine and uridine nucleotides, which are also measured in the enzymatic assay for ATP. Spectral analysis of a deproteinized extract of red cells provides a straightforward means of identifying such nucleotides and is a simple way to screen suspected patients for pyrimidine-5'-nucleotidase deficiency.[8]

A certain amount of caution is necessary in interpreting the results of quantitative assays of enzyme activity. First, only surviving cells are available for sampling in the circulating blood, and the metabolic circumstances of these favored cells cannot necessarily be extrapolated to indicate the status of cells already hemolyzed. Second, assay *in vitro* under optimal conditions of pH, cofactor availability, and substrate concentration may not adequately reflect the performance of an enzyme under less favorable circumstances *in vivo*. Third, the high specific activity of certain enzymes in leukocytes may result in spurious normal values for erythrocyte enzyme activity unless either the leukocytes are removed before assay or their contribution to total activity is compensated for by appropriate calculations. Fourth, transfusion therapy with normal erythrocytes within several months before assay may obscure the presence of an enzyme defect. Finally, the mean enzyme activity that is determined fails to portray distribution of activity within individual erythrocytes. The endowment of intracellular enzymes is fixed with the disappearance of protein synthetic ability at the reticulocyte stage; thereafter, the inevitable dena-

turation of enzyme protein that accompanies cell aging reduces enzymatic activity at a rate characteristic of each enzyme. Transient accentuation of reticulocytosis, therefore, is often accompanied by rising mean enzyme activity. Certain glycolytic enzymes (notably, HK and PK) are strikingly more active in reticulocytes than in post-reticulocyte red cells, and the majority of this excess activity is rapidly lost coincident with reticulocyte maturation.[12–14] The true magnitude of an enzyme deficiency may not be apparent unless comparison is made with equally reticulocyte-rich blood[13] or corrections are applied that separate out the contribution of the reticulocyte subfraction to total enzyme activity.[14]

HEXOKINASE DEFICIENCY

$$\text{Glucose} \xrightarrow[\text{ATP} \quad \text{Mg}^{2+} \quad \text{ADP}]{\text{Hexokinase}} \text{Glucose-6-phosphate}$$

Clinical Manifestations

Twenty-two cases of CNSHA have been attributed to deficient erythrocyte HK activity (Table 17–2). Severely affected individuals may exhibit neonatal hyperbilirubinemia and thereafter require transfusion at regular intervals for intractable anemia, but, in mild cases, hemolysis is fully compensated and anemia is absent. However, jaundice, reticulocytosis, and splenomegaly are usually present in such patients. Gallstones may be evident, even in early childhood.[15] Hyperhemolytic episodes are not a feature of the disorder. Red cell morphology is usually unremarkable, but occasional burr cells, target cells, stippled cells, and densely stained spiculated cells may be observed after splenectomy. The osmotic fragility of fresh erythrocytes is normal, but after incubation at 37°C a fragile population of cells may appear.

Deficient erythrocyte HK activity in association with macrocytic anemia has also been found in a few individuals who had the clinical features of Fanconi's aplastic anemia[16] and thus differed from patients with isolated congenital hemolytic anemia. Thrombocytopenia and leukopenia were present, and both platelet and white cell hexokinase activity were reduced. Other patients with Fanconi's anemia have not been HK deficient. In the setting of Fanconi's anemia, HK deficiency is probably a manifestation of dyserythropoiesis rather than a cause of anemia.

Biochemistry

Hexokinase is the glycolytic enzyme with the lowest activity in normal red cells, and a variety of observations indicate that it plays a rate-limiting role in erythrocyte glycolysis.[17–20] In human red cells, HK is a monomer (molecular weight, 112,000 daltons).[21] Three distinct isozymes, each with identical kinetic properties and molecular weight, can be distinguished in mature red cells, based on differences in isoelectric point.[18] Whether these isozymes are under separate genetic

Table 17-2. HEXOKINASE VARIANTS ASSOCIATED WITH HEMOLYTIC ANEMIA

References	No. of Cases	Clinical Features			Properties of Red Blood Cell Hexokinase			
		Inheritance	Hemolytic Anemia	Other	Activity (% of Normal)	Kinetic Abnormalities	Stability in Vitro	Electrophoretic Mobility
33	1	—	+	Congenital malformations	13–24*	0	—	—
34	1	Recessive	+ +		15–20*	+	Normal	Abnormal
35	1	Recessive	+ +		16*	0	—	Abnormal
36	1	Recessive	+		20*	0	Normal	Normal
37, 38	1	Recessive	+ +	Low platelet and fibroblast hexokinase activity	20*	0	Low	Normal
39	1	Recessive	+ +	Low platelet hexokinase activity	25*	+	Normal	Abnormal
15	1	Recessive	+		25*	0	Low	Normal
40	2	Dominant	+	Spherocytes, ovalocytes	30*	0	Low	Normal
41	1	Recessive	+	Psychomotor retardation	45†	+	Normal	Normal
42	1	Recessive	+		50*	0	Normal	Normal
43	1	—	+	Congenital malformations	33*	+	—	—
29	2	Recessive	+		40–53*	+	Low	Normal
32	1	—	+		50*	+	—	—
44	5	Dominant	+		45–91†	+	Normal	Abnormal
28	2	Dominant	+ +	White blood cell hexokinase activity low	75*	+	Normal	Abnormal

*Maximal enzyme activity (Vmax) compared with reticulocytosis controls.
†Maximal enzyme activity (Vmax) compared with normal red cells.

control or represent post-translational modifications of a single gene product is unknown. Similarly, whether each serves a unique function in the erythrocyte is unclear. HK activity declines as red cells age. Loss of activity is particularly striking during reticulocyte maturation. In human reticulocytes, two major isoenzymes of HK have been identified by chromatographic techniques.[22] One (HK$_R$) has an apparent half-life *in vivo* of only 10 days, whereas the other (HK$_1$) has a longer half-life of 66 days. Differential loss of these two isoenzymes appears to explain the biphasic character of the decay in HK activity during erythrocyte aging. An ATP- and ubiquitin-dependent proteolytic system, capable of degrading about 80% of HK activity, may explain the rapid loss of HK in rabbit reticulocytes,[23] or the loss may be secondary to an intrinsic property of the HK molecule itself.[24] Prior oxidative injury appears to be necessary for recognition and destruction of HK by the ubiquitin-dependent system.[25] Because ATP and ubiquitin-dependent proteolysis is limited to reticulocytes,[23] it cannot be responsible for the loss of HK in aging human red cells.

The maximal activity of erythrocyte HK from deficient patients has varied from 13% to 91% of normal (see Table 17–2). In evaluating these findings, comparisons of enzyme activity must be made between red cell populations of equivalent youth. In the case described by Valentine, for example (Fig. 17–2), although HK activity was 62% of the normal value for mature erythrocytes, it was only 14% of the activity found in high reticulocyte blood. A separation of young and old red cell populations by centrifugation revealed only the expected moderate diminution (to 0.11 mol per minute per 10^{10} red blood cells) of HK activity in older cells from this patient.[26] HK activity was even lower (0.075 mol per minute per 10^{10} red blood cells) in an asymptomatic brother, yet no evidence of undue hemolysis was present. However, Figure 17–2 shows that the brother's cells are actually far less deficient with respect to cell age than are the immature cells of the proposita. It would not be surprising that diminished HK activity might curtail the survival of energetic young cells with increased metabolic needs but have little effect on aged, metabolically indolent cells.[26] As the erythrocyte ages, *in vivo* changes in stability or kinetics peculiar to mutant HK also may render older cells liable to premature hemolysis. In rats and rabbits, HK from immature erythrocytes exhibits a higher K_m (Michaelis constant) glucose than is seen in mature cells, but such is not the case in normal human erythrocytes.[27]

In keeping with their enzymatic defect, HK-deficient erythrocytes have usually demonstrated subnormal glucose consumption and lactate production *in vivo*. Such cells also metabolize fructose poorly but utilize mannose or galactose normally[26] because these substrates are not metabolized by HK. Some HK-deficient erythrocytes are capable of normal glucose consumption at the glucose concentrations (5 mmol/L) customarily found in plasma but utilize glucose poorly or not at all at lower glucose concentrations, either because of an abnormally low affinity for glucose[28] or because of enzyme instability under conditions of low substrate availability.[29] Such erythrocytes may encounter a particularly unfavorable metabolic environment within the spleen. The concentration of glucose in normal splenic homogenates has been found by Necheles and co-workers to be only 5 to 11 μmol per gram of tissue, and in an HK-deficient patient the concentration was even lower (1.1 μmol per gram of tissue).[28] Furthermore, because splenic tissue metabolizes glucose rapidly,[30] prolonged vascular pooling in the spleen is probably accompanied by profound local hypoglycemia. Erythrocytes containing high K_m HK are clearly at a disadvantage competing with voracious reticuloendothelial cells for such a reduced glucose supply. Another disadvantage of the splenic environment is its relative acidity. The pH optimum of erythrocyte HK is approximately 8; at lower pH values, diminished enzyme activity may be expected. Possibly of greater importance, at low pH values, glucose-6-phosphate, a potent inhibitor of HK, accumulates because of PFK inhibition.[31] An erythrocyte whose HK activity is diminished even under optimal pH conditions will be further compromised in the acidic environment of the spleen. The clinical improvement that follows splenectomy attests to the importance of this organ in the pathogenesis of hemolysis. Detailed isotopic studies to define red cell kinetics and sites of hemolysis have yet to be reported. Although in two patients no splenic sequestration of chromated autologous erythrocytes was noted,[15, 32] in another sequestration was present.[16]

Significant alterations in intracellular metabolites are associated with defective HK function. Erythrocyte ATP concentration is sometimes,[16, 32, 40] but not always,[36, 39, 43, 44] subnormal. Glucose-6-phosphate concentration is reduced to approximately half normal concentrations, and other more distal intermediates, most notably 2,3-DPG, are also usually reduced in concentration. These metabolites may exert a significant regulatory influence on glycolysis. For example, Brewer has shown that concentrations of 2,3-DPG in the physiologic range inhibit HK[45] so that the low 2,3-DPG levels in HK-deficient red cells may facilitate the performance of available HK. The increased hemoglobin-oxygen affinity associated with subnormal 2,3-DPG levels has been documented in one anemic HK-deficient patient by Delivoria-Papadopoulos and co-workers[46] and by Oski and associates.[47] This patient, whose hemoglobin oxygen affinity (P_{50}) was 19 mm Hg (normal = 27 ± 1.2), was capable of only minimal exercise on a bicycle ergometer, despite only moderate anemia (hemoglobin = 9.8 g/dL). On exercise, her central venous partial pressure of oxygen promptly fell to minimal levels as oxygen consumption rose. Increased oxygen delivery was achieved primarily by an increase in cardiac output, because the unfavorable oxygen affinity curve precluded any substantial further desaturation of hemoglobin.[47] Thus, the altered concentration of intracellular metabolites induced by HK deficiency may, as in this patient, accentuate the usual clinical manifestations of anemia.

Because of its reactive sulfhydryl group, HK is susceptible to oxidant inactivation in the absence of sufficient glutathione.[48] Both normal and low glutathione levels have been reported in HK deficiency, and, although Lohr and co-workers have discovered Heinz bodies in their patients with Fanconi's anemia,[16] these have not been observed in other enzymopenic individuals. Resting hexose monophosphate (HMP) shunt activity, measured with glucose-1-^{14}C, was quantitatively normal in one patient, despite subnormal glucose consumption, but stimulation with methylene blue produced only a meager 6-fold rise in activity, compared with a 22-fold rise in control blood.[35] Failure of the shunt at low glucose concentrations has also been noted in a high K_m glucose HK mutant.[28] Methylene blue–stimulated methemoglobin reduction was subnormal in the single instance that it was evaluated.[15] When HK-inactivating antibodies are incorporated into normal red cells by the process of hypotonic lysis and isotonic reannealing, enzyme-deficient cells exhibit a greatly impaired response to HMP shunt stimulation by methylene blue.[18] These studies, although not indicating a central role for defective shunt activity in the pathogenesis of hemolysis, do suggest that under unusual circumstances HK-deficient cells might be

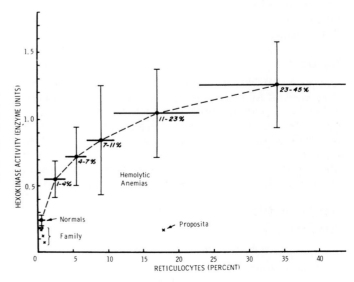

Figure 17-2. Hexokinase activity observed in 54 cases of hemolytic anemia of various causes plotted against reticulocyte percentages in cells assayed. Cases are grouped according to reticulocyte levels. Mean HK activity for each group is plotted against mean reticulocyte percentage in cells of that group. Standard deviations are indicated by *vertical bars*. Values for a single HK-deficient patient (proposita) and her family are designed separately. (From Valentine WH, Oski FA, et al: In Beutler E (ed): Hereditary Disorders of Erythrocyte Metabolism. New York, Grune & Stratton, 1968, p 294.)

compromised by a limited shunt. Such circumstances, for example, might arise on exposure to a potent oxidant in the low glucose environment of the spleen.

Genetics

Inheritance is autosomal recessive. Biochemical identification of asymptomatic carriers is not always possible, because enzyme activity often falls within the low normal range. In a few pedigrees (see Table 17–2), the heterozygous state appears to be severe enough to result in hemolytic anemia. One such heterozygote appeared to be doubly heterozygous for HK and glucose-6-phosphate dehydrogenase (G6PD) deficiency.[49]

The qualitative abnormalities characteristic of variant HK (see Table 17–2) may reflect either a structural or a regulatory gene mutation. On electrophoresis, mutant HK lacks one or more of the normal bands of activity but no bands migrating in an abnormal position have been observed. The various bands represent the presence of several isozymes of HK. Diminished synthesis of one or more isozymes with predominance of the remaining isozyme(s) accounts for the electrophoretic differences observed (see Table 17–2). The kinetic abnormalities noted in many mutant forms of HK undoubtedly reflect as yet undefined structural abnormalities of enzyme protein.

Studies of the tissue distribution of HK deficiency have been performed in blood cells and cultured fibroblasts. Electrophoresis of leukocyte or platelet HK reveals an anodal isozyme (Hk$_3$) distinct from those of the erythrocyte (Hk$_1$, Hk$_2$), as well as a shared isozyme (Hk$_1$).[50, 51] Leukocyte HK activity has been normal in some patients,[26, 29] but the qualitative abnormality of leukocyte HK described by Necheles and colleagues,[28] as well as the case of generalized HK deficiency in all blood cells reported by Rijksen and co-workers,[39] indicate that to some extent the enzyme is under common genetic control in different tissues. When platelet HK activity has been low, platelet function has been normal despite subtle defects in *in vitro* energy metabolism.[52] Cultured fibroblasts from two individuals with different HK mutants contained HK with properties and activity like those found in red cells,[36] suggesting that this source of fetal tissue could be used for prenatal diagnosis.

Therapy

Treatment consists of red cell transfusion as indicated, supplemental folic acid, and close observation for cholelithiasis. Experience with splenectomy has been limited to six patients; none were cured, but all benefited. Pre-existing transfusion requirements were abolished in the five severe cases[26, 28, 34, 37, 39]; in the sixth case,[29] which was milder and did not require transfusion, evidence of diminished hemolysis was obtained.

GLUCOSE PHOSPHATE ISOMERASE DEFICIENCY

Glucose phosphate isomerase

Glucose-6-phosphate $\longleftrightarrow$ Fructose-6-phosphate

Clinical Manifestations

Deficient erythrocyte glucose phosphate isomerase (GPI) has been reported in 46 anemic patients from 34 different pedigrees (Table 17–3). In most cases, hemolytic anemia has first appeared in infancy and has been severe enough to warrant blood transfusion therapy. About 30% of reported patients have exhibited neonatal hyperbilirubinemia.[53] Hydrops fetalis[54, 55] and neonatal death[56] have been described. Several patients have experienced hyperhemolytic crises after infections or drug exposure.[53–63] In some of these individuals, G6PD, as well as GPI, has been deficient.[57, 63]

Red cell morphology generally resembles that seen in other types of CNSHAs. In severely anemic patients, dense, spiculated, or "whiskered" microspherocytes have been noted after splenectomy. In one instance, sufficient numbers of such cells were present before splenectomy to suggest the diagnosis of hereditary spherocytosis.[64] In another, the predominant morphologic abnormality was stomatocytosis.[65] Reticulocytosis may be profound; levels as high as 81% have been observed. The mean corpuscular volume is elevated (97 to 139 fL). When incubated at 37°C, a variable fraction of erythrocytes may exhibit abnormally increased osmotic fragility, whereas fresh cells are usually normal. The survival of chromated autologous red cells is reduced (half-life of 2 to 13 days), often,[66–68] but not invariably,[56, 66, 69] with evidence of splenic sequestration. Hemolytic anemia is usually the sole clinical manifestation of GPI deficiency. The relationship of isolated examples of extraerythrocytic clinical abnormalities (such as priapism[70] or myotonia with mental retardation[71, 72]) to the enzymopathy may, therefore, be fortuitous. In one instance, however (GPI Homburg), neuromuscular abnormalities were correlated with a severe reduction in muscle and cerebrospinal fluid GPI activity.[73] An animal model of GPI deficiency and chronic hemolytic anemia has been developed in the mouse. Clinical and biochemical features of the disease in mice closely resemble those found in humans.[74]

Biochemistry

The metabolic events that precede hemolysis of GPI-deficient erythrocytes are poorly understood. Good evidence exists that erythrocyte glycolysis is impaired *in vivo*, because an increase in the ratio of substrate to product, namely, of glucose-6-phosphate to fructose-6-phosphate, has been a consistent finding in freshly obtained enzymopenic cells.[57, 59, 61, 64, 75–78] Paradoxically, with only occasional exceptions,[58, 64] such cells are fully capable of glycolysis *in vitro*,[57, 69, 79–82] even at the maximal rate imposed by a high phosphate medium (18 mmol/L).[80] In contrast to HK deficiency, in which 2,3-DPG levels are low, sufficient glycolysis usually occurs in GPI deficiency to maintain 2,3-DPG concentration at or above the normal level.[57–59, 76, 81, 83, 84] Except for three patients with diminished ATP, two of whom also exhibited reduced *in vitro* glycolysis for cell age,[57, 64, 69] the erythrocyte ATP concentration has been normal. One such patient[57] was G6PD deficient as well as GPI defi-

Table 17–3. GLUCOSE PHOSPHATE ISOMERASE (GUP) VARIANTS ASSOCIATED WITH HEMOLYTIC ANEMIA

References	Variant	Activity (% of Normal) Red Blood Cells	Activity (% of Normal) White Blood Cells	Electrophoretic Mobility (% of Normal)	Stability in Vitro	Kinetic Abnormalities	pH Optimum	Activity Antigen Ratio*	Apparent Inheritance
Variants Exhibiting Increased Electrophoretic Mobility									
99	Calden	25	20	Fast	Low	0	Normal	—	Compound heterozygote
82	Seattle	29	23	Fast (133, 123)		0	—	—	Compound heterozygote
69, 103	Nordham	22	39	Fast (132)	Low	0	Normal	—	Compound heterozygote
72	—	23	3	Fast (130)	Normal	+	Normal	—	Homozygote
80, 96	Espein	26–32	73	Fast (129)	Low	0	Normal	40	Homozygote
57, 96, 104	Paderborn	29	35	Fast (125)	Low	0	Normal	76	Homozygote
105	Narita	44		Fast (122)	Low	0	Normal	—	Homozygote
77, 98	Kortrijk	25–30	32	Fast (120)	Low	0	Normal	65	Compound heterozygote
65, 97, 98	Barcelona	7–15	20	Fast (116)	Low	0	Acidic	65–70	Compound heterozygote
83	Roma	41	41	Fast (115)	Low	+	Normal	100	Homozygote
Variants Exhibiting Normal Electrophoretic Mobility									
106	Mytho	10	—	Normal	Low	+	Normal	—	Compound heterozygote
78	—	15	55–61	Normal	Low	0	Alkaline	15	Compound heterozygote
76, 105	Matsumoto	15–41	10	Normal	Low	0	Acidic	—	Homozygote
59, 98, 107	Utrecht	15–18	25	Normal	Low	0	Normal	75	Homozygote
55	Tadikonda	19	100	Normal	Low	0	—	—	Homozygote
58	Valle-Hermosa	21	100	Normal	Low	0	Acidic	—	Homozygote
60	Augsberg	22	—	Normal	Low	+	Alkaline	15	Homozygote
67	Johannesburg	24	—	Normal	Low	0	Normal	—	?
56	Kentucky	33	—	Normal	Low	0	Normal	—	Homozygote
108	Hamburg	27	60	Normal	Low	0	Normal		Homozygote
108	Kiel	34	10	Normal	Low	0	Normal		?
Variants Exhibiting Slow Electrophoretic Mobility									
109	Liege enfant	21	—	Slow (96)	Low	0	Normal	—	Homozygote
62	Malades	19	68	Slow (95)	Low	0	Acidic	89	Homozygote
66, 96	Winnipeg	29	—	Slow (95)	Low	0	Normal	50	Compound heterozygote
84	Whitley County	14	—	Slow (90)	—	0	—	—	Homozygote
79	Recklinghausen	15	35	Slow (88)	Low	0	Normal	—	Homozygote
73, 108	Hamburg	7	9	Slow (68)	Normal	+	Normal	—	Compound heterozygote
68, 98	Nijmegen	20	—	Slow (65)	Low	0	Normal	—	Compound heterozygote
62	Paris	23	44	Slow (63)	Low	+	Normal	82	Homozygote
75	Elyria	14	—	Slow (25)	Low	0	Normal	—	Homozygote
66, 96	Los Angeles	14	22	Slow (44.0–28)	Low	0	Normal	35	Compound heterozygote
105	—	39	—	Slow	Low	0	Normal	—	Compound heterozygote
61	Kaiserlautern	9.5	—	Slow	Low	+	Alkaline	—	Compound heterozygote

*GFI enzyme protein (cross-reacting material) determined immunologically. Value shown is percentage of expected activity for amount of GPI protein present.

cient and exhibited unusually high glucose-6-phosphate levels. It was thought that inhibition of HK by the increased concentration of glucose-6-phosphate present might have contributed significantly to the reduced glycolytic rate observed. On the other hand, increased glucose-6-phosphate availability might have favorably influenced the GPI reaction by bringing the enzyme closer to saturation with its substrate.

A profound defect in recycling of fructose-6-phosphate through the pentose phosphate shunt has been observed repeatedly in GPI-deficient red cells.[64, 82, 84] Increased formation of Heinz bodies,[56, 65] as well as glutathione instability,[71, 78] after exposure to acetylphenylhydrazine, an abnormal ascorbate cyanide test, and diminished concentrations of red cell glutathione[65, 69, 75, 76, 78] in fresh erythrocytes all suggest that diminished shunt activity *in vivo* may contribute to hemolysis.

With rare exceptions,[73] mutant forms of red cell GPI exhibit considerable thermal lability *in vitro* (see Table 17–3), raising the possibility that accelerated loss of enzyme activity *in vivo* associated with aging may result in premature metabolic collapse and subsequent

hemolysis. Separation of red cells by centrifugation into young and old subpopulations demonstrated accelerated decay of enzyme activity in two instances[69, 85] but not in a third.[55] Arnold and co-workers attempted to simulate the *in vivo* process of aging by incubating red cells *in vitro* at 37°C for 8 days, frequently changing the incubation medium to ensure that glucose availability and pH remained constant.[85] GPI activity declined by 66% in GPI-deficient red cells during the incubation, reaching a level of only 6% of normal, and lactate production, normal at the onset, was reduced to 11% of normal. In contrast, normal reticulocyte-rich blood lost only 6% of the original GPI activity after 8 days and lactate production fell only 7%. If mannose, rather than glucose, was employed, GPI-deficient and normal red cells made equivalent amounts of lactate, and there was little or no loss in lactate production after 8 days. The normal glycolytic rate noted with mannose, which is isomerized by mannose phosphate isomerase and thus bypasses the GPI reaction, clearly pinpoints defective GPI activity as the cause of glycolytic failure in GPI-deficient cells. ATP depletion with consequent erythrocyte rigidity would be anticipated to follow failure of glycolysis, soon resulting in reticuloendothelial entrapment of the rigid cells. Schroter and Tillmann,[86] using a filtration technique (5-μm nuclepore filters), have demonstrated that GPI-deficient red cells are, indeed, less deformable than normal cells, particularly when comparison is made with young, reticulocyte-rich populations of cells. Similar rheologic findings have been reported by Chilcote and Baehner[87] and by Goulding,[70] who studied a 9-year-old GPI-deficient patient with priapism and concluded that the priapism could well have been the consequence of abnormal erythrocyte deformability. Studies by Coetzer and Zail[88] reveal aggregation of membrane spectrin in GPI-deficient erythrocytes. The extent of aggregation is a function of cell age.

Although hemolysis of GPI-deficient erythrocytes may occur in older cells as a consequence of accelerated loss of enzyme activity, young cells, even reticulocytes, also may be severely enzyme deficient.[89] As described later (see section on pyruvate kinase), reticulocytes become reliant on oxidative phosphorylation for ATP generation when glycolysis is impaired. As in PK deficiency, the acidic, hypoglycemic splenic environment may impair effective oxidative phosphorylation in GPI-deficient reticulocytes, leading to metabolic failure and hemolysis. Large numbers of reticulocytes were found when the spleen of a GPI-deficient patient was examined by transmission electron microscopy.[89] Furthermore, the reticulocyte count often rises after splenectomy.[56, 67, 69, 89] Because hemoglobin levels also rise, this observation suggests survival of a population of reticulocytes that would otherwise be hemolyzed almost immediately after their release from the marrow.

Genetics and Inheritance

Like most other glycolytic enzymopathies, GPI deficiency is inherited as an autosomal recessive trait. Heterozygotes are hematologically normal but exhibit reduced erythrocyte GPI activity (usually to about 50% of normal).

GPI is a dimer[90] composed of two identical subunits, each with a molecular weight of approximately 60,000.[68, 90] Subunit synthesis is directed by a single genetic locus located on chromosome 19.[91] All 9 GPI mutations associated with hemolytic anemia that have been characterized at the molecular level are nucleotide substitutions in the coding region that alter a single amino acid.[92, 93] Heterozygotes inherit one mutant and one normal GPI allele, resulting in the synthesis of two unlike GPI subunits that may combine in one of three ways to form a normal homodimer, a mutant homodimer, or a heterodimer that contains both normal and mutant subunits. Electrophoresis of GPI from the erythrocytes of heterozygotes will demonstrate one to three bands, depending on the extent to which the charge or activity of the mutant subunit is altered. Post-translational events, such as oxidation of enzyme protein, may alter the electrophoretic pattern and confuse its interpretation.[94, 95]

Hemolytic anemia occurs in individuals when GPI activity drops below about 40% of the normal mean activity. The properties of 34 apparently different forms of GPI found in patients with hemolytic anemia are summarized in Table 17–3. Substrate kinetics and the pH optimum of mutant enzymes have almost always been normal, but most mutants have exhibited varying degrees of thermal instability. Thus, the most useful means of classifying such mutants has been on the basis of electrophoretic mobility or residual enzyme activity in red cells and leukocytes. The availability of anti-GPI antibodies has allowed immunologic titration of the amount of residual enzyme protein in erythrocytes. Varying amounts of functionally inactive enzyme protein have been discovered when different mutants have been subjected to immunologic analysis. It can be concluded from these studies that some mutant GPI alleles are "silent" and produce no detectable enzyme protein, whereas others produce structurally altered protein with varying degrees of activity and stability *in vivo*.[96–98] All available evidence indicates that only a single GPI isozyme is present in human tissues.[91] GPI deficiency is usually less severe in nonerythroid tissues than in erythrocytes, because nonerythrocytic tissues retain the ability to synthesize GPI subunits. Clinical abnormalities outside the hematopoietic system are rare. Leukocytes are capable of normal phagocytosis and chemotaxis, despite a reduction in GPI activity to 25%[59] to 73%[80] of normal, but if activity is more severely depressed, granulocyte function is impaired.[73, 99] Similarly, platelet GPI may be only 20% to 30% of normal, but clot formation, platelet aggregation, and other clotting studies are normal.[59, 80] Cultured skin fibroblasts exhibited only half normal GPI activity in one patient.[100] Plasma GPI activity is usually low but may be normal.[58] In one family, amniotic fluid fibroblasts were used to diagnose a severely anemic GPI-deficient infant before birth.[40] In another, chorionic villus trophoblast GPI was obtained at 9 weeks of gestation and used to detect heterozygous GPI deficiency in the fetus.[101]

Blockade of glycolysis at the GPI step may divert the flow of glucose metabolism in the direction of glycogen synthesis. Several GPI-deficient patients have been reported to have increased hepatic glycogen stores,[89, 102] and, in one, complaints of muscular fatigue were severe enough to suggest a diagnosis of glycogen storage disease.[102]

Therapy

Transfusion requirements are usually eliminated by removal of the spleen, but anemia persists.[56, 67, 80, 89] The postsplenectomy hemoglobin levels of 6.7 to 10.3 g/dL and reticulocyte counts of 36% to 73% observed in three siblings by Paglia and co-workers[84] reflect the magnitude of the continued hemolysis that may be present. Attempts by Arnold and colleagues[80] to enhance glycolysis in a GPI-deficient patient by intravenous administration of methylene blue or inorganic phosphate were without lasting benefit.

PHOSPHOFRUCTOKINASE DEFICIENCY

Phosphofructokinase

$$\text{Fructose-6-phosphate} \longleftrightarrow \text{Fructose-1,6-diphosphate}$$

$$\text{ATP} \quad Mg^{2+} \quad \text{ADP}$$

Clinical Manifestations

Inherited deficiency of PFK can involve erythrocytes, muscle, or both tissues, depending on the PFK subunit affected and the nature of the biochemical defect (Table 17–4).

Although low erythrocyte PFK activity and mild hemolytic anemia are commonly found in type VII glycogen storage disease (Tarui's syndrome), the dominant clinical feature of this disorder is exertional myopathy due to deficient muscle PFK activity.[113, 114] Physical activity is limited not by anemia but by weakness, easy fatigability, and severe muscle cramps associated with the myopathy. The disease may manifest at birth and cause death during infancy from respiratory insufficiency and other complications[115] or may be so mild as to present in old age,[116] but most affected individuals are first detected during adolescence or young adulthood. The diagnosis may be suspected if no lactate is produced during an ischemic (anaerobic) forearm exercise test, but confirmation requires muscle biopsy for determination of PFK activity or noninvasive magnetic resonance imaging studies of muscle carbohydrate metabolism.[117]

When PFK deficiency is confined to erythrocytes, there are no symptoms of myopathy and the blood lactate response to anoxic exercise is normal.[118–121] Such patients may be hematologically normal[118, 122, 123] or exhibit mild to moderate hemolytic anemia.[119, 124] In general, red cell morphology is not strikingly abnormal, although prominent basophilic stippling has occasionally been present.

Biochemistry

PFK is one of several glycolytic enzymes that reversibly bind to the inner aspect of the erythrocyte membrane. Binding, which is thought to occur between the amino terminal position of the *trans* membrane protein band 3 and the adenine nucleotide binding site, located in a cleft between the two dimers that comprise the PFK tetramer, may serve both to activate the enzyme and to protect it against proteolytic degradation during erythrocyte aging.[125]

The active form of human erythrocyte PFK is a tetramer (molecular weight, 380,000 daltons) composed in varying combinations of two different subunits, one identical to the M subunit found in muscle PFK and the other identical to the L subunit found in liver PFK.[126, 127] The molecular weight of the M subunit is 85,000 and that of the L subunit is 80,000.[126] Studies of inactivation of human erythrocyte PFK by rabbit anti–human muscle PFK indicate that about 50% of the erythrocyte enzyme is formed from M subunits,[123, 126] whereas muscle PFK is composed entirely of M subunits.[123, 128] A deficiency in M subunits severely depresses muscle PFK activity, resulting in myopathy, but has a lesser effect on erythrocyte PFK because residual L subunits, under separate genetic control, combine to form an active L_4 tetramer of PFK. However, PFK formed entirely from L subunits is unstable to heat or dilution *in vitro* and is more sensitive to ATP inhibition than is muscle (M_4) PFK.[121] At the *in vivo* concentrations of ATP that are present within normal erythrocytes, the enzyme activity of L_4 PFK tetramers is severely inhibited, possibly explaining the presence of hemolytic anemia even when enzyme activity, as measured *in vitro*, is approximately 50% of normal. Most recognized examples of PFK deficiency are the result of either missing[109, 113, 119] or structurally altered[124] M subunits. An interesting exception was found in a clinically normal individual, fortuitously discovered when he volunteered to serve as a "control" during studies of red cell PFK carried out by Vora and colleagues.[122] Normal M subunits but mutant, unstable L subunits were found in his red cells. There was no myopathy, and, although erythrocyte PFK was only 65% of normal, hemolytic anemia was not found, presumably because residual enzyme activity within the red cell was entirely due to the presence of M_4 tetramers of PFK. The relatively greater stability and lesser susceptibility

Table 17–4. VARIOUS FORMS OF HUMAN PHOSPHOFRUCTOKINASE (PFK) DEFICIENCY

Type	No. of Patients	Affected PFK Subunit	Red Blood Cell		Muscle		Other
			Hemolysis	*PFK Activity**	*Myopathy*	*PFK Activity**	
I	18	M (absent or unstable)	+	29–64	+	0–5	Hyperuricemia, arthritis
II	3	NA	NA	17	+	0–6	
III	3	M (unstable)	+	8–62	0	100†	
IVa	2	M (unstable)	0	28–50	0	78†	Asymptomatic
IVb	3	L (unstable)	0	60–65	0	NA	Asymptomatic
V	3	NA	NA	75†	+ +	2–6	Arthritis

NA = data not available.
*Percentage of normal value.
†Studied in only one patient.
Data are from Tani and associates[110, 111] and Vora and co-workers.[113, 124]
Reproduced with permission from Mentzer WC, Glader BE: Disorders of erythrocyte metabolism. In Mentzer WC, Wagner GM (eds): The Hereditary Hemolytic Anemias. New York, Churchill Livingstone, Inc., 1989, pp 267–319.

to ATP inhibition of this form of PFK apparently allowed adequate enzyme activity under conditions normally found within the red cell *in vivo*.

A variety of studies have established the central role of PFK in regulation of erythrocyte metabolism. It is not surprising to find a deficiency of this important enzyme associated with hemolysis. However, little information is thus far available on the mechanism of hemolysis of PFK-deficient red cells. Erythrocyte sodium and potassium concentrations, sodium influx, and lactate production were normal in one patient.[117] Despite their normal glycolytic capabilities *in vitro*, deficient cells were incapable of maintaining normal ATP concentrations *in vivo*. The low (73% of normal) intracellular ATP concentration in these cells, although indicative of an abnormality of cellular metabolism, also may exert a positive influence by partially relieving the inhibitory influence of ATP on PFK.

The complex interaction between metabolites that may dictate actual PFK activity *in vivo* is illustrated by physiologic studies performed on four individuals with Tarui's syndrome.[129] At usual levels of physical activity, the pattern of erythrocyte glycolytic intermediates clearly reflected inhibition at the PFK step, and the concentration of the important downstream metabolite 2,3-DPG was only 50% of the level found in normal red cells. After 2 days of bed rest, red cell 2,3-DPG levels sank to just one third of normal. Subsequently, ergometric exercise on a bicycle eliminated the glycolytic intermediate pattern of PFK inhibition and allowed downstream intermediates, including 2,3-DPG, to rise toward normal. Release of large amounts of inosine and ammonia from exercising enzymopathic muscle into the plasma was observed in these patients. Ammonia is a powerful activator of PFK, and inosine can be metabolized to lactate by glycolytic pathways (i.e., the HMP shunt) that bypass the PFK reaction. Thus, the muscle metabolic abnormalities created by PFK deficiency generate metabolites that alleviated the enzymopathy in erythrocytes. Diversion of the flow of erythrocyte glycolysis through the HMP shunt by the block at PFK also may generate increased amounts of purines and pyrimidines from 5-phosphoribosylpyrophosphate. The hyperuricemia sometimes noted in PFK-deficient individuals (see Table 17–4) may be explained on this basis.[130]

An inherited deficiency of PFK found in English springer spaniels allows interesting comparisons to be made with the human condition.[131–133] As in humans, canine PFK deficiency is an autosomal recessive disorder. Red cell PFK levels are only 7% to 22% of normal in homozygotes, because the muscle subunit, which is lacking, comprises the majority of the available subunits in normal dog red cells.[134] PFK deficiency in dogs is associated with a severe hemolytic anemia. Newborn dogs are not anemic, because there is a greater abundance of L subunits and thus of functional PFK enzymes in their red cells. The hemolytic anemia appears as the normal developmental pattern of replacement of L by M subunit synthesis occurs in a setting where M subunits either are not synthesized or are defective.[135]

A unique feature of dog PFK deficiency is episodic hemolysis induced by hyperventilation during exercise, mating, barking, or other similar activities.[133] Dog red cells exhibit spontaneous hemolysis at alkaline pH, and even the small pH change induced by hyperventilation is sufficient to generate the effect in PFK-deficient animals. Underlying the susceptibility of PFK-deficient dog red cells to hyperventilation induced hemolysis may be their low 2,3-DPG levels, which increase intracellular pH. Raising 2,3-DPG levels to normal *in vitro* normalizes the response to alkalinity.[136] In contrast to humans, even though dog muscle PFK activity is nearly absent,[137] there is little or no evidence of exertional myopathy because dogs do not rely on anaerobic glycolysis for energy generation during exercise.[138]

Erythrocytes from human newborns have PFK activity 50% to 60% that of normal adult cells.[139] Differential centrifugation of cord blood to obtain young and old populations of fetal red cells has shown PFK deficiency to be much more evident in the older cells, perhaps due to accelerated enzyme decay.[140] The existence of an unusually labile fetal type of PFK is suggested by these studies. Antibody neutralization studies with anti-muscle PFK reveal less M subunit in cord red cell PFK than in enzyme from adult red cells.[141] Furthermore, cord red cell PFK exhibits greater sensitivity to ATP inhibition, as would be expected with a predominance of L subunits. Using sensitive chromatographic techniques, Vora and Piomelli have provided evidence that 25% to 30% of newborn erythrocyte PFK is L_4 isozyme, with the remainder being divided equally between three hybrid isozymes of L and M subunits (L_1M_3, L_2M_2, L_3M_1).[142] The L_4 isozyme, not found in normal adult red cells, is unstable, presumably accounting for the reduced PFK activity of older cord red cells. The demonstration that PFK deficiency may result in hemolytic anemia in adults suggests that the enzyme deficiency characteristic of newborn red cells may contribute to their shortened survival.

Genetics and Inheritance

Based on somatic cell hybridization studies, the gene locus for the L subunit of PFK has been assigned to chromosome 21 whereas the M subunit locus is on chromosome 1.[130] The erythrocytes, but not the leukocytes and platelets, of individuals with trisomy 21 consistently contain increased PFK activity.[143] Increased erythrocyte PFK activity is due to increased amounts of L subunit, consistent with a simple gene dosage effect.[130]

Inheritance is autosomal recessive. Type I PFK deficiency (Tarui's disease), which seems to be found predominantly in Ashkenazi Jews and in Japanese, is the result of mutations involving *PFKM*.[144] Splice site mutations involving intron 5[144] and exon 13[145] lead to deletion of exon 5 or of 75 bases within exon 13. A point mutation within exon 4 leads to substitution of leucine for arginine at a position near the PFK active site, apparently interfering with normal tetramer formation.[144] Finally, a frameshift mutation in exon 22 is associated with production of a truncated messenger RNA (mRNA) in low abundance.[144] In PFK-deficient dogs, a stop codon mutation 120 nucleotides from the 3' end of the coding region also produces a truncated mRNA and an unstable M subunit tetramer with altered kinetic properties.[146, 147]

ALDOLASE DEFICIENCY

$$\text{Fructose-1,6-diphosphate} \xrightarrow{\text{Aldolase}} \begin{array}{l} \text{Dihydroxyacetone phosphate} \\ \text{Glyceraldehyde-3-phosphate} \end{array}$$

Clinical Manifestations, Biochemistry, and Genetics

In the initial case of aldolase deficiency associated with CNSHA, enzyme activity was only 16% of normal in erythrocytes and 19% of normal in cultured skin fibroblasts.[148] The patient was mentally retarded, and, because the principal brain aldolase present during early development is the same isozyme ("A") found in red cells, it was suggested that retardation might be due to deficiency of brain aldolase: A variety of other abnormalities were present—mild glycogen storage disease in the liver, intestinal lactase deficiency, growth retardation, and peculiar facial features. No structural abnormality of residual erythrocyte aldolase was detected by electrophoresis, isoelectric focusing, heat stability studies, or kinetic examination. The patient was the offspring of a consanguineous marriage, but both parents were hematologically normal and had normal red cell aldolase activity. Two members of a Japanese family who were severely deficient in red cell aldolase (4.7% to 5.5% of normal activity) have also been reported.[149] These individuals exhibited severe chronic hemolytic anemia, sometimes exacerbated by infections, but displayed none of the other abnormalities noted in the initial case. *In vitro*, glycolysis and HMP shunt activity were depressed, indicating that the deficiency of aldolase was of functional significance. Both parents were hematologically normal but had intermediate reductions in red cell aldolase activity. An autosomal recessive mode of inheritance is suggested by these findings.

The mutant aldolase was strikingly thermolabile. A missense mutation (Gat→Ggt) at position 386 of the coding region encoding a single amino acid substitution (Asp→Gly) at position 128 was present in mutant aldolase A complementary DNA (cDNA) was obtained from a lymphoblastoid cell line derived from one of the patients.[150] Transfection of *Escherichia coli* with an expression plasmid containing normal, mutant, or modified (by site directed mutagenesis) aldolase A cDNA generated functional aldolase molecules that were used to confirm that the amino acid substitution at position 128, a site distant from the catalytic site but within an exposed hinge region, was responsible for enzyme thermolability.[151]

TRIOSE PHOSPHATE ISOMERASE DEFICIENCY

$$\text{Dihydroxyacetone phosphate} \xleftrightarrow{\text{Triose phosphate isomerase}} \text{Glyceraldehyde-3-phosphate}$$

Clinical Manifestations

An association with TPI deficiency has been proved or suspected on clinical and genetic grounds in approximately 30 cases of congenital hemolytic anemia.[152–166] In addition to chronic hemolysis, a severe neurologic disorder, characterized initially by spasticity and psychomotor retardation often progressing to weakness and hypotonia, has been a feature of nearly all patients surviving beyond the neonatal period. Such neurologic abnormalities, which are usually not manifest before 6 to 12 months of age, are almost certainly not related to kernicterus, because most patients have not exhibited neonatal hyperbilirubinemia. The neurologic abnormality may stabilize during childhood[167] or adolescence.[154] In a Hungarian family, one severely TPI-deficient teenage boy had neurologic symptoms whereas his older brother who was equally enzymopenic remained symptom free.[168] Most affected individuals have died before the age of 5 years, often suddenly and without obvious explanation. Increased susceptibility to bacterial infection has been noted in both splenectomized and unsplenectomized patients.

Anemia has ranged from severe to moderate, with most patients requiring at least occasional blood transfusions. Macrocytosis and polychromatophilia are evident on the blood smear, reflecting the presence of reticulocytosis, which may reach 50% on occasion. Aside from occasional small, dense, spiculated cells, no striking changes in erythrocyte morphology are present.

Biochemistry

Triose phosphate isomerase is a homodimer whose two subunits (MW 26750) are the product of a single locus on the short arm of chromosome 12.[169–171] Post-translational modification of one or both subunits may occur by deamidination of aspartines at positions 15 and 71, resulting in multiple forms of the enzyme and creating a complex multibanded pattern on electrophoresis.[172, 173] The 248–amino acid sequence of human (placental) TPI has been determined directly[174] and is nearly but not completely identical to the sequence predicted by nucleotide analysis of adult human liver cDNA.[161]

TPI1 is a classic housekeeping gene, present in all tissues, whose amino acid sequence has been remarkably well conserved during evolution.[175] The eight-stranded αβ barrel structure of the human enzyme has been confirmed at 0.28-nm resolution by x-ray crystallography.[175] TPI has no requirement for cofactors or metal ions, and there is no evidence for cooperativity or allosteric interactions between subunits.

When measured *in vitro*, erythrocyte TPI activity is approximately 1000 times that of HK, the least active glycolytic enzyme. Even deficient erythrocytes with only 2% to 35% of normal TPI activity possess far more TPI than HK activity. In view of the foregoing, it should not be surprising to learn that TPI-deficient erythrocytes are capable of normal glycolysis *in vitro*, even when compared with reticulocyte-rich normal blood.[142] Nonetheless, a striking accumulation of dihydroxyacetone phosphate is present in freshly obtained enzymopenic erythrocytes, and this intermediate accumulates still more on incubation. In addition, erythrocyte ATP concentration is usually low for cell age. Such results indicate the presence of a substantial impairment of glycolysis *in vivo*.

The enzymatic defect can be partially bypassed by means of the HMP shunt, which generates glyceraldehyde-3-phosphate from glucose without the participation of TPI. Methylene blue stimulation of the shunt in TPI-deficient erythrocytes produces a lesser increase in glycolysis relative to the rate found without additives than is found in reticulocyte-rich control blood.[153] This has been interpreted as indicating a markedly greater "resting" shunt rate in the deficient cells, consistent with the proposed reliance of such cells on the shunt. If the shunt is as active as has been suggested, it is difficult to explain the marked susceptibility of one patient's erythrocytes to Heinz body formation after incubation with acetylphenylhydrazine.[156] Reduced glutathione (GSH) levels and stability were normal, however, in the red cells of this patient.

Rare electrophoretic variants of TPI, not associated with reduced enzyme activity or hemolysis, have been described.[173, 175–178] In anemic patients, the characteristics of residual TPI have been evaluated in several pedigrees.[158, 159, 161, 162, 164] Enzyme kinetics and electrophoretic mobility were usually normal, but evidence *in vitro* of enzyme lability after heating was often obtained, suggesting that instability and rapid loss of enzyme protein might play an important role in the pathogenesis of hemolysis *in vivo*.[158, 162] A single amino acid substitution (Glu→Asp) has been found at position 104 in the thermolabile mutant *TPI* from several different pedigrees.[178a] That this mutation induces a thermolabile enzyme was confirmed by introducing normal or mutant *TPI* genes into Chinese hamster cells and evaluating the properties of the expressed human gene product.[179] Computer modeling indicated that a substituted amino acid at position 104, which is buried in a hydrophilic side pocket of the normal enzyme, would reduce the stability of the pocket, promote unfolding, and enhance thermolability.[179]

In the Hungarian pedigree mentioned earlier,[168] a point mutation at codon 240 (Phe→Leu) produced a moderately thermolabile TPI with abnormal substrate kinetics and electrophoretic migration.[180] Phe[240] is near the active site of the enzyme and appears to be essential for maintaining its correct geometry.[175] Coinherited by both anemic brothers in this pedigree was a second *TPI* mutation, as yet uncharacterized, that reduced the output of TPI mRNA from the affected allele by 10- to 20-fold. The red cells of the brothers had less than 10% of the TPI activity found in normal cells.[168, 180]

The enzyme deficiency is manifest not only in red cells but also in leukocytes, platelets, muscle, serum, and cerebrospinal fluid. Histologic examination of muscle from one TPI-deficient girl with myopathy revealed marked degenerative changes of the contractile system, altered mitochondria, and absent TPI by histochemical staining.[181] Brain and nerve tissue have not yet been analyzed, but the cerebrospinal fluid defi-

ciency suggests the possibility that deficient TPI activity in neural tissue may be responsible for the neurologic abnormalities observed in enzymopenic patients. Although increased susceptibility to infection might be the consequence of defective function by TPI-deficient leukocytes,[163] the functional studies carried out on such cells *in vitro* have often been normal.[157, 159, 167] A functional defect in TPI-deficient platelets has been described.[182]

Genetics and Inheritance

Studies of several large pedigrees are consistent with an autosomal recessive mode of inheritance.[157, 162] Obligate heterozygotes are clinically normal, but their erythrocytes contain approximately half the TPI activity of control erythrocytes. As is often the case in other glycolytic enzymopathies, no clear boundary exists between heterozygous-deficient and low normal enzyme activity. The frequency of the heterozygous state in normal newborn populations is surprisingly high: 0.1% to 0.5% in whites, 0.3% in Japanese, and 5.5% in American blacks.[170, 176] The extreme rarity of the homozygous state may be due to early fetal loss as a result of the enzymopathy[170] or to lack of ascertainment.[162] In mice, the homozygous state for a TPI null allele is lethal early in embryogenesis.[183] Segregation patterns in man–Chinese hamster cell hybrids indicate that the locus for *TPI* is situated on the short arm of chromosome 12.[169] The possibility of an additional locus for *TPI* on chromosome 5 was suggested by a study of two children with the cri-du-chat syndrome (partial deletion of chromosome 5) who had only 50% of normal erythrocyte TPI activity.[184] However, 18 other patients with cri-du-chat syndrome studied subsequently had normal levels of TPI activity in erythrocytes.[185, 186] Simultaneous heterozygous inheritance of TPI deficiency and either G6PD deficiency or sickle cell trait has not altered the typical clinical pattern of the disorders when present alone.[156] Prenatal diagnosis of TPI deficiency by analysis of fetal blood cells obtained through cordocentesis is feasible.[165, 166, 187–189] With suitable precautions,[188] cultured amniocytes[164] or trophoblastic cells[189a] also may be used for diagnosis.

Therapy

Aside from transfusions and folic acid supplementation, no other means of therapy is at hand. Splenectomy in one patient did not alter the intensity of hemolysis.[157]

GLYCERALDEHYDE-3-PHOSPHATE DEHYDROGENASE DEFICIENCY

Glyceraldehyde-3-phosphate dehydrogenase

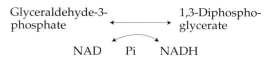

Glyceraldehyde-3-phosphate ⟷ 1,3-Diphosphoglycerate

NAD   Pi   NADH

Clinical Manifestations, Biochemistry, and Genetics

Three males in whom hemolytic anemia was associated with reduced erythrocyte glyceraldehyde-3-phosphate dehydrogenase (G3PD) activity have been briefly described.[190, 191] Differences in erythrocyte osmotic fragility and in G3PD activity indicate that the disorder in one of the patients may not be identical to that in the other two. In the former, infection and an antimalarial drug, dapsone, accelerated hemolysis, yet in all three patients the concentration and stability of GSH were normal. Changes in the pattern of glycolytic intermediates similar to those induced by iodoacetic acid, a known inhibitor of G3PD, were found in the erythrocytes of one patient. Iodoacetic acid inhibited glycolysis more in affected erythrocytes than in control erythrocytes. The disorder is probably hereditary, because both father and son were affected in one pedigree. In one patient, enzyme activity was normal in platelets and reduced in leukocytes.

Study of a large kindred in which three members exhibited a reduction of erythrocyte G3PD activity to 50% of normal levels yet were hematologically normal has clearly established that G3PD deficiency need not result in hemolysis.[192] The gene for hereditary spherocytosis was also present in this kindred, and four members were discovered to have inherited both hereditary spherocytosis and G3PD deficiency. The clinical severity of hemolytic anemia in these spherocytic individuals was not altered by the simultaneous inheritance of G3PD deficiency. Thus, the relationship of G3PD deficiency to hereditary hemolytic anemia cannot yet be considered to be established. Affected members of this kindred were presumed to be heterozygotes, because the amounts of both G3PD enzyme activity and enzyme protein were equally reduced to about 50% of normal and residual G3PD was qualitatively normal. Two of the three anemic G3PD-deficient patients in other kindreds had even lower levels of enzyme activity (20% to 30% of normal) and conceivably are either homozygotes or doubly heterozygous for two mutant G3PD genes.

PHOSPHOGLYCERATE KINASE DEFICIENCY

Phosphoglycerate kinase

1,3-Diphosphoglycerate $\longleftrightarrow$ 3-Phosphoglycerate

ADP $\quad$ Mg^{2+} $\quad$ ATP

Clinical Manifestations

Phosphoglycerate kinase deficiency is a sex-linked disorder in which nearly all individuals with clinical manifestations are male. Those most severely affected usually present with nonspherocytic hemolytic anemia and neurologic abnormalities, which may include seizures, movement disorders, emotional instability, psychomotor retardation, aphasia, and tetraplegia. When PGK deficiency is milder, hemolytic anemia may occur without neurologic deficits; and in one form of mild PGK deficiency (PGK München) no clinical abnormalities exist (Table 17–5). Although neonatal jaundice has sometimes been the initial manifestation of PGK deficiency, neurologic abnormalities have occurred in individuals who were not jaundiced during the newborn period. Another subset of PGK-deficient individuals exhibit myoglobinuria, sometimes after exercise, and rhabdomyolysis. Hemolytic anemia, convulsions, or no other clinical abnormalities may accompany muscle disease (see Table 17–5). In females, erythrocyte PGK activity has been less profoundly depressed than in males, hemolytic anemia has been mild or absent, and neurologic function has been normal (see Table 17–5).

Hematologic findings in anemic PGK-deficient individuals have been those customarily associated with hemolysis, namely, jaundice and reticulocytosis. Erythrocyte morphology has not been remarkable, and osmotic fragility has usually been normal.

Biochemistry

Phosphoglycerate kinase is a monomeric enzyme whose primary structure consists of 417 amino acids.[193] Crystallographic studies of horse muscle PGK, whose primary structure is highly homologous to human PGK, show its tertiary structure to be that of two lobes (the C and N domains) connected by a hingelike structure that allows considerable conformational change to occur during substrate binding (Fig. 17–3).[194] Because the nucleotide (ATP, adenosine diphosphate) combining site is located within the C domain and the phosphoglycerate (1,3-diphosphoglycerate, 3-phosphoglycerate) binding site within the N domain, bending of the enzyme is required to bring into close proximity the several substrates required for the PGK reaction.[194]

PGK-deficient red cells are capable of normal glycolysis *in vitro*.[191, 195, 196] HMP shunt activity is normal under either resting or stimulated conditions.[196a] Intracellular ATP concentrations are normal or slightly low,[195–199] whereas 2,3-DPG concentration is elevated, sometimes to two or three times the normal level.[195–201] These results reflect increased flow through the 2,3-DPG cycle (see Fig. 17–1) at the expense of the ATP generating PGK reaction. Despite the availability of an alternative pathway (the Rapoport-Luebering shunt or 2,3-DPG cycle) to bypass PGK, substantial accumulation of glycolytic intermediates proximal to the enzyme defect is found in fresh red cells, indicating that the normal flow of erythrocyte glycolysis is impeded *in vivo*.

Little is known regarding the mechanism of hemolysis of PGK-deficient red cells. Substantial PGK activity is membrane associated.[202] It has been suggested that ATP for membrane ATPase-mediated cation transport is mostly (or entirely) generated by membrane-bound PGK. Indeed, adenosine diphosphate derived from membrane ATPase exerts an important regulatory influence on glycolysis by its participation in the PGK reaction.[203] However, the implication of a special role for PGK in cation transport has been challenged.[204] The

Table 17-5. CHARACTERISTICS OF REPORTED CASES OF PHOSPHOGLYCERATE KINASE (PGK) DEFICIENCY

References	Variant	Mutation	Red Blood Cell Activity (% of Normal)	Stability in Vitro	Kinetic Abnormalities	Hemolytic Anemia	Neurologic Abnormalities	Other
Hemizygotes (Male): Hemolytic Anemia or Asymptomatic								
197, 228	—		0–4			+	+ +	
199, 219, 204, 229	Amiens	Asp^{163}→Val	2.7	Normal		+	+	Seizures
198, 218, 229	Matsue	Leu^{88}→Pro	5	Low	+			
216, 231	Uppsala	Arg^{205}→Pro	5–10	Low	+	+	+	
200, 207	Cincinnati		8–11			+	+ +	
217	Tokyo	Val^{265}→Met	10	Low	+	+	+	
220	Michigan	Cys^{315}→Arg	10	Low	+	+	+	Behavior disorder
201	San Francisco		12	Normal	+	0	0	
225, 227	Munchen	Asn^{267}→Asp	21	Low	0		0	
Hemizygotes (Male): Muscle Disease								
221	Shizuoka	Gly^{157}→Asp	0.7	Normal	0	+	0	Myoglobinuria
226	Creteil	Asp^{314}→Asn	2–3	Low	+	0	0	Rhabdomyolysis
230	Hammamatsu		8.2	Normal	0	0	+	Myoglobinuria
211	New Jersey		18	Normal	+	0	0	Myoglobinuria
232	Alberta		—	Normal	+	0	0	Myoglobinuria, exercise intolerance, retinitis pigmentosa
Heterozygotes (Female)								
195	Piedmont		27			+	0	
224	Memphis		78			+	0	
197	—		77			+	0	

active transport of sodium and potassium by PGK-deficient red cells with residual PGK activity only 10% to 15% of normal was not impaired, even under the challenge of an increase in intracellular sodium concentration.[205] Thus, it seems unlikely that hemolysis of PGK-deficient red cells is related to premature cation pump failure owing directly to inadequate PGK activity.

PGK activity in leukocytes is consistently subnormal in affected males, but white cell function is not necessarily compromised. In one case, PGK-deficient leukocytes exhibited increased Krebs cycle activity both at rest and during phagocytosis. Abolition of Krebs cycle metabolism with cyanide severely impaired the ingestion of bacteria by such cells but had little or no effect on normal leukocytes.[206] Thus, the PGK-deficient leukocyte appeared to compensate for its glycolytic defect by increased Krebs cycle activity. However, although ingestion of bacteria was normal, deficient leukocytes were unable to kill or iodinate ingested *Staphylococcus aureus* effectively *in vitro*. In contrast to the abnormalities observed in this single case, white cell function has been completely normal in three other PGK-deficient males.[199, 207] Leukocyte function *in vivo* is probably not

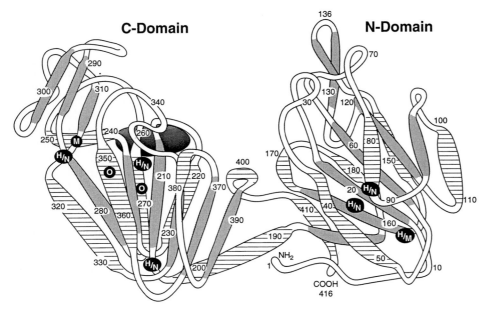

Figure 17-3. Three-dimensional model of human PGK. This figure is based on the three-dimensional model of horse PGK published by Banks and associates.[194] Positions of the amino acid substitutions and the clinical features associated with nine PGK point mutations are indicated by *filled circles*. O = no clinical abnormalities; M = muscle disease; H = hemolytic anemia; N = neurologic manifestations. The *shaded ellipse* in the C-domain indicates the location on the adenosine triphosphate and adenosine diphosphate binding sites. Random coil (*clear*), β strands (*solid*), and α helices (*striped*) are indicated by shading. (Modified from Fujii H, Kanno H, et al: A single amino acid substitution (Gly^{157}→Val) in a phosphoglycerate kinase variant (PGK Shizuoka) associated with chronic hemolysis and myoglobinuria. Blood 1992; 79:1582.)

compromised, because an increased incidence of infection has not been a feature of PGK deficiency.

Genetics and Inheritance

The major structural gene for PGK *(PGK1),* located on the long arm of the X chromosome, is 23 kb and is composed of 11 exons and 10 introns.[208–212] Deficient male hemizygotes have little or no active enzyme and are more symptomatic than heterozygous females with intermediate levels of activity (see Table 17–4). A second functional gene for PGK *(PGK2),* expressed in spermatozoa, is found on chromosome 19.[213] The autosomal *PGK2* lacks introns but is otherwise similar to the X chromosomal *PGK1.* It is thought to have arisen by reverse transcription of PGK mRNA, a gene-processing event conserved during subsequent evolution because it met the need of haploid sperm (devoid of an X chromosome) for a source of PGK to support their metabolic needs.[214]

In 1972, Yoshida and coworkers succeeded in purifying and sequencing both normal erythrocyte PGK and a clinically normal but electrophoretically distinct human mutant PGK, the "New Guinea" variant.[215] The mutant enzyme differed from the normal by the substitution of arginine for threonine at position 352.[193] Subsequently, the structure of 8 of the PGK mutants associated with hemolytic anemia has been determined by peptide or nucleotide sequencing.[216–221] Each differs from the normal wild type enzyme by the substitution of a single amino acid. The position of the substitution in six of the mutants is near the adenosine diphosphate–combining site within the C domain, as shown in Figure 17–3. Most of these mutants (five of six) are thermolabile, and four of six exhibit abnormal substrate kinetics. In contrast, two of the three mutations found in the N domain are thermostable and exhibit normal kinetics. It is not clear how the particular spectrum of clinical abnormalities associated with each mutation is related to its position within the molecule. For example, PGK Michigan, a point mutation at amino acid 315, is associated with hemolytic anemia and neurologic abnormalities whereas individuals with PGK Creteil, a point mutation of the adjacent amino acid at position 314, are free of anemia and neurologic abnormalities but exhibit rhabdomyolysis.[219] Many of the mutants that have not yet been sequenced have kinetic and electrophoretic abnormalities that make it likely that they, too, are due to structural gene mutations.[222] A regulatory gene mutation resulting in diminished synthesis of enzyme protein may be responsible for reduced PGK activity in mutants in which kinetic, electrophoretic, and other studies of the variant enzyme are completely normal.[199] A single isozyme of PGK is found in all human nonhematopoietic tissues except spermatozoa.[223] It is therefore likely that the neurologic disorder found in PGK-deficient males results from an abnormality of this enzyme in neural tissue.

When young and old erythrocytes from two anemic female heterozygotes were separated by centrifugation, greater PGK activity was noted in old cells than in young cells (Fig. 17–4).[197] In contrast, PK activity was

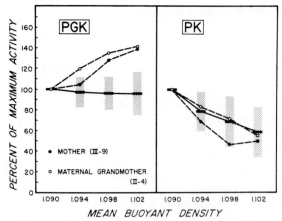

Figure 17–4. Erythrocytes fractionated on the basis of buoyant density. PGK indicates phosphoglycerate activity, and PK represents pyruvate kinase activity. The *solid line* represents the mean activity, and the *shaded bars* indicate the range of activity in four normal controls and 14 unaffected paternal and maternal relatives in the kindred. Comparison is made with the same activities in the affected mother and maternal grandmother. In each, enzyme activity in each fraction is compared with the activity of the least dense red cell fraction. (From Valentine WN, Hsieh HS, et al: Hereditary hemolytic anemia associated with phosphoglycerate kinase deficiency in erythrocytes and leukocytes. N Engl J Med 1969; 280:528. Reprinted, by permission, from the *New England Journal of Medicine.*)

lower in old cells than in young cells, conforming to the normal decline in enzyme activity associated with aging of the red cell. These results have been interpreted as resulting from random inactivation of the X chromosome. Cells possessing an active chromosome dictating the synthesis of normal PGK have normal enzyme activity, whereas those in which the X chromosome for mutant PGK is activated should be markedly enzymopenic. The selective survival of enzyme-replete cells would then result in higher enzyme activity in the population of older erythrocytes.

Random inactivation of the mutant X chromosome may produce differing proportions of enzyme-deficient cells in female heterozygotes. Some may be severely anemic (see Table 17–5), whereas others are clinically and hematologically normal.[224] In the latter, the population of PGK-deficient red cells may be so small that erythrocyte PGK activity will be completely normal.[224]

Therapy

In one patient, splenectomy had no beneficial effect on anemia[224]; but in several others, surgery reduced or eliminated the need for transfusions, reduced the degree of reticulocytosis, and sometimes resulted in a rise of several grams in the hemoglobin level.

2,3-BISPHOSPHOGLYCERATE MUTASE DEFICIENCY

Diphosphoglycerate mutase

1,3-Diphophoglycerate $\longrightarrow$ 2,3-Diphosphoglycerate

3PG   3PG

Clinical Manifestations

The virtually complete absence of erythrocyte 2,3-bis-phosphoglycerate mutase (BPGM) activity need not result in shortening of the red cell life span. In one pedigree, four siblings who completely lacked functional red cell BPGM were polycythemic but otherwise were clinically and hematologically normal. All three children of these individuals had about 50% of the normal amount of red cell BPGM and were hematologically normal except for polycythemia.[233, 234]

In contrast, Schroter[235] described an infant who developed anemia and hepatosplenomegaly in the newborn period, required blood transfusions at increasingly frequent intervals, and died at 3 months of age of overwhelming infection. Erythrocyte BPGM activity and 2,3-DPG concentration were reduced to approximately 50% of normal in both parents, one sister, and one grandmother. These presumed heterozygotes were hematologically normal, despite their enzyme deficiency. It was thought that the infant, whose red cells could not be studied because of the need for frequent transfusions, probably represented the homozygous form of the enzymopathy. A 50% reduction in erythrocyte BPGM was found in a young woman, her father, and her infant daughter by Cartier and coworkers.[236] The infant was jaundiced and anemic at birth, but, in contrast, both affected adults were clinically normal, although the reticulocyte count was elevated in one. Compensated hemolysis was more convincingly demonstrated in two similar patients with moderately reduced red cell BPGM activity, normal hemoglobin level, elevated bilirubin level and reticulocyte count, and reduced survival of chromated autologous red cells.[237, 238] However, in these cases a causal association between BPGM deficiency and hemolysis was not proven.

Biochemistry

Human red cell BPGM is a homodimer whose identical subunits (molecular weight, 29,840 daltons) each consist of 258 amino acids.[239] Nearly all BPG-phosphatase (BPGP) activity also resides in the BPGM molecule, so that 2,3-DPG metabolism is controlled by a single, multifunctional enzyme. In fact, purified BPGM is also capable of performing as a monophosphoglycerate mutase, although at a low rate of activity.[240] Considerable structural homology exists between red cell diphosphoglycerate mutase and monophosphoglycerate mutase,[241, 242] and the enzymes, to some extent, exhibit overlapping functions. However, both biochemical[241] and genetic[243] evidence indicates that they are each unique and under separate genetic control.

The BPGM molecule has been modified in vitro by site-directed mutagenesis in an attempt to model a potential therapeutic approach to sickle cell disease.[244] Substitution of glycine for arginine at codon 13 enhances phosphatase activity at the expense of the mutase. The effect of such an alteration in vivo, achieved by gene therapy or by pharmacologic means, would be to lower erythrocyte 2,3-DPG levels, increase hemo-globin oxygen affinity, and in this way retard the polymerization of hemoglobin S.

BPGM deficiency results in reduced synthesis of 2,3-DPG. In complete BPGM deficiency, virtually no 2,3-DPG exists within the red cell[233, 234] whereas when enzyme activity is less severely depressed, 2,3-DPG levels are generally 30% to 40% of normal.[233, 236, 238] Whole-blood oxygen affinity is increased because of lack of 2,3-DPG, accounting for the polycythemia noted in severely BPGM-deficient individuals.[233-236, 238] The pattern of glycolytic intermediates is disturbed,[233] sometimes exhibiting a crossover at PFK[234, 236] consistent with relief of the inhibitory influence of 2,3-DPG on PFK. Erythrocyte ATP level is usually normal or slightly increased in concentration, compatible with the diversion of 2,3-DPG into the PGK reaction as a consequence of reduced flow through BPGM. Erythrocyte glycolysis[236, 238] and pentose shunt activity have been normal in vitro.[233] Probably as a consequence of the large amount of 1,3-DPG present in BPGM-deficient red cells, hemoglobin A may undergo post-translational modification by glycerylation at alpha 82. The modified hemoglobin, about 3% of the total, has a lower isoelectric-electric point than hemoglobin A_1C and is easily identified by isoelectric focusing.[245]

Genetics and Inheritance

The human genome contains a single locus for BPGM located on chromosome 7.[246] The gene is fully expressed only in erythroid tissue.[247] BPGM deficiency exhibits the expected autosomal recessive mode of inheritance.[233-236, 238]

Individuals with polycythemia and virtually no red cell BPGM activity have been shown to be compound heterozygotes for two different BPGM mutations. One, BPGM Creteil I is a point mutation (Arg[89]→Cys) at or near the BPGM active site[248] and the other, BPGM Creteil II, is a frameshift mutation due to a deletion of nucleotide 205 or 206.[249] Only BPGM Creteil I enzyme protein is found in red cells.[250] It is catalytically inactive, thermolabile in vitro, and exhibits altered electrophoretic mobility.[250] Although BPGM and BPG-phosphatase activities were virtually absent in compound heterozygotes, monophosphoglycerate mutase activity was nearly normal, illustrating the complex nature of this multifunctional enzyme.[248]

Therapy

Polycythemia, if symptomatic, may require phlebotomy.[234]

ENOLASE DEFICIENCY

Enolase

2-Phosphoglycerate $\longleftrightarrow$ Phosphoenol pyruvate

Clinical Manifestations, Biochemistry, Genetics, and Therapy

A woman in whom red cell enolase activity was only 6% of normal exhibited a modest reduction in the survival of ^{51}Cr-labeled autologous erythrocytes (half-life of 18 days; normal, 25 to 30 days) but no overt chronic anemia.[251] A severe, life-threatening acute hemolytic episode occurred when nitrofurantoin was administered for treatment of a urinary tract infection. Poikilocytosis, spherocytosis, and schistocytosis were evident on the peripheral blood smear during the episode of hemolysis, and the same morphologic abnormalities could subsequently be reproduced *in vitro* by incubation of enolase-deficient red cells with nitrofurantoin. The ascorbate-cyanide test and the Heinz body test were positive, but enzymes of the HMP shunt all exhibited normal or increased activity and glutathione stability was normal. Such drug-induced hemolysis is distinctly uncommon in disorders of the Embden-Meyerhof pathway, although theoretically possible in enzyme-deficient reticulocytes.[394] In this case, in which sudden massive hemolysis predominantly involved mature red cells, no biochemical mechanism has yet been defined and the association between enolase deficiency and hemolytic anemia may be coincidental. A sister was hematologically normal, but her red cells were as deficient in enolase activity as were those of the proposita. Leukocyte and platelet enolase activity was normal in both the patient and her sister. Data were insufficient to define the precise mechanism of inheritance.

Partial red cell enolase deficiency was inherited in an autosomal dominant manner by six members of a second pedigree that spanned four generations. With the exception of the propositus, a 13-day-old male newborn with profound hemolytic anemia, affected family members were not anemic and had little or no evidence of hemolysis. Spherocytes were present on the peripheral blood smear, and the mean corpuscular hemoglobin concentration was usually elevated.[252]

Therapy remains undefined, but avoidance of oxidant drugs would seem prudent.

PYRUVATE KINASE DEFICIENCY

Pyruvate kinase

Phosphoenolpyruvate ⟷ Pyruvate

ADP K$^+$ Mg^{2+} ATP

Clinical Manifestations

Pyruvate kinase deficiency is the most frequently encountered glycolytic enzymopathy associated with anemia. Of the approximately 350 human cases thus far reported, the majority have been of Northern European extraction. Sporadic cases have been encountered in blacks, Japanese, Chinese, Mexicans, southern Europeans, and Syrians. A hemolytic anemia resembling that seen in human PK deficiency has also been described in basenji dogs[253, 254] and in beagles[255] that have inherited a mutant, unstable form of erythrocyte PK. Anemia, jaundice, and splenomegaly are regularly present in PK deficiency. Anemia may be profound, presenting *in*

utero[256, 257] or in early infancy[53] and requiring frequent blood transfusion for survival. Conversely, the anemia may be so mild as to evade discovery until adulthood. In a few cases, anemia is absent, hemolysis is fully compensated, and jaundice may be the sole clinical abnormality. When present, anemia is lifelong and usually varies little in intensity, although it may become more severe during pregnancy.[258] Exacerbations of anemia are infrequent and usually result from transient erythroid hypoplasia after infections[259] or, rarely, from increased hemolysis of unknown cause. Manifestations of PK deficiency outside the hematopoietic system are uncommon. In several pedigrees, chronic leg ulcers have been observed in PK-deficient family members with hemolytic anemia.[260, 261]

Hyperbilirubinemia is frequently encountered in PK-deficient newborns and may require exchange transfusions.[53] Serum unconjugated bilirubin levels remain elevated in later life, and gallstones are common. Unconjugated bilirubin levels in excess of 6 mg/dL are occasionally seen[262]; one brother and sister regularly had levels greater than 20 mg/dL.[263] These patients have abnormal hepatic function, in addition to hemolysis. Whether abnormalities of liver PK contribute to hyperbilirubinemia is unknown.[264, 265]

Macrocytosis, occasional shrunken, spiculated erythrocytes, and, rarely, acanthocytes may be observed on examination of the blood smear; these changes may be accentuated by splenectomy. More extreme alterations in erythrocyte morphology are sometimes encountered (Fig. 17–5).[266, 267] Such abnormalities in shape may result from the inadequate ATP synthesis characteristic of PK-deficient erythrocytes.[268] A paradoxical rise in the reticulocyte count often follows splenectomy, despite evidence of a beneficial reduction in the rate of hemolysis. Reticulocyte counts may exceed 90%, and many patients maintain counts of 40% to 70% for years. Conversely, other patients exhibit the expected reduction in reticulocyte count after splenectomy. The osmotic fragility of fresh and incubated erythrocytes is most often normal, although, in occasional patients, minor populations of fragile or resistant cells may be encountered after incubation. The autohemolysis test is usually, but not invariably,[269] abnormal, with hemolysis of as many as 50% of erythrocytes after 48 hours of incubation in saline. Prior addition of glucose may reduce hemolysis in some instances, but more frequently glucose has little or no effect. In fact, if the reticulocyte count exceeds 25%, incubation with glucose regularly accentuates hemolysis. This phenomenon has been attributed to inhibition of oxidative phosphorylation by glucose (Crabtree effect) with unfavorable consequences in PK-deficient reticulocytes because of their reliance on oxidative phosphorylation for ATP synthesis.[270]

Biochemistry

The active form of PK is a homotetramer formed from one of four different tissue-specific subunits. The R subunit is found in red cells; the L subunit in liver; the M$_1$ subunit in muscle, heart, and brain; and the M$_2$

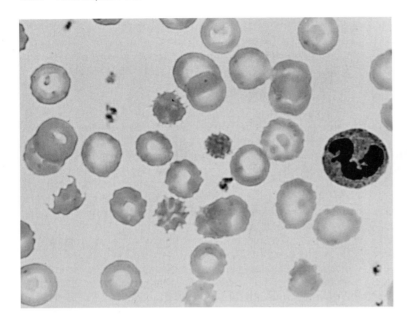

Figure 17-5. Postsplenectomy blood smear from a patient with severe PK deficiency. (From Nathan DG, Oski FA, et al: Extreme hemolysis and red cell distortion in erythrocyte pyruvate kinase deficiency. I. Morphology, erythrokinetics, and family enzyme studies. N Engl J Med 1964; 270:1024. Reprinted by permission of the *New England Journal of Medicine*.)

subunit in all early fetal tissues and most adult tissues, including leukocytes and platelets.[271] R and L subunits derive from a common gene (*PKLR*) located on chromosome 1 (1q21)[272] while M_1 and M_2 subunits are generated by a second gene (*PKM2*), located on chromosome 15 (15q24-q25).[273] In the rat, *PKM2* is 20 kb long and consists of 12 exons and 11 introns.[274] M_1- or M_2-specific mRNA is formed from a common primary transcript by alternate spicing involving the removal of either exon 9 (M_2) or exon 10 (M_1).[275] Because human and rat M_2 cDNAs are highly homologous,[273] alternative splicing probably also accounts for the differences in M_1 and M_2 mRNA in humans. *PKLR* also consists of 12 exons.[276] Tissue-specific expression of one of two different promoters generates a transcript containing either an R or an L exon at the 5′ end.[277, 278] The remaining 10 exons are identical. L-type cDNA encodes a polypeptide of 543 amino acids,[279] whereas R-type cDNA encodes a product longer by 31 amino acids.[271]

The three-dimensional structure of cat muscle PK has been studied by x-ray crystallography.[280] Each M_1 subunit consists of a short N-terminal region and three distinct domains (Fig. 17–6). Domain A is cylindrical, formed by eight parallel strands of β sheet encased by an outer coaxial cylinder of eight α helices; domain B consists of a closed antiparallel β sheet; and domain C is a five-stranded β sheet connected by α helices. The active site lies in a pocket between domains A and B, the monovalent cation (potassium) binding site is in domain A, and allosteric modulation of PK function primarily involves interactions with domain C. Extensive sequence homology exists between species and between M and LR subunits, particularly in the vicinity of the active site,[280] indicating that the enzyme structure has been conserved during evolution.

In erythroid cells, PK is a tetramer (molecular weight, 230,000 daltons)[281, 282] whose subunits may vary in type. In erythroid precursors, M_2 homotetramers are the predominant PK isoenzyme. With erythroid maturation, synthesis of M_2 subunits declines and is replaced by production of R-type subunits.[283–285] The mature red cell enzyme may exist in either of two physical conformations, analogous to the R and T forms proposed by Monod and colleagues for allosteric proteins.[286] Partially purified enzyme preparations usually exhibit sigmoid kinetics in the presence of increasing concentrations of substrate (phospho*enol*pyruvate). Small amounts of this substrate facilitate further bind-

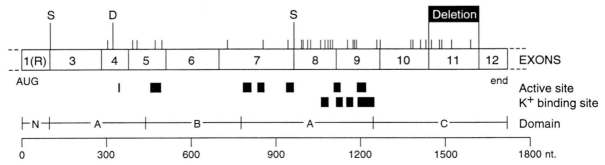

Figure 17-6. Recognized mutations of human *PKLR*. S = splice site mutation; D = deletion (deletion of entire exon 11 is shown as a *solid bar*); vertical tick marks = point mutation or small insertion. Domains of the expressed protein, the active site, and the potassium (K⁺)-binding site are indicated based on analogy to the structure of cat muscle PK.[280]

ing of it by the enzyme in a manner analogous to heme-heme interactions. Fructose diphosphate (FDP) induces a transition from sigmoid to hyperbolic kinetics, probably by acting directly at the phospho*enol*pyruvate binding site.[287]

A number of factors may result in post-translational modification of the enzyme. Transition between an FDP-sensitive conformation with sigmoid kinetics and an insensitive form with hyperbolic kinetics has been achieved by varying pH,[288] temperature,[288–290] and conditions of storage.[281, 289, 291] Aging of the enzyme *in vivo* appears to favor the FDP-sensitive conformation.[292] These transitions may play a significant role in modulation of PK activity *in vivo*. Post-translational modification of enzyme properties mediated by oxidation of exposed thiol groups on the surface of the molecule may explain some abnormalities previously ascribed to genetic or acquired alterations in the primary structure of the enzyme.[293–298] In several instances, using sulfhydryl reagents, it has been possible to restore to normal the altered stability and abnormal kinetics of mutant PK from individuals with hemolytic anemia.[293, 299] On the other hand, it has often not been possible to implicate oxidation of enzyme thiol groups as a cause of abnormal enzyme.[300, 301]

The enzyme is subject to numerous other regulatory influences. ATP is a competitive inhibitor ($K_i = 3.5 \times 10^{-4}$ mol/L)[302]; at physiologic ATP concentrations (approximately 1 mmol/L), erythrocyte PK activity should be significantly constrained by ATP. Both potassium[287, 290] and magnesium[290, 303] activate PK; rubidium or ammonium may substitute for potassium, whereas manganese or cobalt can replace manganese.[295] Activation of purified PK by FDP has been demonstrated at concentrations normally found within the erythrocyte.[304] At higher concentration (0.5 mmol/L), another glycolytic intermediate, glucose-6-phosphate, activates PK, whereas yet other intermediates have no apparent influence on the enzyme.[305] The glycolytic intermediate 2,3-DPG, of particular interest because of its high concentration in PK-deficient erythrocytes, has no influence on PK in hemolysates[306] but has variously been reported to inhibit[307] or activate[305] purified PK. Phosphorylation of PK, mediated by cyclic adenosine monophosphate, alters its kinetic properties and may serve to regulate 2,3-DPG levels and thus oxygen transport by red cells.[308, 309] It is clear that intracellular PK activity will be determined by the complex interplay of a number of regulatory factors and may bear little relation to measures of activity determined *in vitro* under optimal conditions.

When erythrocyte PK (R homotetramer) is abnormal, hepatic PK (L homotetramer) also may be affected because R and L subunits derive from a common gene. In two anemic PK-deficient individuals, liver PK was reduced to 59%[310] and 46%[311] of normal. Residual liver PK, measured in the latter case, was mostly M_2 type. No disorders of hepatic function appear to result from such partial deficiency of PK.[312] In another individual, total liver PK activity was only 22% of normal, virtually no L-type enzyme was detectable, and there were abnormalities in serum aminotransferase values.[264] Par-

adoxically, in still another individual, liver type L PK exhibited entirely normal activity and properties, despite abnormalities in the supposedly identical isoenzyme in the red cells.[265]

PK-deficient erythrocytes vary considerably in their metabolic capabilities *in vitro*. Although resting HMP shunt activity may be slightly to moderately low for cell age,[313] no significant effect on either oxidized or reduced glutathione levels has been observed,[314–318] even after incubation with acetylphenylhydrazine.[270, 316, 317, 319, 320] However, the ascorbate cyanide test is abnormal in PK-deficient patients and stimulated HMP shunt activity is modestly depressed.[318, 321] In many instances, glycolysis, as measured by the glucose consumption or lactate production of incubated erythrocytes, is markedly subnormal.[263, 270, 313] Such diminished glycolysis is relative, rather than absolute, because the glycolytic rate of enzymopenic cells can be increased substantially by incubation in a high inorganic phosphate medium.[270, 322, 323] A reduction of residual PK activity within the erythrocyte to 10% of normal will still leave sufficient enzyme to support normal glycolysis if potential enzyme activity is fully used. Such considerations indicate that intracellular regulators of PK function must play an important role in the reduced glycolysis characteristic of enzymopenic cells. Frequently, particularly in the case of kinetic variants of PK, glycolytic rates characteristic of mature normal erythrocytes are achieved.[291, 317, 324–327] However, such rates are clearly subnormal when compared with those attained by reticulocyte-rich control blood of an equivalent mean cell age.[324] Furthermore, the glucose consumption of incubated normal hemolysate is unchanged when supplemental purified PK is added, whereas addition of supplemental PK to hemolysate from PK-deficient erythrocytes produces a substantial rise in glucose consumption.[324]

Accumulation of glycolytic intermediates proximal to the enzyme defect has customarily,[289, 314, 317, 324, 327] although not invariably,[324] been observed.[326] Detection of elevated 2,3-DPG or 3-phosphoglycerate levels in red cells may help confirm a clinical diagnosis of PK deficiency[328, 329] and the degree of elevation in 2,3-DPG or glucose-6-phosphate levels is directly correlated with clinical severity.[330] In Figure 17–7, the pattern of intermediates obtained in a mildly anemic patient with a high K_m phospho*enol*pyruvate mutant enzyme (patient D. G.) is contrasted to that found in a severely anemic child (patient C. D.) with a low activity PK mutant and a marked reticulocytosis of 50%. Intermediates have accumulated just proximal to PK in both instances, and, in the second patient, a striking accumulation of more distant intermediates is noted as well, extending as far proximal as the triose phosphates, F6P, and G6P. Alteration in the normal ratio of reduced nicotinamide adenine dinucleotide (NADH) to nicotinamide adenine dinucleotide (NAD), as well as complex changes in the substrates governing the rate of PK and 2,3-diphosphoglycerate mutase, appears to be responsible for triose phosphate accumulation when glycolysis is accelerated by inorganic phosphate (Pi) in normal red cells.[331] Such striking elevations in triose

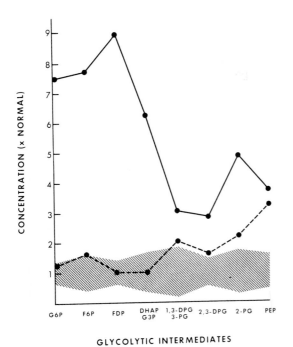

Figure 17-7. Changes in erythrocyte glycolytic intermediates in PK deficiency. Results, expressed as multiples of normal values, are shown for D.G., a patient with mild anemia *(dotted line)* and for C.D. *(solid line)*, whose anemia was severe.

phosphate intermediates can be returned to normal in both control and PK-deficient red cells by the addition of exogenous pyruvate or other oxidant.[323] The concentration of both NAD and NADH is low in PK-deficient erythrocytes,[289, 313, 332] or, if normal in fresh cells, the level of NAD falls with undue rapidity on incubation *in vitro*.[320] The concentration of 2,3-DPG in PK-deficient erythrocytes may exceed three times normal values. The expected rightward shift of the hemoglobin-oxygen dissociation curve associated with such high 2,3-DPG levels is found in PK-deficient blood.[46, 47] The ability to extract a greater percentage of available oxygen from hemoglobin at any given partial pressure of oxygen associated with such a right-shifted curve increases the exercise tolerance of PK-deficient patients.[46] Such patients, although anemic, may exhibit none of the expected symptoms of fatigue and exercise intolerance.

Erythrocyte ATP levels and the formation of phosphoribosylpyrophosphate[333] are often abnormally low in PK deficiency, although patients with reticulocyte counts greater than 25% usually have normal ATP levels. In such high reticulocyte blood, ATP is unstable on incubation with glucose in contrast to normal reticulocyte-rich blood. When incubated, without glucose, however, the PK-deficient reticulocyte conserves ATP more successfully than does the normal cell.[270] The reticulocyte, able to generate ATP from sources other than glucose through oxidative phosphorylation, can circumvent its glycolytic defect. However, in a high glucose environment ATP levels plummet. The PK-deficient reticulocyte is, thus, exquisitely dependent on oxidative phosphorylation for maintenance of ATP, as

was first shown by Keitt.[270] Incubation of PK-deficient blood with cyanide, which inhibits oxidative phosphorylation, produces a striking and rapid decrease in cell ATP content, whereas control reticulocytes are immune to this effect of cyanide. However, fluoride, which inhibits enolase and thus simulates the lesion of PK deficiency, renders normal reticulocytes equally susceptible to the effect of inhibitors of oxidative phosphorylation. The increased oxygen consumption of PK-deficient reticulocytes, compared with normal (3.75 ± 1.55 versus 0.56 ± 0.5 μL O_2 per 10^9 reticulocytes per hour),[263] further demonstrates the reliance of such cells on oxidative phosphorylation. Oxygen consumption is abolished by hypoxia *in vitro* at approximately venous partial pressure of oxygen levels (Fig. 17–8). When exposed to prolonged periods of hypoxia *in vivo*, therefore, or on maturation with consequent loss of mitochondria, the PK-deficient immature erythrocyte will become reliant on its inadequate glycolytic apparatus, with loss of cell ATP the inevitable consequence. In contrast, the reduced ATP needs of the mature erythrocyte may be marginally, but adequately, served for a time by the diminished glycolytic activity of the PK-deficient cell.

ATP depletion greatly increases the cation permeability of PK-deficient erythrocytes.[263] In part, this is the consequence of failure of the ouabain inhibitable ATPase cation pump, which transports 1 to 2 mEq/h of potassium per liter of erythrocytes.[334] Although adequate membrane ATPase is present,[324, 335] a net loss of from 0.2 to 6.3 mEq/h of potassium per liter of cells occurs in freshly obtained PK-deficient blood.[268, 324, 334]

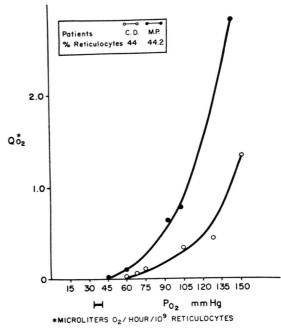

Figure 17-8. Influence of PO_2 on oxygen consumption by PK-deficient reticulocytes. The normal range for venous PO_2 is indicated by the *solid bar*. (From Mentzer WC, Baehner RL, et al: Selective reticulocyte destruction in erythrocyte pyruvate kinase deficiency. J Clin Invest 1971; 50:694, by copyright permission of the American Society for Clinical Investigation.)

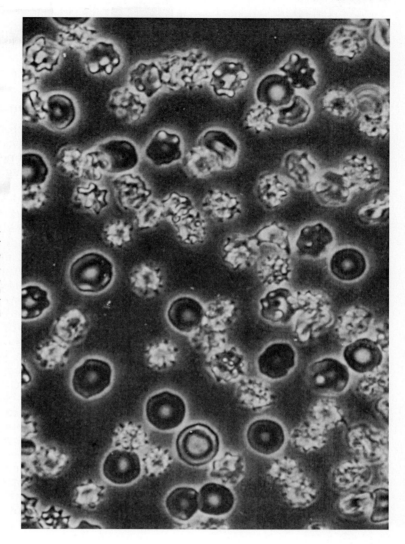

Figure 17-9. Phase contrast photomicrograph of PK-deficient blood (patient C.D. in Figure 17–7) after 2-hour exposure to 5 mM of cyanide to deplete adenosine triphosphate. The spiculated cells are, for the most part, reticulocytes. Magnification: ×6600. (From Mentzer WC, Baehner RL, et al: Selective reticulocyte destruction in erythrocyte pyruvate kinase deficiency. J Clin Invest 1971; 50:695, by copyright permission of the American Society for Clinical Investigation.)

After ATP depletion, net potassium loss may exceed 20 mEq/h per liter of cells.[263] Failure of the cation pump cannot explain such large losses of potassium. The effect of ATP depletion on potassium permeability, first described by Gardos and Straub,[336] is a feature of all metabolically depleted red cells and is not unique to PK deficiency. It is thought to be related to altered binding of membrane-associated calcium and can be partially prevented by ethylenediaminetetraacetic acid or quinine, even though these agents have no direct influence on the rate or extent of ATP depletion.[263, 337]

Initially, in the ATP-depleted cell, potassium loss exceeds sodium gain. The resultant net loss of cations is accompanied by an obligate osmotic loss of water and a reduction in cell volume. The shrunken, crenated cells produced by ATP depletion in PK-deficient reticulocytes are shown in Figure 17–9. These spiculated cells pass, with difficulty, through 8-μm millipore filters, and cell suspensions demonstrate increased viscosity in the Wells-Brookfield viscometer.[263] The destiny of such ATP-depleted erythrocytes, then, is to become dehydrated, rigid "desicytes," whose unfavorable characteristics may well prematurely terminate their existence.[338] Membranes prepared from PK-deficient or normal ATP-depleted red cells are more dense than normal as a result of absorption of cytoplasmic components (in particular an as yet unidentified 50,000-dalton protein) on the inner membrane surface.[339] Such changes in the cell membrane may contribute to the increased rigidity of these cells. There is evidence that membrane abnormalities not related to ATP depletion also may exist in PK-deficient red cells, but the role, if any, of such abnormalities in the hemolytic process is not established.[340] Not all workers have found abnormalities in the red cell membrane protein profile on sodium dodecyl sulfate–polyacrylamide gel electrophoresis,[341] and several other types of membrane analyses (spectrin extractability, membrane fluidity) have been normal.[342]

As enzyme-deficient erythrocytes age, a progressive reduction in glycolysis should accompany the inevitable gradual degradation of enzyme protein. Such deteriorating glycolysis eventually results in ATP depletion and, subsequently, in hemolysis. However, centrifuge studies have not revealed dramatic differences in the PK activity of enzymopenic young and old cells,[263] with the exception of one unstable PK variant[343] in which accelerated denaturation of enzyme protein was present *in vivo* as well as *in vitro*. Deterioration in catalytic efficiency, reported to occur in both normal[292] and variant[344] enzyme on aging *in vivo*, also may hasten the demise of enzymopenic cells.

The normal or near-normal survival of radiolabeled, severely PK-deficient erythrocytes reported by several investigators[263, 289, 325, 326, 345] indicates that diminished PK activity need not significantly curtail the life span of affected erythrocytes. Biphasic erythrocyte survival curves are sometimes obtained[346, 347] and suggest that two populations of cells are present, one destined for almost immediate destruction and the other having a considerably better outlook for survival.

Ferrokinetic studies in 10 patients[263, 347, 348] indicate that destruction of newly made erythrocytes in the bone marrow, spleen, or liver may be the major source of hemolysis in this disorder. Organ monitoring has shown that, as reticulocytes are released from the marrow, some are almost immediately sequestered in the spleen. The paradoxical reticulocytosis that follows splenectomy is probably the consequence of improved survival of this population of reticulocytes.

Spleens removed from anemic PK-deficient patients contain an unduly large number of reticulocytes.[319, 349] Splenic histology contrasts to that seen in hereditary spherocytosis, in that (1) the pulp spaces are empty rather than packed with erythrocytes; (2) erythrophagocytosis of reticulocytes, as well as of mature red cells by reticuloendothelial histiocytes is prominent in PK deficiency but rare in spherocytosis; and (3) many more crenated, deformed cells are seen in PK deficiency.[349, 350] Studies of such cells obtained from the peripheral blood have demonstrated them to be poorly deformable.[351] The hypoxic, acidic environment of the spleen would be expected to produce just such crenation in reticulocytes through the sequence of events outlined earlier—inhibition of oxidative phosphorylation, ATP depletion, selective potassium leakage, loss of cell water, and resultant loss of cell volume. These rigid desicytes should negotiate only with difficulty the 3-μm fenestrations between the splenic cords and sinuses. Thus doomed to a stay of uncertain duration in the metabolically unfavorable splenic environment, further deterioration in cell capabilities would seem inevitable. Isotope studies show that the final *coup de grace* is often administered in the liver.[350, 351]

Splenic destruction of reticulocytes is a variable feature of PK deficiency; in some instances, either bone marrow or liver destruction predominates. Why some reticulocytes are destroyed whereas others survive to reach maturity and thereafter have a near-normal existence despite their enzyme defect is unclear. It is possible that chance determines which reticulocytes will be detained in unfavorable metabolic circumstances. On the other hand, there is some evidence for actual variation in PK activity among reticulocytes.[263] Those most adequately endowed would be more likely to survive.

Although cellular dehydration has been given a central mechanistic role in the destruction of PK-deficient human red cells, it appears to be unimportant in the hemolytic process in PK-deficient basenji dogs. When dog red cells are exposed to cyanide *in vitro*, they

rapidly lose ATP. However, the ensuing potassium loss is balanced by an equivalent sodium gain, so there is no cellular dehydration. Other mechanisms must explain hemolysis in this setting.[352]

Genetics and Inheritance

Autosomal recessive transmission of the enzyme defect is usually observed in PK deficiency. Homozygotes and compound heterozygotes exhibit hemolytic anemia. Although simple heterozygotes usually remain clinically normal despite an approximately 50% reduction in erythrocyte PK activity, some may exhibit evidence of mild hemolysis.[353–355] Population surveys have estimated the incidence of PK heterozygosity to be 6% in Saudi Arabia,[356] 0% to 3.4% in Hong Kong,[357, 358] 2.2% in Canton, China,[359] 1.4% in Germany,[360] and only 0.14% in Ann Arbor, Michigan.[361]

Simple heterozygotes can be distinguished from compound heterozygotes or homozygotes by the degree of reticulocytosis, the extent of accumulation of red cell glucose-6-phosphate, and the *in vitro* properties of the mutant PK enzyme.[362] A transient further reduction in PK activity during the neonatal period was associated with hemolysis in one apparent heterozygote.[355] Such hemolysis in neonates is an exception to the benign nature of the carrier state in later life.

Little correlation exists between severity of anemia in homozygotes and the level of erythrocyte PK activity as measured by the conventional *in vitro* assay system unless enzyme activity is corrected for the degree of reticulocytosis present.[332] Variable clinical severity is explained, at least in part, by the existence of numerous mutant forms of the enzyme whose differing properties result in variable degrees of hemolysis. Such mutants are distinguishable from one another *in vitro* on the basis of maximal activity, electrophoretic mobility, substrate kinetics, stability, immunologic properties, and response to the activator FDP. In general, mutants with unfavorable kinetics are usually associated with more severe hemolysis.[330, 363–365] Diminished thermal stability of the enzyme *in vitro* also seems important in determining clinical severity.[264]

International standards for the characterization of mutant PK phenotypes have facilitated the comparison of mutants studied in different laboratories.[366] In compound heterozygotes, full characterization is difficult because tetramers formed from varying proportions of the two different mutant subunits are present, each with unique properties.[363] The best defined phenotypes are those found in true homozygotes, who are usually the offspring of consanguineous matings (Table 17–6). The kinetic and electrophoretic abnormalities characteristic of each variant PK reflect underlying structural changes in the enzyme owing to point mutations or deletions. At present, a total of 33 mutations in the *PKLR* have been defined at the nucleic acid level (see Fig. 17–6). One is a three-nucleotide insertion, two create stop codons, five are frameshift mutations, and four are deletions. The remainder are single nucleotide substitutions that alter the polypeptide composition by just one amino acid.[367–371] In the basenji, PK deficiency

Table 17-6. ERYTHROCYTE PYRUVATE KINASE (PK) VARIANTS* DESCRIBED IN TRUE HOMOZYGOTES (PRODUCTS OF CONSANGUINEOUS MATINGS) WITH HEMOLYTIC ANEMIA

References	Variant	Mutation	PK Activity (% of Normal)	Phosphoenol-pyruvate (PEP)† K_m	Adenosine Diphosphate (ADP) K_m	F1,6P Activation	Adenosine Triphosphate Inhibition	Nucleotide Specificity	Heat Stability	pH Optimum	Electrophoretic Mobility
High K_m PEP											
364	Itabashi		51	6.0	NL‡	NL	Increased	Abnormal	Very low	NL	Slow (94%)
364, 369	Maebashi	Cys^{1261}→Ala	39	5.5	NL	Low	NL	NL	Very low	NL	NL
364, 369	Fukushima	Cys^{1261}→Ala	92	4.1	NL	Low	Increased	Abnormal	Very low	NL	Slow (93%)
364	Aizu		63	3.85	NL	Low	Increased	Abnormal	Very low	NL	NL
380, 400	Sendai	Cys^{1261}→Ala	48.7	3.44	High	NL	Decreased	NL	Low	NL	Slow (93%)
364, 378	Sapporo	Gly^{1277}→Ala	147	2.81	Low	NL	Increased	Abnormal	NL	NL	Fast (111%)
364	Nagasaki	Cys^{1151}→Thr	136	2.29	Low	NL	NL	NL	Low	Acidic	Slow (83%)
398	Fukien		32	1.97	NL	Low	NL	NL	NL	—	Slow (88%)
364, 377a	Tokyo	Cys^{1151}→Thr	156	1.78	Low	NL	NL	Abnormal	Low	Acidic	Slow (93%)
Normal K_m PEP											
264	—		0–5	NL	—	—	NL	—	Very low	—	Slow (80%)
399	Fresno		—	1.5	NL	NL	NL	NL	NL	NL	Fast (130%)
380, 400	Shinshu	Gly^{1436}→Ala	11.5	1.24	Low	Low	NL	Abnormal	NL	NL	Slow (130%)
403	Beirut	Cys^{1151}→Thr	81	0.71	High	NL	NL	Abnormal	Low	Acidic	Slow (96%)
	Hadano	Cys^{1403}→Thr	40	NL							
Low K_m PEP											
379, 401	Amish	Gly^{1436}→Ala	3.9	0.65	Low	Slightly low	NL	Abnormal	Low	NL	Slow (77.5%)
372, 404	Basenji dogs	Cys^{433}→deleted	212	0.39	NL	—	—	—	Low	—	—
403	Linz	Cys^{487}→Thr	70	0.14	High	Low	Increased	Abnormal	Low	Acidic	Fast (120%)
Abnormal K_m ADP											
402	Westwood		25	0.62	0.30	NL	Decreased	Abnormal	Slightly low	NL	NL

*Characterized by the techniques suggested by the International Committee for Standardization in Haematology.[366]

†mM (normal = 1.31 + 1.13).

‡NL = normal.

is attributable to a frameshift mutation (deletion of cytosine at nucleotide 433).[372] Most PK mutations are extremely rare and usually limited to a single family. Exceptions are the Gly[1529]→Ala substitution, which is common in European PK-deficient patients,[367, 368, 370] and the Cys[1151]→Thr substitution common in Japanese patients.[369] Many of the mutations are located within exon 8 or 9, where components of the active site and the potassium-binding site are located, or in exons 10 or 11, a region responsible for the allosteric regulatory properties of the enzyme. However, the precise way in which each mutation disturbs the structure and function of PK has yet to be worked out. DNA analysis has indicated that several PK variants thought to be unique because of differing enzyme properties are, in fact, due to a single shared mutation (see Table 17–6). For example, PK Maebashi, PK Fukushima, and PK Sendai are each the consequence of a substitution of alanine for cystine at nucleotide 1261. The advent of readily available techniques for DNA analysis of PK mutations will clarify the true number of variant enzymes and will also make possible prenatal diagnosis of affected fetuses, as already demonstrated by Baronciani and Beutler.[373]

When kinetic abnormalities have been discovered in anemic patients, at least one parent has exhibited similar abnormalities. The other parent may also have kinetically aberrant PK[374, 375] or is found to have a low activity variant with normal kinetics.[376] Occasionally, it has not been possible to demonstrate an abnormality of erythrocyte PK in one[374, 377] or both[343] parents of patients with PK activity in the homozygous deficient range. Staal and co-workers[343] have speculated that, in some heterozygotes, a compensatory increase in synthesis of enzyme protein by the normal allele may result in enzyme activity indistinguishable from normal. More complete characterization of PK in these heterozygotes may reveal the presence of mutant enzyme. In at least one instance, increased thermolability was the only abnormality discovered in PK from an obligate heterozygote.[374]

The "classic" form of PK deficiency is associated with severe enzyme deficiency, persistence of the M_2 isoenzyme in mature erythrocytes, and little or no R isozymes. It is thought that the persistence of M_2 isoenzyme represents an attempt to compensate for the lack of R subunit–containing forms of PK.[381] An analogy to the persistence of fetal hemoglobin synthesis in β-thalassemia has been made by Miwa.[382] When M_2 compensation is incomplete, PK activity in mature red cells is low and hemolytic anemia ensues. When M_2 isoenzyme is synthesized at a higher rate, greater than normal amounts of PK activity can accumulate in mature red cells.[284, 383–386] In such patients there is no hemolytic anemia and, in fact, the increased glycolytic flow through PK at the expense of the 2,3-DPG generating pathway may lower 2,3-DPG levels, increase hemoglobin oxygen affinity, and result in erythrocytosis.

A kindred in whom hemolytic anemia occurred in PK heterozygotes was studied by Etiemble and colleagues.[387] PK activity was well below (17% to 45%) the 50% activity usually encountered in the presence of one normal and one mutant PK allele. It was thought that perhaps the presence of only one mutant subunit in the PK tetramer might be sufficient to reduce its catalytic function, with greater impairment accompanying the presence of additional mutant subunits. Similar considerations were raised in another kindred (PK Greensboro) in which heterozygotes exhibited less than 50% of the normal red cell PK activity but no hemolytic anemia.[388] However, in neither kindred was the presence of multiple combinations of mutant and normal subunits (i.e., M_4, M_3N, M_2N_2, M, N_3, N_4, where M = the mutant subunit and N = the normal subunit) actually confirmed.

No evidence suggests interaction between PK deficiency and other disorders of the erythrocyte. The clinical and hematologic presentation of β-thalassemia minor is not altered by the concomitant presence of heterozygous PK deficiency.[389] Although autologous erythrocyte survival was reduced in one woman who was doubly heterozygous for PK and G6PD deficiency, similarly reduced erythrocyte survival was present in a female relative heterozygous for G6PD deficiency only.[266] Reports of spherocytosis or paroxysmal nocturnal hematuria in PK heterozygotes have not mentioned unusual features of either disease in such heterozygotes. Markedly increased involvement of the kidneys was noted at autopsy in a patient with Gaucher's disease who also exhibited hemolytic anemia and deficiency of erythrocyte PK. It was suggested that cerebroside production was enhanced as a result of hemolysis.[390]

Therapy

Although a complete cure is not achieved by splenectomy, elimination or amelioration of transfusion requirements, a fall in bilirubin level, and a rise in hemoglobin concentration are quite often obtained. Whereas in severely anemic individuals splenectomy may be lifesaving,[319, 326] anemia in those with mild cases may be uninfluenced by the procedure. When significant morbidity exists, it would seem reasonable to recommend splenectomy, bearing in mind that the degree of benefit cannot be predicted with certainty. Standard studies of erythrocyte survival and sequestration, using ^{51}Cr-labeled cells, are often not useful in selecting patients for surgery, particularly when hemolysis of newly made cells predominates. Such cells are unavailable for tagging in the circulating blood, and their presence and fate are not reflected in the results obtained. Ferrokinetic studies, with appropriate organ monitoring, may allow a better assessment of the role of the spleen in such circumstances.

Therapeutic intervention with agents that either circumvent the metabolic aberrations induced by the defective enzyme or directly modify enzyme activity is theoretically possible. For example, a redox agent, such as methylene blue or ascorbic acid, might alleviate secondary inhibition of G3PD by increasing the amount of available NAD. Preliminary trials of these agents in one PK-deficient patient produced no change in reticulocyte count or hemoglobin concentration.[391] Activation of a relatively FDP-insensitive mutant form of

PK was apparently achieved in a single patient by intravenous infusion of 20 mmol of inosine and 1 mmol of adenine over 3 hours. Although the induced change in erythrocyte FDP concentration was modest (9×10^{-6} to 5×10^{-5} mol/L), a threefold increase in the survival of labeled red cells, a rise in hemoglobin concentration, and a fall in bilirubin level and reticulocyte count ensued.[392] In one other individual with a different PK mutant, nucleotide therapy was ineffective. Such agents are potentially hazardous, and their use remains experimental and controversial. In another attempt to increase erythrocyte FDP, mannose, galactose, and fructose were given orally to one PK-deficient patient but no increase in PK activity was noted.[343]

Two unrelated individuals, whose abnormalities of PK kinetics and stability could be corrected *in vitro* with sulfhydryl reagents, received a trial of intravenous therapy with 2-mercaptopropionyl glycine. The abnormal enzyme properties were also corrected *in vivo*, and one patient exhibited transient hematologic improvement that did not persist despite continuation of the drug. No hematologic changes occurred in the second patient.[299] Another approach to altering the balance of intraerythrocytic reduced and oxidized sulfhydryl groups was tried in a patient who was deficient in both PK and glutathione reductase activity. In this patient, oral riboflavin therapy for 6 months corrected the glutathione reductase deficiency and resulted in considerable hematologic improvement. PK activity remained low, but enzyme stability and kinetics, previously abnormal, became normal.[393] In this instance, the role of PK in the hemolytic anemia was uncertain and the nature of the effect, if any, of riboflavin on mutant PK was undefined.

Although hemolytic crises are uncommon in PK deficiency and have not been associated with drug ingestion, Glader has demonstrated a potential hazard to the use of large doses of salicylate in severely PK-deficient patients.[394] Salicylates inhibit oxidative phosphorylation and thus cause ATP depletion and cellular dehydration in severely PK-deficient reticulocytes *in vitro*. The salicylate doses used by Glader were high but were equivalent to serum levels achieved in chronic salicylate therapy for disorders such as rheumatoid arthritis. It is prudent to select alternative therapy for such patients when possible or to monitor them carefully for signs of increased hemolysis.

Bone marrow transplantation has permanently corrected the hemolytic anemia seen in PK-deficient basenji and in PK-deficient mice[395, 396] but has not yet been attempted in humans. The potential feasibility of gene therapy has been demonstrated in PK-deficient mice.[397]

LACTATE DEHYDROGENASE DEFICIENCY

Lactate dehydrogenase

$$Pyruvate \longleftrightarrow Lactic\ acid$$
$$NADH \quad NAD$$

Clinical Manifestations, Biochemistry, and Genetics

In one Japanese family, partial or complete absence of the H subunit of lactate dehydrogenase (LDH) in erythrocytes, leukocytes, platelets, and serum was unassociated with anemia or hemolysis.[405] Blood lactate levels were subnormal in all affected family members. Measurement of red cell glycolytic intermediates revealed accumulation of trioses, suggesting insufficient cycling of NADH to NAD by means of LDH to support adequate G3PD activity. It is of interest that such low LDH activity can result in impairment of glycolysis without apparent shortening of the red cell life span. More recently, in four members of another Japanese family the M subunit of LDH was completely lacking. As with H subunit deficiency, no evidence of hemolytic anemia was present.[406] In contrast, mice homozygous for a low activity mutation of the skeletal muscle subunit of LDH have less than 10% of normal enzyme activity in erythrocytes and exhibit severe lifelong hemolytic anemia.[407]

ABNORMALITIES OF ERYTHROCYTE NUCLEOTIDE METABOLISM

In individuals with CNSHA, low erythrocyte ATP levels often play a central role in the pathogenesis of hemolysis. Hemolytic anemia associated with an unusually high erythrocyte ATP level has also been described.[408] In the affected pedigree, red cell PK levels were normal, so that the mechanism for ATP elevation would appear to differ from that found in other families with high red cell ATP, low 2,3-DPG, erythrocytosis, and twofold or greater elevation in PK activity.[384–386] In yet another family, two infants with hemolytic anemia, high erythrocyte ATP, and low 2,3-DPG had reduced DPG phosphatase activity.[409] The relationship of this enzyme abnormality to the unusual elevation of erythrocyte ATP or to hemolysis is uncertain. In the three disorders of erythrocyte nucleotide metabolism to be described in this section, evidence of a relationship between the abnormal enzyme and hemolytic anemia is more convincing, although, even in these disorders, much remains to be learned regarding the pathogenesis of hemolysis.

Pyrimidine-5′-Nucleotidase Deficiency

Pyrimidine-5′-nucleotidase

Cytidine-5′-monophosphate → Cytidine

$$H_2O \qquad\qquad + P_i$$

Uridine-5′-monophosphate → Uridine

Clinical Manifestations

Deficiency of erythrocyte P-5′-N is associated with lifelong chronic hemolytic anemia of moderate severity.[7, 410–418] The half-life survival time of ^{51}Cr-labeled autologous red cells has ranged from 9 to 23 days. Splenomegaly is usually present. Pronounced basophilic stippling, which may occur in as many as 5% of all erythrocytes, is an important and useful finding and stands as an exception to the usual lack of distinguishing morphologic abnormalities in erythroenzymopathies. Erythrocyte osmotic fragility is normal or slightly increased. Definitive diagnosis requires assay of red cell P-5'-N activity.

Biochemistry

Reticulocyte maturation requires disposition of intra-erythrocytic ribosomal RNA, which is no longer required for protein synthesis. The hydrolysis of pyrimidine nucleotides (CMP, UMP) formed by the action of ribonucleases on ribosomal RNA, an essential step in RNA degradation, is catalyzed by pyrimidine-5'-nucleotidase. The cytidine and uridine formed can diffuse across the cell membrane, whereas the pyrimidine nucleotide substrates of the nucleotidase reaction are incapable of diffusion and accumulate within the cell when activity of the nucleotidase is subnormal.[8]

Hirono and associates[419] found two different isoenzymes of P-5'-N in hemolysates from normal or P-5'-N–deficient subjects. Only one isoenzyme, CMP-responsive, was deficient in all five deficient subjects evaluated, while the other, dTMP-responsive, was normal. Kinetic and thermostability abnormalities were seen in the CMP-responsive isoenzyme from deficient subjects but not in the dTMP-responsive isoenzyme. Apparently, the lack of overlapping substrate sensitivities makes it impossible for the residual normal isoenzyme to substitute for its deficient partner in enzymopenic individuals.

The amount of nucleotides in P-5'-N–deficient red cells is increased by 1.3 to 5.0 times, chiefly due to an increase in pyrimidine derivatives (CMP, CDP, CTP, UMP, UDP, UTP).[8, 412, 413, 420, 421] The most abundant derivatives are the diphosphodiesters, CDP-choline and CDP-ethanolamine.[421] Accumulation of pyrimidine derivatives is undoubtedly due in part to RNA degradation[413] but may also reflect *de novo* synthesis of these compounds from uridine and orotic acid transported into the red cell.[422] Classification of P-5'-N deficiency as a high ATP syndrome was based on early observations of unusually high cell ATP levels using an enzymatic assay of ATP content that also reflected the presence of other nucleotide triphosphates, notably CTP and UTP. More specific assays have subsequently shown that cell adenine nucleotide levels are normal[8, 414, 421] or even low[414] rather than elevated.[8]

The extraordinary accumulation of pyrimidine nucleotides within P-5'-N–deficient red cells is easily detected by subjecting cellular extracts to magnetic resonance imaging[423] or to ultraviolet spectroscopy. Extracts from normal cells exhibit an absorbance peak at 255 to 260 nm (almost entirely owing to the presence of adenine nucleotides). In P-5'-N deficiency, a higher absorbance peak slightly shifted in position (266 to 270 nm) is observed, reflecting the presence of large amounts of pyrimidine nucleotides and providing a relatively simple means of screening patients for the disorder.[8, 413]

The secondary effects of P-5'-N deficiency are complex. For example, the concentration of GSH is regularly increased by a factor of 1.5 to 2.3,[413] a finding that may help to confirm the diagnosis in a suspected case of P-5'-N deficiency. Red cell phosphoribosylpyrophosphate synthetase activity is markedly low (15% to 35% of normal) in P-5'-N–deficient red cells.[424, 425] In fact, phosphoribosylpyrophosphate synthetase deficiency was originally thought to be the primary defect responsible for hemolysis. It is now regarded as a secondary phenomenon.[6] Pyrimidine nucleotides have been shown to bind and sequester magnesium, a cofactor required for subunit aggregation and maximal activation of phosphoribosylpyrophosphate synthetase.[426] Magnesium depletion (by the addition of pyrimidine nucleotides) also inhibits PK activity and pentose phosphate shunt activity in hemolysates. On the other hand, red cell magnesium levels are normal or even elevated in P-5'-N–deficient red cells, and incubation of these cells with exogenous magnesium does not reduce their susceptibility to autohemolysis or to Heinz body formation.[427] The role of magnesium deficiency (or unavailability) in the central abnormalities that limit the life span of P-5'-N–deficient red cells is not clear.

In fact, it is not known why P-5'-N–deficient red cells are destroyed prematurely. Perhaps the pyrimidine nucleotides that accumulate interfere with the normal function of key glycolytic enzymes, by competing for available binding sites with the adenine nucleotides that are the normal enzyme substrate. The possible importance of pyrimidine nucleotides in hemolysis is underscored by the report of an individual with chronic hemolysis, basophilic stippling, and normal P-5'-N activity, in whom the only biochemical abnormality detected was a striking elevation in erythrocyte CDP-choline.[428] Pyrimidine nucleotide accumulation has been shown to lower red cell pH in P-5'-N–deficient red cells as a result of shifts in the Donnan equilibrium consequent to the increase in fixed intracellular anion.[417, 420] This drop of 0.1 to 0.2 pH units is sufficient to increase red cell oxygen affinity above the normal range[420] and may also explain the slightly subnormal glycolytic rate of P-5'-N–deficient red cells.[429] Tomoda and colleagues have demonstrated a moderate impairment of stimulated pentose phosphate pathway activity in P-5'-N–deficient erythrocytes, which they attribute to inhibition of G6PD by pyrimidine nucleotides.[417] This impairment in shunt activity is noted in both light and dense red cells separated by centrifugation and is accompanied by a parallel decrease in G6PD activity.[430] It is hard to visualize how pentose phosphate pathway failure could result in the unusually high levels of GSH characteristic of P-5'-N deficiency, because the opposite effect, a deficiency of GSH, would be predicted.[417]

Study of individuals with lead poisoning has confirmed the central role of P-5'-N deficiency in the origin of hemolytic anemia. P-5'-N is markedly inhibited *in vitro* by low concentrations of lead, and the red cells of patients with significant lead poisoning have depressed levels of P-5'-N activity.[431] The basophilic stippling that is present in some patients with lead poisoning has been attributed to nucleotidase deficiency.[381] Although accumulation of pyrimidine nucleotides within erythrocytes is not found in all cases of lead poisoning in which P-5'-N activity is reduced, it is a regular feature of those cases exhibiting acute lead-induced hemolytic anemia.[432, 433] Perhaps because of the shorter duration or less severe character of the enzyme deficiency, the red cells of lead-poisoned individuals do not exhibit ribose-phosphate pyrophosphokinase deficiency.[432] GSH levels are normal[432] or elevated.[413] Despite the less than perfect homology between congenital and acquired P-5'-N deficiency, study of the latter may be expected to provide important insight into the mechanisms of hemolysis in this disorder.

Genetics and Inheritance

More than 40 patients with P-5'-N deficiency and hemolytic anemia have been described.[413] The disorder has been found in whites,[8, 425] blacks,[8, 424] Ashkenazi Jews,[410] Arabs,[434] and Asians.[412, 419, 435] Inheritance is autosomal recessive.[413] Heterozygotes have no clinical manifestations but exhibit a reduction of about 50% in red cell P-5'-N activity.[8, 413] The wide range of enzyme activity encountered in normal individuals makes heterozygote detection difficult in some families.[436] Variation in the severity of disease is, in part, owing to heterogeneity in the molecular nature of the defective enzyme. Several instances of hemolytic anemia in which red cell P-5'-N exhibited abnormal physical properties as well as reduced activity have been recognized.[411, 419, 435] P-5'-N has been found in spleen,[435] kidney, and brain.[414, 437] The presence of the enzyme in brain may be relevant to the mental retardation noted in several P-5'-N–deficient individuals with hemolytic anemia.[414]

Therapy

The congenital form of P-5'-N deficiency must be distinguished from the acquired form associated with lead poisoning, because specific therapy is available for the latter. Splenectomy is not of much benefit in congenital P-5'-N deficiency. Investigational therapeutic use of allopurinol in one affected individual had no effect on hemolysis and actually increased erythrocyte pyrimidine nucleotide levels.[422]

Adenylate Kinase Deficiency

$$2\ ADP \xrightarrow{\text{Adenylate kinase}} ATP + AMP$$

Clinical Manifestations, Biochemistry, and Genetics

Controversy exists regarding the role of adenylate kinase (AK) deficiency in hemolytic anemia. Beutler and colleagues studied two black siblings whose red cells lacked virtually any measurable AK activity. One had hemolytic anemia, but the other did not.[438] It was sug-

gested that in this family, hemolysis was either unrelated to AK deficiency or that another, coexistent defect was required for hemolysis to occur. The latter situation seemed to be the case in an Arab family in which two siblings had severe red cell AK deficiency (less than 5% of normal), but only the sibling who had also inherited severe G6PD deficiency exhibited hemolysis.[439] However, further investigation of this large pedigree disclosed six more individuals with severe AK deficiency (less than 7% of normal) and mental retardation.[440] All had chronic nonspherocytic hemolytic anemia. Three had also inherited G6PD deficiency and were severely anemic, requiring red cell transfusions 6 to 10 times annually. The other three, who were not G6PD deficient, were moderately anemic and only occasionally required transfusions. Family members who had carrier levels of red cell AK activity (50% of normal) either with or without G6PD deficiency and individuals with G6PD deficiency alone did not have chronic hemolytic anemia. These results suggest either a direct role for AK deficiency in hemolysis or that the enzyme defect is a marker for another genetically linked but as yet unidentified defect that is the primary cause of anemia.[441] Two additional cases of AK deficiency associated with hemolytic anemia have been reported in France[442] and Japan,[443] but neither further resolves the question of the role of the enzymopathy in hemolysis. The Japanese subject inherited a point mutation (Arg[128]→Trp) in the coding region of the *AK1* gene from her mother and a normal *AK1* allele from her father. Although both mother and child were heterozygous for AK deficiency, only the child exhibited hemolytic anemia, whereas the mother was hematologically normal.[444] Lachant and colleagues reported undetectably low levels of AK activity in the red cells of a Syrian girl who also had chronic hemolytic anemia.[441] Only modest impairment in the formation of adenosine diphosphate from adenosine monophosphate was observed in intact cells, suggesting that alternative pathways might be available to substitute for the missing AK. Alternatively, it was proposed that AK itself might be present in intact cells but somehow inactivated during the preparation of a hemolysate for assay of enzyme activity.

Therapy

Splenectomy was performed in five of six Arab patients with prompt disappearance of anemia and hemolysis.[440]

Adenosine Deaminase Overproduction

$$\text{Adenosine} + H_2O \xrightarrow{\text{Adenosine deaminase}} \text{Inosine} + H_2O$$

Clinical Manifestations, Biochemistry, and Genetics

Fourteen individuals in three families have been found to have hereditary hemolytic anemia, sharply diminished amounts of intraerythrocytic adenosine nucleotides (to less than 50% of normal), and a remarkable 45- to 110-fold increase in red cell ADA activity.[445–448] In contrast to virtually all other erythroenzymopathies, ADA excess is transmitted as an autosomal dominant trait. Hemolysis is apparently the consequence of diminished red cell ATP content, which is caused by the diversion of nearly all adenosine metabolism through the unusually active ADA reaction at the expense of the competing AK kinase reaction. The former results in irreversible loss of adenosine nucleotides, whereas the latter conserves such nucleotides and preserves cell ATP stores. Abnormalities of lesser magnitude have been found in other enzymes of nucleotide metabolism in affected individuals, suggesting that excess ADA activity may be secondary to an as yet undefined primary defect. The physical properties of the mutant ADA are normal,[447, 449] indicating that the great excess of ADA activity is due to overproduction rather than to an increase in catalytic efficiency. In one subject, an increase in red cell ADA protein equivalent to the striking increase in ADA activity was demonstrated by immunoblotting. Synthesis of ADA by erythroid progenitors grown from bone marrow cells was 11-fold greater in an affected individual.[452] RNase mapping techniques and Northern blotting have revealed at least a 100-fold increase over normal in the ADA mRNA content of affected reticulocytes. Sequencing of ADA cDNA showed no abnormalities in the coding region and 5′ and 3′ untranslated regions of the parent mRNA. Examination of genomic DNA by Southern blotting did not disclose evidence of gene amplification, deletion, or gross rearrangements. Thus, although the basis for ADA excess appears to be an overabundance of apparently normal mRNA, the mechanism underlying this abnormality remains obscure.[451]

Linkage analysis using a polymorphic TAAA repeat located 1.1 kb upstream from the *ADA* gene indicated strongly that the mutation was located in *cis* rather than in *trans*.[453] DNA constructs containing 10.6 kb of 5′ flanking sequences and 12.3 kb of the first intron of the normal or mutant *ADA* gene were linked to a reporter gene (chloramphenicol acyl transferase) and used to study expression in transient transfection assays and in transgenic mice. No difference in expression between wild type and mutant alleles was found. Therefore, the mutation is thought to reside at a more distant 5′ site, within a different intron, or 3′ to the coding region.[454]

Much lesser increases in ADA activity (approximately fourfold) are seen in congenital hypoplastic anemia,[455, 456] arthrogryposis multiplex congenita,[457] the acquired immunodeficiency syndrome,[458] and cartilage-hair hypoplasia.[459] The origin and implications of these increases are obscure, but they are not associated with hemolysis.

ACQUIRED DISORDERS OF ERYTHROCYTE GLYCOLYSIS

Alterations in the external chemical milieu may profoundly influence erythrocyte metabolism. The rate of glycolysis, for example, is governed by the availability of inorganic phosphate. High concentrations of inorganic phosphate augment, and low concentrations impede, the glycolytic synthesis of ATP and 2,3-DPG. Erythrocytes from uremic patients with hyperphosphatemia contain an average of 70% more ATP than do normal erythrocytes, and a lesser, but significant, increase in 2,3-DPG concentration is also found in the hyperphosphatemic cell.[460] Equivalent changes in organic phosphates can be induced in normal erythrocytes by incubation either in hyperphosphatemic uremic plasma or in autologous normal plasma supplemented with inorganic phosphate.[460] Conversely, hypophosphatemia induced by hyperalimentation with low phosphate nutrients[461] or by anion resin therapy for hyperphosphatemia[462] is associated with a reduction in erythrocyte organic phosphates. Organic phosphate depletion consequent to hypophosphatemia may be sufficient to displace the oxyhemoglobin dissociation curve to the left, unfavorably influencing tissue oxygenation. In one patient[463] whose serum inorganic phosphate level was immeasurably low, a transient hemolytic anemia associated with the appearance of spherocytes on the peripheral blood smear, decreased red cell deformability, and an increase in erythrocyte osmotic fragility were attributed to a profound fall in erythrocyte ATP concentration.[464] With correction of hypophosphatemia, the erythrocyte abnormalities disappeared, and red cell survival improved. Klock and co-workers[465] have also observed transient hemolytic anemia and spherocytosis in a hypophosphatemic patient. Red cell membrane phospholipid composition was altered in this patient during the hypophosphatemic interval. Correction of the membrane lipid abnormalities accompanied the return of the serum phosphorus concentration to normal. In hypophosphatemic erythrocytes, a remarkable accumulation of triose phosphate intermediates occurs when the serum phosphorus level falls below 2 mg/dL. This may be attributed to inhibition of G3PD by lack of inorganic phosphorus, a cofactor in the reaction.[461] In addition, the low concentration of ATP and 2,3-DPG that accompanies hypophosphatemia partly relieves inhibition of PFK by these metabolites, accelerating the production of triose phosphate. Overall, in hypophosphatemia, inhibitory influences on glycolysis predominate, and erythrocyte glucose consumption and lactate production are measurably reduced.[466] The opposite effect, acceleration of glycolysis, is observed in hyperphosphatemia. The significant clinical abnormalities of oxygen transport or of erythrocyte shape, rigidity, and life span that attend alterations in the normal level of plasma phosphate are ultimately the consequence of such changes in erythrocyte glycolysis.

Less is known about the influence of other components of the chemical environment on erythrocyte glycolysis. In the hands of some investigators, experimental magnesium deficiency in the rat resembles hypophosphatemia, in that erythrocyte glycolysis is inhibited, ATP and 2,3-DPG levels are subnormal, and red cell rigidity is increased. Spherocytes are evident on the blood smear, and red cell survival is reduced.[467] Magnesium is essential for the normal function of a variety of glycolytic and nonglycolytic enzymes. However, using a different diet to induce magnesium deficiency, Piomelli and co-workers showed that although a hemolytic anemia accompanies magnesium depletion in rats, erythrocyte glycolysis and the activity of red blood cell glycolytic enzymes remain normal.[468] Magnesium deficiency also influences other red cell components, notably the membrane,[469] and the relative contribution of such abnormalities to shortened red cell life span remains undefined. It is not known whether hematologic changes similar to those seen in the rat occur in human magnesium deficiency.

Iron deficiency not only decreases the production of red cells but also accelerates their destruction.[470] Studies of the metabolic properties of iron-deficient red cells have revealed several abnormalities that might reduce cell viability. The activity of both catalase and glutathione peroxidase is reduced in deficient cells[471]; *in vitro* hydrogen peroxide hemolysis is increased; and increased susceptibility to peroxidation of membrane lipids can be inferred from these findings. Although erythrocyte glycolysis *in vitro* is normal for cell age,[472] cell ATP is unstable on incubation. ATP concentration in freshly obtained red cells may either be normal[473] or low.[474, 475] The spontaneous autohemolysis of iron-deficient red cells incubated at 37°C is increased.[476] The increased rigidity characteristic of the ATP-depleted cell is present in iron-deficient cells as well.[476] These findings suggest that a defect in energy metabolism may contribute to the shortened survival of iron-deficient red cells.

Little is known about the possible influence of hormones on erythrocyte glycolytic enzymes. The activity of HK, PFK, PK, and glyceraldehyde-6-phosphate dehydrogenase is often reduced in the erythrocytes of diabetics.[477] The same enzymes were remarkably increased in activity in one patient with an insulinoma before removal of the tumor. The activity of several erythrocyte enzymes is reduced in hypothyroidism and becomes normal after therapy,[478] probably reflecting changes in the mean erythrocyte cell age rather than a direct influence of the hormone on the enzymes. However, Snyder and Reddy[479] have shown that 2,3-DPG synthesis *in vitro* by hemoglobin and membrane-free extracts of erythrocytes is enhanced by thyroid hormone.

Alterations in erythrocyte enzyme activity are often found during the course of either acute or chronic leukemia,[480–484] nonmalignant pancytopenias,[481, 485–487] congenital dyserythropoietic anemia,[488] acquired dyserythropoietic anemia,[481, 489, 490] myeloid metaplasia,[481] and polycythemia vera.[481] One, several, or many enzymes may be involved and activity may be either increased or decreased. For example, the activity of enolase may be elevated as much as threefold to fourfold in erythroleukemia or in monomyelogenous leukemia. These changes do not merely reflect alterations in the mean red cell life span, because enolase activity is normally little different in young and old erythrocytes and because appropriate changes in other enzymes whose activity is clearly related to red cell age do not

occur. In a large group of miscellaneous acquired blood disorders, PK activity was deficient in the red cells of about one third of the patients and PFK activity was deficient in approximately one fifth.[481] Such deficiencies appear not to result in any significant hemolytic anemia,[481] although studies of glycolytic intermediate patterns indicate that there may be adverse effects on erythrocyte metabolism.[491, 492] The unusual pattern of enzyme activities may, on occasion, be useful in diagnosis, as, for example, in distinguishing congenital hypoplastic anemia from transient erythroblastopenia of childhood.[493]

Several quite different processes appear to be responsible for the development of acquired enzymopathies.[494] Reversion to fetal hematopoiesis may alter enzyme function.[495] Post-translational changes in an inherently normal enzyme protein have been demonstrated.[496] In such instances, incubation of affected cells in normal plasma, modification of affected hemolysate by dialysis or treatment with sulfhydryl reagents, or partial purification of the enzyme restores normal enzyme activity and functional properties. In other instances, enzyme-specific activity is normal (measured immunologically) but total activity is low and not enhanced by the measures just described.[496] In these cases, synthesis of enzyme protein by developing erythroid cells is apparently impaired, perhaps as a result of alterations in chromosome number or disorderly and desynchronous nuclear maturation. Although some components of the abnormal pattern of enzymes (such as low PFK or high enolase activity) may suggest a reversion to fetal erythropoiesis, others do not. The possibility that these enzyme abnormalities may be familial and antedate the onset of an acquired blood disorder has not been fully explored.

References

1. Dacie JV, Mollison PL, et al: Atypical congenital hemolytic anemia. Q J Med 1953; 22:79.
2. Valentine WN, Paglia DE: Erythrocyte enzymopathies, hemolytic anemia, and multisystem disease. An annotated review. Blood 1953; 64:583.
3. Selwyn JG, Dacie JV: Autohemolysis and other changes resulting from the incubation *in vitro* of red cells from patients with congenital hemolytic anemia. Blood 1954; 9:414.
4. Robinson MA, Loder PB, et al.: Red cell metabolism in nonspherocytic congenital haemolytic anemia. Br J Haematol 1961; 7:327.
5. Valentine WN, Tanaka KR, et al: A specific erythrocyte enzyme defect (pyruvate kinase) in three subjects with congenital nonspherocytic hemolytic anemia. Trans Assoc Am Physicians 1961; 74:100.
6. Tanaka KR, Zerez CR, et al: Red cell enzymopathies of the glycolytic pathway. Semin Hematol 1990; 27:165.
7. Fujii H, Miwa S: Recent progress in the molecular genetic analysis of erythroenzymopathy. Am J Hematol 1990; 34:301.
8. Valentine WN, Fink K, et al: Hereditary hemolytic anemia with human erythrocyte pyrimidine-5'-nucleotidase deficiency. J Clin Invest 1974; 54:866.
9. Beutler E: Why has the autohemolysis test not gone the way of the cephalin flocculation test? Blood 1978; 51:109.
10. Keitt AS: Diagnostic strategy in a suspected red cell enzymopathy. Clin Haematol 1981; 10:3.
11. Beutler E: Red Cell Metabolism: A Manual of Biochemical Methods, 3rd ed. Orlando, FL, Grune & Stratton, Inc., 1984.
12. Jansen G, Koenderman L, et al: Characteristics of hexokinase,

pyruvate kinase, and glucose-6-phosphate dehydrogenase during adult and neonatal reticulocyte maturation. Am J Hematol 1985; 20:203.

13. Beutler E: Biphasic loss of red cell enzyme activity during *in vivo* aging. In Eaton JW, Konzen DK, White JG (eds): Cellular and Molecular Aspects of Aging: The Red Cell As a Model. New York, Alan R. Liss, Inc., 1985, p 317.

14. Lakomek M, Schroter W, et al: On the diagnosis of erythrocyte defects in the presence of high reticulocyte counts. Br J Haematol 1989; 72:445.

15. Board PG, Trueworthy R, et al: Congenital nonspherocytic hemolytic anemia with an unstable hexokinase variant. Blood 1978; 51:111.

16. Lohr GW, Waller HD, et al: Hexokinasemangel in Blutzellen bei einer Sippe mit familiärer Panmyelopathie (Typ Fanconi). Klin Wochenschr 1965; 43:870.

17. Fornaini G, Dacha M, et al: Role of hexokinase in the regulation of glucose metabolism in human erythrocytes. Ital J Biochem 1986; 35:316.

18. Magnani M, Rossi L, et al: Role of hexokinase in the regulation of erythrocyte hexose monophosphate pathway under oxidative stress. Biochem Biophys Res Commun 1988; 155:423.

19. Magnani M, Rossi L, et al: Improved metabolic properties of hexokinase-overloaded human erythrocytes. Biochim Biophys Acta 1988; 972:1.

20. Magnani M, Rossi L, et al: Human red blood cell loading with hexokinase-inactivating antibodies. An *in vitro* model for enzyme deficiencies. Acta Haematol 1989; 82:27.

21. Magnani M, Serafini G, et al: Hexokinase type I multiplicity in human erythrocytes. Biochem J 1988; 254:617.

22. Murakami K, Blei F, et al: An isozyme of hexokinase specific for the human red blood cell (HKg). Blood 1990; 75:770.

23. Magnani M, Stocchi V, et al: Rabbit red blood cell hexokinase. Decay mechanism during reticulocyte maturation. J Biol Chem 1986; 261:8327.

24. Murakami K, Piomelli S: The isoenzymes of mammalian hexokinase: Tissue specificity and *in vivo* decline. In Magnani M, De Flora A (eds): Red Blood Cell Aging. New York, Plenum Press, 1991, p 277.

25. Thorburn DR, Beutler E: Decay of hexokinase during reticulocyte maturation: Is oxidative damage a signal for destruction? Biochem Biophys Res Commun 1989; 162:612.

26. Valentine WN, Oski FA, et al: Erythrocyte hexokinase and hereditary hemolytic anemia. In Beutler E (ed): Hereditary Disorders of Erythrocyte Metabolism. New York, Grune & Stratton, Inc., 1968, p 288.

27. Gerber GK, Schultz M, et al: Occurrence and function of a high K_m hexokinase in immature red blood cells. Eur J Biochem 1970; 17:445.

28. Necheles TF, Rai US, et al: Congenital nonspherocytic hemolytic anemia associated with an unusual erythrocyte hexokinase abnormality. J Lab Clin Med 1970; 76:593.

29. Keitt AS: Hemolytic anemia with impaired hexokinase activity. J Clin Invest 1969; 48:1997.

30. Jandl JH, Aster RH: Increased splenic pooling and the pathogenesis of hypersplenism. Am J Med Sci 1967; 253:282.

31. Rakitzis ET, Mills GC: Relation of red-cell hexokinase activity to extracellular pH. Biochim Biophys Acta 1967; 141:439.

32. Moser K, Ciresa M, et al: Hexokinasemangel bei hämolytischer Anämie. Med Welt 1970; 21:1977.

33. Gilsanz F, Meyer E, et al: Congenital hemolytic anemia due to hexokinase deficiency. Am J Dis Child 1978; 132:636.

34. Rijksen G, Staal GEJ: Human erythrocyte hexokinase deficiency: characterization of a mutant enzyme with abnormal regulatory properties. J Clin Invest 1978; 62:294.

35. Valentine WN, Oski FA, et al: Hereditary hemolytic anemia with hexokinase deficiency. N Engl J Med 1967; 276:1.

36. Paglia DE, Shende A, et al: Hexokinase "New Hyde Park": a low activity erythrocyte isozyme in a Chinese kindred. Am J Hematol 1981; 10:107.

37. Magnani M, Stocchi V, et al: Hereditary nonspherocytic hemolytic anemia due to a new hexokinase variant with reduced stability. Blood 1985; 66:690.

38. Magnani M, Chiarantini L, et al: Glucose metabolism in fibroblasts from patients with erythrocyte hexokinase deficiency. J Inherited Metab Dis 1986; 9:129.

39. Rijksen G, Akkerman JWN, et al: Generalized hexokinase deficiency in the blood cells of a patient with nonspherocytic hemolytic anemia. Blood 1986; 61:12.

40. Newman P, Muir A, et al: Non-spherocytic haemolytic anaemia in mother and son associated with hexokinase deficiency. Br J Haematol 1980; 46:537.

41. Magnani M, Stocchi V, et al: Human erythrocyte hexokinase deficiency: a new variant with abnormal kinetic properties. Br J Haematol 1985; 61:41.

42. Beutler E, Dyment PG, et al: Hereditary nonspherocytic hemolytic anemia and hexokinase deficiency. Blood 1978; 51:935.

43. Goebel KM, Gassel WD, et al: Hemolytic anemia and hexokinase deficiency associated with malformations. Klin Wochenschr 1972; 50:349.

44. Siimes MA, Rahiala EL, et al: Hexokinase deficiency in erythrocytes: a new variant in 5 members of a Finnish family. Scand J Haematol 1979; 22:214.

45. Brewer GJ: Erythrocyte metabolism and function: hexokinase inhibition by 2,3-diphosphoglycerate and interaction with ATP and Mg^{2+}. Biochim Biophys Acta 1969; 192:157.

46. Delivoria-Papadopoulos M, Oski FA, et al: Oxygen hemoglobin dissociation curves: effect of inherited enzyme defects of the red cell. Science 1969; 165:601.

47. Oski FA, Marshall BE, et al: Exercise with anemia: the role of the left-shifted or right-shifted oxygen hemoglobin equilibrium curve. Ann Intern Med 1971; 74:44.

48. Kosower NS, Vanderhoff GA, et al: Hexokinase activity in normal and glucose-6-phosphate dehydrogenase deficient erythrocytes. Nature 1964; 201:684.

49. Bethenod M, Kissin C, et al: Déficit en hexokinase intraérythrocytaire. Ann Pediatr 1967; 50:825.

50. Rogers PA, Fisher RA, et al: An electrophoretic study of the distribution and properties of human hexokinases. Biochem Genet 1975; 13:857.

51. Povey S, Corney G, et al: Genetically determined polymorphism of a form of hexokinase, HK III, found in human leukocytes. Ann Hum Genet 1975; 38:407.

52. Akkerman JWN, Rijksen G, et al: Platelet function and energy metabolism in a patient with hexokinase deficiency. Blood 1984; 63:147.

53. Matthay KK, Mentzer WC: Erythrocyte enzymopathies in the newborn. Clin Haematol 1981; 10:31.

54. Whitelaw AGL, Rogers PA, et al: Congenital haemolytic anaemia resulting from glucose phosphate isomerase deficiency: genetics, clinical picture, and prenatal diagnosis. J Med Genet 1979; 16:189.

55. Ravindranath Y, Paglia DE, et al: Glucose phosphate isomerase deficiency as a cause of hydrops fetalis. N Engl J Med 1987; 316:258.

56. Hutton JJ, Chilcote RR: Glucose phosphate isomerase deficiency with hereditary nonspherocytic hemolytic anemia. J Pediatr 1974; 85:494.

57. Schroter W, Brittinger G, et al: Combined glucosephosphate isomerase and glucose-6-phosphate dehydrogenase deficiency of the erythrocytes: a new hemolytic syndrome. Br J Haematol 1971; 20:249.

58. Paglia DE, Paredes R, et al: Unique phenotypic expression of glucosephosphate isomerase deficiency. Am J Hum Genet 1975; 27:62.

59. Helleman PW, Van Biervliet JPGM: Haematological studies in a new variant of glucosephosphate isomerase deficiency (GPI Utrecht). Helv Paediatr Acta 1975; 30:525.

60. Arnold H, Lohr GW, et al: Augsburg-type glucosephosphate isomerase deficiency: a new variant causing congenital nonspherocytic hemolytic anemia in a German family. Blut 1980; 40:107.

61. Arnold H, Hasslinger K, et al: Glucosephosphateisomerase type Kaiserslautern: a new variant causing congenital nonspherocytic hemolytic anemia. Blut 1983; 46:271.

62. Kahn A, Bue HA, et al: Molecular and functional anomalies in two new mutant glucose-phosphateisomerase variants with enzyme deficiency and chronic hemolysis. Hum Genet 1978; 40:293.

63. Arnold H, Lohr GW, et al: Combined erythrocyte glucosephosphate isomerase (GPI) and glucose-6-phosphate dehydrogenase (G6PD) deficiency in an Italian family. Hum Genet 1981; 57:226.

64. Oski FA, Fuller E: Glucose-phosphate isomerase (GPI) deficiency associated with abnormal osmotic fragility and spherocytes. Clin Res 1971; 19:427.

65. Vives-Corrons IL, Carrera A, et al: Anemia hemolitica por deficit congenito en fosfohexosaisomerasa. Sangre 1975; 20:197.

66. Blume KG, Hryniuk W, et al: Characterization of two new variants of glucose-phosphate-isomerase deficiency with hereditary nonspherocytic hemolytic anemia. J Lab Clin Med 1972; 79:942.

67. Cayanis E, Penfold GK, et al: Haemolytic anaemia associated with glucosephosphate isomerase (GPI) deficiency in a black South African child. Br J Haematol 1977; 37:363.

68. Van Biervliet JP, Vlug A, et al: A new variant of glucosephosphate isomerase deficiency. Humangenetik 1975; 30:35.

69. Schroter W, Koch HH, et al: Glucose phosphate isomerase deficiency with congenital nonspherocytic hemolytic anemia; a new variant (type Nordhorn). I. Clinical and genetic studies. Pediatr Res 1974; 8:18.

70. Goulding FJ: Priapism caused by glucose phosphate isomerase deficiency. J Urol 1976; 116:819.

71. Van Biervliet JPGM: Glucosephosphate isomerase deficiency in a Dutch family. Acta Paediatr Scand 1975; 64:868.

72. Zanella A, Izzo C, et al: The first stable variant of erythrocyte glucose-phosphate isomerase associated with severe hemolytic anemia. Am J Hematol 1980; 9:1.

73. Schroter W, Eber SW, et al: Generalised glucosephosphate isomerase (GPI) deficiency causing haemolytic anaemia, neuromuscular symptoms and impairment of granulocytic function: a new syndrome due to a new stable GPI variant with diminished specific activity (GPI Homburg). Eur J Paediatr 1985; 144:301.

74. Merkle S, Pretsch W: Glucose-6-phosphate isomerase associated with nonspherocytic hemolytic anemia in the mouse: an animal model for the human disease. Blood 1993; 81:206.

75. Beutler E, Sigalove WH, et al: Glucosephosphateisomerase (GPI) deficiency: GPI Elyria. Ann Intern Med 1974; 80:730.

76. Miwa S, Nakashima K, et al: Three cases in two families with congenital nonspherocytic hemolytic anemia due to defective glucosephosphate isomerase: GPI Matsumoto. Acta Haematol Jpn 1975; 38:238.

77. Staal GEJ, Akkerman JWN, et al: A new variant of glucosephosphate isomerase deficiency: GPI-Kortrijk. Clin Chim Acta 1977; 78:121.

78. Zanella A, Rebulla P, et al: A new mutant erythrocyte glucosephosphate isomerase associated with GSH abnormality. Am J Hematol 1978; 5:11.

79. Arnold H, Engelhardt R, et al: Glucosephosphatisomerase Typ Recklinghausen: eine neue Defektvariante mit hämolytischer Anämie. Klin Wochenschr 1973; 51:1198.

80. Arnold H, Blume KG, et al: Klinische und biochemische Untersuchungen zur Glucosephosphatisomerase normaler menschlicher Erythrocyten und bei Glucosephosphatisosmerase Mangel. Klin Wochenschr 1970; 21:1299.

81. Cartier P, Temkine H, et al: Étude biochimique d'une anémie hémolytique avec déficit familial en phosphohexoisomérase. In Proceedings of the 7th International Congress of Clinical Chemistry, Geneva/Evian, 1969, Vol. 2, Clinical Enzymology. Basel, Karger, 1970, p 139.

82. Baughan M, Valentine WN, et al: Hereditary hemolytic anemia associated with glucosephosphate isomerase (GPI) deficiency—a new enzyme defect of human erythrocytes. Blood 1968; 32:236.

83. Isacchi G, Cotreau D, et al: "GPI Roma," a new glucose phosphate isomerase deficient variant. Hum Genet 1979; 46:219.

84. Paglia DE, Holland P, et al: Occurrence of defective hexosephosphate isomerization in human erythrocytes and leukocytes. N Engl J Med 1969; 280:66.

85. Arnold H, Blume KG, et al: Glucosephosphate isomerase deficiency: evidence for *in vivo* instability of an enzyme variant with hemolysis. Blood 1973; 41:691.

86. Schroter W, Tillmann W: Decreased deformability of erythrocytes in haemolytic anaemia associated with glucosephosphate isomerase deficiency. Br J Haematol 1977; 36:475.

87. Chilcote RR, Baehner RL: Red cell (RBC) glucose phosphate isomerase deficiency (GPI): clinical and laboratory evidence of increased blood viscosity. Pediatr Res 1974; 8:398.

88. Coetzer T, Zail SS: Erythrocyte membrane proteins in hereditary glucose phosphate isomerase deficiency. J Clin Invest 1979; 63:552.

89. Matsumoto N, Ishihara T, et al: Fine structure of the spleen and liver in glucosephosphate isomerase (GPI) deficiency hereditary nonspherocytic hemolytic anemia: selective reticulocyte destruction as a mechanism of hemolysis. Acta Haematol Jpn 1973; 36:46.

90. Tilley BE, Gracy RW: A point mutation increasing the stability of human phosphoglucose isomerase. J Biol Chem 1974; 249:4571.

91. McMorris FA, Chen TR, et al: Chromosome assignments in man of the genes from two hexosephosphate isomerases. Science 1973; 17:1129.

92. Xu W, Beutler E: The characterization of gene mutations for human glucose phosphate isomerase deficiency associated with chronic hemolytic anemia. J Clin Invest 1994; 94:2326.

93. Walker JIH, Layton DM, et al: DNA sequence abnormalities in human glucose-6-phosphate isomerase deficiency. Hum Mol Genet 1993; 2:327.

94. Hopkinson DA: The investigation of reactive sulphydryls in enzymes and their variations by starch-gel electrophoresis: studies on the human phosphohexose isomerase variant PH15-1. Ann Hum Genet 1970; 34:79.

95. Detter IC, Ways PO, et al: Inherited variations in human phosphohexose isomerase. Ann Hum Genet 1968; 31:329.

96. Arnold H, Seiberling M, et al: Immunological studies on glucosephosphate isomerase deficiency: instability and impaired synthesis of the defective enzyme. Klin Wochenschr 1975; 53:1135.

97. Kahn A, Vives-Corrons JL, et al: Glucosephosphate isomerase deficiency due to a new variant (GPI Barcelona) and to a silent gene: biochemical, immunological and genetic studies. Clin Chim Acta 1976; 66:145.

98. Kahn A, Van Biervliet IPGM, et al: Genetic and molecular mechanisms of the congenital defects in glucose phosphate isomerase activity: studies of four families. Pediatr Res 1977; 11:1123.

99. Neubauer BA, Eber SW, et al: Combination of congenital nonspherocytic haemolytic anaemia and impairment of granulocyte function in severe glucose phosphate isomerase deficiency. Acta Haematol 1990; 83:206.

100. Krone W, Schneider G, et al: Detection of phosphohexose isomerase deficiency in human fibroblast cultures. Humangenetik 1970; 10:224.

101. Dallapiccola BH, Novelli G, et al: First trimester monitoring of a pregnancy at risk for glucose phosphate isomerase deficiency. Prenat Diagn 1986; 6:101.

102. Van Biervliet JPGM, Staal EJ: Excessive hepatic glycogen storage in glucosephosphate isomerase deficiency. Acta Paediatr Scand 1977; 66:311.

103. Arnold H, Blume KG, et al: Glucose phosphate isomerase deficiency with congenital nonspherocytic hemolytic anemia: a new variant (type Nordhorn). II. Purification and biochemical properties of the defective enzyme. Pediatr Res 1974; 8:26.

104. Schroter W, Tillmann W: Congenital nonspherocytic hemolytic anemia associated with glucosephosphate isomerase deficiency: variant Paderborn. Klin Wochenschr 1977; 55:393.

105. Nakashima K, Miwa S, et al: Electrophoretic and kinetic studies of glucosephosphate isomerase (GPI) in two different Japanese families with GPI deficiency. Am J Hum Genet 1973; 25:294.

106. Galand C, Torres M, et al: A new variant of glucosephosphate isomerase deficiency with mild haemolytic anaemia (GPI-MYTHO). Scand J Haematol 1978; 20:77.

107. Van Biervliet JPGM, Van Milligen-Boersma L, et al: A new variant of glucosephosphate isomerase deficiency (GPI-Utrecht). Clin Chim Acta 1975; 65:157.

108. Eber SW, Gahr M, et al: Clinical symptoms and biochemical properties of three new glucosephosphate isomerase variants. Blut 1986; 53:21.

109. Arnold H, Dodinval-Versie J, et al: Glucosephosphate isomerase deficiency type Liege: A new variant with congenital nonspherocytic hemolytic anemia. Blut 1977; 35:187.

110. Tani K, Fujii H, et al: Phosphofructokinase deficiency associated with congenital nonspherocytic hemolytic anemia and mild myopathy: biochemical and morphological studies on muscle. Tohoku J Exp Med 1983; 141:287.

111. Tani K, Fujii H, et al: Two cases of phosphofructokinase deficiency associated with congenital hemolytic anemia found in Japan. Am J Hematol 1983; 14:165.

112. Mentzer WC, Glader BE: Disorders of erythrocyte metabolism. In Mentzer WC, Wagner GM (eds): The Hereditary Hemolytic Anemias. New York, Churchill Livingstone, Inc., 1989, pp 267–319.

113. Tarui S, Okuno G, et al: Phosphofructokinase deficiency in skeletal muscle: a new type of glycogenolysis. Biochem Biophys Res Commun 1965; 19:517.

114. Layzer RB, Rowland LP, et al: Muscle phosphofructokinase deficiency. Arch Neurol 1967; 17:512.

115. Servidei S, Bonilla E, et al: Fatal infantile form of phosphofructokinase deficiency. Neurology 1986; 36:1465.

116. Danon MJ, Serenella S, et al: Late-onset muscle phosphofructokinase deficiency. Neurology 1988; 38:956.

117. Duboc D, Jehenson P, et al: Phosphorus NMR spectroscopy study of muscular enzyme deficiencies involving glycogenolysis and glycolysis. Neurology 1987; 37:663.

118. Boulard MR, Meienhofer MC, et al: Red cell phosphofructokinase deficiency. N Engl J Med 1974; 291:978.

119. Miwa S, Sato T, et al: A new type of phosphofructokinase deficiency: hereditary nonspherocytic hemolytic anemia. Acta Haematol Jpn 1972; 35:113.

120. Waterbury L, Frankel EP: Hereditary nonspherocytic hemolysis with erythrocyte phosphofructokinase deficiency. Blood 1972; 39:415.

121. Etiemble J, Kahn A, et al: Hereditary hemolytic anemia with erythrocyte phosphofructokinase deficiency. Hum Genet 1975; 31:83.

122. Vora S, Davidson M, et al: Heterogeneity of the molecular lesions in inherited phosphofructokinase deficiency. J Clin Invest 1983; 72:1995.

123. Etiemble J, Piat C, et al: Inherited erythrocyte phosphofructokinase deficiency: molecular mechanism. Hum Genet 1981; 55:383.

124. Kahn A, Etiemble J, et al: Erythrocyte phosphofructokinase deficiency associated with an unstable variant of muscle phosphofructokinase. Clin Chim Acta 1975; 61:415.

125. Jenkins JD, Kezdy F, et al: Mode of interaction of phosphofructokinase with the erythrocyte membrane. J Biol Chem 1985; 260:10426.

126. Karadsheh NS, Uyeda K, et al: Studies on structure of human erythrocyte phosphofructokinase. J Biol Chem 1977; 252:3515.

127. Vora S, Piomelli S: A fetal isozyme of phosphofructokinase in newborn erythrocytes. Pediatr Res 1977; 11:483.

128. Layzer RB, Rasmussen J: The molecular basis of muscle phosphofructokinase deficiency. Arch Neurol 1984; 31:411.

129. Shimizu T, Kono N, et al: Erythrocyte glycolysis and its marked alteration by muscular exercise in type VII glycogenosis. Blood 1988; 71:1130.

130. Vora S: Isozymes of phosphofructokinase. Isozymes: Curr Top Biol Med Res 1982; 6:119.

131. Giger U, Harvey JW: Hemolysis caused by phosphofructokinase deficiency in English springer spaniels: seven cases (1983–1986). J Am Vet Med Assoc 1987; 191:453.

132. Giger U, Reilly MP, et al: Autosomal recessive inherited phosphofructokinase deficiency in English springer spaniel dogs. Anim Genet 1986; 17:15.

133. Giger U, Harvey JW, et al: Inherited phosphofructokinase deficiency in dogs with hyperventilation-induced hemolysis: increased in vitro and in vivo alkaline fragility of erythrocytes. Blood 1985; 65:345.

134. Vora S, Giger U, et al: Characterization of the enzymatic lesion in inherited phosphofructokinase deficiency in the dog: an animal analogue of human glycogen storage disease type VII. Proc Natl Acad Sci U S A 1985; 82:8109.

135. Harvey JW, Reddy GR: Postnatal hematologic development in phosphofructokinase-deficient dogs. Blood 1989; 74:2556.

136. Harvey JW, Sussman WA, et al: Effect of 2,3-diphosphoglycerate concentration on the alkaline fragility of phosphofructokinase-deficient canine erythrocytes. Comp Biochem Physiol [B] 1988; 89:105.

137. Giger U, Kelly AM, et al: Biochemical studies of canine muscle phosphofructokinase deficiency. Enzyme 1988; 40:24.

138. Giger U, Argov Z, et al: Metabolic myopathy in canine muscle-type phosphofructokinase deficiency. Muscle Nerve 1988; 11:1260.

139. Komazawa M, Oski FA: Biochemical characteristics of "young" and "old" erythrocytes of the newborn infant. J Pediatr 1975; 87:102.

140. Travis SF, Garvin JH: In vivo lability of red cell phosphofructokinase in term infants: the possible molecular basis of the relative phosphofructokinase deficiency in neonatal red cells. Pediatr Res 1977; 11:1159.

141. Kahn A, Boyer C, et al: Immunologic study of the accelerated loss of activity of six enzymes in the red cells from newborn infants and adults—evidence for a fetal type of erythrocyte phosphofructokinase. Pediatr Res 1977; 11:271.

142. Vora S, Piomelli S: Multiple isozymes of human erythrocyte phosphofructokinase and their subunit structural characterization. Blood 1977; 50(Suppl 1):87.

143. Layzer RB, Epstein CJ: Phosphofructokinase and chromosome I. Am J Hum Genet 1972; 24:533.

144. Sherman JB, Raben N, et al: Common mutations in the phosphofructokinase-M gene in Ashkenazi Jewish patients with glycogenesis VII and their population frequency. Am J Hum Genet 1994; 55:305.

145. Nakajima H, Kono N, et al: Genetic defect in muscle phosphofructokinase deficiency. J Biol Chem 1990; 265:9392.

146. Giger U, Smith B, et al: Inherited phosphofructokinase deficiency in an American cocker spaniel. J Am Vet Med Assoc 1992; 201:1569.

147. Mhaskar Y, Giger U, et al: Presence of a truncated M-type subunit and altered kinetic properties of 6-phosphofructo-1-kinase isozymes in the brain of a dog affected by glycogen storage disease type VII. Enzyme 1991; 45:137.

148. Beutler E, Scott S, et al: Red cell aldolase deficiency and hemolytic anemia: a new syndrome. Trans Assoc Am Physicians 1973; 86:154.

149. Miwa S, Fujii H, et al: Two cases of red cell aldolase deficiency associated with hereditary hemolytic anemia in a Japanese family. Am J Hematol 1981; 11:425.

150. Kishi H, Mukai T, et al: Human aldolase A deficiency associated with a hemolytic anemia: thermolabile aldolase due to a single base mutation. Proc Natl Acad Sci U S A 1987; 84:8623.

151. Takasaki Y, Takahashi I, et al: Human aldolase A of a hemolytic anemia patient with asp-128→gly substitution: characteristics of an enzyme generated in E. coli transfected with the expression plasmid pHAAD128G. J Biochem 1990;108:153.

152. Schneider AS, Valentine WN, et al: Triosephosphate isomerase deficiency. A multisystem inherited enzyme disorder: clinical and genetic aspects. In Beutler E (ed): Hereditary Disorders of Erythrocyte Metabolism. New York, Grune & Stratton, Inc., 1968, p 265.

153. Schneider AS, Dunn I, et al: Triosephosphate isomerase deficiency. B. Inherited triosephosphate isomerase deficiency. Erythrocyte carbohydrate metabolism and preliminary studies of the erythrocyte enzyme. In Beutler E (ed): Hereditary Disorders of Erythrocyte Metabolism. New York, Grune & Stratton, Inc., 1968, p 273.

154. Harris SR, Pagha DE, et al: Triosephosphate isomerase deficiency in an adult. Clin Res 1970; 18:529.

155. Kleihauer E, Kleeberg UR, et al: Methylene blue induced hemolytic Heinz body anemia in a newborn infant with glutathione reductase and triosephosphate isomerase deficiency. In Proceedings of the 13th International Congress of Hematology, Munich, 1970.

156. Valentine WN, Schneider AS, et al: Hereditary hemolytic anemia with triosephosphate isomerase deficiency. Am J Med 1966; 41:27.

157. Schneider AS, Valentine WN, et al: Hereditary hemolytic anemia with triose phosphate isomerase deficiency. N Engl J Med 1965; 272:229.

158. Skala H, Dreyfus JC, et al: Triose phosphate isomerase deficiency. Biochem Med 1977; 18:226.

159. Freycon F, Lauras B, et al: Anémie hémolytique congénitale par déficit en triosephosphate-isomérase. Pediatrie 1975; 30:55.

160. Vives-Corrons JL, Rubinson-Skala H, et al: Triosephosphate isomerase deficiency with hemolytic anemia and severe neuromuscular disease: familial and biochemical studies of a case found in Spain. Hum Genet 1978; 42:171.

161. Maquat LE, Chilcote R, et al: Human triosephosphate isomerase cDNA and protein structure. Studies of triosephosphate isomerase deficiency in man. J Biol Chem 1985; 260:3748.

162. Rosa R, Prehu MO, et al: Hereditary triose phosphate isomerase deficiency: seven new homozygous cases. Hum Genet 1985; 71:235.

163. Zanella A, Mariana M, et al: Triosephosphate isomerase deficiency: 2 new cases. Scand J Haematol 1985; 34:417.

164. Clark ACL, Szobolotsky MA: Triose phosphate isomerase deficiency: report of a family. Aust Paediatr J 1987; 22:135.

165. Poinsot J, Parent P, et al: Un cas d'anémie hémolytique congénitale non sphérocytaire, par déficit en triose phosphate isomérase diagnostic prénatal. J Genet Hum 1986; 34:431.

166. Bellingham AJ, Lestas AN, et al: Prenatal diagnosis of a red cell enzymopathy: triosephosphate isomerase deficiency. Lancet 1989; 2:419.

167. Eber W, Pekrun A, et al: Triosephosphate isomerase deficiency: haemolytic anaemia, myopathy with altered mitochondria and mental retardation due to a new variant with accelerated enzyme catabolism and diminished specific activity. J Pediatr 1991; 150:761.

168. Hollan S, Fujii H, et al: Hereditary triosephosphate isomerase (TPI) deficiency: two severely affected brothers, one with and one without neurological symptoms. Hum Genet 1993; 92:486.

169. Jongsma APM, Los WRT, et al: Evidence for synteny between the human loci for triose phosphate isomerase, lactate dehydrogenase-B, and peptidase-B and the regional mapping of these loci on chromosome 12. Cytogenet Cell Genet 1974; 13:106.

170. Mohrenweiser HW, Fielek S: Elevated frequency of carriers for triosephosphate isomerase deficiency in newborn infants. Pediatr Res 1982; 16:960.

171. Yuan PM, Talent JM, et al: A tentative elucidation of the sequence of human triosephosphate isomerase by homology peptide mapping. Biochem Biophys Acta 1981; 671:211.

172. Yuan PM, Talent JM, et al: Molecular basis for the accumulation of acidic isozymes of triosephosphate isomerase on aging. Mech Ageing Dev 1981; 17:151.

173. Peters J, Hopkinson DA, et al: Genetic and nongenetic variation of triose phosphate isomerase isozymes in human tissues. Ann Hum Genet 1973; 36:297.

174. Lu HS, Yuan PM, et al: Primary structure of human triosephosphate isomerase. J Biol Chem 1984; 259:11958.

175. Mande SC, Mainfroid V, et al: Crystal structure of recombinant human triosephosphate isomerase at 2.8 Å resolution. Triosephosphate isomerase-related human genetic disorders and comparison with the trypanosomal enzyme. Protein Science 1994; 3:810.

176. Asakawa J, Sutoh C, et al: Electrophoretic variants of blood proteins in Japanese. III. Triosephosphate isomerase. Hum Genet 1984; 68:185.

177. Asakawa J, Satoh C: Characterization of three electrophoretic variants of human erythrocyte triosephosphate isomerase found in Japanese. Biochem Genet 1986; 24:131.

178. Perry BA, Mohrenweiser HW: Human triosephosphate isomerase: substitution of Arg for Gly at position 122 in a thermolabile electromorph variant, TPI-Manchester. Hum Genet 1992; 88:634.

178a. Schneider A, Westwood B, et al: Triosephosphate isomerase deficiency: Repetitive occurrence of point mutation in amino acid 104 in multiple apparently unrelated families. Am J Hematol 1995; 50:263.

179. Daar IO, Artymiuk PJ, et al: Human triosephosphate isomerase deficiency: a single amino acid substitution results in a thermolabile enzyme. Proc Natl Acad Sci U S A 1986; 83:7903.

180. Chang ML, Artymiuk PJ, et al: Human triosephosphate isomerase deficiency resulting from mutation of Phe-240. Am J Hum Genet 1993; 52:1260.

181. Bardosi A, Eber SW, et al: Myopathy with altered mitochondria due to a triosephosphate isomerase (TPI) deficiency. Acta Neuropathol 1990; 79:387.

182. Pogliani EM, Colombi M, et al: Platelet function defect in triosephosphate isomerase deficiency. Haematologica 1986; 71:349.

183. Merkle S, Pretsch W: Characterization of triosephosphate isomerase mutants with reduced enzyme activity in *Mus musculus*. Genetics 1989; 123:837.

184. Sparkes RS, Carrel RE, et al: Probable localization of a triosephosphate isomerase gene to the short arm of the number 5 human chromosome. Nature 1969; 224:367.

185. Hendrickson RJ, Snapka RM, et al: Studies on human triosephosphate isomerase. III. Characterization of the enzyme from patients with the cri du chat syndrome. Am J Hum Genet 1973; 25:433.

186. Brock DJ, Singer JD: Red cell triosephosphate isomerase and chromosome 5. Lancet 1970; 2:1136.

187. Rosa R, Prehu MO, et al: Possibility of prenatal diagnosis of hereditary triose phosphate isomerase deficiency. Prenat Diagn 1986; 6:231.

188. Bellingham AJ, Lestas AN: Prenatal diagnosis of triose phosphate isomerase deficiency. Lancet 1990; 1:230.

189. Clark ACL, Szobolotzky MA: Triose phosphate isomerase deficiency: prenatal diagnosis. J Pediatr 1985; 106:417.

189a. Arya R, Lalloz MRA, et al: Prenatal diagnosis of triosephosphate isomerase deficiency. Blood 1996; 87:4507.

190. Harkness DR: A new erythrocytic enzyme defect with hemolytic anemia: glyceraldehyde-3-phosphate dehydrogenase deficiency. J Lab Clin Med 1966; 68:879.

191. Oski FA, Whaun J: Hemolytic anemia and red cell glyceraldehyde-3-phosphate dehydrogenase. In Proceedings of the Society for Pediatric Research, 39th annual meeting, Atlantic City, 1969, p 151.

192. McCann SR, Finkel B, et al: Study of a kindred with hereditary spherocytosis and glyceraldehyde-3-phosphate dehydrogenase deficiency. Blood 1976; 47:171.

193. Huang IY, Fujii H, et al: Structure and function of normal and variant human phosphoglycerate kinase. Hemoglobin 1980; 4:601.

194. Banks RD, Blake CC, et al: Sequence, structure and activity of phosphoglycerate kinase: a possible hinge-bending enzyme. Nature 1979; 279:773.

195. Arese P, Bosai A, et al: Red cell glycolysis in a case of 3-phosphoglycerate kinase deficiency. Eur J Clin Invest 1973; 3:86.

196. Cartier P, Habibi B, et al: Anémie hémolytique congénitale associée à un déficit en phosphoglycératekinase dans les globules rouges, les polynucléaires et les lymphocytes. Nouv Rev Fr Hematol 1971; 11:565.

196a. Svirklys L, O'Sullivan WJ: Lack of effect of increased 2,3-diphosphoglycerate on flux through the oxidative pathway in phosphoglycerate kinase deficiency. Clin Chim Acta 1985; 148:167.

197. Valentine WN, Hsieh HS, et al: Hereditary hemolytic anemia associated with phosphoglycerate kinase deficiency in erythrocytes and leukocytes. N Engl J Med 1969; 280:528.

198. Miwa S, Nakashima K, et al: Phosphoglycerate kinase (PGK) deficiency hereditary nonspherocytic hemolytic anemia: report of a case found in Japanese family. Acta Haematol Jpn 1972; 35:571.

199. Boivin P, Hakim J, et al: Erythrocyte and leucocyte 3-phosphoglycerate kinase deficiency. Studies of properties of the polymorphonuclear leucocytes and a review of the literature. Nouv Rev Fr Hematol 1974; 14:495.

200. Konrad PN, McCarthy DJ, et al: Erythrocyte and leukocyte phosphoglycerate kinase deficiency with neurologic disease. J Pediatr 1973; 82:456.

201. Guis MS, Karadsheh N, et al: Phosphoglycerate kinase San Francisco: A new variant associated with hemolytic anemia but not with neuromuscular manifestations. Am J Hematol 1987; 25:175.

202. Schrier SL, Ben-Bassat I, et al: Characterization of erythrocyte membrane-associated enzymes (glyceraldehyde-3-phosphate dehydrogenase and phosphoglyceric kinase). J Lab Clin Med 1975; 85:797.

203. Parker JC, Hoffman JF: The role of membrane phosphoglycerate kinase in the control of glycolytic rate by active cation transport in human red cells. J Gen Physiol 1967; 50:893.

204. Chillar RK, Beutler E: Explanation for the apparent lack of ouabain inhibition of pyruvate production in hemolysates; the "backward" PGK reaction. Blood 1976; 47:507.

205. Segel GB, Feig SA, et al: Energy metabolism in human erythrocytes: the role of phosphoglycerate kinase in cation transport. Blood 1975; 46:271.

206. Baehner RL, Feig SA, et al: Metabolic, phagocytic, and bactericidal properties of phosphoglycerate kinase deficient polymorphonuclear leukocytes. Blood 1971; 38:833.

207. Strauss RG, McCarthy DJ, et al: Neutrophil function in congenital phosphoglycerate kinase deficiency. J Pediatr 1974; 854:341.

208. Chen SH, Malcolm LA, et al: Phosphoglycerate kinase: an X-linked polymorphism in man. Am J Hum Genet 1971; 23:87.

209. Michelson AM, Blake CF, et al: Structure of the human phosphoglycerate kinase gene and the intronmediated evolution and dispersal of the nucleotide binding domain. Proc Natl Acad Sci U S A 1985; 82:6965.

210. Peys BF, Grzeschick KH, et al: Human phosphoglycerate kinase and inactivation of the X chromosome. Science 1972; 175:1002.

211. DiMauro S, Dalakas M, et al: Phosphoglycerate kinase deficiency: another cause of recurrent myoglobinuria. Ann Neurol 1983; 13:11.

212. Michelson AM, Markham AF, et al: Isolation and DNA sequence of a full-length cDNA clone for human X chromosome-encoded phosphoglycerate kinase. Proc Natl Acad Sci U S A 1983; 80:472.

213. Gartler SM, Riley DE, et al: Mapping of human autosomal phosphoglycerate kinase sequence to chromosome 19. Somatic Cell Mol Genet 1986; 12:395.

214. McCarrey JR, Thomas K: Human testis specific PGK gene lacks intron and possesses characteristics of a processed gene. Nature 1987; 326:501.

215. Yoshida A, Watanabe S, et al: Human phosphoglycerate kinase II. Structure of a variant enzyme. J Biol Chem 1972; 247:446.

216. Fujii H, Yoshida A: Molecular abnormality of phosphoglycerate kinase–Uppsala associated with chronic nonspherocytic hemolytic anemia. Proc Natl Acad Sci U S A 1980; 77:5461.

217. Fujii H, Chen SH, et al: Use of cultured lymphoblastoid cells for the study of abnormal enzymes: molecular abnormality of a phosphoglycerate kinase variant associated with hemolytic anemia. Proc Natl Acad Sci U S A 1981; 78:2587.

218. Maeda M, Yoshida A: Molecular defect of a phosphoglycerate kinase variant (PGK Matsue) associated with hemolytic anemia: Leu→Pro substitution caused by T/A→C/G transition in exon 3. Blood 1991; 77:1348.

219. Cohen-Solal M, Valentin C, et al: Identification of new mutations in two phosphoglycerate kinase (PGK) variants expressing different clinical syndromes: PGK Créteil and PGK Amiens. Blood 1994; 84:898.

220. Maeda M, Bawle EV, et al: Molecular abnormalities of a phosphoglycerate kinase variant generated by spontaneous mutation. Blood 1992; 79:2759.

221. Fujii H, Kanno H, et al: A single amino acid substitution (157 Gly→Val) in a phosphoglycerate kinase variant (PGK Shizuoka) associated with chronic hemolysis and myoglobinuria. Blood 1992; 79:1582.

222. Svirklys L, O'Sullivan WJ: Immunochemical studies on phosphoglycerate kinase deficiency. Biochem Med Metab Biol 1986; 36:347.

223. Beutler E: Electrophoresis of phosphoglycerate kinase. Biochem Genet 1969; 3:189.

224. Kraus AP, Langston MF, et al: Red cell phosphoglycerate kinase deficiency. Biochem Biophys Res Commun 1968; 30:173.

225. Fujii H, Krietsch WKG, Yoshida A: A single amino acid substitution (Asp-Asn) in a phosphoglycerate kinase variant (PGK Munchen) associated with enzyme deficiency. J Biol Chem 1980; 255:6421.

226. Rosa R, Geore C, et al: A new case of phosphoglycerate kinase deficiency, PGK Creteil, associated with rhabdomyolysis and lacking hemolytic anemia. Blood 1982; 60:84.

227. Knetsch WKG, Eber SW, et al: Characterization of a phosphoglycerate kinase deficiency variant not associated with hemolytic anemia. Am J Hum Genet 1980; 32:364.

228. Dogson SJ, Lee CS, et al: Erythrocyte phosphoglycerate kinase deficiency: enzymatic and oxygen binding studies. N Z Med J 1980; 10:614.

229. Yoshida A, Miwa S: Characterization of a phosphoglycerate kinase variant associated with a hemolytic anemia. Am J Hum Genet 1974; 26:378.

230. Sugie H, Sugie Y, et al: Recurrent myoglobinuria in a child with mental retardation phosphoglycerate kinase deficiency. J Child Neurol 1989; 4:95.

231. Hjelm M, Wadam B, et al: A phosphoglycerate kinase variant, PGK Uppsala, associated with hemolytic anemia. J Lab Clin Med 1980; 96:1015.

232. Tonin P, Shanske S, et al: Phosphoglycerate kinase deficiency: biochemical and molecular genetic studies in a new myopathic variant (PGK Alberta). Neurology 1993; 43:387.

233. Galacteros F, Rosa R, et al: Déficit en diphosphoglycérate mutase: nouveaux cas associés à une polyglobulie. Nouv Rev Fr Hematol 1984; 26:69.

234. Rosa R, Prehu MO, et al: The first case of a complete deficiency of diphosphoglycerate mutase in human erythrocytes. J Clin Invest 1978; 62:907.

235. Schroter W: Kongenitale nichtesphärocytäre hämolytische Anämie bei 2,3-Diphosphoglyceratemutasemangel der Erythrocyten im frühen Säuglingsalter. Klin Wochenschr 1965; 43:1147.

236. Cartier P, Labie P, et al: Déficit familial en diphosphoglycerate mutase: étude hématologique et biochimique. Nouv Rev Fr Hematol 1972; 12:269.

237. Koler RD, McClung MR, et al: Physiologic and genetic alterations in human red cell DPGM. Hemoglobin 1980; 4:593.

238. Travis SF, Martinez J, et al: Study of a kindred with partial deficiency of red cell 2,3-diphosphoglycerate mutase (2,3-DPGM) and compensated hemolysis. Blood 1978; 51:1107.

239. Joulin V, Peduzzi J, et al: Molecular cloning and sequencing of the human erythrocyte 2,3-bisphosphoglycerate mutase cDNA: revised amino acid sequence. EMBO J 1986; 5:2275.

240. Kappel WK, Hass LF: The isolation and partial characterization of diphosphoglycerate mutase from human erythrocytes. Biochemistry 1976; 15:290.

241. Hass LF, Kappel WK, et al: Evidence for structural homology between human red cell phosphoglycerate mutase and 2,3-bisphosphoglycerate synthase. J Biol Chem 1978; 253:77.

242. Craescu CT, Schaad O, et al: Structural modeling of the human erythrocyte bisphosphoglycerate mutase. Biochimie 1992; 74:519.

243. Chen SH, Anderson JE, et al: Human red cell 2,3-diphosphoglycerate mutase and monophosphoglycerate mutase: genetic evidence for two separate loci. Am J Hum Genet 1977; 29:405.

244. Garel MC, Arous N, et al: A recombinant bisphosphoglycerate mutase variant with acid phosphatase homology degrades 2,3-diphosphoglycerate. Proc Natl Acad Sci U S A 1994; 91:3593.

245. Blouquit Y, Rhoda MD, et al: Glycerated hemoglobin in a2b282 (EF6) N-e-glyceryllysine: a new posttranslational modification occurring in erythrocyte bisphosphoglyceromutase deficiency. Biomed Biochim Acta 1987; 46:S202.

246. Barichard F, Joulin V, et al: Chromosomal assignment of the human 2,3-bisphosphoglycerate mutase gene (BPGM) to region 7q34→7q22. Hum Genet 1987; 77:283.

247. Joulin V, Garel MC, et al: Isolation and characterization of the human 2,3-bisphosphoglycerate mutase gene. J Biol Chem 1988; 263:15785.

248. Rosa R, Blouquit Y, et al: Isolation, characterization, and structure of a mutant 89 Arg→Cys bisphosphoglycerate mutase. Implication of the active site in the mutation. J Biol Chem 1989; 264:7837.

249. Lemarchandel V, Joulin V, et al: Compound heterozygosity in a complete erythrocyte bisphosphoglycerate mutase deficiency. Blood 1992; 80:2643.

250. Rosa R, Galacteros MO, et al: Inactive bisphosphoglycerate mutase variants: new data. Biomed Biochim Acta 1987; 46:S207.

251. Stefanini M: Chronic hemolytic anemia associated with erythrocyte enolase deficiency exacerbated by ingestion of nitrofurantoin. Am J Clin Pathol 1972; 58:408.

252. Lanchant NA, Jennings MA, et al: Partial erythrocyte enolase deficiency: a hereditary disorder with variable clinical expression. Blood 1986; 68:55A.

253. Searcy GP, Miller DR, et al: Congenital hemolytic anemia in the basenji dog due to erythrocyte pyruvate kinase deficiency. Can J Comp Med 1971; 35:67.

254. Nakashima K, Miwa S, et al: Electrophoretic, immunologic and kinetic characterization of erythrocyte pyruvate kinase in the basenji dog with pyruvate kinase deficiency. Tohoku J Exp Med 1975; 117:179.

255. Prasse KW, Crouser D, et al: Pyruvate kinase deficiency anemia with terminal myelofibrosis and osteosclerosis in a beagle. J Am Vet Med Assoc 1975; 166:1170.

256. Ghidini A, Sirtori M, et al: Hepatosplenomegaly as the only prenatal finding in a fetus with pyruvate kinase deficiency anemia. Am J Perinatol 1991; 8:44.

257. Hennekam RCM, Beemer FA, et al: Hydrops fetalis associated with red cell pyruvate kinase deficiency. Genet Couns 1990; 1:75.

258. Fanning J, Hinkle RS: Pyruvate kinase deficiency hemolytic anemia: two successful pregnancy outcomes. Am J Obstet Gynecol 1985; 153:313.

259. Duncan JR, Capellini MD, et al: Aplastic crisis due to parvovirus infection in pyruvate kinase deficiency. Lancet 1983; 2:14.

260. Muller-Soyano Z, de Roura ET, et al: Pyruvate kinase deficiency and leg ulcers. Blood 1976; 47:807.

261. Vives-Corrons JL, Marie J, et al: Hereditary erythrocyte pyruvate kinase (PK) deficiency and chronic hemolytic anemia: clinical, genetic and molecular studies in six new Spanish patients. Hum Genet 1980; 53:401.

262. Morisaki T, Tani K, et al: Ten cases of pyruvate kinase (PK) deficiency found in Japan: enzymatic characterization of the patients' PK. Acta Haematol Jpn 1988; 51:1080.

263. Mentzer WC, Baehner RL, et al: Selective reticulocyte destruction in erythrocyte pyruvate kinase deficiency. J Clin Invest 1971; 50:688.

264. Staal GEJ, Rijksen G, et al: Extreme deficiency of L-type pyruvate kinase with moderate clinical expression. Clin Chim Acta 1982; 118:241.

265. Etiemble J, Picat C, et al: A red cell pyruvate kinase mutant with normal L-type PK in the liver. Hum Genet 1982; 61:256.

266. Oski FA, Nathan DG, et al: Extreme hemolysis and red cell distortion in erythrocyte pyruvate kinase deficiency. I. Morphology, erythrokinetics, and family enzyme studies. N Engl J Med 1964; 270:1023.

267. Leblond PF, Lyonnais J, et al: Erythrocyte populations in pyruvate kinase deficiency anemia following splenectomy. I. Cell morphology. Br J Haematol 1978; 39:55.

268. Nathan DG, Oski FA, et al: Studies of erythrocyte spicule formation in haemolytic anaemia. Br J Haematol 1966; 12:385.

269. Zanella A, Colombo MB, et al: Erythrocyte pyruvate kinase deficiency: 11 new cases. Br J Hematol 1988; 69:399.

270. Keitt AS: Pyruvate kinase deficiency and related disorders of red cell glycolysis. Am J Med 1966; 41:762.

271. Kanno H, Fujii H, et al: cDNA cloning of human R-type pyruvate kinase and identification of a single amino acid substitution (Thr→Met) affecting enzymatic stability in a pyruvate kinase variant (PK Tokyo) associated with hereditary hemolytic anemia. Proc Natl Acad Sci U S A 1991; 88:8218.

272. Tani K, Fujii H, et al: Human liver type pyruvate kinase: cDNA cloning and chromosomal assignment. Biochem Biophys Res Commun 1987; 143:431.

273. Tani K, Yoshida MC, et al: Human M2-type pyruvate kinase: cDNA cloning, chromosomal assignment and expression in hepatoma. Gene 1988; 73:509.

274. Takenaka M, Noguchi T, et al: Rat pyruvate kinase M gene. J Biol Chem 1989; 264:2363.

275. Noguchi T, Inoue H, et al: The M_1- and M_2-type isozymes of rat pyruvate kinase are produced from the same gene by alternative RNA splicing. J Biol Chem 1986; 261:13807.

276. Baronciani L, Beutler E: Analysis of pyruvate kinase deficiency mutations that produce nonspherocytic hemolytic anemia. Proc Natl Acad Sci U S A 1993; 90:4324.

277. Marie J, Simon MP, et al: One gene, but two messenger RNAs encode liver L and red cell L' pyruvate kinase subunits. Nature 1981; 292:7.

278. Noguchi T, Kazuya Y, et al: The L- and R-type isozymes of rat pyruvate kinase are produced from a single gene by use of different promoters. J Biol Chem 1987; 262:14366.

279. Tani K, Fujii H, et al: Human liver type pyruvate kinase: complete amino acid sequence and the expression in mammalian cells. Proc Natl Acad Sci U S A 1988; 85:1792.

280. Muirhead H, Clayden DA, et al: The structure of cat muscle pyruvate kinase. EMBO J 1986; 5:475.

281. Ibsen KH, Schiller KW, et al: Interconvertible kinetic and physical forms of human erythrocyte pyruvate kinase. J Biol Chem 1971; 246:1233.

282. Peterson JS, Chern CJ, et al: The subunit structure of human muscle and human erythrocyte pyruvate kinase isozymes. FEBS Lett 1974; 49:73.

283. Takegawa S, Miwa S: Change of pyruvate kinase (PK) isozymes in classical type PK deficiency and other PK deficiency cases during red cell maturation. Am J Hematol 1984; 16:53.

284. Max-Audit I, Kechemir MT, et al: Pyruvate kinase synthesis and degradation by normal and pathologic cells during erythroid maturation. Blood 1988; 72:1039.

285. Takegawa S, Fujii H, et al: Change of pyruvate kinase isozymes from M2- to L-type during development of the red cell. Br J Haematol 1983; 54:467.

286. Monod J, Wyman J, et al: On the nature of allosteric transitions: a plausible model. J Mol Biol 1964; 12:88.

287. Koler RD, Vanbellinghen P: The mechanism of precursor modulation of human pyruvate kinase I by fructose diphosphate. Adv Enzyme Regul 1968; 6:127.

288. Koster JF, Staal GEJ, et al: The effect of urea and temperature on red blood cell pyruvate kinase. Biochim Biophys Acta 1971; 236:362.

289. Cartier P, Najman A, et al: Les anomalies de la glycolyse au cours de l'anémie hémolytique par déficit du globule en pyruvate kinase. Clin Chim Acta 1968; 22:165.

290. Lakomek M, Scharnetzky M, et al: On the temperature and salt-dependent conformation change in human erythrocyte pyruvate kinase. Hoppe-Seyler's Z Physiol Chem 1983; 364:787.

291. Boivin P, Galand C, et al: Coéxistence de deux types de pyruvate kinase cinétiquement différents dans les globules rouges humains normaux. Nouv Rev Fr Hematol 1972; 12:159.

292. Paglia DE, Valentine WN: Evidence of molecular alteration of pyruvate kinase as a consequence of erythrocyte aging. J Lab Clin Med 1970; 76:202.

293. Van Berkel JC, Staal GEJ, et al: On the molecular basis of pyruvate kinase deficiency. 11. Role of thiol groups in pyruvate kinase from pyruvate kinase–deficient patients. Biochim Biophys Acta 1974; 334:361.

294. Valentine WN, Toohey JI, et al: Modification of erythrocyte enzyme activities by persulfides and methanethiol: possible regulatory role. Proc Natl Acad Sci U S A 1987; 84:1394.

295. Solovonuk PF, Collier HB: The pyruvic phosphoferase of erythrocytes. I. Properties of the enzyme and its activity in erythrocytes of various species. Can J Biochem Physiol 1955; 33:38.

296. Valentine WN, Paglia DE: Studies with human erythrocyte pyruvate kinase (PK): effect of modification of sulfhydryl groups. Br J Haematol 1983; 53:385.

297. Badwey JA, Westhead EW: Post-translational modification of human erythrocyte pyruvate kinase. Biochem Biophys Res Commun 1977; 74:1326.

298. Van Berkel TJ, Koster JF, et al: On the molecular basis of pyruvate kinase deficiency. 1. Primary defect or consequence of increased glutathione disulfide concentration? Biochim Biophys Acta 1973; 321:496.

299. Zanella A, Rebulla P, et al: Effects of sulphydryl compounds on abnormal red cell pyruvate kinase. Br J Haematol 1976; 32:373.

300. Nakashima K: Further evidence of molecular alteration and aberration of erythrocyte pyruvate kinase. Clin Chim Acta 1974; 55:245.

301. Blume KG, Arnold H, et al: On the molecular basis of pyruvate kinase deficiency. Biochim Biophys Acta 1974; 370:601.

302. Koler RD, Bigley RH, et al: Pyruvate kinase: molecular differences between human red cell and leukocyte enzyme. Symp Quant Biol 1964; 29:213.

303. Munro GF, Miller DR: Mechanism of fructose diphosphate activation of a mutant pyruvate kinase from human red cells. Biochim Biophys Acta 1970; 206:87.

304. Blume KG, Hoffbauer RW, et al: Purification and properties of pyruvate kinase in normal and in pyruvate kinase–deficient human red blood cells. Biochim Biophys Acta 1971; 227:364.

305. Staal GEJ, Koster JF, et al: Human erythrocyte pyruvate kinase. Its purification and some properties. Biochim Biophys Acta 1971; 227:86.

306. Srivastava SK, Beutler E: The effect of normal red cell constituents on the activities of red cell enzymes. Arch Biochem Biophys 1972; 148:249.

307. Ponce J, Roth S, et al: Kinetic studies on the inhibition of glycolytic kinases of human erythrocytes by 2,3-diphosphoglycerate acid. Biochim Biophys Acta 1971; 250:63.

308. Westhead EW, Kiener PA, et al: Control of oxygen delivery from

the erythrocyte by modification of pyruvate kinase. Curr Top Cell Regul 1984; 24:21.

309. Fujii S, Nakashima K, et al: Cyclic AMP–dependent phosphorylation of erythrocyte variant pyruvate kinase. Biochem Med 1984; 31:47.

310. Brunetti P, Puxeddu A, et al: Anemia emolitica congenita non sferocitica di carenza di piruvico-chinasi (PK). Haematol Arch 1962; 47:505.

311. Bigley RH, Koler RD: Liver pyruvate kinase (PK) isoenzymes in a PK-deficient patient. Ann Hum Genet 1968; 31:383.

312. Nakashima K, Miwa S, et al: Characterization of pyruvate kinase from the liver of a patient with aberrant erythrocyte pyruvate kinase, PK Nagasaki. J Lab Clin Med 1977; 90:1012.

313. Grimes AJ, Meisler A, et al: Hereditary nonspherocytic haemolytic anaemia. A study of red-cell carbohydrate metabolism in twelve cases of pyruvate kinase deficiency. Br J Haematol 1964; 10:403.

314. Waller HD, Lohr GW: Hereditary nonspherocytic enzymopenic hemolytic anemia with pyruvate kinase deficiency. In Proceedings of IXth Congress of International Society of Hematology, Mexico City, 1962, Vol. 1. Mexico DF, Universidad Nacional Autonoma de Mexico, 1964, p 257.

315. Miwa S, Nagate M: Pyruvate kinase deficiency hereditary nonspherocytic hemolytic anemia. Report of two cases in a Japanese family and review of literature. Acta Haematol Jpn 1965; 28:1.

316. Necheles TF, Finkel HE, et al: Red cell pyruvate kinase deficiency. The effect of splenectomy. Arch Intern Med 1966; 118:75.

317. Busch D: Erythrocyte metabolism in three persons with hereditary nonspherocytic hemolytic anemia, deficient in pyruvate kinase. In Proceedings of IXth Congress of European Society of Hematology, Vol. II. Lisbon, Karger, 1963, p 783.

318. Tomoda A, Lachant NA, et al: Inhibition of the pentose phosphate shunt by 2,3-diphosphoglycerate in erythrocyte pyruvate kinase deficiency. Br J Haematol 1983; 54:475.

319. Bowman HS, Procopio F: Hereditary nonspherocytic hemolytic anemia of the pyruvate-kinase deficient type. Ann Intern Med 1963; 58:567.

320. Oski FA, Diamond LK: Erythrocyte pyruvate kinase deficiency resulting in congenital nonspherocytic hemolytic anemia. N Engl J Med 1963; 269:269.

321. Glader BE: Oxidant-induced injury in pyruvate kinase (PK) deficient erythrocytes. Pediatr Res 1974; 8:401.

322. Jacobasch G, Boese C: Regulation des Kohlenhydratstoff-wechsels roter Blutzellen bei Pyruvatkinasemangel. Folia Haematol 1969; 91:70.

323. Rose IA, Warms JVB: Control of glycolysis in the human red blood cell. J Biol Chem 1966; 241:4848.

324. Oski FA, Bowman H: A low K_m phosphoenolpyruvate mutant in the Amish with red cell pyruvate kinase deficiency. Br J Haematol 1969; 17:289.

325. Paglia DE, Valentine WN, et al: An inherited molecular lesion of erythrocyte pyruvate kinase. Identification of a kinetically aberrant isoenzyme associated with premature hemolysis. J Clin Invest 1968; 47:1929.

326. Zuelzer WW, Robinson AR, et al: Erythrocyte pyruvate kinase deficiency in nonspherocytic hemolytic anemia: a system of multiple genetic markers? Blood 1968; 32:33.

327. Miwa S, Nishina T, et al: Studies on erythrocyte metabolism in various hemolytic anemias: with special reference to pyruvate kinase deficiency. Acta Haematol Jpn 1970; 33:501.

328. Lestas AN, Kay LA, et al: Red cell 3-phosphoglycerate level as a diagnostic aid in pyruvate kinase deficiency. Br J Haematol 1987; 67:485.

329. Colombo MB, Zanella A, et al: 2,3-Diphosphoglycerate and 3-phosphoglycerate in red cell pyruvate kinase deficiency. Br J Haematol 1987; 68:423.

330. Lakomek M, Neubauer B, et al: Erythrocyte pyruvate kinase deficiency: relations of residual enzyme activity, altered regulation of defective enzymes and concentrations of high-energy phosphates with the severity of clinical manifestation. Eur J Haematol 1992; 49:82.

331. Rose IW, Warms JVB: Control of red cell glycolysis. The cause of triose phosphate accumulation. J Biol Chem 1970; 245:4009.

332. Zerez CR, Tanaka KR: Impaired nicotinamide adenine dinucleotide synthesis in pyruvate kinase–deficient human erythrocytes: a mechanism for decreased total NAD content and a possible secondary cause of hemolysis. Blood 1987; 69:999.

333. Zerez CR, Wong MD, et al: Impaired erythrocyte phosphoribosylpyrophosphate formation in hemolytic anemia due to pyruvate kinase deficiency. Blood 1988; 72:500.

334. Nathan DG, Oski FA, et al: Extreme hemolysis and red cell distortion in erythrocyte pyruvate kinase deficiency. II. Measurements of erythrocyte glucose consumption, potassium flux and adenosine triphosphate stability. N Engl J Med 1965; 272:118.

335. Twomey JJ, O'Neal FB, et al: ATP metabolism in pyruvate kinase deficient erythrocytes. Blood 1967; 30:576.

336. Gardos G, Strau FB: Über die Rolle der Adenosintriphosphorsäure (ATP) in der K-Permeabilität der menschlichen roten Blutkörperchen. Acta Physiol Hung 1957; 12:1.

337. Koller CA, Orringer EP, et al: Quinine protects pyruvate-kinase deficient red cells from dehydration. Am J Hematol 1979; 7:193.

338. Nathan DG, Shohet SB: Erythrocyte ion transport defects and hemolytic anemia: "hydrocytosis" and "desicytosis." Semin Hematol 1970; 7:381.

339. Allen DW, Groat JD, et al: Increased adsorption of cytoplasmic proteins to the erythrocyte membrane in ATP depleted normal and pyruvate kinase–deficient mature cells and reticulocytes. J Clin Invest 1981; 70:502.

340. Zanella A, Brovelli A, et al: Membrane abnormalities of pyruvate kinase deficient red cells. Br J Haematol 1979; 42:101.

341. Marik T, Brabec V, et al: Reticulocyte-dependent labeling alterations of red cell membrane in pyruvate kinase deficiency anemia. Biomed Biochim Acta 1987; 46:S192.

342. Marik T, Brabec V, et al: Pyruvate kinase–deficiency anemia: membrane approach. Biochem Med Metab Biol 1988; 39:55.

343. Staal GEJ, Sybesma HB, et al: Familial hemolytic anaemia due to pyruvate kinase deficiency. Folia Med Neerl 1971; 14:72.

344. Staal GEJ, Koster JF, et al: A new variant of red blood cell pyruvate kinase deficiency. Biochim Biophys Acta 1971; 258:685.

345. Mallerme J, Boivin P, et al: L'anémie hémolytique congénitale non sphérocytaire par déficit en pyruvate kinase. Bull Mem Soc Med Hop 1964; 115:483.

346. Nathan DG, Oski FA, et al: Life-span and organ sequestration of the red cells in pyruvate kinase deficiency. N Engl J Med 1968; 278:73.

347. Najean Y, Dresch C, et al: Étude de l'érythrocinétique dans 8 cas de déficit homozygote en pyruvate kinase. Nouv Rev Fr Hematol 1969; 9:850.

348. Gulbis E, Weber A, et al: Contribution à l'étude de l'anémie hémolytique congénitale avec déficit en pyruvate kinase. Arch Fr Pediatr 1970; 27:31.

349. Bowman HS, Oski FA: Splenic macrophage interaction with red cells in pyruvate kinase deficiency and hereditary spherocytosis. Vox Sang 1970; 19:168.

350. Matsumoto N, Ishihara T, et al: Sequestration and destruction of reticulocytes in the spleen in pyruvate kinase deficiency hereditary nonspherocytic hemolytic anemia. Acta Haematol Jpn 1972; 35:525.

351. Leblond PF, Couloumbe L, et al: Erythrocyte populations in pyruvate kinase deficiency following splenectomy. II. Cell deformability. Br J Haematol 1978; 39:63.

352. Muller-Soyano A, Platt O, et al: Pyruvate kinase deficiency in dog and human erythrocytes: effects of energy depletion on cation composition and cellular hydration. Am J Hematol 1986; 23:217.

353. Bossu M, Dacha M, et al: Neonatal hemolysis due to a transient severity of inherited pyruvate kinase deficiency. Acta Haematol 1968; 40:166.

354. Paglia DE, Valentine WN, et al: An isozyme of erythrocyte pyruvate kinase (PK-Los Angeles) with impaired kinetics corrected by fructose-1,6-diphosphate. Am J Clin Pathol 1977; 78:229.

355. Bossu M, Dacha M, et al: Neonatal hemolysis due to a transient severity of inherited pyruvate kinase deficiency. Acta Haematol 1968; 40:166.

356. El-Hazmi MAF, Al-Swailem AR, et al: Frequency of glucose-6-phosphate dehydrogenase, pyruvate kinase and hexokinase deficiency in the Saudi population. Hum Hered 1986; 36:45.

357. Fung RHP, Keung YK, et al: Screening of pyruvate kinase defi-

ciency and G6PD deficiency in Chinese newborns in Hong Kong. Arch Dis Child 1969; 44:373.

358. Feng CS, Tsang SS, et al: Prevalence of pyruvate kinase deficiency among the Chinese: determination by the quantitative assay. Am J Hematol 1993; 43:271.

359. Wu ZL, Yu WD, et al: Frequency of erythrocyte pyruvate kinase deficiency in Chinese infants. Am J Hematol 1985; 20:139.

360. Blume KG, Lohr GW, et al: Beitrag zur Populationsgenetik der Pyruvat-kinase menschlicher Erythrocyten. Humangenetik 1968; 6:261.

361. Mohrenweiser HW: Frequency of enzyme deficiency variants in erythrocytes of newborn infants. Proc Natl Acad Sci U S A 1981; 78:5046.

362. Lakomek M, Winkler H, et al: Erythrocyte pyruvate kinase deficiency: a kinetic method for differentiation between heterozygosity and compound-heterozygosity. Am J Hematol 1989; 31:225.

363. Ishida Y, Miwa S, et al: Thirteen cases of pyruvate kinase deficiency found in Japan. Am J Hematol 1981; 10:239.

364. Miwa S, Fujii H, et al: Seven pyruvate kinase variants characterized by the ICSH recommended methods. Br J Haematol 1980; 45:575.

365. Kahn A, Marie J, et al: Search for a relationship between molecular anomalies of the mutant erythrocyte pyruvate kinase variants and their pathological expression. Hum Genet 1981; 57:172.

366. Miwa S: Recommended methods for the characterization of red cell pyruvate kinase variants. Br J Haematol 1979; 43:375.

367. Lenzner C, Nurnberg P, et al: Mutations in the pyruvate kinase L-gene in patients with hereditary hemolytic anemia. Blood 1994; 83:2817.

368. Baronciani L, Beutler E: Molecular study of pyruvate kinase–deficient patients with hereditary nonspherocytic hemolytic anemia. J Clin Invest 1995; 95:1702.

369. Kanno H, Fujii H, et al: Identical point mutations of the R-type pyruvate kinase (PK) cDNA found in unrelated PK variants associated with hereditary hemolytic anemia. Blood 1992; 79:1347.

370. Lakomek M, Huppke P, et al: Mutations in the R-type pyruvate kinase gene and altered enzyme kinetic properties in patients with hemolytic anemia due to pyruvate kinase deficiency. Ann Hematol 1994; 68:253.

371. Rouger H, Valentin C, et al: Five unknown mutations in the LR pyruvate kinase gene associated with severe hereditary nonspherocytic haemolytic anaemia in France. Br J Haematol 1996; 92:825.

372. Whitney KM, Goodman SA, et al: The molecular basis of canine pyruvate kinase deficiency. Exp Hematol 1994; 22:866.

373. Baronciani L, Beutler E: Prenatal diagnosis of pyruvate kinase deficiency. Blood 1994; 84:2354.

374. Mentzer W, Alpers J: Mild anemia with abnormal RBC pyruvate kinase. Clin Res 1971; 29:209.

375. Sachs JR, Wicker DJ, et al: Familial hemolytic anemia resulting from an abnormal red blood cell pyruvate kinase. J Lab Clin Med 1968; 72:359.

376. Paglia DE, Valentine WN, et al: Defective erythrocyte pyruvate kinase with impaired kinetics and reduced optimal activity. Br J Haematol 1972; 221:651.

377. Busch D, Witt I, et al: Deficiency of pyruvate kinase in the erythrocytes of a child with hereditary nonspherocytic hemolytic anemia. Acta Paediatr Scand 1966; 55:177.

377a. Kanno H, Fujii H, et al: cDNA cloning of human R-type pyruvate kinase and identification of a single amino acid substitution (Thr→Met) affecting enzymatic stability in a pyruvate kinase variant (PK Tokyo) associated with hereditary hemolytic anemia. Proc Natl Acad Sci U S A 1991; 88:8218.

378. Kanno H, Fujii H, et al: Low substrate affinity of pyruvate kinase variant (PK Sapporo) caused by a single amino acid substitution (426 Arg→Gln) associated with hereditary anemia. Blood 1993; 81:2439.

379. Kanno H, Ballas SK, et al: Molecular abnormality of erythrocyte pyruvate kinase deficiency in the Amish. Blood 1994; 83:2311.

380. Kanno H, Wei DC, et al: Hereditary hemolytic anemia caused by diverse point mutations of pyruvate kinase gene found in Japan and Hong Kong. Blood 1994; 84:3505.

381. Takegawa S, Miwa S: Change of pyruvate kinase (PK) isozymes

382. Miwa S: Hereditary disorders of red cell enzymes in the Embem-Meyerhof pathway. Am J Hematol 1983; 14:381.

383. Max-Audit I, Rosa R, et al: Pyruvate kinase hyperactivity genetically determined: metabolic consequences and molecular characterization. Blood 1980; 56:5.

384. Rosa R, Max-Audit I, et al: Hereditary pyruvate kinase abnormalities associated with erythrocytosis. Am J Hematol 1981; 10:47.

385. Staal GEJ, Jansen G, et al: Pyruvate kinase and the "High ATP syndrome." J Clin Invest 1984; 74:231.

386. Kechemir D, Max-Audit I, et al: Comparative study of human M2-type pyruvate kinases isolated from human leukocytes and erythrocytes of a patient with red cell pyruvate kinase hyperactivity. Enzyme 1989; 41:121.

387. Etiemble J, Picat C, et al: Erythrocytic pyruvate kinase deficiency and hemolytic anemia inherited as a dominant trait. Am J Hematol 1984; 17:251.

388. Valentine WN, Herring WB, et al: Pyruvate kinase Greensboro. A four-generation study of a high $K_{0.5s}$ (phosphoenolpyruvate) variant. Blood 1988; 72:1054.

389. Baughan MA, Paglia DE, et al: An unusual hematological syndrome with pyruvate kinase deficiency and thalassemia minor in the kindreds. Acta Haematol 1968; 39:345.

390. Eudlerink F, Cleton FS: Gaucher's disease with severe renal involvement combined with pyruvate kinase deficiency. Pathol Eur 1970; 5:409.

391. Mentzer WC: Unpublished data.

392. Blume KG, Busch D, et al: The polymorphism of nucleoside effect in pyruvate kinase deficiency. Humangenetik 1970; 9:257.

393. Staal GEJ, Van Berkel THJC, et al: Normalization of red blood cell pyruvate kinase in pyruvate kinase deficiency by riboflavin treatment. Clin Chim Acta 1975; 60:323.

394. Glader BE: Salicylate-induced injury of pyruvate-kinase deficient erythrocytes. N Engl J Med 1976; 294:916.

395. Weiden PL, Hackman RC, et al: Long-term survival and reversal of iron overload after marrow transplantation in dogs with congenital hemolytic anemia. Blood 1981; 57:66.

396. Morimoto M, Kanno H, et al: Pyruvate kinase deficiency of mice associated with nonspherocytic hemolytic anemia and cure of the anemia by marrow transplantation without host irradiation. Blood 1995; 86:4323.

397. Tani K, Yoshikubo T, et al: Retrovirus-mediated gene transfer of human pyruvate kinase (PK) cDNA into murine hematopoietic cells: implications for gene therapy of human PK deficiency. Blood 1994; 83:2305.

398. Beutler E, Forman L: Coexistence of β-thalassemia and a new pyruvate kinase variant: PK Fukien. Acta Haematol 1983; 69:3.

399. Shinohara K, Tanaka KR: Pyruvate kinase deficiency hemolytic anemia: enzymatic characterization studies in twelve patients. Hemoglobin 1980; 4:611.

400. Tani K, Tsutsumi H, et al: Two homozygous cases of erythrocyte pyruvate kinase (PK) deficiency in Japan: PK Sendai and PK Shinshu. Am J Hematol 1980; 28:186.

401. Muir WA, Beutler E, et al: Erythrocyte pyruvate kinase deficiency in the Ohio Amish: origin and characterization of the mutant enzyme. Am J Hum Genet 1984; 36:634.

402. Paglia DE, Valentine WN: Molecular lesion affecting the ADP-combining site in a mutant enzyme of erythrocyte pyruvate kinase. Proc Natl Acad Sci U S A 1981; 78:5175.

403. Neubauer B, Lakomek H, et al: Point mutations in the L-type pyruvate kinase gene of two children with hemolytic anemia caused by pyruvate kinase deficiency. Blood 1991; 77:1871.

404. Giger U, Noble N: Determination of erythrocyte pyruvate kinase deficiency in basenjis with chronic hemolytic anemia. J Am Vet Med Assoc 1991; 198:1755.

405. Miwa S, Nishina T, et al: Studies on erythrocyte metabolism in a case with hereditary deficiency of H-subunit of lactate dehydrogenase. Acta Haematol Jpn 1971; 34:228.

406. Kanno T, Sudo K, et al: Hereditary deficiency of lactate dehydrogenase M-subunit. Clin Chim Acta 1980; 108:267.

407. Kremer JP, Datta T, et al: Mechanisms of compensation of hemolytic anemia in a lactate dehydrogenase mouse mutant. Exp Hematol 1987; 15:664.

408. Brewer GJ: A new inherited abnormality of human erythrocytes: elevated erythrocyte adenosine triphosphate. Biochem Biophys Res Commun 1965; 18:430.

409. Jacobasch G, Syllm-Rappoport I, et al: 2,3-PGase-Mangel als mögliche Ursache erhöhten ATP-Gehaltes. Clin Chim Acta 1964; 10:477.

410. Ben-Bassat I, Brok-Simoni F, et al: A family with red cell pyrimidine 5'-nucleotidase deficiency. Blood 1976; 47:919.

411. Rosa R, Rochant H, et al: Electrophoretic and kinetic studies of human erythrocytes deficient in pyrimidine-5'-nucleotidase. Hum Genet 1977; 38:209.

412. Miwa S, Nakashima K, et al: Three cases of hereditary hemolytic anemia with pyrimidine-5'-nucleotidase deficiency in a Japanese family. Hum Genet 1977; 37:361.

413. Paglia DE, Valentine WN: Haemolytic anaemia associated with disorders of the purine and pyrimidine salvage pathways. Clin Haematol 1981; 10:81.

414. Beutler E, Baranko PV, et al: Hemolytic anemia due to pyrimidine-5'-nucleotidase deficiency; report of eight cases in six families. Blood 1980; 56:251.

415. Miwa S, Ishida Y, Kibe A, et al: Two cases of hereditary hemolytic anemia with pyrimidine-5'-nucleotidase deficiency. Acta Haematol Jpn 1981; 44:187.

416. Ozsoylu S, Gurgey A: A case of hemolytic anemia due to erythrocyte pyrimidine-5'-nucleotidase deficiency. Acta Haematol 1981; 66:56.

417. Tomoda A, Noble NA, et al: Hemolytic anemia in hereditary pyrimidine 5'-nucleotidase deficiency: nucleotide inhibition of G6PD and the pentose phosphate shunt. Blood 1982; 60:1212.

418. Willy T, Hansen R, et al: Erythrocyte pyrimidine-5'-nucleotidase deficiency. Scand J Haematol 1983; 31:122.

419. Hirono A, Fujii H, et al: Chromatographic analysis of human erythrocyte pyrimidine-5'-nucleotidase from five patients with pyrimidine-5'-nucleotidase deficiency. Br J Haematol 1987; 65:35.

420. Swanson MS, Angle CR, et al: 31p NMR study of erythrocytes from a patient with hereditary pyrimidine-5'-nucleotidase deficiency. Proc Natl Acad Sci U S A 1983; 80:169.

421. Swanson MS, Markin RS, et al: Identification of cytidine diphosphodiesters in erythrocytes from a patient with pyrimidine nucleotidase deficiency. Blood 1984; 63:665.

422. Harley EH, Heaton A, et al: Pyrimidine metabolism in hereditary erythrocyte pyrimidine-5'-nucleotidase deficiency. Metabolism 1978; 27:12.

423. Kagimoto T, Shirono K: Detection of pyrimidine-5'-nucleotidase deficiency using H- or P-nuclear magnetic resonance. Experimentia 1986; 42:69.

424. Valentine WN, Anderson HM, et al: Studies on human erythrocyte nucleotide metabolism. II. Nonspherocytic hemolytic anemia, high red cell ATP, and ribosephosphate pyrophosphokinase (RPK, EC2.7.6.1) deficiency. Blood 1972; 39:674.

425. Valentine WN, Bennett JM, et al: Nonspherocytic haemolytic anaemia with increased red cell adenine nucleotides, glutathione and basophilic stippling and ribosephosphate pyrophosphokinase (RPK) deficiency: studies on two new kindreds. Br J Haematol 1973; 24:157.

426. Lachant NA, Zerez CR, et al: Pyrimidine nucleotides impair phosphoribosylpyrophosphate (PRPP) synthetase subunit aggregation by sequestering magnesium. A mechanism for the decreased PRPP synthetase activity in hereditary erythrocyte pyrimidine-5'-nucleotidase deficiency. Biochim Biophys Acta 1989; 994:81.

427. Lachant NA, Tanaka KR: Red cell metabolism in hereditary pyrimidine-5'-nucleotidase deficiency: effect of magnesium. Br J Haematol 1986; 63:615.

428. Paglia DE, Valentine WN, et al: Cytosol accumulation of cytidine diphosphate (CDP)-choline as an isolated erythrocyte defect in chronic hemolysis. Proc Natl Acad Sci U S A 1983; 80:3081.

429. Oda S, Tanaka KR: Metabolism studies in erythrocyte pyrimidine 5'-nucleotidase deficiency. Clin Res 1976; 34:149A.

430. David O, Ramenghi U, et al: Inhibition of hexose monophosphate shunt in young erythrocytes by pyrimidine nucleotides in hereditary pyrimidine-5' nucleotidase deficiency. Eur J Haematol 1991; 47:48.

431. Paglia DE, Valentine WN, et al: Effects of low-level lead exposure on pyrimidine-5'-nucleotidase and other erythrocyte enzymes. J Clin Invest 1975; 56:1164.

432. Valentine WN, Paglia DE, et al: Lead poisoning. Association with hemolytic anemia, basophilic stippling erythrocyte pyrimidine-5'-nucleotidase deficiency, and intraerythrocytic accumulation of pyrimidines. J Clin Invest 1976; 58:926.

433. Paglia DE, Valentine WN, et al: Studies on the pathogenesis of lead induced hemolytic anemia. Blood 1977; 50:96.

434. Ghosh K, Abdulrahman HI, et al: Report of the first case of pyrimidine-5' nucleotidase deficiency from Kuwait detected by a screening test. A test report. Haematologia 1991; 24:229.

435. Li JY, Wan SD, et al: A new mutant erythrocyte pyrimidine-5'-nucleotidase characterized by fast electrophoretic mobility in a Chinese boy with chronic hemolytic anemia. Clin Chim Acta 1991; 200:43.

436. Torrance JD, Whittaker D, et al: Erythrocyte pyrimidine-5'-nucleotidase. Br J Haematol 1980; 45:585.

437. Beutler E, West C: Tissue distribution of pyrimidine-5'-nucleotidase. Biochem Med 1982; 27:334.

438. Beutler E, Carson D, et al: Metabolic compensation for profound erythrocyte adenylate kinase deficiency: A hereditary enzyme defect without hemolytic anemia. J Clin Invest 1983; 72:648.

439. Szeinberg A, Kahana D, et al: Hereditary deficiency of adenylate kinase in red blood cells. Acta Haematol 1969; 42:111.

440. Toren A, Brok-Simoni F, et al: Congenital haemolytic anaemia associated with adenylate kinase deficiency. Br J Haematol 1994; 87:376.

441. Lachant NA, Zerez CR, et al: Hereditary erythrocyte adenylate kinase deficiency: a defect of phosphotransferases. Blood 1991; 77:2774.

442. Boivin P, Galand C, et al: Anémie hémolytique congénitale non sphérocytaire et déficit héréditaire en adenylate kinase érythrocytaire. Presse Med 1971; 79:215.

443. Miwa S, Fujii H, et al: Red cell adenylate kinase deficiency associated with hereditary nonspherocytic hemolytic anemia: clinical and biochemical studies. Am J Hematol 1983; 14:325.

444. Matsuura S, Igarashi M, et al: Human adenylate kinase deficiency associated with hemolytic anemia. A single base substitution affecting solubility and catalytic activity of the cytosolic adenylate kinase. J Biol Chem 1989; 264:10148.

445. Valentine WN, Paglia DE, et al: Hereditary hemolytic anemia with increased red cell adenosine deaminase (45- to 70-fold) and decreased adenosine triphosphate. Science 1977; 195:783.

446. Miwa S, Fujii H, et al: A case of red-cell adenosine deaminase overproduction associated with hereditary hemolytic anemia found in Japan. Am J Hematol 1978; 5:107.

447. Perignon JL, Hamet M, et al: Biochemical study of a case of hemolytic anemia with increased (85-fold) cell adenosine deaminase. Clin Chim Acta 1982; 124:205.

448. Kanno H, Tani K, et al: Adenosine deaminase (ADA) overproduction associated with congenital hemolytic anemia: case report and molecular analysis. Jpn J Exp Med 1988; 58:1.

449. Fujii H, Miwa S, et al: Purification and properties of adenosine deaminase in normal and hereditary hemolytic anemia with increased red cell activity. Hemoglobin 1980; 4:693.

450. Chottiner EG, Cloft HJ, et al: Elevated adenosine deaminase activity and hereditary hemolytic anemia. Evidence for abnormal translational control of protein synthesis. J Clin Invest 1987; 79:1001.

451. Chottiner EG, Ginsburg D, et al: Erythrocyte adenosine deaminase overproduction in hereditary hemolytic anemia. Blood 1989; 74:448.

452. Fujii H, Miwa S, et al: Overproduction of structurally normal enzyme in man: hereditary haemolytic anaemia with increased red cell adenosine deaminase activity. Br J Haematol 1982; 51:427.

453. Chen EH, Tartaglia AP, et al: Hereditary overexpression of adenosine deaminase in erythrocytes: evidence for a cis-acting mutation. Am J Hum Genet 1993; 53:889.

454. Chen EH, Mitchell B: Hereditary overexpression of adenosine deaminase in erythrocytes: studies in erythroid cell lines and transgenic mice. Blood 1994; 84:2346.

455. Glader BE, Backer K, et al: Elevated erythrocyte adenosine deaminase activity in congenital hypoplastic anemia. N Engl J Med 1983; 309:1486.

456. Glader BE, Backer K: Comparative activity of erythrocyte adenosine deaminase and orotidine decarboxylase in Diamond-Blackfan anemia. Am J Hematol 1986; 23:135.

457. Novelli G, Stocchi V, et al: Increased erythrocyte adenosine deaminase activity without haemolytic anaemia. Hum Hered 1986; 36:37.

458. Cowan MJ, Brady RO, et al: Elevated erythrocyte adenosine deaminase activity in patients with acquired immunodeficiency syndrome. Proc Natl Acad Sci U S A 1986; 83:1089.

459. Sanchez-Corona J, Garcia-Cruz D, et al: Increased adenosine deaminase activity in a patient with cartilage-hair hypoplasia. Ann Genet 1990; 33:99.

460. Lichtman MA, Miller DR: Erythrocyte glycolysis, 2,3-diphosphoglycerate and adenosine triphosphate concentration in uremic subjects: relationship to extracellular phosphate concentration. J Lab Clin Med 1970; 76:267.

461. Travis SF, Sugarman HJ, et al: Red cell metabolic alterations induced by intravenous hyperalimentation. N Engl J Med 1971; 285:63.

462. Lichtman MA, Miller DR, et al: Energy metabolism in uremic red cells: relationship of red cell adenosine triphosphate concentration to extracellular phosphate. Trans Assoc Am Physicians 1969; 82:331.

463. Jacob HS, Amsden T: Acute hemolytic anemia with rigid red cells in hypophosphatemia. N Engl J Med 1971; 285:1446.

464. Weed RI, LaCelle PL, et al: Metabolic dependence of red cell deformability. J Clin Invest 1969; 48:795.

465. Klock JC, Williams HE, et al: Hemolytic anemia and somatic cell dysfunction in severe hypophosphatemia. Arch Intern Med 1974; 134:360.

466. Lichtman MA, Miller DR, et al: Reduced red cell glycolysis, 2,3-diphosphoglycerate and adenosine triphosphate concentration, and increased hemoglobin oxygen affinity caused by hypophosphatemia. Ann Intern Med 1971; 74:562.

467. Oken MM, Lichtman MA, et al: Spherocytic hemolytic disease during magnesium deprivation in the rat. Blood 1971; 38:468.

468. Piomelli S, Jansen V, et al: The hemolytic anemia of magnesium deficiency in adult rats. Blood 1973; 41:451.

469. Elin RJ, Tan HK: Erythrocyte membrane plaques from rats with magnesium deficiency. Blood 1977; 49:657.

470. MacDougall LG, Judisch JM, et al: Red cell metabolism in iron deficiency anemia. II. The relationship between red cell survival and alterations in red cell metabolism. J Pediatr 1970; 76:660.

471. MacDougall LG: Red cell metabolism in iron deficiency anemia. III. The relationship between glutathione peroxide, catalase, serum vitamin E, and susceptibility of iron deficient red cells to oxidative hemolysis. J Pediatr 1972; 8:775.

472. MacDougall LG: Red cell metabolism in iron deficiency anemia. J Pediatr 1968; 71:303.

473. Slawsky P, Desforge JF: Erythrocyte 2,3-diphosphoglycerate in iron deficiency. Arch Intern Med 1972; 129:914.

474. Brewer GJ: Metabolism of ATP in thalassemic and iron-deficient erythrocytes. J Lab Clin Med 1967; 7:1016.

475. Ramot B, Brok-Simoni F, et al: Glucose-6-phosphate dehydrogenase, hexokinase activities and ATP levels as a function of cell density in thalassemia and iron deficiency anemia. Ann N Y Acad Sci 1968; 165:400.

476. Card RT, Weintraub LR: Metabolic abnormalities of erythrocytes in severe iron deficiency. Blood 1971; 37:725.

477. Kimura H, Horiuchi N, et al: Hormonal response of glycolytic key enzymes of erythrocytes in insulinoma. Metabolism 1971; 20:1119.

478. Butenandt O: Erythrocytic enzyme activities in hypothyroid children. Acta Haematol 1972; 47:335.

479. Snyder L M, Reddy WJ: Thyroid hormone control of erythrocyte 2,3-diphosphoglyceric acid. Science 1970; 169:879.

480. Najman A, Leroux JP, et al: Déficit en pyruvate kinase érythrocytaire au cours des leucémies aigues. Rev Fr Etudes Clin Biol 1969; 14:795.

481. Boivin P, Galand C, et al: Acquired erythroenzymopathies in blood disorders: study of 200 cases. Br J Haematol 1975; 31:531.

482. Emerson PM, Garrow DH: Differences in the two red-cell populations in erythroleukaemia. Lancet 1971; 2:1150.

483. Kahn A, Vroclans M, et al: Differences in the two red cell populations in erythroleukaemia. Lancet 1971; 2:933.

484. Pagnier J, Labie D, et al: Étude biochimique d'un cas d'érythroleucémie. Nouv Rev Fr Hematol 1972; 12:317.

485. Moser K, Fischer M, et al: Glutathionreduktase und Triosephosphatisomerasemangel in Erythrocyten und Thrombocyten bei Pancytopenie (Typ Estren-Damastrek). Klin Wochenschr 1968; 46:995.

486. Schroter W: Chronische idiopathische infantile Panzytopenie. Ein neues Syndrom mit relativem Pyruvatkinase und Glutathionreduktasemangel der Erythrozyten und Hyperplasie des erythropoietischen Gewebes. Schweiz Med Wochenschr 1970; 100:1101.

487. Kleeberg UR, Heimpel H, et al: Relativer Glutathion und/oder Pyruvatkinasemangel in den Erythrocyten bei Panmyelopathien und akuten Leukämien. Klin Wochenschr 1971; 49:557.

488. Valentine WN, Crookston JH, et al: Erythrocyte enzymatic abnormalities in HEMPAS (hereditary erythroblastic multinuclearity with a positive acidified-serum test). Br J Haematol 1972; 23:107.

489. Dreyfus B, Sultan C, et al: Anomalies of blood group antigens and erythrocyte enzymes in two types of chronic refractory anaemia. Br J Haematol 1969; 16:303.

490. Valentine WN, Konrad PN, et al: Dyserythropoiesis, refractory anemia, and "preleukemia": metabolic features of the erythrocytes. Blood 1973; 41:857.

491. Abe S: Secondary red cell pyruvate kinase deficiency. I. Study of 30 subjects with malignant hematological disorder. Acta Haematol Jpn 1976; 9:247.

492. Abe S: Secondary red cell pyruvate kinase deficiency. II. Biochemical studies for the mechanism of pyruvate-kinase deficiency in erythroleukemia. Acta Haematol Jpn 1976; 39:255.

493. Wang WC, Mentzer WC: Differentiation of transient erythroblastopenia of childhood from congenital hypoplastic anemia. J Pediatr 1976; 88:784.

494. Kahn A: Abnormalities of erythrocyte enzymes in dyserythropoiesis and malignancies. Clin Haematol 1981; 10:123.

495. Tani K, Fujii H, et al: Erythrocyte activities in myelodysplastic syndromes: elevated pyruvate kinase activity. Am J Hematol 1989; 30:97.

496. Kahn A, Mane J, et al: Mechanisms of the acquired erythrocyte enzyme deficiencies in blood diseases. Clin Chim Acta 1976; 71:379.

18

Glucose-6-Phosphate Dehydrogenase Deficiency and Hemolytic Anemia

Lucio Luzzatto

Most hemolytic anemias can be neatly categorized, at least in first approximation, as being either inherited or acquired, either due to intracorpuscular or to extracorpuscular causes. Hemolytic anemia associated with deficiency of glucose-6-phosphate dehydrogenase (G6PD) glaringly defies this categorization. Indeed, the majority of persons with inherited G6PD deficiency have no anemia and almost no hemolysis. They develop both only as a result of challenge by exogenous agents. Because the metabolic role of G6PD in red blood cells is primarily related to its reductive potential, the threat to G6PD-deficient red cells is that of oxidative damage. Thus, to understand hemolytic anemia associated with G6PD deficiency we need to define the physiologic role of G6PD[1-3] and to find out why the red cells are G6PD deficient.[4-6]*

G6PD IN RED CELL METABOLISM

The time-honored phrase hexose monophosphate shunt, or pentose phosphate pathway, conveys a some-

what preconceived notion that this sequence of reactions, of which G6PD is the first (Fig. 18–1), is a sideline to glycolysis, contributing little (usually less than 10%) to glucose utilization.[1, 7] It is now clear that the hexose monophosphate shunt is not necessary for glucose utilization; and it is not necessary for pentose synthesis either, because this sugar can be produced through the concerted action of transketolase and transaldolase. In fact, the main role of the so-called pentose phosphate pathway is the production of the reduced form of nicotinamide adenine dinucleotide phosphate (NADPH), which, in turn, is closely related to the metabolism of glutathione (GSH). GSH is of key importance in all cells, for the preservation of sulfhydryl groups in numerous proteins and to prevent oxidative damage in general (Fig. 18–2). This role is particularly crucial in red cells because, being oxygen carriers *par excellence*, they have a literally built-in danger of damage by oxygen radicals, generated continuously in the course of methemoglobin formation.[8] The highly reactive oxygen radicals either decay spontaneously or are converted by superoxide dismutase to hydrogen peroxide (H_2O_2), which is still highly toxic. H_2O_2 detoxification to H_2O is effected by glutathione peroxidase

---

*Only selected references are given in this chapter. For a more extensive bibliography the reader is referred to several reviews that have surveyed extensively the area of G6PD and G6PD deficiency.[4-6, 61, 69]

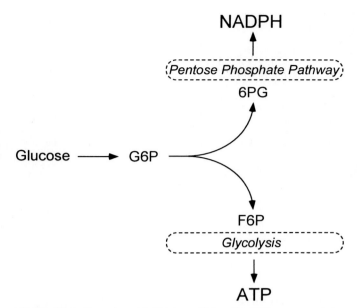

Structure and Biochemistry of G6PD

G6PD is a ubiquitous enzyme that must be quite ancient in evolution because it has been found in all organisms, from prokaryotes to yeasts, to protozoa, to plants and animals.[2, 11] In mammals, G6PD is a typical cytoplasmic enzyme, although some G6PD activity is associated with peroxisomes in liver and kidney cells.[12] This is interesting in view of the fact that these organelles are thought to have evolved as part of the need of early eukaryotes to defend against oxygen, which is germane to the role of G6PD today.

The enzymatically active form of G6PD is either a dimer or a tetramer of a single polypeptide subunit of about 59 kd.[13] The complete primary structure of the human enzyme has been deduced from the sequence of a full-length complementary DNA clone.[14] The amino acid sequence of rat liver G6PD shows 94% homology to the human sequence and provides evidence that the N-terminal amino acid is N-acetylalanine, which must result from post-translational cleavage of the N-terminal methionine. The same is probably true of the human enzyme.[15] The tertiary structure of the molecule has been determined (Fig. 18–3).[15a]

Extensive data are available on the kinetics of G6PD (Table 18–1). The coenzyme specificity is exquisite, in the sense that human G6PD has practically no activity with NAD. The substrate specificity is also very high, because activity on other hexose phosphates (e.g., mannose 6-P or galactose 6-P) is negligible.* By contrast, there is significant activity on substrate analogues, such as desamino-NADP and 2-deoxyglucose 6-P. These compounds, although artificial, have been useful in the characterization of variants (see later). The affinity for NADP is about one order of magnitude higher than the affinity for G6P. There is evidence that the G6P-binding site is near Lys[205], because this residue can be specifically labeled with pyridoxal 5-phosphate and this reaction is prevented by G6P itself.[16] The critical role of this amino acid has been confirmed by showing that its replacement with threonine (produced artifi-

Figure 18-1. The role of G6PD in red blood cell glucose metabolism. As a somewhat crude oversimplification, glucose can be visualized, after phosphorylation to G6P, as being at the bifurcation between two major pathways: glycolysis, producing high-energy phosphate (ATP), and the pentose phosphate pathway, generating reducing power (NADPH). Under ''normal'' conditions, probably less than 1% of G6P enters the pentose phosphate pathway; under maximal oxidative stress, it may probably reach 10%. The G6PD reaction is the first and rate-limiting step of the pentose phosphate pathway. F6P, fructose-6-phosphate.

(GSHPX);[9, 10]* one molecule of GSH is oxidized to GSSG for every molecule of H_2O_2 detoxified, and therefore GSH can only fulfill its functional role if it is continuously and stoichiometrically regenerated to GSH by glutathione reductase. Thus, GSH can be regarded as the key compound in preventing endogenous as well as exogenous oxidative damage (see later).

---

*An alternative to GSHPX in effecting H_2O_2 detoxification is catalase. In first approximation this alternative[173] does not seem to be important in red cells, since acatalasemia is not associated with hemolysis. However, it is interesting that NADPH is an integral constituent of catalase,[9] and it has been suggested that the contribution of catalase to H_2O_2 detoxification may become comparable to that of GSHPX in G6PD-deficient red cells.[10]

---

*Hexose dehydrogenase, active on these compounds and also on nonphosphorylated hexose sugars, is an enzyme encoded by an autosomal gene expressed in the liver,[174] quite different from G6PD.

Figure 18-2. G6PD and the glutathione cycle. The front-line defense against oxidative damage by hydrogen peroxide (H_2O_2) is glutathione (GSH), by means of GSH peroxidase (GSHPX). GSHPX uses up GSH, and its regeneration can be effected only in the red blood cell through GSH reductase (GSSGR) by NADPH, which is ultimately provided by G6PD. (From Luzzatto L, Mehta A: Glucose 6-phosphate dehydrogenase deficiency. In Scriver CR, Beaudet AL, et al (eds): Molecular Basis of Inherited Disease. 7th ed. New York, McGraw-Hill, 1995, pp 3367–3398.)

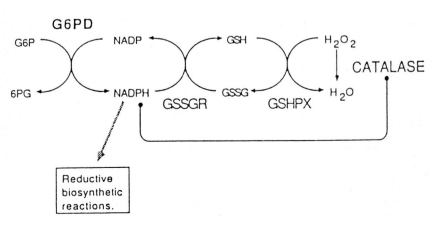

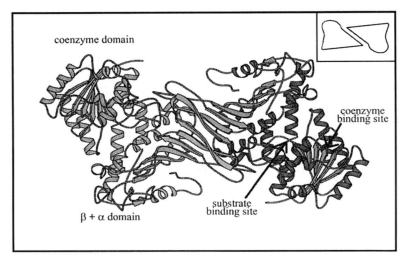

Figure 18-3. Model of the human dimer. In this figure, subunit P is equivalent to subunit A in published illustrations of the dimer of *Leuconostoc mesenteroides* G6PD.[6] The monomer consists of two domains—a smaller coenzyme domain encompassing residues 1 to 198 and a larger β + α domain comprising residues 199 to 515. The sequence GASGDLA (residues 38 to 44) is at the coenzyme binding site *(arrow)*. The G6P binding site includes residues from the perfectly conserved 9-amino acid sequence RIDHYLGKE (198 to 206). Three adjacent strands of the β-sheet of the β + α domain (residues 380 to 425) are in the area of the dimer interface. (From Naylor CD, Rowland P, et al: Glucose 6-phosphate dehydrogenase mutations causing enzyme deficiency in a model of the tertiary structure of the human enzyme. Blood 1996; 87:2974.)

cially by site-directed mutagenesis), nearly abolishes catalytic activity.[17] Moreover, by purifying to homogeneity recombinant human G6PD produced in *Escherichia coli*, it has been shown that Lys[205] is essential for electron transfer rather than for G6P binding.[18]

By contrast, biochemical labeling of the NADP-binding site has proven difficult, and therefore its location remained uncertain. The crystal structure of the G6P from the microorganism *Leuconostoc mesenteroides* has been solved at a resolution of 2.8 Å,[19] and, based on this structure, a model of the human G6PD dimer has been obtained.[20] This analysis has placed the NADP binding site at a fan of β-sheet structures, with a critical G-X-X-G-X-X peptide motif corresponding to amino acids 38 to 43 in exon 3.

Although many natural and non-natural substances can affect the activity of G6PD, it is not certain which ones may be important physiologically. NADPH, one product of the G6PD reaction, is a potent quasi-competitive inhibitor,[21] and because most of the coenzyme in cells is in the reduced form,[22] it can be assumed that G6PD is normally under strong inhibition. Because the K_m values for both G6P and NADP are higher than their normal respective intracellular concentrations, it is likely that these two substrates themselves are the main regulators of intracellular G6PD activity, together with NADPH. Any oxidative event affecting the cell will alter the NADPH/NADP ratio in favor of NADP. The simultaneous increase in NADP and decrease in NADPH act additively to increase G6PD activity by increasing the substrate drive on the reaction rate and decreasing product inhibition.[23] Under most conditions

this may be the most important short-term regulatory signal, although it is, of course, possible that other regulatory effects play a role as well.

Features of G6PD in Red Cells

Biochemical evidence is in keeping with the notion that the G6PD protein in red cells is the same as in other somatic cells. This is supported by genetic evidence. Indeed, there is only one structural gene for G6PD in the human genome (see later); and when red cells are severely G6PD deficient, this deficiency is found to a greater or lesser degree also in other somatic cells.[7] However, a significant difference in the metabolism of G6PD arises from the characteristic inability of mature red cells to synthesize protein. As a result, whereas in most somatic cells G6PD is subject to turnover, in red cells any G6PD molecule undergoing denaturation or proteolytic breakdown cannot be replaced (this is true, of course, not only of G6PD but of most other red cell enzymes as well[24]). In normal red cells, the decay of G6PD approximates an exponential with a half-life of about 60 days,[25] although it has been claimed that it may approximate more closely a two-slope curve with a very fast breakdown when reticulocytes mature to erythrocytes and a much slower breakdown subsequently.[26] The age-dependence of red cell G6PD activity is so characteristic that it can be regarded almost as a marker of red cell age. In normal blood, reticulocytes have about five times more activity than the 10% oldest red cells.[27]

Table 18-1. DISTINCTIVE BIOCHEMICAL PROPERTIES OF INDIVIDUAL G6PD VARIANTS

Variant	Class	Activity (% of Normal)	Electrophoretic Mobility (% of Normal)	K_m of G6P (μmol/L)	Activity on 2d G6P (% of Normal)
Normal (B)	IV	100	100	70	5
A⁻	III	13	110	70	5
Mediterranean	II	3	100	25	50
Harilaou	I	2	95	90	8

Genetics of G6PD

A Note on Terminology

G6PD is the accepted abbreviation for the enzyme glucose-6-phosphate dehydrogenase (E.C. 1.1.1.49). The G6PD gene is designated *Gd*.[4, 11] In this chapter, the terms *G6PD normal* and *G6PD deficient* are used to designate phenotypes of persons; G6PD(+) and G6PD(−) are used to designate the phenotype of individual cells. Because *Gd* is X-linked, males can be only normal hemizygotes (*Gd⁺*) or deficient hemizygotes (*Gd⁻*); females can be normal homozygotes (*Gd⁺/Gd⁺*), deficient homozygotes (*Gd⁻/Gd⁻*), or heterozygotes (*Gd⁺/Gd⁻*). The phenotype of the last group is often referred to as "intermediate," because usually their overall red cell G6PD level lies in between the normal and the deficient range: however, exceptions do occur (see later). Because the majority of G6PD-deficient persons are mostly asymptomatic, their G6PD deficiency is referred to as mild, simple, or common; the minority of persons who have congenital nonspherocytic hemolytic anemia (CNSHA) are referred to as having rare, sporadic, or severe G6PD deficiency.

Cytogenetics and Molecular Genetics

Because G6PD is an oligomer of a single polypeptide chain, its structure is fully specified by a single gene located in the telomeric region of the long arm of the X-chromosome[28–34] (band Xq28) (Fig. 18–4).* The G6PD gene, *Gd*, is genetically and physically closely linked to the genes encoding factor VIII and to those encoding the retinal pigments[35] (whose mutations are responsible for colorblindness). This region of the X chromosome is one of the best mapped in the human genome,[36, 37] with several polymorphic loci being in strong linkage disequilibrium with G6PD itself;[38, 38a] the entire G6PD genomic gene has been fully sequenced,[39] as well as more than 200 kb of DNA surrounding it.†

X-linkage of *Gd* has naturally two important consequences: (1) *Gd* mutations display the typical pattern of mendelian X-linked inheritance. (2) As a result of the phenomenon of X-chromosome inactivation, to which the *Gd* locus is subject, females heterozygous for two different alleles exhibit somatic cell mosaicism.[40] This means that, if one of the alleles entails enzyme deficiency, about one half of the cells will be G6PD(+) and the other half will be G6PD(−). Because of this, G6PD deficiency should not be regarded as a recessive, but rather as a co-dominant, trait.

At the genomic level, the *Gd* gene (Fig. 18–5) consists of 13 exons, the first one of which is noncoding.[41] The total length of the gene, which has been fully sequenced,[39] is about 18.5 kb, much of which (about 12 kb) consists of intron II. The promoter region is highly

*It has been claimed that a portion of the G6PD protein is encoded by an autosomal gene mapped to chromosome 6.[30] However, this latter gene turns out to encode instead guanosine monophosphate reductase,[29] and the claim has been refuted[28, 31] and subsequently retracted.[175]

†GDB accession number X55448, and Chen E: Personal communication, 1994.

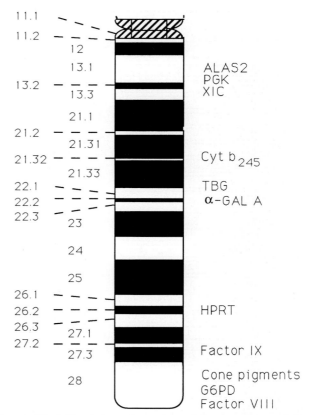

Figure 18–4. The telomeric region of the long arm of the X chromosome. The G6PD gene maps very close to the Xq27.3 fragile site, to colorblindness, and to the hemophilia A (factor VIII) gene. Physical linkage between the G6PD and the factor VIII genes has been established: they are only 400 kb apart from each other.

enriched in guanine and cytosine residues (i.e., GC rich), as found characteristically in other housekeeping genes analyzed so far.[29] Deletion analysis has revealed that the "essential" portion of the promoter is only about 150 bp long.[42] Within this region, two Sp1-binding sites have been identified, either of which is essential for promoter activity.[43] The significance of the large intron is unknown: it may be important for efficient transcription or for processing, because it is still the largest intron even in the compressed version of the G6PD gene found in *Fugu rubripes* (a type of puffer fish).[44]

G6PD Deficiency in Heterozygotes

Gd⁺/Gd⁻ heterozygous women would be expected to have an approximately 1:1 ratio of G6PD(+) to G6PD(−) red cells, with an overall level of G6PD in a whole blood hemolysate equal to about 50% of normal. If a group of heterozygotes is analyzed, this is indeed found to be the modal value of G6PD activity; however, a wide range is observed.[45] The question of why in a heterozygote there may be a wide deviation from the theoretical 1:1 ratio of G6PD(+) to G6PD(−) red cells is incompletely solved. In first approximation it can be assumed that X-inactivation takes place com-

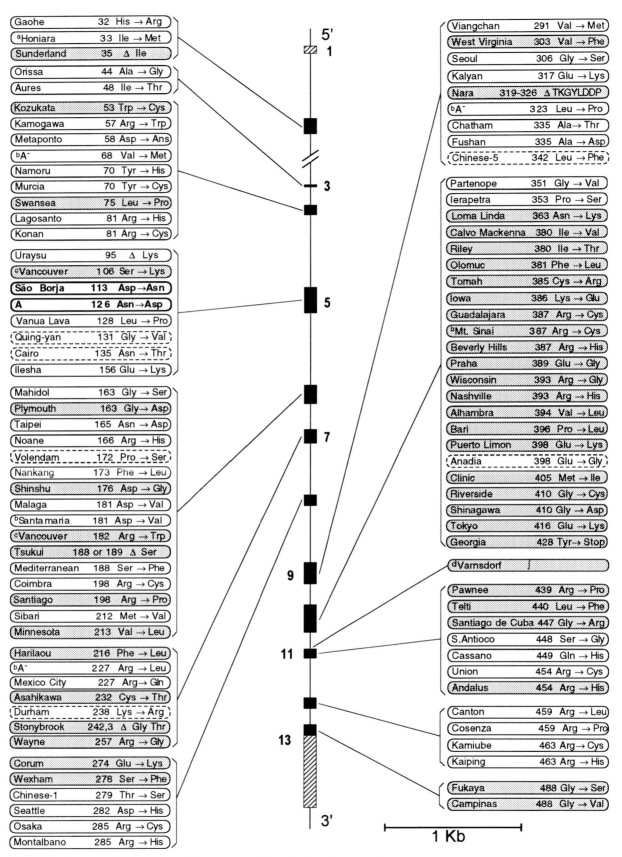

Figure 18-5. The human G6PD gene with a map of structural mutations. Each boxed entry shows a G6PD variant and the corresponding amino acid replacement. All variants shown, except G6PD A, are associated with enzyme deficiency. The shaded boxes indicate CNSHA: these variants belong, by definition, to class I (see Table 18–1). The remaining variants belong to class II or III. Note that G6PD A$^-$ is heterogeneous, because it can result from the combination of the Asn[126]→Asp replacement with any of three additional mutations. However, in the large majority of cases (probably more than 90%), the second mutation of G6PD A$^-$ is Val[68]→Met. This figure includes only the variants for which the molecular basis has been elucidated. For more information see reference 57.

pletely at random, and therefore a binomial distribution would be expected: the width of this depends on the number of cells in the embryo at the time of X-inactivation. If this number is 32-64, a fraction of about 2% of women with an "extreme phenotype" is predicted, that is, with less than 5% of one of the two cell types: this is in good agreement with observation in an unselected sample of Gd^+/Gd^- heterozygotes,[46] although some studies have suggested an even larger proportion.[47] Thus, it seems likely that, in general, unbalanced phenotypes may arise simply by chance, according to the laws of statistics. However, in certain cases there is evidence of selection at the somatic cell level after X-chromosome inactivation. This is well established in women who are heterozygous for hypoxanthine phosphoribosyltransferase (HPRT) deficiency,[48] and it has been observed also in several women heterozygous for severely deficient G6PD variants.[49, 49a] In these cases one has to infer that the G6PD(−) state is a selective disadvantage for hematopoietic stem cells; interestingly, this disadvantage is cell lineage specific, because it does not affect, for instance, fibroblasts.[49] Lastly, it seems reasonable to surmise that if selection can favor certain HPRT and certain G6PD alleles, the same notion can be extrapolated to alleles at other X-linked loci. Thus, heterozygotes exhibiting extreme phenotypes by analysis of G6PD may arise from selection acting on an allele at another locus (a "hitchhiking effect"), as has been suggested in a family with G6PD Ilesha.[50-53]*

Biochemical Basis of G6PD Deficiency

In principle, deficiency of G6PD, like that of any other protein, might be due to deletions or to point mutations affecting transcription, processing, or the primary structure. Careful testing of G6PD-deficient cells has uniformly revealed that the enzyme activity, even when very severely reduced (sometimes to less than 1% of normal), is never completely absent. This essentially rules out large deletions. Further analysis of enzymic properties of the residual G6PD activity has almost invariably revealed deviations from the properties of the normal enzyme,[7] suggesting that G6PD deficiency was due to structural abnormalities (i.e., mutations in the coding region) rather than merely to a decrease in number of normal molecules (as would be expected with transcriptional or processing mutants). Changes in the primary structure (i.e., substitutions of individual amino acids) can cause G6PD deficiency either by affecting its catalytic function or by decreasing the in vivo stability of the protein or by both of these mechanisms. It is likely that one or the other is the main factor responsible for G6PD deficiency in

individual cases. For some variants, an accelerated in vivo breakdown has been demonstrated directly by assaying the activity of G6PD in age-fractionated red cells.[25, 54, 55] In extreme cases, G6PD deficiency can be visualized simply as resulting from a marked change in the exponential decay constant of the enzyme, whereby the half-life becomes, instead of 50 days, 10 days or even less. In such cases the G6PD activity of reticulocytes may be practically normal.

Molecular Basis of G6PD Deficiency

Since the cloning of the G6PD gene,[14] and especially since the introduction of polymerase chain reaction amplification of individual exons or groups of exons,[56] the analysis of G6PD mutations has been relatively easy, and there is now a database of about 100 variants characterized at the molecular level[57] (see Fig. 18–5). From this set of mutants a reasonably clear pattern is beginning to emerge for the molecular basis of G6PD deficiency. First, in nearly all the G6PD variants there is a single amino acid replacement, caused by a single missense point mutation. In a few cases (the three types of "A⁻" variant, G6PD Santamaria and G6PD Mount Sinai) two amino acid replacements are found, and in all of these one of the replacements is that of G6PD A. Because this variant is polymorphic in Africa, the most likely explanation is that a second point mutation has taken place in a Gd^A gene. In one case, three separate amino acid replacements have been reported (G6PD Vancouver): although this finding is thus far unique, one of these replacements is the same as that in G6PD Coimbra, which is polymorphic in the Mediterranean area. Only one mutation affecting splicing has been discovered and only three in-frame deletions—of a single amino acid (G6PD Sunderland), of two adjacent amino acids (G6PD Stonybrook), and of eight amino acids (G6PD Nara), respectively.

Thus, the predictions made by biochemical analysis have been largely validated, in that all mutations are compatible with some residual activity and all have the potential to affect the kinetic properties, the stability of the enzyme, or both. Unlike in many other inherited disorders (e.g., thalassemias, hemophilia, muscular dystrophy), large deletions or major rearrangements have been conspicuous by their absence. An important functional difference between these conditions and G6PD deficiency is that the former result from mutations in tissue-specific genes, whereas G6PD is a housekeeping gene. If a tissue-specific gene is totally inactivated by a mutation, it may not interfere with embryonic development but it may cause severe disease in the respective tissue in the adult. By contrast, at least a low level of G6PD activity may be indispensable for the majority of cells; and, therefore, complete inactivation of the gene (e.g., by a large deletion) may be lethal early in embryonic life, even though it allows the survival of embryonic stem cells.[58]

If G6PD deletions are not encountered because the gene is indispensable, can we identify any rule as to why certain point mutations are seen in preference to

---

*The use of G6PD as a marker to analyze the clonal origin of neoplastic cell populations[50, 51, 176] is discussed elsewhere.[6] "Homogeneous with respect to G6PD" is not synonymous with "monoclonal" because this situation could arise through somatic cell selection rather than common origin from a single cell. By contrast, if a cell population does have a mixed phenotype with respect to G6PD, it cannot be monoclonal.

others? In this respect some speculations can be offered:

1. *Sporadic mutations*. These are probably the majority, and most of them have been detected because they cause clinical manifestations in the form of CNSHA, by causing sufficient loss of activity in red cells to become limiting for their *in vivo* survival. This, in turn, may result, in principle, from two (non–mutually exclusive) mechanisms: (a) severe alterations in the interaction with the substrates, particularly G6P, and (b) marked intracellular instability. Sporadic variants associated with CNSHA are not likely to spread by genetic drift. Thus, the fact that the same variant may be found recurrently and independently in people who are almost certainly not ancestrally related is not trivial. The authors have found, for instance, G6PD Tokyo in Scotland,[59] whereas G6PD Guadalajara has been reported in Japan[60] and in Belfast.[59, 59a] These observations corroborate the notion that subtle constraints make a sporadic variant have a distinctly severe clinical expression while remaining compatible with life.

2. *Polymorphic mutations*. The majority of known mutations in this category are again associated with G6PD deficiency, and there is overwhelming evidence that these have become polymorphic as a result of malaria selection (see later). For these mutations we can visualize more stringent constraints: indeed, although still causing deficiency in red cells, they must not affect them so severely as to outweigh the advantage with respect to malaria. Thus, it is not surprising that nearly all the polymorphic variants fall in classes II or III, and none of them causes CNSHA (class I). Finally, as for other protein polymorphisms, electrophoretically silent, and therefore hitherto undetected, G6PD variants are likely to exist as well.

CLINICAL MANIFESTATIONS OF G6PD DEFICIENCY

The most classic manifestation of G6PD deficiency is acute hemolytic anemia (AHA); in children, however, another syndrome of great clinical and public health importance is neonatal jaundice (NNJ). CNSHA is a much more rare manifestation of G6PD deficiency and a life-long hemolytic process. These different clinical manifestations are now discussed in turn.[1, 61, 62]

Acute Hemolytic Anemia

Clinical Picture. A child with G6PD deficiency is clinically and hematologically normal most of the time, and this can be designated as a steady-state condition.[63] What happens in a situation of "oxidative challenge" has been best characterized after ingestion of fava beans (favism).[64] After a period of hours the child may become fractious and irritable or subdued and even lethargic. Within 24 to 48 hours there is often a moderate elevation of the temperature (up to 38°C). There may be nausea, abdominal pain, and diarrhea and rarely vomiting. In striking contrast to these relatively unspecific symptoms, the patient or a parent will observe, within 6 to 24 hours, the telltale and rather frightening event that the urine is discolored (Fig. 18–6): it will be reported as dark, or red, or brown, or black, or as "passing blood instead of water"; it will be stated, depending on experience, culture, and socioeconomic background, as resembling Coca-Cola or strong tea or port wine. At about the same time jaundice will become obvious. Physical examination may reveal little more than the signs corresponding to these symptoms. The child will be invariably pale and tachycardic; in severe cases there may be evidence of hypovolemic shock or, less likely, of heart failure. The spleen is usually moderately enlarged, and the liver also may be enlarged; either or both may be tender.

Laboratory Findings. Anemia may be from moderate to extremely severe (hemoglobin values of 2.5 g/dL have been recorded). In the absence of other pre-existing hematologic abnormalities the anemia is normocytic and normochromic. The morphology of the red cells may be striking (Fig. 18–7). There is often marked anisocytosis (reflected in a wide red cell size distribution on the electronic counter), owing to the coexistence of large polychromatic cells and of "contracted" cells, some of which can be frankly classified as spherocytes. There is also marked poikilocytosis, with presence of distorted red cells, of "irregularly contracted" red cells, and of red cells with apparently uneven distribution of the hemoglobin inside them (hemighosts[65]). Although some of these appearances are probably smearing artifacts, electron micrographic evidence suggests that in some of the cells opposing surfaces of the membrane have become "cross-linked."[66] Probably the most characteristic poikilocytes are those in which the cell margin appears literally dented, as though a portion has been plucked out or bitten away ("bite cells"; see Fig. 18–7). The reticulocyte count is increased and may reach peaks of 30% or more. Careful inspection of the reticulocyte preparations may reveal inclusion bodies different from those normally seen in reticulocytes, because they are discrete, round, and 1 to 3 μm in diameter, and they usually appear to be leaning, from the interior, against the cell membrane. These inclusions are more clearly displayed by supravital staining with methyl violet, when they are referred to as Heinz bodies. They consist of precipitates of denatured hemoglobin, and they are the vivid manifestation of the oxidative insult that this protein and the cell itself has suffered. Although Heinz bodies are a classic and characteristic finding, it is important to realize that it is a very transient finding, because the Heinz bodies are "pinched off" by the spleen[67] (thus giving rise to the bite cells), and the red cells containing them are very rapidly removed from the circulation. Haptoglobin is reduced to the point of being undetectable. In severe cases it is possible to demonstrate free hemoglobin in the plasma (the somewhat incongruous term of *hemoglobinemia* is used to describe this finding in one word). The white blood cell count is usually moderately elevated, with predominance of granulocytes. The platelet count may be normal, increased, or moderately de-

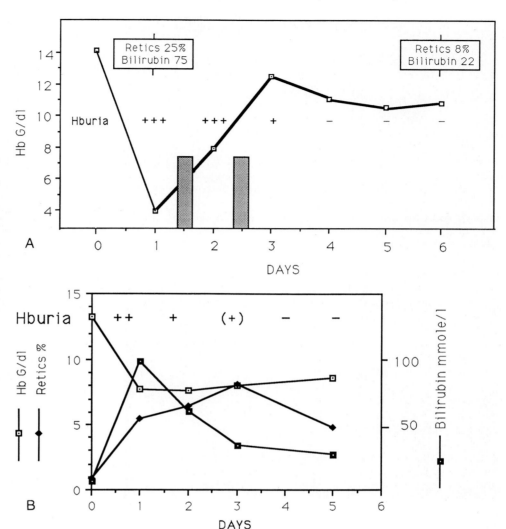

Figure 18–6. Clinical charts of children with acute favism. *A,* A severe attack in a 21-month-old boy, who required two blood transfusions *(hatched bars)* because of life-threatening anemia after ingestion of fava beans. The second blood transfusion was administered because of the persistent hemoglobinuria (Hburia). *B,* A milder attack in a 5-year-old boy. The mother, who is a physician and knows that she is G6PD deficient, reported that the child had eaten fava beans 2 days before admission. Both children had severe G6PD deficiency (red blood cell G6PD activity less than 3% of normal). The values on day 0 are presumed. (Courtesy of Professor Tullio Meloni, Sassari, Sardinia.)

creased. The unconjugated bilirubin level is elevated, but the "liver enzyme" levels are usually normal. The dark urine tests strongly positive for blood. It is easy to demonstrate that this is due to free hemoglobin because after centrifugation the supernatant is as dark as before and in the sediment there are few if any red cells. (Patients are not always alone in confusing hemoglobinuria with hematuria. The importance for the physician of recognizing one from the other in the differential diagnosis of a patient with dark urine cannot be overemphasized) (Table 18–2).

Clinical Course. In the majority of cases the hemolytic attack, even if severe, is self-limited and tends to resolve spontaneously.[68] In the absence of additional or pre-existing pathology the bone marrow response is prompt and effective. Depending on the proportion of red cells that have been destroyed (reflected in the severity of the anemia), the hemoglobin level may be back to normal in 3 to 6 weeks. Although there may be transient elevation of the blood urea level, the development of renal failure in children is exceedingly rare, even in the presence of massive hemoglobinuria (see Fig. 18–6).

Diagnosis. With a history of fava bean ingestion and the finding of hemoglobinuria (clearly reported or directly observed), the diagnosis is almost always straightforward, and it can be made quite confidently even before obtaining the final proof that the patient is G6PD deficient (see later). The differential diagnosis of hemoglobinuria is given in Table 18–2. If hemoglobinuria has already subsided, and the history is uncertain, one is faced instead with the much wider differential diagnosis of an acute hemolytic anemia. The negative direct antiglobulin test will militate against autoimmune hemolytic anemia. In endemic areas it will be important to exclude malaria infection, or the much rarer babesiosis. In the hemolytic-uremic syndrome the red cell morphology is different and there will be evidence of impaired renal function. In all cases the demonstration of G6PD deficiency will be conclusive, and in uncertain cases it will be crucial.

Pathophysiology. The very clinical picture of AHA associated with G6PD deficiency conveys forcefully the impression that, as stated at the beginning of this chapter, hemolysis results from the action of an exogenous factor on intrinsically abnormal red cells.[69] Hemoglo-

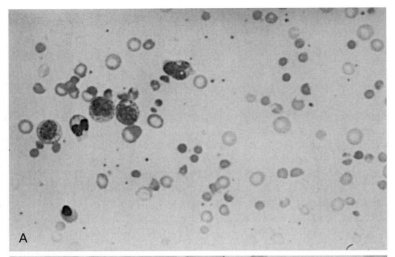

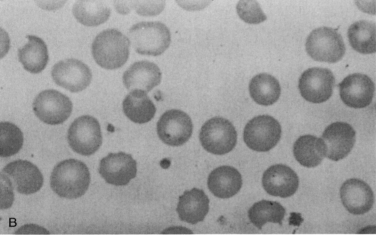

Figure 18-7. Blood smear in G6PD deficiency. *A,* Acute hemolytic anemia (favism). Marked morphologic abnormalities of red blood cells with anisocytosis, polychromasia, bizarre poikilocytes, "bite cells," and "hemighosts." Note the nucleated red blood cell and polymorph leukocytosis with marked shift to the left. *B,* Chronic nonspherocytic hemolytic anemia. The morphologic abnormalities are much less pronounced, but several poikilocytes and the occasional bite cell are seen.

binemia and hemoglobinuria indicate unambiguously that the hemolysis is at least in part intravascular. In first approximation it is easy to visualize the following sequence of events: (1) An oxidative agent causes conversion of GSH to GSSG. (2) Owing to the limited capacity to regenerate GSH of G6PD deficient red cells, their GSH reserve is rapidly depleted. (3) Once GSH is exhausted, the sulfhydryl groups of hemoglobin and probably of other proteins are oxidized to disulfides or sulfoxides. (4) Coarse precipitates of denatured hemoglobin cause irreversible damage to the membrane and the red cells lyse.

Although GSH depletion is a classic *in vitro* finding when red cells are challenged, for instance, with acetyl-phenylhydrazine,[70] not all of these steps have been fully documented *in vivo.* One major difficulty in analyzing the sequential changes that take place in a patient with AHA from the oxidative attack to the final hemolysis is that red cells sampled from the patient are obviously, at any given stage, those that have not yet hemolyzed. However, in one careful study it has been demonstrated that in the course of an episode of favism the first measurable biochemical change is a fall in NADPH, followed by a fall in GSH,[71] in keeping with stages 1 and 2 described earlier. The Heinz bodies are the visible expression of stage 3. Stage 4 is more obscure, because it is not known exactly how the membrane is damaged, although studies suggest that bind-

Table 18-2. HEMOGLOBINURIA IN CHILDREN

Condition	Circumstances	Diagnostic Approach
G6PD deficiency	Exposure to trigger of hemolysis	Test for G6PD activity
Blackwater fever	Relatively rare complication of malaria	Blood slide for malaria parasites
Paroxysmal cold hemoglobinuria	Usually associated with viral infection	Search for Donath-Landsteiner antibody
Mismatched blood transfusion	Usually, ABO incompatibility	Repeat crossmatch
Paroxysmal nocturnal hemoglobinuria	Very rare in children	Ham's test
Clostridium welchii septicemia	Burns; severe open trauma; transfusion of contaminated blood	Culture of blood or appropriate patient material

ing of hemichromes (arising from hemoglobin denaturation) to band 3 molecules may be one intermediate step.[72, 73] Although the diagnostic and pathophysiologic importance of intravascular hemolysis has been emphasized, it is certain that not *all* of the hemolysis is intravascular, as witnessed, for instance, by the enlargement of the spleen. It is not difficult to visualize that the most severely damaged red cells will hemolyze in the blood stream without help, whereas less severely damaged red cells will be recognized as abnormal by macrophages and will undergo extravascular hemolysis in the reticuloendothelial system. This process has been referred to as an example of an "innocent bystander" phenomenon[74] (although the red cells, by virtue of being G6PD deficient, are not that innocent). The role of complement and of immunoglobulins in extravascular hemolysis of damaged G6PD-deficient red cells mediated by macrophages has been discussed in detail.[69]

The clinical picture of AHA impresses one as a sharp transition between the normal steady state and the hemolytic attack, as though the oxidative challenge had tipped the red cell over the hump of a smooth surface leading to a catastrophe. Some chromium-51–labeled red cell survival studies that have been carried out in the *absence* of overt hemolysis in G6PD-deficient subjects have revealed a half-life of 90 to 100 days[75] with some variants but an entirely normal red cell survival with others (A⁻).[76] Because hemolysis of such a low grade, if any, is undetectable on clinical or hematologic grounds, it is reasonable to refer to these subjects as having only acute and not chronic hemolysis.

Finally, it is a very important feature of red cell destruction in AHA associated with G6PD deficiency that it is an orderly function of red cell age. The oldest red cells with the least G6PD are the first to hemolyze, and the hemolytic process progresses upstream toward the cells with more and more G6PD.[77] As a result, there is a selective enrichment in red cells that, although genetically G6PD deficient, have relatively higher levels of G6PD. This phenomenon can be so marked with certain G6PD variants that patients in the posthemolytic state are found to be relatively resistant to further challenge. Under these circumstances, ⁵¹Cr-labeled red cell survival studies will show that this is less than normal, demonstrating that the patient is in a state of compensated hemolysis.[68]

Triggers and Mechanism of Hemolysis. Favism has been used here as a prototypical example of AHA associated with G6PD deficiency, but fava beans are not the only exogenous agent that can cause this manifestation. Indeed, G6PD deficiency was first discovered in the course of investigations on the genetic basis for sensitivity to primaquine. Since that time, numerous other drugs have been reported as potentially dangerous in G6PD-deficient individuals (Table 18–3). There is no obvious relationship in chemical structure among all of these substances, but they have in common the ability to stimulate the pentose phosphate pathway in red cells,[78] which must mean that they are able to oxidize NADPH, directly or indirectly. Extensive stud-

Table 18–3. DRUGS TO BE AVOIDED IN G6PD DEFICIENCY

Antimalarials	*Analgesics*
Primaquine*	Aspirin§
Pamaquine	Phenacetin‖
Chloroquine† (may be used under surveillance when required for prophylaxis or treatment of malaria)	
Sulfonamides and Sulfones	*Anthelminthics*
Sulfanilamide	**β-Naphthol**
Sulfapyridine	**Stibophen**
Sulfadimidine	**Niridazole**
Sulfacetamide	
Sulfisoxazole (Gantrisin)	
Sulfasalazine	
Dapsone‡	
Sulfoxone‖	
Glucosulfone sodium	
Septrin (Glibenclamide)	
Other Antibacterial Compounds	*Miscellaneous*
Nitrofurans	**Vitamin K analogues¶**
Nitrofurantoin	**Naphthalene**
Furazolidone	**Probenecid**
Nitrofurazone	**Dimercaprol (BAL)**
(Nalidixic acid)	**Methylene blue**
Chloramphenicol	
p-Aminosalicylic acid	
(Ciprofloxacin)	

*Reduced dose can be given under surveillance if necessary.
†Can be given under surveillance if necessary.
‡These drugs may cause hemolysis in normal individuals if given in large doses. Many other drugs may produce hemolysis in particular individuals.
§Paracetamol acetaminophen is a safe alternative.
‖Moderate doses probably safe in most cases.
¶Menadiol, 1 mg, parenterally is safe for the prophylaxis of hemorrhagic disease of the newborn.
Drugs in **bold** print should be avoided by people with all forms of G6PD deficiency.
Drugs in normal print should be avoided, in addition, by G6PD-deficient persons of Mediterranean, Middle Eastern, or Asian origin.
Drugs in brackets reflect single case reports or unpublished information.
Modified from WHO Working Group: Glucose 6-phosphate dehydrogenase deficiency. Bull WHO 1989; 67:601.

ies on the components of fava beans responsible for hemolysis have led to the identification of vicine and convicine, two β-glycosides having as aglycones the substituted pyrimidines divicine and isouramil.[79] These compounds, in the course of their auto-oxidation produce free radicals, which, in turn, oxidize GSH, activating the chain reaction of events previously outlined.[80] The drugs listed in Table 18–3, or their metabolites, act in a similar way.

An intriguing feature of AHA associated with G6PD deficiency is its considerably erratic character, which is more conspicuous with certain agents than with others. For instance, it is estimated that in adults ingestion of fava beans does not trigger AHA in more than 25% of cases, and even in the same person favism may occur on one occasion but not on another.[69] Whereas this should not make us complacent, especially with respect to G6PD-deficient children, it poses the question of why this is so. One obvious factor must be the dosage, that is, the amount of fava beans ingested (in relation to body mass). Another is the quality, whereby raw fava beans are more likely to cause favism than cooked, frozen, or canned fava beans. Perhaps even more important is the finding that the glycoside content is a function of the maturity of the beans, with the young, small beans being much richer (as well as more tasty!). Finally, it is possible that β-glycosidases, present in varying amounts both in the beans and in the intestinal mucosa of the consumer, may play an important role in determining the amount and rate of release of active aglycones.[69] As for the drugs, primaquine causes hemolysis regularly but aspirin does so only sometimes.[81] Here it can only be hypothesized that genetic or acquired factors affecting the metabolism of the drug may be responsible.

A rather neglected trigger of hemolysis is bacterial infection (e.g., from pneumococcus).[82] It has been suggested that the mechanism of this may be the release of peroxides during phagocytosis of bacteria by granulocytes.[83] From the clinical point of view it is important to be aware of this complication. Indeed, it is likely that in the past hemolysis has been sometimes attributed to drugs used for treating infection, when it should have been blamed on the infection itself. It is more difficult to imagine a mechanism by which viral infection can trigger hemolysis, but this has been documented in the course of viral hepatitis.[84]

Neonatal Jaundice

Since the elucidation of the mechanism of hemolytic disease of the newborn (HDN) due to rhesus alloimmunization, it has been inevitable that jaundice from any cause developing in the neonatal period would be measured against that yardstick. However, from the epidemiologic point of view it is worth noting that in many populations where G6PD deficiency is prevalent there is a relatively low proportion of pregnancies at risk for rhesus incompatibility.[85, 86] On the other hand, because rhesus-related HDN is disappearing thanks to the implementation of appropriate prophylaxis, one can expect G6PD-related NNJ to be generally on the increase, at least in relative terms.

The clinical picture of NNJ related to G6PD deficiency differs (Fig. 18–8) from the classic rhesus-related NNJ in two main respects: (1) It is very rarely present at birth, and the peak incidence of clinical onset is between day 2 and day 3.[87] (2) There is more jaundice than anemia, and the anemia is very rarely severe.[88] For this reason the terms *HDN* and *NNJ* cannot be regarded as interchangeable, at least in the context of G6PD deficiency.

The severity of NNJ varies enormously from being subclinical to imposing the threat of kernicterus if not treated. Therefore, prompt recognition of the problem is extremely important to avoid crippling neurologic sequelae.[89]

Nature of the Association Between G6PD Deficiency and NNJ. It is not clear why some but not all G6PD-deficient newborns develop NNJ. Indeed, because of this erratic character, one might question whether there is a causal link at all between the two.

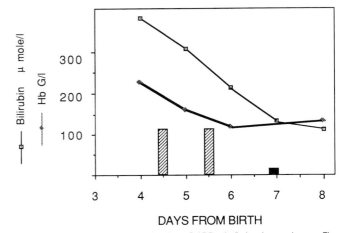

Figure 18–8. Clinical chart of a G6PD-deficient newborn. The newborn was full term (weight at birth, 3200 g). The grandfather was known to have suffered from favism. Clinical jaundice was noted on day 3. The *light hatched bars* represent two full exchange blood transfusions (EBT). Red blood cell G6PD activity was less than 3% of normal. Notice that the newborn was not anemic before EBT. The subsequent anemia was corrected by a "top-up" packed cells transfusion (*dark hatched bar*). The newborn made a full recovery. (Courtesy of Professor Tullio Meloni, Sassari, Sardinia.)

However, several clinical studies have established beyond any possible doubt that the association is statistically much higher than could be expected by chance (Table 18–4).[90] However, because not *all* G6PD-deficient newborns have NNJ, it is likely that some factor in addition to G6PD deficiency is involved and that the same factors that cause NNJ can also, if more extreme, make it severe. There has been an active search for an "additional factor" that may cause NNJ when combined with G6PD deficiency. Several studies have been carried out in an attempt to find such an additional factor. One possibility was that, in view of the marked genetic heterogeneity of G6PD deficiency (see later), NNJ was the prerogative of some but not of others. However, the finding that NNJ is prevalent in widely remote parts of the world (e.g., Sardinia,[91] Nigeria,[90] Singapore,[92] China[93]) does not support this notion. Moreover, NNJ was found among all three different G6PD variants known to be polymorphic in Sardinia.[94]*

*In some cases, variants reported as distinct and assigned different names have turned out to be identical at the molecular level,[120, 177] illustrating the limitations of biochemical analysis or implicating the possibility of postsynthetic modifications.

Table 18–4. ASSOCIATION BETWEEN G6PD DEFICIENCY AND JAUNDICE IN MALE NEWBORNS

	No. Newborns	G6PD Deficiency (%)
Normal	500	22.5
Mild jaundice (bilirubin 150–200 μmol/L)	38	45
Severe jaundice (bilirubin >230 μmol/L)	70	60
Admitted with kernicterus	20	78

Data collected in Ibadan, Nigeria (see reference 90 and Effiong C, Bienzle U, Luzzatto L, unpublished).

Another possibility was that NNJ correlated with the quantitative level of residual G6PD activity in G6PD-deficient newborns, but this was also disproven.[95] Because it is known that fetal red cells differ from those produced after birth in many ways, a third possibility was that in the red cells of some newborns there might be a transient, developmentally related additional enzyme deficiency that, when superimposed on genetically determined G6PD deficiency, would cause NNJ. In this respect, studies have been carried out on glutathione peroxidase, glutathione reductase,[96] and superoxide dismutase,[97] but with negative results. Marked differences in the incidence of NNJ have been demonstrated among different Greek islands;[98] although the study was carried out in the search for an additional genetic factor, thought to be autosomal, it is possible instead that there may be an environmental factor that is different in different islands. In support of the latter possibility, work in Nigeria has revealed that G6PD-deficient newborns with NNJ had had a significantly higher rate of exposure to naphthalene (used in their beddings and clothing) than G6PD-deficient control newborns.[99]

In brief, it is not yet known why some G6PD-deficient newborns develop NNJ, nor are we able to predict which ones will and which ones will not. This, in turn, is related to the question of pathogenesis. Because of the characteristic tendency of G6PD-deficient red cells to hemolyze, and because NNJ is classically the result of HDN, it has been almost taken for granted that NNJ in G6PD-deficient newborns is a manifestation of hemolysis. However, already for some years Meloni and co-workers[88, 91] have called attention to the remarkable dissociation between hyperbilirubinemia and anemia in these newborns; indeed, in one series there was no difference in the distribution of hematocrit values in the cord blood and on day 3 between jaundiced and nonjaundiced G6PD-deficient newborns. They have suggested, therefore, that in a majority of cases this jaundice may be not of hemolytic but of hepatic origin, a view that is still to some extent in dispute, but which has recently received further support.[91a]

In summary, it may be heuristically useful to consider two different types of NNJ associated with G6PD deficiency. (1) A more common type can be best visualized as a marked exaggeration of "physiologic jaundice." This type is not greatly influenced by the environment, and it may result from G6PD deficiency being expressed in the liver. (2) A more rare, frankly hemolytic type, can be visualized as AHA occurring in a newborn because it happened to be exposed to one of the same agents that could cause AHA even in an adult.[100] Here the exogenous agent may be a drug, or infection, or some particular local habit, such as the extensive use of naphthalene ("moth balls" or "camphor balls") in looking after infants.[99] An extreme and preventable example of this type of AHA in the neonatal period, causing severe NNJ, has been reported in a girl heterozygous for G6PD deficiency whose mother had a fava beans meal before delivery. This infant has been described as having favism *in utero*.[101]

Congenital Nonspherocytic Hemolytic Anemia

As stated earlier, all G6PD-deficient individuals have a slightly reduced red cell survival. However, in the steady state the vast majority of them are clinically normal, and their low-grade hemolysis cannot be revealed by any laboratory method short of a chromium-51 study.[61, 102] By contrast, a small minority of G6PD-deficient individuals have a degree of hemolysis that is easily diagnosed by conventional methods and that is sufficiently pronounced to cause them to be anemic. This group of patients is clinically very heterogeneous, for reasons that are explained later; and, therefore, it is not possible to describe any level of expression of this condition as being "typical."

The patient is almost invariably male, and in general he presents because of unexplained jaundice. Frequently the onset is at birth, and a diagnosis is made of NNJ, which may be severe enough to require exchange transfusion. Unfortunately anemia recurs and the jaundice fails to clear completely; this is often the reason for further investigation. In many cases, however, NNJ may become forgotten and the patient is only reinvestigated much later in life (e.g., because of gallstones in a boy or in a young adult). The severity of anemia ranges in different patients from being borderline to being transfusion dependent. The anemia is usually normochromic but somewhat macrocytic, because a large proportion of reticulocytes (up to 20% or more) will cause an increased mean corpuscular volume and a shifted, wider than normal red cell size distribution curve. The red cell morphology is mostly not characteristic, and for this reason it is referred to in the negative as being "nonspherocytic." The bone marrow shows normoblastic hyperplasia, unless the increased requirement of folic acid associated with the high red cell turnover has caused it to become megaloblastic. There is chronic hyperbilirubinemia, decreased haptoglobin, and increased lactate dehydrogenase. Hemoglobinuria is rare, but hemosiderinuria may be detected sometimes. The spleen is usually moderately enlarged in small children, and subsequently it may increase in size sufficiently to cause mechanical discomfort, or hypersplenism, or both.

Pathophysiology. The clinical picture just described is obviously very different from that of AHA seen, for instance, in favism; and it is much more reminiscent of the chronic hemolysis seen in hereditary spherocytosis. Even in severe cases it is different from thalassemia major, because there is no evidence of ineffective erythropoiesis; accelerated destruction is limited to mature circulating red cells. The fact that there is no hemoglobinuria, at least in the steady state, suggests that the hemolysis is mainly extravascular and that therefore its mechanism is different from that of AHA. Indeed, studies of red cell membrane proteins have revealed the presence of high-molecular-weight aggregates,[97, 103] consisting largely of spectrin, which have not been found in asymptomatic G6PD-deficient subjects. These findings suggest that whereas in the latter the reductive potential of residual G6PD is adequate in the steady state, in the former continuous oxidation of sulfhydryl groups takes place, followed by irreversible changes in the configuration of membrane proteins.[104] Naturally this does not mean that the red cells of patients with severe G6PD deficiency are not vulnerable to acute oxidative damage of hemoglobin as well; indeed, the same agents that can cause AHA in persons with the ordinary type of G6PD deficiency will cause severe exacerbations with hemoglobinuria in persons with the severe form of G6PD deficiency. The reason why the severity of CNSHA associated with G6PD deficiency is so variable is that almost every case is due to a different mutation (see later), and each mutation will have a different effect on the stability of the enzyme, on its kinetic properties, or on both.

Diagnosis. The diagnosis of G6PD deficiency is discussed next, but a special problem in relation to CNSHA is to establish firmly the causal link between the former and the latter. If the patient is, for example, a Swede of Swedish ancestry or a Japanese of Japanese ancestry, the link will be taken for granted, and this is generally justified, given the rarity of G6PD deficiency in these populations. On the other hand, if the patient is from a population in which G6PD deficiency is common, its presence in a patient with CNSHA might be a mere coincidence, and the cause of the CNSHA might be something else altogether. In these cases, while other causes of CNSHA are being ruled out, it becomes essential to characterize the G6PD of the patient. If it is a common variant, known to be asymptomatic in other subjects, it can be certainly exonerated, whereas if it is a new unique variant, it is likely to be the culprit.

DIAGNOSIS OF G6PD DEFICIENCY

Although the clinical picture of favism and of other forms of AHA associated with G6PD deficiency is characteristic, the final diagnosis must rely on the direct demonstration of decreased activity of this enzyme in red cells. In NNJ and CNSHA the differential diagnosis is much wider, and therefore this test is even more important. Fortunately, the enzyme assay is very easy, and numerous "screening tests" can be used as substitutes if a spectrophotometer is not available. However, a number of potential pitfalls and sources of error must be understood; and the use of commercial kits is not a substitute for such understanding. Here the value and limitations of the regular quantitative assay are discussed first, and then the use of alternatives is mentioned.

Tests for G6PD Deficiency

G6PD can be assayed by the classic method of Horecker and Smyrniotis,[105] which measures directly the rate of formation of NADPH through its characteristic absorption peak in the near ultraviolet spectrum at 340 nm. The red cell activity is expressed in International Units (micromoles of NADPH produced per minute) per gram of hemoglobin; therefore, it is best to assay the enzyme activity and the hemoglobin concentration in the same hemolysate and work out the ratio. Because

G6PD activity is much higher in leukocytes (particularly in granulocytes) than in erythrocytes, for accurate measurements it is essential to remove all leukocytes by the Ficoll-Hypaque method, or by filtration through cellulose powder,[106] rather than by the cruder approach of sucking off the buffy coat: however, in most cases this is not necessary just for the purpose of diagnosing G6PD deficiency. In normal red cells the range of G6PD activity, measured at 30°C, is 7 to 10 IU/g of hemoglobin.

Several "screening tests" for G6PD deficiency are useful and reliable provided they are properly run and their limitations are understood. The most popular are the dye decolorization tests,[107] the methemoglobin reduction test,[108] and the fluorescence spot test.[109] All of these methods are semi-quantitative, and they are meant to classify a sample simply as "normal" or "deficient." The cutoff point can be set by following the appropriate instructions and by trial and error in the individual diagnostic laboratory: one should aim to classify as deficient any sample having less than 30% of the normal activity, because above this level one is unlikely to encounter clinical manifestations. Screening tests are of course especially useful for testing large numbers of samples. They are also perfectly adequate for diagnostic purposes in patients who are in the steady state but *not* for patients in the post-hemolytic period or with other complications; also, they cannot be expected to identify all heterozygotes. Finally, an ideal screening test ought not to give "false-negative" results (i.e., it should not misclassify a G6PD-deficient subject as normal), but it can be allowed to give a few "false-positive" results (i.e., a G6PD normal subject might be misclassified as G6PD deficient). Ideally, every patient found to be G6PD deficient by screening should be confirmed by the spectrophotometric assay.

Biologic and Technical Problems

The biochemical definition of G6PD deficiency is somewhat arbitrary, because different genetic variants are associated with different degrees of deficiency. However, it seems reasonable to choose as the cutoff point a level that can cause clinical manifestations. As stated earlier, in males there will be no hemolytic complications with a red cell G6PD activity greater than 30% of normal. Thus, from the clinical point of view the demarcation between G6PD-normal and G6PD-deficient males is in principle quite clear-cut. However, two problems deserve consideration (Table 18–5).

1. *The effect of red cell age.* It was mentioned earlier that G6PD decreases gradually as red cells age.[24] Therefore, any condition associated with reticulocytosis will entail an *increase* in G6PD activity. This means that if the subject is genetically G6PD normal the red cell G6PD activity will now be *above* the normal range. This does not affect diagnosis, because G6PD deficiency will be correctly ruled out. However, if the subject is genetically G6PD deficient, the red cell G6PD may now be raised to the extent of being near to or even within

Table 18-5. RED BLOOD CELL G6PD LEVELS IN VARIOUS CLINICAL SITUATIONS

Clinical Condition	Sex	Result of Screening Test	Result of G6PD Assay	Interpretation
Normal	M or F	Normal	8.1	Normal
Normal	M	Abnormal	0.4	G6PD deficiency, steady state
Normal	F	Abnormal	2.1	Heterozygote for G6PD deficiency
Normal	F	Normal	4.9	Heterozygote for G6PD deficiency
Acute hemolysis	M	Abnormal	1.6	Hemolytic attack in G6PD deficiency
Acute hemolysis	F	Normal	7.2	Hemolytic attack in G6PD heterozygote
Chronic hemolysis	M	Normal	15.5	Hemolysis unrelated to G6PD deficiency
Chronic hemolysis	M	Abnormal	1.4	CNSHA, probably due to G6PD deficiency

CNSHA = congenital nonspherocytic hemolytic anemia.

the normal range, and the patient might be therefore misclassified as G6PD normal.[110]

2. *The effect of selective hemolysis.* After a hemolytic attack two circumstances concur to cause the risk of misdiagnosis: first, the older cells have been destroyed selectively; second, the marrow response has caused a sudden outpouring of young cells into the peripheral blood. (A third confusing factor may be admixture of G6PD-normal red cells if the patient has been transfused.) Although the reticulocyte count is a good warning to avoid this mistake, it must be realized that, because reticulocytes turn into morphologically "mature" erythrocytes within 1 to 2 days, their count is not a sensitive index of the mean red cell age: in other words, the mean red cell age may be significantly younger than normal even when the reticulocyte count is normal.

There are several ways to circumvent these problems. First, a G6PD level in the low-normal range (as opposed to higher than normal) in the presence of reticulocytosis is always suspicious. In first approximation, this finding in itself suggests that the patient is actually G6PD deficient. Second, if the patient is suffering or is recovering from AHA, the suspicion generated from the just-mentioned finding can be simply kept in store for a few weeks, when the situation will be evolving toward the steady state, and a repeat test will prove whether the patient is indeed G6PD deficient. Third, if either the urgency of some clinical decision or academic curiosity demands a more prompt solution of the problem, the presence of severely G6PD-deficient red cells can be demonstrated either by enzyme assay of the oldest cells (fractionated by sedimentation) or by a cytochemical method.[111-113]

3. *G6PD deficiency in heterozygotes.* Heterozygote diagnosis by a quantitative test is not difficult in most cases, because the level of G6PD will be intermediate between the normal and the deficient male range: however, in about 10% of cases the G6PD level will "trespass" into either. In addition, the problems outlined for male patients will be compounded in the case of heterozygous females: they can be usually overcome by similar methodologies, particularly by the use of a cytochemical test. With good technique, even only 5% of G6PD-deficient red cells will indicate that the patient is a heterozygote. However, it must be realized that in cases of "extreme phenotypes" (sometimes referred to as arising from "imbalanced lyonization") no test can demonstrate what is not there. In such cases only a family study, if practicable, or DNA analysis, if the mutation involved is known, can prove that the woman is a heterozygote. Fortunately this is not crucial from the clinical point of view. The susceptibility of heterozygotes to develop AHA and its severity are roughly proportional to the percentage of G6PD-deficient red cells. Thus, if this percentage is so low as to be hard to detect, the patient's AHA is most unlikely to be G6PD related.

A special mention should be made of heterozygotes for G6PD variants associated with CNSHA. In the author's experience the mothers of (male) patients with this condition are often G6PD normal either because the variant in the offspring is due to a *de novo* mutation[114] or because the mother is a heterozygote but is phenotypically normal, presumably because somatic selection has favored the hematopoietic progenitor cells with normal G6PD.[49a, 53]

GENETIC VARIATION AND GENETIC POLYMORPHISM OF G6PD

One of the most striking findings in the study of human G6PD has been the high rate of variation that can be revealed in many populations by electrophoretic and quantitative analysis.[11] So many variants have been described, that some kind of classification became desirable.[115, 116] From the point of view of hematology, the most important criterion is, of course, clinical expression. From the biochemical point of view, a simple criterion is the amount of residual enzyme activity that is found even in G6PD-deficient red cells.* A widely accepted classification has been one that combines these two criteria[117] (Table 18-6). In general, not surprisingly, there is a good correlation between the severity of G6PD deficiency and clinical expression. However, there is overlap between the residual enzyme activity in class I variants (which, by definition, are associated with CNSHA) and class II variants (which,

---

*There have been reports in the literature of "complete" G6PD deficiency.[178-180] Naturally what is called complete depends on the sensitivity of the technique used. In fact, if the enzyme is concentrated from a hemolysate after removal of hemoglobin, some G6PD activity is invariably recovered. For the moment, it is safe to assume that complete G6PD deficiency does not exist and it would probably be lethal.

Table 18-6. GENETIC POLYMORPHISM OF G6PD

Class	Clinical Expression	Residual G6PD Activity (% of Normal)	Variants Reported*	No. of Variants†	Electrophoretically Normal (%)
I‡	Severe (CNSHA)	<20‡	94	44	35
II	Mild	<10	114	28	31
III	Mild	10–60	110	16	15
IV	None	100	52	2	10
V	None	>100	2		
			Total 372	90	

*Based on biochemical characterization, before molecular analysis available.
†Based on specific mutations identified by molecular analysis.
‡Class I variants are defined by their clinical phenotype of CNSHA, regardless of the level of residual activity: partly because of reticulocytosis in these patients, they may be associated with enzyme levels higher than some class II variants.

by definition, are only associated with AHA). On the other hand, there is wide overlap in clinical expression between class II and class III variants, because both groups are associated with both AHA and NNJ. Class IV and class V do not entail any known clinical manifestations.

As stated in a previous section, it is reasonable to assume that most of these variants result from point mutations within the coding region of the G6PD gene. Indeed, sequence analysis has largely validated this assumption: in other words, each variant is encoded by a different allele at the G6PD structural locus.* An important characteristic of numerous G6PD variants is that they are so prevalent in certain populations to be regarded as "polymorphisms," rather than pathologic mutants. This distinction is to some extent arbitrary. In classic population genetics the rigorous definition of a polymorphic allele is that its frequency is higher than could be accounted for by recurrent mutation: for convenience, an allele is designated as polymorphic when its frequency is at least 1% (a very conservative approximation of the more rigorous definition). By this criterion, there are an estimated 100 or so polymorphic G6PD alleles already known.

Not surprisingly, individual variants are characteristically found in certain geographic areas. Thus, G6PD Mediterranean is the most prevalent variant in this area and in the Middle East, and it is also found as far as Iran and India.[70] G6PD A⁻ is characteristic of Africa,[118] but it has been found also in southern Italy,[114] Spain,[119] and Mexico.[120] G6PD Mahidol is characteristic of Thailand and may be quite widespread elsewhere in Southeast Asia.[121]

The ratio of subjects having G6PD deficiency associated with CNSHA to those having "simple" G6PD deficiency varies in different populations. For instance, in Japan, where G6PD deficiency is, on the whole, very rare, the majority of patients with G6PD deficiency have been reported to have CNSHA.[122] This suggests

that CNSHA, caused by rare sporadic variants, many of which may result from recent mutations, reflects the intrinsic mutation rate of the human *Gd* gene, which is likely to be uniform throughout the world, whereas "simple" G6PD deficiency results almost always from common variants, which have arisen many generations ago and spread through biologic selection.

G6PD Variants and Clinical Manifestations

The three variants mentioned previously, G6PD A⁻, G6PD Mediterranean, and G6PD Mahidol, are probably those for which the clinical expression has been best characterized.[102] It is conventionally reported that Mediterranean and Mahidol (class II variants) give more severe manifestations than A⁻ (a class III variant). Although this may be true when large series of cases are compared, there is certainly so much overlap among the groups that in an individual case the differences are, in my own view, not very relevant with respect to patient management. For instance, whether hemolysis is "self limited" or not depends on the offending agent, on its dose, and on the time course of exposure at least as much as it depends on the G6PD variant involved. Notably, favism has been unambiguously documented with A⁻ G6PD deficiency.[123, 124]

Genotype-Phenotype Correlations

In terms of clinical expression, the demarcation between class I variants and all others is, by definition, much more clear-cut. Indeed, one of the outstanding questions in the biochemical genetics of G6PD is why a particular variant can cause CNSHA, rather than just AHA. In certain cases the level of residual enzyme activity is not the whole answer: qualitative differences are important, as first suggested by Kirkman.[124a] The most likely way in which a structural change can significantly alter the function of G6PD, *given the same level of deficiency*, is that it affects the binding of one of the main ligands (i.e., G6P, NADP, NADPH). For instance, G6PD Mediterranean and G6PD Coimbra both have mutations near the G6P-binding site, and both have *increased* affinity for G6P. Perhaps because of this, although they are both severely deficient, they belong

*In some cases, variants reported as distinct and assigned different names have turned out to be identical at the molecular level,[120, 177] illustrating the limitations of biochemical analysis or implicating the possibility of postsynthetic modifications. On the other hand, the A⁻ variant has been proven to be heterogenous[119] and the same may turn out to be true of others. Therefore, the figures in Table 18–6 are not necessarily overestimating the genetic variability of human G6PD.

to class II and not to class I. G6PD Orissa, identified very recently as the main polymorphic variant in tribal Indian populations,[125] also belongs to class II, in spite of having a *decreased* affinity for NADP. Thus, the affinity for G6P appears to be of greater importance. Indeed, an analysis of the distribution of K_m^{G6P} values of class I variants, compared with that of class II and III variants, shows that they are significantly lower in the latter group.[7]

However, in most cases the main factor responsible for causing CNSHA is a very low level of residual activity in red cells, which, in turn, is due to marked *in vivo* instability. It is quite remarkable that, although G6PD mutations as a whole are evenly spread throughout the gene's coding sequence, the majority of class I mutations are clustered in exons 10 and 11. The three-dimensional model of the human G6PD dimer has, at long last, provided a reasonable explanation for this finding.[20] Indeed, these two exons encode the protein region that constitutes the interface between the two identical subunits of the enzyme. As a result, any mutation in this region causes the respective amino acid replacements in the two subunits to be quite near each other in the dimer structure, thus potentially increasing their deleterious effects. Even more important, because there is no covalent link between the subunits, it stands to reason that any interference with the shape of the interface surfaces may affect their mutual fit and thus dramatically destabilize the active form of the enzyme.

G6PD Polymorphism and Malaria

The striking correlation between the worldwide distribution of G6PD deficiency (Fig. 18–9) and that of *Plasmodium falciparum* prompted the formulation of the "malaria hypothesis" 30 years ago.[77, 126–129] Since that time, numerous more detailed epidemiologic studies (which can be referred to as "micro-mapping"[130]), as well as clinical studies,[77, 131, 132] have provided additional evidence to support the hypothesis that malaria selects for G6PD deficiency. A more difficult question is to understand the mechanism of this phenomenon. *In vivo* studies have shown that *P. falciparum* parasitemia tends to be lower in G6PD-deficient heterozygous (Gd^+/Gd^-) girls than in G6PD normal subjects;[133] this might protect them from developing those high levels of parasitemia that become life-threatening. However, there are conflicting data on whether this is also the case for G6PD-deficient (Gd^-) hemizygous boys.[133, 133a] *In vitro* studies have shown that invasion by *P. falciparum* of G6PD-deficient red cells takes place normally, but intracellular development of the parasite (i.e., schizogony) is impaired.[134, 135] This impairment is almost completely overcome after the parasite has gone through several schizogonic cycles in G6PD-deficient red cells.[23, 136] This could explain why heterozygotes, who are genetic mosaics, are relatively protected, but hemizygotes are not.[126] However, the precise mechanism whereby growth of the parasite is first inhibited, and whereby the same parasite subsequently adapts to the G6PD-deficient cellular environment remains unexplained. It has been shown conclusively that *P. falci-*

parum has its own G6PD,[137] with properties that are significantly different from those of the host cell enzyme,[138] and it is possible that further investigations of how the parasite's G6PD synthesis is regulated might shed light on the mechanism of protection by G6PD deficiency against malaria and therefore of selection by malaria for G6PD deficiency.

In the meantime, an added strong argument in favor of malaria selection is the genetic heterogeneity of polymorphic *Gd⁻* alleles in itself. Indeed, each one of these alleles, having arisen through an independent mutational event, must have increased in frequency, on its own, in a particular geographic area where malaria was or still is endemic—a good example of convergent evolution driven by the same selective force.

MANAGEMENT OF G6PD DEFICIENCY
Preventive Medicine

Because NNJ and AHA are the most common manifestations of G6PD deficiency, it is most important to consider how they can be prevented. The first step is to identify G6PD-deficient individuals, and this is where screening is most pertinent. Of course, whether population-wide screening is both desirable and feasible depends primarily on the prevalence of G6PD deficiency in any particular community. This will determine the cost-benefit ratio (the main cost being labor, because the reagents and equipment needed are relatively very inexpensive). If screening is done at all, it is best done on cord blood; and this is already practiced, for instance, in Sardinia, in Thailand, and in Malaysia. Once a subject is known to be G6PD deficient, the two main implications are the risk of NNJ and the importance to avoid exposure to agents that can cause AHA. NNJ cannot be prevented as yet, but the awareness of G6PD deficiency must entail surveillance for NNJ until at least day 4 and special recommendations with respect to factors, such as naphthalene, that can cause it or make it worse. By contrast, at least one type of AHA, namely, favism, is completely preventable, if the persons concerned, and their families in the first place, accept the advice to give up eating fava beans (Fig. 18–10). Prevention of infection-induced hemolysis is obviously more difficult. Prevention of drug-induced hemolysis is possible in most cases by choosing alternative drugs, but it may be difficult when there are none. The most common problem is the need to administer primaquine for the eradication of malaria due to *P. vivax* or *P. malariae*. In these cases the administration of a lower dosage for a longer time is the recommended approach. There will still be hemolysis, but under appropriate surveillance it will be of an acceptably mild degree.

A special problem in prevention is what to do about new drugs, the hemolytic potential of which is unknown. Although *in vitro* methods to test drugs in this respect do exist,[139, 140] such tests are not carried out before drugs are released on the market. This is unfortunate, especially when a new drug is introduced in an area where G6PD deficiency is common; and in

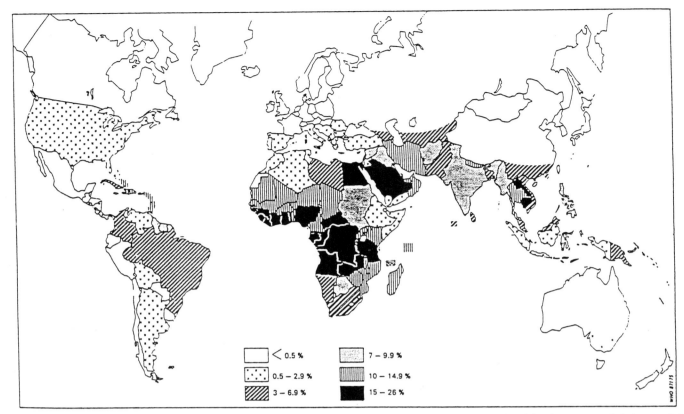

Figure 18–9. World map of G6PD deficiency. (From WHO Working Group: Glucose-6-phosphate dehydrogenase deficiency. Bull WHO 1989; 67:601.)

Legend:
< 0.5 %	7 – 9.9 %
0.5 – 2.9 %	10 – 14.9 %
3 – 6.9 %	15 – 26 %

practice their hemolytic potential will become apparent only from clinical observation.

Treatment

A child with AHA may be a diagnostic problem that, once solved, does not require any specific treatment at all; or he may be a medical emergency requiring immediate action. The most urgent question is whether the child needs a blood transfusion or not. It is difficult to give absolute directives, but the following guidelines may be useful[141]

1. If the hemoglobin level is below 7 g/dL, the child should be transfused forthwith.

2. If the hemoglobin level is below 9 g/dL, and there is evidence of persistent brisk hemolysis (hemoglobinuria), immediate blood transfusion is also indicated.

3. If the hemoglobin level is above 9 g/dL but hemoglobinuria persists, or if the hemoglobin level is between 7 and 9 g/dL but there is no hemoglobinuria, the child is kept under close observation for at least 48 hours and transfused if either condition 1 or 2 develops.

The most important complication that may require treatment is acute renal failure, which is exceedingly rare in children. Apart from a standard renal failure regimen, hemodialysis may be necessary. It has been claimed that haptoglobin administration may help to prevent renal failure in hemolytic anemia associated

with G6PD deficiency,[60] but this anecdotal report does not seem convincing.[142]

Management of NNJ. The management of NNJ due to G6PD deficiency does not differ from that recommended for other causes. Thus, mild cases do not require treatment; intermediate cases require phototherapy; and severe cases require exchange transfusion treatment, just as in NNJ due to "classic" HDN. A "gentler" approach to the management of NNJ has been advocated.[143] Although it is unquestionable that the prompt use of phototherapy has effectively reduced markedly the number of newborns needing exchange transfusion, one should be probably very cautious in avoiding the other extreme. Kernicterus is still an impending threat, especially when severe NNJ is associated with anemia, hypoxia, or infection. In addition, it is not impossible (although entirely speculative) that G6PD deficiency may be expressed in the brain, thus increasing the risk of neurologic damage. For these reasons, the guidelines for the management of NNJ associated with G6PD deficiency still stand.[141] Specifically, it is recommended that, in full-term newborns, exchange transfusion is carried out if the serum bilirubin level exceeds 15 mg/dL in the first 2 days of life, or 20 mg/dL at any time in the first week of life.

Management of CNSHA. In general terms, management of CNSHA from G6PD deficiency does not differ from that of CNSHA due to other causes (e.g., pyruvate kinase deficiency). If the anemia is not severe, regular folic acid supplements and regular hematologic sur-

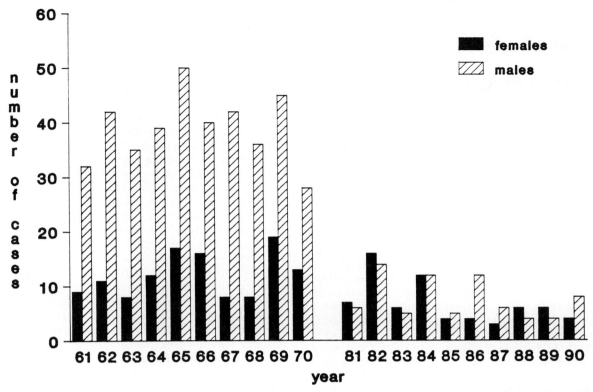

Figure 18-10. Control of favism in a community. The data show the decrease in the number of yearly admissions for favism in the children's department of the main city and university hospitals in Sassari, northern Sardinia. During the 10-year period intervening between the two sets of data, two preventive measures were adopted: (1) education through the media and (2) screening of all newborns for G6PD deficiency. Note the dramatic reduction in the incidence of favism in boys and the more modest decrease in girls. The data suggest that (1) preventive measures are effective; (2) the increased proportion of girls can be attributed to failure of the screening method used to pick out many of the heterozygotes; and (3), in view of (2), the dramatic reduction observed in boys can perhaps be credited to screening more than to the educational campaign. (Courtesy of Professor Tullio Meloni, Sassari, Sardinia.)

veillance suffice. It is important to avoid exposure to potentially hemolytic drugs, and blood transfusion may be indicated when exacerbations occur, mostly in concomitance with intercurrent infection. In rare patients, the anemia is so severe that it must be regarded as transfusion dependent. In these cases blood transfusion will be probably needed at approximately 2-month intervals, to keep the hemoglobin in the 8- to 10-g/dL range. A hypertransfusion regimen aiming to maintain a normal hemoglobin level is not indicated (because there is no ineffective erythropoiesis in the bone marrow). However, depending on the extent of blood transfusion requirement, appropriate iron chelation should be instituted from the age of 2 years onward and must be continued as long as transfusion treatment is necessary; sometimes the transfusion requirement may decrease after puberty.

A special problem is that of splenectomy. There is no evidence of *selective* red cell destruction in the spleen, as in hereditary spherocytosis. However, the fact that the spleen is usually enlarged suggests that its role in hemolysis is not negligible. In practice, there are three indications for splenectomy: (1) if splenomegaly becomes a physical encumbrance; (2) if there is evidence of hypersplenism; and (3) if the anemia is severe, even in the absence of the first two indications. Splenectomy

may reduce the overall rate of hemolysis just enough to make a transfusion-dependent child become transfusion independent. This is doubly important because it will make it possible to dispense with desferrioxamine. The author knows of two patients in whom splenectomy did thus benefit G6PD-deficient patients with severe CNSHA. Of course Pneumovax immunization should be given before splenectomy and penicillin prophylaxis after splenectomy.

When a diagnosis of CNSHA is made, the family must be given genetic counseling, and an effort should be made to establish whether the mother is a heterozygote (this may not be easy by conventional techniques; see earlier). If she is, the chance of recurrence is 1:2 for every subsequent male pregnancy. Prenatal diagnosis can be offered, and it can be carried out by a G6PD assay on amniotic fluid cells, although the expression of G6PD deficiency in these cells varies with each G6PD variant. Nowadays a probably better alternative is to test DNA from chorionic villi with one of the available polymorphic probes that are closely linked to G6PD, and for which the mother is heterozygous. Ideally, the mutation in the G6PD gene of the boy affected by CNSHA could be identified, which will make it possible to establish conclusively whether the mother is heterozygous. Prenatal diagnosis could then be carried out by customized allele-specific oligonucleotide hybridization or by analysis with an appropriate restriction enzyme.[143a]

G6PD DEFICIENCY IN NONERYTHROID CELLS

As mentioned earlier, because nucleated somatic cells have the capability to synthesize G6PD constitutively, they are less affected than red cells by G6PD deficiency.[144] Specifically, if G6PD deficiency is due to instability of a mutant enzyme one would not expect nucleated cells to be severely affected. For instance, subjects with G6PD Mediterranean have less than 5% G6PD activity in red cells but about 30% of normal in granulocytes; subjects with G6PD A⁻ have about 12% G6PD activity in red cells but near-normal activity in granulocytes. On the other hand, if deficiency results from a drastic change in catalytic efficiency, or in substrate affinity, then deficiency may be more universal. In practice, the only well-documented pathologic effect is expressed in granulocytes. Very few of the class I G6PD variants cause not only CNSHA but also granulocyte dysfunction, mainly in the way of impaired killing of phagocytosed bacteria (an example is G6PD Barcelona[145]). Patients with these variants have increased susceptibility to bacterial infection, particularly with *Staphylococcus aureus*. The mechanism whereby G6PD deficiency impairs phagocytosis is a defect of the oxidative burst, due to a shortage in NADPH supply, similar to that observed in chronic granulomatous disease, in which one of the components of the cytochrome-b_{245} system is defective.[146*]

Erythrocytes are not the only non-nucleated cells in the body. Another example is in the eye lens, and juvenile cataracts have been reported occasionally in subjects with G6PD deficiency.[147, 148] Whether G6PD deficiency is more generally associated with higher frequency or earlier onset of cataracts appears to be still controversial.[149–154]

HEMATOLOGIC ASSOCIATIONS OF G6PD DEFICIENCY

Because the epidemiology of G6PD deficiency overlaps with that of other polymorphic red cell traits, it is not surprising that they may occur together in the same person. In several studies, the combination of G6PD deficiency with the sickle cell trait has been no more frequent than could be expected by chance.[155–158] The combination of G6PD deficiency with the β-thalassemia trait has been found to cause a significant increase of the mean corpuscular volume,[159, 160] which remains, however, below the normal range. From the clinical point of view, the most important association is that of G6PD deficiency with homozygous sickle cell

anemia. Some earlier anecdotal reports had suggested that the former might ameliorate the latter. In fact, several studies have shown that there is no significant difference in a variety of clinical and hematologic parameters between two otherwise comparable groups of patients with sickle cell anemia, with and without G6PD deficiency;[110, 157, 161, 162] but it must be born in mind that acute intravascular hemolysis superimposed on chronic severe extravascular hemolysis is an added risk with this association.[163] Association of G6PD deficiency with thalassemia major is unlikely to be a problem, because patients with the latter condition are treated with regular blood transfusion or with bone marrow transplantation. However, the association may be significant in patients with various forms of thalassemia intermedia syndromes (e.g., E-β thalassemia[164]).

Occasionally, G6PD deficiency has been observed in association with much more rare red cell abnormalities, such as pyruvate kinase deficiency,[165, 166] congenital dyserythropoietic anemia type II,[167–169] and hereditary elliptocytosis.[170] In these cases the two abnormalities seem to produce only additive clinical effects, but in at least one family G6PD deficiency was synergistic with hereditary spherocytosis in causing a moderately severe chronic hemolytic anemia.[171]

References

1. Beutler E: Glucose 6-phosphate dehydrogenase deficiency. In Beutler E (ed): Hemolytic Anemia in Disorders of Red Cell Metabolism. New York, Plenum Medical Book Co., 1978, pp 23–167.
2. Levy HR: Glucose 6-phosphate dehydrogenase. In Meister A (ed): Advances in Enzymology. Vol. 48. New York, John Wiley & Sons, Inc., 1979, pp 97–192.
3. Arese P, Mannuzzu L, Turrini F: Pathophysiology of favism. Folia Haematol 1989; 116:745.
4. Beutler E: The genetics of glucose-6-phosphate dehydrogenase deficiency. Semin Hematol 1990; 27:137.
5. Beutler E: Glucose 6-phosphate dehydrogenase deficiency. N Engl J Med 1991; 324:169.
6. Luzzatto L, Mehta A: Glucose 6-phosphate dehydrogenase deficiency. In Scriver CR, Beaudet AL, et al (eds): The Metabolic and Molecular Basis of Inherited Disease. 7th ed. New York, McGraw-Hill Book Co., 1995, pp 3367–3398.
7. Luzzatto L, Testa U: Human erythrocyte G6PD. Structure and function in normal and mutant subjects. In Piomelli S, Yachnin S (eds): Current Topics in Hematology. Vol. 1. New York, Alan R. Liss, Inc., 1978, pp 1–70.
8. Peisach J, Blumberg WE, Rachmilewicz EA: The demonstration of ferrihemochrome intermediates in Heinz body formation following the reduction of oxyhemoglobin A by acetylphenylhydrazine. Biochim Biophys Acta 1975; 393:404.
9. Kirkman HN, Gaetani GF: Catalase: a tetrameric enzyme with four tightly bound molecules of NADPH. Proc Natl Acad Sci U S A 1984; 81:4343.
10. Gaetani GF, Galiano S, et al: Catalase and glutathione peroxidase are equally active in detoxification of hydrogen peroxide in human erythrocytes. Blood 1989; 73:334.
11. Luzzatto L, Battistuzzi G: Glucose 6-phosphate dehydrogenase. Adv Hum Genet 1985; 14:217.
12. Antonenkov VD: Dehydrogenases of the pentose phosphate pathway in rat liver peroxisomes. Eur J Biochem 1989; 183:75.
13. Cohen P, Rosemeyer MA: Human glucose-6-phosphate dehydrogenase: purification of the erythrocyte enzyme and the influence of ions on its activity. Eur J Biochem 1969; 8:1.
14. Persico MG, Viglietto G, et al: Isolation of human glucose-6-phosphate dehydrogenase (G6PD) cDNA clones: primary structure of the protein and unusual 5′ non-coding region. Nucleic Acids Res 1986; 14:2511.

---

*Because chronic granulomatous disease is also X linked, it was thought initially that it was related to G6PD deficiency.[179] In fact, cytochrome-b_{245} has now been mapped to Xq21, and its relationship to G6PD is significant at the metabolic level, rather than at the genetic level.

15. Jeffery J, Soderling-Barros J, et al: Glucose 6-phosphate dehydrogenase. Characteristics revealed by the rat liver enzyme. Eur J Biochem 1989; 186:551.

15a. Naylor CD, Rowland P, et al: Glucose 6-phosphate dehydrogenase mutations causing enzyme deficiency in a model of the tertiary structure of the human enzyme. Blood 1996; 87:2974.

16. Camardella L, Caruso C, et al: Human erythrocyte glucose-6-phosphate dehydrogenase. Identification of a reactive lysyl residue labelled with pyridoxal 5′-phosphate. Eur J Biochem 1988; 171:485.

17. Mason PJ, Vulliamy TJ, et al: The production of normal and variant human glucose-6-phosphate dehydrogenase in *cos* cells. Eur J Biochem 1988; 178:109.

18. Bautista JM, Mason PJ, Luzzatto L: Human glucose-6-phosphate dehydrogenase lysine 205 is dispensable for substrate binding but essential for catalysis. FEBS Lett 1995; 366:61.

19. Rowland P, Basak A, et al: The three-dimensional structure of glucose 6-phosphate dehydrogenase from *Leuconostoc mesenteroides* refined at 2.0 A resolution. Structure 1994; 2:1073.

20. Naylor CE, Rowland P, et al: Glucose 6-phosphate dehydrogenase mutations causing enzyme deficiency in a model of the tertiary structure of the human enzyme. Blood 1996; 87:2974.

21. Luzzatto L: Regulation of the activity of glucose-6-phosphate dehydrogenase by NADP$^+$ and NADPH. Biochim Biophys Acta 1967; 146:18.

22. Kirkman HN, Gaetani GD, et al: Red cell NADP and NADPH in glucose-6-phosphate dehydrogenase deficiency. J Clin Invest 1975; 55:875.

23. Luzzatto L, Sodeinde O, Martini G: Genetic variation in the host and adaptive phenomena in *Plasmodium falciparum* infection. In Evered D, Whelan J (eds): Malaria and the Red Cell, Ciba Foundation Symposium 94. London, Pitman Medical Publishing Co., 1983, pp 159–173.

24. Beutler E: The red cell. In Beutler E (ed): Hemolytic Anemia in Disorders of Red Cell Metabolism. New York, Plenum Medical Book Co., 1978, pp 1–21.

25. Piomelli S, Corash LM, et al: *In vivo* lability of glucose-6-phosphate dehydrogenase in Gd A and Gd Mediterranean deficiency. J Clin Invest 1968; 47:940.

26. Beutler E: The relationship of red cell enzymes to red cell life-span. Blood Cells 1988; 14:69.

27. Marks PA, Johnson AB: Relationship between the age of human erythrocytes and their osmotic resistance: a basis for separating young and old erythrocytes. J Clin Invest 1958; 37:1542.

28. Beutler E, Gelbart T, Kuhl W: Human red cell glucose-6-phosphate dehydrogenase: all active enzyme has sequence predicted by the X chromosome-encoded cDNA. Cell 1990; 62:7.

29. Henikoff S, Smith JM: The human mRNA that provides the N-terminus of chimeric G6PD encodes GMP reductase. Cell 1989; 58:1021.

30. Kanno H, Huang I-Y, et al: Two structural genes on different chromosomes are required for encoding the major subunit of human red cell glucose-6-phosphate dehydrogenase. Cell 1989; 58:595.

31. Mason PJ, Bautista J, et al: Human red cell glucose 6-phosphate dehydrogenase is encoded only on the X-chromosome. Cell 1990; 63:9.

32. Pai GS, Sprenkle JA, et al: Localization of the loci for hypoxanthine phosphoribosyltransferase and glucose-6-phosphate dehydrogenase and biochemical evidence of non-random X-chromosome expression from studies of human X-autosome translocation. Proc Natl Acad Sci U S A 1980; 77:2810.

33. Szabo P, Purrello M, et al: Cytological mapping of the human glucose-6-phosphate dehydrogenase gene distal to the fragile-X site suggests a high rate of meiotic recombination across this site. Proc Natl Acad Sci U S A 1984; 81:7855.

34. Yoshida A, Kan YW: Origin of "fused" glucose-6-phosphate dehydrogenase. Cell 1990; 62:11.

35. Patterson M, Schwartz C, et al: Physical mapping studies on the human X chromosome in the region Xq27-Zqter. Genomics 1987; 1:297.

36. Willard HF, Cremers F, et al: Report and abstracts of the Fifth International Workshop on Human X Chromosome Mapping 1994. Heidelberg, Germany, April 24–27, 1994. Cytogenet Cell Genet 1994; 67:295.

37. Pilia G, Little RD, et al: Isochores and CpG islands in YAC contigs in human Xq26.1-qter. Genomics 1993; 17:456.

38. Vulliamy TJ, Othman A, et al: Polymorphic sites in the African population detected by sequence analysis of the glucose 6-phosphate dehydrogenase gene outline the evolution of the variants A and A−. Proc Natl Acad Sci U S A 1991; 88:8568.

38a. Filosa S, Calabro V, et al: G6PD haplotypes spanning Xq28 from F8C to red/green color vision. Genomics 1993; 17:6.

39. Chen EY, Cheng A, et al: Sequence of human glucose 6-phosphate dehydrogenase cloned in plasmids and a yeast artificial chromosome. Genomics 1991; 10:792.

40. Beutler E, Yeh M, Fairbanks VF: The normal human female as a mosaic of X-chromosome activity: studies using the gene for G6PD deficiency as a marker. Proc Natl Acad Sci U S A 1962; 48:9.

41. Martini G, Toniolo D, et al: Structural analysis of the X-linked gene encoding human glucose 6-phosphate dehydrogenase. EMBO J 1986; 5:1849.

42. Ursini MV, Scalera L, Martini G: High level of transcription driven by a 400 bp segment of the human G6PD promoter. Biochem Biophys Res Commun 1990; 170:1203.

43. Philippe M, Larondelle Y, et al: Promoter function of the human glucose-6-phosphate dehydrogenase gene depends on two GC boxes that are cell specifically controlled. Eur J Biochem 1994; 226:377.

44. Mason PJ, Stevens DJ, et al: Genomic structure and sequence of the *Fugu rubripes* glucose 6-phosphate dehydrogenase gene (G6PD). Genomics 1995; 26:587.

45. Nance WE: Genetic tests with a sex-linked marker: G-6-PD. Cold Spring Harbor Symp Quant Biol 1964; 29:415.

46. Rinaldi A, Filippi G, Siniscalco M: Variability of red cell phenotypes between and within individuals in an unbiased sample of 77 certain heterozygotes for G6PD deficiency in Sardinians. Am J Hum Genet 1976; 28:496.

47. Gale RE, Wheadon H, Linch DC: X-chromosome inactivation patterns using HPRT and PGK polymorphisms in haematologically normal and post-chemotherapy females. Br J Haematol 1991; 79:193.

48. Nyhan WL, Bakay B, et al: Hemixygous expression of glucose 6-phosphate dehydrogenase deficiency in erythrocytes of heterozygotes for the Lesch-Nyhan syndrome. Proc Natl Acad Sci U S A 1970; 65:214.

49. Town M, Athanasiou-Metaxa M, Luzzatto L: Intragenic interspecific complementation of glucose 6-phosphate dehydrogenase in human-hamster cell hybrids. Somatic Cell Mol Genet 1990; 16:97.

49a. Filosa S, Giacometti N, et al: Somatic cell selection is a major determinant of the blood cell phenotype in heterozygotes for glucose 6-phosphate dehydrogenase mutations causing severe enzyme deficiency. Am J Hum Genet 1996; 59:887.

50. Gaetani GF, Ferraris AM: Recent developments on Mediterranean G6PD. Br J Haematol 1988; 68:1.

51. Linder D, Gartler SM: Glucose 6-phosphate dehydrogenase mosaicism. Utilization as a cell marker in the study of leiomyomas. Science 1965; 150:67.

52. Luzzatto L, Mehta A: Glucose-6-phosphate dehydrogenase deficiency. In Scriver CR, Beaudet AL, et al (eds): The Metabolic Basis of Inherited Disease. 6th ed. New York, McGraw-Hill Book Co., 1989, pp 2237–2265.

53. Luzzatto L, Usanga EA, et al: Imbalance in X-chromosome expression: evidence for a human X-linked gene affecting growth of haemopoietic cells. Science 1979; 205:1418.

54. Morelli A, Benatti U, et al: Biochemical mechanisms of glucose-6-phosphate dehydrogenase deficiency. Proc Natl Acad Sci U S A 1978; 75:1979.

55. Viglietto G, Montanaro V, et al: Common glucose 6-phosphate dehydrogenase (G6PD) variants from the Italian population: biochemical and molecular characterization. Ann Hum Genet 1990; 54:1.

56. Poggi V, Town M, et al: Identification of a single base change in the G6PD gene by PCR amplification of the entire coding region from genomic DNA. Biochem J 1990; 271:157.

57. Beutler E, Vulliamy T, Luzzatto L: Hematologically important mutations: glucose 6-phosphate dehydrogenase. Blood Cells Mol Dis 1996; 22:49.

58. Pandolfi PP, Sonati F, et al: Targeted disruption of the housekeeping gene encoding glucose 6-phosphate dehydrogenase (G6PD): G6PD is dispensable for pentose synthesis but essential for defense against oxidative stress. EMBO J 1995; 14:5209.

59. Mason PJ, Sonati MF, et al: New glucose 6-phosphate dehydrogenase mutations associated with chronic anemia. Blood 1995; 85:1377.

59a. Mason PJ: New insights into G6PD deficiency. Br J Haematol 1996; 94:585.

60. Ohga S, Higashi E, et al: Haptoglobin therapy for acute favism: a Japanese boy with glucose-6-phosphate dehydrogenase Guadalajara. Br J Haematol 1995; 89:421.

61. Dacie JV: Hereditary enzyme deficiency haemolytic anaemias. III: Deficiency of glucose-6-phosphate dehydrogenase. In Dacie JV (ed): Haemolytic Anaemias. The Hereditary Haemolytic Anaemias. 3rd ed. London, Churchill Livingstone, Inc., 1985, pp 364–418.

62. Luzzatto L: Inherited haemolytic anaemias. In Hoffbrand AV, Lewis SM (eds): Postgraduate Haematology. 3rd ed. London, Heinemann, 1989, pp 146–182.

63. Sansone G, Piga AM, Segni G. Il Favismo. Torino, Minerva Medica, 1958.

64. Fermi C, Martinetti P: Studio sul favismo. Ann Ig Sper 1905; 15:76.

65. Chan TK, Chan WC, Weed RI: Erythrocyte hemighosts: a hallmark of severe oxidative injury in vivo. Br J Haematol 1982; 50:575.

66. Fischer TM, Meloni T, et al: Membrane cross bonding in red cells in favic crisis: a missing link in the mechanism of extravascular hemolysis. Br J Haematol 1985; 59:159.

67. Rifkind RA: Heinz bodies anaemia: an ultrastructural study. II. Red cell sequestration and destruction. Blood 1965; 26:433.

68. Tarlov AR, Brewer GJ, et al: Primaquine sensitivity. Glucose-6-phosphate dehydrogenase deficiency: an inborn error of metabolism of medical and biological significance. Arch Intern Med 1962; 109:209.

69. Arese P, De Flora A: Pathophysiology of hemolysis in glucose 6-phosphate dehydrogenase deficiency. Semin Hematol 1990; 27:1.

70. Beutler E, Dern RJ, Alving AS: The hemolytic effect of primaquine. VI. An in vitro test for sensitivity of erythrocytes to primaquine. J Lab Clin Med 1955; 45:40.

71. Mareni C, Repetto L, et al: Favism: looking for a autosomal gene associated with glucose-6-phosphate dehydrogenase deficiency. J Med Genet 1984; 21:278.

72. Low PS: Structure and function of the cytoplasmic domain of band 3: center of erythrocyte membrane-peripheral protein interactions. Biochim Biophys Acta 1986; 864:145.

73. Waugh SM, Walder JA, Low PS: Partial characterization of the copolymerization reaction of erythrocyte membrane band 3 with hemichrome. Biochemistry 1987; 26:1777.

74. Kasper ML, Miller WJ, Jacob HS: G6PD deficiency infectious haemolysis: a complement dependent innocent bystander phenomenon. Br J Haematol 1986; 63:85.

75. Bernini L, Latte B, et al: Survival of ^{51}Cr-labelled red cells in subjects with thalassaemia trait, G6PD deficiency or both abnormalities. Br J Haematol 1964; 10:171.

76. McCurdy PR: Discussion. In Yoshida A, Beutler E (eds): Glucose 6-Phosphate Dehydrogenase. New York, Academic Press, 1986, pp 273–278.

77. Beutler E, Dern RJ, Alving AS: The hemolytic effect of primaquine. IV. The relationship of cell age to hemolysis. J Lab Clin Med 1954; 44:439.

78. Szeinberg A, Marks PA: Substances stimulating glucose catabolism by the oxidative reactions of the pentose phosphate pathway in human erythrocytes. J Clin Invest 1961; 40:914.

79. Chevion M, Navok T, et al: The chemistry of favism-inducing compounds. The properties of isouramil and divicine and their reaction with glutathione. Eur J Biochem 1982; 127:405.

80. Winterbourn C, Cowden WB, Sutton HC: Auto-oxidation of dialuric acid, divicine and isouramil. Superoxide dependent and independent mechanisms. Biochem Pharmacol 1989; 38:611.

81. Meloni T, Forteleoni G, et al: Aspirin-induced acute hemolytic anemia in glucose 6-phosphate dehydrogenase deficient children with systemic arthritis. Acta Haematol 1989; 81:208.

82. Tugwell P: Glucose 6-phosphate dehydrogenase deficiency in Nigerians with jaundice associated with lobar pneumonia. Lancet 1973; 1:968.

83. Baehner RL, Nathan DG, Castle WB: Oxidant injury of caucasian glucose-6-phosphate dehydrogenase deficient red blood cells by phagocytosing leukocytes during infection. J Clin Invest 1971; 50:2466.

84. Kattamis CA, Tjortjatou F: The hemolytic process of viral hepatitis in children with normal or deficient glucose 6-phosphate dehydrogenase activity. J Pediatr 1970; 77:422.

85. Valaes T: Severe neonatal jaundice associated with glucose-6-phosphate dehydrogenase deficiency: pathogenesis and global epidemiology. Acta Paediatr 1994; Suppl 394:58.

86. Worlledge S, Luzzatto L, Ogiemudia SE, et al: Rhesus immunization in Nigeria. Vox Sang 1968; 14:202.

87. Doxiadis SA, Valaes F: The clinical picture of glucose 6-phosphate dehydrogenase deficiency in early childhood. Arch Dis Child 1964; 39:545.

88. Meloni S, Costa S, Cutillo S: Haptoglobin, hemopexin, hemoglobin and hematocrit in newborns with erythrocyte glucose 6-phosphate dehydrogenase deficiency. Acta Haematol 1975; 54:284.

89. Singh A: Glucose 6-phosphate dehydrogenase deficiency: a preventable cause of mental retardation. BMJ 1986; 292:397.

90. Bienzle U, Effiong CE, Luzzatto L: Erythrocyte glucose 6-phosphate dehydrogenase deficiency (G6PD type A$^-$) and neonatal jaundice. Acta Paediatr Scand 1976; 65:701.

91. Meloni T, Cagnazzo G, et al: Phenobarbital for prevention of hyperbilirubinemia in glucose 6-phosphate dehydrogenase-deficient newborn infants. J Pediatr 1973; 82:1048.

91a. Kaplan M, Vreman HJ, et al: Contribution of haemolysis to jaundice in Sephardic Jewish glucose-6-phosphate dehydrogenase deficient neonates. Br J Haematol 1996; 93:822.

92. Tan KL, Boey KW: Clinical experience with phototherapy. Ann Acad Med Singapore 1989; 18:43.

93. Yu MW, Hsiao KJ, Wuu KD, et al: Association between glucose-6-phosphate dehydrogenase deficiency and neonatal jaundice: interaction with multiple risk factors. Int J Epidemiol 1992; 21:947.

94. Testa U, Meloni T, et al: Genetic heterogeneity of glucose 6-phosphate dehydrogenase deficiency in Sardinia. Hum Genet 1980; 56:99.

95. Meloni T, Cutillo S, et al: Neonatal jaundice and severity of glucose 6-phosphate dehydrogenase deficiency in Sardinian babies. Early Hum Dev 1987; 15:317.

96. Bienzle U, Effiong CE, et al: Erythrocyte enzymes in neonatal jaundice. Acta Haematol 1976; 55:10.

97. Allen DW, Johnson GJ, et al: Membrane polypeptide aggregates in glucose-6-phosphate dehydrogenase deficient and in vitro aged red blood cells. J Lab Clin Med 1978; 91:321.

98. Doxiadis SA, Valaes T, et al: Risk of severe jaundice in glucose 6-phosphate dehydrogenase deficiency of the newborn. Differences in population groups. Lancet 1964; 2:1210.

99. Owa JA: Relationship between exposure to icterogenic agents, glucose-6-phosphate dehydrogenase deficiency and neonatal jaundice in Nigeria. Acta Paediatr Scand 1989; 78:848.

100. Ifekwunigwe AE, Luzzatto L: Kernicterus in G6PD deficiency. Lancet 1966; 1:667.

101. Corchia C, Balata A, et al: Favism in a female newborn infant whose mother ingested fava beans before delivery. J Pediatrics 1995; 127:807.

102. Luzzatto L: Inherited haemolytic states: glucose-6-phosphate dehydrogenase deficiency. Clin Hematol 1975; 4:83.

103. Johnson GJ, Allen DW, et al: Red cell membrane polypeptide aggregates in glucose-6-phosphate dehydrogenase mutants with chronic haemolytic disease: a clue to the mechanism of haemolysis. N Engl J Med 1979; 301:522.

104. Johnson RM, Ravindranath Y, et al: Oxidant damage to erythrocyte membrane in glucose 6-phosphate dehydrogenase deficiency: correlation with in vivo reduced glutathione concentration and membrane protein oxidation. Blood 1994; 83:1117.

105. Horecker BL, Smyrniotis A: Glucose 6-phosphate dehydrogenase. In Colowick N, Kaplan NO (eds): Methods in Enzymology. Vol. 1. New York, Academic Press, Inc., 1955.

106. Morelli A, Benatti U, et al: The interference of leukocytes and

platelets with measurement of glucose 6-phosphate dehydrogenase activity of erythrocytes with low activity variants of the
enzyme. Blood 1981; 58:642.

107. Motulsky AG, Campbell-Kraut JM: Population genetics of glucose 6-phosphate dehydrogenase deficiency of the red cell. In
Blumberg BS (ed): Proceedings of Conference on Genetic Polymorphisms and Geographic Variations in Disease. New York,
Grune & Stratton, Inc., 1961, pp 159–180.

108. Brewer GJ, Tarlov AR, Alving AS: The methemoglobin reduction test for primaquine-type sensitivity of erythrocytes. A simplified procedure for detecting a specific hypersusceptibility to
drug hemolysis. JAMA 1962; 180:386.

109. Beutler E: Special modifications for the fluorescent screening
test for glucose 6-phosphate dehydrogenase deficiency. Blood
1968; 32:816.

110. Bienzle U, Sodeinde O, et al: G6PD deficiency and sickle cell
anemia: frequency and features of the association in an African
community. Blood 1975; 46:591.

111. Abd-Allah MA, Foda YH, et al: Treatment to reduce total vicine
in Egyptian fava bean (Giza 2 variety). Plant Foods Hum Nutr
1988; 38:201.

112. Fairbanks VF, Lampe LT: A tetrazolium-linked cytochemical
method for estimation of glucose 6-phosphate dehydrogenase
activity in individual erythrocytes: applications in the study of
heterozygotes for glucose 6-phosphate dehydrogenase deficiency. Blood 1968; 31:589.

113. Van Noorden CJF, Vogels IMC, et al: A sensitive cytochemical
staining method for glucose 6-phosphate dehydrogenase activity in individual erythrocytes. Histochemistry 1982; 75:493.

114. Vulliamy TJ, D'Urso M, et al: Diverse point mutations in the
human glucose-6-phosphate dehydrogenase gene cause enzyme
deficiency and mild or severe hemolytic anemia. Proc Natl Acad
Sci U S A 1988; 85:5171.

115. Betke K, Beutler E, et al: Standardisation of procedures for the
study of glucose-6-phosphate dehydrogenase. Report of a WHO
Scientific Group. WHO Tech Rep 1967; 366:5.

116. WHO Working Group: Glucose-6-phosphate dehydrogenase deficiency. Bull WHO 1989; 67:601.

117. Beutler E, Yoshida A: Genetic variation of glucose-6-phosphate
dehydrogenase: a catalog and future prospects. Medicine 1988;
67:311.

118. Luzzatto L: Studies of polymorphic traits for the characterization of populations: African populations south of the Sahara.
Isr J Med Sci 1973; 9:1181.

119. Beutler E, Kuhl W, et al: Molecular heterogeneity of glucose 6-
phosphate dehydrogenase A–. Blood 1989; 74:2550.

120. Beutler E, Kuhl W, et al: Some Mexican glucose 6-phosphate
dehydrogenase (G-6-PD) variants revisited. Hum Genet 1991;
86:371.

121. Panich V: Glucose 6-phosphate dehydrogenase deficiency: II.
Tropical Asia. Clin Haematol 1981; 10:800.

122. Miwa S, Fujii H: Glucose 6-phosphate dehydrogenase variants
in Japan. In Yoshida A, Beutler E (eds): Glucose 6-Phosphate
Dehydrogenase. New York, Academic Press, Inc., 1986, pp 261–
272.

123. Calabro V, Cascone A, et al: Glucose-6-phosphate dehydrogenase (G6PD) deficiency in Southern Italy: a case of G6PD A(–)
associated with favism. Haematologica 1989; 74:71.

124. Galiano S, Gaetani GF, et al: Favism in the African type of
glucose-6-phosphate dehydrogenase deficiency (A–). BMJ
1990; 300:236.

124a. Kirkman HN, Riley HD: Congenital nonspherocytic hemolytic
anemia: studies on a family with a qualitative defect in glucose-
6-phosphate dehydrogenase. Am J Dis Child 1961; 102:313.

125. Kaeda JS, Chootray GP, et al: A new G6PD variant, G6PD
Orissa (44 Ala→Gly), is the major polymorphic variant in tribal
populations in India. Am J Hum Genet 1995; 57:1335.

126. Luzzatto L, O'Brien S, Usanga E, Wanachiwanawin W: Origin
of G6PD polymorphism: malaria and G6PD deficiency. In Yoshida A, Beutler E (eds): Glucose-6-Phosphate Dehydrogenase.
New York, Academic Press, Inc., 1986, pp 181–193.

127. Miller LH: Genetically determined human resistance factors. In
Wernsdorfer WH, McGregor I (eds): Malaria: Principles and
Practice of Malariology. Edinburgh, Churchill-Livingstone, Inc.,
1988, pp 487–500.

128. Allison AC: Glucose 6-phosphate dehydrogenase deficiency in
red blood cells of East Africans. Nature 1960; 186:531.

129. Motulsky AG: Metabolic polymorphisms and the role of infectious diseases in human evolution. Hum Biol 1960; 32:28.

130. Luzzatto L: Genetic factors in malaria. Bull WHO 1974; 50:195.

131. Ruwende C, Khoo SC, et al: Natural selection of hemi- and
heterozygotes for G6PD deficiency in Africa by resistance to
severe malaria. Nature 1995; 376:246.

132. Kar S, Seth S, Seth PK: Prevalence of malaria in Ao Nagas and
its association with G6PD and HbE. Hum Biol 1992; 64:187.

133. Bienzle U, Ayeni O, et al: Glucose-6-phosphate dehydrogenase
deficiency and malaria. Greater resistance of females heterozygous for enzyme deficiency and of males with non-deficient
variant. Lancet 1972; 1:107.

133a. Ruwende C, Khoo SC, et al: Natural selection of hemi- and
heterozygotes for G6PD deficiency in Africa by resistance to
severe malaria. Nature 1995; 376:246.

134. Luzzatto L: Genetics of human red cells and susceptibility to
malaria. In Michal F (ed): Modern Genetic Concepts and Techniques in the Study of Parasites. Basel, Schwabe & Co., 1981,
pp 257–277.

135. Roth EF Jr, Raventos-Suarez C, et al: Glucose 6-phosphate dehydrogenase deficiency inhibits *in vitro* growth of *Plasmodium
falciparum*. Proc Natl Acad Sci U S A 1983; 80:298.

136. Usanga EA, Luzzatto L: Adaptation of *Plasmodium falciparum* to
glucose 6-phosphate dehydrogenase deficient host red cells by
production of parasite-encoded enzyme. Nature 1985; 313:793.

137. Ling IT, Wilson RJM: G6PD activity of the malarial parasite
Plasmodium falciparum. Mol Biochem Parasitol 1988; 31:47.

138. Kurdi-Haidar B, Luzzatto L: Expression and characterization of
glucose-6-phosphate dehydrogenase of *Plasmodium falciparum*.
Mol Biochem Parasitol 1990; 41:83.

139. Gaetani GF, Mareni C, et al: Haemolytic effect of two sulphona-
mides evaluated by a new method. Br J Haematol 1976; 32:183.

140. Magon AM, Leipzig RM, et al: Interactions of glucose 6-phos-
phate dehydrogenase deficiency with drug acetylation and hydroxylation reactions. J Lab Clin Med 1981; 97:764.

141. Luzzatto L, Meloni T: Hemolytic anemia due to glucose 6-
phosphate dehydrogenase deficiency. In Brain MC, Carbone PP
(eds): Current Therapy in Hematology-Oncology: 1985–1986.
Toronto, BC Decker, 1985, pp 21–24.

142. Luzzatto L, Mehta A, Meloni T: Haemoglobinuria and haptoglobin in G6PD deficiency. Br J Haematol 1995; 91:511.

143. Newman TB, Maisels MJ: Evaluation and treatment of jaundice
in the term infant: a kinder, gentler approach. Pediatrics 1992;
89:809.

143a. Beutler E, Kuhl W, et al: Prenatal diagnosis of glucose 6-
phosphate dehydrogenase deficiency. Acta Haematol 1992;
87:103.

144. Morellini M, Colonna-Romano S, et al: Glucose 6-phosphate
dehydrogenase of leukocyte sub-populations in normal and
enzyme-deficient individuals. Haematologica 1985; 70:390.

145. Vives-Corrons JL, Feliu E, et al: Severe glucose-6-phosphate
dehydrogenase (G6PD) deficiency associated with chronic hemolytic anaemia, granulocyte dysfunction and increased susceptibility to infections. Description of a new molecular variant
(G6PD Barcelona). Blood 1982; 59:428.

146. Roos D, deBoer M, et al: Mutations in the X-linked and autosomal recessive forms of chronic granulomatous disease. Blood
1996; 87:1663.

147. Westring DN, Pisciotta AV: Anemia, cataracts and seizures in a
patient with glucose-6-phosphate dehydrogenase deficiency.
Arch Intern Med 1966; 118:385.

148. Harley JD, Agar NS, Yoshida A: Glucose 6-phosphate dehydrogenase variants: Gd(+) Alexandra associated with neonatal
jaundice and Gd(–) Camperdown in a young man with lamel-
lar cataracts. J Lab Clin Med 1978; 91:295.

149. Orzalesi M, Fossarello M, et al: The relationship between glucose 6-phosphate dehydrogenase deficiency and cataracts in
Sardinia. An epidemiological and biochemical study. Doc Ophthalmol 1984; 57:187.

150. Moro F, Gorgone G, et al: Glucose 6-phosphate dehydrogenase
deficiency and incidence of cataract in Sicily. Ophthalmic Paediatr Genet 1985; 5:197.

151. Yuregir G, Varinli I, Donma O: Glucose 6-phosphate dehydroge-

nase deficiency both in red blood cells and lenses of the normal and cataractous native population of Cukurova, the southern part of Turkey. Part I. Ophthalmic Res 1989; 21:155.

152. Meloni T, Carta F, et al: Glucose 6-phosphate dehydrogenase deficiency and cataract of patients in northern Sardinia. Am J Ophthalmol 1990; 110:661.

153. Chen Y, Zeng L, et al: The study of G6PD in erythrocyte and lens in senile and presenile cataract. Yen Ko Hsueh Pao 1992; 8:12.

154. Assaf AA, Tabbara KF, el-Hazmi MA: Cataracts in glucose-6-phosphate dehydrogenase deficiency. Ophthalmic Paediatr Genet 1993; 14:81.

155. Luzzatto L, Allan NC: Relationship between the genes for glucose 6-phosphate dehydrogenase and haemoglobin in a Nigerian population. Nature 1968; 219:1041.

156. Nhonoli AM, Kujwalile JM, et al: Correlation of glucose-6-phosphate dehydrogenase (G6PD) deficiency and sickle cell trait (Hb-AS). Trop Geogr Med 1978; 30:99.

157. Gibbs WN, Wardle J, Serjeant GR: Glucose 6-phosphate dehydrogenase deficiency and homozygous sickle cell disease in Jamaica. Br J Haematol 1980; 45:73.

158. Nieuwenhuis F, Wolf B, et al: Haematological study in Cabo Delgado province, Mozambique; sickle cell trait and G6PD deficiency. Trop Geogr Med 1986; 38:183.

159. Piomelli S, Siniscalco M: The haematological effects of glucose 6-phosphate dehydrogenase deficiency and thalassaemia trait: interaction between the two genes at the phenotype level. Br J Haematol 1969; 16:537.

160. Sanna G, Frau F, et al: Interaction between the glucose-6-phosphate dehydrogenase deficiency and thalassaemia genes at phenotype level. Br J Haematol 1980; 44:555.

161. Steinberg MH, West MS, et al: Effects of glucose-6-phosphate dehydrogenase deficiency upon sickle cell anemia. Blood 1988; 71:748.

162. Awamy BH: Effect of G-6 PD deficiency on sickle cell disease in Saudi Arabia. Indian J Pediatr 1992; 59:331.

163. Smits HL, Oski FA, Brody JI: The hemolytic crisis of sickle cell disease: the role of glucose 6-phosphate dehydrogenase deficiency. J Pediatr 1969; 74:544.

164. Carpentieri U, Haggard ME, et al: Hb E-beta thalassemia associated with G6PD deficiency. South Med J 1980; 73:518.

165. Vives Corrons JL, Garcia AM, et al: Heterozygous pyruvate kinase deficiency and severe hemolytic anemia in a pregnant woman with concomitant, glucose-6-phosphate dehydrogenase deficiency. Ann Hematol 1991; 62:190.

166. Mahendra P, Dollery CT, et al: Pyruvate kinase deficiency: association with G6PD deficiency. BMJ 1992; 305:760.

167. Ventura A, Panizon F, et al: Congenital dyserythropoietic anaemia Type II associated with a new type of G6PD deficiency (G6PD Gabrovizza). Acta Haematol 1984; 71:227.

168. Szeto SC, Ng CS: A case of congenital dyserythropoietic anemia in a male Chinese. Pathology 1986; 18:165.

169. Gangarossa S, Romano V, et al: Congenital dyserythropoietic anemia type II associated with G6PD Seattle in a Sicilian child. Acta Haematol 1995; 93:36.

170. Panich V, Na-Nakorn S, Wasi P: Hereditary elliptocytosis (the first report in Thailand) in association with erythrocyte glucose-6-phosphate dehydrogenase deficiency and hemoglobin E. J Med Assoc Thai 1970; 53:593.

171. Alfinito F, Calabrò V, et al: Glucose 6-phosphate dehydrogenase deficiency and red cell membrane defects: additive or synergistic interaction in producing chronic haemolytic anaemia. Br J Haematol 1994; 87:148.

172. Meloni T, Forteleoni G, Meloni GF: Marked decline of favism after neonatal glucose-6-phosphate dehydrogenase screening and health education: the northern Sardinian experience. Acta Haematol 1992; 87:29.

173. Winterbourn CC, Stern A: Human red cells scavenge extracellular hydrogen peroxide and inhibit formation of hypochlorous acid and hydroxyl radical. J Clin Invest 1987; 80:1486.

174. Hori SH: Glucose-6-phosphate dehydrogenase and hexose-6-phosphate dehydrogenase: an evolutionary aspect. In Yoshida A, Beutler E (eds): Glucose-6-Phosphate Dehydrogenase. Orlando, FL, Academic Press, Inc., 1986.

175. Lux SE, Tse WT, et al: Hereditary spherocytosis associated with deletion of human erythrocyte ankyrin gene on chromosome 8. Nature 1990; 345:736.

176. Fialkow PJ: Clonal origin of human tumors. Biochim Biophys Acta 1976; 458:283.

177. DeVita G, Alcalay M, et al: Two point mutations are responsible for G6PD polymorphism in Sardinia. Am J Hum Genet 1989; 44:233.

178. Escobar MA, Heller P, Trobaugh FE Jr: "Complete" erythrocyte glucose 6-phosphate dehydrogenase deficiency. Arch Intern Med 1964; 113:428.

179. Cooper MR, De Chatelet LR, et al: Complete deficiency of leukocyte glucose 6-phosphate dehydrogenase with defective bactericidal activity. J Clin Invest 1972; 51:769.

180. Gray FR, Klebanoff SJ, et al: Neutrophil dysfunction, chronic granulomatous disease and non-spherocytic haemolytic anemia caused by complete deficiency of glucose-6-phosphate dehydrogenase. Lancet 1973; 2:530.

VI

Disorders of Hemoglobin

Human Hemoglobins: Normal and Abnormal

Sickle Cell Disease

The Thalassemias

Human Hemoglobins: Normal and Abnormal

H. Franklin Bunn

A thorough understanding of human hemoglobin is relevant to a number of biomedical disciplines. Knowledge of hemoglobin's structure and function provides insights into oxygen transport in health and disease, into blood pressure regulation,[1a,b] and even into fish buoyancy.[1c] The thalassemias and other hemoglobinopathies constitute an effective and practical introduction to human genetics and the rapidly expanding field of genetic engineering. In addition, because of acquired alterations in structure, hemoglobin serves as a "reporter molecule," providing cumulative information on metabolic perturbations such as diabetes.

In this chapter the relationship between hemoglobin's structure and function is reviewed first. Second, the various factors in health and disease that can modify hemoglobin's affinity for oxygen are discussed. This background information is useful in the consideration of inherited and acquired disorders of hemoglobin structure and function. Sickle cell disease is covered in Chapter 20, and the thalassemias are described in Chapter 21.

STRUCTURE

Hemoglobin is a tetramer of approximately $5.0 \times 5.5 \times 6.4$ nm, with a molecular weight of 64,400 daltons. It consists of two pairs of unlike globin polypeptide chains designated by Greek letters (e.g., $\alpha_2\beta_2$). A heme group, ferroprotoporphyrin IX, is linked covalently at a specific site to each chain. When heme iron is in the reduced (ferrous) state, it can bind reversibly with gaseous ligands, such as oxygen or carbon monoxide (CO). The ferrihemes of methemoglobin are incapable of oxygenation but can bind tightly to anionic ligands, such as cyanide. Such modifications of hemoglobin cause specific alterations in its color and absorption spectrum.

In developing human erythroblasts, eight genes direct the synthesis of six structurally different globin polypeptide chains, designated α, β, γ, δ, ϵ, and ζ. The α gene is duplicated in humans[1] and other primates and is localized on chromosome 16, adjacent to the ζ gene. Likewise, structural heterogeneity in the γ chain can be explained by gene duplication. The ϵ, γ_1, γ_2, δ and β genes are arranged in sequential order on chromosome 11.1. For a detailed review of globin genetics, see Chapter 21. Strong structural homology between the α and β chains indicates that they arose after duplication of a single gene at an early point in evolution. Their separation onto two different chromosomes is a reflection of the eons that have elapsed in the development of respiratory proteins.

Primary and Secondary Structure

Alpha chains contain 141 amino acids in linear sequence, whereas β chains (as well as δ, γ, and ϵ chains) have 146 residues. The amino acid sequence for each of these polypeptide chains has been established by standard chemical methods and confirmed by analyses of the base sequences of the corresponding genes. In addition, primary structure has been determined on over 50 mammalian hemoglobins as well as on a number of hemoglobins from other classes of vertebrates. This information has helped investigators analyze structural homology of the α chains and β chains among various species. Certain segments of these proteins have specific amino acids in common. Such invariant residues have been shown to be crucial to the molecule's function.

Approximately 80% of hemoglobin in its native state is in the form of an α helix. Each chain consists of either seven or eight helical segments (labeled A through H in Figure 19–1). Figure 19–1 shows the amino acid residues of the α and β chains of human hemoglobin including those that are oriented in an α helix. Individual residues can be assigned to a specific helix, thereby facilitating establishment of homology between globin subunits. Thus, the heme iron is linked covalently to histidines at F8, the eighth residue of the F helix. This is residue number 87 of the α chain and number 92 of the β chain (see Fig. 19–1). All hemoglobins whose primary structures are known have a histidine residue at F8. (Two of the variant M hemoglobins are exceptions. These are discussed in detail later in this chapter.) Residues that have charged side groups, such as lysine, arginine, and glutamic acid, lie on the surface of the molecule in contact with the surrounding water solvent. Uncharged residues are generally oriented toward the hydrophobic interior of the molecule. Unlike many proteins, hemoglobin contains no disulfide bonds.

Tertiary and Quaternary Structure

From x-ray analyses of crystals of horse and human hemoglobins, Max Perutz at the Medical Research Council Laboratory in Cambridge, England, determined the structure of human hemoglobin in three-dimensional space. This remarkable achievement has enabled a thorough understanding of the relationship between structure and function.[2, 3] The hemoglobin tetramer was shown to be a spheroid with a single (dyad) axis of symmetry. The polypeptide chains are themselves folded in such a way that the four heme groups lie in clefts on the surface of the molecule equidistant from one another. Recent x-ray analyses are of sufficiently high resolution that the coordinates of all atoms in the molecule are known to within 0.2 nm.[4, 5] As shown in Figure 19–2, the molecule undergoes a marked change in conformation on deoxygenation. The β chains rotate apart by about 0.7 nm. In contrast, liganded forms, including oxyhemoglobin, carboxyhemoglobin, and cyanmethemoglobin, all appear to be isomorphous. The conformational change that occurs on addition and removal of ligand accounts for the many known differences in physical and chemical properties of oxyhemoglobin and deoxyhemoglobin. Perutz and associates[2, 3] have shown that deoxyhemoglobin is stabilized in a constrained or taut (T) configuration by the presence of intersubunit and intrasubunit salt bonds (Fig. 19–3). These include residues responsible for the Bohr effect and for the binding of 2,3-bisphosphoglycerate (2,3-BPG). On the addition of ligand, such as oxygen, these salt bonds are sequentially broken. The fully liganded hemoglobin is in the so-called relaxed (R) configuration. In this state, there is considerably less bonding energy between subunits and the liganded molecule is able to dissociate reversibly according to the following reaction: $\alpha_2\beta_2 \rightleftharpoons 2\alpha\beta$. The formation of $\alpha\beta$ dimers is required for hemoglobin to bind to haptoglobin and to traverse renal glomeruli. As shown in Figure 19–2, each subunit in the tetramer is oriented toward the two unlike subunits in different ways (i.e., $\alpha^1\beta^1$ and $\alpha^1\beta^2$). The dissociation of the liganded tetramer into dimers occurs at the $\alpha^1\beta^2$ interface. Thus, there is stronger binding energy between α^1 and β^1 subunits than between α^1 and β^2 subunits. Furthermore, during oxygenation and deoxygenation (T $\rightleftharpoons$ R), there is considerable movement along the $\alpha^1\beta^2$ interface. Hemoglobin variants having an amino acid substitution in this region are likely to have markedly abnormal functional properties.

FUNCTION

The oxygenation of hemoglobin, as depicted by the classic sigmoid oxyhemoglobin dissociation curve shown in Figure 19–4, can be characterized by two important properties: oxygen affinity and cooperativity.

A convenient index of oxygen affinity is P_{50}, or the partial pressure of oxygen at which hemoglobin is half saturated. If the oxyhemoglobin dissociation curve is shifted to the right, P_{50} is increased and oxygen affinity is decreased. Thus, P_{50} varies inversely with oxygen affinity. As discussed in detail in this section, P_{50} depends on temperature, pH, organic phosphates, and carbon dioxide tension (P_{CO_2}). Under physiologic conditions (37°C; pH, 7.40; 2,3-BPG, 5 mmol/L; P_{CO_2}, 40 mm Hg), the P_{50} of normal adult blood is 26 mm Hg.

Cooperativity

Data obtained from measurement of oxygen equilibria can be satisfactorily fitted by the empirical Hill equation:

$$\frac{Y}{1-Y} = \left(\frac{P_{O_2}}{P_{50}}\right)^n$$

in which Y is the fractional saturation of hemoglobin with oxygen and n is an index of heme-heme interaction. If such interaction were absent, n would be 1. (This is true for myoglobin and isolated hemoglobin subunits such as Hb H β_4 and Hb Barts γ_4.) If heme-heme interaction were maximal, n would be 4. In pure solutions of phosphate-free Hb A, n is about 3, whereas in whole blood n is somewhat less (2.6 to 2.8).

Cooperativity means that when hemoglobin is partially saturated with oxygen, the affinity of the remaining hemes on the tetramer for oxygen increases markedly. This phenomenon can be considered in terms of two hemoglobin conformations: deoxy (or T) and oxy (or R). The T form has a lower affinity for ligands such as oxygen and CO than the R form has. At some point during the sequential addition of oxygen to the four hemes of the molecule, a transition from the T to the R configuration occurs. At this point, the oxygen affinity of the partially liganded molecule increases markedly. In this way, hemoglobin can be considered a prototype of a more general class of allosteric enzymes, in which the binding of a ligand to a protein alters the affinity for the ligand at a different site on the same macromolecule. How can the oxygenation of one heme cause sufficient alteration in the environment of other heme groups to affect their oxygen affinity? In deoxyhemoglobin, the iron atoms lie outside the plane of the porphyrin ring by about 0.05 nm.[2-5] The trigger that effects this allosteric transition appears to be the decrease in the atomic radius of heme iron with the addition of ligand. The smaller iron atom is now able to snap into the plane of the porphyrin ring. The resulting alteration in heme configuration is amplified by a series of intrasubunit and intersubunit interactions, so that the environments of other hemes within the molecule are perturbed, resulting in increased ligand affinity. It is likely that when deoxyhemoglobin binds oxygen, the α chain hemes are favored. However, there is no information as to which of the remaining three hemes would be oxygenated next. Although the three-dimensional structure of partially liganded hemoglobin is not well understood, there is growing understanding of the mechanism underlying the energetics of the allosteric transition.[6]

Cooperativity (or heme-heme interaction) has considerable physiologic importance. This phenomenon dictates the familiar sigmoid shape of the oxyhemoglobin dissociation curve (see Fig. 19–4). The S-shaped curve allows a considerable amount of oxygen to be released over a relatively small drop in oxygen tension. In contrast, heme proteins, such as myoglobin and hemoglobins H and Bart's, which lack cooperativity, have a hyperbolic curve, which allows much less oxygen unloading.

Inside the red cell, the oxygen affinity of hemoglobin is modulated by varying concentrations of protons, 2,3-BPG, and carbon dioxide (CO_2). These allosteric effectors bind preferentially to deoxyhemoglobin and alter the equilibrium between the T and R quaternary structures.

Bohr Effect

In 1904, Bohr and colleagues[7] discovered that the oxygen affinity of hemoglobin decreased with increasing P_{CO_2}. It was later shown that this phenomenon depends primarily on pH. Thus, over a pH range of 6 to 8.5, oxygen affinity varies directly with pH (see Fig. 19–4). A thermodynamic corollary of this statement is that deoxyhemoglobin binds protons more strongly than oxyhemoglobin does. Under physiologic conditions, a molecule of hemoglobin releases about 2.8 protons upon oxygenation:

$$Hb \cdot H + 4\,O_2 \rightleftharpoons Hb\,(O_2)_4 + 2.8\,H^+$$

High-resolution x-ray data in conjunction with experiments on chemically modified hemoglobins[8] have permitted the identification of specific acid groups on hemoglobin that yield Bohr protons. About half of the Bohr effect is due to an intrasubunit salt bond between the positively charged imidazole of $\beta146$ histidine and the negatively charged carboxyl of $\beta94$ aspartate. This salt bridge is one of the important bonds that stabilize the deoxy conformation (see Fig. 19–3). When hemoglobin is oxygenated, these bonds are broken and protons are released.

The Bohr effect offers a physiologic advantage in facilitating oxygen unloading. At the tissue level, the drop in pH due to CO_2 influx lowers oxygen affinity, thereby enhancing oxygen release (Fig. 19–5). In contrast, during circulation through the lungs, the increase in pH due to the efflux of CO_2 increases oxygen affinity and uptake. As further testimony to its adaptational advantage, the Bohr effect is present in virtually all mammalian species that have been tested as well as in many other animals.

Carbamino Formation

Carbon dioxide affects hemoglobin function in two ways. It readily diffuses into red cells, where, in the presence of a generous supply of carbonic anhydrase, carbonic acid is rapidly formed (see Fig. 19–5). The resulting decrease in pH lowers oxygen affinity (the Bohr effect). In addition, CO_2 can bind free amino groups on hemoglobin to form carbamino complexes according to the following reaction:

$$RNH_2 + CO_2 \rightleftharpoons RNHCOO^- + H^+$$

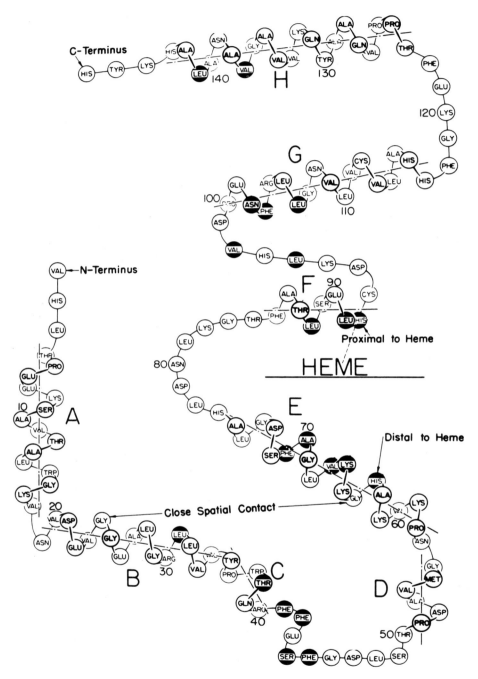

Figure 19-1. *Left,* Primary structure of the α-globin subunit. The helical segments are denoted by large capital letters. The *half black circles* indicate residues in contact with heme. *Right,* Primary structure of the β-globin subunit. (Reprinted from Huisman THJ, Schroeder WA: New Aspects of the Structure, Function, and Synthesis of Hemoglobins. Boca Raton, FL, CRC Press, 1971. Copyright CRC Press, Inc., Boca Raton, FL.)

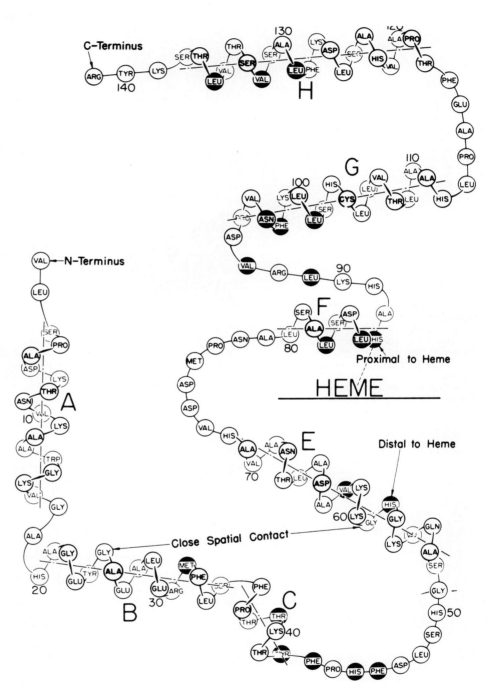

Figure 19-1 *Continued.* See legend on opposite page.

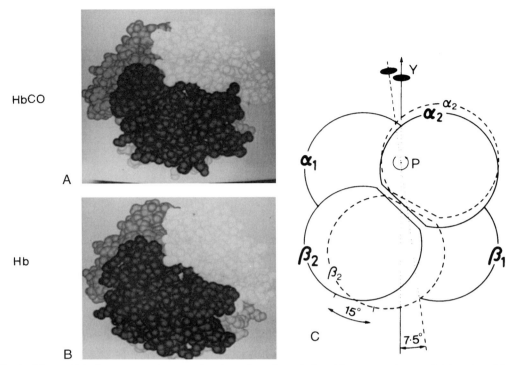

Figure 19-2. Effect of ligand binding on quaternary structure (i.e., the relationship among hemoglobin subunits). *A and B,* Space-filling models comparing three-dimensional structures of human carboxyhemoglobin *(A)* and deoxyhemoglobin *(B)* based on coordinates obtained from x-ray crystallography. Heme groups are not shown. These molecular models were prepared by Richard Feldman, National Institutes of Health. (From Bunn HF, Forget BG: Hemoglobin: Molecular, Genetic and Clinical Aspects. Philadelphia, W.B. Saunders Co., 1986.) *C,* Diagram of the hemoglobin subunits oriented as in *A* and *B,* showing rotation of the $\alpha^2\beta^2$ dimer relative to the $\alpha^1\beta^1$ dimer in deoxyhemoglobin *(solid line)* and carboxyhemoglobin *(broken line).* (From Fermi G, Perutz MF: Haemoglobin and myoglobin. In Phillips PC, Richards FM (eds): Atlas of Molecular Structures in Biology. Oxford, Clarendon Press, 1981.)

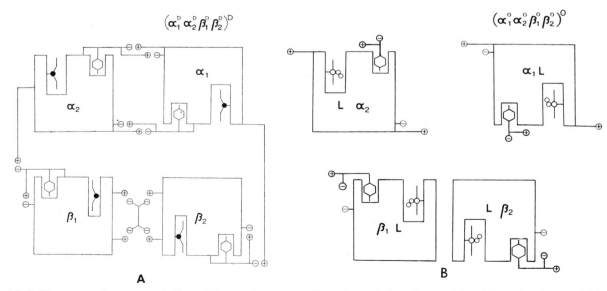

Figure 19-3. Diagrammatic representation of the quaternary configurations of deoxyhemoglobin *(A)* and oxyhemoglobin *(B).* The salt bonds that stabilize the deoxy conformation are broken when the molecule is oxygenated. (Reprinted by permission from Perutz MF: Stereochemistry of cooperative effects of haemoglobin. Nature 1970; 228:726, 1970; Copyright © 1970 Macmillan Magazines Ltd.)

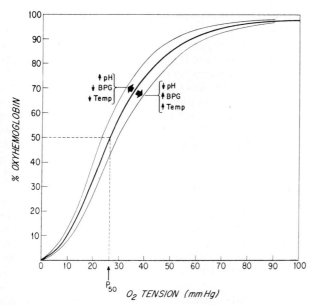

Figure 19-4. The principal factors that influence the position of the oxyhemoglobin dissociation curve. (From Bunn HF, Forget BG: Hemoglobin: Molecular, Genetic and Clinical Aspects. Philadelphia, W.B. Saunders Co., 1986.)

Only nonprotonated amino groups can react with CO_2. The only amino groups in globin whose pKs are low enough to be partially nonprotonated at physiologic pH are at the N termini of the $\alpha\beta$ chains. Deoxyhemoglobin forms carbamino complexes more readily than does oxyhemoglobin. From this, it follows that, at a given pH, CO_2 lowers oxygen affinity. This effect becomes more marked as carbamino formation is fa-

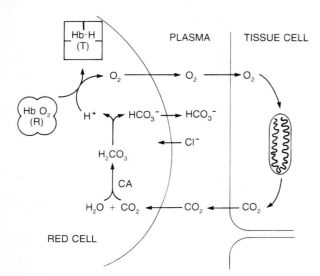

Figure 19-5. The unloading of oxygen (O_2) and the uptake of protons and carbon dioxide (CO_2) during the circulation of the red cell through tissues. The formation of the carbonic acid (H_2CO_3) from CO_2 and water is catalyzed by carbonic anhydrase (CA). The dissociation of O_2 from hemoglobin and the binding of protons are associated with a change from the R to the T quaternary structure. (From Bunn HF, Forget BG: Hemoglobin: Molecular, Genetic and Clinical Aspects. Philadelphia, W.B. Saunders Co., 1986.)

vored at increasing pH. Under physiologic conditions the relatively low pH of the red cell precludes extensive carbamino formation. It is estimated that only about 10% of the CO_2 produced by tissue metabolism is transported to the lungs in the form of carbamino hemoglobin.[9, 10]

Binding of 2,3-Bisphosphoglycerate

The red cell differs metabolically from other tissues in two important ways: It derives its chemical energy almost solely through anaerobic glycolysis, and it contains an unusually high concentration of 2,3-BPG. Normal human erythrocytes contain about 5 mmol of 2,3-BPG per liter (of packed cells), a concentration about fourfold that of the next most abundant organic phosphate, adenosine triphosphate (ATP). The reason for such large amounts of 2,3-BPG in red cells remained elusive until the discovery that this compound is a potent modifier of hemoglobin function.[11, 12] The addition of increasing amounts of 2,3-BPG to a solution of purified Hb A results in a progressive lowering of oxygen affinity. This helps explain the long-known fact that whole blood has a lower oxygen affinity than a solution of dialyzed hemoglobin, studied under comparable conditions. The mechanism by which 2,3-BPG lowers oxygen affinity was clarified when Benesch and Benesch[13] measured its binding to hemoglobin by a modified form of equilibrium dialysis. They showed that at physiologic pH and ionic strength, 2,3-BPG bound to human deoxyhemoglobin rather avidly ($K = 2 \times 10^{-5}$ mol/L) in a 1:1 molar ratio (one molecule 2,3-BPG per hemoglobin tetramer). Furthermore, under these conditions, 2,3-BPG binds only weakly to liganded forms of hemoglobin such as oxyhemoglobin, carboxyhemoglobin, and cyanmethemoglobin.

As shown in Figure 19–6, 2,3-BPG is a strongly anionic compound. At physiologic pH, a molecule of 2,3-BPG has about three and one-half negative charges. A comparison of the reactivities of a number of human and animal hemoglobins of known structure with 2,3-

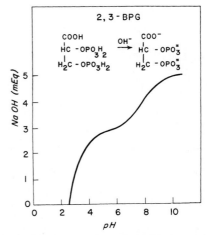

Figure 19-6. Structure of 2,3-bisphosphoglycerate (2,3-BPG). From this titration curve, it is apparent that, at physiologic pH, 2,3-BPG has about 3.5 negative charges per molecule.

BPG suggested that the N-terminal amino groups of the β chains and the imidazoles of β143 histidine are specific residues responsible for 2,3-BPG binding.[14] Model fitting and x-ray diffraction measurements[15] have established these among the sites involved in 2,3-BPG binding. Figure 19–7 shows a cross section of deoxyhemoglobin. The 2,3-BPG is situated in the central cavity between the two β chains. Its negative charges are neutralized by the positively charged groups previously mentioned. In addition, β82 lysine and β2 histidine are also thought to be involved in 2,3-BPG binding.[15] In light of this information on the binding of 2,3-BPG to hemoglobin, the following simple reaction can be written:

$$Hb \cdot DPG + 4\, O_2 \rightleftharpoons Hb\,(O_2)_4 + DPG$$

(Note the similarity of this equation and that for the Bohr effect previously given.) This equilibrium expresses both the preferential binding of 2,3-BPG for deoxyhemoglobin and the 1:1 stoichiometry. Furthermore, changing concentrations of 2,3-BPG shift the oxygen-binding equilibrium in accord with the experimental results cited earlier.

Other red cell phosphates are also able to lower the oxygen affinity of hemoglobin. In their degree of interaction with hemoglobin, these compounds can be ranked as follows: 2,3-BPG > ATP > adenosine diphosphate > adenosine monophosphate > pyrophosphate > inorganic phosphate. Although there is almost one third as much ATP as 2,3-BPG in normal red cells, ATP probably plays an insignificant role in mediating intracellular hemoglobin function. First, it binds to deoxyhemoglobin less avidly than does 2,3-BPG. Second, an appreciable portion of red cell ATP is bound to magnesium ion. This complex does not interact with hemoglobin.

Alterations in Blood Oxygen Affinity

The position of the oxyhemoglobin dissociation curve may be influenced by a number of factors. As depicted in Figure 19–4, the three most important are temperature, pH, and red cell 2,3-BPG. Oxygen affinity varies inversely with temperature. This phenomenon is physiologically appropriate because, during a period of relative hyperthermia, oxygen requirement is likely to be increased. The decrease in oxygen affinity at elevated body temperature would facilitate unloading of oxygen to tissues. The effects of pH and 2,3-BPG on hemoglobin function have already been discussed. Conventionally, whole blood oxygen saturation curves are corrected to pH 7.4, 37°C. Thus, the main variable leading to fluctuation in the position of the standardized oxygen dissociation curve is red cell 2,3-BPG.

Other factors include the transmembrane pH gradient, red cell ATP, P_{CO_2}, and alteration in cell hemoglobin concentration (mean corpuscular hemoglobin concentration). Because of the Bohr effect, any factor that changes the pH of the red cell relative to the plasma affects oxygen affinity. For example, any increase within the cell of an impermeant anion, such as hemoglobin or 2,3-BPG, lowers intracellular pH as a manifestation of the Gibbs-Donnan equilibrium. The effect of 2,3-BPG in lowering intracellular pH is an important factor in the reduction of oxygen affinity inside red cells.[16] Red cell ATP and P_{CO_2} are of much less importance, for reasons mentioned earlier.

How does the oxygen affinity of the blood affect the delivery of oxygen to tissues? This subject is considered in detail in a number of reviews.[17–19] At a given blood flow and hemoglobin concentration, the amount of oxygen that is unloaded depends on the position of the oxyhemoglobin dissociation curve. As shown in Figure 19–8, red cells that are shifted to the right have enhanced oxygen release when going from a normal arterial oxygen tension (PaO_2) (95 mm Hg) to a normal mixed venous oxygen tension ($\bar{P}vO_2$) (40 mm Hg). This is because with this decrease in PO_2, a steeper portion of the oxygen dissociation curve is encompassed. In contrast, if the oxyhemoglobin dissociation curve is shifted to the left, less oxygen is unloaded. From another viewpoint, it is apparent that if the oxygen affin-

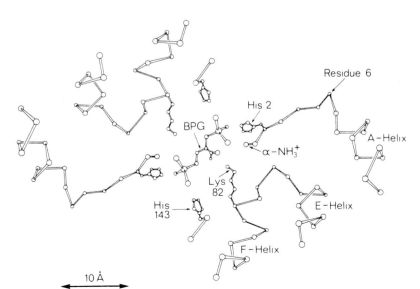

10 Å

Figure 19–7. The site at which 2,3-BPG binds to the β chains of deoxyhemoglobin. This diagram shows a cross section of the molecule, the plane of which is perpendicular to the dyad axis of symmetry. The diagram shows salt bonds between the phosphates of 2,3-BPG and positively charged groups at the β N-terminus, β2 histidine, β82 lysine, and β143 histidine. (Reprinted by permission from Arnone A: X-ray diffraction study of binding of 2,3-diphosphoglycerate to human deoxyhaemoglobin. Nature 1972; 237:146; Copyright © 1972 Macmillan Magazines Ltd.)

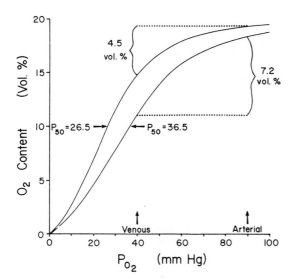

Figure 19–8. Enhancement of O_2 unloading due to a decrease in red cell O_2 affinity. Normal O_2 binding curve: $P_{50} = 26.5$ mm Hg; right-shifted curve: $P_{50} = 36.5$ mm Hg. (From Klocke RA: Oxygen transport and 2,3-diphosphoglycerate (DPG). Chest 1972; 62:79S.)

ity of the blood is increased, a lower oxygen tension will be required to extract a given amount of oxygen. This phenomenon bears on several clinical states to be discussed in detail, including blood transfusion therapy and hemoglobin variants associated with polycythemia.

Decreased Oxygen Affinity: Adaptation to Hypoxia

The uptake of oxygen ($\dot{V}O_2$ [mL/min]) by a given tissue or the whole organism can be expressed in the following equation:

$$\dot{V}O_2 = 1.39 \cdot \dot{Q} \cdot Hb \cdot (SaO_2 - S\bar{v}O_2)$$

Table 19–1. DISPLACEMENT OF THE OXYHEMOGLOBIN DISSOCIATION CURVE IN VARIOUS CLINICAL DISORDERS*

Shift to the Right

Increase in red cell 2,3-biphosphoglycerate (2,3-BPG)
    High altitude adaptation
    Pulmonary hypoxemia
    Cardiac right-to-left shunt
    Severe anemia; decrease in red cell mass
    Congestive heart failure
    Decompensated hepatic cirrhosis
Functional abnormal hemoglobin variants

Shift to the Left

Decrease in red cell 2,3-BPG
    Septic shock
    Severe acidosis
    After transfusion of stored blood
    Hypophosphatemia
    BPG mutase deficiency
Functionally abnormal hemoglobin variants
Methemoglobinemia
Carbon monoxide intoxication

*Connected to pH 7.4.

in which 1.39 is the milliliters of oxygen that can bind to 1 g of hemoglobin; Hb is the hemoglobin concentration of the blood (in grams per deciliter); $\dot{Q}$ is blood flow (in milliliters per minute); and SaO_2 and $S\bar{v}O_2$ are the percentages of saturation of arterial blood and of venous blood, respectively.

During hypoxic stress, $\dot{V}O_2$ may be increased by alteration of one or more of these three variables:

1. Increase in blood flow ($\uparrow \dot{Q}$)
2. Increase in red cell mass ($\uparrow$ Hb)
3. Decrease in whole blood oxygen affinity ($\uparrow [SaO_2 - S\bar{v}O_2]$)

A shift to the right (decreased whole blood oxygen affinity) is encountered in various types of hypoxic states (Table 19–1). In each case, the decreased oxygen affinity can be explained by increased levels of red cell 2,3-BPG. In fact, there is a close correlation between P_{50} (an index of oxygen affinity) and 2,3-BPG in a number of diverse disorders (Fig. 19–9).[17, 18] It is apparent that decreased whole blood oxygen affinity, mediated through increased red cell 2,3-BPG, is a rather general phenomenon in a variety of hypoxic states.

The regulation of the intracellular concentration of 2,3-BPG is poorly understood. In particular, it is not

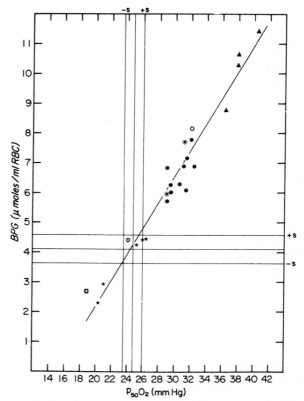

Figure 19–9. Correlation between alterations in red cell 2,3-BPG and P_{50} in a variety of clinical disorders: cyanotic congenital heart disease, ●; pyruvate kinase deficiency, ▲; hexokinase deficiency, □; septic shock, ★; postseptic shock, ⊙; thyrotoxicosis, ⊙ glucose-6-phosphate dehydrogenase deficiency, ○. (From Oski FA, Gottlieb AJ, Miller L: The influences of heredity and environment on the red cells' function of oxygen transport. Med Clin North Am 1970;54:731.)

clear how red cell 2,3-BPG can increase as much as twofold in various hypoxic states. One contributing factor is an increase in intracellular pH. Patients with hypoxia of varying sorts commonly have respiratory alkalosis. Second, if there is an increase in the amount of oxygen extracted per red cell, intracellular pH will increase slightly because of the Bohr effect. Alkalosis not only stimulates glycolysis in general but also may affect the relative degree of 2,3-BPG formation and catabolism by means of the Rapoport-Luebering cycle. A decreased oxygen saturation also may enhance red cell 2,3-BPG because of the specific binding of this organic phosphate to deoxyhemoglobin. The resulting fall in the intracellular concentration of free 2,3-BPG would relieve product inhibition of bisphosphoglycerate mutase, thereby stimulating its own synthesis.[20]

The level of 2,3-BPG falls during *in vivo* cell aging. This may explain why patients with hypoplastic anemia and a relatively old population of red cells have somewhat lower 2,3-BPG concentrations than those with hemolysis and a comparable degree of anemia.

The fact that decreased red cell oxygen affinity is so commonly found in hypoxic states does not constitute proof that the phenomenon is adaptive or beneficial to the organism. Is the position of the oxyhemoglobin dissociation curve an important determinant of tissue oxygenation? This question defies an easy answer. It is a technical challenge to monitor oxygen tension at the cellular level. Clearly, there is a marked P_{O_2} gradient between the red cell and various intracellular organelles, such as mitochondria. Therefore, it is difficult to say what constitutes a critical P_{O_2} for various tissues. Oski and associates[21] investigated this problem by comparing the hemodynamics of two teenagers whose oxygen dissociation curves were abnormally fixed because of congenital red cell enzyme defects. Patient 1, with hexokinase deficiency, had a low red cell 2,3-BPG level and consequently a left-shifted curve. In contrast, patient 2, with pyruvate kinase deficiency, had an elevated red cell 2,3-BPG level and a right-shifted curve. The two individuals were equally anemic. However, patient 1 was a semi-invalid, whereas patient 2 had no appreciable limitations. During graded exercise, the patient with the left-shifted curve (patient 1) experienced a prompt fall in $P\overline{v}_{O_2}$ and a more marked increase in cardiac output.

As Figure 19–10 shows, the decreased oxygen affinity of blood from a patient with anemia provides a marked enhancement of oxygen delivery to tissues. This is not true, however, for individuals with arterial hypoxemia, such as those who have adapted to high altitude or patients with severe chronic obstructive lung disease. As demonstrated in Figure 19–11, when the Pa_{O_2} is significantly decreased, the right-shifted curve provides no significant enhancement in oxygen unloading.[22, 23] Thus, not all types of patients with hypoxia benefit from decreased oxygen affinity. In fact, patients with *increased* oxygen affinity may exhibit less cardiovascular strain than normal individuals when both groups are exposed to high-altitude hypoxia.[23]

The position of the oxygen dissociation curve appears to be one important determinant of red cell mass,

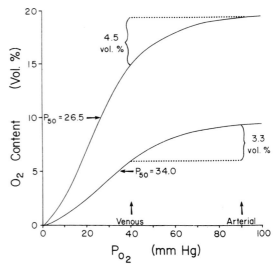

Figure 19–10. Enhancement of O_2 unloading by decreased red cell O_2 affinity in a patient with anemia. Anemic patient with a 50% reduction in hemoglobin concentration has only a 27% reduction in O_2 unloading. (From Klocke RA: Oxygen transport and 2,3-diphosphoglycerate (DPG). Chest 1972; 62:79S.)

presumably through erythropoietin control. A comparison of various hemolytic disorders reveals a correlation between hemoglobin level and oxygen affinity. The polycythemia secondary to high-affinity hemoglobin variants also attests to this relationship.

Increased Oxygen Affinity

From considerations just developed it appears that increased whole blood oxygen affinity may lead to relative tissue hypoxia. In addition to the congenital disorders previously discussed, a "shift to the left" may be encountered in a number of acquired conditions (see

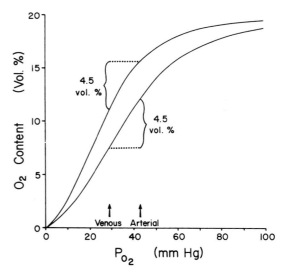

Figure 19–11. Failure of right-shifted O_2 binding curve to enhance O_2 unloading in patients with arterial hypoxemia. (From Klocke RA: Oxygen transport and 2,3-diphosphoglycerate (DPG). Chest 1972; 62:79S.)

Table 19–1). As previously noted, the concentration of 2,3-BPG in the red cell is markedly dependent on pH. Accordingly, patients with severe acidosis generally have low concentrations of 2,3-BPG. The pH-"corrected" oxygen dissociation curve of a patient with acidosis is shifted to the left. However, the *in vivo* curve may be normally placed because the Bohr effect counterbalances the reduction in red cell 2,3-BPG. If metabolic acidosis is rapidly corrected, the prompt rise in blood pH is reflected in a proportional increase in oxygen affinity (the Bohr effect). However, there is a lag of several hours before the red cell 2,3-BPG increases to normal.[24] During this time, there is a shift to the left in both the *in vivo* and the *in vitro* oxygen dissociation curves. This phenomenon may compromise tissue oxygenation in patients who have diminished cardiovascular reserves. Low red cell 2,3-BPG levels have been documented in patients with septic shock. This may be due in part to concomitant metabolic acidosis. The resultant left shift in the oxyhemoglobin dissociation curve probably accounts for the increased mixed venous oxygen content often encountered in this condition. Again, an increase in blood oxygen affinity may have untoward effects in patients who already have severe circulatory dysfunction.

In addition to metabolic acidosis, acquired deficiency of red cell 2,3-BPG (and ATP) may be encountered in patients with pituitary insufficiency as well as those who have hypophosphatemia due either to diarrhea or to inadequate phosphate supplements during hyperalimentation. In all instances, the expected shift to the left has been observed. In contrast, the slight but significant shift to the right encountered in normal children may be due to physiologically increased levels of plasma phosphate, resulting in a marked increase in red cell ATP and a modest increase in red cell 2,3-BPG.[25]

During the first week of storage of blood in acid-citrate-dextrose, red cells become depleted of 2,3-BPG and, as a result, have increased oxygen affinity.[26–28] Thus, patients who are transfused with large amounts of such blood have a left-shifted oxyhemoglobin dissociation curve.[26] The clinical significance of this phenomenon has not been established. At the least, it is safe to say that the recipient does not derive the full physiologic benefit from blood depleted in 2,3-BPG. However, after infusion of such donor cells into normal volunteers, the content of 2,3-BPG returns to normal within 6 to 24 hours.[29–31] Storage media can be effectively modified to preserve red cell 2,3-BPG and normal hemoglobin function.[32, 33]

The oxygen affinity of fetal blood is substantially higher than that of maternal blood (P_{50} = 19 mm Hg compared with 26 mm Hg for normal maternal blood). This difference may be of physiologic importance in facilitating the transport of oxygen across the placenta. The content of 2,3-BPG in the red cells of the newborn is at least as high as that of maternal red cells. Furthermore, phosphate-free Hb A and Hb F have nearly the same oxyhemoglobin dissociation curves. The oxygen affinity of fetal blood is higher because 2,3-BPG binds more weakly with Hb F than it does with Hb A.[34, 35] This can be explained by a comparison of the primary

structure of the β and γ chains. The β143 histidine of Hb A has been shown to be an important binding site for 2,3-BPG (as noted previously). In Hb F, γ143 is serine. This uncharged residue would not participate in electrostatic binding with 2,3-BPG.

The oxygen affinity of the newborn's blood decreases rapidly after birth.[36] During the first week of life, red cell 2,3-BPG increases about 20%. Although this increment in 2,3-BPG would not have much direct interaction with the fetal hemoglobin, it should lower intracellular pH and thereby decrease oxygen affinity. This rapid change in P_{50} seems appropriate for the increased metabolic demands after birth. The postnatal rise in 2,3-BPG is even more marked in healthy premature infants. At 1 to 4 weeks of age, their P_{50} values are close to those of normal adults.[37, 38] During the first 6 months of life, Hb F decreases from 77% to about 5% of the total. This results in a further increase in P_{50}.

In contrast, premature infants with respiratory insufficiency and acidosis have a marked decrease in red cell 2,3-BPG after birth,[37, 38] owing to the marked effect of pH on 2,3-BPG synthesis. Theoretically, such a left-shifted curve could be an advantage to the newborn who has concurrent hypoxemia and low cardiac output.[37] Nevertheless, under most circumstances, the increased oxygen affinity of newborn red cells would result in impaired oxygen delivery to tissues. Oski and associates[39, 40] have found that the mortality of premature newborns with severe respiratory distress syndrome is reduced if these infants are given an exchange transfusion of fresh adult blood having near-normal oxygen affinity. However, one cannot conclude that the enhanced survival was due to a reduction in oxygen affinity. It is possible that the exchange transfusions improved either pulmonary ventilation or pulmonary perfusion.

OTHER HEMOGLOBIN COMPONENTS

This chapter began with a detailed description of the structure and function of Hb A ($\alpha_2\beta_2$). In red cells of adults and children older than 6 months of age, Hb A accounts for more than 90% of the total hemoglobin. However, other globin genes are preferentially expressed during embryonic and fetal development. These different human hemoglobin components are listed in Table 19–2. Several of these hemoglobins provide useful information in the diagnosis of a variety of congenital and acquired hematologic disorders. Furthermore, post-translational modification of hemoglobin by nonenzymatic glycation has proved useful in the monitoring of patients with diabetes mellitus.

Embryonic Hemoglobins

Embryonic hemoglobins are produced in the yolk sac during the third through the eighth weeks of gestation (Fig. 19–12).[41] These components are the products of ε, $^A\gamma$ and $^G\gamma$ genes in combination with α and ζ subunits. Hb Gower 1 is $\zeta_2\epsilon_2$, whereas Hb Gower 2 is $\alpha_2\epsilon_2$. The ε gene is located in the β globin gene complex 5′ to $^A\gamma$. Hb Portland is $\zeta_2\gamma_2$. The ζ gene is located 5′ to α_1 and

Table 19-2. HUMAN HEMOGLOBINS

Hemoglobin	Structure	% of Normal Hemolysate*	Increased In	Decreased In
A	$\alpha_2\beta_2$	92.5	β-Thalassemia (see Table 19–3)	α-Thalassemia (see Table 19–3)
A₂	$\alpha_2\delta_2$	2.5		
A₁ₐ₁	Not known	0.2		
A₁ₐ₂	$\alpha_2(\beta\text{-N-G6P})_2$	0.2	Diabetes mellitus	Hemolytic anemia
A₁ᵦ	$\alpha_2(\beta\text{-N-pyruvate})_2$	0.5		
A₁ᶜ	$\alpha_2(\beta\text{-N-glucose})_2$	4.0		
F	$\alpha\gamma_2$	<1.0	Fetal red cells β-Thalassemia Marrow "stress," (e.g., sickle cell anemia)	
F₁	$\alpha_2(\gamma\text{-N-acetyl})_2$	<1.0		
Gower 1	$\zeta_2\epsilon_2$	0		
Gower 1	$\alpha_2\epsilon_2$	0	Early embryo	
Portland	$\zeta_2\gamma_2$	0		
H	β_4	0	α-Thalassemia	
Bart's	γ_4	0		

*Individuals more than 8 months old.

α_2 globin genes. Trace amounts (~0.3%) of ζ subunits can be encountered in normal fetuses until they are born.[42] These three embryonic hemoglobins serve as physiologic oxygen carriers. Red cells from early embryos in which these hemoglobins predominate have an affinity for oxygen similar to that of cord blood cells, as well as normal cooperativity and Bohr effect.[43]

Hemoglobin F

From 8 to 28 weeks' gestation the liver becomes the major site of erythropoiesis. During the last half of gestation, red cell production gradually shifts from the liver and spleen to the bone marrow. As shown in Figure 19–12, after the eighth week, Hb F becomes the

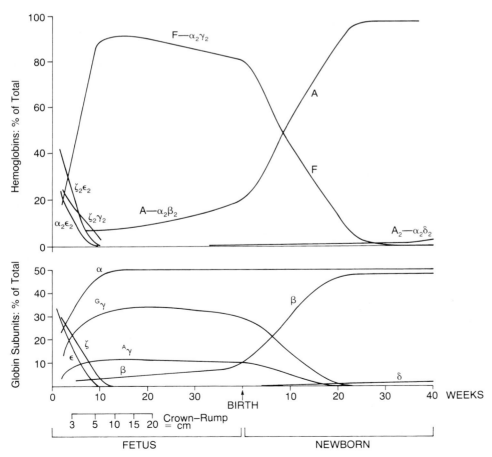

Figure 19-12. Changes in hemoglobin tetramers *(top)* and in globin subunits *(bottom)* during human development from embryo to early infancy. (From Bunn HF, Forget BG: Hemoglobin: Molecular, Genetic and Clinical Aspects. Philadelphia, W.B. Saunders Co., 1986.)

predominant hemoglobin. Other primates and ruminants also have structurally different fetal hemoglobin or hemoglobins. The human γ chain differs from the β chain in 39 of 146 residues. Unlike the other human globin subunits, the γ chain has structural heterogeneity. In newborns, about two thirds of the γ chains have glycine at position 136, whereas the remaining γ chains have alanine.[44] This ratio falls during the switch from γ to β chain production. The $^{G}\gamma$ and $^{A}\gamma$ chains are products of adjacent genes located between ε and δ. In addition, there is structural heterogeneity at position 75, where in certain populations the $^{A}\gamma$ chain contains threonine instead of isoleucine.[45, 46] The incidence of this substitution ranges from 0% to 40%. The determination of these differences in primary sequences has provided new insights into the thalassemias and hereditary persistence of fetal hemoglobin (see Chapter 21).

About 20% of Hb F in the developing fetus has a post-translational modification: the N terminus of the γ chain is acetylated (Hb F).[47] In contrast, no other human globin subunits are acetylated, except for variants that have substitutions of the N-terminal residue.[48]

Hb F has the special property of being remarkably resistant to denaturation at extremes of pH. The measurement of alkali-resistant hemoglobin has proved a very useful, although indirect, way of estimating the content of Hb F within a hemolysate. However, this approach tends to underestimate the amount of Hb F.[49] The percentage of Hb F in a hemolysate can be determined by chromatographic,[50] electrophoretic, and immunologic[51, 52] methods. In general, an immunologic assay is recommended for samples containing less than 2% Hb F; alkali denaturation is suggested for samples containing 2% to 40% Hb F; and chromatography is recommended if the amount of Hb F exceeds 40%.[52] However, high-performance liquid chromatography provides accurate analyses over the whole range of % Hb F. For methodologic details, see the monograph of Schroeder and Huisman.[53]

The red cells of the newborn contain about 80% Hb F, 20% Hb A, and less than 0.5% Hb A₂ (Fig. 19–13). Occasionally, Hb Bart's (γ₄) may be detected in trace amounts in a normal neonate. An increased level of Hb Bart's in a newborn's red cells is useful in the diagnosis of α-thalassemia (see Chapter 21). Shortly before birth there is a switch from γ chain to β chain synthesis. The level of Hb F falls steadily after birth, approaching a nadir at about age 6 months. However, the rate of fall of fetal hemoglobin levels is quite variable. Fetal hemoglobin persists longer in infants born prematurely,[54] with the concentration of Hb F being consistent with age from conception. In addition, the switch from Hb F to Hb A is delayed in infants of diabetic mothers, owing to increased levels of hydroxybutyrate.[55, 56] Conversely, there is a more rapid decline of Hb F in neonates having increased red cell turnover, such as in those with erythroblastosis fetalis.

In red cells of individuals older than 6 months, Hb F constitutes less than 1% of the total hemoglobin. Although alkali denaturation is not sensitive enough to detect Hb F in normal adults, fluorescent antibody labeling has demonstrated this hemoglobin, which is

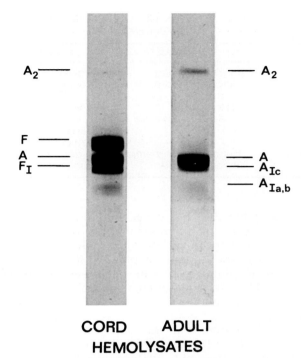

CORD   ADULT
HEMOLYSATES

Figure 19–13. Analysis of human umbilical cord and adult blood hemolysates by gel electrofocusing. The gels have been overloaded to demonstrate Hb A₂. (From Bunn HF, Forget BG: Hemoglobin: Molecular, Genetic and Clinical Aspects. Philadelphia, W.B. Saunders Co., 1986.)

distributed unevenly among red cells.[57–60] Normally, only 0.1% to 7% of red cells contain detectable amounts of fetal hemoglobin. These "F cells" contain about 5 pg of Hb F, approximately 20% of the total hemoglobin in the cell. F cell production is genetically controlled.[61, 62]

Hb F is increased to a variable extent in several hereditary disorders, including β-thalassemia, hereditary persistence of fetal hemoglobin, and sickle cell anemia. In addition, slightly increased levels of fetal hemoglobin may be seen in a variety of acquired hematologic disorders, including megaloblastic anemia, aplastic anemia, and leukemias, particularly chronic myelocytic leukemia in children. The mechanism underlying this return to γ chain synthesis, as well as the normal fetal switch from γ chain to β chain synthesis, is discussed in Chapter 21. In homozygous β-thalassemia and sickle cell anemia, survival of F cells is selectively enhanced, and the circulating concentration of fetal hemoglobin is thereby increased. The production of F cells can be enhanced by administration of several chemotherapeutic drugs such as hydroxyurea[63, 64] and by certain metabolites such as butyrate[65] and high doses of erythropoietin.[66]

Hemoglobin A₂

About 2.5% of the hemoglobin in normal red cells is Hb A₂(α₂δ₂) (see Fig. 19–13). This minor component is evenly distributed among red cells,[67] and its functional behavior is very similar to that of Hb A.[48] The δ and β chains are identical in sequence in all but 10 of 146

Table 19–3. ALTERATIONS IN Hb A_2 IN VARIOUS DISORDERS

	Elevated	Reduced
Congenital	β-thalassemia trait	α-thalassemia
	Unstable hemoglobin variants	δβ-thalassemia
	Sickle trait (AS)	δ-thalassemia
	SS with α-thalassemia	Hereditary persistence of fetal hemoglobin
Acquired	Megaloblastic anemias	Iron deficiency
	Hyperthyroidism	Sideroblastic anemias

residues. Table 19–3 lists congenital and acquired diseases associated with abnormal levels of Hb A_2. The increased percentage of Hb A_2 in β-thalassemia is a useful diagnostic aid (see Chapter 21). In addition, Hb A_2 is slightly increased in megaloblastic anemia. By contrast, Hb A_2 is decreased in α-thalassemia[68–70] as well as in iron deficiency[71] and sideroblastic anemias.[72] The relative rate of synthesis of this minor component is markedly curtailed in the final stages of erythroid development.[73, 74] The level of Hb A_2 appears to depend on the rate of assembly of hemoglobin subunits, as discussed later in this chapter.

Hemoglobin H and Hemoglobin Bart's

Hemoglobin H and Hb Bart's are tetramers of β chains and γ chains, respectively. For hemoglobin to function physiologically, a tetramer must consist of pairs of α and non-α chains. In contrast, Hb H and Hb Bart's have very high oxygen affinity and absent heme-heme interaction and Bohr effect. These hemoglobins are found to a variable extent in patients with the different types of α-thalassemia (see Chapter 21). In addition, high levels of Hb H may occasionally appear in patients who develop erythroleukemia.[75, 76]

Hemoglobins A_{Ia}, A_{Ib}, and A_{Ic}

When the hemoglobin from normal adult red cells is carefully analyzed by column chromatography,[77] several minor components can be detected that have a lower isoelectric point than the main Hb A. These are designated A_{Ia1}, A_{Ia2}, A_{Ib}, and A_{Ic}. On zone electrophoresis at alkaline pH, these components appear as a smear (sometimes designated Hb A_3 or Hb A_1) running anodal to the main component. Hb A_{Ic} accounts for approximately 3% of the hemoglobin in normal adult red cells.[78] Estimates in the literature are often falsely elevated owing to chromatographic or electrophoretic contaminants. Hb A_{Ic} differs from Hb A only at the N-terminal amino group of each β chain where glucose is attached by a ketoamine linkage (Fig. 19–14).[79] In addition, approximately 5% of hemoglobin molecules have glucose linked to certain lysine residues. These adducts cannot be separated from unmodified hemoglobins by ordinary chromatography or electrophoresis (Fig. 19–15) but can be isolated by means of an affinity resin containing phenylboronate, which binds to sugar hydroxyl groups.[78]

Glucose condenses with hemoglobin nonenzymatically. In like manner, sugar phosphates, particularly glucose-6-phosphate, combine with hemoglobin at the β-N terminus to form Hb A_{Ia1} and Hb A_{Ia2}. Hb A_{Ib} is an adduct of pyruvate with the β-N terminus.[80] A small fraction of these adducts can undergo further complex rearrangement reactions to form fluorescent advanced glycation end products.[80A] These hemoglobins are formed slowly and continuously throughout the 120-day life span of the red cell.[81] Consequently, individuals who have increased red cell turnover (hemolysis) have decreased levels of these minor hemoglobin components.[81]

Patients with diabetes mellitus have levels of Hb A_{Ic} that are two to three times higher than normal.[82] The measurement of Hb A_{Ic} has proved a useful independent assessment of the degree of diabetic control, because it is not subject to fluctuations of the blood glucose level.[83, 84] Furthermore, Hb A_{Ic}, along with derivative end products, mentioned earlier, are prototypes of glycosylation of other proteins, which could contribute to the long-term complications of the disease.[85]

Other Post-Translational Modifications

Although glucose adducts are by far the most common and abundant type of chemical modification of hemoglobin, other small molecules also are capable of form-

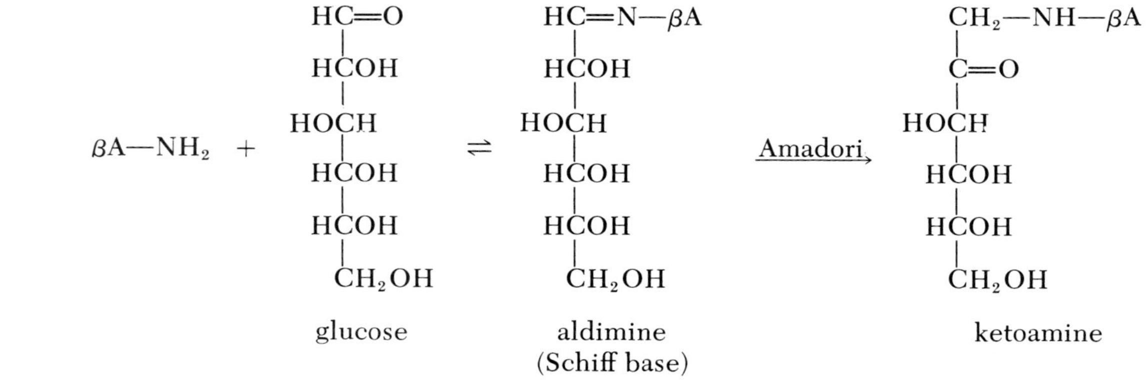

Figure 19–14. Reaction scheme for the formation of Hb A_{Ic}.

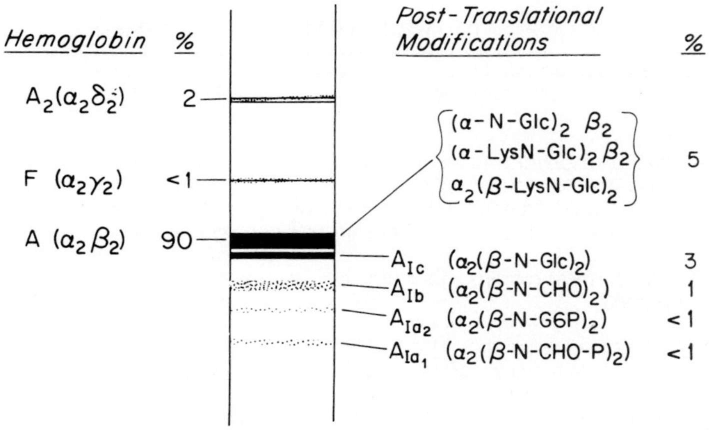

Figure 19-15. Separation of hemoglobin components in a normal hemolysate by means of gel electrofocusing. Glycated hemoglobins are shown on the right, along with the percentage of components in normal individuals. (From Bunn HF, Forget BG: Hemoglobin: Molecular, Genetic and Clinical Aspects. Philadelphia, W.B. Saunders Co., 1986.)

ing covalent linkages and thereby may reflect significant metabolic perturbations.

Carbamylated hemoglobin is formed in patients with uremia who have elevated levels of urea in their plasma and red cells.[86] Urea is in dynamic equilibrium with ammonium ion and cyanate ion. The latter can combine with amino groups or proteins to form irreversible covalent adducts. Increased levels of Hb A_I in uremic patients can be explained by increased carbamylation.

Alcoholics also have an increase of Hb A_I.[87] Although the structure of this modification has not been worked out, it probably involves the first oxidation product of ethanol, acetaldehyde, which is a highly reactive compound.

Children with lead poisoning (see Chapter 13) may have an increase in a hemoglobin component having the electrophoretic and chromatographic behavior of Hb A_{1c}.[88] The abnormal hemoglobin has been more frequently observed in those patients with hypochromic red cells. The hemoglobin does not contain any measurable lead, and, furthermore, does not appear to be a mixed disulfide with glutathione. It is likely to be a hybrid molecule in which at least one of the hemes is replaced by zinc protoporphyrin.[89] Protoporphyrin IX is the immediate precursor of heme and is markedly increased in plumbism. Zinc protoporphyrin can form a stable complex with globin at the heme-binding site (see Chapter 13).

HUMAN HEMOGLOBIN VARIANTS

A number of molecular and genetic mechanisms underlie the hemoglobin variants found in humans (Table 19–4). A detailed discussion of hemoglobin synthesis in general and the thalassemias in particular appears in Chapter 21. Furthermore, certain types of mutations, such as nonhomologous crossing-over and errors in globin-chain termination, are also covered in that chapter.

More than 500 structurally different human hemoglobin variants have been discovered.[90] Most of these constitute a single amino acid replacement in one of the globin polypeptide chains. In each case, the replacement of one residue by another can be accounted for

by a substitution of a single nucleotide base in the DNA or messenger RNA codon, according to the genetic code. In addition, 15 variants have been encountered thus far in which two amino acid replacements have been encountered at separate sites on a given globin subunit (see Table 19–4). There are about 70% more known β chain mutants than α chain mutants. This is somewhat surprising because there are two structural genes for the α chain and one for the β chain. In addition, δ chain and γ chain mutants have been described. The majority of these hemoglobin variants are not associated with any clinical manifestations, and many were discovered during the course of large population surveys. The most useful diagnostic tool for the detection of new hemoglobin variants is zone electrophoresis, which separates hemoglobins that differ in charge. However, recent advances in development of molecular genetic techniques for rapid and accurate diagnosis of hemoglobinopathies have been impressive.[91]

A significant proportion of the hemoglobin variants cannot be explained by a simple amino acid replacement. Some unstable variants contain deletions of from one to five amino acids in sequence (see Table 19–4) and probably arose because of frameshift mutagenesis in the region of reiterated nucleotide sequence.[48] This mechanism is supported by the finding of "mirror image" variants: Hb Gun Hill, which has a 5-residue deletion at position 93–97, and Hb Koriyama, which has a tandem repeat of the same five residues.[92] Frameshift mutagenesis is responsible for other rare variants such as Hb Grady[93] and Hb Zaire[94] in which there is an insertion of 3 and 5 amino acids, respectively. More complex mutations such as Hb Montreal,[94A] Hb Birmingham,[94B] and Hb Galacia[94B] have small in-frame deletions and insertions of novel amino acids, owing to slipped mispairings of short repeats and errors in DNA repair. Several fusion hemoglobins have been encountered in which nonhomologous crossover has occurred between the δ and β chain genes (Lepore and anti-Lepore hemoglobins) or between γ and β chain genes (Hb Kenya). These fusion hemoglobins are discussed in more detail in Chapter 21. Several hemoglobin variants have elongated subunits. As Table 19–4 shows, these mutant hemoglobins have arisen by

Table 19–4. MOLECULAR BASES OF HUMAN HEMOGLOBIN VARIANTS*

I. Single amino acid replacement in subunit (single nucleotide base substitution in codon)	β chain: S, C, D, E, etc. α chain: G-Philadelphia, I, Q, etc. γ chain δ chain
Two amino acid substitutions in subunit (two separate nucleotide base substitutions)	C-Harlem, J-Singapore, C-Ziguinchor, S-Travis, Arlington Park, S-Omen, S-Providence, etc.
II. Amino acid deletions (deletion of corresponding codon(s), probably as a result of frameshift mutagenesis)	Freiburg (1),† Gun Hill (5), Leiden (1), Niteroi (3), Tochigi (4), Leslie (1), Lyons (2), Coventry (1), St. Antoine (2), Tours (1), McKees Rocks (2)‡
III. Fusion hemoglobins (nonhomologous crossover of nearby genes)	δβ: The Lepores βδ: Miyada, P-Congo, P-Nilotic γβ: Kenya
IV. Elongated subunits A. Error in termination of subunit (nucleotide base substitution in termination codon)	α chain: Constant Spring, Icaria, Koya Dora, Seal Rock

B. Frameshift mutation (deletion or addition of one or two bases)
  C. Crossover in phase (tandem repetition of intact triplet codons)
  D. Retention of initiator methionine
	α chain: Wayne
	β chain: Tak, Cranston, Saverne
	Grady, Koriyama
	Long Island, South Florida

*Information collected by International Hemoglobin Information Center, Augusta, GA.
†Figures in parentheses indicate number of residues deleted.
‡May be a chain termination mutation.

one of four genetic mechanisms: base substitution in the UAA chain termination codon, frame shift, crossover in phase, or retention of the initiator methionine.[48, 90] The best known example of a termination codon substitution is Hb Constant Spring. Because this variant is synthesized in such small amounts, it can be considered a form of α-thalassemia and contributes significantly to the overall incidence of Hb H disease in southeast Asia (see Chapter 21). Determination of the primary structure of the elongated subunits provided early information about the structure of the normally nontranslated portion at the 3' end of the α and β globin messenger RNA.

Those abnormal hemoglobins that are of clinical im-

Table 19–5. CLINICALLY IMPORTANT HEMOGLOBIN VARIANTS

I. Sickle syndromes
  A. Sickle cell trait
  B. Sickle cell disease
    1. SS
    2. SC
    3. S/D-Los Angeles
    4. S/O-Arab
    5. S/β Thal
II. Unstable hemoglobins→congenital Heinz body anemia (approx. 100 variants)
III. Hemoglobins with abnormal oxygen affinity
  A. High affinity→familial erythrocytosis (approx. 50 variants)
  B. Low affinity→familial cyanosis (Hbs Kansas, Beth Israel, St. Mandé)
IV. M hemoglobins→familial cyanosis (5 variants)
V. Structural variants that result in a thalassemic phenotype
  A. β-Thalassemia phenotype
    1. Lepore hemoglobins (δβ fusion)
    2. Hb E
    3. Hbs Indianapolis, Showa-Yakushiji, Geneva, etc.
  B. α-Thalassemia phenotype
    Chain termination mutants (e.g., Hb Constant Spring)

portance can be conveniently classified into one of five groups outlined in Table 19–5. Sickle hemoglobin (Hb S, β6 Glu→Val) is the most frequently encountered variant worldwide. Furthermore, sickle cell anemia has the most severe clinical manifestations of any of the hemoglobinopathies. The sickle syndromes and Hb C disease are covered in detail in Chapter 20.

Assembly of Variant Hemoglobins

The proportion of normal and variant hemoglobins in red cells of heterozygotes provides insight into the assembly of human hemoglobins.[95] Because the β-polypeptide chains are encoded on two β-globin genes (one from each parent), individuals heterozygous for a β chain variant would be expected to have approximately equal amounts of normal and variant hemoglobins. A markedly low proportion of β chain variant (less than 25%) is encountered under two circumstances. Some mutations result in unstable hemoglobin variants, which (as explained later) undergo increased catabolism before and after emergence of red cells from the bone marrow. Furthermore, as indicated in Table 19–5, a few variants such as Hb Lepore and Hb Vicksburg are synthesized at a much lower rate than the normal β chain and therefore produce a thalassemic phenotype. However, the great majority of β chain variants investigated are synthesized at the same rate as βᴬ and have normal stability.[96] Nevertheless, even among these variants, the proportion of normal and abnormal hemoglobins in heterozygotes varies widely (Fig. 19–16A). The positively charged variants such as Hb S, Hb D, Hb C, and HB E* constitute significantly less than half of the total hemoglobin in heterozygotes and are reduced further in the presence of α-thalas-

*The proportion of Hb E is further reduced by lowered levels of βᴱ messenger RNA, owing to inefficient splicing. See Chapter 21.

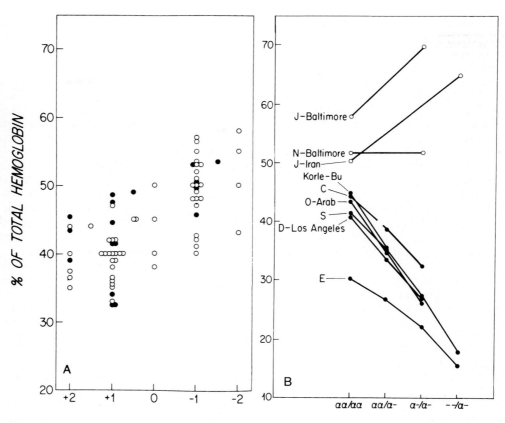

Figure 19-16. *A,* Proportion of variant hemoglobin in red cells of individuals heterozygous for 72 different stable β-chain variants. The horizontal axis shows charge change of the variant. *Solid circles* (●) represent measurements by Huisman[97] employing high-resolution chromatography. (Reprinted by permission from Bunn HF, McDonald MJ: Electrostatic interactions in the assembly of haemoglobin. Nature 1983; 306:498–500. Copyright © 1983 Macmillan Magazines Ltd.) *B,* The effect of α-thalassemia on the proportion of certain variants. ○, negatively charged; ●, positively charged. (Modified by permission from Bunn HF, McDonald MJ: Electrostatic interactions in the assembly of haemoglobin. Nature 1983; 306:498–500. Copyright © 1983 Macmillan Magazines Ltd.)

semia (see Fig. 19–16*B*).[95, 97] In contrast, many of the negatively charged variants are present in amounts exceeding that of Hb A. In two cases involving negatively charged variants (Hb J-Baltimore and Hb J-Iran) in individuals with α-thalassemia, the proportion of the variant hemoglobin was found to be further increased. This analysis of the proportion of β chain variant in heterozygotes suggests that alterations in surface charge contribute to different rates of assembly of the hemoglobin tetramer. Furthermore, *in vitro* mixing experiments on normal and variant β subunits show that when α chains are present in limiting amounts (mimicking α-thalassemia), negatively charged variants are formed much more readily than positively charged variants.[98] Moreover, α chains have a higher affinity for β chains than for γ chains.[98a, 98b]

This electrostatic model of hemoglobin assembly has clinical implications. Differences in rates of assembly explain not only the low proportion of Hb S in sickle trait (AS) but also the higher proportion of Hb S in sickle C (SC) disease. The prominent clinical manifestations of SC disease and their absence in sickle trait can be attributed in part to differences in the intracellular content of Hb S.[99] This model also provides an explanation for differences in the level of Hb A₂ that accompany certain hematologic disorders (see Table 19–3).

Because normal individuals have four α globin genes, α-globin variants usually comprise about 25% of the hemolysate. This fraction increases with concurrent α-thalassemia. The α_2 gene is transcribed more efficiently than the α_1 gene. Accordingly, stable variants expressed by α_2 tend to be relatively more abundant than those expressed by α_1.[100]

The Unstable Hemoglobins (Congenital Heinz Body Hemolytic Anemia)

In 1952, Cathie described a patient with congenital nonspherocytic hemolytic anemia associated with jaundice, splenomegaly, and pigmenturia.[101] Subsequently, other patients with similar clinical findings were suspected of having a structurally abnormal hemoglobin because their hemolysates formed a precipitate readily on heating. In most cases, structural analyses have demonstrated mutant hemoglobins. So-called congenital Heinz body hemolytic anemia (CHBA) constitutes an important type of congenital hemolytic disease. Although the term is widely used, it is a misnomer. Because of its variable severity, clinical manifestations may not appear until later in childhood or in adulthood, and Heinz bodies are not always present.

Unstable hemoglobinopathy has an autosomal dominant pattern of inheritance. Thus, affected individuals are nearly always heterozygotes. Occasionally, unstable α variants are associated with a clinical phenotype only in homozygotes.[101A] Heterozygotes have no detectable abnormalities, owing to the presence of three normal α genes.

In CHBA, the unstable hemoglobin constitutes only a minority (10% to 30%) of the total. As expected in the heterozygous state, the remaining hemoglobin is predominantly normal Hb A. CHBA is more severe when an unstable β chain variant is inherited along with β-thalassemia.[102, 102A] In these individuals, the variant hemoglobin comprises nearly all of the total. Because of the low gene frequency, the homozygous state for this disorder would be a very rare event. In some of the unstable β-globin variants, it would be incompatible with life. Such considerations also apply to erythrocytosis due to a hemoglobin variant with an abnormally high oxygen affinity (discussed later). A sizable minority of cases of unstable hemoglobinopathy appear to have arisen because of a spontaneous mutation, with both parents being unaffected.[48, 103] Viewed another way, of the instances of apparent spontaneous mutations among hemoglobin variants reported to date, approximately two thirds involve patients with unstable hemoglobins. This is not surprising, because many cases are sufficiently severe that medical attention and evaluation are sought. In contrast, the chances are very remote of finding an asymptomatic individual with a hemoglobin variant due to a spontaneous mutation. Furthermore, patients with severe unstable hemoglobinopathy are less likely to have healthy offspring.

One instance of CHBA has been attributed to the presence of Hb F-Poole, an unstable γ chain variant.[104] A significant degree of hemolysis with Heinz body formation and jaundice was noted in an otherwise healthy newborn, but these findings gradually disappeared as Hb F was replaced by Hb A during the first few months of life. There are probably similar cases of hemolytic disease in the newborn due to the presence of other unstable γ chain variants. The diagnosis is challenging because the variant would be present in small amounts and would be transient. Only markedly unstable γ chain variants are likely to produce this syndrome, because the newborn inherits four γ chain genes and therefore the great majority of his fetal hemoglobin would be stable.

Pathogenesis

Over 100 structurally different unstable hemoglobin variants have been documented. Many of these show only mild instability *in vitro* and are not associated with any significant clinical manifestations. About three fourths of these are β chain mutants. Many of them are amino acid replacements in the vicinity of the heme pocket (Fig. 19–17). The majority are neutral replacements, such as Hb Köln (β95 Val→Met). Such an alteration in primary structure may cause considerable perturbations in the hydrophobic interior of the molecule. Considering the nature of such amino acid replacements, it is not surprising that many of these variants have electrophoretic mobility identical with that of Hb A. Others may appear as single or multiple bands having isoelectric points higher than that of Hb A. If these bands are no longer visible after the addition of hemin to the hemolysate, it is likely that the abnormal electrophoretic mobility was due to heme loss (or heme displacement) rather than to an alteration in the charge of a globin subunit. About one fifth of the

unstable variants involve a replacement by proline. Proline residues can prevent the formation of an α helix. Thus, instability may result from disruption of the secondary structure of the subunit.

Much of the red cell destruction in CHBA occurs in the bone marrow.[105] Convincing evidence indicates that normally placed hemes confer considerable stability to their respective globin subunits. In many of the unstable hemoglobin variants, the amino acid substitution prevents a normal heme-globin linkage. Once the heme becomes detached from its normal position in the cleft on the surface of the involved subunit, it probably binds nonspecifically to another site on the globin. Both spectrophotometric and electron spin resonance measurements indicate that formation of hemichrome may be an intermediate step in the denaturation of unstable hemoglobins.[106] After heme displacement, the globin subunits aggregate to form a coccoid precipitate having the morphologic characteristics of a Heinz body. The Heinz bodies and the heat-induced precipitate contain equal amounts of α and β chains and probably a normal complement of heme.[107] Red cells containing Heinz bodies have reduced deformability[108] and are likely to be entrapped in the microcirculation. Morphologically, these Heinz bodies become selectively removed, or "pitted," during circulation through the sinusoids of the spleen.[109] Therefore, it is not surprising that patients who have undergone splenectomy have an increased number of Heinz bodies and, in most cases, a greater percentage of the hemoglobin variant relative to normal Hb A.

The intracellular release of heme from these unstable variants may contribute to decreased deformability of CHBA red cells and therefore to the rate of hemolysis. The production of reactive oxygen species such as hydrogen peroxide, superoxide, and hydroxyl radical may damage the red cell membrane by both lipid peroxidation and cross-linking of membrane proteins.[110, 111] The abnormal heme environment may, in rare instances, cause oxidation of a specific residue in the unstable subunit, such as the post-translational conversion of β141 leucine to hydroxyleucine in Hb Atlanta-Coventry.[111a]

Because the degree of instability of these hemoglobin variants spans a wide range, the extent of hemolysis varies considerably. One patient with particularly severe anemia was shown to have a globin gene (Hb Medicine Lake) with two amino acid replacements: β95 Val→Met, the relatively frequently encountered Hb Köln mutation, and β32 Leu→Gln, which further aggravated the instability.[111b] In some unstable variants, such as Hb Zürich, an additional oxidant stress, such as the ingestion of certain drugs, is required for significant hemolysis. Fever may also increase the hemolytic rate.[112] Many patients, however, have continuous and marked red cell breakdown. The degree of anemia is influenced not only by the severity of the hemolysis but also by the ability of the blood to unload oxygen.[48] Thus, patients having unstable variants of high oxygen affinity, such as Hb Köln, may have a near-normal hemoglobin level (i.e., compensated hemolysis). In contrast, the hemoglobin level is likely to be much lower

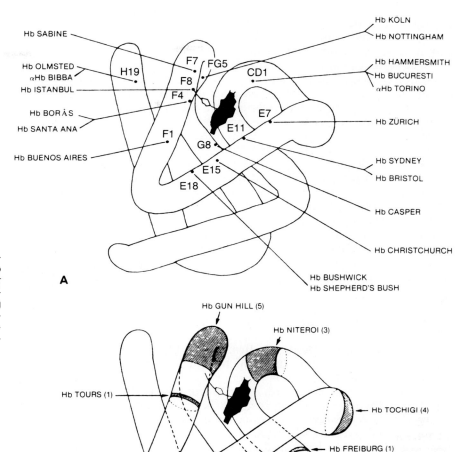

Figure 19-17. A, Three-dimensional representation of β chain showing sites of amino acid substitutions at the heme pocket that cause unstable variants. *B,* Three-dimensional representation of β chain showing sites of amino acid deletions causing unstable hemoglobins. (From White JM: The unstable haemoglobin disorders. Clin Haematol 1974; 3:333–356.)

in patients having variants with decreased oxygen affinity, such as Hb Hammersmith.

The structural alteration in Hb Zürich leads to particularly interesting functional and clinical consequences.[113, 114] The replacement of the distal histidine by arginine at βE7 causes a larger space in the heme pocket where gas ligands bind. Accordingly, CO is able to bind in a nonconstrained fashion and with much higher affinity. Carbon monoxide protects this variant from oxidative denaturation. Individuals with Hb Zürich who smoke tend to accumulate high levels of carboxyhemoglobin and have less hemolysis than affected family members who do not smoke.

A few hemoglobin variants are so unstable that virtually no mutant gene product can be detected in the hemolysate. Examples include Hb Indianapolis,[115] Hb Showa-Yakushiji,[116] Hb Geneva,[117] and Hb Cagliari.[117a] Heterozygotes have a phenotype of thalassemia intermedia with moderate anemia, splenomegaly, microcytic red cells, Heinz bodies, and elevated Hb A2.

Others, such as Hb Mississippi, cause a thalassemia intermedia phenotype when associated with a β+-thalassemia gene *in trans.*[102a] For more information on hemoglobin variants associated with a thalassemic phenotype, see Chapter 21.

Clinical Features

These pathophysiologic considerations explain a number of the clinical features of this disorder. Patients usually present in early childhood with a hemolytic anemia accompanied by jaundice and splenomegaly. In some cases, hemolysis is markedly aggravated by fever or the ingestion of an oxidant-type drug. The red cell morphology is somewhat variable. Often, patients with a functioning spleen have normal-looking red cells. Slight hypochromia and prominent basophilic stippling are common features. Indeed, the intensity of the basophilic stippling may equal or even exceed that noted in pyrimidine 5' nucleotidase deficiency (see Chapters

12 and 17). In both conditions, the stippling may be due to excessive clumping of ribosomes. The blood may have to be incubated to demonstrate Heinz bodies.[118] In some cases, it appears as if a bite had been taken from a margin of the red cells, and it is tempting to speculate that a Heinz body had been pitted at this site. After splenectomy, red cells appear much more abnormal. Heinz bodies are larger and more numerous. Indeed, they may not be detectable until the spleen has been removed. The extent of symptoms varies markedly with the degree of anemia. As mentioned earlier, one of the two parents is affected in about two thirds of the cases. Some patients give a history of passing dark urine. Although this pigment has not been completely characterized, it appears to be a dipyrrole (mesobilifuscin) and may be the consequence of aberrant (perhaps nonenzymatic) heme catabolism. Dipyrroles have also been detected in CHBA red cells by fluorescence microscopy.[119]

Diagnosis

The following studies are valuable in establishing the diagnosis:

Demonstration of Heinz Bodies. Fresh blood is treated with a supravital stain, such as 1% methyl violet. If the patient's spleen is intact, it may be necessary to incubate the blood (either for 60 minutes with acetylphenylhydrazine or for 24 to 48 hours without an additive). A positive test reveals the presence of purple-stained red cell inclusions, often several per cell and measuring up to 1 μm in diameter.

Hemoglobin Instability. Freshly prepared hemolysates of the patient and of a normal control subject are diluted in 0.1 M phosphate buffer, pH 7.4 (final hemoglobin concentration, 0.5 to 1 g/dL). After incubation for 1 hour at 50°C, a precipitate will appear in the solution containing an unstable hemoglobin variant. Hemolysates containing an unstable hemoglobin will also form a flocculent precipitate when incubated in 17% isopropanol, pH 7.4,[120] or in zinc acetate, 3.5 mol per mole of Hb tetramer.[121]

Hemoglobin Electrophoresis. Abnormal patterns have been observed in most patients (see previous discussion on molecular pathogenesis). In some instances, a high-resolution method, such as isoelectric focusing, may be required to demonstrate an abnormal hemoglobin.

Oxyhemoglobin Dissociation Curve. The unstable hemoglobins frequently have abnormal oxygen affinity. The author and his colleagues have studied one patient who presented with compensated hemolysis. Laboratory evaluation included a negative heat instability test and normal hemoglobin electrophoresis (starch gel, pH 8.6) but a positive incubated Heinz body preparation and increased oxygen affinity of both whole blood and a phosphate-free hemoglobin solution. The patient was found to have Hb Buenos Aires (Bryn Mawr) (β85 Phe→Ser).

Treatment

The treatment of unstable hemoglobinopathy is primarily supportive. Anemia is rarely severe enough to warrant blood transfusion. Oxidant drugs should be avoided. Like others with chronic hemolysis, these patients have an increased requirement for folic acid; and those with severe hemolysis may benefit from prophylactic folate therapy. The red cell mass may fall precipitously during a period of bone marrow suppression, such as that resulting from folate deficiency or acute infection. Although patients with severe hemolysis may benefit from splenectomy, this operation is not curative. Because of the risk of bacterial sepsis in infants and young children who have been splenectomized, this treatment should be postponed until the child is older than 5 years of age. The diagnostic tests just cited become more abnormal after splenectomy. For this reason, in some cases the diagnosis may not be definitely established until after the operation.

Hemoglobin Variants with Abnormal Oxygen Binding

In 1966, Charache and coworkers[122] described a family with erythrocytosis due to the presence of a hemoglobin variant, Hb Chesapeake (α92 Arg→Leu). Oxygen equilibria done on both whole blood and the isolated abnormal hemoglobin revealed a marked increase in oxygen affinity and a reduction in subunit cooperativity. Because of the "shift to the left" and consequent reduction in oxygen unloading, individuals with a high-affinity variant have compensatory erythrocytosis through increased production of erythropoietin.[123] More than 50 other stable variants with very high oxygen affinity have been discovered. In each case, affected heterozygous family members have erythrocytosis. An additional 50 stable variants with mildly increased oxygen affinity have been described. Heterozygotes generally do not have significant erythrocytosis, unless coinheritance of β-thalassemia precludes the formation of normal Hb A.[123A] Unlike the unstable hemoglobins, which also may have abnormal oxygen affinity, these variants are not associated with any hemolysis or abnormal red cell morphology.

The location and nature of the amino acid substitutions in these variants have been useful in establishing specific sites on the hemoglobin molecule that are critical to its function. A number of these variants have substitutions at the C terminus of the subunit. Others have substitutions at the α¹β² interface. These structural perturbations may affect the conformational isomerization between the oxy (R) and deoxy (T) forms. For example, there is good experimental evidence that the high oxygen affinity of Hb Bethesda and Hb Kempsey is due to decreased stability of the T form, while the low oxygen affinity of Hb Kansas can be related to decreased stability of the R form.[48] Several variants with high oxygen affinity have substitutions at the 2,3-BPG binding site, which results in impaired binding to 2,3-BPG and increased intracellular oxygen affinity.[48]

Other than erythrocytosis, affected individuals have minimal clinical manifestations. In most cases, the increase in red cell mass is probably appropriate to ensure tissue oxygenation. Hemodynamic studies on these individuals have produced somewhat variable results. Some patients have had increased cardiac output or low $P\overline{v}O_2$ or both when subjected to graded exercise or bled down to a normal red cell mass.[48] Packed cell volumes seldom reach high enough levels so that increased blood viscosity necessitates therapeutic phlebotomy. There are many reports of affected mothers carrying unaffected offspring to term. In these cases, the oxygen affinity of the maternal blood was probably greater than that of the fetus. The lack of any untoward complications[124] argues against the physiologic importance of increased oxygen affinity of fetal blood.

The possibility of a functionally abnormal hemoglobin should be considered in any case of unexplained erythrocytosis. A positive family history and an abnormal hemoglobin electrophoresis are very helpful. However, the author has seen one child in whom neither of these findings was present. She was found to have Hb Bethesda, which apparently arose as a spontaneous mutation. In such cases, a measurement of oxygen affinity is required to establish the diagnosis. Not all familial erythrocytosis is due to a functionally abnormal hemoglobin variant. In some families, mutations of the erythropoietin receptor give rise to enhanced erythroid proliferation. In other cases, increased production of erythropoietin has been documented.[125]

M Hemoglobins

Cyanosis is due to an excess of either deoxyhemoglobin or methemoglobin in the blood. Congenital methemoglobinemia may be due to a deficiency of the enzyme cytochrome-b_5 reductase (also called diaphorase I or NADH-dependent methemoglobin reductase), which enables red cell hemoglobin to be maintained in the reduced form. A more uncommon cause of congenital methemoglobinemia is the presence of one of the M hemoglobins. Like the other two classes of functionally abnormal hemoglobins discussed in detail in this chapter, the M hemoglobins are inherited according to an autosomal dominant pattern. Affected individuals present with cyanosis but are otherwise asymptomatic. Generally, there is no evidence of anemia. The blood has a peculiar mahogany color "like that of Japanese soy sauce."[126] Spectral examination of the hemoglobin shows an abnormal pattern that is similar to that of methemoglobin. Hemoglobin electrophoresis reveals an abnormal band with a slightly anodal mobility. The normal A and abnormal M hemoglobins may be separated more readily if the entire hemolysate is converted to methemoglobin before the electrophoresis.

Seven M hemoglobins have been described (Table 19–6). The α and β chain variants have been detected in unrelated families all over the world. Six of the seven M hemoglobins represent substitution of either the proximal (F8) or distal (E7) histidine by tyrosine. It is likely that the side group of the substituted tyrosine can serve as an internal ligand, stabilizing the heme iron in the ferric form. As anticipated, the M hemoglobins are functionally abnormal. Both α chain variants have decreased oxygen affinity and decreased Bohr effect.[48] The whole blood oxygen affinity of individuals with Hb M may be markedly decreased, owing in part to the intrinsic functional abnormality of the hemoglobin variant and in part to increased 2,3-BPG in the red cell. Furthermore, individuals who have one of the M hemoglobins may have mild hemolysis.[127, 128] However, the M hemoglobins should not be confused with some of the unstable variants such as Hb Freiburg and Hb St. Louis, in which a high proportion of the abnormal subunit oxidizes to methemoglobin. Hb F-M-Osaka (γ63 His→Tyr)[129] and HB F-M-Fort Ripley (γ92 His→Tyr)[130] were discovered in cyanotic newborns. The cyanosis disappeared during the first few months of life as β chains replaced γ chains.

In this disorder, treatment is neither indicated nor possible. The M hemoglobins are perhaps of more interest and concern to molecular biologists than to the individuals affected.

ACQUIRED ABNORMALITIES OF HEMOGLOBIN STRUCTURE AND FUNCTION

The genetic bases for the hemoglobinopathies are well understood (see Table 19–4). However, a number of acquired abnormalities of hemoglobin structure and function also deserve consideration. Some, such as methemoglobinemia (see later) and CO poisoning, involve specific alterations of heme, the prosthetic group of the molecule. In contrast, as discussed earlier, alterations in the distribution of normal globin subunits may accompany such diverse entities as myeloproliferative disorders, iron deficiency, and diabetes mellitus.

Carbon Monoxide Intoxication

Carbon monoxide is an important and widespread industrial pollutant and toxin. This gas may be engen-

Table 19–6. PROPERTIES OF THE M HEMOGLOBINS

M Hemoglobin	Synonyms	Structure	Helical Residue	Oxygen Affinity at P$_{50}$	Bohr Effect
M-Boston	Osaka, Gothenburg	α58 His → Tyr	E7	Decreased	Decreased
M-Iwate	Kankakee, Oldenburg	α86 His → Tyr	F8	Decreased	Decreased
M-Saskatoon	Chicago, Radom, Emory, Kurume	β63 His → Tyr	E7	Normal	Present
M-Hyde Park		β92 His → Tyr	F8	Normal	Present
M-Milwaukee-1		β67 Val → Glu	E11	Decreased	Present

Adapted from Bunn HF, Forget BG, et al: Human Hemoglobins. Philadelphia, W.B. Saunders Co., 1977, p 339.

dered from the combustion of any organic material but, in particular, that of hydrocarbons such as petroleum and tobacco tar. In addition, 1 mole of CO is formed endogenously in the breakdown of heme into bile pigment. Accordingly, individuals with significant hemolysis or ineffective erythropoiesis have a measurably increased amount of circulating carboxyhemoglobin.[131, 132]

Like oxygen, CO is a ligand that binds reversibly to hemoglobin when heme iron is in the reduced (ferrous) state. The toxicity of CO is due to its very high affinity for heme, approximately 210 times that of oxygen. After an acute exposure, CO remains so tightly bound to hemoglobin that about 5 hours are required for an individual with normal ventilation to expel half of it.[133] Because of its slow disappearance time, a toxic level of carboxyhemoglobin may accumulate from continued exposure to a relatively low dose of CO. CO also binds to other heme proteins, such as cytochrome P-450. Whether this contributes significantly to the toxicity of CO is not known.

As expected, the clinical manifestations of CO intoxication are directly related to the duration and extent of exposure. Impaired visual and temporal discrimination have been noted in individuals with carboxyhemoglobin levels of 5%, and alterations in mood and sleep patterns have been noted in volunteers in whom carboxyhemoglobin levels have risen to 8%.[48] At carboxyhemoglobin levels above approximately 20%, more overt and subjective symptoms develop, such as headache and weakness. At levels of 40% to 60%, unconsciousness is followed by death.

The toxic effect of CO is primarily due to increased oxygen affinity of the blood. The mechanism by which CO shifts the oxyhemoglobin dissociation curve to the left is identical with that of methemoglobin (see next section). However, a given percentage of carboxyhemoglobin appears to be more deleterious than a comparable level of methemoglobin. This may be because of a more even distribution of CO among red cells of all ages.

The treatment of CO intoxication is directed primarily toward removal of the source of toxic exposure and facilitation of gas expulsion by the lungs. Thus, maintenance of adequate ventilation is very important. If the patient is treated with an oxygen mask, the disappearance half-time for CO is reduced from 5 hours to 2 hours.[131] Other therapeutic approaches, such as hyperbaric oxygen[134] and exchange transfusion, may have theoretical merit but are not readily available.

METHEMOGLOBINEMIA

Hemoglobin's ability to reversibly bind to oxygen depends on the heme iron being maintained in the ferrous (Fe^{2+}) state. Oxyhemoglobin, when incubated under physiologic conditions, slowly auto-oxidizes to methemoglobin. Moreover, during the prolonged sojourn of the red cell in the circulation, hemoglobin is exposed to a variety of natural and xenobiotic oxidants that enhance the rate of methemoglobin formation. In this section the enzymatic apparatus that effectively maintains intracellular hemoglobin in the Fe^{2+} state is described first and then various clinical conditions are discussed in which this defense is abnormal or inadequate, resulting in methemoglobinemia.

Physiologic Methemoglobin Reduction

The reduction of methemoglobin in the red cell depends primarily on a linked system consisting of two electron carriers, cytochrome-b_5 and the reduced form of nicotinamide-adenine dinucleotide (NADH), along with the enzyme cytochrome-b_5 reductase (Fig. 19–18). Only a small proportion of methemoglobin in red cells is reduced by other means.

In the 1940s, while serving as an obstetrician in Ireland, Quentin Gibson had the opportunity to see two families with congenital methemoglobinemia. His initial investigation of these families led to a classic paper on methemoglobin reduction in red cells.[135] Red cell incubation experiments demonstrated a very slow rate of methemoglobin reduction in affected family members along with decreased accumulation of pyruvate. From these experiments, Gibson concluded that in normal red cells an NADH-dependent enzyme was responsible for methemoglobin reduction and that this enzyme was deficient in individuals with congenital methemoglobinemia. These experiments confirmed and extended prior studies of Kiese,[136] who also demonstrated a relationship between glucose and lactate consumption and methemoglobin reduction. Because of World War II, neither investigator knew of the other's work.

Subsequently, Scott and McGraw[137] began to purify and characterize methemoglobin-reducing enzymes. They were able to distinguish methemoglobin reductases dependent on NADH from those that required the reduced form of nicotinamide-adenine dinucleotide phosphate (NADPH). One species of the NADH-de-

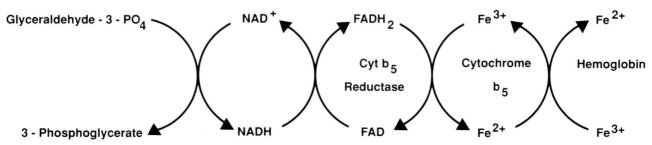

Figure 19–18. Pathway for the physiologic reduction of methemoglobin (Fe^{3+}) to hemoglobin (Fe^{2+}).

pendent enzymes was absent in red cells of Eskimos with hereditary methemoglobinemia,[138] in keeping with the earlier conclusion of Gibson.[135] The fact that the reduction of methemoglobin was very slow in the presence of the purified enzyme and NADH suggested that an additional substance was necessary to transport electrons from the enzyme to methemoglobin.

Cytochrome-b_5

In 1971, Hultquist and Passon[139] isolated a heme protein from red cells that had visible and electron paramagnetic resonance spectra characteristic of cytochrome-b_5 and, indeed, served as a substrate for hepatic microsomal cytochrome-b_5 reductase. This protein greatly accelerated the NADH-dependent enzymatic reduction of methemoglobin, an observation consistent with other studies using hepatic cytochrome-b_5.[140] The cytochrome-b_5 in the erythrocyte and that in the liver were shown to have a common heme-binding peptide.[141] Erythrocyte cytochrome-b_5 corresponds to the N-terminal hydrophilic domain of hepatic cytochrome-b_5.[142] The hydrophobic C-terminal end is embedded in the microsomal membrane. Free cytochrome-b_5 is released by proteolytic cleavage of a parent molecule located in the microsomes of erythroid precursor cells (Fig. 19–19).

Cytochrome-b_5 Reductase

The NADH-dependent methemoglobin reductase isolated from human red cells rapidly reduced erythrocyte cytochrome-b_5 and had properties similar to those of cytochrome-b_5 reductase prepared from hepatic microsomes.[143] Both enzymes contain flavin adenine dinucleotide (FAD) and show the same substrate specificity, pattern of inhibition, and pH dependency as well as immunologic identity.[144–146] These studies provide strong evidence that these enzymes have a common

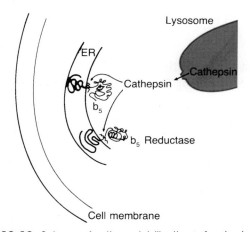

Figure 19-19. Scheme for the solubilization of cytochrome-b_5 and cytochrome-b_5 reductase from precursor proteins in the endoplasmic reticulum of erythroid progenitor cells. (From Hultquist DE, Slaughter SR, et al: Erythrocyte cytochrome-b_5: structure, role in methemoglobin reduction, and solubilization from endoplasmic reticulum. In Brewer G (ed): The Red Cell. New York, Alan R. Liss, Inc., 1978, p 199.)

structure. Like cytochrome-b_5, the soluble erythrocyte cytochrome-b_5 reductase is cleaved, by ATP-dependent proteolysis, from a microsomal precursor protein and is released during erythroid differentiation.[147] Thus, there is compelling evidence that erythrocyte cytochrome-b_5 reductase is the NADH-dependent enzyme responsible for methemoglobin reduction and that erythrocyte cytochrome-b_5 is the physiologic electron carrier. Preliminary information is available on the three-dimensional structure of this enzyme.[148]

The reduction of methemoglobin by reduced cytochrome-b_5 involves the formation of a bimolecular complex.[149–151] In the normal red cell, roughly 20% of cytochrome-b_5 is expected to be bound to the small amount of methemoglobin that is present. The bimolecular complex involves electrostatic interactions between negatively charged groups around the heme group of the cytochrome and positively charged residues around the heme groups in methemoglobin. A comparable interaction has been documented[152] for the cytochrome-b_5/cytochrome-c complex. A comparison of the rates of enzymatic reduction of normal and variant hemoglobins suggests that β66 Lys and β95 Lys are among the residues responsible for binding to cytochrome-b_5.[153]

The rate of methemoglobin reduction in a mixture of enzymes and cofactors simulating that of the red cell (1.1 to 1.4 μmol/mL per hour)[154–156] agrees well with the rate measured in intact red cells (about 1 μmol/mL per hour).[135, 157] The relative concentrations of cytochrome-b_5, cytochrome-b_5 reductase, and NADH in normal red cells suggest that both proteins limit the rate of methemoglobin reduction.[156, 158] The level of the enzyme declines with cell aging.[157, 159–162] Senescent red cells have low levels of enzyme activity. Furthermore, the concentration of cytochrome-b_5 decreases to about 20% of its initial value as red cells age *in vivo* (half-life of 44 days).[162] Thus, young red cells have a much greater capacity for methemoglobin reduction than older red cells. In view of these considerations, it is not surprising that the content of methemoglobin in normal red cells increases during *in vivo* aging.[161, 162]

NADPH-Flavin Reductase

It is unlikely that NADPH-flavin reductase plays any significant physiologic role. Sass and colleagues[163] described an individual who may be presumed to have deficiency of this enzyme. He had neither methemoglobinemia nor any other apparent clinical or hematologic abnormalities. His red cells were unable to reduce methylene blue, even though they contained normal levels of glucose-6-phosphate dehydrogenase and, therefore, could generate adequate amounts of NADPH. Accordingly, methylene blue was unable to accelerate methemoglobin reduction in the red cells of this individual. Except for methylene blue and brilliant cresyl blue, other oxidant compounds were able to stimulate the hexose monophosphate shunt in these red cells.[164] Thus, this individual appears to be deficient in the enzyme that permits flow of electrons from NADPH to certain redox dyes, including methylene blue.

Pathophysiologic Considerations

As normal red cells circulate *in vivo* for 120 days, they are exposed to a variety of endogenous and exogenous agents that are capable of oxidizing hemoglobin. In the absence of an efficient enzymatic reducing system, it is estimated that methemoglobin accumulates at the rate of 2% to 3% per day. However, when the cytochrome-b_5 reducing system is operating and there is no unusual exogenous oxidant exposure, human red cells contain less than 0.6% methemoglobin.[165] Methemoglobin may be somewhat increased in the red cells of normal infants for two reasons. First, newborns,[166, 167] particularly premature ones,[168] have a transient deficiency of enzymatic activity. The level of soluble cytochrome-b_5 reductase is low, even though the membrane bound level is normal.[169] This finding implies that in newborns there is a transient deficiency in the enzymatic cleavage of the parent molecule. In addition, there are conflicting reports on whether Hb F auto-oxidizes somewhat more rapidly than Hb A.[170]

Cyanosis, or a blue-gray appearance of the skin, can be attributed directly to an alteration in the patient's hemoglobin. As shown in Table 19–7, the most common cause of cyanosis is the presence of relatively high levels of deoxyhemoglobin in the blood, most often due to pulmonary or cardiac dysfunction. Less commonly, cyanosis results from an increase in nonphysiologic forms of hemoglobin: methemoglobin or sulfhemoglobin. A concentration of at least 5 g/dL of deoxyhemoglobin in the blood is required to produce recognizable cyanosis, whereas this sign is observed in individuals with 1.5 g/dL of methemoglobin and as little as 0.5 g/dL of sulfhemoglobin.[171]

Congenital methemoglobinemia is due either to one of the M hemoglobins (see previous section) or to impaired enzymatic reduction of methemoglobin. Deficiency of cytochrome-b_5 reductase is relatively common, as discussed in detail subsequently. In contrast, only one family has been reported in whom congenital methemoglobinemia is caused by deficiency of the co-factor, cytochrome-b_5.[172] Acquired methemoglobinemia is caused by oxidant drugs or toxins, described later.

The adverse effect of methemoglobinemia is based on the fact that partial oxidation of hemoglobin results in a marked increase in the oxygen affinity of the remaining hemes in the tetramer. Compare a chronically anemic patient who has a hemoglobin of 7 g/dL with an individual who has a normal hemoglobin concentration (14 g/dL) but a methemoglobin level of 50%. Both patients have a 50% reduction in blood oxygen-carrying capacity. However, the methemoglobinemic individual would be expected to be more symptomatic, because the increased oxygen affinity of the functioning hemoglobin impairs oxygen delivery to tissues.

The effect of methemoglobinemia on physiologic function is difficult to establish with accuracy. Animal studies must be interpreted with caution because of species differences and because the oxidizing agents used to induce methemoglobinemia may have additional metabolic and circulatory effects. Furthermore, the pathophysiologic sequelae of induced methemoglobinemia depend on the relative duration of exposure. As in the case of anemia, acutely induced methemoglobinemia is generally tolerated less well than a comparable degree of chronic methemoglobinemia. It is likely that various modes of adaptation to hypoxia, discussed earlier in this chapter, are called into play.

Individuals with chronic methemoglobinemia due to deficiency of cytochrome-b_5 reductase may be asymptomatic even with methemoglobin levels as high as 50%. In contrast, those with acute toxic methemoglobinemia may develop mild fatigue with 20% methemoglobin. On exercise, methemoglobinemia of this degree leads to excess lactate production. At 30%, acute induction leads to a significant increase in the heart rate but otherwise causes minimal symptoms. As methemoglobin exceeds 50%, patients generally experience more significant symptoms, such as weakness, breathlessness, headache, and confusion. At 70% to 80%, coma and then death may occur. However, newborns exposed to nitrites may survive methemoglobin levels as high as 85%.

Table 19–7. DIFFERENTIAL DIAGNOSIS OF CYANOSIS

Inadequate Oxygenation of Hemoglobin (Common)

Pulmonary disorders
Cardiac right-to-left shunt
Congestive heart failure
Cardiovascular collapse (shock)
Low O_2 affinity Hb variant (rare)

Methemoglobinemia (Rare)

Congenital

Cytochrome-b_5 reductase deficiency
Cytochrome-b_5 deficiency
M hemoglobins

Acquired

Drugs
Industrial environmental toxins, etc.

Sulfhemoglobinemia (Rare)

Acquired: drugs, toxins, etc.

Congenital Methemoglobinemia: Cytochrome-b_5 Reductase Deficiency

Although sporadic families with congenital methemoglobinemia had been noted since 1932, the inheritance pattern of this disorder was not firmly established until Scott's reports[138, 173] on numerous kindred of Eskimos and Native Americans. He documented an autosomal recessive inheritance pattern. Homozygotes had a marked deficiency in the NADH-dependent methemoglobin reductase now known as cytochrome-b_5 reductase, whereas heterozygotes had about half normal levels of the enzyme. From the large population that Scott sampled in Alaska, he obtained a gene frequency of 0.07. The distribution of heterozygotes and homozygotes was in excellent agreement with the Hardy-Weinberg equilibrium. Genetic polymorphisms also occur in Native Americans and Puerto Ricans.[174] In contrast, the gene frequency is much lower in other parts of the world. Individuals with cytochrome-b_5 reductase deficiency are encountered infrequently and sporadically. Because of the autosomal recessive inheritance pattern, often only one member of a family is a clinically recognizable homozygote. In contrast, as discussed earlier, the M hemoglobins have an autosomal dominant mode of inheritance, and as a result, a larger proportion of family members is affected. Because a number of variants of cytochrome-b_5 reductase have been discovered in deficient individuals (see later), it is likely that in many cases, cyanotic individuals with severe enzyme deficiency are not true homozygotes but actually double (or compound) heterozygotes, inheriting a different mutant enzyme from each parent. Indeed, such a doubly heterozygous state has been documented.[175, 176] There are many examples of this phenomenon such as red cell pyruvate kinase deficiency. In kindred in whom there is true homozygosity for a cytochrome-b_5 reductase variant, either consanguinity[176, 177A] or a founder effect is likely.

Methhemoglobinema in heterozygous children and adults generally escapes clinical detection. Even though these persons have approximately half normal levels of enzyme, they have no significant methemoglobinemia. However, on occasion, they may develop methemoglobinemia and cyanosis when exposed to oxidant compounds such as antimalarial agents,[178] nitrites, and phenazopyridine.[179] Heterozygous neonates may be as cyanotic as adult homozygotes,[159, 180] owing to the previously mentioned relative deficiency of the soluble enzyme.

The gene for cytochrome-b_5 reductase has been assigned to human chromosome 22.[181] The complete nucleotide sequence of the gene has been determined.[182] A single gene encodes the microsomal enzyme from which the soluble erythrocyte enzyme is derived.

Recent analyses of the cytochrome-b_5 reductase gene have documented that affected individuals are generally homozygotes. Sequence abnormalities include single amino acid replacements,[183–185] in-frame deletions,[183–186] splicing mutations[187] and a nonsense mutation creating a premature stop codon.[185]

As mentioned above, cytochrome-b_5 deficiency has been reported as a cause of congenital methemoglobinemia.[172] Affected family members have a clinical and hematologic phenotype identical to that of individuals with cytochrome-b_5 reductase deficiency. This important observation adds credence to the pivotal role of cytochrome-b_5 in the physiologic reduction of methemoglobin.

Clinical Features

Individuals with congenital methemoglobinemia are "more blue than sick."[188] Cyanosis is usually noted at birth. In addition to the skin, the mucous membranes also appear dusky, and when examined by an ophthalmologist, the fundus has a mauve hue. The extent of cyanosis varies widely, in proportion to the level of methemoglobin. In milder cases or in pigmented individuals, the abnormality may escape notice until the individual encounters an astute observer or the blood specimen is recognized because of its abnormal color. Understandably, cyanosis is more difficult to detect in black individuals. Nevertheless, two new cytochrome-b_5 reductase variants have been reported in two unrelated black individuals.[189] The vast majority of individuals have no significant symptoms even with deep cyanosis and levels of methemoglobin as high as 40%. Occasional patients have reported nonspecific symptoms, including fatigue, restlessness, and headache. The great majority of patients with cytochrome-b_5 reductase deficiency have no neurologic findings and are sometimes classified as type I.

Of considerably more concern is a subset of individuals with cytochrome-b_5 reductase deficiency who have severe mental retardation.[190] Other neurologic abnormalities may also be present, including microcephaly, opisthotonos, athetoid movements, strabismus, and generalized hypotonia. These patients, classified as type II, have a short life expectancy. Kaplan and colleagues[190, 191] have shown that these individuals have a broad deficiency of cytochrome-b_5 reductase, including both the cytoplasmic and microsomal forms. Accordingly, the enzyme deficiency is noted not only in the red cells but also in leukocytes, platelets, muscle, liver, brain, and fibroblasts.[190–192] The neurologic disorder is probably related to impaired production of unsaturated fatty acids. In fact, the ratio of unsaturated to saturated fatty acids was found to be decreased in myelin, white matter, and gray matter of a patient with generalized enzyme deficiency and mental retardation.[193] In contrast, type I individuals have a deficiency of only the soluble cytoplasmic enzyme. Thus, enzyme activity in tissues other than the red cells is normal.

Several families have been reported to have cytochrome-b_5 reductase deficiency in red cells, white cells, and platelets but not in other tissues.[183, 194, 195] Affected individuals, designated as having type III deficiency, have no neurologic manifestations. The molecular basis of this intermediate phenotype is unknown.

Laboratory Features

Individuals whose cyanosis is due to cytochrome-b_5 reductase deficiency generally have 10% to 35% methemoglobin. They are either homozygotes or compound heterozygotes. Rarely, methemoglobin may reach 50%; such a high level may reflect the superimposition of an oxidant upon severe enzyme deficiency. As mentioned earlier, methemoglobin levels are normal in heterozygotes unless they are challenged with oxidants.

Although some individuals with cyanosis and cytochrome-b_5 reductase deficiency may have mild polycythemia, this finding is often absent. Because the partial oxidation of hemoglobin causes an increase in the affinity of the remaining hemes for oxygen, the resulting impairment in oxygen transport to tissues should result in a compensatory erythrocytosis. The fact that hemoglobin levels are often normal may be explained by the segregation of methemoglobin in the older population of red cells.[157] This phenomenon decreases the interaction between Fe^{3+} subunits and Fe^{2+} subunits, and, therefore, the oxygen affinity of the blood is not as increased as it would be if the methemoglobin were evenly distributed among red cells.

The absorption spectrum of hemolysate from an individual with cytochrome-b_5 reductase deficiency shows the presence of methemoglobin. The spectrum of methemoglobin from such individuals is indistinguishable from that of methemoglobin prepared by oxidation of normal hemoglobin. As shown in Figure 19–20, the decrease in absorption at 630 nm after the addition of cyanide provides a precise measure of methemoglobin. In contrast, when cyanosis is caused by one of the M hemoglobins, the absorption spectrum is abnormal and less affected by the addition of cyanide.

The activity of cytochrome-b_5 reductase is usually measured by the reduction of a dye,[137] or an assay that uses a ferrocyanide-hemoglobin complex as substrate.[196] If a significant decrease in enzyme activity is noted, the defect can be further characterized by electrophoresis, kinetics, pH optimum, and thermal stability. Such investigations have revealed considerable heterogeneity in the variant enzymes of deficient indi-

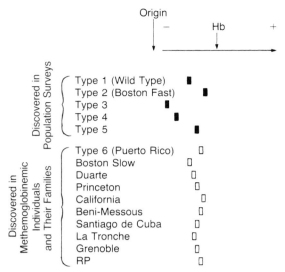

Figure 19–21. Schematic representation of electrophoretic mobilities of variants of cytochrome-b_5 reductase. The normal or wild-type enzyme is designated as type 1. Some variants (e.g., types 2 to 5) encountered in normal, noncyanotic individuals have normal enzyme activity (■). The other variants shown in this figure were encountered in methemoglobinemic individuals. Only one enzyme band was observed, suggesting a homozygous state (□). When present in noncyanotic relatives (heterozygotes), the variant band was much less prominent than that of the wild type, indicating decreased enzymatic activity. (Starch gel electrophoresis, pH 8.6 to 9.3). (From Bunn HF, Forget BG: Hemoglobin: Molecular, Genetic and Clinical Aspects. Philadelphia, W.B. Saunders Co., 1986.)

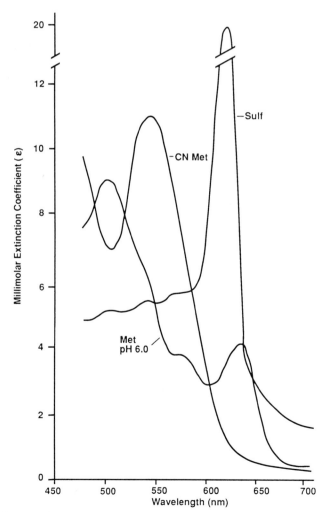

Figure 19–20. Absorption spectra of methemoglobin (Met) (pH 6.0), cyanmethemoglobin (CN Met), and deoxygenated sulfhemoglobin (Sulf).

viduals. A number of cytochrome-b_5 reductase variants have been described that appear to function normally but have abnormal electrophoretic behavior.[48] In addition, at least a dozen variants can be distinguished from one another on the basis of low catalytic activity or instability, accompanied by differences in electrophoretic migration (Fig. 19–21). Some of these have been encountered in specific ethnic groups, such as the Puerto Rico variant. Others are designated according to the location in which they were discovered: California, Duarte, Princeton, Boston Fast, Boston Slow, and Santiago de Cuba. Levels of enzyme in normal and deficient red cells can be accurately quantitated by radioimmunoblotting.[197] Deficiency in immunologically reactive protein generally parallels deficiency in enzyme activity. As mentioned earlier, those individuals with associated neurologic findings may have no detectable enzyme activity in erythrocytes. Heterogeneity among the cytochrome-b_5 reductase variants includes differences in the stability of the enzyme. Extreme instability may be responsible for significant deficiency in all tissues; in contrast, those with a less severe degree of instability may be manifested only in erythrocytes, which are long-lived cells incapable of protein synthesis.

In families who have had a child with the generalized deficiency state and severe mental retardation, the diagnosis can be established in fetuses at risk by culturing amniotic cells and measuring cytochrome-b_5 reductase.[198]

Treatment

Although nearly all enzyme-deficient individuals are asymptomatic, some find their lifelong cyanosis to be a cosmetic handicap. The level of methemoglobin can be reduced to 5% to 10% by the oral administration of methylene blue (100 to 300 mg/d) or ascorbic acid (200 to 500 mg/d). Thus, these agents effectively reverse the cyanosis. As discussed earlier, methylene blue serves as an electron carrier and operates by means of NADPH-flavin reductase. In contrast, ascorbic acid reduces methemoglobin directly. The fact that untreated patients generally have low serum ascorbate levels probably means that the vitamin has been used for methemoglobin reduction. Riboflavin has also been found to be effective in lowering the level of methemoglobin in cytochrome-b_5 reductase–deficient individuals.[177, 199] Reports of decreased glutathione reductase, a flavin enzyme, in individuals with congenital methemoglobinemia[200] raises the possibility that riboflavin is also used for *in vivo* methemoglobin reduction, and, therefore, vitamin stores may become depleted. Of these three agents, methylene blue is probably the most efficient. However, this drug should not be used in individuals with glucose-6-phosphate dehydrogenase deficiency because it is ineffective[201–203] and may cause acute oxidant-type hemolysis.[203]

Toxic Methemoglobinemia

Methemoglobinemia can be induced by a wide range of xenobiotic compounds. Sometimes, in-depth detective work is required to identify the offending agent.[204] Table 19–8 lists drugs and toxins that are well-accepted etiologic agents. The extent of methemoglobinemia depends on the agent, its dose, and the duration of exposure. Furthermore, as mentioned, individuals who are heterozygous for cytochrome-b_5 reductase deficiency are more susceptible than normal individuals when exposed to an equivalent dose.[178, 179]

Newborns and Infants

Newborns and infants appear to be unusually susceptible to the development of toxic methemoglobinemia. As explained earlier, this increased risk is due primarily to decreased amounts of soluble cytochrome-b_5 and cytochrome-b_5 reductase in erythrocytes of newborns.[166, 167] The mean level of enzyme is about 60% of that in adult red cells. Infants are at special risk to develop methemoglobinemia after ingestion of nitrate, such as from well water or plants. If the farmland surrounding a well is treated with large amounts of fertilizer, a significant and sometimes toxic amount of nitrate can seep into the well. Once this contaminated water is ingested, the relatively alkaline pH of an infant's intestine permits the bacterial conversion of nitrate to nitrite,[205] which is, of course, a potent oxidant. In addition, certain vegetables such as spinach have nitrate reductases, which remain active if the food is not adequately cooked. Finally, when infants develop diarrhea, endogenous nitrite production may be enhanced.[206]

Attention must be paid to other potential environmental toxins. Methemoglobinemia in the nursery can be caused by disinfectants or absorption of aniline marker dyes. Because of wide recognition of these potential toxins, the incidence of methemoglobinemia in newborns and infants has decreased markedly in recent years.

Severe methemoglobinemia in infants can be caused by exposure to oxidant drugs such as menadione (vitamin K$_3$) (for prevention of neonatal hemorrhage), over-the-counter teething preparations containing benzocaine[207] or metoclopramide, a derivative of ortho-procaine amide, or methylene blue used for diagnostic tests.[208, 209]

Drug Use and Abuse

The incidence of drug-induced methemoglobinemia depends on the availability of drugs and the frequency of use, factors that vary markedly in time and place. Over-the-counter pain medicines have been responsible for the majority of cases of drug-induced methemoglobinemia. In many instances, the drugs have been used inappropriately and in excess. In the 1940s and 1950s, the widespread use of acetanilid and phenacetin for analgesia was associated with a large number of cases of toxic methemoglobinemia.[210] During the past 10 years, this drug has been supplanted by another nitrobenzene derivative, acetaminophen. Methemoglobinemia generally occurs in those individuals who abuse these agents. Patients often ingest a variety of drugs indiscriminately, so that it may be difficult to establish which were responsible for inducing hemoglobin oxidation. Drug-induced methemoglobinemia and sulfhemoglobinemia are most often due to dapsone or to acetaminophen in conjunction with another nitrobenzene, phenacetin, or phenazopyridine. Phenazopyri-

Table 19–8. AGENTS THAT OXIDIZE HEMOGLOBIN

I. Direct oxidation
   Ferricyanide
   Copper
   Hydrogen peroxide
   Hydroxylamine
   Others: Chromate, chlorate, nitrogen trifluoride,
          tetranitromethane, quinones, dyes
II. Interaction with oxygen
   Nitrites, nitroglycerin
   Hydrazines
   Thiols
   Others: Arsine, aminophenols, arylhydroxylamines,
          N-hydroxyurethane, phenylenediamines
III. Requiring biochemical transformation
   Aniline, dyes (diaper and laundry inks, red wax crayons)
   Sulfonamides
   Procaine derivatives
   4,4'-Diaminodiphenylsulfone (dapsone)
   8-Aminoquinolines: primaquine and pamaquine
   N-Acylarylamines: acetanilid, phenacetin

Adapted from Kiese M: Methemoglobinemia: A Comprehensive Treatise. Cleveland, CRC Press, 1974; reprinted with permission. Copyright CRC Press, Inc., Boca Raton, FL.

dine may also induce hemolytic anemia and impairment of renal function. Furthermore, the drug's oxidant effect is enhanced in the presence of pre-existing renal failure. Among the antibiotics, the sulfa drugs occasionally cause toxic methemoglobinemia. In the past, sulfanilamide was a common offender. In contrast, the sulfa drugs currently in use rarely induce hemoglobin oxidation. The increasing use of nitroprusside for afterload reduction in the treatment of severe congestive heart failure may be associated with sufficient methemoglobinemia to cause cyanosis.[211] This complication can confuse the monitoring and management of these critically ill patients. The therapeutic as well as recreational use of amyl nitrate can also cause toxic methemoglobinemia. A significant proportion of drug-induced methemoglobinemia is caused by the use of local anesthetics. A number of cases have been reported after the use of topical benzocaine before intubation or bronchoscopy. In this setting, cyanosis may be mistakenly attributed to the patient's underlying cardiac or pulmonary condition. Cyanosis can also be induced with prilocaine and lidocaine.

Industrial Toxins

As mentioned in the section on hemoglobin oxidation, a large number of cases of toxic methemoglobinemia occurred during the development of the dye industry in Europe in the early part of this century. The arylamines, especially aniline and its derivatives, were the most common offenders. More recently, rigid standards of employee safety have greatly reduced the incidence of significant methemoglobinemia in industry.

Treatment

Patients whose methemoglobin levels exceed 40% or who appear to be symptomatic from methemoglobinemia should be treated promptly with intravenous methylene blue (1 to 2 mg/kg). The level of methemoglobin should fall to normal within 1 hour after treatment. If not, a second dose of methylene blue can be administered. It is useful but not essential to have spectral documentation of methemoglobinemia either before or soon after treatment is initiated. Failure of the cyanosis to clear promptly may mean that the patient has coexisting glucose-6-phosphate dehydrogenase deficiency[203] or significant amounts of sulfhemoglobin (more than 0.5 g/dL).

Sulfhemoglobinemia

Occasionally, patients who are exposed to oxidant compounds will develop cyanosis that cannot be explained by simple hemoglobin oxidation. The absorbance spectrum differs from that of methemoglobin: there is a broad band at 620 nm that is not altered by the addition of cyanide. Because of its high absorbance in the red region of the visible spectrum, sulfhemoglobinemia causes more cyanosis than an equivalent degree of methemoglobinemia.

Sulfhemoglobin was discovered in 1863 by Hoppe-

Seyler,[212] who observed that when oxyhemoglobin was treated with hydrogen sulfide gas (H_2S), it gradually turned green. Even though it has been investigated with a broad repertoire of analytic techniques, the structure of sulfhemoglobin is not fully established. Indeed, it may not be a single molecular species. The basic problem is that the characteristic sulfhemoglobin spectrum (see Fig. 19–20) can be generated by a variety of compounds, but the relevant chemical reactions are complex and not thoroughly understood. The formation of sulfhemoglobin requires the oxidation of the heme iron followed by the interaction of the heme group with a sulfur-containing compound. The sulfide does not form a coordination complex with the heme iron. Instead, the sulfur atom is incorporated into heme with a 1:1 stoichiometric ratio.[213] The following scheme describes the formation of sulfhemoglobin:

1. In the presence of hydrogen peroxide methemoglobin is converted to ferrylhemoglobin:

$$HbFe^{3+} + H_2O_2 \rightarrow HbFe^{4+}O + H_2O + \epsilon$$

2. On the addition of hydrogen sulfide, the iron in ferrylhemoglobin is reduced to the ferrous state and sulfur is incorporated into the porphyrin ring.

$$HbFe^{4+}O + HS^- + 2\epsilon \rightarrow HbSFe^{2+} + OH^-$$

It is likely that this reaction involves the reduction of a β-carbon double bond in one of the pyrroles in protoporphyrin IX to form a chlorin (Fig. 19–22).

Clinical Features

In the vast majority of cases, sulfhemoglobinemia is associated with exposure to an oxidant compound. The arylamines are the most common offenders. Indeed, when acetanilide and phenacetin were in common use as analgesics, sulfhemoglobinemia was encountered more frequently than it is today.[210] In patients whose cyanosis is induced by acetaminophen, the level of sulfhemoglobin often exceeds that of methemoglobin. Dapsone can also induce increased levels of both hemoglobin derivatives.[214] It is unclear what factors determine the relative proportions of methemoglobin and sulfhemoglobin in these individuals. Direct exposure to lethal doses of hydrogen sulfide does not usually cause sulfhemoglobinemia. Sometimes the gastrointestinal tract plays a critical role in the development of

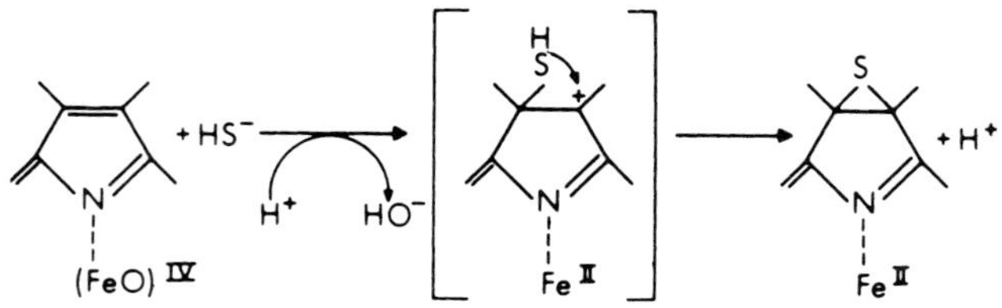

Figure 19-22. Proposed structure of the modified pyrrole in the porphyrin of sulfhemoglobin. One of the pyrroles (left) in protoporphyrin IX is reduced to a chlorin. (From Berzofsky JA, Peisach J, et al: Sulfheme proteins. IV. The stoichiometry of sulfur incorporation and the isolation of sulfhemin, the prosthetic group of sulfmyoglobin. J Biol Chem 1972; 247;3783.)

sulfhemoglobinemia. The association of cyanosis with disturbances of bowel function was recognized by Van den Bergh in 1905 and designated "enterogenous cyanosis."[215] Sulfhemoglobin was often the predominant derivative in patients with constipation, whereas those with diarrhea had predominantly methemoglobin. Van den Bergh[215] described a 9-year-old boy who had a rectal stricture and cyanosis for 2 years. After surgical correction of the obstruction, the cyanosis disappeared. Subsequently, several observers noted the association of cyanosis and constipation in individuals who were exposed to aniline derivatives. It is likely that during bowel stasis, the enhanced production of sulfides by bacterial flora converts methemoglobin to sulfhemoglobin. Red cell glutathione has been suggested as an alternative source of sulfur that may contribute toward the development of sulfhemoglobinemia.[216] Individuals with sulfhemoglobin often have increased glutathione in their red cells. The enzyme β-mercaptopyruvate sulfur transferase, which is abundant in human red cells,[217] may serve in the transfer of HS^- to hemoglobin.

Patients with sulfhemoglobinemia usually have no symptoms other than concern about their skin color. In contrast to methemoglobin, sulfhemoglobin has decreased oxygen affinity and therefore does not impair the unloading of oxygen from the unmodified hemes to tissues.

The diagnosis of sulfhemoglobinemia is established by spectroscopic examination of the patient's hemolysate. As mentioned before, the presence of an absorbance peak at 620 nm after the addition of cyanide indicates the presence of sulfhemoglobin. The percentage of this component can be calculated as follows:

$$\% \text{ SulfHb} = \frac{OD_{620} \times \text{Dil (neutral buffer} + CN^-)}{1.96 \times OD_{540} \times \text{Dil (Drabkins' solution)}}$$

where Dil is the dilution of the hemolysate. The addition of CO causes a characteristic enhancement of the absorbance peak at 620 nm as well as a slight shift to lower wavelength.[218]

When a blood specimen containing sulfhemoglobin is analyzed by isoelectric focusing, a well-defined green band is readily visualized.[219] The fact that its isoelectric point is close to that of deoxyhemoglobin indicates that the sulfhemoglobin has the T quaternary structure.

The formation of sulfhemoglobin appears to be irreversible. The red cell lacks the enzymatic and chemical capability for converting it back to functional hemoglobin. Sulfhemoglobinemia is not usually associated with damage to the red cell membrane or hemolysis. In fact, the disappearance of sulfhemoglobin after withdrawal of the inciting agent parallels normal red cell senescence.[171] Unlike methemoglobinemia, sulfhemoglobinemia cannot be corrected by pharmacologic means. The only treatment is avoidance of oxidant compounds.

References

1. Nienhuis AW, Maniatis T: Structure and expression of globin genes in erythroid cells. In Stamatoyannopoulos G, Nienhuis AW, et al (eds): The Molecular Basis of Blood Diseases. Philadelphia, W.B. Saunders Co., 1987, p 28.
1a. Jia L, Bonaventura C, et al: S-Nitrosohaemoglobin: a dynamic activity of blood involved in vascular control. Nature 1996; 380:221.
1b. Howlett R: Root cause of fish buoyancy. Nature 1996; 380:203.
2. Perutz MF, Fermi G, et al: Stereochemistry of cooperative mechanisms in hemoglobin. Cold Spring Harb Symp Quant Biol 1987; 52:555.
3. Perutz MF: Molecular anatomy, physiology, and pathology of hemoglobin. In Stamatoyannopoulos G, Nienhuis AW, et al (eds): The Molecular Basis of Blood Diseases. Philadelphia, W.B. Saunders Co., 1987, p 127.
4. Shannan B: The structure of human oxyhaemoglobin at 2.1 ÅA resolution. J Mol Biol 1983; 171:31.
5. Fermi G, Perutz MF, et al: The crystal structure of human deoxyhemoglobin at 1.7 ÅA resolution. J Mol Biol 1984; 175:159.
6. Ackers GK, Hazzard JH: Transduction of binding energy into hemoglobin cooperativity. Trends Biochem Sci 1995; 18:385.
7. Bohr C, Hasselbalch K, et al: Über einen in biologischer Beziehung wichtigen Einfluss, den die Kohlensäuerespannung des Blutes auf dessen Sauerstoffbinding übt. Skand Arch Physiol 1904; 16:402.
8. Riggs AF: The Bohr effect. Annu Rev Physiol 1988; 50:181.
9. Rossi-Bernardi L, Roughton FJW, et al: The effect of organic phosphates on the binding of CO_2 to human hemoglobin and CO_2 transport in the circulating blood. In Rorth M, Astrup P (eds): Oxygen Affinity of Hemoglobin and Red Cell Acid-Base Status. Copenhagen, Munksgaard, 1972, p 225.
10. Garby L, Robert M, et al: Proton and carbamino-linked oxygen affinity of normal human blood. Acta Physiol Scand 1972; 84:482.
11. Chanutin A, Curnish RR: Effect of organic and inorganic phosphates on the oxygen equilibrium of human erythrocytes. Arch Biochem Biophys 1967; 121:96.
12. Benesch R, Benesch RE: The effect of organic phosphates from the human erythrocyte on the allosteric properties of hemoglobin. Biochem Biophys Res Commun 1967; 26:162.
13. Benesch R, Benesch RE: Intracellular organic phosphates as regulators of oxygen release by haemoglobin. Nature 1969; 221:618.
14. Bunn HF, Briehl RW: The interaction of 2,3-diphosphoglycerate with various human hemoglobins. J Clin Invest 1970; 49:1088.
15. Arnone A: X-ray diffraction study of binding of 2,3-diphosphoglycerate to human deoxyhaemoglobin. Nature 1972; 237:146.
16. Duhm J: Effects of 2,3-diphosphoglycerate and other organic phosphate compounds on oxygen affinity and intracellular pH of human erythrocytes. Pfluegers Arch 1971; 326:341.
17. Oski FA, Gottlieb AJ: The interrelationship between red cell metabolites, hemoglobin and the oxygen equilibrium curve. Prog Hematol 1971; 7:33.
18. Adamson JW, Finch CA: Hemoglobin function, oxygen affinity and erythropoietin. Ann Rev Physiol 1975; 38:351.
19. Woodson RD: Physiological significance of oxygen dissociation curve shifts. Crit Care Med 1979; 7:368.
20. Oski FA, Gottlieb AJ, et al: The effects of deoxygenation of adult and fetal hemoglobin on the synthesis of red cell 2,3-diphosphoglycerate and its *in vivo* consequences. J Clin Invest 1970; 49:400.
21. Oski FA, Marchall BE, et al: Exercise with anemia. The role of the left-shifted or right-shifted oxygen hemoglobin equilibrium curve. Ann Intern Med 1971; 74:44.
22. Eaton JW, Skelton TD, et al: Survival at extreme altitude: protective effect of increased hemoglobin-oxygen affinity. Science 1974; 183:743.
23. Hebbel RP, Eaton JW, et al: Human llamas: adaptation to altitude in subjects with high hemoglobin oxygen affinity. J Clin Invest 1978; 62:593.
24. Bellingham AJ, Detter JC, et al: The role of hemoglobin oxygen affinity and red cell 2,3-diphosphoglycerate in the management of diabetic ketoacidosis. Trans Assoc Am Phys 1970; 83:113.
25. Card RB, Brain M: The "anemia" of childhood. N Engl J Med 1973; 288:388.
26. Valtis DJ, Kennedy AC: Defective gas transport function of stored red blood cells. Lancet 1954; 1:119.

27. Bunn HF, May MH, et al: Hemoglobin function in stored blood. J Clin Invest 1969; 48:311.

28. Akerblom O, deVerdier CH, et al: Restoration of defective oxygen transport function of stored red blood cells by addition of inosine. Scand J Clin Lab Invest 1968; 21:245.

29. Valeri CR, Hirsch NM: Restoration *in vivo* of erythrocyte adenosine triphosphate, 2,3-diphosphoglycerate, potassium ion and sodium concentrations following the transfusion of acid-citrate-dextrose stored human red blood cells. J Lab Clin Med 1969; 73:722.

30. Beutler E, Wood LA: The in vivo regeneration of red cell 2,3-diphosphoglyceric acid after transfusion of stored blood. J Lab Clin Med 1969; 74:300.

31. Heaton A, Keegan T, et al: *In vivo* regeneration of red cell 2,3-diphosphoglycerate following transfusion of DPG-depleted AS-1, AS-3, and CPDA-1 red cells. Br J Haematol 1989; 71:131.

32. Oski FA, Travis SF, et al: The in vitro restoration of red cell 2,3-diphosphoglycerate levels in banked blood. Blood 1971; 37:52.

33. Wood L, Beutler E: The effect of ascorbate and dihydroxyacetone on the 2,3-diphosphoglycerate and ATP levels of stored human red cells. Transfusion 1974; 14:272.

34. Bauer CI, Ludwig I, et al: Different effects of 2,3-diphosphoglycerate and adenosine triphosphate on the oxygen affinity of adult and fetal human hemoglobin. Life Sci 1968; 7:1339.

35. Tyuma I, Shimizu K: Different response to organic phosphates of human fetal and adult hemoglobins. Arch Biochem Biophys 1969; 129:404.

36. Delivoria-Papadopoulos M, Roncevic NP, et al: Postnatal changes in oxygen transport of term, premature and sick infants. The role of red cell, 2,3-diphosphoglycerate and adult hemoglobin. Pediatr Res 1971; 5:235.

37. Oski FA: Clinical implications of the oxyhemoglobin dissociation curve in the neonatal period. Crit Care Med 1979; 7:412.

38. Wimberley PD: Fetal hemoglobin, 2,3-diphosphoglycerate and oxygen transport in the newborn premature infant. Scand J Clin Lab Invest 1982; 42(Suppl 160):1.

39. Delivoria-Papadopoulos M, Miller L, et al: The role of exchange transfusion in the management of low-birth-weight infants with and without severe respiratory distress syndrome. I. Initial observations. J Pediatr 1976; 89:273.

40. Gottuso M, Williams M, et al: Exchange transfusion in low-birth-weight infants. II. Further observations. J Pediatr 1976; 89:279.

41. Stamatoyannopoulos G, Nienhuis AW: Hemoglobin switching. In Stamatoyannopoulos G, Nienhuis AW, et al (eds): The Molecular Basis of Blood Diseases. 2nd ed. Philadelphia, W.B. Saunders Co., 1994, p 107.

42. Chui DH, Mentzer WC: Human embryonic zeta-globin chains in fetal and newborn blood. Blood 1989; 74:1409.

43. Huehns ER, Farooqui AM: Oxygen dissociation properties of human embryonic red cells. Nature 1975; 254:335.

44. Schroeder WA, Huisman THJ, et al: Evidence of multiple structural genes for γ chain of human fetal hemoglobin. Proc Natl Acad Sci U S A 1968; 60:537.

45. Ricco G, Mazza V, et al: Significance of a new type of human fetal hemoglobin carrying a replacement isoleucine-threonine at position 75 (E 19) of the γ chain. Hum Genet 1976; 32:305.

46. Huisman THJ, Schroeder WA, et al: Evidence for four nonallelic structural genes for the γ chain of human fetal hemoglobin. Biochem Genet 1972; 7:131.

47. Schroeder WA, Cua JT, et al: Hemoglobin F$_1$, an acetyl-containing hemoglobin. Biochem Biophys Acta 1962; 63:532.

48. Bunn HF, Forget BG: Hemoglobin: Molecular, Genetic and Clinical Aspects. Philadelphia, W.B. Saunders Co., 1986.

49. Schroeder WA, Huisman THJ, et al: An improved method for quantitative determination of human fetal hemoglobin. Anal Biochem 1970; 35:235.

50. Huisman THJ, Henson JB, et al: A new high performance liquid chromatographic procedure to quantitate hemoglobin A$_{1c}$ and other minor hemoglobins in blood of normal, diabetic and alcoholic individuals. J Lab Clin Med 1983; 102:163.

51. Garver FA, Jones SC, et al: Specific radioimmunochemical identification and quantitation of hemoglobins A$_2$ and F. Am J Hematol 1976; 1:459.

52. Makler MT, Pesce AJ: ELISA assay for measurement of human hemoglobin A and hemoglobin F. Am J Clin Pathol 1980; 74:673.

53. Schroeder WA, Huisman THJ: The Chromatography of Hemoglobin. New York, Marcel Dekker, Inc., 1980.

54. Garby L, Sjöln S, et al: Studies on erythrokinetics in infancy. II. The relative rate of synthesis of haemoglobin F and haemoglobin A during the first months of life. Acta Paediatr 1962; 51:245.

55. Perrine SP, Rudolph A, et al: Butyrate infusions in the ovine fetus delay the biologic clock for the globin gene switching. Proc Natl Acad Sci U S A 1988; 85:8540.

56. Burns JL, Glauber GJ, et al: Butyrate induces selective transcriptional activation of a hypomethylated embryonic globin gene in adult erythroid cells. Blood 1988; 72:1536.

57. Hosoi T: Studies on hemoglobin F within a single erythrocyte by fluorescent antibody technique. Exp Cell Res 1965; 37:680.

58. Boyer SH, Belding TK, et al: Fetal hemoglobin restriction to few erythrocytes (F cells) in normal human adults. Science 1974; 188:361.

59. Boyer SH, Belding TK, et al: Variations in the frequency of fetal hemoglobin-bearing erythrocytes (F-cells) in well adults, pregnant women and adult leukemics. Johns Hopkins Med J 1975; 137:105.

60. Zago MA, Wood WG, et al: Genetic control of F cells in human adults. Blood 1979; 53:977.

61. Dover GJ, Smith KD, et al: Fetal hemoglobin production is controlled by a gene on the X-chromosome in normal adults and sickle cell patients. Blood 1990; 76:59a.

62. Dover GJ, Boyer SH, et al: F cell production in sickle cell anemia: regulation by genes linked to β-hemoglobin locus. Science 1981; 211:1441.

63. Platt OS, Orkin SH, et al: Hydroxyurea enhances fetal hemoglobin production in sickle cell anemia. J Clin Invest 1984; 74:652.

64. Dover GJ, Humphries RK, et al: Hydroxyurea induction of hemoglobin F production in sickle cell disease: relationship between cytotoxicity and F cell production. Blood 1986; 67:735.

65. Perrine SP, Ginder GD, et al: A short term trial of butyrate to stimulate fetal globin gene expression in the β globin gene disorders. N Engl J Med 1993; 328:81.

66. Al-Khatti A, Veith RW, et al: Stimulation of fetal hemoglobin synthesis by erythropoietin in baboons. N Engl J Med 1987; 317:415.

67. Heller P, Yakulis V: The distribution of hemoglobin A$_2$. Ann N Y Acad Sci 1969; 165:54.

68. Wasi P, Na-Nakorn S, et al: Alpha and beta-thalassemia in Thailand. Ann N Y Acad Sci 1969; 165:60.

69. Alperin JB, Dow PA, et al: Hemoglobin A$_2$ levels in health and various hematologic disorders. Am J Clin Pathol 1977; 67:219.

70. McCormack MK: Quantitation of hemoglobin A$_2$ in alpha thalassemia trait by microcolumn chromatography. Clin Chim Acta 1980; 105:387.

71. Chernoff AK: A method for the quantitative determination of hemoglobin A$_2$. Ann N Y Acad Sci 1964; 119:557.

72. White JM, Brain MC, et al: Globin synthesis in sideroblastic anemia. αβ peptide chain synthesis. Br J Haematol 1971; 20:263.

73. Rieder RF, Weatherall DJ: Studies on hemoglobin biosynthesis: asynchronous synthesis of hemoglobin A and hemoglobin A$_2$ by erythrocyte precursors. J Clin Invest 1965; 44:42.

74. Roberts AV, Weatherall DJ, et al: The synthesis of human hemoglobin A$_2$ during erythroid maturation. Biochem Biophys Res Commun 1972; 47:81.

75. White JC, Ellis M, et al: An unstable haemoglobin associated with cases of leukemia. Br J Haematol 1960; 6:171.

76. Hamilton RW, Schwartz E, et al: Acquired hemoglobin H disease. N Engl J Med 1971; 285:1217.

77. McDonald MJ, Shapiro R, et al: Glycosylated minor components of human adult hemoglobin. I. Purification, identification and structural analysis. J Biol Chem 1978; 253:2327.

78. Garlick RL, Mazer JS, et al: Characterization of glycosylated hemoglobins. Relevance to monitoring of diabetic control and analysis of other proteins. J Clin Invest 1983; 71:1062–1072.

79. Bunn HF, Haney DN, et al: Further identification of the nature and linkage of the carbohydrate in hemoglobin A$_{1c}$. Biochem Biophys Res Commun 1975; 67:103.

80. Prome D, Blouquit Y, et al: Structure of the human adult hemoglobin minor fraction A$_{1b}$ by electrospray and secondary ion mass spectroscopy. Pyruvic acid as amino-terminal blocking group. J Biol Chem 1991; 266:13050.

80a. Makita Z, Vlassara H, et al: Hemoglobin-AGE: A circulating marker of advanced glycosylation. Science 1992; 258:651.

81. Bunn HF, Haney DN, et al: Biosynthesis of human hemoglobin A₁c. Slow glycosylation of hemoglobin *in vivo*. J Clin Invest 1976; 57:1652, 1976.

82. Rahbar S: An abnormal hemoglobin in red cells of diabetics. Clin Chim Acta 1968; 22:296.

83. Koenig RJ, Peterson CM, et al: Correlation of glucose regulation and hemoglobin A₁c in diabetes mellitus. N Engl J Med 1976; 295:417.

84. Larsen ML, Horder M, et al: Effect of long-term monitoring of glycosylated hemoglobin levels in insulin-dependent diabetes mellitus. N Engl J Med 1990; 323:1021.

85. Brownlee M: Glycation and diabetic complications. Diabetes 1994; 43:836.

86. Flückiger R, Harmon W, et al: Hemoglobin carbamylation in uremia. N Engl J Med 1981; 304:823.

87. Hoberman HD: Post-translational modification of hemoglobin in alcoholism. Biochem Biophys Res Commun 1983; 113:1004.

88. Charache S, Weatherall DJ: Fast hemoglobin in lead poisoning. Blood 1966; 28:377.

89. Lamola AA, Piomelli S, et al: Erythropoietic protoporphyria and lead intoxication: the molecular basis for difference in cutaneous photosensitivity. II. Different binding of erythrocyte protoporphyrin to hemoglobin. J Clin Invest 1975; 56:1528.

90. Carver MFH, Kutlar A: International Hemoglobin Information Center variants list. Hemoglobin 1995; 19:37.

91. Camaschella C, Saglio G: Recent advances in diagnosis of hemoglobinopathies. Crit Rev Oncol Hematol 1993; 14:89.

92. Kawata R, Ohba Y, et al: Hyperunstable hemoglobin Koriyama anti-Hb Gun Hill insertion of five residues in the β chain. Hemoglobin 1988; 12:311.

93. Huisman THJ, Wilson JB, et al: Hemoglobin Grady: the first example of a variant with elongated chains due to an insertions of residues. Proc Natl Acad Sci U S A 1974; 71:3270.

94. Wajcman H, Blouquit Y, et al: Two new human hemoglobin variants caused by unusual mutational events: Hb Zaire contains a five residue repetition with the α-chain and Hb Duino has two residues substituted in the β-chain. Hum Genet 1992; 89:676.

94a. Plaseska D, Dimovski A, et al: Hemoglobin Montreal: a new variant with an extended β chain due to a deletion of Asp, Gly, Leu at positions 73, 74, and 75, and an insertion of Ala, Arg, Cys, Gln at the same location. Blood 1991; 77:178.

94b. Wilson JB, Webber BB, et al: Hemoglobin Birmingham and hemoglobin Galicia: the unstable β chain variants characterized by small deletions and insertions. Blood 1990; 75:1883.

95. Bunn HF: Subunit assembly of hemoglobin: an important determinant of hematologic phenotype. Blood 1987; 69:1.

96. Liebhaber S, Cash FE, et al: Evidence for posttranslational control of Hb C synthesis in an individual with Hb C trait and α-thalassemia. Blood 1988; 71:502.

97. Huisman THJ: Percentages of abnormal hemoglobins in adults with a heterozygosity for an α-chain and/or a β-chain variant. Am J Hematol 1983; 14:393.

98. Mrabet NT, McDonald MJ, et al: Electrostatic attraction governs the dimer assembly of dimers of human hemoglobin. J Biol Chem 1986; 261:5222.

98a. Adams JG, Coleman MB, et al: Modulation of fetal hemoglobin synthesis by iron deficiency. N Engl J Med 1985; 313:1402.

98b. Chui DHK, Patterson M, et al: Hemoglobin Bart's disease in an Italian boy. N Engl J Med 1990; 323:179.

99. Bunn HF, Noguchi CT, et al: The molecular and cellular pathogenesis of hemoglobin SC disease. Proc Natl Acad Sci U S A 1982; 79:7527.

100. Cash FE, Monplaisir N, et al: Locus assignment of two α-globin structural mutants from the Caribbean basin: α Fort de France (α⁴⁵ ᴬʳᵍ) and Spanish Town (α²⁷ ⱽᵃˡ). Blood 1989; 74:833.

101. Cathie IAB: Apparent idiopathic Heinz body anemia. Great Ormond St J 1952; 3:43.

101a. Galacteros F, Girodon E, et al: Hb Taybe (α 38 or 39 THR deleted): an α-globin defect, silent in the heterozygous state and producing severe hemolytic anemia in the homozygous. C R Acad Sci III 1994; 317:437.

102. Galacteros F, Loukopoulos D, et al: Hemoglobin Koln occurring in association with a β⁰ thalassemia: hematologic and functional consequences. Blood 1989; 74:496.

102a. Steinberg MH, Adams JG, et al: Hemoglobin Mississippi (β44 Ser-Cys). Studies on the thalassemic phenotype in a mixed heterozygote with a β + thalassemia. J Clin Invest 1987; 79:826.

103. Stamatoyannopoulos G, Nute PE, et al: *De novo* mutations producing unstable hemoglobins or hemoglobins M. Hum Genet 1981; 58:396.

104. Lee-Potter JP, Deacon-Smith RA, et al: A new cause of haemolytic anemia in the newborn. A description of an unstable fetal haemoglobin: F = Poole, α₂Gγ₂¹³⁰ ᵀʳᵖ→ᴳˡʸ. J Clin Pathol 1975; 28:317.

105. Vissers MCM, Winterbourne CC, et al: Rapid proteolysis of unstable globins in human bone marrow. Br J Haematol 1983; 53:417.

106. Rachmilewitz EA: Denaturation of the normal and abnormal hemoglobin molecule. Semin Hematol 1974; 11:441.

107. Winterbourn CC, Carrell RW: Characterization of Heinz bodies in unstable hemoglobins. Nature 1972; 240:150.

108. Jandl JH, Simmons RL, et al: Red cell filtration and the pathogenesis of certain hemolytic anemias. Blood 1961; 18:133.

109. Rivkind RA: Heinz body anemia: an ultrastructural study. II. Red cell sequestration and destruction. Blood 1965; 26:433.

110. Flyn TP, Allen DW, et al: Oxidant damage of the lipids and proteins. J Clin Invest 1983; 71:1215.

111. Allen DW, Burgoyne CF, et al: Comparison of hemoglobin Köln erythrocyte membranes with malondialdehyde-reacted normal erythrocyte membranes. Blood 1984; 64:1263.

111a. Brennan SO, Shaw J, et al: β141 Leu is not deleted in the unstable haemoglobin Atlanta-Coventry but is replaced by a novel amino acid of mass 129 daltons. Br J Haematol 1992; 81:99.

111b. Coleman MB, Lu ZH, et al: Two missense mutations in the β-globin gene can cause severe β thalassemia. Hemoglobin Medicine Lake (β32[B14] leucine-glutamime; 98[FG5] valine-methionine). J Clin Invest 1995; 95:503.

112. Winterbourn CC, Williamson D, et al: Unstable haemoglobin haemolytic crises: contributions of pyrexia and neutrophil oxidants. Br J Haematol 1981; 49:111.

113. Tucker PW, Phillips SEV, et al: Structure of hemoglobins Zürich [His E7(63) β-Arg] and Sydney [Val E11(67) β-Ala] and role of the distal residues in ligand binding. Proc Natl Acad Sci U S A 1978; 75:1076.

114. Zinkham WH, Houtchens RA, et al: Carboxyhemoglobin levels in an unstable hemoglobin disorder (Hb Zurich): effect on phenotypic expression. Science 1980; 209:406.

115. Adams JG III, Boxer LA, et al: Hemoglobin Indianapolis (β112[G14] Arginine). An unstable β-chain variant producing the phenotype of severe β-thalassemia. J Clin Invest 1979; 63:931.

116. Kobayashi Y, Fukumaki Y, et al: A novel globin structural mutant, Showa-Yakushiji (β¹¹⁰ ᴸᵉᵘ⁻ᴾʳᵒ) causing a β-thalassemia phenotype. Blood 1987; 70:1688.

117. Beris P, Miescher PA, et al: Inclusion body β-thalassemia trait in a Swiss family is caused by an abnormal hemoglobin (Geneva) with an altered and extended β chain carboxy-terminus due to a modification in codon β114. Blood 1988; 72:801.

117a. Podda A, Galanello R, et al: Hemoglobin Cagliari (β 60 [E4] Val-Glu); a novel unstable thalassemic hemoglobinopathy. Blood 1991; 77:371.

118. White JM, Dacie JV: The unstable hemoglobins—molecular and clinical features. Prog Hematol 1971; 7:69.

119. Eisinger J, Flores J, et al: Fluorescent cytoplasm and Heinz bodies of hemoglobin Köln erythrocytes: evidence for intracellular heme catabolism. Blood 1985; 65:886.

120. Carrell RW, Kay R: A simple method for the detection of unstable haemoglobins. Br J Haematol 1972; 23:615.

121. Carrell RW, Lehmann H: Zinc acetate as a precipitant of unstable haemoglobins. J Clin Pathol 1981; 34:796.

122. Charache S, Weatherall DJ, et al: Polycythemia associated with a hemoglobinopathy. J Clin Invest 1966; 45:813.

123. Adamson JW, Parer JT, et al: Erythrocytosis associated with hemoglobin Rainier: oxygen equilibria and marrow regulation. J Clin Invest 1969; 48:1376.

123a. Rochette J, Barnetson R, et al: Association of a novel high oxygen affinity haemoglobin variant with δβ thalassemia. Br J Haematol 1994; 86:118.

124. Charache S, Catalano P, et al: Pregnancy in carriers of high-affinity hemoglobins. Blood 1985; 65:713.

125. Adamson JW: Familial polycythemia. Semin Hematol 1975; 12:383.

126. Shibata S, Miyaji T, et al: Hemoglobins M of the Japanese. Bull Yamaguchi Med Sch 1967; 14:141.

127. Josephson AM, Weinstein HG, et al: A new variant of hemoglobin M disease. Hemoglobin M Chicago. J Lab Clin Med 1962; 59:918.

128. Stavem P, Stromme J, et al: Hemoglobin M Saskatoon with slight constant hemolysis increased by sulfonamides. Scand J Haematol 1972; 9:566.

129. Priest JR, Watterson J, et al: Mutant fetal hemoglobin causing cyanosis in a newborn. Pediatrics 1989; 83:734.

130. Hayashi A, Fujita T, et al: A new abnormal fetal hemoglobin, Hb FM Osaka ($\alpha_2\gamma_2^{63His-Tyr}$). Hemoglobin 1980; 4:447.

131. Coburn RF, Forster RD, et al: Considerations of the physiological variables that determine the blood carboxyhemoglobin concentration in man. J Clin Invest 1965; 44:1899.

132. Ostrander CR, Cohen RS, et al: Paired determinations of blood carboxyhemoglobin concentration and carbon monoxide excretion rate in term and preterm infants. J Lab Clin Med 1982; 100:745.

133. Burney RF, Wu SC, et al: Mass carbon monoxide poisoning: clinical effects and results of treatment in 184 victims. Ann Emerg Med 1982; 11:394.

134. Myers RA, Snyder SK, et al: Value of hyperbaric oxygen in suspected carbon monoxide poisoning. JAMA 1981; 246:2478.

135. Gibson QH: The reduction of methaemoglobin in red blood cells and studies on the cause of idiopathic methemoglobinemia. Biochem J 1948; 42:13.

136. Kiese M: Die Reduktion des Hämiglobins. Biochem Zeitschr 1943; 316:264.

137. Scott EM, McGraw JC: Purification and properties of diphosphopyridine nucleotide diaphorase of human erythrocytes. J Biol Chem 1962; 237:249.

138. Scott EM, Hoskins DD: Hereditary methemoglobinemia in Alaskan Eskimos and Indians. Blood 1958; 13:795.

139. Hultquist DE, Passon PG: Catalysis of methaemoglobin reduction by erythrocyte cytochrome-b_5 and cytochrome-b_5 reductase. Nature 1971; 229:252.

140. Sugita Y, Nomura S, et al: Purification of reduced pyridine nucleotide dehydrogenase from human erythrocytes and methemoglobin reduction by the enzyme. J Biol Chem 1971; 246:6072.

141. Hultquist DE, Dean RT, et al: Homogeneous cytochrome-b_5 from human erythrocytes. Biochem Biophys Res Commun 1974; 60:28.

142. Slaughter SR, Williams CH, et al: Demonstration that bovine erythrocyte cytochrome-b_5 is the hydrophilic segment of liver microsomal cytochrome-b_5. Biochim Biophys Acta 1982; 705:228.

143. Passon PG, Hultquist DE: Soluble cytochrome-b_5 reductase from human erythrocytes. Biochim Biophys Acta 1972; 275:62.

144. Kuma F, Prough RA, et al: Studies on methemoglobin reductase: immunologic similarity of soluble methemoglobin reductase and cytochrome-b_5 of human erythrocytes with NADH–cytochrome-b_5 reductase and cytochrome-b_5 of rat liver microsomes. Arch Biochem Biophys 1976; 172:600.

145. Goto-Taura R, Takesue Y, et al: Immunological similarity between NADH–cytochrome-b_5 reductase of erythrocytes and liver microsomes. Biochim Biophys Acta 1976; 423:293.

146. Leroux A, Torlinski L, et al: Soluble and microsomal forms of NADH–cytochrome-b_5 reductase from human placenta. Similarity with NADH-methemoglobin reductase from human erythrocytes. Biochim Biophys Acta 1977; 481:50.

147. Gaetani S, DiGirolamo A, et al: Soluble NADH–cytochrome-b_5 reductase during murine erythroleukemic cell differentiation. Cell Mol Biol 1988; 34:673.

148. Takano T, Ogawa K, et al: Preliminary x-ray data of NADH–cytochrome-b_5 reductase from human erythrocytes. J Mol Biol 1987; 195:749. Letter.

149. Righetti PG, Gacon G, et al: Titration curves of interacting cytochrome-b_5 and hemoglobin by isoelectric focusing. Biochem Biophys Res Commun 1978; 85:1575.

150. Mauk MR, Mauk AG: Interaction between cytochrome-b_5 and human methemoglobin. Biochemistry 1982; 21:4730.

151. Juckett DA, Hultquist DE: Magnetic circular dichroism studies of hemoglobin: the reduction of ferrihemoglobin by ferrocytochrome-b_5 and characterization of the high-spin hydroxy species of mixed-valence hemoglobin. Biophys Chem 1984; 19:321.

152. Ng S, Smith MB, et al: Effect of modification of individual cytochrome-c lysines on the reaction with cytochrome-b_5. Biochemistry 1977; 16:4975.

153. Gacon G, Lostanleu D, et al: Interaction between cytochrome-b_5 and hemoglobin: involvement of β66 (E10) and β95 (FG2) lysyl residues of hemoglobin. Proc Natl Acad Sci U S A 1980; 77:1917.

154. Kuma F, Inomata H: Studies on methemoglobin reductase. II. The purification and molecular properties of reduced nicotinamide adenine dinucleotid-dependent methemoglobin reductase. J Biol Chem 1972; 247:556.

155. Abe K, Sugita Y: Properties of cytochrome-b_5 and methemoglobin reduction in human erythrocytes. Eur J Biochem 1979; 101:423.

156. Sannes LJ, Hultquist DE: Effects of hemolysate concentration, ionic strength and cytochrome-b_5 concentration on the rate of methemoglobin reduction in hemolysates of human erythrocytes. Biochim Biophys Acta 1978; 544:547.

157. Keitt AS, Smith TW, et al.: Red cell "pseudomosaicism" in congenital methemoglobinemia. N Engl J Med 1966; 275:397.

158. Hultquist DE, Sannes LJ, et al: The NADH/NADPH-methemoglobin reduction system of erythrocytes from the red cell. In Brewer G (ed): Fifth Ann Arbor Conference on the Red Cell. New York, Alan R. Liss, Inc., 1981, p 291.

159. Feig SA, Nathan DG, et al: Congenital methemoglobinemia: the result of age-dependent decay of methemoglobin reductase. Blood 1972; 39:407.

160. Schwartz JM, Paress PS, et al: Unstable variant of NADH methemoglobin reductase in Puerto Ricans with hereditary methemoglobinemia. J Clin Invest 1972; 51:1594.

161. Matsuki T, Tamura M, et al: Age dependent decay of cytochromic b_5 and cytochrome-b_5 reductase in human erythrocytes. Biochem J 1981; 194:327.

162. Takeshita M, Tamura M, et al: Exponential decay of cytochrome-b_5 and cytochrome-b_5 reductase during senescence of erythrocytes: relation to the increased methemoglobin content. J Biochem 1983; 93:913.

163. Sass MD, Caruso CJ, et al: TPNH-methemoglobin reductase deficiency. A new red cell enzyme defect. J Lab Clin Med 1967; 70:760.

164. Sass MD: Observation on the role of TPNH-dehydrogenase in human red cells. Clin Chim Acta 1968; 21:101.

165. Kiese M: Methemoglobinemia: A Comprehensive Treatise. Cleveland, CRC Press, 1974.

166. Bartos HR, Desforges JF: Erythrocyte DPNH-dependent diaphorase levels in infants. Pediatrics 1966; 37:991.

167. Ross JD: Deficient activity of DPNH-dependent methemoglobin diaphorase in cord blood erythrocytes. Blood 1963; 21:51.

168. Eng LL, Loo M, et al: Diaphorase activity and variants in normal adults and newborns. Br J Haematol 1972; 23:419.

169. Choury D, Reghis A, et al: Endogenous proteolysis of membrane-bound red cell cytochrome-b_5 reductase in adults and newborns: its possible relevance to the generation of the soluble "methemoglobin reductase." Blood 1983; 61:894.

170. Martin H, Huisman THJ: Formation of ferrihaemoglobin of isolated human hemoglobin types by sodium nitrite. Nature 1963; 200:898.

171. Finch CA: Methemoglobinemia and sulfhemoglobinemia. N Engl J Med 1948; 239:470.

172. Hegesh E, Hegesh J, et al: Congenital methemoglobinemia with a deficiency of cytochrome-b_5. N Engl J Med 1986; 314:757.

173. Scott EM: The relation of diaphorase of human erythrocyte to inheritance of methemoglobinemia. J Clin Invest 1960; 39:1176.

174. Schwartz JM, Jaffe ER: Hereditary methemoglobinemia with deficiency of NADH–cytochrome-b_5 reductase. In Stanbury EJ (ed): The Metabolic Basis of Inherited Disease. New York, McGraw-Hill Book Co., 1978, p 1452.

175. Board PG, Pidcock ME: Methaemoglobinaemia resulting from heterozygosity for two NADH-methaemoglobin reductase variants: characterization as NADH-ferricyanide reductase. Br J Haematol 1981; 47:361.

176. Gonzalez R, Estrada M, et al: Heterogeneity of hereditary met-

haemoglobinaemia: a study of 4 Cuban families with NADH-methaemoglobin reductase deficiency including a new variant (Santiago de Cuba variant). Scand J Haematol 1978; 20:385.

177. Hirano M, Matsuki T, et al: Congenital methaemoglobinaemia due to NADH methemoglobin reductase deficiency: successful treatment with oral riboflavin. Br J Haematol 1981; 47:353.

177a. Posthumus MD, van Berkel W: Cytochrome-b_5 reductase deficiency, an uncommon cause of cyanosis. Neth J Med 1994; 44:136.

178. Cohen RJ, Sachs JR, et al: Methemoglobinemia provoked by malarial chemoprophylaxis in Vietnam. N Engl J Med 1968; 279:1127.

179. Daly JS, Hultquist DE, et al: Phenazopyridine induced methaemoglobinaemia associated with decreased activity of erythrocyte cytochrome-b_5 reductase. J Med Genet 1983; 20:307.

180. Harper MA, Robin H, et al: Transient infantile cyanosis in a diaphorase-deficient male. Aust Paediatr J 1968; 4:144.

181. Fisher RA, Povey S, et al: Assignment of the DIA_1 locus to chromosome 22. Ann Hum Genet 1977; 41:151.

182. Tomatsu S, Kobayashi Y, et al: The organization and the complete nucleotide sequence of the human NADH–cytochrome-b_5 reductase gene. Gene 1989; 80:353.

183. Katsube T, Sakamoto N, et al: Exonic point mutations in NADH–cytochrome-b_5 reductase genes of homozygotes for hereditary methemoglobinemia, types I and III: putative mechanisms of tissue-dependent enzyme deficiency. Am J Hum Genet 1991; 48:799.

184. Kobayashi Y, Fukumaki Y, et al: Serine-proline replacement at residue 127 of NADH–cytochrome-b_5 reductase causes hereditary methemoglobinemia, generalized type. Blood 1990; 75:1408.

185. Vieira LM, Kaplan JC, et al: Four new mutations in the NADH–cytochrome-b_5 reductase gene from patients with recessive congenital methemoglobinemia type II. Blood 1995; 85:2254.

186. Shirabe K, Fujimoto Y, et al: An in-frame deletion of codon 298 of the NADH–cytochrome-b_5 reductase gene results in hereditary methemoglobinemia type II (generalized type). A functional implication for the role of the COOH-terminal region of the enzyme. J Biol Chem 1994; 269:5952.

187. Giordano SJ, Kaftory A, et al: A splicing mutation in the cytochrome-b_5 gene from a patient with congenital methemoglobinemia and pseudohermaphrodism. Hum Genet 1994; 93:568.

188. Jaffe ER, Hultquist DE: Cytochrome-b_5 reductase deficiency and enzymopenic hereditary methemoglobinemia. In Scriver CR, Beaudet AL, et al (eds): The Metabolic Basis of Inherited Disease. 6th ed. New York, McGraw-Hill Book Co., 1989.

189. Prchal JT, Borgese N, et al: Congenital methemoglobinemia due to methemoglobin reductase deficiency in two unrelated American black families. Am J Med 1990; 89:516.

190. Kaplan JC, Leroux A, et al: La lésion enzymatique dans la méthémogobinémie congénitale récessive avec encéphalopathie. Nouv Rev Fr Hematol 1974; 14:755.

191. Leroux A, Junien C, et al: Generalized deficiency of cytochrome-b_5 reductase in congenital methaemoglobinaemia with mental retardation. Nature 1975; 258:619.

192. Tanishima K, Matsuki T, et al: NADH–cytochrome-b_5 reductase in platelets and leukocytes with special reference to normal levels and to levels in carriers of hereditary methemoglobinemia with or without neurological symptoms. Acta Haematol 1980; 63:7.

193. Mirono H: Lipids of myelin, white matter and gray matter in a case of generalized deficiency of cytochrome-b_5 reductase in congenital methemoglobinemia with mental retardation. Lipids 1980; 15:272.

194. Arnold H, Botcher HW, et al: Hereditary methemoglobinemia due to methemoglobin reductase deficiency in erythrocytes and leukocytes without neurological symptoms. Presented before the XVII Congress of the International Society of Hematology, Abstracts (II), Paris, 1978, p 752.

195. Tanishima K, Tanimoto K, et al: Hereditary methemoglobinemia due to cytochrome-b_5 reductase deficiency in blood cells without associated neurologic and mental disorders. Blood 1985; 66:1288.

196. Hegesh E, Avron M: The enzymatic reduction of ferrihemoglobin. I. The reduction of ferrihemoglobin in red blood cells and hemolysates. Biochim Biophys Acta 1967; 146:91.

197. Borgese N, Pietrini G, et al: Concentration of NADH–cytochrome-b_5 reductase in erythrocytes of normal and methemoglobinemic individuals measured with a quantitative radioimmunoblotting assay. J Clin Invest 1987; 80:1296.

198. Kaplan JC, Junien C, et al: Prenatal diagnosis of generalized cytochrome-b_5 reductase deficiency (congenital methemoglobinemia with mental retardation, Type II). Ann Med Interne 1981; 132:93.

199. Kaplan JC, Chirouze M: Therapy of recessive congenital methemoglobinemia by oral riboflavin. Lancet 1978; 2:1043.

200. Das Gupta A, Vaidya MS, et al: Associated red cell enzyme deficiencies and their significance in a case of congenital enzymopenic methemoglobinemia. Acta Haematol 1980; 64:285.

201. Jaffe ER: The reduction of methemoglobin in erythrocytes of a patient with congenital methemoglobinemia, subjects with glucose-6-phosphate dehydrogenase deficiency and normal individuals. Blood 1963; 21:561.

202. Beutler E, Baluda M: Methemoglobin reduction. Studies of the interaction between cell populations and the role of methylene blue. Blood 1963; 22:323.

203. Rosen PJ, Johnson C, et al: Failure of methylene blue treatment in toxic methemoglobinemia associated with glucose-6-phosphate dehydrogenase deficiency. Ann Intern Med 1971; 75:83.

204. Roueche B: Eleven Blue Men. Boston, Little, Brown & Co., Inc., 1947.

205. Cornblath M, Hartmann AF: Methemoglobinemia in young infants. J Pediatr 1948; 33:421.

206. Hegesh E, Shiloah J: Blood nitrates and infantile methemoglobinemia. Clin Chim Acta 1982; 125:107.

207. Gentile DA: Severe methemoglobinemia induced by a topical teething preparation. Pediatr Emerg Care 1987; 3:176.

208. Wilson CM, Bird SG, et al: Case report: Methemoglobinemia following metoclopramide therapy in an infant. J Pediatr Gastroenterol Nutr 1987; 6:640.

209. Kearns GL, Fiser DH: Metoclopramide-induced methemoglobinemia. Pediatrics 1988; 82:364.

210. Brandenburg RO, Smith HL: Sulfhemoglobinemia: a study of 62 clinical cases. Am Heart J 1951; 42:582.

211. Bower PJ, Peterson JN: Methemoglobinemia after sodium nitroprusside therapy. N Engl J Med 1975; 293:865.

212. Hoppe-Seyler F: Einwirkung des Schwefelwasserstoffs aus das Blut. Zentralbl Med Wiss 1863; 1:433.

213. Berzofsky JA, Peisach J, et al: Sulfheme proteins. IV. The stoichiometry of sulfur incorporation and the isolation of sulfhemin, the prosthetic group of sulfmyoglobin. J Biol Chem 1972; 247:3783.

214. Lambert M, Sonnet J, et al: Delayed sulfhemoglobinemia after acute dapsone intoxication. Clin Toxicol 1982; 19:45.

215. van den Bergh AAH, Grutterink A: Enterogene cyanose. Berl Klin Wochenschr 1906; 43:7.

216. Tursz T, Bernard JF, et al: Sulfhemoglobin and glutathione peroxidase deficiency. Nouv Presse Med 1974; 3:1487.

217. Martensson J, Sorbo B: Human β-mercaptopyruvate sulfur transferase: distribution in cellular compartments of the blood and activity in erythrocytes from patients with hematological disorders. Clin Chim Acta 1978; 87:11.

218. Nichol AW, Morell DB: Spectrophotometric determination of mixtures of sulphaemoglobin methaemoglobin in blood. Clin Chim Acta 1968; 22:157.

219. Park CM, Nagel RL: Sulfhemoglobinemia: clinical and molecular aspects. N Engl J Med 1984; 310:1579.

Sickle Cell Disease

George J. Dover • Orah S. Platt

HISTORY

Sickle cell anemia was first described in a West Indian student by Herrick in 1910.[1] Sydenstricker described the first cases in children, recognized the association with a hemolytic anemia, and introduced the term *crisis* to describe periodic acute episodes of pain.[2] The pathologic basis of the disorder and its relation to the hemoglobin molecule were defined in 1927 by Hahn and Gillespie.[3] Shortly after the application of moving-boundary electrophoresis to the separation of sickle from normal hemoglobin by Pauling and co-workers,[4] Beet[5] and Neel[6] defined the genetics of the disorder and clearly distinguished sickle trait—the heterozygous condition (AS)—from sickle cell anemia—the homozygous state (SS). Further understanding of the molecular basis of the disorder was made possible by the finding that normal human hemoglobin is composed of two pairs of globin subunits: one pair that is invariant, the α chain, and another pair that is variable, the ϵ,[7, 8] ζ,[9] γ, β or δ chain. The relative ease with which

sickle hemoglobin could be isolated by chromatography or zone electrophoresis techniques led to Ingram's application of tryptic digestion, high-voltage electrophoresis, and paper chromatography to the isolated sickle hemoglobin, with the result that the amino acid substitution in sickle hemoglobin is now known to be a valine instead of a glutamic acid in the number 6 position of the β chain. The α chain is normal.[10, 11] The chemical nomenclature for sickle hemoglobin is therefore $\alpha_2\beta_2$6Glu$\rightarrow$Val. (See Fig. 20–1 for an overview of pathophysiology of β^s mutation). Excellent reviews of the history of sickle cell anemia are available.[12, 13]

ORIGINS OF MUTATION

The sickle gene is a common mutant that provides some protection to infants who might otherwise succumb to cerebral falciparum malaria, and its incidence parallels the incidence of malaria. The frequency of the sickle gene in a population parallels the historical

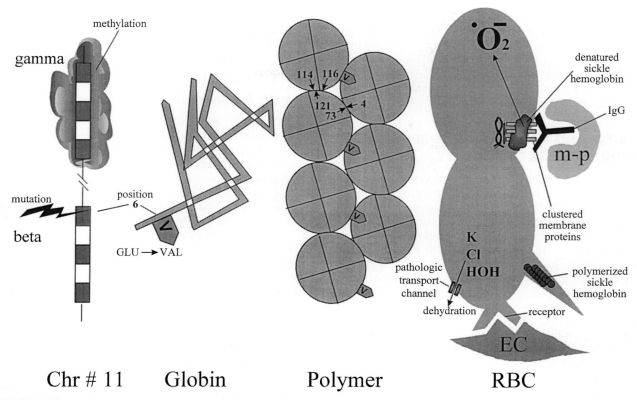

Chr # 11   Globin   Polymer   RBC

Figure 20-1. The pathophysiology of sickle cell disease. Chromosome 11 contains the genes for β and γ globin. Beyond fetal life, the γ gene is highly methylated and barely expressed. The β^s gene contains an A®T mutation in the 6th codon, which results in an abnormal globin with valine instead of glutamic acid in the sixth position. That hydrophobic valine is exposed when the globin assumes the deoxy confirmation and tends to burrow within a hydrophobic pocket in neighboring β chains, forming a polymer. As indicated, other key residues at positions 4, 73, 114, 166, and 121 play roles in stabilizing the polymer. When this process takes place in red blood cells they become distorted and viscous and resist flow. The inherent unstable nature of sickle cell hemoglobin causes it to denature and produce oxidants. A variety of membrane abnormalities appear in the process. The red cells have a short survival, are young, and express receptors that promote adhesion to endothelial cells (EC). Membrane proteins (ankyrin, protein 3) cluster around deposits of denatured hemoglobin, promoting the deposition of immunoglobulin G (IgG), making the cells attractive targets for macrophages (m-p). Pathologic transport channels (Gardos, K–Cl co-transport) are activated, leading to cation and water loss and cell dehydration. RBC = red blood cell; HOH = H$_2$O. (Adapted from Platt OS: Sickle cell paths converge on hydroxyurea. Nature Med 1995; 1:307.)

incidence of malaria.[14–17] Whereas the average incidence of the sickle gene among American blacks is approximately 8%,[18] the frequency is much higher in inhabitants of certain areas of Africa. Polymorphic sites around globin DNA and their linkages to the β^s gene indicate that this mutation may have developed independently and spontaneously at least five times.[19–22] However, analysis of nuclear and mitochondrial DNA from African populations suggests that a single mutation may have occurred 50,000 years ago.[23] In Africa, there are four major sickle haplotypes, each associated with a particular geographic region: "Senegal" (Atlantic West Africa), "Benin" (Central West Africa), "Bantu" (also called "CAR" for Central African Republic), and Cameroon.[21, 24] The Benin type is found not only in Benin but also in Ibadan,[25] Algeria,[21] Sicily,[26] Turkey,[27] Greece,[28] Yemen, and southwest Saudi Arabia.[27] In Caribbean and North American sickle cell patients of African heritage, 50% to 70% of chromosomes are Benin, 15% to 30% are Bantu-CAR, and 5% to 15% are Senegal.[20, 29, 30] In Africa, virtually all patients in a region are homozygous for a given haplotype. Nagel

and co-workers document the different hematologic characteristics of the different homozygote groups.[31, 32] The Benin and Senegalese patients have higher levels of fetal hemoglobin and fewer dense cells compared with Bantu-CAR. The Senegalese have a high proportion of ^{G}γ fetal hemoglobin. In contrast to what is found among Africans in Africa, African Americans are mainly heterozygotes. In Los Angeles, 38% of patients are Benin homozygotes (Benin/Benin); 25% are Benin/Bantu-CAR; 13% are Benin/Senegal; 5% are Bantu-CAR homozygotes, and 3% are Bantu-CAR/Senegal.[29] Less common β^s linked haplotypes are usually recombinations of the common haplotypes occurring 5' to the β globin gene.[33, 34] When patients identified in hospital-based clinics are studied, these haplotypes may be associated with overall clinical severity—the Bantu-CAR being the most severe and the Senegalese being the least severe.[35] However, no study of a cohort of SS patients identified at birth has been done.

A different haplotype is found in India and parts of Saudi Arabia.[25] In the Eastern oases of Saudi Arabia, the African haplotypes are not seen, but a unique "Arabian-Indian" haplotype is found. This haplotype is also seen in patients from Orissa and Poona, India. Patients from these regions have long been recognized as having mild disease and elevated levels of fetal hemoglobin.[36–40] In contrast, in Riyadh, Saudi Arabia, all patients with sickle cell anemia are from southwest Saudi Arabia and Yemen and are homozygous Benin.

MALARIA AND GLUCOSE-6-PHOSPHATE DEHYDROGENASE DEFICIENCY

The physiologic basis for the influence of malaria on the sickle gene (so-called balanced polymorphism) is not well understood.[41] It has been suggested that Hb S may be poorly metabolized by the parasite,[42] that infected cells are more easily sickled and removed from the circulation,[43–45] that the intracellular potassium lost during sickling results in a hostile environment for the parasite,[46] and that increased membrane rigidity inhibits parasite invasion.[47]

Glucose-6-phosphate dehydrogenase (G6PD) deficiency is another genetic variant common in black populations. Originally, because of the unexpectedly high incidence of G6PD deficiency among patients with sickle cell disease, it was concluded that G6PD deficiency conferred a protective effect on sickle cell patients.[48, 49] Subsequent studies reveal no increased incidence of G6PD deficiency in the sickle population.[50, 51] In a survey of 801 SS males, G6PD deficiency did not cause more hemolysis or increased anemic episodes.[52] Because the SS red cell is young, it is difficult to demonstrate the usual A⁻ variety of G6PD deficiency by conventional methods.[34, 50, 51] Episodes of accelerated hemolysis of G6PD-deficient SS red cells have been described.[53] Because of the large population of very young G6PD-rich cells, this accelerated hemolysis is likely to be due to the enzyme abnormality only when the population is shifted toward the oldest cells, that is, during an aplastic episode.

MOLECULAR SICKLING
The Hb S Polymer

In 1927, Hahn and Gillespie[3] showed that sickling, the change from a biconcave disk to the sickle form, was dependent on deoxygenation. Harris[54] subsequently demonstrated that cellular sickling was associated with the formation of "tactoids" of Hb S, which appeared as the hemoglobin became deoxygenated. Electron micrographs of sickled red cells[55–59] reveal long, thin bundles of Hb S fibers that run parallel to the long axis of the cell or the abnormal protuberances. The ultrastructure of these Hb S fibers has been detailed by electron microscopy and image reconstruction. These studies reveal a complex solid-core structure 21 nm in diameter, composed of 14 filaments arranged as seven pairs of double filaments[60, 61]—an inner pair with six peripheral pairs.[62] Each filament pair is half-staggered along the fiber axis and has an inherent polarity. A model with three pairs of one polarity and four pairs of the other polarity is suggested by electron microscope evidence[63] and is compatible with x-ray diffraction analysis of Hb S crystals.[64–66] The radius of the sickle hemoglobin fibers are polymorphic and related to the helical pitch of the double filaments.[67]

Understanding of the fiber structure at the level of specific amino acid residues required additional evidence, obtained with optical dichroism,[68] x-ray diffraction,[64, 69–71] and studies of mutant hemoglobins.[72–78] The detailed crystal structure suggested by Wishner and colleagues[70] identified several critical intermolecular contact sites: β73 Asp, and β121 Glu (see Fig. 20–1). In

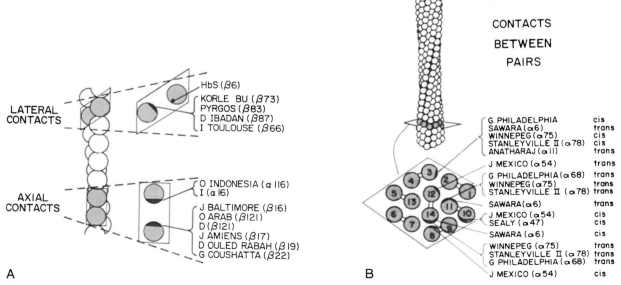

Figure 20-2. Model of the structure of the hemoglobin (Hb) S fiber suggested by Edelstein[79] illustrating the important intermolecular contact points and the associated hemoglobin variants. The notations *cis* and *trans* follow the convention where α₂ = cis and α₁ = trans, with the β6 valine involved in fiber formation in the β₂ subunit. (With thanks to Dr. Edelstein for his review.)

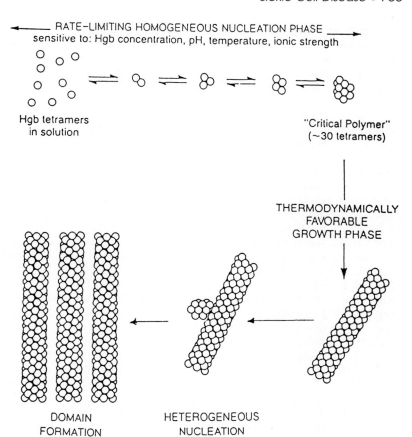

RATE—LIMITING HOMOGENEOUS NUCLEATION PHASE
sensitive to: Hgb concentration, pH, temperature, ionic strength

Hgb tetramers
in solution

"Critical Polymer"
(~30 tetramers)

THERMODYNAMICALLY
FAVORABLE
GROWTH PHASE

DOMAIN
FORMATION

HETEROGENEOUS
NUCLEATION

Figure 20-3. Model for the polymerization and alignment of deoxyhemoglobin S. Hgb = hemoglobin. (Adapted from Hofrichter J, Ross PD, et al: Supersaturations in sickle cell hemoglobin solutions. Proc Natl Acad Sci U S A 1976; 73:303; and Ferrone FA, et al: Kinetics of sickle hemoglobin polymerization: II. A double nucleation mechanism. J Mol Biol 1985; 183:611.)

an elegant synthesis of several lines of evidence, Edelstein has proposed a topographic map of the Hb S fiber,[79] which describes three classes of intermolecular contacts: along the axis of a filament, lateral between filaments of a pair, and lateral between filaments (Fig. 20–2).

With resolution of the crystalline structure of Hb S to 3.0 angstroms this model has been confirmed.[80] The axial contacts are made through both α and β chains and include the following residues where mutants affect fiber formation: β121 (O Arab), β16 (J Baltimore), β17 (J Amiens), β19 (D Ouled Rabah), β22 (G Coushatta), α16 (I), and α116 (O Indonesia). The lateral contacts between filaments of a pair are largely between β chains and include the primary sickle mutation—β6. For each hemoglobin tetramer, one chain contributes the β6 mutation whereas the other contributes a critical receptor region around the β85 Phe residue. In this critical receptor region lie residues where mutants affect fiber formation: β73 (Korle Bu), β66 (I Toulouse), β83 (Pyrgos), and β87 (D Ibadan). The contacts between filament pairs are largely through α chains. Alpha mutations that occur at sites critical for interpair associations influence fiber formation and include the following: J Mexico (α54), Sealy (α47), Winnipeg (α75), Stanleyville II (α78), Sawara (α6), Anantharaj (α11), and G Philadelphia (α68).

Polymer Formation

The polymerization of deoxy-Hb S is a highly complex process that results in the formation of gelled, aggregated Hb S tetramers in equilibrium with hemoglobin tetramers in solution. Pertubations in oxygen levels,[81, 82] temperature,[83–85] pH,[86, 87] ionic strength,[88] 2,3-diphosphoglycerate,[87, 89, 90] and carbon monoxide[91–93] affect the formation of Hb S gels. This sol-gel transition of Hb S is the basic feature that leads to the viscosity changes, distortion of cell morphology, sludging, and organ infarction that are identified as the clinical manifestations of sickle cell disease. The kinetics of Hb S polymerization and the factors that modify this process have been studied with different techniques—light scattering and turbidimetry,[94, 95] sedimentation,[96, 97] optical birefringence,[68, 91, 98, 99] calorimetry,[68, 83] and nuclear magnetic resonance.[100–103] Although data from the various techniques differ somewhat, a representative kinetic model was proposed by Hofrichter, Ross, and Eaton,[83, 91] and was expanded by Ferrone[104] (Fig. 20–3).

The kinetics of Hb S polymerization can be explained by a double nucleation mechanism. Gelation is initiated by a process called "homogeneous nucleation" in which single deoxy-Hb S molecules aggregate. Aggregation of a few molecules is thermodynamically unstable, but once a certain number of molecules aggregate, termed the *critical nucleus*, addition of further molecules produces a more stable aggregate or polymer. Thus, homogeneous nucleation is very highly dependent on the concentration of deoxy-Hb S molecules. The second nucleation phase, termed *heterogeneous nucleation*, takes place on the surface of pre-existing polymer. As polymerization progresses, more surface area becomes available and therefore the reaction becomes autocatalytic. The result of this double nucleation mechanism is a measurable delay time between the initiation of polymerization and the exponential rise in polymer formation. The delay time varies as the 30th power of the hemoglobin concentration:

$$1/t_d = K (C/C_s)^n$$

in which t_d = delay time, C = hemoglobin concentration, C_s = hemoglobin solubility, and n $\cong$ 30 (the number of hemoglobin tetramers in the "critical polymer"). Because n is so large, small changes in hemoglobin concentration have a profound effect on the delay time. For example, decreasing the mean corpuscular hemoglobin concentration (MCHC) from 32 to 30 g/dL will increase the delay time threefold.[105] Alpha-thalassemia in sickle cell anemia patients results in a reduced cellular Hb S content and thus an increased surface-to-volume ratio with a lower MCHC. This magnitude of change in MCHC is seen in SS individuals with four versus two α genes and therefore may explain the longer life span of red cells in individuals with SS disease and α-thalassemia. Gelation is also exquisitely sensitive to changes in temperature and pH. A change from 38.5°C to 37°C or an increase in intracellular pH of 0.03 unit would also double the delay time.

The phenomenon of delayed gelling of Hb S in solution is also seen in cells containing Hb S. Rampling and Sirs[106] studied cellular deformation after immediate deoxygenation and found a delay time of 30 seconds. Messer, Hahn, and Bradley[107, 108] observed changes in rheology and morphology of cells with partial deoxygenation and also demonstrated a delay time. Zarkowsky and Hochmuth[109] studied cell sickling at PO_2 of zero and demonstrated a delay time that is sensitive to cell density, pH, osmolarity, and temperature. Coletta and co-workers examined polymerization in single intact cells[110] and demonstrated that polymerization kinetics of Hb S in these cells was the same as the kinetics of Hb S in solution. Furthermore, the distribution of observed delay times was consistent with the distribution of MCHC in cells from patients with sickle cell anemia. The double nucleation hypothesis provides for the formation of a network of polymers termed a *domain* that is nonuniformly distributed within the cell. Rapid deoxygenation leads to the formation of multiple small domains of polymer and little morphologic deformation of the cell. On the other hand, slow deoxygenation causes large, aligned polymers, which results in significant distortion of cell morphology.[111, 112]

A kinetic model of Hb S gelation that incorporates the concept of a critical delay time has led Eaton and his co-workers to propose that polymerization kinetics play an important role in the pathophysiology of SS disease.[113, 114] The oxygenation and deoxygenation of cells in the circulation take place in a time frame that is of the same order of magnitude as the sickling and unsickling of Hb S *in vitro*. Cells exposed to the high PO_2 of the lungs are quickly "degelled," because Hb S gels melt in less than 0.5 second when exposed to oxygen. The cells are then maintained in the unsickled

state while in the oxygenated environment of the arterial circulation. As the cells enter the capillary circulation, the oxygen saturation decreases rapidly, as does the hemoglobin solubility. The red cell spends an average of 1 second in the capillary circulation, although this is highly variable. If the delay time is less than 1 second, the cell will sickle and occlude the capillary. If the delay time is prolonged, sickling will not take place in the capillary and obstruction will not occur. If the transit time through the capillary is shortened and is less than the delay time, occlusion will not occur. This is presumably the situation in the myocardium, in which sickling and infarction do not occur despite the high oxygen extraction because of the extremely short transit time. Factors such as low pH, high hemoglobin concentration, and high ionic strength, which shorten the delay time *in vitro*, also affect *in vivo* sickling. Patients who become hypoxic, acidotic, dehydrated, and febrile are likely to experience vaso-occlusive episodes. The hypertonic renal medulla and the acidotic, high hematocrit environment of the spleen make these organs prime targets for sickling.

An alternative model relating Hb S polymerization to the pathophysiology of SS disease has been proposed by Noguchi and Schechter.[115] Using nuclear magnetic resonance techniques, they have measured the quantity of Hb S polymer in AS and SS red cells under varying conditions related to MCHC and oxygenation.[103, 116] They have found polymer formation and impaired erythrocyte deformability at oxygen saturations above the level at which cells appear to morphologically sickle.[117] They propose that the amount of Hb S polymer present at equilibrium in SS patients is the major factor determining clinical severity.[118, 119]

Both the kinetic model of Eaton and the equilibrium model of Schechter and Noguchi may be useful in designing therapeutic interventions in SS disease. It appears that decreases in MCHC or increases in non-Hb S (either Hb A or Hb F) have comparable effects on delay times and Hb S polymer content (Fig. 20–4).

Interactions of Hb S with Hb A and Hb F

The study of the interaction with other hemoglobins supports a rational basis for the understanding of the clinical manifestations of the various sickle syndromes. Investigators have extensively studied mixtures of Hb S with Hb F or Hb A to determine the effects on gelation[120–124] and solubility.[120–123, 125–128] In these studies, the nonideal behavior of concentrated hemoglobin solutions[84, 129] was considered—the bulky hemoglobin molecules take up much of the solution volume, making the *effective* concentration of the hemoglobin higher than the *measured* concentration. The kinetic data show that Hb A and Hb F have a profound, dose-related effect, increasing the delay time and decreasing Hb S polymer content in cells (see Fig. 20–4). The effect of Hb F is considerably larger than the effect of Hb A. Sunshine and colleagues demonstrate that compared with pure Hb S solutions (as seen in sickle cell anemia), mixtures with 15% to 30% Hb A (as found in S-β$^+$-thalassemia) have delay times that are 10 to 10^2 longer;

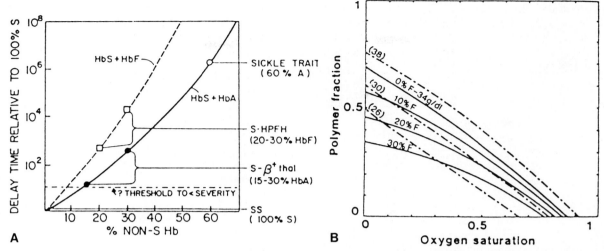

Figure 20–4. *A,* Effect of increasing concentrations of Hb F or Hb A on delay time of polymerization of hemoglobin S. *B,* Sickle hemoglobin polymer formation as a function of oxygen saturation for different levels of fetal hemoglobin and for different concentrations of pure hemoglobin S at concentrations of 26, 30, and 38 g/dL. (*A,* Based on the work of Sunshine HR, Hofrichter J, et al: Requirements for therapeutic inhibition of sickle haemoglobin gelation. Nature 1978; 275:238. *B,* Based on Noguchi CT, et al: Intracellular polymerization of sickle hemoglobin: disease severity and therapeutic goals. Clin Biol Res 1987; 240:390.)

mixtures with 20% to 30% Hb F (as found in S-Hereditary Persistence of Hb F) have delay times that are 10^3 to 10^4 longer; and mixtures with 60% Hb A (as found in sickle trait) have delay times that are 10^6 longer.[120, 122] Hb A and Hb F also increase the solubility of Hb S, with Hb F being more effective than Hb A. Studies of the composition of the gels and supernatant of these mixtures demonstrate that asymmetric hybrids of Hb S and Hb A ($\alpha_2\beta^A\beta^S$) are readily incorporated into the gel. In mixtures of Hb F and Hb S where Hb F concentration is less than 40%, very little if any Hb F is incorporated into polymer, suggesting that asymmetric hybrids of Hb S and Hb F ($\alpha_2\beta^S\gamma$) and Hb F ($\alpha_2\gamma_2$) are not incorporated into polymer under most physiologic conditions.[121, 124, 126, 127, 130] Compared with Hb F, Hb A has a lesser effect on Hb S solubility because the asymmetric hybrids readily copolymerize with Hb S.[130]

Because it is now possible to increase Hb F in patients with sickle cell anemia (see Treatment) and therefore presumably increase delay times and decrease polymer content within cells, it will soon be possible to test the relationship between delay times or polymer content on the clinical severity of sickle cell anemia.

CELLULAR SICKLING

The oxygen-dependent gelation of Hb S described in the previous section has profound effects on the morphology and rheology of the Hb S–containing cell. The time course of cellular events associated with oxygenation and deoxygenation has been investigated by Messer, Hahn, and Bradley,[107, 108] who studied cells from patients with SS disease under physiologic time and oxygen conditions. They described two categories of cells—a fraction of dense cells (MCHC 36 g/dL) that exhibited reversible polymerization and shape change (reversibly sickled cells [RSCs]), and a fraction of very dense cells (MCHC 44 g/dL) that exhibited reversible

polymerization but irreversible shape change (irreversibly sickled cells [ISCs]). Changes in the rheology of the cells paralleled the appearance of polymers in the cytoplasm, a considerable time before any detectable distortion of cell shape.

The RSCs have normal shape and normal viscosity when oxygenated. The vaso-occlusive complications of sickle cell disease may be due to the "Trojan horse performance" of these RSCs, which are able to slip into the microvasculature because of their normal rheologic properties when oxygenated and then become distorted and viscous as they become deoxygenated in the vessel.

The ISCs are the obvious, slender, elongated cells that are visible on an oxygenated peripheral blood smear in sickle cell disease (Fig. 20–5). In 1968, Dobler and Bertles[57] demonstrated unpolymerized hemoglobin in an oxygenated ISC. Numerous investigators have studied this bizarre cell, the membrane of which is frozen in its sickled form. In the Messer, Hahn, and Bradley studies, ISCs underwent hemoglobin polymerization and depolymerization on deoxygenation and reoxygenation. In comparison to the RSC fraction, however, the polymerization took place sooner, was much more highly aligned, and took longer to disappear on deoxygenation.

It is clear from electron microscopic observations and the data relating hemoglobin concentration to polymerization in solution[83] and in cells[110, 117] that the distribution of MCHC in the circulation should have profound clinical implications. A density profile of sickle red cells can be easily determined.[131] Sickle cell individuals have more light cells (reticulocytes) and more dense cells (MCHC >37 mg/dL) than normal individuals. Because of the rigid abnormal shape of dense cells, the MCHC, as estimated electronically, is unreliable.[132] Laser light scattering techniques accurately quantitate the red cell density profile but also tend to underesti-

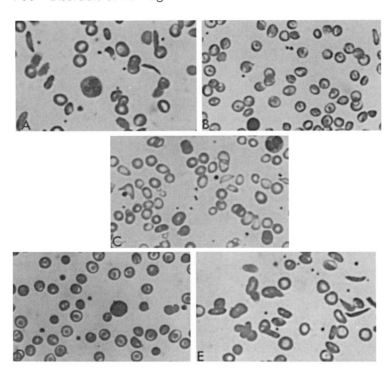

Figure 20-5. Oxygenated peripheral blood smears from individuals with sickle cell anemia *(A)*; hemoglobin SC disease *(B)*; sickle-B⁰ thalassemia *(C)*; homozygous hemoglobin C *(D)*; and hemoglobin SD disease *(E)*.

mate the hemoglobin concentration of very dense sickle cells.[133] The vaso-occlusive nature of these dense cells was reported by Kaul and colleagues, who showed that cells separated by density (and therefore MCHC) from patients with sickle cell anemia obstruct flow in an artificially perfused capillary system in proportion to their MCHC.[134] Although early reports suggested that the percentage of dense cells decreased during vaso-occlusive crises,[135] there is no correlation between the percentage of dense cells and the frequency or onset of crises.[136] The decreased MCHC associated with α-thalassemia leads to a more uniform distribution of red cell densities and a decreased percentage of dense cells.[137, 138] Paradoxically, individuals with Hb SC have milder clinical disease but more dense cells than individuals with homozygous sickle cell anemia (Fig. 20–6).[139]

The heterogeneity of red cell shape and density in sickle cell anemia may be due partially to the heterogeneous distribution of Hb F. In normal and sickle cell individuals Hb F is confined to a subset of red cells called F cells.[140] Because Hb F interferes with Hb S polymerization, F cells survive longer in the circulation than cells with no Hb F[141] and the relative proportions of F cells in the densest cell fractions are very low.[137, 142] Even young reticulocytes poor in Hb F can rapidly dehydrate and be found among the most dense cells in the circulation.[143]

RED CELL MEMBRANE ABNORMALITIES

The basic pathophysiology of sickle cell anemia is directly related to the abnormal hemoglobin, which has the property of polymerizing when deoxygenated. As seen in other genetic diseases, however, secondary effects of the primary lesion may modulate the clinical

expression of the disease. Alterations in the red cell membrane may be one of the important modulators of disease severity for several reasons (see Fig. 20–1). First, the membrane is the structure most intimately associated with the abnormal gene product and is therefore vulnerable to damage. Second, the membrane is largely responsible for maintaining the environment in which this abnormal product resides. Third, the membrane is the face with which the cells presents itself and is recognized by proteins in the plasma, and cells in the circulation, along the vasculature, and in the reticuloendothelium.

Irreversibly Sickled Cells

The ISCs, which are easily identified and studied, have been a focus of attention in the study of the membrane lesion in sickle cell anemia. Bertles and Milner[142] showed that these cells are extremely dense, have little Hb F to dilute their concentrated Hb S, and survive in the circulation for only a few days. These cells provide the most graphic evidence of membrane damage in SS disease. Lux and co-workers demonstrated that the abnormal shape of the ISC is maintained by the membrane (ghost) after hemolysis. Furthermore, when this membrane is treated with nonionic detergent (Triton X-100), all of its lipids and integral membrane are solubilized to maintain the ISC shape[144] (Fig. 20–7). As reviewed in detail in Chapter 16, the red cell skeleton plays a role not only in cell shape but also in permeability, lipid organization, deformability, and control of lateral mobility of integral proteins. ISCs can be formed *in vitro* by prolonged deoxygenation,[145] by incubation of red cells in high calcium buffer,[146] and by repeated oxygenation-deoxygenation cycles.[147] Horiuchi has demonstrated that *in vitro* formation of ISCs is corre-

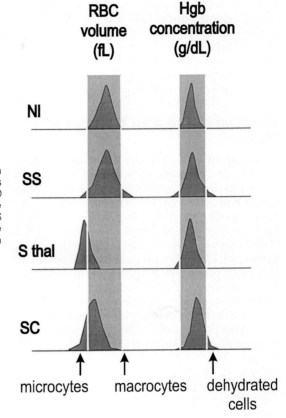

Figure 20-6. Typical distribution patterns of cell volume and hemoglobin concentration in different sickle syndromes. Note that in SS disease, the cells fall below and above both the volume and concentration normal *(shaded)* range. The large (macrocytic) cells are the low-density reticulocytes. The dehydrated population is enriched in ISCs and low fetal hemoglobin. In S thalassemia (s thal) syndromes, the entire volume curve is shifted toward the left, and few dense cells are seen. In SC disease, the microcytes are often spherocytic, very dehydrated cells. NI = normal.

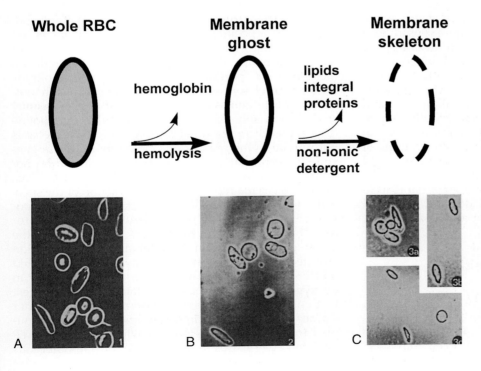

Figure 20-7. *A,* Oxygenated intact red cells from an SS patient showing typical round reversibly sickled cells (RSCs) and elongated irreversibly sickled cells (ISCs). *B,* Same cells as in *A,* lysed to remove all intracellular material, leaving just membrane. Note the retained shape of the RSCs and ISCs. *C,* Same cells as in *B,* extracted with Triton X-100 to remove everything but the integral membrane proteins. Note the retained shape of the RSCs and ISCs. (Adapted from Lux SE, John KM, et al: Irreversible deformation of the spectrin-actin lattice in irreversibly sickled cells. J Clin Invest 1976; 58:955.)

lated with the maximal linear distortion of the red cell diameter under deoxygenated conditions, suggesting that the length of Hb S polymer fibers in SS cells contributes to irreversible membrane damage.[148] As detailed later, ISCs have different cation and water content, which is directly attributable to membrane-mediated events. ISCs vary widely from patient to patient and correspond well with hemolytic rate[149] and spleen size[150] but poorly with vaso-occlusive severity.

The Membrane and the Internal Milieu

Transport and Volume Control. As discussed previously, the concentration of Hb S in the cell has tremendous impact on the amount of polymer, and the speed with which it forms at a given P_{O_2}. The abnormal cation permeability of the sickle red cell allows it to become potassium depleted, calcium loaded, and pathologically dehydrated—enhancing the tendency to sickle. In 1952, Tosteson and colleagues[151, 152] showed that deoxygenation causes a reversible potassium loss and sodium gain in SS cells. Since then, the abnormal water and cation movements across the sickle cell membrane have been shown to be associated with a variety of pumps, channels, and leaks, involving water, potassium (K^+), sodium (Na^+), chloride (Cl^-), calcium (Ca^{2+}), and magnesium (Mg^{2+}) (for a comprehensive review, consult Brugnara[153]). Although the pathogenesis of these pathways remains incompletely understood, they are undoubtedly related to the physical distortion associated with sickling,[154–161] young cell age,[162–165] oxidant damage,[166–170] and the hemoglobin mutation itself.[171–175] The two best characterized dehydrating pathways are the K^+,Cl^--cotransport pathway, and the Gardos channel (see Fig. 20–1). K^+,Cl^- cotransport is stimulated to lose K^+,Cl^- and water when (predominantly young) sickle cells are exposed to a low pH environment, as might occur in areas of poor perfusion.[176] Specific blockade of this channel would be predicted to have beneficial clinical effects; and a search for such an agent is ongoing. Specific blockade of the Gardos channel—the pore that allows K^+ and water loss when stimulated by Ca^{2+}—would also be predicted to have beneficial effects. Clotrimazole, an imidazole antimycotic agent, is a potent inhibitor of this channel and is effective in preventing sickle red cell dehydration *in vitro*,[177] in the SAD mouse model for sickle cell disease *in vivo*,[178] and in a short-term study in patients with sickle cell disease.[179] Clinical studies of this potentially important antisickling agent are underway.

The Membrane and the Outside Surface

Membrane Deformability and Cytoskeletal Defects. There is no doubt that as sickle cells become deoxygenated and fill with polymerized hemoglobin they become less deformable.[180–183] However, even fully oxygenated cells have abnormal rheologic properties.[184] Using the ektacytometer, Clark and colleagues studied the deformability of SS red cells and showed that decreased deformability was directly related to increased MCHC and correcting the elevated MCHC restored normal deformability.[185] Platt, using a high shear/hemolysis assay, also noted a normalization when MCHC was corrected, except in the most dense fraction, where normalization was incomplete.[186] This incomplete normalization suggests the contribution of a membrane lesion. Membrane mechanical properties were measured with micropipette techniques in two studies.[187, 188] In both, it was found that MCHC is the major contributor to cell rigidity but that irreversible membrane changes accompany dehydration and result in increased membrane rigidity.

The clinical significance of membrane rigidity is not immediately obvious but is further evidence that a structural membrane lesion is present. The finding that the cytoskeleton of ISC was permanently distorted led several investigators to analyze the various components. Abnormal ISC skeletal dissociation properties led to the observation that in sickle erythrocytes β actin appears to have abnormally inaccessible cysteine residues, either because of crosslinking or other posttranslational modification.[189] Maintaining the abnormal ISC shape probably requires that the cytoskeleton rearrange during a period of prolonged deformation under conditions that allow spectrin tetramers to dissociate into dimers and re-form with new spectrin partners.[190] The proteins involved in linking the cytoskeleton to the overlying membrane are also abnormal in behavior. Protein 3 and glycophorin are clustered, with abnormal rotational and lateral mobility—especially in the most dehydrated cells (see Fig. 20–1).[191] This disordered mobility may relate to decreased binding of normal ankyrin to sickle protein 3[192] or to binding of normal spectrin to sickle ankyrin.[193]

Lipid Orientation. Although membrane lipid content and composition are relatively normal in SS red cells,[194–196] the organization of these lipids is quite unusual. Normally, the phospholipids of the red cell membrane are partitioned with amino phospholipids (phosphatidyl serine [PS], and phosphatidyl ethanolamine [PE]), sequestered on the inner (cytoplasmic) surface, and sphingomyelin and phosphatidyl choline (PC) exposed on the outer surface. This asymmetry is not unique to the red cell and probably reflects a general structural pattern that keeps the amino phospholipids from activating soluble coagulation factors. This asymmetry is maintained by the interaction of the spectrin[197] with the phospholipids and by a specific adenosine triphosphate (ATP)-dependent translocation process.[198] In RSCs, PS and PE flip back and forth from the inner leaflet to the outer leaflet during oxygenation and deoxygenation. Although early studies suggested that PS was permanently stuck to the outer leaflet in deoxygenated sickle cells,[199, 200] later studies suggest that only small amounts of PS accumulate on the outer surface of sickle cells where the lipid bilayer is uncoupled from the cytoskeleton and when the cell is ATP depleted.[201, 202] Exposure of PS or PE on the outer surface during sickling could accelerate blood coagulation or might alter the adhesiveness of red cells to other membranes.[203, 204] Alteration of the fatty acyl groups in PC results in changes in cell shape and deformability in SS cells, suggesting that the species composition of PC can affect membrane permeability and cellular deformability.[205]

Increased Adhesion to Endothelium. Over 15 years ago, investigators first discovered that sickle erythrocytes have an abnormal propensity to stick to vascular endothelial cells.[206, 207] This observation has taken on increased importance in conceptualizing the pathophysiology of sickle cell disease and has become a major research focus (for a comprehensive review, consult Hebbel and Mohandas[208]). As cells flow through vessels of critical dimension, an increased tendency to linger at the endothelial surface will increase the odds that polymerization and obstruction will occur (Fig. 20–8). Support for this hypothesis comes from studies that suggest a correlation between adhesiveness and clinical severity.[209–211] Adhesive interactions are complex and undoubtedly involve a variety of ligands, receptors, and nonspecific interactions that vary de-

pending on the age and density of the red cell, the type and health of endothelium, the amount of flow, and the composition of the plasma.

Young, light reticulocytes are particularly adherent, at least in part because they retain a variety of surface molecules such as VLA-4[212–214] and fibronectin receptor[215] that are characteristic of red cell precursors. As reticulocytes mature and shed these primitive receptors, they lose the ability to bind to ligands such as vascular cell adhesion molecule-1 (VCAM-1) and fibronectin that are either on or bridge endothelial cells. Older and denser sickle erythrocytes also adhere to endothelium,[216, 217] a difference that is highly dependent on experimental conditions. Cells of varying age and density[218] play different roles as they traverse different endothelial beds at different shear rates, oxygen tensions, and plasma compositions. Under some conditions, deoxygenation-induced erythrocyte-erythrocyte interactions may matter.[219]

Endothelial cells differ as to their repertoire of surface molecules—for example, CD36 is expressed on

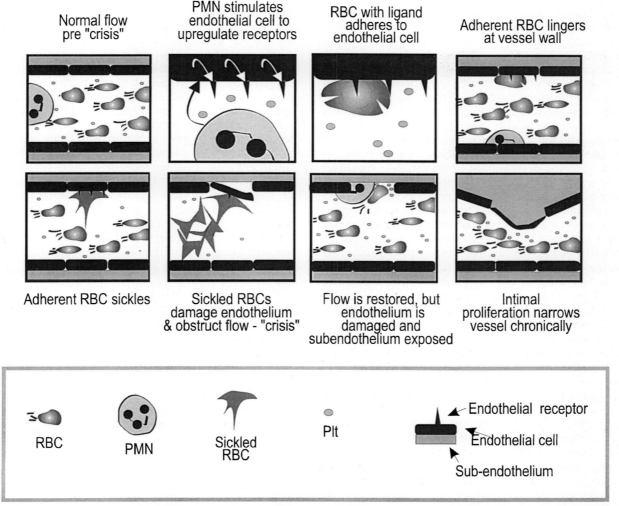

Figure 20–8. Pathophysiology of vessel damage in sickle cell disease. RBCs = red blood cells; PMN = polymorphonuclear neutrophil leukocyte; PIT = platelet. (Adapted from Platt OS: Easing the suffering caused by sickle cell disease. N Engl J Med 1994; 330:783. Adapted, by permission, from *The New England Journal of Medicine*.)

microvascular but not large-vessel endothelium.[220] Endothelial cells also express differing amounts of surface molecules and become more or less adherent depending on environmental stimuli. Cytokines such as interleukin-18 and tumor necrosis factor[221] promote endothelial adherence, largely because of up-regulated VCAM-1 expression. Infected endothelial cells become adhesive by a variety of mechanisms. Herpesvirus-infected cells attract sickle red cells because of increased Fc receptor expression.[222] Endothelial cells exposed to Sendai viral double-stranded RNA become adhesive through up-regulated VCAM-1.[223]

Although over the years, an inconsistent profile of coagulation abnormalities has been described, particularly during crises, a growing body of evidence suggests that procoagulant and anticoagulant proteins and platelets play an important role in sickle vascular disease (reviewed by Francis and Hebbel[224]). This concept is particularly relevant to interactions at the endothelial surface, where von Willebrand factor,[225–229] platelets,[230] and thrombospondin[231, 232] increase adhesiveness.

Mechanism of Membrane Damage

Any pathophysiologically relevant damage to the SS red cell membrane must relate to the Hb S concentrated on its inside surface. Even in normal cells, Hb A has been shown to bind to membranes,[233, 234] at or near the cytoplasmic portion of band 3 protein,[235–239] and with relatively low affinity to PS.[240] Hemoglobin at physiologic concentrations stabilizes the configuration of spectrin heterodimers.[241] Hb S and β^s globin bind to membranes more readily than Hb A.[242–246] Evans and Mohandas demonstrated, using single cell micropipette techniques, that membrane-associated sickle hemoglobin was a major determinant of erythrocyte rigidity.[247] In these experiments, normal deformability was found when normal hemoglobin was reconstituted in sickle or normal membrane ghosts but abnormal deformability was associated with reconstitution of sickle or normal red cell membranes with sickle hemoglobin. Deformability of ISC membranes also improved after the exchange of normal for sickle hemoglobin, although this process was not able to normalize the membrane physical properties. In one study, membrane rigidity was associated with the presence of a small amount of high-molecular-weight spectrin-hemoglobin complex in the membrane.[248]

Sickle hemoglobin is inherently unstable[249, 250] and has an increased tendency to denature and form small aggregates—"micro-Heinz bodies" (see Fig. 20–1). These attach with high affinity to the cytoplasmic portion of band 3 protein at or near the hemoglobin A binding site.[251] This binding on the inside surface of the membrane is translated into changes on the outside surface, because both band 3 protein and glycophorin (the major bearers of the cell's antigens and charge) are found to be clustered above the micro-Heinz bodies.[252] The clustering of band 3 protein is associated with the deposition of specific anti-band 3 protein antibodies on the cell,[251, 253, 254] a process linked to normal cell senescence[255, 256] and perhaps contributing to the short

life span of SS cells.[257] Ankyrin is also abnormally clustered around the denatured Hb S, and, like band 3 protein, may be damaged in the process.[252]

Sickle hemoglobin has an increased tendency to auto-oxidize and form methemoglobin, thereby generating superoxide and losing heme.[258] In fact, sickle cells generate twice the normal amounts of the potent oxidants superoxide, peroxide, and hydroxyl radical.[259] Hebbel discusses the several convincing lines of evidence that suggest that oxidation is a major contributor to the membrane abnormalities of sickle cells.[260] The increased amounts of membrane-associated hemoglobin, heme, and hemichrome[261–265] and the increased nonheme iron[265] may target different vulnerable membrane components.[266–270]

APPROACHES TO ANTISICKLING THERAPY

Replacement of the Defective Gene. The most direct approach to reduction of Hb S polymer is to replace the defective β globin gene with a normal gene. Bone marrow transplants from sickle trait or normal siblings have been successful in a variety of transplant centers around the world.[271–274a] After preparation with various combinations of cyclophosphamide, busulfan, and antithymocyte globulin, and prophylactic treatment for graft-versus-host disease with regimens including cyclosporin A, methotrexate, or prednisone, more than 40 patients have received bone marrow transplants, and a majority have done well. The major transplant complications have included central nervous system (CNS) hemorrhage (particularly in patients with history of stroke),[275] graft rejection, and acute and chronic graft-versus-host disease. Prophylactic anticonvulsant treatment and maintenance of a high platelet count may result in reduced CNS morbidity. The restoration of splenic function in successful transplant recipients holds out the hope that other chronic organ dysfunction may improve with this approach.[276, 277] Selecting patients for this high-risk therapy is particularly problematic because of the unpredictability of clinical course, the paucity of sibling matches,[278] and parental concern.[279]

Stimulation of Hb F Production. As seen in the section on the interactions of Hb S with Hb F, increasing the amount of Hb F will increase the delay time and solubility of Hb S. In sickle cell disease, both 5-azacytidine[280–283] and hydroxyurea[284–288] have been used successfully to increase Hb F in SS individuals. Recombinant human erythropoietin in supraphysiologic doses has also transiently increased Hb F in adult sickle cell patients.[289] Recombinant EPO with hydroxyurea has inconsistently increased Hb F above levels obtained with hydroxyurea alone.[290, 291] Butyric acid analogues also increase fetal hemoglobin production in sickle cell patients, some thalassemia patients, and normal individuals.[292–295a] Charache and colleagues demonstrated that daily hydroxyurea treatment of adult sickle cell patients increased Hb F levels from pretreatment mean levels of 4% to 16% without clinically significant bone marrow toxicity.[286] In addition to increasing Hb F, hydroxyurea has been noted to reduce the proportion of dense cells and increase the mean corpuscular volume (MCV) and mean corpuscular hemoglobin (MCH) of sickle cells.[282-286] On the basis of epidemiologic data that increases in Hb F from 4% to 16% could decrease vaso-occlusive crises by 50%,[296] a multicultured double-blind prospective clinical trial of daily hydroxyurea treatment of SS adults was undertaken.[297] This trial was terminated early when it was obvious that vaso-occlusive crisis, chest syndromes, and transfusions were reduced by almost 50% in the hydroxyurea-treated group compared with controls.[297] Although data analysis from this trial is incomplete, it is clear that reduction in vaso-occlusion begins within 3 months of starting hydroxyurea therapy and persists over the 18 months of follow-up. Preliminary trials in children have begun,[298] but concerns about potential leukemogenesis, teratogenesis, and effects on growth and development preclude immediate use of hydroxyurea in children with SS disease. Patients with SS disease on hydroxyurea with elevations of Hb F have had chest syndromes and strokes,[297, 299] indicating that elevations of Hb F cannot reverse pre-existing organ damage.

Decreased Cell Hb S Concentration. Because the polymerization of Hb S is exquisitely concentration dependent, reduction of the MCHC by swelling the cell with water has been considered as a therapeutic maneuver. Two approaches have been tried: lowering plasma osmolarity and increasing intracellular cations. The first approach was used by Rosa and colleagues,[300] who successfully reduced the duration and frequency of painful crises by lowering the MCHC using dietary salt restriction and desmopressin. Subsequently, others have found this therapy too difficult to maintain, neurologically toxic, and ineffective.[301-303] The second approach has been used primarily *in vitro* and has focused on the property of various membrane-active agents to increase intracellular cations. Some of the interesting agents include the antibiotics monensin[304] and gramicidin[305]; calcium channel blockers nitrendipine, nifedipine, and verapamil[306]; and the peripheral vasodilator cetiedil.[307] As discussed previously, preliminary evidence suggests that blocking the Gardos channel with oral clotrimazole may decrease Hb S concentrations by preventing dehydration.[179]

Increased Hb S Solubility. The most straightforward approach to preventing the polymerization of Hb S is to attack the β6 valine—the key to fiber formation. Unfortunately, this is an extremely unreactive residue, so that efforts to increase the solubility of Hb S have hinged on the importance of the other intermolecular contacts. Reagents that increase deoxy Hb S solubility by noncovalent interactions with Hb S have been recognized. Chang and colleagues[305] have compared the effects of 15 antisickling agents on Hb S solubility, oxygen affinity, and cell sickling. Urea is an effective agent but requires concentrations greater than 200 μM, too high for *in vivo* use. The best studied covalent modifier is cyanate, but clinical trials have not been promising. Unfortunately, despite the encouraging clinical and *in vitro* data, this compound is not usable because of significant neurotoxicity[308] and cataract formation.[309] A major problem with covalent reagents is that they interact with a wide variety of functional groups found in many molecules other than hemoglobin.

Decreased Dwell Time of Cells in Narrow Vessels. Any manipulation that would allow a cell to traverse a vessel faster than its delay time will prevent occlusion of that vessel. Therapy aimed at reducing endothelial adherence may include altering the outer membrane lipids, surface charges, plasma proteins, platelets, white blood cells, or oxidants. An entirely different approach is suggested by the work of Rodgers and co-workers,[310] who showed that microcirculatory flow in patients with sickle cell disease has an unusual periodic pattern, indicating that it may be under vasomotor control and therefore possibly amenable to pharmacologic intervention.

DIAGNOSIS

The Fetus. The ability to perform prenatal diagnosis for sickle cell anemia has progressed rapidly in the past two decades. In 1978, Kan and Dozy described DNA polymorphisms around the β globin gene, which were in linkage disequilibrium with the β-S gene, thereby leading to the first DNA-based method for prenatal diagnosis.[311] Later direct detection of the mutation became possible since the A→T substitution in codon 6 responsible for the glutamic acid–valine change in β globin altered the recognition site of a restriction enzyme.[312-314] Wallace and co-workers showed that specific synthetic oligonucleotides could be used to recognize homologous sequences,[315] leading others to develop radioactive and nonradioactive probes that specifically bind to either the normal β globin gene or to the mutant sickle gene.[316-319] With the advent of polymerase chain reaction amplification of specific DNA sequences, sufficient DNA can be obtained from a very small number of fetal cells, thereby eliminating the necessity for culture of fetal fibroblasts.[320, 321] Chorionic villous biopsy offers an alternative to amniocentesis for obtaining fetal cells as early as 8 to 10 weeks' gestation.[322, 323]

The Newborn. The newborn with sickle cell anemia is generally not anemic and is asymptomatic because of the protective effect of fetal hemoglobin. The "sickle prep" and solubility tests are unreliable during the first few months of life. Mortality due to bacterial sepsis or sequestration crisis is increased in infants with sickle cell anemia after 2 to 3 months of age. Because recognition of the disease in the newborn can lead to prevention of mortality and morbidity, it is now recommended that all newborns at risk be screened for sickle cell anemia.[324] Screening using starch gel electrophoresis and acid or alkaline electrophoresis was first done on a large scale by Schneider and Gilman and their associates.[325, 326] Screening combined with comprehensive follow-up care was first begun by Pearson in New Haven and Serjeant in Jamaica in the 1970s.[327, 328] Present screening methodologies include acid and alkaline electrophoresis, high-performance liquid chromatography, and isoelectric focusing. These tests can be performed on cord blood or on dried blood specimen blotted on filter paper. Diagnosis can also be performed using polymerase chain reaction amplification of DNA extracted from filter paper.[329] Several studies have confirmed that neonatal diagnosis and follow-up can reduce mortality in infants with sickle cell anemia and be cost-effective.[330–333]

The Older Child. After the first few months of life, as β^s globin production increases and Hb F declines, the clinical syndrome of sickle cell anemia emerges (Table 20–1). Although at 1 week of age the hemoglobin level of SS infants is statistically lower than that of AA infants, the overlap between the two groups is considerable and does not diverge much before the second month of life.[327] Anemia and a reticulocytosis is usually evident by 4 months of age.[327, 334] ISCs are frequently absent from the peripheral blood of young children, and the morphology is typical of that of normal newborns—target cells, fragments, and poikilo-

cytes. By 3 years of age, the typical peripheral blood smear is seen, including ISCs, target cells, spherocytes, fragments, biconcave disks, Howell-Jolly bodies, and nucleated red cells. The amount of Hb F decreases with age, as in normal children, but this occurs much more slowly.[327, 335]

CLINICAL MANIFESTATIONS

The clinical manifestations of sickle cell disease are extremely variable. Some patients are entirely asymptomatic and the disease is detected only during population screening, whereas other patients are constantly plagued by painful episodes. Most patients fall between these extremes and have relatively long asymptomatic periods punctuated by occasional clinical crises. The complex nature of the clinical variability from patient to patient and from time to time in each patient has been prospectively studied on a large scale under

Table 20-1. HEMATOLOGY OF INFANTS WITH SS DISEASE, SC DISEASE, AND S-β$^+$-THALASSEMIA

		Age (mo)										
	Percentile	2-3	4-5	6-8	9-11	12-14	15-17	18-23	24-29	30-35	36-47	48-60
SS Disease												
Hemoglobin level (g/dL)	5	7.0	7.0	7.1	7.2	7.2	7.2	7.1	6.9	6.7	6.4	6.6
	50	9.3	9.2	9.2	9.2	9.1	9.0	8.9	8.6	8.3	8.1	8.3
	95	11.4	11.3	11.4	11.5	11.5	11.5	11.3	11.1	10.9	10.5	10.4
Mean corpuscular volume (fL)	5	72	69	68	67	67	67	67	68	69	71	72
	50	84	81	81	82	82	83	84	85	86	88	90
	95	96	94	94	95	96	96	96	97	97	98	100
Fetal hemoglobin level (%)	5	14.6	12.3	10.8	9.1	7.8	6.7	5.6	4.8	4.5	4.4	3.3
	50	43.5	34.1	29.1	24.3	20.6	17.7	14.8	12.8	12.4	12.4	9.0
	95	68.5	59.0	53.0	47.3	42.7	39.1	35.3	32.5	31.2	29.6	21.9
Reticulocyte count (%)	5	1.0	1.1	1.2	1.3	1.4	1.6	1.9	2.3	2.6	2.7	1.8
	50	4.0	5.1	5.9	6.7	7.4	8.0	8.7	9.3	9.8	10.4	11.8
	95	15.5	17.9	19.4	20.7	21.8	22.5	23.2	23.5	23.6	23.6	25.8
SC Disease												
Hemoglobin level (g/dL)	5	8.0	8.2	8.6	8.9	9.2	9.3	9.5	9.5	9.4	9.3	9.6
	50	9.7	9.8	10.1	10.3	10.5	10.6	10.7	10.8	10.7	10.6	10.6
	95	11.6	11.5	11.7	11.8	12.0	12.0	12.1	12.2	12.2	12.1	11.9
Mean corpuscular volume (fL)	5	68	65	64	64	63	63	63	63	64	66	69
	50	81	78	77	75	74	74	74	74	76	77	77
	95	91	88	86	85	84	84	84	84	86	88	87
Fetal hemoglobin level (%)	5	13.6	2.9	2.9	3.1	3.1	2.9	2.4	1.4	0.5	0.0	2.0
	50	31.6	17.9	14.5	11.6	9.3	7.4	5.5	4.2	3.9	4.4	4.2
	95	54.0	39.1	32.1	25.7	20.9	17.6	14.7	13.8	14.7	15.9	8.3
Reticulocyte count (%)	5	0.8	0.8	0.8	0.7	0.7	0.7	0.7	0.7	0.7	0.7	0.9
	50	2.8	2.8	2.7	2.6	2.5	2.5	2.5	2.6	2.7	2.9	2.8
	95	8.2	8.8	8.9	9.0	8.9	8.7	8.4	8.0	7.9	8.8	13.4
S-β$^+$-Thalassemia												
Hemoglobin level (g/dL)	5	9.2	9.4	9.1	8.5	9.1	9.1	9.9	10.0	9.8	9.3	10.0
	50	10.8	10.9	11.0	10.8	10.6	11.2	10.9	11.0	10.7	10.6	10.8
	95	12.4	12.7	13.5	11.8	14.1	12.0	12.0	13.0	11.3	11.6	11.2
Mean corpuscular volume (fL)	5	70	64	61	61	63	82	63	61	66	64	66
	50	80	73	72	69	72	70	70	70	72	76	68
	95	88	83	84	75	84	73	77	79	76	76	76
Reticulocyte count (%)	5	1.1	0.0	1.1	0.9	0.8	0.9	0.7	1.5	1.2	1.0	3.0
	50	2.6	1.8	2.5	2.5	3.0	2.5	2.4	2.2	3.4	2.2	4.1
	95	8.5	6.4	2.5	4.6	5.9	7.4	5.1	6.2	7.4	7.6	5.7

Data from Brown AK, et al: Reference values and hematologic changes from birth to five years in patients with sickle cell disease. Arch Pediatr Adolesc Med 1994; 148:796.

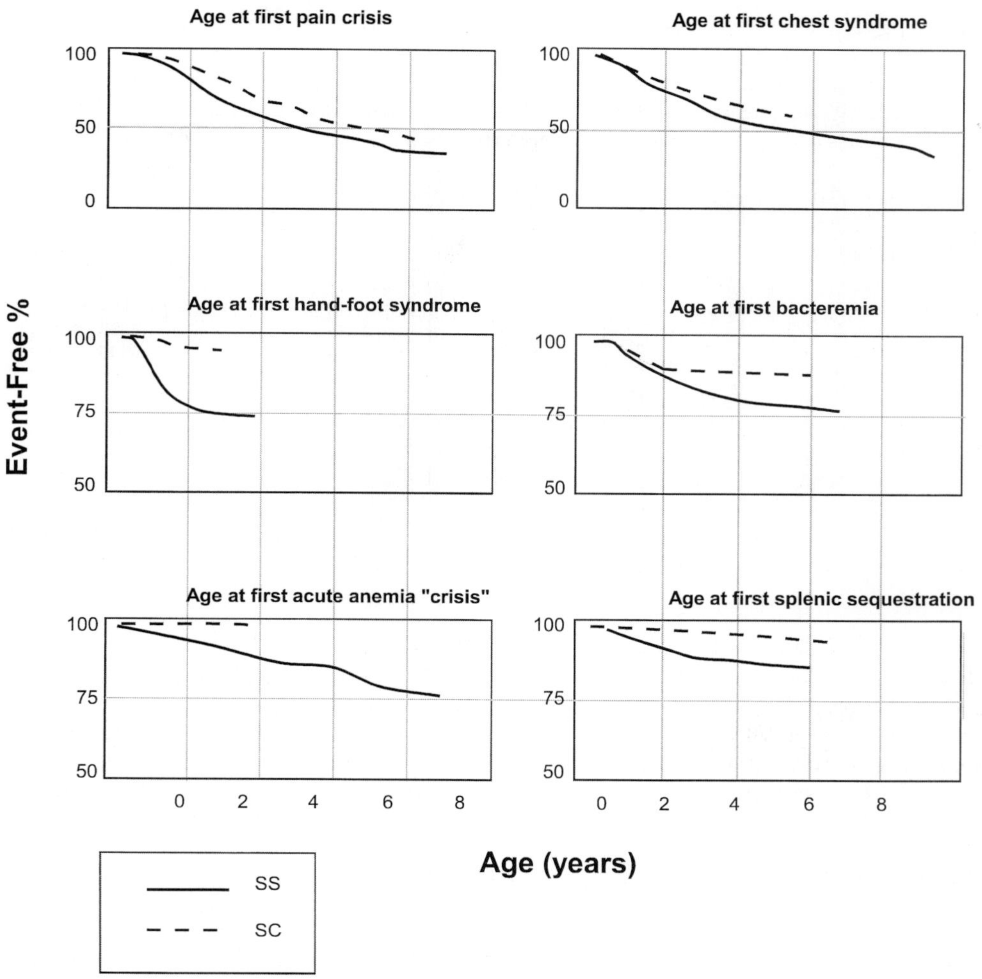

Age at first pain crisis

Age at first chest syndrome

Age at first hand-foot syndrome

Age at first bacteremia

Age at first acute anemia "crisis"

Age at first splenic sequestration

Event-Free %

Age (years)

SS

SC

Figure 20-9. Age at first clinical event in patients with sickle cell disease, from birth to 10 years of age. *A,* Painful event. *B,* Acute chest syndrome. *C,* Hand-foot syndrome (dactylitis). *D,* Bacteremia. *E,* Acute anemic events not including splenic sequestration. *F,* Splenic sequestration. (Adapted from Gill FM, Sleeper LA, Weiner SJ, et al: Clinical events in the first decade in a cohort of infants with sickle cell disease: cooperative study of sickle cell disease. Blood 1995; 86:776–783.)

the auspices of the Sickle Cell Disease Branch of the National Heart, Lung, and Blood Institute.[296, 343]

In the following section the pathophysiology, diagnosis, and management of the acute and chronic complications of sickle cell disease are described. For further general reference on the clinical features of sickle cell disease, the reader is referred to the comprehensive texts by Serjeant[336] and Embury and colleagues.[337] A practical monograph, *Management and Therapy of Sickle Cell Disease*, has been produced under the auspices of the Sickle Cell Disease Branch of the National Heart, Lung, and Blood Institute.[338]

Sickle Cell Crisis

The term *sickle cell crisis* was defined by Diggs[339] as "any new syndrome that develops rapidly in patients with sickle cell disease due to the inherited abnormality." There are three categories of sickle crisis: vaso-occlusive, sequestration, and aplastic, and they are covered individually in the next few sections. The best perspective on how these acute events play out in a typical group of children comes from a report by Gill and colleagues describing the experience of almost 700 infants followed for 10 years as part of the Cooperative

Study of Sickle Cell Disease.[340] The age at first event is displayed in Figure 20–9.

Vaso-occlusive Sickle Crises

Vaso-occlusive crises are acute, often painful episodes due to intravascular sickling and tissue infarction. In a prospective study of children with SS disease followed since birth in Jamaica, painful crisis was the first symptom in more than one fourth of the patients, and the most frequent symptom after the age of 2 years.[341] Painful episodes are such a prominent manifestation of the disease that African tribal names for sickle cell disease are onomatopoeic repetitive descriptions of pain, such as "chwechweechwa" (Ga tribe), "nwiiwii" (Fante tribe), "nucdudui" (Ewe tribe), and "ahotutuo" (Twi tribe). Tribal names translate as "beaten up," "body biting," and "body chewing."[342] Vaso-occlusive episodes are the major clinical manifestations of sickle cell disease and occur most commonly in the bones, lungs, liver, spleen, brain, and penis. Often the differential diagnosis is very difficult because there is no definitive objective hallmark of a vaso-occlusive crisis.

Painful Crisis. The most common acute vaso-occlusive crisis is acute pain. Virtually all patients with SS

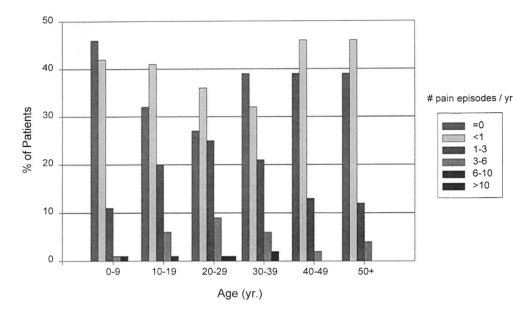

pain episodes / yr

- =0
- <1
- 1-3
- 3-6
- 6-10
- >10

Figure 20-10. Distribution of pain rate among patients with SS disease. (Data from Platt OS, Thorington BD, et al: Pain in sickle cell disease: rates and risk factors. N Engl J Med 1991; 325:11.)

disease experience some degree of acute pain. For many, these episodes are mild and are handled entirely at home, school, or work. Little is known about the extent or nature of pain-coping activities that go on outside the medical environment, but diary studies suggest that it is enormous. The "tip" of the pain "iceberg" is made of those episodes that drive patients to seek medical attention. These episodes vary widely among patients[296] (Fig. 20–10) and represent the most common reason for patients to visit outpatient offices and emergency departments and be admitted for inpatient care. Despite the fact that there is variation in how or why individual patients decide to seek attention for a given episode of pain, epidemiologic evidence strongly indicates that patients with higher rates of medical attention for pain have lower levels of fetal hemoglobin, higher steady-state hemoglobins, and higher mortality.[296, 343] Some studies have suggested that infections,[337] changes in climate,[344, 345] and psychologic factors may precipitate pain episodes, although commonly no precipitating factors can be identified. These patients typically present with rapid onset of deep, gnawing, throbbing pain, usually without any abnormal physical or laboratory findings but sometimes accompanied by local tenderness, erythema, warmth, and swelling. The underlying pathology is bone marrow ischemia, sometimes leading to frank infarction with acute inflammatory infiltrate.[346–348] The most frequently involved areas are the lumbosacral spine, knee, shoulder, elbow, and femur. Less often, the sternum, ribs, clavicles, calcaneus, iliac crest, mandible, zygoma, and mandible are involved.[342] Joint effusions during acute episodes are particularly common in the knees and elbows. Typically, aspiration yields straw-colored fluid, usually with a "noninflammatory" profile. Rarely, sterile purulent exudates are found.[349] Given the range of marrow involvement and inflammatory response, it is not surprising that the patients with the most inflammation mimic the findings of osteomyelitis and those

without findings are at risk of being considered malingerers.

Even in patients with measurable signs of inflammation, the diagnosis of infarction is favored over osteomyelitis. The results of one study suggest that acute long bone infarction is at least 50 times more common than osteomyelitis.[350] In this study of 41 acute long bone infarcts, 38% affected the humerus, 23% affected the tibia, and 19% affected the femur. All patients experienced local tenderness, with swelling in 85%, joint findings in 68%, and local heat in 65%. Fourteen percent appeared "toxic," 21% had a temperature greater than 39°C, and 43% had a temperature less than 38°C. The total white blood cell count ranged between 7200 and 43,000 cells/mm³, with a mean of 17,000 cells/mm³. The mean sedimentation rate was 30.5 mm/h, with a range of 3 to 66 mm/h. Although various radionuclide scans have been suggested as a way of distinguishing between infarction and infection,[351–356] in many studies[350–359] such investigations were inconclusive. Magnetic resonance imaging (MRI) of patients with SS disease shows decreased intensity of short relaxation time/echo time pulse sequence imaging, owing to hyperplastic marrow that converts to high intensity on long relaxation time/echo time images in painful crises,[348] but no definitive series compares infarction with infection. Except for a positive blood or tissue culture, no laboratory test can differentiate acute infection from painful crisis.[347, 360] Needle aspiration and culture of the highly suspicious area is critical in isolating the organism and should be done before initiating empirical antibiotic therapy. The aspirated fluid may be quite purulent even in the patients with sterile infarcts. In most series, the most common organism causing osteomyelitis is *Salmonella*.[361] *Staphylococcus* and *S. pneumoniae* are also common. Initial antibiotic therapy should be chosen to cover these possibilities. Treatment failures are seen when anything but the most aggressive antibiotic regimens are used.

As described earlier, episodes of acute bone pain and impressive signs of inflammation may be difficult to distinguish at outset from osteomyelitis. More common and just as challenging is the evaluation and management of severely painful episodes in patients without signs of inflammation. Some of these patients will show laboratory evidence of acute inflammation such as elevated C-reactive protein,[362] fibrinolysis such as elevated D-dimers,[363, 364] or red cell trapping such as loss of dense cells.[365] These measurements are not helpful in the management of individual cases, nor should they be used as an attempt to "validate" an individual patient's report of symptoms. In a research setting, these measurements done on large numbers of patients with and without symptoms provide clues to potential innovative therapeutic interventions. For example, the common finding of elevated acute phase reactants stimulated a trial of methylprednisolone for treating acute bone pain.[366] This preliminary work showed that a short course of high-dose corticosteroid decreased the duration of severe pain; and a larger-scale trial is underway to confirm the efficacy. Similarly, despite the fact that previous trials of aspirin therapy were not encouraging,[367] a renewed interest in the role of platelets, soluble procoagulants and anticoagulants, and endothelial cells in precipitation or propagation of vaso-occlusion will reopen this potential line of treatment.

In children younger than 5 years of age, the small bones of the hands and feet are frequently affected, and in contrast to most episodes of bone pain in older children, physical findings are common. This painful "hand-foot syndrome" is typically the first clinical manifestation of sickle cell disease. The young child cries with pain, refuses to bear weight, and has puffy, tender, warm feet or hands or both. The child may appear acutely ill, be febrile, and have an impressive leukocytosis, ranging from 20,000 to 60,000 cells/mm³. At the onset of soft tissue swelling, there are usually no bony changes on radiographs. After 1 to 2 weeks, subperiosteal new bone, irregular areas of radiolucency, cortical thinning, or complete destruction of bones can be seen. All the bone changes are usually reversible but may persist for as long as 8 months.[368, 369] A rare complication, permanent shortening of the digits following hand-foot crisis, has been reported.[370]

General supportive care for a patient with an acute painful episode is described later in this chapter.

Acute Chest Syndrome. Episodes of acute chest pain associated with a new infiltrate on chest film are called the "acute chest syndrome." These episodes are second only to acute painful episodes in terms of incidence and need for hospitalization. These episodes are more common in children than adults and, like painful events, are more common in patients with low levels of fetal hemoglobin and high levels of total hemoglobin.[371] Approximately 30% of patients experience at least one episode of acute chest syndrome—and they ultimately have a higher chance of dying at an earlier age.[371] The importance of recognizing and treating these events aggressively is underscored by the observations that it was the leading cause of death among sickle cell patients older than 10 years of age.[372] The extreme vulner-

ability of the patient with acute pulmonary disease reflects the profound effect of hypoxia on sickling. The vagueness of the term *acute chest syndrome* emphasizes that the pulmonary insufficiency, regardless of etiology, is critical. In fact, in most cases, it is difficult to pinpoint a single cause—patients are at high risk for both pneumonia and pulmonary infarction.[373, 374]

Chest pain, infiltrates, effusions, pleural rub, fever, hypoxia, cough, and leukocytosis are features that are common to both infection and infarction.[375, 376] The abnormal radiographic findings typically take several days to appear,[377] and abdominal pain with ileus is frequently the presenting sign in children. Although the incidence of proven bacterial infections in children with acute chest syndrome was thought to be as high as 80% in earlier studies,[373] more recent series suggest that although the incidence of acute chest syndrome is unchanged, bacterial causes may be much rarer.[375-379] Differences may be due to the more widespread use of prophylactic penicillin and bacterial vaccines. The identification of a pathogen is very elusive. Of those confirmed infections, the most common pathogen is pneumococcus, with the others being *Salmonella, Klebsiella, Haemophilus influenzae,* and *Mycoplasma pneumoniae.* In one series, *M. pneumoniae* was the most frequently found infectious agent during the autumn.[375] Pneumonias in patients with SS disease are typically slower to resolve and involve more lobes than the same infection in hematologically normal patients.

A multi-institutional study coordinated by Vichinsky and associates has established pulmonary fat embolization (presumably from the bone marrow) as a prominent cause of acute chest syndrome.[380] In this prospective series of 27 pediatric patients with acute chest syndrome who underwent bronchoscopy, 12 were found to have fat embolus, as determined by the presence of intracellular fat in pulmonary macrophages. The patients with fat emboli were sicker. All had accompanying bone pain in an extremity (compared with 40% of those without fat emboli). Although all 27 patients demonstrated a drop in hemoglobin and platelet count compared with baseline, those with fat embolus had larger drops. The fat emboli patients had more chest pain, more respiratory distress, more lobes involved, more neurologic symptoms, and longer hospitalizations and required more transfusion therapy.

The optimal management of patients with acute chest syndrome requires vigilant monitoring and considered judgment. A few guidelines are presented here, but these should not substitute for consultation and collaboration with a clinician experienced in managing this complex problem.

When to Suspect Acute Chest Syndrome. As described earlier, not all children have chest pain or abnormal chest radiographs at presentation. Even tachypnea is not invariable. Abdominal pain with distention or ileus is a common presentation in children. Extremity pain and rib or sternal pain[381] are also common preludes to full-blown acute chest syndrome. Preliminary evaluation should include a chest radiograph and some measure of oxygenation. The gold standard for assessing oxygenation is the arterial blood gas on room air. In at least one institution, transcutaneous pulse oximetry has been successfully used in the acute setting when patients had been followed formally with serial baseline measurements. In that series, patients with SS disease with acute chest syndrome had O_2 saturation measurements lower than 96% and at least 3 percentage points lower than baseline.[382] Aside from a research setting, however, transcutaneous measurements rarely perform at the 3% confidence level. When the index of suspicion for acute chest syndrome is very low, transcutaneous measurements consistently above 96% on room air can be reassuring. When the suspicion is higher, or the readings are variable or inconsistent, an arterial blood gas measurement is needed. Arterial PO_2 less than 75 mm Hg or a 25% decrease from baseline is highly suggestive of acute chest syndrome. In some hospitals, the careful monitoring of patients suspected of having acute chest syndrome is best accomplished in an intensive care setting.

When to Use Supplemental Oxygenation. Hypoxic patients need supplemental oxygen and usually respond with a rise in arterial PO_2. Liberal use of oxygen in the nonhypoxic child with sickle cell disease can mask the early onset of hypoxia and delay the diagnosis of a chest syndrome. Patients with an increased alveolar-arterial oxygen gradient have a poor prognosis and should have transfusion therapy.[383] Incentive spirometry may prevent progression of pulmonary disease.[384]

How to Manage Analgesics. Because the splinting and atelectasis associated with chest pain may exacerbate or even cause acute chest syndrome, analgesic therapy should not be withheld from patients with chest pain. Guidelines for analgesic usage are described later in this chapter and in the setting of acute chest syndrome should be used with extreme caution. These patients may hover on the brink of hypoventilation from either too little or too much analgesia. Compulsive continuous oxygen saturation monitoring, respiratory rate monitoring, and pain evaluation are critical.

How to Manage Fluids. Fluid overload with congestive failure is easy to achieve in the setting of acute chest syndrome. Once normal hydration is achieved, maintenance fluids should be given.

How to Manage Antibiotics. Empirical coverage for the common pathogens associated with pneumonia typically include a parenteral cephalosporin such as cefuroxime and oral erythromycin.

How to Manage Transfusion. Transfusion therapy is discussed later in this chapter. Patients with acute chest syndrome usually have a hemoglobin level that is 1 to 2 g lower than baseline. This means that they can tolerate a simple transfusion in the case of an episode that is relatively mild—PO_2 >p75 mm Hg, increase to 100 mm Hg with supplemental O_2, one lobe involved, no respiratory distress. With more severe symptoms, or progressing disease, an exchange transfusion is warranted.[385]

Acute Abdominal Pain. Severe acute abdominal pain is a common event that often poses a difficult problem of differential diagnosis. The etiology of this syndrome is unknown, although mesenteric sickling and verte-bral disease with nerve root compression have been suggested. This type of crisis can be accompanied by guarding, tenderness, rebound, fever, and leukocytosis that is indistinguishable from an acute surgical abdomen. Frequently, the patient is the best judge and is aware if the pain is characteristic of a "crisis."

These patients should receive the general supportive measures described later in this chapter, with the omission of high-dose analgesics. Patients should be given nothing by mouth and followed closely by both medical and surgical personnel. Abdominal films, including upright views, may be helpful in identifying a perforated viscus. Usually, the patient with vaso-occlusive pain will remain stable or improve slightly with hydration and mild sedation. In extreme cases, in which the clinical situation is deteriorating, emergency surgical exploration may be necessary. Simple or exchange transfusion should be done if possible before surgery.

Acute right upper quadrant pain with liver enlargement, tenderness, hyperbilirubinemia, and abnormal liver enzyme concentrations may be a result of intrahepatic sickling[386, 387] or acute cholecystitis. Abdominal ultrasonography is an excellent method for detecting the 50% of gallstones that are not radiopaque. Unfortunately, the presence of gallstones and a clinical syndrome characteristic of cholecystitis does not necessarily mean that the symptoms are due to the stones. Many patients and their physicians have been disappointed when their "cholecystitis" returned after cholecystectomy.[388] In a retrospective study of acute abdomen in 28 patients with SS disease,[389] the presence of gallstones evident on ultrasound evaluation did not predict which patients could be managed without surgery. Biliary scans indicated obstruction in 13 patients, of whom 4 improved without surgery. Normal biliary scans were not found in any patient who needed immediate surgery. These patients with acute cholecystitis should be operated on after the gallbladder has had a chance to "cool down." Postoperative management of sickle patients with acute cholecystitis can be fraught with complications.[390] Early experience with laparoscopic cholecystectomy in patients with SS disease appears to be associated with less postoperative complications.

Acute Central Nervous System Event. Acute infarction of the brain can result in a devastating stroke, which occurs in approximately 7% of children with sickle cell disease.[391, 392] The incidence is estimated to be 0.7% per year during the first 20 years of life, with the highest rates in children 5 to 10 years of age.[393] This disaster may occur as an isolated event but also appears in the setting of evolving pneumonia, aplastic crisis, viral illness, painful crisis, priapism, or dehydration.[391-394] The most common underlying lesion is an intracranial arterial stenosis or obstruction, usually in the internal carotid, often in the proximal middle cerebral or anterior cerebral arteries.[394-397] Pathologically, these vessels whose endothelium has presumably been chronically injured by sickle erythrocytes show heaped-up intima with proliferation of fibroblasts and smooth muscle.[398] The lumen may be narrowed or completely obliterated by the vascular lesion, suggesting that *acute* sickling may simply be the "last straw," causing acute infarction in the setting of a chronically damaged vessel. Hemiparesis, speech defects, focal seizures, and gait dysfunction are the most common signs.

A careful discussion of the evaluation of the child with new neurologic symptoms is provided by Adams.[399] He suggests that the best initial diagnostic test is the computed tomographic scan, although it may not be positive for infarction within the first 6 hours of the episode. MRI becomes abnormal in 2 to 4 hours, and this is found in about 90% of patients with stroke.[400] The typical findings are infarcts associated with major vessel obstruction or distal obstruction of smaller vessels leading to infarction in the "border zone" area between the anterior cerebral and middle cerebral vessels.[401, 402] Assessment of the intracranial and cervical artery vasculature can be well visualized using magnetic resonance angiography and is becoming increasingly useful in the early evaluation of the patient with new symptoms.

The standard approach to treating a patient with acute infarction is exchange transfusion (see section on transfusion for details). This approach may limit the amount of acute sickling in poorly perfused areas of the brain and protects the patient from the complications of hypertonic arteriographic dye if such investigation is anticipated. In untreated patients, the mortality rate is approximately 20%, with about 70% of patients experiencing a recurrence within 3 years. In these untreated patients, over 70% were left with permanent motor disabilities and deficit in IQ.[391] Patients treated with exchange transfusion usually show marked improvement in motor function, although the prognosis is considerably worse for those with multiple infarcts. After the initial exchange, a maintenance transfusion program should be carried out (see Transfusion). Prolonged transfusion has a profound influence on the morbidity and mortality of stroke.[394, 396, 404–406] A regular program designed to keep Hb S less than 30% lowers the recurrence rate of stroke to 10%, with only 30% of patients left with residual motor abnormalities and 10% with IQ less than 70. Repeat arteriograms in patients maintained on transfusion generally, but not invariably, show stabilization and smoothing of intimal lesions, whereas untransfused patients demonstrate progression of disease.[394] A study of 12 children with acute strokes revealed a 70% recurrence rate within 5 weeks to 11 months of ending a 1- to 2-year transfusion program.[396] In another follow-up study, recurrences were high even after 5 to 12 years of transfusion in an unusual group of patients with severe encephalomalacia.[407] In one informative series, 15 patients at the Children's Hospital of Philadelphia who had been maintained on a transfusion program that kept the Hb S level less than 30% for 4 years had their regimen liberalized—allowing the pretransfusion Hb S to rise to 50%.[408] With a mean follow-up of 84 months, none had a recurrent infarction. Unfortunately, this program did not prevent hemorrhage—two patients died, one of intraventricular and one of subarachnoid bleeding. Although theoretically beneficial, indefinite maintenance transfusion carries the risks of sensitization, hepatitis, and the acquired immunodeficiency syndrome and the certain problem of iron overload. Bone marrow transplantation, fetal hemoglobin stimulating agents, or antisickling drugs may ultimately prove to be the treatment of choice for patients with stroke.

Application of newer techniques for noninvasive assessment of the brain and its vasculature has focused attention on two new areas—identifying children at high risk for stroke and identifying children with "asymptomatic" brain disease. Adams and his colleagues in Augusta demonstrated that children with abnormal transcranial Doppler measurements had a relative risk of stroke of 44 (95% confidence interval 5.5–346).[409] This observation has stimulated a nationwide collaborative prospective study. The investigators are screening more than 800 children with transcranial Doppler evaluation and randomizing those with an abnormal study to either routine follow-up or prophylactic maintenance transfusion. The results of this study have the potential to alter the routine care of children with sickle cell disease. A systematic study of MRI in asymptomatic children with sickle cell disease has revealed that the finding of unanticipated infarcts is highly predictive of subsequent clinical stroke.[410] These patients may also be appropriate candidates for stroke prevention trials.

Not all acute focal neurologic events in patients with sickle cell anemia are infarcts. Intracranial hemorrhage is the other major category of sickle-related CNS events, although the incidence may be higher in adults than children.[391, 411] These events present as a sudden severe headache, sometimes with neck pain, vertigo, syncope, nystagmus, ptosis, meningismus, or photophobia. Many of these episodes are subarachnoid hemorrhages from small bleeding aneurysms that probably arise from intimal damage during childhood. Multiple aneurysms with extensive collaterals (similar to moyamoya disease) have been found incidentally during angiographic evaluation of children with stroke.[398] Although the mortality in some series approaches 50%,[391] series describe more successful aggressive neurosurgical approaches to these bleeding lesions[403, 404] and suggest that angiography should be done to identify patients with surgically amenable lesions.

Priapism. Priapism is a distressing problem that occurs in males of all ages. The experience in Jamaica[414] suggests that as in many other complications of sickle cell disease, hospital records grossly underestimate the incidence of priapism. In the Jamaican questionnaire study of 104 males aged 10 to 62 years, 42% reported at least one episode of priapism, with a median age at onset of 21 years. Two clinical presentations of acute priapism are seen in children: "stuttering" priapism with multiple short episodes sometimes progresses to "severe prolonged" (>24 hour) episodes. Sexual dysfunction was found in 46% of patients with a history of priapism. In general, however, the young patients with brief episodes are less likely to have involvement of corpora cavernosa *and* spongiosa (tricorporal disease)[415] and to become dysfunctional.[416] Urinary retention requiring catheterization may complicate the acute episode.[417]

Treatment of priapism should include all the basic support measures outlined later in this chapter for the treatment of acute vaso-occlusive episodes, including hydration and analgesia.[417, 418] Extremes of temperatures should be avoided (cold packs increase sickling, and hot packs increase blood flow). If the pain and engorgement persist despite therapy for 24 to 48 hours, transfusion therapy is indicated. Seeler[416] noted marked improvement in priapism with diminution of pain within 24 hours of doubling the hematocrit by transfusion of packed red cells. Automated exchange transfusion has been used to treat several men with priapism. In some patients, marked improvement was noted within hours of the exchange,[419, 420] although some patients also experience acute neurologic complications during the treatment of priapism.[421]

Surgical intervention with procedures ranging from corporal aspiration and irrigation to saphenocorporeal shunts has been advocated.[422–425] The morbidity from these procedures is high, with resultant penile deformities and possible impotence. A different surgical approach involving creation of a temporary fistula between the glans and corpora cavernosa has been successfully used.[426]

Acute Sequestration Crisis

One of the leading causes of death in children with sickle cell anemia is the acute splenic sequestration crisis.[427] Children with SS disease who have not yet undergone autosplenectomy as well as older patients with SC disease or S-β-thalassemia[428] may have sudden, rapid, massive enlargement of the spleen with trapping of a considerable portion of the red cell mass. This complication has been described as early as 8 weeks of age.[429] Emond described the natural history of acute sequestration crisis in a cohort of 308 children with SS disease in Jamaica.[430] Eighty-nine patients experienced 113 attacks, with 67 children having their first attack before the age of 2 years. There were 13 fatalities, 10 of which occurred before the age of 2. The most frequently associated clinical problem was upper respiratory tract infection and acute chest syndrome. Sixteen percent of the patients had positive blood cultures. Recurrences occurred in 49% of survivors of the first attack. A parental education program directed toward teaching parents the technique of spleen palpation and the urgency of seeking medical attention for enlarged spleen and pallor led to an increase in the incidence of cases (from 4.6 to 11.3 per 100 patient-years of observation) and a fatality rate fall (from 29.4 per 100 events to 3.1 per 100 events). Patients suddenly become weak and dyspneic, with rapidly distending abdomen, left-sided abdominal pain, vomiting, and shock. The tempo of this crisis may be so fast that the patient dies before reaching the hospital. On physical examination, there is profound hypotension with cardiac decompensation and massive splenomegaly. The hematocrit is half the patient's usual value, and there is usually a brisk reticulocytosis with increased nucleated red cells and moderate to severe thrombocytopenia.[431] Rao has described a subacute form of sequestration in 11 patients characterized by increased spleen size, 25% drop in hematocrit, less than 100,000 platelets, and reticulocyte count elevation above patient's baseline. All responded to chronic transfusion programs, but 7 patients had recurrent episodes after transfusions were stopped and eventually required splenectomy.[432]

Kinney's review of 23 cases of splenic sequestration from Duke University strengthens the position of those who favor elective splenectomy for children who have had one episode of sequestration.[433] In this series of 23 patients, 4 underwent early splenectomy, 7 were observed carefully, and 12 were placed on a maintenance transfusion program. Of those treated using transfusion, 2 are well and still receiving transfusion, 3 had recurrences while still on transfusion, 4 experienced recurrence within 3 months of the last transfusion, and only 3 remain well at 11 months (3.9 years after the last transfusion). Fourteen percent of children became alloimmunized, and 1 patient developed non-A, non-B hepatitis. Eventually 14 of the 23 patients underwent splenectomy. All were immunized against pneumococcus and were prescribed penicillin for prophylaxis. None has experienced a life-threatening infection 65.6 patient-years later.

Therapy is the emergency restoration of intravascular volume and oxygen-carrying capacity by the immediate transfusion of packed red cells. Once normal cardiovascular status is restored, patients improve rapidly. The spleen usually shrinks within a few days, and the thrombocytopenia resolves. Sequestration may recur, usually within 4 months of the initial episode. In one series,[434] 50% of deaths from splenic sequestration occurred in children with recurrences. To eliminate recurrence, some authors have recommended elective splenectomy after the first episode.[435] However, because of the high incidence of overwhelming sepsis in splenectomized young children, others have suggested splenectomy after two episodes of sequestration.[431] Emergency splenectomy for acute sequestration is not indicated.

Sequestration may also take place in the liver. Liver enlargement and tenderness, with hyperbilirubinemia, increased anemia, and reticulocytosis are the usual clinical features.[386] Because the liver is not as distensible as the spleen, there is rarely pooling of red cells significant enough to cause cardiovascular collapse.

Aplastic Crisis

The clinical characteristics of the aplastic crisis of sickle cell disease have been well characterized.[436–438] In the normal steady state, the patient with sickle cell anemia can compensate for the decreased red cell survival (15 to 50 days) by increasing the bone marrow output sixfold to eightfold. Temporary cessation of bone marrow activity due to suppression by intercurrent viral or bacterial infection causes the hematocrit value to fall as much as 10% to 15% per day with no compensatory reticulocytosis. The short-lived Hb F–poor cells are the first to disappear from the circulation, whereas the high Hb F–containing cells linger.

Table 20-2. BACTEREMIAS AND ASSOCIATED ACUTE EVENTS IN A COHORT OF 694 CHILDREN WITH SICKLE CELL ANEMIA (SS) AND HEMOGLOBIN SC DISEASE FOLLOWED PROSPECTIVELY FROM INFANCY

Organism	Patient	Total No. Cases	Isolated Bacteremia	Acute Chest Syndrome	Meningitis	Bone/Joint
Streptococcus pneumoniae	SS	62	39 (5 dead)	14 (1 dead)	8 (2 dead)	1
	SC	12	9	3	0	0
Haemophilus influenzae	SS	10	6 (2 dead)	3	1	0
	SC	4	2	2	1	0
Staphylococcus aureus	SS	5	2	2	0	1
	SC	1	1	0	0	0
Streptococcus viridans	SS	5	4	1	0	0
	SC	1	1	0	0	0
Escherichia coli	SS	5	3	1	0	1
	SC	2	0	1	0	1
Salmonella species	SS	3	2	0	0	1
	SC	2	1	0	0	1
Other	SS	2	1	1	0	0
	SC	0	0	0	0	0

Data from Gill FM, Sleeper LA, et al: Clinical events in the first decade in a cohort of infants with sickle cell disease. Blood 1995; 86:776.

This natural selection of Hb F–containing cells accounts for the apparent increase in the percentage of Hb F during aplastic episodes.

Spontaneous recovery is usually heralded by a markedly elevated nucleated red blood cell count, followed in 1 or 2 days by a brisk reticulocytosis. This recovery phase, with the characteristic anemia, nucleated red cells, reticulocytosis, and occasional hyperbilirubinemia, is probably responsible for most cases referred to as "hyperhemolytic crisis." Most aplastic episodes are short and mild and require no therapy. Occasionally, a transfusion is necessary if the marrow remains quiescent.

In 1981, Serjeant and colleagues reported an outbreak of aplastic crises that was associated with an epidemic of parvovirus-like agent.[439] Since then, the Jamaican group has documented the epidemiology and follow-up of parvovirus in a cohort of infants identified at birth—308 with sickle cell anemia and 239 controls.[440, 441] They made a number of important observations: (1) the frequency of infection (about 40%) did not differ between sickle and control groups; (2) 20% of infections in the sickle group did *not* result in significant aplasia; (3) 100% of aplastic episodes were associated with parvovirus; (4) no patient had recurrent aplasia; and (5) 45% of infected patients maintained an elevated parvovirus-specific IgG after 5 years. Parvovirus has also been implicated as the etiologic agent in erythema infectiosum (fifth disease).[442, 443] An outbreak of both aplastic crisis and erythema infectiosum occurred in Ohio.[443, 444] All cases of aplastic crises occurred in individuals with hemolytic anemia (25/26 with sickle syndromes), and none of these patients had the classic rash of fifth disease. Since then, the relationship between parvovirus and erythropoiesis has been studied in detail. The virus specifically retards late erythroid precursor differentiation[445] and is responsible for temporary erythroid aplasia in a broad array of hemolytic anemias.[444]

Infections

Infection is the most common cause of death in children with sickle cell anemia.[427, 446] In one study, the risk of acquiring sepsis or meningitis was greater than 15% in children younger than 5 years, with an associated mortality of approximately 30%.[447] In young children, the risk of pneumococcal sepsis appears to be 400 times that of normal children, and *H. influenzae* sepsis appears two to four times as common.[448] In general, the organisms responsible for infection are not unusual pathogens (Table 20–2), but the infections that they cause in such patients are more frequent and severe.

The major risk factor for this increased vulnerability to infection is splenic dysfunction. The spleen normally serves two separate immunologic functions: (1) clearance of particles from the intravascular space and (2) antibody synthesis. Both functions are impaired in sickle cell anemia.

During the first year of life, "functional asplenia," the inability to clear particulate matter from the blood, develops in patients with sickle cell anemia.[449] This is heralded by the appearance of red cells with Howell-Jolly bodies and irregular surface characteristics (pits).[450] When the percent of "pitted" red cells exceeds 3.5%, the spleen is generally nonfunctional.[451] Splenic dysfunction occurs early in life, with 50% of 2068 children with SS disease having greater than 3.5% "pitted" red cells by 2 years of age. Appearance of dysfunction was less rapid and less common in children with Hb SC and S-β-thalassemia. Despite palpable splenomegaly, children with elevated pitted red blood cells have no splenic uptake of technetium-99m (^{99m}Tc) sulfur colloid and are susceptible to the most serious infectious complication of asplenia and pneumococcal sepsis.[452] Repeated infarction results in a nonpalpable, fibrotic, often calcified spleen that may visualize on a ^{99m}Tc-diphosphonate bone scan.[453] Splenic infarction in young children with SS disease appears to be an insidious process—usually without much in the way of symptoms. In older children and adults, however, especially those with SC disease or sickle thalassemia, severe left upper quadrant pain often accompanies infarction. Transfusion[454] and bone marrow transplantation[276] can correct the splenic phagocytic defect; although these treatments are not indicated for splenic dysfunction per se.

Children with functional asplenia fail to respond to intravenously administered antigen,[455] even when the phagocytic function of the spleen has been restored by transfusion. As in other asplenic individuals, however, these children do respond normally to intramuscularly administered antigen, such as pneumococcal vaccine.[456, 457]

Levels of serum immunoglobulins are normal or increased in children with sickle cell anemia.[457–459] However, the serum is deficient in heat-labile opsonizing activity[460] related to an abnormality of the properdin pathway,[461, 462] which is specific for the phagocytosis of pneumococci. There is an increased activation of complement via the alternate pathway[463] and no intrinsic defect in the complement system.[464] Opsonic activity can be reconstituted *in vitro* by addition of only the F(ab')$_2$ fragments of capsular antibodies to *S. pneumoniae*.[465] This abnormal opsonic activity and associated functional asplenia may partially explain the propensity for pneumococcal infections.

Boggs and co-workers[466] have demonstrated that the chronic leukocytosis of sickle cell disease is a reflection of a shift of granulocytes from the marginating to the circulating pool, with a high granulocyte turnover rate. Neutrophil chemotaxis is normal to slightly reduced; and no specific neutrophil abnormality has been found in patients with SS disease.[467–469] Epidemiologic studies have shown a positive correlation between chronic leukocytosis and increased crises rates,[296] early mortality,[343] and frequent chest syndromes.[371]

Treatment. Because of the increased incidence of serious bacterial infections in patients with sickle cell anemia, the index of suspicion for infection should always be high. In general, the higher the temperature[470] and leukocyte count and sedimentation rate,[471] the higher the probability of a serious bacterial infection. Unfortunately, however, the wide variability in the temperature and laboratory values of bacteremic children does not permit an accurate prediction of whether an individual febrile child is bacteremic. The following are guidelines for empirical evaluation and treatment of the febrile child younger than age 12 years:

- Perform complete blood cell count, urinalysis, chest radiography, and cultures of blood, urine, and throat.
- "Toxic" children, or those with temperature over 39.9°C, should be treated with parenteral antibiotics promptly, before radiographs are taken or the results of laboratory tests are available. These children should be admitted to the hospital.
- Lumbar puncture should be performed on "toxic" children and those with any signs of meningitis.
- Nontoxic children with temperatures below 40°C, but with infiltrate on chest radiograph, or with a white blood cell count over 30,000/mm^3 or below 500/mm^3, should be treated parenterally and admitted to the hospital.
- Nontoxic children with temperatures below 40°C, normal chest radiograph, normal leukocyte count,

and reliable parents can be treated with a long-acting antibiotic (e.g., ceftriaxone, 50 mg/kg, parenterally) observed over a period of hours, and be discharged home for follow-up evaluation and repeated antibiotic dosing the next day.[472] Outpatient prophylaxis with long-acting cephalosporins, however, must be re-evaluated with the emergence of penicillin- and cephalosporin-resistant *S. pneumoniae*.

- Antibiotics should be selected based on their ability to kill both pneumococcus and *H. influenzae* and to penetrate the CNS. In areas where β-lactamase–producing *H. influenzae* or penicillin- and cephalosporin-resistant pneumococci are regularly encountered, these issues should be factored into the choice of drug.
- If children do well, and culture results remain negative after 48 to 72 hours, antibiotics can be discontinued.
- Documented sepsis should be treated parenterally for a minimum of 1 week.
- Bacterial meningitis should be treated for a minimum of 10 days parenterally or for at least 1 week after the cerebrospinal fluid has been sterilized.

Patients with infiltrate on the chest radiograph should have cultures of sputum, blood, and stool and be treated as described for acute chest syndrome. Because of the overwhelming incidence of pneumococcal pneumonia, patients should be treated with an appropriate antipneumococcal agent. *M. pneumoniae* infection may present as a lobar infiltrate,[473] and the presence of a positive cold agglutinin, albeit nonspecific,[474] should be an indication for erythromycin. A stool culture positive for *Salmonella* may be the only evidence for a *Salmonella* pneumonia. In most cases, no bacterial confirmation will be available, and the patient should receive at least a 1-week course of antibiotics to cover for pneumococcal and *H. influenzae* infection.

Patients with clinical findings that are highly suggestive of osteomyelitis should have needle aspirate and culture of the lesion. After obtaining cultures, children who appear acutely ill should be started on antibiotics. Antibiotic choice should include agents effective against *Salmonella* and *Staphylococcus aureus*. Antibiotics should be discontinued or modified when culture reports are available.

Prevention. Attempts at preventing pneumococcal disease in patients with sickle cell anemia have focused on prophylactic antibiotics and vaccines. Prophylactic penicillin was first shown to be effective in the prevention of pneumococcal disease by John and associates,[475] who used monthly intramuscular injections of long-acting penicillin. However, if penicillin prophylaxis was terminated after 3 years of age, an increase in pneumococcal infections was noted in the children previously on penicillin. Gaston and co-workers, in a blinded placebo-controlled clinical trial in the United States, showed that 84% of the pneumococcal infections in children younger than the age of 5 years could be prevented with oral penicillin (125 mg bid).[476] As a result of this landmark study, aggressive newborn screening programs have been organized throughout the United States, so that all children with sickle cell anemia can be identified and started on penicillin prophylaxis by 8 weeks of age.[477] Our approach to prophylaxis is as follows:

- Give prophylaxis to all newborns with SS, S-β°–thalassemia, and SC disease. (Some practitioners prefer not to treat infants with SC disease because their splenic dysfunction typically appears later in life.)
- Start as early as possible—optimally by 8 weeks of age.
- Prescribe penicillin, 125 mg orally, twice a day until age 3. At age 3, increase the dose to 250 mg orally, twice a day. A study is underway to determine the optimal time to discontinue prophylaxis. Many practitioners stop at 5 to 6 years of age, with penicillin kept readily available at home, school, daycare, while traveling, and so on, for prompt administration for fever.
- Prescribe erythromycin ethyl succinate, 10 mg/kg orally, twice a day for patients allergic to penicillin.
- Educate families as to the importance of compliance and the early recognition of signs of infection.

In older children (> 4 years old) and adults with sickle cell disease, polyvalent pneumococcal vaccine has been shown to be effective in eliciting a normal antibody response, increases in pneumococcal opsonizing activity, and reducing the incidence of pneumococcal disease.[478, 479] A 24-valent pneumococcal vaccine is commercially available and should be given to patients with sickle cell anemia at 2 years of age. This vaccine represents 90% of the common serotypes of pathogenic pneumococci. Children younger than 2 years of age respond relatively poorly in general to this vaccine[480]; and 2-year-old children respond poorly to two common pneumococcal serotypes, 6A and 19.[481] Revaccination after 4 years improved protective levels of antibody without serious adverse reactions in children.[482] *H. influenzae* vaccine is immunogenic in children with sickle cell disease and should be given on the same schedule used for normal infants.[483, 484]

Although prophylactic penicillin and new vaccines are clearly effective in preventing some overwhelming infections, several children have been documented to have fatal pneumococcal sepsis who were vaccinated and who had been prescribed oral penicillin.[485] The emergence of penicillin-resistant pneumococcus in normal and sickle cell patients will undoubtedly further complicate management of infections in SS children. These examples underscore the need for physicians to emphasize the need for compliance and to continue to have a high index of suspicion of sepsis in the febrile child with sickle cell disease.

Chronic Organ Damage

Cardiovascular System. Abnormal cardiac findings are present in most patients with sickle cell anemia[486–489] and are primarily the result of chronic anemia and the compensatory increased cardiac output.[490] On physical examination, the most common findings are systolic ejection murmur, S_3, split S_1, suprasternal notch thrill, and diastolic murmur.[487] Cardiac findings may closely resemble the findings in rheumatic valvular disease or congenital cardiac anomalies. Frequently, echocardiography is necessary to diagnose abnormal cardiac structure. Cardiomegaly is found in most patients, with electrocardiographic findings of left ventricular hypertrophy in about 50% of patients.[488]

In view of the fact that the hallmark of sickle cell disease is vaso-occlusion, it is remarkable that myocardial infarction is an extremely rare event.[488, 491] In one review of the postmortem literature in sickle cell disease including examination of 153 hearts, only four infarcts were reported.[491] Despite the high oxygen extraction in the coronary circulation, blood in the coronary sinus contains no more sickled forms than does blood in the general circulation,[492] presumably because of the short transit time through the coronary vessels.[490] Atherosclerosis is virtually absent in this population, seen in one study in none of the 100 hearts of patients (55 of whom were 16 to 47 years old, with a median age of 30) examined at autopsy.[491] This is in marked contrast to the Vietnam study,[493] in which atherosclerosis was found in 45% of 105 battle casualties. When injected at autopsy, the sickle cell heart has normal patent coronary arteries, frequently of larger caliber than seen in normal hearts.[494] The cause of this apparent protective effect on atherosclerosis is unknown but may involve genetic or dietary factors or anemia itself.

Although straightforward myocardial infarction is not generally seen,[491] it is not clear whether a more subtle myocardial injury leading to myocardial dysfunction ("sickle myocardiography") is a regular finding.[495] Several studies have documented that the vast majority of patients have normal left ventricular function, as measured at rest by a variety of noninvasive techniques.[496–499] However, several other reports of careful studies of a population of patients in Augusta, Georgia, reported that one third of children demonstrated decreased left ventricular contractility,[500] that 15% developed ischemic electrocardiographic response to exercise,[501] and that those with ischemic responses had abnormal ejection fraction response to exercise.[502] In another study, systemic vascular resistance (afterload) was significantly lower and end-diastolic volume (preload) was significantly higher in sickle cell anemia.[503] The authors point out that these abnormal loading conditions, common compensatory mechanisms in chronic anemia, may mask left ventricular dysfunction as measured by ejection fraction. As the loading conditions were manipulated, left ventricular dysfunction was demonstrated as a decreased end-systolic stress/end-systolic volume index ratio.[503] A comparative study of sickle cell patients and young patients with chronic aortic regurgitation suggests that in sickle cell disease, resting left ventricular function is well preserved, as in other chronic high-output states.[504] The authors emphasize that hypertension, although rare in sickle cell disease,[505] has extremely deleterious effects on left ventricular function. Although it is uncertain how prevalent or important mild left ventricular dysfunction is under normal circumstances, with the stress of volume overload, hypoxemia, hyperthermia, tachycardia, or hypertension, a well-compensated patient can rapidly develop cardiac failure. Elevation of the hematocrit with transfusion can, however, increase exercise capacity and decrease resting heart rate.[506]

Right ventricular dysfunction has been demonstrated by thallium scanning[498] and is thought to be related to chronic volume overload. Pulmonary hypertension and cor pulmonale can be seen in older patients and may be related to a previous history of repeated chest syndromes.[507, 508]

Arrhythmias are rare under usual conditions, although in one study, during the first hour of treatment for painful crisis, 80% of patients had arrhythmias: 67% atrial and 60% ventricular. These were not clinically significant and probably represented response to pain.[509]

Renal System. Hyposthenuria, hematuria, nephrotic syndrome, and uremia are the major renal complications of sickle cell disease.[510] In addition, the production of erythropoietin in response to anemia may be lower in older patients with SS disease, possibly due to primary renal disease.[511]

Hyposthenuria[512, 513] develops early in childhood and, as is the case with functional asplenia, may be temporarily reversed with transfusion.[514, 515] The hypertonic environment of renal medulla promotes sickling even at normal PO_2,[516] which leads to decreased medullary blood flow and derangement of the countercurrent multiplier. Abnormality of the countercurrent multiplier may be the mechanism for hyposthenuria, or, as suggested by Buckalew and Someren,[510] this may be due to decreased flow to nephrons, with long loops of Henle, and preservation of flow to nephrons with short loops. The obligatory water loss results in a tendency toward dehydration and invalidates the use of urine volume or concentration as an indicator of the patient's state of hydration. Nocturia and enuresis are common complaints of these patients, who excrete large volumes of dilute urine.[517] Urinary sodium losses may be high and result in significant hyponatremia.[518] A renal tubular acidification defect,[519, 520] as well as hyporeninemic hypoaldosteronism[521] and impaired potassium excretion,[522] have been identified. In one review, deJong and Van Eps have emphasized that renal vasodilating prostaglandins are increased in sickle cell patients, leading to a compensatory increase in renal blood flow, glomerular filtration rate, and proximal tubular activity.[523]

Although hematuria is usually mild, bleeding is occasionally severe enough to cause significant blood loss.[524, 525] Papillary necrosis is usually the underlying anatomic defect.[526] Epsilon-aminocaproic acid has been suggested to stop severe hematuria that is refractory to transfusion,[527] but this must be used cautiously because of the risk of ureteral or pelvic clotting and obstruction. In patients with long-standing hematuria, supplemental iron may be necessary to prevent iron deficiency.

Uremia is a rare complication in children with sickle cell disease that may follow a symptom-complex of nephrotic syndrome[528] with glomerulonephritis. The nature of the glomerular lesion is unknown and may represent response to iron deposition,[529] antigen–antibody complex,[530] or mesangial phagocytosis of fragmented sickled cells.[531, 532] A study of 381 adults with sickle cell disease demonstrated that 7% had elevated serum creatinine levels and 26% had proteinuria.[533] Ten patients with proteinuria underwent renal biopsy, and the glomerular lesions showed perihilar focal segmental sclerosis and glomerular enlargement similar to findings in an animal model with glomerular hypertension and efferent arteriolar vasoconstriction. To test the animal analogy, these patients were treated with enalapril, an angiotensin-converting enzyme inhibitor that had been shown to decrease efferent arteriolar constriction. In all treated patients, the level of proteinuria fell during treatment and returned toward abnormal after discontinuation. Work is underway to determine whether early and chronic treatment of patients with proteinuria with enalapril can prevent the evolution to renal failure. Bakir and associates estimate that 4% of adult SS patients develop nephrosis and that two thirds of these patients go on to develop renal failure.[532] Renal failure can be managed with peritoneal dialysis, hemodialysis, and transplantation.[534, 535]

Hepatobiliary System. Liver and biliary tract abnormalities are common in sickle cell disease[536–538] and are the result of cholelithiasis, hepatic infarction, and transfusion-related hepatitis.

Bilirubin stones are common.[539, 540] Two large series have studied the incidence of gallstones as detected by ultrasound in children with SS disease.[541, 542] The percentage of gallstones in 226 patients aged 5 to 13 selected randomly from a group of children with SS disease identified at birth was 13%,[536] a value lower than that found in a survey of clinic patients studied by Sarnaik and associates.[541] In this report, the incidence of gallstones was 12% by 2 to 4 years of age.[541] With advancing age, the incidence increased gradually, reaching 42% in the 15- to 18-year-old age group. Fourteen of the 226 patients were noted to have "sludge" in the gallbladder and had repeated ultrasonograms up to 2 years later. Four developed stones, 4 had no further evidence of sludge, and 6 remained unchanged. Fourteen patients were initially symptomatic with biliary tract disease. Ten had stones, 3 had sludge, and 1 had a normal gallbladder. The patients with stones had an average steady-state total bilirubin value (3.8 ± 0.3 mg/dL) that was higher than that of the patients without stones (2.6 ± 0.12 mg/dL). Total hemoglobin and reticulocyte counts did not differ between the two groups. Evidence is good that children tolerate elective cholecystectomy with little morbidity if they are prepared properly for surgery.[543, 544] In contrast, operating during the acute phase carries a significant risk of complication.[545] Persistent *Salmonella* bacteremia is also an indication for elective cholecystectomy in a patient with gallstones.

Intrahepatic sickling can result in massive hyperbilirubinemia,[386] elevated liver enzyme values, and a painful syndrome mimicking acute cholecystitis[387] or viral hepatitis.[546] Fulminant hepatic failure with massive cholestasis and rapidly progressing hepatic encephalopathy and shock has been described as a rare, often fatal, complication of sickle cell disease that may be amenable to exchange transfusion.[547–549]

A review of postmortem liver findings among 70 sickle cell disease patients examined at Johns Hopkins Hospital[550] revealed evidence of unexplained hepatic injury. Hepatic necrosis, portal fibrosis, regenerative nodules, and cirrhosis were common features, thought to be a consequence of recurrent vascular obstruction and repair. In contrast, 19 liver biopsy specimens on symptomatic patients with SS disease failed to show necrosis and more often showed evidence of acute or subacute infection.[551]

Eyes. Tortuosity and sacculation of conjunctival vessels are seen in more than 90% of patients with sickle cell disease. These lesions are best seen in the lower temporal area, disappear after exchange transfusion, and are curiously related to the ISC count in the peripheral blood.[552] They have no deleterious effect on the eye.

Retinopathy is classified as either proliferative or nonproliferative. Nonproliferative retinopathy probably results from retinal arteriolar infarction with adjacent hemorrhage and requires no therapy. Depending on the age, layer, and extension of the hemorrhage, the result can be a salmon patch, schisms cavity, vitreous hemorrhage, or black sunburst.[553] In two patients with documented acute arteriolar occlusion, salmon patches developed in a matter of hours to days, with atrophic schisms cavities evolving in 3 to 4 months.[554] In older patients, angioid streaks are common, but the cause is unknown.[555, 556]

The more serious complication is proliferative retinopathy, which has been classified by Goldberg[557] as stage 1, peripheral arteriolar occlusions; stage 2, arteriolar-venular anastomoses; stage 3, neovascularization; stage 4, vitreous hemorrhages; and stage 5, retinal detachment. Because these lesions may progress to blindness, laser therapy to occlude feeding vessels of advanced proliferative lesions has been advocated. Unfortunately, photocoagulation carries the risks of neovascularization of the choroid[558, 559] and retinal breaks,[560] complications that can result in blindness. The dilemma of choosing potentially blinding therapy for a potentially blinding lesion is complicated by the observation that some proliferative lesions heal spontaneously by autoinfarction. In one study of untreated retinopathy in Jamaica, 567 eyes were observed for 8 years.[561] Proliferative retinopathy was initially present in 12% of the eyes: another 8% developed retinopathy during follow-up. Blindness resulted in 12% of the eyes with retinopathy. In the original group of eyes with retinopathy, 30% developed progressive retinopathy, 10% showed spontaneous regression, and the remaining 30% showed a mix of regression and progression. In another prospective Jamaican study, treatment of retinopathy was compared with no treatment.[562] No statistical difference in visual acuity between the two groups was reported. Macular ischemia and colorblindness have been reported to be prevalent in patients

with SS disease without evidence on ophthalmologic examination of retinal lesions.[563, 564]

Rarely, acute painless loss of vision is the result of central retinal artery occlusion. Although such lesions may resolve spontaneously, exchange transfusion has been recommended for bilateral disease.[565]

Blunt trauma to the eye may result in hyphema (bleeding into the anterior chamber). Because the conditions in this chamber overwhelmingly favor sickling, any hemoglobin-containing red cell will sickle and may cause obstructive glaucoma and blindness. This blood should be evacuated as soon as possible so that vision is preserved.[566] This condition is one of the true ocular emergencies that occurs in patients with sickle trait as well as sickle cell disease.

Skin. Leg ulcers usually do not occur in childhood. In adolescence and adulthood, ulcers may constitute a crippling symptom. This skin lesion is seen on other chronic hemolytic anemias such as hereditary spherocytosis, thalassemia, elliptocytosis, and pyruvate kinase deficiency[567] and therefore may not represent vaso-occlusion. Ulceration may result from increased venous pressure in the legs caused by the expanded blood volume in the hypertrophied bone marrow.[568] In tropical areas in which shoes are not usually worn and insect bites are common, leg ulcers are frequent.[569] In Jamaica, leg ulcers typically start in the 10- to 20-year-old group and eventually appear in 75% of adults. Koshy and colleagues[570] have reported data from the Cooperative Study of Sickle Cell Disease regarding leg ulcers in sickle cell patients. Leg ulcers appear to be less frequent in individuals with two genes than with those with three or four genes. In addition, low steady-state hemoglobin values were associated with a higher incidence of ulcer formation. Finally, leg ulcer frequencies appear to decrease consistently with increases in fetal hemoglobin production.[570] Chronic lesions become a major source of morbidity and have a profound negative impact on educational achievement and employment.[571] Usually present over the medial surface of the lower tibia or just posterior to the medial malleolus, they begin as a small depression with central necrosis and, if unattended, widen to encircle the entire lower leg. Débridement, scrupulous hygiene, topical antibiotics, rest, and elevation of the leg are the mainstays of therapy. In some patients, protection of the ulcer by the application of a soft sponge-rubber doughnut and low pressure elastic bandage seems to be beneficial. One report suggested that an RGD peptide matrix designed to mimic the normal matrix was beneficial.[572] Close attention to improved venous circulation by the use of above-the-knee elastic stockings may prevent ulceration. If ulcers persist despite optimal care, transfusion therapy may be utilized and consideration given to split-thickness skin grafts. Transfusion therapy is sometimes effective, but in many patients the ulcers either do not heal or recur after discontinuation of this therapy. Oral zinc sulfate may promote healing of leg ulcers,[573] and peripheral vasodilator therapy appears ineffective.[574]

Ears. Sensorineural hearing loss at both ends of the auditory spectrum was found in a substantial number of sickle cell patients in Jamaica.[575, 576] In an American study, 12% of children with SS disease had high-frequency sensorineural hearing loss.[577] Interestingly, although there was no increased otitis media or meningitis in the affected group, five of the six children with CNS disease had abnormal hearing. The pathology of the auditory apparatus appears to be sickling in the cochlear vasculature with destruction of hair cells.[578]

Skeleton. Skeletal changes in sickle cell disease are common[349, 579–582] and are due to expansion of the marrow cavity and repeated bone infarction. The expanded marrow is best seen in radiographs of the thickened calvarium with a wide diploic space. Overgrowth of the anterior maxilla may lead to severe orthodontic and cosmetic problems. Vertebrae are generally flattened, with a characteristic biconcave deformity called "codfish vertebrae." In older patients, vertebral disease may cause chronic back pain. These individuals need to be treated as other patients who have chronic back disease—with appropriate exercises, braces, bed rest, muscle relaxants, and moral support. Another major chronic bone complication of sickle cell disease is aseptic necrosis. In children, the most common cause of aseptic necrosis of the femoral head is sickle cell disease. As shown in Figure 20–11 the incidence is relatively low in children and is remarkably increased in patients with SS disease and coexistent α-thalassemia.[583] The patients at highest risk of developing this complication were those with the highest rates of painful crises and those with the highest hematocrits. Milner and colleagues,[583] reporting the findings of the Cooperative Study of Sickle Cell Disease, hypothesize that the pathophysiology of this lesion is sludging in marrow sinusoids, marrow necrosis, healing with increased intramedullary pressure, bone resorption, and eventually collapse. The diagnosis is made radiographically, classically with a spectrum of findings from subepiphyseal lucency and widened joint space to flattening or fragmentation and scarring of the epiphysis. Although roughly half of the patients diagnosed on the basis of screening radiographs were asymptomatic,

significant chronic pain and limited joint mobility plagued the others. Treatment options are limited and often disappointing. Strict bed rest is helpful in a minority of patients,[584] with little or no evidence to support the use of chronic transfusion therapy. Injection of cement[585] and core decompression[586] have been used successfully in some series. It is possible that these procedures might be particularly helpful in patients with very early disease, perhaps those diagnosed using MRI even before deformities are apparent on conventional films. A prospective study in a high-risk population such as young adults with SS disease and α-thalassemia would be helpful in determining the ultimate benefit of such treatment. Unfortunately, total hip replacement may be the only option for severely compromised patients. In the study of Milner and colleagues, 17% of patients underwent hip replacement, 30% of replaced hips required surgical revision within 4.5 years, and more than 60% of patients continued to have pain and limited mobility postoperatively. The epidemiology of aseptic necrosis of the humeral head is virtually identical to that of the femur.[587] In general, however, the patients are less symptomatic, and shoulder arthroplasty was exceedingly rare.

Lungs. In contrast to the acute chest syndrome, chronic lung disease has been difficult to define and quantitate. In general, lung volumes are reduced[588, 589] when compared with those of normal white population but are appropriate when compared with those of a black control population.[590] Resting arterial P_{O_2} in asymptomatic children with sickle cell disease is typically 65 to 85 mm Hg (normal > 87 mm Hg). There are large alveolar-arterial P_{O_2} differences in room air (27 to 42 mm Hg, normal < 16 mm Hg) and on 100% O_2 (186 to 246 mm Hg, normal < 86 mm Hg). These values are consistent with increased pulmonary shunting of 12% to 16% (normal < 7%).[590] The decreased membrane-diffusing capacity observed can be explained on the basis of anemia alone and does not suggest a substantial element of pulmonary vascular occlusion.[591] Cor pulmonale has been described,[507] and in one sur-

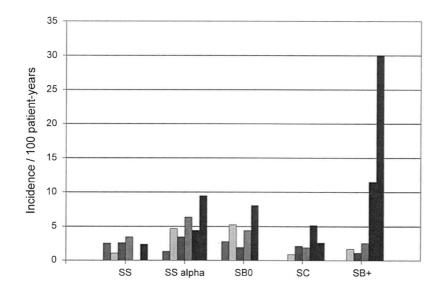

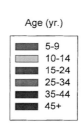

Age (yr.)

■	5-9
■	10-14
■	15-24
■	25-34
■	35-44
■	45+

Figure 20–11. Incidence of osteonecrosis of the femoral head per 100 patient-years by genotype. (Data from Milner PF, Kraus AP, et al: Sickle cell disease as a cause of osteonecrosis of the femoral head. N Engl J Med 1991; 325:1476.)

vey of adults, fatal progressive pulmonary disease may be related to history of previous chest syndromes.[508] However, the relationship between acute episodes of chest syndrome and chronic lung disease has been difficult to establish reproducibly. In a Jamaican study comparing 20 patients with at least six episodes of acute chest syndrome to 20 patients without chest syndrome, no difference in pulmonary artery pressure was found using echocardiography and Doppler evaluation.[592] In another study, patients with SS disease were found to have abnormally small lungs, but this abnormality was not related to episodes of acute chest syndrome.[593] These studies suggest that subtle subacute damage to the lungs proceeds even in the absence of acute disease.

Central Nervous System. Abnormal neurologic findings in sickle cell disease are primarily the result of acute CNS sickling and were discussed earlier. Changes on CT scans may antedate neurologic dysfunction and represent subclinical infarcts.[400–405] Rehabilitation requires the combined skills of physical therapist and speech therapist. An intensive coordinated program tailored to the needs of the individual patients

is essential in the recovery from CNS disease. The transfusion maintenance program described earlier is only one aspect of the care of the patient.

Growth and Development. The birth weight of infants with sickle cell anemia is normal.[594] Subsequently, a pattern of delayed growth emerges. Detailed anthropomorphic measurements of Jamaican children reveal decreased limb length, sitting height, and skinfold thickness, with increased chest anteroposterior diameter[595] possibly related to cardiomegaly.[596] Height and weight growth curves (Fig. 20–12) for individuals with sickle cell disease in the United States were generated as part of the Cooperative Study of Sickle Cell Disease, sponsored by the Sickle Cell Disease Branch of the National Heart, Lung, and Blood Institute.[597] The important features of these curves are that they are different from those for normal black controls, that weight is more affected than height, and that patients with sickle cell anemia and S-β[0] thalassemia experience more delay in growth than patients with Hb SC disease and S-β[+] thalassemia. In general, by the end of adolescence, the patients with sickle cell disease have caught up with controls in height but not weight. The reason

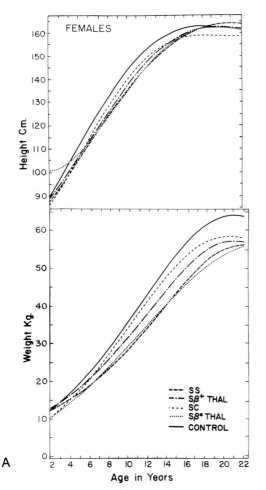

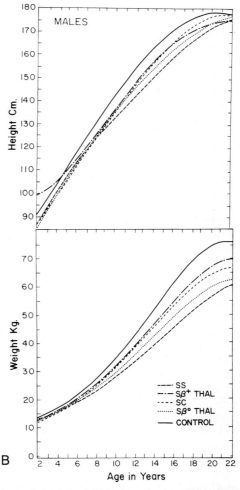

Figure 20-12. Height and weight growth curves for females *(A)* and males *(B)* 2 to 22 years of age, according to type of hemoglobinopathy. Shown are the 50% curves. (From Platt OS, Rosenstock MSPH, et al: Influence of sickle hemoglobinopathies on growth and development. N Engl J Med 1984; 311:7. Reprinted, by permission, from *The New England Journal of Medicine*.)

Table 20-3. ESTIMATED MEDIAN AGE AT ATTAINMENT OF TANNER STAGES, ACCORDING TO HEMOGLOBINOPATHY

	Tanner Stage	Median Age			
		SS	**SC**	**Sβ+**	**Sβ0**
Females					
Breasts	2	11.8	9.8	10.6	11.8
	3	13.5	11.9	12.6	12.8
	4	15	13.9	13.8	14.8
	5	17.3	16	16.5	17.2
Pubic hair	2	12	10.1	10	11.5
	3	13.5	11.8	11.2	12.8
	4	15.2	14	13.8	14.2
	5	19.2	17	17	20.8
Males					
Penis	2	12	10.4	11.9	12.4
	3	14.2	13	13	13.2
	4	16	14.1	13.5	15.5
	5	17.6	16.6	16.6	18.8
Pubic hair	2	13.2	11.5	12	13.2
	3	14.8	13.2	13	13.9
	4	16.2	14.2	13.9	16.2
	5	17.9	16.6	17.1	18.5

Reprinted, with permission from Platt OS, Rosenstock MSPH, et al: Influence of sickle hemoglobinopathies on growth and development. N Engl J Med 1984; 311:7.

for this poor weight gain is not understood but is likely to represent increased caloric requirements in these anemic patients with increased bone marrow activity and cardiovascular compensation.[598] In a second large prospective study in Jamaica, both height and weight were significantly lower than that of age- and sex-matched controls as early as 2 years of age.[599] Zinc deficiency has been suggested as a cause of poor growth in children with SS disease[600, 601] but has not been confirmed.[602] Growth hormone levels and growth hormone stimulation studies appear to be normal in children with SS disease who have impaired growth.[603] A review of nutritional studies in patients with SS disease is available,[604] and one study has suggested that hyperalimentation may be useful in some patients.[605]

Sexual development is also delayed in patients with sickle cell disease.[597] This delay is found in both males and females and follows the same pattern as height and weight in other hemoglobinopathies. The mean age of attainment of Tanner stage for each hemoglobinopathy is listed in Table 20–3. For females (regardless of hemoglobinopathy), menarche status is a function of age and weight. This normal relationship between menarche and weight suggests that in females, delayed sexual maturity is constitutional. This is confirmed in a careful analysis of female fertility in Jamaica, which reveals no difference in interval between sexual exposure and pregnancy between patients and controls.[606] Most males do undergo delayed sexual maturation, also suggesting constitutional delay. However, among males there does seem to be evidence of decreased fertility, with abnormal sperm motility, morphology, and number.[607] Transient primary hypogonadism[608] and hypothalamic hypogonadism responsive to clomiphene[609] also have been described.

Psychologic Aspects. As in any chronic disease, patients require strong, sympathetic support.[610] Most patients with sickle cell anemia handle their illness very well. In one study,[611] patients did not differ from controls in personal, social, or total adjustment. Interestingly, acute anxiety was less in the patients compared with controls, although the patients did demonstrate a lower self concept. Another study points out the pitfalls in interpreting excessive fatigue as depression in these children.[612] Problems of particular concern to patients are coping with chronic pain, inability to keep up with peers, fears of premature death, and delayed sexual maturity. Discussion of prenatal diagnosis and selective abortion, particularly in a patient's own family, increase doubts about self-worth. These issues need to be addressed openly and frankly and with appropriate psychologic support. Self-help groups for patients and families are gaining in effectiveness and popularity throughout the country.

TREATMENT

Routine Health Maintenance

Patients with sickle cell anemia should be followed on a routine basis (Table 20–4). Regular visits with routine laboratory studies when the patient is well help establish both the individual's steady-state normal values

Table 20-4. ROUTINE HEALTH MAINTENANCE FOR PATIENTS WITH SICKLE CELL ANEMIA

	Age (y)			
	<5	**5-10**	**10-20**	**20+**
Issues/Anticipatory Guidance				
Penicillin prophylaxis	──────→			
Splenic sequestration	──────→			
Fever or infection	──────────────────────→			
Coping with pain	──────────────────────→			
Dental care	──────────────────────→			
Groups for parents	───────────→			
Priapism		──────────────→		
Smoking		──────────────→		
Self-esteem, independence		──────────────→		
Education		──────────────→		
Recreation		──────────────→		
Puberty, birth control, genetics			───────→	
Leg ulcer			───────→	
Career planning		──────────────→		
Self-help groups			───────→	
Family planning, fertility				─────→
Prognosis				─────→
Laboratory				
Complete blood count	1–3/y	1–2/y	1–2/y	1–2/y
Red cell antigen typing	Once			
Liver function, renal function		Yearly	Yearly	Yearly
Urinalysis	Yearly	Yearly	Yearly	Yearly
Special studies				
Pulmonary function		q 3–5 y	q 3–5 y	q 3–5 y
Chest radiography		q 3–5 y	q 2–3 y	q 2–3 y
Eye examination		q 3–5 y	Yearly	Yearly
Treatment				
Penicillin prophylaxis	───────────→			
Folate	──────────────────────→			
Pneumococcal vaccine	Age 2	Boosters as recommended		
Haemophilus influenzae vaccine	Infant	Boosters as recommended		
Hepatitis B vaccine	Infant	Boosters as recommended		
Influenza vaccine	Yearly as recommended ─────→			

(e.g., hemoglobin, reticulocytes, white blood cells, differential, platelet count, erythrocyte sedimentation rate, chest film, electrocardiogram) and baseline physical findings (e.g., icterus, cardiomegaly, murmurs, organomegaly). These baseline data are extremely helpful in sorting out the problems when the patient is ill.

Careful evaluation of the interval history may provide insight into factors that provoke painful crises. Continuing education of patients and families as to how to avoid and treat painful episodes will reduce the morbidity and hospitalization rate and will promote the patient's sense of independence. Education should also include genetic counseling of the parents with the goal that they understand the risks of sickle cell disease in future pregnancies.

Careful attention is paid to routine immunization schedules; all patients should receive pneumococcal *H. influenzae,* and hepatitis B vaccines. Prophylactic penicillin should be given to all children younger than 5 years of age.[476] Most important, the patient and family should be educated about the importance of early detection and treatment of infection.

Although folic acid, 1 mg/d, is recommended for prevention of folate deficiency in adults, no definite advantage has been seen in children.[613] Iron deficiency is extremely rare because of the hemolysis-induced increased absorption of gastrointestinal iron. Iron supplements are used only when iron deficiency is documented or when blood loss is chronic (e.g., hematuria).

Ophthalmologic examinations should be started at school age and repeated every few years unless retinopathy is discovered. For patients with retinopathy, more frequent follow-up and fluorescein angiography are necessary to establish the tempo of the lesion and to determine appropriate therapy.

Regular dental care is critical in preventing the intraoral lesions that might predispose to infections, such as mandibular osteomyelitis.[614]

Birth control options should be discussed as with any adolescent patient. Barrier methods and low-dose estrogen oral contraceptives can be used safely.[615]

The Painful Crisis

Most painful crises can be successfully treated at home with increased fluid intake and oral analgesics. If the pain is too severe for oral analgesics or if the patient cannot maintain adequate fluid intake, the episode must be treated in the hospital. Hospital management of painful crisis includes hydration and analgesia. In dehydrated patients, the intravenous fluid rate is usually one and one-half times maintenance (2250 mL/m² per day). Some patients, however, cannot tolerate this expansion of intravascular volume. Frequent monitoring of vital signs during fluid administration is essential to prevention of iatrogenic cardiac failure. Serum electrolyte levels must be checked early and intravenous solutions adjusted appropriately. Although theoretically sound, the use of intravenous bicarbonate has not been shown to be effective.[616] Face-mask oxygen is of little therapeutic value unless the patient is hypoxic. Furthermore, Embury and colleagues have shown that continuous oxygen inhalation can suppress erythropoiesis, with reticulocyte counts falling within days.[617] In addition, painful crisis may result from the rebound marrow activity after the abrupt discontinuation of oxygen therapy or cessation of transfusion programs.[618]

Analgesia must be sufficient to control the pain. "Standard doses" may not be enough for an individual patient. Although narcotic dependence or enhanced narcotic-seeking behavior may be a problem for rare patients, this must not affect the decision to control severe pain. One should choose narcotics with side effects, drug interactions, and serum half-lives in mind. Changes in the route of administration (intravenous, intramuscular, oral) require adjustments for equianalgesic dosages. Serial intramuscular injections can lead to the formation of sterile abscess, and scarring and should be avoided in the treatment of prolonged painful episodes. At the onset of inpatient therapy for severe pain, regular dosage intervals should be used, not "as needed" dosages, thereby avoiding the recurrence of pain and anxiety before the next dose of medicine. High-dose meperidine may cause seizures, particularly in the setting of compromised renal function where toxic levels of normeperidine accumulate.[619] Hypoventilation is the most serious side effect and must be carefully avoided by careful monitoring of oxygen saturations and use of oxygen when the patient is hypoxic. Continuous intravenous narcotic therapy in children has been successfully employed, but chest syndrome may be precipitated by respiratory depression.[620] In one study, epidural anesthesia was successfully used to alleviate pain and maintain or improve oxygenation.[621] The combination of continuous narcotic infusion with patient-controlled boluses is emerging as a particularly effective strategy. Constipation and urinary retention are common problems that should be remedied early. Sometimes it is virtually impossible to make a patient entirely comfortable with safe doses of narcotics. This frustrating situation needs to be approached with care and sensitivity, with involvement of every member of the patient care team.[622, 623] The addition of nonsteroidal anti-inflammatory agents is helpful to some patients. Others have benefitted from adjuncts such as acupuncture,[624] biofeedback, and hypnosis.[625] For the rare patient who is incapacitated by recurrent episodes of pain and who spends more time in the hospital than out, chronic outpatient narcotic therapy may be useful.[626] A maintenance transfusion program can be used as a last resort. Although transfusion (even exchange transfusion) rarely works acutely, a maintenance program for a few months may be enough for the patient to finish the school year or to complete an important project at work.

Vasodilators have been studied as a possible treatment modality in painful crisis without conclusive results. Cetiedil, a vasodilator that inhibits cell dehydration *in vitro,*[627, 628] in a blinded controlled clinical trial reduced the mean duration of days in crisis from 4 to 3 days when given intravenously for the first 4 days of crisis.[629]

Several cases of acute gout mimicking painful crisis

have been reported,[630] even though the increased renal clearance of urate usually prevents this complication.

Transfusion

Patients with sickle cell disease tolerate their chronic anemia well and require transfusions only under certain circumstances—sequestration crisis, CNS infarction, aplastic crisis, preparation for surgery, and hypoxia with acute chest syndrome. In sequestration crisis and aplastic crisis, a standard simple transfusion is necessary to restore a circulating red cell mass. In all other situations, some degree of exchange transfusion is probably preferable so that the increased viscosity due to the higher hematocrit is offset by a reduction in circulating sickle cells. This concept is undergoing considerable scrutiny and debate. As discussed in the preparation for surgery section, simple transfusion compares favorably to exchange transfusion in the preoperative setting. When rapid reduction of Hb S is necessary, as in CNS crisis, an exchange transfusion is preferable. At Johns Hopkins Hospital a routine for exchange transfusions in children with sickle cell disease has been developed. A 60% to 80% reduction of circulating sickle cells can be accomplished in 6 to 12 hours by exchanging two times the red cell mass (2 × blood volume × hematocrit). The total volume or the number of units of blood needed for the exchange must take into consideration the packed red cell mass in a unit of blood (usually 40% of 500 mL of whole blood from a single donation). Initial exchanges can be done with packed red cells but when the hematocrit approaches 35%, packed cell units should be diluted with appropriate electrolyte solutions or plasma. Sickle trait blood should not be used. A similar procedure has been described by Charache.[631] In those centers in which an automated cell separator is available, a two-volume exchange transfusion can be efficiently accomplished in less than 90 minutes.[632, 633]

Maintenance transfusion programs are designed to suppress the patient's production of sickle cells. Indications for chronic transfusion include prevention of further strokes, chronic heart or pulmonary failure, prolonged hematuria, recurrent priapism, unremitting vaso-occlusive crises, and complicated pregnancy. The degree of suppression needed depends on the reason for the chronic transfusion and individual variability in the suppressive effect of the transfusions.[634] Transfusions that keep the percent of sickle hemoglobin less than 30% reduce the frequency of recurrent strokes from 70% to less than 10% and reduce the frequency of vaso-occlusive crises.[635] Iron overload is ultimately unavoidable but can be treated with desferrioxamine.[636, 637] In children who have received multiple transfusions, the rate of alloimmunization is between 7% and 20%.[638–641] The likelihood of alloimmunization is related to the number of transfusions, the racial differences between donor and recipients, and as yet unknown genetic factors that control the responsiveness of the recipient to transfused antigens.[642] Ideally, patients with SS disease should receive antigen-matched red cells to reduce the hazard of sensitization.

Such a strategy has been demonstrated to reduce sensitization,[643–645] although opinions still vary as to the utility of preventing sensitization using expensive antigen-matched cells in contrast to providing those cells after sensitization occurs.[646] Potential benefits from the prevention strategy include prevention of complications from the first delayed transfusion reaction and possibly the prevention of autoantibodies that appear in the same context. Clinically significant autoantibodies do occur in about 10% of patients with sickle cell disease; and the incidence appears to be higher in those with alloantibodies.[641, 644, 645] The most common antibody-provoking antigens are K, C, E, S, Fy^a, Fy^b, and Jk^b. Tahhan and colleagues from North Carolina suggest a modest antibody-preventing strategy: match for K, C, E, and S in all patients; match for Fy^a or Fy^b in Fy (a−b+) or (a+b−) but not (a−b−) patients; match for Jk^b in Jk(a+b−) patients.[643]

Preparation for Surgery

Children with sickle cell disease can be operated on safely if careful attention is paid to oxygenation, hydration, and acid-base balance during the procedure and in the postoperative period.[646–653] Choice of an anesthetic agent is not as critical as the care with which it is delivered.[649] Burrington and Smith[650] suggest some simple rules of procedure: Keep the operating room at 80°F to 85°F, ventilate with 100% oxygen a few minutes before and after intubation or extubation, keep the patient warm in the recovery room (particularly if tremors are present), and take special care of IV boards, casts, dressings and so on to ensure that circulation is maintained. In an analysis of over 1000 surgical procedures from the Cooperative Study of Sickle Cell Disease, the overall mortality rate was 1.1%, but no deaths occurred in children younger than 14 years of age. That same series illustrated comparable complication rates in the SS and SC groups and suggested that patients undergoing regional anesthesia were at higher risk of complication than those undergoing general anesthesia.[653] That prospective "natural history" study did not definitively address the important question of the effectiveness of preoperative transfusion. In a review of records from Dallas Children's Hospital, pulmonary complications were particularly common among patients undergoing laparotomy, thoracotomy, or tonsillectomy and adenoidectomy who were not transfused preoperatively (9/29), compared with those who were transfused for those procedures (0/8).[654] More recently, Vichinsky and colleagues[655] reported the findings of a prospective, multi-institutional study that randomized over 600 preoperative Hb SS patients to receive either simple transfusion designed to increase the total hemoglobin to 10 g/dL or exchange transfusion designed to decrease Hb S percent to less than 30 and increase total hemoglobin to 10 g/dl. Several key points emerged from that study:

- There was no significant difference between the two transfusion strategies in terms of complications; both strategies reported a high 30% postpartum complication rate. Transfusion-related complications were twice as common (14%) in the exchange transfusion arm, compared with the simple transfusion arm (7%).

- The most common and serious complication was the acute chest syndrome, which occurred in 10% of procedures in both arms. The average time at onset was postoperative day 3; the average length of episode was 8 days; 11% of the patients required intubation, and two died.
- Those with higher surgical risk category, history of pulmonary disease, incidence of acute chest syndrome, and frequency of hospitalization were at higher risk of complication.

These data suggest that, at least, a simple transfusion, designed to raise the preoperative hemoglobin to 10 g/dL should be done for all patients with Hb SS disease. Antigen-matched, leukocyte-depleted packed red cells is likely the product of choice. All patients, especially those with prior pulmonary dysfunction or history of multiple hospital admissions should receive a minimum of 12 hours of oxygen treatment and maintenance intravenous hydration and be monitored as high-risk patients, with emphasis on objective markers of oxygenation and compulsive measurement of input, output, and weight.

Management of Pregnancy

Although many women with sickle cell disease have normal pregnancies, pregnancy can be associated with serious problems for both the mother and fetus. Maternal complications may include increase in frequency and severity of painful crises, increase in severity and frequency of chest syndrome, exaggeration of physiologic anemia of pregnancy, toxemia, and death.[656] Because of sickling in the placenta, fetal complications can include spontaneous abortion, prematurity, and intrauterine growth retardation. There has been a tremendous improvement in both maternal and fetal outcomes since the mid 1960s.[657–660] The older literature reports fetal and maternal mortality rates that approach 50%, with some authors suggesting voluntary sterilization of females with SS disease. Charache and colleagues have observed that with modern obstetric management, regular prenatal care, and better nutrition, maternal mortality has been reduced to less than 1% and perinatal deaths have declined to less than 15%.[660] Some authors suggest that pregnancy outcome can be improved further if mothers are prophylactically transfused[661–664] using various transfusion techniques.[665, 666] Results in patients treated with this approach appear to be favorable compared with those observed in historical controls, but benefits of this therapy are not as convincing in contemporary comparisons.[667] Koshy and colleagues[668] were unable to demonstrate any significant benefit of transfusions during pregnancy in the only prospective trial so far published. Hepatitis, alloimmunization, and hemolytic transfusion reactions[668, 669] have been reported in transfused pregnant sickle patients. These pregnancies should be considered as "high risks." At the initial visit, complete red cell typing of both mother and father as well as antibody screening of the mother should be done. Both iron and folate should be prescribed. The early stages of pregnancy should be carefully monitored with serial ultrasonographic studies. A maintenance transfusion program should be initiated if the mother becomes increasingly symptomatic with either vaso-occlusive or anemia-related problems or if there is any sign of fetal distress or poor growth. Blood transfusion should be carefully selected to be compatible in minor group antigens for which the mother is negative and the father positive. This approach minimizes the risk of maternal sensitization against fetal antigens.

DEATH

Leikin and his colleagues from the Cooperative Study of Sickle Cell Disease examined mortality in children with sickle cell disease.[670] They found that the peak incidence of death was between 1 and 3 years of age and was generally caused by infection. The overall mortality rate was 2.6%; and for patients with SS disease, the probability of surviving to age 29 years was about 85%. For those with SC disease, the probability of surviving to age 20 years was about 95%.

As shown in Figure 20–13, when the data on deaths of the children from the Cooperative Study of Sickle Cell Disease are combined with the data in adults, it appears that the median age at death was 42 years for males with SS disease, 48 years for females with SS disease, 60 years for males with SC disease, and 68 years for females with SC disease.[343] Among the adults, those with the lowest levels of fetal hemoglobin, and highest rates of pain and chest syndrome, had the highest risk of dying at an early age. There is an age-related pattern in mortality rates: a peak in the patients younger than 5 years of age and a gradual increase starting in late adolescence. Younger patients die primarily of pneumococcal disease, less often of acute splenic sequestration, acute chest syndrome, or stroke.[372, 427] Older patients die of acute chest syndrome, during pain crises, chronic organ system failure from cancer and other specific diseases of adults, and suddenly without obvious cause.[372] The single largest cause of death in children younger than 4 years old was pneumococcal disease, now a treatable and preventable complication. Through newborn screening, education, prophylactic penicillin treatment, and vaccines, this cause has declined.

OTHER SICKLE SYNDROMES
Sickle Cell Trait $\alpha_2\beta_2$, $\alpha_2\beta_2^{6\ Val}$

Sickle cell trait is a benign condition that is not associated with increased morbidity or mortality.[671–676] Growth, behavior, and educational achievement and pregnancy risks in children with sickle trait are entirely normal.[675–677] Black American professional football players have the same incidence of sickle trait as the general black population.[678] In a retrospective study of

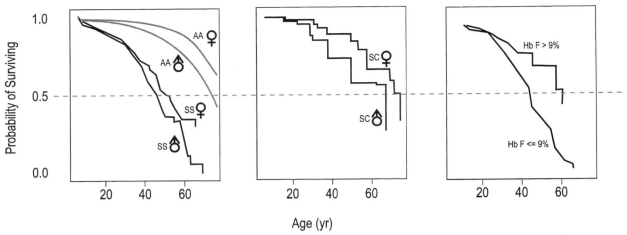

Figure 20-13. Survival of male and female patients with SS disease and SC disease, comparing those in the highest quartile (>9%) of fetal hemoglobin (Hb F) level with the others. African American (AA) controls are shown for comparison. (Adapted from Platt OS, Brambilla DJ, et al: Mortality in sickle cell disease: life expectancy and risk factors for early death. N Engl J Med 1994; 330:1639.)

sudden death during physical training in the U.S. Armed Forces, Kark and colleagues noted a 1/3200 incidence of sudden death among sickle trait recruits, a frequency 27 times greater than non–Hb S controls.[679] All deaths were associated with strenuous physical exertion, and risks increased with age. After this report, modifications in basic training for all recruits have been recommended but follow-up data are not yet available. A subsequent prospective study of 25 sickle trait recruits and non–Hb S controls revealed no difference in exercise tolerance or physical conditioning after 7 weeks of basic training.[680] Several authors have stressed that these data do not justify restriction of sickle trait men from the armed services or organized sports.[681–683] Although anecdotal reports of various severe vaso-occlusive episodes in those with sickle trait appear in the literature,[684] they are extremely rare and not clearly due to sickle trait. Postmortem findings of intravascular sickling are not evidence that the sickling had occurred ante mortem. Under certain extreme conditions, however, sickling and even death may occur in individuals with sickle trait. These include severe pneumonia,[685] unpressurized flying,[686, 687] and exercise at high altitudes.[688, 689] The risk of sickle trait in routine aviation has been overstated.[690] Careful general anesthesia does not carry a great risk for the individual with sickle trait,[691, 692] but tourniquet surgery[693] and deep hypothermia should be avoided. The most consistent abnormality found in sickle trait is the inability to concentrate urine.[694] There is no associated anemia, abnormal morphology, or decreased red cell survival. Most individuals have approximately 40% Hb S and 60% Hb A. A population with 28% to 35% Hb S has been identified and shown to have accompanying α-thalassemia.[695] Decreased levels of Hb S can also be seen in patients with iron[696] and folate[697] deficiencies.

SC Disease $\alpha_2\beta_2^{6\ Val}$, $\alpha_2\beta_2^{6\ Lys}$

Hemoglobin SC disease is a mild chronic hemolytic anemia associated with variable degrees of vaso-occlu-sive complications. As described in Table 20–1, the patient typically has a hemoglobin of 10 to 12 g/dL, a reticulocyte count of 1% to 13%, and a relative microcytosis for the degree of reticulocytosis. The peripheral blood smear (see Fig. 20–5) is more characteristic of Hb C than of Hb S, showing impressive target cells and rare, if any, ISCs. The clinical course is quite variable, with some patients severely affected at an early age and others entirely asymptomatic and identified only as adults on routine screening. Hemolysis is less severe in SC disease than in SS disease,[698] resulting in a higher hematocrit in patients with SC disease.

The major complications of Hb SS disease are not common in SC disease but have been reported, including recurrent painful bone crises, painful abdominal crises, gallstones, pulmonary infarction, priapism, and CNS infarction.[699–702] As shown in Figure 20–9, the pattern of clinical events is different in SC disease, with most events occurring not only less frequently but later in life. Certain complications appear to be more common in the SC disease population: eye disease,[557, 700, 703–705] aseptic necrosis of the femoral heads, renal papillary necrosis,[706] and pregnancy-related problems.[707] Splenomegaly is found in approximately 60% of patients with SC disease and has been associated with splenic infarction[708] and splenic sequestration,[709] particularly at high altitudes. Although infection is not as common in SC disease as in SS disease,[710] splenic hypofunction and an increased risk of pneumococcal and H. influenzae sepsis are found in SC disease.[711] Pneumococcal and H. influenzae vaccines are indicated in SC disease, and some recommend the use of prophylactic penicillin.

Patients with SC disease clearly have more sickling complications than do individuals with sickle trait, who are essentially free of sickling complications. One would therefore assume that mixtures of Hb S and Hb A are less likely to polymerize than mixtures of Hb S and Hb C. Interestingly, Bunn and associates[712] have shown that this is not the case, because the kinetic and equilibrium behaviors of mixtures Hb S and Hb A are essentially identical with the behaviors of mixtures of Hb S and Hb C. One can resolve this apparent paradox by considering how the hemoglobin mixtures are packaged in SC and AS cells. There are two major factors that explain why SC cells sickle more readily than AS cells: (1) There is more Hb S in an SC cell, and (2) there is a higher MCHC in an SC cell. Because of the charge and affinity for α globin differences between β-S globin and β-C globin, individuals with SC disease usually have 50% Hb S and 50% Hb C, whereas those with the sickle trait typically have 60% Hb A and 40% Hb S.[713] This increased Hb S content of SC cells results in an approximately sevenfold increase in the rate of polymerization.[713] The increase in MCHC in SC disease, which is quite obvious on density separation of SC red cells[139, 712, 714] (see Fig. 20–6) and even C trait red cells,[713] is probably due to the activation by the positively charged Hb C molecules of the K^+,Cl^- cotransport system.[173] The cellular dehydration and microcytosis associated with Hb C has been well characterized by Brugnara and colleagues[175] and Ballas and associates.[714]

Hemoglobin SC α-Thalassemia

One patient with Hb SC and α-thalassemia trait has been described.[715] This 7-year-old child had the following laboratory values: hematocrit, 25.8%; Hb, 7.9 g/dL; MCV, 53 μm^3; MCH, 16.2 pg; MCHC, 30.6 g/dL; reticulocytes, 7.2%; Hb S, 50.5%; Hb C, 47.7%; and Hb F, 1.8%. One parent had 27% Hb S with an MCV of 71 μm^3, the other had 24% Hb C with an MCV of 57 μm^3. This patient, like many patients with SC disease, was relatively asymptomatic. Of interest is that her hematocrit level and reticulocyte count are compatible with a considerable degree of hemolysis.

SO Arab $\alpha_2\beta_2^{6\ Val}$, $\alpha_2\beta_2^{121\ Lys}$

SO$_{Arab}$ double heterozygotes are quite rare and have a relatively severe disorder with a chronic hemolytic anemia and vaso-occlusive episodes.[716] As seen in Figure 20–1, the O Arab mutation lies within the area critical to the axial contact in the Hb S fiber. Routine cellulose acetate electrophoresis at 8.6 does not distinguish between Hb C and Hb O$_{Arab}$. Citrate agar electrophoresis at pH 6 does separate Hb C from Hb O and should be done on patients who appear to have Hb SC disease on cellulose acetate electrophoresis but who have particularly severe symptoms.[717]

SD $\alpha_2\beta_2^{6\ Val}$, $\alpha_2\beta_2^{121\ Glu}$

SD double heterozygotes have a severe hemolytic anemia with a peripheral blood smear comparable to that seen in Hb SS (see Fig. 20–5). These rare patients have severe vaso-occlusive complications,[718–720] illustrating, as those with the Hb O$_{Arab}$, the critical nature of the $\beta121$ contact site. Hemoglobin D migrates with Hb S on cellulose acetate electrophoresis at alkaline pH and can be distinguished from Hb S on citrate agar electrophoresis at acid pH. Hemoglobin D is suspected when a hemoglobin appears to be Hb S on cellulose acetate electrophoresis but gives a negative "sickle prep." The

identification of a parent with Hb D is important socially because it may become difficult to explain how a child has "SS disease" and only one parent has a positive sickle prep.

S Korle Bu $\alpha_2\beta_2^{6\ Val}$, $\alpha_2\beta_2^{73\ Asn}$

Hemoglobin Korle Bu is a rare hemoglobin mutant.[721] It is mentioned here only because it illustrates an important pathophysiologic point. Korle Bu participates poorly in sickling.[722] This mutation interferes with the lateral contact between Hb S fibers by blocking the critical receptor area for the $\beta6$ Val. S Korle Bu double heterozygotes are entirely symptom free.

Hemoglobin C$_{Harlem}$ (C$_{Georgetown}$) $\alpha_2\beta_2^{6\ Val,\ 73\ Asn}$

Hemoglobin C$_{Harlem}$ (also known as C$_{Georgetown}$) has two substitutions on the β chain: the sickle mutation $\beta^{6\ Val}$ and the Korle Bu mutation $\beta^{73\ Asn}$.[723] Patients with these mutations are asymptomatic. Patients doubly heterozygous for Hb S and Hb C$_{Harlem}$ have clinical crises resembling SS disease.[723, 724]

Hemoglobin S Antilles $\alpha_2\beta_2^{6\ Val,\ 23\ Ile}$

Hb S Antilles also has two substitutions on the β chain: the sickle mutation $\beta^{6\ Val}$ and a second mutation $\beta^{23\ Ile}$.[725] This mutation results in a low oxygen affinity hemoglobin that in heterozygotes for Hb A and Hb S Antilles results in a mild hemolytic anemia and the presence of 5% to 7% irreversible sickled cells. A transgenic mouse with β^5 Antilles and the β^Dpunjab (see earlier) mutations exhibits many of the clinical features of SS disease.[726]

Sickle Syndromes with Increased Fetal Hemoglobin

Hb F levels in sickle cell anemia may vary over a 60-fold range from 0.5% to 30%. Because of the known ameliorating effect of Hb F in reducing Hb S polymerization, the origin of this marked variability has been of great interest. Because Hb F is heterogeneously distributed among the red cells of SS individuals, the percentage of Hb F is the result of three independent processes; the number of cells containing Hb F (F cells) produced, the amount of Hb F per F cell, and the variable preferential survival of F cells compared with non-F cells in the circulation.[727]

Three broad categories of genetic mutations have been described which increase Hb F in association with Hb S. (See reviews.[728, 729]) Large deletions of the β-globin gene region resulting in δ-β-thalassemia or pancellular hereditary persistence of fetal hemoglobin (HPFH) are rare in the general sickle cell population (see Chapter 21 for more details on these deletions). Hb S-pancellular HPFH patients represent a unique syndrome in which one finds between 24% and 34% Hb F distributed in all red cells, no anemia, minimal microcytosis (MCV 78 $\pm$ 8 μm^3), and no clinical disease.[730–734]

A second group of mutations that increase Hb F in association with Hb S are linked to the β-globin gene region and are termed *nondeletion HPFH*.[735-738] Some linked mutations may be associated with single nucleotide substitutions in the promoter regions of the gamma genes, but these are quite rare among the general SS population.[728-739] Hb F is usually distributed heterogeneously in these disorders, but some have been associated with a pancellular distribution. Another type of linked nondeletion mutation that may increase Hb F is the as yet undefined mutation associated with the Senegal and Arab-Indian (Saudi) β-globin haplotypes.[31, 36-39] These haplotypes are found commonly in genetic isolates in Western Africa, in Shiite Saudi Arabians, and in the Orissa region of India.[740-743] Among U.S. patients with sickle cell anemia, less than 10% have one chromosome with either of these haplotypes and less than 2% are homozygous for the Senegal haplotype.

A third group of genetic disorders that influence Hb F levels in patients with SS disease are not linked to the β-globin region.[744, 745] Boyer and Dover have shown that approximately one third of full siblings each with SS disease have significantly different genetic programs for Hb F production.[746] Because both siblings inherited the same β-globin regions from their sickle trait parents the Hb F program must be separate from the β-globin region. After Myoshi[747] noted that Hb F (defined by F-cell levels) in normal blood donors were inherited in an X-linked pattern, Dover and colleagues showed that F-cell production in sickle cell patients was inherited by a diallelic gene on the short arm of the X-chromosome. They termed this gene the F-cell production (FCP) locus.[748] The FCP locus is likely to account for most of the heterocellular forms of HPFH not linked to the β-globin locus.[748, 749]

In addition to these disorders, it has been shown that α-thalassemia is associated with decreased Hb F levels in SS disease. Although Embury first suggested that the presence of α-thalassemia increased Hb F levels in sickle cell patients,[750] in a much larger study, Higgs and colleagues[751] showed that Hb F levels were indeed lower in SS patients with α-thalassemia. Noguchi[752] and Dover[753] showed that the differences in Hb F levels among SS patients with or without α-thalassemia may be indirectly related to the lowered MCHC of the SS-α-thalassemia red cells[751, 752] (see section on SS-α thalassemia). Preferential survival of F cells compared with non–F cells is less in SS-α-thalassemia because the non–F cells in α-thalassemia have less cation loss and a lower MCHC, which reduces Hb S polymerization and results in a longer life span.

When all known factors responsible for elevated Hb F levels in SS disease were studied in a random population including a cohort of SS patients identified at birth, the following emerged. First, the X-linked FCP locus was responsible for almost 40% of the variation in Hb F levels. Second, β-globin haplotypes, age and sex together accounted for less than 10% of the variation. Third, approximately 50% of the variation remains undefined.[749] Early investigators suggested different "threshold" levels of Hb F (between 10%–20%) were

necessary to ameliorate the clinical severity of SS disease.[754-756] In the natural history study, Platt and co-workers showed that any increment of Hb F above 4% was associated with reduced pain crises[296] and Hb F levels greater than 7% were associated with decreased mortality.[343]

Sickle β-Thalassemia

Patients heterozygous for Hb S and β-thalassemia have clinical severity that depends on the output of the thalassemic β gene.[757-760] If no Hb A is produced ("S-β⁰-thalassemia"), the clinical course is comparable (see Table 20–3 and Fig. 20–11) with that of homozygous sickle cell anemia. Their electrophoresis shows mostly Hb S, with slightly elevated Hb A_2, and variable amounts of Hb F. The features that distinguish these patients from those with sickle cell anemia are that they may be of Mediterranean origin, have microcytosis, and often have splenomegaly. One parent will have classic sickle trait, whereas the other will have β-thalassemia trait. The hemolytic rate is lower, and the patients tend to have a slightly higher hematocrit and lower reticulocyte count. Peripheral blood morphology is notable for target cells, microcytosis, and generally fewer ISCs than in sickle cell anemia. If there is output from the β-thalassemia gene ("S-β⁺-thalassemia"), patients tend to have a milder clinical course, comparable with that of SC disease. These patients have electrophoresis that shows predominantly Hb S, elevated Hb A_2, variable amounts of Hb F, and Hb A. The features that distinguish these individuals from those with sickle cell anemia are Hb A, microcytosis, splenomegaly, and relatively benign clinical course. The ameliorative effects of Hb A (see Tables 20–1 and 20–3 and Fig. 20–11) are apparent. These patients can be distinguished from individuals with sickle trait because of Hb S > Hb A, microcytosis, hemolytic anemia, abnormal peripheral morphology, and splenomegaly. Alpha-thalassemia with Hb S-β⁰-thalassemia results in higher hemoglobin levels, lower reticulocyte counts, and increases in the MCV and MCHC.[761]

SS α-Thalassemia

Homozygous Hb SS disease with accompanying α-thalassemia has been well described.[750-753, 762-773] The diagnosis is based on the following criteria: (1) hemoglobin electrophoresis showing no Hb A, normal Hb A_2, and predominantly Hb S; (2) microcytosis without iron deficiency; (3) both parents with S trait, one with the typical AS α-thalassemia picture (microcytosis and Hb S concentration of less than 35%); (4) elevated Hb Bart's detectable in cord blood; and (5) α gene mapping showing two or three genes. Approximately 30% of American blacks have three α genes, and approximately 2% have two α genes. Alpha-thalassemia in U.S. SS disease patients is usually due to the α-thal-2 haplotype, which is a deletion that spans both α genes.[773] There has been considerable interest in these patients because the α-thalassemia has an effect on some of the hematologic features of sickle cell anemia and may provide insight into the pathophysiology of the disease. The primary effect of α-thalassemia is to decrease the cellular Hb S content that increases the surface to volume ratio, resulting in a reduced MCHC that prolongs the delay time for Hb S polymerization. Patients with α-thalassemia tend to have smaller, lighter cells, with a higher hemoglobin level and fewer reticulocytes.[750, 751, 770, 771] Although the hematologic parameters of sickle cell anemia are clearly improved by coexisting α-thalassemia, the vaso-occlusive severity is not obviously different. One study[751] indicated that leg ulcers and chest syndrome was less frequent with α-thalassemia, but this was not confirmed by others.[772] Avascular necrosis of the femoral head was increased in sickle cell anemia with α-thalassemia (see Fig. 20–11).[773, 774] Alpha-thalassemia does not protect children with SS disease from strokes.[775] Mears has suggested that α-thalassemia is associated with increased life expectancy.[776] Alpha-thalassemia not only reduces the MCV and the MCHC, but it also reduces the percentage of dense cells and ISCs.[752, 777] The cells of patients with α-thalassemia SS disease are more deformable and have less cation fluxes and a greater ratio of membrane surface area to volume.[767] Differences in hemoglobin values between children with SS disease with four and two α genes is not apparent until after the age of 4,[778] but the microcytosis and elevated red cell counts are present at birth.[779]

Hemoglobin C Disease $\alpha_2\beta_2^{6\ Lys}$

Homozygous Hb C disease is a mild disorder characterized by hemolytic anemia, microcytosis, and splenomegaly.[780–786] The tendency of Hb C to aggregate and crystallize[787, 788] is probably responsible for the characteristic target morphology of the stained and dried red cell in homozygous C disease and in Hb C trait, although these crystals are not likely to be directly responsible for the hemolytic anemia. In Hb C trait, target cell formation and mild microcytosis is the only manifestation of the anomaly. Hemolytic anemia is not present.

The basis of the aggregation and crystal formation of Hb C cells is not precisely understood. It is thought that the substantial charge difference between Hb C and Hb A is in some way responsible for the tendency toward aggregation of C molecules, which leads to local increments of hemoglobin concentration in excess of its solubility.[785] The structure of these crystals has been examined by x-ray diffraction analysis.[787–789]

The hemolytic anemia of homozygous Hb C disease is likely due to the fact that these cells are dehydrated. Brugnara and colleagues have demonstrated that CC red cells have decreased water and cation content associated with a large potassium efflux.[175] As discussed in the previous section on membrane abnormalities, this volume-dependent potassium efflux is regulated by the K^+,Cl^- co-transport pathway.

References

1. Herrick JB: Peculiar elongated and sickle-shaped red corpuscles in a case of severe anemia. Arch Intern Med 1910; 6:517.
2. Sydenstricker VP, Mulherin WA, Houseal RW: Sickle cell anemia: report of two cases in children, with necropsy in one case. Am J Dis Child 1923; 26:132.
3. Hahn EV, Gillespie EB: Sickle-cell anemia: report of a case greatly improved by splenectomy. Arch Intern Med 1927; 39:233.
4. Pauling L, Itano H, et al: Sickle cell anemia: a molecular disease. Science 1949; 110:543.
5. Beet EA: Genetics of the sickle cell trait in a Bantu tribe. Ann Eugen 1949; 14:279.
6. Neel JV: Inheritance of the sickling phenomenon with particular reference to sickle-cell disease. Blood 1951; 6:389.
7. Huehns ER, Shooter EM: Human hemoglobins. J Med Gene 1965; 2:1.
8. Huehns ER, Dance N, et al. Human embryonic haemoglobins. Nature 1964; 201:1095.
9. Capp GL, Rigas DA, et al: Evidence for a new haemoglobin chain (ξ chain). Nature 1970; 228:278.
10. Ingram VM: Hemoglobin and Its Abnormalities. Springfield, IL, Charles C Thomas, Publisher, 1961.
11. Ingram VM: Gene mutations in human haemoglobin: the chemical difference between normal and sickle cell haemoglobin. Nature 1957; 180:326.
12. Conley CL: Sickle cell anemia—the first molecular disease. In Wintrobe MW (ed): Blood Pure and Eloquent. New York, McGraw-Hill Co., 1980, p 319.
13. Ranney HM: Historical milestones. In Emburry SH, Hebbel RP, et al (eds): Sickle Cell Disease: Basic Principles and Clinical Practice. New York, Raven Press, 1994, pp 1–5.
14. Allison AC: Recent developments in the study of inherited anemias. Eugen Q 1959; 6:155.
15. Rucknagel DL, Neel JV: The hemoglobinopathies. In Steinberg AG (ed): Medical Genetics. New York, Grune & Stratton, Inc., 1961.
16. Wiesenfeld SL: Sickle-cell trait in human biological and cultural evolution. Science 1967; 157:1134.
17. Konotey-Ahulu FID, Kuma E: Maintenance of high sickling rate in Africa. Role of polygamy. J Trop Med Hyg 1970; 73:19.
18. Motulsky AG: Frequency of sickling disorders in U.S. blacks. N Engl J Med 1973; 288:31.
19. Kan YW, Dozy, AM: Evolution of the hemoglobin S and C genes in the world populations. Science 1980; 209:388.
20. Antonarakis SE, Boehm CD, et al: Origins of the beta^s-globin gene in blacks: the contribution of recurrent mutations or gene conversion or both. Proc Natl Acad Sci U S A 1984; 81:853.
21. Pagnier J, Mears JG, et al: Evidence for the multicentric origin of the sickle cell hemoglobin gene in Africa. Proc Natl Acad Sci U S A 1984; 81:1771.
22. Wainscoat JS, Bell JT, Thien SL, et al: Multiple origins of the sickle mutation: evidence from beta S globin gene cluster polymorphisms. Mol Biol Med 1983; 1:191.
23. Stine OC, Dover GJ, et al: The evolution of two West African populations. J Mol Evol 1992; 34:336.
24. Lapoumeroulie C, Dunda O, et al: A novel sickle gene of yet another origin in Africa: the Cameroon type. Blood 1989; 74(Suppl 1):63a.
25. Kulozik AE, Haque SK, et al: Geographical survey of beta S globin gene haplotypes: evidence for an independent Asian origin of the sickle cell mutation. Am J Hum Genet 1986; 39:239.
26. Ragusa A, Lombardo M, et al: Beta s gene in Sicily is in linkage disequilibrium with the Benin haplotype: implications for gene flow. Am J Hematol 1988; 27:139.
27. Aluoch JR, Kilinc Y, et al: Sickle cell anaemia among Eti-Turks: haematological, clinical and genetic observations. Br J Haematol 1986; 64:45.
28. Boussio M, Christakis J, et al: The origin of the sickle mutation in Greece: evidence from beta s globin gene cluster polymorphisms. Blood 1987; 70(Suppl 1):59a.
29. Schroeder WA, Powars DR, Kay LM, et al: Beta cluster haplotypes, alpha gene status, and hematological data from SS, SC, and S beta thalassemia patients in southern California. Hemoglobin 1989; 13:325.
30. Hattori Y, Kutlar F, et al: Haplotypes of beta S chromosomes among patients with sickle cell anemia from Georgia. Hemoglobin 1986; 10:623.
31. Nagel RL, Fabry ME, et al: Hematologically and genetically

distinct forms of sickle cell anemia in Africa. N Engl J Med 1985; 312:880.

32. Nagel RL, Rai SK, et al: The hematological characteristics of sickle cell anemia bearing the Bantu haplotype. Blood 1987; 69:1026.

33. Srinivas R, Dunda O, et al: Atypical haplotypes linked to the beta S gene in Africa are likely to be the product of recombination. Am J Hematol 1988; 29:60.

34. Antonarakis S, Boehm CD, et al: Non-random association of polymorphic restriction sites in the β-globin gene cluster. Proc Natl Acad Sci U S A 1982; 79:137.

35. Powars, D, Chan L, Schroeder WA: The variable expression of sickle cell disease is genetically determined. Semin Hematol 1990; 27:360.

36. Perrine RP, Brown MJ, et al: Benign sickle-cell anemia. Lancet 1972; 2:1163.

37. Pembrey ME, Wood WG, et al: Fetal haemoglobin production and the sickle gene in the oases of Eastern Saudi Arabia. Br J Haematol 1978; 40:415.

38. Perrine RP, Pembrey ME, et al: Natural history of sickle cell anaemia in Saudi Arabs. A study of 270 subjects. Ann Intern Med 1978; 88:1.

39. Ali SA: Milder variant of sickle-cell disease in Arabs in Kuwait associated with unusually high level of foetal haemoglobin. Br J Haematol 1970; 19:613.

40. Brittenham G, Lozoff B, et al: Sickle cell anemia and trait in Southern India: further studies. Am J Hematol 1979; 6:107.

41. Weatherall DJ: Common genetic disorders of the red cell and the "malaria hypothesis." Ann Trop Med Parasitol 1987; 81:539.

42. Allison AC: Protection afforded by sickle cell trait against subtertian malarial infection. BMJ 1954; 1:290.

43. Miller MJ, Neel JV, et al: Distribution of parasites in the red cell of sickle trait carriers infected with *Plasmodium falciparum*. Trans R Soc Trop Med Hyg 1956; 50:294.

44. Luzzatto L, Nwachuku-Jarrett ES, et al: Increased sickling of parasitized erythrocytes as mechanism of resistance against malaria in the sickle-cell trait. Lancet 1970; 1:319.

45. Roth FF Jr, Friedman M, et al: Sickling rates of human AS red cells infected *in vitro* with *Plasmodium falciparum* malaria. Science 1978; 202:650.

46. Friedman MV, Trager W: The biochemistry of resistance to malaria. Sci Am 1981; 244:154.

47. Pasvol G, Weatherall DJ: A mechanism for the protective effect of hemoglobin S against *P. falciparum* malaria. Nature 1978; 270:171.

48. Lewis RA, Kay RW, et al: Sickle cell disease and glucose-6-phosphate dehydrogenase deficiency. J Pediatr 1969; 74:544.

49. Piomelli S, Reindorf CA, et al: Interactions of G6PD deficiency and sickle cell anemia. N Engl J Med 1972; 287:213.

50. Beutler E, Johnson C, et al: Prevalence of glucose-6-phosphate dehydrogenase deficiency in sickle cell disease. N Engl J Med 1974; 290:826.

51. Steinberg MH, Dreiling BJ: Glucose-6-phosphate dehydrogenase deficiency in sickle cell anemia. Ann Intern Med 1974; 80:217.

52. Steinberg MH, West S, et al: The Cooperative Study of Sickle Cell Disease. Effects of glucose-6-phosphate dehydrogenase deficiency upon sickle cell anemia. Blood 1988; 71:748.

53. Smits HL, Oski FA, et al: The hemolytic crisis of sickle cell disease: the role of glucose-6-phosphate dehydrogenase deficiency. J Pediatr 1969; 74:544.

54. Harris JW: Studies on the destruction of red blood cells: VII. Molecular orientation in sickle-cell hemoglobin solutions. Proc Soc Exp Biol Med 1950; 75:197.

55. Stetson CA Jr: The state of hemoglobin in sickled erythrocytes. J Exp Med 1986; 123:341.

56. White JG: The fine structure of sickled hemoglobin in situ. Blood 1968; 31:561.

57. Dobler J, Bertles JF: The physical state of hemoglobin in sickle cell anemia erythrocytes *in vivo*. J Exp Med 1968; 127:711.

58. Lessin LS: Helical polymerization of hemoglobin molecules in falciform erythrocytes: a study using unmasking by cold. C R Acad Sci [D] (Paris) 1968; 266:1806.

59. Finch JT, Perutz MF, et al: Structure of sickled erythrocytes and of sickle cell hemoglobin fibers. Proc Natl Acad Sci U S A 1973; 70:718.

60. Dykes G, Grepeau RH, et al: Three-dimensional reconstruction of the fibers of sickle cell hemoglobin. Nature 1978; 272:506.

61. Garrell RL, Grepeau RH, et al: Cross-sectional views of hemoglobin S fibers by electron microscopy and computer modeling. Proc Natl Acad Sci U S A 1979; 76:1140.

62. Dykes G, Grepeau RH, et al: Three-dimensional reconstruction of the 14-filament fibers of hemoglobin S. J Mol Biol 1979; 130:451.

63. Edelstein SJ: Patterns in the quinary structures of proteins. Plasticity and inequivalence of individual molecules in helical arrays of sickle cell hemoglobin and tubulin. Biophys J 1980; 32:34.

64. Magdoff-Fairchild B, Chiu CC: X-ray diffraction studies of fibers and crystals of deoxygenated sickle cell hemoglobin. Proc Natl Acad Sci U S A 1979; 76:233.

65. Rodgers DW, Crepeau RH, Edelstein SJ: Pairings and polarities of the 14 strands in sickle cell hemoglobin fibers. Proc Natl Acad Sci U S A 1987; 84:6157.

66. Carragher B, Bluemke DA, et al: Structural analysis of polymers of sickle cell hemoglobin I. Sickle hemoglobin fibers. J Mol Biol 1988; 199:315.

67. Makowski L, Magdoff-Fairchild M: Polymorphism of sickle cell hemoglobin aggregates: structural basis for limited radial growth. Science 1986; 234:1228.

68. Hofrichter J, Hendericker DG, et al: Structure of hemoglobin S fibers: optical determination of the molecular orientation in sickled erythrocytes. Proc Natl Acad Sci U S A 1973; 70:3604.

69. Wellems TE, Vassar RJ, et al: Polymeric assemblies of double strands of sickle cell hemoglobin. J Mol Biol 1981; 153:1011.

70. Wishner BC, Ward KB, et al: Crystal structure of sickle-cell deoxyhemoglobin at 5 A resolution. J Mol Biol 1975; 98:179.

71. Magdoff-Fairchild B, Rosa LS, et al: Triclinic crystals associated with fibers of deoxygenated sickle hemoglobin. Eur Mol Biol Org J 1982; 1:121.

72. Benesch RE, Uung S, et al: α-Chain contacts in the polymerization of sickle cell hemoglobin. Nature 1976; 260:219.

73. Benesch RE, Kwong S, et al: Location and bond type of intermolecular contacts in the polymerization of hemoglobin S. Nature 1977; 369:772.

74. Creapeau RH, Edelstein SJ, et al: Sickle cell hemoglobin fiber structure altered by α-chain mutation. Proc Natl Acad Sci U S A 1984; 78:1406.

75. Nagel RL, Bookchin RM: Areas of interaction in the Hb S polymer. In Caughey W (ed): Biochemical and Clinical Aspects of Hemoglobin Abnormalities. New York, Academic Press, Inc., 1978, p 195.

76. Nagel RL, Johnson J, et al: β-Chain contact sites in the hemoglobin S polymer. Nature 1980; 283:832.

77. Benesch RE, Kwong S, et al.: The effects of β-chain mutations cis and trans to the β-6 mutation on the polymerization of sickle cell haemoglobin. Nature 1982; 299:231.

78. Rhoda M, Martin J, et al: Sickle cell hemoglobin fiber formation strongly inhibited by the Stanleyville II mutation (α→Lys). Biochem Biophys Res Commun 1983; 111:8.

79. Edelstein SJ: Molecular topology in crystals and fibers of hemoglobin S. J Mol Biol 1981; 150:557.

80. Padalan DA, Love WE: Refined crystal structure of deoxyhemoglobin S: II. Molecular interactions in the crystal. J Biol Chem 1985; 260:8280.

81. Gill SJ, Spokane R, et al: Ligand-linked phase equilibria of sickle cell hemoglobin. J Mol Biol 1980; 140:299.

82. Sunshine HR, Hofrichter J, et al: Oxygen binding by sickle cell hemoglobin polymers. J Mol Biol 1982; 158:251.

83. Ross PD, Hofrichter J, Eaton WA: Calorimetric and optical characterization of sickle cell hemoglobin gelation. J Mol Biol 1975; 96:239.

84. Ross PD, Hofrichter J, Eaton WA: Thermodynamics of gelation of sickle deoxyhemoglobin. J Mol Biol 1977; 115:111.

85. Magdoff-Fairchild B, Poillon WN, et al: Thermodynamic studies of polymerization of deoxygenated sickle cell hemoglobin. Proc Natl Acad Sci U S A 1976; 73:990.

86. Goldberg MA, Husson MA, Bunn HF: The participation of hemoglobins A and F in the polymerization of sickle hemoglobin. J Biol Chem 1977; 252:414.

87. Briehl RW: Gelation of sickle cell hemoglobin: IV. Phase transi-

tions in hemoglobin S gels: separate measures of aggregation and solution-gel equilibrium. J Mol Biol 1978; 123:521.

88. Poillon WN, Bertles JF: Deoxygenated sickle hemoglobin: effects of lyotropic salts on its solubility. J Biol Chem 1979; 254:34.

89. Swerdlow PH, Bryan RA, et al: Effect of 2,3-diphosphoglycerate on the solubility of deoxy sickle hemoglobin. Hemoglobin 1977; 1:527.

90. Pollon WN, Kim BC, Walder JA: Deoxygenated sickle hemoglobin: the effects of 2,3-diphosphoglycerate and inositol hexaphosphate on its solubility. In Beuzard Y, Charache S (eds): Approaches to Therapy of Sickle Cell Anemia. Paris, INSERM, 1986, p 89.

91. Hofrichter J, Ross PD, Eaton WA: Supersaturation in sickle cell hemoglobin solutions. Proc Natl Acad Sci U S A 1976; 73:3035.

92. Hofrichter J, Ross PD, Eaton WA: A physical description of gelation of deoxyhemoglobin S. In Hercules JI, Cottman GL, et al (eds): Molecular and Cellular Aspects of Sickle Cell Disease. DHEW publication No. (NIH)76–1007. Bethesda, MD, National Institutes of Health, 1976, p 185.

93. Hofrichter J: Ligand binding and the gelation of sickle cell hemoglobin. J Mol Biol 1979; 128:335.

94. Wilson WW, Luzzana, MR, et al: Pregelation aggregation of sickle cell hemoglobin. Proc Natl Acad Sci U S A 1974; 71:1260.

95. Moffat K, Gibson QH: The rates of polymerization and depolymerization of sickle cell hemoglobin. Biochem Biophys Res Commun 1974; 61:237.

96. Williams RC: Concerted formation of the gel of hemoglobin S. Proc Natl Acad Sci U S A 1973; 70:1506.

97. Briehl RW, Ewert SM: Gelation of sickle cell hemoglobin: II. Methemoglobin. J Mol Biol 1974; 89:759.

98. Mickols W, Maestre MF, et al: Visualization of oriented hemoglobin S in individual erythrocytes by differential extinction of polarized light. Proc Natl Acad Sci U S A 1985; 82:6527.

99. Beach DA, Bustamante C, et al: Differential polarization imaging: III. Theory confirmation. Patterns of polymerization of hemoglobin S in red blood sickle cells. Biophys J 1987; 52:947.

100. Zipp A, James TL, et al: Water proton magnetic resonance studies of normal and sickle erythrocytes. Temperature and volume dependence. Biochim Biophys Acta 1976; 428:291.

101. Lindstrom TR, Koenig SH, et al: Intermolecular interactions of oxygenated sickle hemoglobin molecules in cell and cell-free solutions. Biophys J 1976; 16:679.

102. Cottman GI, Valentine KM, et al: The gelation of deoxyhemoglobin S in erythrocytes as detected by transverse water proton relaxation measurements. Arch Biochem Biophys 1974; 162:487.

103. Noguchi CT, Torchia DA, et al: Determination of deoxyhemoglobin S polymer in sickle erythrocytes upon deoxygenation. Proc Natl Acad Sci U S A 1980; 77:5487.

104. Ferrone FA: Kinetics of sickle hemoglobin polymerization: II. A double nucleation mechanism. J Mol Biol 1985; 183:611.

105. Eaton WA, Hofrichter J: Hemoglobin S gelation and sickle cell disease. Blood 1987; 70:1245.

106. Rampling MW, Sirs JA: The rate of sickling of cells containing sickle cell hemoglobin. Clin Sci Mol Med 1973; 45:6550.

107. Messer MJ, Hahn JA, et al: The kinetics of sickling and unsickling of red cells under physiologic conditions: rheologic and ultrastructural correlations. Symposium on Molecular and Cellular Aspects of Sickle Cell Disease. DHEW publication No. (NIH)76–1007. Bethesda, MD, National Institutes of Health, 1975.

108. Hahn JA, Messer MJ et al: Ultrastructure sickling and unsickling in the time-lapse studies. Br J Haematol 1976; 34:559.

109. Zarkowsky HS, Hochmuth RM: Sickling times of individual erythrocytes at zero Po_2. J Clin Invest 1975; 56:1023.

110. Coletta M, Hofrichter J, et al: Kinetics of sickle haemoglobin polymerization in single red cells. Nature 1982; 300:194.

111. Adachi K, Asakura T: Multiple nature of polymers of deoxy hemoglobin S prepared by different methods. J Biol Chem 1983; 258:304.

112. Asakura T, Mayberry J: Relationship between morphologic characteristics of sickle cells and methods of deoxygenation. J Lab Clin Med 1984; 104:98.

113. Eaton WA, Hofrichter J, et al: Delay time in gelation: a possible determinant of clinical severity in sickle cell disease. Blood 1976; 47:621.

114. Mozzarelli A, Hofrichter J, Eaton WA: Delay time of hemoglobin S polymerization prevents most cells from sickling in vivo. Science 1987; 237:500.

115. Noguchi CT, Schechter AN: Intracellular polymerization of sickle hemoglobin and its relevance to sickle cell disease. Blood 1981; 58:1057.

116. Noguchi CT, Torchia DA, et al: The intracellular polymerization of sickle hemoglobin: effects of cell heterogeneity. J Clin Invest 1983; 72:846.

117. Green MA, Noguchi CT, Keidan AJ, et al: Polymerization of sickle cell hemoglobin at arterial oxygen saturation impairs erythrocyte deformability. J Clin Invest 1988; 81:1667.

118. Brittenham GM, Schechter AN: Hemoglobin S polymerization: primary determinant of the hemolytic and clinical severity of the sickling syndromes. Blood 1985; 65:183.

119. Keidan AJ, Sowter MC, Johnson CS, et al: Effect of polymerization tendency on hematological, rheological and clinical parameters in sickle cell anaemia. Br J Haematol 1989; 71:551.

120. Sunshine HR, Hofrichter J, et al: Requirements for therapeutic inhibition of sickle haemoglobin gelation. Nature 1978; 275:238.

121. Sunshine HR, Hofrichter J, et al: Gelation of sickle cell hemoglobin in mixtures with normal adult and fetal hemoglobins. J Mol Biol 1979; 133:435.

122. Behe MJ, Englander SW: Mixed gelation theory: kinetics, equilibrium and gel incorporation in sickle hemoglobin mixtures. J Mol Biol 1979; 133:137.

123. Adachi K, Ozguc M, et al: Nucleation-controlled aggregation of deoxyhemoglobin S. J Biol Chem 1980; 255:3092.

124. Adachi K, Segal R, et al: Nucleation-controlled aggregation of deoxyhemoglobin S. J Biol Chem 1980; 255:7595.

125. Cheetham RC, Heuhns ER, et al: Participation of haemoglobins A, F, A2 and C in polymerization of haemoglobin S. J Mol Biol 1979; 129:45.

126. Goldberg MA, Husson MA, et al: Participation of hemoglobins A and F in polymerization of sickle cell hemoglobin. J Biol Chem 1977; 252:3414.

127. Benesch RE, Edalji R, et al: Solubilization of hemoglobin S by other hemoglobins. Proc Natl Acad Sci U S A 1980; 77:5130.

128. Jones MM, Steinhardt J, et al: Evidence of the incorporation of normally non-aggregating hemoglobins into crystalline aggregates of deoxyhemoglobin S. J Biol Chem 1982; 257:1913.

129. Minton AP: Non-ideality and the thermodynamics of sickle-cell hemoglobin gelation. J Mol Biol 1977; 110:89.

130. Sunshine HR: Effects of other hemoglobins on gelation of sickle cell hemoglobin. Tex Rep Biol Med 1981; 40:233.

131. Rodgers GP, Schechter AN, Noguchi CT: Cell heterogeneity in sickle cell disease: quantitation of the erythrocyte density profile. J Lab Clin Med 1985; 106:30.

132. Mohandas N, Kim YR, et al: Accurate and independent measurement of volume and hemoglobin concentration of individual red cells by laser light scattering. Blood 1986; 68:506.

133. Mohandas N, Johnson A, et al: Automated quantitation of cell density distribution and hyperdense cell fraction in RBC disorders. Blood 1990; 75:1192.

134. Kaul DK, Fabry ME, et al: Erythrocytes in sickle cell anemia are heterogeneous in their rheological and hemodynamic characteristics. J Clin Invest 1983; 72:22.

135. Billett HH, Fabry ME, Nagel RL: Hemoglobin distribution width: a rapid assessment of dense red cell in the steady state and during painful crisis in sickle cell anemia. J Lab Clin Med 1988; 112:339.

136. Billett HH, Kim K, et al: The percentage of dense red cells does not predict incidence of sickle cell painful crisis. Blood 1986; 68:301.

137. Noguchi CT, Dover GJ, et al: Alpha thalassemia changes erythrocyte heterogeneity in sickle cell disease. J Clin Invest 1985; 75:1632.

138. Baudin V, Pagnier J, et al: Heterogeneity of sickle cell disease as shown by density profiles: effects of fetal hemoglobin and alpha thalassemia. Haematologica 1986; 19:177.

139. Fabry ME, Kaul DK, et al: SC erythrocytes have an abnormally high intracellular hemoglobin concentration: pathophysiological consequences. J Clin Invest 1982; 70:1315.

140. Boyer SH, Belding TK, et al: Fetal hemoglobin restriction to a few erythrocytes (F cells) in normal human adults. Science 1975; 188:361.

141. Dover GJ, Boyer SH, et al: Individual variation in the production and survival of F cells in sickle cell anemia. N Engl J Med 1978; 299:1428.

142. Bertles JF, Milner PF: Irreversibly sickled erythrocytes: a consequence of the heterogeneous distribution of hemoglobin types in sickle cell anemia. J Clin Invest 1968; 47:1731.

143. Franco RS, Barker-Geor R, et al: Fetal hemoglobin and potassium in isolated transferrin receptor-positive dense sickle reticulocytes. Blood 1994; 84:2013.

144. Lux SE, John KM, et al: Irreversible deformation of the spectrin-actin lattice in irreversibly sickled cells. J Clin Invest 1976; 58:955.

145. Jensen M, Shohet SB, Nathan DG: The role of red cell energy metabolism in the generation of irreversibility sickled cells *in vitro*. Blood 1973; 42:835.

146. Glader BE, Nathan DG: Cation permeability alterations during sickling: relation to cation composition and cellular hydration or irreversibility sickled cells. Blood 1978; 51:983.

147. Ohnishi ST, Horiuchi KY, Horiuchi K: The mechanism *in vitro* formation of irreversibly sickled cells and modes of action of its inhibitors. Biochim Biophys Acta 1986; 886:119.

148. Horiuchi K, Ballas SK, Asakura T: The effect of deoxygenation rate on the formation of irreversibly sickled cells. Blood 1988; 71:46.

149. Serjeant GR, Serjeant BE, et al: The irreversible sickled cell: a determinant of haemolysis in sickle cell anemia. Br J Haematol 1969; 17:527.

150. Serjeant GR: Irreversibly sickled cells and splenomegaly in sickle cell-anemia. Br J Haematol 1970; 19:635.

151. Tosteson DC, Carlsen F, et al: The effects of sickling on ion transport: I. Effect of sickling on potassium transport. J Gen Physiol 1955; 39:31.

152. Tosteson DC: The effects of sickling on ion transport: II. The effect of sickling on sodium and cesium transport. J Gen Physiol 1955; 39:55.

153. Brugnara C: Cation hemostasis. In Embury S, et al (eds): Sickle Cell Disease: Basic Principles and Clinical Practice. New York, Raven Press, 1994, p 173.

154. Mohandas N, Rossi ME, et al: Association between morphologic distortion of sickle cells and deoxygenation-induced cation permeability increase. Blood 1986; 68:450.

155. Joiner CH, Dew A, et al: Deoxygenation-induced cation fluxes in sickle cells: relationship between net potassium efflux and net sodium influx. Blood Cells 1988; 13:339.

156. Joiner CH: Deoxygenation-induced cation fluxes in sickle cells: II. Inhibition by stilbene disulfonates. Blood 1990; 76:212.

157. Clark MR, Rossi ME: Permeability characteristics of deoxygenated sickle cells. Blood 1990; 76:2139.

158. Joiner CH, Morris CL, Cooper ES: Deoxygenation-induced cation fluxes in sickle cells: III. Cation selectivity and response to pH and membrane potential. Am J Physiol 1993; 264:C734.

159. Johnson RM, Gannon SA: Erythrocyte cation permeability induced by mechanical stress: a model for sickle cell cation loss. Am J Physiol 1990; 259:C746.

160. Bookchin RM, Lew VL: Effect of a "sickling pulse" on calcium and potassium transport in sickle cell trait red cells. J Physiol 1981; 312:265.

161. Etzion Z, Tiffert JT, et al: Effects of deoxygenation on active and passive Ca^{2+} transport and on the cytoplasmic Ca^{2+} levels of sickle cell anemia red cells. J Clin Invest 1993; 92:2489.

162. Bookchin RM, Ortiz OE, Lew VL: Evidence for a direct reticulocyte origin of dense red cells in sickle cell anemia. J Clin Invest 1991; 87:113.

163. Fabry M, Romero JR, et al: Rapid increase in red blood cell density driven by the KCl cotransport in a subset of sickle cell anemia reticulocytes and discocytes. Blood 1991; 78:217.

164. Canessa M, Fabry M, et al: Volume-stimulated, Cl-dependent K^+ efflux is highly expressed in young human red cells containing normal hemoglobin of HbS. J Membr Biol 1987; 97:98.

165. Sugihara T, Hebbel RP: Exaggerated cation leak from oxygenated sickle red blood cells during deformation: evidence for a unique leak pathway. Blood 1992; 80:2374.

166. Hebbel RP, Mohandas N: Reversible deformation-dependent erythrocyte cation leak: extreme sensitivity conferred by minimal peroxidation. Biophys J 1991; 60:712.

167. Ney PA, Christopher MM, Hebbel RP: Synergistic effects of oxidation and deformation on erythrocyte monovalent cation leak. Blood 1990; 75:1192.

168. Sugihara T, Rawciz W, et al: Lipid hydroperoxides permit deformation-dependent leak of monovalent cations from erythrocytes. Blood 1991; 77:2757.

169. Hebbel RP, Shalev O, et al: Inhibition of erythrocyte Ca^{2+}-ATPase by activated oxygen through thiol- and lipid-dependent mechanisms. Biochim Biophys Acta 1986; 862:8.

170. Leclerc L, et al: The calmodulin-stimulated (Ca^{2+} + Mg^{2+})-ATPase in hemoglobin S erythrocyte membranes: effects of sickling and oxidative agents. Biochim Biophys Acta 1987; 897:33.

171. Brugnara C, Bunn HF, Tosteson DC: Ion content and transport and the regulation of volume in sickle cells. Ann N Y Acad Sci 1989; 565:96.

172. Olivieri O, Vitoux D, et al: Hemoglobin variants and activity of the (K^+Cl^-) cotransport system in human erythrocytes. Blood 1992; 79:793.

173. Orringer EP, et al: Okadaic acid inhibits activation of K–Cl cotransport in red blood cells containing hemoglobin S and C. Am J Physiol 1991; 261:C591.

174. Caness M, Spalvin A, Nagel RL: Volume-dependent and NEM-stimulated K^+Cl^- transport is elevated in SS, SC and CC human red cells. FEBS Lett 1986; 200:197.

175. Brugnara C, Kopin AK, et al: Regulation of cation content and cell volume in erythrocytes from patients with homozygous hemoglobin C disease. J Clin Invest 1985; 75:1608.

176. Brugnara C, Van Ha T, Tosteson DC: Acid pH induces formation of dense cells in sickle erythrocytes. Blood 1989; 74:487.

177. Brugnara C, deFranceschi L, Alper SL: Inhibition of $Ca(^{2+})$-dependent K^+ transport and cell dehydration in sickle erythrocytes by clotrimazole and other imidazole derivatives. J Clin Invest 1993; 92:520.

178. de Franceschi L, et al: Treatment with oral clotrimazole blocks Ca^+-activated K^+ transport and reverses erythrocyte dehydration in transgenic SAD mice. Blood 1994; 93:1670.

179. Brugnara C, Gee B, Armsby C, et al: Therapy with oral clotrimazole induces inhibition of the Gardos channel and reduction of erythrocyte dehydration in patients with sickle cell disease. J Clin Invest 1996; 97:1227.

180. Itoh T, Chien S, Usami S: Deformability measurements on individual sickle cells using a new system with P_{O_2} and temperature control. Blood 1992; 79:2141.

181. Mackie LH, Hochmuth RM: The influence of oxygen tension, temperature, and hemoglobin concentration on the rheological properties of sickle erythrocytes. Blood 1990; 76:1256.

182. Nash GB, Johnson CS, Meiselman H: Influence of oxygen tension on the viscoelastic behavior of red blood cells in sickle cell disease. Blood 1986; 67:110.

183. Sorette MP, Lavenant MG, Clark MR: Ektacytometric measurement of sickle cell deformability as a continuous function of oxygen tension. Blood 1987; 69:316.

184. Chien S, Usami S, et al: Abnormal rheology of oxygenated blood in sickle cell anemia. J Clin Invest 1970; 49:623.

185. Clark MR, Mohandas N, et al: Deformability of oxygenated irreversibly sickled cells. J Clin Invest 1980; 65:189.

186. Platt OS: Exercise-induced hemolysis in sickle cell anemia: shear sensitivity and erythrocyte dehydration. Blood 1982; 59:1055.

187. Evans E, Mohandas N, et al: Static and dynamic rigidities of normal and sickle erythrocytes, major influence of cell hemoglobin concentration. J Clin Invest 1984; 73:477.

188. Nash GB, Johnson CS, et al: Mechanical properties of oxygenated red blood cells in sickle (HbSS) disease. Blood 1984; 63:73.

189. Shartava A, et al: Posttranslational modification of β–actin contributes to the slow dissociation of the spectrin-protein 4.1-actin complex of irreversibly sickled cells. J Cell Biol 1995; 128:805.

190. Liu SC, Derick LH, Palek J: Dependence of the permanent deformation of red blood cell membranes on spectrin dimer-tetramer equilibrium: implication for permanent membrane deformation of irreversibly sickled cells. Blood 1993; 81:522–28.

191. Corbett JD, Golan DE: Band 3 and glycophorin are progressively aggregated in density-fractionated sickle and normal red blood cells. Evidence from rotational and lateral mobility studies. J Clin Invest 1993; 91:208.

192. Platt OS, Falcone JF: Membrane protein interactions in sickle

red cells: evidence of abnormal protein 3 function. Blood 1995; 85:1992.

193. Platt O, Falcone JF, Lux SE: Molecular defect in the sickle erythrocyte skeleton. Abnormal spectrin binding to sickle inside-out vesicles. J Clin Invest 1985; 75:266.

194. Clark MR, Unger RC, et al: Monovalent cation composition and ATP and lipid content of irreversibly sickled cells. Blood 1978; 51:1169.

195. Westerman MP, Diloy-Puray M, et al: Membrane components in the red cells of patients with sickle cell anemia. Biochem Biophys Acta 1979; 557:149.

196. Sasaki J, Waterman MR, et al: Plasma and erythrocyte lipids in sickle cell anemia. Clin Lab Haematol 1983; 5:35.

197. Haest CWM, Williamson PJ, et al: Interaction between membrane skeleton proteins and the intrinsic domain of the erythrocyte membrane. Biochim Biophys Acta 1982; 694:331.

198. Seigneuret M, Devaux PF: ATP-dependent asymmetric distribution of spin-labeled phospholipids in the erythrocyte membrane: relation to shape changes. Proc Natl Acad Sci U S A 1984; 81:3751.

199. Chiu D, Lubin B, et al: Erythrocyte membrane lipid reorganization during the sickling process. Br J Haematol 1979; 41:223.

200. Lubin B, Chiu D, et al: Abnormalities in membrane phospholipid organization in sickled erythrocytes. J Clin Invest 1981; 67:1643.

201. Franck PFH, Bevers EM, et al: Uncoupling of the membrane skeleton from the lipid bilayer: the cause of accelerated phospholipid flip-flop leading to an enhanced procoagulant activity of sickled cells. J Clin Invest 1985; 75:183.

202. Middlekoop E, Lubin BH, et al: Studies on sickled erythrocytes provide evidence that the asymmetric distribution of phosphatidylserine in the red cell membranes is maintained by both ATP-dependent translocation and interaction with membrane skeletal proteins. Biochim Biophys Acta 1988; 937:281.

203. Chiu D, Lubin B, et al: Sickled erythrocytes accelerate clotting *in vitro:* an effect of abnormal membrane lipid asymmetry. Blood 1981; 58:398.

204. Schwartz RS, Duzgunes N, et al: Interaction of phosphatidylphosphatidycholine liposomes with sickle erythrocytes. J Clin Invest 1982; 71:1570.

205. Kuypers FA, Chiu D, et al: The molecular species composition of phosphatidylcholine affects cellular properties in normal and sickle erythrocytes. Blood 1987; 70:1111.

206. Hoover R, Rubin R, et al: Adhesion of normal and sickle erythrocytes to endothelial monolayer cultures. Blood 1979; 54:872.

207. Hebbel RP, Yamada O, et al: Abnormal adherence of sickle erythrocytes to cultured vascular endothelium: possible mechanism for microvascular occlusion in sickle cell disease. J Clin Invest 1980; 65:154.

208. Hebbel RP, Mohandas N: Sickle cell adherence. In Embury SH, Hebbel RP, et al: (eds): Sickle Cell Disease: Basic Principles and Clinical Practice. New York, Raven Press, 1984, p 217.

209. Hebbel RP, Boogaerts MAB, et al: Erythrocyte adherence to endothelium in sickle-cell anemia: a possible determinant of disease severity. N Engl J Med 1980; 302:992.

210. Wautier JL, Galacteros F, et al: Clinical manifestations and erythrocyte adhesion to endothelium in sickle cell syndrome. Am J Hematol 1985; 19:121.

211. Smith BD, La Celle PL: Erythrocyte-endothelial cell adherence in sickle cell disorders. Blood 1986; 68:1050.

212. Joneckis CC, Ackley RL, et al: Integrin α4β 1 and glycoprotein IV (CD36) are expressed on circulating reticulocytes in sickle cell anemia. Blood 1993; 82:3548.

213. Swerlick RA, Eckman JR, et al. α4αβ1-integrin expression on sickle reticulocytes: vascular cell adhesion molecule-1-dependent binding to endothelium. Blood 1993; 82:1891.

214. Gee B, Platt OS: Sickle reticulocytes adhere to VCAM-1. Blood 1995; 85:268.

215. Patel VP, Ciehanover A, et al: Mammalian reticulocytes lose adhesion to fibronectin during maturation to erythrocytes. Proc Natl Acad Sci U S A 1985; 82:440.

216. Mohandas N, Evans E: Adherence of sickle erythrocytes to vascular endothelial cells: requirement for both cell membrane changes and plasma factors. Blood 1984; 64:282.

217. Mohandas N, Evans E: Sickle erythrocyte adherence to vascular endothelium. J Clin Invest 1985; 76:1605.

218. Kaul DK, Chen D, Zhan J: Adhesion of sickle cells to vascular endothelium is critically dependent on changes in density and shape of the cells. Blood 1994; 83:3006.

219. Morris CL, Rucknagel DL, Joiner CH: Deoxygenation-induced changes in sickle cell–sickle cell adhesion. Blood 1993; 81:3138.

220. Swerlick RA, et al. Human dermal microvascular endothelial but not human umbilical vein endothelial cells express CD36 *in vivo* and *in vitro.* J Immunol 1992; 148:78.

221. Vordermeier S, Singh S, et al: Red blood cells from patients with sickle cell disease exhibit an increased adherence to cultured endothelium pretreated with tumor necrosis factor (TNF). Br J Haematol 1992; 81:591.

222. Hebbel RP, Visser MR, et al: Potentiated adherence of sickle erythrocytes to endothelium infected by virus. J Clin Invest 1987; 80:1503.

223. Smolinski PA, Offerman MK, et al: Double-stranded RNA induces sickle erythrocyte adherence to endothelium: a potential role for viral infection in vaso-occlusive pain episodes in sickle cell anemia. Blood 1995; 85:2945.

224. Francis RB, Hebbel RP: Hemostasis in sickle cell disease. In Embury SH, Hebbel RP, et al: (eds): Basic Principles and Clinical Practice. New York, Raven Press, 1984, p 299.

225. Wick TM, Moake JL, et al: Unusually large von Willebrand factor multimers increase adhesion of sickle erythrocytes to human endothelial cells under controlled flow. J Clin Invest 1987; 80:905.

226. Brittain HA, Eckman JR, Wick TM: Sickle erythrocytes adherence to large vessel and microvascular endothelium under physiologic flow is qualitatively different. J Lab Clin Med 1992; 120:538.

227. Kaul DK, et al: Sickle erythrocyte-endothelial interactions in the microcirculation; the role of von Willebrand factor. Blood 1993; 81:24299.

228. Fabry ME, et al: Demonstration of endothelial adhesion of sickle cells *in vivo:* a distinct role for deformable sickle cell discocytes. Blood 1992; 79:1602.

229. Tsai H-M, Sussman II, et al: Desmopressin induces adhesion of normal human erythrocytes to the endothelial surface of a perfused microvascular preparation. Blood 1990; 75:261.

230. Antonucci R, Walker R, et al: Enhancement of sickle erythrocyte adherence to endothelium by autologous platelets. Am J Hematol 1990; 34:44.

231. Sugihara K, Sugihara T, et al: Thrombospondin mediates adherence of CD36 + sickle reticulocytes to endothelial cells. Blood 1992; 80:2634.

232. Brittain HA, Eckman JR, et al: Thrombospondin from activated platelets promotes sickle erythrocyte adherence to human microvascular endothelium under physiologic flow: a potential role for platelet activation in sickle cell vaso-occlusion. Blood 1993; 81:2137.

233. Shaklai N, Yguerabide J, et al: Interaction of hemoglobin with red blood cell membranes as shown by a fluorescent chromophore. Biochemistry 1977; 16:5585.

234. Shaklai N, Yguerabide J, et al: Classification and localization of hemoglobin binding sites on the red blood cell membrane. Biochemistry 1977; 16:5593.

235. Eisinger J, Flores J: Cytosol membrane interface of the human erythrocyte. A resonance energy transfer study. Biophys J 1983; 41:367.

236. Eisinger J, Flores J, et al: Association of cytosol hemoglobin with the membrane in intact erythrocytes. Proc Natl Acad Sci U S A 1982; 79:408.

237. Cassoly R: Quantitative analysis of the association of human hemoglobin with the cytoplasmic portion of band 3 protein. J Biol Chem 1983; 258:3859.

238. Salhany JM, Cordes KA, et al: Light scattering measurements of hemoglobin binding to the erythrocyte membrane. Evidence for transmembrane effects related to a disulfic stilbene binding to band 3. Biochemistry 1980; 19:1447.

239. Sayare M, Schuster TM: Association of hemoglobins A and S with the cytoplasmic surface of the erythrocyte membrane. Fed Proc Am Soc Exp Biol 1980; 39:1916.

240. Szundi I, Szeleny JG, et al: Interactions of hemoglobin with erythrocyte phospholipids in monomolecular lipid layers. Biochim Biophys Acta 1980; 595:41.

241. Liu SC, Palek J: Hemoglobin enhances spectrin dimer association at physiological conditions. Blood 1982; 60:22a.
242. Fischer S, Nagel RL, et al: The binding of hemoglobin to membranes of normal and sickle erythrocytes. Biochem Biophys Acta 1975; 375:422.
243. Klipstein FA, Ranney HM: Electrophoretic components of the hemoglobin of red cell membranes. J Clin Invest 1960; 39:1894.
244. Bank A, Mears G, et al: Preferential binding of S globin chains associated with stroma in sickle cell disorder. J Clin Invest 1974; 54:805.
245. Shaklai N, Ranney MH: Interaction of sickle cell hemoglobin with erythrocyte membranes. Proc Natl Acad Sci U S A 1981; 78:65.
246. Fung LWM, Litvin SD, et al: Spin-label detection of sickle hemoglobin-membrane interaction at physiological pH. Biochemistry 1983; 22:864.
247. Evans EA, Mohandas H: Membrane-associated sickle hemoglobin: A major determinant of sickle erythrocyte rigidity. Blood 1987; 70:1443.
248. Fortier N, Snyder M, Garver F, et al: The relationship between in vivo generated hemoglobin skeletal protein complex and increased red cell membrane rigidity. Blood 1988; 71:1427.
249. Asakura T, Agarwal PL, et al: Mechanical instability of the sickle hemoglobin. Nature 1973; 244:437.
250. Asakura T, Minakata K, et al: Denatured hemoglobin in sickle erythrocytes. J Clin Invest 1977; 59:633.
251. Schluter K, Drenckhahn D: Co-clustering of denatured hemoglobin with band 3: its role in binding autoantibodies against band 3 to abnormal and aged erythrocytes. Proc Natl Acad Sci U S A 1986; 83:6137.
252. Waugh SM, Willardson BM, Kannan R, et al: Heinz bodies induce clustering of band 3, glycophorin, and ankyrin in sickle cell erythrocytes. J Clin Invest 1986; 78:1155.
253. Green GA, Kalra VK: Sickling-induced binding of immunoglobulin to sickle erythrocytes. Blood 1988; 71:636.
254. Petz LO, Yam P, et al: Increased IgG molecules bound to the surface of red blood cells of patients with sickle cell anemia. Blood 1984; 64:301.
255. Kay MM: Mechanisms of removal of senescent cells by human macrophages in situ. Proc Natl Acad Sci U S A 1975; 72:3521.
256. Kay MM, Sorenson BK, et al: Antigenicity, storage, and aging: physiologic autoantibodies to cell membrane and serum proteins and the senescent cell antigen. Mol Cell Biochem 1982; 49:65.
257. Hebbel RP, Miller WJ: Phagocytosis of sickle erythrocytes: immunologic and oxidative determinants of hemolytic anemia. Blood 1984; 64:733.
258. Hebbel RP, Morgan WT, et al: Accelerated autoxidation and heme loss due to instability of sickle hemoglobin. Proc Natl Acad Sci U S A 1988; 85:237.
259. Hebbel RP, Eaton JW, et al: Spontaneous oxygen radical generation by sickling erythrocytes. J Clin Invest 1982; 70:1253.
260. Hebbel RP: The sickle erythrocyte in double jeopardy: autoxidation and iron decompartmentalization. Semin Hematol 1990; 27:51.
261. Schneider RG, Takeda I, et al: Intraerythrocytic precipitations of haemoglobins S and C. Nature 1972; 235:88.
262. Kim HC, Friedman S, et al: Inclusions in red blood cells containing HbS or HbC. Br J Haematol 1980; 44:547.
263. Liu S-C, Zhai S, Palek J: Detection of hemin release during hemoglobin S denaturation. Blood 1988; 71:1755.
264. Campwala HQ, Desforges JF: Membrane-bound hemochrome in density-separated cohorts of normal (AA) and sickled (SS) cells. J Lab Clin Med 1982; 99:25.
265. Kuross SA, Hebbel RP: Nonheme iron in sickle erythrocyte membranes: association with phospholipids and potential role in lipid peroxidation. Blood 1988; 72:1278.
266. Das SK, Nair RC: Superoxide dismutase, glutathione peroxidase, catalase, and lipid peroxidation of normal and sickled erythrocytes. Br J Haematol 1963; 44:87.
267. Jain SK, Shohet SB: A novel phospholipid in irreversibly sickled cells: evidence for in vivo peroxidative membrane damage in sickle cell disease. Blood 1984; 63:362.
268. Repka T, Shalev O, et al: Nonrandom association of free iron with membranes of sickle and beta-thalassemic erythrocytes. Blood 1993; 82:3204.
269. Sugihara T, Repka T, Hebbel RP: Detection, characterization, and bioavailability of membrane-associated iron in the intact sickle red cell. J Clin Invest 1992; 90:2327.
270. Repka T, Hebbel RP: Hydroxyl radical formation by sickle erythrocyte membranes: role of pathologic iron deposits and cytoplasmic reducing agents. Blood 1991; 78:2753.
271. Johnson FL, Look AT, et al: Bone marrow transplantation in a patient with sickle cell anemia. N Engl J Med 1987; 31:964.
272. Vermylen C, Ninane J, et al: Bone marrow transplantation in five children with sickle cell anemia. Lancet 1988; 2:1427.
273. Johnson FL, Mentzer WC, et al: The United States experience. Am J Pediatr Hematol Oncol 1994; 16:22.
274. Vermylen C, Cornu G: Bone marrow transplantation for sickle cell disease. The European experience. Am J Pediatr Hematol Oncol 1994; 16:18.
274a. Walters MC, Patience M, et al: Bone marrow transplantation for sickle cell disease. N Engl J Med 1996; 335:369.
275. Walters MC, Sullivan KM, et al: Neurologic complications after allogeneic marrow transplantation for sickle cell anemia. Blood 1995; 85:879.
276. Abboud MR, Jackson SM, et al: Bone marrow transplantation for sickle cell anemia. Am J Pediatr Hematol Oncol 1994; 16:86.
277. Ferster A, Bujan W, et al: Bone marrow transplantation corrects the splenic reticuloendothelial dysfunction in sickle cell anemia. Blood 1993; 81:1102.
278. Mentzer WC, Heller S, et al: Availability of related donors for bone marrow transplantation in sickle cell anemia. Am J Pediatr Hematol Oncol 1994; 16:27.
279. Kodish E, Lantos J, et al: Bone marrow transplantation for sickle cell disease. A study of parents' decisions. N Engl J Med 1991; 325:1349.
280. Ley TJ, De Simone J, et al: 5-Azacytidine selectively increases gamma-globin synthesis in a patient with β+ thalassemia. N Engl J Med 1982; 307:1469.
281. Charache S, Dover G, et al: Treatment of sickle cell anemia with 5-azacytidine results in increased fetal hemoglobin production and is associated with non-random hypomethylation of DNA around the gamma-delta-beta-globin gene complex. Proc Natl Acad Sci U S A 1983; 80:4842.
282. Ley TJ, De Simone J, et al: 5-Azacytidine increases gamma globin synthesis and reduces the proportion of dense cells in patients with sickle cell anemia. Blood 1983; 62:370.
283. Dover GJ, Charache SH, et al: 5-Azacytidine increases HbF production and reduces anemia in sickle cell disease. Dose response and analysis of subcutaneous and oral dosage regimens. Blood 1985; 66:527.
284. Platt OS, Orkin SH, et al: Hydroxyurea enhances fetal hemoglobin production in sickle cell anemia. J Clin Invest 1984; 74:652.
285. Dover GJ, Humphries RK, et al: Hydroxyurea induction of hemoglobin F production in sickle cell disease: relationship between cytotoxicity and F cell production. Blood 1986; 67:735.
286. Charache SH, Dover GJ, et al: Hydroxyurea-induced augmentation of fetal hemoglobin production in patients with sickle cell anemia. Blood 1987; 69:109.
287. Bunn HF: Reversing ontogeny. N Engl J Med 1993; 328:129.
288. Rodgers GP, Dover GJ, et al: Hematological responses of sickled cell patients treated with hydroxyurea. N Engl J Med 1990; 322:1037.
289. Stamatoyannopoulos G, Umemura T, et al: Modulation of fetal hemoglobin production by erythropoietin. In Stamatoyannopoulos G, Nienhuis AW (eds): Hemoglobin Switching Part B: Cellular and Molecular Mechanisms. New York, Alan R. Liss, Inc., 1989, p 269.
290. Goldberg MA, Brugnara C, et al: Treatment of sickle cell anemia with hydroxyurea and erythropoietin. N Engl J Med 1990; 323:366.
291. Rogers EP, Dover GJ, et al: Augmentation by erythropoietin of fetal hemoglobin response to hydroxyurea in sickle cell disease. N Engl J Med 1993; 328:73.
292. Perrine SP, Ginder GD, Faler DV, et al: A short term trial of butyrate to stimulate fetal globin-gene expression in the β-globin disorders. N Engl J Med 1993; 328:81.
293. Dover GJ, Brusilow SW, Charrache S: Induction of HbF production in subjects with sickle cell anemia by oral sodium phenylbutyrate. Blood 1994; 84:339.

294. Collins AF, Dover GJ, Luban NLC: Increased fetal hemoglobin production in patients receiving valponic acid for epilepsy. Blood 1995; 85:1690.

295. Sher GD, Oliveri NF: Rapid healing of chronic leg ulcers during arginine butyrate therapy. Blood 1995; 85:2398.

295a. Bunn HF: Reversing ontogeny. N Engl J Med 1993; 328:129.

296. Platt OS, et al: Pain in sickle cell diseases: rate and risk factors. N Engl J Med 1991; 325:11.

297. Charache S, Terrin ML, et al: Controlled clinical trials. Effect of hydroxyurea on the frequency of painful crises in sickle cell anemia. N Engl J Med 1995; 332:1317.

298. Scott JP, Hillery CA, et al: Hydroxyurea therapy in children severely affected with sickle cell disease. J Pediatr 1996; 128:820.

299. Vichinsky EP, Lubin BH: A cautionary note regarding hydroxyurea in sickle cell disease. Blood 1994; 83:1124.

300. Rosa R, Bierer BE, et al: A study of hyponatremia in the prevention and treatment of sickle cell crises. N Engl J Med 1980; 303:1138.

301. Leary M, Abramson N: Induced hyponatremia for sickle cell crisis. N Engl J Med 1981; 304:844.

302. Charache S, Walker WG: Failure of desmopressin to lower serum sodium or prevent crisis in patients with sickle cell anemia. Blood 1981; 58:892.

303. Charache S, Moyer MA, et al: Treatment of acute sickle cell crises with a vasopressin analogue. Am J Hematol 1983; 15:315.

304. Clark MR, Mohandas N, et al: Hydration of sickle cells using the sodium ionophore monensin. J Clin Invest 1982; 70:1074.

305. Chang H, Nagel RL, et al: Comparative evaluation of fifteen anti-sickling agents. Blood 1983; 61:693.

306. Ohnishi TS, Horiuchi KY, et al: Nitrendipine, nifedipine and verapamil inhibit the *in vitro* formation of irreversible sickled cells. Pharmacology 1986; 32:248.

307. Schmidt WF, Asakura T, et al: Effect of cetiedil on cation and water movements in erythrocytes. J Clin Invest 1982; 69:589.

308. Peterson CM, Tsairis P, et al: Sodium cyanate–induced polyneuropathy in patients with sickle cell disease. Ann Intern Med 1974; 81:152.

309. Charache S, Duffy TR, et al: Toxic-therapeutic ratio of sodium cyanate. Arch Intern Med 1975; 135:1043.

310. Rogers GP, Schechter A, et al: Microcirculatory adaptation in sickle cell anemia. Am J Physiol 1990; 258:113.

311. Kan YW, Dozy AM: Polymorphism of DNA sequence adjacent to human β-globin structural gene: relationship to sickle mutation. Proc Natl Acad Sci U S A 1978; 75:5631.

312. Wilson JT, Milner PF, et al: Use of restriction endonucleases for mapping the beta-s-allele. Proc Natl Acad Sci U S A 1982; 79:3628.

313. Chang JC, Kan YW: A sensitive new prenatal test for sickle cell anemia. N Engl J Med 1982; 307:30.

314. Orkin SH, Little PFR, et al: Improved detection of the sickle mutation by DNA analysis. N Engl J Med 1982; 307:32.

315. Wallace RB, Schold M, et al: Oligonucleotide-directed mutagenesis of the human beta-globin gene: a general method for producing specific point mutations in cloned DNA. Nucleic Acids Res 1981; 9:3647.

316. Conner BJ, Reyes AA, et al: Detection of sickle cell beta-s-globin allele by hybridization with synthetic oligonucleotides. Proc Natl Acad Sci U S A 1983; 80:278.

317. Studencki AB, Conner BJ, et al: Prenatal diagnosis of beta-thalassemia: detection of a single mutation in DNA. N Engl J Med 1983; 309:284.

318. Saiki RK, Chang CA, et al: Diagnosis of sickle cell anemia and beta-thalassemia with enzymatically amplified DNA and non-radioactive allele specific oligonucleotides probes. N Engl J Med 1988; 319:537.

319. Cheehbab FF, Kan YW: Detection of sickle cell anemia by colour DNA amplification. Lancet 1990; 335:15.

320. Saiki RK, Scharf S, et al: Enzymatic amplification of beta-globin genomic sequences and restriction site analysis for diagnosis of sickle cell anemia. Science 1985; 230:1350.

321. Embury SH, Scharf SJ, et al: Rapid prenatal diagnosis of sickle cell anemia by a new method of DNA analysis. N Engl J Med 1987; 316:656.

322. Gossens M, Dumez Y, et al: Prenatal diagnosis of sickle-cell anemia in the first trimester of pregnancy. N Engl J Med 1983; 309:831.

323. Old JM, Fitches A, et al: First-trimester fetal diagnosis for haemoglobinopathies: report on 200 cases. Lancet 1986; 2:763.

324. Newborn Screening for Sickle Cell Disease and Other Hemoglobinopathies. Consensus Development Conference Statement. Bethesda, MD, National Institutes of Health, 1987.

325. Schneider RG, Gustafson LP, Haggard ME: The incidence of genetically determined abnormalities in 11,427 cord blood samples. Presented at the 13th International Congress of Haematology, Munich, August 1970.

326. Gilman PA, McFarlane JM, Huisman TJ: Natural history of sickle cell anemia: re-evaluation of a 15 year cord blood testing program. Pediatr Res 1976; 10:376.

327. Serjeant G, Grandison Y, et al: The development of hematological changes in homozygous sickle cell disease: a cohort study from birth to six years. Br J Haematol 1981; 48:533.

328. Pearson HA: A neonatal program for sickle cell anemia. Adv Pediatr 1986; 33:381.

329. Jinks DC, Minter M, et al: Molecular genetic diagnosis of sickle cell disease using dried blood specimens on blotters used for newborn screening. Hum Genet 1989; 81:363.

330. Powars D: Diagnosis at birth improves survival of children with sickle cell anemia. Pediatrics 1989; 83:830.

331. Grover R: Program effects on decreasing morbidity and mortality: newborn screening in New York City. Pediatrics 1989; 83:819.

332. Gill FM, Brown A, et al: Newborn experience in the cooperative study of sickle cell disease. Pediatrics 1989; 83:827.

333. Sprinkle RH, Hynes DM, Knorad TR: Is universal neonatal Hemoglobinopath screening cost effective? Arch Pediatr Adolesc Med 1994; 148:461.

334. Brown AK, Sleeper LA, et al: Reference values and hematologic changes from birth to 5 years in patients with sickle cell disease. Arch Pediatr Adolesc Med 1994; 148:796.

335. O'Brien RT, McIntosh S, et al: Prospective study of sickle cell anemia in infancy. J Pediatr 1976; 89:205.

336. Serjeant GR: Sickle Cell Disease. Oxford, Oxford University Press, Inc., 1985.

337. Embury SH, Hebbel RP, et al: Sickle Cell Disease: Basic Principles and Clinical Practice. New York, Raven Press, 1994.

338. Charache S, Lubin B, Reid C (eds): Management and Therapy of Sickle Cell Disease. NIH publication No. 89–2117. Bethesda, MD, National Institutes of Health, 1989.

339. Diggs LW: Sickle cell crises. Am J Clin Pathol 1965; 441:1.

340. Gill FM, Sleeper LA, et al: Clinical events in the first decade in a cohort of infants with sickle cell disease. Blood 1995; 86:776.

341. Bainbridge R, Higgs DR, et al: Clinical presentation of homozygous sickle cell disease. J Pediatr 1985; 106:881.

342. Konotey-Ahulu FI: The sickle cell diseases. Arch Intern Med 1974; 133:611.

343. Platt OS, et al: Mortality in sickle cell disease. Life expectancy and risk factors for early death. N Engl J Med 1994; 330:1639.

344. Redwood AM, Williams EM, et al: Climate and painful crises of sickle cell disease in Jamaica. BMJ 1976; 1:66.

345. Ibrahim AS: Relationship between meteorological changes and occurrence of painful sickle cell crises in Kuwait. Trans R Soc Trop Med Hyg 1980; 74:159.

346. Milner PF, Brown M, et al: Bone marrow infarction in sickle cell anemia: correlation with hematologic profiles. Blood 1982; 60:1411.

347. Charache S, Page DL: Infarction of bone marrow in the sickle cell disorders. Ann Intern Med 1967; 67:1195.

348. Mankad VN, Williams JP, et al: Magnetic resonance imaging of bone marrow in sickle cell disease: clinical, hematologic, and pathologic correlations. Blood 1990; 75:274.

349. Diggs LW: Bone and joint lesions in sickle-cell disease. Clin Orthop 1967; 51:119.

350. Keeley K, Buchanan GR: Acute infarction of long bones in children with sickle cell anemia. J Pediatr 1982; 101:170.

351. Sain A, Sham R, et al: Bone scan in sickle cell crisis. Clin Nucl Med 1978; 3:85.

352. Alavi A, Schumacher HR, et al: Bone marrow scan evaluation of arthropathy in sickle cell disorders. Arch Intern Med 1976; 136:436.

353. Hammel CF, DeNardo SJ, et al: Bone marrow and bone mineral scintigraphic studies in sickle cell disease. Br J Haematol 1973; 25:593.

354. Lutzker LG, Alavi A: Bone and marrow imaging in sickle cell disease: diagnosis of infarction. Semin Nucl Med 1976; 6:83.

355. Kahn CE, Ryan JW, et al: Combined bone marrow and gallium imaging differentiation of osteomyelitis and infarction in sickle hemoglobinopathy. Clin Nucl Med 1988; 13:433.

356. Fernadez-Ulloa M, Vasavada PJ, Black RR: Detection of acute osteomyelitis with indium-111 labeled white blood cells in a patient with sickle cell disease. Clin Nucl Med 1989; 14:97.

357. Rao VM, Solomon N, et al: Scintigraphic differentiation of bone infarction from osteomyelitis in children with sickle cell disease. J Pediatr 1985; 107:685.

358. Kim HC, Alavi A, et al: Differentiation of bone marrow infarcts from osteomyelitis in sickle cell disorders. Clin Nucl Med 1989; 14:249.

359. Guze BH, Hawkins RA, Marcus CS: Technetium-99m white blood cell imaging: false-negative results in Salmonella osteomyelitis associated with sickle cell disease. Clin Nucl Med 1989; 14:104.

360. Cole TB, Smith SJ, Buchanan GR: Hematologic alterations during acute infection in children with sickle cell disease. Pediatr Infect Dis J 1987; 6:454.

361. Syrogiannopoulos GA, McCracken GH, Nelson JD: Osteoarticular infections in children with sickle cell disease. Pediatrics 1986; 78:1090.

362. Stuart J, Stone PC, et al: Monitoring the acute phase response to vaso-occlusive crisis in sickle cell disease. J Clin Pathol 1994; 47:166.

363. Devine D, Kinney T, et al: Fragment D-dimer levels: an objective marker of vaso-occlusive crisis and other complications of sickle cell disease. Blood 1986; 68:317.

364. Francis RB Jr: Elevated fibrin D-dimer fragment in sickle cell anemia: evidence for activation of coagulation during the steady state as well as in painful crisis. Haemostasis 1989; 19:105.

365. Ballas SK, Smith ED: Red blood cell changes during the evolution of the sickle cell painful crisis. Blood 1992; 79:2154.

366. Griffin TC, McIntire D, Buchanan GR: High-dose intravenous methylprednisolone therapy for pain in children and adolescents with sickle cell disease. N Engl J Med 1994; 330:733.

367. Greenberg J, Ohene-Frempong K, et al: Trial of low doses of aspirin as prophylaxis in sickle cell disease. J Pediatr 1983; 102:781.

368. Watson RJ, Burko H, et al: The hand-foot syndrome in sickle-cell disease in young children. Pediatrics 1963; 45:975.

369. Worrell VT, Batera V: Sickle cell dactylitis. J Bone Joint Surg [Am] 1976; 58:1161.

370. Serjeant GR, Ashcroft MT: Shortening of the digits in sickle cell anemia: a sequela of the hand-foot syndrome. Trop Geogr Med 1971; 23:341.

371. Castro O, Brambilla DJ, et al: The acute chest syndrome in sickle cell disease: incidence and risk factors. Blood 1994; 84:643.

372. Thomas AN, Pattison C, Serjeant GR: Causes of death in sickle-cell disease in Jamaica. BMJ [Clin Res] 1982; 285:633.

373. Barrett-Connor E: Acute pulmonary disease and sickle cell anemia. Am Rev Respir Dis 1971; 104:159.

374. Barrett-Connor E: Acute pulmonary infarction in sickle cell anemia. JAMA 1973; 224:997.

375. Poncz M, Kane E, Gill FM: Acute chest syndrome in sickle cell disease: etiology and clinical correlates. J Pediatr 1985; 107:861.

376. Petch MC, Serjeant GR: Clinical features of pulmonary lesions in sickle cell anemia. BMJ 1970; 3:31.

377. Davies SC, Luce PJ, et al: Acute chest syndrome in sickle cell disease. Lancet 1984; 1:36.

378. DeCeulaer K, McMullen KW, et al: Pneumonia in young children with homozygous sickle cell disease: risk and clinical features. Eur J Pediatr 1985; 144:255.

379. Sprinkle RH, Cole T, et al: Acute chest syndrome in children with sickle cell disease. Am J Pediatr Hematol Oncol 1986; 8:105.

380. Vichinsky E, Williams R, et al: Pulmonary fat embolism: a distinct cause of severe acute chest syndrome in sickle cell anemia. Blood 1994; 83:3107.

381. Gelfand MJ, Shashikant AD, et al: Simultaneous occurrence of rib infarction and pulmonary infiltrates in sickle cell disease patients with acute chest syndrome. J Nucl Med 1993; 34:614.

382. Rackoff WR, Kunkel N, et al: Pulse oximetry and factors associated with hemoglobin oxygen desaturation in children with sickle cell disease. Blood 1993; 81:3422.

383. Emre U, Miller ST, et al: Alveolar-arterial oxygen gradient in acute chest syndrome of sickle cell disease. J Pediatr 1993; 123:272.

384. Bellet PS, Kalinyak RA, et al: Incentive spirometry to prevent acute pulmonary complications in sickle cell disease. N Engl J Med 1995; 333:699.

385. Lanzkowsky P, Sherde A, et al: Partial exchange transfusion in sickle cell anemia: use in children with serious complications. Am J Dis Child 1978; 132:1286.

386. Buchanan GR, Glader BE: Benign course of extreme hyperbilirubinemia in sickle cell anemia. Analysis of six cases. J Pediatr 1977; 91:21.

387. Sheehy TW: Sickle cell hepatopathy. South Med J 1977; 70:533.

388. Mintz AA, Church G, et al: Cholelithiasis in sickle cell anemia. J Pediatr 1955; 47:171.

389. Serafini AN, Spoilansky G, et al: Diagnostic studies in patients with sickle cell anemia and acute abdominal pain. Arch Intern Med 1987; 147:1061.

390. Stephens CG, Scott RB: Cholelithiasis in sickle cell anemia: surgical or medical management. Arch Intern Med 1980; 140:648.

391. Powars D, Wilson B, et al: The natural history of stroke in sickle cell disease. Am J Med 1978; 65:461.

392. Balkaran B, Char G, et al: Stroke in a cohort of patients with homozygous sickle cell disease. J Pediatr 1992; 120:360.

393. Frempong KO: Stroke in sickle cell disease: demographic, clinical and therapeutic considerations. Semin Hematol 1991; 28:213.

394. Russell, MO, Goldberg HI, et al: Effect of transfusion therapy on arteriographic abnormalities and on recurrence of stroke in sickle cell disease. Blood 1984; 63:162.

395. Stockman JA, Nigro MA, et al: Occlusion of large cerebral vessels in sickle cell anemia. N Engl J Med 1972; 287:846.

396. Wilimas J, Goff JR, et al: Efficacy of transfusion theory for one to two years in patients with sickle cell disease and cerebrovascular accidents. J Pediatr 1980; 96:205.

397. Boros L, Thomas C, et al: Large cerebral vessel disease in sickle cell anemia. J Neurol Neurosurg Psychiatry 1976; 39:1236.

398. Merkel KH, Ginsberg PL, et al: Cerebrovascular disease in sickle cell anemia: a clinical, pathological and radiological correlation. Stroke 1978; 9:45.

399. Adams RJ: Neurologic complications. In Embury SH, Hebbel RP, et al (eds): Sickle Cell Disease: Basic Principles and Clinical Practice. New York, Raven Press, 1984, p 599.

400. Pavlakis SG, Bellos J, et al: Brain infarction in sickle cell anemia: magnetic resonance imaging correlates. Ann Neurol 1988; 23:125.

401. Adams RJ, Nichols FT, et al: Cerebral infarction in sickle cell anemia: mechanism based on CT and MRI. Neurology 1988; 38:1012.

402. Herold S, Brozovic M, et al: Measurement of regional cerebral flow, blood volume and oxygen metabolism in patients with sickle cell disease using position emission tomography. Stroke 1986; 17:692.

403. Wiznitzer M, Masaryk TJ: Cerebrovascular abnormalities in pediatric stroke: assessment using parenchymal and angiographic magnetic resonance imaging. Ann Neurol 1991; 29:585.

404. Russell MO, Goldberg HI, et al: Transfusion therapy for cerebrovascular abnormalities in sickle cell disease. J Pediatr 1976; 88:382.

405. Lusher JM, Haghighat H, et al: A prophylactic transfusion program for children with sickle cell anemia complicated by CNS infarction. Am J Hematol 1976; 1:265.

406. Seeler RA, Royal JE: Commentary: Sickle cell anemia, stroke, and transfusion. J Pediatr 1980; 96:243.

407. Wang WC, Kavaar EH, et al: High risk of recurrent stroke after discontinuance of five to twelve years of transfusion therapy in patients with sickle cell disease. J Pediatr 1991; 118:377.

408. Cohen AR, Martin MB, et al: A modified transfusion program for prevention of stroke in sickle cell disease. Blood 1992; 79:1657.

409. Adams R, McKie V, et al: The use of transcranial ultrasonography to predict stroke in sickle cell disease. N Engl J Med 1992; 326:605.

410. Kugler S, Anderson B, et al: Abnormal cranial magnetic resonance imaging scans in sickle-cell disease. Neurological correlates and clinical implications. Arch Neurol 1993; 50:629.

411. Van Hogg J, Ritchey AK, Shaywitz BA: Intracranial hemorrhage in children with sickle cell disease. Am J Dis Child 1985; 139:1120.

412. Oyesiku NM, Barrow DL, et al: Intracranial aneurysms in sickle cell anemia: clinical features and pathogenesis. J Neurosurg 1991; 75:552.

413. Anson JA, Koshy M, et al: Subarachnoid hemorrhage in sickle cell disease. J Neurosurg 1991; 75:552.

414. Emond AM, Holman R, et al: Priapism and impotence in homozygous sickle cell disease. Arch Intern Med 1980; 140:1434.

415. Sharpstein JR, Powars D, et al: Multisystem damage associated with tricorporal priapism in sickle cell disease. Am J Med 1993; 94:289.

416. Seeler RA: Intensive transfusion therapy for priapism in boys with sickle cell anemia. J Urol 1973; 110:360.

417. Grace DA, Winter CC: Priapism: an appraisal of management of twenty-three patients. J Urol 1968; 99:301.

418. Karayalcin G, Imran M, et al: Priapism in sickle cell disease: report of five cases. Am J Med Sci 1972; 264:289.

419. Rifkind S, Waisman J, et al: RBC exchange pheresis for priapism in sickle cell disease. JAMA 1979; 242:2317.

420. Walker EM Jr, Mitchum EN, et al: Automated erythrocytapheresis for relief of priapism in sickle cell hemoglobinopathies. J Urol 1969; 101:71.

421. Rackoff WR, Ohene-Frempong K, et al: Neurologic events after partial exchange transfusion for priapism in sickle cell disease. J Pediatr 1992; 120:882.

422. Campbell JH, Cummings SD: Priapism in sickle cell anemia. J Urol 1969; 101:71.

423. Kinney TR, Harris MB, et al: Priapism in association with sickle hemoglobinopathies in children. J Pediatr 1975; 86:241.

424. Howe GE, Prentiss RJ, et al: Priapism: a surgical emergency. J Urol 1969; 101:576.

425. Hasen HB, Raines SL: Priapism associated with sickle cell disease. J Urol 1962; 88:71.

426. Noe HN, Wilimas J, et al: Surgical management of priapism in children with sickle cell anemia. J Urol 1981; 126:770.

427. Seeler RA: Deaths in children with sickle cell anemia: a clinical analysis of 19 fatal instances in Chicago. Clin Pediatr 1972; 11:634.

428. Pearson HA: Hemoglobin S thalassemia syndrome in Negro children. Ann N Y Acad Sci 1969; 165:83.

429. Pappo A, Buchanan GR: Acute splenic sequestration in a 2-month-old infant with sickle cell anemia. Pediatrics 1989; 84:578.

430. Emond AM, Collis R, et al: Acute splenic sequestration in homozygous sickle cell disease: natural history and management. J Pediatr 1985; 107:201.

431. Seeler RA, Shiwiaki MZ: Acute splenic sequestration crises (ASSC) in young children with sickle cell anemia. Clin Pediatr 1972; 11:701.

432. Rao S, Gooden S: Splenic sequestration in sickle cell disease: role of transfusion therapy. Am J Pediatr Hematol Oncol, Brief Reports, Fall 1985, pp 298–301.

433. Kinney TR, Ware RE, et al: Long-term management of splenic sequestration in children with sickle cell disease. J Pediatr 1990; 117:194.

434. Simmons JF, Gilani D, et al: The pattern of mortality in sickle cell disease. Presented at the National Sickle Cell Conference. San Juan, Puerto Rico, November 1978.

435. Jenkins ME, Scott RB, et al: Studies in sickle cell anemia: XVI. Sudden death during sickle cell anemia crises in young children. J Pediatr 1960; 56:30.

436. MacIver JE, Parker-Williams EJ: Aplastic crisis in sickle-cell anemia. Lancet 1961; 1:1086.

437. Singer K, Motulsky AG, et al: Aplastic crisis in sickle cell anemia. J Lab Clin Med 1950; 35:721.

438. Leikin SL: The aplastic crisis of sickle cell disease: occurrence in several members of families within a short period of time. Am J Dis Child 1957; 93:128.

439. Serjeant GR, Manson K, et al: Outbreak of aplastic crises in sickle cell anemia associated with parvovirus-like agent. Lancet 1981; 1:595.

440. Goldstein AR, Anderson MJ, Serjeant GR: Parvovirus associated aplastic crisis in homozygous sickle cell disease. Arch Dis Child 1987; 62:585.

441. Serjeant GR, Serjeant BE, et al: Human parvovirus infection in homozygous sickle cell disease. Lancet 1993; 341:1237.

442. Plummer FA, Hammond GW, et al: An erythema infectiosum–like illness caused by human parvovirus infection. N Engl J Med 1985; 313:74.

443. Chorba T, Coccia P, et al: The role of parvovirus B19 in aplastic crisis and erythema infectiosum (fifth disease). J Infect Dis 1986; 154:383.

444. Saarinen UM, Chorba TL, et al. Human parvovirus B19–induced epidemic acute red cell aplasia in patients with hereditary hemolytic anemia. Blood 1986; 67:1411.

445. Mortimer PP, Humphries RK, et al: A human parvovirus-like virus inhibits haematopoietic colony formation *in vitro*. Nature 1983; 302:426.

446. Barrett-Connor E: Bacterial infection and sickle cell anemia. An analysis of 25 infections in 166 patients and a review of the literature. Medicine 1971; 50:97.

447. Overturf GD, Powars D, et al: Bacterial meningitis and septicemia in sickle cell disease. Am J Dis Child 1977; 131:784.

448. Powars D, Overturf G, et al: Is there an increased risk of *Haemophilus influenzae* septicemia in children with sickle cell anemia? Pediatrics 1983; 71:927.

449. Pearson HA, Spencer RP, et al: Functional asplenia in sickle-cell anemia. N Engl J Med 1969; 281:923.

450. Pearson HA, McIntosh S, et al: Interference phase microscopic enumeration of pitted RBC and splenic hypofunction in sickle cell anemia. Pediatr Res 1978; 12:471.

451. Pearson HA, Gallagher D, et al: Cooperative Study of Sickle Cell Disease. Developmental pattern of splenic dysfunction in sickle cell disorders. Pediatrics 1985; 76:392.

452. Seeler RA, Metzger W, et al: *Diplococcus pneumoniae* infections in children with sickle cell anemia. Am J Dis Child 1972; 123:8.

453. Fischer KC, Shapiro S, et al: Visualization of the spleen with a bone-seeking radionuclide in a child with sickle cell anemia. Radiology 1977; 122:398.

454. Pearson HA, Cornelius EA, et al: Transfusion-reversible functional asplenia in young children with sickle cell anemia. N Engl J Med 1970; 283:334.

455. Schwartz AD, Pearson HA: Impaired antibody response to intravenous immunization in sickle cell anemia. Pediatr Res 1972; 6:145.

456. Ammann AJ, Addrego J, et al: Polyvalent pneumococcal-polysaccharide immunization of patients with sickle cell anemia and patients with splenectomy. N Engl J Med 1977; 297:897.

457. Overturf GD, Rigau-Perez JG, et al: Pneumococcal polysaccharide immunization of children with sickle cell disease: I. Clinical reactions to immunization and relationship to preimmunization antibody. Am J Pediatr Hematol Oncol 1982; 4:19.

458. Evans HE, Reindorf C: Serum immunoglobulin levels in sickle cell disease and thalassemia major. Am J Dis Child 1968; 16:586.

459. De Ceular K, Pagliuca A, et al: Recurrent infections in sickle cell disease: haematological and immune studies. Clin Chim Acta 1985; 148:161.

460. Winkelstein JA, Drachman RH: Deficiency of pneumococcal serum opsonizing activity in sickle-cell disease. N Engl J Med 1968; 279:459.

461. Johnston RB Jr, Newman SL, et al: Serum opsonins and the alternate pathway in sickle cell disease. N Engl J Med 1973; 288:803.

462. Wilson WA, Hughes GRV, et al: Deficiency of factor 13 of the complement systems in sickle cell anemia. BMJ 1967; 1:367.

463. Chudwin DS, Korenbilt AD, et al: Increased activation of the alternative complement pathway in sickle cell disease. Clin Immunol Immunopathol 1985; 37:93.

464. Bjornson AB, Lobel JS, Kathleen SH: Relation between serum opsonic activity for *Streptococcus pneumoniae* and complement function in sickle cell disease. J Infect Dis 1985; 152:701.

465. Bjornson AB, Lobel JS: Lack of requirement for the Fc region of IgG in restoring pneumococcal opsonization via the alternative complement pathway in sickle cell disease. J Infect Dis 1986; 154:760.

466. Boggs DR, Hyde F, et al: An unusual pattern of neutrophil kinetics in sickle cell anemia. Blood 1973; 41:59.

467. Dimitrov NV, Douwes FR, et al: Metabolic activity of polymorphonuclear leukocytes in sickle cell anemia. Acta Haematol 1972; 47:283.

468. Strauss RG, Johnson RB Jr, et al: Neutrophil oxidative metabolism in sickle cell disease. J Pediatr 1976; 89:391.

469. Boghossian SH, Wright G, et al: Investigations of host defense in patients with sickle cell disease. Br J Haematol 1985; 59:523.

470. McIntosh S, Rooks Y, et al: Fever in young children with sickle cell disease. J Pediatr 1980; 96:199.

471. Buchanan GR, Glader BE: Leukocyte counts in children with sickle cell disease. Arch Dis Child 1978; 132:396.

472. Wilimas JA, Flynn PM, et al: A randomized study of outpatient treatment with ceftriaxone for selected febrile children with sickle cell disease. N Engl J Med 1993; 329:472.

473. Shulman ST, Bartlett J, et al: The unusual severity of mycoplasmal pneumonia in children with sickle-cell disease. N Engl J Med 1972; 287:164.

474. McSweeney JEJ, Mermann AC, Wagley PF: Cold hemagglutinins in sickle cell anemia. Am J Med Sci 1947; 214:542.

475. John AB, Ramlal A, et al: Prevention of pneumococcal infection in children with homozygous sickle cell disease. BMJ [Clin Res] 1984; 288:1567.

476. Gaston MH, Verter JI, et al: Prophylaxis with oral penicillin in children with sickle cell anemia: a randomized trial. N Engl J Med 1986; 314:1593.

477. Sickle Cell Disease: Screening, Diagnosis, Management, and Counseling in Newborns and Infants. Clinical Practice Guideline No. 6. AHCPR publication No. 93–0562. Washington, DC, U.S. Department of Health and Human Services, Agency for Health Care Policy and Research, 1993.

478. Chudwin DS, Wara DW, et al: Increases in serum opsonic activity and antibody concentration in patients with sickle cell disease after pneumococcal polysaccharide immunization. J Pediatr 1983; 102:51.

479. Wong WY, Powars DR, et al: Polysaccharide encapsulated bacterial infection in sickle cell anemia: a 30-year epidemiologic experience. Am J Hematol 1992; 39:176.

480. Buchanan GR, Schiffman G: Antibody responses to polyvalent pneumococcal vaccine in infants with sickle cell anemia. J Pediatr 1980; 96:264.

481. Kaplan J, Frost H, et al: Type-specific antibodies in children with sickle cell anemia given polyvalent pneumococcal vaccine. J Pediatr 1982; 100:404.

482. Kaplan J, Sarnaik S, Schiffman G: Revaccination with polyvalent pneumococcal vaccine in children with sickle cell anemia. Am J Pediatr Hematol Oncol 1986; 8:80.

483. Frank AL, Laborka RJ, et al: *Haemophilus influenzae* type b immunization of children with sickle cell diseases. Pediatrics 1988; 82:571.

484. Gigliotti F, Feldman S, et al: Immunization of young infants with sickle cell disease with a *Haemophilus influenzae* type b saccharide-diphtheria CRM197 protein conjugate. J Pediatr 1989; 114:1006.

485. Buchanan GR, Smith SJ: Pneumococcal septicemia despite pneumococcal vaccine and prescription of penicillin prophylaxis in children with sickle cell anemia. Am J Dis Child 1986; 140:428.

486. Ng ML, Liebman J, et al: Cardiovascular findings in children with sickle cell anemia. Dis Chest 1967; 52:748.

487. Lindsey J Jr, Meshel JC, et al: The cardiovascular manifestations of sickle cell disease. Arch Intern Med 1974; 133:643.

488. Shubin H, Kaufman R, et al: Cardiovascular findings in children with sickle cell anemia. Am J Cardiol 1960; 6:8875.

489. Chung EE, Dianzumba SB, et al: Cardiac performance in children with homozygous sickle cell disease. J Am Coll Cardiol 1987; 9:1038.

490. Finch CA: Pathophysiologic aspects of sickle cell anemia. Am J Med 1972; 53:1.

491. O'Neill B Jr, Saunders DE Jr, et al: Myocardial infarction in sickle cell anemia. Am J Hematol 1984; 16:139.

492. Jensen WN, Rucknagel DL, et al: *In vivo* study of the sickle cell phenomenon. J Clin Med 1960; 56:854.

493. McNamara JJ, Molot MA Jr, et al: Coronary artery disease in combat casualties in Vietnam. JAMA 1971; 216:1185.

494. Gerry JL, Bulkley BH, et al: Clinicopathologic analysis of cardiac dysfunction in 52 patients with sickle cell anemia. Am J Cardiol 1978; 42:211.

495. Falk RH, Hood WB Jr: The heart in sickle cell anemia. Arch Intern Med 1982; 142:1680.

496. Gerry JL, Baird MG, et al: Evaluation of left ventricular function in patients with sickle cell anemia. Am J Med 1976; 60:967.

497. Val-Mejias J, Lee WK, et al: Left ventricular performance during and after sickle cell crises. Am Heart J 1979; 97:585.

498. Manno BV, Burka ER, et al: Biventricular function in sickle-cell anemia: radionuclide angiographic and thallium-201 scintigraphic evaluation. Am J Cardiol 1983; 52:584.

499. Covarrubias EA, Sheikh MU, et al: Left ventricular function in sickle cell anemia: a noninvasive evaluation. South Med J 1980; 73:342.

500. Rees AH, Stefadouros MA, et al. Left ventricular performance in children with homozygous sickle cell anaemia. Br Heart J 1978; 40:690.

501. Alpert BS, Gilman PA, et al. Hemodynamic and ECG responses to exercise in children with sickle cell anemia. Am J Dis Child 1981; 135:362.

502. Covits W, Eubig C, et al: Exercise-induced cardiac dysfunction in sickle cell anemia. A radionuclide study. Am J Cardiol 1983; 51:570.

503. Deneberg BS, Criner G, et al: Cardiac function in sickle cell anemia. Am J Cardiol 1983; 51:1674.

504. Willens HJ, Lawrence C, et al: A noninvasive comparison of left ventricular performance in sickle cell anemia and chronic aortic regurgitation. Clin Cardiol 1983; 6:542.

505. Johnson CS, Giorgio AJ: Arterial blood pressure in adults with sickle cell disease. Arch Intern Med 1981; 141:891.

506. Charache S, Bleecher ER, et al: Effects of blood transfusion on exercise capacity in patients with sickle cell anemia. Am J Med 1983; 74:757.

507. Moser KM, Shea JC: The relationship between pulmonary infarction, cor pulmonale and the sickle states. Am J Med 1957; 22:561.

508. Powars D, Weidman JA, et al: Sickle cell chronic lung disease: prior morbidity and the risk of pulmonary failure. Medicine 1988; 67:66.

509. Maisel A, Friedman H, et al: Continuous electrocardiographic monitoring in patients with sickle-cell anemia during pain crisis. Clin Cardiol 1983; 6:339.

510. Buckalew VM, Someren A: Renal manifestations of sickle cell disease. Arch Intern Med 1974; 133:660.

511. Sherwood JB, Goldwasser E, et al: Sickle cell anemia patients have low erythropoietin levels for their degree of anemia. Blood 1986; 67:46.

512. Whitten CF, Younes AA, et al: Comparative study of renal concentrating ability in children with sickle cell anemia and in normal children. J Lab Clin Med 1960; 55:400.

513. Hatch FF, Culbertson JW, et al: Nature of the renal concentrating defect in sickle cell disease. J Clin Invest 1967; 46:336.

514. Statius van Eps LW, Schouten H, et al: The influence of red blood cell transfusions on the hyposthenuria and renal hemodynamics of sickle cell anemia. Clin Chim Acta 1967; 17:449.

515. Statius van Eps LW, Pinedo-Veels C, et al: Nature of concentrating defect in sickle-cell nephropathy. Lancet 1970; 1:450.

516. Perillie PE, Epstein F II: Sickling phenomenon produced by hypertonic solutions: a possible explanation for the hyposthenuria of sicklemia. J Clin Invest 1963; 42:570.

517. Noll JB, Newman AJ, et al: Enuresis and nocturia in sickle cell disease. J Pediatr 1967; 70:965.

518. Radel EG, Kochen JA, et al: Hyponatremia in sickle cell disease. A renal salt losing state. Pediatrics 1976; 88:800.

519. Goossens JP, Statius van Eps LW, et al: Incomplete renal tubular acidosis in sickle cell disease. Clin Chim Acta 1972; 41:149.

520. Oster JR, Lespier IE, et al: Renal acidification in sickle cell disease. J Lab Clin Med 1976; 88:389.

521. Yoshino M, Amerian R, et al: Hyporeninemic hypoaldosteronism in sickle cell disease. Nephrologie 1982; 31:242.

522. Oster JR, Lanier DC, et al: Renal response to potassium loading in sickle cell trait. Arch Intern Med 1980; 140:534.

523. deJong PE, van Eps LWS: Sickle cell nephropathy: new insights into pathophysiology. Kidney Int 1985; 27:711.

524. Lucas WM, Bullock W: Hematuria in sickle cell disease. J Urol 1960; 83:733.

525. Allen TD: Sickle cell disease and hematuria: a report of 29 cases. J Urol 1964; 91:177.

526. Diggs LW: Anatomic lesions in sickle cell disease. In Abramson

H, Bertles JF (eds): Sickle Cell Disease, Diagnosis, Management, Education and Research. St. Louis, C. V. Mosby Co., 1973.

527. Bilinsky RT, Kandel GL, et al: Epsilon aminocaproic acid therapy of hematuria due to heterozygous sickle cell diseases. J Urol 1969; 102:93.

528. Nicholson GD, Amin UF, Aleyne GA: Proteinuria and the nephrotic syndrome in homozygous sickle cell anaemia. West Indian Med J 1980; 29:239.

529. McCoy RC: Ultrastructural alterations in the kidney of patients with sickle cell disease and the nephrotic syndrome. Lab Invest 1969; 21:85.

530. Pardo V, Strauss J, et al: Nephropathy associated with sickle cell anemia: an autologous immune complex nephritis. Am J Med 1975; 59:650.

531. Elfenbein B, Patchefsky A, et al: Pathology of the glomerulus in sickle cell anemia with and without nephrotic syndrome. Am J Pathol 1974; 77:374.

532. Bakir AA, Hathiwala SC, et al: Prognosis of the nephrotic syndrome in sickle glomerulopathy. Am J Nephrol 1987; 7:110.

533. Falk RJ, Scheinman J, et al: Prevalence and pathologic features of sickle cell nephropathy and response to inhibition of angiotensin-converting enzyme. N Engl J Med 1992; 326:910.

534. Chatterjee SN: National study on natural history of renal allografts in sickle cell disease or trait. Nephrologie 1980; 25:199.

535. Gonzalez-Carrillo M, Rudge CJ, et al: Renal transplantation in sickle cell disease. Clin Nephrol 1982; 18:209.

536. Green TW, Conley CL, et al: Liver in sickle cell anemia. Bull Johns Hopkins Hosp 1953; 92:99.

537. Bogosh A, Casselman WGB, et al: Liver disease in sickle cell anemia: a correlation of clinical, biochemical and histochemical observations. Am J Med 1955; 19:583.

538. Alli AF, Lewis FA: The liver in sickle cell disease: pathological aspects based on a report on the pathological study of 77 necropsy and 5 biopsy specimens of liver. Ghana Med J 1969; 8:119.

539. Barrett-Connor E: Cholelithiasis in sickle cell anemia. Am J Med 1968; 45:889.

540. Rennels MB, Dunne MG, et al: Cholelithiasis in patients with major sickle hemoglobinopathies. Am J Dis Child 1983; 138:66.

541. Sarnaik S, Slovis TL, et al: Incidence of cholelithiasis in sickle cell anemia using the ultrasonic gray-scale technique. J Pediatr 1980; 96:1005.

542. Webb DKH, Darby JS, et al: Gallstones in Jamaican children with homozygous sickle cell disease. Arch Dis Child 1989; 64:693.

543. Ware R, Filston HC, et al: Elective cholecystectomy in children with sickle hemoglobinopathies. Successful outcome using a perioperative transfusion regimen. Ann Surg 1988; 208:17.

544. Malone BS, Werlin SL: Cholecystectomy and cholelithiasis in sickle cell anemia. Am J Dis Child 1988; 142:799.

545. Stephens CG, Scott RB: Cholelithiasis in sickle cell anemia: surgical or medical management. Arch Intern Med 1980; 140:648.

546. Barrett-Connor E: Sickle cell disease and viral hepatitis. Ann Intern Med 1968; 69:517.

547. Sheey TW, Law DE, et al: Exchange transfusion for sickle cell intrahepatic cholestasis. Arch Intern Med 1980; 140:1364.

548. Klion FM, Weiner MJ, et al: Cholestasis in sickle cell anemia. Am J Med 1964; 37:829.

549. Schubert TT: Hepatobiliary system in sickle cell disease. Gastroenterology 1986; 90:2013.

550. Bauer TN, Moore GW, et al: The liver in sickle cell disease. A clinicopathologic study of 70 patients. Am J Med 1980; 69:833.

551. Omata M, Johnson CS, et al: Pathological spectrum of liver diseases in sickle cell disease. Dig Dis Sci 1986; 31:247.

552. Armaly MF: Ocular manifestations in sickle cell disease. Arch Intern Med 1974; 133:670.

553. Asdourian G, Nagpal KC, et al: Evolution of the retinal black sunburst lesion in sickling haemoglobinopathies. Br J Ophthalmol 1975; 59:710.

554. Jampol LM, Condon PI, et al: Salmon-patch hemorrhages after central retinal artery occlusion in sickle cell disease. Arch Ophthalmol 1981; 99:237.

555. Condon PI, Serjeant GR: Ocular findings in elderly cases of homozygous sickle cell disease in Jamaica. Br J Ophthalmol 1976; 60:361.

556. Hamilton AM, Pope FM, et al: Angioid streaks in Jamaican patients with homozygous sickle cell disease. Br J Ophthalmol 1981; 65:341.

557. Goldberg MF: Natural history of untreated proliferative sickle retinopathy. Arch Ophthalmol 1971; 85:428.

558. Dizon-Moore RV, Jampol LM, et al: Chorioretinal and choriovitreal neovascularization. Their presence after photocoagulation of proliferative sickle cell retinopathy. Arch Ophthalmol 1981; 99:842.

559. Condon PI, Serjeant GR: An important complication of photocoagulation for proliferative sickle cell retinopathy. Trans Ophthalmol Soc U K 1981; 101:429.

560. Jampol LM, Goldberg MF: Retinal breaks after photocoagulation of proliferative sickle cell retinopathy. Arch Ophthalmol 1980; 98:676.

561. Condon PI, Serjeant GR: Behavior of untreated proliferative sickle retinopathy. Br J Ophthalmol 1980; 64:404.

562. Condon PI, Serjeant GR: Photocoagulation in proliferative sickle retinopathy: results of a 5 year study. Br J Ophthalmol 1980; 64:832.

563. Roy MS, Rodgers G, Gunkel R, et al: Color vision defects in sickle cell anemia. Arch Ophthalmol 1987; 105:1676.

564. Lee CM, Charles HC, et al: Quantification of macular ischemia in sickle cell retinopathy. Br J Ophthalmol 1987; 71:540.

565. Weissman II, Nadel AJ, et al: Simultaneous bilateral retinal arterial occlusions treated by exchange transfusions. Arch Ophthalmol 1979; 97:2151.

566. Goldberg MF: Sickled erythrocytes, hyphema, and secondary glaucoma: I. The diagnosis and treatment of sickled erythrocytes in human hyphemas. Ophthalmic Surg 1979; 10:17.

567. Peachey R: Leg ulceration and haemolytic anaemia: an hypothesis. Br J Dermatol 1978; 98:245.

568. Thrall JH, Rucknagel DL: Increased bone marrow blow flow in sickle cell anemia demonstrated by thallium-201 and Tc-99m human albumin microspheres. Radiology 1978; 127:817.

569. Wolfort FG, Krizek TJ: Skin ulceration in sickle cell anemia. Plast Reconstr Surg 1969; 43:71.

570. Koshy M, Entsuah R, et al: Leg ulcers in patients with sickle cell disease. Blood 1989; 74:1403.

571. Alleye S, Wint E, et al: Social effect of leg ulceration in sickle cell anemia. South Med J 1977; 702:213.

572. Wethers DL, Ramirez GM, et al: Accelerated healing of chronic sickle cell leg ulcers treated with RGD peptide matrix. Blood 1994; 84:1777.

573. Serjeant GR, Galloway RE, et al: Oral zinc sulfate in sickle cell ulcers. Lancet 1970; 2:89.

574. Serjeant GR, Howard C: Isoxsuprine hydrochloride in the therapy of sickle cell leg ulceration. West Indian Med J 1977; 26:164.

575. Todd GB, Serjeant GR, et al: Sensorineural hearing loss in Jamaicans with SS disease. Acta Otolaryngol 1973; 76:268.

576. Serjeant GR, Norman W, et al: The internal auditory canal and sensorineural hearing loss in homozygous sickle cell disease. J Laryngol Otolarynol 1975; 98:453.

577. Friedman EM, Luban NLC, et al: Sickle cell anemia and hearing. Ann Otol Rhinol Laryngol 1980; 89:342.

578. Morganstein KM, Manace CD: Temporal bone histopathology in sickle cell disease. Laryngoscope 1969; 79:2172.

579. Reynolds J: Roentgenological Features of Sickle Cell Disease and Related Hemoglobinopathies. Springfield, IL, Charles C Thomas, Publisher, 1971.

580. Bohrer SP: Acute long bone diaphyseal infarcts in sickle cell disease. Br J Radiol 1970; 43:685.

581. Golding JSR, MacIver JE, et al: Bone changes in sickle-cell anemia and its genetic variants. J Bone Joint Surg Br 1959; 41:711.

582. Reynolds J: Radiologic manifestations of sickle cell hemoglobinopathy. JAMA 1977; 238:247.

583. Milner PF, Kraus AP, et al: Sickle cell disease as a cause of osteonecrosis of the femoral head. N Engl J Med 1991; 325:1476.

584. Washington ER, Root L: Conservative treatment of sickle cell avascular necrosis of the femoral head. J Pediatr Orthop 1985; 5:192.

585. Hernigou P, Bachir D, Galacteros F: Avascular necrosis of the femoral head in sickle-cell disease. Treatment of collapse by the injection of acrylic cement. J Bone Joint Surg [Br] 1993; 75:875.

586. Hungerford DS: The role of core decompression in the treatment of ischemic necrosis of the femoral head. Arthritis Rheum 1989; 32:801.

587. Milner PF, Kraus AP, et al: Osteonecrosis of the humeral head in sickle cell disease. Clin Orthop Rel Res 1993; 289:136.

588. Miller GJ, Serjeant GR: An assessment of lung volumes and gas transfer in sickle cell anemia. Thorax 1971; 26:309.

589. Femi-Pearse D, Gazioglu KM, et al: Pulmonary function studies in sickle cell disease. J Appl Physiol 1970; 28:574.

590. Wall MA, Platt OS, et al: Lung function in children with sickle cell anemia. Am Rev Respir Dis 1979; 120:210.

591. Bromberg PA: Pulmonary aspects of sickle cell disease. Arch Intern Med 1974; 133:652.

592. Denbow CE, Chung EE, Serjeant GR: Pulmonary artery pressure and the acute chest syndrome in homozygous sickle cell disease. Br Heart J 1993; 69:536.

593. Pianosi P, D'Souza SJ, et al: Pulmonary function abnormalities in childhood sickle cell disease. J Pediatr 1993; 122:366.

594. Booker CR, Scott RB, et al: Studies in sickle cell anemia: XXII. Clinical manifestations during the first two years of life. Clin Pediatr 1964; 3:111.

595. Stevens MCG, Hayes RJ, et al: Body shape in young children with homozygous sickle cell disease. Pediatrics 1983; 71:610.

596. Morais PV, Clarke WF, et al: Heart size and chest shape in homozygous sickle cell disease. West Indian Med J 1983; 32:157.

597. Platt OS, Rosenstock W, et al: Influence of sickle hemoglobinopathies on growth and development. N Engl J Med 1984; 311:7.

598. Singhal A, Davies P, et al: Resting metabolic rate in homozygous sickle cell disease. Am J Clin Nutr 1993; 57:32.

599. Stevens MCG, Maude GH, et al: Prepubertal growth and skeletal maturation in children with sickle cell disease. Pediatrics 1986; 70:124.

600. Prasad AS, Cossack ZT: Zinc supplementation and growth in sickle cell disease. Ann Intern Med 1984; 100:367.

601. Phebus CK, Maciak BJ, et al: Zinc status of children with sickle cell disease: Relationship to poor growth. Am J Hematol 1988; 29:67.

602. Abshire TC, English JL, et al: Zinc status in children and young adults with sickle cell disease. Am J Dis Child 1988; 142:1356.

603. Oberfield SE, Wethers DL, et al: Growth hormone response to growth hormone releasing factor in sickle cell disease. Am J Pediatr Hematol Oncol 1987; 9:331.

604. Reed JD, Redding-Lallinger R, Orringer EP: Nutrition and sickle cell disease. Am J Hematol 1987; 24:441.

605. Heyman MB, Vichinsky E, et al: Growth retardation in sickle-cell disease treated by nutritional support. Lancet 1985; 1:903.

606. Alleyne SI, Rauseo RD, et al: Sexual development and fertility of Jamaican female patients with homozygous sickle cell disease. Arch Intern Med 1981; 141:1295.

607. Osegbe DN, Akinyanju O, et al: Fertility in males with sickle cell disease. Lancet 1981; 2:275.

608. Olambiwonnu NO, Penny R, et al: Sexual maturation in subjects with sickle cell anemia. Studies of serum gonadotropin concentration, height, weight, and skeletal age. J Pediatr 1975; 87:459.

609. Landefeld M, Schambelau M, et al: Clomiphine-responsive hypogonadism in sickle cell anemia. Ann Intern Med 1983; 99:480.

610. Scott RB, Ferguson AD: Studies in sickle cell anemia: XIV. Management of the child with sickle-cell anemia. Am J Dis Child 1960; 100:85.

611. Kumars D, Allen J, et al: Anxiety, self-concept, and personal and social adjustments in children with sickle cell disease. J Pediatr 1976; 88:859.

612. Yand YM, Cepeda M, et al: Depression in children and adolescents with sickle cell disease. Arch Pediatr Adolesc Med 1994; 148:457.

613. Rabb LM, Grandison Y, et al: A trial of folate supplementation in children with homozygous sickle cell disease. Br J Haematol 1983; 54:589.

614. Snager RG, Greer RO, et al: Differential diagnosis of some simple osseous lesions associated with sickle-cell anemia. Oral Surg 1977; 43:538.

615. Freie HM: Sickle cell diseases and hormonal contraception. Acta Obstet Gynecol Scand 1983; 62:211.

616. Cooperative Urea Trial Group: Clinical trials of therapy for sickle cell vaso-occlusive crises. JAMA 1974; 228:1120.

617. Embury SH, Garcia JF, et al: Effects of oxygen inhalation on endogenous erythropoietin kinetics, erythropoiesis and properties of blood cells in sickle cell anemia. N Engl J Med 1984; 311:291.

618. Keidan AJ, Marwah SS, et al: Painful sickle cell crises precipitated by stopping prophylactic exchange transfusions. J Clin Pathol 1987; 40:505.

619. Szeto HH, Inturrisi CE, et al: Accumulation of normeperidine, an active metabolite of meperidine, in patients with renal failure or cancer. Ann Intern Med 1977; 85:73.

620. Cole TB, Sprinkle RH, et al: Intravenous narcotic therapy for children with severe sickle cell pain crisis. Am J Dis Child 1986; 140:1255.

621. Yaster M, Tobin JR, et al: Epidural anesthesia in the management of severe vaso-occlusive crises. Pediatrics 1994; 93:310.

622. Vichinsky EP, Johnson R., et al: Multidisciplinary approach to pain management in sickle cell disease. Am J Pediatr Hematol Oncol 1982; 4:328.

623. Shapiro BS: The management of pain in sickle cell disease. Pediatr Clin North Am 1989; 36:1029.

624. Co LL, Schmitz TH, et al: Acupuncture: an evaluation in painful crises of sickle cell anaemia. Pain 1979; 7:181.

625. Zeltzer L, Dash J, et al: Hypnotically induced pain control in sickle cell anemia. Pediatrics 1979; 64:533.

626. Portenoy RK, Foley M: Chronic use of opioid analgesics in nonmalignant pain: report of 38 cases. Pain 1986; 25:171.

627. Berkowitz LR, Orringer EP: Effect of cetiedil, an in vitro antisickling agent, on erythrocyte membrane cation permeability. J Clin Invest 1981; 68:1215.

628. Stuart J, Stone PCW, et al: Oxpentifylline and cetiedil citrate improve deformability of dehydrated sickle cells. J Clin Pathol 1987; 40:1182.

629. Benjamin LJ, Berkowitz LR, et al: A collaborative, double-blind randomized study of citrate in sickle cell crisis. Blood 1986; 67:1442.

630. Leff RD, Aldo-Benson MA, et al: Tophaceous gout in a patient with sickle-cell thalassemia: case report and review of the literature. Arthritis Rheum 1983; 26:928.

631. Charache S: The treatment of sickle cell anemia. Arch Intern Med 1974; 133:698.

632. Rifkind S, Waisman J, et al: RBC exchange pheresis for priapism in sickle cell disease. JAMA 1979; 242:2317.

633. Walker EM Jr, Mitchum EN, et al: Automated erythrocytapheresis for relief of priapism in sickle cell hemoglobinopathies. J Urol 1983; 130:912.

634. Quattlebaum TG, Pierce MM: Estimates of need for transfusions during hypertransfusion therapy in sickle cell disease. J Pediatr 1986; 109:456.

635. Styles LA, Vichinsky E: Effects of a long-term transfusion regimen on sickle cell-related illnesses. J Pediatr 1994; 125:909.

636. Cohen A, Schwartz E: Excretion of iron in response to deferoxamine in sickle cell anemia. J Pediatr 1978; 92:659.

637. Wang WC, Ahmed N, Hanna M: Non–transferrin-bound iron in long-term transfusion in children with congenital anemias. J Pediatr 1986; 108:552.

638. Davies SC, McWilliam AC, et al: Red cell alloimmunization in sickle cell disease. Br J Haematol 1986; 63:241.

639. Reisner EG, Kostyu DD, et al: Alloantibody responses in multiply transfused sickle cell patients. Tissue Antigens 1987; 30:161.

640. Sarnaik S, Schornack J, Lusher JM: The incidence of development of irregular red cell antibodies in patients with sickle cell anemia. Transfusion 1986; 26:249.

641. Vichinsky EP, Earles A, et al: Alloimmunization in sickle cell anemia and transfusion of racially unmatched blood. N Engl J Med 1990; 322:1617.

642. Rosse WF, Gallagher D, et al: Transfusion and alloimmunization in sickle cell disease. Blood 1990; 76:1431.

643. Tahhan HR, Holbrook CT, et al: Antigen-matched donor blood in the transfusion management of patients with sickle cell disease. Transfusion 1994; 34:562.

644. Ambruso DR, Githens JH, et al: Experience with donors matched for minor group antigens in patients with sickle cell anemia who are receiving chronic transfusion therapy. Transfusion 1987; 27:94.

645. Orlina AR, Sosler SD, Koshy M: Problems of chronic transfusions in sickle cell disease. J Clin Apheresis 1991; 6:234.

646. Ness PM: To match or not to match: the question for chronically transfused patients with sickle cell anemia. Transfusion 1994; 34:558.

647. Speigelman A, Warden MJ: Surgery in patients with sickle cell disease. Arch Surg 1972; 104:761.

648. Howells TH, Huntsman RG: Anaesthesia in sickle cell states. BMJ 1973; 1:174.

649. Searle JF: Anesthesia in sickle state. Anesthesia 1973; 28:48.

650. Burrington JD, Smith MD: Elective and emergency surgery in children with sickle cell disease. Surg Clin North Am 1976; 56:55.

651. Janik JS, Seeler RA: Surgical procedures in children with sickle hemoglobinopathy. J Pediatr 1977; 91:505.

652. Bentley PG, Howard ER: Surgery in children with homozygous sickle cell anaemia. Ann R Coll Surg Engl 1979; 61:55.

653. Koshy M, Weiner SJ, et al: Surgery and anesthesia in sickle cell disease. Cooperative study of sickle cell diseases. Blood 1995; 86:3676.

654. Griffin TC, Buchanan GR: Elective surgery in children with sickle cell disease without preoperative blood transfusion. J Pediatr Surg 1993; 28:681.

655. Vichinsky EP, Haberkern C, et al: A comparison of conservative and aggressive transfusion regimens in the perioperative management of sickle cell disease. The Preoperative Transfusion in Sickle Cell Disease Study Group. N Engl J Med 1995; 333:206.

656. Freeman MG, Ruth GU: SS disease, SC disease and CC disease-obstetric considerations and treatment. Clin Obstet Gynecol 1969; 12:134.

657. Morrison JC, Fort AT, et al: The modern management of pregnant sickle cell patients. South Med J 1972; 65:533.

658. Pritchard JA: The effects of maternal sickle cell hemoglobinopathies and sickle cell trait on reproductive performance. Am J Obstet Gynecol 1973; 117:662.

659. Milner PF, Jones BR: Outcome of pregnancy in sickle cell anemia and sickle cell-hemoglobin C disease. An analysis of 181 pregnancies in 98 patients, and a review of the literature. Am J Obstet Gynecol 1980; 138:239.

660. Charache S, Scott J, et al: Management of sickle cell disease in pregnant patients. Obstet Gynecol 1980; 55:407.

661. Cunningham FG, Pritchard JA, et al: Pregnancy and sickle cell hemoglobinopathies: results with and without prophylactic transfusions. Obstet Gynecol 1983; 62:419.

662. Cunningham FG, Pritchard JA, et al: Prophylactic transfusions of normal red blood cells during pregnancies complicated by sickle cell hemoglobinopathies. Am J Obstet Gynecol 1979; 135:1994.

663. Morrison JC, Schneider JM, et al: Prophylactic transfusions in pregnant patients with sickle hemoglobinopathies: benefit versus risk. Obstet Gynecol 1980; 56:274.

664. Morrison JC, Wiser W: The effect of maternal partial exchange transfusion on the infants of patients with sickle cell anemia. J Pediatr 1976; 89:286.

665. Nagey DA, Alawode NA, et al: Isovolumetric partial exchange transfusion in the management of sickle cell disease in pregnancy: II. Simplified ambulatory technique. Am J Obstet Gynecol 1983; 147:693.

666. Key TC, Horger EO III, et al: Automated erythrocytapheresis for sickle cell anemia during pregnancy. Am J Obstet Gynecol 1980; 138:731.

667. Miller JM Jr, Horger EO Jr, et al: Management of sickle hemoglobinopathies in pregnant patients. Am J Obstet Gynecol 1981; 141:237.

668. Koshy M, Burd L, et al: Prophylactic red-cell transfusions in pregnant patients with sickle cell disease: a randomized cooperative study. N Engl J Med 1988; 319:1447.

669. Brumfield CG, Huddleston JF, et al: A delayed hemolytic transfusion reaction after partial exchange transfusion for sickle cell disease in pregnancy: a case report and review of the literature. Obstet Gynecol 1985; 63:139.

670. Leiken SL, Gallagher D, Kinney TR, et al: Mortality in children and adolescents with sickle cell disease. Pediatrics 1989; 84:500.

671. Boyle E Jr, Thompson C, et al: Prevalence of sickle cell trait in adults of Charleston County. Arch Environ Health 1968; 17:891.

672. Ashcroft MT, Miall WE, et al: Comparison between characteristics of Jamaican adults with normal hemoglobin and those with sickle cell trait. Am J Epidemiol 1969; 90:236.

673. Ashcroft MT, Desai P: Mortality and morbidity in Jamaican adults with sickle-cell trait and with normal haemoglobin followed up for twelve years. Lancet 1976; 2:784.

674. Sears DA: The morbidity of sickle cell trait. A review of the literature. Am J Med 1978; 64:1021.

675. Ashcroft MT, Desai P, et al: Growth, behaviour, and educational achievement of Jamaican children with sickle cell trait. BMJ 1976; 1:1371.

676. Kramer MS, Rooks Y, et al: Growth and development in children with sickle cell trait. N Engl J Med 1978; 299:686.

677. Blattner P, Dar H, et al: Pregnancy outcome in women with sickle cell trait. JAMA 1977; 238:1392.

678. Murphy JR: Sickle cell hemoglobin (Hb AS) in black football players. JAMA 1973; 225:981.

679. Kark JA, Posey DM, et al: Sickle-cell trait as a risk factor for sudden death in physical training. N Engl J Med 1987; 317:782.

680. Weisman IM, Zeballos RJ, et al: Effect of army basic training in sickle-cell trait. Arch Intern Med 1988; 148:1140.

681. Charache S: Sudden death in sickle trait. Am J Med 1988; 84:459.

682. Sullivan LW: The risk of sickle-cell trait: caution and common sense. N Engl J Med 1987; 317:830.

683. Pearson HA: Sickle cell trait and competitive athletics: is there a risk? Pediatrics 1989; 83:613.

684. Harris JW, Kellermeyer RN (eds): Globin biosynthesis and the hemoglobinopathies. In The Red Cell. Cambridge, MA, Harvard University Press, 1970, p 173.

685. Ober WB, Bruno MS, et al: Fatal intravascular sickling in a patient with sickle cell trait. N Engl J Med 1960; 263:947.

686. McCormick WF: Abnormal hemoglobins: II. The pathology of sickle cell trait. Am J Med Sci 1961; 241:329.

687. Smith EW, Conley CL: Clinical features of the genetic variants of sickle cell disease. Bull Johns Hopkins Hosp 1954; 94:289.

688. Jones SR, Binder RA, et al: Sudden death in sickle-cell trait. N Engl J Med 1970; 282:323.

689. O'Brien RT, Pearson HA, et al: Splenic infarct and sickle cell trait. N Engl J Med 1970; 287:720.

690. Long ID: Sickle cell trait and aviation. Aviat Space Environ Med 1982; 53:1921.

691. Atlas SA: The sickle trait and surgical complications. A matched-pair patient analysis. JAMA 1974; 229:1078.

692. Metras D, Quezzin A, et al: Open-heart surgery in sickle-cell haemoglobinopathies: report of 15 cases. Thorax 1982; 37:486.

693. Searle JF: Anesthesia and sickle-cell haemoglobin. Br J Anesthesiol 1972; 44:1335.

694. Schlitt LE, Keital HG: Renal manifestations of sickle cell disease. A review. Am J Med Sci 1960; 239:773.

695. Huisman THJ: Trimodality in the percentages of β-chain variants in heterozygotes: the effect of the number of active HB structural loci. Hemoglobin 1977; 1:349.

696. Levere RD, Lichtman HS, et al: Effect of iron deficiency anaemia on the metabolism of the heterogenic haemoglobins in sickle cell trait. Nature 1964; 202:499.

697. Heller P, Yakulis V, et al: Variation in the amount of hemoglobins in sickle cell trait and megaloblastic anemia. Blood 1963; 21:479.

698. McCurdy PR: Erythrokinetics in abnormal hemoglobin syndromes. Blood 1962; 20:686.

699. Tuttle AH, Koch B: Clinical and hematological manifestations of hemoglobin C-S disease in children. J Pediatr 1960; 56:331.

700. Serjeant GR, Ashcroft MT, et al: The clinical features of haemoglobin SC disease in Jamaica. Br J Haematol 1973; 24:491.

701. Rowley PT, Enlander D: Hemoglobin S-C disease presenting as acute cor pulmonale. Am Rev Respir Dis 1968; 98:492.

702. Fabian RH, Peters BH: Neurological complications of hemoglobin SC disease. Arch Neurol 1984; 41:289.

703. Ryan SJ, Goldberg MF: Anterior segment ischemia following scleral bucking in sickle cell hemoglobinopathy. Am J Opthalmol 1971; 72:35.

704. Goldberg MF: Treatment of proliferative sickle retinopathy. Trans Am Acad Ophthalmol Otolaryngol 1971; 75:532.

705. Barton CJ, Cockshott WP: Bone changes in hemoglobin SC disease. AJR 1962; 88:523.

706. Kay CJ: Renal papillary necrosis in hemoglobin SC disease. Radiology 1968; 90:897.

707. Pritchard JA: The effects of maternal sickle cell hemoglobinopa-

thies and sickle cell trait on reproductive performance. Am J Obstet Gynecol 1973; 117:662.

708. Yeung KY, Lessin LS: Splenic infarction in sickle cell hemoglobin C disease. Arch Intern Med 1976; 1236:905.

709. Githens JH, Gross GP, et al: Splenic sequestration syndrome at mountain altitudes in sickle/hemoglobin C disease. J Pediatr 1977; 90:203.

710. Barrett-Connor E: Infection and sickle cell C disease. Am J Med Sci 1971; 262:162.

711. Buchanan GR, Smith SJ, et al: Bacterial infection and splenic reticuloendothelial function in children with hemoglobin SC disease. Pediatrics 1983; 72:93.

712. Bunn HF, Noguchi CT, et al: Molecular and cellular pathogenesis of hemoglobin SC disease. Proc Natl Acad Sci U S A 1982; 79:7527.

713. Bunn HF, McDonald MJ: Electrostatic interactions in the assembly of haemoglobin. Nature 1983; 306:498.

714. Ballas SK, Larner J, et al: The xerocytosis of Hb SC disease. Blood 1987; 69:124.

715. Honig GR, Gunay U, et al: Sickle syndromes: I. Hemoglobin SC-α thalassemia. Pediatr Res 1976; 10:613.

716. Milner PF, Miller C, et al: Hemoglobin O Arab in 4 Negro families and its interaction with hemoglobin S and hemoglobin C. N Engl J Med 1970; 283:1417.

717. Charache S, Zinkham WH, et al: Hemoglobin SC, SS/G, Philadelphia, and SOArab disease. Am J Med 1977; 62:439.

718. Sturgeon P, Itano HA, et al: Clinical manifestations of inherited abnormal hemoglobins: VI. The interaction of hemoglobin S with hemoglobin D. Blood 1955; 10:389.

719. Schneider RG, Veda S, et al: Hemoglobin D Los Angeles in two Caucasian families: hemoglobin SD disease and hemoglobin D thalassemia. Blood 1968; 32:250.

720. Cawein MJ, Lappat EJ, et al: Hemoglobin SD disease. Ann Intern Med 1966; 64:62.

721. Konotey-Ahulu FID, Gallo E, et al: Haemoglobin Korle-Bu (β73 aspartic acid (asparagine) showing one of the two amino acid substitutions of haemoglobin C Harlem. J Med Genet 1968; 5:107.

722. Bookchin RM, Nagel RL, et al: Ligand-induced conformation dependence of hemoglobin in sickling interactions. J Molec Biol 1971; 60:262.

723. Bookchin RM, Nagel RL, et al: Structure and properties of hemoglobin C Harlem, a human hemoglobin variant with amino acid substitutions in 2 residues of the β polypeptide chain. J Biol Chem 1967; 242:248.

724. Moo-Penn W, Bechtel K, et al: The presence of hemoglobin S and C Harlem in an individual in the United States. Blood 1975; 46:363.

725. Monplasir N, Merault E, et al: Hemoglobin S Antilles: a variant with lower solubility than hemoglobin S and producing sickle cell in heterozygotes. Proc Natl Acad Sci 1986; 83:9363.

726. Trudel M, Depaipe ME, et al: Sickle cell disease of transgenic SAD mice. Blood 1994; 84:3189.

727. Dover GJ, Boyer SH, et al: Individual variation in the production and survival of F cells in sickle-cell disease. N Engl J Med 1978; 299:1428.

728. Boyer SH: The emerging complexity of genetic control of persistent fetal hemoglobin biosynthesis in adults. Ann Acad Sci 1989; 565:23.

729. Stamatoyannopoulos G, Nienhuis AW: Hemoglobin switching. In Stamatoyannopoulos G, Nienhuis AW, et al (eds): Molecular Basis of Blood Diseases. Philadelphia, W. B. Saunders Co., 1987, p 66.

730. Charache S, Conley CL: Hereditary persistence of fetal hemoglobin. Ann N Y Acad Sci 1969; 165:37.

731. Bradley TB Jr, Brawner JN III, et al: Further observations of an inherited anomaly characterized by persistence of fetal hemoglobin. Bull Johns Hopkins Hosp 1961; 108:242.

732. Jacob GF, Raper AB: Hereditary persistence of foetal hemoglobin production and its interaction with the sickle cell trait. Br J Haematol 1958; 4:138.

733. Weatherall DJ, Clegg JB: The Thalassemia Syndromes, 2nd ed. Oxford, Blackwell Scientific Publications, Inc., 1972, p 195.

734. Murray N, Serjeant BE, Serjeant GR: Sickle cell-hereditary persistence of fetal haemoglobin and its differentiation from other sickle cell syndromes. Br J Haematol 1988; 69:89.

735. Old JM, Ayyub H, et al: Linkage analysis of non-deletion hereditary persistence of fetal hemoglobin. Science 1982; 215:981.

736. Milner PF, Leibfarth JD, et al: Increased Hb F in sickle cell anemia is determined by a factor linked to the βs gene from one parent. Blood 1984; 63:64.

737. Stamatoyannopoulos G, Wood WG, et al: A new form of hereditary persistence of fetal hemoglobin in blacks and its association with sickle cell trait. Blood 1975; 46:683.

738. Makler MT, Berthrog M, et al: A new variant of sickle cell disease with high levels of foetal haemoglobin homogeneously distributed within red cells. Br J Haematol 1974; 26:519.

739. Economou EP, Antonarakis SE, et al: The variation in Hb F production among normal adults or SS subjects is not related to nucleotide substitutions in the gamma promoter regions. Blood 1991; 77:1.

740. Miller B, Salameh M, et al: Analysis of Hb F production in Saudi Arabian families with sickle cell anemia. Blood 1987; 70:716.

741. Kar BC, Kulozik AE, et al: Sickle cell disease in Orissa state, India. Lancet 1986; 2:1198.

742. Miller B, Salameh M, et al: High fetal hemoglobin production in sickle cell anemia in the eastern province of Saudi Arabia is genetically determined. Blood 1986; 67:1404.

743. Kulozik AE, Kar BC, et al: Fetal hemoglobin levels and Beta-S globin haplotypes in an Indian population with sickle cell disease. Blood 1987; 69:1742.

744. Gianni AM, Bregni M, et al: A gene controlling fetal hemoglobin expression in adults is not linked to the non-α-globin cluster. EMBO J 1983; 2:921.

745. Wood WG, Weatherall DJ, Clegg JB: Interaction of heterocellular hereditary persistence of foetal haemoglobin with β thalassaemia and sickle cell anaemia. Nature 1976; 264:247.

746. Boyer SH, Dover GJ, et al: Production of F cells in sickle cell anemia. J Clin Invest 1984; 74:652.

747. Miyoshi K, Koneto Y, et al: X-linked dominant control of F cells in normal adult life. Blood 1988; 72:1854.

748. Dover GJ, Smith KD, et al: Fetal hemoglobin levels in sickle cell disease and normal individuals are partially controlled by an X-linked gene located at Xp22.2. Blood 1992; 80:816.

749. Chang YC, Smith KD, et al: An analysis of fetal hemoglobin variation in sickle cell disease: the relative contribution of the X-linked factors, B globin haplotype, X-globin gene number, gender, and age. Blood 1995; 85:111.

750. Embury SH, Dozy AM, et al: Concurrent sickle cell anemia and alpha-thalassemia: effect on severity of anemia. N Engl J Med 1982; 306:270.

751. Higgs DR, Aldridge BE, et al: The interaction of alpha-thalassemia and homozygous sickle cell disease. N Engl J Med 1982; 306:1441.

752. Noguchi CT, Dover GJ, et al: Alpha thalassemia changes erythrocyte heterogeneity in sickle cell disease. J Clin Invest 1985; 75:1632.

753. Dover GJ, Chang VT, et al: The cellular basis for different fetal hemoglobin levels among sickle cell individuals with two, three, and four-globin genes. Blood 1987; 69:341.

754. Powars DR, Schroeder WN, et al: Lack of influence of fetal hemoglobin levels or erythrocyte indices on the severity of sickle cell anemia. J Clin Invest 1980; 65:732.

755. Powars DR, Weiss JN, et al: Is there a threshold level of fetal hemoglobin that ameliorates morbidity in sickle cell anemia. Blood 1984; 63:9921.

756. Rucknagel DL, Saranik SA, et al: Fetal hemoglobin concentration predicts severity in children with sickle cell anemia. In Stamatoyannopoulos G, Nienhuis AW (eds): Developmental Control of Globin Gene Expression. New York, Alan R. Liss, Inc., 1987, p 487.

757. Fabian, RH, Peters BH: Neurological complications of hemoglobin SC disease. Arch Neurol 1984; 41:289.

758. Weatherall DJ: Biochemical phenotypes of thalassemia in the American Negro population. Ann N Y Acad Sci 1964; 119:450.

759. Pearson HA: Hemoglobin S-thalassemia syndrome in Negro children. Ann N Y Acad Sci 1969; 165:83.

760. Serjeant GR, Ashcroft MT, et al: The clinical features of sickle cell/β thalassemia in Jamaica. Br J Haematol 1973; 24:19.

761. Vyas P, Higgs DR, et al: The interaction of alpha thalassemia and sickle cell–beta thalassemia. Br J Haematol 1988; 70:449.

762. Honig GR, Koshy M, et al: Sickle cell syndromes: II. The sickle cell anemia-α thalassemia syndrome. J Pediatr 1978; 92:556.

763. Sergeant BE, Mason KP, et al: Effect of α-thalassemia on the rheology of homozygous sickle cell disease. Br J Haematol 1983; 55:479.

764. Higgs DR, Presley L, et al: The genetics and molecular basis of α-thalassemia in association with HbS in Jamaican Negroes. Br J Haematol 1981; 47:43.

765. Steinberg MH, Rosenstock W, et al: Effects of thalassemia and microcytosis on the hematological and vaso-occlusive severity of sickle cell anemia. Blood 1984; 63:1353.

766. DeCeulaer K, Higgs DR, et al: α-Thalassemia reduces the hemolytic rate in homozygous sickle cell disease. N Engl J Med 1983; 309:189.

767. Embury SH, Clarke MR, et al: Concurrent sickle cell anemia and α-thalassemia. J Clin Invest 1984; 74:116.

768. Kulozik AE, Kar BC, et al: The molecular basis of α-thalassemia in India. Its interaction with sickle cell gene. Blood 1988; 71:467.

769. Steinberg MH, Embury SH: Alpha-thalassemia in blacks: genetic and clinical aspects and interactions with sickle hemoglobin gene. Blood 1986; 68:985.

770. Milner PF, Garbutt GJ, et al: The effect of Hb F and alpha-thalassemia on the red cell indices in sickle cell anemia. Am J Hematol 1986; 21:383.

771. Embury SH: The interaction of alpha-thalassemia with sickle cell anemia. Hemoglobin 1988; 12:509.

772. Steinberg MH, Rosenstock W: Effects of thalassemia and microcytosis on the hematological and vaso-occlusive severity of sickle cell anemia. Blood 1984; 63:1353.

773. Steinberg MH, Embury SH: Alpha-thalassemia in blacks: genetic and clinical aspects and interactions with the sickle hemoglobin gene. Blood 1986; 68:985.

774. Hawker H, Neilson H, et al: Haematological factors associated with avascular necrosis of the femoral head in homozygous sickle cell disease. Br J Haematol 1982; 50:29.

775. Miller ST, Rieder RF, et al: Cerebrovascular accidents in children with sickle cell disease and alpha-thalassemia. J Pediatr 1988; 113:847.

776. Mears JG, Lachman H, et al: Alpha thalassemia is related to prolonged survival in sickle cell anemia. Blood 1983; 62:286.

777. Fabry ME, Mears JG, et al: Dense cells in sickle cell anemia: the effects of gene interaction. Blood 1984; 64:1042.

778. Felice AE, McKie KM, et al: Effects of alpha thalassemia-2 on the developmental changes of hematological values in children with sickle cell disease from Georgia. Am J Hematol 1987; 25:389.

779. Stevens MCG, Maude GH, et al: Alpha-thalassemia and the hematology of homozygous sickle cell disease in childhood. Blood 1986; 67:411.

780. Itano HA: A third abnormal hemoglobin associated with hereditary hemolytic anemia. Proc Natl Acad Sci U S A 1951; 37:775.

781. Thomas ED, Motulsky AG, et al: Homozygous hemoglobin C disease. Am J Med 1955; 18:832.

782. Jensen WN, Schoefield RA, et al: Clinical and necropsy findings in hemoglobin C disease. Blood 1957; 12:74.

783. Charache C, Conley CL, et al: Pathogenesis of hemolytic anemia in homozygous hemoglobin C disease. J Clin Invest 1967; 46:1795.

784. Kraus AP, Diggs LW: *In vitro* crystallization of hemoglobin occurring in citrated blood from patients with hemoglobin C. J Clin Med 1965; 47:700.

785. Smith EW, Krevans JR: Clinical manifestations of hemoglobin C disorders. Bull Johns Hopkins Hosp 1959; 104:17.

786. Redetzki JE, Bickers JN, et al: Homozygous hemoglobin C disease. Clinical review of fifteen patients. South Med J 1968; 61:238.

787. Fitzgerald PMD, Love WE: Structure of deoxy hemoglobin C (β6Glu→Lys) in two crystal forms. J Mol Biol 1979; 132:603.

788. Houston C: A disease with intra-erythrocytic crystals. Biochim Biophys Acta 1979; 576:497.

789. Girling RL, Houston TE, et al: An x-ray determination of the molecular interactions in hemoglobin C: a disease characterized by intraerythrocytic crystals. Biochem Biophys Res Commun 1979; 88:768.

CHAPTER
21

The Thalassemias

Stuart H. Orkin • David G. Nathan

The thalassemias are a heterogeneous group of inherited anemias caused by mutations affecting the synthesis of hemoglobin.[1-3] Milder forms are among the most frequent genetic disorders in humans, whereas less frequent, yet severe forms lead to significant morbidity and mortality worldwide (Fig. 21–1).

Study of the thalassemias traces the history of the application of recombinant DNA methods to analysis of inherited diseases and underscores how naturally occurring mutations in humans illuminate genetic principles. In this chapter the genetics of hemoglobin genes are reviewed as background for discussion of the molecular basis of the thalassemia syndromes, their clinical phenotypes, prenatal diagnosis, and current management.

HUMAN HEMOGLOBINS: COMPOSITION AND GENETICS

Normal hemoglobins are tetramers of two α-like and two β-like globin polypeptides. The predominant hemoglobin in normal adult red blood cells is Hb A, $\alpha_2\beta_2$.[4,5] The α- and β-globins contain 141 and 146 amino acids, respectively. In addition to Hb A, adult red cells normally contain two minor hemoglobins, Hb A_2 ($\alpha_2\delta_2$) and Hb F ($\alpha_2\gamma_2$). The γ and δ polypeptides are related to the β polypeptide, but differ in their primary amino acid sequences; hence, they are referred to as β-like globins. Hb A_2 normally comprises 2% to 3.5% of total hemoglobin. Although it is a minor component in adult red cells, Hb F is the predominant hemoglobin in fetal red cells during the latter two trimesters of gestation. Because it does not bind 2,3-diphosphoglycerate, its affinity for oxygen is higher than that of Hb A.[6] As such, Hb F enhances the ability of the fetus to extract oxygen from the placenta. Hb F constitutes a small fraction of total hemoglobin in adult red cells (0.3%–1.2%), where it is largely restricted to a small subset of circulating erythrocytes (0.2%–7% of total cells) referred to as F cells.[7,8] Production of Hb F in normal adults appears to be genetically controlled by several loci, including at least one on the X chromosome[9] and another on the long arm of chromosome 6.[10] During the first trimester *in utero*, embryonic hemoglobins with differing subunit composition are found in the yolk sac–derived macrocytic (or primitive) red cells.[1]

The genes that encode the globin polypeptides are organized into two small clusters.[2,4,5,11,12] The α-like genes are located near the telomere of the short arm of chromosome 16 (16p13.3), whereas the β-like genes reside on chromosome 11 at band 11p15.5.[13,14] A schematic diagram of the human globin genes and the compositions of the various hemoglobins are shown in Figure 21–2.

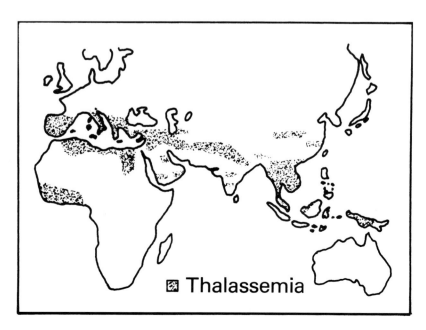

Figure 21–1. Geographic distribution of thalassemia.

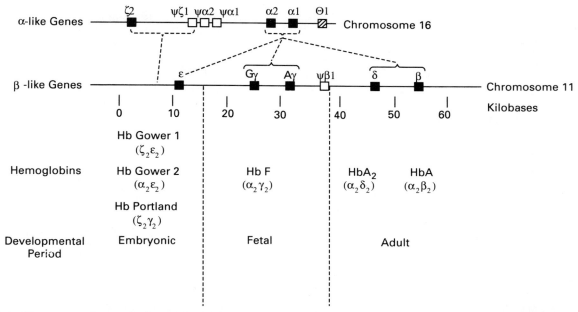

Figure 21-2. Chromosomal organization of the globin genes and their expression during development. The solid boxes indicate functional globin genes, whereas the open boxes indicate pseudogenes (see text). The scale of the depicted chromosomal segments is in kilobases of DNA (kb). The switch from embryonic to fetal hemoglobin occurs between 6 and 10 weeks of gestation, and the switch from fetal to adult hemoglobin occurs at about the time of birth.

The α-globin gene cluster contains three functional genes, ζ, α1, and α2, oriented in the 5′ to 3′ direction along the chromosome.[2, 12, 15, 16] Zeta-globin, encoded by the ζ gene, is found in two embryonic hemoglobins: Hb Gower I ($\zeta_2\epsilon_2$) and Portland ($\zeta_2\gamma_2$).[17] The duplicated α-globin genes (α1 and α2) encode identical polypeptides. DNA sequence analysis has revealed three additional globin gene–like sequences in the cluster: pseudo-ζ (ψζ1), pseudo-α1 (ψα1), and pseudo-α2 (ψα2).[2, 12] Although these resemble the functional genes, sequence differences in coding or critical regulatory regions render these genes inactive; hence, they are referred to as pseudogenes. Such crippled genes are postulated to be derived from previously functional genes that became dispensable during evolution.

Five functional genes, ε, $^G\gamma$, $^A\gamma$, δ, and β, are present within the β-like cluster and arranged 5′ to 3′ as they are expressed during development.[18–21] The product of the embryonic ε gene is found in the embryonic hemoglobins, Hb Gower 1 ($\zeta_2\epsilon_2$) and Hb Gower 2 ($\alpha_2\epsilon_2$). The fetal γ genes are duplicated but encode globins that differ only at position 136 in the polypeptide chain; $^G\gamma$-globin and $^A\gamma$-globin have a glycine or alanine residue, respectively. The $^G\gamma$- and $^A\gamma$-globins are both normally found in Hb F ($\alpha_2\gamma_2$). The δ-globin gene encodes a polypeptide differing in only 10 of 146 residues from β, and yet it is expressed at a very low level in adult red cells (<3% of β). The poor expression of δ-globin is attributed to differences in critical regulatory sequences,[22] sequences within the gene that appear to inhibit messenger RNA (mRNA) processing,[23] and inherent instability of δ mRNA.[24] Only a single functional β-globin gene is present in the cluster. Beta-globin is the predominant β-like globin in adult red cells in which Hb A ($\alpha_2\beta_2$) comprises more than 95% of the total hemoglobin.

The relative synthesis of individual globin chains and the major sites of erythropoiesis during development are depicted in Figure 21–3.[1, 4, 25–27] Embryonic hemoglobins are expressed nearly exclusively in primitive, nucleated red cells differentiating in the yolk sac blood islands. Fetal hemoglobin is produced during the next wave of erythropoiesis, which takes place in the fetal liver. Fetal liver-derived red cells lose their nuclei as terminal maturation occurs, whereas the primitive, yolk sac–derived cells remain nucleated. The transition from Hb F to Hb A coincides approximately with the switch from fetal liver to bone marrow erythropoiesis. Despite this correlation between the site of erythropoiesis and the hemoglobins expressed, careful analysis of tissues derived from experimental animals and human fetuses has shown that embryonic hemoglobins are synthesized in the liver as well as the yolk sac and fetal hemoglobins are produced in the bone marrow as well as the liver. The developmental switches in hemoglobin expression are related to time of gestation rather than to anatomic site of erythropoiesis *per se*.

Globin Gene Structure

The globin genes were among the first eukaryotic genes to be isolated by recombinant DNA cloning methods in the late 1970s. Subsequent work has provided the entire DNA sequences of the human α- and β-globin gene clusters and extensive sequences of other vertebrate globin complexes. These data have been invaluable for determining mutations underlying thalassemia syndromes and for manipulating gene regulatory regions.

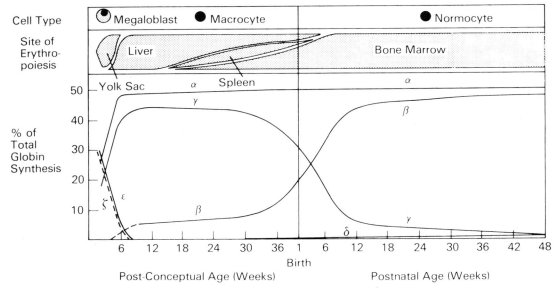

Figure 21–3. The sites of erythropoiesis and the pattern of globin biosynthesis during development. Nucleated megaloblasts are produced predominantly in the yolk sac. These are replaced by macrocytic fetal red cells produced in the liver and subsequently in the spleen and bone marrow. The height of the shaded area approximates the proportion of circulating red cells produced by each organ. Globin biosynthetic measurements were made to obtain the data shown in the lower part of the figure through incubation of intact cells in the presence of radioactive amino acids followed by globin chain separation. (From Weatherall DG, Clegg JB: The Thalassemia Syndromes. Oxford, England, Blackwell Scientific Publications, Inc., 1981, p 54.)

Intervening Sequences or Introns

A remarkable finding was made on initial study of globin genes: the coding region, rather than organized in a single continuous unit, is interrupted by noncoding DNA, known as intervening sequences (IVS) or introns. It is now recognized that the majority of eukaryotic genes contain one or more introns. As indicated in Figure 21–4, globin genes are interrupted at two positions. In the α-globin gene family, introns are present between the codons for amino acids 31 and 32 and between codons 99 and 100. In the β-globin gene family, introns are found between codons 30 and 31 and between codons 104 and 105.

The discontinuous nature of the coding region of globin genes poses a formidable problem for the formation of mRNA that must be translated into globin polypeptides on cytoplasmic ribosomes. Transcription of a globin gene generates a precursor mRNA containing introns. Formation of mature mRNA is accomplished

by post-transcriptional processing, termed *RNA splicing*. The pathway of RNA processing is depicted in Figure 21–5.

RNA splicing must be executed with exquisite precision for functional mRNA to be generated. Because translation of mRNA proceeds by the reading of triplets (codons), excision of introns needs to be accurate to the nucleotide; otherwise, shifts in the reading frame of the translated polypeptide result. RNA processing is guided by specific sequences, known as splice site consensus sequences, located at the 5' and 3' boundaries of the introns. The donor site, which marks the 5' end of the intron, generally conforms to the sequence 5' (C/A)AG'GT(A/G)AGT, where the prime sign indicates the position of splicing and GT is an essentially invariant dinucleotide at the 5' end of the intron. The acceptor site, which defines the 3' end of the intron, usually fits the consensus 5' (T/C)ₙN(C/T)AG'G, where n is greater than or equal to 11, N is any nucleotide, the prime sign indicates the site of splicing, and AG is an essentially invariant dinucleotide. Although excision of introns generally occurs between the dinucleotides GT and AG (the GT-AG rule), rare examples have been reported in which GT is replaced by GC. As reviewed later, mutations in thalassemia that disturb the normal pattern of RNA splicing of globin precursor mRNAs underscore the importance of the splice site consensus sequences.

Conserved Features of Mature Globin mRNAs

Sequences of human globin genes represented in processed globin mRNAs include additional segments located before (5') and after (3') the coding region. These

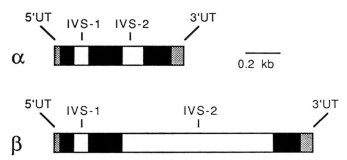

Figure 21-4. Structure of the human α- and β-globin genes. Untranslated regions, exon, and intervening sequences (introns) are depicted by stippled, solid, and open boxes, respectively.

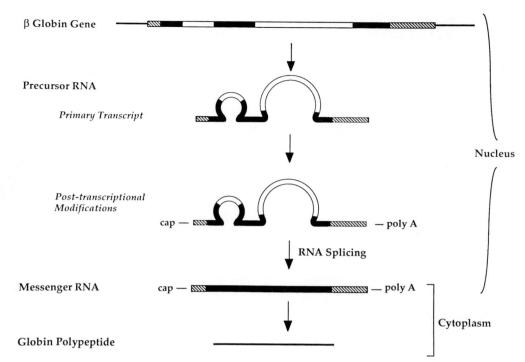

Figure 21–5. Expression of the β-globin gene. Transcription of the gene generates the precursor RNA, which is processed by RNA splicing to form messenger RNA.

untranslated regions are depicted in Figure 21–5. In addition, the mature mRNA is modified at both its termini. At the 5' end a methylated guanylic acid (m⁷G) cap structure is present. A variable number of adenylic acid residues are added at the 3' end and constitute a poly(A) tail. The 5'-cap structure appears important for efficient initiation of mRNA translation, whereas the poly(A) tail contributes to mRNA stability.

Overlapping the beginning of the mRNA sequence in genomic DNA are sequences that aid in directing the initiation of transcription to the proper site. In some eukaryotic genes these sequences conform to an initiator (or Inr) consensus element.[28] Characterization of potential initiator sequences in globin genes is incomplete. However, the human β-globin gene has been shown to possess an Inr element that is functional in transcription reactions performed *in vitro*.[29]

Polyadenylation at the 3' end of mRNA precursors is dependent on a signal in the 3'-untranslated region, generally AAUAAA (AATAAA in genomic DNA). The mechanism of 3'-end modification is complex and involves not only polyadenylation but also cleavage of the precursor RNA, because the primary RNA transcript extends several hundred nucleotides past what becomes the position at which the poly(A) tail is added.

Translation of mRNA into a polypeptide proceeds by the reading of triplets (codons) on cytoplasmic ribosomes. The first AUG codon (specifying methionine) present in the mRNA specifies the start site for translation of the mRNA into protein and is embedded in a sequence context (the Kozak consensus sequence, typically CC(A/G)CCATGG) that signals the binding of translation initiation factors and ribosomes to the

RNA. Usually the amino-terminal methionine residue is removed from the growing polypeptide chain even before its synthesis is completed. Termination of polypeptide chain translation is directed by termination codons UAA, UAG, or UGA. Mutation of these codons allows for continued translation into the 3'-untranslated sequences of mRNA, as occurs in selected α-globin chain variants associated with α-thalassemia (see later).

As briefly reviewed earlier, formation of functional mature mRNA demands extraordinary precision and is dependent on highly conserved sequence elements. As exemplified by the thalassemia syndromes, point (or other) mutations in these signals lead to reduced or absent polypeptide chain synthesis, the hallmark of thalassemia. Mutations causing thalassemia involve all phases of gene expression, including gene transcription, RNA splicing, integrity of the coding sequence, 3'-polyadenylation, and translation initiation (see later).

Regulation of Globin Gene Expression

Globin genes in all vertebrates are expressed in both a tissue-specific and developmentally programmed manner. Their transcription is activated only within developing erythroid precursor cells. Moreover, individual globin genes are expressed at different developmental stages. Hence, within the genes of the β-cluster, globins are expressed at embryonic (ε), fetal (γ), or adult (βδ) stages; whereas within the α-cluster, embryonic (ζ) and adult (α) chain expression is seen. A central problem posed by the organization of the globin gene clusters, recognized more than a decade ago, is how these patterns of tissue- and developmental-stage specificity are achieved. Findings suggest that interactions between regulatory regions and their chromatin-bound proteins located near the genes (the proximal regulatory elements) and more distant control regions provide the means by which transcription is orchestrated in globin gene clusters.

Proximal Regulatory Sequences and Transcription Factors

Several conserved sequence elements (motifs) in the 5'-flanking sequences of globin genes contain the promoter, a region required for accurate and efficient transcription of genes by RNA polymerase II.[30–33] Promoters of vertebrate globin genes are similar in overall configuration and subset of motifs present but differ in their detailed organization and sequences. Promoters generally cooperate with more distant regulatory elements termed *enhancers* to stimulate transcription.[34–36] Globin gene promoters appear to interact in a synergistic fashion with very powerful distant elements, known as locus control regions (LCRs), that may be considered particularly powerful enhancers.

The TATA (or ATA)-box, also referred to as the Hogness box, is one motif that is seen in numerous promoters, including those of all globin genes. The TATA box, which is typically located 20 to 30 base pairs upstream from the transcription start site, constitutes the binding site for a general transcription factor, the TATA-binding protein (TBP).[37–39] Binding of TBP to the TATA box is the first step in the assembly of a basal transcription complex (often termed TFIID) that includes many additional proteins (e.g., TFIIA, TFIIB, TFIIE/F, TFIIH) and RNA polymerase II.[33] Mutations within the TATA box, as occur in some types of β-thalassemia,[40–46] decrease the binding of TBP to the promoter and decrease transcription.[37, 38, 47]

DNA sequence motifs located upstream of the TATA box bind proteins that interact with the general transcription machinery through protein/protein contacts with the TFIID complex and other associated proteins.[32, 34, 35, 39] These promoter-bound proteins may either increase (activate) or decrease (repress) the rate of transcription. A relatively small set of motifs is consistently present in globin gene, as well as many other gene, promoters. These include the CCAAT box, the CACC box, and GATA-consensus sequences. Each motif may be viewed as a potential binding site for one or multiple transcription factors, which are either tissue restricted or ubiquitous in their cellular distribution.

Transcription factors are typically viewed as modular proteins made up of two broad domains that fulfill different functions: a DNA-binding domain responsible for sequence-specific DNA recognition and activation (or repression) domain(s) that interact with components of the basal complex to modulate transcription. The multiplicity of transcription factors, even within a single cell type, able to bind an individual motif provides for fine-tuned regulation while complicating assignment of specific *in vivo* functions to specific proteins. It is believed that overall transcriptional specificity is achieved by functional cooperation and interaction between cell-restricted and general transcription factors. As background for understanding globin gene control, the presently characterized erythroid-enriched transcription factors are reviewed here. For additional discussion of these proteins, readers are referred elsewhere.[48]

The consensus motif (A/T)GATA(A/G), the GATA-motif, is found in the promoter region of most vertebrate globin genes and binds an abundant erythroid-restricted transcription factor GATA-1. GATA motifs have been identified in the regulatory elements of virtually all erythroid-expressed genes, consistent with the notion that GATA-1 should serve a critical role in erythroid gene expression. Multiple GATA sites are also present within distant regulatory elements. The essential role of GATA-1 in erythroid development was formally demonstrated through gene targeting experiments in mouse embryonic stem (ES) cells. Disruption of the single X chromosome *GATA-1* gene in totipotent ES cells prevents their development into normal erythroid cells both *in vivo* and *in vitro*. The GATA-1 protein is a member of a small family of related "GATA factors" that are distinguished by a novel zinc-finger DNA-binding domain. In addition to merely specifying DNA recognition, this domain also mediates protein/protein interactions. Accordingly, GATA-1 is able to interact physically with other GATA-1 molecules or with other types of zinc-finger proteins, including the ubiquitous CACC- or GC-binding factor Sp1 and the erythroid transcription factor EKLF (see later). It is envisioned that through its multiple physical interactions GATA-1 may cooperate with other transcription factors, perhaps bound to DNA at distant sites, to program erythroid-specific transcription.

CACC motifs, which are represented by diverse sequences within globin and other gene promoters, bind a variety of transcription factors. Many CACC sequences are recognized by Sp1, a ubiquitous zinc-finger, activator protein.[49] A particular CACC motif, CCACCCT, is found in the adult β-globin gene promoter and is recognized with high affinity by the erythroid-specific protein EKLF (erythroid Krüppel-like factor). The functional relevance of this binding site has been established through naturally occurring mutations that lead to β-thalassemia (see later). In addition, gene targeting (or knockout) experiments in mice have formally established the requirement for EKLF for efficient β-globin transcription *in vivo*.

A third erythroid transcription factor, known as NFE2, binds to an extended motif {(T/C)TGCTGA(C/G)TCA(T/C)} that is found within some distant regulatory elements (see later) and a small subset of erythroid promoters, but not within globin gene promoters. NFE2 is a heterodimer of two polypeptides of the basic domain-leucine zipper (or b-zip) class of transcription factors.[50, 51] One subunit of NFE2 is tissue restricted, whereas the other is ubiquitous. Although NFE2 is essential for globin gene expression in mouse erythroleukemia cells in tissue culture,[52, 53] its role *in vivo* appears to overlap with that of one or more unknown factors that may act through the same target sites in DNA.[54]

Locus Control Regions and Chromatin Domains

How is globin gene transcription activated and developmentally controlled? Inspection of the DNA sequences of globin gene promoters in the early 1980s failed to provide substantive insights. Initial attempts to dissect control elements involved introducing globin genes into the germline of mice by oocyte injection but were plagued by low level and erratic transgene expression. Nonetheless, it was possible to show that some stage specificity was imparted by the human β- and γ-globin gene promoters. For example, when the human β-globin promoter is introduced into transgenic mice, it directs gene expression only in adult erythroid cells,[55–58] whereas the human γ-globin promoter is active only in embryonic erythroid cells (mice do not have a fetal hemoglobin stage).[59, 60] Although indicative of some specificity inherent in the promoters, the significance of these findings needs to be reconsidered in light of the low level expression of these transgenes and more recent findings regarding the dominant role of distant regulatory elements.

These early globin gene regulation studies suggested that critical regulatory elements were missing from the immediate vicinity of the genes themselves. When sensitivity to digestion by the enzyme DNase I was employed as an indicator of chromatin structure in the mid 1980s, regions of extreme sensitivity (hypersensitivity sites [HSs]) were identified far upstream (~30–50 kb) of the adult human β-globin gene[61, 62] (Fig. 21–6). Four subregions were delimited that are present in the chromatin of erythroid, but not nonerythroid, cells. An additional site located even farther upstream was found in all tissues. In a formal test of their functional relevance, the HSs were linked to a human β-globin and introduced into the germline of mice. Remarkably, transgenic mice then expressed the human β-globin gene at a level equivalent to that of the endogenous mouse β-gene.[63] Further studies showed the transgene is expressed not only in a tissue-specific manner but also in a copy-number–dependent fashion independent of the chromosomal site of integration. These HSs comprise an essential distal regulatory domain, now referred to as the locus control region (LCR).[48]

An LCR appears to resemble other regulatory sequences first termed *enhancers*. These sequences, initially characterized in viral genomes, function in an orientation- and position-independent manner to enhance expression from a linked gene. Often enhancers are associated with the appearance of DNase I hypersensitivity in chromatin. Not all enhancers, however, allow for the copy-number–dependent, position-independent activity characteristic of the β-locus LCR in transgenic mice. It is believed that the LCR serves to decondense or "open" the chromatin domain to permit expression of the downstream globin genes. Consistent with this notion, deletion of the human β-LCR alters chromosomal properties over a large distance (perhaps >200 kb), including a change in timing of replication of the locus.

Other globin gene clusters also contain erythroid-specific DNase I hypersensitive sites. A segment of extreme DNase I hypersensitivity (known as HS-40) located far upstream of the human α-globin genes serves as an enhancer for the α-locus. HS-40, however, does not display the full properties of an LCR, because it does not direct copy-number–dependent transgene expression.[64] Nonetheless, the *in vivo* relevance of both the β-LCR and HS-40 is underscored by the discovery of thalassemia patients with specific deletions in these regions that abolish expression of the downstream globin genes (see later).

The human β-LCR, HS-40, and analogous regions studied in other species are composed of cores, each encompassing a DNase I–hypersensitive site. Cores are 200 to 300 bp in length. Remarkably, within the cores three major protein binding sites are consistently found: GATA, AP-1 (NFE2), and CACC sequences. The position-independent activity of the β-LCR correlates best with the presence of GATA and CACC motifs, particularly within the subregion known as HS 3. Enhancer activity of the LCR, particularly within subregion HS 2, requires the NFE2 motif. The protein-binding motifs within the LCR are also found in globin and other erythroid-expressed gene promoters. No protein-binding sites unique to LCR elements have been identified. Hence, the distinctive properties of the LCR (or HS-40) appear to reflect the synergistic interactions of more typical transcription factors rather than the action of a new set of regulatory proteins.

The discovery of distant control elements, marked by DNase I hypersensitivity, emphasizes the relationship between chromatin structure and globin gene regulation, an association solidified by the unraveling of a rare syndrome, α-thalassemia with X-linked mental retardation.[65] This condition results from mutations in a gene designated XH2 that encodes a member of the

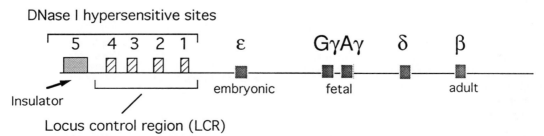

Figure 21–6. Schematic representation of the human β-globin gene locus. The hatched boxes depict the core DNase I hypersensitive subregions of the locus control region. The individual globin genes are indicated with their stage of expression.

helicase superfamily.[66] Such proteins, which are often involved in DNA recombination and repair and in the regulation of transcription in *Drosophila* and yeast, appear to influence transcription in a global manner by altering chromatin structure.

Regulation at a Distance: Globin Gene Switching

How do LCR sequences influence globin gene transcription over large distances (>50 kb)? How are the individual globin genes developmentally regulated? Intensive research has been devoted to these questions. Two formal possibilities have been considered. On the one hand, the LCR might merely provide an environment conducive for activation of the downstream globin genes; the globin genes would be autonomously regulated, that is, the developmental profile of their expression would be intrinsic to the individual genes (and presumably determined by their promoters). The "influence" of the LCR is most simply viewed as reflecting physical association of the LCR with globin genes brought into apposition by chromosomal looping. On the other hand, sequential activation of the particular genes might depend (at least in part) on competition of each gene for the influence of LCR, such that only one gene-LCR interaction would be productive on a single chromosome at any time. The outcome of the competition would be dependent on the array of proteins bound not only at each promoter but also at specific sites in the LCR. Data in favor of both autonomous and competitive mechanisms of regulation have been obtained.[48]

The human embryonic ζ- and ε-globin genes appear to be largely autonomously regulated. LCR-containing transgenes are expressed during embryonic erythropoiesis (the yolk sac stage) and then extinguished during the fetal liver stage. The information required for shutoff is contained nearby the globin genes, and competition by adjacent globin genes is not required. Shutoff is hypothesized to reflect the action of repressors, or silencer proteins, that bind the gene promoters. Motifs within the human ε-globin promoter involved in silencing bind GATA-1 and a ubiquitous factor, YY1.[67]

The competitive model of gene regulation is based on experiments in chicken erythroid cells demonstrating competition between the chicken β- and ε-globin gene promoters for a single enhancer located between the genes.[68] In the chicken it has been proposed that an adult stage-specific factor (NFE4) favors the interaction of the β-promoter with the enhancer to the exclusion of the ε-promoter. In an analogous fashion, data suggest that the human β-globin gene may be negatively regulated in a competition fashion by the γ-globin gene. Whereas the γ-globin gene is largely autonomously regulated, the β-globin gene is silenced in the embryonic and early fetal stage by a linked γ-globin gene (a γ gene in *cis* to β). Shutoff of the γ-globin gene, presumably due to repressors (or silencers), allows the adult β-globin to be expressed. It has been suggested that a protein complex, known as stage-selector protein (SSP), which binds to a site in the proximal γ-promoter, serves a function analogous to that proposed for chicken NFE4 and tips the balance to γ-globin transcription at early stages.[69] Of interest, both NFE4 and SSP complexes appear to contain the ubiquitous transcription factor CP2.[70] The additional protein or proteins in these complexes remain to be fully characterized. How these complexes function *in vivo* is poorly understood.

Although other models are theoretically possible, the capacity of the LCR to act at a distance in regulating activation of globin genes is most compatible with the formation of physical contacts between the LCR (or subregions thereof) and their associated proteins with regulatory elements that are neighbors to the genes themselves. Stage-specific and competitive regulation would, therefore, reflect the engagement of the LCR with genes one at a time. LCR/gene interactions likely have intrinsic stabilities and off-rates, such that a single erythroid cell might express more than one globin over time, even from a single chromosome. Experiments examining nascent human globin RNAs along the β-gene complex tend to support such speculations and lend credence to the notion that chromosomal looping brings the LCR and individual genes in apposition. The dynamic interactions between the β-LCR and the γ and β-globin genes appear to underlie the reciprocal expression of these genes in erythroid cells and provide hope that subtle alterations in the nuclear environment may facilitate reactivation of γ-globin genes in patients with hemoglobinopathies such as sickle cell anemia or with β-thalassemia.

CLASSIFICATION OF THE THALASSEMIAS

The hallmark of thalassemia syndromes is decreased or absent synthesis of one or more globin chains. Alpha- and β-thalassemias refer to deficits in α- and β-globin production, respectively. The α- and β-thalassemias include several clinical syndromes of varying severity (Table 21–1). Knowledge of the molecular genetics of the thalassemias provides a framework in which to consider their clinical heterogeneity.

Because the structural gene for α-globin is duplicated on chromosome 16, each diploid human cell contains

Table 21–1. CLINICAL CLASSIFICATION OF THE THALASSEMIAS

Silent carrier (α or β)	Hematologically normal
Thalassemia trait (α or β)	Mild anemia with microcytosis and hypochromia
Hb H disease (α-thal)	Moderately severe hemolytic anemia, icterus, and splenomegaly
Hydrops fetalis (α-thal)	Death *in utero* caused by severe anemia
Severe β-thalassemia (Cooley's anemia)	Severe anemia, growth retardation, hepatosplenomegaly, bone marrow expansion, and bone deformities
Thalassemia major	Transfusion dependent
Thalassemia intermedia	No regular transfusion requirement

four copies of the α-globin gene. The four α-thalassemia syndromes—silent carrier, α-thalassemia trait, Hb H disease, and hydrops fetalis (Table 21–2)—reflect the inheritance of molecular defects affecting the output of 1, 2, 3, or 4 of the α-globin genes, respectively. More than 30 different mutations affecting one or both α-globin genes on a chromosome have been described.[2, 16] Some mutations abolish expression of an α-globin gene (α^0), whereas others reduce expression of the gene to a variable degree (α^+). Within the four general categories of α-thalassemia there is marked genetic and clinical heterogeneity. Heterogeneity arises because the syndrome in any given individual may represent the combination (or so-called interaction) of 2 of the 30 or more mutations that have been described.

The β-thalassemias also include four clinical syndromes of increasing severity: silent carrier, thalassemia trait, thalassemia intermedia, and thalassemia major (see Table 21–1).[1, 3, 71, 72] In contrast to the α-thalassemias, the four classes of β-thalassemia are not correlated with the number of functioning genes. Because a single functional β-globin gene resides on each chromosome 11, a diploid cell normally has two β-globin genes. The clinical heterogeneity of the β-thalassemias represents the diversity of specific mutations that variably affect β-globin gene expression. Almost exclusively, these mutations involve the β-globin gene rather than an unlinked genetic determinant. Many mutations eliminate β-globin gene expression (β^0), whereas others cause a variable decrease in the level of β-globin gene expression (β^+).[3, 72] The capacity of individual patients to synthesize γ-globin modulates clinical severity. Such is the case because the severity of thalassemias is determined by the degree of globin chain imbalance rather than the absolute level of either α- or β-globin synthesis *per se*.[73–77] Substantial synthesis of γ-globin in the marrow cells of β-thalassemic individuals tends to lessen the extent of chain imbalance and, therefore, improve red cell production.[78–80] Particular mutations of the β-globin gene in β-thalassemia mutations appear to affect γ-globin gene expression directly. However, some individuals with otherwise severe β-thalassemia may co-inherit additional genetic determinants that enhance fetal hemoglobin synthesis. Coincident inheritance of an α-thalassemia mutation also reduces chain imbalance in patients with homozygous or heterozygous β-thalassemia.[81] Clinical severity

in any individual patient represents the outcome of these complex genetic interactions.

Origin of Thalassemia Mutations: The Influence of Malaria

Mutations causing thalassemia have arisen spontaneously. The nearly exclusive distribution of lethal red blood cell disorders, such as thalassemia, sickle cell disease, and glucose-6-phosphate deficiency, in tropical and subtropical regions led Haldane in 1949 to propose that the heterozygous carrier state for these conditions confers a selective advantage where malaria is endemic.[82] The frequency of these genes in a population, then, is determined by the balance between the premature death of the homozygote and the increased fitness of the heterozygote. Beta-thalassemia mutations achieve high gene frequencies (>0.01) in regions such as the Mediterranean basin, northern Africa, Southeast Asia, India, and Indonesia but are uncommon in northern Europe, Korea, Japan, and northern China.[3, 83, 84] The incidence of β-thalassemia trait may exceed 20% in some villages in Greece.[85] Alpha-thalassemia is perhaps the most common single gene disorder in the world.[2] The frequency of α^+-thalassemia alleles ranges from 5% to 10% in the Mediterranean basin,[86] from 20% to 30% in portions of West Africa,[87] and up to 68% in the Southwest Pacific.[88] The frequency of α-thalassemia is less than 0.01% in Great Britain, Iceland, and Japan.[89, 90]

Additional epidemiologic studies have provided evidence for the validity of the "malaria hypothesis" in both α-thalassemia and β-thalassemia.[88, 91–95] Siniscalco and co-workers showed that β-thalassemia is uncommon in the mountainous areas of Sardinia, where malaria is rare, as compared with coastal populations.[91] In Melanesia, α-thalassemia is correlated with malaria across both latitude and altitude.[88] Beta-thalassemia in Melanesia is also associated with malarious coastal regions.[95]

The cellular mechanisms responsible for the selective advantage of thalassemia heterozygotes remain incompletely defined. Cultured erythrocytes containing high concentrations of Hb F retard the growth and development of *Plasmodium falciparum*.[96] Beta-thalassemia heterozygotes have a delayed disappearance of fetal hemoglobin in the first year of life.[1] This might be

Table 21–2. α-THALASSEMIA SYNDROMES

Syndrome	Clinical Features	Hemoglobin Pattern	α-Globin Genes Affected by Thal Mutation
Silent carrier (α-thal-2)	No anemia, normal red cells	1%–2% Hb Bart's (γ_4) at birth; may have 1%–2% Hb CS; remainder Hb A	1
Thalassemia trait (α-thal-1)	Mild anemia, hypochromic and microcytic red cells	5%–10% Hb Bart's (γ_4) at birth; may have 1%–2% Hb CS; remainder Hb A	2
Hb H disease	Moderate anemia; fragmented, hypochromic, and microcytic red cells; inclusion bodies may be demonstrated	5%–30% Hb H (β_4); may have 1%–2% Hb CS; remainder Hb A	3
Hydrops fetalis	Death *in utero* caused by severe anemia	Mainly Hb Bart's, small amounts of Hb H and Hb Portland also present	4

protective from potentially fatal cerebral malaria early in life, because passive immunity acquired *in utero* wanes. Until recently, however, investigators were unable to document decreased invasion or growth of *P. falciparum* in red blood cells from thalassemia heterozygotes except under conditions of unusual oxidant stress.[84, 97] Using modified tissue culture conditions, Brockelman and colleagues demonstrated decreased parasite multiplication in red cells of β-thalassemia heterozygotes.[98] They theorized that *P. falciparum* resistance was a consequence of the inability of the parasite to acquire sufficient nutrients from the digestion of hemoglobin in thalassemic red cells. In one study α-β-thalassemia trait red cells bound greater levels of antibody than controls. This could lead to greater removal of parasitized red cells and hence provide protection.[99] Erythrocytes from individuals with Hb H disease also appear to inhibit *P. falciparum in vitro*,[98, 100] but a similar effect has not been found in erythrocytes from individuals with α-thalassemia trait. It has been suggested that rosette formation, the binding of uninfected red cells to *P. falciparum*–infected red cells, is decreased in thalassemia due to reduced red cell size

and may hinder the development of cerebral malaria by lessening sequestration.[101]

The difficulty in documenting the cellular mechanism of *P. falciparum* resistance in thalassemic erythrocytes *in vitro* suggests that the heterozygote advantage may be small. The high mortality associated with malaria in endemic regions is a powerful selective force that may be sufficient to amplify a small increase in fitness.

Classes of Mutations That Cause Thalassemia

Thalassemia is the consequence of mutations that diminish (or abolish) the production of either the α or β chain of hemoglobin. Molecular cloning, DNA sequencing, and functional analysis of cloned genes have provided the tools with which to dissect the thalassemia syndromes. This analysis has revealed remarkable heterogeneity in the specific alterations in DNA that lead to these clinical syndromes.

Typically single nucleotide mutations associated with thalassemia interfere with one of the critical steps in mRNA production (Fig. 21–7 and Table 21–3). Base

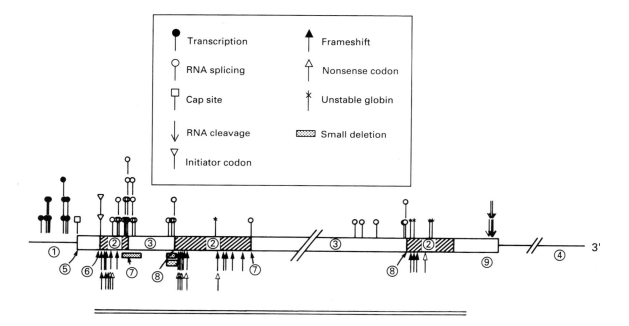

Figure 21-7. The location of various classes of point mutations that cause β-thalassemia, with respect to important structural elements present in the β-globin gene. (Adapted from Kazazian HH Jr, Boehm CD: Molecular basis and prenatal diagnosis of beta-thalassemia. Blood 1988; 72:1107.)

Table 21-3. POINT MUTATIONS THAT CAUSE THALASSEMIA

Gene		Position*	Mutation	Classification	Ethnic Group†	Detection‡	References
A. Transcription Mutations							
β:	1	−101	C-T	β+	Turkish		102
					Bulgarian		
					Italian		
	2	−92	C-T	β+	Mediterranean		3
	3	−88	C-T	β+	American black	(+) Fok I	103
					Asian Indian		
	4	−88	C-A	β+	Kurdish		104
	5	−87	C-G	β+	Mediterranean	(−) Avr II	105
	6	−86	C-G	β+	Lebanese		3
	7	−31	A-G	β+	Japanese		40
	8	−30	T-A	β+	Turkish		41
					Bulgarian		
	9	−30	T-C	β+	Chinese		42
	10	−29	A-G	β+	American black	(+) Nla III	43
					Chinese		44
	11	−28	A-C	β+	Kurdish		45
	12	−28	A-G	β+	Chinese		46
B. Cap Site Mutation							
β:	1	1	A-C	β+	Asian Indian		106
C. RNA Splicing Mutations							
1. Splice junction change in:							
a. 5′ donor site							
α2:	1	IVS-1 n. 2–6	5 bp deletion	α0	Mediterranean		107, 108
β:	1	IVS-1 n. 1	G-A	β0	Mediterranean	(−) Bsp M1	105
	2	IVS-1 n. 1	G-T	β0	Asian Indian	(−) Bsp M1	109
					Chinese		
	3	IVS-1 n. 2	T-G	β0	Tunisian		110
	4	IVs-1 n. 2	T-C	β0	Black		189
	5	IVS-1 5′ end	44 bp deletion	β0	Mediterranean		111
	6	IVS-2 n. 1	G-A	β0	Mediterranean	(−) Hph I	112
					Tunisian		110
					American black		113
b. 3′ acceptor site							
β:	1	IVS-1 n. 130	G-C	β0	Italian		3
	2	IVS-1 n. 130	G-A	β0	Egyptian		3
	3	IVS-1 3′ end	17 bp deletion	β0	Kuwaiti		111
	4	IVS-1 3′ end	25 bp deletion	β0	Asian Indian		114
	5	IVS-2 n. 849	A-G	β0	American black		43
	6	IVS-2 n. 849	A-C	β0	American black		115
2. Splice consensus sequence change in:							
a. 5′ donor site							
β:	1	IVS-1 n. −3 (codon 29)	C-T	?	Lebanese		117
	2	IVS 1 n. − 1 (codon 30)	G-C	Hb Monroe	Tunisian		110
					American black		118
	3	IVS 1 n. − 1 (codon 30)	G-A	?	Bulgarian		119
	4	IVS-1 n. 5	G-C	β+	Asian Indian		109
					Chinese		120
	5	IVS-1 n. 5	G-T	β+	Melanesian		95
					Mediterranean		121
					American black		122
	6	IVS-1 n. 5	G-A	β+	Algerian	(+) Eco RV	123
					Mediterranean		
	7	IVS-1 n. 6	T-C	β+	Mediterranean	(+) Sfa NI	105
b. 3′ acceptor site							
β:	1	IVS-1 n. 128	T-G	β+	Saudi Arabian		124
	2	IVS-2 n. 843	T-G	β+	Algerian		125
	3	IVS-2 n. 848	C-A	β+	Iranian		124
					Egyption		
					American black		122
3. Mutations within exons that affect processing							
β:	1	Codon 19 (Asn-Ser)	A-G	Hb Malay	Malaysian		126
	2	Codon 24 (silent)	T-A	β+	American black		127
	3	Codon 26 (Glu-Lys)	G-A	Hb E	S.E. Asian	(−) Mnl I	72, 128
					European		
	4	Codon 27 (Ala-Ser)	G-T	Hb Knossos	Mediterranean		129

Table continued on following page

Table 21-3. POINT MUTATIONS THAT CAUSE THALASSEMIA *(Continued)*

Gene		Position*	Mutation	Classification	Ethnic Group†	Detection‡	References
4. Internal IVS change							
β:	1	IVS-1 n. 110	G-A	β+	Mediterranean		130, 131
	2	IVS-1 n. 116	T-G	β0	Mediterranean		132
	3	IVS-2 n. 654	C-T	β0	Chinese		120
	4	IVS-2 n. 705	T-G	β+	Mediterranean		133
	5	IVS-2 n. 745	C-G	β+	Mediterranean	(+) Rsa I	105
D. RNA Cleavage and Polyadenylation Mutations							
α2:	1	Cleavage Signal	AATAAA-AATAAG	α+	Middle East		134, 135
					Mediterranean		
β:	1	Cleavage Signal	AATAAA-AACAAA	β+	American black		136
	2	Cleavage Signal	AATAAA-AATAAG	β+	Kurdish		104
	3	Cleavage Signal	AATAAA-AATGAA	β+	Mediterranean		137
	4	Cleavage Signal	AATAAA-AATAGA	β+	Malaysian		137
	5	Cleavage Signal	AATAAA-A (-AATAA)	β+	Arab		3
E. Initiation Consensus Sequence Mutations							
α2:	1	Initiation Codon	ATG-ACG	α0	Mediterranean	(−) Nco I	138
α1:	2	Initiation Codon	ATG-GTG	α0	Mediterranean	(−) Nco I	139
−α:	3	Initiation Codon	ATG-GTG	α0	Black	(−) Nco I	140
−α3.7II:	4	Initiation Consensus	CCACCATGG-CC . . . CATGG	α+	Algerian		141
					Mediterranean		142
β:	1	Initiation Codon	ATG-AGG	β0	Chinese		3
	2	Initiation Codon	ATG-ACG	β0	Yugoslavian		137
	3	Initiation Codon	ATG-ATA	β0	Swedish		
F. Premature Termination Mutations							
1. Substitutions							
α2:	1	Codon 116	GAC-TAG	α0	Black		144
B:	1	Codon 15	G-A	β0	Asian Indian		109
	2	Codon 17	A-T	β0	Chinese	(+) Mae I	145
	3	Codon 35	C-A	β0	Thai		146
	4	Codon 37	G-A	β0	Saudi Arabian		147
	5	Codon 39	C-T	β0	Mediterranean	(+) Mae I	148
	6	Codon 43	G-T	β0	European		149
	7	Codon 61	A-T	β0	Chinese	(−) Hinf I	150
					Black		122
2. Frameshifts							
−α:	1	Codons 30/31	−2 bp (− AG)	α0	Black		151
β:	1	Codon 1	−1 bp (− G)	β0	Mediterranean		3
	2	Codon 5	−2 bp (− CT)	β0	Mediterranean		152
	3	Codon 6	−1 bp (− A)	β0	Mediterranean	(−) Cvn I	122
					American black		153
	4	Codon 8	−2 bp (− AA)	β0	Turkish		154
	5	Codons 8/9	+1 bp (+ G)	β0	Asian Indian		109
	6	Codon 11	−1 bp (− T)	β0	Mexican		3
	7	Codons 14/15	+1 bp (+ G)	β0	Chinese		155
	8	Codon 16	−1 bp (− C)	β0	Asian Indian		109
	9	Codons 27/28	+1 bp (+ C)	β0	Chinese		3
	10	Codon 35	−1 bp (− C)	β0	Indonesian		126
	11	Codons 36/37	−1 bp (− T)	β0	Iranian		104
	12	Codon 37	−1 bp (− G)	β0	Kurdish		104
	13	Codons 37–39	−7 bp (− GACCCAG)	β0	Turkish		156
	14	Codons 41/42	−4 bp (− CTTT)	β0	Asian Indian		109
					Chinese		157
	15	Codon 44	−1 bp (− C)	β0	Kurdish		158
	16	Codon 47	+1 bp (+ A)	β0	Surinamese black		3
	17	Codon 64	−1 bp (− G)	β0	Swiss		159
	18	Codon 71	+1 bp (+ T)	β0	Chinese		3
	19	Codons 71/72	+1 bp (+ A)	β0	Chinese		120
	20	Codon 76	−1 bp (− C)	β0	Italian		160
	21	Codons 82/83	−1 bp (− G)	β0	Azerbaijani		3
	22	Codons 106/107	+1 bp (+ G)	β0	American black		106
G. Termination Codon Mutations							
α2:	1	Codon 142 (ter-Gin)	TAA-CAA	Hb Constant Spring	Chinese		161, 162
	2	Codon 142 (ter-Lys)	TAA-AAA	Hb Icaria	Mediterranean		163
	3	Codon 142 (ter-Ser)	TAA-TCA	Hb Koya Dora	Indian		164
	4	Codon 142 (ter-Glu)	TAA-GAA	Hb Seal Rock	Black		165
β:	1	Codon 147 (ter-Gin)		Hb Tak	Thai		166

822

Table 21–3. POINT MUTATIONS THAT CAUSE THALASSEMIA *(Continued)*

Gene		Position*	Mutation	Classification	Ethnic Group†	Detection‡	References
H. Unstable Hemoglobin Chains							
1. Amino acid substitutions							
−α:	1	Codon 14 (Trp-Arg)		Hb Evanston	Black		167
α2:	2	Codon 109 (Leu-Arg)	T-G	Hb Suan Dok	Southeast Asian		168, 169
α:	3	Codon 110 (Ala-Asp)	T-C	Petah Tikvah	Middle Eastern		170
α2:	4	Codon 125 (Leu-Pro)		Hb Quong Sze	Southeast Asian		171, 172
β:	1	Codon 60 (Val-Glu)	T-A	β⁺	Italian		173
	2	Codon 110 (Leu-Pro)	T-C	Hb Showa-Yakushiji	Japanese		174
	3	Codon 112 (Cys-Arg)		Hb Indianapolis	European		175
	4	Codon 127 (Gln-Pro)		Hb Houston	British		176
	5	Codons 127/128 (Gln, Ala-Pro)	−3 bp (− AGG)	β⁺	Japanese		177
2. Frameshift, extended chain							
β:	1	Codon 94	+2 bp (+TG)	Hb Agnana (Inclusion body)	Italian		178
	2	Codons 109/110	−1 bp (−G)	Hb Manhattan	Lithuanian		3, 176
	3	Codon 114					
			−2, + 1 (− CT, + G)	Hb Geneva (Inclusion body)	French-Swiss		179
	4	Codons 128–135	Net − 10 bp	β⁺ (inclusion body)	Irish		180
3. Premature termination:							
β:	1	Codon 121	G-T	β⁰ (inclusion body)	Greek-Polish French-Swiss British		180, 181, 182

*The position specifies the location in the gene at which the point mutation occurs. Positions are specified with reference to the start site for transcription (Cap site), the position within the intron (IVS), or the position of the codon.

†Where more than one ethnic group is indicated, the mutation has had more than one origin.

‡Loss (−) or gain (+) of a restriction enzyme site with mutation is indicated; the remainder of the mutations can be detected with allele specific oligonucleotides (see Direct Detection of Thalassemia Mutations).

We are grateful to Drs. Halg Kazazian and Titus Huisman and his colleagues for providing us with their detailed lists of β-thalassemia point mutations. (From Kazazian H: The thalassemia syndromes: molecular basis and prenatal diagnosis in 1990. Semin Hematol 1990; 27:209, and reprinted from Huisman TH: Beta-thalassemia repository. Hemoglobin 1990; 14:661, by courtesy of Marcel Dekker, Inc.)

substitutions alter promoter function, RNA processing, or mRNA translation or modify a codon into a "nonsense codon" that leads to premature termination of translation or to the substitution of an incorrect amino acid. Insertion or deletion mutations within the coding region of the mRNA create "frameshifts" that prevent the synthesis of a complete, normal globin polypeptide. Large deletions within the α- or β-globin clusters may remove one or more genes and alter the regulation of the remaining genes in the cluster. The phenotype that results from the diverse mutations found in thalassemia is determined by the degree of inactivation of the affected gene or genes and the extent of associated increases in expression of other genes within the cluster.

Mutations Affecting Gene Transcription

Point mutations within promoter sequences recognized by transcription factors tend to reduce the affinity with which these proteins bind. Typically this leads to reduced gene transcription. Analysis of the promoter for the β-globin gene in patients with β-thalassemia has identified a variety of mutations clustered in the ATA and CACC motifs (see Table 21–3 and Fig. 21–8).[3, 40–46, 102–105] These mutations are associated with preservation of some β-globin expression and hence are customarily associated with the phenotype of thalassemia intermedia. The C→T substitution at position −101, which results in a particularly mild defect, is associated with the "silent carrier" phenotype in heterozygous carriers.[102, 183] Although the CCAAT box is highly conserved in globin genes, no mutations within this motif have been identified in thalassemia. At present, mutations in transcription factors that result in thalassemia have not been identified, although exceedingly rare families have been identified in which a thalassemia mutation is unlinked to the globin clusters (see later).

Mutations of the ATA box presumably reduce binding of TBP and, therefore, lead to decreased transcription initiation. Substitutions in the CACC motifs decrease the affinity of binding by several transcription factors, including the erythroid-specific factor EKLF and the ubiquitous protein Sp1. Studies showing that mice engineered to lack EKLF suffer from lethal β-thalassemia at the fetal liver stage establish EKLF as

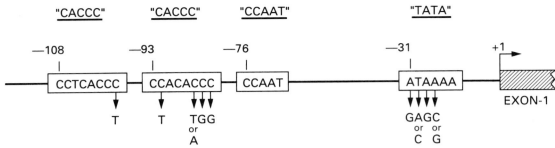

Figure 21-8. Point mutations in the β-globin gene promoter. The sequences of conserved motifs within the promoter and their distance from the transcription start site are indicated. Single base substitution at the indicated positions results in β⁺-thalassemia.

a β-globin activator protein *in vivo*.[184, 185] Human β-thalassemias resulting from mutation of a single CACC motif are presumably mild owing to the presence of one normal CACC motif within the promoter.

In addition to the protein binding sites in the promoter, proper transcription is dependent on sequences surrounding the start site of transcription (known as +1). These sequences often display functional activity in *in vitro* assays, heralding the binding of specific protein complexes to this type of element, termed the *initiator* (Inr). Mild β-thalassemia has been associated with a base substitution (A→C) at +1. This substitution has been shown to impair the β-globin Inr.[29] The proteins that mediate this effect are unknown.

RNA Processing Defects in Thalassemia

The importance of RNA splicing for formation of functional mRNA cannot be overemphasized. As discussed earlier, removal of introns must be accurate to the nucleotide for a continuous, translatable mRNA to be generated from an mRNA precursor. As soon as introns were discovered, it was hypothesized that mutations affecting RNA splicing would likely be involved in the thalassemia syndromes. Apart from its role in constructing a functional mRNA, RNA splicing also appears to be a determinant of mRNA stability[186, 187] and possibly coupled to RNA transport from nucleus to cytoplasm.[188]

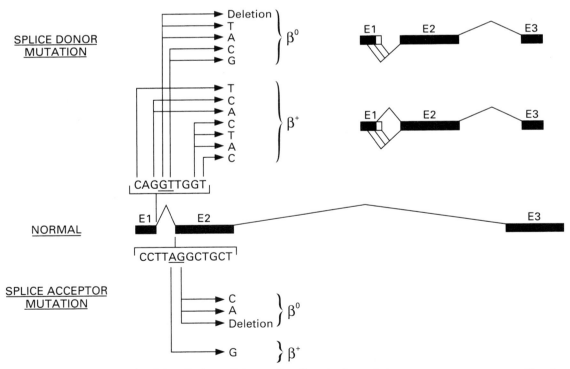

Figure 21-9. Examples of abnormal splicing that result from alterations in the splicing consensus sequences. The three β-globin gene exons are symbolized by solid boxes, the normal splicing pattern is illustrated by lines that project above the exons, and the splice donor and splice acceptor sequences of the first intron are shown. Mutations in the invariant GT dinucleotide of the splice donor site abolish normal splicing of the first intron and result in β⁰-thalassemia, whereas mutations elsewhere in the consensus sequence preserve some normal splicing and cause β⁺-thalassemia. Changes in the splice donor site are associated with abnormal splicing from three cryptic splice donors *(lines that project below the exons)*; one site is within the first intron and results in the addition of intron sequences to Exon 1 *(open box)*. Similarly, changes in the invariant AG dinucleotide of the splice acceptor sequence are associated with β⁰-thalassemia, whereas a mutation in an adjacent nucleotide causes β⁺-thalassemia.

Mutations That Alter Splice Junctions or Splice Consensus Sequences

Mutations of the 5' donor site (GT)[105, 107–113, 189] or at the 3' splice acceptor site (AG)[3, 43, 111, 114–116] abolish proper splicing of the pre-mRNA transcript and result in α[0]- or β[0]-thalassemia (see Table 21–3 and Fig. 21–9). Substitutions at other sites within the splice junction consensus sequence have varied effects; as some correctly spliced RNA, albeit a reduced amount, is produced, a β[+]-thalassemia phenotype ensues.[95, 105, 109, 110, 117–125]

Mutations within the splice site, or the splice site consensus sequences, favor improper processing of the mRNA precursor. These secondary splicing events, which are not seen under normal circumstances, occur at positions that resemble splice site consensus sequences. Splicing at these "cryptic" sites generates aberrantly processed, nonfunctional globin mRNAs (see Fig. 21–9). Mutations within the β-globin IVS-1 splice donor site activate two cryptic donor sites in exon 1 and a third site in IVS-1,[105, 112, 190] whereas mutation in the IVS-2 splice donor activates a cryptic donor site in IVS-2.[112] Mutation of the IVS-2 splice acceptor site activates an upstream cryptic splice acceptor at position 579 in IVS-2.[43] These incorrectly spliced mRNAs suffer either insertions or deletions in the coding region and also shifts in the translational reading frame downstream of the cryptic splice site. The polypeptide synthesized beyond this point bears no resemblance to the globin chain and is often prematurely shortened by a termination codon encountered in the new reading frame.

Mutations Within Exons That Create an Alternative Splice Site

RNA from β-thalassemia genes with mutations in the IVS-1 donor splice site may be processed using a cryptic splice donor site GTGGTGAGG in exon 1 (codons 24–27). Four independent mutations have been identified that activate this cryptic site in the presence of a *normal* IVS-1 splice donor site (see Table 21–3 and Fig. 21–10).[72, 127–129] These mutations appear to enhance the ability of the cryptic site to compete with the normal site for binding of the splicing complex. A T→A mutation at codon 24 is "silent" at the translational level, yet approximately 80% of RNA transcripts are spliced at this incorrect site; hence, mild β[+]-thalassemia ensues.[127] Two mutations—GAG→AAG in codon 26[72, 128]

and GCC→TCC in codon 27[129]—lead to amino acid replacements that produce the hemoglobin variants Hb E and Hb Knossos, respectively, in normally processed mRNA. Because a proportion of transcripts are aberrantly spliced, mild β[+]-thalassemia results. An analogous mutation in codon 19 produces β[+]-thalassemia with the hemoglobin variant Hb Malay.[126] These represent mutations that lead to thalassemic hemoglobinopathies.

Mutations Within Introns That Create an Alternative Splice Site

Mutations within β-globin IVS-1 may create a new splice acceptor sequence (see Table 21–3 and Fig. 21–10).[130–132] In the first of this class of mutations to be characterized, a G→A substitution at position 110 (19 nucleotides upstream of the normal intron/exon boundary), the majority of globin mRNA precursors are spliced at this alternative site.[130, 131, 191, 192] Because the incorrectly spliced mRNA contains 19 nucleotides from IVS-1, a shift in the reading frame leads to premature termination of translation. A T→G mutation at position 116 of IVS-1 creates a new acceptor site that is used exclusively, leading to little or no normal β mRNA production and β[0]-thalassemia.[132]

Three mutations in IVS-2 create new donor sites and activate an upstream cryptic donor site located 579 nucleotides from the exon 2/IVS-2 boundary (see Table 21–3 and Fig. 21–10).[105, 120, 133] The consequence of these mutations is the insertion of a fourth "exon" derived from sequences within IVS-2. Although the normal donor and acceptor sites are unaffected, little or no correctly spliced β-globin mRNA may be produced.[105, 120, 133]

RNA Cleavage and Polyadenylation Defects

Proper cleavage at the 3'-end of the pre-mRNA and subsequent poly(A) addition depend on the integrity of the AAUAAA signal in the 3'-untranslated region. The importance of the polyadenylation signal for the efficient production of globin mRNA was first demonstrated in α-thalassemia.[134, 135, 193] Mutation of AAUAAA→AAUAAG in the α2 gene reduces the efficiency of cleavage-polyadenylation of precursor RNAs and leads to "run-on" transcripts that terminate downstream of the gene (Fig. 21–13). Mutations in the AAU-

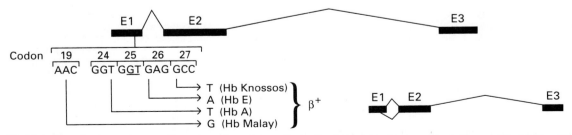

Figure 21–10. Mutations that create an alternate splice donor site in the first exon decrease but do not abolish the frequency of normal splicing *(pattern that projects above the exons)* and are associated with splicing from the new site in the first exon *(pattern that projects below the exons)*. Three of these mutations lead to the incorporation of a different amino acid into the β-globin chain derived from the decreased quantity of correctly spliced β-globin mRNA and generate variant hemoglobins.

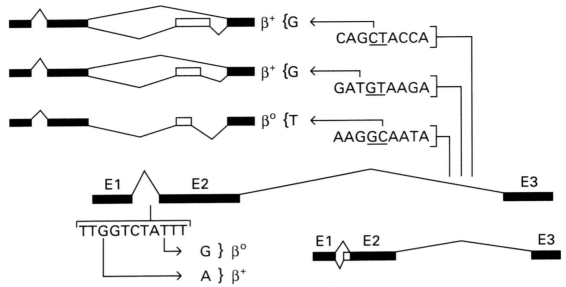

Figure 21-11. Mutations within introns that create a new splice site. Three mutations in the second intron create a new splice acceptor site (the invariant GT is underlined) and activate the identical cryptic splice donor site located just upstream. Abnormal splicing from these sites *(pattern that projects below the exons)* leads to the creation of a fourth exon *(open box)* derived from sequences within the second intron. Two mutations in the first intron create a new splice acceptor site with the conserved AG dinucleotide, and abnormal splicing from this site *(pattern that projects below the exons)* adds sequences from the first intron to the beginning of the second exon.

AAA element have also been described in β-thalassemia,[104, 136, 137] in which the presence of the elongated *in vivo* transcripts has been demonstrated.[136] The transcripts appear to terminate at the next AAUAAA signal, which is present about 900 nucleotides downstream of the normal cleavage site. These mutations lead to a moderate reduction in the level of β-globin mRNA and a β⁺-phenotype.

Mutations Affecting mRNA Translation Initiation

Translation begins at an AUG codon that usually lies within a consensus sequence, (GCC)GCC(A/G)-

CCATGG.[194] Substitutions within the AUG codon abolish translation, whereas those in the other positions of the consensus often result in less efficient translation initiation.

Four mutations in α-globin genes alter the consensus sequence and impair translation (see Table 21–3). Three of these affect the AUG initiator.[138–140] No globin polypeptide is produced, because the next downstream initiator is in a different reading frame. The fourth α-globin mutation in this class, found on a chromosome in which one α-globin gene was deleted, alters the consensus sequence by the deletion of two base pairs and reduces mRNA translation to 50% of normal.[141, 142] Two AUG initiator mutations of the β-globin gene have

		31	32	33	34	35	36	37	38
· · · · · · ·	CTTAGG	CTG	CTG	GTG	GTC	TAC	CCT	TGG	ACC
	Intron I	Leu	Leu	Val	Val	Tyr	Pro	Trp	Thr

Deleted in β⁰ - 44 Gene
↑
| | | | | | Ser | Leu | Gly | Ile | Cys | Pro | Leu |

39	40	41	42	43	44	45	46	47	48	49	50
CAG	AGG	TTC	TTT	GAG	TCC	TTT	GGG	GAT	CTG	TCC	ACT
Gln	Arg	Phe	Phe	Glu	Ser	Phe	Gly	Asp	Leu	Ser	Thr

T in β⁰ - 39 Gene (7)
↓
Ter

| Leu | Met | Leu | Leu | Trp | Ala | Thr | Leu | Arg | Ter |
51	52	53	54	55	56	57	58	59	60	61
CCT	GAT	GCT	GTT	ATG	GGC	AAC	CCT	AAG	GTG	AAG	· ·
Pro	Asp	Ala	Val	Met	Gly	Asn	Pro	Lys	Val	Lys

Figure 21-12. Two of the several thalassemia mutations that destroy gene function by introduction of a premature translation termination codon in β-globin mRNA. The numbers above the individual codons refer to the encoded amino acid's position in the β-globin mRNA. Replacement of C with T in codon 39 introduces the terminator UAG in β-globin mRNA. Another β⁰ gene has a deletion of the third nucleotide (C) in codon 41. This results in a shift in the reading frame of the mRNA; the new amino acid sequence is shown above the line. This new reading frame has an in-phase terminator (UGA) in a position corresponding to codon 60-61. (From Nienhuis AW, Anagnou NP, Ley TJ: Advances in thalassemia research. Blood 1984; 63:738.)

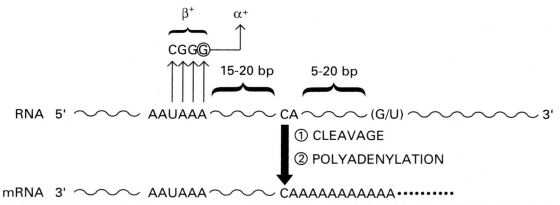

Figure 21-13. RNA cleavage and polyadenylation occurs 15 to 20 bp downstream from the AAUAAA polyadenylation signal. Mutational analysis in the rabbit β-globin gene has established that sequences located downstream from the polyadenylation site, called the G/U cluster, are also required for efficient cleavage and polyadenylation. Individual point mutations at one of several nucleotides within the AAUAAA polyadenylation signal result in β⁺-thalassemia. The same A to G mutation in the last position that causes β-thalassemia has been observed in the α2-globin gene and results in α⁺-thalassemia.

been described, and both are of the β⁰ type (see Table 21–3).[3, 137]

Premature Termination (Nonsense) Mutations

Nucleotide substitutions within the coding region are innocuous if they occur in the third position of a codon and do not alter the amino acid inserted during translation. Substitutions that alter codons from one amino acid to another lead to hemoglobin structural variants. Some substitutions change a triplet coding for an amino acid to a stop codon (UAG, UUA, UGA). Such chain-termination (or nonsense) mutations abort mRNA translation and lead to synthesis of a truncated polypeptide. Moreover, nonsense mutations also reduce the amount of stable mRNA generated, reflecting coupling between mRNA biogenesis and mRNA translation.[195]

Chang and Kan described the first nonsense mutation in β-thalassemia in which a lysine codon at amino acid position 17 was converted to a stop codon (AAG→UAG).[145] Although no β-globin chains were produced *in vivo*, complete translation of the abnormal mRNA could be achieved in a cell-free extract capable of protein synthesis by the addition of a "suppressor" transfer RNA (tRNA) that inserts a serine at the UAG codon.[196] Several other nonsense mutations causing thalassemia have been described (see Table 21–3 and Fig. 21–13).[109, 122, 146–150] In addition, single or dinucleotide insertions or deletions have been observed that alter the translational reading frame and introduce a premature stop codon as a consequence.* Two termination mutations have been described in the α-globin genes, one which introduces a stop codon [144] and the other a frameshift.[151] In addition, frameshift mutations have been described that result in abnormal elongation of globin chains (see Unstable β-Globin Chains).

mRNAs with termination mutations often do not accumulate to a normal level *in vivo*.[195, 197] The extent of this effect is variable and dependent on the specific mutations; deletion of the third nucleotide (C) from codon 41 (Fig. 21–14) leads to complete absence of globin mRNA,[198] whereas a single substitution in the β-39 codon allows accumulation of 5% to 10% of the normal amount of globin mRNA.[197] The basis for this quantitative deficiency of these mRNA species is of considerable interest. Speculation that abnormal mRNAs are unstable because impaired translation exposes such molecules to cytoplasmic nucleases has not been experimentally verified. Rather, data suggest that such mutations lead to intranuclear degradation of abnormal globin RNA molecules and suggest a link between mRNA translation and nuclear RNA processing or nuclear to cytoplasmic transport of mRNA.[199, 200] Experimental studies in tissue culture systems have shown that the deficiency in β-globin mRNA accumulation is specific for nonsense mutations and is not observed with missense mutations[195]; a suppressor tRNA that allows the abnormal mRNA molecule to be translated completely will correct the quantitative deficiency in globin mRNA.[200] The specific mechanisms responsible for the defect in mRNA accumulation remain unclear.

Termination Codon Mutations

UAA is the normal termination codon for both α- and β-globin mRNA translation. The 3' untranslated regions are 109 and 132 nucleotides for α- and β-mRNAs, respectively. A single nucleotide substitution in the termination codon could create either another stop codon (UAG) or permit incorporation of an amino acid at this position and the translation of the otherwise untranslated 3'-sequences until the next in-frame stop codon. Four termination codon mutations involving the α2 gene have been reported (see Table 21–3).[161–166] These mutants differ only in the specific amino acid incorporated at the terminator codon position (see Fig. 21–14). Translation terminates in each instance at a UAA codon in the polyadenylation signal (AAUAAA) downstream, producing a 172 amino acid polypeptide.

---

*See references 3, 104, 106, 109, 120, 122, 126, and 152 through 160.

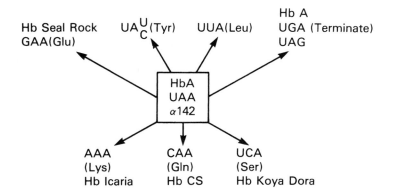

Figure 21-14. Point mutations in the terminator codon of the α-globin gene that lead to synthesis of elongated α-globins. The normal terminator, UAA, of α-globin mRNA is shown in the center. Each of the nine possible single nucleotide substitutions is depicted; two would result in formation of another terminator codon, whereas the other seven would lead to insertion of an amino acid at this position and continued synthesis of the globin chain. Four such mutations have been described; that which causes synthesis of Hb Constant Spring (CS) is the most common. (Adapted from Weatherall DJ, Clegg JB: The Thalassemia Syndromes. Oxford, England, Blackwell Scientific Publications, Inc., 1981, p 578.)

The first of these elongated α chains to be described was found in Hb Constant Spring.[161, 162] The α chain in this hemoglobin has a glycine substituted at codon 142. Hb Constant Spring produces an associated thalassemia phenotype owing to a marked reduction of α2-globin mRNA stability.[201–203]

Mutations that give rise to elongated β-globin chains have also been described. Hb Tak is a 157 amino acid product of a β-globin mRNA molecule containing two inserted nucleotides in the terminator codon 147.[166] An analogous elongated β-globin with 157 amino acids found in Hb Cranston reflects a two-nucleotide insertion in codon 147, but red cells containing Hb Cranston are morphologically normal.[204] The mechanism by which the β[Tak] mutation causes thalassemia has not been elucidated.

Mutations Affecting Globin Chain Stability

Hemoglobin Assembly. Shortly after synthesis is completed, α- and β-globin chains bind a heme moiety and rapidly associate into $\alpha_1\beta_1$ dimers in a noncovalent reaction that is nearly irreversible under physiologic conditions.[205] The majority of the heme contact points are present in the portion of the globin chains encoded by exon 2, whereas most $\alpha_1\beta_1$ contacts are located within the exon 3 domain (Fig. 21–15).[6, 206] These dimers may then reversibly associate with other dimers to form the hemoglobin tetramer. The formation of the $\alpha_1\beta_1$ dimer, therefore, is the principal controlling step in the assembly of hemoglobin.

Hemoglobin assembly is an important determinant of the final hemoglobin composition of the erythrocyte.[205, 207, 208] The rate constant of dimer formation is highly dependent on the surface electrostatic charge of the subunits.[205] Alpha-globin has a net positive surface charge, whereas β-globin has a net negative surface charge. The other normal β-like globin chains, γ-globin and δ-globin, dimerize with the α chain at a lower rate. Delta-globin has a lower net negative surface charge than β-globin, whereas the significant structural differences between γ- and β-globins presumably account for the differing dimerization rates. Where β-globin chains are in limited supply (i.e., β-thalassemia), Hb A_2 and Hb F levels may rise owing to enhanced dimerization with α chains, independent of changes in the production of δγ chains. In α-thalassemia or iron deficiency, Hb A_2 and Hb F levels will fall because of competition with β chains for the limited number of α chains. Similarly, β chain variants may have decreased (β^S, β^E) or increased ($\beta^{Baltimore}$) affinity for α chains based on their net surface charge. The net hemoglobin composition of the cell is determined by these simple rules of competition based on the relative affinity of hemoglobin subunits.

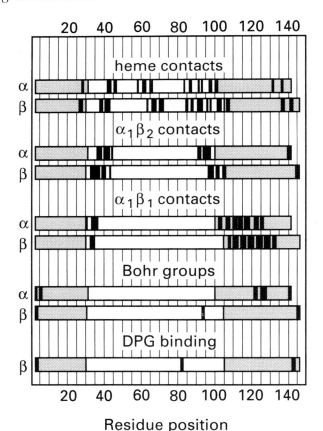

Figure 21-15. Schematic representation of the α- and β-globin chains, indicating the location of residues involved in different hemoglobin functions (*solid vertical bars*). Heme contact sites and $\alpha_1\beta_2$ contacts are concentrated in the second exon (*unshaded*), while $\alpha_1\beta_1$ contacts are principally located in the third exon (*shaded*). (Adapted from Eaton WA: The relationship between coding sequences and function in haemoglobins. Nature 1980; 284:183. Reprinted by permission from Nature, copyright © 1980 Macmillan Magazines Limited.)

An efficient, energy-dependent proteolytic system is present in erythrocytes that rapidly degrades free globin chains, while leaving chains incorporated into dimers or tetramers unaffected.[205] Changes in globin chain structure that result from amino acid substitutions, premature chain termination, or chain elongation may slow or block the formation of stable $\alpha_1\beta_1$ dimers and lead to rapid degradation of the globin chain. In some instances, as discussed later, mutations may also enhance association of the free globin chain with the cell membrane, promoting oxidative damage to the membrane and shortened red cell survival.

Unstable α-Globin Chains

One such unstable variant was identified on sequencing of a mutant α-globin gene (see Table 21–3).[171] Alpha[Quong Sze], which contains a Leu→Pro substitution at position 125, is so unstable that the mutant globin chain cannot be detected by biosynthetic studies in intact cells or by conventional hemoglobin electrophoresis.[172] The $\alpha^{Quong Sze}$ chain appears to be stable once it is incorporated into the hemoglobin tetramer. Three other similar unstable α-globin chain mutations have been described (see Table 21–3).[167–170]

Unstable β-Globin Chains

Several unstable β-globin chains have been associated with thalassemia (see Table 21–3). Five mutations lead to amino acid substitutions in the β-globin chain.[173–177] Four frameshift mutations in the third exon result in synthesis of an elongated β-globin chain with a novel carboxy-terminus.[3, 176, 178–180] A premature termination mutation in exon 3 has also been described.[180–182] Many of the unstable β-globin chain mutations in exon 3 are associated with a dominantly inherited form of thalassemia.[176, 180] Thein and associates have proposed that alterations of β-globin structure in exon 3 interfere with $\alpha_1\beta_1$ dimer formation yet may permit binding of heme to the mutant globin chain through contacts in the exon-2 domain. These free, heme-associated β-globin chains may be more resistant to proteolysis and associate with the cell membrane, forming "inclusion bodies" and inducing oxidative damage.[180]

Thalassemic Hemoglobinopathies

The mutations described in this section, taken together with the RNA processing mutants Hb E, Hb Knossos, and Hb Malay and the termination mutant Hb Tak, comprise a distinctive set characterized by structural changes in the hemoglobin molecule *and* a thalassemia phenotype. These mutations are often referred to as "thalassemic hemoglobinopathies" (see Thalassemic Hemoglobinopathies)[209] and are characterized clinically by a syndrome of ineffective erythropoiesis. Other globin variants may be associated with mild hypochromia, microcytosis, and chronic hemolysis because of instability and degradation of hemoglobin tetramers and are discussed in detail in Chapter 19. Because thalassemia is the consequence of an imbalance in α- and β-globin chains, these variants are not considered part of the spectrum of thalassemia.

Identification, Characterization, and Ethnic Distribution of β-Thalassemia Mutations

The disorders of hemoglobin serve as a paradigm for the molecular analysis of genetic disease. The dissection of β-thalassemia was aided by the introduction of now widely used methods for identifying and characterizing mutant alleles. Accordingly, the identification of β-thalassemia mutations in many ethnic groups is nearly complete.[3, 111]

In this section, the molecular techniques that have been applied to the characterization of β-thalassemia mutations are briefly outlined. An understanding of these methods is important not only because of their broad use in the study of other genetic diseases but also because they are directly relevant to strategies for genetic screening and prenatal diagnosis of β-thalassemia.

Haplotype Analysis

The first several β-thalassemia mutations were identified by the cloning and sequencing of β-globin genes isolated from individuals with β thalassemia major.* Because certain mutations are extremely common, a nondirected strategy is inefficient: β-globin genes with common mutations will be repeatedly studied. For example, 95% of the β-thalassemia alleles on the island of Sardinia contain the codon 39 nonsense mutation.[214]

To facilitate the search for new β-thalassemia mutations, Orkin, Kazazian, and their colleagues introduced the concept of haplotype analysis to the study of thalassemia.[105, 215, 216] Naturally occurring, genetically neutral, nonselected sequence differences among individuals constitute polymorphisms, which are estimated to occur roughly once every 100 base pairs.[217] These sequence differences are heritable, and those residing close to one another on a chromosome tend to be inherited together, a property known as *linkage*. A subset of polymorphisms will alter the cleavage site for a restriction enzyme or create a site where one did not exist. Therefore, when DNA from unrelated individuals is digested with a restriction enzyme and analyzed by Southern blotting, polymorphisms in the restriction enzyme digest pattern may be observed; these are referred to as restriction fragment length polymorphisms (RFLP).[218] Within the 60 kb of the human β-globin cluster, more than 20 such RFLPs are known[5, 219]; at least 13 have been identified in the α-globin cluster.[2, 220] The pattern of these RFLPs (each based on the presence [+] or absence [−] of a restriction enzyme cutting site) along the chromosome defines a haplotype of associated or linked polymorphisms. Seven RFLPs were employed initially to define nine distinct haplotypes (I–IX) of the β-globin gene cluster in the analysis

---

*See references 112, 130, 131, 145, 148, 154, and 210 through 213.

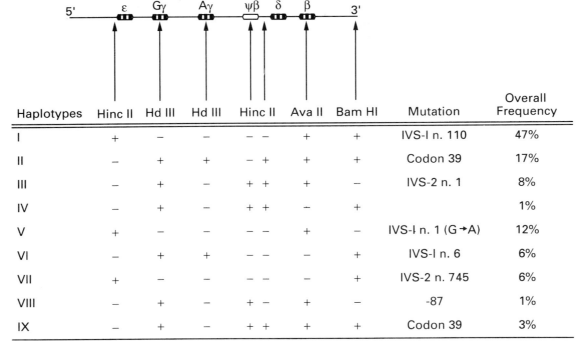

Figure 21-16. Linkage of chromosomal haplotypes to specific β-thalassemia mutations in Mediterranean populations. A haplotype is defined by the sequential pattern of restriction enzyme sites (present ``+'' or absent ``−'') along a chromosome. In this example, seven restriction enzymes were used to classify nine haplotypes. Overall frequency refers to the prevalence of the specific haplotype as found in all individuals, with or without thalassemia. (Adapted from Orkin SH, Kazazian HH Jr, et al: Linkage of beta thalassemia mutations and beta-globin gene polymorphisms with DNA polymorphisms in the human beta-globin gene cluster. Nature 1982; 296:627. Reprinted by permission from Nature, copyright © 1982 Macmillan Magazines Limited.)

of thalassemia mutations in Greek and Italian populations from the Mediterranean basin (Fig. 21–16).[105]

Close inspection of these haplotypes revealed a nonrandom association of restriction digest patterns within the β-gene cluster (Fig. 21–17).[215, 221] The pattern of restriction sites upstream of the δ globin gene is inherited as a group, whereas restriction sites downstream (including the β-globin gene) track as another set. In all populations, only a few haplotypes predominate.[222] The full spectrum of haplotypes is derived from random association over evolutionary time between the 5' and the 3' subhaplotypes, presumably reflecting the presence of a recombination "hot spot" lying between these regions.[109, 221, 223, 224]

The generation of haplotypes appears to be an ancient event predating racial dispersion. Consequently, a specific haplotype may be found in diverse ethnic and racial groups from different geographic locations. The introduction of malaria as a selective pressure for

certain random mutations is a more recent phenomenon. A mutation leading to thalassemia would be under positive selection and amplified within a population; accordingly, the mutation would be expected to be found on the haplotype background in which it originated in that ethnic group. Several conclusions can be derived from the study of different racial groups.[72] Within a single population both normal and thalassemia β-globin genes are found on the same haplotype, but specific thalassemia mutations tend to be linked to a single haplotype. Individual thalassemia mutations are generally restricted to a single population (see Table 21–3). In circumstances in which specific mutations are found in different populations, the identical thalassemia mutation may have occurred and been selected for independently and will be found on a different haplotype background.[44, 113, 225] This observation has provided a sound genetic basis for the belief that thalassemia has had multiple distinct origins throughout

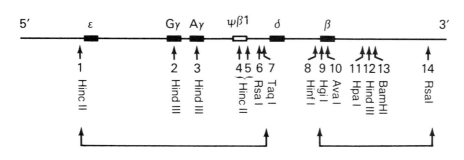

Figure 21-17. Restriction endonuclease sites for which RFLP have been identified in the β-globin gene cluster. A recombinational hot spot has been identified between the two brackets; the RFLP enclosed in each bracket must often remain associated during recombination (see text).

the world. In circumstances in which a specific mutation is found on more than one haplotype within a population, the 3' subhaplotype (where the β-globin gene resides) may be identical whereas the 5' subhaplotypes differ due to recombination between the two subhaplotypes (for an example, see codon 39 mutation, Fig. 21–16). By this mechanism, specific mutations can be distributed to new haplotypes within an ethnic group and an independent origin of the mutation need not be invoked.

New thalassemia mutations were identified by cloning thalassemia β-globin genes from distinct haplotypes within a population, thereby avoiding the likelihood of repeated cloning of the same common mutation.[105] In this way, the great diversity of thalassemia mutations was elucidated.[111]

Direct Detection of Thalassemia Mutations

Restriction Enzyme Analysis. Several thalassemia mutations fortuitously result in the creation or destruction of a restriction enzyme cleavage site within the α- or β-globin gene. The change in the restriction digest pattern can be detected in a Southern blot of digested genomic DNA or can be visualized directly when the analysis is performed on DNA amplified by the polymerase chain reaction (PCR, see later).[226–228] A list of mutations that alter restriction enzyme sites is provided in Table 21–3. Although approximately 50% of the common thalassemia mutations in Mediterranean populations may be detected in this manner, this approach is of less utility in other groups.[3, 111]

Allele Specific Oligonucleotide Hybridization. Specific synthetic oligonucleotide probes of about 19 nucleotides in length extend the capacity to detect specific thalassemia mutations directly in genomic DNA or DNA amplified by PCR.[229, 230] Single nucleotide mismatches between a probe of this length and a target DNA sequence destabilize hybridization.[231] To study a given mutation or allele, two probes are generally used, one identical in sequence to the normal gene and the other identical to the mutant sequence. To facilitate detection of a mutation, probes are generally designed to position the difference in the center of the probe. In Southern blot analysis, such probes can be shown to be highly specific for cloned DNA fragments containing particular mutations (Fig. 21–18). When the target is DNA amplified by PCR, low specific activity probes or nonradioactive probes can be utilized to detect the presence of the mutation.[232–235] Although there are many β-thalassemia mutations, relatively few predominate in each ethnic group (see Ethnic Distribution). Hence, a small panel of oligonucleotides can be used to identify the majority of potential mutations in any given population.[236, 237]

Denaturing Gradient Electrophoresis. The use of restriction enzyme analysis or allele-specific oligonucleotide hybridization requires prior knowledge of the mutation to be studied at the DNA sequence level. Other methods have been developed that permit detection of differences before nucleotide sequencing. DNA

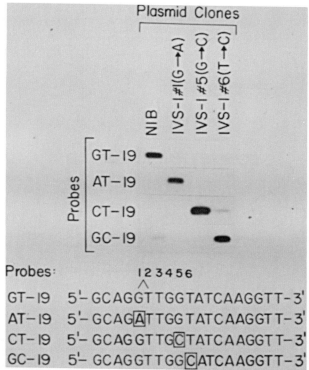

Figure 21-18. Detection of thalassemia point mutations using synthetic oligonucleotide probes. Southern blots of cloned DNA fragments were hybridized to a series of specific probes. The first probe shown below (GT-19) has the sequence of the normal β-globin gene at the exon 1–intron 1 boundary. The obligatory GT is indicated, above which appear the numbers that designate the first several nucleotides in intron 1. The three probes below, AT-19, CT-19, and GC-19, correspond to point mutations at the indicated positions that have been described in β-thalassemia genes. Cloned DNA fragments derived either from the normal gene or from a gene having one of the three point mutations underwent electrophoresis in agarose and were transferred to nitrocellulose by the Southern blotting method. The results show that each probe is nearly completely specific for the DNA fragment containing the corresponding point mutation. (With permission from Orkin SH: Prenatal diagnosis of hemoglobin disorders by DNA analysis. Blood 1984; 63:249.)

heteroduplexes containing single base pair mismatches electrophorese differently from DNA homoduplexes on denaturing gradient acrylamide gels[238, 239] or under neutral gel conditions. With such a strategy, multiple mutations in Chinese individuals[240] were described. This approach is of increasing utility, although it remains unclear if all potential single nucleotide substitutions can be detected by available methods.

Polymerase Chain Reaction. The introduction of PCR in 1985[241] and the subsequent modification of the procedure with the use of thermostabile *Taq* polymerase[242] have revolutionized molecular biology and the ease with which specific mutations can be identified in DNA.[243, 244] The application of PCR to the analysis of thalassemia facilitated the rapid identification of new, and quite rare, mutations.[111] A schematic diagram of the PCR is provided in Figure 21–19. Several features of the PCR method are of particular relevance.[242–244] First, only minute quantities of relatively impure geno-

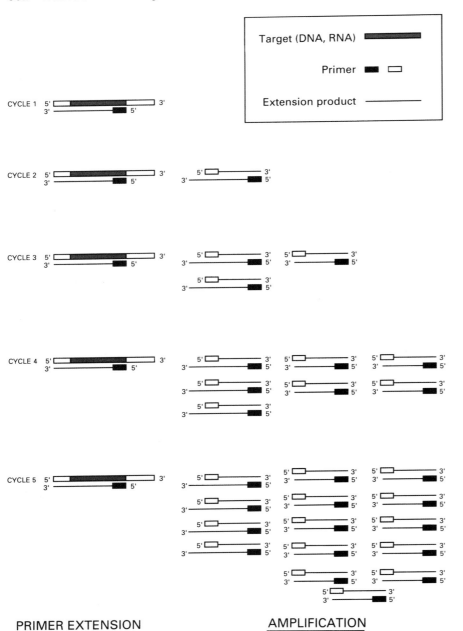

CYCLE 1

CYCLE 2

CYCLE 3

CYCLE 4

CYCLE 5

Target (DNA, RNA)

Primer

Extension product

Figure 21-19. Polymerase chain reaction (PCR). The direct target for PCR is single-stranded DNA that can be derived from denaturation of double-stranded DNA or from RNA after reverse transcription. The amplification is carried out by hybridizing the target DNA with two short synthetic oligonucleotide "primers" that are complementary to sequences at either end of the segment of the target DNA to be amplified. The primers are "extended" by a DNA polymerase, in the presence of excess deoxynucleotide triphosphates, to the end of the molecule. After denaturation, these primer extension products become targets for hybridization and extension. After just several rounds of amplification, there is a dramatic accumulation of DNA products whose length and ends are delimited by the two oligonucleotide primers. Typical PCR protocols continue amplification for 25 to 40 cycles, in which each cycle encompasses one round of denaturation, hybridization, and extension.

PRIMER EXTENSION

AMPLIFICATION

mic DNA are required as starting material; in fact, the DNA of a single cell may be sufficient. Fragments ranging from 50 to several thousand base pairs can be rapidly amplified over 10^6-fold *in vitro*. Second, the product of PCR, double-stranded DNA, can be readily subcloned, subjected to restriction enzyme analysis,[227, 228] hybridized to allele-specific probes,[232–235] or directly sequenced.[106] As discussed earlier, the combination of PCR with restriction enzyme analysis or oligonucleotide hybridization lessens the need to work with high-specific activity radioactive probes to detect mutations. Third, the technique is easily automated. Finally, the analysis, including DNA sequencing if required, can be completed within several days of obtaining tissue for DNA preparation.

Ethnic Distribution

Determining the frequencies of specific β-thalassemia mutations in different ethnic groups is particularly relevant to strategies for prenatal diagnosis of thalassemia.[3] Nearly complete surveys of thalassemia mutations have been performed in Greek and Italian,[216] Asian Indian,[109, 245] American black,[43, 122] Sardinian,[214] Chinese,[246, 247] Lebanese,[117] Turkish,[248] Spanish,[249] Sicilian,[160] Thai,[146] Kurdish Jewish,[104] and Japanese[177] populations. From these studies, several general conclusions can be made. First, in each ethnic group a small subset of mutations (as few as four or six) account for more than 90% of the mutant alleles. This is particularly striking on the island of Sardinia, where the codon 39 nonsense mutation accounts for 95% of the β-thalassemia genes, whereas a codon 6 frameshift represents another 4%.[214] Second, the remaining 5% to 10% of mutant alleles in an ethnic group are divided among a larger number of rarer alleles. For example, four alleles comprise 90% of the β-thalassemia genes in Chinese, whereas 11 rare alleles account for the remaining 10%.[3, 246] Third, several mutations appear to have originated independently in different ethnic groups and are present on different haplotype backgrounds as discussed earlier. For example, the IVS-2 number 1 (G→A) mutation is present in Mediterranean, Tunisian, and American black populations[110, 112, 113]; the IVS-1 number 5 (G→C) substitution is present in Asian Indians, Chinese, and Melanesians.[95, 109, 120] Finally, as a consequence of the large number of mutations present in each population, most individuals with severe β-thalassemia are genetic compound heterozygotes for two different thalassemia mutations.

Mutations That Affect β-Globin Gene Regulation

Deletions within the β-globin gene cluster often lead to thalassemia. Many of these are associated with a significant increase in Hb F, a finding that distinguishes them from the common varieties of β-thalassemia. Ordinarily, heterozygous carriers of β-thalassemia have an increase in Hb A_2 (to >3% of total Hb) and, at most, a slight increase in Hb F. Before detailed molecular analysis, these conditions were broadly grouped into two categories, hereditary persistence of fetal hemoglobin (HPFH) and δβ-thalassemia[1, 4, 250] (Table 21–4). HPFH heterozygotes have normocytic, normochromic red cells, whereas δβ-thalassemia heterozygotes have hypochromic and microcytic cells. Many HPFH heterozygotes have high levels of Hb F (up to 30%) with a uniform or pancellular distribution in circulating erythrocytes, whereas in δβ-thalassemia heterozygotes, Hb F is less abundant and present in an uneven or heterocellular distribution among red cells. In rare individuals homozygous for either condition, only Hb F is found. HPFH homozygotes have normal or slightly elevated total hemoglobin concentration; their red cells are slightly hypochromic and microcytic; and globin synthesis is modestly imbalanced.[251, 252] Thus, these mutations are appropriately considered along with the thalassemia mutations.

Deletion mutations of the β-globin gene cluster represent *in vivo* experiments of nature useful in developing and validating experimental models of gene regulation. Multiple regulatory elements are present within the cluster and the clinical phenotypes observed with specific deletions relate to removal of one or more such regulatory elements. Over 30 deletion mutations have been described (Table 21–5 and Fig. 21–20)[253]; these are highly variable, ranging from a few hundred base pairs of the β-globin gene to more than 100 kb with loss of the entire cluster. In addition to deletion mutations, significant elevations of fetal hemoglobin in adults may arise on account of single base substitutions within the γ-globin gene promoters (Table 21–6). Such mutations, also classified as nondeletion HPFH, appear to enable the γ-globin genes to "capture" the influence of the LCR at the adult stage. Individuals with these HPFH mutations have Hb F values ranging from only slightly elevated to over 20%, typically distributed in a heterocellular fashion.

The HPFH mutations and δβ-thalassemias are infrequent, and individuals who inherit these mutations are asymptomatic or have mild disease. Their importance relates to the insights they provide into globin gene regulation and the role of Hb F in modulating disease severity in patients with severe β-thalassemia or sickle cell anemia.

Isolated point mutations of the δ-globin gene, similar to those in β-thalassemia, may lead to δ-thalassemia. This is a benign condition with no clinical significance that when inherited with a β-thalassemia mutation may lead to a normal or low Hb A_2 thalassemia phenotype in heterozygotes.[254, 255]

Crossover Globins: Hemoglobin Lepore and Hemoglobin Kenya

Deletion mutations in both the α- and β-globin gene clusters arise through unequal homologous recombination or through nonhomologous (illegitimate) recombination. In contrast to the α-globin cluster, in which there are long blocks of tandemly duplicated sequences (see later discussion), the only directly repeated homologous segments of DNA in the β cluster are the globin genes themselves. Hence, mutations arising from homologous, but unequal, crossing-over in the β-globin cluster are relatively infrequent and usually involve two globin genes directly (Fig. 21–21). Two such crossover hemoglobins, Hb Lepore and Hb Kenya, are associated with thalassemia.

In 1958, Gerald and Diamond identified a minor hemoglobin component by starch gel electrophoresis in the blood of parents of a patient with thalassemia major.[317] Structural analysis revealed that the hemoglobin was composed of α-globin and a heretofore undescribed globin, consisting of a fusion of the 80 and 100 amino-terminal amino acids of δ-globin with the carboxyl-portion of β-globin.[279–282, 318] This "chimeric" globin polypeptide, named Lepore after the family in which it was first described, arose from an unequal, homologous recombination event between the δ-globin and β-globin genes (see Fig. 21–21). It is poorly expressed because transcription of the fusion gene is under control of the δ-gene promoter. Other Lepore-

Table 21–4. PHENOTYPES OF $^G\gamma^A\gamma$ HPFH AND $^G\gamma^A\gamma$ $(\delta\beta)^0$ THALASSEMIA HETEROZYGOTES

	HPFH	δβ-Thalassemia
Red cell morphology	Normal	Abnormal
MCH	Nearly normal	Decreased
Hematocrit	Normal	Slightly decreased
Hb F (%)	15–30	1–15
Hb F distribution in red cells	Pancellular	Heterocellular

Table 21-5. DELETION MUTATIONS OF THE β-GLOBIN GENE CLUSTER

Type	Ethnic Group	Deletion Size (kb)	Deletion Coordinates	Hb F Level in Heterozygotes (%)	Other Information	References
A. Aγ⁰:						
1		2.5	37.7–40.2	0.2	"Silent"	256
B. δ⁰:						
1	Corfu	7.20	48.9–56.1	1.1 to 1.6	δ⁰-thalassemia	257, 258
C. β⁰:						
1	Indian	0.619	63.?–64.0	Normal	β⁰-Thalassemia	109, 210–212, 259
2	American black	1.393	61.6–63.0	7.0 to 7.9	β⁰-Thalassemia	260, 261
3	Dutch	12.6	59.7–72.3	4 to 11	β⁰-Thalassemia	262, 263
4	Turkish	0.29	62.1–62.4	2.7 to 3.3	β⁰-Thalassemia	264, 265
	Jordanian			9.4	β⁰-Thalassemia	266
5	Czech Canadian	4.237	58.9–63.1	3.3 to 5.7	β⁰-Thalassemia	267
D. (δβ)⁰:						
1	Sicilian	13.377	56.0–69.4	5 to 15		253, 268, 270
2	Spanish	≃114	52.2–?	5 to 15		271, 272, 273
3	American black	12.0	52.3–64.1	25	Pancellular*	274
4	Japanese	>130	43.1–?	5 to 7		275, 276
5	Laotian	12.5	56.0–68.5	11.5		277
6	Macedonian	18–23	54–74	7 to 14		278
7	Mediterranean	7.4	55.3–62.7	1 to 5	Hb Lepore	279–283
E. Gγ⁺(AγδβΒ)⁰:						
1	Indian	Total 8.3 Kb	40.1–40.9	10 to 15		284, 285
	Iranian	Deleted	55.5–63.0			
	Kuwaiti	14.6 kb inverted	40.9–55.5			
2	American black	35.7	40.7–76.4	6 to 16		253, 286
3	Turkish	36.22	37.1–73.3	10 to 15		253, 287, 288
	American black					
4	Malaysian (1)	>27	37.0–?	Unknown		289
5	Malaysian (2)	>40	39.1–?	Unknown		290
6	Chinese	≃100	40.5–?	10 to 15		291, 292
7	German	53.0	37.6–90.6	9.9 to 12.5		293
8	Cantonese	>43	37.0–?	20		294
F. (γδβ)⁰:						
1	Hispanic	39.5	−19.5–10.0			295
2	English	>100	?–35.9			296
3	Dutch	99.4	?–59.8			297–299
4	Anglo-Saxon	95.9	?–62.6			288, 298, 300
5	Mexican	>105	?–?			301
6	Scotch-Irish	>105	?–64 to 71			302
7	Yugoslavian	>148	?–?			303
8	Canadian	>185	?–?			303
H. HPFH:						
1	American black	≃106	51.2–?	20 to 30 (5% G)†	HPFH-1	273, 288, 304, 307
2	Black (Ghana)	≃105	47–?	20 to 30 (30% G)†	HPFH-2	253, 273, 304–308
3	Indian	48.5	45.0–93.5	22 to 23 (70% G)†	HPFH-3	308–310
4	Italian	40.0	50.0–90.0	14 to 30	HPFH-4	311
5	Italian	12.9	51.6–64.5	16 to 20 (15% G)†		312
6	Kenyan	22.8	40.0–62.8	5 to 8	Hb Kenya	313–316

*In a compound δβ thalassemia/Hb S heterozygote.
†Percentage Gγ of total γ(Gγ/Gγ + Aγ).
40% Gγ is the normal value for an adult.

type globins have been characterized in which the relative contribution of the δ-globin and β-globin genes to the fusion protein varies as a result of a different point of crossing-over. Homozygotes for Hb Lepore have 90% Hb F and approximately 10% Hb Lepore but no Hb A or Hb A₂, whereas heterozygotes have mainly Hb A, 2% to 4% Hb Lepore, and 3% to 5% Hb F.[319, 320] In heterozygotes, red cells are very heterogeneous with regard to their Hb F content. Anti-Lepore globins having the amino-terminal sequence of β-globin and the carboxyl-sequence of δ-globin have also been described (see Fig. 21–21).[321–324] Individuals with anti-Lepore genes also have two normal δ-globin genes and two normal β-globin genes; hence, their red cells lack any stigmata of thalassemia. The anti-Lepore globins are produced in very low amounts, perhaps owing to sequences within the large intron of the δ-globin gene that may reduce mRNA production.[23]

Hb Kenya, another important crossover hemoglobin, contains a non–α-globin composed of amino-sequences of γ-globin and carboxyl-sequences of β-globin[313, 314, 316, 325] (see Fig. 21–21). Molecular analysis demonstrated that the Aγ globin gene was involved in the crossover. The crossover occurred approximately at the position of amino acid codon 100. Hb Kenya was first observed in an individual who was heterozygous for a βS gene.

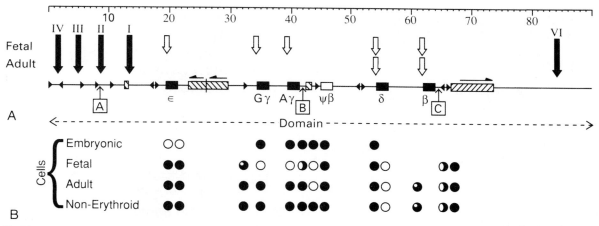

Figure 21-20. *A,* Organization and chromatin structure of the human β-globin cluster. The expressed genes are shown as solid boxes, and the single pseudogene in the cluster as an open box. The arrowheads in the line figure indicate the location and orientation of *Alu* repetitive DNA sequences, while the hatched boxes represent members of the L1 family of repetitive DNA. The solid downward arrows mark developmentally stable, erythroid-specific hypersensitive sites that constitute the locus-activating region (LAR), flanking the cluster. The true boundaries of the "active" chromatin domain established by these sites are unknown and extend beyond the cluster. Hypersensitive sites are also found over the promoters of the expressed genes *(open downward arrows).* The location of the three enhancers in the cluster are marked by letters: A = hypersensitive site II enhancer, B = 3' ^Aγ enhancer; C = 3'β enhancer. *B,* The methylation pattern of the locus at different stages of ontogeny is depicted. Open circles show an unmethylated site, closed circles a totally methylated site, and partially filled circles degree of site methylation. The coordinates refer to distance in kb. (Adapted from Stamatoyannopoulos G, Nienhuis AW: Hemoglobin switching. In Stamatoyannopoulos G, Nienhuis AW, et al [eds]: *The Molecular Basis of Blood Diseases.* Philadelphia, WB Saunders, 1987, p 79.)

This patient had increased Hb F (up to 6%), that was uniformly distributed in all his red cells. The Hb F was entirely of the ^Gγ type. Hb Kenya accounted for 17% to 20% of the total hemoglobin. Individuals who are heterozygous for Hb Kenya without Hb S are clinically well. Approximately 10% Hb Kenya and 6% to 10% Hb F of the ^Gγ type are found homogeneously distributed in their red cells, in contrast to the distribution of Hb F with the Lepore type deletion.[315] It was originally hypothesized that the deletion removes a regulatory element that suppresses γ synthesis in adult life, leading to a pancellular or uniform increase of Hb F in the

Table 21-6. NONDELETION HPFH MUTATIONS

	Molecular Defect	γ Gene	Ethnic Group	Percent Hb F in Heterozygotes	Chains Gγ, Aγ	Distribution of Hb F	References
1	C to G at −202	G	Black	15 to 20	G only	Pancellular	333, 334
2	C to T at −202	A	Black	2 to 3	93% A	Heterocellular	335
3	T to C at −198	A	British*	4 to 12	90% A	Heterocellular	336–338
4	C to T at −196	A	Chinese	10 to 15	90% A	Heterocellular#	339, 340
			Italian**	10 to 20	95% A	Pancellular	342, 343
5	T to C at −175	G	Italian	20 to 30	90% G		344
			Black	30#§	G only	Pancellular	345
6	T to C at −175	A	Black	35 to 40‖	80% A	Pancellular	346
7	G to A at −161	G	Black	1 to 2		Heterocellular	347
8	G to T at −158†	G	Saudi***	2 to 4	G > A	Heterocellular	348–354
9	G to A at −117	A	Mediterranean****	10 to 20	95% A	Pancellular	355–357
			Black	10 to 20	85% A	Pancellular	340
10	Deletion −114 to −102	A	Black	30#§	85% A††		358
11	X-Linked	G	"Swiss"*****	0.8 to 3.4		Heterocellular	9, 359
12	Unknown‡	G	German	5 to 8	A and G	Heterocellular	360
13	Unknown	G	"Georgia"	2.6 to 6	G > A	Heterocellular	361, 362
14	Unknown	G	"Seattle"	3.7 to 7.8	G = A	Heterocellular	363, 364

*Also found in whites in North America.
**Also found in cis to codon 39 mutation (Sardinian δβ-thalassemia).
***Identified in Greek and Sardinian families.
****Also found in several other ethnic groups.
*****Found in all ethnic groups.
†This determinant appears to increase Hb F only in patients with erythropoietic stress.
‡Associated with a translocation involving chromosome 11.
§In a β-S heterozygote.
‖In a β C heterozygote with the −158 T to C substitution in the ^Ggamma promoter.
#More than 80% of the red cells contain fetal hemoglobin.
††Ratio varies in different families.

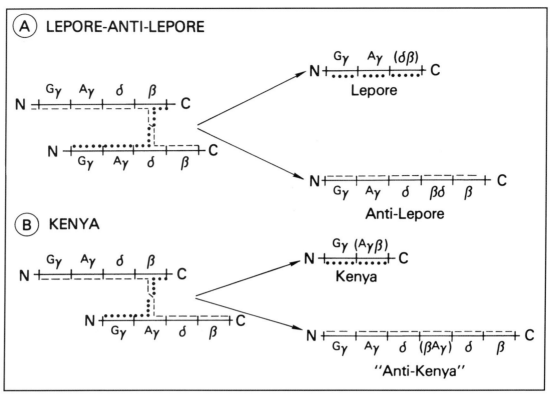

Figure 21-21. Schematic representation of the unequal crossover events that occurred during meiosis and resulted in formation of the Lepore and anti-Lepore *(A)* and Kenya *(B)* genes. (From Nienhuis AW, Benz EJ Jr: Regulation of hemoglobin synthesis during the development of the red cell. N Engl J Med 1977; 297:1318. Reprinted, by permission, from The New England Journal of Medicine.)

red cells of individuals with the Kenya fusion gene.[326] Even before the discovery of the LCR and other regulatory elements within the β cluster, this hypothesis was disproven by analysis of several other deletion mutations (see later). Current models of hemoglobin switching posit that increased expression and pancellular distribution of the ᴬγβ fusion gene and the adjacent ᴳγ gene result from deletion of the adult stage δ- and β-globin genes and their promoters, which serves to eliminate competition for the LCR. In addition, the deletion repositions an enhancer 3' to the β-globin gene immediately downstream of the γ-globin genes and may also contribute to their increased expression.

Silent Deletions

Deletions that eliminate a single γ-globin gene or the δ-globin gene are unlikely to result in a phenotype that would be detected in hematologic screening. Thus, few of these mutations have been detected and described. A clinically silent deletion of the ᴬγ-globin gene was identified through extensive molecular screening of chromosomes in Melanesia.[256] A 7.2-kb deletion involving the δ-, but not the γ- or β-, globin gene was reported in Corfu (δβ)⁰-thalassemia in cis to the G→A substitution at IVS-1 position 5.[257] Homozygotes for the IVS-1 position 5 mutation ordinarily exhibit a mild β⁺-thalassemia intermedia phenotype with 10% to 20% Hb A,[123] but homozygotes for Corfu (δβ)⁰-thalassemia

display the clinical phenotype of β⁰-thalassemia intermedia with 100% Hb F. This has been interpreted as evidence that sequences in the deleted region are important in activating the β-globin gene and potentially in suppressing γ-globin gene expression. Subsequently, however, the identical deletion was identified in *cis* to a normal β-globin gene.[258] In this circumstance, the deletion leads to failure of δ-globin gene expression but has no demonstrable effect on expression of the γ- and β-globin genes on the same chromosome. Hence, the basis for the lack of β-globin gene expression in Corfu (δβ)⁰-thalassemia remains unresolved.

β⁰-Thalassemia Deletion Mutations

Several deletions remove the β-globin gene and are associated with typical high Hb A₂ β⁰-thalassemia (see Table 21–5). Interestingly, deletions that remove the promoter region are associated with somewhat higher Hb F levels than are usually seen in β⁰-thalassemia heterozygotes.[327] The Hb F is distributed in a heterocellular pattern. In contrast, a 0.6-kb deletion at the 3'-end of the β-globin gene seen in Asian Indians, which spares the β-globin promoter, is not associated with increased Hb F in heterozygotes.[109, 210–212, 259] A possible explanation for the different phenotypes relates to the possibility that an intact β-globin gene promoter may interact productively with the LCR and thereby effectively compete with an incompletely silenced γ-globin gene at the adult stage. Removal of the promoter may alleviate competition and favor persistent γ-globin expression.

δβ-Thalassemia

Individuals heterozygous for these deletions generally have 5% to 15% Hb F, composed of both ^{G}γ and ^{A}γ globins, distributed in a heterocellular fashion (see Table 21–5). The erythrocytes are typically hypochromic and microcytic.[1] Hb A_2 is characteristically low, in contrast to the modest elevations observed in most individuals with β-thalassemia trait. Homozygotes for these deletions produce only Hb F, yet exhibit a mild β[0]-thalassemia intermedia phenotype with hemoglobin levels of about 10 g/dL. The most common of these deletions is referred to as the Sicilian type.[253, 268–270] The deletion extends from within the δ-globin gene to just beyond the β-globin gene (see Table 21–5).

The 5' breakpoint junctions of δβ-thalassemia deletions generally lie between the pseudo-β-globin gene and the δ-globin gene. Located within this region are moderately repetitive sequences, known as Alu sequences.[328] Although the function of such sequences elements is unknown, their preservation in δβ-thalassemia deletions and their deletion in HPFH encouraged speculation that the Alu elements might be involved in modulating Hb F production during development.[272, 326] Based on analysis of additional deletion mutations, this hypothesis seems unlikely (see Table 21–5). For example, the 7.2-kb Corfu deletion removes both Alu elements and the δ-globin gene yet is not associated with increased γ-globin gene expression.[257, 258] Moreover, the Japanese type of deletion, which also removes the Alu elements, is associated with a heterocellular distribution of Hb F and thalassemic red cell indices.[275, 276] The increase in fetal hemoglobin expression may be more appropriately explained by the deletion of local δ- and β-globin gene regulatory elements, leaving the γ-globin genes to interact with the LCR unopposed by competition from the adult genes.

^{A}γδβ-Thalassemia

The phenotype of these deletions in heterozygotes is identical to that of δβ-thalassemia: hypochromic microcytic red cells with low Hb A_2 and moderately increased in ^{G}γ-Hb F (5%–15%) with a heterocellular distribution (see Table 21–5). Homozygotes have β[0]-thalassemia intermedia with 100% ^{G}γ-Hb F. The 5' breakpoints in these instances lie between the two γ-globin genes or within the body of the ^{A}γ-globin gene, thereby resulting in silencing of the ^{A}γ-globin gene together with the δ- and β-globin genes.[253, 284–290, 292–294] The 3' endpoints of several of these deletions have been precisely mapped. Other deletions are very large and extend well beyond the boundary of the β-globin gene complex (see Table 21–5). One interesting mutation of this type, the Indian form (see Table 21–5), has two deletions, one involving the γ-globin gene and the second involving a portion of the δ-globin and β-globin

genes and intragenic DNA. The segment of DNA between the two deletions is inverted so that the 5' ends of the γ and δ genes come to be adjacent but in an inverted orientation.[284, 285]

γδβ-Thalassemia

The diagnosis of γδβ-thalassemia should be considered in cases of hemolytic disease in newborns associated with hypochromic red cells. In adults, it is also a cause of normal Hb A_2, normal Hb F β-thalassemia trait. The syndrome was first identified in a newborn with a microcytic, hemolytic anemia.[329] Heterozygous β-thalassemia associated with normal levels of Hb A_2 and Hb F was identified in the father and many relatives. Decreased γ and β chain synthesis was demonstrated in the infant's reticulocytes. The anemia was self-limited; as the infant grew older, hemolytic anemia disappeared and the child developed the phenotype of simple heterozygous β-thalassemia.

The syndrome of γδβ-thalassemia results from large deletions within the β-globin gene cluster (see Table 21–5). They can be divided into two categories: extremely large deletions that remove the entire β-globin gene cluster or all of the structural genes[301–303]; or deletions such as the Hispanic, English, Dutch, and Anglo-Saxon forms that leave structural genes intact but remove LCR elements.[288, 295–300] The remaining genes on the chromosome are not expressed and are found in inactive chromatin that is methylated and resistant to nuclease digestion. Study of these deletions has provided the most convincing evidence that the LCR is required in normal erythroid cells for transcription of the β-like globin genes *in vivo*. Homozygous γδβ-thalassemia is anticipated to be incompatible with survival and has not been observed.

Hereditary Persistence of Fetal Hemoglobin

Individuals heterozygous or homozygous for mutations that enhance Hb F are entirely asymptomatic. They are generally identified incidentally in routine screening programs or during investigation of family members with hematologic disease because of interaction of these variants with other mutations in the β-globin gene cluster. Homozygotes for deletion forms of HPFH have normal hemoglobin concentrations, but their red cells are slightly hypochromic and microcytic.[251, 252] Minimal globin-chain biosynthetic imbalance may be demonstrated. No symptoms or physiologic impairment has been associated with exclusive production of Hb F, despite its high oxygen affinity.

HPFH Deletion Mutations

Several deletions produce the HPFH phenotype of increased Hb F in otherwise normal red cells (see Table 21–5).[253, 273, 288, 304–316] The 5' breakpoints lie between the ^{A}γ-globin gene and the δ-globin gene, and in all cases (with the exception of Hb Kenya) an enhancer 3' to the ^{A}γ gene is unaffected by the mutation. Two of the deletions (HPFH-1 and HPFH-2) are very large and extend beyond the 3' end of the cluster (see Table 21–5). The Kenya mutation is also included in this category because of the pancellular distribution of Hb F that is characteristic of this mutation.

Heterozygotes for these deletions produce up to 30% Hb F, containing both $^G\gamma$ and $^A\gamma$ chains, in a pancellular distribution. Differences in the relative percentage of $^G\gamma$ and $^A\gamma$ chains can be detected between different types of HPFH deletions (see Table 21–5). Heterozygotes have normocytic red cells. The red cells of homozygotes contain exclusively Hb F. The higher oxygen affinity of Hb F may lead to slightly elevated hemoglobin levels in such individuals. Although homozygotes are clinically well, the α/γ-globin chain biosynthetic ratio may be slightly imbalanced and mild microcytosis and hypochromia may be observed. This suggests that γ chain synthesis occurs at levels below the output of the normal β-globin gene on these chromosomes.

Several hypotheses have been put forward to account for the increased expression and pancellular distribution of Hb F in the deletion HPFH syndromes, particularly as compared with the moderate increase and heterocellular distribution in $\delta\beta$-thalassemia. Sequence analysis has confirmed that the γ-globin genes linked to the HPFH-1 deletion do not contain additional mutations responsible for the increased Hb F expression.[330] As discussed earlier, deletion of postulated inhibitory sequences[272, 326] has not been substantiated by the effects of other mutations that remove similar elements. Because several mutations extend far beyond the 3' end of the β-globin cluster, it has been suggested that introduction of a distant enhancer into the locus might lead to activation of the γ-globin genes. Some evidence is consistent with this model. Sequences located immediately 3' of the HPFH-1 deletion breakpoint, which are translocated into the cluster by the deletion event, display transient enhancer activity when tested in erythroid cell lines.[273] In addition, the DNA in the vicinity of this enhancer is hypomethylated and nuclease sensitive in normal erythroid cells and contains a long open reading frame,[273, 331] suggesting that the enhancer may belong to a distinct gene that is also transcribed in erythroid cells. RNA transcripts from this putative gene have been detected in erythroid cell lines.[332] In Spanish $\delta\beta$-thalassemia, a deletion nearly identical to that in HPFH-1, the 3' breakpoint is located approximately 9-kb downstream of HPFH-1, and therefore the putative distant enhancer is not imported into the locus.[273]

In another type of deletion HPFH observed in an Italian family, a 12.9-kb deletion removes the $\delta\beta$-globin genes and brings the enhancer 3' of the β-globin gene closer to the γ-globin genes.[312] Analogous to the comparisons between HPFH-1 and Spanish $\delta\beta$-thalassemia, deletions similar in size and location to the 12.9-kb Italian HPFH deletion that remove the 3'β enhancer result in $\delta\beta$-thalassemia rather than HPFH.[312] The Kenyan deletion also brings the 3'β-globin gene enhancer closer to the γ-globin genes. Although distributed in a pancellular pattern, the level of Hb F is lower in the Kenyan deletion than the other HPFH syndromes. It is also the only deletion mutation that does not spare the 3' $^A\gamma$-globin enhancer.

Nondeletion HPFH Mutations

Individuals with nondeletion HPFH mutations exhibit elevated levels of Hb F with normal red cell indices and are identified through hemoglobin screening programs or by study of families in which a segregating high Hb F allele modulates severity of sickle cell disease or β-thalassemia.[78, 79] (The role of nondeletion HPFH mutations in modifying the course of sickle cell disease is discussed in more detail in Chapter 20.[118]) In many instances, single base changes have been discovered within the promoter region of either the $^G\gamma$- or $^A\gamma$-globin gene.[333–358] These mutations are postulated to alter the binding of nuclear regulatory proteins and lead to a more favorable interaction of the promoter with the LCR at the adult stage.[355, 356, 365–370] Typically, only increased expression of the γ-globin gene in which the mutation is found occurs. In cases of the nondeletion HPFH syndrome, no mutation has been characterized. As discussed in a later section, the Swiss HPFH determinant may segregate with the X chromosome.[9]

The level of Hb F observed in patients with this syndrome is extremely variable and ranges from 1% to 4% in Swiss HPFH[9, 359] to 30% in the −175 T→C substitution found in either the $^G\gamma$- or $^A\gamma$-globin gene.[344–346] Similar to the deletion forms of HPFH, the Hb F may be found in either a heterocellular or pancellular distribution (see Table 21–6; Fig. 21–22). The −158 C→T substitution in the $^G\gamma$-globin gene is associated with a normal level of Hb F in otherwise normal heterozygotes but with a high level in the presence of erythropoietic stress.[348–354] For example, in Saudi Arabia, patients with sickle cell anemia often have high Hb F levels (25% or greater) and mild disease, whereas their sickle cell trait parents have normal, or only slightly elevated, levels.[348] Identification of individuals with this mutation (or polymorphism) has been aided by the finding that it is linked to a rare subhaplotype.[349, 351] The −158 HPFH substitution also improves the clinical course of β-thalassemia. A Chinese individual homozygous for the −29 promoter mutation has transfusion-dependent β-thalassemia,[44] yet black patients homozygous for the same mutation who coinherit the −158 HPFH mutation in the $^G\gamma$ promoter have mild β-thalassemia.[43, 80]

The evidence that the base substitutions in the promoter region are the cause of increased γ chain synthesis rather than associated random DNA polymorphisms is based on several lines of evidence.[371] As mentioned earlier, they are generally associated with overexpression of the gene in which the mutation is found and typically represent the only sequence change. None of the mutations listed, with the exception of the −158 mutation, has been observed in individuals with normal Hb F levels. Haplotype analysis in some HPFH pedigrees has demonstrated that the HPFH determinant is linked to the β-globin cluster. The British type of nondeletion HPFH is quite informative in this regard. The gene has been followed through

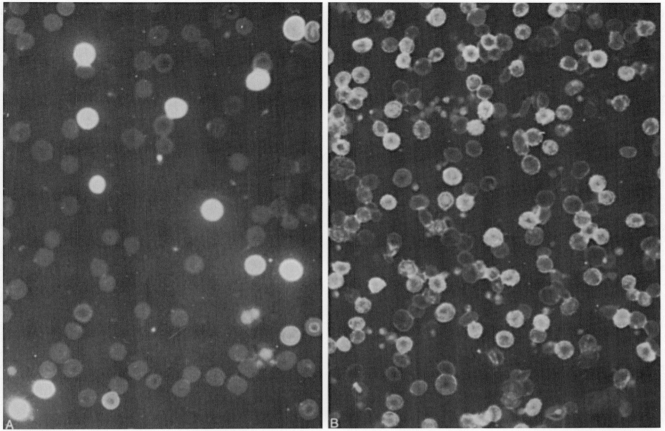

Figure 21–22. *A,* Immunofluorescence stain of erythrocytes with antibody directed against Hb F shows distribution of Hb F in a heterocellular pattern. *B,* Immunofluorescence stain of erythrocytes with Hb F distributed in a pancellular pattern. (Courtesy of Dr. George Stamatoyannopoulos.)

three generations, and three homozygous individuals have been observed.[336–338, 372] Haplotype analysis using restriction enzyme polymorphisms has established linkage of the British HPFH phenotype to the β-globin gene locus.[337] More than 90% of the γ chains are of the ^{G}γ type, whereas there is an associated mutation at −198 of the ^{G}γ-globin gene.[337] Even the three homozygotes, with approximately 20% Hb F, have heterogeneous distribution of the Hb F among their red cells. Two homozygotes for the −117 ^{A}γ HPFH have also been described and had 24% Hb F in a pancellular pattern.[373] More recent transgenic experiments unequivocally demonstrate that single base substitutions seen in HPFH lead to enhanced γ-globin expression into adult life.

An interesting aspect of this syndrome is a balanced α- to non–α- globin chain synthetic ratio, even in homozygotes,[373] which implies that increased γ-globin synthesis is offset by decreased β-globin synthesis.[357] Expression of the β-globin gene in *cis* to the mutation may be reduced by 20% to 30%.[333, 345, 346, 358, 374] It has also been observed that Hb A$_2$ levels are uniformly low in the nondeletion HPFH syndromes and generally correlate inversely with Hb F levels.[1] The reduction in δ- and β-globin gene expression in *cis* to the HPFH mutations is compatible with models of competitive regulation of β-globin expression by the linked γ-globin gene.

Mutations That Alter α-Globin Gene Regulation

In contrast to the β-globin cluster, where single nucleotide substitutions are the most frequent cause of thalassemia, large deletions within the α-globin cluster are the predominant basis of α-thalassemia. The overall impairment in α-globin chain synthesis that results from defects in the α-globin cluster is determined by the number of genes inactivated (either by deletion or mutation), the type of lesion (deletion or mutation), and whether the lesion affects the αα1 gene.

The α-globin cluster on chromosome 16[13, 375, 376] contains three functional genes (ζ, α1, and α2), an expressed gene of no apparent significance (θ), and three pseudogenes[2, 12] (see Fig. 21–2). Transcription of the genes depends on the integrity of the distant regulatory element, HS-40. An α-thalassemia deletion mutation (αα^{RA}/) has been reported that removes a large segment of DNA upstream of the ζ2 gene but spares the remainder of the cluster.[377] In heterozygotes, no expression of the ζ- and α-globin genes from this chromosome is detected in heterozygotes. These findings are formally analogous to those in Hispanic and English γδβ-thalassemias (see Table 21–5),[295, 296] where upstream LCR elements of the β-globin cluster are deleted.

The two human α-globin genes are thought to have

been generated through a gene duplication event about 60 million years ago.[378] The nucleotide sequences of the $\alpha 2$ and $\alpha 1$ genes have remained remarkably similar and represent an example of concerted evolution,[379–381] where the two genes have exchanged genetic information through crossover fixation and gene conversion events. The coding regions of the two genes are virtually identical and encode identical polypeptides.[379, 382] The genes differ only in minor respects within IVS-2, whereas the sequences diverge significantly in the 3' untranslated region.

The α-globin genes are expressed in embryonic, fetal, and adult stage erythroid cells. Initially, it was believed that the two α genes were expressed at similar levels, but subsequent RNA analysis relying on sequence differences in their 3'-untranslated regions revealed that the $\alpha 2$ RNA predominates over $\alpha 1$ RNA by a ratio of 3:1.[201, 383–385] Because two α-globin mRNAs have the same intrinsic stability, the higher level of $\alpha 2$ RNA reflects increased transcription of the $\alpha 2$ gene. "Transcriptional interference" of the $\alpha 1$ gene by the upstream $\alpha 2$ gene has been proposed as an explanation for this observation.[386] Ribosome loading studies suggest that $\alpha 1$ and $\alpha 2$ transcripts are translated at equivalent rates.[387] The systematic characterization of the expression of α-globin structural variants at both the $\alpha 1$ and $\alpha 2$ locus confirmed that the $\alpha 2$ gene has a predominant role in α-globin chain production.[384, 385] A direct prediction of this model is that mutations altering the $\alpha 2$ gene would result in a greater deficiency in α-globin chain production than mutations of the $\alpha 1$ gene. Clinical support for this prediction is provided by a study of Sardinian patients with Hb H disease heterozygous for one chromosome with a deletion of both α genes ($- -/$) and a chromosome with a nondeletion mutation affecting the initiator codon of either the $\alpha 2$ gene ($\alpha^T\alpha/$) or the $\alpha 1$ gene ($\alpha\alpha^T/$).[139] Patients with the mutation in the $\alpha 2$ gene ($\alpha^T\alpha/$) are clinically more severe. Consistent with its predominance, the majority of the reported mutations of the α-globin genes involve the $\alpha 2$ gene (see Table 21–3).

Deletion Mutations Within the α-Globin Gene Cluster

Mutations That Remove One α-Globin Gene

The two α-globin genes are embedded in highly homologous, tandemly repeated sequence blocks (called X, Y, and Z) that are separated by nonhomologous segments (Fig. 21–23).[15] Unequal, homologous recombination through the X and the Z blocks generates a chromosome with a single α-globin gene and another with three α-globin genes. Recombination in the small Y box of homology has not been observed. The most common type of deletion in this class removes 3.7 kb as a result of misalignment of the Z boxes and is known as the "rightward deletion." The products of this crossover are the $(-\alpha^{3.7}/)$[388, 389] and $(\alpha\alpha\alpha^{anti3.7}/)$ haplotypes.[390, 391] The $-\alpha^{3.7}$ products may be further subdivided into types I, II, and III by the precise location of recombination within the Z box.[381] Unequal crossover events through the X box leads to the "leftward deletion" of 4.2 kb of DNA and the $-\alpha^{4.2}$ chromosome[389] and its triplicated antitype.[392, 393] The frequency of the observed recombination products appears to reflect the size of the homologous target sequence within the boxes, because the $-\alpha^{3.7I}$ (1436 bp) is most common, followed by $-\alpha^{4.2}$ (1339 bp), $-\alpha^{3.7II}$ (171 bp), and $-\alpha^{3.7III}$ (46 bp).[2, 379, 380, 394] Unequal α-globin gene recombination through the X and Z boxes has been reproduced in both prokaryotic and eukaryotic experimental systems using episomal vectors.[15, 395, 396]

The $-\alpha^{3.7I}$ deletion is extremely common and is seen in all populations where α-thalassemia is prevalent, whereas the $-\alpha^{4.2}$ deletion is most common in Asian populations.[2, 12] Frequencies of 80% to 90% for the single deletion chromosome have been reported in some populations.[88] The association of these mutations with a variety of α-globin cluster haplotypes and α-globin variants in different populations suggests that they have arisen through numerous independent mutational events.[88, 397]

Deletion of one α-globin gene does not affect expression of the ζ-globin gene[398] but has unanticipated consequences on expression of the remaining α-globin gene. The $\alpha 1$ gene that remains on the $-\alpha^{3.7}$ chromosome is expressed approximately 1.8 times higher than the $\alpha 1$ gene on a normal chromosome.[384] Individuals homozygous for the leftward deletion ($-\alpha^{4.2}/-\alpha^{4.2}$), who carry two copies of the $\alpha 1$ gene, express more α-globin than the anticipated 25% of normal.[399] Homozygotes for the $\alpha^{3.7III}$ deletion ($-\alpha^{3.7III}/-\alpha^{3.7III}$), who carry two $\alpha 2$ genes, express less than the anticipated 75% of normal.[399] The increased expression of the $\alpha 1$ gene on the $-\alpha^{3.7}$ and $-\alpha^{4.2}$ chromosomes may be secondary to a release of transcriptional interference from the upstream $\alpha 2$ gene,[386] whereas the lower expression of the $\alpha 2$ gene in the $-\alpha^{3.7III}$ deletion remains to be explained. An important consequence of this observation, however, is that the common mutations that delete the $\alpha 2$ gene ($\alpha^{3.7I}$ and $\alpha^{4.2}$) may lead to increased expression of the remaining $\alpha 1$ gene and a less severe clinical phenotype than predicted from the expression studies of the native α-globin genes.[399] Single nucleotide substitutions that inactivate the $\alpha 2$ gene do not affect $\alpha 1$ expression and consequently lead to a more severe clinical phenotype than single gene deletions.[2, 12]

Triplicated α-globin gene chromosomes are observed in populations where the $\alpha^{3.7I}$ and $\alpha^{4.2}$ chromosomes are present. The third gene is expressed, leading to a slight increase in the $\alpha:\beta$ chain ratio in homozygotes for the triplication, but this is generally of no clinical consequence.[400, 401] However, if a triplicated α gene chromosome is co-inherited with a β-thalassemia gene, thalassemia intermedia may be noted.[402, 403]

Mutations That Remove Both α-Globin Genes

Illegitimate, nonhomologous recombination within the α-globin cluster results in the partial or complete deletion of both α-globin genes and generates an α^0 chro-

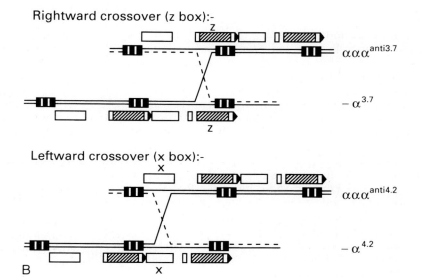

Figure 21–23. *A,* Deletion mutations that give rise to α-thalassemia. The two α-globin genes are embedded in a duplicated segment of DNA with homologous (X, Y, Z boxes) and nonhomologous (I, II, III) regions. The extent of specific mutations that delete a single α-globin gene are indicated by solid boxes and the limits of the breakpoints as solid lines. These deletions, and the reciprocal chromosomes containing three functional α-globin genes, result from misalignment and unequal recombination mediated by the homologous blocks. *B,* Unequal crossing over through the Z box deletes 3.7 kb of DNA and produces the α³·⁷ chromosome and its antitype, whereas recombination through the X box produces the −α⁴·² chromosome and its antitype. The −α³·⁷ deletion can be further subdivided (I to III) by the exact location within the Z box where recombination occurs (see panel A). (From Higgs DR, Vickers MA, et al: A review of the molecular genetics of the human alpha-globin gene cluster. Blood 1989; 73:1081.)

mosome.[2, 377, 404–408] (Note that the terms α⁺ and α⁰ may refer to the expression α-globin from a single gene or may refer to the presence or absence of an intact α-globin gene on a chromosome.) In some circumstances, the ζ-globin gene may also be encompassed by the deletion. The boundaries of many of the deletions that have been characterized are summarized in Figure 21–24. The geographic distribution of these lesions is more restricted than that of the α⁺ thalassemia deletions, the most common being the −−^SEA (Southeast Asia) and −−^MED (Mediterranean) deletions, suggesting that they are infrequent genetic events. Theories concerning the mechanisms of these deletions are summarized elsewhere.[2]

Homozygotes for α⁰ chromosomes (−−/−−) suffer from hydrops fetalis, whereas individuals heterozygous for an α⁺ chromosome and an α⁰ chromosome (−−/−α, or −−/αᵀα) exhibit Hb H disease. In-

creased expression of minute quantities of ζ-globin into adulthood may accompany some of the mutations in which the ζ-globin gene is left intact by the deletion.[398] Sensitive radioimmunologic assays for the presence of ζ-globin chains in heterozygous adult carriers of these mutations have been devised[409] and may prove useful in areas such as Southeast Asia where the gene frequency of the −−^SEA chromosome is as high as 3%.[410]

Mutations Not Linked to the Globin Gene Clusters That Alter Globin Gene Expression

Acquired Hemoglobin H Disease

A particularly severe, acquired form of Hb H disease has been described in elderly men with clonal myeloproliferative disorders.[411–414] In this setting, levels of Hb

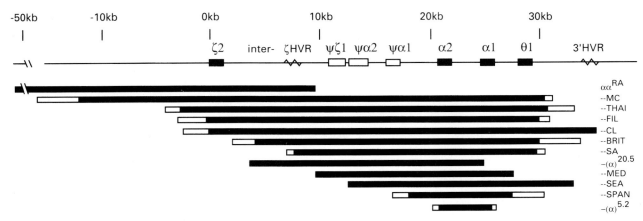

Figure 21-24. Deletion mutations that give rise to α⁰-thalassemia. The organization of the α-globin cluster is shown. Expressed genes are represented by solid boxes, whereas pseudogenes are shown as open boxes. Two hypervariable regions (HVR) are indicated as zigzag lines. Coordinates are in kilobase pairs. The extent of each deletion is defined by a solid box and the uncertainty of the breakpoints by open boxes. The designation of the genotype is indicated to the right of each deletion. (From Higgs DR, Vickers MA, et al: A review of the molecular genetics of the human alpha-globin gene cluster. Blood 1989; 73:1081.)

H approaching 60% Hb H may be seen.[412] Extremely low α:β chain synthesis ratios and low α-globin mRNA levels have been documented in bone marrow cells from affected individuals.[412, 413] Residual α mRNA expression may be derived from nonclonal erythroid cells. A bimorphic population of cells is present on examination of the peripheral blood smear. Hemolytic disease caused by the Hb H may wax and wane with the clinical course of the myeloproliferative disorder.[412]

Available evidence suggests that the absence of a positive regulatory factor in the clonal population, or the presence of an inhibitory factor, is responsible for the lack of α-globin gene expression. Extensive molecular analysis of the α-globin gene cluster in patients with acquired Hb H disease indicates that it is structurally intact and hypomethylated in these individuals.[412, 413] Human α-globin gene expression can be detected in somatic cell hybrids derived by fusion of bone marrow cells from patients with acquired Hb H disease to murine erythroleukemia cells,[415] further suggesting that the transcriptional defect is not linked to the α-globin cluster. Further study of this unusual condition may provide important information about factors regulating the α-globin gene cluster.

X-linked α-Thalassemia Associated with Mental Retardation (ATR-X Syndrome)

Rare instances of α-thalassemia occurring in Anglo-Saxon individuals with phenotypically normal parents first drew attention to a new syndrome.[416] Further investigation revealed the frequent association of profound mental retardation, facial anomalies, and genital abnormalities.[65] Important studies demonstrate mutation of the AH2 genes, a member of the SNF2 superfamily and presumed global transcriptional regulator, as the underlying basis of this syndrome.[66]

Silent β-Thalassemia

Hematologically normal "silent carriers" of β-thalassemia are identified through family studies.[1, 6, 417–420]

Some cases of "silent" β-thalassemia may be attributed to mutations that cause a very modest reduction in β-globin gene expression: the −101 promoter mutation[102, 183] and the +1 cap site mutation[109]; or to the inheritance of triplicated α-globin gene chromosomes.[402, 403] In an Albanian family in which the father was a silent carrier, the mother had high Hb A₂ β thalassemia trait, and two children had β-thalassemia, the silent carrier determinant did not appear to segregate with either of the paternal β-globin gene clusters.[421–424] This family illustrates the rare circumstance in which determinants not linked to the β-globin gene cluster appear to regulate β-globin gene expression.

Swiss HPFH

Ordinarily, Hb F constitutes less than 1% of the total hemoglobin in normal adult erythrocytes and is restricted to a subpopulation of erythrocytes (F cells) that represent between 3% and 7% of the total number of red cells.[7, 8] Both the percentage of F cells present in the circulation and the amount of Hb F per F cell are under genetic control, and evidence suggests that the determinants are not linked to the β-globin gene cluster.[425]

In the Swiss type of nondeletion HPFH (see Table 21–6), Hb F is distributed in a heterocellular fashion with levels of Hb F of 0.8% to 3.4% in heterozygotes.[1, 9, 78, 359, 425] Interpretation of earlier studies of Swiss HPFH was complicated by the small size of the pedigrees, overlap of Hb F levels in heterozygotes and normal subjects, varying age of the research subjects (Hb F levels tend to fall with age), and concomitant inheritance of β-globin gene alleles that can also influence Hb F levels.

Several studies have been published in which linkage analysis clearly demonstrates that the HPFH determinant segregates independently from the β-globin gene cluster. In the first, a large Sardinian pedigree,[426, 427] and the second, a large Asian Indian pedigree,[428] nondeletion HPFH and β⁰-thalassemia genes were segregating in each family. Studies of normal individuals in Japan with Swiss HPFH, using F-cell percentage to define HPFH rather than Hb F levels, have demonstrated that the "high F-cell trait" segregates as an X-linked determinant.[9] Researchers in one study have also localized a genetic determinant for Hb F production in another large family to the long arm of chromosome 6 in a large HPFH pedigree.[10] Further mapping of these HPFH determinants may provide important insights into the mechanisms regulating hemoglobin switching.

CLINICAL HETEROGENEITY OF THALASSEMIA DUE TO DIVERSITY OF MUTATIONS

In the previous sections, the extraordinary array of mutations associated with the clinical syndrome of thalassemia have been described. In populations in which thalassemia is prevalent, different types of mutations, affecting genes of either the α- or β- or both globin clusters, may coexist. Frequently, patients are compound heterozygotes for these mutations. The relative degree to which globin chain synthesis is impaired reflects this genetic heterogeneity and determines the clinical phenotype. In the following clinical descriptions of the thalassemia syndromes, such genetic interrelationships are emphasized.

α-Thalassemia

Genetics of α-Thalassemia

Alpha-thalassemias are divided into four clinical subsets that reflect the extent of impairment in α-globin chain production: silent carrier, α-thalassemia trait, hemoglobin H disease, and hydrops fetalis. Before the introduction of molecular analysis, these syndromes were classified on the basis of red blood cell parameters (hemoglobin level, mean corpuscular volume [MCV], mean corpuscular hemoglobin [MCH], globin biosynthetic ratio, presence of inclusions, and Hb H [β_4] levels) as well as the manner in which they interacted genetically to produce different phenotypes. Much of this early work relied on the study of Asian populations, in which α-thalassemia is particularly common.[1] Thus, the "silent" carrier state for α-thalassemia in which a single α-globin gene on a chromosome was inactivated has traditionally been designated as α-thalassemia-2. Homozygosity for α-thalassemia-2, or heterozygosity for a more severe allele in which both α-globin genes were inactivated, leads to α-thalassemia trait, also termed α-thalassemia-1. By the historical nomenclature, Hb H disease reflects heterozygosity for α-thalassemia-2 and α-thalassemia-1, whereas hydrops fetalis results from heterozygosity for α-thalassemia-1.

Advances in the molecular characterization of the α-globin gene cluster clarified the genetic basis of these phenotypes. Weatherall and colleagues proposed a more informative nomenclature for these mutations.[1, 2] Each chromosome may be designated as α^+ or α^0 to indicate the presence or absence of any α-globin chain

production derived from that chromosome. This is referred to as a haplotype and should be distinguished from the usage of the term *haplotype* in describing the linkage of DNA polymorphisms on a chromosome. Haplotypes are further subdivided by the status of each α-globin gene on a chromosome. As discussed previously, mutations may be of the deletion or nondeletion type. Normal individuals are designated ($\alpha\alpha/\alpha\alpha$) to indicate the presence of four active α genes, two on each chromosome 16, where the first position corresponds to the $\alpha2$ gene and the second position to the $\alpha1$ gene. Deletion of a single α-globin gene on a chromosome is designated as ($-\alpha/$), whereas deletion of both genes is indicated as ($--/$). A further refinement of this nomenclature includes the designation of the specific mutation; for example ($--^{SEA}/$) signifies the α^0 deletion mutation that is common in the southeastern Asian populations (see Fig. 21–24), whereas ($-\alpha^{3.7}/$) symbolizes the α^+ rightward α-globin gene deletion that is extremely common in the American black population (see Fig. 21–24). Nondeletion mutations in a haplotype are designated in this scheme by a superscript T ($\alpha\alpha^T$) and can be more precisely described by symbols for the specific mutation and the gene affected. For example, ($\alpha^{CS}\alpha$) designates a chromosome bearing the Constant Spring chain termination mutation affecting the $\alpha2$ gene (see Table 21–3), and $\alpha^{QS}\alpha$ designates a chromosome bearing the α-globin gene with a substitution in codon 125 that leads to synthesis of an unstable globin (see Table 21–3). This shorthand nomenclature is extremely useful when a patient's genotype is known in detail, and it has simplified the description of the many genotypes that interact to generate the heterogeneous clinical syndromes.

The silent carrier state, or α-thalassemia-2 defect, is due to the presence of a mutation affecting only one α-globin gene. Most often this occurs due to a deletion mutation ($-/\alpha\alpha\alpha$). Two genotypes, ($--/\alpha\alpha$) and ($-\alpha/-\alpha$), are associated with α-thalassemia trait and reflect the inactivation of two α-globin genes. Substitution mutations that affect the predominant $\alpha2$ gene $\alpha^T\alpha/\alpha\alpha$ may also lead to α thalassemia trait. The extent of the observed changes in red cell indices mirrors the reduction in α-globin production with each genotype with the ($-\alpha/-\alpha$) less affected than the ($--\alpha\alpha$) genotype.

Hb H disease occurs in individuals who have only a single fully functional α-globin gene. Genotypes leading to Hb H disease are diverse.[2] Most common is heterozygosity for the single and double deletion chromosomes ($--/-\alpha$). As a result, Hb H disease is observed most often in Southeast Asia ($--^{SEA}/-\alpha^{3.7}$) and the Mediterranean basin ($--^{MED}/-\alpha^{3.7}$) where both the α^+ and α^0 haplotypes are present at significant frequency. Nondeletion mutations may also interact to cause Hb H disease. As discussed earlier, the $\alpha2$ genes are responsible for the production of about 75% of the total α-globin chains. Mutations that decrease expression from the $\alpha2$ gene $\alpha^T\alpha$ result in an α^+ haplotype that produces fewer α-globin chains than a deletion α^+ haplotype ($-\alpha/$). Thus, homozygosity for mutations in both $\alpha2$ genes $\alpha^T\alpha/\alpha^T\alpha$ is phenotypically equivalent to deletion of three genes and is associated with Hb H disease and not α-thalassemia trait.[2, 12] Consistent with this observation, nondeletion α⁺-thalassemia haplotypes that are paired with α⁰-thalassemia haplotypes ($- - /\alpha^T\alpha$) lead to more severe Hb H disease than the interaction of the deletion α⁺ haplotypes ($- - /-\alpha$).

Homozygosity for the α⁰ haplotype ($- - /- -$) leads to hydrops fetalis, a disorder that is particularly common in Southeast Asia where the frequency of the α⁰ haplotype is appreciable. In rare infants from Greece and Southeast Asia, hydrops fetalis has been shown to result from the interaction of α⁰ haplotypes with nondeletion α⁺ haplotypes.[429–431]

Because there are at least 30 mutations that may inactivate one or both α-globin genes, the different combinations of chromosomes bearing α-thalassemia mutations number more than 200. The frequency of the different genotypes and haplotypes defines the spectrum of disease observed in a given ethnic group. For example, severe forms of α-thalassemia (Hb H disease and hydrops fetalis) are uncommon in blacks. In this group, the single deletion chromosome is very common,[432, 433] whereas chromosomes with two defective α-globin genes are quite rare.[434–436] In some circumstances, the phenotype of Hb H disease is not readily related to genotype. Indeed, there is a significant spectrum of disease severity in individuals from the Southeast Asian area with the same genotype ($-\alpha^{3.7}/- -^{SEA}$).[397] The observed phenotype may be further complicated by the inheritance of another hemoglobin disorder (β-thalassemia) or the influence of environmental factors, such as iron or other nutritional deficiency.

Silent Carrier

One parent of an individual with Hb H disease (severe α-thalassemia) usually has the features of thalassemia trait, whereas the other has normal-appearing red cells and no anemia (see Table 21–2).[1] Offspring of individuals with Hb H disease fall into two groups: (1) thalassemia trait and (2) nearly normal hemoglobin synthesis. These findings suggested that a silent carrier state for α-thalassemia existed. Patients with silent carrier α-thalassemia have three rather than four functional α-globin genes.[389, 437] As such, impairment in α-globin synthesis is very mild. There is significant overlap of their globin biosynthetic ratio both with normal subjects and with individuals having only two functional α-globin genes (Fig. 21–25). Similarly, the mean MCV of patients with three functional genes is slightly lower than for normal subjects, but significant overlap between the two groups exists.[2] Despite these differences that become apparent on comparison of groups with different numbers of α-globin genes, there is no reliable way to diagnose silent carriers of α-thalassemia by hematologic criteria. Diagnosis has been reported by detection of small amounts of Hb Bart's in cord blood,[1] but additional studies indicate that this approach is unreliable in ascertaining the presence of the silent carrier state.[438, 439]

Hb Constant Spring—Elongated α-Globins

Some silent carriers for α-thalassemia produce small quantities of slowly migrating hemoglobins (Fig. 21–26), which contain elongated α-globin chain variants resulting from termination codon mutations[161–165] (see Table 21–3 and Fig. 21–14). The original elongated α chain variant, Hb Constant Spring, was named for the small Jamaican town in which the Chinese family in whom these hemoglobins were first discovered resided.[162] The family had three children with Hb H disease; each had a small amount of the abnormal hemoglobins. One parent had typical thalassemia trait, whereas the other had normal red cells but, in addition, had approximately 1% of the abnormal hemoglobin. Similar slowly migrating hemoglobins have been found in other racial groups in Thailand and Greece.[440] Individuals homozygous for the α^CSα mutation α^CSα/α^CSα have a clinical syndrome similar to Hb H disease, though their erythrocytes contain Hb Bart's (γ₄) rather than Hb H, and the degree of anemia and the extent of abnormalities in red cell indices are more mild than in most cases of Hb H disease.[441] Compound heterozygotes for α⁰ and α^CS haplotypes ($- -\alpha^{CS}\alpha$) exhibit typical Hb H disease.

α-Thalassemia Trait

Alpha-thalassemia trait is characterized by marked microcytosis and hypochromia of red cells in conjunction with mild anemia and erythrocytosis (see Table 21–2). Levels of Hb A₂ and Hb F are generally normal or low. Diagnosis of this condition is typically made by family studies or by excluding iron deficiency and β-thalassemia trait. The frequency is particularly high among Asian populations and less among African, Mediterranean, and American black populations. Even in the neonatal period, the red cells appear hypochromic and microcytic. Hb Bart's may be found in up to 1% in the blood of normal neonates but reaches levels of 4% to 6% in infants who are later shown to have α-thalassemia trait[1] (see Table 21–2). Beyond the neonatal period, biochemical markers, such as Hb A₂ and Hb F in β-thalassemia, are not particularly helpful in confirming the diagnosis of α-thalassemia trait. The one exception occurs in circumstances in which the expression of ζ-globin is increased owing to deletion of both α-globin genes on a chromosome.[398, 409, 442] In Southeast Asia, where the $- -^{SEA}$ allele is common, a sensitive radioimmunoassay allows detection of ζ-globin chains in adult carriers of this mutation.

Measurement of the β:α biosynthetic ratio has little place in the routine diagnosis of α-thalassemia trait. Although detection of impaired α-globin synthesis has been reported,[443, 444] the measurement is technically difficult to perform, because these individuals have a low reticulocyte count and the measured values overlap with those found in normal individuals (see Table 21–2). Iron deficiency may raise the measured βα biosynthetic ratio, further complicating interpretation.[445, 446] Thus, in most cases, the diagnosis of α-thalassemia trait

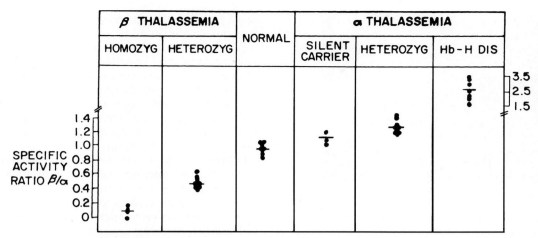

Figure 21-25. The α:β globin biosynthetic ratio in various forms of thalassemia. Peripheral blood cells were incubated with (^{14}C)-leucine for 2 hours in autologous plasma. The globin chains were isolated by ion exchange chromatography. The specific activity of the chains and the ratio of their radioactivities were then calculated. (With permission from Nathan DG: Thalassemia. The New England Journal of Medicine 1972; 286:586. Copyright 1972, Massachusetts Medical Society.)

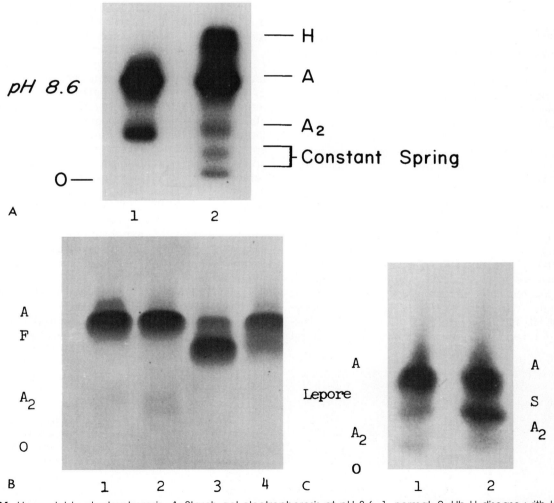

Figure 21-26. Hemoglobin electrophoresis. *A,* Starch gel electrophoresis at pH 8.6; 1, normal; 2, Hb H disease with Hb Constant Spring. *B,* Agarose electrophoresis at pH 8.6; 1, normal; 2, β-thalassemia trait with increased Hb A₂; 3 and 4, homozygous β-thalassemia with different relative amounts of Hb A and Hb F. *C,* Starch gel electrophoresis at pH 8.6; 1, Hb Lepore trait; 2, sickle cell trait. ''O'' indicates the origin. The anode is at the top of the page.

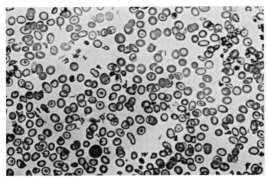

Figure 21–27. Peripheral blood smear from a patient with Hb H disease.

is established by red cell morphology and parameters, coupled with exclusion of β-thalassemia trait and iron deficiency. Gene deletions responsible for deficient α-globin production can be demonstrated by restriction endonuclease mapping; this technique may be applied in special instances in which an accurate diagnosis is critical.

Hemoglobin H Disease

Hemoglobin Pattern. An anemia of moderate severity characterized by hypochromia, microcytosis, striking red cell fragmentation (Fig. 21–27), and the presence of a fast migrating hemoglobin, Hb H β_4, on electrophoresis (see Fig. 21–26)[447, 448] may be shown to be an α-thalassemia syndrome by measurement of the β:α biosynthetic ratio.[443, 449, 450] Incubation of peripheral blood reticulocytes with ³H-leucine and subsequent chromatographic resolution of the globins indicate that such patients have a twofold to fivefold excess of β chain synthesis (see Table 21–2 and Fig. 21–25). These excess β chains form Hb H, which comprises 5% to 30% of the total hemoglobin in patients with Hb H disease.[451] In approximately 50% of individuals with Hb H disease in Southeast Asia, small quantities of Hb Constant Spring are found (see Fig. 21–26). Hemoglobin H disease may be suspected in anemic neonates in whom all the red cells are severely hypochromic. At birth, patients with Hb H disease also have large amounts of Hb Bart's (γ_4). In patients with Hb H disease with an intact spleen, incubation of the peripheral

blood cells in brilliant cresyl blue produces many small inclusions in most red cells (Fig. 21–28). The dye induces precipitation of Hb H by a redox reaction. In contrast, large and usually single preformed inclusions (Heinz bodies) may be visualized with methyl violet in red cells of splenectomized patients (see Fig. 21–28).[76, 452] These inclusions are composed of precipitated β globin, rendered insoluble by hemichrome formation or by interaction of the β-globin sulfhydryl groups with the red cell membrane.[76, 453]

Pathophysiology. Hb H exhibits no Bohr effect or heme-heme interaction and thus is ineffective for oxygen transport under physiologic conditions.[454] Consequently, patients with appreciable amounts of Hb H have a more severe deficit in functional hemoglobin and oxygen-carrying capacity than the measured hemoglobin concentration might suggest. Red cells containing Hb H are sensitive to oxidative stress, accounting for the enhanced red cell destruction that may occur on administration of oxidant drugs such as the sulfonamides.[455] As erythrocytes age and lose their capacity to withstand oxidant stress, Hb H precipitates, leading to premature destruction of circulating red cells.[76] Thus, Hb H is primarily a hemolytic disorder.[452, 456] Inclusions of Hb H are rarely seen in bone marrow cells,[457] and erythropoiesis is fairly effective.[456]

Clinical Features and Therapy. Typical patients with Hb H disease live quite normally. Generally, anemia is moderate with a hemoglobin concentration of 7 to 10 g/dL, although occasional patients may have hemoglobin levels as low as 3 to 4 g/dL.[1] The complications of Hb H disease are those related to chronic hemolysis. Jaundice and hepatosplenomegaly are commonly present. Folic acid deficiency, pigment gallstones, leg ulcers, and increased susceptibility to infection are also observed. Hemolytic episodes may be precipitated by drugs or infection. Iron overload is uncommon but may occur in transfused patients and those older than the age of 45.[458] Development of characteristic thalassemic facies, reflecting expansion of marrow space equivalent to that seen in patients with severe β-thalassemia, is rare. Usually only moderate bone marrow erythroid hyperplasia is evident.[448]

Consistent with its benign course, treatment of Hb H disease is primarily supportive. Therapy includes supplementation with folic acid, avoidance of oxidant drugs and iron salts, prompt treatment of infectious

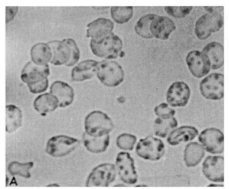
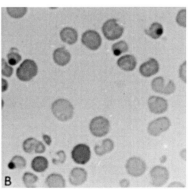

Figure 21–28. Red cell inclusions in Hb H disease. *A,* Inclusions induced by incubation of peripheral blood in 1% brilliant cresyl blue (BCB) and 0.4% citrate for 30 minutes at 37°C. (Patient not splenectomized.) *B,* Preformed inclusions in peripheral blood of a splenectomized patient stained by new methylene blue reticulocyte stain.

episodes, and judicious use of transfusions. Splenectomy should be contemplated in patients with Hb H disease only if hypersplenism is present, as reflected by leukopenia, thrombocytopenia, and worsening anemia or development of a transfusion requirement in a previously stable patient. In contrast to β-thalassemia, thrombocytosis in severe Hb H disease after splenectomy may be complicated by a clotting diathesis and recurrent pulmonary emboli, particularly in patients with a fairly normal hematocrit.[459, 460] Measurement of red cell survival and splenic sequestration by chromium-51 labeling of red cells is controversial in making clinical decisions regarding splenectomy, because the label binds selectively to β-globin chains and may, by virtue of selective removal of Hb H inclusions from red cells in the spleen, give a falsely high index of splenic destruction.[461] Other studies, however, suggest that the chromium-51 labeling technique may be valid.[462]

α-Thalassemia with Mental Retardation Syndrome. Patients have been described with a syndrome characterized by mental retardation and a form of α-thalassemia that cannot be explained by simple mendelian inheritance of an α-thalassemia gene.[416, 463] In rare patients, the mutation arises as a *de novo* event in a paternal germ cell. These patients can be divided into having two distinct syndromes (deletion and nondeletion) on the basis of their clinical features and the results of molecular analysis of their α-globin gene clusters.

Patients have been described with extensive deletions involving chromosome band 16p3.3 or, alternatively, deletions resulting from unbalanced chromosome translocations that also led to aneuploidy in a second chromosome. Patients with deletion mutations exhibit mild to moderate mental retardation and a broad spectrum of dysmorphic features. Other rare patients are characterized by more severe mental retardation and a uniform pattern of dysmorphic features including genital abnormalities but no detectable deletions involving the α-globin gene cluster.[65] This X-linked condition is now known as X-linked α-thalassemia/mental retardation syndrome (ATR-X). As noted earlier, the affected gene is a putative global regulator (XH2).[66]

Although these disorders are infrequent, they may be underrecognized. This is particularly true of ethnic groups in which α-thalassemia is uncommon, and the mild hematologic findings in patients who do not inherit a second α-thalassemia gene might be overlooked. Infants with uncharacterized mental retardation should be studied with techniques suitable for detection of a deficiency in α-globin synthesis.

Acquired Hb H Disease. Hb H is also found rarely in the red cells of patients with erythroleukemia or a myeloproliferative syndrome.[411–413] The disorder may be clonal and displays a striking male predisposition (85% of confirmed cases).[416] The clinical features manifested by these patients are those of their primary disorder; the finding of Hb H is incidental to the outcome of the disease, although striking red cell abnormalities and active hemolysis may be present. The genetic mechanism of this syndrome appears to involve abnormal regulation of α-globin gene expression because of a mutation affecting a distant genetic locus (see earlier).

Hydrops Fetalis. The birth of stillborn infants to α-thalassemia trait parents reflects the most severe form of α-thalassemia.[464, 465] Infants are grossly edematous or hydropic secondary to congestive heart failure induced by severe anemia. They are unable to synthesize any α-globin, and thus their blood contains only Hb Bart's (γ_4), Hb H (β_4), and small amounts of Hb Portland ($\zeta_2\gamma_2$), present within red cells displaying morphologic changes characteristic of severe thalassemia.[466, 467] The blood smear is characterized by large hypochromic macrocytes and numerous nucleated red cells. Although the hemoglobin concentration averages 6.2 g/dL, both Hb H and Hb Bart's have high oxygen affinity and no subunit cooperativity. Therefore, the hydropic infant has very little functional hemoglobin. Viability *in utero* is maintained by the presence of small quantities of Hb Portland I and Hb Portland II. Generally, affected infants are delivered stillborn at 30 to 40 weeks' gestation or die shortly after delivery at term.[410, 466] At autopsy, extensive extramedullary hematopoiesis and placental hypertrophy are seen.

A high incidence of toxemia of pregnancy and postpartum hemorrhage is observed in mothers of hydropic infants,[448, 468] presumably as a consequence of the massive placenta. Hence, early recognition of the disorder in at-risk pregnancies by prenatal diagnosis should lead to consideration of termination of the pregnancy. At least five infants born prematurely with hydrops fetalis have survived after chronic transfusion regimens.[469, 470] Intrauterine transfusion of fetuses with hydrops fetalis should also be considered if treatment after delivery is contemplated.[471]

Mild β-Thalassemia

Silent Carrier

A silent carrier state for β-thalassemia was recognized through study of families in which affected children had a more severe β-thalassemia syndrome than a parent with typical β-thalassemia trait.[1, 6, 417–420] Study of the "normal" parent often revealed mild microcytosis or a slight impairment in β-globin synthesis on radiolabeling of the globin chains in peripheral blood reticulocytes. Characteristically, silent carriers of β-thalassemia have normal levels of Hb A_2. These silent carriers must be distinguished from individuals whose red cells have all the stigmata of β-thalassemia trait but have normal Hb A_2. Several patients who are homozygous for the silent carrier β-thalassemia gene have been described.[1] Anemia is moderate (6–7.0 g/dL), and these patients rarely require transfusion. Hepatosplenomegaly may be significant. The Hb F values range from 10% to 15%, and the Hb A_2 is elevated to the range normally seen in individuals with thalassemia trait.

The silent carrier state of β-thalassemia appears to be a distinct clinical and biochemical entity. The underlying molecular defects cause only a modest reduction in β-globin synthesis. Two point mutations in the β-globin gene region have been linked to the silent carrier phenotype. The −101 promoter mutation appears to be a common cause of silent β-thalassemia in the Italian population[183] and has been observed in Bulgarian and Turkish individuals,[102] whereas the +1 cap site Inr mutation is associated with a silent carrier phenotype in an Indian family.[109] As noted earlier, rare instances of silent β-thalassemia due to mutations unlinked to the β-globin gene cluster have been reported.

β-Thalassemia Trait

Clinical Features

In 1925, Rietti[472] described mild anemic Italian patients whose red cells exhibited increased resistance to osmotic lysis. A similar syndrome was later recognized in American patients of Italian descent by Wintrobe and co-workers,[473] who noted that both parents of a patient with Cooley's anemia also had this syndrome. Detailed analysis of several pedigrees by Valentine and Neel[474] and others[475, 476] established that this form of thalassemia occurs in individuals who are heterozygous for a mutation that affects β-globin synthesis.

The peripheral blood smear in β-thalassemia trait is shown in Figure 21–29. Microcytosis, hypochromia, targeting, basophilic stippling, and elliptocytosis may be striking features, although in occasional patients the red cells may be nearly normal. The bone marrow is characterized by mild to moderate erythroid hyperplasia; red cell survival is modestly decreased, and slight ineffective erythropoiesis is present.[477] Inclusions in bone marrow cells and peripheral red cells are rare. Similar hematologic parameters appear to characterize Thai, Chinese, Greek, British, and Italian populations

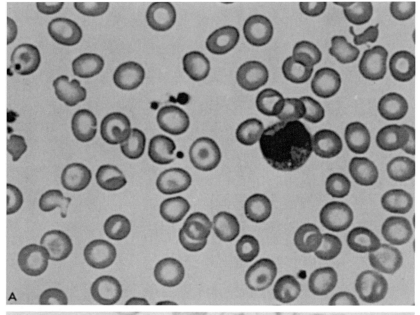
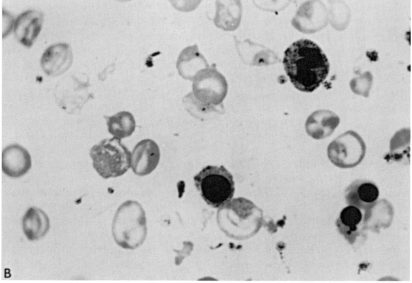

Figure 21-29. Peripheral blood smears in heterozygous β-thalassemia (A) and homozygous β-thalassemia (B) after splenectomy.

with β-thalassemia trait,[478–481] whereas American blacks appear to have a milder syndrome.[482] Hepatomegaly and splenomegaly have been reported in 10% to 19% of Italian and Greek patients but are less common in other groups.[480, 481] Iron or folic acid deficiency, pregnancy, or intercurrent illness may exacerbate the anemia in patients with thalassemia trait.

Globin Biosynthetic Ratio. In peripheral blood reticulocytes, the measured β:α biosynthetic ratio varies from 0.5 to 0.7, as predicted for the inactivation of a single β-globin gene (see Fig. 21–25). However, when bone marrow cells are incubated with ^{3}H-leucine, the measured β:α biosynthetic ratio is often 1:1 in patients with heterozygous β-thalassemia.[483–487] The capacity of bone marrow cells to degrade free α-globin by proteolysis may explain why it is difficult to demonstrate unbalanced synthesis of β- and α-globin chains in the marrow cells of heterozygotes. The measured β:α ratio approximates 0.5 in pulses of 10 to 20 minutes, but if the incubation of bone marrow cells is prolonged, proteolysis apparently destroys the excess newly synthesized α-globin.[488, 489] Fractionation of bone marrow cells after incubation in ^{3}H-leucine demonstrated that proteolysis is most efficient in the earliest erythroid cells, namely, proerythroblasts and basophilic erythroblasts.[489] The impairment in β-globin synthesis becomes easier to detect as erythroid cells mature, accounting for the reduced β:α globin biosynthetic ratio that is usually found in peripheral blood reticulocytes.

Classification and Genetics. Individuals with thalassemia trait are heterozygous for β-thalassemia. Expression of one β gene is impaired by mutation whereas that of the other gene is normal. Characteristically, Hb A_2 or Hb F or both are elevated in patients with β-thalassemia trait, although occasionally normal levels are observed. The relative amounts of Hb A_2 or Hb F have been used to classify thalassemia trait that has relevance to the molecular lesion in certain instances and also to the severity of the disease in homozygous offspring.

δ-Globin synthesis. Among inherited anemias, the elevation in Hb A_2 level is unique to β-thalassemia. The absolute quantity of Hb A_2 present in red cells is a complex function of the inherent capacity for δ-globin chain synthesis and factors regulating rates of hemoglobin dimer and tetramer assembly. As discussed earlier, δ-globin is normally expressed at a low level, about 2.5% that of the β-globin. The level may be further reduced by mutations that affect δ-globin expression. Heterozygous[490, 491] and homozygous[492] states have been described. Delta-thalassemias reflect point mutations that completely silence the already defective δ-globin genes.[254, 255, 258, 420, 493–495]

In heterozygous β-thalassemia, the observed increase in Hb A_2 represents an absolute increase in the quantity of Hb A_2 per red cell from the normal level of 0.6 to 0.7 pg to 1.0 pg.[1] The increased Hb A_2 contains δ-globin chains derived from the δ-globin gene adjacent to the mutant β-globin gene as well as from the δ-globin gene on the opposite chromosome. This has been inferred from study of β-thalassemia heterozygotes who also have a variant δ-globin chain.[496] The increase in Hb A_2 can be accounted for by enhanced incorporation of δ-globin chains into hemoglobin dimers as a consequence of deficient β-globin chain production (see earlier discussion of hemoglobin assembly).[205]

Environmental factors also influence the absolute level of Hb A_2. Iron deficiency leads to a decrease in Hb A_2, which may normalize its level in thalassemia heterozygotes and, therefore, mask the diagnosis of β-thalassemia trait. In such instances, the level of Hb A_2 becomes elevated on iron repletion.[497] An increase in Hb A_2 may be seen in acquired megaloblastic disorders secondary to either folic acid or vitamin B_{12} deficiency.[497]

High A_2 β-Thalassemia. This is the most common form of β-thalassemia trait. Hb A_2 levels vary from 3.5% to 8.0%, whereas the Hb F level varies from less than 1% to 5%.[1, 478–482] The vast majority of single base mutations leading to β-thalassemia (see Table 21–3) lead to typical high Hb A_2 β-thalassemia trait. Although individual mutations variably reduce β-globin synthesis, efforts to differentiate the effect of specific mutations in heterozygous individuals have largely been unrewarding.[1, 480, 498, 499] In blacks, β[0] and β[+] mutations can often be distinguished in individual families owing to the frequency of double heterozygotes for a β-thalassemia mutation and the β[S] mutation. In this population, the mean MCV and MCH are higher in β[+] heterozygotes than in β[0] heterozygotes, but the circulating hemoglobin concentrations are nearly equivalent.[482, 500] The common mutations found in American blacks, most notably residing in the ATA-box of the promoter (see Table 21–3), only modestly impair β-globin gene expression,[43, 122] perhaps accounting for the relatively mild phenotype of many individuals with heterozygous or homozygous β[+] thalassemia in this population.

Homozygous offspring of two individuals with high Hb A_2 β-thalassemia trait usually suffer from transfusion-dependent anemia but may sometimes show a thalassemia intermedia phenotype. The precise nature of the mutation or mutations in homozygous individuals is one factor in determining the clinical phenotype.

δβ-Thalassemia. Individuals heterozygous for these mutations have increased levels of Hb F (5%–15%) and low Hb A_2 levels. This phenotype is most often generated by deletions that remove most or all of the coding sequences of the δ- and β-globin genes (see Table 21–5). The propensity of these deletion mutations to enhance the expression of the γ-globin genes contributes to a relatively mild phenotype in homozygous individuals or in those in whom a δβ-thalassemia deletion is inherited along with a thalassemia allele having a typical substitution mutation.

High A_2 High F β-Thalassemia. A distinct variant of β-thalassemia trait has been described in which Hb A_2 is elevated and Hb F is also elevated (5%–20%).[262, 263, 501] This form of thalassemia trait is associated with deletions of the β-globin gene that leave the δ- and γ-globin genes intact (see Table 21–5).

Normal A_2 β-Thalassemia. This form of β-thalassemia trait should be distinguished from the silent carrier state. Although both are characterized by low

Table 21-7. HEMATOLOGIC PARAMETERS IN THALASSEMIA TRAIT AND IRON DEFICIENCY

Parameter	α-Thal	β-Thal	Iron Deficiency
Hemoglobin concentration (g/dL)	12.6 ± 1.1 (651)* 12 ± 0.7	†M—12.6 ± 1.4 (626–629) F—10.8 ± 0.9 (626–629) C—11.3 ± 1 (626–629) *Adults*—12 ± 1.3	10.2 ± 1.6 (656)
Red cell count (× 10⁶/μL)	5.6 ± 0.5	M—5.8 ± 0.6 (626–629) F—5.1 ± 0.9 (626–629) C—4.7 ± 0.6 (626–629) *Adults*—6 ± 0.48	4.67 ± 0.43 (656)
Mean corpuscular volume (88.7 ± 5.3) (651) (4 m³/red cell)	72.2 ± 3.3 (651) 65.2 ± 3 (653)	64.7 ± 4.3 (651) 60.8 ± 5.6 (656)	67 ± 6.6 (656)
Mean corpuscular hemoglobin (pg/red cell)	23.2 + 3.3 (651) 21 ± 1 (653)	20.3 ± 2.2 (651) 20.2 ± 1.9 (656)	21.8 ± 2.9 (656)
Hemoglobin A₂ (2%–3.5%)	Normal or decreased	5.2 ± 0.8 (626–629)	Normal or decreased
Hemoglobin F (Less than 1%)	Less than 1%	2.1 ± 1.2 (626–629)	Less than 1%

*Numbers in parentheses are reference citations.
†M = males, F = females, C = children.

or normal Hb A₂, the red cells in individuals with normal Hb A₂ β-thalassemia are characteristically hypochromic and microcytic,[419, 502] in contrast to silent carriers whose red cells appear near normal.[417, 418] Individuals who co-inherit this type of β-thalassemia allele from one parent along with a high Hb A₂ β-thalassemia allele from the other usually have severe transfusion-dependent β-thalassemia.

This phenotype is thought to represent co-inheritance of mutations that decrease β- and δ-globin gene function. The mutations in the δ-globin gene may be present on the same chromosome or on the opposite chromosome from the β-thalassemia gene.[254, 255, 258, 420, 493–495]

Differential Diagnosis of Thalassemia Trait. In clinical practice, thalassemia trait must be distinguished from iron deficiency (see Chapter 11 for additional discussion of the differential diagnosis of microcytosis and iron deficiency). Often the differential diagnosis may be suspected from red blood cell indices; mild erythrocytosis and marked microcytosis are characteristic of thalassemia trait (Table 21–7).[503–505] The red cell count is usually decreased in patients with iron deficiency, whereas the MCV may be normal or decreased, depending on whether the iron deficiency anemia is acute or chronic,[506–509] but the MCV is rarely as low as in thalassemia trait. The mean corpuscular hemoglobin concentration (MCHC) is usually normal in thalassemia trait and iron deficiency; in both syndromes the hypochromic appearance of the red cells reflects their small size, diminished hemoglobin content, and high surface-to-volume ratio. The red cell distribution width (RDW), a parameter available in modern automated cell counters, was originally believed to distinguish between iron deficiency and other causes of microcytosis.[510, 511] However, the RDW is also increased in the thalassemias and other hemoglobinopathies and is not a useful independent discriminator.[512–516] The absence of stainable iron in a bone marrow specimen is highly suggestive of iron deficiency, but the presence of iron does not necessarily exclude an iron-responsive anemia.

Several formulas have been developed to assist in the diagnosis of thalassemia trait during the assessment of microcytic hypochromic anemia (Table 21–8).[507, 517, 518] None of the discriminant functions are infallible. Nonetheless, the Mentzer index[507] is useful as an office screening test. More accuracy in separating thalassemia trait from iron deficiency may be available from the England and Fraser function[518–520]; but when both conditions exist simultaneously all indices are subject to error. Additional discriminant functions and automated protocols have been proposed that may also prove useful.[521–523] The free erythrocyte protoporphyrin, often incorporated into the initial workup of hypochromic microcytic anemia in childhood to screen for lead exposure, is an additional useful test in screening patients suspected of having thalassemia trait.[524, 525] This technique has been especially useful in evaluating newly arrived Southeast Asian refugees to the United States.[526] Of course, measurement of transferrin saturation or ferritin may also be used to verify or exclude the diagnosis of iron deficiency.

In office practice the distinction between thalassemia trait and iron deficiency usually rests on examination of peripheral blood smears, evaluation of the color of serum (pale in iron deficiency), and, above all, the clinical history. It is worth remembering that patients with thalassemia trait are not immune to iron deficiency. In these patients, iron deficiency may mask the

Table 21-8. FORMULAS FOR DIFFERENTIATION OF THALASSEMIA TRAIT FROM IRON DEFICIENCY

	Thalassemia Trait	Iron Deficiency
Mentzer index (655)* MCV/RBC	<13	>13
Shine and Lal (665) (MCV) 2 × MCH	<1530	>1530
England and Fraser (666) MCV − RBC − (5 × Hb) − 8.4	Negative values	Positive values

*Numbers in parentheses are reference citations.

increases in Hb A_2 and Hb F that would otherwise suggest a diagnosis of β-thalassemia.

Once iron deficiency is excluded, the differential diagnosis between α- and β-thalassemia traits rests on the measurement of Hb A_2 and Hb F levels (see Table 21–7) and rarely on more sophisticated tests, such as the measurement of the αβ biosynthetic ratio in peripheral blood reticulocytes. In patients with microcytosis, hypochromia, and erythrocytosis but without evidence of iron deficiency or altered Hb A_2 and Hb F levels, α-thalassemia is most probable. When both α- and β-thalassemia co-exist, the changes in Hb F and Hb A_2 characteristic of β thalassemia trait may not be present[81] (see later). Molecular genetic analysis and family studies are often necessary to define these complex interactions.

Severe β-Thalassemia

Historical Perspective

It was not until Thomas Cooley, a Detroit pediatrician, first described the clinical entity that was to bear his name that thalassemia major was recognized as a distinct disease.[527, 528] Cooley recognized similarities in the appearance and clinical course in four children of Greek and Italian ancestry. These children exhibited severe anemia (hemoglobin concentrations of 3 to 7 g/dL), massive hepatosplenomegaly, and severe growth retardation. In addition, bony deformities, such as frontal bossing and maxillary prominence, gave the patients a characteristic facies. Deformities of the long bones of the legs were also commonly seen and thought to reflect severe osteoporosis. Thalassemia major, or "Cooley's anemia," is far more common in Greece and Italy than in the United States, and descriptions of the disease in these countries soon followed Cooley's original report.[529]

Autopsy studies revealed extraordinary expansion of bone marrow at the expense of the bony structures. Extramedullary hematopoiesis is often a striking feature, presenting either as isolated massive hepatosplenomegaly or as hepatosplenomegaly in association with intrathoracic or intra-abdominal masses.[527–530] Children were also noted to have significant iron deposition in almost all organs, the significance of which was not initially appreciated.[530] Before the institution of regular blood transfusions, these changes progressed inexorably and were invariably fatal during the first few years of life. Patients died of the effects of their anemia: congestive heart failure, intercurrent infection, or complications resulting from all too frequent pathologic fractures.

Initial transfusion regimens were mainly palliative; transfusions were recommended only when anemia interfered significantly with a patient's ability to function on a daily basis. In defense of this regimen, it must be appreciated that the pathophysiology of the disease was not understood and that clinicians first attempted to minimize the transfusional iron administered because they feared that the iron, seen ubiquitously in these patients at autopsy, might itself be the causative agent of the disease.[530] Palliative therapy enabled affected persons to live somewhat longer than untransfused patients, but the bony deformities and severe anemia forced them to lead markedly restricted lives.

In an attempt to improve the quality of life for these patients, trials used routine transfusion schedules to maintain hemoglobin levels greater than or equal to 8.5 g/dL.[531–533] Patients improved dramatically, showing fewer overt side effects of anemia and more normal growth.[534, 535] Clinical improvement proved transient, however, because regular transfusions led to the complications of chronic iron overload, including growth retardation due to endocrine disturbances, diabetes mellitus, and delayed sexual maturation. Death invariably ensued in the second or early third decade of life, most often from cardiac arrhythmias or intractable congestive heart failure.[536]

Pathophysiology

Imbalance in Globin Biosynthesis. That severe β-thalassemia was caused by impaired production of β-globin was established in the mid 1960s by direct measurement of globin biosynthesis in reticulocytes.[537–541] Soon thereafter, impaired production of α chains was demonstrated in the α-thalassemia syndromes.[443] Decreased hemoglobin production is reflected in the peripheral blood smear by hypochromia, microcytosis, and target cells (that reflect the severe impairment in total hemoglobin production) and frequent teardrops, fragments, and microspherocytes (see Fig. 21–29). Red cell fragmentation is a direct consequence of unbalanced globin chain synthesis. Excess α chains, that have no complementary non–α chains with which to pair, form insoluble inclusions, demonstrable on methyl violet staining of the peripheral blood of asplenic β-thalassemia patients (Fig. 21–30). In nonsplenectomized individuals, these inclusions are difficult to demonstrate, because they are efficiently removed during passage of red cells through the splenic sinusoids, generating fragments and teardrops (Fig. 21–31).

Alpha-globin inclusions in the erythrocytes and nucleated erythroid cells of patients with thalassemia major were first demonstrated by Fessas and associ-

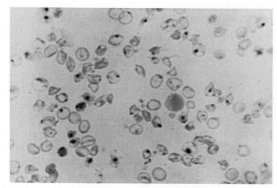

Figure 21–30. Supervital stain (methyl violet) of the peripheral blood cells from a patient with homozygous β-thalassemia after splenectomy.

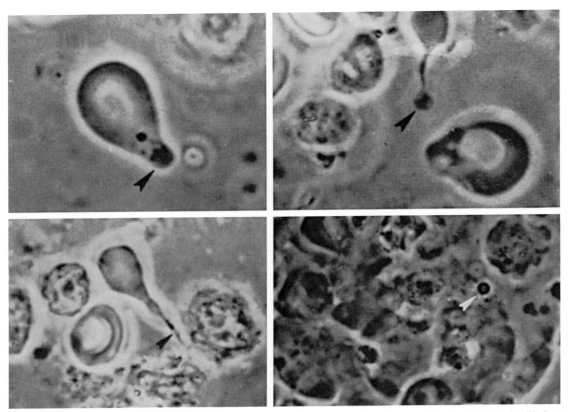

Figure 21-31. Phase-contrast microscopy of a wet preparation of scrapings from the spleen of a patient with homozygous β-thalassemia. Note the chain inclusion bodies *(black arrows)* within teardrop-shaped red cells, inclusions being pulled out, or ``pitted,'' from the red cell by reticuloendothelial cell action *(lower left)*, and inclusions free in the splenic pulp *(white arrow)*.

ates[542–544] and by Nathan and colleagues.[545] The frequency of the inclusions parallels the degree of impairment in β-globin synthesis. Inclusions have several deleterious effects on erythroid cells and are believed to lead to severe ineffective erythropoiesis. Electron microscopy has made it possible to visualize intranuclear α-globin inclusions, which have been hypothesized to interfere with cell division.[546, 547] Intracytoplasmic inclusions damage cell membranes, perturb the internal ionic environment, and thereby contribute to intramedullary death of erythroid cells. Moreover, α-inclusions reduce red cell deformability and very likely interfere with egress from the bone marrow spaces. The combined effects of ineffective erythropoiesis and severe anemia account for the extraordinary marrow expansion seen in patients with thalassemia major. In fact, these individuals have a nonfunctional cell mass that approximates the 10^{12} tumor cells present in patients with fatal leukemia and is associated with a profound hypermetabolic state including fever, wasting, and hyperuricemia.[545]

The Red Cell Membrane. Numerous membrane abnormalities of thalassemic erythrocytes have been described.[455, 548, 549] Many are attributable to oxidative damage from excess globin chains and association of heme and iron with the cell membrane after degradation of precipitated hemoglobin chains.[548, 550] Other abnormalities may result from selective interaction of excess α or β chains with the membrane cytoskeleton. After oxidation, globin chains, as well as trace metals such as iron and copper, generate free oxygen radicals that foster oxidative injury of the membrane.[551] Peroxidation of lipids in the red cell membrane is reflected in altered membrane lipid composition and distribution; polymerization of membrane components secondary to lipid peroxidation leads to cation loss and dehydration, decreased cell deformability, and increased rigidity of the phospholipid bilayer.[75, 76, 552] Similar changes are observed in normal red cells forced to engulf excess α chains.[553] Observed reductions in the level of serum and red cell vitamin E, a natural antioxidant, may be secondary to accelerated consumption from oxidant stress. The abnormal lipid distribution may contribute to enhanced clearance by macrophages. Increased binding of autologous IgG with an α-antigalactosyl specificity, originally proposed to reflect a decrease in sialic acid content of the membrane, may also promote clearance of thalassemic red cells from the circulation. Increased calcium content of thalassemic red cells is yet another manifestation of membrane damage.

Electrophoresis of red cell membrane proteins readily demonstrates increased association of globin chains with the red cell membranes (up to 11% of total protein), and similar findings can be reproduced in nonthalassemic erythrocytes by exposure to experimental oxidative stress.[554] Alpha- and β-globin chains interact differently with components of the cytoskeletal components.[555-557] The specificity of these interactions may contribute to the different phenotypic manifestations of the disorders. Membrane protein 4.1 of β-thalassemia erythrocytes is diminished in its capacity to enhance binding of spectrin to actin. In Hb H disease, protein 4.1 appears to be normal, but the binding of spectrin to inside-out vesicles is decreased, potentially because of oxidative damage of ankyrin promoted by binding of Hb H to protein band 3 with which ankyrin interacts. Spectrin binding is normal in β-thalassemia erythrocytes.

Schrier and colleagues reported differences in the rheologic properties of erythrocytes obtained from patients with Hb H disease and β-thalassemia intermedia.[558] Erythrocytes from both groups had a normal surface area but decreased cellular volume and increased membrane rigidity that is manifested by decreased cellular deformability under conditions of hypertonic osmotic stress. Although Hb H erythrocytes exhibit an increase in mechanical stability and a decrease in cell density, β-thalassemia erythrocytes are prone to cellular dehydration and have markedly decreased mechanical stability. In a murine model of β thalassemia, these cellular abnormalities are correlated with the extent of α-globin association with the membrane; small increases in β-globin chain expression through the introduction of a β-globin transgene resulted in a marked decrease in membrane-associated globin and a significant reversal of rheologic abnormalities.[559] Thus, slight improvements in chain synthetic balance that accompany increased expression of γ-globin or decreased expression of α-globin may result in dramatic improvements in membrane integrity in patients with β-thalassemia. A more detailed understanding of the red cell membrane abnormalities in thalassemia may facilitate the development of novel therapies in the future.

Genetic Heterogeneity. In current hematologic parlance, the term *thalassemia major* refers to patients with severe β-thalassemia requiring regular blood transfusions to sustain life. In the vast majority of such patients, both β-globin genes are affected by a thalassemia mutation; hence they have homozygous β-thalassemia. Other patients who also appear to be homozygous for β-thalassemia mutations, based on family studies, may be able to maintain a hemoglobin concentration of 6 to 10 g/dL without blood transfusions except during periods of infection, surgery, or other stresses.[1, 560] Such patients are said to have thalassemia intermedia. *Thalassemia intermedia* is a clinical term that describes the transfusion status of the patient. The term *Cooley's anemia* is still often used and applied somewhat indiscriminately to individual patients with either the major or the intermedia clinical syndromes.

Although other acquired and genetic modifiers exist, disease severity in the β-thalassemias is most directly related to the degree of imbalance between α- and total non–α-globin synthesis. Three major factors emerge as important determinants of the biosynthetic ratio in individual patients: (1) the nature of the specific mutation or mutations, (2) the presence of abnormalities in the α-globin cluster that increase or decrease α-globin expression, and (3) the genetic capacity for Hb F synthesis. Proteolysis of excess α chains, evident on comparison of the α to non-α biosynthetic ratio by short- and long-term incubations of bone marrow cells,[483-487] is also likely to modulate disease severity, although no meaningful quantitative studies of this mechanism have appeared.

Nature of Specific Mutations. The capacity of an individual with thalassemia to produce β-globin chains is directly determined by the specific mutations involving the β-globin gene. Because several different mutations are commonly found in populations with a high incidence of β-thalassemia, most patients with clinical homozygous β-thalassemia are heterozygous for two different mutations. The effect of specific mutations may range from total loss to only a mild impairment in β-globin synthesis, and thus the potential interactions based on the many different mutations is extraordinary. Indeed, disease severity may be viewed as a continuum, the extremes of which have been shown to correlate with specific mutations.

The mutations in the IVS-1 splice donor site (see Table 21–3 and Fig. 21–11) provide a particularly illustrative example of the variable consequences of specific mutations on β chain synthesis. These mutations lead to either a complete block in correct splicing of β globin mRNA or merely a reduction in the abundance of normal mRNA. Patients homozygous for a mutation in the conserved GT splice junction dinucleotide, who have not co-inherited an α-thalassemia gene or a determinant that increases Hb F synthesis, display severe transfusion-dependent β[0]-thalassemia.[105, 109, 110, 189] Substitutions of C or T at position 5 of the splice donor consensus sequence result in severe β[+] thalassemia,[95, 109, 120-122] whereas substitution of A at the same position results in a more mild phenotype.[123] The T→C substitution at position 6 is also associated with a mild β[+] thalassemia.[105]

Dominant β-Thalassemia. In rare circumstances, the heterozygous state of β thalassemia may be associated with severe disease rather than typical thalassemia trait. Several pedigrees with severe heterozygous β-thalassemia characterized by splenomegaly, cholelithiasis, and leg ulcers have been described.[561, 562] A striking association has been noted between mutations involving the exon 3 of the β-globin gene and these unusual cases of dominantly inherited β-thalassemia.[176, 180] Third exon mutations typically lead to the production of an unstable β-globin chain. A subset of third exon β-thalassemia mutations are associated with the presence of inclusion bodies in the normoblasts of affected heterozygotes (see Table 21–3)[178-182] and were first reported as "inclusion-body β-thalassemia," originally defined as a dominantly inherited dyserythropoietic anemia.[563, 564] The inclusion bodies, which may contain both α-globin and β-globin, represent aggregation of precipitated α-globin and unstable β-globin chains with the cell membrane, where they presumably potentiate oxidative damage. The dominantly inherited β-thalassemias are relatively rare and found in ethnic groups from nonmalarious regions.[176, 180] Presumably there is little selective pressure for these mutations owing to the decreased fitness of heterozygous individuals.

Increased production of α-globin chain above normal levels may exacerbate chain imbalance in β-thalassemia heterozygotes; co-inheritance of triplicated α-globin gene chromosomes is another potential cause of severe heterozygous β-thalassemia, usually with the phenotype of thalassemia intermedia.[402, 403, 565-567]

Interaction with Genetic Determinants That Increase Hb F Synthesis. Deletions within the β-globin gene cluster and mutations in the γ-globin promoters are sometimes associated with increased expression of γ-globin (see earlier discussion). Relatively small, genetically determined heterocellular increases in Hb F ameliorate the clinical course of thalassemia,[78, 79, 337, 348, 426, 501] thereby raising the prospect that pharmacologic therapy augmentation of γ chain production may be of particular benefit in the management of thalassemia (see later).

Readily demonstrated in thalassemic patients is an apparent amplification of the capacity for Hb F synthesis during erythroid maturation. In the earliest erythroid precursor cells, γ-globin may be synthesized at a level less than that of β, and at only a few percent of that of α, yet the final proportion of Hb F in untransfused patients may be quite high.[1, 75] This occurs because the subset of cells expressing γ-globin have less overall globin chain imbalance, and therefore preferentially survive in both bone marrow and peripheral blood. Hence, measurement of steady-state Hb F levels provides an imperfect measure of the capacity for γ-globin synthesis in individual patients. A more accurate assessment of the Hb F program is achieved by measurement of Hb F accumulated in progenitor-derived erythroid colonies produced in vitro.[568]

Interaction of α- and β-Thalassemia Mutations. Because the clinical severity of α- and β-thalassemias correlates with the degree of imbalance in the production of α and non-α chains, co-inheritance of α- and β-thalassemia mutations would be anticipated to yield syndromes of intermediate severity.[569-575] This principle has been validated by clinical experience.[81, 576, 577] One striking example is the influence of the number of functional α-globin genes in individuals with β-thalassemia trait in Sardinia.[81] As shown in Table 21-9, the MCV and MCH improve in a stepwise fashion as α-globin production decreases and the α/β-globin ratio approaches 1 but then deteriorates as the ratio drops to less than 1. This analysis provides conclusive evidence that the degree of chain synthesis imbalance determines the red cell phenotype. As such, a higher frequency of α-globin gene deletions ($-\alpha/\alpha\alpha$ or $-\alpha/-\alpha$) has been found in those patients with thalassemia intermedia as compared with those with thalassemia. Further evidence for the effect of α-globin gene number on clinical phenotype is the occurrence of thalassemia intermedia in a subset of individuals doubly heterozygous for β-thalassemia and triplicated α genes ($\alpha\alpha\alpha/\alpha\alpha$)[402, 403, 565-567] or severe β-thalassemia trait in individuals also heterozygous for triplicated α genes.[556, 557, 578-584] Individuals heterozygous for β-thalassemia but homozygous for triplicated α genes invariably have thalassemia intermedia.

Clinical Features and Laboratory Values on Presentation. Patients with severe β-thalassemia are most often diagnosed between 6 months and 2 years of age when the normal physiologic anemia of the neonate fails to improve. Gamma-globin production is not impaired in utero; therefore, only when β-globin becomes the predominant β-like globin does anemia ensue. Occasionally, the disease is not recognized until 3 to 5 years of age owing to prolonged Hb F synthesis compensating for the lack of Hb A. On presentation, affected infants usually display pallor, poor growth, and abdominal enlargement from hepatosplenomegaly.

Children with severe β-thalassemia are readily distinguished from those with other congenital hemolytic anemias. At presentation, untransfused patients show 20% to 100% Hb F, 2% to 7% Hb A₂, and 0% to 80% Hb A (see Fig. 21-26), depending on the precise genotype.[1] Consistent with severe ineffective erythropoiesis and splenomegaly, the reticulocyte count is characteristically low (often less than 1%), whereas the nucleated red cell count is elevated. Erythrocytes are severely microcytic (MCV = 50 to 60 μm^3) with a hemoglobin content as low as 12 to 18 pg per cell. Hb F can be shown to be heterogeneously distributed among the red cells either by the Betke-Kleihauer acid elution technique or by anti-Hb F fluorescent staining (see Fig. 21-22).

Bone marrow examination reveals marked erythroid hyperplasia often with an erythroid:myeloid ratio of greater than or equal to 20:1. Before the onset of hypersplenism, the accelerated rate of hematopoiesis may also be reflected in elevated white cell and platelet counts in peripheral blood. The serum iron value is markedly elevated, but the total iron binding capacity is usually only slightly increased, resulting in a trans-

Table 21-9. EFFECT OF SUCCESSIVE α-GLOBIN GENE DELETION ON HEMATOLOGIC PARAMETERS IN A HOMOGENEOUS POPULATION OF β-THALASSEMIA TRAIT

Group/ Genotype	Hb (g/dL)	MCV (μm^3)	MCH (pg)	Hb A₂ (%)	Hb F (%)	Ratio
αα/αα (n = 20)	12.4 ± 1.2	66.2 ± 3.7	21.2 ± 1.2	4.8 ± 0.7	1.4 ± 1.3	2.2 ± 0.3
α−/αα (n = 12)	12.8 ± 1.3	67.3 ± 3.4	22.1 ± 1.1	5.2 ± 0.7	1 ± 0.3	1.3 ± 0.1
α−/α− (n = 4)	14.1 ± 1.1	76 + 3.4	24.8 ± 1.4	4.8 ± 0.6	1.3 ± 0.7	0.8 ± 0.1
α−/−− (n = 4)	11.7 ± 0.8	54.7 ± 2.5	18.4 ± 0.8	4.6 ± 0.2	—	0.5 ± 0.05

Adapted from Kanavakis E, Wainscoat JS, et al: The interaction of alpha thalassemia with beta thalassemia. Br J Haematol 1982; 52:465.

ferrin saturation of more than or equal to 80%. Serum ferritin levels are generally elevated for age.

If laboratory parameters fail to establish the diagnosis of thalassemia on presentation, measurement of globin biosynthetic ratios in peripheral blood reticulocytes or bone marrow cells will unequivocally permit an accurate diagnosis. Unfortunately, the procedure is not routine and requires a well-equipped laboratory and personnel familiar with the procedure. Most often, demonstration of a mild microcytic and hypochromic anemia, indicating the presence of thalassemia trait in both parents, allows the diagnosis to be made with confidence.

Complications

Radiologic Changes

To appreciate the spectrum of bony changes of severe β-thalassemia, one must examine patients who receive infrequent blood transfusions.[527, 528] Bony disease is related to erythroid expansion and not to iron overload or abnormalities in vitamin D metabolism.[585, 586] Maintenance of near-normal hemoglobin levels results in suppression of erythropoiesis and prevents, or partially reverses, bony abnormalities.[556, 557, 578–584, 587–589]

Radiologic abnormalities may be present during the first 6 months of life but are usually not marked until about 1 year of age.[590] In the small bones of the hands and feet the trabecular pattern is coarse, cystic abnormalities are present, and the bones are tubular. The long bones of the extremities exhibit thinning of the cortices and marked dilatation of the medullary cavities. Accordingly, they become extremely fragile and prone to pathologic fractures.[591] The skull is also classically involved with marked widening of the diploic space and arrangement of the trabeculae in vertical rows, tending to give a "hair on end" appearance to the skull radiograph (Fig. 21–32). Other radiologic abnormalities in the skull include failure of pneumatization of the maxillary sinuses and overgrowth of the maxilla. These changes lead to maxillary overbite, prominence of the upper incisors, and separation of the orbits—changes that contribute to the classic "thalassemic facies."

Other bony changes consequent to the medullary overgrowth include widening of the ribs with notching and development of masses of extramedullary hematopoietic tissue that may present as tumors in the chest and mediastinum. The vertebrae are square with coarse trabeculae. Osteoporosis is common, and associated bone pain may be relieved by calcitonin therapy.[592] Calcium bilirubinate gallstones due to excessive excretion of the products of heme catabolism are frequent in older patients.

Computed tomography has been used to demonstrate iron overload in thalassemic patients by detection of increased density of the liver.[593–595] It has also shown increased density of the spleen, pancreas, adrenal glands, and lymph nodes in the abdomen of these patients,[596] while also offering another assessment of extramedullary hematopoiesis[597, 598] and bony abnor-

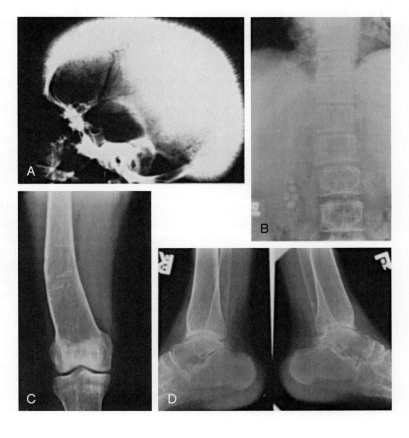

Figure 21–32. Radiologic abnormalities in a patient with homozygous β-thalassemia who receives blood transfusions infrequently (thalassemia intermedia). *A,* Skull radiograph illustrates typical "hair-on-end" appearance of the diploë and failure of pneumatization of the frontal sinus. *B,* Abdominal film illustrates the coarse trabeculation and osteoporosis within the vertebrae. Multiple calcified gallstones also are seen. *C,* Severe osteoporosis, pseudofractures, thinning of the cortex, and bowing of the femur are illustrated. *D,* Degenerative arthritis affecting particularly the tibiotalar joint is reflected by loss of the cartilage space and sclerosis in the adjacent bone.

malities.[599] Magnetic resonance imaging has also been used to evaluate these abnormalities.[600]

Clinical Consequences of Iron Deposition

Mechanisms of Toxicity. The pathology of thalassemia as originally described[530, 601] was concerned with conditions extant in the untreated state and is not relevant to that seen in today's chronically transfused and iron-overloaded patients. In countries where transfusion is widely available, patients demonstrate few of the stigmata that characterized the disease during the first few years of life in untransfused patients. Depending on the level of hemoglobin maintained, most patients fortunately no longer have difficulty with the marked erythroid hyperplasia that causes extensive medullary expansion and its consequent pathology.[531] However, patients are now confronted with consequences of chronic iron overload that accompany routine transfusion therapy.[602] In a study of British Cypriot patients at autopsy, Modell[603] found evidence of marked iron deposition in the liver, pancreas, thyroid, parathyroid, adrenal zona glomerulosa, renal medulla, heart, bone marrow, and spleen. Such parenchymal iron loading and the accumulation of "free" iron in the blood remain the major causes of morbidity and mortality in severe β-thalassemias.

Although the contribution of transfusional iron is easily appreciated, anemic thalassemic patients also have markedly enhanced gastrointestinal iron absorption.[604] This seems paradoxical, because one might expect suppression of iron absorption in the presence of iron overload. In normal individuals, a portion of dietary iron presented to the gut lumen is transported across the brush border of the gut epithelium and is available for transfer to the plasma iron transport protein, transferrin. The individual's iron status should then determine the amount of iron eventually presented to the serum pool.[605] The observation that anemic patients with thalassemia major have increased iron absorption remains an enigma. Elegant calculations by Modell and Berdoukas[606] suggested that the kinetic requirement of the expanded bone marrow for iron to make new red cells exceeds the rate at which the reticuloendothelial system is able to salvage iron from senescent red cells and replenish the erythron with iron. On this basis they argue that the bone marrow is relatively iron deficient on a kinetic basis, leading to enhanced gastrointestinal absorption. Increased absorption is variable (range, 2%–40%)[604] and appears to be directly related to erythroid activity,[607] measured either by morphologic observation of patient bone marrow[608] or enumeration of nucleated red cells in the peripheral blood.[604] Experimental studies in animals suggest that hypoxia, even in the absence of increased erythropoiesis, may increase iron absorption.[609]

Most modern transfusion regimens significantly decrease iron absorption but increase iron loading as transfused red cells become senescent and their iron is deposited in the reticuloendothelial system. Reticuloendothelial cells relinquish iron directly to transferrin.

Although the erythron usually claims most of this circulating iron, a certain amount is also delivered to other cells according to their individual needs. Cellular uptake may normally depend on the number of transferrin receptors on the cell membrane.[610] As iron accumulates in the body, individual tissues accelerate their production of apoferritin molecules to store the iron in a nontoxic form as ferritin or hemosiderin.[611, 612]

Apoferritin production can be monitored by measurement of serum ferritin concentration by radioimmunoassay. In multiply transfused patients[613] and in untransfused thalassemia patients with increased gastrointestinal iron absorption,[614] serum ferritin levels correlate well with total body iron stores during the first several years of iron loading, but less well at later stages.[615] Serum ferritin is an acute phase reactant, as well as a product of hepatocellular damage. Infection, congestive heart failure, and hepatitis may elevate serum ferritin levels. Thus, in patients with marked iron overload, the serum ferritin correlates poorly with liver iron concentration.

The human body is extremely conservative in its handling of iron (see Chapter 11). Under normal conditions, iron is always in the presence of a chelating protein with a high affinity constant. Serum transferrin binds iron with an association constant of 10 to 20 mol/L.[616–618] When transferrin arrives at its surface receptor, the complex is transferred to the "labile iron pool"[619] by receptor-mediated endocytosis.[618, 620–622] This pool supplies iron to cytosolic proteins. The remaining iron is directed to apoferritin for storage as ferritin. When ferritin molecules accumulate, the protein moiety is apparently cleaved, leaving smaller, but more heavily iron-concentrated hemosiderin granules.[623] Theoretically, these storage forms of iron are inert and do not exert any pathologic damage. However, accumulated hemosiderin granules appear to cause release of hydrolytic enzymes from lysosomes that are toxic to the cell.[624, 625]

As iron stores increase both from transfusions and gastrointestinal absorption, transferrin becomes saturated to more than 90% with iron. In parallel, a pool of non–transferrin-bound or "free" serum iron is found in iron-overloaded individuals.[626–628] Its source is uncertain but presumably reflects an expansion of the intracellular labile iron pool, and it is thought to be particularly cardiotoxic.

Cell damage likely occurs as a result of iron-related catalysis leading to oxidation of membrane components.[629, 630] Unbound iron produces lipid peroxidation in vitro.[631–633] Peroxidation of mitochondrial membranes and hepatocyte microsomes has been demonstrated in vivo in rats overloaded with iron by parenteral or oral administration[634] and in the spleens of thalassemic patients.[635] Lysosomal leakage of hemosiderin and hydrolytic enzymes may also occur.[636, 637] Cultured rat myocardial cells have been used to study the effects of iron deposition.[638] Peroxidation of membrane lipids induces functional abnormalities in cultured myocardial cells that are exacerbated by ascorbic acid (see later) and corrected in part by the antioxidant vitamin E and markedly suppressed by desferrioxamine.[639]

Further evidence in support of the free radical hypothesis stems from measurement of substances that defend against free-radical attack. Vitamin E, a potent antioxidant, is decreased in serum and red cells of iron-overloaded thalassemic patients.[548, 640] Both vitamin E levels[641] and serum total antioxidant activity bear strong inverse correlations to the degree of iron overload.[642] Perhaps most intriguing is a correlation between superoxide production in resting neutrophils and serum ferritin in multiply transfused patients. The observed superoxide generation approaches five times normal in some patients.[643]

Indirect data also suggest that the route of accumulation (i.e., gastrointestinal absorption versus parenteral red cell transfusion) may be an important determinant of iron toxicity.[644, 645] Attention must be paid to the contribution of gastrointestinal iron absorption.[604, 608] Experiments in rats suggest that oral iron loading leads to more global hepatocyte damage than parenteral loading.[634] Patients with hereditary hemochromatosis and untransfused thalassemia intermedia sustain parenchymal damage entirely from gastrointestinal absorption.[608, 646, 647] On the other hand, extensive transfusions in patients with hypoplastic anemia is associated with a lower incidence of cirrhosis.[644] Nonetheless, the view that reticuloendothelial iron derived from transfused red cells is innocuous is overly simplistic. There is little reason to believe that current transfusion protocols, designed to maintain a normal hemoglobin level and reduce gastrointestinal iron absorption, will be free of the complications of iron overload.

Assessment of Body Iron Burden. Most longitudinal studies of iron overload have used serum iron, iron binding capacity, and ferritin as noninvasive measures of stored iron. As mentioned previously, these parameters are easily perturbed by effects of other diseases (e.g., hepatitis) or are not highly quantitative (iron/iron binding capacity). The poor correlation between serum ferritin and total body iron in heavily transfused thalassemic patients[648] may be improved by measuring the glycosylated form.[649] Grading of stainable iron in liver biopsy specimens also offers a better assessment of parenchymal iron stores.

Nonetheless, the study of iron loading in patients would be significantly advanced by noninvasive methods for establishing parenchymal iron burden. Computed tomography, as mentioned previously, may be useful for longitudinal assessment of hepatic iron.[593, 595, 650] The paramagnetic properties of iron have also been used to make accurate measurements that correlate well with liver iron measured in biopsy specimens by atomic absorption spectroscopy,[651] but this is presently only a research tool.

Cardiac Abnormalities

Patients with thalassemia major have traditionally succumbed to the cardiac complications of iron overload.[536] Recurrent pericarditis distinguished by characteristic pain, fever, and a friction rub may be the initial manifestation of myocardial iron deposition and occasionally requires pericardectomy to relieve constriction.

Ventricular tachycardia and fibrillation or severe refractory congestive heart failure often prove fatal.[652]

Pathology. Cardiac iron deposition has been studied in autopsies of patients with transfusional hemosiderosis and idiopathic hemochromatosis.[653] Patients with a history of more than 100 units of transfused red cells without chronic blood loss generally exhibit significant cardiac iron deposition. Cardiac hemosiderosis is not observed unless significant iron accumulation has occurred in other organs. Patients with grossly visible cardiac iron at autopsy experience cardiac dysfunction during life. Gross anatomic changes include dilatation of the atrial and ventricular cavities and thickening of the muscle layer, resulting in a twofold to threefold increase in heart weight. Microscopic evaluation suggests that iron is first deposited in the ventricular myocardium and later in the conduction tissue.[653] It is therefore not surprising that intracavitary endomyocardial biopsy is not useful in these patients as a means to evaluate cardiac iron.[654, 655] Supraventricular arrhythmias correlate well with the extent of iron deposition in the atrial myocardium. Cardiac abnormalities seem to be a function of both the quantity of iron deposited per fiber and the absolute number of fibers affected. Link and Pinson[656] have shown that myocardial cells in culture take up iron if there is no physiologic or pharmacologic chelator present. As iron loading takes place, peroxidation products accumulate and contractility and rhythm are disturbed.[639] This *in vitro* model parallels concepts developed from clinical findings.

Noninvasive Studies of Cardiac Function. Echocardiography, radionuclide cineangiography, and 24-hour recording of cardiac rhythm have been used to assess the effects of iron deposition in the heart and evaluate results of chelation therapy.[657] In general, echocardiography may reveal changes in cardiac anatomy but little change in cardiac function until clinically evident cardiomyopathy develops.[658–660] Radionuclide cineangiography offers the ability to observe dynamic cardiac function during exercise and may reveal changes in function before clinical disease.[660–663] Twenty-four-hour recordings of cardiac rhythm in patients with iron overload have demonstrated marked disturbances in most patients older than 12 years of age regardless of clinical symptoms.[657, 664] In one large series, Beirman and coworkers demonstrated abnormalities in more than 75% of patients, ranging from occasional premature beats to runs of ventricular tachycardia.[664]

Table 21–10 summarizes the clinical course of patients before the onset of aggressive chelation programs. The efficacy of future transfusion and chelation programs must be assessed in this context. Considerable data have demonstrated the benefits of chelation therapy, both for prophylaxis and treatment of cardiac disease in iron overloaded patients (see later).

Hepatic Abnormalities

Liver enlargement, long viewed as a hallmark of thalassemia, is prominent with contemporary transfusion regimens only in patients older than 10 years of age. Hepatomegaly is due to progressive engorgement of

Table 21–10. CARDIAC DISEASE IN PATIENTS WITH
IRON OVERLOAD

Stage I (<100 units transfusion)

Asymptomatic
Echocardiogram: slight left-ventricular wall thickening
Radionuclide cineangiogram: normal
24-hour ECG: normal

Stage II (100—400 units transfusion)

Asymptomatic or mild-fatigue
Echocardiogram: left-ventricular wall thickening; left
    ventricular dilatation but normal ejection fraction
Radionuclide cineangiogram: normal at rest but no increase
    or fall in ejection fracture with exercise
24-hour ECG: atrial and ventricular premature beats

Stage III

Palpitations and/or congestive heart failure
Echocardiogram: decreased ejection fraction
Radionuclide cineangiogram: normal or decreased ejection
    fraction at rest but a fall in ejection fraction during
    exercise
24-hour ECG: atrial and ventricular premature beats, often
    in pairs or runs

Adapted from Nienhuis AW, Griffith P, et al: Evaluation of cardiac
    function in patients with thalassemia major. Ann NY Acad Sci 1980;
    344:384.

hepatic parenchymal and phagocytic cells with hemo-siderin deposits, rather than extramedullary hemato-poiesis.[665] In addition, iron deposition induces intralo-bular fibrosis.[666, 667] Intercurrent episodes of hepatitis may lead to marked liver dysfunction and contribute to development of fibrosis and cirrhosis.[668–670] Liver enzymes levels are rarely elevated in the absence of hepatitis. Total bilirubin in adequately transfused patients is seldom more than 2 mg/dL. Fifty percent or less of the total bilirubin is typically indirect. Data clearly demonstrate that chelation therapy reduces liver iron concentration[665, 671–673] and forestalls iron-induced liver damage. Progressive liver disease in patients managed with an adequate program is often due to viral hepatitis.[674]

Endocrine Abnormalities

Endocrine disorders commonly associated with thalassemia in the United States today are generally thought to be secondary to the effects of chronic iron loading.[602, 606, 675, 676] Most of the pathologic processes develop slowly and usually are not apparent until the second decade of life. In untransfused patients, these abnormalities develop more slowly.

Growth and Development. Growth retardation, historically considered a typical finding in thalassemia major,[675] is generally associated with moderate retardation in bone age. Patients undergoing chronic transfusion therapy may be spared growth retardation, which is seen in less than 50% of cases and then not until the second decade of life.[606] Growth retardation is less evident in well-chelated patients,[677] although excessive desferrioxamine can also impair growth.[678] Alternative causes should be sought in young, adequately trans-fused thalassemic children who exhibit significant growth retardation.

Growth retardation may also be associated with evidence of endocrine dysfunction. Impaired growth hormone production has been reported in some patients[679] but not confirmed in others.[680] A subset of patients with normal growth hormone production have low serum levels of somatomedin,[681] a factor produced by the liver in response to growth hormone that promotes cartilage growth. Failure of adrenal androgen production may also contribute to growth failure.[682] Thyroid deficiency is an additional potential contributing factor (see later). A thorough search for endocrine dysfunction is warranted in growth-retarded patients, because a favorable response to specific replacement therapy may be anticipated.

Puberty. Puberty will occur normally in about a third of patients with β-thalassemia, typically those with the least growth retardation. Variable sexual maturation is observed in other patients. In transfused patients, failure of sexual maturation may be the first indication of iron toxicity. Breast development in females tends to begin normally, but menarche is frequently delayed until the late teenage years. Eventually, many female patients who progress through puberty normally will develop secondary amenorrhea due to progressive iron accumulation.

Failure of sexual development is usually not related to primary end-organ unresponsiveness.[683, 684] Although males tend to have low baseline testosterone levels, response to human chorionic gonadotropin is usually normal.[684] Moreover, spermatogenesis correlates directly with the stage of sexual maturation of the patient.[685] Gonadotropins, on the other hand, have been implicated in a number of studies as the primary lesion in the hypothalamic pituitary gonadial axis.[684, 686–689] Although defective ovarian function has been described in some patients,[690] patients who fail to attain puberty or who have experienced regression of secondary sexual characteristics demonstrate blunted responses to luteinizing hormone–releasing factor and to follicle-stimulating hormone. Prolactin levels respond normally to thyroid-releasing factor stimulation. Failure of sexual maturation, therefore, appears most often related to hypothalamic-pituitary dysfunction.

Although one report suggested preservation of normal gonadotropin production in young, heavily chelated patients,[685] modification of transfusion schedules and chelation has yet to preserve normal function in many patients. This constitutes a problem of increasing severity as the long-term clinical prognosis for patients improves. In approaching such patients, Modell and Berdoukas have likened the attainment of puberty as a trophy in a race between a patient's physical growth and iron overload.[606] Patients with a constitution that favors tall stature and a rapid growth rate and who have been on high transfusion programs and adequate chelation regimens are likely to attain puberty. Those who do not require transfusion in the first year of life may also have an advantage. Constitutionally short children or those with inadequate transfusion and chelation frequently fail to "win the race."

For patients with delayed puberty, initial effort should be devoted to assessment of nutritional status, general health (i.e., presence of hepatitis), and the adequacy of transfusion and chelation. In addition, attention should be paid to the availability of calcium for growth (see later). For those on maximal therapy with delayed puberty and also biochemical evidence of hypothalamic-pituitary dysfunction, pulsatile gonadotropin-releasing hormone infusions have been used to artificially induce puberty and growth,[691] although this approach may not succeed.[688] More conventional management includes testosterone or estrogen supplementation after the age of 14 or 15 for those who failed to achieve puberty or have developed secondary hypogonadism, either clinically or based on loss of response to luteinizing hormone–releasing factor.

Thyroid. Even though iron deposition in thyroid parenchymal tissue is often extensive, dysfunction is usually limited to primary subclinical hypothyroidism. In one large series in which simultaneous serum thyroxine and thyroid-stimulating hormone levels were obtained in 31 thalassemic patients, mean thyroxine levels were significantly lower (6.2 vs. 9.5 μg/dL) and thyroid-stimulating hormone levels significantly higher (3.2 vs. 1.0 μU/mL) than in age-matched controls.[686] On longitudinal study, serum thyroxine levels declined, whereas thyroid-stimulating hormone secretion increased. Although the means were significantly different, individual thalassemic patients could not be reliably distinguished from controls. Androgen replacement in males may correct abnormalities in thyroid function.[692]

Adrenal. Adrenal pathologic processes in patients with thalassemia are historically characterized by iron deposition limited primarily to the zona glomerulosa,[601] the site of mineralocorticoid production. Iron deposition in the zona fasciculata may also occur.[606] In one series, normal aldosterone production in response to salt deprivation was achieved only at the expense of a marked increase in serum renin concentration.[681] Basal morning adrenocorticotropic hormone levels measured in prepubertal thalassemic patients were 3 to 10 times normal.[693] Basal glucocorticoid production and response to adrenocorticotropic hormone and insulin provocation are generally normal in younger patients, although older patients often demonstrate a blunted provocative response.

Pancreas. Diabetes mellitus is a frequent and often underrecognized complication of thalassemia, which is due both to pancreatic hypoproduction[694] and (at least in some cases) to insulin resistance.[695] Even in patients between 5 and 10 years of age whose iron burden is 5 to 20 g, fasting blood glucose levels are significantly elevated.[693] When glucose tolerance tests are performed, as many as 50% of thalassemic patients have "chemical diabetes," defined by glucose tolerance testing; the majority of these patients have normal, or elevated, circulating insulin levels.[695] Insulin resistance may predate the onset of glucose intolerance, as revealed by the euglycemic clamp method.[696] In contrast, untransfused thalassemic patients display accelerated insulin clearance and normal tissue sensitivity.[697] As diabetes becomes symptomatic, insulin output decreases, as is the case in most patients with juvenile diabetes. Glucose intolerance generally correlates with the number of transfusions received, age of the patient, and genetic predisposition.[698]

Parathyroid. Symptomatic parathyroid disease, presenting as classic tetany, hypocalcemia, and hyperphosphatemia, is an uncommon complication of iron overload.[686, 694, 698–700] Subclinical deficiency of parathyroid function is difficult to diagnose. The provocative use of calcium chelates to identify subclinical deficiency of parathormone has been described.[701] Patients with thalassemia major have been reported to show diminished response to a challenge.[701] Although symptomatic parathyroid disease may be rare, more common defects may affect the mobilization of calcium for growth and the preservation of normal serum ionized calcium—important in patients with cardiomyopathy or arrhythmia. To complicate matters, deficiency of activated vitamin D may occur, perhaps partially as a consequence of parathormone deficiency. Case reports have been described of symptomatology due to deficiency of 25-hydroxytachysterol,[702, 703] which is relieved either by iron chelation or vitamin D supplementation. Therefore, careful attention should be paid to calcium, phosphate, and vitamin D in patients with growth disturbances and cardiac disease.

Arterial Hypoxemia

In 1981, Fucharoen and co-workers[704] reported significant arterial hypoxemia in patients with Hb E-β^0-thalassemia, especially in those who had been splenectomized. These authors found circulating platelet aggregates in such patients and successfully used aspirin and dipyridamole to improve oxygenation. Other groups have reported hypoxemia in thalassemia major[705–711] but have related it to changes in ventilatory mechanics, obstructive airway disease, or iron deposition in the lungs. Pulmonary hypertension, possibly secondary to thrombocytosis, may contribute to right ventricular dysfunction in these patients.[712–717]

Therapy for β-Thalassemia[718–721]

Transfusion

Choice of Transfusion Regimen. The mainstay of management of severe β-thalassemia remains blood transfusion.[718, 722] Several aims are addressed in a transfusion program. By increasing the hemoglobin content, transfusion enhances the oxygen-carrying capacity of the blood and thereby decreases tissue hypoxia. The concomitant fall in erythropoietin levels blunts the massive erythroid expansion associated with the anemia. Furthermore, improved tissue oxygenation and the reversal of the hypercatabolic state promote more normal growth and development. Suppression of erythropoiesis is associated with decreased intestinal iron absorption. These benefits must be weighed against the prospects of excessive iron loading, particularly with more intensive transfusion protocols.

A major debate in the management of thalassemia centers on the optimal maintenance level of hemoglobin targeted by transfusion programs. Wolman and Ortalani first recommended a pretransfusion hemoglobin level of 8.5 g/dL.[531, 675] This approach improved survival, but chronic illness, bone disease, and anemic cardiomyopathy persisted. To enhance the quality of life, Piomelli and associates suggested maintaining the hemoglobin level at more than 10 g/dL with a mean of 12 g/dL.[535] Such "hypertransfusion," if initiated in the first year of life, promotes normal initial growth and development, limits development of hepatosplenomegaly, prevents disfiguring bone abnormalities, reduces intestinal iron absorption, and decreases cardiac work.[723–726]

In 1980, Propper and associates[727] proposed that maintenance of a pretransfusion hemoglobin level greater than 12 g/dL with a mean of 14 g/dL would more effectively eliminate chronic tissue hypoxia. By continued suppression of endogenous erythropoiesis, this "supertransfusion" program was predicted to further decrease intestinal iron absorption, eliminate bone disease, and decrease hypercatabolism, thereby improving growth and development. Initial studies reported that the quantity of blood required to maintain a higher hemoglobin level was no greater than that required for maintenance of a lower level due to a decrease in intravascular volume.[727–729] Data from other centers, however, suggested that increasing the pretransfusion hemoglobin level may simply increase the quantity of transfused blood and thus increase iron loading.[606, 730] As a result of the conflicting clinical experience, "supertransfusion" has not been widely used in patient management. If it is to be implemented, iron balance parameters should be carefully monitored.[721]

Red cells senesce as a function of cell age. Because the iron content of transfused erythrocytes is independent of cell age, attempts have been made to improve the "quality" of transfused blood by infusing the youngest third of red cells present in whole blood ("neocytes").[727, 731] Administration of these cells would be predicted to decrease the transfusion requirement. Neocytes can be readily prepared with automated cell separators,[732–736] but 3 or more units are required to prepare the equivalent of 1 unit of blood. Although prolonged survival of neocytes has been documented in vivo, the observed sparing of transfusions with such therapy has been disappointing.[737–740] Similarly, methods to remove "gerocytes" (old red cells) from the recipient's circulation at the time of transfusion, though technically feasible, have not been widely applied.[739, 741] These approaches should be considered experimental.

Although specific practices will differ among clinical centers, transfusion is indicated both to correct anemia and to suppress erythropoiesis.[718] After diagnosis, a period of observation should be initiated to determine if transfusion is required to maintain the hemoglobin level greater than or equal to 7 g/dL. Patients with thalassemia intermedia will be stable without transfusion. If the hemoglobin level falls below 7 g/dL, a transfusion program should be initiated to maintain the hemoglobin level at 9.5 to 11.5 g/dL. During the

first decade of life, normal growth provides reassurance that the transfusion regimen is adequate. Because the rate of iron absorption parallels the number of nucleated red cells in the peripheral blood,[604] adequate transfusion should suppress the nucleated cell count to less than 5/100 white blood cells[718]; however, in older patients who received inadequate transfusion early in life, it may not be possible to achieve this level. During the teenage years, growth failure may reflect endocrine dysfunction rather than inadequate transfusion; laboratory investigation and appropriate replacement therapy are then indicated. After epiphyses are fused and growth is complete, a hemoglobin level of 8.0 to 9.0 g/dL may be well tolerated. If the transfusion requirement exceeds 200 mL of packed red cells/kg per year, splenectomy should be considered (see further discussion later).[718] The authors' current transfusion procedure is outlined in Table 21–11.

Complications of Blood Transfusion. The primary long-term complication of blood transfusion is iron loading and resulting parenchymal organ toxicity, as discussed previously. Febrile reactions to leukocyte antigenic determinants and allergic reactions to plasma components are commonly encountered in chronically transfused patients. Washing of red cells in saline or the use of microaggregate filtration to remove leukocytes can be beneficial.[742] Alternatively, frozen-deglycerolized cells may be used in severely sensitized patients but may be associated with an increase in

Table 21–11. CHRONIC TRANSFUSION GUIDELINES FOR PATIENTS WITH THALASSEMIA

1. Determine the blood type of the patient completely to identify minor red cell antigens before first transfusion.
2. Keep the pretransfusion hemoglobin level between 9.5 and 11.5 mg/dL as needed for suppressing ineffective erythropoiesis and maintaining a reasonable sense of well-being.
3. Give 10 to 20 mL/kg of leukopoor, washed, and filtered red blood cells with a maximum infusion rate of 10 mL/kg over 2 hours, transfusing more slowly in patients with heart disease.
4. Avoid raising the post-transfusion hemoglobin above 16 g/dL.
5. Choose a transfusion interval to maintain pretransfusion levels as outlined above (3–5 weeks depending on individual patient needs). (*Comment:* Some patients tolerate slightly lower pretransfusion hemoglobin levels and need 5 weeks between transfusions, whereas others feel best coming every 4 weeks. Some prefer getting fewer units and coming every 3 weeks. Some of the younger patients whose weights would require between 1 and 2 units receive a transfusion every 3 or 4 weeks and alternate between 1 and 2 units per transfusion.
6. Pretransfusion laboratory tests include a complete blood cell count, differential, crossmatch, and red cell antibody screen.
7. Height and weight is recorded at least every 3 months.
8. Liver function (AST, ALT, bilirubin, LDH) is evaluated every 3 months and serum ferritin every 3 to 6 months. A deferoxamine (Desferal) challenge test is performed at irregular intervals to measure appropriate Desferal dosage and chelatable iron stores.

AST = aspartate transaminase; ALT = alanine transaminase; LDH = lactate dehydrogenase.

transfusion requirements.[743] These strategies should be employed only in patients with documented transfusion reactions.

Alloimmunization to minor blood group antigens occurs in 20% to 30% of patients[744-746] and may present as delayed hemolysis. In rare circumstances, this may pose a potentially life-threatening complication in patients with transfusion-dependent β-thalassemia. Alloimmunization is often a less significant problem in patients in whom transfusion is initiated before the age of 3.[744-746] The benefits of extended red cell phenotyping to minimize alloimmunization have been debated in the literature,[747, 748] but crossmatching for Rhesus and Kell systems from the time of initial transfusion may decrease the incidence of alloimmunization.[745] Detailed red cell phenotyping should be performed in all newly diagnosed patients before transfusion.

The transmission of viral infections by transfusion is a serious problem in chronically transfused patients. In one study, about 25% of transfusion-dependent patients with thalassemia demonstrated exposure to hepatitis B, 80% of whom had clinical evidence of hepatitis.[749] Exposure to hepatitis C, with an incidence of approximately 6% per transfusion, is nearly inevitable in regularly transfused thalassemia patients, and this agent may account for active hepatitis in some patients. The recent identification of the hepatitis C agent and the development of a serologic test to screen donors may minimize this risk.[750, 751] A minority of patients with thalassemia have become infected with human immunodeficiency virus, and the rate of progression to symptomatic acquired immunodeficiency syndrome has been proportionately lower than in most infected populations.[752] Although death and complications from these illnesses are uncommon in this patient population, it is prudent to exercise precautions. The most important consideration is the use of blood products screened for the presence of potential infectious agents. Patients should be immunized against hepatitis B on diagnosis or if they have not acquired immunity. When practical, exposure to multiple donors or units should be minimized. In this regard, it is important to recognize that the use of washed or frozen red cells may lead to an increase in the number of transfused units.

Splenectomy. The role of the spleen must be considered in patients who are treated with transfusion or iron chelation programs. The spleen serves both as a scavenger by increasing red cell destruction and iron redistribution and as a storage depot by sequestrating the released iron in a potentially nontoxic pool. Unfortunately, splenic iron may equilibrate with other iron pools throughout the body. In one uncontrolled study, three splenectomized patients exhibited cirrhosis and massive iron deposition, whereas slightly younger patients with an intact spleen had only iron deposition.[753] Risdon and associates, however, observed no difference between splenectomized and nonsplenectomized patients with regard to liver pathology.[665] If the spleen acts primarily as a storage depot for excess iron, premature removal could theoretically be detrimental. On the other hand, if the splenic pool is a particular target for desferrioxamine, the beneficial effects of aggressive chelation therapy might be diminished by preferential removal of iron from this relatively innocuous pool. Perhaps most important is the feasibility of achieving negative iron balance with conventional chelation regimens (see later). Eventually, an increased transfusion requirement due to hypersplenism perturbs the balance and contributes to iron loading.[754]

Splenectomy is often indicated in the management of patients with severe β-thalassemia. Massive splenomegaly with hypersplenism causing leukopenia, thrombocytopenia, and an increasing transfusion requirement is frequent in young patients on sporadic or moderate transfusion regimens. Early splenectomy is often required. The development of splenomegaly is delayed in patients maintained on a high transfusion regimen. The decision to remove the spleen must take several factors into consideration. Modell[606, 755, 756] carefully documented the annual blood requirement for splenectomized patients with thalassemia major and suggested that the spleen be removed if the observed requirement exceeds that predicted by 50%. Data from other investigators suggest that the benefits of splenectomy on iron balance are realized if the transfusion requirement exceeds 200 to 250 mL packed red cells/kg per year with a minimum hemoglobin level of 10 g/dL.[754, 757] Because a huge spleen, irrespective of functional hypersplenism, may account for a large fraction of the total blood volume, its removal often leads to a marked, although transient, reduction in blood requirement.[758, 759] Most patients achieve a moderate, but significant, reduction in requirement to the predicted 200 mL of packed red cells/kg per year[755, 756] that remains stable over many years.[760]

The surgical risk accompanying splenectomy is minimal in experienced hands. The potential of overwhelming *Streptococcus pneumoniae, Haemophilus influenzae,* or *Neisseria meningitidis* infection[761-763] should always loom in the mind of the attending physician. Because removal of the spleen may blunt the primary immune response to encapsulated organisms, delay of splenectomy until older than age 5 years is preferable. Patients should be immunized with polyvalent pneumococcal, meningococcal, and *H. influenzae* vaccines.[764-767] Supplemental prophylactic oral penicillin may also be used to prevent colonization by strains not covered by vaccines,[718] particularly in young children. Illnesses accompanied by high fever of uncertain etiology should be aggressively treated with parenteral antibiotics until bacterial culture results are available. Patients in endemic regions should be treated prophylactically for malaria.[756]

Red cell survival usually increases immediately after splenectomy.[758] The peripheral blood smear may reveal increased numbers of hypochromic, microcytic, and nucleated red cells. Platelet counts greater than $10^6/mm^3$ are often seen, although correction of anemia by transfusion usually results in suppression of platelet production.[459] White cell counts of 15,000 to $20,000/mm^3$ are common; the differential is usually normal.

As discussed in more detail later, arterial hypoxemia and evidence of pulmonary vascular disease have been reported in patients with thalassemia, and it has been suggested that splenectomy may exacerbate these problems.[704, 712] Accordingly, splenectomized patients should be examined carefully for these findings. Because thrombocytosis may be an inciting factor,[713, 768] prophylaxis with low dose aspirin may be considered, although effective transfusion to correct anemia is probably the best form of preventive therapy.

Chelation Therapy

Progressive iron overload is the life-limiting complication of transfusion therapy. In the absence of adequate chelation, cardiac dysfunction ends the life of the transfused thalassemic patient during the teenage years. Regular chelation with the drug desferrioxamine has proved remarkably effective in reducing the iron burden of transfused patients. Cardiac disease is delayed or prevented, susceptibility to infection is reduced,[769] and life expectancy is significantly extended; nonetheless, endocrine dysfunction may develop and persist. Unfortunately, effective use of the drug requires strict compliance to subcutaneous administration by means of a mechanical pump. Lack of oral absorption of the drug and its short serum half-life dictates this cumbersome route of administration. An equally effective oral alternative remains to be discovered, as discussed below.

Desferrioxamine. Desferrioxamine is a complex hydroxylamine with a remarkable affinity for iron. Desferrioxamine binds metal iron stochiometrically with a weight ratio of desferrioxamine to iron of approximately 11:1. Desferrioxamine enters cells, chelates iron, and appears in serum and bile as the iron chelate product feroxamine.[629]

Humans have no intrinsic mechanism for excreting excess iron. Iron available for chelation is thought to be derived from the "labile iron pool"[619]; the size of this pool is directly related to the total body iron burden.[770, 771] Non–transferrin-bound plasma iron should also be available for chelation.[627, 628] A fraction of reticuloendothelial iron salvaged from red cells may also be chelated,[772] perhaps only when stored as ferritin.[773] Urinary iron excretion appears to be proportional to marrow erythroid activity and is diminished by transfusion.[774] Net iron loss, however, is not compromised because the diminution of urinary iron excretion is balanced by an increased fecal excretion of iron.[773, 774] In patients with primary hemochromatosis in whom iron deposition is predominantly in parenchymal cells and erythropoiesis is normal, desferrioxamine administration results primarily in enhanced fecal iron excretion.[629] Thus the site of iron removal is influenced by the transfusion schedule, but there are no data available regarding the influence of the hemoglobin level on the prevention or removal of cardiac iron deposits.

Chelation Regimens. Desferrioxamine is active when administered by the intramuscular, subcutaneous, or intravenous routes. After its introduction in 1962, the drug was given by intramuscular route until the late 1970s. This regimen was only partially successful in that iron removal was insufficient to achieve a negative net iron balance in most patients.[775] Supplemental oral ascorbic acid enhanced urinary excretion (see later),[776] but only 14 to 16 mg of iron could be removed per day even from severely hemosiderotic patients. Adults on full transfusion support require removal of more than 35 mg/d to achieve negative net iron balance.[775] Furthermore, little iron excretion could be obtained by this regimen in patients whose iron stores were less than 10 times normal.[777]

The efficacy of intramuscular injections is limited by the rapid clearance of desferrioxamine from plasma by means of metabolism and biliary and urinary excretion.[629] Continuous intravenous infusion significantly enhances iron excretion,[775, 777] presumably due to exchange between desferrioxamine and tissue iron pools. Significant plasma and tissue drug concentrations can be attained by continuous subcutaneous administration.[778] Iron excretion is markedly enhanced compared with the intramuscular route,[775, 778–780] and net negative iron balance can be achieved in most patients older than the age of 3 or 4 with an iron burden of 4 to 5 g.[723, 730, 778]

A typical regimen involves administration of 30 to 40 mg/kg of drug overnight (8–12 hours), thereby avoiding the need to carry the pump during the daytime hours. Patients are advised to use the drug at least 5 or 6 days per week. Obviously, such a program is a compromise in that optimal management demands drug infusion every hour of every day, a schedule met with poor compliance, particularly among teenagers. Data now show that regular use of desferrioxamine forestalls significant iron overload if started by the age of 3 or 4. It also promotes elimination of excess iron in patients if started after a significant transfusional iron burden has already developed.[673, 781–785] There is general agreement that treatment should be initiated by age 5 years in transfusion-dependent patients; some advocate treatment by age 3 years.[721, 730, 786–788] It has been argued that irreversible tissue damage, particularly to endocrine glands, occurs at a very low iron burden during the first years of life. However, the toxicity of desferrioxamine is most significant in patients with a low iron burden (see later). Indeed, growth retardation and other toxicity has been documented in children younger than age 3 given high doses of the drug.[789] A test infusion of desferrioxamine may be used to determine if mobilizable iron is present.[718, 721]

Periodic intravenous administration of desferrioxamine may also be used to accelerate the rate of iron removal in symptomatic patients with substantial iron burdens. Intravenous administration allows for use of higher doses (6 to 10 g/d); local reactions at the site of administration limit the tolerable subcutaneous dose to 2.0 to 2.5 g/d. By extending the time of infusion and increasing the drug dose, iron removal can be greatly enhanced over that achievable with conventional subcutaneous therapy. This approach is indicated in attempts to reverse established cardiac dysfunction in multiply transfused patients (see later).

Efficacy of Chelation. Clinical experience has shown subcutaneous desferrioxamine administration to be effective in preventing cardiac disease and prolonging the life of transfused thalassemic patients.[673, 784, 790–792] Life expectancy previously was about 16 years, with rare patients surviving into their mid 20s.[536, 652, 793] Subsequent to the introduction of subcutaneous desferrioxamine therapy, the projected life expectancy extends into the middle fourth decade.[794] Several studies have also documented sparing of cardiac disease in well-chelated patients.[673, 784, 795, 796] Figure 21–33 shows a striking comparison between two groups of patients; one group was well chelated, whereas the other group was poorly compliant. Onset of cardiac disease in chelated patients who achieved negative iron balance has been observed,[795] but the dose of the drug used was relatively low.

High-dose chelation by the intravenous route is capable of reversing established cardiac disease in some patients who continue to require transfusion.[662, 797, 798] This regimen must be instituted while the patient is still compensated either with or without cardiac medications. Individuals with refractory congestive heart failure or hypotension due to cardiac disease are poor candidates for intravenous desferrioxamine.

Unfortunately, the cohort of patients in whom subcutaneous desferrioxamine was initiated in their late first decade of life after accumulation of significant iron continue to exhibit endocrine dysfunction and growth retardation.[785] Glucose intolerance and diabetes are observed even in well-chelated patients,[799] although the incidence is reduced.[673] There is scant evidence that desferrioxamine can reverse established endocrine dysfunction. It remains to be determined whether patients started on subcutaneous desferrioxamine at a very young age will fair better with respect to growth, sexual development, and endocrine function. Because this cohort of patients is just now entering their teenage years, information on this point may become available in the near future.

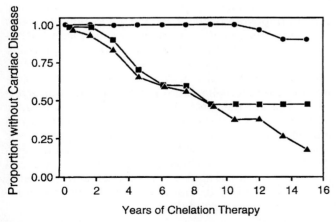

Figure 21–33. Cardiac disease-free survival of patients with respect to serum ferritin level. The circles depict cardiac disease-free survival assay patients with less than 33% of ferritin measurements > 2500 ng/mL; squares: those patients with 33% to 67% > 2500 ng/mL; triangles: patients with > 67% measurements > 2500 ng/mL. (From Olivieri NF, Nathan DG, et al: Survival in medically treated patients with homozygous beta-thalassemia. N Engl J Med 1994; 331:574. Copyright 1994, Massachusetts Medical Society.)

Toxicity of Desferrioxamine. At high doses of desferrioxamine, significant side effects are seen.[629, 718] Local erythema may occur at the site of infusion and contribute to an inflammatory response characterized by multiple subcutaneous nodules. These local reactions can be partially suppressed by inclusion of 5 to 10 mg of hydrocortisone in the desferrioxamine solution.

Of particular concern is neurosensory toxicity observed at high dose. Several large series report a 30% to 40% incidence of high frequency hearing loss, which may become symptomatic.[800–804] Reversal with discontinuation of the drug has been reported, although other patients have experienced persistent hearing loss. Ocular toxicity has also been reported.[800, 805] Progressive visual failure with night blindness and colorblindness and field loss are also described[806] but may be independent of chelation.[807] Reversal after discontinuation of desferrioxamine has also been reported.

The neurosensory complications of desferrioxamine are dose related and inversely correlated with the body iron burden. Heavily loaded patients are relatively protected, but aggressively chelated individuals with lower iron burdens may be more susceptible to these toxicities.[803, 808, 809] Administration of desferrioxamine to patients with rheumatoid arthritis with normal iron stores has induced neurologic deficits including confusion, nausea and vomiting, and coma.[808, 810] These findings suggest that the toxicity is caused by free drug, which may chelate other metal irons.[804] Alternatively, desferrioxamine may reduce the concentration of iron in neurosensory cells below a threshold needed for normal function. These serious complications necessitate careful monitoring of patients receiving the drug. Young children and individuals from whom the majority of iron has been removed by chelation are particularly susceptible to these effects. Complications are most likely in patients on continuous intravenous infusions of more than 50 mg/kg per day. Formal audiometry and ophthalmologic examination should be performed at 6-month intervals. The use of a test infusion to access the ability of desferrioxamine to mobilize iron, as advocated by Fosburg and Nathan,[718] may help in avoiding toxicity.

Desferrioxamine is normally used by microorganisms to facilitate iron uptake.[629, 811] *Yersinia enterocolitica*, for example, employs desferrioxamine in this manner.[769] Although it is associated with low virulence in humans, serious *Y. enterocolitica* infections have been reported in treated patients.[812, 813] Mucormycosis has also been reported in hemodialysis patients receiving desferrioxamine.[814] Of interest is the observation that iron chelators have profound *in vitro* effects on T-lymphocyte function.[718, 815–820] Whether these effects can be put to practical use is not known.[819]

Additional rare complications have been associated with high doses of desferrioxamine. Pulmonary infiltrates and respiratory insufficiency have been reported in eight patients[821, 822] and in iron-loaded mice.[823] Curiously, desferrioxamine also protects the developing lung[824]; therefore, the view that the drug causes pulmonary toxicity in the treatment of iron overload is controversial.[825] Indeed, iron overload is thought to contribute to pulmonary disease in thalassemia,[712] although the latter is complex and probably related as well to pulmonary vascular obstruction secondary to chronic thrombocytosis.[713, 768] Acute and chronic renal decompensation has also been described.[713, 768, 826–828] Growth failure and skeletal changes have been reported.[829, 830]

The array of potential side effects should not obscure the finding that desferrioxamine has proved to be very safe in the vast majority of patients. Many of the side effects have been seen only at higher intravenous doses. Although careful follow-up of patients is warranted, patients can be reassured that the desferrioxamine therapy is both remarkably effective and generally quite safe. Indeed, methods have been designed to permit chronic intravenous infusion[831–833] and a twice-daily subcutaneous regimen that obviates a pump is being explored.[834, 834a]

Oral Chelators. The availability of effective oral chelators would be a major clinical advance. Of those examined thus far, only one, L1 (1,2-dimethyl-3-hydroxy-pyridin-4-one; deferiprone), has proved efficacious[672, 835–849]; oral chelation is appropriate, in principle, for noncompliant patients or those for whom desferrioxamine treatment is impractical or unavailable. At a sufficient dose (75–100 mg/kg per day) L1 administration removes hepatic and reticuloendothelial cell iron stores in iron-overloaded patients. In contrast to desferrioxamine, its affinity for iron is dependent on drug concentration; it is, therefore, uncertain that its administration will maintain a blood level of effective chelator adequate to protect against long-term iron cardiotoxicity.[848] Administration of L1 is associated with several adverse side effects, including idiosyncratic agranulocytosis in nearly 2% of cases.[846, 849] Other complications include arthropathy, zinc deficiency, gastrointestinal symptoms, and abnormal liver function tests.[842] Until the risk-benefit ratio of L1 administration is established by additional clinical trials, compliant patients should be advised to remain on an effective desferrioxamine chelation program. Indeed, unpublished observations suggest that L1 is considerably less effective than previously thought.[849a]

Vitamin Supplementation

Ascorbic Acid. The role of ascorbic acid in iron metabolism and chelation therapy is complex and controversial.[629, 850] Hemosiderotic patients often develop tissue deficiency of vitamin C owing to accelerated catabolism; frank scurvy is documented in individuals with marginal dietary intake.[851–854] Administration of vitamin C significantly augments iron excretion in response to desferrioxamine, particularly in patients who are vitamin C deficient. Serum iron and ferritin levels may also rise.[774, 854, 855] Ascorbic acid retards the rate of conversion of ferritin to hemosiderin[856, 857] and presumably allows more iron to remain in a chelatable form. Unfortunately, ascorbic acid also enhances iron-mediated peroxidation of membrane lipids[858, 859] and has been shown to enhance iron-induced membrane damage in cultured myocardial cells.[639] It has also been observed that iron-overloaded patients receiving vita-

min C may experience cardiac dysfunction, which is reversed when supplementation is discontinued.[860, 861]

Some investigators have suggested giving low doses of ascorbic acid (3 mg/kg) at the start of each subcutaneous infusion of desferrioxamine. The chelator should be able to block the deleterious effects of ascorbic acid on lipid peroxidation of cellular organelles *in vitro*. Others avoid using vitamin C in iron-overloaded patients, arguing that iron depletion can be achieved without supplemental vitamin C. Patients with significant iron burden should be cautioned against self-administration of substantial amounts of ascorbic acid, because abrupt cardiac deterioration has been observed in this setting.[798]

Vitamin E. Deficiency of vitamin E has been noted in many chronically transfused patients with thalassemia major.[641, 642, 777, 862, 863] It may contribute to hemolysis due to red cell membrane damage.[548, 640] Alpha-tocopherol has long been considered to be a potent antioxidant that protects membrane lipids from attack by free radicals, formed when excess iron is present. Deficiency in the neonatal period[864] or secondary to malnutrition is associated with varying degrees of hemolysis. Hemolysis and the characteristic increased red cell susceptibility to *in vitro* hydrogen peroxide are readily reversed by administration of supplemental vitamin E. Of interest, supplemental iron administration increases the hemolytic rate, even among nonthalassemic patients with vitamin E deficiency.[864] In iron-overloaded patients, supplemental vitamin E may lessen iron-mediated cellular toxicity. One study in experimental animals suggests that vitamin E may also inhibit desferrioxamine-induced urinary iron excretion,[865] although this effect has not been demonstrated in humans.

Folic Acid. Megaloblastic anemia, which is almost invariably due to folic acid deficiency, may occur in patients with severe β-thalassemia.[866–868] In contrast, vitamin B$_{12}$ deficiency is extremely rare in thalassemic patients.[868] Folic acid deficiency is thought to develop due to decreased absorption, low dietary intake, and the enormous demand of an expanded bone marrow. Most patients benefit from daily folic acid administration (1 mg), although well-transfused patients probably do not require supplementation.

Trace Metals. Trace metal deficiency is not commonly observed secondary to thalassemia or aggressive chelation therapy.[629, 869] A case of zinc deficiency (acrodermatitis enteropathica) has been reported in a patient chelated with diethylenetetraminepentaacetic acid (DTPA).[870] Reversible toxicities seen with high-dose desferrioxamine chelation may reflect trace metal deficiency or intracellular chelation of a trace metal. Newer techniques to analyze trace metal concentrations may yet reveal subtle deficiencies.

Allogeneic Bone Marrow Transplantation

Successful cure of β-thalassemia by bone marrow transplantation was first reported by Thomas and associates in 1982.[871] Subsequently, a number of centers have explored this modality as a therapy for β-thalassemia. The most extensive published experience with bone marrow transplantation in β-thalassemia is from Lucarelli and co-workers in Italy.[872–876] The results of their early attempts at transplantation in this patient population were discouraging.[873] The preparative regimens used were frequently ineffective and associated with failure to engraft, toxicity, and high mortality. Their recent experience is considerably more promising.[876] In 222 patients (ages 1 to 15 years) who underwent transplantation between 1983 to 1988 with five different preparative regimens, overall and event-free survivals were 82% and 75%, respectively. The longest surviving patient was alive and free of disease 6 years after transplantation. Their current preparative protocol, which has been used in 116 patients since 1985, includes oral busulfan and intravenous cyclophosphamide. Patients were analyzed to identify clinically important variables predictive of transplant outcome. The probability of survival was decreased in the presence of poor chelation status, hepatomegaly (>2 cm), and portal fibrosis. The probability of event-free survival was reduced in the presence of hepatomegaly. The risk factors of hepatomegaly and portal fibrosis were used to divide the patients into three classes. Patients in class 1 (absence of both risk factors) had 3-year probabilities of survival, event-free survival, and graft rejection of 94%, 94%, and 0% respectively. In class 2 (one risk factor), the 3-year probabilities were 80%, 77%, and 9%; in class 3 (two risk factors) they were 61%, 53%, and 16%. However, such subsetting of patients may be difficult to reproduce (viz., hepatomegaly of 2 cm or more and a history of chelation adherence). It is probably wise to consider the likely event-free survival to be closer to 75%, even though some small series can vary above or below that estimate.[877–879]

One of the major reasons for failure of bone marrow transplantation in thalassemia may be unpredictable pharmacology of busulfan used in most preparative regimens. Hyperabsorption of the drug is associated with hepatic veno-occlusive disease; hypoabsorption with recurrent thalassemia. Improved control of busulfan levels during induction may offer better clinical results.[880] Whatever the event-free survival estimates, bone marrow transplantation is the only viable option for patients who cannot, or will not, adhere to a well-administered transfusion and chelation program.[881]

On the basis of available data, bone marrow transplantation may be recommended to well-chelated patients without evidence of liver disease. Many of these patients can be cured. Although most such patients are very young, age does not appear to be a significant variable in determining outcome. Chronic graft-versus-host disease is still a potential long-term complication of successful allogeneic transplantation. A current limitation to the general applicability of this therapy is the availability of a related, HLA-matched donor. Only one in four siblings on average will be HLA identical. Improved management of graft-versus-host disease and the development of technologies for bone marrow transplantation from unrelated donors may expand the pool of potential donors in the near future.

Pharmacologic Manipulation of Hb F Synthesis

The interaction between β-thalassemia and genetic syndromes that increase γ-globin synthesis has illustrated how even small increases in γ-globin production lead to a significant improvement in the effectiveness of red blood cell production in patients with thalassemia. Although steady-state production of Hb F is a genetically determined trait,[9] perturbations in erythropoiesis may be associated with increased capacity for Hb F synthesis. Treatment of experimental animals or patients with a variety of cytoreductive agents, including 5-azacytidine, hydroxyurea, vinblastine, and cytarabine, leads to an increase in production of Hb F.[882–890] Although the precise mechanism of action of these drugs remains incompletely defined, the increased capacity for γ-globin synthesis appears to be linked to rapid erythroid regeneration. Consistent with this hypothesis, hematopoietic growth factors that promote the expansion and maturation of the erythroid precursors have also been shown to enhance Hb F synthesis in primate models; these include erythropoietin (Epo),[891–893] interleukin-3 (IL-3),[892–894] and granulocyte-macrophage colony-stimulating factor (GM-CSF).[892] Of particular interest is the observation that infants delivered of diabetic mothers exhibit a delayed γ-β-switch.[895] Butyric acid derivatives are elevated in the serum of these mothers and their infants before birth. Similarly, patients with metabolic disorders associated with increased levels of short-chain fatty acids also have elevated Hb F levels.[896] Infusions of sodium butyrate or α-aminobutyric acid into fetal sheep markedly delay the perinatal switch,[897] whereas infusions in primates lead to activation of the γ-globin gene.[898–900] It has been proposed that butyrate, proprionate, or the metabolite acetate promotes increased γ gene expression by acetylation of histones and altering chromatin structure, but other mechanisms cannot be excluded.[901, 902] A flurry of articles have described results of treatment of patients with butyrate or its derivatives.[903–908] With the exception of one patient,[904] none has had a sustained rise in hemoglobin, although healing of leg ulcers without an increment in circulating hemoglobin has been observed.[907] Caution must be exercised, because high doses of butyrate are associated with neurotoxicity in simians.[909]

The most extensive experience with pharmacologic manipulation of Hb F synthesis in patients has involved use of hydroxyurea to patients with sickle cell disease.[888, 910–914] In this population, the majority of patients appear to respond to the drug with a twofold or higher increase in Hb F over their baseline. Many patients achieve Hb F levels between 10% and 15% of total hemoglobin. This increase reflects both augmented production and enhanced survival of Hb F–containing cells. The clinical results in sickle cell anemia are impressive (see Chapter 20), but results in thalassemia are so far disappointing.[890]

Several patients with thalassemia have been shown to respond to 5-azacytidine (Fig. 21–34).[883, 915, 916] The dramatic increases in Hb F associated with administra-

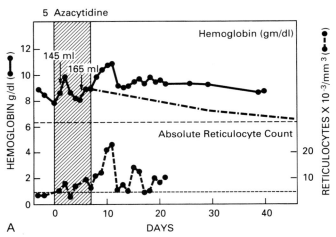

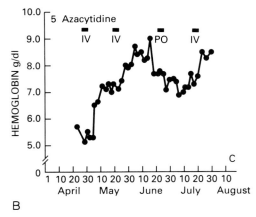

Figure 21-34. *A*, The effects of 5-azacytidine on erythropoiesis in a patient with severe homozygous β-thalassemia after a single administration of the drug by continuous infusion over 7 days. Two small blood transfusions were administered on days 2 and 5. The dashed lines indicate the projected hemoglobin concentration and reticulocyte count in this patient without treatment, based on clinical records. *B*, The effects of sequential courses of treatment with 5-azacytidine in a β-thalassemia patient with severe cardiomyopathy and alloimmunization. (*A* adapted from information appearing in Ley TJ, DeSimone J, et al: 5-Azacytidine selectively increases gamma-globin synthesis in a patient with beta thalassemia. N Engl J Med 1982; 307:1469. Reprinted by permission, from The New England Journal of Medicine.) (*B* from Dunbar C, Travis W, et al: 5-Azacytidine treatment in a beta⁰-thalassemic patient unable to be transfused due to multiple alloantibodies. Br J Haematol 1989; 72:467.)

tion of this drug may result from a combination of cytotoxicity and inhibition of post–synthetic methylation of DNA.[917–920] After administration of 5-azacytidine, global demethylation of DNA, including the γ-globin gene, is observed. Despite its effectiveness, the use of 5-azacytidine in the treatment of the hemoglobinopathies has been limited by concerns regarding its known carcinogenic potential,[921–923] as well as the demonstrated effectiveness and safety of current treatment strategies involving transfusion and chelation. Because the response to the drug is short lived, chronic therapy would be required.

Treatment of β-thalassemia with busulfan has been reported in two patients in China.[924] Combinations of agents, notably erythropoietin and hydroxyurea, often enhance Hb F production in experimental animals[893, 925] and have shown promise in preliminary trials in sickle cell patients.[926] Undoubtedly, the response of individual patients to these medications will be influenced by their endogenous, genetically determined capabilities for γ and β chain synthesis.[927]

Gene Therapy

As a result of advances in molecular biology, treatment of hematologic disease through the introduction of new genetic material into bone marrow stem cells is a foreseeable future goal.[928–930] Application of somatic gene therapy to the treatment of hematologic diseases requires improved efficiency of gene delivery, regulated and sustained expression of introduced genes, and biologic studies demonstrating expression of the foreign gene. Although active research is ongoing, experimental shortcomings in all these aspects presently preclude use of gene therapy in the management of thalassemia or sickle cell anemia.

Correction of thalassemia by gene transfer will neces-

sitate introduction of a normal β-globin gene into pluripotent hematopoietic stem cells.[928–930] Recombinant retroviral vectors provide the most efficient delivery system. These vectors take advantage of normal cellular mechanisms facilitating viral entry and incorporation of new genetic information into host cell chromosomes. Once integrated within the genome of the target cell, the viral sequences, lacking structural genes necessary to produce infectious virus, are stably maintained in the host cell genome. Experimental studies in mice have demonstrated that retroviral vectors are capable of transferring foreign sequences to hematopoietic stem cells.[931, 932] Expression of transferred genes has been more problematic but has been reported. The efficiency with which primate (or human) stem cells are infected by retroviral vectors appears to be lower than that observed with murine cells. Nonetheless, transfer of foreign sequences to long-term repopulating hematopoietic cells of primates and humans has been demonstrated.[933] Many human experimental studies are ongoing to determine how best to transfer and express genes in hematopoietic cells.

If gene therapy is to be useful in the management of β-thalassemia, it will be necessary to design vectors that not only deliver a normal β-globin gene to hematopoietic stem cells but also provide for high-level, regulated expression during erythroid development. This is a particularly challenging problem. Although regulated expression of the β-globin gene is achieved in transgenic mice using the complete β-LCR, it has been difficult thus far to generate high titer retroviruses containing appropriate LCR sequences.[934, 935] New vector designs, or different viral vectors, are being investigated to overcome these limitations. Gene expression may not need to match that of a normal β-globin gene precisely, because relatively low-level expression might allow for substantial clinical improvement and lessen the demand for transfusion. Expression of a β-globin transgene at 10% to 20% of normal endogenous levels is adequate to achieve a dramatic phenotypic improvement in a thalassemic mouse model.[559]

Interaction of Thalassemia with Globin Structural Variants

In geographic areas where thalassemia mutations and structural variants of α- and β-globin genes are both frequent (such as Africa and Southeast Asia), compound heterozygotes with a thalassemia mutation and a structural variant are common.[1] In such double heterozygotes, disease may be more or less severe than that seen in individuals who are heterozygous for only the structural variant. For example, heterozygotes for a β^S-globin gene have 30% to 45% Hb S and are usually clinically well, whereas patients with a β^S-globin gene and a β-thalassemia mutation (in the *trans* β-gene) have 60% to 95% Hb S and may suffer a severe sickling disorder. Individuals with a β^S-globin gene and α-thalassemia trait generally have less Hb S than those with sickle trait[936, 937] and are asymptomatic.[938, 939] The interaction of α- and β-thalassemia mutations and the HPFH mutations with the β^S-globin gene have been described in detail in Chapter 20.

Hemoglobin E-β-Thalassemia

This syndrome is particularly common in Southeast Asia.[940, 941] As a result of immigration from Southeast Asia, Hb E-β-thalassemia is now a commonly encountered form of transfusion-dependent thalassemia in certain areas of the United States.[942, 943] Untransfused double heterozygotes have hemoglobin levels of 2.3 to 7 g/dL, depending primarily on the output of the β-thalassemia gene. Because α-thalassemia is common in Southeast Asia, more complex phenotypes may be observed.[944] Nucleated red blood cells are found on the peripheral blood smear, whereas they are absent in patients homozygous for β^E. Hb E and Hb A$_2$ account for 50% to 70% of total hemoglobin (5% A$_2$ by HPLC).[943, 945] Small quantities of Hb A are found in association with a β$^+$-thalassemia gene. Patients with Hb E-β-thalassemia are usually transfusion dependent and have clinical features of thalassemia major. In areas where intensive treatment is unavailable, the disease resembles classic thalassemia major with massive hepatosplenomegaly, hypersplenism, severe skeletal disease, and death from infection in childhood. Iron loading occurs either from transfusion or enhanced intestinal absorption.[946] Proper treatment is that recommended for thalassemia major or intermedia, depending on the requirement for regular blood transfusion.

Hemoglobin C-β-Thalassemia

The β^C-globin gene, which encodes a variant β chain with a lysine-glutamic acid substitution at position 6,[947] is common in blacks of West African origin. The only hematologic consequence of simple heterozygosity for the β^C gene is increased target cells on the peripheral smear. Double heterozygotes with β^C gene and β-thalassemia genes exhibit a moderately severe hemolytic anemia with splenomegaly. The peripheral blood smear reveals hypochromia and microcytosis with many target cells. Hb C comprises 65% to 95% of total hemoglobin, depending on whether the thalassemia mutation is of the β$^+$ or β^0 variety. In the black population the disease is generally mild, reflecting the prevalence of mild β-thalassemia genes (see earlier),[482] whereas in Italian,[948] North African,[949] and Turkish patients[950] the disease is more severe, particularly in those who have a β^0-thalassemia mutation.

Thalassemic Hemoglobinopathies

As discussed in detail in earlier sections, several variant polypeptides can be described as thalassemic hemoglobinopathies. With the exception of Hb E and the elongated α chain variants, these mutations are very infrequent. Interest in these mutations arises from the unique mechanisms by which they produce the thalassemia phenotype.[209, 951] The most common thalassemic hemoglobinopathy is Hb E disease.

Hemoglobin E Disease

As described earlier, the β^E mutation activates a cryptic splice site in exon 1 (see Fig. 21–10). Because the correct splice site is less efficiently utilized, decreased production of functional β-globin mRNA that codes for the variant ensues.[128] The frequency or the β^E-globin gene is extraordinarily high in some populations (~30% in Laos, Cambodia, and Thailand).[940, 952] The gene frequencies observed in immigrants from Southeast Asia to the United States reflect these origins.[943]

In the heterozygous form, patients are largely asymptomatic with a hemoglobin of greater than or equal to 12 g/dL, no reticulocytosis, an MCV of 74 ± 10.6 μm, and an MCH of 25 ± 2.5 pg. The peripheral blood smear is distinguished by mild microcytosis and occasional target cells. Hemoglobin electrophoresis reveals Hb E co-migrating with Hb A$_2$ in the range of 19% to 34%. The α/β biosynthetic ratio is usually greater than or equal to 0.8, hence the mild nature of Hb E trait.

Patients with homozygous Hb E disease are also asymptomatic.[941, 945] The hemoglobin is rarely less than 10 g/dL, and significant reticulocytosis is uncommon. The red cells, however, are markedly microcytic (MCV = 50 to 66 μm) and hypochromic (MCH = 20.1 pg). Targeting and occasional coarse stippling are evident on smear. Hb E comprises 90% or more of the total hemoglobin with varying levels of Hb F.

The differential diagnosis of microcytic anemias in the Southeast Asian population initially requires exclusion of iron deficiency. When Hb E is present, electrophoresis will identify it. However, its level may be diminished in the presence of α-thalassemia or iron deficiency, because the affinity of normal β chains for α-globin exceeds that of β^E chains. The interaction of α-thalassemia mutations with the β^E-globin gene is fre-

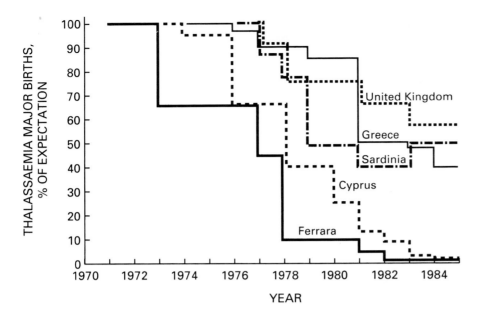

Figure 21–35. Decrease in the birth rate of infants with thalassemia major in Great Britain and several Mediterranean regions after the introduction of effective prenatal diagnosis. (Adapted, by permission of the World Health Organization, from Modell B, Bulyzhenkov V: Distribution and control of some genetic disorders. World Health Stat Q 1988; 41:209.)

quently seen due to high incidence of each in the Southeast Asian population.[944]

Prenatal Diagnosis of Thalassemia

The morbidity and mortality associated with severe forms of thalassemia prompted efforts to develop effective prenatal diagnosis more than two decades ago. For the vast majority of β-thalassemias for which point mutations are usually responsible, early efforts focused on the determination of globin-chain synthesis in fetal blood cells obtained by aspiration of placental vessels or direct visualization of fetal vessels.[956–958] The risk of fetal blood sampling at 18 to 20 weeks' gestation proved acceptably low in the hands of experienced personnel (fetal loss rate ~3%; error rate <0.5%), such that between 1975 and 1985 more than 7900 pregnancies were studied.[959] As molecular methods and the knowledge of mutations leading to thalassemias improved, strategies for prenatal detection of these conditions evolved.

Successful prenatal diagnosis of α-thalassemia of the hydrops fetalis variety using solution hybridization methods to detect deficiency of α-globin genes in amniotic fluid cell DNA was first reported by Kan and associates in 1975.[953] Southern blot analysis rapidly supplanted this approach for the detection of gene deletion in either α- or β-thalassemias.[954, 955]

Detection of mutations in DNA rapidly became the preferred strategy for prenatal diagnosis as mutations became defined in β-thalassemias.[3] The introduction of PCR methods further facilitated mutation detection and also permitted the use of nonradioactive tests.[960] Coupled with chorionic villus biopsy, accurate and safe diagnoses can be accomplished within the first trimester of pregnancy.

Besides molecular biology, prenatal diagnosis of thalassemia has relied on identification of couples at risk, widespread public education, and genetic counseling.

In countries where the incidence of β-thalassemia is high and the burden of disease to the overall population great, such as on the island of Sardinia and in Greece, intensive prevention programs have been established and proved to be extraordinarily successful. For example, the births of children with β-thalassemia in these area have been reduced by more than 90% in recent years (Fig. 21–35).[879, 961–965] These represent major achievements in the prevention of genetic disease and paradigms for other disorders.

References

1. Weatherall DJ, Clegg JB: The Thalassemia Syndromes. 3rd ed. Oxford, Blackwell Scientific Publications, Inc., 1981.
2. Higgs DR, Vickers MA, et al: A review of the molecular genetics of the human alpha-globin gene cluster. Blood 1989; 73:1081.
3. Kazazian HH Jr: The thalassemia syndromes: molecular basis and prenatal diagnosis in 1990. Semin Hematol 1990; 27:209.
4. Karlsson S, Nienhuis AW: Developmental regulation of human globin genes. Annu Rev Biochem 1985; 54:1071.
5. Collins FS, Weissman SM: The molecular genetics of human hemoglobin. Prog Nucl Acid Res Mol Biol 1984; 31:315.
6. Bunn HF, Forget BG: Hemoglobin: Molecular, Genetic and Clinical Aspects. Philadelphia, W.B. Saunders Co., 1986.
7. Boyer SH, Belding TK, et al: Fetal hemoglobin restricted to a few erythrocytes (F-cells) in normal human adults. Science 1975; 188:361.
8. Wood WG, Stamatoyannopoulos G, et al: F-cells in the adult: normal values and levels in individuals with hereditary and acquired elevations of Hb F. Blood 1975; 46:671.
9. Miyoshi K, Kaneto Y, et al: X-linked dominant control of F-cells in normal adult life: characterization of the Swiss type as hereditary persistence of fetal hemoglobin regulated dominantly by gene(s) on X chromosome. Blood 1988; 72:1854.
10. Craig JE, Rochette J, et al: Dissecting the loci controlling fetal haemoglobin production on chromosomes 11p and 6q by the regressive approach. Nat Genet 1996; 12:58.
11. Maniatis T, Fritsch EF, et al: The molecular genetics of human hemoglobins. Annu Rev Genet 1980; 14:145.
12. Liebhaber SA: Alpha thalassemia. Hemoglobin 1989; 13:685.
13. Deisseroth A, Nienhuis AW, et al: Localization of the human alpha-globin structural gene to chromosome 16 in somatic cell hybrids by molecular hybridization assay. Cell 1977; 12:205.
14. Deisseroth A, Nienhuis AW, et al: Chromosomal localization of

the human beta-globin gene on chromosome 11 in somatic cell hybrids. Proc Natl Acad Sci U S A 1978; 75:1459.

15. Lauer J, Shen CKJ, et al: The chromosomal arrangement of human alpha-like globin genes: sequence homology and alpha-globin gene deletions. Cell 1980; 20:119.

16. Liebhaber SA, Goossens M, et al: Homology and concerted evolution at the alpha-1 and alpha-2 loci of human alpha-globin. Nature 1981; 290:26.

17. Proudfoot NJ, Gil A, et al: The structure of the human zeta-globin gene and a closely linked nearly identical pseudogene. Cell 1982; 31:553.

18. Fritsch EF, Lawn RM, et al: Molecular cloning and characterization of the human beta-like globin gene cluster. Cell 1980; 19:959.

19. Efstradiatis A, Posakony JW, et al: The structure and evolution of the human beta-globin gene family. Cell 1980; 21:653.

20. Slightom JL, Blechl AE, et al: Human fetal gamma and gamma globin genes: complete nucleotide sequences suggest that DNA can be exchanged between these duplicated genes. Cell 1980; 21:627.

21. Baralle FE, Shoulders CC, et al: The primary structure of the human epsilon-globin gene. Cell 1980; 21:621.

22. Humphries RK, Ley T, et al: Differences in human alpha-, beta- and delta-globin gene expression in monkey kidney cells. Cell 1982; 30:173.

23. Kosche KA, Dobkin C, et al: DNA sequences regulating human beta globin gene expression. Nucleic Acids Res 1985; 13:7781.

24. Ross J, Pizarro A: Human beta and delta globin messenger RNAs turn over at different rates. J Mol Biol 1983; 167:607.

25. Pataryas HA, Stamatoyannopoulos G: Hemoglobins in human fetuses: evidence for adult hemoglobin production after the 11th gestational week. Blood 1972; 39:688.

26. Henri A, Testa U, et al: Disappearance of Hb F and i antigen during the first year of life. Am J Hematol 1980; 9:161.

27. Terrenato L, Bertilaccio C, et al: The switch from haemoglobin F to A: the time course of qualitative and quantitative variations of haemoglobins after birth. Br J Haematol 1981; 47:31.

28. Smale ST, Baltimore D: The "initiator" as a transcriptional control element. Cell 1989; 57:103.

29. Lewis BA, Orkin SH: A functional initiator element in the human β-globin promoter. J Biol Chem 1995; 270:28139.

30. Dynan WS, Tjian R: Control of eukaryotic messenger RNA synthesis by sequence-specific DNA-binding proteins. Nature 1985; 316:774.

31. McKnight S, Tjian R: Transcriptional selectivity of viral genes in mammalian cells. Cell 1986; 46:795.

32. Maniatis T, Goodbourn S, et al: Regulation of inducible and tissue-specific gene expression. Science 1987; 236:1237.

33. Saltzman AG, Weinmann R: Promoter specificity and modulation of RNA polymerase II transcription. FASEB J 1989; 3:1723.

34. Dynan WS: Modularity in promoters and enhancers. Cell 1989; 58:1.

35. Guarente L: UASs and enhancers: common mechanism of transcriptional activation in yeast and mammals. Cell 1988; 52:303.

36. Muller MM, Gerster T, et al: Enhancer sequences and the regulation of gene transcription. Eur J Biochem 1988; 176:485.

37. Peterson MG, Tanese N, et al: Functional domains and upstream activation properties of cloned human TATA binding protein. Science 1990; 248:1625.

38. Kao CC, Lieberman PM, et al: Cloning of a transcriptionally active human TATA binding factor. Science 1990; 248:1646.

39. Lewin B: Commitment and activation at pol II promoters: a tail of protein-protein interactions. Cell 1990; 61:1161.

40. Takihara Y, Nakamura T, et al: A novel mutation in the TATA box in a Japanese patient with beta$^+$-thalassemia. Blood 1986; 67:547.

41. Fei YJ, Stoming TA, et al: Beta-thalassemia due to a T→A mutation within the ATA box. Biochem Biophys Res Commun 1988; 153:741.

42. Cai SP, Zhang JZ, et al: A new TATA box mutation detected at prenatal diagnosis for beta-thalassemia. Am J Hum Genet 1989; 45:112.

43. Antonarakis SE, Irkin SH, et al: Beta thalassemia in American blacks: Novel mutations in the TATA box and an acceptor splice site. Proc Natl Acad Sci U S A 1984; 81:1154.

44. Huang S-Z, Wong C, et al: The same TATA box beta thalassemia mutation in Chinese and U.S. Blacks: another example of independent origins of mutation. Hum Genet 1986; 74:152.

45. Poncz M, Ballantine M, et al: Beta thalassemia in a Kurdish Jew. J Biol Chem 1983; 257:5994.

46. Orkin SH, Sexton JP, et al: ATA box transcription mutation in beta-thalassemia. Nucleic Acids Res 1983; 11:4727.

47. Hoey T, Dynlacht BD, et al: Isolation and characterization of the *Drosophila* gene encoding the TATA box binding protein, TFIID. Cell 1990; 61:1179.

48. Orkin SH: Regulation of globin gene expression in erythroid cells. Eur J Biochem 1995; 231:271.

49. Kadonaga JT, Carner KR, et al: Isolation of cDNA encoding transcription factor Sp1 and functional analysis of the DNA binding domain. Cell 1987; 51:1079.

50. Andrews NC, Erdjument-Bromage H, et al: Erythroid transcription factor NF-E2 is a haematopoietic-specific basic-leucine zipper protein. Nature 1993; 362:722.

51. Andrews NC, Kotkow KJ, et al: The ubiquitous subunit of erythroid transcription factor NF-E2 is a small basic-leucine zipper protein related to the v-*maf* oncogene. Proc Natl Acad Sci U S A 1993; 90:11488.

52. Lu S-J, Rowan S, et al: Retroviral integration within the *Fli-2* locus results in inactivation of the erythroid transcription factor NF-E2 in Friend erythroleukemias: evidence that NF-E2 is essential for globin expression. Proc Natl Acad Sci U S A 1994; 91:8398.

53. Kotkow KJ, Orkin SH: Dependence of globin gene expression in mouse erythroleukemia cells on the NF-E2 heterodimer. Mol Cell Biol 1995; 15:4640.

54. Shivdasani RA, Orkin SH: Erythropoiesis and globin gene expression in mice lacking the transcription factor NF-E2. Proc Natl Acad Sci U S A 1995; 92:8690.

55. Chada K, Magram J, et al: Specific expression of a foreign beta-globin gene in erythroid cells of transgenic mice. Nature 1985; 314:377.

56. Magram J, Chada K, et al: Developmental regulation of a cloned adult beta-globin gene in transgenic mice. Nature 1985; 315:338.

57. Townes TM, Lingrel JB, et al: Erythroid-specific expression of human beta-globin genes in transgenic mice. EMBO J 1985; 4:1715.

58. Costantini F, Radice G, et al: Developmental regulation of human globin genes in transgenic mice. Cold Spring Harb Symp Quant Biol 1985; 50:361.

59. Chada K, Magram J, et al: An embryonic pattern of expression of a human fetal globin gene in transgenic mice. Nature 1986; 319:685.

60. Kollias G, Wrighton N, et al: Regulated expression of human A gamma-, beta-, and hybrid gamma beta-globin genes in transgenic mice: manipulation of the developmental expression patterns. Cell 1986; 46:89.

61. Tuan D, Solomon W, et al: The "beta-like-globin" gene domain in human erythroid cells. Proc Natl Acad Sci U S A 1985; 82:6384.

62. Tuan DY, Solomon WB, et al: An erythroid-specific, developmental-stage-independent enhancer far upstream of the human "beta-like globin genes. Proc Natl Acad Sci U S A 1989; 86:2554.

63. Grosveld F, van Assendelft GB, et al: Position-independent, high-level expression of the human beta-globin gene in transgenic mice. Cell 1987; 51:975.

64. Higgs DR, Wood WG, et al: A major positive regulatory region is located far upstream of the human α-globin gene locus. Genes Dev 1990; 4:1588.

65. Gibbons RJ, Brueton L, et al: Clinical and hematologic aspects of the X-linked α-thalassemia/mental retardation syndrome (ATR-X). Am J Med Genet 1995; 55:288.

66. Gibbons RJ, Picketts DJ, et al: Mutations in a putative global transcriptional regulator cause X-linked mental retardation with alpha-thalassemia (ATR-X syndrome). Cell 1995; 80:837.

67. Raich N, Clegg CH, et al: GATA1 and YY1 are developmental repressors of the human ε-globin gene. EMBO J 1995; 14:801.

68. Choi OR, Engel JD: Developmental regulation of beta-globin gene switching. Cell 1988; 55:17.

69. Jane SM, Ney PA, et al: Identification of a stage selector element in the human γ-globin gene promoter that fosters preferential interaction with the 5' HS2 enhancer when in competition with the β-promoter. EMBO J 1992; 11:2961.

70. Jane SM, Nienhuis AW, et al: Hemoglobin switching in man and chicken is mediated by a heteromeric complex between the ubiquitous transcription factor CP2 and a developmentally specific protein. EMBO J 1995; 14:97.

71. Nienhuis AW, Anagnou NP, et al: Advances in thalassemia research. Blood 1984; 63:738.

72. Orkin SH, Kazazian HH Jr: Mutation and polymorphism of the human beta-globin gene and its surrounding DNA. Annu Rev Genet 1984; 18:131.

73. Benz EJ Jr, Nathan DG: Pathophysiology of the anemia in thalassemia. In Weatherall DJ (ed): Congenital Disorders of Erythropoiesis. Amsterdam, Elsevier Science Publishing Co., 1976, p 205.

74. Fessas P, Loukopoulos D: The beta-thalassemias. Clin Haematol 1974; 3:411.

75. Nathan DG, Gunn RB: Thalassemia: the consequences of unbalanced hemoglobin synthesis. Am J Med 1966; 41:815.

76. Nathan DG, Stossel TB, et al: Influence of hemoglobin precipitation on erythrocyte metabolism in alpha and beta thalassemia. J Clin Invest 1969; 48:33.

77. Nathan DG: Thalassemia. N Engl J Med 1972; 286:586.

78. Wood WG, Weatherall DJ, et al: Interaction of heterocellular hereditary persistence of fetal hemoglobin with beta thalassemia and sickle cell anemia. Nature 1976; 264:247.

79. Prchal J, Stamatoyannopoulos G: Two siblings with unusually mild homozygous beta thalassemia: a didactic example of non-allelic modifier gene on the expressivity of a monogenic disorder. Am J Med Genet 1981; 10:291.

80. Safaya S, Rieder RF, et al: Homozygous beta-thalassemia without anemia. Blood 1989; 73:324.

81. Kanavakis K, Wainscoat JS, et al: The interaction of alpha thalassemia with beta thalassemia. Br J Haematol 1982; 52:465.

82. Haldane JBS: The rate of mutation of human genes. In Proceedings of the VIII International Congress on Genetics and Heredity, supplement No. 35, 1949, p 267.

83. Livingstone FB: Frequency of Hemoglobin Variants. New York, Oxford University Press, Inc., 1985.

84. Weatherall DJ: Common genetic disorders of the red cell and the "malaria hypothesis." Ann Trop Med Parasitol 1987; 81:539.

85. Frazer GR, Kitsos C, et al: Thalassemias, abnormal hemoglobins, and glucose-6-phosphate dehydrogenase deficiency in the Arta area of Greece: diagnostic and epidemiologic aspects of complete village studies. Ann N Y Acad Sci 1964; 119:415.

86. Kanavakis E, Tzotzos S, et al: Molecular basis and prevalence of alpha-thalassemia in Greece. Birth Defects 1988; 23:377.

87. Falusi AG, Esan GJ, et al: Alpha-thalassaemia in Nigeria: its interaction with sickle-cell disease. Eur J Haematol 1987; 38:815.

88. Flint J, Hill AV, et al: High frequencies of alpha-thalassaemia are the result of natural selection by malaria. Nature 1986; 321:744.

89. Flint J, Hill AV, et al: Alpha globin genotypes in two North European populations. Br J Haematol 1986; 63:796. Letter.

90. Shimizu K, Harano T, et al: Abnormal arrangements in the alpha- and gamma-globin gene clusters in a relatively large group of Japanese newborns. Am J Hum Genet 1986; 38:45.

91. Siniscalco M, Bernini L, et al: Population genetics of haemoglobin variants, thalassemia and glucose-6-phosphate dehydrogenase deficiency, with particular reference to malaria hypothesis. Bull WHO 1966; 34:379.

92. Willcox M, Bjorkman A, et al: Falciparum malaria and beta-thalassaemia trait in northern Liberia. Ann Trop Med Parasitol 1983; 77:335.

93. Oppenheimer SJ, Higgs DR, et al: Alpha thalassaemia in Papua New Guinea. Lancet 1984; 1:424.

94. Teo CG, Wong HB: The innate resistance of thalassemia to malaria: a review of the evidence and possible mechanisms. Singapore Med J 1985; 26:504.

95. Hill AV, Bowden DK, et al: Beta thalassemia in Melanesia: association with malaria and characterization of a common variant (IVS-1 nt 5 G→C). Blood 1988; 72:9.

96. Pasvol G, Weatherall DJ, et al: Effects of foetal haemoglobin on susceptibility of red cells to Plasmodium falciparum. Nature 1977; 270:171.

97. Nagel RL, Roth EF: Malaria and red cell genetic defects. Blood 1989; 74:1213.

98. Brockelman CR, Wongsattayanont B, et al: Thalassemic erythrocytes inhibit in vitro growth of Plasmodium falciparum. J Clin Microbiol 1987; 25:56.

99. Luzzi GA, Merry AH, et al: Surface antigen expression on Plasmodium falciparum–infected erythrocytes is modified in alpha- and beta-thalassemia. J Exp Med 1991; 173:785.

100. Ifediba TC, Stern A, et al: Plasmodium falciparum in vitro: diminished growth in hemoglobin H disease erythrocytes. Blood 1985; 65:452.

101. Carlson J, Nash GB, et al: Natural protection against severe Plasmodium falciparum malaria due to impaired rosette formation. Blood 1994; 84:3909.

102. Gonzalez-Redondo JM, Stoming TA, et al: A C→T substitution at nt–101 in a conserved DNA sequence of the promotor region of the beta-globin gene is associated with "silent" beta-thalassemia. Blood 1989; 73:1705.

103. Orkin SH, Antonarakis SE, et al: Base substitution at position −88 in a beta-thalassemic globin gene. Further evidence for the role of distal promoter element ACACCC. J Biol Chem 1984; 259:8679.

104. Rund D, Filon D, et al: Molecular analysis of beta thalassemia in Kurdish Jews: novel mutations and expression studies. Blood 1989; 74:821A.

105. Orkin SH, Kazazian HH Jr, et al: Linkage of beta thalassemia mutations and beta-globin gene polymorphisms with DNA polymorphisms in the human beta-globin gene cluster. Nature 1982; 296:627.

106. Wong C, Dowling CE, et al: Characterization of beta-thalassaemia mutations using direct genomic sequencing of amplified single copy DNA. Nature 1987; 330:384.

107. Orkin SH, Goff SC, et al: Mutation in an intervening sequence splice junction in man. Proc Natl Acad Sci U S A 1981; 78:5041.

108. Felber BK, Orkin SH, et al: Abnormal RNA splicing causes one form of alpha thalassemia. Cell 1982; 29:895.

109. Kazazian HH Jr, Orkin SH, et al: Molecular characterization of seven beta-thalassemia mutations in Asian Indians. EMBO J 1984; 3:593.

110. Chibani J, Vidaud M, et al: The peculiar spectrum of beta-thalassemia genes in Tunisia. Hum Genet 1988; 78:190.

111. Kazazian HH Jr, Boehm CD: Molecular basis and prenatal diagnosis of beta-thalassemia. Blood 1988; 72:1107.

112. Treisman R, Proudfoot NJ, et al: A single base change at a splice site in a beta thalassemia gene causes abnormal RNA splicing. Cell 1982; 29:903.

113. Wong C, Antonarakis SE, et al: On the origin and spread of beta-thalassemia: recurrent observation of four mutations in different ethnic groups. Proc Natl Acad Sci U S A 1986; 83:6529.

114. Orkin SH, Sexton JP, et al: Inactivation of an acceptor RNA splice site by a short deletion in beta-thalassemia. J Biol Chem 1983; 258:7249.

115. Atweh GF, Anagnou NP, et al: Beta-thalassemia resulting from a single nucleotide substitution in an acceptor splice site. Nucleic Acids Res 1985; 13:777.

116. Padanilam BJ, Huisman TH: The beta zero-thalassemia in an American black family is due to a single nucleotide substitution in the acceptor splice junction of the second intervening sequence. Am J Hematol 1986; 22:259.

117. Chehab FF, Der KV, et al: The molecular basis of beta-thalassemia in Lebanon: application to prenatal diagnosis. Blood 1987; 69:1141.

118. Gonzalez-Redondo JM, Stoming TA, et al: Hb Monroe or alpha2beta2 30(B12)Arg→Thr, a variant associated with beta-thalassemia due to A G→C substitution adjacent to the donor splice site of the first intron. Hemoglobin 1989; 13:67.

119. Kalydjieva L, Eigel A, et al: The molecular basis of thalassemia in Bulgaria. Presented before the Third International Conference on Thalassemia and the Hemoglobinopathies, Sardinia, 1989, p 43.

120. Cheng TC, Orkin SH, et al: Beta thalassemia in Chinese: use of in vivo RNA analysis and oligonucleotide hybridization in systematic characterization of molecular defects. Proc Natl Acad Sci U S A 1984; 81:2821.

121. Atweh GF, Wong C, et al: A new mutation in IVS-1 of the human beta globin gene causing beta thalassemia due to abnormal splicing. Blood 1987; 70:147.

122. Gonzalez-Redondo JM, Stoming TA, et al: Clinical and genetic

heterogeneity in black patients with homozygous beta-thalassemia from the southeastern United States. Blood 1988; 72:1007.

123. Lapoumeroulie C, Pagnier J, et al: Beta thalassemia due to a novel mutation in IVS 1 sequence donor site consensus sequence creating a restriction site. Biochem Biophys Res Commun 1986; 139:709.

124. Wong C, Antonarakis SE, et al: Beta-thalassemia due to two novel nucleotide substitutions in consensus acceptor splice sequences of the beta-globin gene. Blood 1989; 73:914.

125. Beldjord C, Lapoumeroulie C, et al: A novel beta thalassemia gene with a single base mutation in the conserved polypyrimidine sequence at the 3' end of IVS 2. Nucleic Acids Res 1988; 16:4927.

126. Yang KG, Kutlar F, et al: Molecular characterization of beta-globin gene mutations in Malay patients with Hb E-beta-thalassaemia and thalassaemia major. Br J Haematol 1989; 72:73.

127. Goldsmith ME, Humphries RK, et al: Silent nucleotide substitution in a beta⁺-thalassemia globin gene activates splice site in coding sequence RNA. Proc Natl Acad Sci U S A 1983; 80:2318.

128. Orkin SH, Kazazian HH Jr, et al: Abnormal RNA processing due to the exon mutation of the beta E globin gene. Nature 1982; 300:768.

129. Orkin SH, Antonarakis SE, et al: Abnormal processing of beta Knossos RNA. Blood 1984; 64:311.

130. Spritz RA, Jagadeeswaran P, et al: Base substitution in an intervening sequence of a beta⁺ thalassemic human globin gene. Proc Natl Acad Sci U S A 1981; 78:2455.

131. Westaway D, Williamson R: An intron nucleotide sequence variant in a cloned beta⁺ thalassemia globin gene. Nucleic Acids Res 1981; 9:1777.

132. Metherall JE, Collins FS, et al: Beta zero thalassemia caused by a base substitution that creates an alternative splice acceptor site in an intron. EMBO J 1986; 5:2551.

133. Dobkin C, Pergolizzi RG, et al: Abnormal splice in a mutant human beta-globin gene not at the site of a mutation. Proc Natl Acad Sci U S A 1983; 80:1184.

134. Higgs DR, Goodbourn SE, et al: Alpha-thalassaemia caused by a polyadenylation signal mutation. Nature 1983; 306:398.

135. Thein SL, Wallace RB, et al: The polyadenylation site mutation in the alpha-globin gene cluster. Blood 1988; 71:313.

136. Orkin SH, Cheng TC, et al: Thalassemia due to a mutation in the cleavage-polyadenylation signal of the human beta-globin gene. EMBO J 1985; 4:453.

137. Jankovic L, Efremov GD, et al: Three novel mutations leading to beta thalassemia. Blood 1989; 74:226A.

138. Pirastu M, Saglio G, et al: Initiation codon mutation as a cause of alpha thalassemia. J Biol Chem 1984; 259:12315.

139. Moi P, Cash FE, et al: An initiation codon mutation (AUG→GUG) of the human alpha 1-globin gene. Structural characterization and evidence for a mild thalassemic phenotype. J Clin Invest 1987; 80:1416.

140. Olivieri NF, Chang LS, et al: An alpha-globin gene initiation codon mutation in a black family with Hb H disease. Blood 1987; 70:729.

141. Morle F, Starck J, et al: Alpha-thalassemia due to the deletion of nucleotides −2 and −3 preceding the AUG initiation codon affects translation efficiency both *in vitro* and *in vivo*. Nucleic Acids Res 1986; 14:3279.

142. Morle F, Lopez B, et al: Alpha thalassaemia associated with the deletion of two nucleotides at position −2 and −3 preceding the AUG codon. EMBO J 1985; 4:1245.

143. Landin B, Rudolphi O, et al: Initiation codon mutation (ATG→ATA) of the beta-globin gene causing beta-thalassemia in a Swedish family. Am J Hematol 1995; 48:158.

144. Liebhaber SA, Coleman MB, et al: Molecular basis for nondeletion alpha-thalassemia in American blacks: Alpha 2(116GAG→UAG). J Clin Invest 1987; 80:154.

145. Chang JC, Kan YW: Beta zero thalassemia, a nonsense mutation in man. Proc Natl Acad Sci U S A 1979; 76:2886.

146. Fucharoen S, Fucharoen G, et al: A novel ochre mutation in the beta-thalassemia gene of a Thai. Identification by direct cloning of the entire beta-globin gene amplified using polymerase chain reactions. J Biol Chem 1989; 264:7780.

147. Boehm CD, Dowling CE, et al: Use of oligonucleotide hybridization in the characterization of a beta zero-thalassemia gene (beta 37 TGG→TGA) in a Saudi Arabian family. Blood 1986; 67:1185. Published erratum appears in Blood 1986; 68:323.

148. Trecartin RF, Liebhaber SA, et al: Beta zero thalassemia in Sardinia is caused by a nonsense mutation. J Clin Invest 1981; 68:1017.

149. Chehab FF, Honig GR, et al: Spontaneous mutation in beta-thalassaemia producing the same nucleotide substitution as that in a common hereditary form. Lancet 1986; 1:3.

150. Atweh GF, Brickner HE, et al: New amber mutation in a beta-thalassemic gene with nonmeasurable levels of mutant messenger RNA *in vivo*. J Clin Invest 1988; 82:557.

151. Safaya S, Rieder RF: Dysfunctional alpha-globin gene in hemoglobin H disease in blacks. A dinucleotide deletion produces a frameshift and a termination codon. J Biol Chem 1988; 263:4328.

152. Kollia P, Gonzalez-Redondo JM, et al: Frameshift codon 5 [Fsc-5 (-CT)] thalassemia; a novel mutation detected in a Greek patient. Hemoglobin 1989; 13:597.

153. Kazazian HH Jr, Orkin SH, et al: Beta thalassemia due to a deletion of the nucleotide which is substituted in the beta S-globin gene. Am J Hum Genet 1983; 35:1028.

154. Orkin SH, Goff SC: Nonsense and frameshift mutations in beta thalassemia detected in cloned beta globin genes. J Biol Chem 1981; 256:9782.

155. Chan V, Chan TK, et al: A novel beta-thalassemia frameshift mutation (codon 14/15), detectable by direct visualization of abnormal restriction fragment in amplified genomic DNA. Blood 1988; 72:1420.

156. Schnee J, Griese EU, et al: Beta-thalassemia gene analysis in a Turkish family reveals a 7-bp deletion in the coding region. Blood 1989; 73:2224. Letter.

157. Kimura A, Matsunaga E, et al: Structural analysis of a beta-thalassemia gene found in Taiwan. J Biol Chem 1983; 258:2748.

158. Kinniburgh AJ, Maquat LE, et al: mRNA-deficient beta zero thalassemia results from a single nucleotide deletion. Nucleic Acids Res 1982; 10:5421.

159. Chehab FF, Winterhalter KH, et al: Characterization of a spontaneous mutation in beta-thalassemia associated with advanced paternal age. Blood 1989; 74:852.

160. DiMarzo R, Dowling CE, et al: The spectrum of beta-thalassaemia mutations in Sicily. Br J Haematol 1988; 69:393.

161. Clegg JB, Weatherall DJ, et al: Haemoglobin Constant Spring—a chain termination mutant? Nature 1971; 234:337.

162. Milner PF, Clegg JB, et al: Haemoglobin H disease due to a unique haemoglobin variant with an elongated alpha chain. Lancet 1971; 1:729.

163. Clegg JB, Weatherall DJ, et al: Haemoglobin Icaria, a new chain termination mutant which causes alpha thalassemia. Nature 1974; 251:245.

164. De Jong WW, Khan PM, et al: Hemoglobin Koya Dora: high frequency of a chain termination mutant. Am J Hum Genet 1975; 27:81.

165. Bradley TB, Wohl RC, et al: Elongation of the alpha globin chain in a black family: interaction with Hb G Philadelphia. Clin Res 1975; 23:1314.

166. Lehmann H, Casey R, et al: Hemoglobin Tak: a beta chain elongation. Br J Haematol 1975; 31:119.

167. Honig GR, Shamsuddin M, et al: Hemoglobin Evanston (alpha 14 Trp→Arg): an unstable alpha-chain variant expressed as alpha-thalassemia. J Clin Invest 1984; 73:1740.

168. Sanguansermsri T, Matragoon S: Hemoglobin Suan-Dok (alpha 2 109[G16] Leu-Arg beta 2): an unstable variant associated with alpha thalassemia. Hemoglobin 1979; 3:161.

169. Steinberg MH, Coleman MB, et al: Thalassemic expression of an alpha-2 globin structural mutant. Blood 1987; 70:80A.

170. Honig GR, Shamsuddin M, et al: Hemoglobin Petah Tikvah (alpha110 Ala→Asp): a new unstable variant with alpha-thalassemia-like expression. Blood 1981; 57:705.

171. Goossens M, Lee KY, et al: Globin structural mutant alpha125 Leu→Pro is a novel cause of alpha thalassemia. Nature 1982; 296:864.

172. Liebhaber SA, Kan YW: Alpha thalassemia caused by an unstable alpha-globin mutant. J Clin Invest 1983; 71:461.

173. Podda A, Galanello R, et al: A new unstable hemoglobin variant producing a beta-thalassemia-like phenotype. Presented before the Third International Conference on Thalassemia and the Hemoglobinopathies, Sardinia, 1989, p 51.

872 • Disorders of Hemoglobin

174. Kobayashi Y, Fukumaki Y, et al: A novel globin structural mutant, Showa-Yakushiji (beta 110 Leu-Pro) causing a beta-thalassemia phenotype. Blood 1987; 70:1688.

175. Adams JG, Steinberg MH, et al: The structure of hemoglobin Indianapolis (beta112[G14] Arginine): an unstable variant detectable only by isotopic labelling. J Biol Chem 1979; 254:3479.

176. Kazazian HH Jr, Dowling CE, et al: Thalassemia mutations in exon 3 of the beta globin gene often cause a dominant form of thalassemia and show no predilection for malarial-endemic regions of the world. Am J Hum Genet 1989; 45:A242.

177. Hattori Y, Yamane A, et al: Characterization of beta-thalassemia mutations among the Japanese. Hemoglobin 1989; 13:657.

178. Ristaldi MS, Pirastu M, et al: A spontaneous mutation produced a novel elongated beta-globin chain structural variant (Hb Agnana) with a thalassemia-like phenotype. Blood 1990; 75:1378. Letter.

179. Beris P, Miescher PA, et al: Inclusion body beta-thalassemia trait in a Swiss family is caused by an abnormal hemoglobin (Geneva) with an altered and extended beta chain carboxy-terminus due to a modification in codon beta 114. Blood 1988; 72:801.

180. Thein SL, Hesketh C, et al: Molecular basis for dominantly inherited inclusion body beta thalassemia. Proc Natl Acad Sci U S A 1990; 87:3924.

181. Kazazian HH Jr, Orkin SH, et al: Characterization of a spontaneous mutation to a beta-thalassemia allele. Am J Hum Genet 1989; 38:860.

182. Fei YJ, Stoming TA, et al: One form of inclusion body beta-thalassemia is due to a GAA→TAA mutation at codon 121 of the beta chain. Blood 1989; 73:1075.

183. Ristaldi MS, Murru S, et al: The C→T substitution in the distal CACCC box of the beta-globin gene promoter is a common cause of silent beta thalassemia in the Italian population. Br J Haematol 1990; 74:480.

184. Nuez B, Michalovich D, et al: Defective haematopoiesis in fetal liver resulting from inactivation of the *EKLF* gene. Nature 1995; 375:316.

185. Perkins AC, Sharpe AH, et al: Lethal β-thalassaemia in mice lacking the erythroid CACCC-transcription factor EKLF. Nature 195; 375:318.

186. Brinster RL, Allen JM, et al: Introns increase transcriptional efficiency in transgenic mice. Proc Natl Acad Sci U S A 1988; 85:836.

187. Buchman AR, Berg P: Comparison of intron-dependent and intron-independent gene expression. Mol Cell Biol 1988; 8:4395.

188. Chang DD, Sharp PA: Messenger RNA transport and HIV rev regulation. Science 1990; 249:614.

189. Gonzalez-Redondo JM, Stoming TA, et al: Severe Hb S-beta zero-thalassaemia with a T→C substitution in the donor splice site of the first intron of the beta-globin gene. Br J Haematol 1989; 71:113.

190. Treisman R, Orkin SH, et al: Specific transcription and RNA splicing defects in five cloned beta-thalassaemia genes. Nature 1983; 302:591.

191. Busslinger M, Moschonas N, et al: Beta-thalassemia: aberrant splicing results from a single point mutation in an intron. Cell 1981; 27:289.

192. Fukumaki Y, Ghosh PK, et al: Abnormally spliced messenger RNA in erythroid cells from patients with beta thalassemia and monkey kidney cells expressing a cloned beta-thalassemia gene. Cell 1982; 28:585.

193. Whitelaw E, Proudfoot N: Alpha-thalassaemia caused by a poly(A) site mutation reveals that transcriptional termination is linked to 3′ end processing in the human alpha 2 globin gene. EMBO J 1986; 5:2915.

194. Kozak M: An analysis of 5′-noncoding sequences from 699 vertebrate messenger RNAs. Nucleic Acids Res 1987; 15:8125.

195. Baserga SJ, Benz EJ: Nonsense mutations in the human beta-globin gene affect mRNA metabolism. Proc Natl Acad Sci U S A 1988; 85:2056.

196. Chang JC, Temple GF, et al: Suppression of the nonsense mutation in homozygous beta thalassemia. Nature 1979; 281:602.

197. Benz EJ Jr, Forget BG, et al: Variability in the amount of beta-globin mRNA in beta thalassemia. Cell 1978; 14:299.

198. Maquat LE, Kinniburgh AJ, et al: Unstable beta-globin mRNA in mRNA-deficient beta-thalassemia. Cell 1981; 27:543.

199. Humphries RK, Ley TJ, et al: Beta-39-thalassemia gene: a premature termination codon causes beta-mRNA deficiency without changing cytoplasmic beta-mRNA stability. Blood 1984; 23:64.

200. Takeshita K, Forget BG, et al: Intranuclear defect in beta-globin mRNA accumulation due to a premature translation termination codon. Blood 1984; 64:13.

201. Liebhaber SA, Kan YW: Differentiation of the mRNA transcripts originating from the alpha-1 and alpha-2 globin loci in normals and alpha thalassemics. J Clin Invest 1981; 68:439.

202. Hunt DM, Higgs DR, et al: Haemoglobin Constant Spring has an unstable alpha chain messenger RNA. Br J Haematol 1982; 51:405.

203. Derry S, Wood WG, et al: Hematologic and biosynthetic studies in homozygous hemoglobin Constant Spring. J Clin Invest 1984; 73:1673.

204. Bunn HF, Schmidt GJ, et al: Hemoglobin Cranston, an unstable variant having an elongated beta chain due to non-homologous cross over between two normal beta chain genes. Proc Natl Acad Sci U S A 1975; 72:3609.

205. Bunn HF: Subunit assembly of hemoglobin: an important determinant of hematologic phenotype. Blood 1987; 69:1.

206. Eaton WA: The relationship between coding sequences and function in haemoglobins. Nature 1980; 284:183.

207. Adams JG III, Coleman MB, et al: Modulation of fetal hemoglobin synthesis by iron deficiency. N Engl J Med 1985; 313:1402.

208. Chui DHK, Patterson M, et al: Hemoglobin Bart's disease in an Italian boy. N Engl J Med 1990; 323:179.

209. Adams HGI, Coleman MB: Structural hemoglobin variants that produce the phenotype of thalassemia. Semin Hematol 1990; 27:229.

210. Flavell RA, Bernards R, et al: The structure of the human beta-globin gene in beta-thalassaemia. Nucleic Acids Res 1979; 6:2749.

211. Orkin SH, Old JM, et al: Partial deletion of beta-globin gene DNA in certain patients with beta-thalassemia. Proc Natl Acad Sci U S A 1979; 76:2400.

212. Orkin SH, Kolodner R, et al: Cloning and direct examination of a structurally abnormal human beta-thalassemia globin gene. Proc Natl Acad Sci U S A 1980; 77:3558.

213. Moschonas N, deBoer E, et al: Structure and expression of a cloned beta thalassemia globin gene. Nucleic Acids Res 1982; 9:4391.

214. Rosatelli C, Falchi AM, et al: Prenatal diagnosis of beta-thalassaemia with the synthetic-oligomer technique. Lancet 1985; 1:241.

215. Antonarakis SE, Boehm CD, et al: Nonrandom associations of polymorphic restriction sites in the beta-globin gene cluster. Proc Natl Acad Sci U S A 1982; 79:137.

216. Kazazian HH Jr, Orkin SH, et al: Quantification of the close association between DNA haplotypes and specific beta-thalassaemia mutations in Mediterraneans. Nature 1984; 310:152.

217. Jeffreys AJ: DNA sequence variants in the G gamma-, A gamma-, delta-, and beta-globin genes of man. Cell 1979; 18:1.

218. Kan YW, Dozy AM: Polymorphism of DNA sequence adjacent to human beta-globin structural gene: Relationship to sickle mutation. Proc Natl Acad Sci U S A 1978; 75:5631.

219. Antonarakis SE, Kazazian HH Jr, et al: DNA polymorphism molecular pathology of the human globin gene clusters. Hum Genet 1985; 69:1.

220. Higgs DR, Wainscoat JS, et al: Analysis of the human alpha-globin gene cluster reveals a highly informative genetic locus. Proc Natl Acad Sci U S A 1986; 83:5165.

221. Chakravarti A, Buetow KH, et al: Nonuniform recombination within the human beta-globin gene cluster. Am J Hum Genet 1984; 36:1239.

222. Wainscoat JS, Hill AVS, et al: Evolutionary relationships of human populations from an analysis of nuclear DNA polymorphisms. Nature 1986; 319:491.

223. Gerhard DS, Kidd KK, et al: Identification of a recent recombination event within the human beta-globin gene cluster. Proc Natl Acad Sci U S A 1984; 81:7875.

224. Old JM, Heath C, et al: Meiotic recombination between two polymorphic restriction sites within the beta globin gene cluster. J Med Genet 1986; 23:14.

225. Antonarakis SE, Orkin SH, et al: Evidence for multiple origins

of the beta E-globin gene in Southeast Asia. Proc Natl Acad Sci U S A 1982; 79:6608.

226. Chehab FF, Doherty M, et al: Detection of sickle cell anaemia and thalassaemias. Nature 1987; 329:293. Letter. Published erratum appears in Nature 1987; 329:678.

227. Kulozik AE, Lyons J, et al: Rapid and non-radioactive prenatal diagnosis of beta thalassaemia and sickle cell disease: application of the polymerase chain reaction (PCR). Br J Haematol 1988; 70:455.

228. Pirastu M, Ristaldi MS, et al: Prenatal diagnosis of beta thalassaemia based on restriction endonuclease analysis of amplified fetal DNA. J Med Genet 1989; 26:363.

229. Pirastu M, Kan YW, et al: Prenatal diagnosis of beta-thalassemia. Detection of a single nucleotide mutation in DNA. N Engl J Med 1983; 309:284.

230. Orkin SH, Markham AF, et al: Direct detection of the common Mediterranean beta-thalassemia gene with synthetic DNA probes. An alternative approach for prenatal diagnosis. J Clin Invest 1983; 71:775.

231. Wallace RB, Schold M, et al: Oligonucleotide directed mutagenesis of the human beta-globin gene: a general method for producing specific point mutations in cloned DNA. Nucleic Acids Res 1981; 9:3647.

232. Saiki RK, Chang CA, et al: Diagnosis of sickle cell anemia and beta-thalassemia with enzymatically amplified DNA and nonradioactive allele-specific oligonucleotide probes. N Engl J Med 1988; 319:537.

233. Cai SP, Zhang JZ, et al: A simple approach to prenatal diagnosis of beta-thalassemia in a geographic area where multiple mutations occur. Blood 1988; 71:1357.

234. Cai SP, Chang CA, et al: Rapid prenatal diagnosis of beta thalassemia using DNA amplification and nonradioactive probes. Blood 1989; 73:372.

235. Ristaldi MS, Pirastu M, et al: Prenatal diagnosis of beta-thalassaemia in Mediterranean populations by dot blot analysis with DNA amplification and allele specific oligonucleotide probes. Prenat Diagn 1989; 9:629.

236. Sutcharitchan P, Saiki R, et al: Reverse dot-blot detection of Thai beta-thalassaemia mutations. Br J Haematol 1995; 90:809.

237. Giambona A, Lo Gioco P, et al: The great heterogeneity of thalassemia molecular defects in Sicily. Hum Genet 1995; 95:526.

238. Myers RM, Lumelsky M, et al: A new strategy for detecting point mutations in genomic DNA. Nature 1985; 313:495.

239. Myers RM, Fischer SG, et al: Nearly all single base substitutions in DNA fragments joined to a GC-clamp can be detected by denaturing gradient gel electrophoresis. Nucleic Acids Res 1985; 13:3131.

240. Cai SP, Kan YW: Identification of the multiple beta-thalassemia mutations by denaturing gradient gel electrophoresis. J Clin Invest 1990; 85:550.

241. Saiki RK, Scharf S, et al: Enzymatic amplification of beta-globin genomic sequences and restriction site analysis for diagnosis of sickle cell anemia. Science 1985; 230:1350.

242. Saiki RK, Gelfand DH, et al: Primer-directed enzymatic amplification of DNA with a thermostable DNA polymerase. Science 1988; 239:487.

243. Erlich HA, Gelfand DH, et al: Specific DNA amplification. Nature 1988; 331:461.

244. Eisenstein BI: The polymerase chain reaction: a new method of using molecular genetics for medical diagnosis. N Engl J Med 1990; 322:178.

245. Thein SL, Hesketh C, et al: The molecular basis of thalassaemia major and thalassaemia intermedia in Asian Indians: application to prenatal diagnosis. Br J Haematol 1988; 70:225.

246. Kazazian HH Jr, Dowling CE, et al: The spectrum of beta-thalassemia genes in China and Southeast Asia. Blood 1986; 68:964.

247. Zhang JZ, Cai SP, et al: Molecular basis of beta thalassemia in south China: Strategy for DNA analysis. Hum Genet 1988; 78:37.

248. Diaz-Chico JC, Yang KG, et al: Mild and severe beta-thalassemia among homozygotes from Turkey: Identification of the types by hybridization of amplified DNA with synthetic probes. Blood 1988; 71:248.

249. Amselem S, Nunes V, et al: Determination of the spectrum of beta-thalassemia genes in Spain by use of dot-blot analysis of amplified beta-globin DNA. Am J Hum Genet 1988; 43:95.

250. Weatherall DJ, Wood WG, et al: The developmental genetics of human hemoglobin. In Stamatoyannopoulos G, Nienhuis AW (eds): Experimental Approaches for the Study of Hemoglobin Switching. New York, Alan R. Liss, Inc., 1985, p 3.

251. Charache S, Clegg JB, et al: The Negro variety of hereditary persistence of fetal hemoglobin is a model form of thalassemia. Br J Haematol 1976; 34:527.

252. Friedman S, Schwartz E, et al: Variation in globin chain synthesis in hereditary persistence of fetal hemoglobin. Br J Haematol 1976; 32:357.

253. Henthorn PS, Smithies O, et al: Molecular analysis of deletions in the human beta-globin gene cluster: deletion junctions and locations of breakpoints. Genomics 1990; 6:226.

254. Oggiano L, Pirastu M, et al: Molecular characterization of a normal Hb A2 beta-thalassaemia determinant in a Sardinian family. Br J Haematol 1987; 67:225.

255. Moi P, Paglietti E, et al: Delineation of the molecular basis of delta- and normal HbA2 beta-thalassemia. Blood 1988; 72:530.

256. Tate VE, Hill AV, et al: A silent deletion in the beta-globin gene cluster. Nucleic Acids Res 1986; 14:4743.

257. Kulozik AE, Yarwood N, et al: The Corfu delta beta zero thalassemia: a small deletion acts at a distance to selectively abolish beta globin gene expression. Blood 1988; 71:457. Published erratum appears in Blood 1988; 71:1509.

258. Galanello R, Podda A, et al: Interaction between deletion delta-thalassemia and beta zero-thalassemia (codon 39 nonsense mutation) in a Sardinian family. Prog Clin Biol Res 1989; 316B:113.

259. Spritz RA, Orkin SH: Duplication followed by deletion accounts for the structure of an Indian deletion beta thalassemia. Nucleic Acids Res 1982; 10:8025.

260. Padanilam BJ, Felice AE, et al: Partial deletion of the 5' beta-globin gene region causes beta zero-thalassemia in members of an American black family. Blood 1984; 64:941.

261. Anand R, Boehm CD, et al: Molecular characterization of a beta zero-thalassemia resulting from a 1.4 kilobase deletion. Blood 1988; 72:636.

262. Gilman JG, Huisman TH, et al: Dutch beta°-thalassaemia: a 10 kilobase DNA deletion associated with significant gamma-chain production. Br J Haematol 1984; 56:339.

263. Gilman JG: The 12.6 kilobase DNA deletion in Dutch beta zero-thalassaemia. Br J Haematol 1987; 67:369.

264. Diaz-Chico JC, Yang KG, et al: An approximately 300 bp deletion involving part of the 5' beta-globin gene region is observed in members of a Turkish family with beta-thalassemia. Blood 1987; 70:583.

265. Spiegelberg R, Aulehla SC, et al: A beta-thalassemia gene caused by a 290-base pair deletion: analysis by direct sequencing of enzymatically amplified DNA. Blood 1989; 73:1695.

266. Aulehla-Scholz C, Spiegelberg R, et al: A beta-thalassemia mutant caused by a 300-bp deletion in the human beta-globin gene. Hum Genet 1989; 81:298.

267. Popovich BW, Rosenblatt DS, et al: Molecular characterization of an atypical beta-thalassemia caused by a large deletion in the 5' beta-globin gene region. Am J Hum Genet 1986; 39:797.

268. Ottolenghi S, Giglioni B: Delta beta thalassemia is due to a gene deletion. Cell 1976; 9:71.

269. Ramirez F, O'Donnell JV, et al: Abnormal or absent beta mRNA in beta Ferrara and gene deletion in delta beta thalassemia. Nature 1976; 263:471.

270. Bernards R, Kooter JM, et al: Physical mapping of the globin gene deletion in delta beta thalassemia. Gene 1979; 6:265.

271. Ottolenghi S, Giglioni B: The deletion in a type of delta beta thalassemia begins in an inverted Alu I repeat. Nature 1982; 300:770.

272. Ottolenghi S, Giglioni B, et al: Molecular comparison of delta beta thalassemia and hereditary persistence of fetal hemoglobin DNAs: evidence of a regulatory area? Proc Natl Acad Sci U S A 1982; 79:2347.

273. Feingold EA, Forget BG: The breakpoint of a large deletion causing hereditary persistence of fetal hemoglobin occurs within an erythroid DNA domain remote from the beta-globin gene cluster. Blood 1989; 74:2178.

274. Anagnou NP, Papayannopoulou T, et al: Structurally diverse molecular deletions in the beta-globin gene cluster exhibit an identical phenotype on interaction with the beta S-gene. Blood 1985; 65:1245.

275. Matsunaga E, Kimura A, et al: A novel deletion in delta beta-thalassemia found in Japan. Biochem Biophys Res Commun 1985; 126:185.

276. Shiokawa S, Yamada H, et al: Molecular analysis of Japanese delta beta-thalassemia. Blood 1988; 72:1771.

277. Zhang JW, Stamatoyannopoulos G, et al: Laotian (delta-beta)°-thalassemia: molecular characterization of a novel deletion associated with increased production of fetal hemoglobin. Blood 1988; 72:983.

278. Efremov GD, Nikolov N, et al: The 18- to 23-kb deletion of the Macedonian delta beta-thalassemia includes the entire delta and beta globin genes. Blood 1986; 68:971.

279. Baglioni C: The fusion of two peptide chains in hemoglobin Lepore and its interpretation as a genetic deletion. Proc Natl Acad Sci U S A 1962; 48:1880.

280. Flavell RA, Kooter JM, et al: Analysis of the beta delta globin gene loci in normal and Hb Lepore DNA: direct determination of gene linkage and intergene distance. Cell 1978; 15:25.

281. Baird M, Driscoll C, et al: Localization of the site of recombination in formation of the Lepore Boston globin gene. J Clin Invest 1981; 68:560.

282. Mavilio F, Giampaolo A, et al: The delta-beta crossover region in Lepore Boston hemoglobinopathy is restricted to a 59 base pair region around the 5' splice junction of the large globin gene intervening sequence. Blood 1983; 62:230.

283. Dobkin C, Clyne J, et al: Expression of a cloned Lepore globin gene. Blood 1986; 67:168.

284. Jones RW, Old JM, et al: Major rearrangement in the human beta globin gene cluster. Nature 1981; 291:39.

285. Jennings MW, Jones RW, et al: Analysis of an inversion within the human beta globin gene cluster. Nucleic Acids Res 1985; 13:2897.

286. Henthorn PS, Smithies O, et al: (A gamma delta beta)-Thalassaemia in blacks is due to a deletion of 34 kbp of DNA. Br J Haematol 1985; 59:343.

287. Orkin SH, Alter BP, et al: Deletion of the A gamma-globin gene in G gamma-delta beta-thalassemia. J Clin Invest 1979; 64:866.

288. Tuan D, Feingold E, et al: Different 3' end points of deletions causing delta beta-thalassemia and hereditary persistence of fetal hemoglobin: implications for the control of gamma-globin gene expression in man. Proc Natl Acad Sci U S A 1983; 80:6937.

289. Trent RJ, Jones RW, et al: (A gamma delta beta) thalassaemia: similarity of phenotype in four different molecular defects, including one newly described. Br J Haematol 1984; 57:279.

290. George E, Faridah K, et al: Homozygosity for a new type of G gamma (A gamma delta beta)°-thalassemia in a Malaysian male. Hemoglobin 1986; 10:353.

291. Jones RW, Old JM, et al.: Restriction mapping of a new deletion responsible for G gamma(delta-beta)° thalassemia. Nucleic Acids Res 1981; 9:6813.

292. Mager DL, Henthorn PS, et al: A Chinese G gamma + (A gamma delta beta)° thalassemia deletion: comparison to other deletions in the human beta-globin gene cluster and sequence analysis of the breakpoints. Nucleic Acids Res 1985; 13:6559.

293. Anagnou NP, Papayannopoulou T, et al: Molecular characterization of a novel form of (A gamma delta beta)°-thalassemia deletion with a 3' breakpoint close to those of HPFH-3 and HPFH-4: Insights for a common regulatory mechanism. Nucleic Acids Res 1988; 16:6057.

294. Zeng YT, Huang SZ, et al: Hereditary persistence of fetal hemoglobin or (delta beta)°-thalassemia: three types observed in South-Chinese families. Blood 1985; 66:1430.

295. Driscoll MC, Dobkin CS, et al: Gamma delta beta-thalassemia due to a de novo mutation deleting the 5' beta-globin gene activation-region hypersensitive sites. Proc Natl Acad Sci U S A 1989; 86:7470.

296. Curtin P, Pirastu M, et al: A distant gene deletion affects beta-globin gene function in an atypical gamma delta beta-thalassemia. J Clin Invest 1985; 76:1554.

297. Kioussis D, Vanin E, et al: Beta-globin gene inactivation by DNA translocation in gamma beta-thalassaemia. Nature 1983; 306:662.

298. Vanin EF, Henthorn PS, et al: Unexpected relationships between four large deletions in the human beta-globin gene cluster. Cell 1983; 35:701.

299. Wright S, Taramelli R, et al: DNA sequences required for regulated expression of the human beta-globin gene. Prog Clin Biol Res 1985; 191:251.

300. Orkin SH, Goff SC, et al: Heterogeneity of the DNA deletion in gamma-delta-beta thalassemia. J Clin Invest 1981; 67:878.

301. Pirastu M, Kan YW, et al: Hemolytic disease of the newborn caused by a new deletion of the entire beta-globin cluster. J Clin Invest 1983; 72:602.

302. Fearon ER, Kazazian HJ, et al: The entire beta-globin gene cluster is deleted in a form of gamma delta beta-thalassemia. Blood 1983; 61:1269.

303. Diaz-Chico JC, Huang HJ, et al: Two new large deletions resulting in epsilon gamma delta beta-thalassemia. Acta Haematol 1988; 80:79.

304. Fritsch EF, Lawn RM, et al: Characterization of deletions which affect the expression of fetal globin genes in man. Nature 1979; 279:598.

305. Bernards R, Flavell RA: Physical mapping of the globin gene deletion in hereditary persistence of foetal hemoglobin (HPFH). Nucleic Acids Res 1980; 8:1521.

306. Jagadeeswaran P, Tuan D, et al: A gene deletion ending at the midpoint of a repetitive DNA sequence in one form of hereditary persistence of fetal hemoglobin. Nature 1982; 296:469.

307. Tuan D, Murnane MJ, et al: Heterogeneity in the molecular basis of hereditary persistence of fetal hemoglobin. Nature 1980; 285:335.

308. Kutlar A, Gardiner MB, et al: Heterogeneity in the molecular basis of three types of hereditary persistence of fetal hemoglobin and the relative synthesis of the G gamma and A gamma types of gamma chains. Biochem Genet 1984; 22:21.

309. Wainscoat JS, Old JM, et al: Characterization of an Indian (delta beta)0 thalassaemia. Br J Haematol 1984; 58:353.

310. Henthorn PS, Mager D, et al: A gene deletion ending within a complex array of repeated sequences 3' to the human beta-globin gene cluster. Proc Natl Acad Sci U S A 1986; 83:5194.

311. Saglio G, Camaschella C, et al: Italian type of deletional hereditary persistence of fetal hemoglobin. Blood 1986; 68:646.

312. Camaschella C, Serra A, et al: A new hereditary persistence of fetal hemoglobin deletion has the breakpoint within the 3' beta-globin gene enhancer. Blood 1990; 75:1000.

313. Huisman THJ, Wrightstone RN, et al: Hemoglobin Kenya: the product of fusion of alpha- and beta-polypeptide chains. Arch Biochem Biophys 1972; 152:850.

314. Kendall AG, Ojwang PJ, et al: Hemoglobin Kenya, the product of a gamma-beta fusion gene: studies of the family. Am J Hum Genet 1973; 25:548.

315. Nute PE, Wood WG, et al: The Kenya form of hereditary persistence of fetal hemoglobin: structural studies and evidence for homogeneous distribution of haemoglobin F using fluorescent anti-haemoglobin F antibodies. Br J Haematol 1976; 32:55.

316. Ojwang PJ, Nakatsuji T, et al: Gene deletion as the molecular basis for the Kenya-G gamma-HPFH condition. Hemoglobin 1983; 7:115.

317. Gerald PS, Diamond LK: The diagnosis of thalassemia trait by starch block electrophoresis of the hemoglobin. Blood 1958; 13:61.

318. Mears JG, Ramirez F, et al: Changes in restricted human cellular DNA fragments containing globin gene sequences in thalassemia related disorders. Proc Natl Acad Sci U S A 1978; 75:1222.

319. Fessas P, Karaklis A: Two-dimensional paper-agar electrophoresis of hemoglobin. Clin Chim Acta 1962; 7:133.

320. Duma H, Efremov G, et al: Study of nine families with hemoglobin Lepore. Br J Haematol 1978; 15:161.

321. Lehmann H, Charlesworth D: Observations on hemoglobin P (Congo type). Biochem J 1970; 119:43.

322. Ohta Y, Yamaoka K, et al: Hemoglobin Miyada, a beta-delta fusion peptide (anti-Lepore) type discovered in a Japanese family. Nature (New Biol) 1971; 234:218.

323. Baird FM, Lorkin PA, et al: Hemoglobin P Nilotic containing a beta-delta chain. Nature (New Biol) 1973; 242:107.

324. Kimura A, Ohta Y, et al: A fusion gene in man: DNA sequence analysis of the abnormal globin gene of hemoglobin Miyada. Biochem Biophys Res Commun 1984; 119:968.

325. Huisman THJ, Shroeder WA, et al: Hemoglobin Kenya, the product of non-homologous crossing-over of gamma and beta genes. Blood 1972; 40:947.

326. Huisman THJ, Schroeder WA, et al: The present status of the heterogeneity of fetal hemoglobin in beta-thalassemia: an attempt to unify some observations in thalassemia and related conditions. Ann N Y Acad Sci 1974; 232:107.

327. Oner C, Oner R, et al: A new Turkish type of beta-thalassaemia major with homozygosity for two non-consecutive 7.6 kb deletions of the psi beta and beta genes and an intact delta gene. Br J Haematol 1995; 89:306.

328. Schmid CW, Jelinek WR: The Alu family of dispersed repetitive sequences. Science 1982; 216:1065.

329. Kan YW, Forget BG, et al: Gamma-beta thalassemia: a cause of hemolytic disease of newborns. N Engl J Med 1972; 286:129.

330. Stolle CA, Penny LA, et al: Sequence analysis of the gamma-globin gene locus from a patient with the deletion form of hereditary persistence of fetal hemoglobin. Blood 1990; 75:499.

331. Elder JT, Forrester WC, et al: Translocation of an erythroid-specific hypersensitive site in deletion-type hereditary persistence of fetal hemoglobin. Mol Cell Biol 1990; 10:1382.

332. Feingold EA, Forget BG: The breakpoint of a large deletion causing hereditary persistence of fetal hemoglobin occurs within an erythroid DNA domain remote from the beta-globin gene cluster. Blood 1989; 74:2178.

333. Collins FS, Stoeckert CJJ, et al: G gamma beta+ hereditary persistence of fetal hemoglobin: cosmid cloning and identification of a specific mutation 5' to the G gamma gene. Proc Natl Acad Sci U S A 1984; 81:4894.

334. Collins FS, Boehm CD, et al: Concordance of a point mutation 5' to the gamma globin gene with G gamma beta hereditary persistence of fetal hemoglobin in the Black population. Blood 1984; 64:1292.

335. Gilman JG, Mishima N, et al: Upstream promoter mutation associated with a modest elevation of fetal hemoglobin expression in human adults. Blood 1988; 72:78.

336. Weatherall DJ, Cartner R, et al: A form of hereditary persistence of fetal haemoglobin characterized by uneven cellular distribution of haemoglobin F and the production of haemoglobins A and A2 in homozygotes. Br J Haematol 1975; 29:205.

337. Old JM, Ayyub H, et al: Linkage analysis of nondeletion hereditary persistence of fetal hemoglobin. Science 1982; 215:981.

338. Tate VE, Wood WG, et al: The British form of hereditary persistence of fetal hemoglobin results from a single base mutation adjacent to an S1 hypersensitive site 5' to the A gamma globin gene. Blood 1986; 68:1389.

339. Farquhar M, Gelinas R, et al: Restriction endonuclease mapping of gamma-delta-beta-globin region in G gamma (beta)+ HPFH and a Chinese A gamma HPFH variant. Am J Hum Genet 1983; 35:611.

340. Gelinas R, Bender M, et al: C to T at position −196 of the A gamma gene promoter. Blood 1986; 67:1777.

341. Yang KG, Stoming TA, et al: Identification of base substitutions in the promoter regions of the A gamma- and G gamma-globin genes in A gamma- (or G gamma-) beta+-HPFH heterozygotes using the DNA-amplification-synthetic oligonucleotide procedure. Blood 1988; 71:1414.

342. Giglioni B, Casini C, et al: A molecular study of a family with Greek hereditary persistence of fetal hemoglobin and beta-thalassemia. EMBO J 1984; 3:2641.

343. Ottolenghi S, Giglioni B, et al: Sardinian delta beta zero-thalassemia: a further example of a C to T substitution at position −196 of the A gamma globin gene promoter. Blood 1987; 69:1058.

344. Ottolenghi S, Nicolis S, et al: Sardinian G gamma-HPFH: a T→C substitution in a conserved "octamer" sequence in the G gamma-globin promoter. Blood 1988; 71:815.

345. Surrey S, Delgrosso K, et al: A single-base change at position −175 in the 5'-flanking region of the G gamma-globin gene from a black with G gamma-beta+ HPFH. Blood 1988; 71:807.

346. Stoming TA, Stoming GS, et al: An A gamma type of nondeletional hereditary persistence of fetal hemoglobin with a T→C mutation at position −175 to the cap site of the A gamma globin gene. Blood 1989; 73:329.

347. Gilman JG, Kutlar F, et al: A G to A nucleotide substitution 161 base pairs 5' of the G gamma globin gene cap site (−161) in a high G gamma non-anemic person. Prog Clin Biol Res 1987; 251:383.

348. Pembrey ME, Wood WG, et al: Fetal hemoglobin production and the sickle gene in the oases of Eastern Saudi Arabia. Br J Haematol 1978; 40:415.

349. Wainscoat JS, Thein SL, et al: A genetic marker for elevated levels of hemoglobin F in homozygous sickle cell disease? Br J Haematol 1985; 60:261.

350. Gilman JG, Huisman THJ: DNA sequence variation associated with elevated fetal G gamma globin production. Blood 1985; 66:783.

351. Labie D, Pagnier J, et al: Common haplotype dependency of high G gamma-globin gene expression and high Hb F levels in beta-thalassemia and sickle cell anemia patients. Proc Natl Acad Sci U S A 1985; 82:2111.

352. Labie D, Dunda BO, et al: The −158 site 5' to the G gamma gene and G gamma expression. Blood 1985; 66:1463.

353. Miller BA, Salameh M, et al: High fetal hemoglobin production in sickle cell anemia in the eastern province of Saudi Arabia is genetically determined. Blood 1986; 67:1404.

354. Miller BA, Olivieri N, et al: Molecular analysis of the high-hemoglobin-F phenotype in Saudi Arabian sickle cell anemia. N Engl J Med 1987; 316:244.

355. Collins FS, Metherall JE, et al: A point mutation in the A gamma-globin gene promoter in Greek hereditary persistence of fetal haemoglobin. Nature 1985; 313:325.

356. Gelinas R, Endlich B, et al: G to A substitution in the distal CCAAT box of the A gamma-globin gene in Greek hereditary persistence of fetal haemoglobin. Nature 1985; 313:323.

357. Ottolenghi S, Camaschella C, et al: A frequent A gamma-hereditary persistence of fetal hemoglobin in northern Sardinia: its molecular basis and hematologic phenotype in heterozygotes and compound heterozygotes with beta-thalassemia. Hum Genet 1988; 79:13.

358. Gilman JG, Mishima N, et al: Distal CCAAT box deletion in the A gamma globin gene of two black adolescents with elevated fetal A gamma globin. Nucl Acids Res 1988; 16:10635.

359. Marti HR: Normale und Anormale Menschliche Hemoglobine. Berlin, Springer Verlag, 1963, p 81.

360. Jensen M, Wirtz A, et al: Hereditary persistence of fetal haemoglobin (HPFH) in conjunction with a chromosomal translocation involving the haemoglobin beta locus. Br J Haematol 1984; 56:87.

361. Sukumaran PK, Huisman THJ, et al: A homozygote for the gamma type of fetal hemoglobin in India: a study of two Indians and four Negro families. Br J Haematol 1972; 23:403.

362. Boyer SH, Margolet L, et al: Inheritance of F cell frequency in heterocellular hereditary persistence of fetal hemoglobin: an example of allelic exclusion. Am J Hum Genet 1977; 29:256.

363. Stamatoyannopoulos G, Wood WG, et al: A new form of hereditary persistence of fetal hemoglobin in blacks and its association with sickle cell trait. Blood 1975; 46:683.

364. Gelinas RE, Rixon M, et al: Gamma gene promoter and enhancer structure in Seattle variant of hereditary persistence of fetal hemoglobin. Blood 1988; 71:1108.

365. Gumucio DL, Rood KL, et al: Nuclear proteins that bind the human gamma-globin gene promoter: alterations in binding produced by point mutations associated with hereditary persistence of fetal hemoglobin. Mol Cell Biol 1988; 8:5310.

366. Superti-Furga G, Barberis A, et al: The −117 mutation in Greek HPFH affects the binding of three nuclear factors to the CCAAT region of the gamma-globin gene. EMBO J 1988; 7:3099.

367. Martin DI, Tsai SF, et al: Increased gamma-globin expression in a nondeletion HPFH mediated by an erythroid-specific DNA-binding factor. Nature 1989; 338:435.

368. Mantovani R, Superti FG, et al: The deletion of the distal CCAAT box region of the A gamma-globin gene in black HPFH abolishes the binding of the erythroid specific protein NFE3 and of the CCAAT displacement protein. Nucleic Acids Res 1989; 17:6681.

369. Sykes K, Kaufman R: A naturally occurring gamma globin gene mutation enhances SP1 binding activity. Mol Cell Biol 1990; 10:95.

370. Ronchi A, Nicolis S, et al: Increased Sp1 binding mediates erythroid-specific overexpression of a mutated (HPFH) gamma-globulin promoter. Nucleic Acids Res 1989; 17:10231.

371. Ottolenghi S, Mantovani R, et al: DNA sequences regulating

human globin gene transcription in nondeletional hereditary persistence of fetal hemoglobin. Hemoglobin 1989; 13:523.

372. Wood WG, MacRae IA, et al: The British type of non-deletion HPFH: characterization of developmental changes *in vivo* and erythroid growth *in vitro*. Br J Haematol 1982; 30:401.

373. Camaschella C, Oggiano L, et al: The homozygous state of G to A–117A gamma hereditary persistence of fetal hemoglobin. Blood 1989; 73:1999.

374. Friedman S, Schwartz E: Hereditary persistence of foetal haemoglobin with beta-chain synthesis in *cis* position (Ggamma-beta+-HPFH) in a Negro family. Nature 1976; 259:138.

375. Nicholls RD, Jonasson JA, et al: High resolution gene mapping of the human alpha globin locus. J Med Genet 1987; 24:39.

376. Simmers RN, Mulley JC, et al: Mapping the human alpha globin gene complex to 16p13.2-pter. J Med Genet 1987; 24:761.

377. Nicholls RD, Fischel-Ghodsian N, et al: Recombination at the human alpha-globin gene cluster: sequence features and topological constraints. Cell 1987; 49:369.

378. Sawada I, Schmid CW: Primate evolution of the alpha-globin gene cluster and its Alu-like repeats. J Mol Biol 1986; 192:693.

379. Michelson AM, Orkin SH: Boundaries of gene conversion within the duplicated human alpha-globin genes. Concerted evolution by segmental recombination. J Biol Chem 1983; 258:15245.

380. Hess JF, Schmid CW, et al: A gradient of sequence divergence in the human adult alpha-globin duplication units. Science 1984; 226:67.

381. Higgs DR, Hill AV, et al: Independent recombination events between the duplicated human alpha globin genes; implications for their concerted evolution. Nucl Acids Res 1984; 12:6965.

382. Foldi J, Cohen-Solal M, et al: The human alpha-globin gene. The protein products of the duplicated genes are identical. Eur J Biochem 1980; 109:463.

383. Orkin SH, Goff SC: The duplicated human alpha-globin genes: their relative expression as measured by RNA analysis. Cell 1981; 24:345.

384. Liebhaber SA, Cash FE, et al: Compensatory increase in alpha 1-globin gene expression in individuals heterozygous for the alpha-thalassemia-2 deletion. J Clin Invest 1985; 76:1057.

385. Liebhaber SA, Cash FE, et al: Human alpha-globin gene expression. The dominant role of the alpha 2-locus in mRNA and protein synthesis. J Biol Chem 1986; 261:15327.

386. Proudfoot NJ: Transcriptional interference and termination between duplicated alpha-globin gene constructs suggests a novel mechanism for gene regulation. Nature 1986; 322:562.

387. Shakin SH, Liebhaber SA: Translational profiles of alpha 1-, alpha 2-, and beta-globin messenger ribonucleic acids in human reticulocytes. J Clin Invest 1986; 78:1125.

388. Orkin SH, Old J, et al: The molecular basis of alpha thalassemias: frequent occurrence of dysfunctional alpha loci among non-Asians with Hb H disease. Cell 1979; 17:33.

389. Embury SH, Miller JA, et al: Two different molecular organizations account for the single alpha-globin gene of the alpha-thalassemia-2 genotype. J Clin Invest 1980; 66:1319.

390. Goossens M, Dozy AM, et al: Triplicated alpha-globin loci in humans. Proc Natl Acad Sci U S A 1980; 77:518.

391. Higgs DR, Old JM, et al: A novel alpha-globin gene arrangement in man. Nature 1980; 284:632.

392. Lie-Injo LE, Herrera AR, et al: Two types of triplicated alpha-globin loci in humans. Nucleic Acids Res 1981; 9:3707.

393. Trent RJ, Higgs DR, et al: A new triplicated alpha-globin gene arrangement in man. Br J Haematol 1981; 49:149.

394. Hess JF, Fox M, et al: Molecular evolution of the human adult alpha-globin-like gene region: insertion and deletion of Alu family repeats and non-Alu DNA sequences. Proc Natl Acad Sci U S A 1983; 80:5970.

395. Hu WS, Shen CK: Reconstruction of human alpha thalassemia-2 genotypes in monkey cells. Nucleic Acids Res 1987; 15:2989.

396. Gomez-Pedrozo M, Hu WS, et al: Recombinational resolution in primate cells of two homologous human DNA segments with a gradient of sequence divergence. Nucleic Acids Res 1988; 16:11237.

397. Winichagoon P, Higgs DR, et al: The molecular basis of alpha-thalassaemia in Thailand. EMBO J 1984; 3:1813.

398. Chui DH, Wong SC, et al: Embryonic zeta-globin chains in adults: a marker for alpha-thalassemia-1 haplotype due to a greater than 17.5-kb deletion. N Engl J Med 1986; 314:76.

399. Bowden DK, Hill AV, et al: Different hematologic phenotypes are associated with the leftward (-alpha 4.2) and rightward (-alpha 3.7) alpha+-thalassemia deletions. J Clin Invest 1987; 79:39.

400. Galanello R, Ruggeri R, et al: A family with segregating triplicated alpha globin loci and beta thalassemia. Blood 1983; 62:1035.

401. Trent RJ, Mickleson KN, et al: Alpha globin gene rearrangements in Polynesians are not associated with malaria. Am J Hematol 1985; 18:431.

402. Kulozik AE, Thein SL, et al: Thalassaemia intermedia: interaction of the triple alpha-globin gene arrangement and heterozygous beta-thalassaemia. Br J Haematol 1987; 66:109.

403. Camaschella C, Bertero MT, et al: A benign form of thalassaemia intermedia may be determined by the interaction of triplicated alpha locus and heterozygous beta-thalassaemia. Br J Haematol 1987; 66:103.

404. Fischel-Ghodsian N, Vickers MA, et al: Characterization of two deletions that remove the entire human zeta-alpha globin gene complex (− −THAI and − −FIL). Br J Haematol 1988; 70:233.

405. Fortina P, Delgrosso K, et al: A large deletion encompassing the entire alpha-like globin gene cluster in a family of northern European extraction. Nucleic Acids Res 1988; 16:11223.

406. Drysdale HC, Higgs DR: Alpha-thalassaemia in an Asian Indian. Br J Haematol 1988; 68:264. Letter.

407. Gonzalez-Redondo JM, Diaz-Chico JC, et al: Characterization of a newly discovered alpha-thalassaemia-1 in two Spanish patients with Hb H disease. Br J Haematol 1988; 70:459.

408. Gonzalez-Redondo JM, Gilsanz F, et al: Characterization of a new alpha-thalassaemia-1 deletion in a Spanish family. Hemoglobin 1989; 13:103.

409. Luo HY, Clarke BJ, et al: A novel monoclonal antibody based diagnostic test for alpha-thalassaemia-1 carriers due to the (−SEA/) deletion. Blood 1988; 72:1589.

410. Liang ST, Wong VC, et al: Homozygous alpha-thalassaemia: clinical presentation, diagnosis and management. A review of 46 cases. Br J Obstet Gynaecol 1985; 92:680.

411. Keuh YK: Acute lymphoblastic leukemia with brilliant cresyl blue erythrocyte inclusions-acquired hemoglobin H? N Engl J Med 1982; 307:193.

412. Higgs DR, Wood WG, et al: Clinical features and molecular analysis of acquired hemoglobin H disease. Am J Med 1983; 75:181.

413. Anagnou NP, Ley TJ, et al: Acquired alpha-thalassemia in preleukemia is due to decreased expression of all four alpha-globin genes. Proc Natl Acad Sci U S A 1983; 80:6051.

414. Abbondanzo SL, Anagnou NP, et al: Myelodysplastic syndrome with acquired hemoglobin H disease. Evolution through megakaryoblastic transformation into myelofibrosis. Am J Clin Pathol 1988; 89:401.

415. Helder J, Deisseroth A: S1 nuclease analysis of alpha-globin gene expression in preleukemic patients with acquired hemoglobin H disease after transfer to mouse erythroleukemia cells. Proc Natl Acad Sci U S A 1987; 84:2387.

416. Wilkie AO, Zeitlin HC, et al: Clinical features and molecular analysis of the alpha thalassemia/mental retardation syndromes. II. Cases without detectable abnormality of the alpha globin complex. Am J Hum Genet 1990; 46:1127.

417. Schwartz E: The silent carrier of beta thalassemia. N Engl J Med 1969; 281:1327.

418. Aksoy M, Dincol G, et al: Different types of beta-thalassemia intermedia. Acta Haematol (Basel) 1978; 59:178.

419. Kattamis C, Metaxotou-Mavromati A, et al: The heterogeneity of normal Hb A2 beta thalassemia in Greece. Br J Haematol 1979; 42:109.

420. Kanavakis E, Metaxotou-Mavromati A, et al: Globin gene mapping in normal Hb A2 types of beta thalassemia. Br J Haematol 1982; 51:59.

421. Semenza GL, Delgrosso K, et al: The silent carrier allele: beta thalassemia without a mutation in the beta-globin gene or its immediate flanking regions. Cell 1984; 39:123.

422. Wong SC, Stoming TA, et al: High frequencies of a re-

arrangement (+ATA; -T) at -530 to the beta-globin gene in different populations indicate the absence of a correlation with a silent beta-thalassemia determinant. Hemoglobin 1989; 13:1.

423. Berg PE, Williams DM, et al: A common protein binds to two silencers 5' to the human beta-globin gene. Nucl Acids Res 1989; 17:8833.

424. Berg PE, Trabuchet G, et al: Is polymorphism 0.5 kb 5' to the beta-globin gene relevant to beta S gene expression? Blood 1989; 74:143a.

425. Boyer SH: The emerging complexity of genetic control of persistent fetal hemoglobin biosynthesis in adults. Ann N Y Acad Sci 1989; 565:23.

426. Cappellini MD, Fiorelli G, et al: Interaction between homozygous beta zero thalassemia and the Swiss type of hereditary persistence of fetal haemoglobin. Br J Haematol 1981; 48:561.

427. Gianni AM, Bregni M, et al: A gene controlling fetal hemoglobin expression in adults is not linked to the non-alpha globin cluster. EMBO J 1983; 2:921.

428. Thein SL, Weatherall DJ: A non-deletion hereditary persistence of fetal hemoglobin (HPFH) determinant not linked to the beta-globin gene complex. In Stamatoyannopoulos G, Nienhuis AW (eds): Hemoglobin Switching, Part B: Cellular and Molecular Mechanisms. New York, Alan R. Liss, Inc., 1989, p 97.

429. Sharma RS, Yu V, et al: Haemoglobin Bart's hydrops fetalis syndrome in an infant of Greek origin and prenatal diagnosis of alpha thalassemia. Med J Aust 1979; 2:433.

430. Trent RJ, Wilkinson T, et al: Molecular defects in 2 examples of severe Hb H disease. Scand J Haematol 1986; 36:272.

431. Chan V, Chan TK, et al: Hydrops fetalis due to an unusual form of Hb H disease. Blood 1985; 66:224.

432. Dozy AM, Kan YW, et al: Alpha-globin gene organization in Blacks precludes the severe form of alpha-thalassemia. Nature 1979; 280:605.

433. Higgs DR, Pressley L, et al: Alpha thalassemia in Black populations. Johns Hopkins Med J 1980; 146:300.

434. Higgs DR, Pressley L, et al: The genetics and molecular basis of alpha thalassemia in association with HbS in Jamaican Negroes. Br J Haematol 1981; 47:43.

435. Felice AE, Cleek MP, et al: The rare alpha-thalassemia-1 of blacks is a zeta alpha-thalassemia-1 associated with deletion of all alpha- and zeta-globin genes. Blood 1984; 63:1253.

436. Steinberg MH, Embury SH: Alpha-thalassemia in blacks: genetic and clinical aspects and interactions with the sickle hemoglobin gene. Blood 1986; 68:985.

437. Phillips JAI, Vik TA, et al: Unequal crossing-over: a common basis of single alpha-globin genes in Asians and American Blacks with hemoglobin-H disease. Blood 1980; 55:1066.

438. Galanello R, Maccioni L, et al: Alpha thalassaemia in Sardinian newborns. Br J Haematol 1984; 58:361.

439. Kanavakis E, Tzotzos S, et al: Frequency of alpha-thalassemia in Greece. Am J Hematol 1986; 22:225.

440. Weatherall DJ, Clegg JB: The alpha-chain-termination mutants and their relation to the alpha thalassemias. Philos Trans R Soc Lond 1975; 271:411.

441. Pootrakul P, Winichagoon P, et al: Homozygous haemoglobin Constant Spring: a need for revision of concept. Hum Genet 1981; 59:250.

442. Chui DH, Luo HY, et al: Potential application of a new screening test for alpha-thalassemia-1 carriers. Hemoglobin 1988; 12:459.

443. Kan YW, Schwartz E, et al: Globin chain synthesis in alpha-thalassemia syndromes. J Clin Invest 1968; 47:2515.

444. Pootrakul S, Sapprapa S, et al: Hemoglobin synthesis in 28 obligatory cases for alpha-thalassemia trait. Humangenetik 1975; 29:121.

445. Ben-Bassat I, Mozel M, et al: Globin synthesis in iron-deficiency anemia. Blood 1974; 44:451.

446. El-Hazmi MAF, Lehmann H: Interaction between iron deficiency and alpha thalassaemia: the in vitro effect of haemin on alpha chain synthesis. Acta Haematol (Basel) 1978; 60:1.

447. Rigas DA, Koler RD, et al: New hemoglobin possessing a higher electrophoretic mobility than normal adult hemoglobin. Science 1955; 121:372.

448. Wasi P, Na-Nakorn S, et al: Alpha and beta-thalassemia in Thailand. Ann N Y Acad Sci 1969; 165:60.

449. Clegg JB, Weatherall DJ: Hemoglobin synthesis in alpha-thalassemia (hemoglobin H disease). Nature (Lond) 1967; 215:1241.

450. Benz EJ, Swerdlow PS, et al: Globin messenger RNA in Hb H disease. Blood 1973; 42:825.

451. Jones RT, Schroeder WA: Chemical characterization and subunit hybridization of human hemoglobin H and associated compounds. Biochemistry 1963; 2:1357.

452. Rigas DA, Koler RD: Decreased erythrocyte survival in hemoglobin H disease as a result of the abnormal properties of hemoglobin H: the benefit of splenectomy. Blood 1961; 18:1.

453. Rachmilewitz EA: Formation of hemichromes from oxidized hemoglobin subunits. Ann N Y Acad Sci 1969; 165:171.

454. Benesch RE, Ranney HM, et al: The chemistry of the Bohr effect: II. Some properties of hemoglobin H. J Biol Chem 1961; 236:2926.

455. Shinar E, Rachmilewitz EA: Oxidative denaturation of red blood cells in thalassemia. Semin Hematol 1990; 27:70.

456. Pearson HA, McFarland W: Erythrokinetics in thalassemia: II. Studies in Lepore trait and hemoglobin H disease. J Lab Clin Med 1962; 59:147.

457. Fessas P, Yataganas X: Intra-erythroblastic instability of hemoglobin beta (HbH). Blood 1968; 31:323.

458. Tso SC, Loh TT, et al: Iron overload in patients with haemoglobin H disease. Scand J Haematol 1984; 32:391.

459. Hirsh J, Dacie JV: Persistent post-splenectomy thrombocytosis and thromboembolism: a consequence of continuing anemia. Br J Haematol 1966; 12:45.

460. Tso SC, Chan TK, et al: Venous thrombosis in haemoglobin H disease after splenectomy. Aust N Z J Med 1982; 12:635.

461. Lubin BH, Shohet BG, Nathan DG: Changes in fatty acid metabolism after erythrocyte peroxidation: stimulation of membrane repair process. J Clin Invest 1972; 49:911.

462. Tso SC: Red cell survival studies in hemoglobin H disease using [51 Cr] chromate and [32 P] di-isopropyl phosphofluoridate. Br J Haematol 1972; 23:621.

463. Wilkie AOM, Buckle VJ, et al: Clinical features and molecular analysis of the alpha thalassemia/mental retardation syndromes: I. Cases due to deletions involving chromosome band 16p13.3. Am J Hum Genet 1990; 46:1112.

464. Lie-Injo LE, Jo BH: A fast-moving hemoglobin in hydrops fetalis. Nature (Lond) 1960; 185:698.

465. Kan YW, Allen A, et al: Hydrops fetalis with alpha thalassemia. N Engl J Med 1967; 276:18.

466. Weatherall DJ, Clegg JB, et al: The hemoglobin constitution of infants with haemoglobin Bart's hydrops foetalis syndrome. Br J Haematol 1970; 18:357.

467. Todd D, Lai MCS, et al: The abnormal hemoglobins in homozygous alpha thalassaemia. Br J Haematol 1970; 19:27.

468. Wasi P, Na-Nakorn S, et al: The alpha thalassemias. Clin Haematol 1974; 3:383.

469. Beaudry MA, Ferguson DJ, et al: Survival of a hydropic infant with homozygous alpha-thalassemia-1. J Pediatr 1986; 108:713.

470. Bianchi DW, Beyer EC, et al: Normal long-term survival with alpha-thalassemia. J Pediatr 1986; 108:716.

471. Carr S, Rubin L, et al: Intrauterine therapy for homozygous alpha-thalassemia. Obstet Gynecol 1995; 85:876.

472. Rietti F: Ittero emolitico primitivo. Atti Accad Sci Med Nat Ferrara 1925; 2:14.

473. Wintrobe MM, Mathews E, et al: Familial hematopoietic disorder in Italian adolescents and adults resembling Mediterranean disease (thalassemia). JAMA 1940; 114:1530.

474. Valentine WN, Neel JV: Hematologic and genetic study of transmission of thalassemia (Cooley's anemia: Mediterranean anemia). Arch Intern Med 1944; 74:185.

475. Smith CH: Detection of mild types of Mediterranean (Cooley's anemia). Am J Dis Child 1948; 75:505.

476. Silvestroni E, Bianco I: Microcytemia, constitutional microcytic anemia and Cooley's anemia. Am J Hum Genet 1949; 1:83.

477. Pearson HA, McFarland W, et al: Erythrokinetic studies in thalassemia trait. J Lab Clin Med 1960; 56:866.

478. Mazza U, Saglio G, et al: Clinical and hematological data on 254 cases of beta-thalassemia trait in Italy. Br J Haematol 1976; 33:91.

479. Malamos B, Fessas P, et al: Types of thalassemia-trait carriers as revealed by a study of their incidence in Greece. Br J Haematol 1962; 8:5.

480. Pootrakul P, Wasi P, et al: Hematological data in 312 cases of beta-thalassemia trait in Thailand. Br J Haematol 1973; 24:703.

481. Knox-Macaulay WHM, et al: Thalassaemia in the British. BMJ 1973; 3:150.

482. Weatherall DJ: Biochemical phenotypes of thalassemia in the American Negro population. Ann N Y Acad Sci 1964; 119:450.

483. Braverman AS, Bank A: Changing rates of globin chain synthesis during erythroid cell maturation in thalassemia. J Mol Biol 1969; 42:57.

484. Schwartz E: Heterozygous beta-thalassemia: Balanced globin synthesis in bone marrow cells. Science 1970; 167:1513.

485. Kan YW, Nathan DG, et al: Equal synthesis of alpha- and beta-globin chains in erythroid precursors in heterozygous beta-thalassemia. J Clin Invest 1972; 51:1906.

486. Freidman S, Oski FA, et al: Bone marrow and peripheral blood globin synthesis in an American Black family with beta thalassemia. Blood 1972; 39:785.

487. Nienhuis AW, Canfield PH, et al: Hemoglobin messenger RNA from human bone marrow: isolation and translation in homozygous and heterozygous beta thalassemia. J Clin Invest 1973; 52:1735.

488. Chalevelakis G, Clegg JB, et al: Imbalanced globin synthesis in heterozygous beta-thalassemia bone marrow. Proc Natl Acad Sci U S A 1975; 72:3853.

489. Wood W, Stamatoyannopoulos G: Globin synthesis in fractionated normoblasts of beta thalassemia heterozygotes. J Clin Invest 1975; 55:567.

490. Fessas P, Stamatoyannopoulos G: Absence of haemoglobin A2 in an adult. Nature 1962; 195:1215.

491. Thompson RB, Odom J, et al: Thalassemia with complete absence of hemoglobin A2 in adult. Acta Haematol 1965; 33:186.

492. Ohta Y, Yamaoka K, et al: Homozygous delta-thalassemia first discovered in a Japanese family with hereditary persistence of fetal hemoglobin. Blood 1971; 37:706.

493. Kimura A, Matsunaga E, et al: Structure of cloned delta-globin genes from a normal subject and a patient with delta-thalassemia: sequence polymorphisms found in the delta-globin gene region of Japanese individuals. Nucleic Acids Res 1982; 10:5725.

494. Taramelli R, Giglioni B, et al: Delta thalassemia: a non-deletion defect. Eur J Biochem 1983; 129:589.

495. Pirastu M, Galanello R, et al: Delta +-thalassemia in Sardinia. Blood 1983; 62:341.

496. Huisman TJH, Punt K, et al: Thalassemia minor associated with hemoglobin B heterozygosity. A family report. Blood 1961; 17:747.

497. Alperin JB, Dow PA, et al: Hemoglobin A levels in health and various hematologic disorders. Am J Clin Pathol 1977; 67:219.

498. Pootrakul S, Assayamunkong S, et al: Beta-thalassemia trait: hematologic and hemoglobin synthesis studies. Hemoglobin 1976; 1:75.

499. Agraphiotis A, Fessas P, et al: Hematological, biochemical and biosynthetic differences between beta and beta thalassemia heterozygotes. In Proceedings of the XVII Congress of the International Society of Hematology, Paris, 1978, p 435.

500. Millard DP, Mason K, et al: Comparison of hematological features of the beta and beta thalassemia traits in Jamaican Negroes. Br J Haematol 1977; 36:161.

501. Schokler RC, Went LN, et al: A new genetic variant of beta-thalassemia. Nature 1966; 209:44.

502. Kalpsoya-Tassopoulos A, Zoumbos N, et al: "Silent" beta thalassemia and normal HbA2 beta thalassemia. Br J Haematol 1980; 45:177.

503. Pearson HA, O'Brien RT, et al: Screening for thalassemia trait by electronic measurement of means corpuscular volume (MCV). N Engl J Med 1973; 288:351.

504. Torlontano G, Tata A, et al: A rapid screen test for thalassemia trait. Acta Haematol 1972; 48:234.

505. Hedge UM, White JM, et al: Diagnosis of alpha thalassemia trait from Coulter counter "S" indices. J Clin Pathol 1977; 30:884.

506. Conrad ME, Crosby WH: The natural history of iron deficiency induced by phlebotomy. Blood 1962; 20:173.

507. Mentzer WC: Differentiation of iron deficiency from thalassemia trait. Lancet 1973; 1:882.

508. England JM, Fraser PM: Differentiation of iron deficiency from thalassemia trait by routine blood count. Lancet 1973; 1:449.

509. England JM, Ward SM, et al: Microcytosis, anisocytosis, and the red cell indices in iron deficiency. Br J Haematol 1976; 34:589.

510. Bessman JB, Gilmer PR, et al: Improved classification of anemias by MCV and RDW. Am J Clin Pathol 1983; 80:322.

511. McClure S, Custer E, et al: Improved detection of early iron deficiency in nonanemic subjects. JAMA 1985; 253:1021.

512. Ghionni A, Miotti TC, et al: Differential erythrocyte parameters in thalassemia minor and hyposideremic syndromes. Minerva Med 1985; 76:1143.

513. Roberts GT, El-Badawi SB: Red blood cell distribution width in some hematologic diseases. Am J Clin Pathol 1985; 83:222.

514. Flynn MM, Reppun TS, et al: Limitations of red blood cell distribution width (RDW) in evaluation of microcytosis. Am J Clin Pathol 1986; 85:445.

515. Marti HR, Fischer S, et al: Can automated haematology analysers discriminate thalassaemia from iron deficiency? Acta Haematol (Basel) 1987; 78:180.

516. Miguel A, Linares M, et al: Red cell distribution width analysis in differentiation between iron deficiency and thalassemia minor. Acta Haematol (Basel) 1988; 80:59.

517. Shin I, Lal S: Strategy to detect beta thalassemia minor. Lancet 1977; 1:692.

518. England JM, Fraser P: Discrimination between iron deficiency and heterozygous-thalassemia syndromes in the differential diagnosis of microcytosis. Lancet 1979; 1:145.

519. Rowley PT: The diagnosis of beta thalassemia trait: a review. Am J Hematol 1976; 1:129.

520. Chalevelakis G, Tsi Royannis K, et al: Screening for thalassemia and/or iron deficiency. Scand J Clin Lab Invest 1984; 44:l.

521. Bessman JD, McClure S, et al: Distinction of microcytic disorders: comparison of expert, numerical-discriminant, and microcomputer analysis. Blood Cells 1989; 15:533.

522. Green R, King R: A new red cell discriminant incorporating volume dispersion for differentiating iron deficiency anemia from thalassemia minor. Blood Cells 1989; 15:481.

523. Makris PE: Utilization of a new index to distinguish heterozygous thalassemic syndromes: comparison of its specificity to five other discriminants. Blood Cells 1989; 15:497.

524. Piomelli S, Brickman A, et al: Rapid diagnosis of iron deficiency by measurement of free erythrocyte porphyrins and hemoglobins: the FEP/hemoglobin ratio. Pediatrics 1976; 57:136.

525. Meloni T, Gallisai D, et al: Free erythrocyte porphyrin (REP) in the diagnosis of beta thalassemia trait and iron deficiency anemia. Haematologica 1982; 67:341.

526. Hurst D, Tittle B, et al: Anemia and hemoglobinopathies in Southeast Asian refugee children. J Pediatr 1983; 102:692.

527. Cooley TB, Lee P: Series of cases of splenomegaly in children with anemia and peculiar bone changes. Trans Am Pediatr Soc 1925; 37:29.

528. Cooley TB, Witwer ER, et al: Anemia in children with splenomegaly and peculiar changes in the bones. Report of cases. Am J Dis Child 1927; 34:347.

529. Castagnari G: Intorno ad una particolare sindrome osteopatica diffusa in una caso di anemia eritroblastica dell'infanzia. Boll Sci Med (Bologna) 1933; 1:399.

530. Whipple GH, Bradford WL: Racial or familial anemia of children associated with fundamental disturbances of bone and pigment metabolism (Cooley-von Jaksch). Am J Dis Child 1932; 44:336.

531. Wolman LJ: Transfusion therapy in Cooley's anemia: growth and health as related to long-range hemoglobin levels. A progress report. Ann N Y Acad Sci 1964; 119:736.

532. Schorr JB, Radel E: Transfusion therapy and its complications in patients with Cooley's anemia. Ann N Y Acad Sci 1964; 119:703.

533. Modell CB: High transfusion treatment of a case of thalassemia major. Trans R Soc Trop Med Hyg 1967; 61:1967.

534. Beard ME, Necheles TF, et al: Intensive transfusion therapy in thalassemia major. Pediatrics 1967; 40:911.

535. Piomelli S, Danoff SJ, et al: Prevention of bone malformation and cardiomegaly in Cooley's anemia by early hypertransfusion regimen. Ann N Y Acad Sci 1969; 165:427.

536. Engle MA: Cardiac involvement in Cooley's anemia. Ann N Y Acad Sci 1964; 119:694.

537. Heywood JD, Karon M, et al: Amino acid incorporation into alpha- and beta-chains of hemoglobin by normal and thalassemic reticulocytes. Science 1964; 146:530.

538. Heywood JD, Karon M, et al: Asymmetric incorporation of

amino acids into alpha and beta chains of hemoglobin synthesized in thalassemic reticulocytes. J Lab Clin Med 1965; 66:476.

539. Weatherall DJ, Clegg JB, et al: Globin synthesis in thalassemia: an *in vitro* study. Nature (Lond) 1965; 208:1061.

540. Bank A, Marks PA: Excess alpha chain synthesis relative to beta chain synthesis in thalassemia major and minor. Nature 1966; 212:1198.

541. Bargellesi A, Pontremoli S, et al: Absence of beta-globin synthesis in homozygous beta thalassemia. Eur J Biochem 1967; 1:73.

542. Fessas P: Inclusions of hemoglobin in erythroblasts and erythrocytes of thalassemia. Blood 1963; 21:21.

543. Fessas P, Loukopoulos D, et al: Absorption spectra of inclusion bodies in beta-thalassemia. Blood 1965; 25:105.

544. Fessas P, Loukopoulos D, et al: Peptide analysis of the inclusions of erythroid cells in beta thalassemia. Biochem Biophys Acta 1966; 124:430.

545. Nathan DG: Thalassemia as a proliferative disorder. Medicine 1964; 43:779.

546. Polliack A, Yataganas P, et al: An electron-microscopic study of the nuclear abnormalities and erythroblasts in beta-thalassemia major. Br J Haematol 1974; 26:203.

547. Wichramsinghe SN: The morphology and kinetics of erythropoiesis in homozygous beta thalassemia. In Weatherall DJ (ed): Congenital Disorders of Erythropoiesis. Amsterdam, Elsevier North-Holland, 1975, p 221.

548. Rachmilewitz E, Shiner E, et al: Erythrocyte membrane alterations in beta-thalassemia. Clin Hematol 1985; 14:163.

549. Shinar E, Rachmilewitz EA: Haemoglobinopathies and red cell membrane function. Baillieres Clin Haematol 1993; 6:357. Review.

550. Schrier SL: Thalassemia: pathophysiology of red cell changes. Annu Rev Med 1994; 45:211.

551. Yuan J, Bunyaratvej A, et al: The instability of the membrane skeleton in thalassemic red blood cells. Blood 1995; 86:3495.

552. Gabuzda TG, Nathan DG, et al: The metabolism of the individual C14-labelled hemoglobins in patients with H-thalassemia, with observations on radiochromate binding to the hemoglobins during red cell survival. J Clin Invest 1965; 44:315.

553. Scott MD: Entrapment of purified alpha-hemoglobin chains in normal erythrocytes as a model for human beta thalassemia. Adv Exp Med Biol 1992; 326:139.

554. Shinar E, Shalev O, et al: Erythrocyte membrane skeleton abnormalities in severe beta-thalassemia. Blood 1987; 70:158.

555. Shinar E, Rachmilewitz EA, et al: Differing erythrocyte membrane skeletal protein defects in alpha and beta thalassemia. J Clin Invest 1989; 83:404.

556. Advani R, Rubin E, et al: Oxidative red blood cell membrane injury in the pathophysiology of severe mouse beta-thalassemia. Blood 1992; 79:1064.

557. Olivieri O, DeFranceschi L, et al: Oxidative damage and erythrocyte membrane transport abnormalities in thalassemias. Blood 1994; 84:315.

558. Schrier SL, Rachmilewitz E, et al: Cellular and membrane properties of alpha and beta thalassemic erythrocytes are different: implication for differences in clinical manifestations. Blood 1989; 74:2194.

559. Sorensen S, Rubin E, et al: The role of membrane skeletal-associated alpha-globin in the pathophysiology of beta-thalassemia. Blood 1990; 75:1333.

560. Wainscoat JS, Thein SL, et al: Thalassaemia intermedia. Blood Rev 1987; 1:273.

561. McCarthy GM, Temperley IJ, et al: Thalassemia in an Irish family. Irish J Med Sci 1968; 1:303.

562. Friedman S, Ozsoylu S, et al: Heterozygous beta-thalassemia of unusual severity. Br J Haematol 1976; 32:65.

563. Weatherall DJ, Clegg JB, et al: A genetically determined disorder with features both of thalassemia and congenital dyerythropoietic anaemia. Br J Haematol 1973; 24:679.

564. Stamatoyannopoulos G, Woodson R, et al: Inclusion-body-beta-thalassemia trait. N Engl J Med 1974; 290:939.

565. Kanavakis E, Metaxotou MA, et al: The triplicated alpha gene locus and beta thalassaemia. Br J Haematol 1983; 54:201.

566. Sampietro M, Cazzola M, et al: The triplicated alpha-gene locus and heterozygous beta thalassaemia: a case of thalassaemia intermedia. Br J Haematol 1983; 55:709.

567. Thein SL, Al-Hakim I, et al: Thalassaemia intermedia: a new molecular basis. Br J Haematol 1984; 56:333.

568. Friedman AD, Linch DC, et al: Determination of the hemoglobin F program in human progenitor-derived erythroid cells. J Clin Invest 1985; 75:1359.

569. Pearson HA: Alpha-beta-thalassemia disease in a Negro family. N Engl J Med 1969; 281:1327.

570. Kan YW, Nathan DG: Mild thalassemia: the result of interactions of alpha and beta thalassemia genes. J Clin Invest 1970; 49:635.

571. Knox-McAulay HHM, Weatherall DJ, et al: The clinical and biosynthetic characterization of alpha beta-thalassemia. Br J Haematol 1972; 22:497.

572. Ozsoylu S, Hicsonmez C, et al: Hemoglobin H-beta-thalassemia. Acta Haematol 1973; 50:184.

573. Altay C, Say B, et al: Alpha-thalassemia and beta-thalassemia in a Turkish family. Am J Hematol 1977; 2:1.

574. Bate CM, Humphries G: Alpha-beta-thalassemia. Lancet 1977; 1:1031.

575. Furbetta M, Galanello R, et al: Interaction of alpha and beta thalassemia genes in two Sardinian families. Br J Haematol 1979; 41:203.

576. Wainscoat JS, Kanavakis E, et al: Thalassaemia intermedia in Cyprus: the interaction of alpha and beta thalassaemia. Br J Haematol 1983; 53:411.

577. Winichagoon P, Fucharoen S, et al: Concomitant inheritance of alpha-thalassemia in beta-thalassemia/Hb E disease. Am J Hematol 1985; 20:217.

578. Villegas A, Lopez Rubio M, et al: Primer caso de talasemia intermedia descrito en Espana debido a la interaccion de tres gene alpha con beta talasemia minor. Rev Clin Espanol 1993; 192:268.

579. Camaschella C, Cappellini MD: Thalassemia intermedia. Haematologica 1995; 80:58.

580. Oron V, Filon D, et al: Severe thalassaemia intermedia caused by interaction of homozygosity for alpha-globin gene triplication with heterozygosity for beta zero-thalassemia. Br J Haematol 1994; 86:377.

581. Garewal G, Fearon CW, et al: The molecular basis of beta thalassaemia in Punjabi and Maharashtran Indians includes a multilocus aetiology involving triplicated alpha-globin loci. Br J Haematol 1994; 86:372.

582. Oggiano L, Rimini E, et al: Haematological phenotypes in a family with triplicated alpha-globin gene, beta zero 39 and delta + 27 thalassaemia mutations. Clin Lab Haematol 1992; 14:289.

583. Villegas A, Perez-Clausell C, et al: A new case of thalassemia intermedia: interaction of a triplicated alpha-globin locus and beta-thalassemia trait. Hemoglobin 1992; 16:99.

584. Leoni GG, Rosatelli C, et al: Molecular basis of beta-thalassemia intermedia in a southern Italian (Puglia). Acta Haematol 1991; 86:174.

585. Dandona P, Menon RK, et al: Serum 1,25 dihydroxyvitamin D and osteocalcin concentrations in thalassaemia major. Arch Dis Child 1987; 62:474.

586. Rioja L, Girot R, et al: Bone disease in children with homozygous beta-thalassemia. Bone Mineral 1990; 8:69.

587. Lawson JP, Ablow RC, et al: The ribs in thalassemia. Radiology 1981; 140:663.

588. Williams BA, Morris LL, et al: Limb deformity and metaphyseal abnormalities in thalassaemia major. Am J Pediatr Hematol Oncol 1992; 14:197.

589. Orvieto R, Leichter I, et al: Bone density, mineral content, and cortical index in patients with thalassemia major and the correlation to their bone fractures, blood transfusions, and treatment with desferrioxamine. Calcif Tissue Int 1992; 50:397.

590. Baker DH: Roentgen manifestations of Cooley's anemia. Ann N Y Acad Sci 1964; 119:641.

591. Michelson J, Cohen A: Incidence and treatment of fractures in thalassemia. J Orthop Trauma 1988; 2:29.

592. Canatan D, Akar N, et al: Effects of calcitonin therapy on osteoporosis in patients with thalassemia. Acta Haematol 1995; 93:20.

593. Mills SR, Doppman JL, et al: Computed tomography in the diagnosis of disorders of excessive iron storage of the liver. J Comput Assist Tomogr 1977; 1:101.

594. Babiker MA, Patel PJ, et al: Comparison between serum ferritin and computed tomographic densities of liver, spleen, kidney and pancreas in beta-thalassaemia major. Scand J Clin Lab Invest 1987; 47:715.

595. Olivieri NF, Grisaru D, et al: Computed tomography scanning of the liver to determine efficacy of iron chelation therapy in thalassemia major. J Pediatr 1989; 114:427.

596. Long JA Jr, Doppmann JL, et al: Computed tomographic analysis of beta-thalassemic syndromes with hemochromatosis: pathologic findings with clinical and laboratory correlations. J Comput Assist Tomogr 1980; 4:165.

597. Long JA Jr, Doppman JL, et al: Computed tomographic studies of thoracic extramedullary hematopoiesis. J Comput Assist Tomogr 1980; 4:67.

598. Papavasiliou C, Gouliamos A, et al: The marrow heterotopia in thalassemia. Eur J Radiol 1986; 6:92.

599. Singcharoen T: Unusual long bone changes in thalassaemia: findings on plain radiography and computed tomography. Br J Radiol 1989; 62:168.

600. Papavasiliou C, Trakadas S, et al: Magnetic resonance imaging of marrow heterotopia in haemoglobinopathy. Eur J Radiol 1988; 8:50.

601. Ellis JT, Schulman I, et al: Generalized siderosis with fibrosis of liver and pancreas in Cooley's (Mediterranean) anemia with observations on the pathogenesis of the siderosis and fibrosis. Am J Pathol 1954; 30:287.

602. Fink H: Transfusion hemochromatosis in Cooley's anemia. Ann N Y Acad Sci 1964; 119:680.

603. Modell B: A Guide to the Management of Thalassemia. EMBO Conference on Thalassemia, 1978.

604. de Alarcon PA, Donovan ME, et al: Iron absorption in the thalassemia syndromes and its inhibition by tea. N Engl J Med 1979; 300:5.

605. Worwood M: The clinical biochemistry of iron. Semin Hematol 1977; 14:30.

606. Modell B, Berdoukas V: The Clinical Approach to Thalassemia. Grune & Stratton, 1984.

607. Cazzola M, Finch CA: Iron balance in thalassemia. Prog Clin Biol Res 1989; 309:93.

608. Pippard MJ, Weatherall DJ: Iron absorption in non-transfused iron loading anemias: prediction of risk for iron loading and response to iron chelation treatment in beta thalassemia intermedia and congenital sideroblastic anemias. Haematologica 1984; 17:17.

609. Peters TJ, Raja KB, et al: Mechanisms and regulation of intestinal iron absorption. Ann N Y Acad Sci 1988; 526:141.

610. Bridges K, Cudkowicz A: Effect of iron chelators on the transferrin receptor in K562 cells. J Biol Chem 1984; 259:12970.

611. Harrison PM: Ferritin: an iron storage molecule. Semin Hematol 1977; 14:55.

612. Drysdale JW, Adelman TG, et al: Human isoferritins in normal and disease states. Semin Hematol 1977; 14:71.

613. Letsky EA, Miller F, et al: Serum ferritin in children with thalassemia regularly transfused. J Clin Pathol 1974; 27:652.

614. Logos P, Lagona E, et al: Serum ferritin in beta-thalassemia intermedia. Lancet 1980; 1:204.

615. Kaltwassen T, Werner E: Assessment of iron burden. Bailliers Clin Hematol 1989; 2:370.

616. Morgan EH: Transferrin biochemistry, physiology and clinical significance. Mol Aspects Med 1981; 4:1.

617. Aisen P: The role of transferrin in iron transport. Br J Haematol 1974; 26:159.

618. Huebers HA, Finch CA: Transferrin: physiological behaviour and clinical implications. Blood 1984; 64:763.

619. Jacobs A: Low molecular weight intracellular iron transport compounds. Blood 1977; 50:433.

620. van Renswonde J, Bridges KR, et al: Receptor-mediated endocytosis of transferrin and the uptake of Fe in K562 cells: identification of a nonlysosomal acidic compartment. Proc Natl Acad Sci U S A 1982; 79:6186.

621. Dautry-Varsat A, Ciechanover A, et al: pH and the recycling of transferrin during receptor-mediated endocytosis. Proc Natl Acad Sci U S A 1983; 80:2258.

622. Klausner RD, Ashwell G, et al: Binding of apo transferrin to K562 cells: explanation of the transferrin cycle. Proc Natl Acad Sci U S A 1983; 80:2263.

623. Seligman PA: The biochemistry of proteins involved in iron transport and storage. In Stamatoyannopoulos G, Nienhuis AW, Leder P, Majerus P (eds): The Molecular Basis of Blood Diseases. Philadelphia, WB Saunders Co., 1987.

624. Seymour CA, Peters TJ: Organelle pathology in primary and secondary hemochromatosis with special reference to lysosomal changes. Br J Haematol 1978; 40:239.

625. Roifman CM, Eytan GD, et al: Ferritin-phospholipid interaction: a model system for intralysosomal ferritin segregation in iron-overloaded hepatocytes. J Ultrastruc Res 1982; 79:307.

626. Richter GW: The iron-loaded cell—the cytopathology of iron storage: a review. Am J Pathol 1978; 91:363.

627. Hershko C, Graham G, et al: Non-specific serum iron fraction of potential toxicity. Br J Haematol 1978; 40:255.

628. Anuwajanakulchai M, Pootrakul P, et al: Non-transferrin plasma iron in beta-thalassemia/Hb E and hemoglobin H diseases. Scand J Haematol 1984; 32:153.

629. Hershko C, Weatherall DJ: Iron-chelating therapy. Crit Rev Clin Lab Sci 1988; 26:303.

630. Herbert V, Shaw S, et al: Most free-radical injury is iron-related: it is promoted by iron, hemin, holoferritin and vitamin C, and inhibited by desferoxamine and apoferritin. Stem Cells 1994; 12:289.

631. Willis ED: Effects of iron overload on lipid peroxide formation and oxidative demethylation by the liver endoplasmic reticulum. Biochem Pharmacol 1972; 21:239.

632. Tong Mak I, Weglicki WB: Characterization of iron-mediated peroxidative injury in isolated hepatic lysosomes. J Clin Invest 1985; 75:58.

633. Bacon BR, Park CH, et al: Hepatic mitochondrial oxidative metabolism in rats with chronic dietary iron overload. Hepatology 1985; 5:789.

634. Bacon BR, Tavill AS, et al: Hepatic lipid peroxidation in vivo in rats with chronic iron overload. J Clin Invest 1983; 71:429.

635. Heys AD, Dormandy TL: Lipid peroxidation in iron-overloaded spleens. Clin Sci 1981; 60:295.

636. Peters TJ, Seymour CA: Acid hydrolase activities and lysosomal integrity in liver biopsies from patients with iron overload. Clin Sci Mol Med 1978; 50:75.

637. O'Connell MJ, Ward RJ, et al: The role of iron in ferritin- and haemosiderin-mediated lipid peroxidation in liposomes. Biochem J 1985; 229:135.

638. Hershko C, Link G, et al: Modification of iron uptake and lipid peroxidation by hypoxia, ascorbic acid, and alpha-tocopherol in iron-loaded rat myocardial cell cultures. J Lab Clin Med 1987; 110:355.

639. Link G, Athias P, et al: Effect of iron loading on transmembrane potential, contraction, and automaticity of rat ventricular muscle cells in culture. J Lab Clin Med 1989; 113:103.

640. Rachmilewitz EA, Lubin BH, et al: Lipid membrane peroxidation in beta-thalassemia major. Blood 1976; 47:495.

641. Miniero R, Piga A, et al: Vitamin E and beta thalassemia. Haematologica 1983; 68:562.

642. Cranfield M, Gollan JL, et al: Serum antioxidant activity in normal and abnormal subjects. Ann Clin Biochem 1979; 16:299.

643. de Martino M, Rossi ME, et al: Change in superoxide anion production in neutrophils from multiply transfused beta thalassemia patients. Acta Haematol 1984; 71:289.

644. Bothwell TJ, Finch CA: Iron Metabolism. Boston, Little, Brown & Co., 1962.

645. Fawwaz RA, Winchell HS, et al: Hepatic iron deposition in humans: I. First-pass hepatic deposition of intestinally absorbed iron in patients with low plasma latent iron-binding capacity. Blood 1967; 30:417.

646. Buonanno G, Valente A, et al: Serum ferritin in beta thalassemia intermedia. Scand J Haematol 1984; 83:32.

647. Pippard MJ, Callender ST, et al: Iron absorption and loading in beta thalassemia intermedia. Lancet 1979; 2:819.

648. de Virgiliis S, Sanna G, et al: Serum ferritin, liver iron stores, and liver histology in children with thalassemia. Arch Dis Child 1980; 55:43.

649. Worwood M, Cragg SJ, et al: Binding of serum ferritin to concanavalin A: patients with homozygous beta thalassemia and transfusional iron overload. Br J Haematol 1980; 46:409.

650. Houang MTW, Skalicka A, et al: Correlation between computed

tomographic values and liver iron content in thalassemia major with iron overload. Lancet 1979; 1:1322.

651. Brittenham GM, Farrell DE, et al: Magnetic-susceptibility measurement of human iron stores. N Engl J Med 1982; 307:1671.

652. Engle MA, Erlandson M, et al: Late cardiac complications of chronic, severe, refractory anemia with hemochromatosis. Circulation 1964; 30:698.

653. Buja LM, Roberts WC: Iron in the heart. Etiology and clinical significance. Am J Med 1971; 51:209.

654. Lixi M, Montaldo P: Cardiological aspects and thalassemia syndrome in the past pediatric age: instrumental findings, intracavitary cardiac biopsy reports and autopsy findings. Boll Soc Ital Cardiol 1979; 24:637.

655. Fitchett DH, Coltart DJ, et al: Cardiac involvement in secondary hemochromatosis: a catheter biopsy study and analysis of myocardium. Cardiovasc Res 1980; 14:719.

656. Link G, Pinson A: Heart cells in culture: a model of myocardial iron overload and chelation. J Lab Clin Med 1985; 106:147.

657. Nienhuis AW, Griffith P, et al: Evaluation of cardiac function in patients with thalassemia major. Ann N Y Acad Sci 1980; 80:384.

658. Henry WL, Nienhuis AW, et al: Echocardiographic abnormalities in patients with transfusion-dependent anemia and secondary myocardial iron deposition. Am J Med 1978; 64:547.

659. Valdez-Cruz LM, Reinecke C, et al: Preclinical abnormal segmental cardiac manifestations of thalassemia major in children on transfusion-chelation therapy: echographic alterations of left ventricular posterior wall contraction and relaxation patterns. Am Heart J 1982; 103:505.

660. Kremastinos DT, Toutouzas PK, et al: Iron overload and left ventricular performance in beta thalassemia. Acta Cardiol 1984; 39:29.

661. Leon MB, Borer JS, et al: Detection of early cardiac dysfunction in patients with severe beta-thalassemia and chronic iron overload. N Engl J Med 1979; 301:1143.

662. Freeman AP, Giles RW, et al: Early left ventricular dysfunction and chelation therapy in thalassemia major. Ann Intern Med 1983; 99:450.

663. Canale C, Terrachini V, et al: Thalassemic cardiomyopathy: echocardiographic difference between major and intermediate thalassemia at rest and during isometric effort: yearly follow-up. Clin Cardiol 1988; 11:563.

664. Beirman J, Propper R, et al: Unpublished observations.

665. Risdon RA, Barry M, et al: Transfusional iron overload: the relationship between tissue iron concentration and hepatic fibrosis in thalassemia. J Pathol 1975; 116:83.

666. Iancu TL, Neustein HB: Ferritin in human liver cells of homozygous beta thalassemia: ultrastructural observations. Br J Haematol 1977; 37:527.

667. Weintraub LR, Goral A, et al: Pathogenesis of hepatic fibrosis in experimental iron overload. Br J Haematol 1985; 59:321.

668. Masera G, Jean G, et al: Role of chronic hepatitis in development of thalassemic liver disease. Arch Dis Child 1976; 51:680.

669. Masera G, Jean G, et al: Sequential study of liver biopsy in thalassaemia. Arch Dis Child 1980; 55:800.

670. de Virgiliis S, Cornacchia G, et al: Chronic liver disease in transfusion-dependent thalassemia: liver iron quantitation and distribution. Acta Haematol 1981; 65:32.

671. Barry M, Flynn DM, et al: Long-term chelation therapy in thalassemia major: effect on liver iron concentration, liver histology, and clinical progress. BMJ 1974; 2:16.

672. Cohen A: Current status of iron chelation therapy with deferoxamine. Semin Hematol 1990; 27:86.

673. Brittenham GM, Griffith PM, et al: Efficacy of deferoxamine in preventing complications or iron overload in patients with thalassemia major. N Engl J Med 1994; 331:567.

674. Aldouri MA, Wonke B, et al: Iron state and hepatic disease in patients with thalassaemia major, treated with long term subcutaneous desferrioxamine. J Clin Pathol 1987; 40:1353.

675. Wolman IJ, Ortalani M: Some clinical features of Cooley's anemia patients as related to transfusion schedules. Ann N Y Acad Sci 1969; 105:407.

676. De Sanctis V, Vullo C, et al: Endocrine complications in thalassaemia major. Prog Clin Biol Res 1989; 309:77.

677. Garcia-Mayor RV, Andrade Olivie A, et al: Linear growth in thalassemic children treated with intensive chelation therapy. A longitudinal study. Horm Res 1993; 40:189.

678. Benso L, Gambotto S, et al: Growth velocity monitoring of the efficacy of different therapeutic protocols in a group of thalassaemic children. Eur J Pediatr 1995; 154:205.

679. Pintor C, Cella SG, et al: Impaired growth hormone (GH) response to GH-releasing hormone in thalassemia major. J Clin Endocrinol Metab 1986; 62:263.

680. Leheup BP, Cisternino M, et al: Growth hormone response following growth hormone releasing hormone injection in thalassemia major: influence of pubertal development. J Endocr Invest 1991; 14:37.

681. Saenger D, Schwartz E, et al: Depressed serum somatomedin activity in beta-thalassemia. J Pediatr 1980; 96:214.

682. Sklar CA, Lew LQ, et al: Adrenal function in thalassemia major following long-term treatment with multiple transfusions and chelation therapy. Evidence for dissociation of cortisol and adrenal androgen secretion. Am J Dis Child 1987; 141:327.

683. Anoussakis CH, Alexiou D, et al: Endocrinological investigation of pituitary gonadal axis in thalassemia major. Acta Paediatr Scand 1977; 66:49.

684. Nienhuis AW, Henry W, et al: Evaluation and treatment of chronic iron overload. In Zaino EC, Roberts RH (eds): Chelation Therapy in Chronic Iron Overload. Miami, Symposium Specialists, Inc., 1977, p 1.

685. Masala A, Melan T, et al: Endocrine functioning in multi-transfused prepubertal patients with homozygous beta thalassemia. J Clin Endocrinol Metab 1984; 58:667.

686. Flynn DM, Fairney A, et al: Hormonal changes in thalassaemia major. Arch Dis Child 1976; 51:828.

687. De Sanctis V, Vullo C, et al: Hypothalamic-pituitary-gonadal axis in thalassemia patients with secondary amenorrhea. Obstet Gynecol 1988; 72:643.

688. Wang C, Tso SC, et al: Hypogonadotropic hypogonadism in severe beta-thalassemia: effect of chelation and pulsatile gonadotropin-releasing hormone therapy. J Clin Endocrinol Metab 1989; 68:511.

689. Valenti S, Giusti M, et al: Delayed puberty in males with beta-thalassemia major: pulsatile gonadotropin-releasing hormone administration induced changes in gonadotropin isoform profiles and an increase in sex steroids. Eur J Endocr 1995; 133:48.

690. De Sanctis V, Vullo C, et al: Gonadal function in patients with beta thalassemia major. J Clin Pathol 1988; 41:133.

691. Chaterjee B: Personal communication.

692. Spitz IM, Hirsch HJ, et al: TSH secretion in thalassemia. J Endocrinol Invest 1984; 7:495.

693. McIntosh N: Endocrinopathy in thalassemia major. Arch Dis Child 1976; 51:195.

694. Suadek CD, Hemm RM, et al: Abnormal glucose tolerance in beta-thalassemia major. Metabolism 1977; 26:43.

695. Lassman MN, Genel M, et al: Carbohydrate homeostasis and pancreatic islet function in thalassemia. Ann Intern Med 1974; 80:65.

696. Merkel PA, Simonson DC, et al: Insulin resistance and hyperinsulinemia in patients with thalassemia major treated by hypertransfusion. N Engl J Med 1988; 318:809.

697. Brianda S, Maioli M, et al: The euglycemic clamp in patients with thalassaemia intermedia. Horm Metab Res 1987; 19:319.

698. Lassman MN, O'Brien RT, et al.: Endocrine evaluation in thalassemia major. Ann N Y Acad Sci 1974; 232:226.

699. Christenson RA, Pootrakul P, et al: Patients with thalassemia develop osteoporosis, osteomalacia, and hypoparathyroidism, all of which are corrected by transfusion. Birth Defects 1987; 23:409.

700. DeSanctis V, Vullo C, et al: Hypoparathyroidism in beta-thalassemia major. Acta Haematol 1992; 88:105.

701. Gerfner J, Boadus A, et al: Impaired parathyroid response to induced hypocalcemia in thalassemia major. J Pediatr 1979; 95:210.

702. Mautalen CA, Kuicala R, et al: Hypoparathyroidism and iron storage disease. Am J Med Sci 1979; 276:363.

703. Aloia JF, Ostuni JA, et al: Combined vitamin D parathyroid defect in thalassemia major. Arch Intern Med 1982; 142:831.

704. Fucharoen S, Youngchaiyud P, et al: Hypoxaemia and the effect of aspirin in thalassemia. Southeast Asian J Med Publ Health 1981; 12:90.

705. Keens T, O'Neal M, et al: Pulmonary function abnormalities in

thalassemia patients on a hypertransfusion program. Pediatrics 1981; 65:1013.

706. Cooper D, Mangell A, et al: Low lung capacity and hypoxemia in children with thalassemia major. Am Rev Respir Dis 1980; 121:639.

707. Grant GP, Mansell AL, et al: The effect of transfusion on lung capacity, diffusing capacity, and arterial oxygen saturation in patients with thalassemia major. Pediatr Res 1986; 20:20.

708. Hoyt RW, Scarpa N, et al: Pulmonary function abnormalities in homozygous beta-thalassemia. J Pediatr 1986; 109:452.

709. Fung KP, Chow OK, et al: Pulmonary function in thalassemia major. J Pediatr 1987; 111:534.

710. Songkhla SN, Fucharoen S, et al: Lung perfusion in thalassemia. Birth Defects 1987; 23:371.

711. Youngchaiyud P, Suthamsmai T, et al: Lung function tests in splenectomized beta-thalassemia/Hb E patients. Birth Defects 1987; 23:361.

712. Factor JM, Pottipati SR, et al: Pulmonary function abnormalities in thalassemia major and the role of iron overload. Am J Respir Crit Care Med 1994; 149:1570.

713. Eldor A, Maclouf J, et al: A chronic hypercoagulable state and life-long platelet activation in beta thalassemia major. Southeast Asian J Trop Med Public Health 1993; 24:92.

714. Koren A, Garty I, et al: Right ventricular cardiac dysfunction in beta-thalassemia major. Am J Dis Child 1987; 141:93.

715. Giardini C, Angelucci E, et al: Bone marrow transplantation for thalassemia. Experience in Pesaro, Italy. Am J Pediatr Hematol Oncol 1994; 16:6.

716. Giardini C, Galimberti M, et al: Bone marrow transplantation in thalassemia. Annu Rev Med 1995; 46:319.

717. Lucarelli G, Galimberti M, et al: Bone marrow transplantation in thalassemia. Hematol Oncol Clin North Am 1991; 5:549.

718. Fosburg MT, Nathan DG: Treatment of Cooley's anemia. Blood 1990; 76:435.

719. Giardina PJ, Hilgartner MW: Update on thalassemia. Pediatr Rev 1992; 13:55.

720. Dover GJ, Valle D: Therapy for beta-thalassemia—a paradigm for the treatment of genetic disorders. N Engl J Med 1994; 331:609.

721. Piomelli S, Loew T: Management of thalassemia major (Cooley's anemia). Hematol Oncol Clin North Am 1991; 5:557.

722. Rebulla P, Modell B: Transfusion requirements and effects in patients with thalassaemia major. Lancet 1991; 337:277.

723. Weiner M, Kartpatkin M, et al: Cooley's anemia: high transfusion regimen and chelation therapy. Results and perspective. J Pediatr 1978; 92:653.

724. Necheles TF, Chang S, et al: Intensive transfusion therapy in thalassemia major: an eight-year follow-up. Ann N Y Acad Sci 1974; 232:179.

725. Brook CG, Thompson EN, et al: Growth in children with thalassemia major—an effect of two different transfusion regimens. Arch Dis Child 1969; 44:612.

726. Kattamis C, Touliadts N, et al: Growth of children with thalassemia: effect of different transfusion regimens. Arch Dis Child 1970; 45:502.

727. Propper RD, Button LN, et al: New approaches to the transfusion management of thalassemia. Blood 1980; 55:55.

728. Masera G, Terzoli S, et al: Evaluation of the super-transfusion regimen in homozygous beta thalassemia children. Br J Haematol 1982; 52:11.

729. Gabutti V, Piga A, et al: Hemoglobin levels and blood requirement in thalassemia. Arch Dis Child 1982; 57:156.

730. Piomelli S, Graziano J, et al: Chelation therapy, transfusion requirement and iron balance in young thalassemia patients. Ann N Y Acad Sci 1980; 344:409.

731. Piomelli S, Seamon C, et al: Separation of younger red cells with improved survival in vivo. An approach to chronic transfusion therapy. Proc Natl Acad Sci U S A 1978; 75:3474.

732. Graziano JH, Piomelli S, et al: A simple technique for preparation of young red cells for transfusion from ordinary blood units. Blood 1982; 59:865.

733. Bracey AW, Klein HG, et al: Ex-vivo selective isolation of young red blood cells using the IBM-2991 cell washer. Blood 1983; 61:1068.

734. Hogan VA, Blanchette VS, et al: A simple method for preparing neocyte-enriched leukocyte-poor blood for transfusion dependent patients. Transfusion 1986; 26:253.

735. Kevy SV, Jacobson MS, et al: A new approach to neocyte transfusion: preliminary report. J Clin Apheres 1988; 4:194.

736. Simon TL, Sohmer P, et al: Extended survival of neocytes produced by a new system. Transfusion 1989; 29:221.

737. Cohen AR, Schmidt JM, et al: Clinical trial of young red cell transfusions. J Pediatr 1984; 104:865.

738. Marcus RE, Wonke B, et al: A prospective trial of young red cells in 48 patients with transfusion-dependent thalassaemia. Br J Haematol 1985; 60:153.

739. Wolfe LC, Sallan D, et al: Current therapy and new approaches to the treatment of thalassemia major. Ann N Y Acad Sci 1985; 45:248.

740. Piomelli S, Hart D, et al: Current strategies in the management of Cooley's anemia. Ann N Y Acad Sci 1985; 445:256.

741. Propper RD: Neocytes and neocyte-gerocyte exchange. Prog Clin Biol Res 1982; 88:227.

742. Meryman HT, Hornblower M: The preparation of red cells depleted of leukocytes. Transfusion 1986; 26:101.

743. Piomelli S, Karpatkin MH, et al: Hypertransfusion regimen in patients with Cooley's anemia. Ann N Y Acad Sci 1974; 232:186.

744. Coles SM, Klein HG, et al: Alloimmunization in two multitransfused patient populations. Transfusion 1981; 21:462.

745. Michail-Merianou V, Pamphili-Panousopoulou L, et al: Alloimmunization to red cell antigens in thalassemia: comparative study of usual versus better-match transfusion programmes. Vox Sang 1987; 52:95.

746. Spanos T, Karageorga M, et al: Red cell alloantibodies in patients with thalassemia. Vox Sang 1990; 58:50.

747. Diamond WJ, Brown FL, et al: Delayed hemolytic transfusion reaction presenting a sickle cell crisis. Ann Intern Med 1980; 93:231.

748. Blumberg N, Ross K, et al: Should chronic transfusion be matched for antigens other than ABO and Rh(o)D? Vox Sang 1984; 47:205.

749. Moroni GA, Piacentini G, et al: Hepatitis B or non-A, non-B virus infection in multitransfused thalassaemic patients. Arch Dis Child 1984; 59:1127.

750. Choo Q, Kuo G, et al: Isolation of a cDNA clone derived from a blood-borne non-A non-B hepatitis genome. Science 1989; 244:359.

751. Kuo G, Choo Q, et al: An assay for circulating antibodies to a major etiologic virus of human non-A non-B hepatitis. Science 1989; 244:362.

752. Manconi PE, Dessi C, et al: Human immunodeficiency virus infection in multi-transfused patients with thalassaemia major. Eur J Pediatr 1988; 147:304.

753. Okon E, Levij S, et al: Splenectomy, iron overload, and liver cirrhosis in beta-thalassemia major. Acta Haematol 1976; 56:142.

754. Graziano JH, Piomelli S, et al: Chelation therapy in beta-thalassemia major: III. The role of splenectomy in achieving iron balance. J Pediatr 1981; 99:695.

755. Modell B: Management of thalassemia major. Br Med Bull 1976; 32:270.

756. Modell CB: Total management of thalassaemia major. Arch Dis Child 1977; 52:489.

757. Cohen A, Markenson AL, et al: Transfusion requirements and splenectomy in thalassemia major. J Pediatr 1980; 97:100.

758. Blendis LM, Modell CB, et al: Some effects of splenectomy in thalassemia major. Br J Haematol 1974; 28:77.

759. Engelhard D, Cividalli G, et al: Splenectomy in homozygous beta-thalassemia: a retrospective study of thirty patients. Br J Haematol 1975; 31:391.

760. Cohen A, Gayer R, et al: Long-term effect of splenectomy on transfusion requirements in thalassemia major. Am J Hematol 1989; 30:254.

761. Eraklis AJ, Kevy SV, et al: Hazard of overwhelming infection after splenectomy in childhood. N Engl J Med 1967; 276:1225.

762. Erickson WD, Burgert EO, et al: The hazard of infection following splenectomy in children. Am J Dis Child 1968; 116:l.

763. Ein SH, Shandling V, et al: The morbidity and mortality of splenectomy in childhood. Ann Surg 1977; 185:307.

764. Aommann AJ, Addiego J, et al: Polyvalent pneumococcal polysaccharide immunization of patients with sickle cell anemia and patients with splenectomy. N Engl J Med 1977; 297:897.

765. Kafidi KT, Rotschafer JC: Bacterial vaccines for splenectomized patients. Drug Intell Clin Pharm 1988; 22:192.

766. Recommendations of the advisory committee on immunization practices (ACIP): use of vaccines and immune globulins in persons with altered immunocompetence. MMWR 1993; 42:1.

767. Ambrosino DM, Molrine DC: Critical appraisal of immunization strategies for prevention of infection in the immunocompromised host. Hematol Oncol Clin North Am 1993; 7:1027.

768. Rostagno C, Prisco D, et al: Pulmonary hypertension associated with long-standing thrombocytosis. Chest 1991; 99:1303.

769. Green NS: *Yersinia* infections in patients with homozygous beta-thalassemia associated with iron overload and its treatment. Pediatr Hematol Oncol 1992; 9:247.

770. Karabus C, Fielding J: Desferrioxamine chelatable iron in hemolytic, megaloblastic and sideroblastic anemia. Br J Haematol 1967; 13:924.

771. White GP, Bailey-Wood R, et al: The effect of chelating agents on cellular iron metabolism. Clin Sci Mol Med 1976; 50:152.

772. Hershko C, Rachmilewitz EA: Mechanism of deferrioxamine-induced iron excretion in thalassemia. Br J Haematol 1979; 42:125.

773. Bianco I, Graziani B, et al: A study of the mechanisms and sites of action of deferrioxamine in thalassemia major. Acta Haematol (Basel) 1984; 71:100.

774. Pippard M, Callendar ST, et al: Ferrioxamine excretion in iron-loaded man. Blood 1982; 60:288.

775. Propper RD, Shurin SB, et al: Reassessment of the use of desferrioxamine B in iron overload. N Engl J Med 1976; 294:1421.

776. O'Brien RT: Ascorbic acid enhancement of desferrioxamine-induced urinary iron excretion in thalassemia major. Ann N Y Acad Sci 1974; 232:221.

777. Modell CB, Beck J: Long-term desferrioxamine therapy in thalassemia. Ann N Y Acad Sci 1974; 232:201.

778. Propper RD, Cooper B, et al: Continuous subcutaneous administration of desferrioxamine in patients with iron overload. N Engl J Med 1977; 297:418.

779. Hussain MAM, Green N, et al: Subcutaneous infusion and intramuscular injection of desferrioxamine in patients with transfusional iron overload. Lancet 1976; 2:1278.

780. Graziano JH, Markenson A, et al: Chelation therapy in beta-thalassemia major: I. Intravenous and subcutaneous desferrioxamine. J Pediatr 1978; 92:648.

781. Hoffbrand AV, Gorman A: Improvement in iron status and liver function in patients with transfusional iron overload with long-term subcutaneous desferrioxamine. Lancet 1979; 1:947.

782. Cohen A, Martin M, et al: Response to long-term deferoxamine therapy in thalassemia. J Pediatr 1981; 99:689.

783. Modell B, Letsky E, et al: Survival and desferrioxamine in thalassemia major. BMJ 1982; 284:1081.

784. Wolfe L, Olivieri N, et al: Prevention of cardiac disease by subcutaneous deferoxamine in patients with thalassemia major. N Engl J Med 1985; 312:1600.

785. Maurer HS, Lloyd SJ, et al: A prospective evaluation of iron chelation therapy in children with severe beta-thalassemia. A six-year study. Am J Dis Child 1988; 142:287.

786. de Virgiliis S, Cossu P, et al: Effect of subcutaneous desferrioxamine on iron balance in young thalassemia patients. Am J Pediatr Hematol Oncol 1983; 5:73.

787. Fargion S, Taddei MT, et al: Early iron overload in beta thalassemia major. When to start chelation therapy. Arch Dis Child 1982; 57:929.

788. Russo G, Romeo MA, et al: Early iron chelation therapy in thalassemia major. Haematologica 1983; 68:69.

789. de Virgiliis S, Congia M, et al: Deferoxamine-induced growth retardation in patients with thalassemia major. J Pediatr 1988; 113:661.

790. Freeman AP, Giles RW, et al: Sustained normalization of cardiac function by chelation therapy in thalassaemia major. Clin Lab Haematol 1989; 11:299.

791. Olivieri NF, Nathan DG, et al: Survival in medically treated patients with homozygous beta-thalassemia. N Engl J Med 1994; 331:574.

792. Ehlers KH, Giardina PJ, et al: Prolonged survival in patients with beta-thalassemia major treated with deferoxamine. J Pediatr 1991; 118:540.

793. Ehlers KH, Levin AR, et al: Longitudinal study of cardiac function in thalassemia major. Ann N Y Acad Sci 1980; 344:397.

794. Matthew R, Brain M, et al: Thalassemia: Current Therapy in Hematology/Oncology-3. Philadelphia, B.C. Decker, Inc., 1988, p 39.

795. Giardina PJ, Ehlers KH, et al: The effect of subcutaneous deferoxamine on the cardiac profile of thalassemia major: a five-year study. Ann N Y Acad Sci 1985; 445:282.

796. Lerner N, Blei F, et al: Chelation therapy and cardiac status in older patients with thalassemia major. Am J Pediatr Hematol Oncol 1990; 12:56.

797. Marcus RE, Davies SC, et al: Desferrioxamine to improve cardiac function in iron overloaded patients with thalassemia major. Lancet 1984; 1:392.

798. Nienhuis AW: Unpublished observations.

799. De Sanctis V, D'Ascola G, et al: The development of diabetes mellitus and chronic liver disease in long-term chelated beta thalassaemic patients. Postgrad Med J 1986; 62:831.

800. Olivieri NF, Bunic JR, et al: Visual and auditory neurotoxicity in patients receiving subcutaneous deferoxamine infusions. N Engl J Med 1986; 314:869.

801. Barratt PS, Toogood IR: Hearing loss attributed to desferrioxamine in patients with beta-thalassaemia major. Med J Aust 1987; 147:177.

802. Albera R, Pia F, et al: Hearing loss and desferrioxamine in homozygous beta-thalassemia. Audiology 1988; 27:207.

803. Porter JB, Jaswon MS, et al: Desferrioxamine ototoxicity: evaluation of risk factors in thalassaemic patients and guidelines for safe dosage. Br J Haematol 1989; 73:403.

804. de Virgiliis S, Congia M, et al: Depletion of trace elements and acute ocular toxicity induced by desferrioxamine in patients with thalassaemia. Arch Dis Child 1988; 63:250.

805. Davies SC, Marcus RE, et al: Ocular toxicity of high-dose intravenous desferrioxamine. Lancet 1983; 2:181.

806. Marciani MG, Cianciulli P, et al: Toxic effects of high-dose deferoxamine treatment in patients with iron overload: an electrophysiological study of cerebral and visual function. Haematologica 1991; 76:131.

807. Rinaldi M, Della Corte M, et al: Ocular involvement correlated with age in patients affected by major and intermedia beta-thalassemia treatment or not with desferrioxamine. Metab Pediatr Syst Ophthalmol 1993; 16:23.

808. Polson RJ, Jawed A, et al: Treatment of rheumatoid arthritis with desferrioxamine: relation between stores of iron before treatment and side effects. BMJ 1985; 291:448.

809. Bentur Y, Koren G, et al: Comparison of deferoxamine pharmacokinetics between asymptomatic thalassemic children and those exhibiting severe neurotoxicity. Clin Pharmacol Ther 1990; 47:478.

810. Blake DR, Winyard P, et al: Cerebral and ocular toxicity induced by desferrioxamine. Q J Med 1985; 56:345.

811. Peto TEA, Hershko C: Iron and infection. Bailliere's Clin Hematol 1989; 2:435.

812. Robins-Browne RM, Prpic JK: Effects of iron and desferrioxamine on infections with *Yersinia enterocolitica*. Infect Immun 1985; 47:774.

813. Gallant T, Freedman MH, et al: *Yersinia* sepsis in patients with iron overload treated with deferoxamine. N Engl J Med 1986; 314:1643.

814. Goodhill JJ, Abuelo JG: Mucormycosis—a new risk of deferoxamine therapy in dialysis patients with aluminum or iron overload? N Engl J Med 1987; 317:54.

815. Bowern N, Ramshaw IA, et al: Effect of an iron-chelating agent on lymphocyte proliferation. Aust J Exp Biol Med Sci 1984; 62:743.

816. Bowern N, Ramshaw IA, et al: Inhibition of autoimmune neuropathological process by treatment with an iron-chelating agent. J Exp Med 1984; 160:1536.

817. Bierer BE, Nathan DG: The effect of desferrithiocin, an oral iron chelator, on T cell function. Blood 1990; 76:2052.

818. Carotenuto P, Pontesilli O, et al: Desferoxamine blocks IL 2 receptor on T lymphocytes. J Immunol 1986; 136:2342.

819. Estrov Z, Tawa A, et al: *In vitro* and *in vivo* effects of deferoxamine in neonatal acute leukemia. Blood 1987; 69:757.

820. Lederman HM, Cohen A, et al: Deferoxamine: a reversible S-

phase inhibitor human lymphocyte proliferation. Blood 1984; 64:748.

821. Freedman MH, Grisaru D, et al: Pulmonary syndrome in patients with thalassemia major receiving intravenous deferoxamine infusions. Am J Dis Child 1990; 144:565.

822. Tenenbein M, Kowalski S, et al: Pulmonary toxic effects of continuous desferrioxamine administration in acute iron poisoning. Lancet 1992; 339:699.

823. Adamson IY, Sienko A, et al: Pulmonary toxicity of deferoxamine in iron-poisoned mice. Toxicol Appl Pharmacol 1993; 120:13.

824. Frank L: Hyperoxic inhibition of newborn rat lung development: protection by deferoxamine. Free Radical Biol Med 1991; 11:341.

825. Shannon M: Desferrioxamine in acute iron poisoning. Lancet 1992; 339:1601.

826. Koren G, Bentur Y, et al: Acute changes in renal function associated with deferoxamine therapy. Am J Dis Child 1989; 143:1077.

827. Koren G, Kochavi-Atiya Y, et al: The effects of subcutaneous deferoxamine administration on renal function in thalassemia major. Int J Hematol 1991; 54:371.

828. Cianciulli P, Sollecito D, et al: Early detection of nephrotoxic effects in thalassemic patients receiving desferrioxamine therapy. Kidney Int 1994; 46:467.

829. Hartkamp MJ, Babyn PS, et al: Spinal deformities in deferoxamine-treated homozygous beta-thalassemia major patients. Pediatr Radiol 1993; 23:525.

830. Olivieri NF, Koren G, et al: Growth failure and bony changes induced by deferoxamine. Am J Pediatr Hematol Oncol 1992; 14:48.

831. Olivieri NF, Berriman AM, et al: Reduction in tissue iron stores with a new regimen of continuous ambulatory intravenous deferoxamine. Am J Hematol 1992; 41:61.

832. Tamary H, Goshen J, et al: Long-term intravenous deferoxamine treatment for noncompliant transfusion-dependent beta-thalassemia patients. Isr J Med Sci 1994; 30:658.

833. deMontalembert M, Jan D, et al: Intensification du traitement chelateur pu fer par la desferrioxamine a l'aide d'une chambre implantable d'acces veineux (Port-A-Cath). Arch Fr Pediatr 1992; 49:159.

834. Jensen PD, Jensen FT, et al: Evaluation of transfusional iron overload before and during iron chelation by magnetic resonance imaging of the liver and determination of serum ferritin in adult non-thalassaemic patients. Br J Haematol 1995; 89:880.

834a. Borgna-Pignatti C, Cohen A: Evaluation of a new method of administration of the iron chelating agent deferoxamine. J Pediatr 1997; 130:86.

835. Nathan DG, Piomelli S: Introduction: oral iron chelators. Semin Hematol 1990; 27:83.

836. Hershko C, Link G, et al: Principles of iron chelating therapy. Semin Hematol 1990; 27:91.

837. Porter JB, Hilder RC, et al: Update on the hydroxypyridinone oral iron-chelating agents. Semin Hematol 1990; 27:95.

838. Olivieri NF, Koren G, et al: Studies of the oral chelator 1,2-dimethyl-3-hydroxypyrid-4-one in thalassemia patients. Semin Hematol 1990; 27:101.

839. Grady RW, Hershko C: An evaluation of the potential of HBED as an orally effective iron-chelating drug. Semin Hematol 1990; 27:105.

840. Brittenham GM: Pyridoxal isonicotinoyl hydrazone: an effective iron-chelator after oral administration. Semin Hematol 1990; 27:112.

841. Wolfe LC: Desferrithiocin. Semin Hematol 1990; 27:117.

842. Hoffbrand AV: Oral iron chelation. Semin Hematol 1996; 33:1.

843. Olivieri NF, Brittenham GM, et al: Iron-chelation therapy with oral deferiprone in patients with thalassemia major. N Engl J Med 1995; 332:918.

844. Olivieri NF, Koren G, et al: Reduction of tissue iron stores and normalization of serum ferritin during treatment with the oral iron chelator L1 in thalassemia intermedia. Blood 1992; 79:2741.

845. Shalev O, Repka T, et al: Deferiprone (L1) chelates pathologic iron deposits from membranes of intact thalassemic and sickle red blood cells both in vitro and in vivo. Blood 1995; 86:2008.

846. al-Refaie FN, Hoffbrand AV: Oral iron-chelating therapy: the L1 experience. Bailliereres Clin Haematol 1994; 7:941.

847. Matsui D, Klein J, et al: Relationship between the pharmacokinetics and iron excretion pharmacodynamics of the new oral iron chelator 1,2-dimethyl-3-hydroxypyrid-4-one in patients with thalassemia. Clin Pharmacol Ther 1991; 50:294.

848. Nathan DG: An orally active iron chelator. N Engl J Med 1995; 332:953.

849. al-Refaie FN, Wonke B, et al: Efficacy and possible adverse effects of the oral iron chelator 1,2-dimethyl-3-hydroxypyrid-4-one (L1) in thalassemia major. Blood 1992; 80:593.

849a. Olivieri NF, Brittenham GM: Iron-chelating therapy and the treatment of thalassemia. Blood 1997; 89:739.

850. Roesner HP: The role of ascorbic acid in the turnover of storage iron. Semin Hematol 1983; 20:91.

851. Lynch SR, Seftel HC, et al: Accelerated oxidative catabolism of ascorbic acid in sideretic Bantu. Am J Clin Nutr 1967; 20:641.

852. Lipschitz DA, Bothwell TH, et al: The role of ascorbic acid in the metabolism of storage iron. Br J Haematol 1972; 20:155.

853. Wapnick AA, Bothwell TH, et al: The relationship between serum iron levels and ascorbic acid stores in sideretic Bantu. Br J Haematol 1970; 19:271.

854. Cohen A, Cohen IJ, et al: Scurvy and altered iron stores in thalassemia major. N Engl J Med 1981; 304:158.

855. Nienhuis AW, Delea C, et al: Evaluation of desferrioxamine and ascorbic acid for the treatment of chronic iron overload. In Bergsma D, Cerami A, et al (eds): Birth Defects: Iron Metabolism and Thalassemia. New York, Alan R. Liss, Inc., 1976, p 177.

856. Bridges KR, Hoffman KE: The effects of ascorbic acid on the intracellular metabolism of iron and ferritin. J Biol Chem 1986; 261:14273.

857. Bridges KR: Ascorbic acid inhibits lysosomal autophagy of ferritin. J Biol Chem 1987; 262:14773.

858. Miller DM, Aust SD: Studies of ascorbate-dependent, iron-catalyzed lipid peroxidation. Arch Biochem Biophys 1989; 271:113.

859. Burkitt MJ, Gilbert BC: The control of iron-induced oxidative damage in isolated rat-liver mitochondria by respiration state and ascorbate. Free Radic Res Commun 1989; 5:333.

860. Henry W: Echocardiographic evaluation of the heart in thalassemia major. In Nienhuis AW (moderator): Thalassemia major: Molecular and Clinical Aspects. Ann Intern Med 1979; 91:883.

861. Nienhuis AW: Vitamin C and iron. N Engl J Med 1981; 304:170.

862. Hyman CB, Landing B, et al: dl-alpha-Tocopherol, iron, and lipofuscin in thalassemia. Ann N Y Acad Sci 1974; 232:211.

863. Zannos-Mariolea L, Papagregoriou-Theodoridou M, et al: Relationship between tocopherols and serum lipid levels in children with beta-thalassemia major. Am J Clin Nutr 1978; 31:259.

864. Oski FA, Barnes LA: Vitamin E deficiency: a previously unrecognized cause of hemolytic anemia in the premature infant. J Pediatr 1967; 70:211.

865. Hershko C, Rachmilewitz EA: The inhibitory effect of vitamin E on desferrioxamine-induced iron excretion in rats. Proc Soc Exp Biol Med 1976; 152:249.

866. Lubhy AL, Cooperman JM, et al: Folic acid deficiency as a limiting factor in the anemia of thalassemia major. Blood 1961; 18:786.

867. Robinson MG, Watson RJ: Megaloblastic anemia complicating thalassemia major. Am J Dis Child 1963; 105:275.

868. Lubhy AL, Cooperman JM, et al: Vitamin B₁₂ metabolism in thalassemia major. Ann N Y Acad Sci 1969; 165:443.

869. Zaino E: Deferoxamine and trace metal excretion. In Zaino E, Roberts R (eds): Chelation Therapy in Chronic Iron Overload. Miami, Symposia Specialists, 1977, p 95.

870. Ridley CM: Zinc deficiency developing in treatment for thalassemia. J R Soc Med 1982; 75:38.

871. Thomas ED, Buckner CD, et al: Marrow transplantation for thalassemia. Lancet 1982; 11:8292.

872. Lucarelli G, Polchi P, et al: Allogenic marrow transplantation for thalassemia. Exp Hematol 1984; 12:676.

873. Piomelli S, Lerner N, et al: Bone marrow transplantation for thalassemia. N Engl J Med 1987; 317:964. Correspondence.

874. Lucarelli G, Polchi P, et al: Marrow transplantation for thalassemia following busulphan and cyclophosphamide. Lancet 1985; 1:1355.

875. Lucarelli G, Galimberti M, et al: Marrow transplantation in patients with advanced thalassemia. N Engl J Med 1987; 316:1050.

876. Lucarelli G, Galimberti M, et al: Bone marrow transplantation in patients with thalassemia. N Engl J Med 1990; 322:417.

877. Walters MC, Sullivan KM, et al: Bone marrow transplantation for thalassemia. The USA experience. Am J Pediatr Hematol Oncol 1994; 16:11.

878. Vellodi A, Picton S, et al: Bone marrow transplantation for thalssaemia: experience of two British centres. Bone Marrow Transplant 1994; 13:559.

879. Cao A, Galanello Renzo M, et al: Clinical experience of management of thalassemia: the Sardinian experience. Semin Hematol 1996; 33:66.

880. Shulman HM, Hinterberger W: Hepatic veno-occlusive disease-liver toxicity syndrome after bone marrow transplantation. Bone Marrow Transpl 1992; 10:197.

881. Apperley JF: Bone marrow transplant for the haemoglobinopathies: past, present and future. Baillieres Clin Haematol 1993; 6:299.

882. DeSimone J, Heller P, et al: 5-Azacytidine stimulates fetal hemoglobin synthesis in anemia baboons. Proc Natl Acad Sci U S A 1982; 79:4428.

883. Ley TJ, DeSimone J, et al: 5-Azacytidine selectively increases gamma-globin synthesis in a patient with beta thalassemia. N Engl J Med 1982; 307:1469.

884. Charache S, Dover G, et al: Treatment of sickle cell anemia with 5-azacytidine results in increased fetal hemoglobin production and is associated with nonrandom hypomethylation of DNA around the gamma-delta-beta-globin gene complex. Proc Natl Acad Sci U S A 1983; 80:4842.

885. Ley TJ, DeSimone J, et al: 5-Azacytidine increases gamma-globin synthesis and reduces the proportion of dense cells in patients with sickle cell anemia. Blood 1983; 62:370.

886. Letvin NL, Linch DC, et al: Augmentation of fetal-hemoglobin production in anemic monkeys by hydroxyurea. N Engl J Med 1984; 310:869.

887. Papayannopoulou T, de Ron AT, et al: Arabinosylcytosine induces fetal hemoglobin in baboons by perturbing erythroid cell differentiation kinetics. Science 1984; 224:617.

888. Platt O, Orkin SH, et al: Hydroxyurea enhances fetal hemoglobin production in sickle cell anemia. J Clin Invest 1984; 74:652.

889. Lavelle D, DeSimone J, et al: Fetal hemoglobin reactivation in baboon and man: a short perspective. Am J Hematol 1993; 42:91.

890. Hajjar FM, Pearson HA: Pharmacologic treatment of thalassemia intermedia with hydroxyurea. J Pediatr 1994; 125:490.

891. Al-Khatti A, Veith RW, et al: Stimulation of fetal hemoglobin synthesis by erythropoietin in baboons. N Engl J Med 1987; 317:415.

892. McDonagh KT, Dover GJ, et al: Manipulation of HbF production with hematopoietic growth factors. In Stamatoyannopoulos G, Nienhuis AW (eds): Hemoglobin Switching, Part B: Cellular and Molecular Mechanisms. New York, Alan R. Liss, Inc., 1989, p 307.

893. McDonagh KT, Dover GJ, et al: Hydroxyurea-induced HbF production in anemic primates: augmentation by erythropoietin, hematopoietic growth factors, and sodium butyrate. Exp Hematol 1992; 20:1156.

894. Umemura T, al-Khatti A, et al: Effects of interleukin-3 and erythropoietin on in vivo erythropoiesis and F-cell formation in primates. Blood 1989; 74:1571.

895. Perrine SP, Greene MF, et al: Delay in the fetal globin switch in infants of diabetic mothers. N Engl J Med 1985; 312:334.

896. Little JA, Dempsey NJ, et al: Metabolic persistence of fetal hemoglobin. Blood 1995; 75:1712.

897. Perrine SP, Rudolph A, et al: Butyrate infusions in the ovine fetus delay the biologic clock for globin gene switching. Proc Natl Acad Sci U S A 1988; 85:8540.

898. Constantoulakis P, Papayannopoulou T, et al: Alpha-Amino-N-butyric acid stimulates fetal hemoglobin in the adult. Blood 1988; 72:1961.

899. Constantoulakis P, Knitter G, et al: On the induction of fetal hemoglobin by butyrates: in vivo and in vitro studies with sodium butyrate and comparison of combination treatments with 5-AzaC and AraC. Blood 1989; 74:1963.

900. McDonagh KT: Unpublished observations.

901. Burns LJ, Glauber JG, et al: Butyrate induces selective transcriptional activation of a hypomethylated embryonic globin gene in adult erythroid cells. Blood 1988; 72:1536.

902. Stamatoyannopoulos G, Blau CA, et al: Fetal hemoglobin induction by acetate, a product of butyrate catabolism. Blood 1944; 84:3198.

903. Dover GJ, Brusilow S, et al: Induction of fetal hemoglobin production in subjects with sickle cell anemia by oral sodium phenylbutyrate. Blood 1994; 84:339.

904. Perrine SP, Ginder GD, et al: A short-term trial of butyrate to stimulate fetal-globin-gene expression in the beta-globin disorders. N Engl J Med 1993; 328:81.

905. Perrine SP, Olivieri NF, et al: Butyrate derivatives. New agents for stimulating fetal globin production in the beta-globin disorders. Am J Pediatr Hematol Oncol 1994; 16:67.

906. Collins AF, Pearson HA, et al: Oral sodium phenylbutyrate therapy in homozygous beta thalassemia: a clinical trial. Blood 1995; 85:43.

907. Sher GD, Olivieri NF: Rapid healing of chronic leg ulcers during arginine butyrate therapy in patients with sickle cell disease and thalassemia. Blood 1994; 84:2378.

908. Sher GD, Ginder GD, et al: Extended therapy with intravenous arginine butyrate in patients with beta-hemoglobinopathies. N Engl J Med 1995; 332:1606.

909. Blau CA, Constantoulakis P, et al: Fetal hemoglobin induction with butyric acid: efficacy and toxicity. Blood 1993; 81:529.

910. Veith R, Galanello R, et al: Stimulation of F-cell production in patients with sickle-cell anemia treated with cytarabine or hydroxyurea. N Engl J Med 1985; 313:1571.

911. Dover GJ, Humphries RK, et al: Hydroxyurea induction of hemoglobin F production in sickle cell disease: relationship between cytotoxicity and F-cell production. Blood 1986; 67:735.

912. Charache S, Dover GJ, et al: Hydroxyurea-induced augmentation of fetal hemoglobin production in patients with sickle cell anemia. Blood 1987; 69:109.

913. Rodgers GP, Dover GJ, et al: Hematologic responses of patients with sickle cell disease to treatment with hydroxyurea. N Engl J Med 1990; 322:1037.

914. Dover GJ: Personal communication.

915. Dunbar C, Travis W, et al: 5-Azacytidine treatment in a beta⁰-thalassaemic patient unable to be transfused due to multiple alloantibodies. Br J Haematol 1989; 72:467.

916. Lowrey CH, Nienhuis AW: Brief report: treatment with azacytidine of patients with end-stage beta-thalassemia. N Engl J Med 1993; 329:845.

917. Riggs AD: 5-Methylcytosine, gene regulation, and cancer. Adv Cancer Res 1983; 40:1.

918. Santi DV, Garrett CE, et al: On the mechanism of inhibition of DNA-cytosine methyltransferases by cytosine analogs. Cell 1983; 33:9.

919. Cooper DN: Eukaryotic DNA methylation. Hum Genet 1983; 64:315.

920. Jones PA: Altering gene expression with 5-azacytidine. Cell 1985; 40:485.

921. Landolph JR, Jones PA: Mutageneticity of 5-azacytidine and related nucleosides in C3H/10Tl/a clone 8 and V79 cells. Cancer Res 1982; 42:817.

922. Harrison JJ, Anisowicz A, et al: Azacytidine-induced tumorigenesis of CHEF/18 cells: Correlated DNA methylation and chromosome changes. Proc Natl Acad Sci U S A 1983; 80:6606.

923. Darmon M, Nicolas J-F, et al: 5-Azacytidine is able to induce the conversion of teratocarcinoma-derived mesenchymal cells into epithelial cells. EMBO J 1984; 3:961.

924. Liu DP, Liang CC, et al: Treatment of severe beta-thalassemia (patients) with Myleran. Am J Hematol 1990; 33:50.

925. Al-Khatti A, Papayannopoulou T, et al: Cooperative enhancement of F-cell formation in baboons treated with erythropoietin and hydroxyurea. Blood 1988; 72:817.

926. Rodgers GP: Personal communication.

927. Stamatoyannopoulos JA: Future prospects for treatment of hemoglobinopathies. West J Med 1992; 157:631.

928. Anderson WF: Prospects for human gene therapy. Science 1984; 226:401.

929. Friedmann T: Progress toward human gene therapy. Science 1989; 244:1275.

930. Cournoyer D, Caskey CT: Gene transfer into humans: a first step. N Engl J Med 1990; 323:601.

931. Nienhuis AW, McDonagh KT, et al: Gene transfer into hematopoietic stem cells. Cancer 1991; 67:2700.

932. Friedmann T: The promise and overpromise of human gene therapy. Gene Ther 1994; 1:217.

933. Brenner MK, Rill DR, et al: Gene-marking to trace origin of relapse after autologous bone-marrow transplantation. Lancet 1993; 341:85.

934. Novak U, Harris EA, et al: High-level beta-globin expression after retroviral transfer of locus activation region-containing human beta-globin gene derivatives into murine erythroleukemia cells. Proc Natl Acad Sci U S A 1990; 87:3386.

935. Sadelain M, Wang CH, et al: Generation of a high-titer retroviral vector capable of expressing high levels of the human beta-globin gene. Proc Natl Acad Sci U S A 1995; 92:6728.

936. Huisman THJ: Trimodality in the percentages of beta chain variants in heterozygotes. The effect of the number of active Hb alpha structural loci. Hemoglobin 1977; 1:239.

937. Higgs DR, Pressley L, et al: The genetics and molecular basis of alpha thalassemia in association with HbS in Jamaican Negroes. Br J Haematol 1981; 47:43.

938. Steinberg MH, Adams JG, et al: Alpha thalassemia in adults with sickle-cell trait. Br J Haematol 1975; 30:31.

939. Shaeffer JR, DeSimone J, et al: Hemoglobin synthesis in a family with alpha-thalassemia trait and sickle cell trait. Biochem Genet 1975; 13:783.

940. Wasi P: Hemoglobinopathies including thalassemia: I. Tropical Asia. Clin Haematol 1981; 10:707.

941. Cunningham TM: Hemoglobin E in Indochinese refugees. West J Med 1982; 137:186.

942. Monzon CM, Fairbanks VF, et al: Hereditary red cell disorders in Southeast Asian refugees and the effect on the prevalence of thalassemia disorders in the United States. Am J Med Sci 1986; 292:147.

943. Anderson HM, Ranney HM: Southeast Asian immigrants: the new thalassemias in Americans. Semin Hematol 1990; 27:239.

944. Sicard D, Lieurzou Y, et al: High genetic polymorphism of hemoglobin disorders in Laos; complex phenotypes due to associated thalassemic syndromes. Hum Genet 1979; 50:327.

945. Marsh WL, Rogers RS, et al: Hematologic findings in Southeast Asian immigrants with particular reference to hemoglobin E. Ann Clin Lab Sci 1983; 13:299.

946. Bhamarapravati N, Na-Nakorn S, et al: Pathology of abnormal hemoglobin diseases seen in Thailand: I. Pathology of beta-thalassemia hemoglobin E disease. Am J Clin Pathol 1967; 47:745.

947. Itano HA: A new inherited abnormality of human hemoglobin. Proc Natl Acad Sci U S A 1950; 36:613.

948. Perosa L, Manganelli G, et al: Il primo caso di Hb C-thalassemia descritto in Italia. Haematologica 1961; 46:211.

949. Portier A, Traverse P, et al: L'hemoglobinose C-thalassemia. Presse Med 1960; 68:1760.

950. Goksel V, Tartaroglu N: Haemoglobin-C-thalassemia bei zwei Geschwistern von Weisser Rasse. In Lehmann H, Betke K (eds): Haemoglobin Colloquium. Stuttgart, Georg Thieme Verlag, 1961, p 55.

951. Steinberg MH, Adams JG: Thalassemic hemoglobinopathies. Am J Pathol 1983; 113:396.

952. Flatz G: Hemoglobin E: distribution and population genetics. Hum Genetik 1967; 3:189.

953. Kan YW, Golbus MS, et al: Successful application of prenatal diagnosis in a pregnancy at risk for homozygous beta-thalassemia. N Engl J Med 1975; 292:1099.

954. Orkin SH, Alter BP, et al: Application of endonuclease mapping to the analysis and prenatal diagnosis of thalassemias caused by globin-gene deletion. N Engl J Med 1978; 299:166.

955. Dozy AM, Forman EN, et al: Prenatal diagnosis of homozygous alpha thalassemia. JAMA 1969; 241:1610.

956. Kan YW, Valenti C, et al: Fetal blood-sampling in utero. Lancet 1974; 1:79.

957. Rodeck C: Fetoscopy guided by real-time ultrasound for pure fetal blood samples, fetal skin samples, and examination of the fetus in utero. Br J Obstet Gynaecol 1980; 87:449.

958. Daffos F, Capella-Pavlovsky M, et al: Fetal blood sampling via the umbilical cord using a needle guided by ultrasound. Prenat Diagn 1983; 3:271.

959. Alter BP: Prenatal diagnosis: general introduction, methodology, and review. Hemoglobin 1988; 12:763.

960. Saiki RK, Walsh PS, et al: Genetics analysis of amplified DNA with immobilized sequence-specific oligonucleotide probes. Proc Natl Acad Sci U S A 1989; 86:6230.

961. Modell B, Petrou M, et al: Effect of fetal diagnostic testing on birth-rate of thalassaemia major in Britain. Lancet 1984; 2:1383.

962. Loukopoulos D: Prenatal diagnosis of thalassemia and of the hemoglobinopathies; a review. Hemoglobin 1985; 9:435.

963. Modell B, Bulyzhenkov V: Distribution and control of some genetic disorders. World Health Stat Q 1988; 41:209.

964. Cao A, Rosatelli C, et al: The prevention of thalassemia in Sardinia. Clin Genet 1989; 36:277.

965. Loukopoulos D: Current status of thalassemia and the sickle cell syndromes in Greece. Semin Hematol 1996; 33:76.

VII

The Phagocyte System

The Phagocyte System and Disorders of
Granulopoiesis and Granulocyte Function

The Phagocyte System and Disorders of Granulopoiesis and Granulocyte Function

Mary C. Dinauer

DEFINITION AND CLASSIFICATION OF PHAGOCYTES

Phagocytic leukocytes are bone marrow-derived cells that have the capacity to engulf and digest particulate matter. Phagocytes are essential for the host response to infection and inflammation and are equipped with specialized machinery enabling them to seek out, ingest, and kill microorganisms. Other functions include the synthesis and secretion of cytokines, pyrogens, and other cellular mediators, as well as the digestion of senescent cells and debris.

The phagocyte system has two principal limbs: granulocytes (neutrophils, eosinophils, and basophils) and mononuclear phagocytes (monocytes and tissue macrophages). Neutrophils circulate in the blood stream until encountering specific chemotactic signals that promote adhesion to the vascular endothelium, diapedesis into tissues, and migration to sites of microbial invasion. In contrast, mononuclear phagocytes function primarily as resident cells in certain tissues, such as lung, liver, spleen, and peritoneum, where they perform a surveillance role and also interact closely with lymphocytes to promote specific immune responses. Both groups of phagocytes dispose of appropriately opsonized targets by engulfment and sequestration within intracellular vacuoles, followed by the release of digestive lysosomal enzymes and bactericidal antibiotic proteins from storage granules and by the generation of highly reactive oxidants from the respiratory burst pathway.

This chapter is divided into three major sections. In the first section the distribution and functional properties of the granulocytic and mononuclear phagocytes are summarized. In the second section, clinical disorders associated with a deficiency or excess of phagocytic leukocytes in the circulation or tissues are reviewed. The third section focuses on disorders of phagocyte function, including those due to intrinsic phagocyte defects as well as those secondary to other disease processes.

PHAGOCYTE MORPHOLOGY, DISTRIBUTION, AND STRUCTURE

Regulation of Myelopoiesis

Granulocytes and monocytes are produced in the bone marrow in a complex, highly regulated, and dynamic process that requires both specific hematopoietic growth factors and an appropriate bone marrow microenvironment. As reviewed in Chapter 6, multipotent, self-renewing hematopoietic stem cells give rise to lineage-restricted progenitor cells that divide and further differentiate in the bone marrow before their release into the intravascular compartment. Cytokines important for promoting the proliferation and differentiation of neutrophils and monocytes from primitive precursor cells include interleukin (IL)-3, IL-6, granulocyte-macrophage colony-stimulating factor (GM-CSF), macrophage colony-stimulating factor (M-CSF), and granulocyte colony-stimulating factor (G-CSF).[1-3] M-CSF and G-CSF are relatively specific for the monocyte and neutrophil lineages, respectively. During infections, activated macrophages release cytokines such as IL-1, IL-6, and tumor necrosis factor (TNF), which activate stromal cells and T lymphocytes to produce additional amounts of colony-stimulating factors and increase the production of myeloid cells. IL-5 appears to play an important role in inducing eosinophil differentiation,[4-6] and IL-3 is the principal cytokine inducing human basophil growth and differentiation.[7] In addition to their regulatory role in hematopoiesis, hematopoietic growth factors can act on mature myeloid cells

Table 22-1. NEUTROPHIL AND MONOCYTE KINETICS

	Transit Time Range (h)	Total Cells (×10⁹/kg)
Neutrophils		
Marrow mitotic compartment		
Myeloblast	23	0.14
Promyelocyte	26–78	0.51
Myelocyte	17–1266	1.95
Marrow maturation—storage compartment		
Metamyelocyte	8–108	2.7
Band	12–96	3.6
Neutrophil	0–120	<u>2.5</u>
Total marrow storage		8.8
Vascular compartment		
Circulating neutrophils	4–10	0.3
Marginated neutrophils	4–10	<u>0.4</u>
Total blood neutrophils		0.7
Tissue compartments	0–3 days (?)	Not known
Neutrophil turnover rate	1.6 × 10⁹/kg per d	
Monocytes		
Marrow mitotic compartment: promonocyte	~160	0.006
Marrow nonmitotic compartment: monocyte	24	0.10
Vascular compartment	36–104	0.024
Tissue compartment	Days–months	Not known
Blood monocyte turnover rate	6 × 10⁶/kg per d	

Neutrophil and monocyte kinetics based on references 15 through 18 and 91.

$$\text{×10}^9\text{/kg}$$

$$\text{Transit Time Range (h)}$$

Table 22-2. CONTENT OF HUMAN NEUTROPHIL GRANULES AND SECRETORY ORGANELLES

Primary: Azurophil Granules	Secondary: Specific Granules	Tertiary: Gelatinase Granules	Secretory Vesicles
Membranes	**Membranes**	**Membranes**	**Membranes**
CD63	CD15 antigens (Lewis X)	Mac-1 (CD11b/CD18)	Alkaline phosphatase
CD68	Cytochrome b_{558}	Formyl peptide receptor	Cytochrome b_{558}
Matrix	Formyl peptide receptor	Diacylglycerol-deacylating enzyme	Formyl peptide receptor
Acid mucopolysaccharide	Fibronectin receptor		Mac-1 (CD11b/CD18)
Alpha$_1$-antitrypsin	G-protein α subunit	**Matrix**	Uroplasminogen activator-receptor
Alpha-mannosidase	Laminin receptor	Gelatinase	
Azurocidin	Mac-1 (CD11b/CD18)	Acetyltransferase	**Matrix**
Bactericidal permeability-increasing protein	Rap 1, Rap 2		Plasma protein
Beta-glycerophosphatase	Thrombospondin receptor		
Beta-glucuronidase	Tumor necrosis factor receptor		
Cathepsins	Vitronectin		
Defensins	**Matrix**		
Elastase	Beta$_2$-microglobulin		
Heparin binding protein	Collagenase		
Lysozyme	Gelatinase		
Myeloperoxidase	Histaminase		
N-Acetyl-β-glucosaminidase	Heparanase		
Proteinase-3	Lactoferrin		
Sialidase	Lysozyme		
	Plasminogen activator		
	Vitamin B$_{12}$–binding protein (transcobalamin I)		

Adapted from Borregaard N, Lollike K, Kjeldsen L, et al: Human neutrophil granules and secretory vesicles. Eur J Haematol 1993: 51:187–198. © 1993 Munksgaard International Publishers Ltd., Copenhagen, Denmark.

and stimulate their functional activities. For example, circulating phagocytes become "primed" to undergo an enhanced respiratory burst on exposure to GM-CSF.[8]

Myeloid differentiation also appears to be modulated by retinoic acid through specific retinoic acid receptors,[9, 10] which are members of the steroid–thyroid hormone receptor superfamily.[11] The participation of retinoic acid in myeloid development was originally surmised from its ability to induce differentiation of myeloid leukemia cell lines and, more recently, leukemic promyelocytes in patients with acute promyelocytic leukemia, which is distinguished by a t(15:17) translocation.[12] This rearrangement results in a fusion gene of the retinoic acid receptor and a putative transcription factor.[13, 14]

Granulocytes

Neutrophils

The neutrophil life span is traditionally divided into the bone marrow, circulating, and tissue phases. Approximately 14 days are spent in the bone marrow, where proliferation and the early stages of neutrophil differentiation are followed by the final stages of maturation and retention in a large, nonmitotic, storage pool that is manyfold larger than the circulating and tissue neutrophil populations (Table 22–1).[15–18] Once released into the blood stream, neutrophils have a half-life of 6 to 10 hours and move between circulating and marginated pools in a reversible fashion. Neutrophils then exit by diapedesis between endothelial cells into tissue sites of infection or inflammation. Once in the tissues,

neutrophils are believed to live for another 1 to 2 days before undergoing apoptosis and engulfment by macrophages.[19–21]

Myeloblasts are the earliest morphologically recognizable granulocyte precursors in the marrow and are identified by their relatively undifferentiated appearance with a large, oval nucleus, several prominent nucleoli, and few or no granules in a gray-blue cytoplasm in Wright-stained preparations. This stage of neutrophil differentiation is followed by the promyelocyte and myelocyte stages, which are distinguished by the appearance of distinct neutrophil granule populations[22] (Table 22–2). Azurophilic, or primary, granules are formed during the promyelocyte stage and contain myeloperoxidase, bactericidal peptides, and lysosomal enzymes. The subsequent myelocyte stage is distinguished by the formation of peroxidase-negative specific, or secondary, granules containing lactoferrin. No further cell divisions occur after the myelocyte stage. The metamyelocyte, band, and mature neutrophil exhibit progressive nuclear condensation, accumulation of glycogen, and development of a third granule population that has a high content of gelatinase.[23]

In Wright-stained blood smears, the mature neutrophil is 10 to 15 μm, with a multilobed, polymorphic nucleus with highly condensed chromatin and a yellow-pink cytoplasm containing numerous granules as well as clumps of glycogen. Circulating neutrophils appear round with some cytoplasmic projections and surface ruffling. A scaffold of cytoskeletal filaments, composed largely of actin microfilaments and microtubules, plays a key role in mediating neutrophil locomotion on surfaces, phagocytosis, and exocytosis.[24–26] Microtubules radiate from the centriole in the perinuclear cytoplasm near the Golgi region, whereas actin tends to be located more peripherally, where it forms an organelle-excluding meshwork. Actin is associated with a variety of actin-binding proteins that regulate the structure of this meshwork and link the actin cytoskeleton to the plasma membrane.

The numerous intracellular granules and vesicles in the neutrophil cytoplasm function as storage pools for cell surface receptors and as reservoirs of sequestered digestive and microbicidal proteins. The older classification of granules as either peroxidase-positive (azurophilic or primary) and peroxidase-negative (specific or secondary) has proven to be too simplistic, based on recent subcellular fractionation, immunoelectron microscopy, and biosynthetic studies.[23] A current classification of neutrophil granules is shown in Table 22–2, which summarizes the composition of their membranes and luminal (matrix) contents. On neutrophil activation by inflammatory signals, granule fusion can result in vacuolization and toxic granulation (prominent azurophilic granules). The degree of these changes in peripheral blood neutrophils has some correlation with the presence of bacterial infection.[27] Döhle bodies can also be seen in infection. These inclusion bodies represent strands of rough endoplasmic reticulum that are retained from a more immature stage and stain bluish owing to their high content of RNA.

Azurophilic granules are defined histochemically by their peroxidase positivity, which is due to myeloperoxidase, an important enzyme in the respiratory burst-dependent killing pathway. Azurophilic granules also contain defensins and bactericidal permeability-increasing protein, which are cytotoxic polypeptides that participate in oxygen-independent killing of microbes. Other components of the azurophilic granule matrix include neutral serine proteases, such as cathepsin and elastase, and other digestive enzymes. Lactoferrin, an iron-binding protein believed to have bactericidal activity, is a marker for secondary granules, which are uniquely found in neutrophils. The membrane of the secondary granules contains a major store of the neutrophil's supply of cytochrome-b_{558}, the electron carrier in the respiratory burst oxidase.[28, 29] Specific granule membranes also contain a pool of receptors for adhesive proteins, TNF, and chemotactic formyl peptides. Although specific granules contain some gelatinase, most of the neutrophil's store of this metalloproteinase is localized to tertiary granules. Tertiary granules are formed relatively late in neutrophil differentiation and are smaller and more easily mobilized for exocytosis than secondary granules.[23] Secretory vesicles are other small granules that are formed in bands and mature neutrophils by endocytosis of the plasma membrane and serve as an important store of the adhesive protein Mac 1 (CD11b/CD18) and other membrane receptors.

The morphologic changes seen with neutrophil differentiation are accompanied by temporally coordinated changes in gene expression and protein synthesis.[30, 31] For example, transcription and translation of messenger RNAs (mRNAs) for myeloperoxidase and cathepsin, which are both primary granule constituents, are restricted to myeloblasts and promyelocytes.[30, 32–34] In contrast, expression of the secondary granule proteins lactoferrin and transcobalamin I occurs in myelocytes and metamyelocytes.[33–35] Gelatinase expression occurs even later in maturation and is first detected in bands and bone marrow neutrophils.[33] The leukocyte β-integrin subunit CD11b is first detectable in myelocytes, and its level increases throughout the later stages of neutrophil differentiation.[30] The gp91[phox] subunit of the respiratory burst oxidase complex is expressed relatively late in neutrophil maturation,[36] consistent with the observation that respiratory burst activity is not detected until the metamyelocyte stage.[37]

The primary function of the mature neutrophil is to move rapidly into tissue sites to destroy invading microbes and clear inflammatory debris. To respond to inflammatory stimuli, the neutrophil is equipped with an array of cell surface receptors for adhesive ligands, chemoattractants, and cytokines that can be divided into groups based on their structure and the major intracellular signaling pathway to which they are linked (Table 22–3). The signal transduction pathways of phagocytes are complex and overlapping.[38, 39] A common early downstream event in transmembrane signaling is the activation of membrane phospholipid metabolism to generate two important second messengers, diacylglycerol and inositol 1,4,5-triphosphate,[40, 41] which in turn cause release of calcium from intracellular stores and activate protein kinase C. Changes in intracellular calcium concentration are important for neutrophil degranulation and secretion and for phagolysosome fusion during phagocytosis.[42] Neutrophil activation is also accompanied by alterations in the phosphorylation status of intracellular proteins, as regulated by protein kinase C,[43] tyrosine kinases and phosphatases,[44, 45] and serine and threonine kinases of the mitogen-activated kinase family.[46, 47] Guanine nucleotide binding proteins play important roles in neutrophil signal transduction. These include the heterotrimeric guanosine triphosphate (GTP)-binding proteins that are coupled to the seven transmembrane-spanning domain (serpentine) receptors for chemoattractants and chemokines[48] and the low-molecular-weight GTPases of the Ras superfamily. The latter category includes Ras p21 itself, which can be activated by means of chemoattractant receptors[49] and Rac proteins, which regulate activity of the respiratory burst nicotinamide-adenine dinucleotide phosphate (NADPH) oxidase.[50]

The mature neutrophil, previously thought of as an "end-stage" cell, retains the capacity for inducible gene expression and protein synthesis even after release from the marrow cavity. For example, expression of mRNA transcripts encoding respiratory burst oxidase components increases in response to inflammatory cytokines such as interferon gamma (IFN-γ).[51] Mature neutrophils can also synthesize and secrete a variety of cytokines, including IL-1, IL-6, TNF-α, GM-CSF, M-CSF, and IL-8, which may promote recruitment and activation of both phagocyte and lymphocyte populations in the inflammatory response.[52, 53]

Table 22–3. RECEPTORS IN NEUTROPHILS

Receptor Grouping	Examples	Structural Characteristics
G-protein linked	FMLP, C5a, PAF, LTB$_4$, IL-8, chemokines	Seven transmembrane spanning domains (serpentine); linked to heterotrimeric guanosine triphosphate binding proteins
Membrane tyrosine kinases	PDGF	Integral membrane protein, intrinsic tyrosine kinase activity; ligation leads to receptor dimerization and cross (``auto'') phosphorylation.
Tyrosine kinase linked	FcγRIIA, GM-CSF	FcγRII is a member of the immunoglobulin family of receptors The GM-CSF receptor is an 84-kd transmembrane protein related to receptors of IL-2 and IL-6. Ligation of receptor activates cytosolic tyrosine kinases.
GPI linked	FcγRIIIB, DAF	These receptors have no intracellular domain. FcγRIIIB may be linked to FcγRIIA.
Adhesion molecules	Beta$_2$ integrins (CD11a/CD18, CD11b/CD18, CD11c/CD18)	Beta-integrins are heterodimers structured with relatively long cytoplasmic tails. L-Selectin has an extracellular lectin-binding domain and a very short cytoplasmic tail.
	L-Selectin	Ligation results in potentiation of the oxidative burst and phagocytosis in adherent cells, calcium signaling, actin cytoskeletal changes, and up-regulation of gene expression.
Ceramide linked	TNF	Two TNF receptors have been cloned; both are single membrane-spanning glycoproteins; ligation activates membrane-bound sphingomyelinase with generation of ceramide, which in turn activates a 96-kd protein kinase.

DAF = decay-accelerating factor; FMLP = *N*-formyl-methionyl-leucyl-phenylalanine; GM-CSF = granulocyte-macrophage colony-stimulating factor; GPI = glycosyl phosphatidylinositol; IL = interleukin; LTB$_4$ = leukotriene B$_4$; PAF = platelet-activating factor; PDGF = platelet-derived growth factor; TNF = tumor necrosis factor.
Adapted from Downey G: Signalling mechanisms in human neutrophils. Curr Opin Hematol, 1995; 2:76–88.

Eosinophils

Like the neutrophil, the eosinophil is compartmentalized in the bone marrow into mitotic and storage pools that constitute up to no more than 0.3% of the nucleated bone marrow cells.[54] Eosinophils arise from a progenitor cell, the CFC-Eo, that is committed at a relatively early stage to differentiate into eosinophils instead of neutrophils and monocytes. Morphologic differentiation and maturation of the eosinophil parallel that of the neutrophil series, and the characteristic eosin-staining specific granules of this granulocyte lineage are prominent by the myelocyte stage. IL-5 plays a key role in regulating eosinophil proliferation, differentiation, and functional activation, and IL-5 levels can be elevated in patients with eosinophilia of diverse causes.[4–6, 55, 56] The mature eosinophil is slightly larger than the neutrophil, with a diameter of 12 to 17 μm. The nucleus is characteristically bilobed, although multiple lobes can be seen in patients with eosinophilia of diverse causes. The cytoplasm has prominent and morphologically distinctive granules that stain strongly with acid aniline dyes, owing to their high content of basic proteins.

Once released from the bone marrow, eosinophils have a half-life in the blood stream similar to neutrophils.[57] After leaving the circulation, eosinophils typically localize in areas exposed to the external environment, such as the tracheobronchial tree, gastrointestinal tract, mammary glands, and vagina and cervix.[58] They are also found in connective tissue immediately below the epithelial layer. As discussed in a later section, eosinophils have both immunoenhancing and immu-

nosuppressive functions and play a role in helminthic infection, allergy, and the responses to certain tumors.[58–60] The majority of mature eosinophils reside in tissues, with a blood-to-tissue ratio of 1:300 to 1:500. The life span of tissue eosinophils is not known but may be several weeks.[58] The number of circulating eosinophils tends to be highest late at night, decreases during the morning, and begins to rise at midafternoon. These changes correlate with the diurnal variation in adrenal glucocorticoid levels, to which circulating eosinophils are very sensitive.[61]

Like the neutrophil, the mature eosinophil is endowed with the capacity for chemotaxis, phagocytosis, degranulation, and the synthesis of reactive oxidants and arachidonate metabolites[58, 62–64] (Table 22–4). Eosinophil cell surface membranes have a variety of receptors for adhesive proteins, immunoglobulin and complement fragments, and numerous chemotactic molecules.[58, 59] The latter includes the tetrapeptides that constitute the eosinophil chemotactic factor of anaphylaxis,[65] which may be responsible for the accumulation of eosinophils at sites of anaphylactic allergies.[59, 60]

Mature eosinophil granules are membrane-bound organelles, 0.15 to 1.5 μm long and 0.3 to 1 μm wide, that contain a variety of enzymes and cytotoxic proteins (see Table 22–4).[66] The small granules are round and homogeneous by electron microscopy. These include the primary granules, which develop early in eosinophilic maturation,[67] and a smaller population appearing in late eosinophils that contain arylsulfatase and other enzymes.[68] The more numerous eosin-staining secondary (specific) granules are large ovoid bodies that contain an electron-dense crystalloid core sur-

Table 22-4. COMPARISON OF EOSINOPHILS AND BASOPHILS

	Eosinophils	Basophils
Chemoattractants	C5a FMLP LTB_4 PAF Histamine IL-3	Eosinophil chemotactic factor of anaphylaxis (ECFA) C5a FMLP LTB_4 Monocytic chemoattractant protein-1 IL-8
Stimulants for Degranulation	LTB_4 ECFA TNF PAF IgG, IgA, IgE IL-3, IL-5 Histamine CSF-GM	IgE C3a, C5a IL-1, IL-5 Insect venoms Cold exposure Some drugs Some hormones CSF-GM
Arachidonic Acid Products Produced by Cells	LTB_4 LTC_4	Leukotriene C_4 (LTC_4) LTD_4 (slow-reacting substance of anaphylaxis (SRS-A)) PAF
Colony-Stimulating Factors for Cells	IL-3 IL-5 GM-CSF	IL-1 IL-3 GM-CSF
Granule Contents	Major basic protein (dense core) Eosinophil peroxidase (matrix) Eosinophil-derived neurotoxin Arginine-rich cationic proteins Acid phosphatase Aryl sulfatase Lysophospholipase	Histamine Kallikrein Toluene-sulfo-trypsin arginine methyl esterase (TAME) Sulfated glycosaminoglycans (heparin, chondroitin sulfate) Trypsin Chymotrypsin
Membrane	NADPH-dependent oxidase Fc receptor for IgA, IgG, and IgE	Fc receptor for IgE Lysophospholipase

Adapted from Shurin S: Eosinophil and basophil structure and function. In Hoffman R, Benz EJ, et al (eds): Hematology: Basic Principles and Practice. New York, Churchill Livingstone, 1995, pp 762–769.

rounded by a less dense matrix.[66] Hydrolytic enzymes, cathepsin, and an eosinophil-specific peroxidase are located in the matrix. The eosinophil peroxidase plays an important role in the anthelminthic function of eosinophils[69, 70] and uses bromate to generate hypobromous acid from hydrogen peroxide.[71] The specific granule matrix also contains eosinophilic cationic protein and eosinophil-derived neurotoxin, which are cationic proteins with ribonuclease activity.[58] The eosinophil major basic protein makes up about 50% of the dense crystalloid core of the eosinophilic specific granule, along with other basic proteins rich in lysine, arginine, and phospholipids.[59, 72] Major basic protein strongly absorbs to membranes, precipitates DNA, and neutralizes heparin. It is toxic to schistosomules of *Schistosoma mansoni* and larvae of *Trichinella spiralis*[59, 73] and induces histamine release from basophils and mast cells.[74]

Both eosinophils and basophils have a lysophospholipase in their plasma membranes and primary granules that can polymerize to form the bipyramidal hexagons known as Charcot-Leyden crystals.[75, 76] Charcot-Leyden crystals are typically found in areas of eosinophil degeneration, such as the nasal mucus of patients with allergies, the stools of patients with parasitic infections, and the pleural fluid of patients with pulmonary eosinophilic infiltrates. The lysophospholipase of the Charcot-Leyden crystals, whose protein sequence is distinct from other eukaryotic or prokaryotic lysophospholipases,[60] catalyzes the hydrolysis and inactivation of lysophospholipids generated by phospholipase A_2, thus preventing the generation of proinflammatory arachidonic acid metabolites. The Charcot-Leyden crystal protein composes about 5% of the total protein in eosinophils.[58]

Basophils

Basophils, like other granulocytes, differentiate and mature in the bone marrow over 7 days before their release into the blood stream and are not normally found in the connective tissues.[77] Basophils account for 0.5% of the total circulating leukocytes and 0.3% of nucleated marrow cells.[78] Mature basophils have a bilobed nucleus and contain prominent metachromatic granules that stain purple or bluish with Wright's stain owing to their high content of sulfated glycosaminoglycans. These granules are rich in heparin, chondroitin sulfate, histamine, and kallikrein but lack acid hydrolases, alkaline phosphatase, and peroxidase[79] (see Table 22–4). The heparin of basophils appears to have poor anticoagulant activity. Basophil granules also contain small amounts of major basic protein as well as serine proteases. Receptors expressed on the plasma membrane for basophils include a high-affinity receptor for the Fc portion of IgE, which is an important trigger for release of granule contents and production of arachidonic acid metabolites in anaphylactic degranulation[80] (see Table 22–4). Hence, basophils are key effector cells in certain hypersensitivity reactions. Basophils can synthesize and secrete IL-4, which is the only known cytokine to be produced by human basophils.[81–83]

Basophils share certain morphologic and functional features with mast cells, which appear to be derived from a common marrow progenitor cell.[84] Similar to basophils, mast cells contain histamine-laden metachromatic granules, express high-affinity IgE receptors, and participate in immediate and cutaneous hypersensitivity.[85] However, mast cells lack receptors for IL-2, IL-3, and CD11b/CD18, which are present on basophils.[7] Receptors for KIT (stem cell factor) are present on mast cells but are absent on the majority of basophils.[85, 86] Murine mast cells can secrete a wide variety of mitogenic or inflammatory cytokines, including many interleukins (1, 3, 4, 5, and 6), chemokines, GM-CSF, and TNF-α, that are likely to play an important role in leukocyte recruitment and inflammation in IgE-dependent reactions.[85]

The fate of the basophil in the tissues is unknown. Mast cells are ordinarily distributed throughout normal connective tissue, where they are often situated adjacent to blood and lymphatic vessels, near or within nerve sheaths, and beneath epithelial surfaces that are exposed to environmental antigens, such as the respiratory and gastrointestinal tracts.[87] Mast cells do not circulate in the blood and retain a limited proliferative capacity in the tissue compartment.[88] In contrast to monocytes and macrophages, a transformation between the circulating and tissue forms of basophils and mast cells has not been observed.

Mononuclear Phagocytes

The blood monocyte is derived from a bone marrow progenitor cell, the colony-forming unit–granulocyte-macrophage, shared with the neutrophil, and undergoes similar stages of differentiation as monoblasts and promonocytes in the marrow cavity. However, the transit time in the marrow compartment is briefer, and the mature monocyte is released into the circulation only 24 hours after the last mitosis (see Table 22–1).[89–91] Consequently, a relative peripheral blood monocytosis commonly precedes the return of granulocytes during recovery from bone marrow aplasia or hypoplasia. The monocyte may spend several days in the intravascular compartment in either circulating or marginated pools.[92] Monocytes then migrate into tissues and body cavities to participate in inflammatory processes as exudate macrophages and to replenish the resident tissue macrophages, which have a relatively long life span. In patients receiving allogeneic bone marrow transplants, host tissue macrophages disappear gradually and are replaced by donor macrophages approximately 3 months after transplantation.[93]

The circulating monocyte in Wright-stained blood smears is 10 to 18 μm in diameter with a convoluted surface, a gray-blue cytoplasm, and an indented or kidney-shaped, foamy nucleus. However, some monocytes can be as small as 7 μm in diameter[94] and can be difficult to distinguish morphologically from lymphocytes.[91] In contrast to neutrophils, monocytes contain a single class of granules with lysosomal characteristics.[95–97] After leaving the circulation, monocytes become larger and take on the appearance of tissue macrophages characteristic of the organ in which they reside. The macrophage nucleus is typically oval with more prominent nucleoli, and the cytoplasm stains blue owing to an increase in RNA content. Monocytes and macrophages are distinguished by the presence of a fluoride-inhibitable nonspecific esterase, which can help in differentiating these cells from other mononuclear cells (e.g., lymphocytes) at inflammatory sites. Monoclonal antibodies specific for mononuclear phagocytes (e.g., the human CD14 antigen, a receptor for endotoxin)[98] are also available.[92]

Monocytes and macrophages share many structural and functional features with neutrophils and are capable of sensing chemotactic gradients, migrating to inflamed sites, ingesting bacteria, and killing them using a variety of cytocidal products. However, compared with neutrophils, the mononuclear phagocytes have a large and diverse developmental potential. In addition to their protective function as phagocytic cells in host defense, mononuclear phagocytes play a central role in the immune response by presenting antigens to lymphocytes; elaborate growth factors and cytokines important for lymphocyte function, wound repair, and hematopoiesis; and participate in a variety of scavenger and homeostatic pathways.

Factors modifying the enzymatic, antigenic, and functional profile of mononuclear phagocytes are incompletely understood and involve a combination of tissue-specific signals as well as the release of inflammatory cytokines and toxins.[98–101] Mononuclear phagocytes at inflammatory sites become "activated," displaying morphologic alterations and a variety of enhanced functions. These include a more pronounced ruffling of the plasma membrane and pseudopod formation, an increased capacity for adherence and migration to chemotactic factors, increased microbicidal and tumoricidal activity, and enhanced ability to release cytokines.[99] IFN-γ is one of the principal macrophage-activating factors and is secreted by T lymphocytes as well as by macrophages and neutrophils.[53, 97, 102, 103] IFN-γ induces changes in macrophage gene expression through a pathway that is often referred to as the Jak-STAT pathway, whose general features are shared by many other cytokines, including IL-2, IL-6, and G-CSF.[31, 104–106] Binding of IFN-γ to its cell surface receptor activates cytoplasmic protein tyrosine kinases of the Janus kinase (Jak) family, which then phosphorylate and activate a family of transcription factors known as STATs (for signal transducers and activators of transcription). On phosphorylation, STAT proteins translocate into the nucleus to bind to specific regulatory sequences in interferon-responsive genes. Endotoxin, the bacterial lipopolysaccharide derived from gram-negative bacteria, is another important trigger of macrophage activation.[98] Signals from the microenvironment in which tissue macrophages reside can also produce phenotypic changes. For example, although monocytes and macrophages are generally facultative anaerobes, pulmonary macrophages are entirely dependent on aerobic metabolism.[107]

In keeping with their broad range of activities, mononuclear phagocytes possess a variety of cell surface receptors not found in neutrophils. These include receptors for coagulation factors VII, VIIa, and thrombin[108, 109] and for low and very low density lipoproteins.[110] Macrophages and monocytes are also active secretory cells and are capable of secreting over 100 defined substances,[97] many of which are listed in Table 22–5. These include molecules important in control of microbial pathogens, such as lysozyme, neutral prote-

Table 22–5. PRODUCTS SECRETED BY MONONUCLEAR PHAGOCYTES

Enzymes
Acid ceramidase, lipase, phosphatase, DNase, RNase
Alpha-iduronidase, α-L-fucosidase, α-mannosidase, α-neuraminidase
Alpha-naphthylesterase
Angiotensin-converting enzyme
Arginase
Aspartylglycosaminidase
Beta-glucuronidase, β-glucosidase, β-galactosidase
Cathepsins, collagenase, elastase
Leucine-2-naphthylaminidase
Lipoprotein lipase
Lysozyme
N-Acetyl-β-galactosaminidase, N-acetyl-β-glucosaminidase
Phospholipase A_2
Sphingomyelinase
Sulfatases

Oxidants
Hydroxyl radical, hydrogen peroxide, hypohalous acids, nitric oxide, peroxynitrate, and superoxide anion

Binding Proteins
Avidin, apolipoprotein E, acidic isoferritins, gelsolin, haptoglobin, transcobalamin II, transferrin

Coagulation System Proteins
Factors V, VII, IX, X, XIII
Tissue factor/procoagulant activity, plasminogen activator, urokinase, thrombospondin, plasminogen activator inhibitors, plasmin inhibitors

Lipid Metabolites
Prostaglandin (PG) E_2, PGF_2, PGI, thromboxane A_2; leukotrienes B, C, D, and E; malonyldialdehyde; mono-diHETEs; PAF

Complement System Proteins
C1, 2, 3, 4, 5; factors B, D, H; properdin; C3b inactivator

Cytokines and Growth Factors
Interferon (INF)-α, INF-β, INF-γ
Interleukin-1α, IL-1β, IL-6, IL-8
TNF-α
Fibroblast growth factor, platelet-derived growth factor (PDGF), transforming growth factor-β
G-CSF, GM-CSF, M-CSF
Macrophage inflammatory proteins (MIP)-1α, MIP-1β, MIP-2
Monocyte chemoattractant proteins (MCP)-1, 2, 3
Thymosin B_4

Matrix Proteins
Fibronectin, proteoglycans, thrombospondin

Other Metabolites, Peptides, and Proteins
Glutathione, purines, pyrimidines
Sterol hormones, including 1α, 25-dihydroxyvitamin D_3

---

mono-diHETEs = mono- and dihydroxyeicosatetraenoic acids.
Adapted from Nathan CF: Secretory products of macrophages. J Clin Invest 1987; 79:319, by copyright permission of the Society for Clinical Investigation.

ases, acid hydrolases and reactive oxidants, components of the complement cascade, and coagulation factors. Mononuclear phagocytes also secrete a large array of cytokines and hormones that regulate the proliferation and function of other cells that participate in the immune response, inflammation, wound repair, and hematopoiesis.

Monocytes and tissue macrophages are considered to make up a *mononuclear phagocyte system.* This term has replaced *reticuloendothelial system,* which referred to the filtering function performed by mononuclear phagocytes in concert with nonspecific trapping mechanisms within lymphatics and blood vessels.[92] Resident tissue macrophages were formerly referred to as *histiocytes,* an imprecise and often loosely applied term that can be confusing. Tissue macrophages are widely distributed and are found both at portals of entry, such as the pulmonary alveoli, and in sterile sites, such as the bone marrow.

Spleen. Macrophages are distributed in all parts of the spleen, including the germinal centers, where they are associated with lymphocytes. Splenic macrophages located in the red pulp and sinuses serve a clearance function, in which a sluggish blood circulation maximizes the interaction between blood elements and the macrophages lining the sinus walls.

Liver. The portal circulation percolates through a labyrinthine system, the spaces of Disse, before exiting via the hepatic venous system. This hepatic circulation, although less sluggish than that of the spleen, provides considerable contact between the blood and the resident liver macrophages, known as Kupffer cells, that reside within these vascular sinuses.

Lymph Nodes. As in the spleen, macrophages exist in all regions of peripheral lymph nodes. They are most abundant in the medullary zone close to efferent lymphatic and blood capillaries. This location is likely related to the important role macrophages play in the presentation of antigens to T lymphocytes.[111]

Lungs. Pulmonary macrophages reside both in the interstitium of alveolar sacs and free in the air spaces, where they participate in the clearance of inhaled microorganisms and particulate matter. The number of lung macrophages increases in many chronic pulmonary inflammatory disorders. Pulmonary macrophages are easily seen in lungs of smokers, where black inclusions within macrophage vacuoles are noted.[112] Hemosiderin-laden alveolar macrophages can be indicative of recurrent pulmonary hemorrhage, such as in idiopathic hemosiderosis or Goodpasture's syndrome. Gastric aspiration to detect ingested iron-laden macrophages is a useful test for these disorders.

Bone Marrow. Macrophages are found throughout the bone marrow cavity. They are particularly abundant within hematopoietic islands and on the walls of the marrow sinuses. Bone marrow macrophages may have a clearance function in normal or pathologic states of ineffective hematopoiesis.[113] The clearance function of marrow macrophages is dramatically illustrated by the lysosomal storage diseases such as Gaucher's disease.[114] Large inclusions build up within marrow macrophages (as well as hepatic and splenic macrophages), because of the inability of these cells to break down lysosomal contents. This can lead to a "myelophthisic" process with displacement of normal immature hematopoietic cells into the peripheral blood (leukoerythroblastosis) and, in Gaucher's disease, to a weakening of bone osteoid matrix.[99]

Other Sites. Mononuclear phagocytes associated with lymphoid cells reside throughout the alimentary tract, particularly in the submucosal tissues and small intestinal villi. They are present in the central nervous system, especially after injury, and may contribute to the pathogenesis of the central nervous system manifestations of infection with the human immunodeficiency virus.[115] Mammary gland macrophages released into milk during lactation have been implicated as a potential source of postnatal transmission of the human immunodeficiency virus.[116]

The Langerhans cell of the epidermis, the veiled cells in lymph, and the interdigitating cells in lymph nodes are related to mononuclear phagocytes and share some of their antigenic characteristics, but they may be derived from a different progenitor cell in the bone marrow.[92]

Osteoclasts. Osteoclasts are large, multinucleated cells that resorb mineralized cartilage and bone and are closely related to mononuclear phagocytes.[117] Rodent transplantation studies have shown osteoclasts can be derived from granulocyte-macrophage progenitor cells.[118] Defects in osteoclast function result in osteopetrosis, a genetically heterogeneous group of disorders characterized by progressive obliteration of the marrow space by the unchecked formation of new bone. The *op/op* osteopetrotic mouse mutant lacks M-CSF, which results in deficiencies of both osteoclasts and tissue macrophages.[119] M-CSF levels and osteoclast numbers are normal in human infantile ("malignant") osteopetrosis,[120] a disorder correctable by bone marrow transplantation.[121] Administration of IFN-γ, a major activator of macrophage function, can produce a clinically significant increase in bone resorption in children with infantile osteopetrosis.[122] Increases in both urinary hydroxyproline and urinary calcium excretion were observed during IFN-γ therapy, with associated decreases in trabecular bone area, widening of cranial nerve foramina, and improvement in bone marrow function and peripheral blood cell counts.

FUNCTION OF PHAGOCYTES
Overview

Phagocytic leukocytes play a central role in the acute phases of the inflammatory response, where they are rapidly mobilized into sites of tissue infection or injury and release an array of cytotoxic molecules to quickly but nonspecifically eliminate the offending substance or microbe. Phagocytes are also essential for normal repair of tissue injury, as evidenced by the impairment in wound healing in patients with deficits in leukocyte function or number.

The classic signs of the inflammatory response were described by the Roman writer Celsus as "rubor et tumor, cum calore et dolore"—redness and swelling with heat and pain.[123] However, it was not until the late 19th century that the importance of the inflammatory process for host defense and wound healing was generally recognized.[124] The beneficial role of phagocytes in this process was championed by Metchnikov. Much of his work, for which he received a Nobel Prize,[124, 125] involved studies on the wandering ameboid mesenchymal cells of marine organisms like the larval starfish, for which he coined the term *phagocyte*, after the Greek word, *phagein*, meaning "to eat."

In this section, the principal functions of granulocytes and mononuclear phagocytes in the inflammatory process are reviewed. Although these functions are discussed as individual components, it is important to recognize that many occur either simultaneously or in rapid succession. Moreover, many of the cellular structures or secreted molecules participating in the inflammatory process have multiple functions. For example, phagocyte cell surface proteins that act as adhesive ligands for receptors on the vascular endothelium can also trigger phagocytosis and activation of the phagocyte respiratory burst.

Humoral Mediators of the Inflammatory Response

The inflammatory response reflects an ongoing collaboration between tissue macrophages and mast cells, vascular endothelial cells, and circulating phagocytes. The release of soluble inflammatory mediators plays a crucial role in activating and coordinating this process. These molecules can be generated from serum proteins (e.g., the complement-derived protein fragment C5a), secreted by endothelial cells or inflammatory leukocytes (e.g., lipid metabolites, histamine, cytokines), or derived from invading microbes (e.g., endotoxin or formulated chemotactic peptides).

The proinflammatory cytokines TNF-α and IL-1 have a broad range of activities in the acute inflammatory response.[126–130] Both IL-1 and TNF can cause fever and muscle breakdown and are involved in the cachexia associated with chronic infection and malignancy. The synthesis of acute-phase reactants by the liver is induced by IL-6, whose synthesis and secretion is stimulated by IL-1. Proinflammatory cytokines also induce a proadhesive state on the surface of endothelium and increase the production of the chemotactic cytokines (chemokines). IFN-γ is another important proinflammatory mediator that enhances the responsiveness of phagocytes to inflammatory stimuli.[102, 103] Counterbalancing the activities of these polypeptides are IL-4, IL-10, and transforming growth factor-β, which tend to down-regulate the acute inflammatory response.[131–133]

Vasodilation and increased vascular permeability are two early responses to an inflammatory insult that are elicited, in large part, by products secreted by granulocytes and mononuclear phagocytes. Activated basophils and tissue mast cells release histamine, which leads to vasodilation of tissue arterioles and microvascular beds through H_1-type receptors.[134–136] The lipid metabolite platelet activating factor (PAF), which is secreted by activated macrophages, mast cells, and endothelial cells, induces platelet degranulation and the release of additional histamine and also serotonin, another vasoactive amine.[137, 138] Prostaglandin E and other arachidonic acid metabolites secreted by activated neutrophils and macrophages are another group of potent vasodilators.[139] Finally, vasodilation can be triggered by the release of nitric oxide from endothelial and smooth muscle cells as well as perhaps activated macrophages, which may be particularly important in the hypotension noted in patients with gram-negative septicemia.[140, 141] The increased vascular permeability that produces the edema of acute inflammation allows plasma proteins such as immunoglobulins and complement to enter tissues to promote phagocyte activation and opsonize microbes. Agents that increase vascular permeability include histamine, serotonin, PAF, and leukotrienes C_4, D_4, and E_4.[137, 142] Bradykinin, which is generated as the result of Hageman factor (factor XII) cleavage, also induces enhanced vascular permeability.

A wide variety of chemoattractants for neutrophils and other circulating phagocytes are generated at sites of inflammation (Table 22–6).[40, 143–145] These molecules are chemically diverse and are derived from many different sources in response to bacterial products and inflammatory mediators released as a result of tissue necrosis. This diversity provides a functional redundancy and ensures that leukocytes will be attracted to sites of injury or infection. In addition to molecules generated by the activation of complement (C5a) or bacteria themselves (formylated peptides), many are secreted by activated phagocytes; this acts as a positive feedback loop for additional recruitment and activation of inflammatory cells. The phospholipid PAF, released by both activated phagocytes and endothelial cells, triggers platelet activation and granule release in addi-

tion to acting as a potent chemoattractant for neutrophils and eosinophils.[137, 138] Activation of phagocytes also stimulates the phospholipase A_2–mediated cleavage of membrane phospholipids to generate arachidonic acid, which is then converted into a variety of eicosanoid metabolites, including the chemoattractant leukotriene B_4.[139]

Phagocyte chemoattractants include a recently discovered family of small (8–10 kd) basic heparin-binding proteins known as chemokines (for their combined *chemo*tactic and cyto*kine* properties).[134, 145] Chemokines interact relatively specifically with subsets of inflammatory leukocytes and are therefore believed to play an important role in mediating the sequential influx of neutrophils, monocytes, and, finally, lymphocytes into an inflamed tissue site. Members of this family, which have a conserved structure containing two cysteine pairs, have been divided into two groups based on the disulfide sequence pattern. The α family, in which the first cysteine pair is separated by an intervening amino acid (C—X—C), includes IL-8, the GRO peptides, and neutrophil-activating peptide (NAP)-2, which are all potent neutrophil activators and, except for NAP-2, chemoattractants. NAP-2 is generated by the cleavage of platelet secretory proteins by cathepsin G released from monocytes and neutrophils,[146] whereas IL-8 and GRO chemokines are released from phagocytes and mesenchymal cells (including endothelial cells) in response to inflammatory mediators such as IL-1 and TNF.[134, 147] The β intercrine family, in which the first two cysteines are adjacent to each other (C—C), includes two important inducers of mononuclear phagocyte migration, monocyte chemoattractant protein (MCP)-1 and RANTES (*r*egulated upon *a*ctivation, *n*ormal *T* cell *e*xpressed and presumably *s*ecreted).[134, 147–150] Monocyte chemoattractant protein-1 is produced by a

Table 22–6. GRANULOCYTE AND MONOCYTE CHEMOATTRACTANTS IN HUMANS

Chemoattractant	Source	Up-Regulators	Target Cells
Lipids			
PAF	N, E, B, P, M Endothelium (phosphatidyl choline metabolism)	Calcium ionophores	N, E
LTB$_4$	N, M (arachidonate metabolism)	Microbial pathogens, *N*-formyl peptides	N, M, E
Intercrines (α Subfamily)			
IL-8	M, endothelium, many other cells	LPS, IL-1, TNF, IL-3	N, B
GRO α, β, γ	M, endothelium, many other cells	IL-1, TNF	N
NAP-2	P*	Platelet activators	N
Intercrines (β Subfamily)			
MCP-1 (MCAF)	M, endothelium, many other cells	IL-1, TNF, LPS, PDGF	M, B
RANTES	M	IL-1, TNF, anti-CD3	M, B
Other			
N-formyl peptides	Bacteria Mitochondria	—	N, M, E, B
C5a	Complement activation	Complement activation	N, M, E, B

*Platelets, when activated, secrete platelet basic protein (PBP) and connective tissue–activating peptide-III (CTAP-III), which are cleaved to NAP-2 by cathepsin.
B = Basophil; E = eosinophil; F = fibroblast; GRO = growth-related gene; K = keratinocyte; LPS = lipopolysaccharide; M = monocyte; MCAF = monocyte chemotactic and activating factor; N = neutrophil; NAP-2 = neutrophil-activating peptide-2; P = platelet; RANTES = regulated upon activation, normal T cell expressed and presumably secreted; T = T lymphocyte.
Adapted from Curnutte JT, Orkin SH, Dinauer MC: Genetic disorders of phagocyte function. In Stamatoyannopoulos G, Nienhuis AW, et al (eds): The Molecular Basis of Blood Disease. 2nd ed. Philadelphia, W.B. Saunders Co., 1993, pp 493–522.

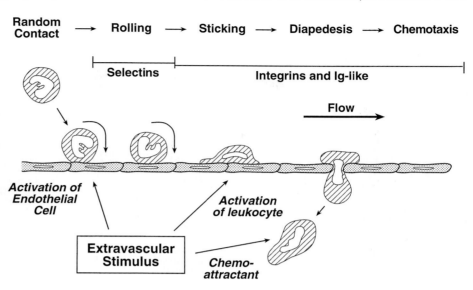

Figure 22-1. Adhesive interactions during phagocyte emigration. Under conditions of flow within postcapillary venules, leukocytes are first observed to roll along the endothelium adjacent to the extravascular site of inflammation. Subsequently, some of the rolling leukocytes adhere firmly, diapedese between endothelial cells, and then migrate into subendothelial tissue. Studies *in vitro* and *in vivo* indicate that rolling is mediated by multiple low-affinity interactions between selectin receptors and carbohydrate counter-receptors, and firm adhesion and diapedesis are largely dependent on integrin and immunoglobulin (Ig)-like adhesion proteins. (From Carlos TM, Harlan JM: Leukocyte-endothelial adhesion molecules. Blood 1994; 84:2068.)

wide variety of cells, whereas RANTES is secreted only by macrophages. RANTES is chemotactic for memory T cells as well as monocytes,[134, 150] and both MCP-1 and RANTES induce histamine release from basophils.[135, 136, 150] The heparin-binding sites on chemokines may bind to negatively charged proteoglycans on endothelial cells or in the subendothelial matrix to facilitate the production of locally high chemokine concentrations at an inflamed site.[151–153]

In addition to their role as chemoattractants, the molecules listed in Table 22–6 induce the activation of many other phagocyte functions on binding to their cognate cell surface receptors. These include the up-regulation and increased affinity of integrin adhesion receptors to promote firm attachment to the endothelium, rearrangement of the actin cytoskeleton, degranulation, and activation of the phagocyte respiratory burst.[38, 134, 139, 143, 144] These responses generally require higher ligand concentrations compared with those that elicit chemotaxis, which can be as low as 10^{-9} mol/L.[154]

Despite the diverse chemical structures of phagocyte chemoattractants listed in Table 22–6, all of the corresponding receptors that have been cloned to date belong to the seven transmembrane-domain family of receptors, also known as the serpentine receptors.[48, 145, 155] The transduction of signals through serpentine receptors is mediated by heterotrimeric G proteins, which bind to specific intracellular domains of the receptor.[156–160] Ligand binding to the receptor promotes the exchange of GTP for guanosine diphosphate (GDP) bound to the G protein α subunit, which in turns leads to the dissociation of the β-γ subunits and their interaction with downstream signaling effectors.[38] These include a phosphatidylinositol-specific phospholipase C that generates diacylglycerol and inositol 1,4,5-triphosphate, which then activate protein kinase C and induce release of intracellular calcium stores, respectively. Binding of formylated peptides to neutrophils also activates the Ras p21–macrophage activated kinase pathway.[49] Certain G protein α subunits appear to be expressed preferentially in leukocytes and may be important in signaling through the phagocyte serpentine receptors.[161, 162]

Adhesion and Migration into Tissues

The discovery that leukocytes migrate from the blood stream into extravascular sites of inflammation, described by Cohnheim in 1867, was a major milestone in the conceptualization of the inflammatory process.[124] Cohnheim, who used intravital microscopy to study the microvasculature in the frog tongue and mesentery after tissue injury, also proposed that inflammatory stimuli induce a molecular change in the blood vessel wall that promoted the increased adherence of leukocytes, a concept that was finally proven a century later.

To move from the blood stream into inflamed sites, leukocytes must attach to the vascular endothelium, migrate between adjacent endothelial cells in a process referred to as diapedesis, and penetrate the basement membrane. The molecular mechanisms underlying these events have been the subject of intense study in recent years and involve a series of sequential adhesive interactions between chemoattractant-activated leukocytes and endothelial cells that are activated by inflammatory mediators (Fig. 22–1).[144, 163–166]

The initial step in emigration from postcapillary venules is a low-affinity interaction between the neutrophil and the endothelium that is often referred to "rolling," based on its appearance in intravital microscopy. This transient adherence, also called "tethering," is mediated by the up-regulation of selectin expression on endothelial cells. The selectin family of adhesion molecules are membrane-spanning glycoproteins (Fig. 22–2) that bind to fucosylated structures such as Lewis X (Galβ1→4[Fucα1→3]GlcNac→R), sialyl-Lewis X, and other specific carbohydrates.[167–170] P-selectin appears to be the most important for the initial steps of neutrophil adhesion to the endothelium and is stored in the Weibel-Palade bodies and α granules of endothelial cells and platelets, respectively.[164, 167] On endothelial cell activation by histamine, thrombin, and other inflammatory molecules, these cytoplasmic storage granules fuse with the cell membrane to increase rapidly the surface expression of P-selectin. E-selectin is expressed on endothelial cells at low levels but is up-regulated by

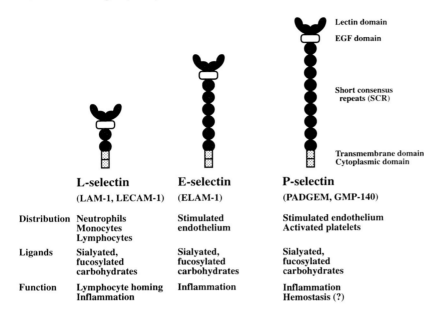

Figure 22-2. The selectin family of adhesion molecules. EGF = epidermal growth factor. (Adapted from Kishimoto TK, Rothlein R: Integrins, ICAMS, and selectins: Role and regulation of adhesion molecules in neutrophil recruitment to inflammatory sites. Adv Pharmacol 1994; 25:117.)

transcriptional activation and *de novo* protein synthesis in response to inflammatory cytokines.[171] L-selectin is expressed constitutively on the surface of neutrophils, mononuclear phagocytes, and lymphocytes and is shed within minutes of leukocyte activation by a proteolytic cleavage event near the external membrane surface insertion site.[172, 173] Circulating L-selectin may modulate leukocyte adhesion during inflammation.[174]

Rolling neutrophils can detach and return to the circulation. Others will come to a halt and, within seconds, adopt a flattened, adherent morphology and attach firmly to the vessel wall.[164] This firm attachment appears in large part to be mediated by leukocyte integrin adhesion receptors binding to intracellular adhesion molecules (ICAMs) on the endothelium.[144, 163, 164, 166] In addition, complement fragments are found on the endothelial surface at inflamed sites and also may function as integrin binding sites.[175] Leukocyte activation by chemoattractants is critical to the development of these strong adhesive interactions, because it leads to the up-regulation of the number and avidity of cell surface integrins. Exposure to locally high concentrations of chemoattractants may be enhanced by selectin-mediated tethering and by the retention of chemokines on the extracellular matrix.[151–153]

The integrins are a large family of adhesion proteins that are glycosylated heterodimers of a noncovalently linked α and a β chain and can be classified into subfamilies according to the type of β subunit.[166, 168, 176–178] Many integrins mediate attachment to extracellular matrices by serving as receptors for matrix proteins. Others are involved in hemostasis, such as glycoprotein IIb/IIIa on platelets. The leukocyte β₂ integrins (Fig. 22–3) play a critical role in mediating adhesive interactions in inflammation, including the attachment of leukocytes to endothelial cells and as opsonic receptors for complement fragment-coated particles.

There are three different leukocyte β₂ integrins, each having a common 95-kd β subunit (CD18) but different α subunits, CD11a (177 kd), CD11b (165 kd), and CD11c

(150 kd) (see Fig. 22–3). CD11a/CD11b (LFA-1) is expressed by all leukocytes, including lymphocytes. Mac-1 and p150,95 are expressed by granulocytes, mononuclear phagocytes, some activated T lymphocytes, and large granular lymphocytes.[164, 168] Mutations in the common β subunit result in an inherited defect in phagocyte function, leukocyte adhesion deficiency type I (LAD I), which is discussed in a later section. All three β₂ integrins are absent in LAD I, indicating that the stability of each α subunit requires association with the chain, which normally occurs in the Golgi compartment.[166] The β subunit has a large, glycosylated extracellular domain, a single transmembrane-spanning domain, and a short cytoplasmic tail.[179] The extracellular domain has two regions that are conserved among other β subunits.[164, 166, 177] There are four cysteine-rich tandem repeats that appear to be important for the tertiary structure of the β subunit. Another conserved

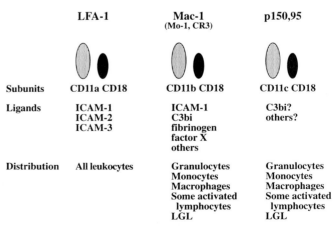

Figure 22-3. The β₂ (CD18) family of leukocyte integrins. ICAM = intercellular adhesion molecule; LGL = large granular lymphocytes. (Adapted from Kishimoto TK, Rothlein R: Integrins, ICAMS, and selectins: Role and regulation of adhesion molecules in neutrophil recruitment to inflammatory sites. Adv Pharmacol 1994; 25:117.)

region, located near the N-terminus, is critical for maintenance of the α/β heterodimer. Point mutations in these conserved regions have been reported in LAD I.[164] The α subunit is also a glycosylated integral membrane protein with a single membrane-spanning segment and a short cytoplasmic tail. The external domain contains three divalent cation-binding motifs that must be occupied for ligand binding to occur.[177, 178] The intracellular domain of the α subunit includes a conserved sequence that is critical for the modulation of integrin avidity (see later).[180] The cytoplasmic tails of both the αβ integrin subunits also interact with the cytoskeletal proteins.[168, 181] The endoparasite hookworm *Ancylostoma caninum* produces a heavily glycosylated protein called NIF that binds to CD11b/CD18 to inhibit neutrophil spreading and attachment to the endothelium.[182, 183]

Although β₂ integrins are constitutively expressed on the neutrophil cell surface, a large pool is also stored in intracellular secretory vesicles (see Table 22–2). These vesicles are rapidly mobilized on neutrophil activation by chemoattractants and fuse with the membrane to increase the cell surface expression of β₂ integrins by about 10-fold.[23, 144, 184] Signaling through chemoattractant receptors also markedly increases the avidity of β₂ integrins for their ligands, which plays an even more important role in rapidly up-regulating integrin activity and promoting firm attachment to the blood vessel wall.[166, 177] The increased adhesiveness of the β₂ integrins appears to involve a conformational change in integrin structure on cellular activation.

The major counter-receptors for the β₂ integrins are the ICAMs (Fig. 22–4), which are members of the immunoglobulin superfamily.[163, 164, 166] These transmembrane proteins contain anywhere from two to six immunoglobulin domains and are present on endothelial cells, T cells, and a variety of other cell types. ICAM-1 and ICAM-2 are of particular importance in mediating binding of neutrophils and other leukocytes to the endothelium. Endothelial cell expression of ICAM-1 increases in response to inflammatory cytokines, which promotes increased cell-cell interactions with leukocytes at inflamed sites. Vascular cell adhesion molecule 1 (VCAM-1) is another immunoglobulin superfamily member expressed on endothelial cells that is inducible by cytokines.[164] VCAM-1 is the counter-receptor for the β1 integrin very late activation antigen (VLA)-4 and appears to be important in promoting the adherence of monocytes and eosinophils during inflammation. The β₂ integrin Mac-1 (CD11b/CD18) also has an important role as an opsonic receptor for the complement fragment, C3bi, as discussed later.

Although leukocyte β₂ integrin–mediated adhesion is clearly important for neutrophil recruitment from the systemic microvasculature into inflammatory sites, neutrophil emigration out of the pulmonary circulation can also be mediated by an alternative pathway, depending on the inflammatory stimulus.[185, 186] Whether the alternative pathway in pulmonary capillaries involves selectins or other adhesion molecules remains to be defined. Neutrophil emigration from the bone marrow storage pool into the circulation is also a poorly understood process and appears to involve ad-

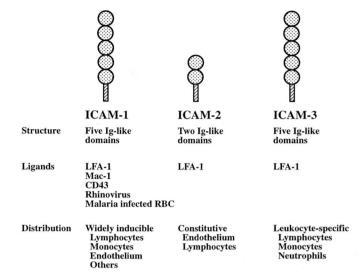

Structure	ICAM-1	ICAM-2	ICAM-3
	Five Ig-like domains	Two Ig-like domains	Five Ig-like domains
Ligands	LFA-1 Mac-1 CD43 Rhinovirus Malaria infected RBC	LFA-1	LFA-1
Distribution	Widely inducible Lymphocytes Monocytes Endothelium Others	Constitutive Endothelium Lymphocytes	Leukocyte-specific Lymphocytes Monocytes Neutrophils

Figure 22–4. The intercellular adhesion molecules (ICAMs). (Adapted from Kishimoto TK, Rothlein R: Integrins, ICAMS, and selectins: Role and regulation of adhesion molecules in neutrophil recruitment to inflammatory sites. Adv Pharmacol 1994; 25:117.)

hesion molecules distinct from the β₂ integrins and L-selectin.[187]

The final steps in emigration of neutrophils from the blood vessel lumen into inflamed tissue involve squeezing between adjacent endothelial cells (diapedesis) and penetrating the basement membrane (see Fig. 22–1). The presence of a chemotactic gradient is required to induce the directional migration of neutrophils.[151, 188, 189] Adhesive interactions between the β₂ integrins and ICAM-1 are essential for neutrophil diapedesis, whereas VCAM-1 and E-selectin can mediate the transmigration of monocytes and eosinophils.[164] Transendothelial migration of neutrophils is also dependent on homologous binding events between neutrophil and endothelial cell platelet-endothelial cell adhesion molecule-1 (PECAM-1) (CD31) adhesion receptors.[190, 191] PECAM-1, another member of the immunoglobulin superfamily, is expressed on leukocytes, platelets, and endothelial cells, where it is localized at the junctions between cells.[163] Migrating neutrophils also may induce an increase in endothelial intracellular calcium levels that facilitates the opening of spaces between endothelial cells by means of a still undefined mechanism.[192] Finally, chemoattractant-induced degranulation of neutrophil secretory vesicles results in the release of digestive enzymes, including collagenase, elastase, and gelatinase, which facilitate basement membrane penetration.[23, 193]

Chemotaxis is the directional movement of a cell along a concentration gradient.[194] Defects in neutrophil cellular motility or other steps in chemotaxis can result in decreased resistance to bacterial and fungal infections, as discussed later in this chapter. The neutrophil chemotactic response occurs at chemoattractant concentrations that approximate the dissociation constants of the chemotactic factors for their receptors, which are much lower than those that elicit degranulation and activation of the respiratory burst.[26] Cells respond to a chemotactic gradient by sensing constantly across their surface, and bound chemotactic receptors are continuously internalized.[194] A migrating neutrophil has a polarized appearance, with the leading edge extending pseudopodia or lamellepodia, thin structures rich in actin filaments and lacking intracellular organelles.[25] The pseudopods appear to glide forward, pulling the cell body behind them. The nucleus tends to remain at the posterior half of the moving leukocyte. Neutrophil movement requires reversible adhesion to the underlying substrate; and proteases localized at the neutrophil surface, such as urokinase-type plasminogen activator, may be involved in successive breaking of attachments to the extracellular matrix.[195–198] The glycosyl phosphatidylinositol (GPI)-linked receptor for urokinase-type plasminogen activator has also been shown to play a role in monocyte chemotaxis that is distinct from its role in localizing urokinase-type plasminogran activator–mediated proteolysis at the cell surface.[199]

Neutrophil movement is dependent on the dynamic assembly and disassembly of filamentous actin, which is coordinated by various actin-binding proteins whose activity is regulated by intracellular signaling molecules.[25, 26, 198] Hence, leukocyte motility is inhibited by the cytochalasins, which block actin assembly. Actin can exist as either a soluble monomer (globular actin) or in needle-like helical filaments (filamentous actin). Actin filaments align spontaneously in parallel bundles, but in the cell they are organized into a branching network due to the presence of actin filament crosslinkers such as actin-binding protein.[200] Another class of actin regulatory proteins sequesters actin monomers and thus can control the availability of globular actin for filament formation. Prophyllin and thymosin B_4 are two major actin monomer-binding proteins in neutrophils.[201] Other actin-binding proteins, such as gelsolin, cap the fast-growing barbed end of the actin filament or sever filamentous actin into shorter pieces.[25, 26] Agonists acting through receptors on the cell membrane trigger the generation of second messengers, which interact with actin-binding proteins to control dynamic local cycles of filamentous actin assembly.[25] For example, increased local calcium concentrations activate gelsolin, promoting actin disassembly by cleaving actin filaments and capping its barbed ends. On the other hand, actin assembly is stimulated by the accumulation of phosphoinositols liberated from membrane phospholipids around an activated receptor. Phosphoinositols, such as phosphatidyl inositol-4,5-bisphosphate, interact both with actin-sequestering proteins to liberate actin monomers and with gelsolin to uncap the barbed ends of filamentous actin. The Ras-related GTP-binding proteins, Rho and Rac, also appear to participate in signal transduction events that lead to actin remodeling.[50, 202]

During pseudopod extension in chemoattractant-activated neutrophils, new actin polymerization occurs at the site of membrane protrusion while the filamentous actin in the rear of the cell disassembles.[203–205] How actin assembly-disassembly results in membrane extension and formation of pseudopodia is not fully understood but may involve localized changes in osmotic pressure owing to changes in actin polymerization.[25, 26] Membrane movement also may be mediated in part by contractile proteins such as myosin 1, but this has not been well studied in leukocytes.

Opsonization and Phagocytosis

The ingestion and disposal of microbes, foreign particulate matter, and damaged cells constitutes a major aspect of phagocyte function. To facilitate their recognition by phagocytes, these targets are coated with serum opsonins (Gr., *opsonein*, "to prepare for dining"), which include proteolytic fragments derived from the complement cascade as well as specific immunoglobulins. Tissue macrophages, which are often the first cell to encounter invading microbes, also have receptors capable of recognizing ligands even in the absence of opsonins. These include the mannose receptor and the scavenger receptor.[206–209] The macrophage mannose receptor in the mouse, for example, recognizes *Pneumocystis carinii* and mediates its ingestion. The scavenger receptor has broad binding specificities and likely participates in the clearance of diverse foreign materials.[206]

The key humoral opsonins are the opsonic antibodies, IgM, IgG_1, and IgG_3 as well as the proteolytic cleavage products of C3 (C3b and C3bi). Targets are opsonized by the deposition of the IgG onto their surfaces through the specific (Fab) portion of the antibody or by deposition of C3b and C3bi. Antibacterial IgM antibodies, while not opsonic by themselves, play an important role in phagocytosis by activating complement. Opsonins are recognized by phagocyte cell surface glycoprotein receptors for immunoglobulin and C3 cleavage products (Table 22–7). Inherited deficiencies of either immunoglobulins or complement can result in increased susceptibility to bacterial infections, as discussed in a following section. In contrast, primary defects in phagocyte receptors for these opsonins appear to be an uncommon cause of recurrent infections.

Immunoglobulins are recognized by Fc receptors, which are members of the immunoglobulin gene superfamily. Fc receptors bind to the "constant domain" of the antibody molecule, these being specific to each class of immunoglobulins (IgA, IgE, IgG, and IgM).[210–214] The most important from the standpoint of microbial opsonization are those Fc receptors that recognize IgG (see Table 22–7). The Fc receptors for IgG include three distinct classes, FcγRI, FcγRII, and FcγRIII, which are encoded by at least eight genes that have evolved through gene duplication and alternative splicing.[213] The low-affinity FcγR genes (FcγRIIB and FcγRIIIB families) and two of the genes for the high-affinity IgE receptor are clustered on chromosome 1q22. The high-affinity IgG Fc receptors map to other sites on chromosome 1. The FcγR proteins have a single transmembrane domain and are all associated with at least one other polypeptide chain important for their stable expression and function.[213] An exception is FcγRIIIB, which is anchored in the membrane by a GPI moiety.

Each FcγR is expressed at different levels, depending on the type of phagocytic cell (see Table 22–7), and

Table 22-7. HUMAN PHAGOCYTE Fc RECEPTOR FOR IMMUNOGLOBULIN G AND COMPLEMENT RECEPTORS

	FcγRIA	FcγRIIA, B	FcγRIIIB	CR1	CR3 (CD11b/CD18)
Alleles	2	2 for FcγRIIA	2 (NA-1, NA-2)	10	1/1
Cell Distribution	Monocytes Macrophages IFN-γ–treated neutrophils	Monocytes Neutrophils Macrophages Eosinophils B lymphocytes Platelets	Neutrophils	Monocytes Macrophages Neutrophils Erythrocytes B lymphocytes	Monocytes Macrophages Monocytes
Inducers	IFN-γ G-CSF	—	—	—	—
Ligands	Monomeric IgG (G1=G3>G4>>G2)	Complexed IgG (G1=G3>>G2,G4)	Complexed IgG (G1=G3>>G2,G4)	C3b C4b	C3bi ICAM-1 ICAM-2
Affinity	High	Low	Low	Moderate	Moderate
Function	Trigger respiratory burst Phagocytosis ADCC	Trigger respiratory burst Exocytosis ADCC	Immune complex clearance Phagocytosis Exocytosis	Phagocytosis	Phagocytosis Cell adherence Activation

ADCC = Antibody-dependent cellular cytoxicity; G-CSF = granulocyte colony stimulating factor; IFN-γ = interferon gamma; FcγR = Fc receptor for IgG; CR = complement receptor; ICAM = intracellular adhesion molecule.
See text for references.

some FcγRII and FcγRIII family members are also expressed on lymphocytes, platelets, thymocytes, natural killer cells, and mast cells.[210, 211, 213] The FcγRI class includes the products of three highly homologous genes, denoted A, B, and C, although the protein products of the latter two have not been localized *in vivo*. The FcγRIA receptors are expressed by monocytes and neutrophils stimulated by IFN-γ or G-CSF and have a high affinity for monomeric IgG.[210, 211] Members of the FcγRII (A, B, and C) and FcγRIII (A and B) families have a low affinity for monomeric IgG but a high affinity for clusters of IgG (e.g., several antibodies bound to the same particle) and immune complexes. Only neutrophils appear to express FcγRIIIB, and polymorphisms in this receptor correspond to the serologically defined NA1/NA2 antigen system, which is a common antibody target in alloimmune and autoimmune neutropenia.[211, 215]

The specific functions of the different phagocyte Fc receptors for IgG have not been clearly delineated, although all can function as opsonins. Binding of IgG to FcγRI and FcγRII activates the respiratory burst, whereas secretion of granular contents is promoted by binding to FcγRII and FcγRIIIB.[210] Although the ligand-binding domains of different Fcγ receptors all bind IgG, the specificity of the cellular response is governed by the unique transmembrane and cytoplasmic domains of a particular Fcγ receptor subtype.[213] Ligation of Fcγ receptors initiates a cascade of biochemical signals that appear to be initiated by activation of nonreceptor protein tyrosine kinases linked to specific receptors or their associated subunits.[211]

The human phagocyte C3b receptor (CR1) is a high-molecular-weight, single-subunit glycoprotein that shows a substantial heterogeneity in size because of the presence of four distinct alleles in the human population that encode proteins ranging from 160 to 250 kd. CR1 is responsible for the binding of C3b-opsonized

particles and for initiating their ingestion. The other major opsonic receptor, CR3, recognizes particles opsonized with C3bi. This receptor is the same as the β2 integrin Mac-1 (CD11b/CD18) discussed in detail in an earlier section (see Fig. 22–3). Binding of C3bi-opsonized particles to CD11b/CD18 triggers both phagocytosis and the respiratory burst.

The opsonization of microbes with secretory IgA antibodies is likely to be important in the clearance of microbes from the mucosal surfaces of the respiratory, gastrointestinal, and urogenital tracts. Neutrophils and monocytes have an Fc receptor for IgA (Fcα receptor), which has close structural similarities with other members of the Fc receptor family.[216] Ligation of the phagocyte Fcα receptor can trigger phagocytosis, degranulation, and superoxide release.[217, 218]

Engagement of any of the opsonic receptors initiates phagocytosis of an opsonized particle, which involves the simultaneous invagination of the membrane and extension of pseudopodia to form a phagocytic vacuole that encloses the particle. The molecular details of this process are incompletely understood but are likely to involve the regulated assembly and disassembly of the actin cytoskeleton, in a fashion analogous to the mechanisms that result in cell movement when chemotactic receptors are engaged.

Cytocidal and Digestive Activity

The binding of ligands to phagocyte chemoattractant and opsonic receptors ultimately leads to the mobilization of phagocyte granules that contain cytotoxic and hydrolytic proteins and to the activation of enzymatic reactions that generate toxic oxygen metabolites. These complementary processes are designed to modify or destroy the inciting object and are often classified as oxygen-independent and oxygen-dependent pathways.

Neutrophil granules are secretory organelles that can

be divided into four general classes, as discussed in a preceding section (see Table 22–2). Degranulation (also referred to as mobilization), the fusion of granule membranes with the plasma or phagosome membrane, results in the transfer of granule membrane constituents to a new membrane compartment and the discharge of the granule contents into the extracellular fluid or phagocytic vacuole. Degranulation is triggered by increases in intracellular calcium concentration when neutrophils are activated through chemoattractant and other receptors. There are marked differences between different granule classes in their responsiveness to this signal, which leads to the mobilization of different granule classes depending on the calcium concentration, which, in turn, is in proportion to receptor occupancy.[23] Secretory vesicles, whose membranes are storage pools for β_2 integrin adhesion proteins and other receptors, are mobilized with relatively low concentrations of calcium. The degranulation of secretory vesicles provides a rapid way of up-regulating the cell surface expression of these receptors. Gelatinase (tertiary) granules are also easily mobilized for exocytosis at the cell surface, and the release of gelatinase facilitates migration of neutrophils through the extracellular matrix.[193] In contrast, azurophil (primary) granules, which contain cytotoxic proteins and hydrolytic enzymes, are mobilized very slowly. Azurophil granules generally do not undergo exocytosis, fusing instead with phagocytic vacuoles to deliver their contents into a sequestered compartment.[219, 220]

Certain microorganisms can become intracellular parasites because they have developed mechanisms to prevent granule fusion with the phagocytic vacuole or otherwise evade the phagocyte digestive and oxidative armamentarium. For example, although mycobacteria exist intracellularly within the phagosome, they produce compounds that inhibit their fusion of phagocyte granules.[221–223] *Legionella pneumophila* and *Toxoplasma* may inhibit lysosomal acidification.[224, 225] *Salmonella* may not activate the oxidase on ingestion.[226] *Listeria monocytogenes* escapes from the phagocytic vacuole altogether to avoid attack by lysosomal products and can survive in the cytoplasm of relatively quiescent macrophages and hepatocytes.[227]

Oxygen-Independent Toxicity

Phagocyte granules supply preformed cytotoxic and digestive compounds that play a key role in oxygen-independent killing and digestion of microbes, senescent cells, and particulate debris. Oxygen-independent pathways complement those dependent on the respiratory burst (see next section) and are also important for phagocyte antimicrobial activity under the adverse conditions of hypoxia and acidosis often encountered locally at the site of infection.

Numerous cationic antimicrobial proteins are contained within neutrophil azurophilic granules.[219, 220, 228] Defensins are small (25–29 amino acid residue) basic peptides that constitute more than 5% of the total cellular protein of human neutrophils, although they are absent in murine neutrophils.[229, 230] These peptides exhibit antimicrobial effects against a broad range of gram-positive and gram-negative organisms, fungi, mycobacteria, and some enveloped viruses. Defensins are also cytotoxic to mammalian cells. Defensins kill target cells by insertion into the cellular membrane and formation of voltage-regulated channels. Defensin-like peptides have also been found in small intestinal Paneth cells and in tracheal epithelium.[228] Bactericidal permeability-increasing protein is a 55-kd cationic protein that has potent cytotoxic effects toward gram-negative bacteria.[231] It binds avidly to lipopolysaccharide, leading to both bacterial killing by damaging the cell membrane and to the neutralization of endotoxin associated with the bacterial cell wall and in serum. Serpocidins are a family of 25- to 29-kd glycoproteins that are homologous to members of the serine protease superfamily and include azurocidin and three serine proteases (cathepsin G, elastase, and proteinase 3).[228] In human neutrophils, serpocidins are even more potent than the defensins in antimicrobial activity and have a broad spectrum of cytotoxicity that is, with few exceptions, unrelated to proteolytic activity. Cathepsin G, elastase, and proteinase 3 are often referred to as neutral proteases because the pH optima for their proteolytic activity is about pH 7. The CAP37 protein has been shown to bind endotoxin, which appears to account for its microbacterial activity for gram-negative bacteria.[232] Azurocidin is also a potent chemoattractant for monocytes.[232]

Both azurophilic and specific granules contain lysozyme, which hydrolyzes the cell wall of saprophytic gram-positive organisms and also may assist in the nonlytic killing of other organisms.[219] Specific (secondary) granules contain the iron-binding glycoprotein lactoferrin, which has direct bactericidal activity both related and unrelated to the chelation of iron compounds required for bacterial metabolism.[233] Lactoferrin may also catalyze the nonenzymatic formation of hydroxide radicals during the respiratory burst (see next section). Vitamin B_{12} (cobalamin)-binding protein has been proposed to bind the analogous family of compounds found in bacteria to exert an antimicrobial effect.[234]

Azurophilic granules contain a variety of hydrolases (see Table 22–2) that have a lower pH optimum (less than 6), consistent with the lysosomal character of these granules. Studies using indicator dyes and biochemical techniques suggest that after a transient rise, the pH of the phagocytic vacuole falls below 6, which would enhance the activity of these enzymes on their discharge into the vacuole.[235, 236] The acid hydrolases serve primarily a digestive rather than a microbicidal function.[237] Azurophilic granules also contain myeloperoxidase, which is an important enzyme in the microbicidal oxygen-dependent reactions described in the following section. Inherited partial or complete deficiency of myeloperoxidase, which occurs in 0.05% of the population, can occasionally result in increased susceptibility to infection (see later in this chapter). Specific deficiencies in other neutrophil granule proteins have not yet been described, but a few rare disorders involving defects in granule formation or degranulation are associated with recurrent bacterial infections.

Oxygen-Dependent Toxicity

The resting neutrophil relies primarily on glycolysis for energy and hence consumes relatively little oxygen.[238] However, within seconds after contacting opsonized microbes or high concentrations of chemoattractants, oxygen consumption increases dramatically, often by more than 100-fold. This "extra respiration of phagocytosis" was first observed in 1933,[239] but it was almost 30 years before it was appreciated that this process was insensitive to mitochondrial poisons and thus not related to increased energy demands.[240] The enzyme complex responsible for this phenomenon, referred to as NADPH or respiratory burst oxidase, is associated with the plasma and phagolysosomal membranes and catalyzes the transfer of an electron from NADPH to molecular oxygen, thereby forming the superoxide radical (O_2^-) (Fig. 22–5).[241–248] Superoxide, although not an important microbicidal agent by itself, is the precursor to a family of potent oxidants that are essential for the killing of many microorganisms (see Fig. 22–5).[238, 247, 249] The importance of the respiratory burst to normal host defense is underscored by the recurrent and often life-threatening infections seen in patients with chronic granulomatous disease (CGD), who are genetically deficient in respiratory burst oxidase activity.

The respiratory burst oxidase is a multisubunit enzyme complex assembled from membrane-bound and soluble proteins on phagocyte activation (Fig. 22–6). The identification of the components of this enzyme has benefited greatly from the biochemical and molecular genetic analysis of patients with CGD. Four polypeptides that are essential for respiratory burst function have been identified (Table 22–8), and mutations in the corresponding genes are responsible for the four different genetic subgroups of CGD. The oxidase subunits have been given the designation *phox*, for *phagocyte oxidase*.

An unusual b-type cytochrome, located in the plasma membranes and specific granules of resting neutrophils, mediates electron transfer in the oxidase complex. This cytochrome is a heterodimer that contains a 91-kd glycosylated protein, gp91*phox*, and a nonglycosylated subunit, p22*phox*.[241, 243, 244] The gene for gp91*phox*, which is the site of mutations in the X-linked form of CGD, was one of the first to be identified by positional cloning.[250] The respiratory burst oxidase cytochrome has been referred to as cytochrome-b_{558}, for its spectral peak of light absorbance at 558 nm, or as cytochrome-b_{-245}, in reference to its midpoint potential of −245 mV, which is the lowest reported for any mammalian cytochrome.[251] In addition to two heme prosthetic groups per heterodimer[252] that are embedded in the membrane, the oxidase cytochrome-*b* has been reported to contain a flavin group and an NADPH-binding site.[242–244, 253] The gp91*phox* subunit has regions of similarity with the ferredoxin-NADP+-reductase family of flavoproteins[254] and with a ferric iron reductase in yeast involved in transmembrane iron transport.[255] Based on the redox properties of the cytochrome, the following pathway has been proposed for transfer of electrons from NADPH to O_2 (reaction 1 in Fig. 22–5):

$$NADPH \atop -330mV \rightarrow {flavin \atop -256mV} \rightarrow {heme \atop -245mV} \rightarrow {O_2 \atop -160mV} \rightarrow O_2^-$$

The cytochrome spans membrane, so that NADPH is oxidized at the cytoplasmic surface and oxygen is reduced to form O_2^- on the outer surface of the plasma membrane (or inner surface of the phagosomal membrane).[241, 243, 244, 247]

Activation of electron transfer requires the participation of two soluble oxidase subunits, p47*phox* and p67*phox*, which translocate from the cytoplasm of unstimulated cells to the membrane on oxidase activation, where they form a complex with the cytochrome.[243, 244] Oxidase assembly is associated with the phosphorylation of p47*phox* and is in part mediated by associations between SH3 (*src* homology domain 3) domains in p47*phox* and p67*phox*, with proline-rich target SH3-binding domains in p22*phox*, p47*phox*, and p67*phox*.[256–259] The activity of the respiratory burst oxidase is also modulated by the small GTPases, Rac and Rap1a.[50]

Oxidase assembly is triggered by receptor-mediated binding of many soluble chemoattractants (see Table 22–6), which requires higher concentrations of these molecules compared with the initiation of chemotaxis.

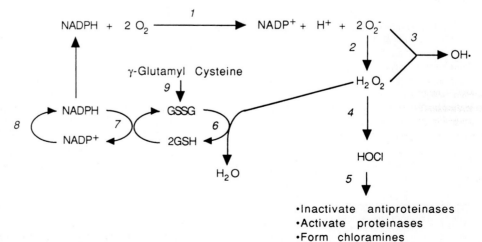

Figure 22-5. Reactions of the respiratory burst pathway. The enzymes responsible for reactions 1 through 9 are as follows: (1) the respiratory burst oxidase (NADPH oxidase); (2) superoxide dismutase or spontaneous; (3) nonenzymatic, Fe^{2+}-catalyzed; (4) myeloperoxidase; (5) spontaneous; (6) glutathione peroxidase; (7) glutathione reductase; (8) glucose-6-phosphate dehydrogenase; and (9) glutathione synthetase. GSSG = oxidized glutathione; GSH = reduced glutathione. (Reproduced from Curnutte J, Orkin S, Dinauer M: Genetic disorders of phagocyte function. In Stamatoyannopoulos G (ed): The Molecular Basis of Blood Diseases. 2nd ed. Philadelphia, W.B. Saunders Co., 1994, p 493.)

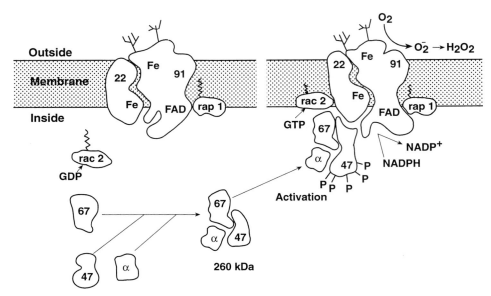

Figure 22-6. Hypothetical model of NADPH oxidase activation. Current knowledge suggests that the oxidase in its dormant state *(left side of figure)* is composed of both membrane-bound and cytosolic components. The former include the gp91^{phox} and p22^{phox} subunits of cytochrome-*b* (and possibly Rap1A). The flavin and heme groups (Fe) that mediate the transfer of electrons from NADPH to molecular oxygen are localized in the cytochrome. The cytosolic components p47^{phox} and p67^{phox} may exist as a preformed complex of 260 kd, which may also include a third protein (α), possibly p40^{phox}. The small GTPase Rac2 also is present in the cytosol in its inactive guanosine diphosphate (GDP)-bound state. On phagocyte activation, the cytosolic complex translocates to the membrane, which may be under the control of the active (guanosine triphosphate (GTP)-bound) form of Rac2 and further regulated by phosphorylation of p47^{phox}. (Adapted with permission from Curnutte J, Orkin S, Dinauer M: Genetic disorders of phagocyte function. In Stamatoyannopoulos G (ed): The Molecular Basis of Blood Diseases. 2nd ed. Philadelphia, W.B. Saunders Co., 1994, p 493.)

Table 22-8. PROPERTIES OF THE PHAGOCYTE RESPIRATORY BURST OXIDASE COMPONENTS

	gp91^{phox}	p22^{phox}	p47^{phox}	p67^{phox}
Synonyms	Beta chain Heavy chain	Alpha chain Light chain	NCF-1 SOC II	NCF-2 SOC III
Amino acids	570	195	390	526
Molecular weight (kd)				
Predicted	65.0	20.9	44.6	60.9
As seen by PAGE	91	22	47	67
Glycosylation	Yes (N-linked)	No	No	No
pI	9.7	10.0	9.5	5.8
Gene locus	gp91^{phox} Xp21.1	p22^{phox} 16q24	p47^{phox} 7q11.23	p67^{phox} 1q25
Cellular location in resting neutrophil	Specific granule membrane; plasma membrane	Specific granule membrane; plasma membrane	Cytosol	Cytosol
Tissue specificity	Myeloid, B lymphocytes	mRNA in all cells tested; protein only in myeloid and B cells	Myeloid, B lymphocytes	Myeloid, B lymphocytes
Functional domains	Heme- and FAD-binding domain; carboxy-terminus may bind cytosolic oxidase components	Heme-binding domain (?); SH3-binding domains	Six to 9 potential serine phosphorylation sites; SH3 domains, SH3-binding domains	SH3 domains, SH3-binding domains
Homologies	Ferredoxin-NADP$^+$ reductase, yeast ferric iron reductase	Polypeptide I of cytochrome *c* oxidase (weak homology)	—	—

phox = phagocyte oxidase component; NCF = neutrophil cytosol factor; SOC = soluble oxidase component; FAD = flavin adenine dinucleotide; PAGE = polyacrylamide gel electrophoresis; pI = isoelectric point; SH3 = *src* homology domain 3.
Modified from Curnutte JT: Molecular basis of the autosomal recessive forms of chronic granulomatous disease. Immunodef Rev 1992; 3:149.

The binding of opsonized microbes to Fc and complement receptors is another major physiologic trigger of the respiratory burst that is activated at sites of microbial contact.[260, 261] The specific molecules in the signal transduction cascade that activate oxidase assembly are still unknown but may involve serine-threonine kinases that phosphorylate p47^{phox}.[262] The functional oxidase complex is assembled at the plasma membrane and is also incorporated into phagosomes during ingestion. Because release of O_2^- occurs largely at the extracellular side of the membrane, oxidants are released at sites of microbial contact or within the phagocytic vacuole, where they can interact with granule contents to potentiate their microbicidal effects. The degranulation and membrane fusion of specific granules, which contain the majority of cytochrome-*b* in neutrophils,[23] may contribute to a sustained respiratory burst.

Once formed, the O_2^- radical is first converted, either spontaneously or by means of superoxide dismutase, into H_2O_2 (reaction 2 in Fig. 22–5). Myeloperoxidase, in the presence of halides, catalyzes the conversion of H_2O_2 to hypochlorous acid (HOCl), the active agent in household bleach (reaction 4 in Fig. 22–5). Hydrogen peroxide also may be converted into the hydroxyl radical (OH·) in a nonenzymatic reaction with O_2^- catalyzed by either iron or copper ions (reaction 3 in Fig. 22–5). Hydrogen peroxide, HOCl, and OH· are all strong oxidants that participate in microbial killing within the phagocytic vacuole.[249] Reactive oxidants also regulate phagocyte proteolytic activity by activating latent phagocyte metalloproteinases (such as collagenase and gelatinase) and inactivating plasma antiproteinases.[193] Enhanced phagocyte proteolysis at localized sites may be important for facilitating cellular migration into inflamed tissues, destruction of microbes, and removal of cellular debris.

Other enzymatic pathways related to oxidant generation include the detoxification of H_2O_2 by glutathione peroxidase and reductase (reactions 6 and 7, Fig. 22–5).[249] Glutathione is produced from γ-glutamyl cysteine by the enzyme glutathione synthetase (reaction 9, Fig. 22–5). Other important antioxidant systems in phagocytes and other tissues include catalase, which catalyzes the conversion of H_2O_2 into oxygen and water; ascorbic acid; and α-tocopherol (vitamin E).[263] The generation of NADPH is important in providing a source of reducing equivalents for the glutathione detoxification pathway as well as the respiratory burst itself. NADPH is replenished from the oxidized form of nicotinamide-adenine dinucleotide phosphate (NADP$^+$) by leukocyte glucose-6-phosphate dehydrogenase (G6PD; reaction 8, Fig. 22–5) in the hexose monophosphate shunt.

A second oxygen-dependent pathway with antimicrobial effects, at least in the mouse, is the generation of nitric oxide (NO) from the oxidation of L-arginine to L-citrulline. This reaction is catalyzed by nitric oxide synthase (NOS), with molecular oxygen supplying the oxygen in NO.[140, 264, 265] There are three different nitric oxide synthases, two of which are constitutively expressed in a variety of tissues, including endothelium,

brain, and neutrophils. Expression of an iNOS is inducible by inflammatory stimuli in a variety of cells, including macrophages and neutrophils, where it has a wide spectrum of antitumor and antimicrobial activity against bacteria, parasites, helminths, and viruses.[140, 265, 266] Mice with genetic absence of iNOS, generated by targeted disruption of iNOS in murine embryonic stem cells, have increased susceptibility to infection with *Listeria monocytogenes*.[267] High levels of iNOS-catalyzed nitric oxide production are readily elicited in normal mouse macrophages by exposure, for example, to INF-γ and endotoxin. However, there has been widespread difficulty in consistently documenting a similar phenomenon in human macrophages, casting doubt on a role for the inducible production of NO in human host defense. The expression of functional iNOS in human macrophages has been elicited with either the cross-linking of CD69, a member of the natural killer cell family of signal transducing receptors,[268] or in activated human immunodeficiency virus–infected macrophages.[269]

Although the precise role of NO in host defense in humans remains to be defined, it is clear that in the mouse NO cannot substitute for oxidants derived from the respiratory burst pathway. A murine model of X-linked chronic granulomatous disease has been produced by gene targeting of the X-linked gene encoding gp91^{phox}.[270] Affected male mice exhibit delayed clearance of *Staphylococcus aureus* associated with abscess formation and develop a fatal pneumonia when exposed to the opportunistic fungus *Aspergillus fumigatus*. Both organisms are common causes of infections in patients with CGD, as discussed in a later section.

Specialized Functions of Mononuclear Phagocytes

Mononuclear phagocytes, particularly tissue macrophages, participate in a broad range of activities important for tissue homeostasis and repair, as well as in the host defense against viruses, bacteria, fungi, and protozoa (Table 22–9).[102, 271–275] From the standpoint of antimicrobial function, activated macrophages play a key role in the ingestion and killing of intracellular parasites, such as *Mycobacterium*, *Listeria*, *Leishmania*, *Toxoplasma*, and some fungi.[276] Both oxygen-independent and oxygen-dependent systems are involved in this process, as described earlier. Activated macrophages also exhibit cytotoxicity against tumor cells, although the importance of this process *in vivo* remains to be determined. Tumor cell killing can be mediated by an antibody-dependent process (antibody-dependent cellular cytotoxicity), which requires reactive oxygen intermediates for cytocidal effects.[101] Alternatively, macrophage tumoricidal activity can be mediated by an antibody-independent process, which involves the participation of TNF-α and a neutral serine protease secreted only by fully activated macrophages.[101]

Interactions of macrophages with T and B cells are essential for the development of cellular and humoral immunity.[111] Macrophages are involved in the proc-

Table 22-9. FUNCTIONS OF MONONUCLEAR PHAGOCYTES

Tissue Homeostasis and Repair

Wound repair
    Débridement and phagocytosis
    Secretion of growth factors for endothelial cells and
        fibroblasts
Hematopoiesis
    Secretion of growth factors
Participation in iron and lipid metabolism
Scavenger function
    Phagocytosis of debris
    Removal of senescent cells
    Detoxification

Immune Regulation

Antigen processing and presentation
Secretion of cytokines

Inflammatory Response and Pathogen Control

Secretion of cytokines, eicosanoids, proteases, coagulation
    factors, and other products
Antimicrobial activity
Antiviral activity
Antitumor activity

essing of exogenous antigens, which are taken up by endocytosis and degraded by proteases in the endosomal or lysosomal compartments into small peptides.[111, 277] Some of these peptides bind to major histocompatibility class II molecules and are transported to the plasma membrane for presentation to T lymphocytes, which stimulates inflammatory and antibody responses. Macrophages also produce IL-1, which supports B-cell proliferation and stimulates the production of IL-2 and other lymphokines by T cells.[126] Subsequent interactions between T and B cells result in the production of specific immunoglobulins.[111, 277]

Macrophages participate in many aspects of wound repair.[278–281] The early phases of this process are dominated by an influx of neutrophils, followed by the migration of monocytes that differentiate into activated macrophages, and, finally, by the appearance of T lymphocytes. Proliferating fibroblasts secrete collagen and other matrix proteins important for wound closure and tissue remodeling, and migrating keratinocytes regenerate the epithelial surface. Both neutrophils and macrophages protect against infection and dispose of phagocytosed debris. Mononuclear phagocytes also elaborate fibroblast, epithelial, and angiogenic growth factors (see Table 22–5), which stimulate the normal progression of tissue repair and neovascularization that characterize the later phases of wound healing.[97, 279, 282]

Resident tissue macrophages, including those lining the sinusoids of the spleen, ingest aged erythrocytes and other senescent cells. Mechanisms involved in the recognition of such cells are not fully defined. In the process of breaking down hemoglobin, iron is removed and incorporated into ferritin and hemosiderin, where it accounts for about two thirds of the body's store of reserve iron. Iron in this macrophage storage pool is constantly turning over and returned in a transferrin-bound form to the bone marrow for new red blood cell synthesis.[283, 284]

Monocytes and macrophages take up native very low density lipoproteins as well as denatured (oxidized or otherwise modified) low density lipoproteins by receptor-mediated endocytosis.[110, 285] The low density lipoproteins enter the lysosomal compartments, and free cholesterol is liberated and esterified in the cytoplasm. The scavenger receptor for denatured low density lipoproteins is not subject to down-regulation during uptake of high amounts of cholesterol, and cells exposed to sufficient quantities can acquire the appearance of foam cells, possibly contributing to a role in atherogenesis.[110, 286, 287]

Specialized Functions of Eosinophils and Basophils

Eosinophils and basophils, while sharing many of the functional characteristics of neutrophils and mononuclear phagocytes, participate in distinctive aspects of the inflammatory response, and interact with each other in the context of certain allergic reactions. Eosinophils and mast cells are often situated beneath epithelial surfaces exposed to environmental antigens, such as the respiratory and gastrointestinal tracts, where they may be actively involved in mucosal immune responses. However, the role of eosinophils, basophils, and mast cells is better known in pathologic settings than in normal homeostasis.

Eosinophils appear to have both immunoenhancing and immunosuppressive functions (Table 22–10).[58, 60, 288, 289] Although capable of ingesting and killing bacteria, eosinophils are not particularly efficient at this task. Rather, they possess an unusual ability to destroy invasive metazoan parasites, especially helminthic parasites. Eosinophils bind to the surface of both adult and larval helminths and inflict damage through release of cationic granule proteins and by the generation of reactive oxidants, including the eosinophil peroxidase-catalyzed formation of hypohalous acids through the ac-

Table 22-10. EOSINOPHIL FUNCTION

Function	Mechanism
Defense against helminths (both larval and adult forms)	1. Binding of eosinophils to surface 2. Peroxidation of larval surface mediated by eosinophil peroxidase 3. Toxicity to larval surface by released major basic protein
Immunosuppression of immediate hypersensitivity reactions	1. Engulfment of mast cell granules 2. Release of prostaglandin E_1/E_2 to suppress basophil degranulation 3. Release of histaminase 4. Oxidation of slow-reacting substance of anaphylaxis 5. Release of phospholipase D to inactivate mast cell platelet-activating factor 6. Release of major basic protein that binds mast cell heparin 7. Release of plasminogen to reduce local thrombus formation

tion of the respiratory burst and eosinophil peroxidase (see Table 22–4).[60, 71, 290, 291]

Eosinophil production of the lipid inflammatory mediators, leukotriene C_4 and PAF, play a role in the pathogenesis of allergic diseases.[292, 293] PAF and leukotriene C_4 can induce smooth muscle contraction and promote the secretion of mucus, and PAF itself is a potent activator of eosinophils. The release of eosinophil granule contents may also contribute to localized tissue damage. Purified eosinophil major basic protein, for example, can cause cytopathic changes in tracheal epithelium *in vitro* that are similar to the changes observed in asthmatic patients.[294]

Eosinophils may also perform an immunosuppressive function in immediate hypersensitivity reactions (see Table 22–10).[295] IgE-activated basophils or mast cells release eosinophil chemotactic factor of anaphylaxis, which recruits eosinophils to the site. Subsequent eosinophil degranulation releases products that can inactivate inflammatory mediators. For example, histaminase inactivates histamine, phospholipase B inactivates PAF, major basic protein inactivates mast cell heparin, and lysophospholipase prevents the generation of arachidonic acid metabolites.[60]

Basophils and mast cells are central participants in a variety of inflammatory and immunologic disorders, particularly immediate hypersensitivity diseases. Basophils and mast cells express plasma membrane receptors that specifically bind with high affinity the Fc portion of the IgE antibody (Fcε receptors).[213] After active or passive sensitization with IgE, exposure to specific multivalent antigen triggers an almost immediate release of granule contents (anaphylactic degranulation) and the synthesis and release of newly generated chemical mediators such as leukotriene C_4, which stimulates smooth muscle contraction, mucus secretion, and vasoactive changes.[296] Degranulation can also be triggered in response to insect venoms, radiocontrast dye, and other nonspecific agents. Studies on mutant mice engineered by gene targeting to lack Fcγ or Fcε receptors have shown that mast cell FcγRIII receptors are essential in activating the inflammatory response to immune complexes (Arthus reaction), heretofore an unrecognized role for the mast cell.[297]

Pathologic Consequences of Phagocyte Activation and Inflammatory Response

Although normally serving a protective function, the inflammatory response can also result in damage to host tissues. The release of proteases, oxygen radicals, and proinflammatory cytokines by activated phagocytes appears to play a major role in the generation of tissue injury in a wide variety of pathologic inflammatory processes (Table 22–11).[193, 298–301] For example, neutrophil elastase has been implicated in the pathogenesis of emphysema in both adult smokers and individuals with α_1-antitrypsin deficiency. Neutrophil granule proteases may contribute to the joint destruction in rheumatoid arthritis and other chronic arthropathies.[302]

Table 22–11. SELECTED PATHOLOGIC INFLAMMATORY REACTIONS ASSOCIATED WITH PHAGOCYTE-INDUCED TISSUE INJURY

Arthus reaction
Systemic inflammatory response syndrome
Nephrotoxic and immune-complex nephritis
Postischemic myocardial damage
Adult respiratory distress syndrome
Atherosclerosis
Bronchiectasis
Acute and chronic allograft rejection
Malignant transformation with chronic inflammation
Rheumatoid arthritis

See references 299, 300, 301, and 617.

Neutrophils are also believed to play a key role in the *systemic inflammatory response syndrome*, a term that has been created to encompass the host response to both infectious (e.g., gram-negative sepsis) and noninfectious (e.g., pancreatitis, trauma) etiologies, and can lead to organ dysfunction and tissue damage.[301] Sequestration of activated neutrophils in the pulmonary capillary bed and subsequent release of tissue-damaging agents is an important component in the development of adult respiratory distress syndrome.[209] Activation of the complement cascade by artificial membrane surfaces during hemodialysis and cardiopulmonary bypass can also result in neutrophil activation, intrapulmonary sequestration, and lung injury. In addition to their cytotoxic effects, oxidative products released by activated phagocytes are also mutagenic, as documented by plasmid mutagenesis, sister chromatid exchange, and transformation of cells in culture.[299, 303] Hence, the increased risk of malignancy observed with certain chronic inflammatory states, such as ulcerative colitis or chronic hepatitis, has been postulated to be in part related to oxidant-induced carcinogenesis.

The development of anti-inflammatory interventions based on agents that block leukocyte adhesion or inhibit the action of specific phagocyte products has been an area of intense interest. Protective effects of monoclonal antibodies directed against either β_2 integrins, ICAM-1, or selectins have been demonstrated in various animal models of inflammation, including ischemia-reperfusion injury, endotoxic shock, and acute arthritis.[168] Furthermore, a phase 1 trial in which anti-ICAM-1 monoclonal antibodies were given to renal allograft recipients demonstrated improved function of cadaveric renal allografts and a reduced incidence of graft rejection.[303a] This approach may be less useful in other clinical settings in which the leukocyte-endothelial cell inflammatory cascade has already been activated. The contributions of nonphagocytic cells to inflammatory tissue injury must also be kept in mind. For example, the adult respiratory distress syndrome can occur in the presence of severe neutropenia.[304] Finally, despite the adverse consequences of the acute inflammatory process, these events are also important for the normal healing process. For example, the use of anti-inflammatory agents in myocardial infarction, which can decrease infarct size acutely, results in impaired healing of the myocardium and the formation of fragile scar tissue.[300, 305, 306]

QUANTITATIVE GRANULOCYTE DISORDERS

Overview

Abnormally high or low numbers of circulating granulocytes or monocytes are frequently seen in pediatrics. In this section, the clinical disorders associated with disturbances in granulocyte numbers are reviewed. Particular emphasis is placed on those syndromes in which the granulocyte abnormality is a central feature. The clinical conditions discussed here, in general, are poorly understood at the molecular level, and most of what is known about their pathophysiology is descriptive. This section of the chapter therefore is organized along those lines.

Neutropenia

Definition and Classification

Neutropenia is defined as an absolute decrease in the number of circulating neutrophils in the blood. Normal neutrophil levels should be stratified for age, race, and other factors. For whites, the lower limit for normal neutrophil counts (neutrophils and bands) is 1000 cells/μL in infants between 2 weeks and 1 year of age. After infancy, the corresponding value is 1500 cells/μL. Blacks have somewhat lower neutrophil counts, and the lower limits of normal can tentatively be considered to be from 200 to 600 cells/μL less relative to whites.[307–309] The basis for this observation is probably due to a relative decrease of neutrophils in the bone marrow storage compartment. Note that falsely low white blood cell counts can result when counts are done long after blood is drawn or after excessive leukocyte clumping in the presence of certain paraproteins.

Neutropenia can be due to disturbances in production, a shift of neutrophils from the circulating to marginated or tissue pools, increased peripheral utilization or destruction, or a combination of these causes. From the clinical standpoint, assays of leukokinetics and myelopoiesis are not routinely available. Classifications based on biochemical or functional studies are also difficult because of the paucity of neutrophils in the circulation of neutropenic patients. Therefore, the neutropenic syndromes discussed in this section are grouped according to whether the underlying cause of neutropenia is due to intrinsic defects in the myeloid progenitors or whether neutropenia is acquired as a result of extrinsic factors, such as drugs, infections, or autoantibodies (Table 22–12).

Individual patients may be characterized as having mild neutropenia with neutrophil counts of 1000 to 1500 cells/μL, moderate neutropenia with counts of 500 to 1000 cells/μL, and severe neutropenia with counts generally fewer than 500 cells/μL. This stratification is useful for predicting the risk of pyogenic infections, because only patients with severe neutropenia have increased susceptibility to life-threatening

Table 22–12. CLASSIFICATION OF NEUTROPENIA

Neutropenia Caused by Intrinsic Defects in Myeloid Cells or Their Progenitors
Reticular dysgenesis
Severe congenital neutropenia (Kostmann's syndrome)
Cyclic neutropenia
Myelokathexis
Shwachman's syndrome
Dyskeratosis congenita
Chédiak-Higashi syndrome
Familial benign neutropenia
Fanconi's anemia
Bone marrow failure syndromes

Neutropenia Caused by Extrinsic Factors
Infection
Drug-induced neutropenia
Autoimmune neutropenia
Chronic benign neutropenia of childhood (autoimmune neutropenia of childhood)
Immune neonatal neutropenia
Neutropenia associated with immune dysfunction
Neutropenia associated with metabolic diseases
Nutritional deficiencies
Reticuloendothelial sequestration
Bone marrow infiltration
Chronic idiopathic neutropenia

infection, particularly if the neutropenia persists for more than a few days. Endogenous bacteria are the most frequent invaders, but colonization with a variety of organisms of nosocomial origin is also common.

Susceptibility to bacterial infection, even with severe neutropenia, is quite variable. For example, some patients with chronic neutropenia due to autoantibodies do not experience serious infections over a period of many years even with neutrophil counts as low as 200 cells/μL (or even lower), most likely because these individuals have normocellular bone marrow. Many patients with chronic neutropenia also have normal to increased numbers of circulating monocytes.[310] However, the recruitment of monocytes to inflammatory sites is delayed relative to neutrophils, and monocytes are not as efficient as neutrophils in ingesting bacteria.[311, 312] Thus, monocytes appear to provide only marginal protection against pyogenic organisms in severely neutropenic patients. It is likely that the humoral, cell-mediated, and tissue macrophage immune systems also play critical roles preventing infection in these individuals.

The most frequent types of pyogenic infections in patients with significant neutropenia are cutaneous cellulitis, superficial or deep cutaneous abscesses, furunculosis, pneumonia, and septicemia.[310, 313–315] Stomatitis, gingivitis, periodontitis, perirectal inflammation, and otitis media (especially in children) occur as well. However, neutropenia in and of itself does not heighten susceptibility of patients to viral, fungal, and parasitic infections or to bacterial meningitis. The most commonly isolated organisms from neutropenic patients are *S. aureus* and gram-negative bacteria. The usual symptoms and signs of local infection—such as exudates, fluctuation, ulceration, and regional adenopathy—are much less evident in neutropenic patients than they are in non-neutropenic individuals.[316]

Neutropenia Caused by Intrinsic Defects in Myeloid Cells or Their Progenitors

Reticular Dysgenesis

The selective failure of stem cells committed to myeloid and lymphoid development leads to reticular dysgenesis.[317-322] Affected infants have severe neutropenia and moderate to severe lymphopenia associated with the absence of lymph nodes, tonsils, and Peyer's patches and splenic follicles. Erythroid and megakaryocyte development is normal. Because of the combined effects of neutropenia, agammaglobulinemia, and lymphopenia, such infants are highly vulnerable to fatal bacterial or viral infections. Reticular dysgenesis may be an inherited disorder, and both males (some who were siblings) and females have been reported. Bone marrow transplantation has been successful in treating this disorder in at least two cases.[322, 323]

Severe Congenital Neutropenia

This disease was first described by Kostmann in 1956 as an autosomal recessive disorder associated with severe neutropenia that was identified in the population of an isolated northern parish of Sweden.[324] Affected patients usually died of pyogenic infection during infancy and childhood. Other congenital disorders have since been identified that appear related to Kostmann's disease.[325-327] Affected patients chronically maintain an absolute neutrophil count of fewer than 200 cells/μL, which has been documented on the first day of life in several cases.[324] In spite of an accompanying monocytosis and moderate eosinophilia, these patients develop frequent episodes of fever, skin infections (including omphalitis), stomatitis, and perirectal abscesses that typically appear during the first months of life. Infections often disseminate to the blood, meninges, and peritoneum and are usually caused by *S. aureus*, *Escherichia coli*, and *Pseudomonas* species. Bone marrow findings have been variable but usually show normal neutrophil development up to the promyelocyte or myelocyte stage with a marked depletion of mature neutrophils.[324] Ultrastructural abnormalities in granules of neutrophilic cells have been observed in some cases.[326] Monocytes, eosinophils, macrophages, and reactive plasma cells are typically increased.

Culture of bone marrow cells *in vitro* has generally demonstrated normal numbers of colony-forming granulocyte-monocyte progenitor cells that are capable of generating neutrophils in the presence of exogenous G-CSF.[326, 328-330] G-CSF[331, 332] and GM-CSF[333] production in patients with Kostmann's syndrome appears to be normal, if not elevated. The underlying cause of the disease appears to be heterogeneous. In the majority of patients, including three Swedish patients with known familial disease, the G-CSF receptor itself appears to be normal,[327, 334, 335, 335a] suggesting that the downstream signaling pathway may be abnormal. However, three unrelated patients have been found to have mutations that truncate the C-terminal cytoplasmic portion of the G-CSF receptor that is involved in intracellular signaling.[327, 335] In all three cases the mutation involved only one allele and appeared to be an acquired (somatic) mutation. Additional studies in cell lines have suggested that the mutant receptors can interfere in a dominant negative manner with the function of wild-type G-CSF receptors and thereby inhibit G-CSF induction of neutrophil maturation.[327, 335]

The severe neutropenia of this disorder eventually leads to fatal infections in the majority of patients. Splenectomy, corticosteroids, and androgens have had no effect. Supportive care of these patients has included the use of prophylactic trimethoprim-sulfamethoxazole and the judicious use of antibiotics at the time of documented infections, along with scrupulous attention to oral hygiene. Bone marrow transplantation has resulted in partial and complete correction of the agranulocytosis.[323, 336, 337]

Almost all patients with severe congenital neutropenia have increases in the absolute neutrophil count and reduced infections when treated with G-CSF.[330, 338, 339] In contrast, GM-CSF treatment results in large increases in eosinophils and monocytes but not neutrophils.[329] These data have suggested that putative defects in the transduction of signals through the G-CSF receptor can be overridden *in vivo* by pharmacologic doses of this growth factor. G-CSF has become a widely used treatment modality for severe congenital neutropenia. In one report summarizing data on patients treated for 4 to 6 years, 40 of 44 patients had a sustained increase in peripheral neutrophil counts in response to G-CSF that was associated with a greatly improved quality of life due to decreased infections.[339] Two patients required increasing doses to maintain this response, and in one patient the condition became refractory. The effective dose of G-CSF has varied from patient to patient, ranging from 3 to 60 μg/kg per day.[330, 338] Side effects are usually mild and include headache, bone pain, and rashes. Adverse events noted in 44 patients treated for 4 or more years include osteopenia (15 patients), splenomegaly (12), bone marrow fibrosis (2), myelodysplastic syndrome and leukemia (3), and transient inverted chromosome 5q with excess blasts (1).[339] The development of myeloid leukemia has also been reported in 2 other children with severe congenital neutropenia undergoing treatment with G-CSF.[340, 341] The relationship of these events to G-CSF treatment, particularly the development of myelodysplasia and leukemia, is unclear, because these patients already have an increased risk of developing myeloid leukemia.[342, 343] Two of the 3 patients with mutations that result in truncation of the C-terminal region of the G-CSF receptor have developed leukemias.[335] The mutation was documented in the neutropenic phase in 1 patient. Patients with severe congenital neutropenia and C-terminal mutations in the G-CSF receptor may represent a subgroup with a higher risk of leukemic transformation. Before G-CSF therapy is started, a bone marrow examination with cytogenetic analysis should be performed; how frequently these studies should be undertaken in patients on G-CSF treatment is unclear.

Cyclic Neutropenia

Cyclic neutropenia is a rare disorder characterized by regular periodic oscillations approximately every 21 days in the number of peripheral blood neutrophils, with a nadir of less than 200 cells/µL (Fig. 22–7).[344, 345] In most cases, reticulocytes, platelets, and other leukocytes also cycle. In 1910, Leale[346] described a case of recurrent furunculosis in an infant who showed a cyclical variation in peripheral blood cell counts, which is probably the first recorded report of human cyclic neutropenia. During the neutropenic period, the majority of patients suffer from malaise, fever, oral ulcers, gingivitis and periodontitis, and pharyngitis associated with lymph node enlargement. More serious complications can occasionally occur, including mastoiditis, pneumonia, or recurrent ulcerations of vaginal or rectal mucosa. The severity of the infections tends to parallel the severity of the neutropenia, but some patients escape infections entirely during the neutropenic period. Many patients experience improvement in symptoms as they grow older. In these individuals, the cycles tend to become less noticeable as the hematologic picture begins to resemble chronic neutropenia.

Although cyclic neutropenia is frequently viewed as a benign condition, 10% of patients in historical reviews have died of infectious complications.[345, 347] Pneumonias and peritonitis-sepsis (*Clostridium perfringens* is a notable pathogen) have been the most frequent causes of death.[344, 345] In about one fourth of families, cyclic neutropenia appears to be inherited in an autosomal dominant fashion. Cyclic neutropenia has not been associated with an increased risk of developing myeloid leukemia, in contrast to severe congenital neutropenia.

Oscillations in the rate of bone marrow production of neutrophils result in neutropenia with nadirs at intervals of 21 ± 3 days in the majority of patients, although the cycles can be as long as 28 to 36 days and as short as 14 days.[347] Neutrophil counts typically fall to 0 at some time during the nadir and remain below 200 cells/µL for at least 3 to 5 days. In some patients, monocytosis and eosinophilia occur when neutrophil counts are at their lowest. In the recovery phase, the neutrophil counts often remain less than 1900 cells/µL, and cycles in which neutrophil counts do not rise above 1000 cells/µL are seen in many patients. When seen, oscillations in reticulocyte and platelet counts parallel those seen for neutrophils but range between

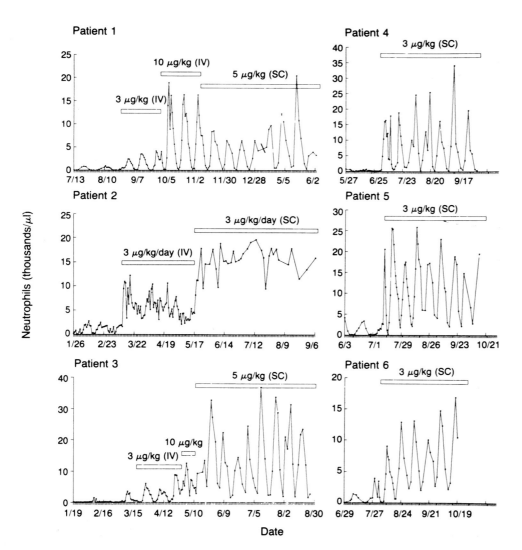

Figure 22-7. Cyclic neutropenia and the response to clinical administration of granulocyte colony-stimulating factor (G-CSF) in 6 patients. The cycling of neutrophil counts before and during therapy with various doses of G-CSF is shown. The rectangles represent the duration of G-CSF treatment, with the corresponding dose shown above each rectangle. Note the approximately 21-day cycle before therapy in patients 1, 5, and 6 that is characteristic of cyclic neutropenia. The cycle shortened to approximately 14 days during G-CSF therapy, whereas the peak neutrophil counts increased approximately 10-fold. (Reprinted with permission from Hammond WP IV, Price TH, et al: Treatment of cyclic neutropenia with granulocyte colony-stimulating factor. N Engl J Med 1989; 320:1307.)

normal and elevated levels.[345, 348] Marrow aspirates obtained during periods of neutropenia have shown either hypoplasia or an arrest at the myelocyte stage.

A variety of studies have suggested that cyclic neutropenia occurs because of a regulatory abnormality involving early hematopoietic precursor cells.[334, 344] Studies of autosomal recessive cyclic neutropenia in collies have shown that transplantation of marrow from normal dogs to affected animals abolishes the blood cell count fluctuations, whereas the converse experiment results in cyclic neutropenia in the previously normal animal.[344, 349] In both dogs and humans it can be demonstrated that there are oscillations of hematopoietic activity involving all hematopoietic lineages. In humans, cyclic neutropenia has been transferred by allogeneic bone marrow transplantation from a sibling with the disorder to another sibling undergoing treatment for leukemia.[349] Thus, it has been presumed that cyclic neutropenia involves a regulatory defect in hematopoietic stem cells.

Cyclic neutropenia must be distinguished from cyclic fevers without neutropenia[350] and from other causes of neutropenia. To establish the diagnosis of cyclic neutropenia, neutrophil counts must be monitored at least two times a week for 6 to 8 weeks.

The management of patients with cyclic neutropenia includes careful attention to the identification and treatment of infections acquired when these patients are neutropenic. In general, fevers, upper respiratory tract symptoms, and cervical lymphadenopathy occurring during neutropenic episodes require no specific therapy. However, the physician must remain alert to symptoms suggesting a specific infection or an abdominal crisis. Careful attention to oral and dental hygiene is important to minimize periodontal disease and ameliorate the discomfort of mouth sores. G-CSF has been effective in improving peripheral blood neutrophil counts in cyclic neutropenia. In one report, six patients were treated with G-CSF (3 to 10 μg/kg per day) for 3 to 15 months.[351] As shown in Figure 22–7, one patient (patient 2) no longer experienced cycles while taking G-CSF. The other five continued to experience cycles, but the duration of each period decreased from 21 to 14 days and the mean neutrophil nadir increased to approximately 1400 cells/μL. These hematologic changes were associated with markedly decreased symptoms and infections.[351] The dose of G-CSF required to maintain this effect in individual patients can usually be reduced to 1 to 3 g/kg per day, and daily doses are not always required.[339, 351] No cases of leukemia were observed in a group of 10 patients with cyclic neutropenia treated with G-CSF for a total of 4 to 6 years.[339, 351] As is the case for severe congenital neutropenia, the ever-present risk of developing a life-threatening infection in patients with cyclic neutropenia merits serious consideration of prophylactic G-CSF therapy.

Myelokathexis

Myelokathexis is an uncommon form of moderate to severe neutropenia with bizarre morphologic disturbances of the granulocyte nucleus.[352–356] Most of the blood neutrophils have cytoplasmic vacuoles and abnormal nuclei with very thin filaments connecting the nuclear lobes. The marrow appears hyperplastic and contains degenerating hypersegmented granulocytes. Leukokinetic and morphologic studies suggest increased intramedullary destruction of neutrophils as the basis of the neutropenia. Increased numbers of apoptotic bone marrow neutrophils have also been observed.[356a] Neutrophil motility is also abnormal in many patients, and the disorder was associated with hypogammaglobulinemia in one family.[357] One patient has been successfully treated with G-CSF, with resolution of her severe gingivitis and periodontitis.[358]

Shwachman's Syndrome

Shwachman's syndrome is a rare multiorgan disease of unknown cause that is inherited as an autosomal recessive trait.[359, 360] Metaphyseal chondrodysplasia, dwarfism, pancreatic exocrine insufficiency, and neutropenia have been noted.[361–365] Diarrhea, weight loss, failure to thrive, eczema, otitis media, and pneumonia may occur in affected neonates. Skin infections, osteomyelitis, and sepsis can also be seen. Almost all infants develop malabsorption by 4 months of age. Growth failure and dwarfism are usually noted during the first or second year of life, and puberty is often delayed. Normal gait can become impaired because of hip discomfort secondary to metaphyseal chondrodysplasia. The skeletal abnormalities can also result in pathologic fractures, coxa vara, kyphosis, and scoliosis.[366] Dysmorphic features include cutaneous syndactyly, a bifid uvula, a short soft palate, and hypertelorism.

Virtually all patients with Shwachman's syndrome have neutropenia, and the neutrophil count is below 1000 cells/μL in approximately two thirds. The neutrophil counts tend to be constant, with no reciprocal monocytosis. Some patients also have a moderately severe defect in motility that can contribute to the increased susceptibility to pyogenic infection.[361] Mild to moderate thrombocytopenia and anemia can be present. Bone marrow studies have generally shown some degree of myeloid hypoplasia[364, 367] but are nondiagnostic. The underlying cause of the hematopoietic defect has not been identified. Patients also have evidence of pancreatic exocrine insufficiency by laboratory testing. Histologic studies of the pancreas have shown acinar degeneration with fatty replacement.

Treatment includes pancreatic enzyme replacement, which does not improve the neutropenia or dwarfism. Steatorrhea tends to diminish with time, although pancreatic insufficiency persists.[362] The frequency of bacterial infections can vary between patients, which generally respond to the appropriate antibiotics. Administration of G-CSF increases the neutrophil count to the normal range[330, 368] and should be considered as adjunctive therapy in the setting of serious infection. In approximately 25% of cases, aplastic anemia develops. As is the case for other congenital bone marrow failure syndromes, leukemic transformation can also occur.[363]

Dyskeratosis Congenita

Dyskeratosis congenita is an X-linked recessive disorder characterized by nail dystrophy, leukoplakia, and reticulated hyperpigmentation of the skin.[369] Many of these patients have associated marrow hypoplasia, including 35% with neutropenia. Most of the patients have little in the way of serious infections and survive into adulthood.

Chédiak-Higashi Syndrome

Chédiak-Higashi syndrome (CHS) is a rare genetic disorder characterized by partial oculocutaneous albinism, giant lysosomes in many cell types, including granulocytes, and neuropathy.[370–373] Most patients have a moderate neutropenia, apparently due to ineffective granulopoiesis. This disorder is described in detail in a later section.

Familial Benign Neutropenia

Familial benign neutropenia is characterized by a mild neutropenia and no tendency to increased infection. An autosomal dominant transmission has been identified in some familial cases.[374] Familial benign neutropenia has been described in Yemenite Jews,[375] American and African blacks,[376] and Germans, French, Americans, and South Africans.[377]

Other Causes of Neutropenia Due to Intrinsic Defects in Myelopoiesis

Other bone marrow failure syndromes can occasionally present as isolated neutropenia, including Fanconi's anemia, aplastic anemia, and myelodysplastic syndromes.

Neutropenia Caused by Extrinsic Factors

Infection

The most common cause of transient neutropenia in childhood is viral infection. Viruses commonly causing neutropenia include hepatitis A and B, respiratory syncytial virus, influenza A and B, measles, rubella, and varicella.[96, 378–381] Neutropenia develops during the first 24 to 48 hours of the illness and may persist for 3 to 6 days. This usually corresponds to the period of acute viremia and may relate to virus-induced redistribution of neutrophils from the circulating to the marginated granulocyte pool, sequestration, or increased neutrophil utilization after tissue damage by the viruses.[382, 383] Several human viruses, including measles and herpes simplex virus, have been demonstrated to replicate in human endothelial cells and lead to the expression of receptors on endothelium for immune complexes containing IgG and C3, which potentially might promote enhanced neutrophil adhesion to the endothelium.[384, 385] Acute transient neutropenia often occurs during the early stages of infectious mononucleosis.[386, 387]

In most of these cases, the basis of the neutropenia is unknown, but in some it may be related to accelerated destruction of neutrophils by antineutrophil antibodies.[388, 389]

Leukopenia is commonly seen in patients with the acquired immunodeficiency syndrome.[390] In the pediatric population with this syndrome, neutropenia can be caused by antiviral drugs, vitamin B_{12} or folate deficiency, or cellular immune dysfunction.[391] Neutropenia in human immunodeficiency virus infection can also be associated with hypersplenism and antineutrophil antibodies.[392, 393]

Significant neutropenia may occur during typhoid, paratyphoid, tuberculosis, brucellosis, tularemia, and rickettsial infections.[378, 379, 394–396] The mechanisms responsible for neutropenia in these conditions remain ill defined. During periods of relapsing fever caused by acute vivax malaria, the apparent neutropenia may be secondary to increased neutrophil margination in the intravascular compartment.[397]

Sepsis is one of the more serious causes of neutropenia. The neutropenia in patients with bacteremia and endotoxemia may result from excessive destruction of neutrophils. This can occur after phagocytosis of microbes, from the release of metabolites of arachidonic acid, or from activation of the complement system through either the alternate or classic pathway leading to the generation of C5a. C5a, in turn, induces neutrophil aggregation and leads to the formation of leukoemboli in the pulmonary capillary bed, which adhere to endothelial surfaces. This process is probably accelerated as a result of "priming" of neutrophils by endotoxin and by TNF and IL-1 released by macrophages.[398] The adherent, activated neutrophils may release noxious substances that can cause acute cardiopulmonary complications. C5a neutropenia occurs transiently during hemodialysis, during continuous-flow leukapheresis, and after burn injury.[399–402]

Significant neutropenia can occur in neonatal bacterial sepsis. Newborns can exhaust their neutrophil reserves during overwhelming bacterial infection, because the neutrophil storage pool is small and neutrophil production is already near a maximum.[403] Septic newborns may benefit from granulocyte transfusion[404–406] or G-CSF,[407–409] both of which are under clinical investigation for this indication.

Drug-Induced Neutropenia

Drug-induced neutropenia is a disorder characterized by severe and selective reduction in the levels of circulating blood neutrophils (usually to levels of fewer than 200 cells/μL) and is due to an idiosyncratic reaction to the offending drug (Table 22–13).[410–422] This definition thus excludes disorders in which other cell lines are perturbed (such as in aplastic anemia), those in which drug administration is not a feature, and the predictable neutropenias observed with anticancer therapy. Implicit in this definition is the unpredictability of the condition. Drug-induced neutropenia is a serious disorder, with mortality rates reported to be as high as 32% in one series.

Table 22–13. PARTIAL LIST OF DRUGS ASSOCIATED WITH IDIOSYNCRATIC NEUTROPENIA

Drug	Possible Mechanism		
	Direct Suppression	Metabolite Suppression	Immune Destruction
Analgesics/ Anti-inflammatory Agents			
Aminopyrine			X
Ibuprofen			X
Indomethacin	X		
Phenylbutazone	X		
Antibiotics			
Chloramphenicol	X		
Penicillins	X		X
Sulfonamides	X		
Anticonvulsants			
Phenyloin			X
Carbamazepine		X	
Antithyroid Agents			
Propylthiouracil			X
Cardiovascular Agents			
Hydralazine			X
Procainamide			X
Quinidine			X
Hypoglycemic Agents			
Chlorpropamide			X
Tranquilizers			
Chlorpromazine	X		
Phenothiazines	X		
Other			
Cimetidine, ranitidine	X		
Levamisole			X

The partial list of agents capable of causing idiosyncratic drug-induced neutropenia is summarized from references 410 through 422.

Idiosyncratic reactions tend to develop more frequently in women than in men and more often in older than in younger persons.[416] Drugs reported to have been associated with agranulocytosis have been extensively reviewed.[410-412, 420-422] These include antimicrobial agents, particularly sulfonamides and penicillins; antithyroid drugs; phenothiazines; antipyretics, including aspirin, acetaminophen, and phenylbutazone; antirheumatics, including gold, levamisole, and penicillamine; and sedatives, including barbiturates and benzodiazepines (see Table 22–13).

Although the underlying mechanisms for most drug-induced neutropenias are unknown, studies with certain drugs have suggested at least three major mechanisms.[411, 413, 421, 422] First, differences in drug pharmacokinetics can lead to toxic levels of the drug or metabolites in the marrow microenvironment. An example is the neutropenia induced by sulfasalazine. Whereas neutropenia can be observed in any patient taking this drug, those individuals who are slow acetylators show much greater toxicity than do those who are fast acetylators.[418] Second, myeloid precursors may be abnormally sensitive to typical drug concentrations. Phenothi-

azines and perhaps nitrous oxide induce neutropenia by this mechanism in that myeloid precursors in the marrow are particularly sensitive to these agents.[411, 422, 423] The toxic damage by phenothiazines manifests itself as a neutropenia that appears 20 to 40 days after the patient has received 10 to 12 g of the drug. Third, drugs can induce an immune-mediated neutropenia in two ways. In one, the drug serves as a hapten in promoting the synthesis of antibodies that are capable of destroying mature neutrophils. Aminopyrine, penicillin, propylthiouracil, and gold can cause neutropenia by this mechanism.[411, 415, 419, 422] In the other way, the drug causes the formation of circulating immune complexes that presumably attach to the surface of the neutrophil and lead to its destruction, as in the case of quinidine. In addition, immunologic changes induced by drugs can suppress granulopoiesis. For example, activation of both cellular and humoral immune responses has been reported to impair myelopoiesis after therapy with quinidine and phenytoin, respectively.[413, 422] Drug-induced immune neutropenia is characterized by its unpredictability. It normally begins abruptly 7 to 14 days after the first exposure to the drug or immediately after re-exposure. Fever, chills, and severe prostration are common in these patients.

The duration of drug-induced neutropenia is highly variable. Acute idiosyncratic drug reactions may last only a few days, whereas chronic idiosyncratic reactions may last for months or years. By contrast, immune-mediated neutropenia usually lasts for 6 to 8 days. Once neutropenia occurs, the most important therapeutic action is, of course, to withdraw all drugs that are not absolutely essential, particularly those suspected to be myelotoxic. During recovery from drug-induced neutropenia, a rebound leukocytosis can occur, accompanied by marrow and peripheral blasts.

Autoimmune Neutropenia

Autoimmune neutropenia (AIN) can be seen as an isolated phenomenon, in association with other autoimmune diseases or otherwise secondary to infection, drugs, or malignancy.[215, 424] Many cases of chronic idiopathic neutropenia in children and adults are now recognized as secondary to autoimmune antibodies directed against neutrophils. In primary AIN, low circulating neutrophil counts are the only hematologic finding and associated diseases or other factors that cause neutropenia are absent. The peak incidence of AIN occurs in infants and young children,[215] where it is a generally benign disorder that remits spontaneously, as discussed in the following section. Immune-mediated neutropenias are also seen in association with other disorders (Table 22–14), where it is often referred to as secondary AIN.

Patients with AIN generally have neutrophil counts of 250 cells/μL or lower, and neutrophils can be absent entirely. Monocytosis is common. Bone marrow examination shows normal to increased cellularity and decreased to normal numbers of mature neutrophils, although maturation arrest at earlier stages of neutrophil differentiation can also be seen.[215, 315, 425, 426] Mild spleno-

Table 22-14. DISORDERS ASSOCIATED WITH IMMUNE-MEDIATED NEUTROPENIA

Autoimmune Disorders
Autoimmune hemolytic anemia
Autoimmune thrombocytopenia
Evans' syndrome
Systemic lupus erythematosus
Felty's syndrome (arthritis, splenomegaly, leukopenia)
Sjögren's syndrome
Scleroderma
Primary biliary cirrhosis

Infection
Infectious mononucleosis
Human immunodeficiency virus infection

Malignancy
Leukemia
Lymphoma
Hodgkin's disease

Hypogammaglobulinemias

Angioimmunoblastic Lymphadenopathy (Castleman's Disease)

Drug Reaction

megaly is occasionally present. The incidence of pyogenic infection is not always related to the degree of neutropenia and is generally limited to cutaneous and respiratory infections. Serious infections are generally uncommon. Spontaneous remissions can occasionally occur but are much less frequent compared with what is observed in younger patients (see following section).

Neutrophil-specific cell surface antigens are a frequently identified target of the autoantibodies identified in AIN, including NA1 and NA2, NB1, ND1, and NE1.[215] The NA1 and NA2 antigens are glycosylated isoforms of the neutrophil opsoninic X FcγRIII receptor[210] (see Table 22–7), and the NB1 antigen is a 58- to 64-kd GPI-anchored membrane glycoprotein on the plasma membrane and on secondary granules.[427] Mechanisms that trigger autoantibody production are unknown.

A combination of the granulocyte immunofluorescence test and granulocyte agglutination test appears to result in optimal sensitivity and specificity for detection of antineutrophil antibodies.[215, 424, 428, 429] In the granulocyte immunofluorescence test, heterologous granulocytes are incubated with serum or plasma from patients and controls and bound immunoglobulins are detected by a fluorescent dye-labeled antihuman immunoglobulin antibody. The granulocyte agglutination test is based on the observation that neutrophils coated with autoantibodies bound through their F(ab) domain will move toward each other and agglutinate by means of binding to their all-surface Fc receptors. These assays detect IgG and IgM antibodies, both of which have been identified in AIN.[215] Neutrophil-binding immune complexes may also give positive results in these assays and may be important in the pathogenesis of neutropenia in Felty's syndrome.[424] Sera containing HLA antibodies require preabsorption to determine whether there is specific antineutrophil activity. Several adult patients with AIN have been found to have auto-

antibodies directed against the leukocyte adhesion β2 integrin Mac-1 (CD11b/CD18).[430] Laboratory demonstration of antineutrophil antibodies may not always be necessary to make the diagnosis of AIN, and its utility depends on the specific clinical setting.

The neutropenia of AIN is presumed primarily due to the peripheral destruction of antibody-coated neutrophils, which also may be augmented by the deposition of C3. Phagocytosis of neutrophils in the spleens of patients with AIN has been noted.[431] In some cases, antineutrophil antibodies also appear to interfere with myelopoiesis.[215, 424, 432] Impairment of phagocytosis, respiratory burst activity, and adhesion by neutrophil-directed antibodies has also been observed, which may contribute to the risk of infection in AIN.[215, 424, 430]

Treatment of patients with immune neutropenia includes the judicious use of appropriate antibiotics for bacterial infections and, in patients with occasional mouth sores or gingivitis, antibacterial mouthwashes and regular dental hygiene. Infections tend to be less frequent in immune neutropenia than with the corresponding degree of neutropenia from other causes, probably because granulopoiesis in most cases is intact. Corticosteroid and intravenous gamma globulin administration can result in normalization of the neutrophil count, but efficacy is variable and often short-lived.[215, 424] Splenectomy appears to be of only transient benefit and further predisposes the patients to life-threatening bacterial infections. The daily administration of G-CSF in doses of 1 to 2 μg/kg has been successful in increasing the neutrophil count to the normal range or even higher within 2 weeks in patients with primary AIN, Evans' syndrome, and Felty's syndrome.[424] Hence, G-CSF therapy should be considered as part of the management of serious or recurrent infections in patients with immune neutropenias. Prophylactic administration of trimethoprim-sulfamethoxazole also may be helpful for management of recurrent minor infections, although there are no controlled studies addressing the efficacy of this approach.

Chronic Benign Neutropenia and Autoimmune Neutropenia of Childhood

Most cases of what was termed *chronic benign neutropenia of infancy and childhood* are now believed to represent an AIN that has parallels to childhood idiopathic thrombocytopenic purpura and autoimmune hemolytic anemia.[215, 315, 433–436] The handful of cases reported as the "lazy leukocyte syndrome,"[437–439] characterized by profound neutropenia, a normal-appearing bone marrow, and little increase in the peripheral blood neutrophil count in response to steroids or epinephrine, are also likely to have been AIN of childhood.

AIN of childhood occurs predominantly in children younger than 3 years (Table 12–15). The median age at presentation is 8 to 11 months, with a range of 2 to 54 months.[215, 433, 434] There is a slight female predominance. The mean absolute neutrophil count at presentation is 150 to 250 cells/μL and often approaches zero. A relative monocytosis or eosinophilia can occur. Transient increases in circulating neutrophil counts can occur in

Table 22-15. SUMMARY OF AUTOIMMUNE NEUTROPENIA OF CHILDHOOD

Incidence	Most common cause of chronic neutropenia in infancy and childhood; greater than or equal to 1 per 100,000 children per year.
Clinical features	Median age at diagnosis is 8 to 11 months of age (range, 3–38 months). Slight female predominance (56% F; 44% M). Relatively minor infections (otitis media, gingivitis, upper respiratory tract, skin) occur with an increased incidence in some patients and respond well to antimicrobial therapy. Occasional patients have pneumonia or sepsis (usually infants).
Laboratory evaluation	Median absolute neutrophil count at time of diagnosis is about 200 neutrophils/μL (range, 0–500 cells/μL). Hemoglobin value and platelet count are generally normal. Antineutrophil antibodies can be detected in majority of patients and are often directed to NA1 antigen (neutrophil FcγRIII receptor). Bone marrow is normocellular to hypercellular, often with a decrease in mature neutrophils, although maturation arrest at earlier stages is noted occasionally.
Differential diagnosis	Other causes of autoimmune neutropenia (e.g., Evans' syndrome, drug reaction), transient postinfectious neutropenia, immunodeficiency syndromes, aminoacidopathies, intrinsic defects in myelopoiesis (e.g., severe congenital neutropenia, cyclic neutropenia, Shwachman's syndrome)
Therapy	Antibiotics for acute infection; prophylactic antibiotics may be helpful in some patients with recurrent otitis media. Consider use of G-CSF in the event of serious infection.
Prognosis	Excellent. Although the absolute neutrophil count often remains below 500 cells/μL for 12 or more months, spontaneous remission occurs in almost all patients (median of 20 months, range, 6–54 months).

response to infection. Other peripheral counts are normal for age, although mild thrombocytopenia (greater than or equal to 100,000 cells/μL) has been reported.[434] There is no family history of neutropenia.

Antineutrophil antibodies can be detected in almost all patients when a combination of immunofluorescent and agglutination assays are used; however, absence of detectable antibody does not exclude the diagnosis. As in AIN in adults, antibodies are typically directed against neutrophil-specific antigens of the NA, NB, and ND loci. Antibody specificity to NA1, an allele of the neutrophil FcγRIII opsonin receptor, is seen in about one fourth of cases.[215, 433, 434] No correlation exists between the strength of the antibody and the severity of clinical manifestations; however, as neutropenia resolves, antibodies gradually become undetectable. Results of bone marrow examination generally show a normal to hypercellular marrow, with reduction in mature neutrophils or bands, although a maturation arrest can occur in earlier stages.[215, 315, 434] Some patients manifest an increase in the peripheral neutrophil count in response to hydrocortisone or prednisone.

Bacterial infections during the neutropenic period are often increased in frequency but mild (e.g., skin infections, upper respiratory tract infections, otitis media, gingivitis) and responsive to standard antibiotics.[215, 315, 433] Cellulitis involving the labia majora was seen in 23% of 26 girls with AIN in one series, often due to *P. aeruginosa*.[315] Pneumonia, sepsis, and meningitis have been seen occasionally in infants with AIN.[215] Spontaneous remission occurs in almost all patients, with neutropenia persisting for a median duration of 20 months.[433] Children younger than 9 months of age at the time of diagnosis may recover normal peripheral neutrophil counts more rapidly.[434] With increasing age, spontaneous remission becomes less likely.

The diagnosis of AIN of childhood is generally straightforward if the presentation is within the first 2 years of life, there is no history of serious infections over several months of observation, and neutrophil morphology and other peripheral counts are otherwise normal. Demonstration of an antineutrophil antibody is not necessary for diagnosis in the patient with the typical clinical features of childhood AIN (see Table 22–15). Evaluation of immunoglobulin levels should be performed to exclude hypogammaglobulinemias, in addition to T-cell studies if clinical signs of cell-mediated immunodeficiency are present. A bone marrow examination should be performed if hematologic abnormalities other than neutropenia are present and if the child is older than the typical patient with AIN of childhood. Other laboratory tests to consider are outlined later in this section.

Febrile episodes should be managed conservatively in the first few months after the diagnosis of childhood AIN is suspected and include the use of broad-spectrum parenteral antibiotics. However, if during this initial observation period the patient has either no infections or responds promptly to antibiotics, subsequent infectious illnesses can be managed as for any other child. Prophylactic trimethoprim-sulfamethoxazole can be helpful in the child with recurrent otitis media. Administration of G-CSF results in an increased peripheral neutrophil count in childhood AIN.[440] Steroids and intravenous gamma globulin are also effective in some cases. However, these interventions should be reserved for the rare child who manifests severe or very recurrent infections.

Although AIN of childhood is the most common cause of chronic neutropenia in the pediatric age group, it is still a relatively infrequent diagnosis, with an incidence of approximately 1 in 100,000 children per year.[315, 435] However, this figure may be an underestimate because of the generally benign course of this disorder.

Immune Neonatal Neutropenia

Neonatal alloimmune neutropenia is analogous to Rh hemolytic disease and results from maternal sensitiza-

tion to fetal neutrophils bearing antigens that differ from the mother's. Maternal IgG antibodies cross the placenta and result in an immune-mediated neutropenia that can be severe and last for several weeks to as long as 6 months.[441–443] During the neutropenic phase, the bone marrow demonstrates myeloid hyperplasia with depletion of mature neutrophil forms.

Neutrophil antibodies are found in the serum of the mother and the infant and are frequently directed to the neutrophil-specific NA antigen system. The NA1 and NA2 antigens are two isotypes of the neutrophil FcγRIIIB receptor (see Table 22–7). Affected infants can be asymptomatic or develop omphalitis, other cutaneous infections, pneumonia, sepsis, and meningitis. Because neonatal sepsis can be associated with profound neutropenia, the underlying immune-mediated neutrophil destruction may not be appreciated immediately in affected newborns who present with sepsis.

The initial management of neonatal alloimmune neutropenia should include parenteral antibiotics even if signs of infection are absent, due to the association of neutropenia with neonatal sepsis. Intravenous gamma globulin is not always effective in increasing the neutrophil counts.[444, 445] However, the administration of three daily doses of G-CSF (5 μg/kg dose) resulted in normalization of the neutrophil count within 4 days in two infants with alloimmune neutropenia.[445] Thus, treatment with G-CSF should be considered when serious infections develop in infants with alloimmune neutropenia.

Neonatal immune neutropenia can also occur in infants whose mother has AIN. Transplacental passage of an IgG antineutrophil antibody can react with the infant's neutrophils bearing the inciting antigen and result in a profound neutropenia lasting 2 to 4 weeks.[446] Leukoagglutinating antibodies have often been found in multiparous women, and these antibodies have been observed in their newborn children's sera without any corresponding neutropenia.[447, 448] The antibodies are directed against human leukocyte antigens found on neutrophils and other tissues and are presumably absorbed by the placenta, various plasma antigens, and tissues in the fetus. As a result, serum concentrations of these antibodies are insufficient to induce neutropenia. It appears that only antibodies directed specifically against neutrophils can produce immune-mediated neonatal neutropenia.

Neutropenia Associated with Immune Dysfunction

Disorders of immunoglobulin production have been associated with neutropenic syndromes. One third of males with X-linked agammaglobulinemia have neutropenia at some time during the course of their disease.[449] Persistent or cyclic neutropenia is common in patients with the hyper-IgM immunodeficiency syndrome, which in many instances appears to be secondary to the formation of autoantibodies.[450, 451] Gamma globulin abolished the neutropenia in some of these patients.[452] AIN and other autoimmune cytopenias can

also be seen in common variable immunodeficiency and isolated IgA deficiency.[451, 453]

Cartilage-hair hypoplasia, an autosomal recessive disorder found frequently in the Amish population, is characterized by short-limbed dwarfism, fine hair, moderate neutropenia (100 to 2000 neutrophils/μL), and impaired cell-mediated immunity.[454, 455] Bone marrow transplantation has corrected both the immunologic defect and neutropenia.[456, 457]

Neutropenia can be seen with a variety of other disorders of the immune system. A syndrome of severe neutropenia associated with eczema, polyarthralgias, recurrent bacterial infections, eosinophilia, and depressed cellular immunity has been reported in four siblings (three girls and a boy).[458] Serum IgA levels were markedly elevated, but antibody responses to tetanus and poliomyelitis vaccines were depressed. A case of severe granulocytic hypoplasia in a girl with defects in T-cell function has been reported that failed to improve with corticosteroid treatment but responded to serial infusions of antithymocyte globulin.[459] This patient had previously developed autoimmune thrombocytopenia and a Coombs-positive hemolytic anemia, both of which responded to prednisone. Autoimmune disorders, such as systemic lupus erythematosus, can be associated with antibody- or immune complex–mediated destruction of neutrophils and, in some cases, their precursors, as discussed previously. Finally, neutropenia is common in patients with the acquired immunodeficiency syndrome; its causes can be multifactorial and include cellular immune dysfunction, ineffective hematopoiesis, antiviral drugs, antineutrophil antibodies, and hypersplenism.[390–393]

Neutropenia Associated with Metabolic Diseases

Children suffering from hyperglycinemia, isovaleric acidemia, propionic acidemia, methylmalonic acidemia, and tyrosinemia may have significant neutropenia.[460–466, 466a] Significant neutropenia is also seen in Barth's syndrome, a distinctive X-linked disorder also associated with dilated cardiomyopathy, growth retardation, and 3-methylglutaconic aciduria.[467–469] A relative monocytosis is common. Affected boys develop symptoms in infancy or childhood, and neutropenia can precede the development of cardiac abnormalities. The mechanisms underlying the neutropenia associated with disorders of organic acid metabolism are not known, although the finding that propionate and isovalerate impair the development of myeloid colonies in vitro suggests that altered levels of metabolites in vivo may suppress myelopoiesis.[470]

Neutropenia is common in glycogen storage disease type IB, and neutrophil counts of less than 500 cells/μL are not infrequent.[464, 465, 471, 472] Multiple abnormalities in neutrophil function are also common, including chemotaxis, respiratory burst activity, and bacterial killing.[464, 466] Recombinant G-CSF has been effective in correcting the neutropenia in glycogen storage disease type IB patients, in association with reducing serious infections.[471, 472] Decreased monocyte superoxide produc-

tion and chemotaxis have been reported in Gaucher's disease, which may contribute to the infections occasionally seen in patients with this disease.[473, 474]

Nutritional Deficiencies

Ineffective granulopoiesis is part of the megaloblastic marrow pathology observed in patients with nutritional deficiencies of vitamin B_{12} or folic acid.[475] As a reflection of the increased neutrophil turnover due to ineffective myelopoiesis, serum muramidase levels are often elevated.[475] Neutropenia also occurs with starvation in such conditions as anorexia nervosa[476] and marasmus in infants, and occasionally in patients on parenteral feeding. Neutropenia and marrow megaloblastosis have also been observed in patients thought to have copper deficiency, because these patients have responded promptly to copper replacement.[477, 478]

Reticuloendothelial Sequestration

Splenic enlargement due to portal hypertension, intrinsic splenic disease, or splenic hyperplasia can lead to neutropenia. The usual picture is one of moderate neutropenia that may be accompanied by a similar degree of thrombocytopenia and anemia. The reduced neutrophil survival corresponds with the size of the spleen, and the extent of neutropenia is proportional to bone marrow compensatory mechanisms.[479] The neutropenia is usually mild and may be ameliorated by successful treatment of the underlying disease. Bed rest alone may lead to restoration of the neutrophil counts owing to reduction in portal pressure. In selected situations, splenectomy may be necessary to restore the neutrophil count to normal. Malignant histiocyte disorders may also cause reticuloendothelial hyperplasia, leading to neutropenia and anemia secondary to ingestion of neutrophils and red cells by the malignant cells.[410]

Bone Marrow Infiltration

Malignancies, such as leukemia or lymphoma, that infiltrate the bone marrow result in a myelophthisic picture, producing leukoerythroblastic peripheral blood smears. Tumor-induced myelofibrosis may further accentuate the neutropenia.[480] Myelofibrosis can also result from granulomatous infections, Gaucher's disease, osteopetrosis, benzol drugs, fluoride, or x-ray exposure.[481–483]

Chronic Idiopathic Neutropenia

Chronic idiopathic neutropenia represents a group of disorders that, by definition, are poorly understood and cannot be placed in any of the previously discussed categories.[310, 313, 315] Investigation of granulopoiesis has suggested that, in some cases, decreased or ineffective production of neutrophils may be the principal mechanism of neutropenia. The underlying cause of the defective myelopoiesis is not well characterized.[313, 484, 485]

Overall, the clinical features, bone marrow findings, and natural history of chronic idiopathic neutropenia are variable.[310, 313, 315] Many patients rarely have serious infections relative to their degree of neutropenia; it is likely that many of the cases described in older studies had antibody-mediated neutrophil destruction and normal bone marrow reserve.[486] Treatment should be based on the severity of symptoms. Corticosteroids, cytotoxic agents, and G-CSF have each been reported to be successful in individual cases.[313, 487]

Evaluation of the Patient with Neutropenia

The basic approach to a patient with neutropenia includes a history and physical examination with emphasis on (1) related phenotypic abnormalities; (2) determination of whether bacterial infection is present (including evaluation of gingiva and rectum); (3) evaluation of lymphadenopathy, hepatosplenomegaly, and any other signs of an underlying associated chronic illness; and (4) history of recent infection and drug exposure. The frequency and duration of symptoms is important, and a history of periodontitis, dental abscesses, or tooth loss is particularly suspicious for significant chronic or recurrent neutropenia. The family history may reveal other individuals with recurrent infection. Unexplained deaths in children younger than 1 year of age, and the race and ethnic group of each patient should be noted.

The duration and severity of the neutropenia and the presence or absence of significant other symptoms or physical findings greatly influence the speed and extent of laboratory evaluation. If the patient has isolated neutropenia and is asymptomatic and if other findings are absent, clinical observation for several weeks is usually the best approach. Any medications known to be associated with neutropenia should be discontinued. If an acute bacterial infection is suspected, prompt evaluation and treatment should be initiated, including the use of intravenous antibiotics in the patient with moderate to severe neutropenia and fever.

Patients with persistent neutropenia should have white blood cell counts and differential counts obtained twice weekly for 6 weeks to evaluate periodicity suggestive of cyclic neutropenia. A Coombs test and serum immunoglobulins should also be performed to evaluate for the presence of a red cell autoantibody and for possible associated hypogammaglobulinemia syndromes, respectively. T-cell studies or human immunodeficiency virus testing also may be indicated in certain cases. Bone marrow aspirate with cytogenetics and bone marrow biopsy should be performed on selected patients. If anemia, macrocytosis, or thrombocytopenia is present, these studies should be performed immediately. Other laboratory tests that should be considered, depending on the clinical situation, include investigation for antineutrophil antibodies, evaluation for collagen vascular disease and for metabolic and exocrine pancreatic disease, acid hemolysis test, radiographic studies of long bones and chest, and measure-

ment of vitamin B_{12}, folate, and copper levels. Assessing whether the peripheral neutrophil count increases in response to steroid or epinephrine is of little clinical utility.

Principles of Therapy for Neutropenia

The management of neutropenia depends on the underlying cause and severity of the neutropenia. The major concern in neutropenic patients is the development of serious pyogenic infection. Patients with severe neutropenia (absolute neutrophil count less than or equal to 500 cells/μL) with poor marrow reserve secondary to, for example, severe congenital neutropenia, aplastic anemia, or chemotherapy, are at highest risk for developing progressive infection and septicemia. Fever may often be the only indication of infection, because the usual signs and symptoms of inflammation are often diminished in the presence of neutropenia. Organisms involved are usually from the skin or gastrointestinal tract. Thus, febrile patients with neutropenia due to poor marrow function should be treated promptly with broad-spectrum antimicrobial agents after blood and other appropriate cultures are obtained. If there is a defervescence response and blood cultures do not reveal any growth, the antibiotics should be continued for at least 3 days after the patient is afebrile. However, if the patient continues to have fevers to 38°C or higher in the presence of negative blood cultures, antimicrobial therapy should be continued. A large percentage of febrile patients with neutropenia receiving antibiotics for 7 days develop fungal infections, and empiric treatment with amphotericin B should be considered in this setting. Neutropenic patients with documented fungal or gram-negative bacterial sepsis who have responded poorly to appropriate therapy are candidates for neutrophil transfusions.[488, 489]

Neutropenic patients with normal to increased marrow cellularity, for example, in the setting of AIN, often have a minimal history of pyogenic infection and respond more briskly to appropriate antibiotics. A less aggressive course may be a reasonable approach to a febrile illness in such patients who clinically look well, even if the absolute neutrophil count is below 500 cells/μL. A child in whom the diagnosis of AIN of childhood has been established who develops fever or infection can generally be managed as an outpatient, unless the infection is severe.

An important component in management of all patients with chronic or cyclic neutropenia is close attention to oral hygiene. Chronic gingivitis and periodontitis can be a persistent source of morbidity and result in tooth loss. All patients should receive regular dental care, along with regular use of antibiotic mouthwash.

Therapy directed at increasing the neutrophil count in patients with either intrinsic defects in myelopoiesis or with acquired neutropenia have included the use of corticosteroids and intravenous gamma globulin. These treatments, in general, have been only variably successful. The advent of recombinant G-CSF and of other hematopoietic growth factors has the potential to revolutionize therapy for neutropenias.[490] As discussed in previous sections, G-CSF has been used successfully to increase the neutrophil count in a wide variety of neutropenic conditions, including severe congenital neutropenia, cyclic neutropenia, and immune-mediated neutropenias. In some cases, chronic prophylactic use of G-CSF has been recommended, for example, in severe congenital neutropenia, in which patients have poor marrow production of neutrophils and a high risk of developing serious infection. Several of these latter patients have also developed myelodysplasia or leukemia while on G-CSF[335, 339–341]; how this is related to their underlying disease is still unknown. For other causes of neutropenia in which patients tend to have fewer problems with infection, such as AIN, G-CSF therapy should be reserved for specific clinical indications such as serious or progressive infection.

Neutrophilia

Neutrophilia refers to an alteration in the total number of blood neutrophils that is in excess of about 7500 cells/μL in adults (Table 22–16). During the first few days of life the upper limit of the normal neutrophil count ranges from 7000 to 13,000 cells/μL for neonates born prematurely and at term gestation, respectively.[491] A decrease to adult levels occurs within the first few weeks of life and is maintained thereafter.

An increase in circulating neutrophils is the result of a disturbance of the normal equilibrium involving neutrophil bone marrow production, movement in and out of the marrow compartments into the circulation, and neutrophil destruction (see Table 22–16). Three mechanisms, either alone or in combination, largely

Table 22-16. CLASSIFICATION OF NEUTROPHILIA

Increased Production
Chronic infection
Chronic inflammation
    Ulcerative colitis
    Rheumatoid arthritis
Tumors (perhaps with necrosis)
Postneutropenia rebound
Myeloproliferative disease
Drugs (lithium, occasionally ranitidine)
Chronic idiopathic neutrophilia
Familial cold urticaria
Leukemoid reactions

Enhanced Release from Marrow Storage Pool
Corticosteroids
Stress
Hypoxia
Acute infection
Endotoxin

Decreased Egress from Circulation
Corticosteroids
Splenectomy
Leukocyte adhesion deficiency

Reduced Margination
Stess
Infections
Exercise
Epinephrine

For references, see text.

account for neutrophilia.[16, 492] First, increased numbers of neutrophils may be mobilized from either the bone marrow storage compartment or the peripheral marginating pools into the circulating pool. Second, there may be increased blood neutrophil survival owing to impaired neutrophil egress into tissue. Finally, there may be expansion of the circulating neutrophil pool as a result of (1) increased progenitor cell proliferation and terminal differentiation through the neutrophilic series, (2) increased mitotic activity of neutrophilic cell precursors, or (3) shortening of the cell mitotic cycle in neutrophil precursors.

Acute neutrophilia occurs rapidly within minutes in response to exercise or epinephrine-induced reactions and has been attributed to mobilization of the marginating pool of neutrophils into the circulating pool.[493] It has been postulated that epinephrine stimulates β receptors on endothelial cells to induce the release of cyclic adenosine monophosphate, which affects the adhesive properties of neutrophils and might account for the release of neutrophils from the marginating pool.[494] Slower onset of acute neutrophilia can occur after glucocorticoid administration or with inflammation or infection associated with the generation of endotoxin, TNF, IL-1, and a cascade of growth factors.[1, 2, 495, 496] Maximal response usually occurs within 4 to 24 hours after exposure to these agents and is probably due to the release from the marrow storage compartment of neutrophils into the circulation. The mechanisms that underlie the release of neutrophils from the marrow pool are unknown but may involve neutrophil activation through chemoattractant or cytokine receptors.[187] Glucocorticoids may also slow the egress of neutrophils from the circulation into tissue.[497] Less well understood mechanisms leading to delayed-onset acute neutrophilia have been reported after electric shock trauma, anesthesia, and surgery.[498–500]

Chronic neutrophilia is usually associated with continued stimulation of neutrophil production, possibly through perturbation of marrow feedback mechanisms. Chronic neutrophilia may follow the prolonged administration of glucocorticoids, persistent inflammatory reactions, infection, chronic blood loss, or chronic anxiety.[501–505] Most reactions of this type last for days or weeks, but some may persist for many months. Pyogenic microorganisms, leptospiral infection, and certain viruses (including herpes simplex, varicella, rabies, and poliomyelitis) all may produce neutrophilia.[506] Significant neutrophilic leukocytosis has also been reported with both Kawasaki's disease and infectious mononucleosis.[507, 508] Occasionally, extreme neutrophilia has been observed in tuberculosis, usually in seriously ill patients with widespread necrotizing inflammatory disease.[509] Chronic inflammation is frequently responsible for persistent neutrophilia, especially in patients with juvenile rheumatoid arthritis.[510]

Sustained moderate neutrophilia invariably follows either surgical or functional asplenia.[511] It probably arises because of a failure to remove circulating neutrophils (a normal function of the spleen) rather than from an increase in granulopoiesis.[17] Similarly, neutrophilia has been reported in functional disorders of neutro-

phils associated with impaired adhesion or motility, such as that found in patients with LAD or actin dysfunction (see later).

In the autosomal dominant form of hereditary neutrophilia the patients maintain an absolute granulocyte count between 14,000 and 164,000 cells/μL.[512] These patients have hepatosplenomegaly and increased alkaline phosphatase level along with Gaucher-type histiocytes. Neutrophilia also occurs in familial cold urticaria, in which elevated neutrophil counts, fever, urticaria, and a rash characterized histologically by a neutrophil infiltrate occur beginning about 7 hours after cold exposure.[513, 514]

Leukemoid Reactions

The elevation of the total leukocyte counts to greater than 50×10^3 cells/μL is referred to as a leukemoid reaction. The peripheral blood often has increased numbers of immature myeloid cells, including occasional myeloblasts and promyelocytes. Chronic myelogenous leukemia can be differentiated from a leukemoid reaction by the frequent finding of splenomegaly, a low leukocyte alkaline phosphatase score, and the presence of the Philadelphia chromosome on cytogenetic analysis of bone marrow. Basophil numbers are almost always elevated in chronic myelogenous leukemia and normal in reactive neutrophilia.[505] Juvenile myelogenous leukemia, which presents in the first few years of life, is also generally easily distinguished from a leukemoid reaction by the findings of lymphadenopathy, rash, and thrombocytopenia.

Leukemoid reactions can be triggered by pyogenic infections, especially those secondary to *S. aureus* or *Streptococcus pneumoniae*. Tuberculosis, brucellosis, and toxoplasmosis have also been associated with leukemoid reactions.[515] Leukemoid reactions can also occur in inflammatory syndromes such as acute glomerulonephritis, acute rheumatoid arthritis, liver failure, or diabetic acidosis or after the administration of iron-containing complexes.[505, 516, 517] Tumor or granulomatous infiltration of bone marrow can also result in the appearance of immature myeloid cells in the peripheral circulation, along with teardrop-shaped erythrocytes and nucleated red blood cells (leukoerythroblastic response).

Infants with Down's syndrome may develop a transient myeloid leukemoid reaction that appears to arise from an intrinsic intracellular defect in the regulation of neutrophil proliferation and maturation within the bone marrow.[518] Large numbers of circulating blast cells can be present. Leukemoid reactions have also been identified in neonates in association with decreased numbers of megakaryocytes, thrombocytopenia, and congenital skeletal defects.[519]

Clinical States Associated with Alterations of Eosinophil Numbers

Eosinophilia

Eosinophil stimulation most commonly occurs after repetitive or prolonged antigen exposure, especially when the antigens are deposited in the tissues and elicit hypersensitivity reactions, whether of the immediate (IgE-mediated) or delayed (T lymphocyte–mediated) type. Unlike the case with the neutrophil, stimulation of eosinophilia is T lymphocyte dependent and underlies the immune response to metazoan parasites.[58, 520]

Eosinophils obtained from normal individuals are different from those obtained from patients with eosinophilia.[58, 60, 521] "Resting" eosinophils from patients with eosinophilia and normal eosinophils stimulated *in vitro* both demonstrate a reduced cell surface charge, enhanced transport of glucose into the cell, and an activation of demonstrable acid phosphatase in the specific granules. Also, whereas oxidative metabolism of normal eosinophils is similar to that of normal neutrophils, eosinophils from patients with eosinophilia demonstrate a significant enhancement of oxidative metabolism in both resting cells and cells stimulated during phagocytosis. Thus, eosinophils from patients with eosinophilia appear significantly activated when compared with normal eosinophils. A multilobulated eosinophil nucleus can be seen in patients with eosinophilia.

Allergy is the most common cause of eosinophilia in children in the United States[522] (Table 22–17). Acute allergic reactions may cause leukemoid eosinophilic responses, with eosinophil counts exceeding 20,000 cells/μL, whereas chronic allergy is rarely associated with eosinophil counts of more than 2000 cells/μL.[523] During an immediate hypersensitivity reaction, mast cells and basophils release ECF-A, which is chemotactic for eosinophils[65] and may be related to the observation that tissues rich in mast cells, as those found in the respiratory and gastrointestinal tracts, are particularly common sites for eosinophil tissue invasion. A variety of skin diseases have been associated with eosinophilia,[524, 525] the best documented being atopic dermatitis, eczema, pemphigus, acute urticaria, and toxic epidermal necrolysis. Gastrointestinal disorders also may be associated with eosinophilia,[524] including ulcerative colitis, which usually involves large numbers of tissue eosinophils associated with a slight elevation of blood eosinophils. Crohn's disease during symptomatic phases is usually associated with a slight elevation of the number of blood eosinophils.[526] Both eosinophilic gastroenteritis and milk precipitin disease are associated with a modest elevation of circulating eosinophils.[527] About one third of patients with chronic hepatitis have eosinophilia in excess of 5%. Nearly 40% of patients being treated for intra-abdominal neoplasms exhibit eosinophilia during the first few weeks after initiation of radiation therapy.

Eosinophilia is found in a significant proportion of most of the immunodeficiency syndromes, especially Wiskott-Aldrich syndrome.[527] Approximately 10% of patients with rheumatoid arthritis will develop a mild eosinophilia during the course of their disease. About one third of patients undergoing chronic hemodialysis develop blood eosinophilia without an apparent cause.[528] Similarly, chronic peritoneal dialysis may cause an eosinophilic peritoneal effusion and occasion-

Table 22–17. CAUSES OF EOSINOPHILIA

Allergic Disorders
Asthma
Hay fever
Acute urticaria
Drug reaction
Allergic bronchopulmonary aspergillosis

Dermatitis
Pemphigus
Pemphigoid
Atopic dermatitis

Parasitic and Other Infections
Metazoan infection
Pneumocystis carinii infection
Toxoplasmosis
Amebiasis
Malaria
Scabies
Coccidioidomycosis

Tumors
Brain tumors
Hodgkin's and non-Hodgkin's lymphoma
Myeloproliferative disorders

Hereditary Disorders
Hereditary eosinophilia

Gastrointestinal Disorders
Radiation therapy for intra-abdominal neoplasms
Regional enteriits
Milk precipitin disease
Chronic active hepatitis

Hypereosinophilic Syndromes
Löffler's syndrome
Eosinophilic leukemia
Polyarteritis nodosa

Miscellaneous
Immunodeficiency disorders
Peritoneal dialysis
Thrombocytopenia with absent radius
Familial reticuloendotheliosis
Episodic angioedema associated with
  eosinophilia

ally an elevated number of eosinophils in the blood.[529] Eosinophilia has been described in a significant proportion of patients with congenital heart disease, usually in those types with stenotic lesions.[527] Eosinophilia is also frequently present in the syndromes of thrombocytopenia with absent radii and familial reticuloendotheliosis with eosinophilia. A mild eosinophilia may accompany Hodgkin's disease in 20% of patients; however, on occasion, marked eosinophilia with counts of up to 98% can occur.

In general, fungal diseases do not cause eosinophilia, but one dramatic exception is coccidioidomycosis.[527] Although not an invasive infection, allergic bronchopulmonary aspergillosis may be the most frequent cause of eosinophilia due to a fungal pathogen. In contrast to viral exanthems, scarlet fever is frequently associated with modest degrees of eosinophilia. Eosinophilia is also observed in cytomegalovirus pneumonia of infancy, cat-scratch disease, infectious lymphocytosis, and, occasionally, infectious mononucleosis. Many patients with acute pulmonary tuberculosis show decreased numbers of circulating eosinophils followed by an increase in eosinophil numbers during the convalescent phase.

Outside the United States, parasitic infections are the most common causes of eosinophilia.[530] Infestations by certain parasites, including helminths, induce greater degrees of eosinophilia than do protozoan infestations.[527] Although some parasite antigens appear to be potent immunogens, the eosinophilia resulting from parasitic infection is not due to some unique component of the parasites themselves but rather to a tissue granulomatous response requiring the participation of intact parasites. Other parasites, such as *Giardia lamblia*, *Enterobius vermicularis*, and *Trichuris trichiuria*, fail to elicit an eosinophilic response, probably because they remain localized to the intestinal tract and do not enter the systemic circulation. When parasites invade systemic organs, they may incite clinical symptoms and signs related to the involved organs, such as hepatomegaly and pulmonary infiltrates. These features are further associated with eosinophilic leukocytosis, anemia, and hyperglobulinemia, as are commonly seen in visceral larva migrans from *Toxocara canis*.[531, 532] The patient may be brought for medical attention because of fever, cough, and wheezing. Complications include seizures, encephalitis, myocarditis, retinal lesions (that are often difficult to distinguish from retinoblastoma), and skin nodules on the palms of the hands and soles of the feet. Leukocyte counts may exceed 100,000 cells/μL, with marked eosinophilia persisting from months to years after resolution of symptoms. Polyclonal hypergammaglobulinemia is frequent. Increased anti-A and anti-B titers are commonly observed because of crossed reactivity between red cell and parasitic antigens. No specific therapy is available to eradicate the invading parasites responsible for visceral larva migrans, but the condition generally subsides spontaneously within weeks to months. The broad-spectrum anthelminthic agent thiabendazole may relieve symptoms and shorten convalescence.[533]

An elevated blood eosinophil level has been observed in several families with no specific association of illness or congenital abnormalities noted.[534] This disorder appears to be a benign one in which the normal regulation of eosinophil production is disturbed. Another syndrome associated with eosinophilia is episodic angioedema.[288, 289] Affected patients have recurrent attacks of fever, urticaria, and angioedema with up to approximately 90,000 eosinophils/μL of blood. Symptoms generally respond to corticosteroid therapy.

Hypereosinophilic Syndrome

The term *hypereosinophilic syndrome* (HES) has been used to include a broad continuum of illnesses varying from the self-resolving Löffler's pulmonary syndrome to severe chronic (and ultimately fatal) syndromes. HES is now defined as a persistent eosinophilia in patients with the following criteria: (1) eosinophilia of at least 1500 cells/μL for longer than 6 months (or fatal termination within 6 months), (2) lack of other diagnoses to explain the eosinophilia, and (3) signs and symptoms of organ involvement by infiltrating

eosinophils.[535] HES probably represents a heterogeneous group of disorders, some of which have some resemblance to myeloproliferative states[535-537]; the relationship of HES to "eosinophilic leukemia" has been controversial, but the latter appears to be more appropriately considered a subgroup of acute myeloid leukemia,[536] as discussed later.

The majority of patients with HES are male, with the greatest incidence occurring in the fourth decade of life, although there are rare instances of affected children.[535] The total leukocyte count is typically 10,000 to 30,000 cells/μL, of which 30% to 70% are eosinophils. Leukocyte alkaline phosphatase levels can be normal, decreased, or increased. The bone marrow is usually hypercellular with a predominance of eosinophils. Although dysplastic changes are occasionally seen, expansion of lineages other than eosinophils are rare, as is myelofibrosis. The presence of increased myeloblasts or numerous dysplastic cells suggests an alternative diagnosis, such as acute myelogenous leukemia or a myelodysplastic syndrome. However, chromosomal abnormalities have been reported in some patients with clinical features of HES.[538, 539] Clinical manifestations result from tissue infiltration by eosinophils and the release of eosinophil granule products that cause tissue damage. Symptoms include nonspecific findings of fever, weight loss, and fatigue. Hepatosplenomegaly can be seen. Cardiac damage is the major cause of morbidity and mortality in HES and includes endocardial fibrosis and formation of mural thrombi with infiltrating eosinophils. These findings can also be seen from eosinophilia of multiple other causes, including parasitic infection, drug reactions, or secondary to malignancies. Pulmonary and skin involvement with urticarial or nodular lesions is common. Neuropathies, encephalopathy, and central nervous system thromboemboli can also occur. Corticosteroids are used as first-line therapy for symptomatic patients, and hydroxyurea has been beneficial in those patients who do not respond to corticosteroids.

The underlying causes of HES are unknown and are probably heterogeneous. Elevations in IL-5, considered to be the dominant cytokine in stimulating eosinophil production, have been reported in HES, but also in patients with eosinophilia of other causes.[536] Transgenic mice expressing high IL-5 levels exhibit chronic marked eosinophilia but do not have evidence of cardiac or other organ damage, suggesting that other factors are involved in producing the tissue injury seen in HES.[536]

HES can generally be distinguished from the M4Eo variant of AML, which is characterized by myelomonocytic blasts with eosinophilia and has been referred to in the past as eosinophilic leukemia.[540] In acute leukemia, typically there is a marked increase in the number of immature eosinophils in the blood, marrow or both, tissue infiltration with immature cells of predominantly an eosinophilic type, and secondary anemia and thrombocytopenia. The eosinophils in M4Eo leukemia have an additional granule population that stains with periodic acid–Schiff and chloroacetate esterase that are lacking in normal eosinophils. Almost all patients in the M4Eo leukemia subgroup have abnormalities in chromosome 16.[541]

Eosinopenia

Eosinopenia is not uncommon but is seldom recognized clinically, because its diagnosis requires an absolute eosinophil count.[542] The potential diagnostic usefulness of identifying eosinopenia is rarely appreciated. Because it occurs in relatively limited circumstances, the finding of eosinopenia can be of value clinically. Eosinopenia may be produced by at least two mechanisms: (1) acute stress, with resultant stimulation of adrenocorticoids or release of epinephrine (or both), and (2) acute inflammatory states. The immediate eosinopenia that occurs after administration of glucocorticoids appears to be due to reversible sequestration of eosinophils at an unknown site, presumably in the marginating pool within the vascular compartment. The mechanism underlying this effect is unknown. Acute inflammation is associated with alterations in eosinophil distribution and production that resemble those observed after corticosteroid administration. Thus, there is an initial peripheral sequestration and an initial increase in marrow eosinophils, followed after 36 hours by a decrease in marrow production. At least part of this response occurs independently of adrenocorticoid release. Acute infections associated with marked inflammatory response, including all invasive bacteria and most acute viral infections, are often associated with eosinopenia persisting during the period of the fever. Administration of appropriate antimicrobial therapy is followed by a return of the eosinophil count to normal levels. Persistent infections cause a less predictable eosinophil reaction.

Basophilia and Basophilopenia

Basophilia is commonly associated with hypersensitivity reactions of the immediate type[543] (Table 22–18). Basophil levels may be elevated in ulcerative colitis,

Table 22–18. DISORDERS ASSOCIATED WITH BASOPHILIA AND BASOPHILOPENIA

Basophilia
Hypersensitivity reactions
Drug and food hypersensitivity
Urticaria
Inflammation and infection
Ulcerative colitis
Rheumatoid arthritis
Influenza
Chickenpox
Smallpox
Tuberculosis
Myeloproliferative diseases
Chronic myelogenous leukemia
Myeloid metaplasia
Basophilopenia
Glucocorticoid administration
Thyrotoxicosis

See references 543, 546, 547, 551, and 552.

juvenile rheumatoid arthritis, iron deficiency, and chronic renal failure and after radiation therapy.[544-547] Frequently, basophil levels are increased in the chronic myeloproliferative disorders, particularly chronic myelogenous leukemia. In this disorder, basophils may appear abnormal both morphologically and ultrastructurally. Basophil counts exceeding 30% can occur during the course of chronic myelogenous leukemia; marked basophilia often heralds the terminal phase.[548] Occasionally, patients with chronic myelogenous leukemia may develop circulating basophil counts as high as 40% to 80% of the total leukocyte count at the beginning of the disease. Many of these patients will have developed symptoms attributed to the release of biogenic amines or heparin-like material released from degranulated basophils.[549] Such individuals may benefit from the administration of antihistamines. Increased numbers of marrow basophils may occur in myelodysplastic syndromes and sideroblastic anemia, where it appears to reflect disruption of normal maturational controls.

Basophilopenia occurs in conditions that are associated with eosinophilopenia, such as during acute infection or after the administration of glucocorticoids or epinephrine.[550-552] Also, basophil counts are diminished in thyrotoxicosis and after treatment with thyroid hormones, and, conversely, they may be increased in myxedema.[550]

Monocytosis and Monocytopenia

The average absolute blood monocyte count varies with the age of the patient, and this must be taken into account when assessing monocytosis. During the first 2 weeks of life, the absolute monocyte count is more than 1000 cells/μL.[553] With increasing age there is a gradual decline in the monocyte count until it reaches a plateau of 400 cells/μL in adulthood. *Monocytosis* may therefore be defined as a total monocyte count of more than 500 cells/μL. Given the widespread importance of monocytes, as previously described, it is not surprising that many clinical disorders give rise to monocytosis (Table 22–19). Typically, monocytosis is associated with certain bacterial, protozoal, and rickettsial infections such as subacute bacterial endocarditis, tuberculosis, syphilis, Rocky Mountain spotted fever, and kala-azar.[554] Monocytosis also can be observed in malignant disorders such as preleukemia, acute myelogenous leukemia, chronic myelogenous leukemia, and lymphomas.[554, 555] Approximately 25% of all patients with Hodgkin's disease have monocytosis, although its presence does not correlate with prognosis.[556] Monocytosis has also been noted in a wide variety of inflammatory and immune disorders, including collagen vascular diseases, sarcoidosis, and gastrointestinal disorders such as ulcerative colitis and regional enteritis.[554] Finally, monocytosis occurs in some forms of neutropenia and in postsplenectomy states. As mentioned earlier, patients recovering from myelosuppressive chemotherapy exhibit monocytosis before the return of their neutrophil count to normal.

Monocytopenia has been observed after glucocorti-

Table 22-19. DISORDERS ASSOCIATED WITH MONOCYTOSIS AND MONOCYTOPENIA

Monocytosis
Hematologic disorders and lymphomas
  Preleukemia
  Acute myelogenous leukemia
  Lymphoma (Hodgkin's and non-Hodgkin's)
  Chronic neutropenia
  Histiocytic medullary reticulosis
Collagen vascular disease
  Systemic lupus erythematosus
  Rheumatoid arthritis
  Myositis
Granulomatous diseases
  Ulcerative colitis
  Regional enteritis
  Sarcoidosis
Infection
  Subacute bacterial endocarditis
  Tuberculosis
  Syphilis
  Same protozoal and rickettsial infections (e.g., Rocky Mountain spotted fever, kala-azar)
  Fever of unknown origin
Malignant disease (usually carcinoma)
Miscellaneous disorders
  Postsplenectomy state
  Tetrachlorethane poisoning

Monocytopenia
Glucocorticoid administration
Infections associated with endotoxemia

For review see reference 558, as well as references 554 through 556.

coid administration and in infections associated with endotoxemia.[557, 558] In the latter case, systemic activation of complement occurs with the deposition of C5a on the surface of monocytes, leading to their aggregation and clearance. In contrast to the profound granulocytopenia and lymphopenia associated with irradiation or cytotoxic chemotherapy, noncirculating monocytes and tissue macrophages are relatively resistant to these agents.[559] Monocytopenia is associated with a poor prognosis in aplastic anemia.[559a]

Besides the lysosomal storage diseases, there is one disorder in which an important qualitative abnormality in a specialized tissue macrophage has been described. This is congenital osteopetrosis, an autosomal recessive disease seen in infants and characterized by the progressive obliteration of the bone marrow space by the formation of new bone.[117] The disorder is caused by a failure of the osteoclast to resorb bone matrix. As discussed in a preceding section, human infantile osteopetrosis is associated with normal numbers of dysfunctional osteoclasts and not an absence of M-CSF, as is the case for the *op/op* osteopetrotic mouse. Recombinant INF-γ has been shown to increase bone resorption and improve hematopoietic marrow function in children with congenital osteopetrosis.[122]

DISORDERS OF GRANULOCYTE FUNCTION
Overview

Inherited and acquired clinical disorders have been identified that are caused by abnormalities in one or more steps of phagocyte function and adhesion, chemotaxis, ingestion, degranulation, and oxidative metabolism. Consistent with the critical role of phagocyte function in host defense, patients afflicted with these disorders often suffer from recurrent, difficult-to-treat bacterial and fungal infections. This group of disorders can be classified according to a scheme based on the phagocyte function primarily affected. Some of the disorders manifest abnormalities in several phagocyte functions. In these instances, the primary functional defect is used to classify the disorder.

During the past 25 years, numerous papers have been published that describe abnormalities in phagocyte function, often associated with other diseases. In many of these reports, marginal abnormalities were noted using *in vitro* phagocyte assays, with little evidence that the observed defects were responsible for the clinical predisposition toward infection. In this section, those disorders in which good correlations exist between the phagocyte abnormality and the clinical condition are emphasized. In several of these disorders, particularly LAD and CGD, the molecular basis for the functional abnormality is well understood. Because these conditions serve as prototypes for understanding the less well characterized phagocyte disorders, the underlying biochemical and molecular genetic aspects of these conditions are reviewed in some depth.

One final point should be emphasized at this time. In clinical practice, most physicians encounter a large number of patients who suffer from recurrent bacterial infections. Although it is true that nearly all patients with well-characterized phagocyte abnormalities have recurrent infections, the converse is seldom the case. Most patients with impressive histories of persistent and repeated infections do not have identifiable qualitative or quantitative phagocyte abnormalities. Therefore, the major disorders described below account for only a small fraction of patients with recurrent infections. This point is discussed further in the section describing the laboratory evaluation of phagocyte function.

Disorders of Adhesion
Leukocyte Adhesion Deficiency Type I

Leukocyte adhesion deficiency type I is a rare, autosomal recessive disorder in which phagocyte adhesion, chemotaxis, and ingestion of C3bi-opsonized microbes are impaired owing to mutations in the gene for CD18, the β subunit of the β₂ integrins. As a result, the expression of β₂ integrins on leukocyte cell surfaces is reduced or absent.[178, 560-563] Approximately 70 patients with this disorder have been described in the literature. The hallmark of LAD I is the occurrence of repeated, frequently severe bacterial and fungal infections without the accumulation of pus despite a persistent granulocytosis (Table 22–20). The clinical syndrome is heterogeneous and is related to the severity of the reduction in β₂ integrin expression. A severe clinical phenotype is seen when fewer than 0.3% of the normal amount of β₂ integrins are present, whereas a more moderate

Table 22-20. CLINICAL PRESENTATIONS OF LEUKOCYTE ADHESION DEFICIENCY TYPE I

Chronic Conditions	Acute Infections	Infecting Organisms	Other
Persistent granulocytosis (12,000–100,000 cells/mm³) Gingivitis Periodontitis Stomatitis Impaired wound healing	Omphalitis Cutaneous abscesses and cellulitis (possibly invasive) Perirectal abscesses and cellulitis (possibly invasive) Facial cellulitis Sepsis Pneumonia Laryngotracheitis Peritontitis Necrotizing enterocolitis Sinusitis Esophagitis Erosive gastritis Appendicitis Otitis media	*Staphylococcus aureus* *Escherichia coli* *Pseudomonas aeruginosa* *Pseudomonas* species *Proteus* *Klebsiella* *Candida albicans* *Aspergillus* species Viral (slightly increased risk)	Delayed umbilical cord separation

Each list is arranged in approximate order of frequency based on reviews summarizing various series of patients with leukocyte adhesion deficiency (see text for references).

phenotype is observed with levels of 2.5% to 11% of normal. Patients with the severe form of LAD I, which is more common, generally present in early infancy with omphalitis and delayed separation of the umbilical cord. Skin and perirectal abscesses and cellulitis are common, which often heal poorly. An aggressive form of gingivitis and periodontitis is characteristic, and ulcerative lesions of the tongue and pharynx can be seen. Otitis media and pneumonia are also often encountered. The majority of infections are caused by *S. aureus* and gram-negative enteric bacteria. Fungal infections also occur, particularly those from *Candida albicans* and *Aspergillus* species.

The molecular basis for LAD I was first suggested by Crowley and colleagues,[564] who found that neutrophils from a patient with this clinical syndrome lacked a high-molecular-weight membrane glycoprotein. Because the patient's neutrophils neither adhered to plastic surfaces nor underwent an oxidative burst when exposed to serum-opsonized particles, it was hypothesized that the missing glycoprotein was responsible for both adhesion and cell-particle interactions. A similar glycoprotein was also found to be missing in several other patients,[565, 566] which proved to be the subunit (CD11b) of the Mac-1 β₂ integrin (CD11b/CD18).[567] It was subsequently recognized that the levels of all three leukocyte β₂ integrins, LFA-1, Mac-1 and p150,95 (see Fig. 22–3) were absent or severely deficient in LAD I.[178, 560–562]

Deficient β₂ integrin expression impairs a variety of leukocyte adhesion-dependent activities, with neutrophil function being the most significantly affected.[560–562, 564, 565, 568] One of the striking findings in LAD I is the failure of neutrophils to migrate to sites of inflammation. The initial phases of neutrophil adhesion to the endothelium (see Fig. 22–1), which is mediated by selectins and their sialylated counter-receptors, is normal in LAD. However, because of the absence or marked deficiency in Mac-1 (CD11b/CD18) expression, LAD I neutrophils are neither able to attach firmly to the endothelium nor undergo transendothelial migration.[164, 569] Neutrophil intravascular survival is prolonged,[570] presumably related to deficient adhesion and migration. *In vitro* assays of neutrophil adhesion to glass or to cultured endothelial cells and of neutrophil chemotaxis also exhibit marked abnormalities. An exception to these observations is neutrophil adhesion and emigration in the pulmonary capillary bed, which can be mediated by CD11/CD18-independent mechanisms under some circumstances.[185] In autopsy tissue from a patient with severe LAD I, no neutrophils were observed in infected appendiceal and skin lesions, whereas many neutrophils were seen within the alveolar spaces.[185] In contrast to neutrophils, other leukocytes (monocytes, eosinophils, and lymphocytes) express the β₁ integrin VLA-4 and are able to use this adhesion molecule to emigrate into inflammatory sites throughout the body.[164, 571]

The other major defect in LAD I is the inability of neutrophils and monocytes to recognize microorganisms coated with the opsonic complement fragment C3bi, because Mac-1 is the C3bi receptor.[561, 562, 564, 568, 572] The binding of C3bi normally triggers neutrophil degranulation, phagocytosis, and activation of the respiratory burst, but these responses are diminished or absent in neutrophils from patients with LAD I. Control experiments have consistently demonstrated, however, that these functions are normal in LAD I when neutrophils are activated with opsonins (e.g., IgG, C3b) that have different cell surface receptors or by soluble agonists that bypass Mac-1.[564]

Defects in lymphocyte functions dependent on LFA-1 (CD11a/CD18) have been observed in many LAD I patients *in vitro*. These include proliferative responses to mitogens, natural killer cell function, and lymphocyte-mediated killing.[573–575] Nevertheless, most patients with LAD I manifest few problems related to lymphocyte dysfunction *in vivo*. Cutaneous hypersensitivity reactions are normal, and patients are not unusually susceptible to viral infections.

Molecular Basis

That LAD I involves a deficiency of all three leukocyte CD11/CD18 integrins focused attention on the common β_2 chain (CD18 gene) of this integrin family as the site of the molecular defect. This hypothesis has proved to be correct. Expression of the leukocyte integrin α subunits is normal in LAD I, but these are not transported to the cell surface because the β_2 chain is absent or contains mutations that disrupt β_2 structure or its interaction with the α subunit.[576–579] More than 20 patients with LAD I have now been characterized at the molecular genetic level, and all have mutations in the gene for β_2, which is localized on chromosome 21q22.3. A heterogenous group of mutations has been identified. Many patients are compound heterozygotes for two different mutant alleles, whereas others are homozygous for a single mutant allele. About one half of patients with LAD I with characterized genetic defects have point mutations that result in single amino acid substitutions in CD18, which almost invariably reside between amino acids 111 and 361.[580–587] This protein domain is highly conserved among all β subunits and appears to be important for interaction with the α subunit. In this LAD I subgroup, approximately one half exhibit a low level of CD11/CD18 cell-surface expression and moderate disease, with the remainder having absent expression and the severe phenotype. Messenger RNA splicing abnormalities resulting in either deletion or insertion of amino acids in the conserved extracellular domain of CD18 have also been described in two kindreds.[587, 588] Finally, small deletions within the coding sequences of the CD18 gene disrupting the reading frame[585, 586, 589] or a nucleotide substitution resulting in a premature termination signal[589] have been reported.

There are several animal models of LAD I. These include the occurrence of a severe form of the disease in an Irish setter born of a mother-son mating[590, 591] and in Holstein cattle.[592–594] In the latter case, affected calves could be traced to a common sire and have been shown to be homozygous for a point amino acid substitution in the conserved extracellular domain of CD18.[595] Finally, a CD18-deficient mouse with 2% to 6% of normal β_2 integrin expression has been produced by gene targeting.[596]

Diagnosis and Treatment

The diagnosis of LAD I should be suspected in any infant or child who presents with unusually severe or recurrent infections or with periodontitis accompanied by persistently elevated peripheral blood neutrophil counts. Although this laboratory finding may simply represent a leukemoid reaction in an otherwise immunologically normal infant, the diagnosis of LAD I should nonetheless be considered, particularly if there is a paucity of neutrophils at affected sites or there is a delayed separation of the umbilical cord. The diagnosis of LAD I is established by flow cytometric analysis to assess cell surface expression of any of the three β_2 integrin α (CD11) subunits or the shared CD18 subunit.

Monoclonal antibodies to each are commercially available. Although not necessary to establish the diagnosis of LAD I, *in vitro* functional assays of neutrophils obtained from these patients demonstrate striking defects in adherence, chemotaxis, and C3bi-mediated phagocytosis and respiratory burst activation. Carriers of LAD I can also generally be identified by flow cytometry, because they typically express approximately 50% of the normal level of β_2 integrins on leukocyte cell surfaces.[561, 597] Prenatal diagnosis of LAD I can be made by one of two methods. In those families in which the mutations in the two CD18 alleles are known, chorionic villus or amniocyte DNA can be analyzed for the presence of the mutations. Alternatively, fetal blood granulocytes can be assayed for expression of β_2 integrin expression using flow cytometry.[563, 598]

Treatment of LAD I depends on the clinical severity of the disorder. In patients with the moderate clinical phenotype, who typically have some residual β_2 integrin expression, cutaneous and oral infections should be treated aggressively as they occur. The use of prophylactic trimethoprim-sulfamethoxazole appears to be beneficial. Aggressive prophylactic treatment of periodontal disease is also advisable in the form of frequent dental cleanings and the use of antimicrobial oral rinses such as chlorhexidine gluconate. The clinical management of patients with moderate phenotype should be guided by the observation that these patients are still at risk for dying of overwhelming infection, with 75% succumbing between the ages of 12 and 32 years.[563] Patients with severe LAD I have the even grimmer prognosis of a high incidence of death due to infection before the age of 2 years.[178, 562, 599] Bone marrow transplantation is recommended for these patients if a suitable donor can be found and has been successful in at least six cases.[562, 563, 600]

Because LAD I is caused by a defect in a single gene, transfer of a normal CD18 sequence into a patient's hematopoietic stem cells using retroviral or other vectors could, in principle, correct the defect. Preliminary *in vitro* studies using Epstein-Barr virus–transformed B-lymphocyte cell lines from patients with LAD I and *in vivo* using a mouse system have shown the feasibility of this approach.[576, 601–603] High-level expression of the transferred CD18 sequence may not be necessary to confer substantial clinical benefits, based on the observed milder course of patients with some residual β_2 integrin expression. At present, a major obstacle in applying this approach to clinical use is the development of techniques that achieve high-level gene transfer into human hematopoietic stem cells.[604, 605]

Leukocyte Adhesion Deficiency Type II

A clinical syndrome similar to LAD but associated with defective selectin-mediated adhesion has been reported in two unrelated boys of Moslem Arab origin and has been termed *leukocyte adhesion deficiency type II* (LAD II).[606] Both patients were offspring of consanguineous marriages, suggesting an autosomal recessive inheritance. As in CD11/CD18-deficient LAD, these children suffered from recurrent cellulitis, otitis media, periodontitis, and pneumonia without the formation of pus despite peripheral leukocyte counts of 30,000 to 150,000 cells/μL. However, neutrophils from these patients had normal levels of CD18 and were able to phagocytose C3bi-opsonized particles. Also, in distinction from classic LAD, the two boys had short stature, a distinctive facial appearance, severe mental retardation, and the Bombay (hh) blood phenotype and were secretor negative and Lewis antigen negative.

The underlying basis for LAD II appears to be due to a fundamental defect in fucose metabolism. The Bombay and nonsecretor phenotypes are caused by deficient formation of Fucα1→2 Gal linkages in ABO blood group core antigens, whereas the Lewis antigen-negative phenotype is due to failure to synthesize Fucα1→4 GlcNAc and Fucα1→3 GlcNAc moieties. Neutrophils from both boys were found to lack immunoreactive sialyl-Lewis X structures, which also contain fucose, and were unable to adhere to activated human umbilical cord endothelial cells that expressed E-selectin.[606] Thus, the functional defect in LAD II neutrophils appears to be caused by the absence of neutrophil sialyl-Lewis X structures that serve as selectin counter-receptors.

Other studies on LAD II neutrophils have included the use of intravital microscopy to demonstrate a significant decrease in neutrophil rolling in postcapillary venules *in vivo*,[569] consistent with the role of selectin-mediated adhesion in this process (see Fig. 22–1). Under static conditions, however, chemoattractant-induced tight adhesion and emigration of LAD II neutrophils were observed, both of which were absent in CD18-deficient neutrophils.[569] Despite the peripheral blood neutrophilia, the half-life of circulating neutrophils in an LAD II patient was found to be approximately one half of normal.[607] The explanation of this latter observation is unknown.

Acquired Disorders of Adherence

Neutrophils may exhibit decreased adhesiveness after exposure to a variety of drugs, the most common being corticosteroids and epinephrine.[494, 608, 609] Clinically, the diminished adhesiveness induced by these drugs is manifested by a dramatic rise in the total neutrophil count in the blood as cells from the marginated pool are quickly released into the circulating pool. Although the mechanism by which corticosteroids alter adherence is not known, epinephrine and other β-adrenergic agonists exert their effect indirectly by causing endothelial cells to release cyclic adenosine monophosphate, which in turn impairs the ability of neutrophils to adhere.[494, 610]

The adhesiveness in neutrophils can be dramatically increased in a variety of clinical conditions that have in common the formation of biologically active complement fragments: gram-negative bacterial sepsis, severe thermal injury, pancreatitis, trauma, and exposure of neutrophils to artificial membrane surfaces during hemodialysis and cardiopulmonary bypass.[399, 400, 611–613] In these various conditions, the generation of complement fragments leads to activation of neutrophils and enhanced adhesiveness, possibly owing to enhanced expression of β₂ integrins. Under these conditions, neutrophils undergo increased aggregation with each other and become trapped within capillary beds, such as those in the lungs.[614] It is believed that the aggregated neutrophils then generate toxic oxygen radicals and release proteases that conspire to damage structural protein such as collagen and elastin.[193]

Amphotericin B has been associated with increased neutrophil aggregation, particularly when administered in conjunction with the transfusions of granulocytes that have been harvested by filtration (rather than by centrifugation).[615, 616] It is possible that the enhanced aggregation is medicated by up-regulation of surface β₂ integrins induced both by the amphotericin B and by the filters used to harvest the cells.

Disorders of Chemotaxis

The directed migration into sites of infection and inflammation involves a complex series of events. As reviewed in the beginning of this chapter, the generation of chemotactic signals and their binding to specific receptors on the phagocyte surface leads to the generation of intracellular second messengers. These intracellular signals, in turn, trigger changes in adhesiveness and in the actin cytoskeleton that result in adhesion to the endothelium and chemotaxis into the inflamed tissue site. Given the numerous cellular functions involved in chemotaxis, it is perhaps not surprising that impaired phagocyte chemotaxis has been observed in a large number of clinical conditions.[617] Some of the more important syndromes are listed in Table 22–21. These disorders have been classified according to the mechanisms thought to be responsible for defective chemotaxis, which are related to either abnormalities in the production or inhibition of chemotactic factors or to defects in the phagocyte itself involving adhesiveness and locomotion. In some cases, abnormal chemotaxis is one component of a disorder that involves multiple defects.

In many of the reports describing defective *in vitro* chemotaxis of neutrophils from various clinical conditions, it is not clear whether the increased number of infections observed clinically is due to the observed chemotactic abnormality or to medical complications of the underlying disorder (such as malnutrition or exposure to nosocomial infection). Further complicating the interpretation of these reports is that the *in vitro* assays for chemotaxis are subject to laboratory artifacts and may not accurately reflect the *in vivo* extracellular environment. These limitations apply to the micropore filter method developed by Boyden[618, 619] as well as to the under-agarose technique.[620] The former assay system consists of a chamber with a horizontal filter membrane separating two compartments. The upper compartment contains phagocytes that migrate through the micropore filter in response to chemotactic solutions that fill the lower compartment. The under-agarose assay uses a similar principle in that neutrophils in one agarose well migrate toward a chemoattractant in another. Phagocyte motility *in vivo* can be measured by

Table 22–21. CLINICAL CONDITIONS ASSOCIATED WITH IMPAIRED NEUTROPHIL CHEMOTAXIS

Defect in Generation of Chemotactic Agents
Familial deficiency of C1r, C2, C4
Familial deficiency of C3, C5
Other abnormalities of complement pathways (e.g., systemic lupus erythematosus, immature complement system in neonates, diabetes mellitus, C5 dysfunction, chronic hemodialysis, glomerulonephritis)

Excessive Production of Normal Chemotactic Factor Inactivators
Hodgkin's disease
Cirrhosis of the liver
Sarcoidosis
Lepromatous leprosy

Inhibitors of the Neutrophil Response to Chemotactic Factors
Hyperimmunoglobulin E syndrome
Localized juvenile periodontitis
Immune complex diseases (rheumatoid arthritis)
IgA paraproteinemia states
Solid tumors
Bone marrow transplantation
Drugs (ethanol, antithymocyte globulin)

Deactivation (Down-Regulation) by Increased Levels of Chemotactic Factors
Wiskott-Aldrich syndrome
C5a generation in plasma (hemodialysis)
Bacterial sepsis

Phagocyte Defects
Neutrophil actin dysfunction
Localized juvenile periodontitis
Neonatal neutrophils
Leukocyte adhesion deficiency
Chédiak-Higashi syndrome
Specific granule deficiency

Miscellaneous Defects
Hypophosphatemia
Shwachman's syndrome
Burn patients

---

the skin window technique of Rebuck and Crowley, in which a superficial dermal abrasion is produced in the patient and the appearance of inflammatory cells in the lesion is monitored over a 24-hour period.[621] Because of difficulties in standardizing the dermal lesion, variable results may be obtained with this method. Moreover, the assay can measure only the response of phagocytes to the chemotactic signals generated by this type of sterile injury.

As outlined in Table 22–21, several of the conditions associated with impaired neutrophil chemotaxis are due to complement deficiencies and other immunodeficiency syndromes (e.g., Wiskott-Aldrich syndrome). These disorders are discussed elsewhere in this text. In addition, several disorders of phagocyte function (LAD, CHS, and specific granule deficiency) are reviewed in other sections of this chapter. This section focuses on clinical conditions in which there is evidence that a chemotactic defect plays a major contribution in decreased resistance to bacterial and fungal infections.

Hyperimmunoglobulin E Syndrome

The hyperimmunoglobulin E syndrome (see also Chapter 25) is a relatively rare disorder characterized by markedly elevated serum levels of IgE (often greater than 2000 IU/mL), serious recurrent staphylococcal infections of the skin and lower respiratory tract, pneumatoceles, and chronic pruritic dermatitis.[622–626] The key features of hyper-IgE syndrome are summarized in Table 22–22. Neutrophils from patients with this syndrome exhibit a variable, but at times severe, chemotactic defect.[622, 627–629] This syndrome was originally known as "Job's syndrome" when it was first reported in 1966 in two red-haired, fair-skinned females who had hyperextensible joints and "cold" abscesses that lacked the usual characteristics of inflammation.[623] It is now appreciated that only a small fraction of patients with hyper-IgE syndrome have red hair or hyperextensible joints, and it may be that Job's syndrome is a variant subset of hyper-IgE syndrome. Based on larger series of patients, it is now clear that the disease can occur in both males and females and that other ethnic groups, including blacks and Asians, can be affected. The mode of inheritance has not been firmly established, although familial patterns have suggested autosomal dominant inheritance with incomplete penetrance.[622, 624, 626]

The molecular basis of the hyper-IgE syndrome is unknown. It has been proposed by some investigators that there is an underlying defect in the T lymphocytes[630, 631] that is manifested, at least in part, by the greatly reduced production of IFN-γ and TNF.[632, 633] This putative T-cell defect would then explain the hyperproduction of IgE (perhaps caused by the deficiency of IFN-γ) as well as the abnormal antibody responses that have been documented in some patients in response to various vaccines.[634] This latter abnormality could directly contribute to the enhanced susceptibility of these patients to infection, while the former may reflect an imbalance in the production of various types of immunoglobulin. Patients with hyper-IgE syndrome produce excessive amounts of IgE directed against *S. aureus* at the expense of protective antistaphylococcal IgG.[176, 622] Finally, the recurrent bacterial infections in hyper-IgE syndrome also may be aggravated by the chemotactic defect that is periodically observed in these patients. The underlying T-cell defect also may be responsible for this chemotactic defect by causing the release of chemotactic inhibitors from mononuclear cells.[622, 635, 636]

The clinical manifestations of the hyper-IgE syndrome are often severe and usually become apparent during infancy. Staphylococcal furuncles of the head and neck as well as chronic dermatitis are seen most frequently in younger patients. Recurrent staphylococcal pneumonia is a common problem as patients grow older and can be complicated by the formation of persistent pneumatoceles that can become superinfected with *Haemophilus influenzae*, gram-negative bacteria, or *Aspergillus*.[637] Chronic infections of the ears, sinuses, and eyes (keratoconjunctivitis) are seen in many patients, while septic arthritis and osteomyelitis have been observed in a few individuals. Bone abnormalities are also a common feature of the hyper-IgE syndrome. Osteopenia of unknown etiology is observed in most patients and results in an increased risk of fractures of the long bones and the vertebral bodies.[626] Coarse facial

Table 22-22. SUMMARY OF HYPERIMMUNOGLOBULIN E SYNDROME

Incidence	Approximately 50 cases have been reviewed in the literature; single institution series of 6, 13, and 23 cases have been described
Inheritance	Autosomal (? dominant) with incomplete penetrance
Molecular defect	Unknown; putative T-lymphocyte defect, in part manifested by diminished production of IFN-γ, which affects regulation of IgE production as well as other immune functions
Pathogenesis	The following may contrubute to the increased risk of infection: high levels of antistaphylococcal IgE and low levels of antistaphylococcal IgG; fluctuating neutrophil chemotactic defect possibly due to an inhibitor from mononuclear cells; poor antibody response in some patients
Clinical manifestations	Staphylococcal pneumonia
	Pneumatoceles
	Fungal superinfection of lung cysts
	``Cold'' cutaneous skin abscesses and furuncles
	Chronic eczematoid dermtitis
	Mucocutaneous candidiasis
	Coarse facies, growth retardation, osteopenia
	Sinusitis keratoconjunctivitis
Laboratory evaluation	Serum IgE > 2500 IU/mL
	Peripheral blood eosinophilia
Differential diagnosis	Atopic dermatitis
	Wiskott-Aldrich syndorme, DiGeorge's syndrome
	Hypergammaglobulinemia
	Chronic granulomatous disease
Therapy	Prophylactic antibiotics for *Staphylococcus aureus*
	Aggressive treatment of acute infections with parenteral antibiotics
	Surgical drainage of deep infections and resection of lung cysts
	Plasmapheresis in severe cases (experimental)
	IFN-γ (experimental)
Prognosis	Generally good if managed aggressively; some patients develop lymphoid malignancies

features characterized by a broad nasal bridge and a prominent nose have been noted in a majority of patients. Craniosynostosis can also occur.

The diagnosis of hyper-IgE syndrome should be considered in any child with the aforementioned clinical history. A markedly elevated polyclonal serum IgE and a peripheral blood eosinophilia are constant laboratory findings. Despite the impressive elevations in serum IgE, this laboratory finding alone is not diagnostic, because comparably high serum levels of IgE can be seen in patients with atopic dermatitis.[622] Because many patients with atopic dermatitis suffer from superficial skin infections and eczema, this disorder must be considered in the differential diagnosis of hyper-IgE syndrome. The two can be distinguished from each other because of the severe and recurrent nature of the staphylococcal furuncles and pneumonias seen in patients with hyper-IgE syndrome.

One of the mainstays of therapy for hyper-IgE syndrome is the use of prophylactic antibiotics, such as dicloxacillin or trimethoprim-sulfamethoxazole. These drugs can help prevent staphylococcal infections and should be prescribed at the time of diagnosis. Pneumonias and other deep-seated infections should be treated aggressively with parenteral antibiotics. Patients with hyper-IgE syndrome are unusually predisposed to developing pneumatoceles as a result of staphylococcal lung infections. If these lesions persist, they should be surgically resected to prevent superinfection by fungal and gram-negative organisms. If infections and their complications are managed aggressively, the prognosis for patients with hyper-IgE syndrome is good.

Recombinant human IFN-γ has been proposed as a therapeutic modality for hyper-IgE syndrome based on the observations that this cytokine can suppress IgE synthesis[638, 639] and that IFN-γ production by mononuclear leukocytes from patients with hyper-IgE syndrome is low or absent.[633, 640] In 9 of 13 patients with hyper-IgE syndrome in one report, IgE production by peripheral blood mononuclear cells was inhibited by 67% to 93% *in vitro* in the presence of 10^4 units of IFN-γ/mL.[641] Five of these patients were treated for 2 weeks with IFN-γ (50 μg/m² subcutaneously three times per week), and all were found to have decreased IgE production *in vitro*. In another report, neutrophils from 5 patients with hyper-IgE syndrome exhibited an average threefold increase in chemotaxis after *in vitro* incubation with IFN-γ.[642] Formal clinical trials have not been conducted to test the efficacy of IFN-γ in ameliorating the clinical manifestations of hyper-IgE syndrome. Studies on IFN-γ in the treatment of CGD suggest that this cytokine may reduce the frequency of infections by mechanisms that do not necessarily reverse the underlying defect in respiratory burst oxidase function.[643] IFN-γ may therefore be of general benefit in other immunodeficiencies, such as hyper-IgE syndrome. Finally, several case reports have described dramatic improvements in the eczematous skin lesions of hyper-IgE syndrome using either interferon alfa or high-dose intravenous gamma globulin.[644, 645]

Neutrophil Actin Dysfunction

Primary defects in neutrophil actin polymerization are exceedingly rare. The first such case, described by Boxer and colleagues in 1974, occurred in a male infant who suffered from recurrent skin infections due to *S. aureus* and a cutaneous-cecal fistula complicated by *S.*

faecalis sepsis.[646] Despite a marked neutrophilia, sites of infections were devoid of neutrophils and healed slowly. The patient's neutrophils showed markedly diminished chemotaxis and a decreased capacity to ingest serum-opsonized particles. He underwent a bone marrow transplantation with transient engraftment of normally functioning neutrophils but died of infectious complications. The underlying defect in this patient appeared to involve neutrophil actin or an actin-binding protein. Neutrophils from his parents and a sibling had actin that polymerized *in vitro* half as well as that of control subjects.[647] Neutrophils from family members also had intermediate levels of surface expression of the Mac-1 integrin (CD11b/CD18),[648] raising the question of whether the neutrophil actin dysfunction in the proband was due to a primary defect in the leukocyte β2 integrins and hence represented a subgroup of LAD. However, actin filament assembly has been found to be normal in LAD I patients.[648] Alternatively, a primary actin-associated defect might alter cell surface expression of the integrins, which have binding sites in their cytoplasmic domains for cytoskeletal proteins.[166]

Coates and co-workers have reported a single case of a male infant of Tongan descent who was afflicted with severe skin and mucosal infections.[649] At the age of 2 months, he was found to have hepatosplenomegaly, moderate thrombocytopenia, recurrent pulmonary infiltrates, and a lingual ulcer that grew *C. tropicalis*. Two siblings had previously died in infancy with a similar clinical picture. Neutrophils from this patient, which had normal cell surface expression of CD11b, exhibited abnormalities in a wide range of motile behaviors, including chemotaxis, phagocytosis, and spreading on glass. Morphologically, the neutrophils displayed thin, filamentous projections of membrane with an underlying abnormal cytoskeletal structure. Biochemical studies revealed markedly defective actin polymerization, and a severe deficiency of an 89-kd protein along with a markedly elevated level of a 47-kd protein. Hence, this disorder has been referred to as neutrophil actin dysfunction with 47- and 89-kd protein abnormalities (NAD 47/89). The 47-kd protein has been identified as LSP1 (lymphocyte-specific protein),[650] which is an actin-binding protein present in normal neutrophils. Overexpression of LSP1 has been proposed to result in defective actin polymerization, defective cytoskeletal structure, and motility defects in NAD 47/89 neutrophils. The identity of the 89-kd protein and its relationship to LSP1 is unknown. Neutrophils from the patient's mother and father showed a partial defect in actin polymerization and intermediate abnormalities in the levels of LSP1 and the 89-kd protein. These observations, along with the history of previously affected siblings, suggest that NAD 47/89 is an autosomal recessive disorder. The patient has received an allogeneic bone marrow transplantation at the age of 7 months and no longer suffers from thrombocytopenia or the neutrophil motility disorder.

Localized Juvenile Periodontitis

Localized juvenile periodontitis (LJP) is a disorder of unknown etiology characterized by severe alveolar bone loss localized to the first molars and incisors, with an onset around the time of puberty.[651–655] Defective neutrophil chemotaxis has been identified *in vitro* in approximately 70% of patients with LJP.[651, 653, 656–662] The observation that not all patients with LJP exhibit abnormal chemotaxis may be due to the intrinsic variability in *in vitro* chemotaxis assays (see earlier) or to a fundamental heterogeneity in this disorder. Some support for the latter comes from studies showing that the spectrum of neutrophil defects may vary from patient to patient. For example, whereas most individuals with LJP showed defective chemotaxis in response to both formyl peptides and C5a,[651, 657, 659] others may show an abnormality only with formyl peptides.[658] Further support for the heterogeneity of LJP is provided by studies showing that factors elaborated by periodontopathic bacteria may secondarily alter leukocyte function and depress chemotaxis (e.g., *Capnocytophaga* species, *Actinobacillus actinomycetemcomitans*, and *Bacteroides* species).[599, 663, 664] Whether these factors are the same as the chemotactic inhibitors identified in the sera from some patients with LJP remains to be determined.[659, 660] In one report, the serum chemotaxis inhibitor from 18 patients with LJP was partially neutralized by antibodies to TNF and IL-1.[660] In the subset of patients with LJP who have abnormal chemotaxis, phagocytosis has generally been found to be abnormal, whereas degranulation (of specific granules) and superoxide generation have been found to be normal.[657]

Based on the aforementioned considerations, it appears that LJP is a heterogeneous group of disorders. In the subset with a chemotactic defect, evidence exists that at least some of these patients may have an intrinsic, inherited neutrophil defect. A 40% to 50% decrease in the total number of receptors for formyl peptides and C5a has been reported for some patients with LJP.[651, 658] The cloning of the normal human neutrophil receptors for formyl peptides, C5a, and IL-8[665–669] will permit the putative receptor defector defects in LJP to be examined at the molecular level. The observations that LJP tends to cluster in families and that the neutrophil chemotactic activity is not restored *in vitro* or after the patient is treated for periodontal infection also lend support to the hypothesis that certain patients with LJP may have an inherited disorder in chemotactic receptor function.

The diagnosis of LJP should be suspected in any adolescent in whom there is unusually severe and destructive alveolar bone loss involving the first molars and incisors. From a diagnostic point of view, it is important to bear in mind that many qualitative and quantitative neutrophil disorders are associated with periodontal disease that, at times, may be severe.[655] The differential diagnosis should include LAD, CGD, CHS, leukemia, chronic neutropenia, and cyclic neutropenia.

Neonatal Neutrophils

Although most infants are able to defend themselves successfully against microbial challenges, they are nonetheless at increased risk for development of severe bacterial infections—particularly sepsis, pneumonia, and meningitis caused by group B streptococci.[670] The risk of infection and the rate of mortality from pyogenic infections are even greater in premature infants. As a result, phagocyte function in neonates has been the subject of intense investigation for many years.[670, 671] It is generally agreed that neonates have defects in various aspects of specific immunity (immune cellular cytotoxic mechanisms and cytokine generation) as well as nonspecific (phagocyte-mediated) immunity. In the second category, defects in neutrophil adherence, chemotaxis, phagocytosis, and bacterial killing all have been reported.[671] Compounding these functional defects in neonates is a deficiency of antibodies directed against organisms that typically infect infants. Furthermore, neonates can easily exhaust bone marrow reserves of granulocytes and develop neutropenia in the midst of severe pyogenic infections, as discussed in the previous section.

It appears that the most important of the functional defects, at least from a clinical point of view, is the depressed chemotactic ability of neonatal neutrophils that itself appears to be due to a combination of factors. Compared with adult cells, the directed migration of neonatal neutrophils toward a variety of chemotactic agents (C5a, formyl peptides, and bacterial extracts) is reduced by approximately 50% for the first several weeks of life.[671–675] The biochemical basis for the diminished chemotaxis does not appear to be related to abnormalities in the number or affinity of either the C5a or formyl peptide receptor.[671, 674] Instead, there appears to be a defect in the chemotaxis-induced up-regulation of cell adhesion molecules. Baseline expression of the two subunits of the β_2 integrin Mac-1 (CD11b and CD18) was found to be normal in neonatal neutrophils but failed to increase normally after exposure to chemotactic concentrations of C5a and formyl peptides.[676, 677] Fetal, preterm, and term infant neutrophils expressed levels of Mac-1 in stimulated neutrophils that were only 40% to 60% of those seen in adult cells. This defect, in turn, appears to be due to diminished fusion of neutrophil granules with the plasma membrane after stimulation. Because the specific granule membranes serve as an intracellular pool for Mac-1 (see Table 22–3), abnormal mobilization of these granule populations could explain the diminished up-regulation of Mac-1 seen in neonatal cells after stimulation. Another underlying biochemical defect that may contribute to the chemotaxis defect is a diminished polymerization of F-actin in neonatal neutrophils after stimulation.[678] Finally, Hill[671] has found that neonatal neutrophils fail to increase the intracellular concentration of free calcium to normal levels in response to chemotactic factors. It is possible that this signal transduction defect could be responsible for both the diminished levels of Mac-1 up-regulation and the F-actin polymerization.

Other Disorders of Neutrophil Chemotaxis

A new syndrome of severe neutrophil dysfunction, characterized by a selective abnormality in chemoat-

tractant-induced neutrophil functions, has been reported by Roos and co-workers.[679] The patient, a female, was the first child of nonconsanguineous healthy parents, both originating from India, who suffered from chronic omphalitis and otitis media secondary to *S. aureus*, buccal candidiasis, and an internal cecal fistulation that ultimately led to death from gram-negative sepsis at 8 months of age. The peripheral neutrophil counts were markedly elevated, and leukocyte β_2 integrin expression was normal. Neutrophils from the patient were defective in chemoattractant-induced chemotaxis, actin polymerization, exocytosis of azurophilic granules, and superoxide generation. However, actin polymerization and superoxide generation in response to other stimuli were normal, as were adherence and phagocytosis of serum-opsonized particles. Stimulation of patient neutrophils with formyl-methionyl-leucyl-phenylalanine induced a normal increase in free intracellular calcium but a decreased formation of diglycerides. Actin polymerization in T cells was normal in response to the chemokine. Hence, the patient appeared to have a selective defect in signaling through neutrophil chemoattractant receptors that affects multiple neutrophil functions.

A study of 240 patients with a significant history of recurrent infection, generally requiring at least one hospitalization, identified 10 patients, all children, with a consistent marked reduction in chemotactic activity *in vitro* that was not associated with any other neutrophil abnormalities.[680] In 6 of these patients, a partial reduction in chemotactic activity was also seen in either the mother or a sibling. However, other than for the disorders discussed earlier, well-defined clinical entities in which defective neutrophil chemotaxis plays a predominant role in impaired host resistance to bacteria and fungi have not been established or the underlying mechanisms identified. In part, this is related to the difficulties in performing and interpreting *in vitro* assays of adhesion and chemotaxis except in specialized research settings. Biochemical approaches to delineating a specific abnormality are also difficult owing to the complex nature of the chemotactic response.

Disorders of Opsonization and Ingestion

Clinical disorders of recognition fall into two major categories: humoral and cellular. In the former, plasma-derived opsonins are deficient or absent and result in incomplete opsonization. In contrast, the cellular disorders are characterized by defective receptors for opsonins or by abnormalities in the actin cytoskeletal system responsible for microbial ingestion.

Humoral Disorders of Opsonization

Primary B cell deficiencies result in the decreased or absent production of immunoglobulins, most commonly IgG. Patients afflicted with these antibody-deficiency syndromes suffer from recurrent infections with pyogenic bacteria such as *S. aureus*, pneumococci, and *H. influenzae*. One of the major functional abnormalities in these disorders is the defective opsonization of pathogenic microorganisms. As a result, these microbes are not efficiently cleared by the host phagocytic system. A variety of clinical disorders may lead to an antibody deficiency; these are discussed elsewhere in this text.

Complement deficiencies can also result in recurrent infections, particularly when they involve those factors shared by both the classic and the alternative pathways. Therefore, patients with deficiencies of C1, C2, or C4 have relatively minor problems with infections, because the alternative pathway remains intact. In the case of C3, on the other hand, recurrent infections are much more common, because this is the protein that is the direct precursor of two major complement opsonins—C3b and C3bi. Two forms of C3 deficiency have been described, and both are rare. In one, a congenital deficiency of C3 is inherited in an autosomal recessive manner.[681-684] Heterozygotes contain half the normal levels of C3 but do not suffer from infections. In at least one case, the molecular genetic basis of the C3 deficiency has been identified.[682] The patient had an unusual RNA splicing abnormality that resulted in a 61-bp deletion in exon 18, with a premature stop codon 17 bp downstream from the abnormal splice site (the C3 gene is located on human chromosome 19 and consists of 41 exons that span approximately 41 kb. As a result of this splice mutation, the patient had no detectable levels of C3. A second type of C3 deficiency is caused by unchecked catabolism of C3 due to the absence of a C3 protease inhibitor.[685] In both types of C3 deficiencies, the majority of patients suffer from recurrent pyogenic infections caused by encapsulated bacteria such as pneumococci. Patients with deficiencies of the terminal complement components (C5, C6, C7, C8, or C9) are particularly susceptible to infections with meningococci or gonococci. Infections in complement-deficient individuals should be treated with the aggressive use of antibiotics, and immunization against *H. influenzae*, *S. pneumoniae*, and *Neisseria meningitidis* may be helpful.

Approximately 5% of the population have low serum levels of mannose binding protein (MBP), a serum lectin secreted by the liver that binds mannose sugars present on the surface of bacteria, fungi, and some viruses.[686] Bound MBP activates the complement cascade, and hence functions as an opsonin of broad specificity. The incidence of MBP deficiency is higher in infants with frequent unexplained infections, chronic diarrhea, and otitis media; and it has been proposed that MBP is an important defense mechanism during the time period when maternal antibody levels have waned yet the antibody repertoire of the infant is still immature.[686] MBP deficiency is associated with autosomal dominant inheritance of point mutations in a collagen-like domain of the MBP polypeptide.[687-689] These mutations appear to interfere with the normal polymerization of MBP subunits to form an oligomeric structure required for complement activation. Clinical illness associated with MBP deficiency may not be limited to infants. In one report, MBP deficiency was the only identifiable immune defect in four adults with recurrent infections as well as in one patient who also had IgA deficiency.[690] The spectrum of illness included recurrent skin abscesses, chronic cryptosporidial diarrhea, meningococcal meningitis with recurrent herpes simplex, and fatal *Klebsiella* pneumonia. Three of the five adults were homozygotes for mutant MBP alleles.

Cellular Disorders of Ingestion

Patients with LAD I show a marked abnormality in phagocytosis of C3bi-opsonized particles, because the Mac-1 β_2 integrin (CD11b/CD18) that is deficient in LAD I functions as the C3bi receptor (see Table 22–7 and Fig. 22–3). Patients with neutrophil actin dysfunction also show abnormal ingestion, because actin assembly plays a critical role in the formation of phagosomes.

A deficiency of FcγRIA has been described in four members of a Dutch family.[691] The monocytes from the affected family members did not bind IgG with high affinity. Interestingly, these individuals did not show an increased susceptibility to infection despite this receptor deficiency. The incidence is 4 in 3377 in the French population for the complete absence of FcγRIIIB, and neutrophils from affected individuals type as NA-null.[692] None of these individuals exhibit any increased incidence of infection, although infants of women with the NA-null phenotype can develop alloimmune neutropenia due to placental transmission of anti-FcγRIIIB antibodies. Similar findings were also reported in a study of 21 individuals from 14 families with FcγRIIIB deficiency in the Netherlands.[693] Three of the women who had multiple pregnancies lacked antineutrophil antibodies, suggesting that neonatal alloimmune neutropenia does not always develop in this setting. Complete absence of FcγRIIIB was found in all kindreds studied.[693] Marked deficiency in neutrophil FcγRIIIB has also been observed in patients with paroxysmal nocturnal hemoglobinuria,[694] an acquired stem cell disorder caused by a defect in the biosynthesis of GPI membrane anchors. Because neutrophil FcγRIIIB is linked to the plasma membrane by means of a GPI anchor,[695] this receptor is unable to insert in the cell membranes in patients with paroxysmal nocturnal hemoglobinuria. Decay-accelerating factor and acetylcholinesterase are also deficient in the membranes of patients with paroxysmal nocturnal hemoglobinuria, because these two proteins are also anchored by GPI moieties.[214] Neutrophils from patients with paroxysmal nocturnal hemoglobinuria undergo a normal oxidative burst in response to IgG-coated latex particles.[695] Thus, there appears to be sufficient redundancy in the function of Fc and complement receptors to permit normal phagocytic function in these cases of FcγRI and FcγRIIIB deficiencies.

There are two allelic polymorphisms in FcγRIIA and in FcγRIIIB that may each contribute to a subtle defect in the host response to encapsulated microorganisms, particularly in individuals with terminal complement deficiencies.[696] Patients who are homozygous for both the FcγRIIA allele with an arginine at position 131 and the FcγRIIIB*NA2 allele also appear to be at higher risk for meningococcal meningitis.

Disorders of Degranulation

Phagocytes can kill microorganisms using a variety of cytotoxic compounds, as reviewed earlier in this chapter. These include a host of preformed antimicrobial polypeptides that are stored within intracellular granules and released into the phagocytic vacuole on phagocytosis. The importance of granule contents in host defense is attested to by two clinical syndromes associated with disorders of degranulation: Chédiak-Higashi syndrome and specific granule deficiency.

Chédiak-Higashi Syndrome

The Chédiak-Higashi syndrome is a rare, multiorgan disease characterized by partial oculocutaneous albinism, frequent bacterial infections, giant lysosomes in granulocytes, and (in many patients) a mild bleeding diathesis as well as peripheral and cranial neuropathies associated with decussation defects at the optic chiasm[370-373] (Table 22–23). Ten types of oculocutaneous albinism have been described in humans, and CHS is one of the tyrosinase-positive forms that has been designated as type VIB.[370]

Patients with CHS have defects in lysosomes or lysosome-like organelles in a variety of tissues. In melanocytes, giant melanosomes prevent the even distribution of melanin, which results in hypopigmentation of the hair, skin, iris, and ocular fundus.[370] Giant granules are also seen in Schwann cells, leukocytes, and certain cells in the liver, spleen, pancreas, gastric mucosa, kidney, adrenal gland, and pituitary gland.[370] Approximately 200 CHS cases have been reported. Based on careful histopathologic studies in humans[697-699] and in animals with a homologous type of disorder (Aleutian mink, beige mice, blue foxes, cats, killer whales, and Hereford cattle[370, 371, 700]), it appears that CHS is caused by a fundamental defect in granule morphogenesis that results in abnormally large granules in multiple tissues. The most extensively studied of the affected cells are the neutrophils. In the early stages of myelopoiesis, some of the normal-size azurophil granules coalesce to form giant granules that later fuse with some of the specific granules to form huge secondary lysosomes that contain constituents of both granule types.[701-704] In addition to this uncontrolled fusion of granules, CHS neutrophils are markedly deficient in neutral proteases,[705] including two azurophil granule enzymes: cathepsin G and elastase.[706] Some evidence suggests that the genetic defect may affect fundamental biochemical properties of the membrane or microtubules. Elevated levels of cyclic adenosine monophosphate, disordered assembly of microtubules, defective interaction of microtubules with lysosomal membranes, and increased fluidity of CHS neutrophil membranes have been observed and provide support for this view.[707-713] A gene locus termed *bg* for the granule defect in beige mice has been identified and mapped to the proximal end of mouse chromosome 13, which is syntenic with human chromosome 1q.[714] This is consistent with the well-documented autosomal recessive pattern of inheritance observed in humans with CHS as well as the high incidence of consanguinity in these families. Recently, it has been learned that a regulatory gene called LYST appears to be mutated in CHS and its murine counterpart, beige.[714a]

Some of the most dramatic examples of the lysosome defect in CHS are manifested in the various blood cells and are summarized in Table 22–24. As discussed previously, a few to a large majority of circulating neutrophils contain giant coalesced azurophil-specific granules. These giant granules are often more prominent in the bone marrow than in the peripheral blood, because many of the abnormal myeloid precursors are destroyed before they ever leave the marrow. Extensive

Table 22–23. SUMMARY OF CHÉDIAK-HIGASHI SYNDROME

Incidence	Approximately 200 cases described
Inheritance	Autosomal recessive
Molecular defect	A putative defect in granule morphogenesis resulting in abnormally large granules in multiple tissues
Pathogenesis	Giant coalesced azurophil/specific granules in neutrophils resulting in ineffective granulopoiesis and neutropenia, delayed and incomplete degranulation, and defective chemotaxis
Clinical manifestations	Partial oculocutaneous albinism
	Recurrent severe bacterial infections (usually *Staphylococcus aureus*)
	Gingivitis and periodontitis
	Cranial and peripheral neuropathies (muscle weakness, ataxia, sensory loss, nystagmus)
	Hepatosplenomegaly and complications of pancytopenia in the accelerated phase
Laboratory evaluation	Giant granules in peripheral blood granulocytes and in bone marrow myeloid progenitor cells
	Widespread lymphohistiocytic infiltrates in accelerated phase
Prenatal diagnosis	Demonstration of giant granules in fetal blood neutrophils or cultured amniotic cells. Detection methods for carrier state have not been reported.
Differential diagnosis	Other genetic forms of oculocutaneous albinism
	Giant granules can be seen in acute and chronic myelogenous leukemias
Therapy	Prophylactic trimethoprim-sulfamethoxazole
	Parenteral antibiotics for acute infections
	Ascorbic acid (200 mg/d for infants; 6 g/d for adults)
	Bone marrow transplantation before or at beginning of accelerated phase
Prognosis	Most patients die of infection or complications of the accelerated phase during the first or second decade of life. A few patients have survived into their thirties.

Table 22-24. HEMATOLOGIC MANIFESTATIONS OF CHÉDIAK-HIGASHI SYNDROME

Stable Phase
Neutrophils
1. Giant, coalesced azurophil/specific granules
2. Vacuolization of marrow neutrophils (ineffective myelopoiesis)
3. Neutropenia (intramedullary destruction)
4. Decreased bactericidal activity
   a. Decreased chemotaxis *in vivo* and *in vitro*
   b. Delayed and incomplete degranulation
Monocytes/Macrophages
1. Ring-shaped lysosomes
2. Decreased chemotaxis
Lymphocytes/Natural Killer (NK) Cells
1. Giant cytoplasmic granules
2. Diminished NK function
3. Diminished antibody-dependent cell-mediated cytolysis of tumor cells
Platelets
1. Giant cytoplasmic granules may be seen
2. Normal platelet count
3. Increased bleeding time due to abnormal aggregation caused by storage pool deficiency of adenosine diphosphate and serotonin

Accelerated Phase
1. Hepatosplenomegaly
2. Bone marrow infiltration
3. Hemophagocytosis by histiocytes
4. Worsening neutropenia, thrombocytopenia, and anemia due to 1, 2, and 3

myeloid cell vacuolization, enhanced marrow cellularity, and elevated levels of serum lysozyme all reflect this process of intramedullary granulocyte destruction.[715] As a result, most patients with CHS have a moderate neutropenia, with absolute neutrophil counts ranging between 500 and 2000 cells/mm[3].[372, 373] Monocytes are also affected in CHS and have similar, but not identical, cytoplasmic inclusions that appear to be ring-shaped lysosomes.[716] Lymphocytes can also contain giant cytoplasmic granules that may contribute to abnormalities in specific immunity (see later). Finally, CHS platelets have a decreased number of dense granules and a storage pool deficiency of adenosine diphosphate and serotonin.[717–720] This abnormality leads to a defect in platelet aggregation and an increased bleeding time, manifested clinically as easy bruising, intestinal bleeding, and epistaxis. Most patients with CHS do not have thrombocytopenia until they enter the accelerated phase of the disease (see later).

The infections usually encountered with CHS involve the skin, respiratory tract, and mucous membranes and are caused by both gram-positive and gram-negative bacteria as well as by fungi. The most common organism is *S. aureus*. These infections are often recurrent and may result in death at any time. Gingivitis and periodontitis are common. The skin is also susceptible to severe sunburns, and photosensitivity in bright light is common.

The phagocytes are primarily responsible for the propensity to infection. In addition to the moderate neutropenia, several defects in neutrophil function lead to impaired bactericidal activity. First, chemotaxis is markedly depressed, whether measured *in vivo* by the Rebuck skin window or *in vitro* by the method of Boyden.[372, 721] The large granules appear to interfere with the ability of neutrophils to travel through narrow passages, such as those between endothelial cells. Second, degranulation is delayed and incomplete in CHS neutrophils.[711, 722–724] Third, the marked deficiency of antimicrobial proteins such as cathepsin G probably contributes to the diminished bactericidal potency of CHS neutrophils.[711] Finally, decreased expression of Mac-1 (CD11b/CD18) in CHS neutrophils may also play a role.[725]

Contributing to the enhanced susceptibility to infection are abnormalities in monocytes, lymphocytes, and natural killer cells. Monocytes, such as neutrophils, exhibit decreased chemotaxis.[219] Peripheral blood CHS lymphocytes demonstrate diminished antibody-dependent cellular cytotoxicity of tumor cells.[726] Perhaps most important, natural killer cell function is profoundly abnormal in CHS.[726–731] This defect not only contributes to the recurrent infection problem but also may be involved in the development of the accelerated phase of CHS.

Those patients who survive the infectious and neurologic problems of the stable phase of CHS have a high risk of progressing to the accelerated phase of the disease.[373] This transition generally occurs during the first or second decade of life.[373, 697] The accelerated phase is characterized pathologically by a diffuse lymphohistiocytic infiltration of the liver, spleen, lymph nodes, and bone marrow. This infiltration is not lymphomatous or neoplastic by histopathologic criteria, although the outcome for the patient is uniformly fatal.[697] The accelerated phase is heralded by hepatosplenomegaly, bone marrow infiltration, and hemophagocytosis, which leads to a worsening of the neutropenia and an ever-increasing risk of infection. Thrombocytopenia likewise develops and intensifies the bleeding disorder already present in the platelets.

The diagnosis of CHS should be suspected in any child who presents with one or more of the following findings: (1) recurrent bacterial infections of unknown etiology; (2) hypopigmentation of the hair, skin, and eyes; (3) the presence of giant peroxidase-positive lysosomal granules in granulocytes from peripheral blood or bone marrow; (4) easy bruising or nasal hemorrhage despite a normal platelet count; and (5) unexplained hepatosplenomegaly (associated with the accelerated phase of the disease). CHS is usually manifested in infancy or early childhood but may present later when the child is in the accelerated phase of the disease. In some patients, the disease may be suspected on the basis of neurologic abnormalities, which include ataxia, muscle weakness, decreased deep tendon reflexes, sensory loss, a diffusely abnormal electroencephalogram, and abnormal visual and auditory evoked potentials indicative of optic and otic neuronal tract misrooting.[732, 733] The physician should not be dissuaded from considering the diagnosis of CHS if the patient does not show clear-cut oculocutaneous albinism. Depending on the skin coloration in the family, the only manifestations of the albinism may be a metallic sheen in the hair (which can vary from blond to dark brown) and a lighter skin color than that seen in siblings. In younger patients, a cartwheel distribution of pigment in the iris and an abnormal red reflex is likely.

The diagnosis of CHS is made on the basis of giant lysosomal granules found in blood or bone marrow myeloid cells. In some cases, relatively few abnormal granulocytes are seen in the peripheral blood, presumably because of extensive intramedullary destruction of myeloid precursors. In these cases, a bone marrow aspirate may be necessary to identify the large lysosomes. Microscopic examination of the hair reveals giant melanin granules. An affected fetus with CHS diagnosed by fetal blood sampling, which showed large abnormal granules in neutrophils, was also found to have significantly larger than normal acid phosphatase lysosomes in cultured amniotic and chorionic villus cells.[734] This suggests that prenatal diagnosis of CHS might be accomplished using the latter techniques, which is less risky than fetal blood sampling. At present, the carrier state in CHS cannot be reliably diagnosed. In the accelerated phase, biopsy specimens of the liver, spleen, and lymph nodes reveal diffuse infiltrates of lymphohistiocytic cells. The differential diagnosis for CHS includes other genetic forms of partial albinism.[370] Giant granules resembling those seen in CHS can be seen in both acute and chronic myelogenous leukemias[735-737] and should not be confused with those seen in CHS.

The management of the stable phase of CHS primarily involves treatment of infectious complications. Prophylactic trimethoprim-sulfamethoxazole may be beneficial. Infections should be treated vigorously with appropriate intravenous antibiotics. Treatment with high doses of ascorbic acid (20 mg/kg per day) has been reported to cause clinical improvement as well as improved function of neutrophils in vitro (neutrophil chemotaxis or bactericidal function).[710, 738] Although in the literature some disagreement exists regarding the efficacy of ascorbic acid,[739] it would seem prudent to try this medication in all patients, given its safety in moderate doses. Natural killer cell function appears to remain abnormal even after ascorbate therapy.

The treatment of the accelerated phase is extremely difficult and is usually modeled after treatment used for other forms of lymphoid malignancy. Vincristine and corticosteroids have been effective in inducing temporary remissions.[373, 697, 715] The only curative therapy is bone marrow transplantation.[323, 740–743] This procedure is ideally performed before the onset of the accelerated phase. Five of the six patients with CHS who have received bone marrow transplantation were free of disease and still alive at the time of this report. It is possible that the accelerated phase of CHS can be prevented or delayed by vaccines against Epstein-Barr virus.[219] It has been hypothesized that the accelerated phase may be triggered by the inability of patients with CHS to control this virus.[697, 744]

Specific Granule Deficiency

Specific granule deficiency is an extremely rare congenital disorder of neutrophil function characterized by recurrent bacterial infections and multiple abnormalities in neutrophil structure and composition.[745] Despite its rarity, specific granule deficiency is an important part of the differential diagnosis in patients with suspected phagocyte immunodeficiencies. Moreover, the disorder provides important insights into the functional roles of lactoferrin, vitamin B_{12}–binding protein, and other specific granule constituents in phagocyte-mediated host defense. Five patients have been reported with specific granule deficiency: a 13-year-old girl (age at the time of the latest report),[746, 747] a 29-year-old man,[706, 748–754] a 15-year-old boy,[706, 755–758] a 5-year-old girl,[326] and a 43-year-old man[759] (who may have had an acquired form of specific granule deficiency, based on his age at the time of diagnosis). The occurrence of this disorder in both males and females, the parental consanguinity in one case,[756, 757] and the death due to severe infection in a female sibling of one of the male patients[756] all suggest that this disorder is inherited in an autosomal recessive manner.

The key features of specific granule deficiency are summarized in Table 22–25. Clinically, patients with this disorder suffer from indolent, smoldering cutaneous infections punctuated by episodes (sometimes prolonged) of severe infections involving the lungs, ears, lymph nodes, and the deeper structures of the skin. Lung abscesses and mastoiditis have been reported as complications of these infections. S. aureus, P. aeruginosa, Proteus species, other enteric gram-negative bacteria, and C. albicans appear to be the major pathogens. Further complicating the clinical course in some of the patients is the presence of neutropenia that is either intermittent and mild[746, 748] or prolonged and severe.[326]

The clinical picture of specific granule deficiency is consistent with the functional defects identified in patient neutrophils. A marked abnormality in chemotaxis is observed both in vivo by the Rebuck skin window technique and in vitro in the Boyden chamber assay.[746, 748, 749, 757] The indolent nature of some infections in specific granule deficiency may be attributable to this chemotactic defect. In vitro measurements of neutrophil killing of E. coli and S. aureus show a moderate impairment despite the presence of a normal respiratory burst.[746–749, 757, 759] Patient neutrophils adhere normally to plastic surfaces[747, 757] but exhibit slightly diminished sticking to nylon fibers and endothelial cells.[749] Degranulation of both azurophil and (to the extent that they are present) specific granules also appears to be normal.[747, 749, 757]

The molecular defect responsible for specific granule deficiency has not been identified nor has the possibility of genetic heterogeneity in this disorder been ruled out. At least three cellular compartments are affected by the underlying defect or defects: nucleus, specific granules, and azurophil granules. Approximately half or more of the peripheral blood neutrophils in specific granule deficiency have nuclei that resemble those seen in the Pelger-Huët anomaly. The nucleus has a kidney-shaped, bilobed configuration that is flawed by a series of microlobulations and clefts apparent by electron microscopy.[748, 749, 757] As the name of the disorder indicates, neutrophils from these patients show a severe defi-

Table 22-25. SUMMARY OF NEUTROPHIL-SPECIFIC GRANULE DEFICIENCY

Incidence	Five cases reported
Inheritance	Autosomal recessive
Molecular defect	Although the precise defect is unknown, protein deficiencies in azurophil granules (defensins), specific granules (lactoferrin, vitamin B_{12}-binding protein, gelatinase), and secretory vesicles (alkaline phosphatase) suggest a common defect in the regulation of the production of these proteins in myeloid cells. Eosinophil-specific granules are also deficient in protein contents.
Pathogenesis	Recurrent infections result from the combined effect of deficiencies in microbicidal granule protein (e.g., defensins and lactoferrin) and abnormal chemotaxis, perhaps due to a failure to up-regulate surface β_2 integrins and chemotactic peptide receptors from granule stores
Clinical manifestations	Recurrent (sometimes indolent) pyogenic infections of the skin, ears, lungs, and lymph nodes that may have diminished neutrophil infiltration; onset usually during infancy
Laboratory evaluation	Absent or empty specific granules or vesicles in neutrophils by electron microscopy (by light microscopy, granules appear absent) Bilobed nuclei resembling the Pelger-Huët anomaly frequently seen in neutrophils Severe deficiency of neutrophil lactoferrin, vitamin B_{12}-binding protein, defensins, and alkaline phosphatase (by histochemical assay)
Differential diagnosis	Acquired specific granule deficiency (e.g., thermal burns or myeloproliferative syndromes)
Therapy	Prophylactic antibiotics Parenteral antibiotics for acute infections Surgical drainage or resection of refractory infections
Prognosis	With appropriate medical management, patients can survive into their adult years.

ciency in normal specific granules.[748, 749] On a Wright-stained specimen of peripheral blood, neutrophils appear to be devoid of the pink-staining specific granules. By electron microscopic analysis, however, it is apparent that the specific granules are not actually absent but are instead present as empty, elongated vesicles that retain their characteristic trilamellar membrane structure and positive staining for complex carbohydrates.[748,750,752,756] Biochemical measurements of specific granule contents parallel the morphologic studies. Lactoferrin, vitamin B_{12}–binding protein, and gelatinase[760] are present at levels that are only 3% to 10% of normal.[747, 749, 757] Thus, there appears to be an abortive and incomplete formation of normal specific granules.

Azurophil granules in this disorder are also strikingly abnormal. Although they contain a normal (if not slightly elevated) amount of myeloperoxidase and are present in normal numbers, they are severely deficient in defensins.[706] A severe deficiency of alkaline phosphatase activity is also evident in peripheral blood neutrophils, as determined by standard histochemical techniques employing naphthol AS phosphate as substrate.[746, 748, 757] This enzyme activity is localized to secretory vesicles, and its deficiency probably represents yet another organelle abnormality in this disorder.[752] Finally, granule formation also appears to be abnormal in eosinophils. These cells are deficient in three eosinophil-specific granule proteins (eosinophil cationic protein, major basic protein, and eosinophil-derived neurotoxin), although the corresponding mRNA transcripts are present.[761]

In view of the multiple deficits in granule matrix contents, it seems unlikely that the underlying defect involves a mutation in an individual specific granule protein. Instead, studies suggest that there may be an abnormality in the transcriptional regulation of a series of granule (and probably nongranule) proteins.[755] Lomax and colleagues[755] have shown that lactoferrin mRNA was of normal size but was greatly diminished in abundance in the nucleated marrow cells from one patient with specific granule deficiency. In contrast, the levels of lactoferrin and its transcript were normal in nasal glandular epithelia in the same patient.[755] It is possible, therefore, that there is a defect in a myeloid-specific, *trans*-acting factor that controls transcription of a group of genes whose products are necessary for normal neutrophil function. In this regard, it is interesting that the syndrome of specific granule deficiency also involves a severe deficiency of defensins. Defensins, in contrast to other azurophilic granule proteins that are synthesized at the promyelocyte stage, are produced during the subsequent myelocyte stage, along with the specific granule matrix proteins.

The molecular defects previously described can explain, at least in part, the observed clinical problems in specific granule deficiency. The markedly abnormal specific granules and secretory vesicles, which contain intracellular stores of both β_2 integrins[762–764] and a chemotactic peptide receptor,[765] fail to support normal up-regulation of these two types of receptors[754, 757] and may thereby contribute to the chemotactic defect. Furthermore, the severe deficiency of key bactericidal proteins such as lactoferrin and the defensins renders the cell less efficient in killing bacteria. Neutropenia, when it does occur, also impairs host defense and appears to be caused by intramedullary destruction of the abnormal neutrophils, as evidenced by their ingestion by marrow macrophages.[756]

The diagnosis of specific granule deficiency can be made by light microscopic examination of Wright-stained peripheral blood neutrophils. Electron microscopic studies can confirm the presence of empty specific granule vesicles. Bilobed nuclei and greatly diminished levels of alkaline phosphatase by histochemical analysis also support the diagnosis. In conjunction with these morphologic studies, biochemical and immunologic measurements of lactoferrin, vitamin B_{12}–binding protein, and defensins can be made. As discussed previously, all three of these granule proteins are severely deficient in this disorder. Acquired specific granule deficiency is observed in myeloproliferative syndromes and after thermal burns.[745, 766] In these acquired disorders, however, at least a few intact specific granules are still observed microscopically, and the deficiencies of the various granule enzymes are less profound. As with other neutrophil disorders, prophylactic antibiotics appear to be beneficial, based on anecdotal experience. Parenteral antibiotics should be used aggressively for acute infections. With appropriate medical management, patients can survive into their adult years. Malignant transformation of the dysmorphic myeloid cells in this disorder has not been reported.

Disorders of Oxidative Metabolism

The elimination of many pathogens requires oxygen-derived microbicidal compounds that are generated by the phagocyte respiratory burst pathway in response to inflammatory stimuli (see Fig. 22–5). Five clinically significant defects have been identified in this series of reactions. These include deficiencies in NADPH oxidase (reaction 1 in Fig. 22–5), glucose-6-phosphate dehydrogenase (G6PD, reaction 8), myeloperoxidase (reaction 4), glutathione reductase (reaction 7), and glutathione synthetase (reaction 9).

Chronic Granulomatous Disease

Chronic granulomatous disease is an inherited disorder of phagocyte function in which the generation of superoxide by the respiratory burst oxidase (see Fig. 22–6) in neutrophils, monocytes, macrophages, and eosinophils is absent or markedly deficient.[241, 243–245] The disorder is relatively rare, occurring with an incidence of approximately 1 in 500,000 individuals,[246] and is due to mutations in any one of four essential subunits of the respiratory burst oxidase complex (see Tables 22–8 and 22–9). Although originally described as an X-linked recessive disorder affecting boys,[767–771] approximately 40% of CGD is inherited as an autosomal recessive trait[772, 773] (Table 22–26). In more than 90% of patients, superoxide production by activated phagocytes is undetectable. A respiratory burst of 1% to 10% of normal is observed in the remaining patients, who are often referred to as having "variant" CGD.[241, 772, 774–776] Other aspects of phagocyte function are normal in CGD, including adherence, ingestion, and degranulation.[777–779]

Clinical Manifestations

The distinctive clinical syndrome of CGD provides clear evidence for the importance of the phagocyte respiratory burst in host defense and the inflammatory response.[246, 780–787] Patients suffer from recurrent, often severe purulent bacterial and fungal infections, which can be caused by organisms not ordinarily considered pathogens. The other hallmark of this disorder is the propensity to develop chronic inflammatory granulomas that can be of widespread tissue distribution. The majority of patients with CGD manifest symptoms within the first year of life,[785] although some may remain relatively symptom free until later in childhood or even adult life.[788–792]

Table 22–27 summarizes the types of infections and infecting organisms most frequently encountered in CGD.[782, 783, 785–787, 793–795] The major sites of infection are those that come into contact with the external environment—lungs, skin, gastrointestinal tract (including the liver, which can often develop abscesses), and the lymph nodes that drain these organs. The most common pathogens include *S. aureus, Aspergillus* species (most often *A. fumigatus* but occasionally *A. nidulans*),[795] and a variety of gram-negative bacilli, including *Serratia marcescens* and various *Salmonella* species. Of particular note is that *P. cepacia* has been increasingly identified as a potentially lethal pathogen in CGD.[788, 796–798] In many cases, no organism can be identified despite extensive culturing. In these cases, it is important to look carefully for the presence of unusual

Table 22–26. CLASSIFICATION OF CHRONIC GRANULOMATOUS DISEASE

Component Affected	Inheritance	Subtype*	Cytochrome *b* Spectrum	Nitroblue Tetrazolium Test Score (% Positive)	Frequency (% of Cases)	Immunoblot Levels†				Activity in Cell-Free System	
						gp91	*p22*	*p47*	*p67*	*Membrane*	*Cytosol*
gp91*phox*	X	X91⁰	0	0	57	0	0–trace	N	N	0	N
		X91⁻	Low	80–100 (weak)	3	Low	Low	N	N	Trace	N
		X91⁺	0	0	2	N	N	N	N	0	N
p22*phox*	A	A22⁰	0	0	5	0	0	N	N	0	N
		A22⁺	N	0	1	N	N			0	N
p47*phox*	A	A47⁰	N	0	27	N	N	0	N	N	0
p67*phox*	A	A67⁰	N	0	5	N	N	N	0	N	0

*In this nomenclature, the first letter represents the mode of inheritance (X-linked (X) or autosomal recessive (A)), and the number indicates the *phox* component that is genetically affected. The superscript symbols indicate whether the level of protein of the affected component is undectable(⁰), diminished (⁻), or normal (⁺) as measured by immunoblot analysis.
†Defined by immunoblotting with component-specific antibodies.
N, normal level of protein; 0, undetectable level of protein activity.
Adapted from Curnutte JT: Molecular basis of the autosomal recessive forms of chronic granulomatous disease. Immunodef Rev 1992; 3:149; see also references 772, 773, and 881.

Table 22–27. INFECTIONS IN CHRONIC GRANULOMATOUS DISEASE

Infections	Infections (%)	Infecting Organisms	Isolates (%)
Pneumonia	70–80	*Staphylococcus aureus*	30–50
Lymphadenitis*	60–80	*Aspergillus* species	10–20
Cutaneous infections/impetigo*	60–70	*Escherichia coli*	5–10
Hepatic/perihepatic abscesses*	30–40	*Klebsiella* species	5–10
Osteomyelitis	20–30	*Salmonella* species	5–10
Perirectal abscesses/fistulae*	15–30	*Pseudomonas cepacia* and *P. aeruginosa*	5–10
Septicemia	10–20	*Serratia marcescens*	5–10
Otitis media*	≈20	*Staphylococcus epidermidis*	5
Conjunctivitis	≈15	*Streptococcus* species	4
Enteric infections	≈10	*Enterobacter* species	3
Urinary tract infections/pyelonephritis	5–15	*Proteus* species	3
Sinusitis	<10	*Candida albicans*	3
Renal/perinephric abscesses	<10	*Nocardia* species	2
Brain abscesses	<5	*Haemophilus influenzae*	1
Pericarditis	<5	*Pneumocystis carinii*	<1
Meningitis	<5	*Mycobacterium fortuitum*	<1
		Chromobacterium violaceum	<1
		Francisella philomiragia	<1
		Torulopsis glabrata	<1

*Those infections most frequently seen at the time of presentation.
The relative frequencies of different types of infections in CGD are estimated from data pooled from several large series of patients in the United States, Europe, and Japan. See text for references. These series encompass approximately 550 patients with CGD after accounting for overlap between reports. The list of infecting organisms is also arranged according to the data in these reports and is not paired with the entries in the first column.

microbes that can occasionally cause serious infections in CGD[789, 795, 799–806] (see Table 22–27).

Pneumonia is most frequently caused by *S. aureus*, *Aspergillus* species, and enteric bacteria. It is common for an organism not to be identified even in lung biopsy specimens. Complications of pneumonia include empyema or lung abscess. Suppurative lymphadenitis, usually involving the cervical nodes, is especially common in younger patients and is typically caused by *S. aureus* and enteric bacilli such as *Serratia* and *Klebsiella*. Staphylococcal skin infections are also common. Hepatic and perihepatic abscesses, usually caused by *S. aureus*, are surprisingly frequent and should suggest the diagnosis of CGD if it has not already been made.[807, 808] Bone infections can be particularly problematic in CGD and arise either from direct spread of infections from contiguous sites or from hematogenous spread from more distant locations.[809, 810] The former type of osteomyelitis is usually seen in ribs and vertebral bodies as a result of invasion by pulmonary *Aspergillus*.[809] The latter type is more frequently seen in peripheral long and small bones and is typically caused by *Serratia marcescens*, *Nocardia* species, and *S. aureus*.[809] Perirectal infections are extremely difficult to treat in CGD and can lead to fistula formation.[807] Other important, but less commonly seen, infections in CGD are summarized in Table 22–27.

It has long been recognized that patients with CGD are particularly susceptible to organisms that contain catalase, which prevents the CGD phagocyte from scavenging microbial-generated H_2O_2 for phagosomal killing.[811] Another possible link among the organisms with increased virulence in CGD is that they are resistant to nonoxidative killing mechanisms of the phagocyte mediated by antibiotic proteins contained within the various granule compartments.[220, 812–814]

Chronic conditions associated with CGD are responsible for many of the major complications seen with this disorder and are summarized in Table 22–28. These include the formation of granulomas, which are believed to reflect a chronic inflammatory response to inadequate phagocyte killing or digestion. These lesions contain a mixture of lymphocytes and inflammatory macrophages, some of which may have a foamy lipoid cytoplasm that has a characteristic yellow-brown color. Although not pathognomonic of CGD, the pres-

Table 22–28. CHRONIC CONDITIONS ASSOCIATED WITH CHRONIC GRANULOMATOUS DISEASE

Condition	Cases (%)
Lymphadenopathy	98
Hypergammaglobulinemia	60–90
Hepatomegaly	50–90
Splenomegaly	60–80
Anemia of chronic disease	Common
Underweight	70
Chronic diarrhea	20–60
Short stature	50
Gingivitis	50
Dermatitis	35
Hydronephrosis	10–25
Ulcerative stomatitis	5–15
Pulmonary fibrosis	<10
Esophagitis	<10
Gastric antral narrowing	<10
Granulomatous ileocolitis	<10
Granulomatous cystitis	<10
Chorioretinitis	<10
Glomerulonephritis	<10
Discoid lupus erythematosus	<10

The relative frequencies of the chronic conditions associated with CGD were estimated from the series of reports listed in Table 22–27. See also reference 910.

ence of such macrophages in granulomas or other tissue sites should suggest the diagnosis of CGD.[767, 770, 771, 815] Granuloma formation can lead to obstructive symptoms in the upper gastrointestinal tract, including gastric outlet obstruction that can be confused clinically with pyloric stenosis.[807, 816–818] A chronic ileocolitis syndrome resembling Crohn's disease is seen in 5% to 10% of patients and can lead to a debilitating syndrome of diarrhea and malabsorption.[819, 820] Chronic inflammatory lesions have been identified in the urinary bladder walls of some patients and can cause a chronic cystitis that can present as dysuria, penile pain, and decreased urine volume.[821–824] In one study of 60 patients with CGD, 11 cases of granulomatous inflammation of the bladder wall lesions, ureters, or urethra were reported, accompanied by stricture formation in the latter two sites.[825] Hydronephrosis can occur as a complication of obstruction.

Other chronic inflammatory complications of CGD include lymphadenopathy, hepatosplenomegaly, and an eczematoid dermatitis,[783, 785, 826] along with hypergammaglobulinemia, anemia of chronic disease, and short stature (see Table 22–28). Gingivitis and ulcerative stomatitis may occur.[827] Chorioretinitis[828, 829] and destructive white matter lesions in the brain also have been described.[830, 831] Glomerulonephritis due to immune complex deposition has been reported.[832] Rarely, patients may develop either discoid or systemic lupus erythematosus[833–836] or juvenile rheumatoid arthritis.[837]

The severity and pattern of complications of CGD is heterogeneous, which may partly reflect the heterogeneity of molecular defects (see later) and whether any residual respiratory burst oxidase function is present. However, a severe clinical course can be seen in patients in the latter "variant" category that is indistinguishable from what is observed in patients with complete absence of phagocyte superoxide production.[776, 838] On the other hand, some individuals with undetectable levels of respiratory burst activity experience relatively few symptoms and have intervals of years between severe infections.

Heterozygous carriers of the CGD trait are generally asymptomatic except for two important exceptions. Carriers of the autosomal recessive forms of CGD have a normal phagocyte respiratory burst and are free from infection. Carriers of X-linked CGD, on the other had, typically have two populations of circulating neutrophils and monocytes—some with normal respiratory burst activity and others with none[839–845]—due to random X chromosome inactivation.[846, 847] In most X-linked carriers, these two populations are approximately equal in number, but occasionally individuals have an unusually small percentage of either abnormal or normal cells. If the percentage of functioning cells is less than 10, the carrier may suffer from some of the infectious complications of CGD.[776, 790, 839, 848] The other major clinical problem occasionally seen in female carriers of X-linked CGD is discoid lupus erythematosus. In a 1991 review of the literature,[835] 22 cases were summarized from 11 reports. Clinically, the carriers had discoid-like skin lesions (13 of 22 patients), photosensitivity (13 patients), and recurrent apthous stomatitis (12

patients). In a few, polyarthritis, arthralgia, and Raynaud's phenomenon were also observed. Serologic testing for lupus was generally negative, as were immunofluorescence studies of sampled lesions. Interestingly, all the reported cases were carriers of X-linked CGD. Discoid lupus–like lesions have also been reported in 5 patients with autosomal recessive CGD.[833, 834, 849] Because the lupus skin lesions do not appear to develop unless there is at least a subpopulation of nonfunctioning phagocytes, it has been hypothesized that autoantibodies to antigens from incompletely destroyed microbes may be responsible for the syndrome.[835]

Molecular Basis

Classification of CGD is according to the respiratory burst oxidase subunit that is affected (see Table 22–26). Nomenclature has also been adopted for an abbreviated designation within each major genetic subgroup and includes the mode of inheritance and level of *phox* protein expression. The genes or corresponding complementary DNAs of all four subunits have been cloned and their chromosomal locations mapped (see Table 22–8).[250, 850–852] In two large studies of 140 pedigrees in the United States and Europe, defects in the X-linked gene for the gp91*phox* subunit of cytochrome-*b* accounted for approximately 62% of cases, with the remainder due to autosomal recessive inheritance of defects in p47*phox* (27%), p67*phox* (5%), and p22*phox* (6%).[773, 782] However, deficiency of p47*phox* has been reported to account for only 7% of CGD in Japan.[853]

Mutations in Cytochrome-*b*. More than a decade ago, it was reported that neutrophils obtained from the majority of patients with CGD lacked a low-potential cytochrome-*b*.[854–856] This finding focused attention on the role of this cytochrome in the respiratory burst. It is known that the phagocyte cytochrome-*b* is composed of two subunits and contains both flavin and heme groups that mediate the transfer of electrons from NADPH to molecular oxygen to generate superoxide.[243, 244] The cytochrome has two subunits, a 91-kd glycoprotein, gp91*phox*, which is the site of mutations in X-linked CGD, and a 22-kd polypeptide, p22*phox*, which is defective in a rare subgroup of patients with autosomal recessive inheritance of CGD. Formation of the gp91*phox*/p22*phox* heterodimer appears to be important to stabilize each subunit within the phagocyte, and absent expression of both subunits is typically seen in both forms of cytochrome-negative CGD.[857–859]

The gene encoding gp91*phox* was mapped to Xp21.1 by its linkage to the X-linked form of CGD[860] and was the first human gene to be cloned on the basis of its chromosomal location,[250] an approach often referred to as "positional cloning" or "reverse genetics." The gp91*phox* gene contains 13 exons and spans approximately 30 kb in the Xp21.1 region of the X chromosome.[250, 860, 861] Mechanisms that regulate the phagocyte-specific transcription of this gene include a repressor protein, CCAAT displacement protein (CDP), that binds to multiple sites upstream of the transcription start site in nonphagocytic or undifferentiated myeloid cells.[861] However, other regulatory elements appear to be located relatively long distances from the coding portion of gp91[phox].[861, 862]

Defects in the gene for gp91[phox] in X-linked CGD have proved to be very heterogeneous[243, 250, 792, 848, 860, 863–874] and, with few exceptions, are associated with absence of both the cytochrome heterodimer (X91°) and respiratory burst activity. Identification of the specific mutation in gp91[phox] has now been reported in more than 40 patients with X-linked CGD. In general, each mutation is unique to a given kindred, although a few have been seen in several unrelated pedigrees.[244] Up to 20% of X-linked CGD is caused by new germ line mutations. A small percentage of patients with X-linked CGD express a small amount of residual cytochrome-b (X91[-]) associated with low levels of superoxide production. In addition, individuals have been reported who have normal levels of a dysfunctional cytochrome-b (X91[+]).[243, 257, 792, 869, 874–876]

Relatively large deletions in Xp21.1 involving gp91[phox] and adjacent loci have been described in a few rare patients.[250, 860, 863–866] These individuals have complex phenotypes that include CGD and McLeod's syndrome (a mild hemolytic anemia associated with depressed levels of Kell antigens due to defects in the red cell antigen Kx), with or without concomitant Duchenne muscular dystrophy and retinitis pigmentosa. Partial deletions of gp91[phox] have also been reported.[244, 877]

The majority of patients with X-linked CGD have mutations limited to only one or several nucleotides, so that the gp91[phox] appears grossly intact by Southern blot hybridization. These include missense mutations resulting in nonconservative amino acid substitutions, mutations of mRNA splicing sites, point deletions or insertions that disrupt the reading frame, and nonsense mutations that create a premature stop codon. Amino acid substitutions or in frame insertions or deletions are generally associated with markedly reduced or absent expression of the gp91[phox] protein.[579] Some of the mutations that result in normal levels of a dysfunctional cytochrome have involved gp91[phox] domains that appear to either participate in oxidase assembly[876, 878] or are involved in its redox function.[242, 243, 875, 879]

Mutations affecting the regulation of gp91[phox] transcription are rare and have been identified in two unusual phenotypes. In one type, described in two unrelated kindreds, affected males have two distinct populations of phagocytic cells.[838] One subset has normal respiratory burst activity and accounts for 5% to 15% of circulating phagocytes and myeloid progenitor cells, whereas the other subset, accounting for the remainder of the cells, entirely lacks a respiratory burst. Affected males had a severe clinical course.[838] Sequencing of the gp91[phox] gene identified a point mutation in the promoter sequence that was located 57 bp upstream of the normal transcription initiation site in one kindred and 54 bp upstream in the other.[880] These mutations were both associated with the inability of an as yet uncharacterized DNA-binding protein to interact with this region of the promoter.[880] These observations suggest that gp91[phox] expression is dependent on this region of the promoter in all but a subset of neutrophils. Another patient with X-linked CGD has been reported who had normal levels of gp91[phox] expression and function in circulating eosinophils, but whose neutrophils, monocytes, and B lymphocytes had markedly reduced levels of gp91[phox].[872] The molecular basis of this phenotype has not yet been determined but is likely to involve abnormal regulation of gp91[phox] transcription.

Mutations in the gene for the p22[phox] subunit of cytochrome β are an uncommon cause of autosomal recessive CGD (see Table 22–26). This locus has been mapped to chromosome 16q24 and contains 6 exons that span 8.5 kb.[850] The genetic defects that have been identified in this cytochrome subunit are also heterogeneous and range from a large interstitial gene deletion[850] to point mutations associated with missense, frameshift, or RNA splicing defects.[850, 868, 881] The majority of patients are the offspring of consanguineous marriages. A single amino acid substitution (Pro→Glu) in a cytoplasmic domain of p22[phox] has been reported that is associated with normal levels of cytochrome-b and a dysfunctional oxidase (A22[+] CGD).[881] This mutation disrupts a proline-rich sequence in p22[phox] that normally interacts with an *src* homology domain 3 (SH3) in p47[phox] during assembly of the active oxidase complex.[258, 259, 882] SH3 motifs, first described in the *src* tyrosine kinase family, mediate protein-protein interactions by binding to proline-rich sequences in target proteins.[883, 884] The proline substitution in p22[phox] is the second example of a genetic disease caused by disruption of protein-protein interactions mediated by means of SH3 domains. A kindred with X-linked agammaglobulinemia due to deletion of the SH3 region of Bruton's tyrosine kinase has also been reported.[885]

Mutations in Cytosolic Factors. One of the key discoveries in unraveling the molecular basis of the different genetic subgroups in CGD was the observation that both the plasma membrane and cytosol were required to reconstitute a catalytically active oxidase in a cell-free assay.[886–889] Complementation analysis using this assay identified two different subgroups of CGD in which the defect involved a cytosolic protein rather than the membrane-bound cytochrome-b.[890, 891] Mutations in the gene encoding the cytosolic phosphoprotein *neutrophil cytosolic factor 1* (p47[phox]) account for approximately one fourth of all cases of CGD, whereas inherited defects in the gene for neutrophil cytosolic factor 2 (p67[phox]) account for a small subgroup of autosomal recessive CGD (see Table 22–26). In both of these two subgroups, the genetic defects result in absence of detectable protein. The function of p47[phox] and p67[phox] in the respiratory burst oxidase is not well understood but is believed to involve activation of the electron transport function of cytochrome-b.

p47[phox] resides on chromosome 7[892] and contains 9 exons spanning 18 kb.[893] In contrast to other forms of CGD, the majority of cases of p47[phox]-deficient CGD are due to a single type of mutation, a GT deletion at the beginning of exon 2 that results in a frameshift and premature translational termination.[893, 894] The majority of patients appear to be homozygous for this mutation without any history of consanguinity, although a few compound heterozygotes have been described with a missense mutation accompanying the GT deletion. The high frequency of the GT deletion mutation now appears to be because humans have at least one highly conserved pseudogene for p47[phox] that contains the GT deletion.[895] Recombination events between the authentic p47[phox] and its pseudogene or pseudogenes result in the creation of a mutant p47[phox] allele containing the GT deletion.[896]

p67[phox], which has been mapped to the long arm of chromosome 1,[897] spans 37 kb and contains 16 exons.[898] Mutations identified in p67[phox]-deficient CGD have included missense mutations[868] and splice junction mutations affecting mRNA processing.[899]

Diagnosis

A diagnosis of CGD is suggested by the characteristic clinical features (see Tables 22–27 and 22–28) or by a family history of the disease. Because the severity and onset of the disease can vary considerably among different patients, CGD should still be considered in adolescents and adults who present with an unusual site of infection or organism typical of CGD (see Table 22–27). The diagnosis of CGD is established by demonstrating an absent or greatly diminished neutrophil respiratory burst.

Many different methods have been used to monitor respiratory burst activity.[900] These include assays using probes that exhibit either chemiluminescence or fluorescence when superoxide is released from activated phagocytes.[842, 843] However, one of the simplest and most accurate techniques is the nitroblue tetrazolium (NBT) test, in which neutrophils are stimulated to undergo a respiratory burst in the presence of NBT.[840, 841, 901, 902] When reduced by electrons donated from superoxide, the water-soluble, yellow tetrazolium dye is converted into deep blue, insoluble formazan deposits that precipitate on any cell that undergoes a respiratory burst. NBT reduction can be evaluated quantitatively using cells in suspension[902] or, preferably, by examination of neutrophils and monocytes that have adhered to a microscope slide (the NBT slide test).[840, 841] As shown in the NBT slide test in Figure 22–8, a striking difference is evident between resting neutrophils and monocytes (panel A) and those that have been stimulated (panel B), particularly if a strong respiratory burst agonist is used, such as phorbol myristate acetate

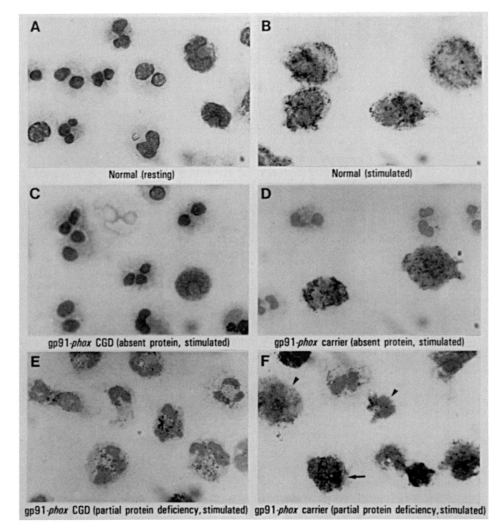

Figure 22-8. Evaluation of chronic granulomatous disease (CGD) using the nitroblue tetrazolium (NBT) test. Photomicrographs are shown of NBT tests performed on normal cells (at rest and after phorbol myristate acetate (PMA) stimulation) and on PMA-stimulated cells from X91° and X91⁻ CGD patients and their mothers (who are carriers). Dense formazan crystals are seen in all the normal phagocytes after stimulation (B) but are absent from resting cells (A). The CGD patients are seen to have homogeneous populations of cells that either do not respond (X91° (C)) or respond only minimally (X91⁻ (E)) to PMA. In contrast, the NBT tests on the CGD carriers show heterogeneous populations of cells that respond either normally or in a fashion similar to that of the abnormal cells from their offspring (D and F). In the case of the maternal carrier shown in F, the cells with normal deposits of formazan (arrow) are intermixed with cells containing minimal amounts of formazan (arrowheads) identical to those seen in her affected male child (E). (Reprinted from Smith RM, Curnutte JT: Molecular basis of chronic granulomatous disease. Blood 1991; 77:681.)

Normal (resting)

Normal (stimulated)

gp91-*phox* CGD (absent protein, stimulated)

gp91-*phox* carrier (absent protein, stimulated)

gp91-*phox* CGD (partial protein deficiency, stimulated) gp91-*phox* carrier (partial protein deficiency, stimulated)

(PMA). Cells from patients with X91°, A22°, A47°, and A67 fail to stain with NBT (an X91° patient is shown in C), whereas patients with variant forms of the disease show light staining of all their neutrophils and monocytes (an X91$^-$ patient is shown in E). The NBT slide test is also very useful in diagnosing the carrier states of either X91° or X91$^-$ CGD, because a mixed population of NBT-positive and NBT-negative (or NBT-weakly stained) cells is observed (see Figs. 22–8D and F). Failure to detect a mixed population of formazan-staining cells does not necessarily rule out the X-linked carrier state, because nonrandom inactivation of cells with the mutant X chromosome can occur by chance. A normal maternal NBT test may also indicate that there has been a *de novo* mutation in the germ line of a parent[892] or that the patient has one of the autosomal recessive forms of CGD. Intermediate levels of NBT reduction are not seen in phagocytes of autosomal recessive carriers.

With the exception of classic X-linked disease in a male, determining the specific oxidase gene affected in a given CGD patient (see Table 22–26) requires techniques at present available only in research laboratories. These include immunoblot analysis of neutrophil extracts, cytochrome-*b* spectroscopy, and functional analysis of membrane and cytosol fractions in the cell-free oxidase assay. In a male with absent cytochrome-*b* without clear evidence for a maternal carrier, it is necessary to search for the mutation in both gp91*^{phox}* and p22*^{phox}* by DNA sequencing or another method of analysis.

Identification of the specific genetic subgroup for a patient is useful primarily for purposes of genetic counseling and prenatal diagnosis, although it may also become increasingly important when successful approaches to somatic gene therapy are developed. In cases of suspected X-linked CGD, further analysis is not necessary if the fetus is first determined to be a 46,XX female. Fetal blood sampling and NBT slide test analysis of fetal neutrophils can be used for prenatal diagnosis of CGD.[903–906] However, even when the blood sample is successfully obtained, a low number of neutrophils adherent to the slide or contamination of the sample by maternal blood can complicate the interpretation of this test. DNA analysis of amniotic fluid cells or chorionic villus biopsy is an option for earlier prenatal diagnosis of CGD. Restriction fragment length polymorphisms have been identified for gp91*^{phox}*[867, 907, 908] and p67*^{phox}*,[909] and they can be useful for diagnosis in informative families. The most specific approach to prenatal diagnosis is to first determine the family-specific mutation or mutations and then analyze fetal DNA for the presence of the mutant alleles using polymerase chain reaction–based technology.[910] These latter techniques are presently available only in a few specialized research laboratories.

Prognosis and Treatment

The prognosis for patients afflicted with CGD has continued to improve since the disorder was first described in the 1950s, at which time almost all patients died in childhood.[769–771] In one retrospective review of 38 patients followed between 1964 and 1989, actuarial analysis showed 50% survival through the third decade of life.[780] In another retrospective study of 48 patients followed between 1969 and 1985 in Paris, the actuarial survival rate was 50% at 10 years of age, with a prolonged plateau thereafter.[786] Further refinements in treatment, coupled with the introduction of IFN-γ therapy, appear to have further improved the prognosis. Although no recent data are available that examine the long-term impact of these newer treatments, it is generally agreed that a large majority of patients should survive well into their adult years. Patients with defects in cytosolic oxidase components have often been noted to exhibit a milder disease compared with those with cytochrome-negative CGD.[745, 783, 911, 912]

A multifaceted therapeutic approach has been responsible for the greatly improved prognosis in CGD. The cornerstones of current therapy include (1) prevention and early treatment of infections; (2) use of prophylactic trimethoprim-sulfamethoxazole or dicloxacillin; (3) early use of parenteral antibiotics, including antifungal drugs, augmented by surgical drainage or resection of recalcitrant abscesses; (4) granulocyte transfusions for poorly responding infections; and (5) the use of prophylactic recombinant human IFN-γ (rIFN-γ).

Several approaches can be used to prevent infections. Patients with CGD should receive all routine immunizations (including live-virus vaccines) on schedule and an influenza vaccine yearly. Cuts and skin abrasions should be promptly cleansed with soap and water and rinsed with a 2% solution of hydrogen peroxide. The frequency and severity of rectal infections can be greatly reduced by avoiding constipation and soaking early lesions in warm, soapy water. Flossing and professional dental cleaning can help prevent gingivitis and periodontitis. The risk of *Aspergillus* infection can be decreased by avoiding marijuana smoke[913] and decaying plant material (e.g., rotting wood, mulch, hay), both of which often contain numerous *Aspergillus* spores.

Retrospective studies have shown that chronic prophylaxis with trimethoprim-sulfamethoxazole (5 mg/kg per day of trimethoprim given in one or two doses) can decrease the number of bacterial infections in patients with CGD. In one series of 36 patients followed at the National Institutes of Health, this regimen decreased the incidence of bacterial infections from 7.1 to 2.4 per 100 patient-months in patients with autosomal CGD and from 15.8 to 6.9 infections per 100 patient-months in X-linked patients.[912] Similar conclusions were reached in a review of 48 European patients.[786] Dicloxacillin (25 to 50 mg/kg per day) can be used in sulfa-allergic patients, although there are relatively few data documenting its efficacy. Although ketoconazole was found not to provide any protection against *Aspergillus* infections,[786] oral itraconazole may prove to be useful in this regard. One prospective study of 30 patients found an incidence of 3.4 *Aspergillus* infections (lung) per 100 patient-years compared with 11.5 in a historical control group that did not receive any prophylaxis.[914]

A frequent shortcoming in the treatment of patients with CGD is the failure to treat potentially serious infections promptly or long enough with the appropriate parenteral antibiotics. Therapy should be directed initially at characteristic pathogens. In the absence of a diagnostic culture, broad-spectrum gram-negative coverage (e.g., an aminoglycoside or one of the newer cephalosporins with antipseudomonal activity) should be administered in conjunction with a potent antistaphylococcal agent (e.g., oxacillin or vancomycin). If the site of infection or offending pathogen is not known, and if the patient is severely ill and is not responding to the initial therapy, an aggressive search for the underlying infection should be conducted. In these cases, therapy for fungi, *Nocardia* species, and *P. cepacia* may have to be given empirically. Even when appropriate antibiotics are used, infections often respond slowly, and some may require months of therapy (particularly *Aspergillus* infections but *Staphylococcus* infections as well). Surgical drainage or resection can play a key role in the management of lymphadenitis, osteomyelitis, and abscesses of the liver, lungs, kidney, brain, and rectum.[807, 915] Finally, granulocyte transfusions may be helpful in the treatment of recalcitrant or life-threatening infections.[793, 916]

Recombinant human IFN-γ has been shown to be an effective and well-tolerated treatment that reduces the frequency of serious infection in patients with CGD.[917, 918] IFN-γ enhances many aspects of normal phagocyte function, including microbial killing and rates of hydrogen peroxide production.[102, 919] The latter appears, in part, related to increased levels of gp91*phox* mRNA[920] and prompted attempts to use rIFN-γ to correct the functional defect in the respiratory burst in CGD. These initial studies showed that rIFN-γ improved both superoxide production and bacterial killing by CGD neutrophils both *in vitro* and *in vivo*.[920–922] This effect was most dramatic in some of the patients with variant X-linked CGD (X91⁻ in Table 22–26). One site of action of rIFN-γ, at least in X91⁻ patients, appears to be granulocyte-monocyte precursor cells in the bone marrow. A single injection of rIFN-γ resulted in increased superoxide production by circulating phagocytes 2 weeks later, an effect that persisted for 28 days.[921] Peripheral blood progenitor cells isolated 7 days after rIFN-γ injection and then cultured *in vitro* also gave rise to NBT-positive colonies.[922a]

The encouraging results of the preclinical studies led to a double-blinded, placebo-controlled phase III trial conducted over 12 months to evaluate whether rIFN-γ could be of benefit in CGD.[643] The findings in this study established this cytokine as an effective and well-tolerated treatment that reduces the infectious complications of CGD in all four genetic subgroups, a result that has continued to be supported by longer follow-up studies.[918] The main conclusions of the original study are summarized in Table 22–29. Patients receiving rIFN-γ had a significant reduction in the number of serious infections during the study period and in total number of days in the hospital. These beneficial

Table 22-29. SUMMARY OF THE PHASE III STUDY ESTABLISHING THE EFFICACY OF RECOMBINANT INTERFERON GAMMA (rIFN-γ) FOR INFECTION PROPHYLAXIS IN CHRONIC GRANULOMATOUS DISEASE

Variable	Treatment Group		
	Interferon	**Placebo**	**P Value**
Number of patients	63	65	
Age ± Sd (y)	14.3 ± 10.1	15.0 ± 9.6	
Number of patients with at least one serious infection (%)	14 (22%)	30 (46%)	0.0006
Total number of serious infections	20	56	<0.0001
Total hospital days	497	1493	0.02
Average hospital stay (days)	32	48	
Percentage Without Serious Infection*			
Age			
<10 y (52 patients)	81	20	
≥10 y (76 patients)	73	34	
Inheritance			
X-linked (86 patients)	79	33	
Autosomal (42 patients)	71	39	
Prophylactic antibiotics			
Yes (111 patients)	78	33	
No (17 patients)	69	28	

*The bottom portion of the table shows the Kaplan-Meler estimates of the cumulative proportion of patients free from serious infections at 12 months (after randomization) with adjustment for stratification factors.

The table shows a summary of the final results of a phase III randomized, double-blind, placebo-controlled study in which 128 patients with CGD received either recombinant IFN-γ (50 μg/M² per dose) or placebo by subcutaneous injections three times per week for an average duration of 8.9 months.[99] The major endpoints of the study were the time to the first serious infection and the number of such infections. A serious infection was defined as an event requiring hospitalization and parenteral antibiotics.

effects were independent of age, mode of inheritance, and concomitant use of prophylactic antibiotics. However, patients younger than 10 years of age had the most pronounced reduction in infectious complications. Treatment (50 μg/m² three times a week subcutaneously) was well tolerated and easy to administer. The most common side effects were fever and headache. In contrast to what was observed in the initial studies of patients with variant CGD, there was no difference in neutrophil superoxide production and killing of *S. aureus* between the rIFN-γ and placebo groups.[643, 923] Hence, the beneficial effect of rIFN-γ in most patients with CGD appears to be achieved by enhancing nonoxidative microbicidal mechanisms or other aspects of phagocyte function. This observation has raised the possibility of a more general role for rIFN-γ as an adjunct to conventional antimicrobial therapy in other settings.

Granulomatous inflammation in the esophagus, gastric antrum, and bladder can result in symptoms of obstruction, and lesions in the bowel wall can cause a syndrome resembling inflammatory bowel disease. These complications can cause considerable morbidity in some patients with CGD and are generally managed with a combination of antibiotics and corticosteroids.[818,

[824, 924–927] Although the anti-inflammatory effects of corticosteroids are often beneficial in this setting, their use should be carefully monitored because of their additional immunosuppressive effects. Cyclosporine has also been used successfully to treat a case of intractable gastrointestinal disease, although the patient did develop a serious fungal pneumonia secondary to *Paecilomyces variotii* while on cyclosporine.[928] IFN-γ has had no clear role in the management of the chronic inflammatory complications of CGD, although anecdotal reports suggest that it may be beneficial in some patients.

Allogeneic bone marrow transplantation can be used to treat CGD and has been successfully employed in several cases.[323, 456, 929, 930] However, because of the risks associated with this procedure, marrow transplantation is generally considered only for those patients who have frequent and severe infections despite aggressive medical management.

Because CGD results from single gene defects in proteins expressed in myeloid cells, patients with this disorder are excellent candidates for gene replacement therapy targeted at hematopoietic stem cells. Based on the lack of symptoms observed in female carriers of X-linked CGD with as few as 10% to 20% NBT-positive neutrophils, significant clinical benefit may result even if a fraction of the phagocyte population is successfully corrected. For the X-linked gene product, gp91*phox*, it also appears that expression of even modest amounts of recombinant protein in a cultured myeloid cell model of X-linked CGD can lead to considerable reconstitution of superoxide-generating capacity.[931, 932] However, patients with variant X-linked CGD with residual respiratory burst activity in either a subpopulation or all of their circulating neutrophils can have a severe clinical course.[776, 838] Mouse models of X-linked and A47° CGD that have been developed by gene targeting are useful in evaluating these questions in the preclinical setting.[270, 933] Affected mice have a phenotype that resembles CGD in humans, with increased susceptibility to serious infections due to *S. aureus* and *A. fumigatus*.[270]

Several groups have reported using gene transfer technology to successfully reconstitute respiratory burst oxidase activity in all four genetic subgroups using Epstein-Barr virus–transformed B lymphocytes from patients with CGD, a cultured myeloid X-CGD cell line, or peripheral blood myeloid progenitor cells from all four genetic subgroups.[932, 934–940] Both plasmid-based and retroviral vectors have been used. The major barrier to the future clinical use of gene replacement therapy for CGD, however, relates to achieving efficient vector-mediated gene transfer into long-lived human hematopoietic stem cells.[604, 605]

Glucose-6-Phosphate Dehydrogenase Deficiency

The substrate for the respiratory burst oxidase, NADPH, is generated by the first two reactions of the hexose monophosphate shunt, glucose-6-phosphate dehydrogenase (G6PD) (see Fig. 22–5, reaction 8) and 6-phosphogluconate dehydrogenase (6PGD). Because G6PD is the first enzyme in this pathway, its absence results in greatly diminished shunt activity and thus a severe decrease in the availability of NADPH. As would be expected, severe G6PD deficiency in neutrophils results in attenuated respiratory burst and, in some cases, a clinical picture somewhat similar to that observed in CGD.[941–944] The key features of G6PD deficiency are summarized in Table 22–30. The organisms causing infection in severely deficient patients are similar to those observed in CGD and are predominately catalase-positive bacteria.

In light of the relative high frequency of G6PD mutations in the American black and Mediterranean populations,[945] as well as the fact that leukocyte and erythrocyte G6PD are encoded by the same gene,[946] it might be expected that clinically significant neutrophil G6PD deficiency would occur more often than it does (fewer

Table 22–30. SUMMARY OF NEUTROPHIL GLUCOSE-6-PHOSPHATE DEHYDROGENASE (G6PD) DEFICIENCY

Incidence	Extremely rare
Inheritance	X-linked
Molecular defect	Poorly characterized family of mutations that cause congenital nonspherocytic hemolytic anemia (CNSHA) in erythrocytes and functional failure of G6PD in neutrophils (possibly kinetic mutants); other rare mutants may also be responsible
Pathogenesis	Severe functional failure of neutrophil G6PD (<5% of normal), leading to an extremely low steady-state concentration of NADPH, which serves as the substrate for NADPH oxidase
Clinical manifestations	CNSHA (hemolytic anemia that occurs even in the absence of redox stress)
	CGD-like syndrome with recurrent bacterial infections
Laboratory evaluation	Neutrophil G6PD activity <5% of normal
	Severely diminished respiratory burst and abnormal nitroblue tetrazolium test
	Associated CNSHA with elevated reticulocyte count and diminished erythrocyte G6PD activity
Differential diagnosis	CGD
	Glutathione reductase or synthetase deficiency
Therapy	Prophylactic trimethoprim-sulfamethoxazole
	Aggressive use of parenteral antibiotics
	Transfusion support for severe anemia
Prognosis	Not clear, because too few patients have been reported
	May be as severe as CGD

Reprinted from Curnutte JT: Disorders of phagocyte function. In Hoffman R, Benz EJ, et al (eds): Hematology: Basic Principles and Practice. New York, Churchill Livingstone, 1991, p 577.

than 10 cases have been reported in the literature). One of the reasons it does not is that neutrophils must have a severe deficiency (less than 5% of normal) before respiratory burst function is adversely affected. Even low levels of G6PD are apparently sufficient to recycle NADP$^+$ back to NADPH at a rate that permits reasonable levels of respiratory burst activity. Furthermore, it is apparent from studies on patients with variant CGD that surprisingly low levels of respiratory burst activity (5% to 10% of normal) can still provide adequate protection against microbial infection (see earlier). Therefore, the frequency with which these critically low levels of neutrophil G6PD are encountered is very low. In most types of G6PD deficiency, neutrophil levels are in the range of 20% to 75% of normal.[947, 948] Because most G6PD mutations cause the enzyme to decay over a period of days and weeks, levels in the short-lived neutrophil usually do not become critically low, even in some of the more unstable G6PD variants. Hence, it appears that only a rare (and poorly understood) group of mutations causes extremely low levels of G6PD in neutrophils.

The diagnosis of G6PD deficiency should be considered in any patient with congenital nonspherocytic hemolytic anemia in whom the erythrocyte G6PD level is unusually low or the frequency of infections is high. The diagnosis is established by measuring the level of G6PD activity in neutrophil homogenates. Although not necessary for the diagnosis, neutrophil function tests show a diminished respiratory burst (5% to 30% of normal).[944, 949] The treatment of neutrophil G6PD deficiency is similar to that of CGD except that the efficacy of rIFN-γ has not been demonstrated in the former. In general, G6PD deficiency appears to be somewhat milder than CGD, although recurrent pneumonias and a fatal infection with *Chromobacterium violaceum* have been described.[944, 949]

Myeloperoxidase Deficiency

Deficiency of myeloperoxidase is the most common inherited disorder of phagocytes. A complete deficiency is seen in approximately 1 in 4000 individuals, and partial deficiencies occur in 1 in 2000 persons.[950, 951] The enzymatic deficiency is seen in neutrophils and monocytes. Peroxidase levels in eosinophils, on the other hand, are normal, because eosinophil peroxidase is encoded by a different gene.[60, 952]

Myeloperoxidase plays a pivotal role in amplifying the toxicity of hydrogen peroxide generated by the respiratory burst and catalyzes the formation of hypochlorous acid (HOCl) from chloride and hydrogen peroxide (see Fig. 22–5, reaction 4).[193, 953] HOCl, in turn, reacts with a variety of primary and secondary amines to form chloramines, some of which can be toxic.[193] Moreover, HOCl is capable of activating latent metalloproteinases.[193] Based on these considerations, one would expect that severe myeloperoxidase deficiency should attenuate important antimicrobial reactions catalyzed by HOCl. Neutrophils from myeloperoxidase-deficient patients show markedly abnormal *in vitro* killing of *C. albicans* and hyphal forms of *A. fumiga-*

Table 22–31. SUMMARY OF MYELOPEROXIDASE DEFICIENCY

Incidence	1 in 2000 (partial deficiency)
	1 in 4000 (total deficiency)
Inheritance	Autosomal recessive with variable expression; myeloperoxidase gene on chromosome 17 at q22–q23
Molecular defect	Defective post-translational processing of an abnormal myeloperoxidase precursor polypeptide due to at least four genetic lesions; eosinophil peroxidase encoded by different gene, and levels normal
Pathogenesis	Partial or complete myeloperoxidase deficiency leads to diminished production of HOCl and HOCl-derived chloramines; myeloperoxidase products are necessary for rapid killing of microbes (especially *Candida*) but not absolutely required
Clinical manifestations	Usually clinically silent
	Rarely disseminated candidiasis/fungal disease (usually in conjunction with diabetes mellitus); acquired deficiency in M2, M3, and M4 acute myeloid leukemias (AML) and myelodysplasia
Laboratory evaluation	Deficiency of neutrophil/monocyte peroxidase by histochemical analysis (eosinophil peroxidase normal)
	Delayed, but eventually normal, killing of bacteria *in vitro*
	Failure to kill *C. albicans* and hyphal forms of *Aspergillus fumigatus in vitro*
Differential diagnosis	Acquired partial myeloperoxidase deficiency seen in AML (M2, M3, and M4), myelodysplastic syndromes, and Batten's disease
Therapy	None in asymptomatic patients
	Aggressive treatment of fungal infections when they occur
	Control of blood glucose levels in diabetes
Prognosis	Usually excellent

Reprinted from Curnutte JT: Disorders of phagocyte function. In Hoffman R, Benz EJ, et al (eds): Hematology: Basic Principles and Practice. New York, Churchill Livingstone, 1991, p 578.

tus.[950, 954, 955] Curiously, however, these *in vitro* abnormalities are rarely reflected in an increased incidence of infection in patients except for rare individuals who also suffer from diabetes mellitus.[950, 954, 956] In these individuals, disseminated candidiases can be noted (Table 22–31).

Myeloperoxidase deficiency is inherited in an autosomal recessive manner,[951, 952, 956, 957] and variable expression of the defect has been reported.[957] The myeloperoxidase gene has been localized to the long arm of chromosome 17 at position q21.3–q23.[958, 959] Myeloperoxidase-deficient cells can also be seen in the M2, M3, and M4 forms of acute myeloid leukemia as well as in approximately 25% of patients with myelodysplastic syndrome and chronic myeloid leukemia.[951, 960, 961]

The molecular basis of congenital myeloperoxidase

deficiency is heterogeneous. Myeloperoxidase encodes a 90-kd protein that undergoes proteolytic cleavage to heavy and light chains, which oligomerize to form a tetramer composed of two heavy and two light chains.[951] One cause of complete absence of immunoreactive myeloperoxidase is a point mutation that results in an arginine to tryptophan substitution at codon 569, which was found in 6 of 12 patients with this phenotype.[962, 963] This mutation also creates a new Bgl II restriction site that can be detected by Southern blotting of genomic DNA. Other patients appear to have defects affecting myeloperoxidase processing.[964–966]

Several possible reasons exist for the surprisingly mild clinical phenotype of myeloperoxidase deficiency. First, neutrophils contain such a large amount of myeloperoxidase that appreciable levels may be left in the cell even in cases of severe deficiency. These residual stores, coupled with normal levels of eosinophil peroxidase, may provide at least some degree of peroxidative activity at sites of infection. Second, the respiratory burst in myeloperoxidase-deficient neutrophils is substantially augmented in terms of velocity and duration.[967, 968] This may be due to the enhanced stability of the respiratory burst oxidase made possible by the absence of HOCl, which normally inactivates the oxidase.[969] Finally, other oxidants produced by the respiratory burst may work together with the various granule antimicrobial proteins to provide sufficient protection against most microorganisms.

Given the mild clinical nature of myeloperoxidase deficiency, no treatment is generally required. Infections, when they occur, are treated as in normal individuals. The clinician must be aware of the increased risk of *Candida* infections in myeloperoxidase-deficient patients and to treat them aggressively when they do occur.

Disorders of Glutathione Metabolism

As shown in Figure 22–5 (reaction 6), glutathione peroxidase protects neutrophil proteins (including NADPH oxidase) from the harmful effects of hydrogen peroxide generated in the course of the respiratory burst by degrading it to water. The reducing equivalents for this reaction are carried by the reduced form of glutathione (GSH), the intracellular levels of which are maintained by recycling oxidized glutathione (GSSG) back to GSH by means of glutathione reductase (see Fig. 22–5, reaction 7). Glutathione levels are also maintained through *de novo* synthesis catalyzed by glutathione synthetase (see Fig. 22–5, reaction 9). Severe deficiencies of glutathione reductase and glutathione synthetase in neutrophils have been reported and found to cause moderately severe abnormalities in the respiratory burst.[970–974] The key features of each of these extremely rare disorders are summarized in Table 22–32.

Glutathione reductase deficiency has been reported in one family in which three siblings were found to have a marked deficiency of this enzyme in their neutrophils (10% to 15% of normal).[970, 972] The inheritance appeared to be autosomal recessive, because the parents of the children were first cousins and their neutrophils contained 50% of the normal levels of glutathione reductase. The mutation responsible for the enzyme deficiency in this family has not been reported. It is known that the gene for glutathione reductase is located on chromosome 8 at position p21.1.[975]

Clinically, none of the affected patients showed signs of increased infection. Their erythrocytes were also deficient in glutathione reductase and therefore were prone to hemolysis in the presence of oxidant stress. Two siblings did suffer from juvenile cataracts and deafness. The structure and function of the neutrophil

Table 22–32. DISORDERS OF GLUTATHIONE METABOLISM

Disease Aspect	Glutathione Reductase Deficiency	Glutathione Synthetase Deficiency
Incidence	One family: three siblings	Several reported cases
Inheritance	Autosomal recessive	Autosomal recessive
Molecular defect	Diminished glutathione reductase levels in neutrophils (10–15% of normal) and erythrocytes; mutation not known	Severe deficiency of glutathione synthetase activity (5–10% of normal); mutation(s) not known
Pathogenesis	Brief respiratory burst truncated by toxic accumulation of H_2O_2 in neutrophil caused by diminished catabolism of H_2O_2 by glutathione	Same as with glutathione reductase deficiency except that the respiratory burst is normal; elevated 5-oxoproline levels due to lack of feedback inhibition by glutathione
Clinical manifestations	No history of repeated infection Hemolysis with oxidant stress	Metabolic acidosis due to elevated 5-oxoproline Otitis media Intermittent neutropenia Hemolysis with oxidant stress Severe decrease in glutathione synthetase level
Laboratory evaluation	Glutathione reductase level diminished Premature cessation of O_2^- production by neutrophils	Normal respiratory burst
Differential diagnosis	CGD Glucose-6-phosphate dehydrogenase deficiency	Glutathione reductase deficiency
Therapy	None required	Vitamin E for hemolysis and infections Treatment of metabolic acidosis
Prognosis	Benign disorder	Relatively benign disorder

Reprinted with permission from Curnutte JT: Disorders of phagocyte function. In Hoffman R, Benz EJ, et al (eds): Hematology: Basic Principles and Practice. New York, Churchill Livingstone, 1991, p 578.

in vitro were normal except for a premature termination of the respiratory burst after about 5 minutes.[970] The probable reason for this defect is that NADPH oxidase is inactivated by the products of the myeloperoxidase reaction.[969] If glutathione reductase is deficient, the neutrophils cannot maintain a level of GSH sufficient to detoxify hydrogen peroxide. After several minutes of the respiratory burst, toxic levels of hydrogen peroxide accumulate and lead to deactivation of the oxidase.

This explanation is supported by experiments showing that glutathione reductase–deficient neutrophils pre-exposed to exogenous hydrogen peroxide fail to undergo even an abbreviated respiratory burst. One important insight gained from the study of these patients is that only a brief respiratory burst appears to be necessary for adequate microbial killing.

The diagnosis of glutathione reductase deficiency is made by measuring the levels of this enzyme in neutro-

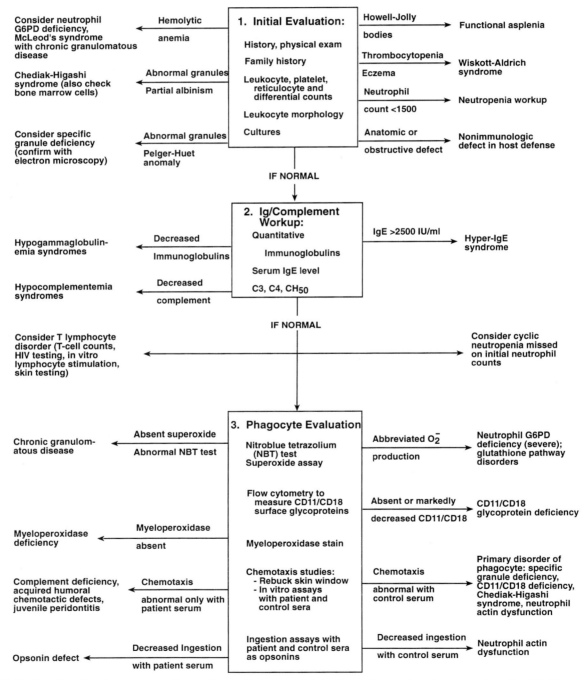

Figure 22-9. Algorithm for the workup of a patient with recurrent infections. The various tests are described in the appropriate sections of the chapter. G6PD = glucose-6-phosphate dehydrogenase; O_2^- = superoxide. The units for the neutrophil count *(box 1)* are neutrophils/mm³. (Adapted from Lehrer RI, Ganz T, Selsted ME, et al: Neutrophils and host defense. Ann Intern Med 1988; 109:127. Clinical conference.)

phil homogenates. The finding of a truncated respiratory burst provides supporting evidence, although a similar abnormality can be seen in G6PD deficiency. No therapy is required.

Several forms of congenital glutathione synthetase deficiency have been described, all of which are inherited in an autosomal recessive fashion. Specific mutations have not been reported. Only in those cases in which the glutathione synthetase activity is severely deficient in neutrophils (5% to 10% of normal) is a phagocytic abnormality detected.[971, 973, 974] In contrast to glutathione reductase deficiency, neutrophils deficient in glutathione synthetase have a normal respiratory burst.[971, 974] However, for reasons that are uncertain, *in vitro* bacterial killing is decreased. Despite this microbicidal defect, patients with glutathione synthetase deficiency have only a relatively mild problem resolving infections. They do suffer from a severe metabolic acidosis resulting from elevated levels of 5-oxoproline, a metabolite formed in one of the early steps in the pathway of glutathione synthesis. This acidosis may be responsible for the intermittent neutropenia observed in glutathione synthetase–deficient patients.[971] Because the erythrocytes in these patients are also deficient in glutathione synthetase, a hemolytic anemia brought on by oxidant stress is noted. Therapy with vitamin E (400 IU/day) has been found to be beneficial in patients who suffer from hemolysis and infection.[971]

Glutathione peroxidase (see Fig. 22–5, reaction 6) was found to be decreased to levels 25% of normal in three unrelated patients with a clinical syndrome resembling CGD.[976, 977] Although this enzyme plays an important role in removing hydrogen peroxide, it has not been established whether the degree of deficiency seen in these patients is sufficient to cause functional abnormalities in neutrophils. Two of the affected kindreds have been restudied, and a severe deficiency of the respiratory burst oxidase cytochrome-*b* has been identified in affected members of each.[848] It thus appears that in at least two of these previously reported cases, CGD is the underlying problem, not glutathione peroxidase deficiency.

Evaluation of the Patient with Recurrent Infections

The patient who presents with recurrent infections can be a diagnostic challenge. Many of the phagocyte disorders have similar clinical manifestations that can overlap those seen in inherited or acquired disorders of lymphocyte function. Furthermore, the majority of patients with recurrent infections do not have an identifiable granulocyte or monocyte defect. Given this low yield and the lack of ability to characterize many aspects of phagocyte function in routine laboratory studies, physicians are faced with the difficult question of which patients merit a complete evaluation. Those who have at least one of the following clinical features are more likely to have a phagocyte defect: (1) an unusually high frequency of bacterial and fungal infections; (2) the presence of an infection at an unusual site (e.g., a hepatic or brain abscess); (3) infections with atypical

pathogens (e.g., *Aspergillus* pneumonia, disseminated candidiasis, lymphadenitis due to *Serratia* or *Klebsiella*); (4) infections of exceptional severity; and (5) childhood periodontal disease. Certain other clinical findings can also be helpful. For example, a child with nystagmus, fair skin, and recurrent staphylococcal infections should be evaluated for CHS, whereas an infant with bacterial infections and delayed separation of the umbilical cord should be tested for LAD. Once the physician has decided that a phagocyte evaluation is warranted, the algorithm present in Figure 22–9 may be helpful in organizing the workup. When coupled with a thorough clinical history and physical examination, the laboratory tests outlined in Figure 22–9 should allow the physician to establish the diagnosis and formulate an appropriate therapeutic plan.

References

1. Sieff CA: Hematopoietic growth factors. J Clin Invest 1987; 79:1549.
2. Metcalf D: The molecular control of cell division, differentiation, commitment and maturation of hematopoietic stem cells. Blood 1989; 339:27.
3. Lieschke GJ, Burgess AW: Granulocyte colony-stimulating factor and granulocyte-macrophage colony-stimulating factor (part II). N Engl J Med 1992; 327:99.
4. Clutterbuck EF, Hirst EM, Sanderson CG: Human interleukin-5 (IL-5) regulates the production of eosinophils in human bone marrow cultures: Comparison and interaction with IL-1, IL-3, IL-6, and GMCSF. Blood 1989; 73:1504.
5. Warren DJ, Moore MA: Synergism among interleukin 1, interleukin 3, and interleukin 5 in the production of eosinophils from primitive hematopoietic stem cells. J Immunol 1988; 140:94.
6. Sanderson CJ: Interleukin-5, eosinophils, and disease. Blood 1992; 79:3101.
7. Denburg JA: Basophil and mast cell lineages *in vitro* and *in vivo*. Blood 1992; 79:846.
8. Halett MB, Lloyds D: Neutrophil priming: The cellular signals that say "amber" but not "green." Immunol Today 1995; 16:264.
9. Tsai S, Collins SJ: A dominant negative retinoic acid receptor blocks neutrophil differentiation at the promyelocyte stage. Proc Natl Acad Sci U S A 1993; 90:7153.
10. Jacobsen SEW, Fahlman C, et al: *All-trans*- and 9-*cis*-retinoic acid: Potent direct inhibitors of primitive murine hematopoietic progenitors *in vitro*. J Exp Med 1994; 179:1665.
11. Evans R: The steroid and thyroid hormone receptor superfamily. Science 1988; 240:889.
12. Lo Coco F, Avvisati G, et al: Molecular evaluation of response to *all-trans* retinoic acid therapy in patients with acute promyelocytic leukemia. Blood 1991; 77:1657.
13. Borrow J, Goddard AD, et al: Molecular analysis of acute promyelocytic leukemia breakpoint cluster region on chromosome 17. Science 1990; 249:1577.
14. De The H, Lavau C, et al: The PML-RAR fusion mRNA generated by the t(15;17) translocation in acute promyelocytic leukemia encodes a functionally altered RAR. Cell 1991; 66:675.
15. Athens JW, Haab OP, et al: Leukokinetic studies: IV. The total blood, circulating and marginal granulocyte pools and the granulocyte turnover rate in normal subjects. J Clin Invest 1961; 40:989.
16. Cronkite EP: Kinetics of granulopoiesis. Clin Haematol 1979; 8:351.
17. Dancey JT, Deubelbeiss KA: Neutrophil kinetics in man. J Clin Invest 1976; 58:705.
18. Donohue DM, Reiff RH: Quantitative measurement of the erythrocytic and granulocytic cells of the marrow and blood. J Clin Invest 1958; 37:1571.
19. Fadok VA, Savill JS, et al: Different populations of macrophages use either the vitronectin receptor or the phosphatidylserine

receptor to recognize and remove apoptotic cells. J Immunol 1992; 149:4029.

20. Savill JS, Wyllie AH, et al: Macrophage phagocytosis of aging neutrophils in inflammation. Programmed cell death in the neutrophil leads to recognition by macrophages. J Clin Invest 1989; 83:865.

21. Squier MKT, Sehner AJ, Cohen JJ: Apoptosis in leukocytes. J Leukoc Biol 1995; 57:2.

22. Bainton DF: Neutrophilic leukocyte granules: From structure to function. Adv Exp Med Biol 1993; 336:17.

23. Borregaard N, Lollike K, et al: Human neutrophil granules and secretory vesicles. Eur J Haematol 1993; 51:187.

24. Hoffstein S, Weissmann G: Microtubules in calcium ionophore induced secretion of lysosomal enzymes from human polymorphonuclear leukocytes. J Cell Biol 1978; 78:78.

25. Stossel TP: On the crawling of animal cells. Science 1993; 260:1086.

26. Howard TH, Watts RG: Actin polymerization and leukocyte function. Curr Opin Hematol 1994; 1:61.

27. Liu CH, Lehan C, et al: Degenerative changes in neutrophils: An indicator of bacterial infection. Pediatrics 1984; 74:823.

28. Borregaard N, Tauber AI: Subcellular localization of the human neutrophils NADPH oxidase, b-cytochrome and associated flavoprotein. J Biol Chem 1984; 259:47.

29. Jesaitis AJ, Buescher ES, et al: Ultrastructural localization of cytochrome b in the membranes of resting and phagocytosing human granulocytes. J Clin Invest 1990; 85:821.

30. Lubbert M, Herrmann F, Koeffler P: Expression and regulation of myeloid-specific genes in normal and leukemic myeloid cells. Blood 1991; 77:909.

31. Shapiro LH, Look AT: Transcriptional regulation in myeloid cell differentiation. Curr Sci 1995; 2:3.

32. Grisolano JL, Sclar GM, Ley TJ: Early myeloid-specific expression of the human cathepsin G gene in transgenic mice. Proc Natl Acad Sci U S A 1994; 91:8989.

33. Borregaard N, Sehested M, et al: Biosynthesis of granule proteins in normal human bone marrow cells. Gelatinase Ia a marker of terminal neutrophil differentiation. Blood 1995; 85:812.

34. Berliner N, Hsing A, et al: Granulocyte colony-stimulating factor induction of normal human bone marrow progenitors results in neutrophil-specific gene expression. Blood 1995; 85:799.

35. Fouret P, Du Bois RM, et al: Expression of the human elastase gene during human bone marrow cell differentiation. J Exp Med 1989; 169:833.

36. Orkin SH: Molecular genetics of chronic granulomatous disease. Annu Rev Immunol 1989; 7:277.

37. Zakhireh B, Root R: Development of oxidase activity by human bone marrow granulocytes. Blood 1979; 54:429.

38. Downey GP, Fukushima T, Fialkow L: Signaling mechanisms in human neutrophils. Curr Opin Hematol 1995; 2:76.

39. Bokoch GM: Chemoattractant signaling and leukocyte activation. Blood 1995; 86:1649.

40. Lew PD: Receptors and intracellular signaling in human neutrophils. Am Rev Respir Dis 1990; 141:5127.

41. Thelen M, Wirthmueller U: Phospholipases and protein kinases during phagocyte activation. Curr Opin Immunol 1994; 6:106.

42. Lew DP: Receptor signalling and intracellular calcium in neutrophil activation. Eur J Clin Invest 1989; 19:338.

43. Huang C-K: Protein kinases in neutrophils: A review. Membr Biochem 1989; 8:61.

44. Berkow RI, Dodson RW: Tyrosine-specific protein phosphorylation during activation of human neutrophils. Blood 1990; 75:2445.

45. Rollet E, Caon AC, et al: Tyrosine phosphorylation in activated human neutrophils: Comparison of the effects of different classes of agonists and identification of signalling pathways involved. J Immunol 1994; 153:353.

46. Grinstein S, Furuya W, et al: Receptor-mediated activation of multiple serine/threonine kinases in human leukocytes. J Biol Chem 1993; 268:20223.

47. Ding J, Bawdwey JA: Stimulation of neutrophils with a chemoattractant activates several novel protein kinases that can catalyze the phosphorylation of the 47-kDa protein component of the phagocyte oxidase and the myristoylated alanine-rich C kinase substrate. J Biol Chem 1993; 268:17326.

48. Perez HD: Chemoattractant receptors. Curr Opin Hematol 1994; 1:40.

49. Worthen GS, Avdi N, et al: FMLP activates Ras and Raf in human neutrophils: Potential role in activation of MAP kinase. J Clin Invest 1994; 94:815.

50. Bokoch GM, Knaus UG: Ras-related GTP-binding proteins and leukocyte signal transduction. Curr Opin Hematol 1994; 1:53.

51. Newburger PE, Dai Q, Whitney C: In vitro regulation of human phagocyte cytochrome b heavy and light chain gene expression by bacterial lipopolysaccharide and recombinant human cytokines. J Biol Chem 1991; 266:16171.

52. Lloyd AR, Oppenheim JJ: Poly's lament: The neglected role of the polymorphonuclear neutrophil in the afferent limb of the immune response. Immunol Today 1992; 13:169.

53. Cassatella MA: The production of cytokines by polymorphonuclear neutrophils. Immunol Today 1995; 16:21.

54. Anderson V, Bro-Rasmussen F: Autoradiographic studies of eosinophil kinetics. Cell Tissue Kinet 1969; 2:139.

55. Enokihara H, Furusawa S, et al: T cells from eosinophilic patients produce interleukin-5 with interleukin-2 stimulation. Blood 1989; 73:1809.

56. Carlson M, Peterson C, Venge P: The influence of IL-3, IL-5, and GM-CSF on normal human eosinophil and neutrophil C3b-induced degranulation. Allergy 1993; 48:437.

57. Parwaresch MR, Walle AJ: The peripheral kinetics of human radiolabelled eosinophils. Virchows Arch 1976; 1321:57.

58. Weller PF: The immunobiology of eosinophils. N Engl J Med 1991; 324:1110.

59. Gleich GJ, Adolphson CR: The eosinophilic leukocyte: Structure and function. Adv Immunol 1986; 39:177.

60. Shurin SB: Pathologic states associated with activation of eosinophils and with eosinophilia. Hematol Oncol Clin North Am 1988; 2:171.

61. Thevathason OI, Gordon AS: Adrenocorticomedullary interactions on the blood eosinophils. Acta Haematol 1958; 19:162.

62. Baehner RL, Johnston RB Jr: Metabolic and bactericidal activities of human eosinophils. Br J Haematol 1971; 20:277.

63. Klebanoff SJ, Durack DT: Functional studies on human peritoneal eosinophils. Infect Immun 1977; 17:167.

64. Tauber AI, Goetzl EF, Babior BM: Unique characteristics of superoxide production by human eosinophils in eosinophilic states. Inflammation 1979; 3:261.

65. Goetzl EJ, Austin KF: Purification and synthesis of eosinophilotactic tetrapeptides of human lung tissue: Identification as eosinophil chemotactic factor of anaphylaxis. Proc Natl Acad Sci U S A 1975; 72:4123.

66. Dvorak AM, Ackerman SJ, Weller PF: Subcellular morphology and biochemistry of eosinophils. In Harris JR (ed): Blood Cell Biochemistry. London, Plenum Publishing Corp., 1990, p 237.

67. Bainton D, Farquhar MG: Segregation and packaging of granule enzymes in eosinophilic leukocytes. J Cell Biol 1970; 45:54.

68. Parmley RT, Spicer SS: Cytochemical and ultrastructural identification of a small type granule in human late eosinophils. Lab Invest 1974; 30:557.

69. Jong EC, Henderson WR, Klebanoff SR: Bactericidal activity of eosinophil peroxidase. J Immunol 1980; 124:1378.

70. Magler R, DeChatelet LR, Bass DA: Human eosinophil peroxidase: Role in bactericidal activity. Blood 1978; 51:445.

71. Weiss SJ, Test ST, et al: Brominating oxidants generated by human eosinophils. Science 1986; 234:200.

72. Olsson I, Venge P: Arginine-rich cationic proteins of human eosinophil granules. Comparison of the constituents of eosinophilic and neutrophilic leukocytes. Lab Invest 1977; 36:493.

73. Butterworth AE, Wassom DL, et al: Damage to schistosomula of Schistosoma mansoni induced directly by eosinophil major basic protein. J Immunol 1979; 122:221.

74. O'Donnell MC, Ackerman SJ, et al: Activation of basophil and mast cell histamine release by eosinophil major basic protein. J Exp Med 1983; 257:1981.

75. Weller PF, Bach D, Austen KF: Human eosinophil lysophospholipase: The sole protein component of Charcot-Leyden crystals. J Immunol 1982; 128:1346.

76. Dvorak AM, Letourneau L, et al: Ultrastructural location of the Charcot-Leyden crystal proteins (lysophospholipase) to a distinct crystalloid-free granule population in mature human eosinophils. Blood 1988; 72:150.

77. Murakami I, Ogawa M, et al: Studies on kinetics of human leukocytes *in vivo* with ³H-thymidine autoradiography: II. Eosinophils and basophils. Acta Haematol Jpn 1969; 32:384.

78. Juhlin L: Basophil leukocyte differential in blood and bone marrow. Acta Haematol 1963; 29:89.

79. Dvorak HF, Dvorak AM: Basophilic leukocytes: Structure, function, and role in disease. Clin Haematol 1975; 4:651.

80. Kinet J-P: The high-affinity receptor for IgE. Curr Opin Immunol 1989; 2:499.

81. Seder RA, Paul WE, et al: Mouse splenic and bone marrow cell populations that express high-affinity Fce receptors and produce interleukin-4 are highly enriched in basophils. Proc Natl Acad Sci U S A 1991; 88:2835.

82. Brunner T, Heusser CH, Dahinden CA: Human peripheral blood basophils primed by interleukin-3 (IL-3) produce IL-4 in response to immunoglobulin E receptor stimulation. J Exp Med 1993; 177:605.

83. Schroeder JT, MacGlashan DW, et al: Cytokine generation by human basophils. J Allergy Clin Immunol 1994; 94:1189.

84. Hatanaka K, Kitamura Y, Nishimune Y: Local development of mast cells from bone marrow–derived precursors in the skin of mice. Blood 1979; 53:142.

85. Galli SJ: New concepts about the mast cell. N Engl J Med 1993; 328:257.

86. Columbo M, Horowitz EM, et al: The human recombinant *c-kit* receptor ligand, rhSCF, induces mediator release from human cutaneous mast cells and enhances IgE-dependent mediator release from both skin mast cells and peripheral blood basophils. J Immunol 1992; 149:599.

87. Galli SJ, Dvorak AM, Dvorak HF: Basophils and mast cells: Morphologic insights into their biology, secretory patterns, and function. Prog Allergy 1984; 34:1.

88. Kuriu A, Sonoda S, et al: Proliferative potential of degranulated murine peritoneal mast cells. Blood 1989; 74:925.

89. Whitelaw DM: The intravascular lifespan of monocytes. Blood 1966; 28:445.

90. Whitelaw DM: Observations on human monocyte kinetics after pulse labeling. Cell Tissue Kinet 1972; 5:311.

91. Van Furth R, Raeburn JA: Characteristics of human mononuclear phagocytes. Blood 1979; 54:485.

92. Van Furth R: Development and distribution of mononuclear phagocytes. In Gallin JI, Goldstein IM, Snyderman R (eds): Inflammation: Basic Principles and Clinical Correlates. New York, Raven Press, 1992, p 325.

93. Thomas ED, Ramberg RE, et al: Direct evidence for a bone marrow origin of the alveolar macrophage in man. Science 1976; 192:1016.

94. Arenson EB, Epstein MB, Seeger RC: Monocyte subsets in neonates and children. Pediatrics 1979; 64:740.

95. Cohn ZA, Wiener E: The particulate hydrolases of macrophages. I. Comparative enzymology, isolation, and properties. J Exp Med 1963; 118:991.

96. Nagaraju M, Weitzman S, Baumann G: Viral hepatitis and agranulocytosis. Am J Dig Dis 1973; 18:247.

97. Nathan CF: Secretory products of macrophages. J Clin Invest 1987; 79:319.

98. Raetz CR, Ulevitch RJ, et al: Gram-negative endotoxin: An extraordinary lipid with profound effects on eukaryotic signal transduction. FASEB J 1991; 5:2652.

99. Johnston RB: Monocytes and macrophages. N Engl J Med 1988; 318:747.

100. Beutler B, Cerami A: The biology of cachectin/TNF—a primary mediator of the host immune response. Annu Rev Immunol 1989; 7:625.

101. Adams DO, Hamilton TA: Macrophages as destructive cells in host defense. In Gallin J, Goldstein I, Snyderman R (eds): Inflammation: Basic Principles and Clinical Correlates. New York, Raven Press, 1992, p 637.

102. Murray HW: Interferon gamma: The activated macrophage, and host defense against microbial challenge. Ann Intern Med 1988; 108:595.

103. Hill HR: Modulation of host defenses with interferon-γ in pediatrics. J Infect Dis 1993; 167:S23.

104. Williams BRG: Transcriptional regulation of interferon-stimulated genes. Eur J Biochem 1991; 200:1.

105. Darnell JE Jr, Kerr IM, Stark GR: Jak-STAT pathways and transcriptional activation in response to IFNs and other extracellular signaling proteins. Science 1994; 264:1415.

106. Ihle JN, Kerr IM: Jaks and Stats in signaling by the cytokine receptor superfamily. Trends Genet 1995; 11:69.

107. Simon LD, Robin ED, et al: Enzymatic basis for bioenergetic differences of alveolar versus peritoneal macrophages and enzyme regulation by molecular oxygen. J Clin Invest 1977; 59:443.

108. Bar-Shavit R, Kahn A, et al: Monocyte chemotaxis: Stimulation by specific exosite region in thrombin. Science 1983; 220:728.

109. Broze G: Binding of human factor VII and VIIa to monocytes. J Clin Invest 1982; 70:526.

110. Brown MS, Goldstein JL: Lipoprotein metabolism in the macrophage: Implications for cholesterol deposition in atherosclerosis. Annu Rev Biochem 1983; 52:223.

111. Unanue ER, Allen PM: The basis for the immunoregulatory role of macrophages and other accessory cells. Science 1987; 236:551.

112. Hocking WG, Golde DW: The pulmonary alveolar macrophage. N Engl J Med 1979; 301:580.

113. Tavassoli M: Intravascular phagocytosis in the rabbit bone marrow: A possible fate of normal senescent red cells. Br J Haematol 1977; 36:323.

114. Beutler E: Gaucher's disease. N Engl J Med 1991; 325:1354.

115. Ho D, Pomerantz R, Kaplan JC: Pathogenesis of infection with human immunodeficiency virus. N Engl J Med 1987; 317:278.

116. Friedland GH, Klein RS: Transmission of the human immunodeficiency virus. N Engl J Med 1987; 317:1125.

117. Marks SC: Osteoclast biology: Lessons from mammalian mutations. Am J Med Genet 1989; 34:43.

118. Schneider GB, Relfson M: The effects of transplantation of granulocyte-macrophage progenitors on bone resorption in *ia* osteopetrotic rats. J Bone Miner Res 1988; 3:225.

119. Suda T, Takahashi N, Martin T: Modulation of osteoclast differentiation. Endocr Rev 1992; 13:66.

120. Orchard PJ, Dahl N, et al: Circulating macrophage colony-stimulating factor is not reduced in malignant osteopetrosis. Exp Hematol 1992; 20:103.

121. Coccia PF, Krivit W, et al: Successful bone-marrow transplantation for infantile malignant osteopetrosis. N Engl J Med 1980; 302:701.

122. Key LL, Rodriguiz RM, et al: Long-term treatment of osteopetrosis with recombinant human interferon gamma. N Engl J Med 1995; 332:1594.

123. Majino G: The Healing Hand: Man and Wound in the Ancient World. Cambridge, MA, Harvard University Press, 1975.

124. Craddock CG: Defenses of the body: The initiators of defense, the ready reserves, and the scavengers. In Wintrobe M (ed): Blood, Pure and Eloquent. New York, McGraw-Hill Book Co., 1980.

125. Metchnikov I: Immunity in Infective Diseases. New York, Dover Publications, Inc., 1968.

126. Dinarello CA: Interleukin-1 and interleukin-1 antagonism. Blood 1991; 77:1627.

127. Dinarello CA, Wolff SM: The role of interleukin-1 in disease. N Engl J Med 1993; 328:106.

128. Fiers W: Tumor necrosis factor. FEBS Lett 1991; 285:199.

129. Strieter RM, Kunkel SL: Acute lung injury: The role of cytokines in the elicitation of neutrophils. J Invest Med 1994; 42:640.

130. Warren JS: Interleukins and tumor necrosis factor in inflammation. Crit Rev Clin Lab Sci 1990; 28:37.

131. Moore KW, O'Garra A, et al: Interleukin-10. Annu Rev Immunol 1993; 11:165.

132. Kulkarni AB, Huh CG, et al: Transforming growth factor beta-1 null mutation in mice causes excessive inflammatory response and early death. Proc Natl Acad Sci U S A 1993; 90:770.

133. Wahl SM: Transforming growth factor beta: The good, the bad, and the ugly. J Exp Med 1994; 180:1587.

134. Oppenheim JJ, Zachariae CO, et al: Properties of the novel proinflammatory supergene "intercrine" cytokine family. Annu Rev Immunol 1991; 9:617.

135. Kuna P, Reddigari SR, et al: RANTES, a monocyte and T lymphocyte chemotactic cytokine releases histamine from human basophils. J Immunol 1992; 149:636.

136. Alam R, Lett-Brown MA, et al: Monocyte chemotactic and activating factor is a potent histamine-releasing factor for basophils. J Clin Invest 1992; 89:723.

137. Snyder F: Biochemistry of platelet-activating factor: A unique class of biologically active phospholipids. Proc Soc Exp Biol Med 1989; 190:125.

138. Prescott SM, Zimmerman GA, McIntyre TM: Platelet-activating factor. J Biol Chem 1992; 120:17381.

139. Serhan CN: Eicosanoids in leukocyte function. Curr Opin Hematol 1994; 1:69.

140. Nathan C: Nitric oxide as a secretory product of mammalian cells. FASEB J 1992; 6:3051.

141. Lowenstein CJ, Snyder SH: Nitric oxide, a novel biologic messenger. Cell 1992; 70:705.

142. Lewis RA, Austen KF, Soberman RJ: Leukotrienes and other products of the 5-lipoxygenase pathway. Biochemistry and relation to pathobiology in human disease. N Engl J Med 1990; 323:645.

143. Baggiolini M, Clark-Lewis I: Interleukin-8, a chemotactic and inflammatory cytokine. FEBS Lett 1992; 307:97.

144. Springer TA: Traffic signals for lymphocyte recirculation and leukocyte emigration: The multistep paradigm. Cell 1994; 76:310.

145. Murphy PM: The molecular biology of leukocyte chemoattractant receptors. Annu Rev Immunol 1994; 12:593.

146. Walz A, Baggiolini M: Generation of the neutrophil-activating peptide NAP-2 from platelet basic protein or connective tissue-activating peptide III through monocyte proteases. J Exp Med 1990; 171:449.

147. Baggiolini M, Walz A, Kunkel SL: Neutrophil-activating peptide-1/interleukin 8, a novel cytokine that activates neutrophils. J Clin Invest 1989; 84:1045.

148. Zachaiae CO, Anderson AO, et al: Properties of monocyte chemotactic and activating factor (MCAF) purified from a human fibrosarcoma cell line. J Exp Med 1990; 171:2177.

149. Rollins BJ, Walz A, Baggiolini M: Recombinant human MCP-1/JE induces chemotaxis, calcium flux, and the respiratory burst in human monocytes. Blood 1991; 78:1112.

150. Schall TJ, Bacon K, et al: Selective attraction of monocytes and T lymphocytes of the memory phenotype by cytokines RANTES. Nature 1990; 347:669.

151. Huber AR, Kunkel SL, et al: Regulation of transendothelial neutrophil migration by endogenous interleukin-8. Science 1991; 254:99.

152. Rot A: Endothelial cell binding of NAP-1/IL-8: Role in neutrophil emigration. Immunol Today 1992; 13:291.

153. Tanaka Y, Adams DH, et al: T-cell adhesion induced by proteoglycan-immobilized cytokine MIp-1. Nature 1993; 361:79.

154. Zigmond S: The ability of polymorphonuclear leukocytes to orient in gradients of chemotactic factors. J Cell Biol 1977; 117:606.

155. Gerard C, Gerard NP: The pro-inflammatory seven-transmembrane segment receptors of the leukocyte. Curr Opin Immunol 1994; 6:140.

156. Gilman AG: Transducers of receptor-generated signals. Annu Rev Biochem 1987; 56:615.

157. Kaziro Y, Itoh H, et al: Structure and function of signal-transducing GTP-binding proteins. Annu Rev Biochem 1991; 60:349.

158. Polakis PG, Uhing RJ, Snyderman R: The formylpeptide chemoattractant receptor copurifies with a GTP-binding protein containing a distinct 40 kDa pertussis toxin substrate. J Biol Chem 1988; 263:4969.

159. Wu D, LaRosa GJ, Simon MI: G protein-coupled signal transduction pathways for interleukin-8. Science 1993; 261:101.

160. Gierschik P, Sidiropoulos D, Jakobs KH: Two distinct Gi-proteins mediate formyl peptide receptor signal transduction in human leukemia (HL-60) cells. J Biol Chem 1989; 264:21470.

161. Amatruda TT, Steele DA, et al: G alpha 16, a G protein alpha subunit specifically expressed in hematopoietic cells. Proc Natl Acad Sci U S A 1991; 88:5587.

162. Amatruda TT, Gerard NP, et al: Specific interactions of chemoattractant factor receptors with G-proteins. J Biol Chem 1993; 268:10139.

163. Albelda SM, Smith CW, Ward PA: Adhesion molecules and inflammatory injury. FASEB J 1994; 8:504.

164. Carlos TM, Harlan JM: Leukocyte-endothelial adhesion molecules. Blood 1994; 84:2068.

165. Lasky LA: Combinatorial mediators of inflammation? Curr Biol 1993; 3:366.

166. Springer TA: Adhesion receptors of the immune system. Nature 1990; 346:425.

167. Lasky LA: Selectins: Interpreters of cell-specific carbohydrate information during inflammation. Science 1992; 258:964.

168. Kishimoto TK, Rothlein R: Integrins, ICAMS, and selectins: Role and regulation of adhesion molecules in neutrophil recruitment to inflammatory sites. Adv Pharm 1994; 25:117.

169. McEver RP: Selectins. Curr Opin Immunol 1994; 6:75.

170. Varki A: Selectin ligands. Proc Natl Acad Sci U S A 1994; 91:7390.

171. Bevilacqua MP, Stengelin S, et al: Endothelial leukocyte adhesion molecule 1: An inducible receptor of neutrophils related to complement regulatory proteins and lectins. Science 1989; 243:1160.

172. Kishimoto TK, Jutila MA, et al: Neutrophil Mac-1 and MEL-14 adhesion proteins inversely regulated by chemotactic factors. Science 1989; 245:1238.

173. Jung TM, Dailey MO: Rapid modulation of homing receptors (gp90MEL-14) induced by activators of protein kinase C: Receptor shedding due to accelerated proteolytic cleavage at the cell surface. J Immunol 1990; 144:3130.

174. Gearing AJH, Newman W: Circulating adhesion molecules in disease. Immunol Today 1993; 14:506.

175. Jutila MA: Leukocyte traffic to sites of inflammation. Acta Pathol Microbiol Immunol Scand 1992; 100:191.

176. Ruoslahti E: Integrins. J Clin Invest 1991; 87:1.

177. Larson RS, Springer TA: Structure and function of leukocyte integrins. Immunol Rev 1990; 114:181.

178. Arnaout MA: Structure and function of the leukocyte adhesion molecules CD11/CD18. Blood 1990; 75:1037.

179. Kishimoto TK, O'Connor K, et al: Cloning of the β subunit of the leukocyte adhesion proteins: Homology to an extracellular matrix receptor defines a novel supergene family. Cell 1987; 48:681.

180. O'Toole TE, Katagiri Y, et al: Integrin cytoplasmic domains mediate inside-out signal transduction. J Cell Biol 1994; 124:1047.

181. Clark EA, Brugge JS: Integrins and signal transduction pathways: The road taken. Science 1995; 268:233.

182. Rieu P, Ueda T, et al: The A-domain of b2 integrin CR3 (CD11b/CD18) is a receptor for the hookworm-derived neutrophil adhesion inhibitor NIF. J Cell Biol 1994; 127:2081.

183. Moyle M, Foster DL, et al: A hookworm glycoprotein that inhibits neutrophil function is a ligand of the integrin CD11b/CD18. J Biol Chem 1994; 269:10008.

184. Sengelov H, Kjeldsen L, et al: Subcellular localization and dynamics of Mac-1 (αβ2) in human neutrophils. J Clin Invest 1993; 92:1467.

185. Doerschuk CM, Winn RK, et al: CD18-dependent and independent mechanisms of neutrophil adherence in the pulmonary and systemic microvasculature of rabbits. J Immunol 1990; 144:2327.

186. Hogg JC, Doerschuk CM: Leukocyte traffic in the lung. Annu Rev Physiol 1995; 57:97.

187. Jagels MA, Hugli TE: Mechanisms and mediators of neutrophilic leukocytosis. Immunopharmacology 1994; 28:1.

188. Hechtman DH, Cybulsky MI, et al: Intravascular IL-8: Inhibitor of polymorphonuclear leukocyte accumulation at sites of acute inflammation. J Immunol 1991; 147:883.

189. Rosengren S, Olofsson AM, et al: Leukotriene B4-induced neutrophil-mediated endothelial leakage in vitro and in vivo. J Appl Physiol 1991; 71:1322.

190. Vaporciyan AA, DeLisser HM, et al: Involvement of platelet-endothelial cell adhesion molecule-1 in neutrophil recruitment in vivo. Science 1993; 262:1580.

191. Muller WA, Weigl SA, et al: PECAM-1 is required for transendothelial migration of leukocytes. J Exp Med 1993; 178:449.

192. Huang AJ, Manning JE, et al: Endothelial cell cytosolic free calcium regulates neutrophil migration across monolayers of endothelial cells. J Cell Biol 1993; 120:1371.

193. Weiss SJ: Tissue destruction by neutrophils. N Engl J Med 1989; 320:365.

194. Devreotes PN, Zigmond SH: Chemotaxis in eukaryotic cells: A focus on leukocytes and Dictyostelium. Annu Rev Cell Biol 1988; 4:649.

195. Hebert C, Baker J: Linkage of extracellular plasminogen activator to the fibroblast cytoskeleton: colocalization of cell surface urokinase with vinculi. J Cell Biol 1988; 156:1241.

196. Pepper M, Vassalli J, et al: Urokinase type plasminogen activator is induced in migrating capillary endothelial cells. J Cell Biol 1987; 105:23.

197. Estreicher A, Muhlhauser J, et al: The receptor for urokinase type plasminogen activator polarizes expression of the protease to the leading edge of migrating monocytes and promotes degradation of enzyme inhibitor complexes. J Cell Biol 1990; 111:783.

198. Zigmond SH: Cell locomotion and chemotaxis. Curr Opin Cell Biol 1989; 1:80.

199. Gyetko MR, Todd RF, et al: The urokinase receptor is required for human monocyte chemotaxis *in vitro*. J Clin Invest 1994; 93:1380.

200. Hartwing JH, Shevlin P: The architecture of actin filaments and the ultrastructural location of actin-binding protein in the periphery of lung macrophages. J Cell Biol 1986; 103:1007.

201. Cassimeris L, Safer D, et al: Thymosin B4 sequesters the majority of G-actin in resting human polymorphonuclear leukocytes. J Cell Biol 1992; 119:1261.

202. Ridley A, Hall A: The small GTP-binding protein Rac regulates growth factor-induced membrane ruffling. Cell 1992; 70:401.

203. Coates TD, Watts RG, et al: Relationship of F-actin distribution to development of polar shape in human polymorphonuclear neutrophils. J Cell Biol 1992; 117:765.

204. Cortese JD, Schwab B III, et al: Actin polymerization induces a shape change in actin-containing vesicles. Proc Natl Acad Sci U S A 1989; 86:5773.

205. Tilney LG, DeRosier DJ, Tilney MS: How listeria exploits host cell actin to form its own cytoskeleton. I. Formation of a tail and how that tail might be involved in movement. J Cell Biol 1992; 118:71.

206. Krieger M: Molecular flypaper and atherosclerosis: Structure of the macrophage scavenger receptor. Trends Biochem Sci 1992; 17:141.

207. Sastry K, Zahedi K, et al: Molecular characterization of the mouse mannose-binding proteins. The mannose-binding protein A but not C is an acute phase reactant. J Immunol 1991; 147:692.

208. Ezekowitz RA, Sastry K, et al: Molecular characterization of the human macrophage mannose receptor: Demonstration of multiple carbohydrate recognition-like domain and phagocytosis of yeasts in Cos-I cells. J Exp Med 1990; 172:1785.

209. Ezekowitz RA, Williams DJ, et al: Uptake of *Pneumocystis carinii* is mediated by the macrophage mannose receptor. Nature 1991; 351:155.

210. Huizinga TWJ, Roos D, van dem Borne AE: Neutrophil Fc-γ receptors: A two-way bridge in the immune system. Blood 1990; 75:1211.

211. McKenzie SE, Schreiber AD: Biological advances and clinical applications of Fc receptors for IgG. Curr Opin Hematol 1994; 1:45.

212. Metzger H: Handicapping the immune response. Curr Biol 1994; 4:644.

213. Ravetch JV: Fc receptors: Rubor redux. Cell 1994; 78:553.

214. Unkeless JC: Function and heterogeneity of human Fc receptors for immunoglobulin G. J Clin Invest 1989; 83:355.

215. Bux J, Mueller-Eckhardt C: Autoimmune neutropenia. Semin Hematol 1992; 29:45.

216. Maliszewski CR, March CJ, et al: Expression cloning of a human Fc receptor for IgA. J Exp Med 1990; 172:1665.

217. Kerr MA: The structure and function of human IgA. Biochem J 1990; 271:285.

218. Albrechtsen M, Yeaman GR, Kerr MA: Characterization of the IgA receptor from human polymorphonuclear leucocytes. Immunology 1988; 64:201.

219. Boxer LA, Smolen JE: Neutrophil granule constituents and their release in health and disease. Hematol Oncol Clin North Am 1988; 2:101.

220. Spitznagel JK: Antibiotic proteins of human neutrophils. J Clin Invest 1990; 86:1381.

221. D'Arcy Hart P, Young MR: Ammonium chloride, an inhibitor of phagosome-endosome fusion in macrophages, concurrently induces phagosome-endosome fusion and opens a novel pathway: studies of a pathogenic mycobacterium and a nonpathogenic yeast. J Exp Med 1991; 174:881.

222. Goren MB, D'Arcy Hart P, et al: Prevention of phagosome-lysosome fusion in cultured macrophages by sulfatides of *Mycobacterium* tuberculosis. Proc Natl Acad Sci U S A 1976; 73:2510.

223. Sibley LD, Hunter SW, et al: Mycobacterial lipoarabinomannan inhibits gamma interferon mediated action of macrophages. Infect Immunol 1988; 56:1232.

224. Horwitz MA, Maxfield FR: *Legionella pneumophila* inhibits acidification of its phagosome in human monocytes. J Cell Biol 1984; 99:1936.

225. Joiner KA, Fuhrman SA, et al: *Toxoplasma gondii*: Fusion competence of parasitophorous vacuoles in Fc receptor–transfected fibroblasts. Science 1990; 249:641.

226. Groisman EA, Saier MH: *Salmonella* virulence: New clues to intramacrophage survival. Trends Biochem Sci 1990; 15:30.

227. Kaufmann SHE: Immunity to intracellular bacteria. Annu Rev Immunol 1993; 11:129.

228. Weiss J: Leukocyte-derived antimicrobial proteins. Curr Opin Hematol 1994; 1:78.

229. Lehrer RI, Lichtenstein AK, Ganz T: Defensins: Antimicrobial and cytotoxic peptides of mammalian cells. Annu Rev Immunol 1993; 11:105.

230. Kagan BL, Ganz T, Lehrer RI: Defensins: A family of antimicrobial and cytotoxic peptides. Toxicology 1994; 87:131.

231. Elsbach P, Weiss J: Oxygen-independent antimicrobial systems of phagocytes. In Gallin JI, Goldstein IM, Snyderman R (eds): Inflammation: Basic Principles and Clinical Correlates. New York, Raven Press, 1992, p 603.

232. Pereira HA: CAP37, a neutrophil-derived multifunctional inflammatory mediator. J Leukoc Biol 1995; 57:805.

233. Arnold RR, Cole MF, McGhee JR: A bactericidal effect for human lactoferrin. Science 1977; 197:263.

234. Murphy MF, Sourial NA, et al: Megaloblastic anemia due to vitamin B_{12} deficiency caused by small intestinal bacterial overgrowth: Possible role of vitamin B_{12} analogues. Br J Haematol 1986; 62:7.

235. Cech P, Lehrer RI: Phagolysosomal pH of human neutrophils. Blood 1984; 63:88.

236. Segal AW, Geisow M, et al: The respiratory burst of phagocytic cells is associated with a rise in vacuolar pH. Nature 1981; 290:406.

237. Welsh IRH, Spitznagel JK: Distribution of lysosomal enzymes, cationic proteins, and bactericidal substances and subcellular fractions of human polymorphonuclear leukocytes. Infect Immun 1971; 4:97.

238. Babior BM: Oxygen-dependent microbial killing by phagocytes. N Engl J Med 1978; 298:659.

239. Baldridge CW, Gerard RW: The extra respiration of phagocytosis. Am J Physiol 1933; 103:235.

240. Sbarra AJ, Karnovsky ML: The biochemical basis of phagocytosis. I. Metabolic changes during the ingestion of particles by polymorphonuclear leukocytes. J Biol Chem 1959; 234:1355.

241. Smith RM, Curnutte JT: Molecular basis of chronic granulomatous disease. Blood 1991; 77:673.

242. Segal A: Cytochrome b_{-245} is a flavocytochrome containing FAD and the NADPH-binding site of the microbicidal oxidase of phagocytes. Biochem J 1992; 284:781.

243. Thrasher A, Keep N, et al: Review: Chronic granulomatous disease. Biochim Biophys Acta 1994; 1227:1.

244. Dinauer M: The respiratory burst oxidase and the molecular genetics of chronic granulomatous disease. Crit Rev Clin Lab Sci 1993; 30:329.

245. Gallin J, Leto T, et al: Delineation of the phagocyte NADPH oxidase through studies of chronic granulomatous diseases of childhood. Curr Opin Immunol 1992; 4:53.

246. Curnutte JT, Babior BM: Chronic granulomatous disease. In Harris H, Hirschhorn K (eds): Advances in Human Genetics. New York, Plenum Publishing Corp., 1987, p 229.

247. Cross AR, Jones OTG: Enzymic mechanisms of superoxide production. Biochim Biophys Acta 1991; 1057:281.

248. Babior BM, Kipnes RS, Curnutte JT: Biological defense mechanisms: The production by leukocytes of superoxide, a potential bactericidal agent. J Clin Invest 1973; 52:741.

249. Klebanoff SJ: Oxygen metabolites from phagocytes. In Gallin JI, Goldstein IM, Snyderman R (eds): Inflammation Basic Principles and Clinical Correlates. New York, Raven Press, 1992, p 541.

250. Royer-Pokora B, Kunkel LM, et al: Cloning the gene for an inherited human disorder—chronic granulomatous disease—on the basis of its chromosomal location. Nature 1986; 322:32.

251. Cross AR, Jones OTG, et al: Oxidation-reduction properties of the cytochrome *b* found in the plasma-membrane fraction of human neutrophils. Biochem J 1981; 194:599.

252. Parkos CA, Allen RA, et al: Purified cytochrome *b* from human granulocyte plasma membrane is comprised of two polypeptides with relative molecular weights of 91,000 and 22,000. J Clin Invest 1987; 80:732.

253. Rotrosen D, Yeung C, et al: Cytochrome *b558*: the flavin-binding component of the phagocyte NADPH oxidase. Science 1992; 256:1459.

254. Karplus PA, Daniels MJ, Herriott JR: Atomic structure of ferredoxin-NADT+ reductase: Prototype for a structurally novel flavoenzyme family. Science 1991; 251:60.

255. Roman DG, Dancis A, et al: The fission yeast ferric reductase gene frp1+ is required for ferric iron uptake and decodes a protein that is homologous to the gp91-phox subunit of the human NADPH phagocyte oxidoreductase. Molec Cell Biol 1993; 13:4342.

256. McPhail LC: SH3-dependent assembly of the phagocyte NADPH oxidase. J Exp Med 1994; 180:2011.

257. Leusen JHW, Bolscher GJM, et al: 156Pro→Gln substitution in the light chain of cytochrome. J Exp Med 1994; 180:2011.

258. Sumimoto H, Kage Y, et al: Role of Src homology 3 domains in assembly and activation of the phagocyte NADPH oxidase. Proc Natl Acad Sci U S A 1994; 91:5345.

259. Leto T, Adams A, De Mendez I: Assembly of the phagocyte NADPH oxidase: Binding of Src homology 3 domains to proline-rich targets. Proc Natl Acad U S A 1994; 91:10650.

260. Ohno YI, Hirai KI, et al: Subcellular localization of hydrogen peroxide production in human polymorphonuclear leukocytes stimulated with lectins, phorbol myristate acetate, and digitonin: An electron microscope study using CeCl3. Blood 1982; 60:1195.

261. Robinson JM, Badwey JA: The NADPH oxidase complex of phagocytic leukocytes: A biochemical and cytochemical view. Histochemistry 1995; 103:163.

262. Knaus U, Morris S, et al: Regulation of human leukocyte p21-activated kinases through G protein-coupled receptors. Science 1995; 269:221.

263. Bast A, Haenen GRMM, Doelman CJA: Oxidants and antioxidants: State of the art. Am J Med 1991; 91(Suppl 3):2.

264. Prince R, Gunson D: Rising interest in nitric oxide synthase. Trends Biochem Sci 1993; 18:35.

265. Marletta M: Nitric oxide synthase: Aspects concerning structure and catalysis. Cell 1994; 78:927.

266. Nathan C, Xie Q: Nitric oxide synthases: Roles, tolls, and controls. Cell 1994; 78:915.

267. MacMicking J, Nathan C, et al: Altered responses to bacterial infection and endotoxic shock in mice lacking inducible nitric oxide synthase. Cell 1995; 81:641.

268. De Maria R, Cifone MG, et al: Triggering of human monocyte activation through CD69, a member of the NKC family of signal transducing receptors. J Exp Med 1994; 180:1999.

269. Bukrinsky MI, Nottet HSLM, et al: Regulation of nitric oxide synthase activity in HIV-1–infected monocytes: Implications for HIV-associated neurological disease. J Exp Med 1995; 181:735.

270. Pollock J, Williams D, et al: Mouse model of X-linked chronic granulomatous disease, an inherited defect in phagocytes superoxide production. Nat Genet 1995; 9:202.

271. Green SJ, Meltzer MS, et al: Activated macrophages destroy intracellular *Leishmania major* amastigotes by an L-arginine–dependent killing mechanism. J Immunol 1990; 144:278.

272. Nathan CF: Mechanisms of macrophage antimicrobial activity. Trans R Soc Trop Hyg 1983; 77:620.

273. Edelson PJ: Intracellular parasites and phagocytic cells: Cell biology and pathophysiology. Rev Infect Dis 1982; 4:124.

274. Lowrie DB, Andrew PW: Macrophage antimycobacterial mechanisms. Br Med Bull 1988; 44:624.

275. Nelson DS: Macrophages as effectors of cell-mediated immunity. In Laskin AI, LeChevalier H (eds): Macrophages and Cellular Immunity. Cleveland, CRC Press, 1972, p 45.

276. Sharma SD, Remington JS: Macrophage activation and resistance to intracellular infection. Lymphokines 1981; 3:181.

277. Perlmutter RM: Antigen processing and T-cell effector mechanisms. In Stamatoyannopoulos G, Nienhuis AW, et al (eds): The Molecular Basis of Blood Diseases. Philadelphia, W.B. Saunders Co., 1994, p 463.

278. Knighton DR, Fiegel VD: Macrophage-derived growth factors in wound healing. Am Rev Respir Dis 1989; 140:1108.

279. Barbul A: Immune aspects of wound repair. Clin Plast Surg 1990; 17:433.

280. Cromack DT, Porras-Reyes B, Mustoe TA: Current concepts in wound healing: Growth factor and macrophage interaction. J Trauma 1990; 30:S129.

281. Leibovich SK, Ross R: The role of the macrophage in wound repair: A study with hydrocortisone and antimacrophage serum. Am J Pathol 1975; 78:71.

282. Sunderkotter C, Goebler M, et al: Macrophage-derived angiogenesis factors. Pharmacol Ther 1991; 51:195.

283. Uchida T, Akitsuki T, et al: Relationship among plasma iron, plasma iron turnover, and reticuloendothelial iron release. Blood 1983; 61:799.

284. Deiss A: Iron metabolism in reticuloendothelial cells. Semin Hematol 1983; 20:81.

285. Kraemer FB, Chen YD, et al: Characterization of the binding site on thioglycolate-stimulated mouse peritoneal macrophages that mediates uptake of very low density lipoproteins. J Biol Chem 1983; 258:12190.

286. Ross R: The pathogenesis of atherosclerosis: An update. N Engl J Med 1986; 314:488.

287. Steinberg D, Parthasrathy S, et al: Beyond cholesterol. Modifications of low-density lipoprotein that increase its atherogenicity. N Engl J Med 1989; 320:915.

288. Gleich GJ, Loegering DA: Immunobiology of eosinophils. Ann Rev Immunol 1984; 2:429.

289. Abu-Ghazaleh RI, Kita H, Gleich GJ: Eosinophil Activation and Function in Health. Rochester, MN, Mayo Clinic and Mayo Foundation, 1992.

290. Butterworth AE: Cell-mediated damage to helminths. Adv Parasitol 1984; 23:143.

291. Jong EC, Klebanoff SJ: Eosinophil-mediated mammalian tumor cell cytotoxicity: Role of the peroxidase system. J Immunol 1980; 124:1949.

292. Henderson WR Jr: Lipid-derived and other chemical mediators of inflammation in the lung. J Allergy Clin Immunol 1987; 79:543.

293. Kay AB: Biological properties of eosinophils. Clin Exp Allergy 1991; 21:23.

294. Frigas E, Loegering DA: Cytotoxic effects of the guinea pig eosinophil major basic protein on tracheal epithelium. Lab Invest 1980; 42:35.

295. Gleich GJ, Olson GM, Loegering DA: The effect of ablation of eosinophils on immediate-type hypersensitivity. Arch Pathol Lab Med 1975; 99:1.

296. Marone G, Casolaro V, et al: Pathophysiology of human basophils and mast cells in allergic disorders. Clin Immunol Immunopathol 1989; 50:524.

297. Sylvestre DL, Ravetch JV: Fc receptors initiate the Arthus reaction: Redefining the inflammatory cascade. Science 1994; 265:1095.

298. Henson PM, Johnston RB: Tissue injury in inflammation. J Clin Invest 1987; 79:669.

299. Jackson H, Cochrane C: Leukocyte-induced tissue injury. Hematol Oncol Clin North Am 1988; 2:317.

300. Lehr HA, Arfors KE: Mechanisms of tissue damage by leukocytes. Curr Opin Hematol 1994; 1:92.

301. Members of American College of Chest Physicians/Society of Critical Care Medicine Consensus Conference: Definition for sepsis and organ failure and guidelines for the use of innovative therapies in sepsis. Crit Care Med 1992; 20:864.

302. Brown KA: The polymorphonuclear cell in rheumatoid arthritis. Br J Rheumatol 1988; 27:150.

303a. Haug CE, Colvin RB, et al: A phase 1 trial of immunosuppression with anti-ICAM-1 (CD54) mAB in renal allograft recipients. Transplantation 1993; 55:766.

303. Weitzman SA, Gordon LI: Inflammation and cancer: Role of phagocyte-generated oxidants in carcinogenesis. Blood 1990; 76:655.

303a. Haug CE, Colvin RB, et al: A phase 1 trial of immunosuppression with anti-ICAM-1 (CD54) mAB in renal allograft recipients. Transplantation 1993; 55:766.

304. Ognibene FP, Martin SE: Adult respiratory distress syndrome in patients with severe neutropenia. N Engl J Med 1986; 315:547.

305. Brown EJ, Kloner RA, et al: Scar thinning due to ibuprofen administration after experimental myocardial infarction. Am J Cardiol 1983; 51:877.

306. Bulkley BH, Roberts WC: Steroid therapy during acute myocardial infarction. A cause of delayed healing and of ventricular aneurysm. Am J Med 1974; 56:244.

307. Sadowitz PO, Oski FA: Differences in polymorphonuclear cell counts between healthy white and black infants: Response to meningitis. Pediatrics 1983; 72:405.

308. Reed WW, Diehl LF: Leukopenia, neutropenia, and reduced hemoglobin levels in healthy American blacks. Arch Intern Med 1991; 151:501.

309. Karayalcin G, Rosner F, Sawitsky A: Pseudoneutropenia in American negroes. Lancet 1972; 1:387.

310. Pincus SH, Boxer LA, Stossel TP: Chronic neutropenia in childhood. Analysis of 16 cases and a review of the literature. Am J Med 1976; 61:849.

311. Baehner RL, Johnston RB Jr: Monocyte function in children with neutropenias and chronic infections. Blood 1972; 40:31.

312. Greenwood MF, Jones EA Jr, Holland P: Monocyte functional capacity in chronic neutropenia. Am J Dis Child 1978; 132:131.

313. Dale DC, Guerry D, et al: Chronic neutropenia. Medicine 1979; 58:128.

314. Howard MW, Strauss RG, Johnston RB: Infections in patients with neutropenia. Am J Dis Child 1977; 131:788.

315. Jonsson OG, Buchanan GR: Chronic neutropenia during childhood: A 13-year experience in a single institution. Am J Dis Child 1991; 145:232.

316. Sickles EA, Greene WH, Wiernik PH: Clinical presentation of infection in granulocytopenic patients. Arch Intern Med 1975; 135:715.

317. De Vaal OM, Seynhaeve V: Reticular dysgenesis. Lancet 1959; 2:1123.

318. Gitlin D, Vawter G, Craig JM: Thymic alymphoplasia and congenital aleukocytosis. Pediatrics 1964; 33:184.

319. Ownby DR, Pizzo S, et al: Severe combined immunodeficiency with leukopenia (reticular dysgenesis) in siblings: Immunologic and histopathologic findings. J Pediatr 1976; 89:382.

320. Roper M, Parmley RT, et al: Severe congenital leukopenia (reticular dysgenesis): Immunologic and morphologic characterizations of leukocytes. Am J Dis Child 1985; 139:832.

321. Alonso K, Dew JM, Starke WR: Thymic alymphoplasia and congenital aleukocytosis (reticular dysgenesis). Arch Pathol 1972; 94:179.

322. Levinsky RJ, Tiedeman K: Successful bone-marrow transplantation for reticular dysgenesis. Lancet 1983; 1:671.

323. Fischer A, Friedrich W, et al: Bone-marrow transplantation for immunodeficiencies and osteopetrosis: European survey, 1968–1985. Lancet 1986; 1:1080.

324. Kostmann R: Infantile genetic agranulocytosis. A review with presentation of ten new cases. Acta Paediatr Scand 1975; 64:362.

325. Parmley RT, Crist WM, et al: Congenital dysgranulopoietic neutropenia: Clinical, serologic, ultrastructural, and in vitro proliferative characteristics. Blood 1980; 56:465.

326. Parmley RT, Ogawa M, et al: Congenital neutropenia: Neutrophil proliferation with abnormal maturation. Blood 1975; 56:723.

327. Dong F, Hoefsloot LH, et al: Identification of a nonsense mutation in the granulocyte-colony-stimulating factor receptor in severe congenital neutropenia. Proc Natl Acad Sci U S A 1994; 91:4480.

328. Wriedt K, Kauder E, Mauer AM: Defective myelopoiesis in congenital neutropenia. N Engl J Med 1970; 283:1072.

329. Vadhan-Raj S, Jeha SS, et al: Stimulation of myelopoiesis in a patient with congenital neutropenia: Biology and nature of response to recombinant human granulocyte-macrophage colony-stimulating factor. Blood 1990; 75:858.

330. Bonilla MA, Gillio AP, et al: Effects of recombinant human granulocyte colony-stimulating factor on neutropenia in patients with congenital agranulocytosis. N Engl J Med 1989; 320:1574.

331. Pietsch T, Buhrer C, et al: Blood mononuclear cells from patients with severe congenital neutropenia are capable of producing granulocyte colony-stimulating factor. Blood 1991; 77:1234.

332. Mempel K, Pietsch T, et al: Increased serum levels of granulocyte colony-stimulating factor in patients with severe congenital neutropenia. Blood 1991; 77:1919.

333. Glasser L, Duncan BR, Corrigan JJ Jr: Measurement of serum granulocyte colony-stimulating factor in a patient with congenital agranulocytosis (Kostmann's syndrome). Am J Dis Child 1991; 145:925.

334. Moore MAS: Clinical implications of positive and negative hematopoietic stem cell regulators. Blood 1991; 78:1.

335. Dong F, Brynes RK, et al: Mutations in the gene for the granulocyte colony-stimulating-factor receptor in patients with acute myeloid leukemia preceded by severe congenital neutropenia. N Engl J Med 1995; 333:487.

335a. Guba SC, Sartor CA, et al: Granulocyte colony-stimulating factor (G-CSF) production and G-CSF receptor structure in patients with congenital neutropenia. Blood 1994; 83:1486.

336. Pahwa RN, O'Reilly RJ, et al: Partial correction of neutrophil deficiency in congenital neutropenia following bone marrow transplantation (BMT). Exp Hematol 1977; 5:45.

337. Rappeport JM, Parkman R, et al: Correction of infantile agranulocytosis (Kostmann's syndrome) by allogeneic bone marrow transplantation. Am J Med 1980; 68:605.

338. Welte K, Zeidler C, et al: Differential effects of granulocyte-macrophage colony-stimulating factor and granulocyte colony-stimulating factor in children with severe congenital neutropenia. Blood 1990; 75:1056.

339. Bonilla MA, Dale D, et al: Long-term safety of treatment with recombinant human granulocyte colony-stimulating factor (r-metHug-CSF) in patients with severe congenital neutropenias. Br J Haematol 1994; 88:723.

340. Weinblatt ME, Scimeca P, et al: Transformation of congenital neutropenia into monosomy 7 and acute nonlymphoblastic leukemia in a child treated with granulocyte colony-stimulating factor. J Pediatr 1995; 126:263.

341. Imashuku S, Hibi S, et al: Myelodysplasia and acute myeloid leukaemia in cases of aplastic anaemia and congenital neutropenia following G-CSF administration. Br J Haematol 1995; 89:188.

342. Rosen RB, Kang SJ: Congenital agranulocytosis terminating in acute myelomonocytic leukemia. J Pediatr 1979; 94:406.

343. Gilman PA, Jackson DP, Guild HG: Congenital agranulocytosis: Prolonged survival and terminal acute leukemia. Blood 1970; 36:576.

344. Dale DC, Hammond WP: Cyclic neutropenia: A clinical review. Blood Rev 1988; 2:178.

345. Wright DG, Dale DC, et al: Human cyclic neutropenia: Clinical review and long-term follow-up of patients. Medicine 1981; 60:1.

346. Leale M: Recurrent furunculosis in an infant showing an unusual blood picture. JAMA 1910; 54:1845.

347. Lange RO: Cyclic hematopoiesis: Human cyclic neutropenia. Exp Hematol 1983; 11:435.

348. Engelhard D, Landreth KS, et al: Cycling of peripheral blood and marrow lymphocytes in cyclic neutropenia. Proc Natl Acad Sci U S A 1983; 80:5734.

349. Krance RA, Spruce WE, et al: Human cyclic neutropenia transferred by allogeneic bone marrow grafting. Blood 1982; 60:1263.

350. Marshall G, Edwards K, et al: Syndrome of periodic fever, pharyngitis, and aphthous stomatitis. J Pediatr 1987; 110:43.

351. Hammond WP, Price TH, et al: Treatment of cyclic neutropenia with granulocyte colony-stimulating factor. N Engl J Med 1989; 320:1306.

352. Zuelzer WW: Myelokathexis—A new form of chronic granulocytopenia. N Engl J Med 1970; 282:231.

353. O'Regan S, Newman AJ, Graham RC: "Myelokathexis": Neutropenia with narrow hyperplasia. Am J Dis Child 1977; 131:655.

354. Rassam SMB, Roderick P, et al: A myelokathexis-like variant of myelodysplasia. Eur J Haematol 1989; 42:99.

355. Plebani A, Cantu-Rajnoldi A, et al: Myelokathexis associated with multiple congenital malformations: Immunological study on phagocytic cells and lymphocytes. Eur J Haematol 1988; 40:12.

356. Mamlok RJ, Juneja HS, et al: Neutropenia and defective chemotaxis associated with binuclear, tetraploid myeloid-monocytic leukocytes. J Pediatr 1987; 111:555.

356a. Liles WC, Park JR, et al: Myelokathexis—a congenital form of neutropenia characterized by accelerated apoptosis and defective expression of BCL-X in neutrophil precursors. Blood 1995; 86:259a.

357. Mentzer WC, Johnston RB Jr, et al: An unusual form of chronic neutropenia in a father and daughter with hypogammaglobulinemia. Br J Haematol 1977; 36:313.

358. Weston B, Axtell RA, et al: Clinical and biologic effects of granulocyte colony stimulating factor in the treatment of myelokathexis. J Pediatr 1991; 118:229.

359. Shmerling DH, Prader A, et al: The syndrome of exocrine pancreatic insufficiency, neutropenia, metaphyseal dysostosis and dwarfism. Helv Paediatr Acta 1969; 24:547.

360. Shwachman H, Diamond LK: The syndrome of pancreatic insufficiency and bone marrow dysfunction. J Pediatr 1964; 65:645.

361. Aggett PJ, Harries JT, et al: An inherited defect of neutrophil mobility in Shwachman's syndrome. J Pediatr 1979; 94:391.

362. Hill RE, Durie PR, et al: Steatorrhea and pancreatic insufficiency in Shwachman syndrome. Gastroenterology 1982; 83:22.

363. Huijgens PC, Van Der Veen EA, Muntinghe OG: Syndrome of Shwachman and leukaemia. Scand J Haematol 1977; 18:20.

364. Saunders EF, Gall G, Freedman MH: Granulopoiesis in Shwachman's syndrome (pancreatic insufficiency and bone marrow dysfunction). Pediatrics 1979; 64:515.

365. Tada H, Yoshida TR, et al: A case of Shwachman syndrome with increased spontaneous chromosome breakage. Hum Genet 1987; 77:289.

366. Bodian M, Sheldon W, Lightwood RI: Congenital hypoplasia of the exocrine pancreas. Acta Paediatr 1964; 53:282.

367. Aggett PJ, Cavanagh NPC, et al: Shwachman's syndrome. Arch Dis Child 1980; 55:331.

368. Paley C, Murphy S, et al: Treatment of neutropenia in Shwachman diamond syndrome (SDS) with recombinant human granulocyte colony stimulating factor (RH-GCSF). Blood 1991; 78:3a.

369. Trowbridge AA, Sirinavin CC, Linman JW: Dyskeratosis congenita: Hematologic evaluation of a sibship and review of the literature. Am J Hematol 1977; 3:143.

370. Witkop CJ Jr, Quevedo WC Jr, et al: Albinism. New York, McGraw-Hill Book Co., 1989.

371. Windhorst DB, Padgett G: The Chédiak-Higashi syndrome and the homologous trait in animals. J Invest Dermatol 1973; 60:529.

372. Wolff SM, Dale DC, et al: The Chédiak-Higashi syndrome: Studies of host defenses. Ann Intern Med 1972; 76:293.

373. Blume RS, Wolff SM: The Chédiak-Higashi syndrome: Studies in four patients and a review of the literature. Medicine 1972; 51:247.

374. Cutting HO, Lang JE: Familial benign chronic neutropenia. Ann Intern Med 1964; 61:876.

375. Mintz U, Sachs L: Normal granulocyte-forming cells in the bone marrow of yemenite Jews with genetic neutropenia. Blood 1973; 41:745.

376. Shaper AG, Lewis P: Genetic neutropenia in people of African origin. Lancet 1971; 1:1021.

377. Jacobs P: Familial benign chronic neutropenia. S Afr Med J 1975; 49:692.

378. Horsfall FL, Tamm L: Viral and Rickettsial Infections of Man. 4th ed. Philadelphia, J.B. Lippincott Co., 1965.

379. Murdoch JM, Smith CC: Hematological aspects of systemic disease: Infection. Clin Haematol 1972; 1:619.

380. Holbrook AA: The blood picture in chicken pox. Arch Intern Med 1941; 68:294.

381. Benjamin B, Ward SM: Leukocytic responses to measles. Am J Dis Child 1932; 44:921.

382. MacGregor RR, Friedman HM, et al: Virus infection of endothelial cells increased granulocyte adherence. J Clin Invest 1980; 65:1469.

383. Downie AW: Pathway of virus infection. In Smith E (ed): Mechanisms of Virus Infection. New York, Academic Press, Inc., 1963.

384. Ryan US, Schultz DR, Ruan JW: Fc and C3b receptors on pulmonary endothelial cells: Induction by injury. Science 1981; 214:557.

385. Cines DB, Lyss AP, et al: Fc and C3 receptors induced by herpes simplex virus on cultured human endothelial cells. J Clin Invest 1982; 69:123.

386. Habib MA, Babka JC, Burningham RA: Profound granulocytopenia associated with infectious mononucleosis. Am J Med Sci 1973; 265:339.

387. Hammond WP, Harlan JM, Steinberg SE: Severe neutropenia in infectious mononucleosis. West J Med 1979; 131:92.

388. Stevens DL, Everett ED, et al: Infectious mononucleosis with severe neutropenia and opsonic antineutrophil activity. South Med J 1979; 72:519.

389. Schooley RT, Densen P, et al: Antineutrophil antibodies in infectious mononucleosis. Am J Med 1984; 76:85.

390. Zon L, Groopman J: Hematologic manifestations of the human deficiency virus (HIV). Semin Hematol 1988; 25:208.

391. Israel DS, Plaisance KI: Neutropenia in patients infected with human immunodeficiency virus. Clin Pharmacol 1991; 10:268.

392. McCance-Katz E, Hoecker J, Vitale N: Severe neutropenia associated with anti-neutrophil antibody in a patient with acquired immunodeficiency syndrome–related complex. Pediatr Infect Dis 1987; 6:417.

393. Fronteira M, Myers A: Peripheral blood and bone marrow abnormalities in the acquired immunodeficiency syndrome. West J Med 1987; 147:157.

394. Dietrich HS: Typhoid fever in children. A study of 60 cases. J Pediatr 1937; 10:191.

395. Ball K, Jones H: Acute tuberculosis septicemia with leukopenia. BMJ 1951; 2:869.

396. Pullen RL, Stuart BM: Tularemia. JAMA 1945; 129:495.

397. Dale DC, Wolff SM: Studies of the neutropenia of acute malaria. Blood 1973; 41:197.

398. Nathan CF: Neutrophil activation on biological surfaces. J Clin Invest 1987; 80:1550.

399. Wolach B, Coates TD, et al: Plasma lactoferrin reflects granulocyte activation via complement in burn patients. J Lab Clin Med 1984; 103:284.

400. Chenoweth DE, Cooper SW, et al: Complement activation during cardiopulmonary bypass: Evidence for generation of C3a and C5a anaphylatoxins. N Engl J Med 1981; 304:497.

401. Craddock PR, Hammerschmidt DE, et al: Granulocyte aggregation as a manifestation of membrane interactions with complement: Possible role in leukocyte margination, microvascular occlusion, and endothelial damage. Semin Hematol 1979; 16:140.

402. Ivanovich P, Chenoweth DE, et al: Symptoms of activation of granulocytes and complement with two dialysis membranes. Kidney Int 1983; 24:758.

403. Strauss RG: Granulopoiesis and neutrophil function in the neonate. In Stockman JA, Pochedley CE (eds): Developmental and Neonatal Hematology. New York, Raven Press, 1988.

404. Cairo M: The use of granulocyte transfusions in neonatal sepsis. Trans Med Rev 1990; 4:14.

405. Christensen RD, Bradley PP, Rothstein G: The leukocyte left shift in clinical and experimental neonatal sepsis. Fetal Neonatal Med 1981; 98:101.

406. Christensen RD, Rothstein G, et al: Granulocyte transfusions in neonates with bacterial infection, neutropenia, and depletion of mature marrow neutrophils. Pediatrics 1982; 70:1.

407. Cairo M: Review of G-CSF and GM-CSF: Effects on neonatal neutrophil kinetics. Am J Pediatr Hematol Oncol 1989; 11:238.

408. Roberts RL, Szelc CM, et al: Neutropenia in an extremely premature infant treated with recombinant human granulocyte colony-stimulating factor. Am J Dis Child 1991; 145:808.

409. Gillan E, Christensen R, et al: A randomized, placebo-controlled trial of recombinant human granulocyte colony-stimulating factor administration in newborn infants with presumed sepsis: Significant induction of peripheral and bone marrow neutrophilia. Blood 1994; 84:1427.

410. The International Agranulocytosis and Aplastic Anemia Study Group: Risks of agranulocytosis and aplastic anemia: A first report of their relation to drug use and special reference to analgesics. JAMA 1986; 256:1749.

411. Pisciotta AV: Drug induced agranulocytosis peripheral destruction of polymorphonuclear leukocytes and their marrow precursors. Blood Rev 1990; 4:226.

412. Vincent PC: Drug-induced aplastic anemia and agranulocytosis: Incidence and mechanisms. Drugs 1986; 31:52.

413. Salama A, Schutz B, et al: Immune-mediated agranulocytosis related to drugs and their metabolites: Mode of sensitization and heterogeneity of antibodies. Br J Haematol 1989; 72:127.

414. Mamus SW, Burton JD, et al: Ibuprofen-associated pure white-cell aplasia. N Engl J Med 1986; 314:624.

415. Weitzman SA, Stossel TP: Drug-induced immunological neutropenia. Lancet 1978; 1:1068.

416. Pisciotta AV: Immune and toxic mechanisms in drug-induced agranulocytosis. Semin Hematol 1973; 10:291.

417. Heit WFW: Hematologic effects of antipyretic analgesics. Drug induced agranulocytosis. Am J Med 1983; 74:65.

418. Schroder H, Evans DAP: Acetylator phenotype and adverse effects of sulfasalazine in healthy subjects. Gut 1972; 13:278.

419. Murphy MF, Riordon T, et al: Demonstration of an immune-mediated mechanism of penicillin-induced neutropenia and thrombocytopenia. Br J Haematol 1983; 55:155.

420. Hartl PW: Drug-induced agranulocytosis. In Girdwood RH (ed): Blood Disorders Due to Drugs and Other Agents. Amsterdam, Excerpta Medica, 1973, p 147.

421. Uetrecht J: Drug metabolism by leukocytes and its role in drug-induced lupus and other idiosyncratic drug reactions. Crit Rev Toxicol 1990; 20:213.

422. Young GA, Vincent PC: Drug-induced agranulocytosis. Clin Haematol 1980; 9:438.

423. Editorial: Nitrous oxide and the bone-marrow. Lancet 1978; 2:613.

424. Shastri KA, Logue GL: Autoimmune neutropenia. Blood 1993; 81:1984.

425. Logue GL, Shimm DS: Autoimmune granulocytopenia. Annu Rev Med 1980; 31:191.

426. Currie MS, Weinberg JB, et al: Antibodies to granulocyte precursors in selective myeloid hypoplasia and other suspected autoimmune neutropenias: Use of HL-60 cells as targets. Blood 1987; 69:529.

427. Stroneck DF, Skubitz KM, et al: Biochemical characterization of the neutrophil specific antigen NB1. Blood 1990; 75:744.

428. Lucas GF, Carrington PA: Results of the First International Granulocyte Serology Workshop. Vox Sang 1990; 59:251.

429. Von Dem Borne AE: Neutrophil alloantigens: nature and clinical relevance. Vox Sang 1994; 67:105.

430. Hartman KR, Wright DG: Identification of autoantibodies specific for the neutrophil adhesion glycoproteins CD11b/CD18 in patients with autoimmune neutropenia. Blood 1991; 78:1096.

431. Boxer LA, Greenberg MS, et al: Autoimmune neutropenia. N Engl J Med 1975; 293:748.

432. Duckham DJ, Rhyne RL Jr, et al: Retardation of colony growth of *in vitro* bone marrow culture using sera from patients with Felty's syndrome, disseminated lupus erythematosus (DLE), rheumatoid arthritis and other disease states. Arthritis Rheum 1975; 18:323.

433. Lalezari P, Khorshidi M, Petrosova M: Autoimmune neutropenia in infancy. J Pediatr 1986; 109:764.

434. Neglia JP, Watterson J, et al: Autoimmune neutropenia of infancy and early childhood. Pediatr Hematol Oncol 1993; 10:369.

435. Lyall EGH, Lucas GF, Eden OB: Autoimmune neutropenia of infancy. J Clin Pathol 1992; 45:431.

436. Conway LT, Clay ME, et al: Natural history of primary autoimmune neutropenia in infancy. Pediatrics 1987; 79:728.

437. Miller ME, Oski FA, Harris MB: Lazy-leucocyte syndrome: A new disorder of neutrophil function. Lancet 1971; 1:665.

438. Yoda S, Morosawa H, et al: Transient "Lazy-Leukocyte" syndrome during infancy. Am J Dis Child 1980; 134:467.

439. Aggarwal J, Khan AJ, et al: Lazy leukocyte syndrome in a black infant. J Natl Med Assoc 1985; 77:928.

440. Komiyama A, Ishigura A, et al: Increases in neutrophil counts by purified human urinary colony-stimulating factor in chronic neutropenia of childhood. Blood 1988; 71:41.

441. Boxer LA: Immune neutropenias. Clinical and biological implications. Am J Pediatr Hematol Oncol 1981; 3:89.

442. Lalezari P, Radel E: Neutrophil antigens: Immunology and clinical implications. Semin Hematol 1974; 11:231.

443. Levine D, Madyastha P: Isoimmune neonatal neutropenia. Am J Perinatol 1986; 3:231.

444. Cartron J, Tchernia G, et al: Alloimmune neonatal neutropenia. Am J Pediatr Hematol Oncol 1991; 13:21.

445. Gilmore M, Stroncek D, Korones D: Treatment of alloimmune neonatal neutropenia with granulocyte colony-stimulating factor. J Pediatr 1994; 125:948.

446. Van Leeuwen EF, Roord JJ, et al: Neonatal neutropenia due to maternal autoantibodies against neutrophils. BMJ 1983; 287:94.

447. Payne R: Neonatal neutropenia and leukoagglutinins. Pediatrics 1964; 33:194.

448. Abilgaard H, Jensen KG: The influence of maternal leukocyte antibodies in infants. Scand J Haematol 1964; 1:47.

449. Buckley RH, Rowlands DJ: Agammaglobulinemia, neutropenia, fever and abdominal pain. J Allergy Clin Immunol 1973; 51:308.

450. Kozlowski C, Evans DI: Neutropenia associated with X-linked agammaglobulinaemia. J Clin Pathol 1991; 44:388.

451. Rosen FS, Cooper MD, Wedgwood RJP: The primary immunodeficiencies. N Engl J Med 1995; 333:431.

452. Rieger CHL, Moohr JW, Rothberg RM: Correction of neutropenia associated with dysgammaglobulinemia. Pediatrics 1974; 54:508.

453. Schaeffer FM, Monteiro RC, et al: IgA deficiency. In Rosen FS, Seligmann M (eds): Immunodeficiencies. Chur, Switzerland, Harwood Academic, 1993, p 77.

454. Lux SE, Johnston RB Jr, et al: Chronic neutropenia and abnormal cellular immunity in cartilage-hair hypoplasia. N Engl J Med 1970; 282:231.

455. McKusick VA, Eldridge R: Dwarfism in the Amish. II. Cartilage hair hypoplasia. Bull Johns Hopkins Hosp 1965; 116:285.

456. O'Reilly RJ, Brochstein J, et al: Marrow transplantation for congenital disorders. Semin Hematol 1984; 21:188.

457. Amman AJ, Hang F: Disorders of T cell system. In Steinham RF, Fulginiti VA (eds): Immunological Disorders in Infants and Children. Philadelphia, W.B. Saunders Co., 1980, p 286.

458. Bjorksten B, Lundmark KM: Recurrent bacterial infections in four siblings with neutropenia, eosinophilia, hyperimmunoglobulinemia A, and defective neutrophil chemotaxis. J Infect Dis 1976; 133:63.

459. Chudwin DS, Cowan MJ, et al: Response of agranulocytosis to prolonged antithymocyte globulin therapy. J Pediatr 1983; 103:223.

460. Soriano JR, Taitz LS, et al: Hyperglycinemia with ketoacidosis and leukopenia: Metabolic studies on the nature of the defect. Pediatrics 1967; 39:818.

461. Rosenberg LE, Fenton WA: Disorders of propionate and methylmalonate metabolism. In Scriver CR, Beaudet AL, et al (eds): The Metabolic Basis of Inherited Disease. New York, McGraw-Hill Book Co., 1989, p 821.

462. Sweetman L: Branched chain organic acidurias. In Scriver CR, Beaudet AL, et al (eds): The Metabolic Basis of Inherited Disease. New York, McGraw-Hill Book Co., 1989, p 791.

463. Childs B, Nyhan W, et al: Idiopathic hyperglycinemia and hyperglycinuria: A new disorder of amino acid metabolism. Pediatrics 1961; 27:522.

464. Beaudet AL, Anderson DC, et al: Neutropenia and impaired neutrophil migration in type 1B glycogen storage disease. J Pediatr 1980; 97:906.

465. Ambruso DR, McCabe ERB, et al: Infectious and bleeding complications in patients with glycogenosis Ib. Am J Dis Child 1985; 139:691.

466. Couper R, Kapelushnik J, Griffiths AM: Neutrophil dysfunction in glycogen storage disease Ib: Association with Crohn's-like colitis. Gastroenterology 1991; 100:549.

466a. Lindstedt S, Holme E, et al: Treatment of hereditary tyrosinaemia type I by inhibition of 4-hydroxyphenylpyruvate dioxygenase. Lancet 1992; 340:813.

467. Barth PG, Scholte HR, et al: An X-linked mitochondrial disease affecting cardiac muscle, skeletal muscle and neutrophil leucocytes. J Neuro Sci 1983; 62:327.

468. Kelley RI, Cheatham JP, et al: X-linked dilated cardiomyopathy with neutropenia, growth retardation, and 3-methylglutaconic aciduria. J Pediatr 1991; 119:738.

469. Ades LC, Gedeon AK, et al: Barth syndrome: Clinical features and confirmation of gene localisation to distal Xq28. Am J Med Genet 1993; 45:327.

470. Hutchinson RJ, Bunnell K, Thoene JG: Suppression of granulo-

poietic progenitor cell proliferation by metabolites of the branched chain amino acids. J Pediatr 1985; 106:62.

471. Wang WC, Crist WM, et al: Granulocyte colony-stimulating factor corrects the neutropenia associated with glycogen storage disease type. Leukemia 1991; 5:347.

472. Schroten H, Wendel U, et al: Colony-stimulating factors for neutropenia in glycogen storage disease Ib. Lancet 1991; 337:736.

473. Liel Y, Rudich A, et al: Monocyte dysfunction in patients with Gaucher disease: Evidence for interference of glucocerebroside with superoxide generation. Blood 1994; 83:2646.

474. Aker M, Zimran A, et al: Abnormal neutrophil chemotaxis in Gaucher disease. Br J Haematol 1993; 83:187.

475. Perillie PE, Kaplan SS, Finch SC: Significance of changes in serum muramidase activity in megaloblastic anemia. N Engl J Med 1967; 277:10.

476. Pearson HA: Marrow hypoplasia in anorexia nervosa. J Pediatr 1967; 71:211.

477. Zidar BL, Shadduck RK, et al: Observations on the anemia and neutropenia of human copper deficiency. Am J Hematol 1977; 3:177.

478. Al-Rashid RA, Spangler J: Neonatal copper deficiency. N Engl J Med 1971; 285:841.

479. Natelson EA, Lynch EC, et al: Histiocytic medullary reticulosis: The role of phagocytosis in pancytopenia. Arch Intern Med 1968; 122:223.

480. Boxer LA, Camitta BM, et al: Myelofibrosis-myeloid metaplasia in childhood. Pediatrics 1975; 55:861.

481. Crail HW, Alt HL, Nadler WH: Myelofibrosis associated with tuberculosis—a report of four cases. Blood 1948; 3:1426.

482. Erf LA, Herbut PA: Primary and secondary myelofibrosis: A clinical and pathological study of thirteen cases of fibrosis of the bone marrow. Ann Intern Med 1945; 21:863.

483. Ward H, Block MH: The natural history of agnogenic myeloid metaplasia and a critical evaluation of its relationship with the myeloproliferative syndrome. Medicine 1971; 50:357.

484. Price TH, Lee MY, et al: Neutrophil kinetics in chronic neutropenia. Blood 1979; 54:581.

485. Greenburg PL, Mara B, et al: The chronic idiopathic neutropenic syndrome: Correlation of clinical features with in vitro parameters of granulocytopoiesis. Blood 1980; 55:915.

486. Logue GL, Shastri KA, et al: Idiopathic neutropenia: Antineutrophil antibodies and clinical correlations. Am J Med 1991; 90:211.

487. Jakabowski AA, Souza L, et al: Effects of human granulocyte colony-stimulating factor in a patient with idiopathic neutropenia. N Engl J Med 1989; 320:38.

488. Strauss RG: Therapeutic granulocyte transfusions in 1993. Blood 1993; 31:1675.

489. Huestis DW, Glasser L: Neutrophil in transfusion medicine. Transfusion 1994; 34:630.

490. Dale DC: Potential role of colony-stimulating factors in the prevention and treatment of infectious diseases. Clin Infect Dis 1994; 18:S180.

491. Coulombel L, Dehan M, et al: The number of polymorphonuclear leukocytes in relation to gestational age in the newborn. Acta Paediatr Scand 1979; 68:709.

492. Cartwright GE, Athens JW: Blood granulocyte kinetics in conditions associated with granulocytosis. Ann NY Acad Sci 1964; 113:963.

493. Athens JW: Leukocyte physiology. JAMA 1966; 198:38.

494. Boxer LA, Allen JM, Baehner RL: Diminished polymorphonuclear leukocyte adherence. Function dependent on release of cyclic AMP by endothelial cells after stimulation of beta-receptors by epinephrine. J Clin Invest 1980; 66:268.

495. Ostlund RE, Bishop CR, Athens JW: Evaluation of non-steady-state neutrophil kinetics during endotoxin-induced granulocytosis. Proc Soc Exp Biol Med 1968; 137:461.

496. Dale DC, Fauci AS, et al: Comparison of agents producing a neutrophilic leukocytosis in man. J Clin Invest 1975; 56:808.

497. Bishop CR, Athens JW, et al: Leukokinetic studies: XIII. A non-steady-state evaluation of the mechanism of cortisone-induced granulocytosis. J Clin Invest 1968; 47:249.

498. Rey JJ, Wolf PL: Extreme leukocytosis in accidental electric shock. Lancet 1968; I:18.

499. Watkins J, Ward AM: Changes in peripheral blood leukocytes following I.V. anaesthesia and surgery. Br J Anaesthesiol 1977; 49:953.

500. Ryhanen P: Effects of anesthesia and operative surgery on the immune response of patients of different ages. Ann Clin Res 1977; 9(Suppl):19.

501. Walker RI, Willemze R: Neutrophil kinetics and the regulation of granulopoiesis. Rev Infect Dis 1980; 2:282.

502. Shoenfeld Y, Gurewich Y: Prednisone-induced leukocytosis. Influence of dosage, method, and duration of administration on the degree of leukocytosis. Am J Med 1981; 71:773.

503. Milhout AT, Small SM: Leukocytosis during various emotional states. Arch Neurol Psychiatry 1942; 47:779.

504. Craddock CG, Perry S: Dynamics of leukopoiesis and leukocytosis, as studied by leukapheresis and isotopic techniques. J Clin Invest 1956; 35:285.

505. Peterson LA, Hrisinko MA: Benign lymphocytosis and reactive neutrophilia. Clin Lab Med 1993; 13:863.

506. Holland P, Mauer AM: Myeloid leukemoid reactions in children. Am J Dis Child 1963; 105:568.

507. Calabro JJ, Williamson P: Kawasaki syndrome. N Engl J Med 1982; 306:237.

508. Finch SC: Laboratory findings in infectious mononucleosis. In Carter RL, Penman HG (eds): Infectious Mononucleosis. Oxford, Blackwell Scientific Publications, 1969, p 57.

509. Skarberg KO: Leukaemia, leukaemoid reaction and tuberculosis. Acta Med Scand 1967; 182:427.

510. Schaller J, Wedgewood R: Juvenile rheumatoid arthritis: A review. Pediatrics 1970; 50:940.

511. McBride JA, Dacie JV: The effect of splenectomy on the leukocyte count. Br J Haematol 1968; 14:225.

512. Herring WB, Smith LB, et al: Hereditary neutrophilia. Am J Med 1974; 56:729.

513. Tindall JP, Beeker SK, Rosse WF: Familial cold urticaria. A generalized reaction involving leukocytosis. Arch Intern Med 1969; 124:129.

514. Hendrik M, Doeglas M, Bleumink E: Familial cold urticaria. Clinical findings. Arch Dermatol 1974; 110:382.

515. MacDougall LG, Strickwold B: Myeloid leukemoid reactions in South African blacks. S Afr Med J 1978; 53:14.

516. Tullis JL: A cause of leukocytosis in diabetic acidosis: Effects of experimental hypertonia on circulating leukocytes. J Clin Invest 1947; 26:1098.

517. Nettleship A: Leukocytosis associated with acute inflammation. Am J Clin Pathol 1938; 8:398.

518. Engel RR, Hammond D: Transient congenital leukemia in seven children with mongolism. J Pediatr 1964; 65:303.

519. Dignan PS, Mauer AM, Frantz C: Phocomelia with congenital hypoplastic thrombocytopenia and myeloid leukemoid reactions. J Pediatr 1967; 70:561.

520. Basten A, Beeson PB: Mechanisms of eosinophilia: II. Role of the lymphocyte. J Exp Med 1970; 131:1288.

521. Bass DA, Lewis JC: Biochemistry and metabolism of human eosinophils. Trans R Soc Trop Med Hyg 1980; 74(Suppl):11.

522. Stickney JM, Heck FJ: The clinical occurrence of eosinophilia. Med Clin North Am 1944; 28:914.

523. Lowell FC: Clinical aspects of eosinophilia in atopic diseases. JAMA 1967; 202:109.

524. Lecka HI, Kravis L: The allergist and the eosinophil. Pediatr Clin North Am 1969; 16:125.

525. Donohugh DL: Eosinophils and eosinophilia. Calif Med 1966; 104:421.

526. Haeberle MG, Griffen WO Jr: Eosinophilia and regional enteritis. A possible diagnostic aid. Am J Digest Dis 1972; 17:200.

527. Beeson PB, Bass DA: The Eosinophil. Philadelphia, W.B. Saunders Co., 1977.

528. Hoy WE, Castero RVM: Eosinophilia in maintenance hemodialysis patients. J Dialysis 1979; 3:73.

529. Lee S, Schoen I: Eosinophilia and peritoneal fluid and peripheral blood associated with chronic peritoneal dialysis. Am J Clin Pathol 1967; 47:638.

530. Conrad ME: Hematologic manifestations of parasitic infections. Semin Hematol 1971; 8:267.

531. Huntley CC, Costas MD, Lyerly A: Visceral larvae migrans syndrome. Clinical characteristics in immunologic studies in 51 patients. Pediatrics 1965; 36:523.

532. Mok CH: Visceral larvae migrans: A discussion based on review of the literature. Clin Pediatr 1968; 7:565.

533. Aur JA, Pratt CB, Johnson WW: Thiabendazole and visceral larvae migrans. Am J Dis Child 1971; 121:226.

534. Naiman JL, Oski FA, et al: Hereditary eosinophilia. Report on a family and review of literature. Am J Hum Genet 1971; 16:195.

535. Chusid MJ, Dale DC, et al: The hypereosinophilic syndrome: Analysis of fourteen cases with review of the literature. Medicine 1975; 54:1.

536. Weller PF, Bubley GJ: The idiopathic hypereosinophilic syndrome. Blood 1994; 83:2759.

537. Spry CJ: The hypereosinophilic syndrome: Clinical features, laboratory findings and treatment. Allergy 1982; 37:539.

538. Fauci A, Harley J, et al: The idiopathic hypereosinophilic syndrome. Clinical, pathophysiologic, and therapeutic considerations. Ann Intern Med 1982; 97:78.

539. da Silva M, Heerema N, et al: Evidence for the clonal nature of hypereosinophilic syndrome. Cancer Genet Cytogenet 1988; 32:109.

540. Bennett J, Catovsky D, Daniel M: Proposed revised criteria for the classification of acute myeloid leukemia. A report of the French-American-British cooperative group. Ann Intern Med 1985; 103:626.

541. Liu PP, Hajra A, et al: Molecular pathogenesis of the chromosome 16 inversion in the M4Eo subtype of acute myeloid leukemia. Blood 1995; 85:2289.

542. Bass DA: Eosinopenia. In Mahmoud AAF, Austen KF (eds): The Eosinophil in Health and Disease. New York, Grune & Stratton, Inc., 1980, p 275.

543. Shelley WB, Parnes HM: The absolute basophil count. JAMA 1965; 192:108.

544. Juhlin L: Basophil leukocytes in ulcerative colitis. Acta Med Scand 1963; 173:351.

545. Fredericks RE, Maloney WC: The basophilic granulocyte. Blood 1959; 14:571.

546. May ME, Waddell CC: Basophils in peripheral blood and bone marrow. A retrospective review. Am J Med 1984; 76:509.

547. Athreya BH, Moser G, Raghaven TES: Increased circulating basophils in juvenile rheumatoid arthritis. Am J Dis Child 1975; 129:935.

548. Lennert K, Koster E, et al: Über die Mastzellen-leukaemie. Acta Haematol 1956; 16:255.

549. Rosenthal S, Schwartz JH, Canellos GP: Basophilic chronic granulocytic leukemia with hyperhistaminemia. Br J Haematol 1977; 36:367.

550. Juhlin L: Basophil and eosinophil leukocytes in various internal disorders. Acta Med Scand 1963; 174:249.

551. Galli SJ, Colvin RB, et al: Patients without basophils. Lancet 1977; 2:409.

552. Juhlin L, Michaelsson G: A new syndrome characterized by absence of eosinophils and basophils. Lancet 1977; 1:1233.

553. Kato K: Leukocytes in infancy and childhood: A statistical analysis of 1,081 total and differential counts from birth to fifteen years. J Pediatr 1935; 7:7.

554. Maldonado JE, Hanlon DG: Monocytosis: A current appraisal. Mayo Clin Proc 1965; 40:248.

555. Koeffler HP, Golde DW: Human preleukemia. Ann Intern Med 1980; 93:347.

556. Ultmann JE: Clinical features and diagnosis of Hodgkin's disease. Cancer 1966; 9:297.

557. Scully FJ: The reaction after intravenous injections of foreign protein. JAMA 1917; 69:20.

558. Thompson J, Van Furth R: The effect of glucocorticoids on the proliferation and kinetics of promonocytes and monocytes of the bone marrow. J Exp Med 1973; 137:10.

559. Valkmann A, Gowans JL: The production of macrophages in the rat. Br J Exp Pathol 1965; 46:50.

559a. Twomey CC, Douglass CC, Sharkey O Jr: The monocytopenia of aplastic anemia. Blood 1973; 41:187.

560. Anderson DC, Springer TA: Leukocyte adhesion deficiency: An inherited defect in the Mac-1, LFA-1 and p150, 95 glycoproteins. Annu Rev Med 1987; 38:175.

561. Anderson DC, Schmalsteig FC, et al: The severe and moderate phenotypes of heritable Mac-1, LFA-1 deficiency: Their quantitative definition and relation to leukocyte dysfunction and clinical features. J Infect Dis 1985; 152:668.

562. Todd RF III, Freyer DR: The CD11/CD18 leukocyte glycoprotein deficiency. Hematol Oncol Clin North Am 1988; 2:13.

563. Fischer A, Lisowska-Grospierre B, et al: Leukocyte adhesion deficiency: Molecular basis and functional consequences. Immunodefic Rev 1988; 1:39.

564. Crowley CA, Curnutte JT, et al: An inherited abnormality of neutrophil adhesion: Its genetic transmission and its association with a missing protein. N Engl J Med 1980; 302:1163.

565. Arnaout MA, Pitt J, et al: Deficiency of a granulocyte-membrane glycoprotein (gp150) in a boy with recurrent bacterial infections. N Engl J Med 1982; 306:693.

566. Bowen TJ, Ochs HD, et al: Severe recurrent bacterial infections associated with defective adherence and chemotaxis in two patients with neutrophils deficient in a cell-associated glycoprotein. J Pediatr 1982; 101:932.

567. Dana N, Todd RF III, et al: Deficiency of a surface membrane glycoprotein (Mo1) in man. J Clin Invest 1984; 73:153.

568. Arnaout MA: Leukocyte adhesion molecules deficiency: Its structural basis, pathophysiology and implications for modulating the inflammatory response. Immunol Rev 1990; 114:145.

569. von Andrian UH, Berger EM, et al: In vivo behavior of neutrophils from two patients with distinct inherited leukocyte adhesion deficiency syndromes. J Clin Invest 1993; 91:2893.

570. Davies KA, Toothill VJ, et al: A 19-year-old man with leukocyte adhesion deficiency. In vitro and in vivo studies of leucocyte function. Clin Exp Immunol 1991; 84:223.

571. Hemler M, Lobb R, Phil D: The leukocyte 1 integrins. Curr Opin Hematol 1995; 2:61.

572. Beller DI, Springer TA, Schreiber RD: Anti-Mac 1 selectively inhibits the mouse and human type three complement receptor. J Exp Med 1982; 156:1000.

573. Krensky AM, Sanchez-Madrid F, et al: The functional significance, distribution, and structure of LFA-1, LFA-2, LFA-3: Cell surface antigens associated with CTL-target interactions. J Immunol 1983; 131:611.

574. Kohl S, Springer TA, et al: Defective natural killer cytotoxicity and polymorphonuclear leukocyte antibody-dependent cellular cytotoxicity in patients with LFA-1/OKM-1 deficiency. J Immunol 1984; 133:2972.

575. Kohl S, Loo LS, et al: The genetic deficiency of leukocyte surface glycoprotein Mac-1, LFA-1, p150, 95 in humans is associated with defective antibody-dependent cellular cytotoxicity in vitro and defective protection against herpes simplex virus infection in vivo. J Immunol 1986; 137:1688.

576. Hibbs ML, Wardlaw AJ, et al: Transfection of cells from patients with leukocyte adhesion deficiency with an integrin β subunit (CD18) restores lymphocyte function-associated antigen-1 expression and function. J Clin Invest 1990; 85:674.

577. Springer TA, Thompson WS, et al: Inherited deficiency of the Mac-1, LFA-1, p150, 95 glycoprotein family and its molecular basis. J Exp Med 1984; 160:1901.

578. Marlin SD, Morton CC, et al: LFA-1 immunodeficiency disease: Definition of the genetic defect and chromosomal mapping of alpha and beta subunits by complementation in hybrid cells. J Exp Med 1986; 164:855.

579. Curnutte J, Orkin S, Dinauer M: Genetic disorders of phagocyte function. In Stamatoyannopoulos G (ed): The Molecular Basis of Blood Diseases. 2nd ed. Philadelphia, W.B. Saunders Co., 1994, p 493.

580. Ohashi Y, Yambe T, et al: Familial genetic defect in a case of leukocyte adhesion deficiency. Hum Mutat 1993; 2:458.

581. Back AL, Kerkering M, et al: A point mutation associated with leukocyte adhesion deficiency type 1 of moderate severity. Biochem Biophys Res Commun 1993; 193:912.

582. Corbi AL, Vara A, et al: Molecular basis for a severe case of leukocyte adhesion deficiency. Eur J Immunol 1992; 22:1877.

583. Arnaout MA, Dana N, et al: Point mutations impairing cell surface expression of the common β subunit (CD18) in a patient with leukocyte adhesion molecule (Leu-CAM) deficiency. J Clin Invest 1990; 85:977.

584. Wardlaw AJ, Hibbs ML, et al: Distinct mutations in two patients with leukocyte adhesion deficiency and their functional correlates. J Exp Med 1990; 172:335.

585. Sligh JE Jr, Hurwitz MY, et al: An initiation codon mutation in CD18 in association with the moderate phenotype of leukocyte adhesion deficiency. J Biol Chem 1992; 267:714.

586. Back AL, Hickstein DD: Two different CD18 mutations in a child with severe leukocyte adhesion deficiency (LAD). Blood 1990; 76:176a. Abstract.

587. Nelson C, Rabb H, Arnaout MA: Genetic cause of leukocyte adhesion molecule deficiency. Abnormal splicing and a missense mutation in a conserved region of CD18 impair cell surface expression of 2 integrins. J Biol Chem 1992; 267:3351.

588. Kishimoto TK, O'Connor K, Springer TA: Leukocyte adhesion deficiency: Aberrant splicing of a conserved integrin sequence causes a moderate deficiency phenotype. J Biol Chem 1989; 264:3588.

589. Lopez RC, Nueda A, et al: Characterization of two new CD18 alleles causing severe leukocyte adhesion deficiency. Eur J Immunol 1993; 23:2792.

590. Giger U, Boxer LA, et al: Deficiency of leukocyte surface glycoproteins Mo1, LFA-1, and Leu M5 in a dog with recurrent bacterial infections: An animal model. Blood 1987; 69:1622.

591. Renshaw HW, Davis WC: Canine granulocytopathy syndrome: An inherited disorder of leukocyte function. Am J Pathol 1979; 95:731.

592. Hagemoser WA, Roth JA, et al: Granulocytopathy in a Holstein heifer. J Am Vet Med Assoc 1983; 183:1093.

593. Kehrli ME, Ackermann MR, et al: Animal model of human disease. Bovine leukocyte adhesion deficiency. β2 integrin deficiency in young Holstein cattle. Am J Pathol 1992; 140:1489.

594. Kehrli ME, Schmalstieg FC, et al: Molecular definition of the bovine granulocytopathy syndrome: Identification of deficiency of the Mac-1 (CD11b/CD18) glycoprotein. Am J Vet Res 1990; 51:1826.

595. Shuster D, Kehrli M, et al: Identification and prevalence of a genetic defect that causes leukocyte adhesion deficiency in Holstein cattle. Proc Natl Acad Sci U S A 1992; 89:9225.

596. Wilson RW, Ballantyne CM, et al: Gene targeting yields a CD18-mutant mouse for study of inflammation. J Immunol 1993; 151:1571.

597. Arnaout MA, Spits H, et al: Deficiency of a leukocyte surface glycoprotein (LFA-1) in two patients with Mo1 deficiency. Effects of cell activation on Mo1/LFA-1 surface expression in normal and deficient leukocytes. J Clin Invest 1984; 74:1291.

598. Weisman SJ, Mahoney MJ, et al: Prenatal diagnosis for Mo1 (CDw18) deficiency. Clin Res 1987; 35:435a. Abstract.

599. Anderson DC, Smith CW, Springer TA: Leukocyte adhesion deficiency and other disorders of leukocyte motility. In Scriver CR, Beaudet AL (eds): The Metabolic Basis of Inherited Disease. New York, McGraw-Hill Book Co., 1989, p 2751.

600. Fischer A, Descamps-Latscha B, et al: Bone marrow transplantation for inborn error of phagocytic cells associated with defective adherence, chemotaxis and oxidative response during opsonized particle phagocytosis. Lancet 1983; 2:473.

601. Krauss J, Mayo-Bond L, et al: An in vivo animal model of gene therapy for leukocyte adhesion deficiency. J Clin Invest 1991; 88:1412.

602. Wilson JM, Ping AJ, et al: Correction of CD18-deficient lymphocytes by retrovirus-mediated gene transfer. Science 1990; 248:1413.

603. Back AL, Kwok WW, et al: Retroviral-mediated gene transfer of the leukocyte integrin CD18 subunit. Biochem Biophys Res Commun 1990; 171:787.

604. Mulligan R: The basic science of gene therapy. Science 1993; 260:926.

605. Karlsson S: Treatment of genetic defects in hematopoietic cell function by gene transfer. Blood 1991; 78:2481.

606. Etzioni A, Frydman M, et al: A syndrome of leukocyte adhesion deficiency (LAD II) due to deficiency of Sialyl-Lewis-X, a ligand for selectins. N Engl J Med 1992; 327:1789.

607. Price TH, Ochs HD, et al: In vivo neutrophil and lymphocyte function studies in a patient with leukocyte adhesion deficiency type II. Blood 1994; 84:1635.

608. Oseas RS, Allen J, et al: Mechanism of dexamethasone inhibition of chemotactic factor-induced granulocyte aggregation. Blood 1982; 59:265.

609. Skubitz KM, Craddock PR, et al: Corticosteroids block binding of chemotactic peptide to the receptor on granulocytes and cause disaggregation of granulocyte aggregates in vitro. J Clin Invest 1981; 68:13.

610. Bryant RE, Sutcliff MC: The effect of 3′, 5′-adenosine monophosphate on granulocyte adhesion. J Clin Invest 1974; 54:1241.

611. Craddock PR, Fehr J, et al: Complement-and leukocyte-mediated pulmonary dysfunction in hemodialysis. N Engl J Med 1977; 196:769.

612. Heflin AC Jr, Brigham KL: Prevention by granulocyte depletion of increased vascular permeability of sheep lung following endotoxemia. J Clin Invest 1981; 68:1253.

613. Craddock PR, Hammerschmidt D, White JG: Complement (C5a)-induced granulocyte aggregation in vitro: A possible mechanism of complement-mediated leukostasis and leukopenia. J Clin Invest 1977; 60:260.

614. Tate RM, Repine JE: Neutrophils and the adult respiratory distress syndrome. Am Rev Respir Dis 1983; 128:552.

615. Wright DG, Robiechaud KJ, et al: Lethal pulmonary reactions associated with the combined use of amphotericin B and leukocyte transfusions. N Engl J Med 1981; 304:1185.

616. Boxer LA, Ingraham LM, et al: Amphotericin B promotes leukocyte aggregation of nylon wool fiber-treated polymorphonuclear leukocytes. Blood 1981; 58:518.

617. Brown CC, Gallin JI: Chemotactic disorders. Hematol Oncol Clin North Am 1988; 2:61.

618. Boyden S: The chemotactic effect of mixtures of antibody and antigen on polymorphonuclear leukocytes. J Exp Med 1962; 115:453.

619. Smith CW, Hollers JC, et al: Motility and adhesiveness in human neutrophils: Effects of chemotactic factors. J Clin Invest 1979; 63:221.

620. Nelson RD, Quie PG, Simmons RL: Chemotaxis under agarose: A new and simple method for measuring chemotaxis and spontaneous migration of human polymorphonuclear leukocytes and monocytes. J Immunol 1975; 115:1650.

621. Rebuck JW, Crowley JH: A method of studying leukocytic functions. Ann N Y Acad Sci 1955; 59:757.

622. Leung DYM, Geha RS: Clinical and immunologic aspects of the hyperimmunoglobulin E syndrome. Hematol Oncol Clin North Am 1988; 2:81.

623. Davis SD, Schaller J, Wedgwood RJ: Job's syndrome: Recurrent, "cold," staphylococcal abscesses. Lancet 1966; 1:1013.

624. Donabedian H, Gallin JI: The hyperimmunoglobulin E recurrent-infection (Job's) syndrome. A review of the NIH experience and the literature. Medicine 1983; 62:195.

625. Buckley RH, Wray BB, Belmaker EZ: Extreme hyperimmunoglobulinemia E and undue susceptibility to infection. Pediatrics 1972; 49:59.

626. Buckley RH: Immunodeficiency, hyper IgE type. In Buyse ML (ed): Birth Defects Encyclopedia. Cambridge, England, Blackwell Scientific Publications, Inc., 1990, p 953.

627. Hill HR, Estensen RD, et al: Severe staphylococcal disease associated with allergic manifestation, hyperimmunoglobulinemia E, and defective neutrophil chemotaxis. J Lab Clin Med 1976; 88:796.

628. Hill HR, Ochs HD, et al: Defect in neutrophil granulocyte chemotaxis in Job's syndrome of recurrent "cold" staphylococcal abscesses. Lancet 1974; 2:617.

629. Mawhinney H, Killen M, et al: The hyperimmunoglobulin E syndrome: A neutrophil chemotactic defect reversible by histamine H2 receptor blockade? Clin Immunol Immunopathol 1980; 17:483.

630. Buckley RH, Becker WG: Abnormalities in the regulation of human IgE synthesis. Immunol Rev 1978; 41:288.

631. Geha RS, Reinherz E, et al: Deficiency of suppressor T cells in hyperimmunoglobulin E syndrome. J Clin Invest 1981; 68:783.

632. Martricardi PM, Capobianchi MR: Interferon production in primary immunodeficiencies. J Clin Immunol 1984; 4:388.

633. Del Prete G, Tiri A, et al: Defective in vitro production of gamma interferon and tumor necrosis factor-alpha by circulating T cells from patients with the hyper-immunoglobulin E syndrome. J Clin Invest 1989; 84:1830.

634. Sheerin KA, Buckley RH: Antibody responses to protein, polysaccharide, and phi X174 antigens in the hyperimmunoglobulinemia E (hyper-IgE) syndrome. J Allergy Clin Immunol 1991; 87:803.

635. Donabedian H, Gallin JI: Two inhibitors of neutrophil chemotaxis are produced by hyperimmunoglobulin E recurrent infec-

tion syndrome mononuclear cells exposed to heat-killed staphylococci. Infect Immun 1983; 40:1030.

636. Donabedian H, Gallin JI: Mononuclear cells from patients with the hyperimmunoglobulin E–recurrent infection syndrome produce an inhibitor of leukocyte chemotaxis. J Clin Invest 1982; 69:115.

637. Merten DF, Buckley RH, et al: Hyperimmunoglobulinemia E syndrome: Radiographic observations. Radiology 1979; 132:71.

638. Snapper CM, Paul WE: Interferon-gamma and B cell stimulatory factor-1 reciprocally regulate Ig isotype production. Science 1987; 236:944.

639. Coffman RL, Carty J: A T-cell activity that enhances polyclonal IgE production and its inhibition by interferon-gamma. J Immunol 1986; 136:949.

640. Matricardi PM, Capobianchi MR, et al: Interferon production in primary immunodeficiencies. J Clin Immunol 1984; 4:388.

641. King CL, Gallin JI, et al: Regulation of immunoglobulin production in hyperimmunoglobulin E recurrent-infection syndrome of interferon gamma. Proc Natl Acad Sci U S A 1989; 86:10085.

642. Jeppson JD, Jaffe HS, Hill HR: Use of recombinant human interferon gamma to enhance neutrophil chemotactic responses in Job syndrome of hyperimmunoglobulinemia E and recurrent infections. J Pediatr 1991; 118:383.

643. The International Chronic Granulomatous Disease Cooperative Study Group: A controlled trial of interferon gamma to prevent infection in chronic granulomatous disease. N Engl J Med 1991; 324:509.

644. Pung YH, Vetro SW, Bellanti JA: Use of interferons in atopic (IgE-mediated) diseases. Ann Allergy 1993; 71:234.

645. Kimata H: High-dose intravenous gamma-globulin treatment for hyperimmunoglobulinemia E syndrome. J Allergy Clin Immunol 1995; 95:771.

646. Boxer LA, Hedley-Whyte ET, Stossel TP: Neutrophil actin dysfunction and abnormal neutrophil behavior. N Engl J Med 1974; 291:1093.

647. Southwick FS, Dabiri GA, Stossel TP: Neutrophil actin dysfunction is a genetic disorder associated with partial impairment of neutrophil actin assembly in three family members. J Clin Invest 1988; 82:1525.

648. Southwick FS, Howard TH, et al: The relationship between CR3 deficiency and neutrophil actin assembly. Blood 1989; 73:1973.

649. Coates TD, Torkildson JC, et al: An inherited defect of neutrophil motility and microfilamentous cytoskeleton associated with abnormalities in 47-Kd and 89-Kd proteins. Blood 1991; 78:1338.

650. Howard T, Li Y, et al: The 47-kD protein increased in neutrophil actin dysfunction with 47- and 89-kD protein abnormalities is lymphocyte-specific protein. Blood 1994; 83:231.

651. Van Dyke TE: Role of the neutrophil in oral disease: Receptor deficiency in leukocytes from patients with juvenile periodontitis. Rev Infect Dis 1985; 7:419.

652. Van Dyke TE, Vaikuntam J: Neutrophil function and dysfunction in periodontal disease. Curr Opin Periodontol 1994:19.

653. Van Dyke TE, Schweinebraten M, et al: Neutrophil chemotaxis in families with localized juvenile periodontitis. J Periodontol Res 1985; 20:503.

654. Donly KJ, Ashkenazi M: Juvenile periodontitis: A review of pathogenesis, diagnosis and treatment. J Clin Pediatr Dent 1992; 16:73.

655. Van Dyke TE, Hoop GA: Neutrophil function and oral disease. Crit Rev Oral Biol Med 1990; 1:117.

656. Van Dyke TE, Horoszewicz HU, et al: Neutrophil chemotaxis dysfunction in human periodontitis. Infect Immun 1980; 27:124.

657. Van Dyke TE, Zinney W, et al: Neutrophil function in localized juvenile periodontitis. Phagocytosis, superoxide production and specific granule release. J Periodontol 1986; 57:703.

658. Perez HD, Kelly E, et al: Defective polymorphonuclear leukocyte formyl peptide receptor(s) in juvenile periodontitis. J Clin Invest 1991; 87:971.

659. Clark RA, Page RC, Wilde G: Defective neutrophil chemotaxis in juvenile periodontitis. Infect Immun 1977; 18:694.

660. Agarwal S, Suzuki JB: Altered neutrophil function in localized juvenile periodontitis: Intrinsic cellular defect or effect of immune mediators? J Periodontol Res 1991; 26:276.

661. Suzuki JB, Colison C, et al: Immunologic profile of juvenile periodontitis. II. Neutrophil chemotaxis, phagocytosis and spore germination. J Periodontol 1984; 55:461.

662. Cianciola LJ, Genco RJ, et al: Defective polymorphonuclear leukocyte function in a human periodontal disease. Nature 1977; 265:445.

663. Tsai C-C, McArthur WP, et al: Extraction and partial characterization of a leukotoxin from a plaque-derived gram-negative microorganism. Infect Immun 1979; 25:427.

664. Shurin SB, Socransky SS, et al: A neutrophil disorder induced by capnocytophaga, a dental micro-organism. N Engl J Med 1979; 301:849.

665. Gerard NP, Gerard C: The chemotactic receptor for human C5a anaphylatoxin. Nature 1991; 349:614.

666. Boulay F, Mery L, et al: Expression cloning of a receptor for C5a anaphylatoxin on differentiated HL-60 cells. Biochemistry 1991; 30:2993.

667. Holmes WE, Lee J, et al: Structure and functional expression of a human interleukin-8 receptor. Science 1991; 253:1278.

668. Murphy PM, Tiffany HL: Cloning of complementary DNA encoding a functional human interleukin-8 receptor. Science 1991; 253:1280.

669. Boulay F, Tardif M, et al: The human N-formyl peptide receptor. Characterization of two cDNA isolates and evidence for a new subfamily of G-protein-coupled receptors. Biochemistry 1990; 29:11123.

670. Wilson CB: Immunologic basis for increased susceptibility of the neonate to infection. J Pediatr 1986; 108:1.

671. Hill HR: Biochemical, structural, and functional abnormalities of polymorphonuclear leukocytes in the neonate. Pediatr Res 1987; 22:375.

672. Hill HR, Augustin NH, Jaffe HS: Human recombinant interferon gamma enhances neonatal polymorphonuclear leukocyte activation and movement, and increases free intracellular calcium. J Exp Med 1991; 173:767.

673. Klein RB, Fischer TJ, et al: Decreased mononuclear and polymorphonuclear chemotaxis in human newborns, infants, and young children. Pediatrics 1977; 60:467.

674. Anderson DC, Hughes BJ, Smith CW: Abnormal motility of neonatal polymorphonuclear leukocytes: Relationship to impaired redistribution of surface adhesion sites by chemotactic factor or colchicine. J Clin Invest 1981; 68:863.

675. Anderson DC, Hughes BJ, et al: Impaired motility of neonatal PMN leukocytes: Relationship to abnormalities of cell orientation and assembly of microtubules in chemotactic gradients. J Leukoc Biol 1984; 36:1.

676. Anderson DC, Becker Freeman KL, et al: Abnormal stimulated adherence of neonatal granulocytes: Impaired induction of surface MAC-1 by chemotactic factors or secretagogues. Blood 1987; 70:740.

677. Smith JB, Campbell DE, et al: Expression of the complement receptors CR1 and CR3 and the Type III Fc-gamma receptor on neutrophils from newborn infants and from fetuses with Rh disease. Pediatr Res 1990; 28:120.

678. Sacchi F, Rondini G, et al: Clinical and laboratory observations: Different maturation of neutrophil chemotaxis in term and preterm newborn infants. J Pediatr 1982; 101:273.

679. Roos D, Kuijpers TW, et al: A novel syndrome of severe neutrophil dysfunction: Unresponsiveness confined to chemotaxin-induced functions. Blood 1993; 81:2735.

680. Brenneis H, Schmidt A, et al: Chemotaxis of polymorphonuclear neutrophils (PMN) in patients suffering from recurrent infection. Eur J Clin Invest 1993; 23:693.

681. Alper CA, Colten HR, et al: Homozygous deficiency of C3 in a patient with repeated infections. Lancet 1972; 2:1179.

682. Botto M, Fong KY, et al: Molecular basis of hereditary C3 deficiency. J Clin Invest 1990; 86:1158.

683. Roord JJ, Daha M, et al: Inherited deficiency of the third component of complement associated with recurrent pyogenic infections, circulating immune complexes, and vasculitis in a Dutch family. N Engl J Med 1983; 71:81.

684. Borzy MS, Gewurz A, et al: Inherited C3 deficiency with recurrent infections and glomerulonephritis. Am J Dis Child 1988; 142:79.

685. Alper CA, Abramson N, et al: Studies in vivo and in vitro on an abnormality in the metabolism of C3 in a patient with increased susceptibility to infection. J Clin Invest 1970; 49:1975.

686. Super M, Thiel S, et al: Association of low levels of mannan-

binding protein with a common defect of opsonisation. Lancet 1989; 2:1236.

687. Sumiya M, Super M, et al: Molecular basis of opsonic defect in immunodeficient children. Lancet 1991; 337:1569.

688. Turner MW, Lipscombe RJ, et al: Mutations in the human mannose binding protein gene: Their frequencies in three distinct populations and relationship to serum levels of the protein. Immunodeficiency 1993; 4:285.

689. Madsen HO, Garred P, et al: A new frequent allele is the missing link in the structural polymorphism of the human mannan-binding protein. Immunogenetics 1994; 40:37.

690. Summerfield JA, Ryder S, et al: Mannose binding protein gene mutations associated with unusual and severe infections in adults. Lancet 1995; 345:886.

691. Ceuppens JL, Bloemmen FJ, Van Wauwe JP: T-cell unresponsiveness to the mitogenic activity of OKT3 antibody results from a deficiency of the monocyte Fc-gamma receptors for murine IgG2a and inability to cross-link the T3-Ti complex. J Immunol 1985; 135:165.

692. Fromont P, Bettaib A, et al: Frequency of the polymorphonuclear neutrophil Fc-gamma receptor III deficiency in the French population and its involvement in the development of neonatal alloimmune neutropenia. Blood 1992; 79:2131.

693. de Haas M, Kleijer M, et al: Neutrophil FcRIIIb deficiency, nature, and clinical consequences: A study of 21 individuals from 14 families. Blood 1995; 86:2403.

694. Selvaraj P, Rosse WF, et al: The major Fc receptor in blood has a phosphatidylinositol anchor and is deficient in paroxysmal nocturnal haemoglobinuria. Nature 1988; 333:565.

695. Huizinga TW, van der Schoot CE, et al: The PI-linked receptor FcR III is released on stimulation of neutrophils. Nature 1988; 333:667.

696. Van De Winkel JGJ, Capel PJA: Human IgG Fc receptor heterogeneity: Molecular aspects and clinical implications. Immunol Today 1993; 14:215.

697. Rubin CM, Burke BA, et al: The accelerated phase of Chédiak-Higashi syndrome. An expression of the virus-associated hemophagocytic syndrome? Cancer 1985; 56:524.

698. Padgett GA, Reiquam CW, et al: Comparative studies of the Chédiak-Higashi syndrome. Am J Pathol 1967; 51:553.

699. Ito J, Tokumaru M, Okazaki T: Chédiak-Higashi syndrome: Report of a case with autopsy and electron microscopic studies. Acta Pathol Jpn 1972; 22:755.

700. Sjaastad OV, Blom AK, et al: Adenine nucleotides, serotonin and aggregation properties of the platelets of blue foxes (Alopex lagopus) with the Chédiak-Higashi syndrome. Am J Med Genet 1990; 35:373.

701. White JG, Clawson CC: The Chédiak-Higashi syndrome: The nature of the giant neutrophil granules and their interactions with cytoplasm and foreign particulates. I. Progressive enlargement of the massive inclusions in mature neutrophils. II. Manifestations of cytoplasmic injury and sequestration. III. Interactions between giant organelles and foreign particulates. Am J Pathol 1980; 98:151.

702. Rausch PG, Pryzwansky KB, Spitznagel JK: Immunocytochemical identification of azurophilic and specific granule markers in the giant granules of Chédiak-Higashi neutrophils. N Engl J Med 1978; 298:693.

703. Davis WC, Douglas SD: Defective granule formation and function in the Chédiak-Higashi syndrome in man and animals. Semin Hematol 1972; 9:431.

704. Davis WC, Spicer SS, et al: Ultrastructure of cells in bone marrow and peripheral blood of normal mink and mink with the homologue of the Chédiak-Higashi trait of humans. II. Cytoplasmic granules in eosinophils, basophils, mononuclear cells and platelets. Am J Pathol 1971; 63:411.

705. Vassali JD, Piperno-Granelli A, et al: Specific protease deficiency in polymorphonuclear leukocytes of Chédiak-Higashi syndrome and beige mice. J Exp Mice 1978; 149:1285.

706. Ganz T, Metcalf JA, et al: Microbicidal/cytotoxic proteins of neutrophils are deficient in two disorders: Chédiak-Higashi syndrome and "specific" granule deficiency. J Clin Invest 1988; 82:552.

707. Ingraham LM, Burns CP, et al: Fluidity properties and lipid composition of erythrocyte membranes in Chédiak-Higashi syndrome. J Cell Biol 1981; 89:510.

708. Ostlund RE Jr, Tucker RW, et al: The cytoskeleton in Chédiak-Higashi syndrome fibroblasts. Blood 1980; 56:806.

709. Haak RA, Ingraham LM, et al: Membrane fluidity in human and mouse Chédiak-Higashi leukocytes. J Clin Invest 1979; 64:138.

710. Boxer LA, Watanabe AM, et al: Correction of leukocyte function in Chédiak-Higashi syndrome by ascorbate. N Engl J Med 1976; 295:1041.

711. Root RK, Rosenthal AS, Balestra DJ: Abnormal bactericidal, metabolic, and lysosomal functions of Chédiak-Higashi syndrome leukocytes. J Clin Invest 1972; 51:649.

712. Nath J, Flavin M, Gallin JI: Tubulin tyrosinolation in human polymorphonuclear leukocytes: Studies in normal subjects and in patients with the Chédiak-Higashi syndrome. J Cell Biol 1982; 95:519.

713. Wilson DW, Whiteheart SW, et al: Intracellular membrane fusion. Trends Biochem Sci 1991; 16:334.

714. Jenkins NA, Justice MJ, et al: Nidogen/entactin (Nid) maps to the proximal end of mouse chromosome 13 linked to beige (bg) and identifies a new region of homology between mouse and human chromosomes. Genomics 1991; 9:401.

714a. Barbosa MDFS, Nguyen QA, et al: Identification of the homologous beige and Chédiak-Higashi syndrome genes. Nature 1996; 382:262.

715. Blume RS, Bennett JM, et al: Defective granulocyte regulation in the Chédiak-Higashi syndrome. N Engl J Med 1968; 279:1009.

716. White JG, Clawson CC: The Chédiak-Higashi syndrome. Ring-shaped lysosomes in circulating monocytes. Am J Pathol 1979; 96:781.

717. Novak EK, McGarry MP, Swank RT: Correction of symptoms of platelet storage pool deficiency in animal models for Chédiak-Higashi syndrome and Hermansky-Pudlak syndrome. Blood 1985; 66:1196.

718. Buchanan GB, Handin RI: Platelet function in the Chédiak-Higashi syndrome. Blood 1976; 47:941.

719. Boxer GJ, Holmsen H, et al: Abnormal platelet functions in Chédiak-Higashi syndrome. Br J Haematol 1977; 35:521.

720. Bell TG, Meyers KM, et al: Decreased nucleotide and serotonin storage associates with defective function in Chédiak-Higashi syndrome cattle and human platelets. Blood 1976; 48:175.

721. Clark RA, Kimball HR: Defective granulocyte chemotaxis in the Chédiak-Higashi syndrome. J Clin Invest 1971; 50:2645.

722. Clawson CC, Repine JE, White JG: Chédiak-Higashi syndrome: Quantitative defect in bactericidal capacity. Blood 1971; 38:814.

723. Clawson CC, Repine JE, White JG: The Chédiak-Higashi syndrome. Quantitation of a deficiency in maximal bactericidal capacity. Am J Pathol 1979; 94:539.

724. Clawson CC, Repine JE, White JG: Quantitation of bactericidal capacity in normal and abnormal human neutrophils. Pediatr Res 1972; 6:367.

725. Cairo MS, Vandeven C, et al: Fluorescent cytometric analysis of polymorphonuclear leucocytes in Chédiak-Higashi syndrome: Diminished C3bi receptor expression (OKM-1) with normal granular cell density. Pediatr Res 1988; 24:673.

726. Klein M, Roder J, et al: Chédiak-Higashi gene in humans. II. The selectivity of the defect in natural-killer and antibody dependent cell–mediated cytotoxicity function. J Exp Med 1980; 151:1049.

727. Abo T, Roder JC, et al: Natural killer (HNK-1+) cells in Chédiak-Higashi patients are present in normal numbers but are abnormal in function and morphology. J Clin Invest 1982; 70:193.

728. Haliotis T, Roder J, et al: Chédiak-Higashi gene in humans. I. Impairment of natural-killer function. J Exp Med 1980; 151:1039.

729. Targan SR, Oseas R: The "lazy" NK cells of Chédiak-Higashi syndrome. J Immunol 1983; 130:2671.

730. Nair MPN, Gray RH, et al: Deficiency of inducible suppressor cell activity in the Chédiak-Higashi syndrome. Am J Hematol 1987; 26:55.

731. Merino F, Klein GO, et al: Elevated antibody titers to Epstein-Barr virus and low natural killer cell activity in patients with Chédiak-Higashi syndrome. Clin Immunol Immunopathol 1983; 27:326.

732. Creel D, Boxer LA, Fauci AS: Visual and auditory anomalies in Chédiak-Higashi syndrome. Electroencephalogr Clin Neurophysiol 1983; 55:252.

733. Pettit RE, Berdal KG: Chédiak-Higashi syndrome: Neurologic appearance. Arch Neurol 1984; 41:1001.

734. Diukman R, Tanigawara S, et al: Prenatal diagnosis of Chédiak-Higashi syndrome. Prenat Diagn 1992; 12:877.

735. Van Slyck E, Rebuck JW: Pseudo-Chédiak-Higashi anomaly in acute leukemia. Am J Clin Pathol 1974; 62:673.

736. Gorman AM, O'Connell LG: Pseudo-Chédiak-Higashi anomaly in acute leukemia. Am J Clin Pathol 1976; 65:1030. Letter to the editor.

737. Tulliez M, Vernant JP, et al: Pseudo-Chédiak-Higashi anomaly in a case of acute myeloid leukemia: Electron microscopic studies. Blood 1979; 54:863.

738. Weening RS, Schoorel EP, et al: Effect of ascorbate on abnormal neutrophil, platelet, and lymphocyte function in a patient with the Chédiak-Higashi syndrome. Blood 1981; 57:856.

739. Gallin JI, Elin RJ, et al: Efficacy of ascorbic acid in Chédiak-Higashi syndrome (CHS): Studies in humans and mice. Blood 1979; 53:226.

740. Kazmierowski JA, Elin RJ, et al: Chédiak-Higashi syndrome: Reversal of susceptibility to infection by bone marrow transplantation. Blood 1976; 47:555.

741. Virelizier JL, Lagrue A, et al: Reversal of natural killer defect in a patient with Chédiak-Higashi syndrome after bone-marrow transplantation. N Engl J Med 1981; 306:1055.

742. Colgan SP, Hull-Thrall MA, et al: Restoration of neutrophil and platelet function in feline Chédiak-Higashi syndrome by bone marrow transplantation. Bone Marrow Transplant 1991; 7:365.

743. Griscelli C, Virelizier J-L: Bone marrow transplantation in a patient with Chédiak-Higashi syndrome. In Wedgwood RJ, Rosen F, et al (eds): Primary Immunodeficiency Diseases. New York, Alan R. Liss, Inc., 1983, p 333.

744. Merino F, Henle W, Ramirez Duque P: Chronic active Epstein-Barr virus infection in patients with Chédiak-Higashi syndrome. J Clin Immunol 1986; 6:299.

745. Gallin JI: Neutrophil specific granule deficiency. Annu Rev Med 1985; 36:263.

746. Komiyama A, Morosawa H, et al: Abnormal neutrophil maturation in a neutrophil defect with morphologic abnormality and impaired function. J Pediatr 1979; 94:19.

747. Ambruso DR, Sasada M, et al: Defective bactericidal activity and absence of specific granules in neutrophils from a patient with recurrent bacterial infections. J Clin Immunol 1984; 4:23.

748. Strauss RG, Bove KE, et al: An anomaly of neutrophil morphology with impaired function. N Engl J Med 1974; 290:278.

749. Boxer LA, Coates TD, et al: Lactoferrin deficiency associated with altered granulocyte function. N Engl J Med 1982; 307:404.

750. Parmley RT, Tzeng DY, et al: Abnormal distribution of complex carbohydrates in neutrophils of a patient with lactoferrin deficiency. Blood 1983; 62:538.

751. Borregaard N, Boxer LA, et al: Anomalous neutrophil granule distribution in a patient with lactoferrin deficiency: Pertinence to the respiratory burst. Am J Hematol 1985; 18:255.

752. Parmley RT, Gilbert CS, Boxer LA: Abnormal peroxidase-positive granules in "specific granule" deficiency. Blood 1989; 73:838.

753. Lomax KJ, Leto TL, et al: Recombinant 47-kD cytosol factor restores NADPH oxidase in chronic granulomatous disease. Science 1989; 245:409.

754. Petty HR, Francis JW, et al: Neutrophil C3bi receptors: Formation of membrane clusters during cell triggering requires intracellular granules. J Cell Physiol 1987; 133:235.

755. Lomax KJ, Gallin JI, et al: Selective defect in myeloid cell lactoferrin gene expression in neutrophil specific granule deficiency. J Clin Invest 1989; 83:514.

756. Breton-Gorius J, Mason DY, et al: Lactoferrin deficiency as a consequence of a lack of specific granules in neutrophils from a patient with recurrent infections. Detection by immunoperoxidase staining for lactoferrin and cytochemical electron microscopy. Am J Pathol 1980; 99:413.

757. Gallin JI, Fletcher MP, et al: Human neutrophil-specific granule deficiency: A model to assess the role of neutrophil-specific granules in the evolution of the inflammatory response. Blood 1982; 59:1317.

758. O'Shea JJ, Brown EJ, et al: Evidence for distinct intracellular pools of receptors for C3b and C3bi in human neutrophils. J Immunol 1985; 134:2580.

759. Spitznagel JK, Cooper MR, et al: Selective deficiency of granules associated with lysozyme and lactoferrin in human polymorphs (PMN) with reduced microbicidal capacity. J Clin Invest 1972; 51:92a.

760. Hibbs MS, Bainton DF: Human neutrophil gelatinase is a component of specific granules. J Clin Invest 1989; 84:1395.

761. Rosenberg HF, Galin JI: Neutrophil-specific granule deficiency includes eosinophils. Blood 1993; 82:268.

762. Miller LJ, Bainton DF: Stimulated mobilization of monocyte Mac-1 and p150, 95 adhesion proteins from an intracellular vesicular compartment to the cell surface. J Clin Invest 1987; 80:535.

763. Todd RF III, Arnaout MA, et al: Subcellular localization of the large subunit of Mo1 (Mo1; formerly gp110), a surface glycoprotein associated with adhesion. J Clin Invest 1984; 74:1280.

764. Petrequin PR, Todd RF III, et al: Association between gelatinase release and increased plasma membrane expression of the Mo1 glycoprotein. Blood 1987; 69:605.

765. Fletcher MP, Gallin JI: Human neutrophils contain an intracellular pool of putative receptors for the chemoattractant N-formyl-methionyl-leucyl-phenylalanine. Blood 1987; 62:792.

766. Kuriyama K, Tomonaga M, et al: Diagnostic significance of detecting pseudo-Pelger-Huët anomalies and micro-megakaryocytes in myelodysplastic syndrome. Br J Haematol 1986; 63:665.

767. Johnston RB, McMurry JS: Chronic familial granulomatosis: Report of five cases in the literature. Am J Dis Child 1967; 114:370.

768. Windhorst DB, Holmes B, Good RA: A newly defined X-linked trait in man with demonstration of the Lyon effect in carrier females. Lancet 1967; 1:737.

769. Berendes H, Bridges RA, Good RA: Fatal granulomatosis of childhood: Clinical study of new syndrome. Minn Med 1957; 40:309.

770. Bridges RA, Berendes H, Good RA: A fatal granulomatous disease of childhood. The clinical, pathological, and laboratory features of a new syndrome. Am J Dis Child 1959; 97:387.

771. Landing BH, Shirkey HS: Syndrome of recurrent infection and infiltration of viscera by pigmented lipid histiocytes. Pediatrics 1957; 20:431.

772. Casimir C, Chetty M, et al: Identification of the defective NADPH-oxidase component in chronic granulomatous disease: A study of 57 European families. Eur J Clin Invest 1992; 22:403.

773. Clark RA, Malech HL, et al: Genetic variants of chronic granulomatous disease: Prevalence of deficiencies of two cytosolic components of the NADPH oxidase system. N Engl J Med 1989; 321:647.

774. Curnutte JT: Molecular basis of the autosomal recessive forms of chronic granulomatous disease. Immunodefic Rev 1992; 3:149.

775. Newburger PE, Luscinskas FW, et al: Variant chronic granulomatous disease: Modulation of the neutrophil by severe infection. Blood 1986; 68:914.

776. Roos D, de Boer M, et al: Chronic granulomatous disease with partial deficiency of cytochrome b558 and incomplete respiratory burst: Variants of the X-linked, cytochrome b558–negative form of the disease. J Leukoc Biol 1992; 51:164.

777. Stossel TP, Root RK: Phagocytosis in chronic granulomatous disease and the Chédiak-Higashi syndrome. N Engl J Med 1972; 286:120.

778. Gaither TA, Medley SR, et al: Studies of phagocytosis in chronic granulomatous disease. Inflammation 1987; 11:211.

779. Hasui M, Hirabayashi Y, et al: Increased phagocytic activity of polymorphonuclear leukocytes of chronic granulomatous disease as determined with flow cytometric assay. J Lab Clin Med 1991; 117:291.

780. Finn A, Hadzic N, et al: Prognosis of chronic granulomatous disease. Arch Dis Child 1990; 65:942.

781. Bohler MC, Seger RA, et al: A study of 25 patients with chronic granulomatous disease: A new classification by correlating respiratory burst, cytochrome b, and flavoprotein. J Clin Immunol 1986; 6:136.

782. Tauber AI, Borregaard N, et al: Chronic granulomatous disease: A syndrome of phagocyte oxidase deficiencies. Medicine 1983; 62:286.

783. Forrest CB, Forehand JR, et al: Clinical features and current management of chronic granulomatous disease. Hematol Oncol Clin North Am 1988; 2:253.

784. Babior BM, Woodman RC: Chronic granulomatous disease. Semin Hematol 1990; 27:247.

785. Johnston RB Jr, Newman SL: Chronic granulomatous disease. Pediatr Clin North Am 1977; 24:365.

786. Mouy R, Fischer A, et al: Incidence, severity, and prevention of infections in chronic granulomatous disease. J Pediatr 1989; 114:555.

787. Hayakawa H, Kobayashi N, Yata J: Chronic granulomatous disease in Japan: A summary of the clinical features of 84 registered patients. Acta Paediatr Jpn 1985; 27:501.

788. Styrt B, Klempner MS: Late-presenting variant of chronic granulomatous disease. Pediatr Infect Dis 1984; 3:556.

789. Chusid MJ, Parrillo JE, Fauci AS: Chronic granulomatous disease: Diagnosis in a 27-year-old man with Mycobacterium fortuitum. JAMA 1975; 233:1295.

790. Cazzola M, Sacchi F, et al: X-linked chronic granulomatous disease in an adult woman. Evidence for a cell selection favoring neutrophils expressing the mutant allele. Haematologica 1985; 70:291.

791. Dilworth JA, Mandell GL: Adults with chronic granulomatous disease of "childhood." Am J Med 1977; 63:233.

792. Schapiro BL, Newburger PE, et al: Chronic granulomatous disease presenting in a 69-year-old man. N Engl J Med 1991; 325:1786.

793. Gallin JI, Buescher ES, et al: Recent advances in chronic granulomatous disease. Ann Intern Med 1983; 99:657.

794. Hitzig WH, Seger RA: Chronic granulomatous disease, a heterogeneous syndrome. Hum Genet 1983; 64:207.

795. Cohen MS, Isturiz RE, et al: Fungal infection in chronic granulomatous disease. Am J Med 1981; 71:59.

796. Speert DP, Bond M, et al: Infection with Pseudomonas cepacia in chronic granulomatous disease—role of nonoxidative killing by neutrophils in host defense. J Infect Dis 1994; 170:1524.

797. O'Neil KM, Herman JH: Pseudomonas cepacia: An emerging pathogen in chronic granulomatous disease. J Pediatr 1986; 108:940.

798. Clegg HW, Ephros M, Newburger PE: Pseudomonas cepacia pneumonia in chronic granulomatous disease. Pediatr Infect Dis 1986; 5:111.

799. Phillips P, Forbes JC, Speert DP: Disseminated infection with Pseudallescheria boydii in a patient with chronic granulomatous disease: Response to gamma-interferon plus antifungal chemotherapy. Pediatr Infect Dis 1991; 10:536.

800. Schwartz DA: Sporothrix tenosynovitis—differential diagnosis of granulomatous inflammatory disease of the joints. J Rheumatol 1989; 16:550.

801. Sorensen RU, Jacobs MR, Shurin SB: Chromobacterium violaceum adenitis acquired in the northern United States as a complication of chronic granulomatous disease. Pediatr Infect Dis 1985; 4:701.

802. Macher AM, Casale TB, Fauci AS: Chronic granulomatous disease of childhood and Chromobacterium violaceum infections in the southeastern United States. Ann Intern Med 1982; 97:51.

803. Wenger JD, Hollis DG, et al: Infection caused by Francisella philomiragia (formerly Yersinia philomiragia). A newly recognized human pathogen. Ann Intern Med 1990; 110:888.

804. Kenney RT, Kwon-Chung KJ, et al: Invasive infection with Sarcinosporon inkin in a patient with chronic granulomatous disease. Am J Clin Pathol 1990; 94:344.

805. Pedersen FK, Johansen KS, et al: Refractory Pneumocytis carinii infection in chronic granulomatous disease: Successful treatment with granulocytes. Pediatrics 1979; 64:935.

806. Adinoff AD, Johnston RB Jr, et al: Chronic granulomatous disease and Pneumocytis carinii pneumonia. Pediatrics 1982; 69:133.

807. Mulholland MW, Delaney JP, Simmons RL: Gastrointestinal complications of chronic granulomatous disease of childhood: Surgical implications. Surgery 1983; 94:569.

808. Garel LA, Pariente DM, et al: Liver involvement in chronic granulomatous disease: The role of ultrasound in diagnosis and treatment. Radiology 1984; 153:117.

809. Sponseller PD, Malech HL, et al: Skeletal involvement in children who have chronic granulomatous disease. J Bone Joint Surg Am 1991; 73:37.

810. Wolfson JJ, Kane WJ, et al: Bone findings in chronic granulomatous disease of childhood: A genetic abnormality of leukocyte function. Surgery 1969; 51:1573.

811. Mandell GL, Hook EW: Leukocyte bactericidal activity in chronic granulomatous disease: Correlation of bacterial hydrogen peroxide production and susceptibility in intracellular killing. J Bacteriol 1969; 100:531.

812. Lehrer RI, Ganz T: Antimicrobial polypeptides of human neutrophils. Blood 1990; 76:2169.

813. Gabay JE, Scott RW, et al: Antibiotic proteins of human polymorphonuclear leukocytes. Proc Natl Acad Sci U S A 1989; 86:5610.

814. Odell EW, Segal AW: Killing of pathogens associated with chronic granulomatous disease by the non-oxidative microbicidal mechanisms of human neutrophils. J Med Microbiol 1991; 34:129.

815. Johnston RB Jr, Baehner RL: Chronic granulomatous disease: Correlation between pathogenesis and clinical findings. Pediatrics 1971; 48:730.

816. Renner WR, Johnson JF, et al: Esophageal inflammation and stricture: Complication of chronic granulomatous disease of childhood. Radiology 1991; 178:189.

817. Griscom NT, Kirkpatrick JA Jr, et al: Gastric antral narrowing in chronic granulomatous disease of childhood. Pediatrics 1974; 54:456.

818. Hiller N, Fisher D, et al: Esophageal involvement in chronic granulomatous disease. Pediatr Radiol 1995; 25:308.

819. Ament ME, Ochs HD: Gastrointestinal manifestations of chronic granulomatous disease. N Engl J Med 1973; 288:382.

820. Isaacs D, Wright VM, et al: Case report: Chronic granulomatous disease mimicking Crohn's disease. J Pediatr Gastroenterol Nutr 1985; 4:498.

821. Aliabadi H, Gonzalez R, Quie PG: Urinary tract disorders in patients with chronic granulomatous disease. N Engl J Med 1989; 321:706.

822. Bauer SB, Kogan SJ: Vesical manifestations of chronic granulomatous disease in children. Its relation to eosinophilic cystitis. Urology 1991; 37:463.

823. Cyr WL, Johnson H, Balfour J: Granulomatous cystitis as a manifestation of chronic granulomatous disease of childhood. J Urol 1973; 110:357.

824. Southwick FS, Van der Meer JWM: Recurrent cystitis and bladder mass in two adults with chronic granulomatous disease. Ann Intern Med 1988; 109:118.

825. Walther M, Malech H, et al: The urological manifestations of chronic granulomatous disease. J Urol 1992; 147:1314.

826. Windhorst DB, Good RA: Dermatologic manifestations of fatal granulomatous disease of childhood. Arch Dermatol 1971; 103:351.

827. Cohen MS, Leong PA, Simpson DM: Phagocytic cells in periodontal defense: Periodontal status of patients with chronic granulomatous disease of childhood. J Periodontol 1985; 56:611.

828. Martyn LJ, Lischner HW, et al: Chorioretinal lesions in familial chronic granulomatous disease of childhood. Am J Ophthalmol 1972; 73:403.

829. Valluri S, Chu FC, Smith ME: Ocular pathologic findings of chronic granulomatous disease of childhood. Am J Ophthalmol 1995; 120:120.

830. Hadfield MG, Ghatak NR, et al: Brain lesions in chronic granulomatous disease. Acta Neuropathol 1991; 81:467.

831. Walker DH, Okiye G: Chronic granulomatous disease involving the central nervous system. Pediatr Pathol 1983; 1:159.

832. Van Rhenen DJ, Koolen MI, et al: Immune complex glomerulonephritis in chronic granulomatous disease. Acta Med Scand 1979; 206:233.

833. Stalder JF, Dreno B, et al: Discoid lupus erythematosus-like lesions in an autosomal form of chronic granulomatous disease. Br J Dermatol 1986; 114:251.

834. Smitt JHS, Bos JD, et al: Discoid lupus erythematosus-like skin changes in patients with autosomal recessive chronic granulomatous disease. Arch Dermatol 1990; 126:1656.

835. Manzi S, Urbach AH, et al: Systemic lupus erythematosus in a boy with chronic granulomatous disease: Case report and review of the literature. Arthritis Rheum 1991; 34:101.

836. Schmitt CP, Scharer K, et al: Glomerulonephritis associated with chronic granulomatous disease and systemic lupus erythematosus. Nephrol Dial Transplant 1995; 10:891.

837. Lee BW, Yap HK: Polyarthritis resembling juvenile rheumatoid

arthritis in a girl with chronic granulomatous disease. Arthritis Rheum 1994; 37:773.

838. Woodman RC, Newburger PE, et al: A new X-linked variant of chronic granulomatous disease characterized by the existence of a normal clone of respiratory burst-competent phagocytic cells. Blood 1995; 85:231.

839. Johnston RB, Harbecker RJ, Johnston RB Jr: Recurrent severe infections in a girl with apparently variable expression of mosaicism for chronic granulomatous disease. J Pediatr 1985; 106:50.

840. Ochs HD, Igo RP: The NBT slide test: A simple screening method for detecting chronic granulomatous disease and female carriers. J Pediatr 1973; 83:77.

841. Meerhof LJ, Roos D: Heterogeneity in chronic granulomatous disease detected with an improved nitroblue tetrazolium slide test. J Leukoc Biol 1986; 39:699.

842. Roesler J, Hecht M, et al: Diagnosis of chronic granulomatous disease and of its mode of inheritance by dihydrorhodamine 123 and flow microcytofluorometry. Eur J Pediatr 1991; 150:161.

843. Rothe G, Emmendorffer A, et al: Flow cytometric measurements of the respiratory burst activity of phagocytes using dihydrorhodamine 123. J Immunol Methods 1991; 138:133.

844. Hassan NF, Campbell DE, Douglas SD: Phorbol myristate acetate induced oxidation of 2', 7'-dichlorofluorescein by neutrophils from patients with chronic granulomatous disease. J Leukoc Biol 1988; 43:317.

845. Windhorst DB, Page AR, Holmes B, et al: The pattern of genetic transmission of the leukocyte defect in fatal granulomatous cause of childhood. J Clin Invest 1968; 47:1026.

846. Lyon MF: Sex chromatin and gene action in the mammalian X-chromosome. Am J Hum Genet 1962; 14:135.

847. Beutler E, Yeh M, Fairbans VF: The normal human female as a mosaic of X-chromosome activity: Studies using the gene for G-6-PD deficiency as a marker. Proc Natl Acad Sci U S A 1962; 48:9.

848. Newburger PE, Malawista SE, et al: Chronic granulomatous disease and glutathione peroxidase deficiency, revisited. Blood 1994; 84:3861.

849. Strate M, Brandup F, Wang P: Discoid lupus erythematosus-like skin lesions in a patient with autosomal recessive chronic granulomatous disease. Clin Genet 1986; 30:184.

850. Dinauer MC, Pierce EA, et al: Human neutrophil cytochrome b light chain (p22-phox): Gene structure, chromosomal location, and mutations in cytochrome-negative autosomal recessive chronic granulomatous disease. J Clin Invest 1990; 86:1729.

851. Volpp BD, Nauseef WM, et al: Cloning of the cDNA and functional expression of the 47-kilodalton cytosolic component of the human neutrophil respiratory burst oxidase. Proc Natl Acad Sci U S A 1989; 86:7195.

852. Leto TL, Lomax KJ, et al: Cloning of a 67-kDa neutrophil oxidase factor with similarity to a non-catalytic region of p60^{c-src}. Science 1990; 248:727.

853. Iwata M, Nunoi H, et al: Homologous dinucleotide (GT or TG) deletion in Japanese patients with chronic granulomatous disease with p47-phox deficiency. Biochem Biophys Res Commun 1994; 199:1372.

854. Segal AW, Jones OTG, et al: Absence of a newly described cytochrome b from neutrophils of patients with chronic granulomatous disease. Lancet 1978; 2:446.

855. Borregaard N, Staehr-Johansen K, et al: Cytochrome b is present in neutrophils from patients with chronic granulomatous disease. Lancet 1979; 1:949.

856. Segal AW, Cross AR, et al: Absence of cytochrome b-245 in chronic granulomatous disease: A multicenter European evaluation of its incidence and relevance. N Engl J Med 1983; 308:245.

857. Dinauer MC, Orkin SH, et al: The glycoprotein encoded by the X-linked chronic granulomatous disease locus is a component of the neutrophil cytochrome b complex. Nature 1987; 327:717.

858. Segal AW: Absence of both cytochrome b$_{-245}$ subunits from neutrophils in X-linked chronic granulomatous disease. Nature 1987; 326:88.

859. Parkos CA, Dinauer MC, et al: Absence of both the 91-kD and 22-kD subunits of human neutrophil cytochrome b in two genetic forms of chronic granulomatous disease. Blood 1989; 73:1416.

860. Baehner RL, Kunkel LM, et al: DNA linkage analysis of X

chromosome–linked chronic granulomatous disease. Proc Natl Sci Acad U S A 1986; 83:3398.

861. Skalnik DG, Strauss EC, Orkin SH: CCAAT displacement protein as a repressor of the myelomonocytic-specific gp91-phox gene promoter. J Biol Chem 1991; 266:16736.

862. Lee YS, Lien L, Orkin SH: Regulated expression of the human myeloid-specific gp91-phox gene following yeast artificial chromosome (YAC) transfer into mouse embryonic stem (ES) cells. Blood 1993; 82:321a.

863. Francke U, Ochs HD, et al: Minor Xp21 chromosome deletion in a male associated with expression of Duchenne muscular dystrophy, chronic granulomatous disease, retinitis pigmentosa, and McLeod syndrome. Am J Hum Genet 1985; 37:250.

864. Kousseff B: Linkage between chronic granulomatous disease and Duchenne's muscular dystrophy. Am J Dis Child 1981; 135:1149.

865. Frey D, Machler M, et al: Gene deletion in a patient with chronic granulomatous disease and McLeod syndrome: Fine mapping of the Xk gene locus. Blood 1988; 71:252.

866. De Saint-Basile G, Bohler MC, et al: Xp21 DNA microdeletion in a patient with chronic granulomatous disease, retinitis pigmentosa, and McLeod phenotype. Hum Genet 1988; 80:85.

867. Pelham A, O'Reilly MAJ, et al: RFLP and deletion analysis for X-linked chronic granulomatous disease using the cDNA probe: Potential for improved prenatal diagnosis and carrier determination. Blood 1990; 76:820.

868. De Boer M, Bolscher BGJM: Splice site mutations are a common cause of X-linked chronic granulomatous disease. Blood 1992; 80:1553.

869. Dinauer MC, Curnutte JT, et al: A missense mutation in the neutrophil cytochrome b heavy chain in cytochrome-positive X-linked chronic granulomatous disease. J Clin Invest 1989; 84:2012.

870. Bolscher BGJM, De Boer M, et al: Point mutations in the β-subunit of cytochrome b$_{558}$ leading to X-linked chronic granulomatous disease. Blood 1991; 7:2482.

871. Ariga T, Sakiyama Y, Matsumoto S: A 15-base pair (bp) palindromic insertion associated with a 3-bp deletion in exon 10 of the gp91-phox gene, detected in two patients with X-linked chronic granulomatous disease. Hum Genet 1995; 96:6.

872. Kuribayashi F, Kumatori A, et al: Human peripheral eosinophils have a specific mechanism to express gp91-phox, the large subunit of cytochrome b$_{558}$. Biochem Biophys Res Commun 1995; 2009:146.

873. Curnutte J: Chronic granulomatous disease: the solving of a clinical riddle at the molecular level. Clin Immunol Immunopathol 1993; 67:S2.

874. Ariga T, Sakiyama Y, et al: A newly recognized point mutation in the cytochrome b$_{558}$ heavy chain gene replacing alanine^{57} by glutamic acid, in a patient with cytochrome b positive X-linked chronic granulomatous disease. Eur J Pediatr 1993; 152:469.

875. Cross A, Heyworth P, et al: A variant X-linked chronic granulomatous disease patient (X91$^+$) with partially functional cytochrome b*. J Biol Chem 1995; 270:8194.

876. Azuma H, Oomi H, et al: A new mutation on exon 12 of the gp91-phox gene leading to cytochrome b-positive X-linked chronic granulomatous disease. Blood 1995; 85:3274.

877. Ariga T, Sakiyama Y, Matsumoto S: A 15-base pair (bp) palindromic insertion associated with a 3-bp deletion in exon 10 of the gp91-phox gene, detected in two patients with X-linked chronic granulomatous disease. Hum Genet 1995; 96:6.

878. Leusen J, de Boer M, et al: A point mutation in gp91-phox of cytochrome b$_{558}$ of the human NADPH oxidase leading to defective translocation of the cytosolic proteins p47-phox and p67-phox. J Clin Invest 1994; 93:2120.

879. Dinauer M, Curnutte J, et al: A missense mutation in the neutrophil cytochrome b heavy chain in X-linked chronic granulomatous disease. J Clin Invest 1989; 84:2012.

880. Newburger P, Skalnik D, et al: Mutations in the promoter region of the gene gp91-phox in X-linked chronic granulomatous disease with decreased expression of cytochrome b$_{558}$. J Clin Invest 1994; 94:1205.

881. Dinauer MC, Pierce EA, et al: Point mutation in the cytoplasmic domain of the neutrophil p22-phox cytochrome b subunit is associated with a nonfunctional NADPH oxidase and chronic

granulomatous disease. Proc Natl Acad Sci U S A 1991; 88:11231.

882. Leusen J, Bolscher B, et al: ^{156}Pro→Gln substitution in the light chain of cytochrome b_{558} of the human NADPH oxidase (p22-*phox*) leads to defective translocation of the cytosolic proteins p47-*phox* and p67-*phox*. J Exp Med 1994; 180:2329.

883. McPhail L: SH3-dependent assembly of the phagocyte NADPH oxidase. J Exp Med 1994; 180:2011.

884. Ren R, Mayer BJ, et al: Identification of a 10-amino acid proline-rich SH3 binding site. Science 1993; 259:1157.

885. Zhu Q, Zhang M, et al: Detection within the Src homology domain 3 of Bruton's tyrosine kinase resulting in X-linked agammaglobulinemia (XLA). J Exp Med 1994; 180:461.

886. Bromberg Y, Pick E: Unsaturated fatty acids stimulate NADPH-dependent superoxide production by cell-free system derived from macrophages. Cell Immunol 1984; 88:213.

887. Heyneman RA, Vercauteren RE: Activation of a NADPH oxidase from horse polymorphonuclear leukocytes in a cell-free system. J Leukoc Biol 1984; 36:751.

888. Curnutte JT: Activation of human neutrophil nicotinamide adenine dinucleotide phosphate, reduced (triphosphopyridine nucleotide, reduced) oxidase by arachidonic acid in a cell-free system. J Clin Invest 1985; 75:1740.

889. McPhail LC, Shirley PS, et al: Activation of the respiratory burst enzyme from human neutrophils in a cell-free system. J Clin Invest 1985; 75:1735.

890. Nunoi H, Rotrosen D, et al: Two forms of autosomal chronic granulomatous disease lack distinct neutrophil cytosol factors. Science 1988; 242:1298.

891. Curnutte JT, Scott PJ, Mayo LA: Cytosolic components of the respiratory burst oxidase: Resolution of four components, two of which are missing in complementing types of chronic granulomatous disease. Proc Natl Acad Sci U S A 1989; 86:825.

892. Francke U, Ochs HD, et al: Origin of mutations in two families with X-linked chronic granulomatous disease. Blood 1990; 76:602.

893. Chanock SJ, Barrett DM, et al: Gene structure of the cytosolic component, *phox*-47 and mutations in autosomal recessive chronic granulomatous disease. Blood 1991; 78:165a.

894. Casimir CM, Bu-Ghanim HN, et al: Autosomal recessive chronic granulomatous disease caused by deletion at a dinucleotide repeat. Proc Natl Acad Sci U S A 1991; 88:2753.

895. Gorlach A, Roesler J, et al: The p47-*phox* gene has a pseudogene carrying the most common mutation for p47-*phox* deficient chronic granulomatous disease. Blood 1995; 86:260a.

896. Roesler J, Gorlach A, et al: Recombination events between the normal p47-*phox* gene and a highly homologous pseudogene are the main cause of autosomal recessive chronic granulomatous disease (CGD). Blood 1995; 86:260a.

897. Francke U, Hsieh CL, et al: Genes for two autosomal recessive forms of chronic granulomatous disease assigned to 1q25 (NCF2) and 7q11.23 (NCF1). Am J Hum Genet 1990; 47:483.

898. Kenney RT, Malech HL, Leto TL: Structural characterization of the p67-*phox* gene. Clin Res 1992; 40:261a. Abstract.

899. Tanugi-Cholley LC, Issartel JP, et al: A mutation located at the 5' splice junction sequence of intron 3 in the p67^{phox} gene causes the lack of p67^{phox} mRNA in a patient with chronic granulomatous disease. Blood 1995; 85:242.

900. Curnutte JT: Classification of chronic granulomatous disease. Hematol Oncol Clin North Am 1988; 20:241.

901. Segal AW: Nitroblue-tetrazolium tests. Lancet 1974; 2:1248.

902. Baehner RL, Nathan DG: Quantitative nitroblue tetrazolium test in chronic granulomatous disease. N Engl J Med 1968; 278:971.

903. Newburger PE, Cohen HJ, et al: Prenatal diagnosis of chronic granulomatous disease. N Engl J Med 1979; 300:178.

904. Matthay KK, Golbus MS, et al: Prenatal diagnosis of chronic granulomatous disease. Am J Med Genet 1984; 17:731.

905. Huu TP, Dumez Y, et al: Prenatal diagnosis of chronic granulomatous disease (CGD) in four high risk male fetuses. Prenat Diagn 1987; 7:253.

906. Borregaard N, Bang J, et al: Prenatal diagnosis of chronic granulomatous disease. Lancet 1982; 1:114.

907. Battat L, Francke U: Nsi I RFLP at the X-linked chronic granulomatous disease locus (*CYBB*). Nucleic Acids Res 1989; 18:4966.

908. Muhlebach TJ, Robinson W, et al: A second NsiI RFLP at the *CYBB* locus. Nucleic Acids Res 1990; 18:4966.

909. Kenney R, Leto T: A HindIII polymorphism in the human *NCF2* gene. Nucleic Acids Res 1990; 18:7193.

910. Hopkins PJ, Bemiller LS, Curnutte JT: Chronic granulomatous disease: Diagnosis and classification at the molecular level. Clin Lab Med 1992; 12:277.

911. Weening RS, Corbeel L, et al: Cytochrome b deficiency in an autosomal form of chronic granulomatous disease. A third form of chronic granulomatous disease recognized by monocyte hybridization. J Clin Invest 1985; 75:915.

912. Margolis DM, Melnic DA, et al: Trimethoprim-sulfamethoxazole prophylaxis in the management of chronic granulomatous disease. J Infect Dis 1990; 162:723.

913. Chusid MJ, Gelfand JA, et al: Pulmonary aspergillosis, inhalation of contaminated marijuana smoke, chronic granulomatous disease. Ann Intern Med 1975; 82:682.

914. Mouy R, Veber F, et al: Long-term itraconazole prophylaxis against *Aspergillus* infections in thirty-two patients with chronic granulomatous disease. J Pediatr 1994; 125:998.

915. Roback SA, Weintraub WH, et al: Chronic granulomatous disease of childhood: Surgical considerations. J Pediatr Surg 1971; 6:601.

916. Emmerndorffer A, Lohmann-Mathes ML, Roesler J: Kinetics of transfused neutrophils in peripheral blood and BAL fluid of a patient with variant X-linked chronic granulomatous disease. Eur J Haematol 1991; 47:246.

917. Gallin JI, Malech HL, et al: A controlled trial of interferon gamma to prevent infection in chronic granulomatous disease. N Engl J Med 1991; 324:509.

918. Weening RS, Leitz GJ, Seger RA: Recombinant human interferon-gamma in patients with chronic granulomatous disease—European follow up study. Eur J Pediatr 1995; 154:295.

919. Nathan CF, Murray HW, et al: Identification of interferon gamma as the lymphokine that activates human macrophage oxidative metabolism and antimicrobial activity. J Exp Med 1983; 158:670.

920. Ezekowitz RAB, Orkin SH, Newburger PE: Recombinant interferon gamma augments phagocyte superoxide production and X-chronic granulomatous disease gene expression in X-linked variant chronic granulomatous disease. J Clin Invest 1987; 80:1009.

921. Ezekowitz RA, Dinauer MC, et al: Partial correction of the phagocyte defect in patients with X-linked chronic granulomatous disease by subcutaneous interferon gamma. N Engl J Med 1988; 319:146.

922. Sechler JMG, Malech HL, et al: Recombinant human interferon-gamma reconstitutes defective phagocyte function in patients with chronic granulomatous disease. Proc Natl Acad Sci U S A 1988; 85:4374.

922a. Ezekowitz RA, Sieff CA, et al: Restoration of phagocyte function by interferon-γ in X-linked chronic granulomatous disease occurs at the level of progenitor cell. Blood 1990; 76:2443.

923. Woodman R, Erickson R, et al: Prolonged recombinant interferon-γ therapy in chronic granulomatous disease: Evidence against enhanced neutrophil oxidase activity. Blood 1992; 79:1558.

924. Chin TW, Stiehm ER, et al: Corticosteroids in treatment of obstructive lesions of chronic granulomatous disease. J Pediatr 1987; 111:349.

925. Quie PG, Belani KK: Corticosteroids for chronic granulomatous disease. J Pediatr 1987; 111:393.

926. Fischer A, Segal AW, Weening RS: The management of chronic granulomatous disease. Eur J Pediatr 1993; 152:896.

927. Danziger RN, Goren AT, et al: Outpatient management with oral corticosteroid therapy for obstructive conditions in chronic granulomatous disease. J Pediatr 1993; 122:303.

928. Rosh JR, Tang HB, et al: Treatment of intractable gastrointestinal manifestations of chronic granulomatous disease with cyclosporine. J Pediatr 1995; 126:143.

929. Schettini F, De Mattia D, et al: Bone marrow transplantation for chronic granulomatous disease associated with cytochrome b deficiency. Pediatr Hematol Oncol 1987; 4:277. Letter to the editor.

930. Kamani N, August CS, et al: Marrow transplantation in chronic granulomatous disease: An update, with 6-year follow-up. J Pediatr 1988; 113:697.

931. Kume A, Dinauer MC: Retrovirus-mediated reconstitution of respiratory burst activity in X-linked chronic granulomatous disease cells. Blood 1994; 84:331.

932. Zhen L, King A, et al: Gene targeting of X-linked chronic granulomatous disease locus in a human myeloid leukemia cell line and rescue by expression of recombinant gp91^{phox}. Proc Natl Acad Sci U S A 1993; 90:9832.

933. Jackson SH, Gallin JI, Holland SM: The p47^{phox} mouse knockout model of chronic granulomatous disease. J Exp Med 1995; 182:751.

934. Porter C, Parkar M, et al: X-linked chronic granulomatous disease: Correction of NADPH oxidase defect by retrovirus-mediated expression of gp91-phox. Blood 1993; 82:2196.

935. Kume A, Dinauer M: Retrovirus-mediated reconstitution of respiratory burst activity in X-linked chronic granulomatous disease cells. Blood 1994; 84:3311.

936. Li F, Linton G, et al: CD34$^+$ peripheral blood progenitors as a target for genetic correction of the two flavocytochrome b_{558} defective forms of chronic granulomatous disease. Blood 1994; 84:53.

937. Sekhsaria S, Gallin J, Malech H: Retrovirus mediated correction of superoxide production by gene transfer into peripheral blood hematopoietic progenitors (PBHP) from patients with p47^{phox} deficient chronic granulomatous disease. Clin Res 1993; 41:213A.

938. Volpp B, Lin Y: In vitro molecular reconstitution of the respiratory burst in B lymphoblasts from p47-phox-deficient chronic granulomatous disease. J Clin Invest 1993; 91:201.

939. Thrasher A, Chetty M, et al: Restoration of superoxide generation to a chronic granulomatous disease–derived B-cell like by retrovirus mediated gene transfer. Blood 1992; 80:1125.

940. Chanock SJ, Faust LRP, et al: O$_2$ production by B-lymphocytes lacking the respiratory burst oxidase subunit p47-phox after transfection with an expression vector containing a p47-phox cDNA. Proc Natl Acad Sci U S A 1992; 89:10174.

941. Baehner RL, Johnston RB, Nathan DG: Comparative study of the metabolic and bactericidal characteristics of severely glucose-6-phosphate dehydrogenase deficient polymorphonuclear leukocytes and leukocytes from children with chronic granulomatous disease. J Reticuloendothel Soc 1972; 12:150.

942. Gray GR, Stamatoyannopoulos G, et al: Neutrophil dysfunction, chronic granulomatous disease, and non-spherocytic haemolytic anaemia caused by complete deficiency of glucose-6-phosphate dehydrogenase. Lancet 1973; 2:530.

943. Cooper MR, Dechatelet LR, et al: Leukocyte G-6-PD deficiency. Lancet 1970; 2:110.

944. Vives Corrons JL, Feliu E, et al: Severe glucose-6-phosphate dehydrogenase (G6PD) deficiency associated with chronic hemolytic anemia, granulocyte dysfunction, and increased susceptibility to infections: Description of a new molecular variant (G6PD Barcelona). Blood 1982; 59:428.

945. Beutler E: G6PD deficiency. Blood 1994; 84:3613.

946. Yoshida A, Stamatoyannopoulos G, Motulsky A: Biochemical genetics of glucose-6-phosphate dehydrogenase variation. Ann N Y Acad Sci 1968; 155:868.

947. Justice P, Shih L-Y, et al: Characterization of leukocyte glucose-6-phosphate dehydrogenase in normal and mutant human subjects. J Lab Clin Med 1966; 68:552.

948. Ramot B, Fisher S, et al: A study of subjects with erythrocyte glucose-6-phosphate dehydrogenase deficiency. II. Investigation of leukocyte enzymes. J Clin Invest 1959; 38:2234.

949. Mamlok RJ, Mamlok V, et al: Glucose-6-phosphate dehydrogenase deficiency, neutrophil dysfunction and Chromobacterium violaceum sepsis. J Pediatr 1987; 111:852.

950. Parry MF, Root RK, et al: Myeloperoxidase deficiency: Prevalence and clinical significance. Ann Intern Med 1981; 95:293.

951. Nauseef WM: Myeloperoxidase deficiency. Hematol Oncol Clin North Am 1988; 2:135.

952. Salmon SE, Cline MJ, et al: Myeloperoxidase deficiency. Immunological study of a genetic leukocyte defect. N Engl J Med 1970; 282:250.

953. Nauseef WM, Metcalf JA, Root RK: Role of myeloperoxidase in the respiratory burst of human neutrophils. Blood 1983; 61:483.

954. Lehrer RI, Cline MJ: Leukocyte myeloperoxidase deficiency and disseminated candidiasis: The role of myeloperoxidase in resistance to Candida infection. J Clin Invest 1969; 48:1478.

955. Diamond RD, Clark RA, Haudenschild CC: Damage to Candida albicans hyphae and pseudohyphae by the myeloperoxidase system and oxidative products of neutrophil metabolism in vitro. J Clin Invest 1980; 66:908.

956. Cech P, Stalder H, et al: Leukocyte myeloperoxidase deficiency and diabetes mellitus associated with Candida albicans liver abscess. Am J Med 1979; 66:149.

957. Kitahara M, Eyre HJ, et al: Hereditary myeloperoxidase deficiency. Blood 1981; 57:888.

958. Chang KS, Schroeder W, et al: The localization of the human myeloperoxidase gene is in close proximity to the translocation breakpoint in acute promyelocytic leukemia. Leukemia 1987; 1:458.

959. Van Tuinen P, Johnson KR, et al: Localization of myeloperoxidase to the long arm of human chromosome 17: Relationship to the 15, 17 translocation of acute promyelocytic leukemia. Oncogene 1987; 1:319.

960. Bendix-Hansen K, Kerndrup G: Myeloperoxidase-deficient polymorphonuclear leukocytes (V): Relation to FAB classification and neutrophil alkaline phosphatase activity in primary myelodysplastic syndromes. Scand J Haematol 1985; 35:197.

961. Bendix-Hansen K, Kerndrup G, Pedersen B: Myeloperoxidase-deficient polymorphonuclear leukocytes (VI): Relation to cytogenetic abnormalities in primary myelodysplastic syndromes. Scand J Haematol 1986; 36:3.

962. Kizaki M, Miller CW, et al: Myeloperoxidase (MPO) gene mutation in hereditary MPO deficiency. Blood 1994; 83:1935.

963. Nauseef WM, Brigham S, Cogley M: Hereditary myeloperoxidase deficiency due to a missense mutation of arginine 569 to tryptophan. J Biol Chem 1994; 269:1212.

964. Nauseef WM: Aberrant restriction endonuclease digests of DNA from subjects with hereditary myeloperoxidase deficiency. Blood 1989; 73:290.

965. Tobler A, Selsted ME, et al: Evidence for a pretranslational defect in hereditary and acquired myeloperoxidase deficiency. Blood 1989; 73:1980.

966. Selsted ME, Miller CW, et al: Molecular analysis of myeloperoxidase deficiency shows heterogeneous patterns of the complete deficiency state manifested at the genomic, mRNA, and protein levels. Blood 1993; 82:1317.

967. Stendahl O, Coble B-I, et al: Myeloperoxidase modulates the phagocytic activity of polymorphonuclear leukocytes. Studies with cells from a myeloperoxidase-deficient patient. J Clin Invest 1984; 73:366.

968. Rosen H, Klebanoff SJ: Chemiluminescence and superoxide production by myeloperoxidase-deficient leukocytes. J Clin Invest 1976; 58:50.

969. Jandl RC, Andre-Schwartz J, et al: Termination of the respiratory burst in human neutrophils. J Clin Invest 1978; 61:1176.

970. Roos D, Weening RS, et al: Protection of phagocytic leukocytes by endogenous glutathione: Studies in a family with glutathione reductase deficiency. Blood 1979; 53:851.

971. Boxer LA, Oliver JM, et al: Protection of granulocytes by vitamin E in glutathione synthetase deficiency. N Engl J Med 1979; 301:901.

972. Loos JA, Roos D, et al: Familial deficiency of glutathione reductase in human blood cells. Blood 1976; 48:53.

973. Spielberg SP, Kramer LI, et al: S-Oxoprolinuria: Biochemical observations and case report. J Pediatr 1977; 91:237.

974. Spielberg SP, Boxer LA, et al: Oxidative damage to neutrophils in glutathione synthetase deficiency. Br J Haematol 1979; 42:215.

975. Nevin NC, Morrison PJ, et al: Inverted tandem duplication of 8p12–p23.1 in a child with increased activity of glutathione reductase. J Med Genet 1990; 27:135.

976. Holmes B, Park BH, et al: Chronic granulomatous disease in females: A deficiency of leukocyte glutathione peroxidase. N Engl J Med 1970; 283:217.

977. Matsuda I, Oka Y, et al: Leukocyte glutathione peroxidase deficiency in a male patient with chronic granulomatous disease. J Pediatr 1976; 88:581.

Appendices

Reference Values in Infancy and Childhood

Carlo Brugnara

Appendix 1. HEMATOLOGIC VALUES IN NORMAL FETUSES AT DIFFERENT GESTATIONAL AGES

Week of Gestation	Hemoglobin (g/dL)	RBCs (× 10⁶/μL)	Hematocrit (%)	Mean Corpuscular Volume (fL)	Total WBCs (× 10⁶/μL)	Corrected WBCs (× 10⁶/μL)	Platelets (× 10⁶/μL)
18–21 (n = 760)	11.69 ± 1.27	2.85 ± 0.36	37.3 ± 4.32	131.1 ± 11.0	4.68 ± 2.96	2.57 ± 0.42	234 ± 57
22–25 (n = 1200)	12.2 ± 1.6	3.09 ± 0.34	38.59 ± 3.94	125.1 ± 7.8	4.72 ± 2.82	3.73 ± 2.17	247 ± 59
26–29 (n = 460)	12.91 ± 1.38	3.46 ± 0.41	40.88 ± 4.4	118.5 ± 8.0	5.16 ± 2.53	4.08 ± 0.84	242 ± 69
>30 (n = 440)	13.64 ± 2.21	3.82 ± 0.64	43.55 ± 7.2	114.4 ± 9.3	7.71 ± 4.99	6.4 ± 2.99	232 ± 87

Hematologic data obtained with a Coulter S plus II instrument. Total WBC count included nucleated red blood cells. Corrected WBC count included only WBCs, after subtracting the nucleated red cell component, based on a 100-cell manual differential.
From Forestier F, Daffos F, et al: Developmental hematopoiesis in normal human fetal blood. Blood 1991; 77:2360.

Appendix 2. WHITE CELL MANUAL DIFFERENTIAL COUNTS IN NORMAL FETUSES AT DIFFERENT GESTATIONAL AGES

Week of Gestation	Lymphocytes (%)	Neutrophils (%)	Eosinophils (%)	Basophils (%)	Monocytes (%)	Nucleated Red Cells (% of WBC)
18–21 (n = 186)	88 ± 7	6 ± 4	2 ± 3	0.5 ± 1	3.5 ± 2	45 ± 86
22–25 (n = 230)	87 ± 6	6.5 ± 3.5	3 ± 3	0.5 ± 1	3.5 ± 2.5	21 ± 23
26–29 (n = 144)	85 ± 6	8.5 ± 4	4 ± 3	0.5 ± 1	3.5 ± 2.5	21 ± 67
>30 (n = 172)	68.5 ± 15	23 ± 15	5 ± 3	0.5 ± 1	3.5 ± 2	17 ± 40

From Forestier F, Daffos F, et al: Developmental hematopoiesis in normal human fetal blood. Blood 1991; 77:2360.

Appendix 3. HEMATOLOGIC PARAMETERS IN NORMAL, FULL-TERM CORD BLOOD

	Paterakis et al. (1993)*	Diagne et al. (1995)†	Boulot et al. (1993)‡
Hemoglobin (g/dL)	15.6 ± 1.2	15.3 ± 1.3	13.9 ± 1.6
RBCs (× 10⁶/μL)	4.42 ± 0.35	4.30 ± 0.4	—
Hematocrit (%)	51.0 ± 4.5	49 ± 5	41.3 ± 4.9
Mean Corpuscular Volume (fL)	119.1 ± 4.8	112 ± 6	109 ± 9.8
Mean Corpuscular Hemoglobin (pg)	36.4 ± 1.6	36.2 ± 2.2	38.7 ± 4.0
Mean Corpuscular Hemoglobin Concentration (g/dL)	30.6 ± 1.3	30.9 ± 1.3	33.3 ± 1.4

Data are expressed as mean ± SD.
*Paterakis GS, Lykopoulou L, et al: Flow-cytometric analysis of reticulocytes in normal cord blood. Acta Haematol 1993; 90:182. Data obtained in 35 specimens with H*1 Technicon analyzer.
†Diagne I, Archambeaud MP, et al: Parametres erythrocytaires et reservés en fer dans le sang du cordon. Arch Fr Pediatr 1995; 2:208. Data obtained in 142 specimens with H*2 Technicon analyzer.
‡Boulot P, Cattaneo A, et al: Hematologic values of fetal blood obtained by means of cordocentesis. Fetal Diagn Ther 1993; 8:309.

Appendix 4. ERYTHROBLAST AND LEUKOCYTE COUNTS IN UMBILICAL CORD BLOOD

Type of Delivery	Erythroblast Count ($\times 10^9$/L)	Leukocyte Count ($\times 10^9$/L)
Spontaneous, vaginal (n = 55)	0.75 (0.0–5.3)	13.8 (7.25–48.0)
Elective cesarean section (n = 39)	0.30 (0.0–0.49)	10.6 (6.2–17.7)
Emergency cesarean section (n = 55)	1.10 (0.0–15.9)	13.5 (4.2–40.3)

Values are expressed as mean (range). Erythroblast counts were significantly higher in the spontaneous vaginal and emergency cesarean section groups compared with the elective cesarean delivery group.
From Thilaganathan B, Athanasiou S, et al: Umbilical cord blood erythroblast count as an index of intrauterine hypoxia. Arch Dis Child 1994; 70:F192.

Appendix 5. HEMATOLOGIC VALUES FOR NORMAL CORD BLOOD

	Mean ± SD
Red Blood Cells	
Hb (g/dL)	15.3 ± 1.3
Hct (%)	49 ± 5
RBC ($\times 10^6$/μL)	4.3 ± 0.4
MCV (fL)	112 ± 6
MCH (pg)	36.2 ± 2.2
MCHC (g/dL)	30.9 ± 1.3
CHCM (g/dL)	30.4 ± 1.2
% HYPO (MCHC < 28 g/dL)	17.3 ± 11.9
% HYPER (MCHC > 41 g/dL)	0.6 ± 0.3
% MICRO (MCV < 61 fL)	0.8 ± 0.3
% MACRO (MCV > 120 fL)	31.8 ± 9.7
Reticulocytes	
%	3.63 ± 1.11
Absolute reticulocytes ($\times 10^9$/L)	156.1 ± 47.7
MCVr (fL)	125.8 ± 7.3
CHCMr (g/dL)	25.6 ± 1.2
CHr (pg)	31.3 ± 1.4

MCV = mean corpuscular volume; MCHC = mean corpuscular hemoglobin concentration; MCH = mean corpuscular hemoglobin; CHCM = cell hemoglobin concentration mean; % HYPO = % hypochromic red cells; % HYPER = % hyperchromic red cells; % MICRO = % microcytic red cells; % MACRO = % macrocytic red cells; MCVr = reticulocyte mean corpuscular volume; CHCMr = reticulocyte cell hemoglobin concentration mean; CHr = reticulocyte hemoglobin content. Values obtained with Technicon H*2 and H*3 Hematology analyzers (Bayer Diagnostics) in neonates delivered at term with weight ≥ 2500 g.
Adapted from Diagne I, Archambeaud MP, et al: Parametres erythrocytaires et reservés en fer dans le sang du cordon. Arch Fr Pediatr 1995; 2:208, and from G Tchernia, personal communication. Data obtained in 142 specimens with H*2 Technicon analyzer.

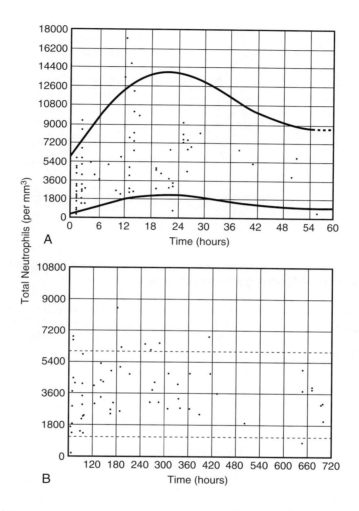

Appendix 6. Reference range for circulating neutrophil counts in healthy very-low-birth-weight neonates.

Based on 160 neutrophil counts obtained in 63 infants without perinatal complications at 0 to 60 hours of age. Birth weight was 1220 ± 203 g, gestational age 29.9 ± 2.3 weeks ($\pm$SD). *A,* Neutrophil count at birth to 60 hours of life. *B,* Neutrophil count at 61 hours to 28 days of life. Bold *(A)* and dotted *(B)* lines represent the envelopes bounding these data, respectively. (From Mouzinho A, Rosenfeld CR, et al: Revised reference ranges for circulating neutrophils in very-low-birth-weight neonates. Pediatrics 1994; 94:76. Reproduced by permission of *Pediatrics,* Copyright 1994.)

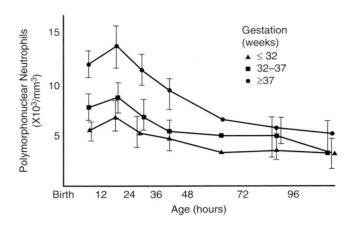

Appendix 7. Changes in polymorphonuclear neutrophils after birth in three groups with different gestational ages.

Total WBC counts were obtained with a Coulter S analyzer; manual differential counts were performed on 200 nucleated cells. (From Coulombel L, Dehan M, et al: The number of polymorphonuclear leukocytes in relation to gestational age in the newborn. Acta Paediatr Scand 1979; 68:709.)

Appendix 8. NORMAL HEMATOLOGIC VALUES DURING THE FIRST 2 WEEKS OF LIFE IN THE TERM INFANT*

Value	Cord Blood	Day 1	Day 3	Day 7	Day 14
Hemoglobin (g/dL)	16.8	18.4	17.8	17.0	16.8
Hematocrit (%)	53.0	58.0	55.0	54.0	52.0
Red cells (mm³)	5.25	5.8	5.6	5.2	5.1
MCV (fL)	107	108	99.0	98.0	96.0
MCH (pg)	34	35	33	32.5	31.5
MCHC (g/dL)	31.7	32.5	33	33	33
Reticulocytes (%)	3–7	3–7	1–3	0–1	0–1
Nucleated RBCs (/mm³)	500	200	0–5	0	0
Platelets (1000's/mm³)	290	192	213	248	252

MCV = mean corpuscular volume; MCH = mean corpuscular hemoglobin; MCHC = mean corpuscular hemoglobin concentration.
*During the first 2 weeks of life a venous hemoglobin value below 13.0 g/dL or a capillary hemoglobin value below 14.5 g/dL should be regarded as anemic.
From Oski FA, Naiman JL: Hematologic Problems in the Newborn. 2nd ed. Philadelphia, W.B. Saunders Co., 1972, p 13.

Appendix 9. NORMAL HEMATOLOGIC VALUES DURING THE FIRST YEAR OF LIFE IN HEALTHY TERM INFANTS*

n	Age (mo)						
	0.5 (N = 232)	1 (N = 240)	2 (N = 241)	4 (N = 52)	6 (N = 52)	9 (N = 56)	12 (N = 56)
Hemoglobin (mean ± SE)	16.6 ± 0.11	13.9 ± 0.10	11.2 ± 0.06	12.2 ± 0.14	12.6 ± 0.10	12.7 ± 0.09	12.7 ± 0.09
−2 SD	13.4	10.7	9.4	10.3	11.1	11.4	11.3
Hematocrit (mean ± SE)	53 ± 0.4	44 ± 0.3	35 ± 0.2	38 ± 0.4	36 ± 0.3	36 ± 0.3	37 ± 0.3
−2 SD	41	33	28	32	31	32	33
RBC count (mean ± SE)	4.9 ± 0.03	4.3 ± 0.03	3.7 ± 0.02	4.3 ± 0.06	4.7 ± 0.05	4.7 ± 0.04	4.7 ± 0.04
−2 SD +2 SD	3.9–5.9	3.3–5.3	3.1–4.3	3.5–5.1	3.9–5.5	4.0–5.3	4.1–5.3
MCH (mean ± SE)	33.6 ± 0.1	32.5 ± 0.1	30.4 ± 0.1	28.6 ± 0.2	26.8 ± 0.2	27.3 ± 0.2	26.8 ± 0.2
−2 SD	30	29	27	25	24	25	24
MCV (mean ± SE)	105.3 ± 0.6	101.3 ± 0.3	94.8 ± 0.3	86.7 ± 0.8	76.3 ± 0.6	77.7 ± 0.5	77.7 ± 0.5
−2 SD	88	91	84	76	68	70	71
MCHC (mean ± SE)	314 ± 1.1	318 ± 1.2	318 ± 1.1	327 ± 2.7	350 ± 1.7	349 ± 1.6	343 ± 1.5
−2 SD	281	281	283	288	327	324	321

MCH = mean corpuscular hemoglobin; MCV = mean corpuscular volume; MCHC = mean corpuscular hemoglobin concentration.
*These values were obtained from a selected group of 256 healthy term infants followed at the Helsinki University Central Hospital who were receiving continuous iron supplementation and who had normal values for transferrin saturation and serum ferritin.
Values at the ages of 0.5, 1, and 2 months were obtained from the entire group, and those at the later ages were obtained from the iron-supplemented infant group after exclusion of iron deficiency.
From Saarinen UM, Siimes MA: Developmental changes in red blood cell counts and indices of infants after exclusion of iron deficiency by laboratory criteria and continuous iron supplementation. J Pediatr 1978; 92:414.

Appendix 10. HEMOGLOBIN CONCENTRATION DURING THE FIRST 6 MONTHS OF LIFE IN IRON-SUFFICIENT PRETERM INFANTS*

Age	No.	Birth Weight	
		1000–1500 g	1501–2000 g
2 wk	17, 39	16.3 (11.7–18.4)	14.8 (11.8–19.6)
1 mo	15, 42	10.9 (8.7–15.2)	11.5 (8.2–15.0)
2 mo	17, 47	8.8 (7.1–11.5)	9.4 (8.0–11.4)
3 mo	16, 41	9.8 (8.9–11.2)	10.2 (9.3–11.8)
4 mo	13, 37	11.3 (9.1–13.1)	11.3 (9.1–13.1)
5 mo	8, 21	11.6 (10.2–14.3)	11.8 (10.4–13.0)
6 mo	9, 21	12.0 (9.4–13.8)	11.8 (10.7–12.6)

*These infants were admitted to the Helsinki Children's Hospital during a 15-month period. None had a complicated course during the first 2 weeks of life or had undergone an exchange transfusion. All infants were iron sufficient, as indicated by a serum ferritin ≥ 10 ng/mL.
From Lundstrom U, Siimes MA, et al: At what age does iron supplementation become necessary in low birth weight infants? J Pediatr 1977; 91:882.

Appendix 11. NORMAL HEMATOLOGIC VALUES IN CHILDREN*

Age	Hemoglobin (g/dL) Mean	Hemoglobin (g/dL) − 2 SD	Hematocrit (%) Mean	Hematocrit (%) − 2 SD	Red Cell Count (10¹²/L) Mean	Red Cell Count (10¹²/L) − 2 SD	MCV (fL) Mean	MCV (fL) − 2 SD	MCH (pg) Mean	MCH (pg) − 2 SD	MCHC (g/dL) Mean	MCHC (g/dL) − 2 SD
Birth (cord blood)	16.5	13.5	51	42	4.7	3.9	108	98	34	31	33	30
1 to 3 days (capillary)	18.5	14.5	56	45	5.3	4.0	108	95	34	31	33	29
1 week	17.5	13.5	54	42	5.1	3.9	107	88	34	28	33	28
2 weeks	16.5	12.5	51	39	4.9	3.6	105	86	34	28	33	28
1 month	14.0	10.0	43	31	4.2	3.0	104	85	34	28	33	29
2 months	11.5	9.0	35	28	3.8	2.7	96	77	30	26	33	29
3 to 6 months	11.5	9.5	35	29	3.8	3.1	91	74	30	25	33	30
0.5 to 2 years	12.0	10.5	36	33	4.5	3.7	78	70	27	23	33	30
2 to 6 years	12.5	11.5	37	34	4.6	3.9	81	75	27	24	34	31
6 to 12 years	13.5	11.5	40	35	4.6	4.0	86	77	29	25	34	31
12 to 18 years												
Female	14.0	12.0	41	36	4.6	4.1	90	78	30	25	34	31
Male	14.5	13.0	43	37	4.9	4.5	88	78	30	25	34	31
18 to 49 years												
Female	14.0	12.0	41	36	4.6	4.0	90	80	30	26	34	31
Male	15.5	13.5	47	41	5.2	4.5	90	80	30	26	34	31

*These data have been compiled from several sources. Emphasis is given to studies employing electronic counters and to the selection of populations that are likely to exclude individuals with iron deficiency. The mean ± 2 SD can be expected to include 95% of the observations in a normal population.
From Dallman PR: In Rudolph A (ed): Pediatrics, 16th ed. New York, Appleton-Century-Crofts, 1977, p 1111.

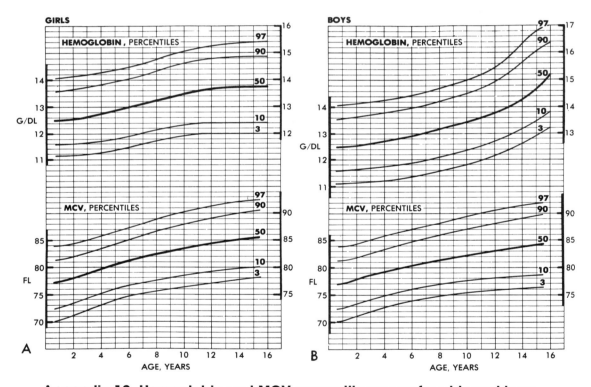

Appendix 12. Hemoglobin and MCV percentile curves for girls and boys.

A, Hemoglobin and MCV percentile curves for girls. *B,* Hemoglobin and MCV percentile curves for boys. These figures were obtained from populations of nonindigent white children residing in either northern California or Finland. Hemoglobin values were derived from a total of 9946 children and MCV values from 2314 children. The reference population excluded subjects with laboratory evidence of iron deficiency, thalassemia minor, and hemoglobinopathy. (New curves based on HANES III should be published soon. They show lower values in infants for hemoglobin.) (From Dallman PR, Siimes MA: Percentile curves for hemoglobin and red cell volume in infancy and childhood. J Pediatr 1979; 94:28.)

Appendix 13. HEMOGLOBIN CONCENTRATION IN WHITE, BLACK, AND EAST ASIAN CHILDREN*

Age	Males No.	Median	2.5 to 97.5 Percentile Range	Females No.	Median	2.5 to 97.5 Percentile Range
5 to 9 years						
White	305	13.0	11.6–14.3	291	12.9	11.5–14.4
Black	87	12.6	11.1–14.1	104	12.5	11.2–13.6
East Asian	50	13.1	11.9–14.4	64	13.0	11.6–14.2
10 to 14 weeks						
White	447	13.7	12.3–15.5	484	13.4	12.0–14.9
Black	143	13.1	11.5–15.2	150	12.9	11.2–14.3
East Asian	87	13.7	12.1–15.6	79	13.5	12.2–14.7

*Hemoglobin concentration in subjects with hemoglobin AA, normal glucose-6-phosphate-dehydrogenase screen, and mean corpuscular volume 95% or more of median value for whites of same age and sex. The data strengthen the impression that blacks normally have a concentration of hemoglobin averaging about 0.5 g/dL less than whites.
From Dallman PR, Barr GD, et al: Hemoglobin concentration in white, black, and Oriental children: is there a need for separate criteria in screening for anemia? Am J Clin Nutr 1978; 31:379. © Am. J. Clin. Nutr., American Society for Clinical Nutrition.

Appendix 14. HEMOGLOBIN, SERUM TRANSFERRIN SATURATION, SERUM FERRITIN, AND RED CELL INDICES IN ADOLESCENTS (15–16 YEARS OF AGE)

	Mean ± SD	Percentile 10th	25th	50th	75th	90th
Boys						
Hb (g/dL)	14.7 ± 0.831	135	14.2	14.7	15.2	15.7
Transferrin saturation (%)	32.7 ± 10.25	21.2	25.7	31.7	38.6	46.3
Serum ferritin (µg/L)	26.4 ± 17.71	13.2	22	29	40.8	52
MCV (fl)	88.4 ± 3.87	83.5	85.5	88.1	90.9	93.2
RDW (%)	13.0 ± 0.95	12.3	12.5	12.9	13.2	13.5
MCH (pg)	29.4 ± 1.43	27.7	28.6	29.2	30.2	31.0
Girls						
Hb (g/dL)	13.4 ± 0.763	12.3	12.9	13.4	13.9	14.3
Transferrin saturation (%)	29.9 ± 10.7	17.2	22.8	29	35.2	43.4
Serum ferritin (µg/L)	18.2 ± 1.98	7.5	12	18.2	28.5	41.5
MCV (fl)	90.1 ± 3.86	84.8	87.6	90.3	92.8	94.8
RDW (%)	12.8 ± 0.71	12.1	12.4	12.7	13.2	13.6
MCH (pg)	29.6 ± 1.43	27.8	28.8	29.5	30.6	31.3

Data for serum ferritin are presented as geometric means ± antilog of logarithmic values. Data collected in 197 to 207 boys and 215 to 220 girls, aged 15–16.
From Hallberg L, Hultén L, et al: Prevalence of iron deficiency in Swedish adolescents. Pediatr Res 1993; 34:680–687.

Appendix 15. VALUES OF SERUM IRON (SI), TOTAL IRON-BINDING CAPACITY (TIBC), AND TRANSFERRIN SATURATION (S%) FROM INFANTS DURING THE FIRST YEAR OF LIFE*

			Age (mo) 0.5	1	2	4	6	9	12
SI	Median	µmol/L	22	22	16	15	14	15	14
	95% range		11–36	10–31	3–29	3–29	5–24	6–24	6–28
		µg/dL	120	125	87	84	77	84	78
			63–201	58–172	15–159	18–164	28–135	34–135	35–155
TIBC (mean ± SD)		µmol/L	34 ± 8	36 ± 8	44 ± 10	54 ± 7	58 ± 9	61 ± 7	64 ± 7
		µg/dL	191 ± 43	199 ± 43	246 ± 55	300 ± 39	321 ± 51	341 ± 42	358 ± 38
S%	Median		68	63	34	27	23	25	23
	95% range		30–99	35–94	21–63	7–53	10–43	10–39	10–47

*These data were obtained from a group of healthy, full-term infants who were born at the Helsinki University Central Hospital. Infants received iron supplementation in formula and cereal throughout the 12-month period. Infants with hemoglobin below 110 g/dL, mean corpuscular volume of red blood cells below 71 µ³, or serum ferritin below 10 ng/mL, were excluded from the study. The 95% range of the transferrin saturation values indicates that the lower limit of normal is about 10% after 4 months of age.
From Saarinen UM, Siimes MA: Serum iron and transferrin in iron deficiency. J Pediatr 1977; 91:876.

Appendix 16. ACTIVITIES OF RED CELL ENZYMES

Enzyme	Activity at 37°C (mean ± SD)
Acetylcholinesterase	36.93 ± 3.83
Adenosine deaminase	1.11 ± 0.23
Adenylate kinase	258 ± 29.3
Aldolase	3.19 ± 0.86
Bisphosphoglyceromutase (2,3-diphosphoglyceromutase)	4.78 ± 0.65
Catalase	$15.3 ± 2.4 \times 10^4$
Enolase	5.39 ± 0.83
Epimerase	0.23 ± 0.06
Galactokinase	0.029 ± 0.004
Galactose-1-phosphate uridyl transferase	28.4 ± 6.94
Glucose phosphate isomerase	60.8 ± 11.0
Glucose-6-phosphate dehydrogenase	8.34 ± 1.59
WHO method	12.1 ± 2.09
Glutamic oxaloacetic transaminase without PLP	3.02 ± 0.67
Glutamic oxaloacetic transaminase with PLP	5.04 ± 0.90
γ-Glutamyl-cysteine synthetase	0.43 ± 0.04
Glutathione peroxidase*	30.82 ± 4.65
Glutathione reductase without FAD	7.18 ± 1.09
Glutathione reductase with FAD	10.4 ± 1.50
Glutathione-S-transferase	6.66 ± 1.81
Glyceraldehyde phosphate dehydrogenase	226 ± 41.9
Hexokinase	1.78 ± 0.38
Hypoxanthine phosphoribosyl-transferase	1.72 ± 0.30
Lactate dehydrogenase	200 ± 26.5
Methemoglobin reductase	2.60 ± 0.71
Monophosphoglyceromutase	37.71 ± 5.56
NADH-methemoglobin reductase	19.2 ± 3.85 (30°)
NADPH diaphorase	2.26 ± 0.16
Phosphofructokinase	11.01 ± 2.33
Phosphoglucomutase	5.50 ± 0.62
Phosphoglycerate kinase	320 ± 36.1
Phosphoglycolate phosphatase	1.23 ± 0.10
Pyrimidine 5′ nucleotidase	0.11 ± 0.03
Pyruvate kinase	15.0 ± 1.99
6-Phosphogluconate dehydrogenase	8.78 ± 0.78
Triose phosphate isomerase	2111 ± 397

From Beutler E, Blum KG: In Altman PL, Dittmer DS (eds): Human Health and Disease. Bethesda, MD, Federation of American Societies for Experimental Biology. 1977, p 156; and Beutler E. Red cell metabolism: a manual of biochemical methods. 3rd Ed. Orlando, FL, Grune & Stratton, 1984.

Appendix 17. LEVELS OF INTERMEDIATE METABOLITES IN NORMAL ADULT ERYTHROCYTES

Metabolite	Abbreviation	Concentration (mean ± 1 SD)		
		nmol/g Hb	nmol/mL Red Cells	μmol/L in Whole Blood
Adenosine-5′-diphosphate	ADP	6635 ± 105	216 ± 36	—
Adenosine-5′-monophosphate	AMP	62 ± 10	21.1 ± 3.4	—
Adenosine-5′-triphosphate	ATP	4230 ± 290 (whites)	1438 ± 99	—
		3530 ± 301 (blacks)	1200 ± 102	—
2,3-Diphosphoglycerate	2,3-DPG	1227 ± 1870	4171 ± 636	—
Glutathione	GSH	6570 ± 1040	2234 ± 354	—
Glutathione (oxidized)	GSSG	12.3 ± 4.5	4.2 ± 1.53	—
Glucose-6-phosphate	G6P	82 ± 22	27.8 ± 7.5	—
Fructose-6-phosphate	F6P	27 ± 5.8	9.3 ± 2.0	—
Fructose-6-diphosphate	FDP	5.6 ± 1.8	1.9 ± 0.6	—
Dihydroxyacetone phosphate	DHAP	27.6 ± 8.2	9.4 ± 2.8	—
3-Phosphoglyceric acid	3-PGA	132 ± 15.0	44.9 ± 5.1	—
2-Phosphoglyceric acid	2-PGA	21.5 ± 7.35	7.3 ± 2.5	—
Phosphoenolpyruvate	PEP	35.9 ± 6.47	12.2 ± 2.2	—
Creatine		1310 ± 310 (male)	445 ± 105	—
		1500 ± 250 (female)	510 ± 85	—
Lactate		—	—	932 ± 211
Pyruvate		—	—	53.3 ± 21.5

From Beutler E: Red Cell Metabolism: A Manual of Biochemical Methods. 3rd ed. Orlando, FL, Grune & Stratton, Inc., 1984.

Appendix 18. RED CELL ENZYME ACTIVITY IN ADULTS AND TERM INFANTS*

Enzyme	Adults (20)	Infants (10)
Hexokinase	12.9 ± 2.1	34.0 ± 6.0
Phosphoglucose isomerase	406 ± 37	560 ± 112
Phosphofructokinase	148 ± 24.5	84.5 ± 24
Aldolase	24.5 ± 3.7	42.0 ± 10.0
Glyceraldehyde-3-phosphate dehydrogenase	885 ± 127	884 ± 245
Triosephosphate isomerase	26,323 ± 3240	29,111 ± 4100
Phosphoglycerate kinase	2795 ± 144	3926 ± 528
Phosphoglycerate mutase	751 ± 99	1049 ± 160
Enolase	252 ± 54	517 ± 121
Pyruvate kinase	179 ± 16	256 ± 50
Lactic dehydrogenase	2033 ± 287	2756 ± 425
Glucose-6-phosphate dehydrogenase	215 ± 18	328 ± 40

*Infant samples were obtained from newborns weighing more than 2800 g whose gestational age was 39 weeks or greater. Blood was drawn within 24 hours of birth. All the newborns were clinically healthy. Adult samples were obtained from healthy, normal volunteers.
From Oski FA: Red cell metabolism in the newborn infant: V. Glycolytic intermediates and glycolytic enzymes. Pediatrics 1969; 44:89. Reproduced by permission of *Pediatrics,* Copyright 1969.

Appendix 19. RED CELL GLYCOLYTIC INTERMEDIATE METABOLITES IN NORMAL ADULTS, TERM INFANTS, AND PREMATURE INFANTS*

Metabolite	Normal Adults (10)	Term Infants (10)	Premature Infants (11)	Normals (5)
Glucose-6-phosphate	24.8 ± 9.8	45.2 ± 8.7	66.8 ± 34.8	27 ± 2.4
Fructose-6-phosphate	5.4 ± 1.0	9.9 ± 2.3	20.5 ± 8.9	11 ± 2.5
Fructose, 1,6-diphosphate	4.6 ± 1.0	3.8 ± 0.7	3.6 ± 0.8	5 ± 0.9
Dihydroxyacetone phosphate	4.9 ± 3.5	11.9 ± 5.0	18.6 ± 10.7	12 ± 3.7
Glyceraldehyde-3-phosphate	2.6 ± 0.7	1.9 ± 1.6	6.5 ± 3.2	4 ± 1.5
3-Phosphoglycerate	61.6 ± 12.4	58.2 ± 14.4	47.5 ± 14.2	48 ± 16.1
2-Phosphoglycerate	4.3 ± 1.8	4.9 ± 1.6	4.4 ± 2.5	7 ± 1.7
Phosphoenolpyruvate	8.8 ± 2.6	7.6 ± 2.9	7.4 ± 3.0	12 ± 0.9
Pyruvate	73.5 ± 33.1	70.4 ± 32.3	78.4 ± 4.15	71 ± 17.7
2,3-Diphosphoglycerate	4423 ± 1907	3609 ± 800	3152 ± 2133	4000

*Samples from normal adults and term infants were identical to those described in Appendix 18. Premature infants had birth weights below 2200 g and gestational age less than 37 weeks. These premature infants were healthy at the time of investigation.
From Oski FA: Red cell metabolism in the newborn infant: V. Glycolytic intermediates and glycolytic enzymes. Pediatrics 1969; 44:87. Reproduced with permission of *Pediatrics,* Copyright 1969.

Appendix 20. RED CELL ENZYME ACTIVITY LEVELS IN CORD BLOOD AND 4th-DAY BLOOD

	Cord	4th Day	P
Glucose-6-phosphate dehydrogenase	8.51 ± 1.20	6.23 ± 1.45	.005
Glutathione peroxidase	12.73 ± 1.32	14.01 ± 1.10	.001
Glutathione reductase	5.27 ± 1.21	6.49 ± 1.15	.004
Catalase	11.36 ± 1.28	12.73 ± 1.12	.025
Superoxide dismutase	1.21 ± 0.09	1.20 ± 0.08	NS

Data expressed in IU/g Hb as mean ± SD; n = 36.
From Buonocore G, Berni S, et al: Characteristics and functional properties of red cells during the first days of life. Biol Neonate 1991; 60:137. Reproduced with permission of S. Karger AG, Basel.

Appendix 21. HEMOGLOBIN A CONCENTRATION IN MALE AND FEMALE NEWBORNS ACCORDING TO BIRTH WEIGHT

Birth Weight (g)	Males Hb A (%)	Females Hb A (%)
<1501	7.1 ± 1.3 (9)	13.2 ± 11.3 (14)
1501–2000	12.2 ± 8.2 (36)	13.1 ± 10.4 (44)
2001–2500	12.6 ± 5.2 (139)	14.9 ± 6.5 (206)*
2501–3000	15.8 ± 6.4 (635)	17.8 ± 6.2 (776)*
3001–3500	18.2 ± 6.5 (1289)	19.9 ± 6.8 (1204)*
3501–4000	20.0 ± 6.6 (803)	20.9 ± 7.2 (590)*
4001–4500	19.7 ± 6.3 (200)	22.6 ± 8.6 (94)*
>4500	21.7 ± 7.0 (45)	20.9 ± 7.2 (20)

*P < .05 between males and females.
From Galacteros F, Guilloud-Bataille M, Feingold J: Sex, gestational age, and weight dependency of adult hemoglobin concentration in normal newborns. Blood 1991; 78:1121.

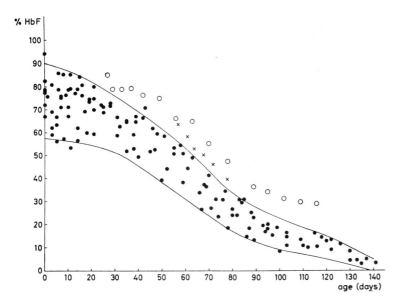

Appendix 22. Relative concentration of hemoglobin F in infants and its variation with age.

The region between the curved lines contains 120 observations in 17 normal children. (From Garby L, Sjolin S: Development of erythropoiesis. Acta Paediatr 1962; 51:245.)

Appendix 23. PERCENTAGE OF HEMOGLOBINS F AND A2 IN THE NEWBORN AND ADULT*

	% Hb F (Gα:Aα ratio)	% Hb A2
Newborn	60–90 (3:1)	<1.0
Adult	<1.0 (2:3)	1.6–3.5

*The α chains of fetal hemoglobin contain either a glycyl residue or an alanyl residue at position 136. The Gα:Aα ratio in the newborn undergoes a considerable change between the third and fourth months of life, at which time it approximates that of the Hb F of adults.
From Charache S: In Altman PL, Dittmer DS (eds): Human Health and Disease. Bethesda, MD, Federation of American Societies for Experimental Biology, 1977, p 159.

Appendix 24. METHEMOGLOBIN LEVELS IN NORMAL CHILDREN*

	No. Cases	No. Det.	Methemoglobin (g/dL)			No. Cases	No. Det.	Methemoglobin as Per Cent of Total Hemoglobin		
			Mean	Range	Standard Dev.			Mean	Range	Standard Dev.
Prematures (birth–7 days)	29	34	0.43	(0.02–0.83)	±0.07	24	28	2.3	(0.08–4.4)	±1.26
Prematures (7–72 days)	21	29	0.31	(0.02–0.78)	±0.19	18	23	2.2	(0.02–4.7)	±1.07
Prematures (total)	50	63	0.38	(0.02–0.83)	±0.10	42	51	2.2	(0.08–4.7)	±1.10
Cook County Hospital, prematures (1–14 days)	8	8	0.52	(0.18–0.83)	±0.08	—	—	—	—	—
Newborns (1–10 days)	39	39	0.22	(0.00–0.58)	±0.17	25	30	1.5	(0.00–2.8)	±0.81
Infants (1 month–1 year)	8	8	0.14	(0.02–0.29)	±0.09	8	8	1.2	(0.17–2.4)	±0.78
Children (1–14 years)	35	35	0.11	(0.00–0.33)	±0.09	35	35	0.79	(0.00–2.4)	±0.62
Adults (14–78 years)	30	30	0.11	(0.00–0.28)	±0.09	27	27	0.82	(0.00–1.9)	±0.63

*The premature and full-term infants were free of known disease. None had respiratory distress or cyanosis. Analysis of milk and water ingested by these infants revealed a nitrate level less than 0.027 ppm. The premature infants routinely received vitamin C orally each day from the seventh day of life.
From Kravitz H, Elegant LD, et al: Methemoglobin values in premature and mature infants and children. Am J Dis Child 1956; 91:2. Copyright 1956, American Medical Association.

Appendix 25. MEMBRANE LIPID COMPOSITION OF FETAL ERYTHROCYTES

	G1 20–25 wk n = 8	G2 28–35 wk n = 7	G3 38–41 wk n = 7	G4 Adults n = 10
Cholesterol (μg/μg prot.)	0.22 ± 0.01	0.23 ± 0.01	0.22 ± 0.01	0.23 ± 0.01
Phospholipids (μg/μg prot.)	0.70 ± 0.14	0.81 ± 0.07	0.89 ± 0.16	0.93 ± 0.11
CH/PL	0.36 ± 0.05	0.30 ± 0.03	0.26 ± 0.02	0.27 ± 0.02
Phospholipids				
Sphingomyelin (%)	30.11 ± 0.91	30.64 ± 0.65	31.97 ± 0.62	30.83 ± 0.3
Phosphatidylcholine (%)	30.30 ± 0.48	30.17 ± 1.0	26.78 ± 0.30*	26.88 ± 0.4*
Phosphatidylinositol (%)	3.76 ± 0.29	3.70 ± 0.24	3.39 ± 0.2	3.38 ± 0.21
Phosphatidylserine (%)	11.75 ± 1.24	11.87 ± 0.8	12.73 ± 0.31	12.02 ± 0.81
Phosphatidic acid (%)	2.98 ± 0.11	2.99 ± 0.22	2.79 ± 0.12	2.81 ± 0.18
Phosphatidylethanolamine (%)	20.93 ± 0.6	20.68 ± 1.33	22.25 ± 0.63	21.82 ± 0.43
Fatty Acids				
16:0 (%)	22.51 ± 0.92	25.31 ± 0.78*	22.95 ± 0.73	23.02 ± 0.79
18:0 (%)	17.74 ± 0.92	17.52 ± 0.51	18.18 ± 0.33	17.92 ± 0.46
18:1w9 (%)	13.03 ± 0.21	11.74 ± 0.38*	10.70 ± 0.30*	10.57 ± 0.33*
18:1bw7 (%)	1.75 ± 0.12	1.57 ± 0.07	1.73 ± 0.08	1.59 ± 0.07
18:2w6 (%)	4.81 ± 0.36	4.85 ± 0.42	4.38 ± 0.31	4.18 ± 0.32
20:3w6 (%)	2.40 ± 0.14	2.79 ± 0.11	3.42 ± 0.11*†	3.59 ± 0.11*
20:4w6 (%)	21.95 ± 0.5	23.13 ± 0.4	22.36 ± 0.46	22.47 ± 0.48
22:4w6 (%)	3.76 ± 0.34	4.28 ± 0.19	4.98 ± 0.23*	5.31 ± 0.40*
22:5w3 (%)	1.29 ± 0.19	1.45 ± 0.04	1.76 ± 0.17	1.63 ± 0.15
22:6w3 (%)	9.41 ± 0.71	8.79 ± 0.26	9.49 ± 0.46	9.48 ± 0.52
Fatty Acids of Phosphatidylcholine				
16:0 (%)	40.40 ± 2.10	40.78 ± 1.74	35.75 ± 2.76	32.12 ± 2.58
18:0 (%)	9.36 ± 0.48	9.32 ± 0.53	12.27 ± 0.57*	13.07 ± 0.51*
18:1w9 (%)	20.10 ± 0.82	15.96 ± 0.65*	14.63 ± 0.56*	12.23 ± 0.88*
18:1bw7 (%)	3.51 ± 0.15	3.05 ± 0.15	3.62 ± 0.21	3.45 ± 0.18
18:2w6 (%)	6.37 ± 0.47	6.94 ± 0.5	8.71 ± 0.78*	10.42 ± 0.9*
20:3w6 (%)	1.97 ± 0.15	2.92 ± 0.20*	4.89 ± 0.28*	6.05 ± 0.21*
20:4w6 (%)	16.23 ± 0.98	17.18 ± 14.2	14.21 ± 1.17	14.12 ± 1.74
22:4w6 (%)	0.54 ± 0.06	0.57 ± 0.07	0.73 ± 0.09	0.73 ± 0.08
22:5w3 (%)	0	0.35 ± 0.07	0.42 ± 0.03	0.22 ± 0.03
22:6w3 (%)	1.93 ± 0.16	2.6 ± 0.47	3.73 ± 0.43*	4.37 ± 0.49*
Fatty Acids of Phosphatidylethanolamine				
16:0 (%)	29.83 ± 0.83	30.19 ± 1.71	30.20 ± 1.44	28.55 ± 1.23
18:0 (%)	11.62 ± 0.68	10.36 ± 0.64	9.16 ± 0.57*	7.63 ± 0.58*
18:1w9 (%)	17.25 ± 1.20	16.44 ± 0.22	17.36 ± 0.33	16.17 ± 0.62
18:1bw7 (%)	1.63 ± 0.08	1.22 ± 0.05	1.59 ± 0.15	1.28 ± 0.13
18:2w6 (%)	3.01 ± 0.2	2.71 ± 0.15	3.11 ± 0.20	4.52 ± 0.26*
20:3w6 (%)	1.61 ± 0.11	1.82 ± 0.16	2.16 ± 0.14*	2.4 ± 0.12*
20:4w6 (%)	22.85 ± 0.68	24.22 ± 1.4	21.60 ± 0.98	23.6 ± 1.5
22:4w6 (%)	3.95 ± 0.29	4.92 ± 0.52	5.14 ± 0.27*	5.5 ± 0.43*
22:5w3 (%)	1.52 ± 0.16	1.37 ± 0.09	1.65 ± 0.17	1.72 ± 0.12
22:6w3 (%)	7.81 ± 0.30	7.27 ± 0.45	8.01 ± 0.42	9.00 ± 0.88

Results are expressed as mean ± SEM; $P < .05$ versus G1(*) or G2(†).
From Colin FC, Gallois Y, et al: Impaired fetal erythrocytes' filterability: relationship with cell size, membrane fluidity, and membrane lipid composition. Blood 1992; 79:2148.

Appendix 26. GEOMETRIC DATA FOR UNFRACTIONATED, TOP AND BOTTOM NEONATAL AND ADULT ERYTHROCYTES

	Neonatal	Adult
Volume (fL)		
Unfractionated	107.3 ± 5.6*†	90.5 ± 4.4†
Top	130.8 ± 13.1*†	99.2 ± 6.3†
Bottom	89.4 ± 5.9*	80.3 ± 4.0
Surface Area (μm²)		
Unfractionated	153.5 ± 7.0*†	137.1 ± 6.7†
Top	186.1 ± 10.6*†	150.6 ± 8.4†
Bottom	108.5 ± 8.2*	118.6 ± 6.2
Surface area/volume		
Unfractionated	1.43 ± 0.04*†	1.51 ± 0.04
Top	1.43 ± 0.05*	1.51 ± 0.03
Bottom	1.21 ± 0.05*	1.49 ± 0.04
Diameter (μm)		
Unfractionated	8.8 ± 0.4†	7.9 ± 0.4
Top	9.8 ± 0.4*†	8.6 ± 0.5†
Bottom	6.9 ± 0.5	7.5 ± 0.4
Mean thickness (μm)		
Unfractionated	1.76 ± 0.10†	1.84 ± 0.13
Top	1.70 ± 0.11	1.71 ± 0.11†
Bottom	2.39 ± 0.13*	1.83 ± 0.14
Surface area index		
Unfractionated	1.40 ± 0.05†	1.41 ± 0.04†
Top	1.49 ± 0.07†	1.46 ± 0.05†
Bottom	1.12 ± 0.04*	1.33 ± 0.04

Data are presented as mean ± SD for 10 neonatal and 10 adult samples.
*Significant difference ($P < .05$, unpaired t test) between adult and neonatal erythrocytes.
†Significant difference ($P < .05$, paired t test) between top or bottom fraction and unfractionated erythrocytes.
From Linderkamp O, Friederichs E, Meiselman HJ: Mechanical and geometrical properties of density-separated neonatal and adult erythrocytes. Pediatr Res 1993; 34:688.

Appendix 27. ESTIMATED BLOOD VOLUMES

Age	Plasma Volume (mL/kg) (PV)	Red Cell Mass (mL/kg) (RCM)	Total Blood Volume (mL/kg) From PV	Total Blood Volume (mL/kg) From RCM
Newborn	41.3	43.1	82.1	86.1
	46.0			84.7
1–7 days	51–54	37.9	78.0	77.8
			82–86	
1–12 months	46.1	25.5	78.1	72.8
1–3 years	44.4	24.9	73.8	69.1
	47.2		81.8	
4–6 years	48.5	25.5	80.0	67.5
	49.6		85.6	
7–9 years	52.2	24.3	87.6	67.5
	49.0		86.1	
10–12 years	51.9	26.3	87.6	67.4
	46.2		83.2	
13–15 years	51.2		88.3	
16–18 years	50.1		90.2	
Adults	39–44	25–30	68–88	55–75

From Price DC, Ries C: In Handmaker H, Lowenstein JM (eds): Nuclear Medicine in Clinical Pediatrics. New York, Society of Nuclear Medicine, 1975, p 279.

Appendix 28. REFERENCE RANGES FOR LEUKOCYTE COUNTS IN CHILDREN*

Age	Total Leukocytes Mean	Total Leukocytes Range	Neutrophils Mean	Neutrophils Range	%	Lymphocytes Mean	Lymphocytes Range	%	Monocytes Mean	%	Eosinophils Mean	%
Birth	18.1	9.0–30.0	11.0	6.0–26.0	61	5.5	2.0–11.0	31	1.1	6	0.4	2
12 hours	22.8	13.0–38.0	15.5	6.0–28.0	68	5.5	2.0–11.0	24	1.2	5	0.5	2
24 hours	18.9	9.4–34.0	11.5	5.0–21.0	61	5.8	2.0–11.5	31	1.1	6	0.5	2
1 week	12.2	5.0–21.0	5.5	1.5–10.0	45	5.0	2.0–17.0	41	1.1	9	0.5	4
2 weeks	11.4	5.0–20.0	4.5	1.0–9.5	40	5.5	2.0–17.0	48	1.0	9	0.4	3
1 month	10.8	5.0–19.5	3.8	1.0–9.0	35	6.0	2.5–16.5	56	0.7	7	0.3	3
6 months	11.9	6.0–17.5	3.8	1.0–8.5	32	7.3	4.0–13.5	61	0.6	5	0.3	3
1 year	11.4	6.0–17.5	3.5	1.5–8.5	31	7.0	4.0–10.5	61	0.6	5	0.3	3
2 years	10.6	6.0–17.0	3.5	1.5–8.5	33	6.3	3.0–9.5	59	0.5	5	0.3	3
4 years	9.1	5.5–15.5	3.8	1.5–8.5	42	4.5	2.0–8.0	50	0.5	5	0.3	3
6 years	8.5	5.0–14.5	4.3	1.5–8.0	51	3.5	1.5–7.0	42	0.4	5	0.2	3
8 years	8.3	4.5–13.5	4.4	1.5–8.0	53	3.3	1.5–6.8	39	0.4	4	0.2	2
10 years	8.1	4.5–13.5	4.4	1.8–8.0	54	3.1	1.5–6.5	38	0.4	4	0.2	2
16 years	7.8	4.5–13.0	4.4	1.8–8.0	57	2.8	1.2–5.2	35	0.4	5	0.2	3
21 years	7.4	4.5–11.0	4.4	1.8–7.7	59	2.5	1.0–4.8	34	0.3	4	0.2	3

*Numbers of leukocytes are in thousands per mm³, ranges are estimates of 95% confidence limits, and percentages refer to differential counts. Neutrophils include band cells at all ages and a small number of metamyelocytes and myelocytes in the first few days of life.
From Dallman PR: In Rudolph AM (ed): Pediatrics, 16th ed. New York, Appleton-Century-Crofts, 1977, p 1178.

Appendix 29. REFERENCE RANGES FOR PEDIATRIC LYMPHOCYTE SUBSETS AT DIFFERENT AGES

Age		Total Lymphocytes	CD4	CD8	CD2	CD3	CD19	Helper/ Suppressor Ratio
0–6 mo	%	.62–.72	.50–.57	.08–.31	.55–.88	.55–.82	.11–.45	1.17
(n = 10)	A	5.4–7.2	2.8–3.9	0.35–2.5	3.9–5.3	3.5–5.0	0.43–3.3	6.22
6–12 mo	%	.60–.69	.49–.55	.08–.31	.55–.88	.55–.82	.11–.45	1.17
(n = 9)	A	5.3–6.7	2.6–3.5	0.35–2.5	3.8–4.9	3.4–4.6	0.43–3.3	6.22
12–18 mo	%	.56–.63	.46–.51	.08–.31	.55–.88	.55–.82	.11–.45	1.17
(n = 9)	A	4.9–5.9	2.3–2.9	0.35–2.5	3.5–4.2	3.2–3.9	0.43–3.3	6.22
18–24 mo	%	.52–.59	.42–.48	.08–.31	.55–.88	.55–.82	.11–.45	1.17
(n = 10)	A	4.4–5.5	1.9–2.5	0.35–2.5	3.1–3.9	2.8–3.5	0.43–3.3	6.22
24–30 mo	%	.45–.57	.38–.46	.08–.31	.55–.88	.55–.82	.11–.45	1.17
(n = 9)	A	3.9–5.2	1.5–2.2	0.35–2.5	2.6–3.6	2.3–3.3	0.43–3.3	6.22
30–36 mo	%	.39–.53	.33–.44	.08–.31	.55–.88	.55–.82	.11–.45	1.17
(n = 10)	A	3.3–5.1	1.2–2.0	0.35–2.5	2.2–3.5	1.9–3.1	0.43–3.3	6.22
3 years	%	.22–.69	.27–.57	.14–.34	.65–.84	.55–.82	.09–.29	0.98
(n = 73)	A	1.6–5.4	0.56–2.7	0.33–1.4	1.2–4.1	1.0–3.9	0.20–1.3	3.24

Values are expressed as 95th percentile reference range; %, relative %; A, Absolute cell count × 10⁹/L.
From Kotylo PK, Finenberg NS, et al: Reference ranges for lymphocyte subsets in pediatric patients. Am J Clin Pathol 1993; 100:111. See also Denny T, Yogev R, et al: Lymphocyte subsets in healthy children during the first 5 years of life. JAMA 1992; 267:1484.

Appendix 30. LYMPHOCYTE SUBSETS IN TERM AND PREMATURE NEONATES IN THE FIRST WEEK OF LIFE

		Term (n = 21)	Premature (n = 104)	Healthy Premature (n = 36)	Sick Premature (n = 68)
Total leukocytes	—	15.44 ± 1.42	13.63 ± 0.94	13.81 ± 1.12	13.54 ± 1.32
Lymphocytes	—	3.51 ± 0.38	5.47 ± 0.23	6.04 ± 0.36	5.18 ± 0.28
CD2	%	67 ± 4	72 ± 1.5	77 ± 3	70 ± 2
	A	2.65 ± 0.34	3.97 ± 0.20	4.61 ± 0.33	3.63 ± 0.24
CD4	%	45 ± 2	47 ± 1.5	52 ± 2	45 ± 2
	A	1.56 ± 0.20	2.58 ± 0.14	3.16 ± 0.14	2.29 ± 0.17
CD8	%	13 ± 1	12 ± 0.5	12.6 ± 0.7	12 ± 0.6
	A	0.57 ± 0.13	0.67 ± 0.04	0.73 ± 0.07	0.64 ± 0.05
CD20	%	5.3 ± 0.4	6.4 ± 0.4	5.6 ± 0.4	6.8 ± 0.6
	A	0.18 ± 0.03	0.34 ± 0.03	0.34 ± 0.04	0.34 ± 0.03
CD21	%	9.1 ± 0.6	8.6 ± 0.5	6.8 ± 0.6	9.5 ± 0.7
	A	0.33 ± 0.06	0.44 ± 0.03	0.39 ± 0.04	0.47 ± 0.05

Values are expressed as mean ± SEM; %, relative %; A, Absolute cell count × 10⁹/L.
From Series IM, Pichette J, et al: Quantitative analysis of T and B cell subsets in healthy and sick premature infants. Early Hum Develop 1991; 26:143.

Appendix 31. BONE MARROW CELL POPULATIONS OF NORMAL INFANTS*

Cell Type	Month				
	0(n = 57)†	1(n = 71)	2(n = 48)	3(n = 24)	4(n = 19)
Small lymphocytes	14.42 ± 5.54	47.05 ± 9.24	42.68 ± 7.90	43.63 ± 11.83	47.06 ± 8.77
Transitional cells	1.18 ± 1.13	1.95 ± 0.94	2.38 ± 1.35	2.17 ± 1.64	1.64 ± 1.01
Proerythroblasts	0.02 ± 0.06	0.10 ± 0.14	0.13 ± 0.19	0.10 ± 0.13	0.05 ± 0.10
Basophilic erythroblasts	0.24 ± 0.25	0.34 ± 0.33	0.57 ± 0.41	0.40 ± 0.33	0.24 ± 0.24
Early erythroblasts	0.27 ± 0.26	0.44 ± 0.42	0.71 ± 0.51	0.50 ± 0.38	0.28 ± 0.30
Polychromatic erythroblasts	13.06 ± 6.78	6.90 ± 4.45	13.06 ± 3.48	10.51 ± 3.39	6.84 ± 2.58
Orthochromatic erythroblasts	0.69 ± 0.73	0.54 ± 1.88	0.66 ± 0.82	0.70 ± 0.87	0.34 ± 0.30
Extruded nuclei	0.47 ± 0.46	0.16 ± 0.17	0.26 ± 0.22	0.19 ± 0.12	0.16 ± 0.17
Late erythroblasts	14.22 ± 7.14	7.60 ± 4.84	13.99 ± 3.82	11.40 ± 3.43	7.34 ± 2.54
Early/late erythroblasts ratio‡	1:50	1:15	1:18	1:22	1:23
Fetal erythroblasts	14.48 ± 7.24	8.04 ± 5.00	14.70 ± 3.86	11.90 ± 3.52	7.62 ± 2.56
Blood reticulocytes	4.18 ± 1.46	1.06 ± 1.13	3.39 ± 1.22	2.90 ± 0.91	1.65 ± 0.73
Neutrophils					
Promyelocytes	0.79 ± 0.91	0.76 ± 0.65	0.78 ± 0.68	0.76 ± 0.80	0.59 ± 0.51
Myelocytes	3.95 ± 2.93	2.50 ± 1.48	2.03 ± 1.14	2.24 ± 1.70	2.32 ± 1.59
Early neutrophils	4.74 ± 3.43	3.27 ± 1.94	2.81 ± 1.62	3.00 ± 2.18	2.91 ± 2.01
Metamyelocytes	19.37 ± 4.84	11.34 ± 3.59	11.27 ± 3.38	11.93 ± 13.09	6.04 ± 3.63
Bands	28.89 ± 7.56	14.10 ± 4.63	13.15 ± 4.71	14.60 ± 7.54	13.93 ± 6.13
Mature neutrophils	7.37 ± 4.64	3.64 ± 2.97	3.07 ± 2.45	3.48 ± 1.62	4.27 ± 2.69
Late neutrophils	55.63 ± 7.98	29.08 ± 6.79	27.50 ± 6.88	31.00 ± 11.17	31.30 ± 7.80
Early/late neutrophil ratio	1:12	1:9	1:9	1:9	1:11
Total neutrophils	60.37 ± 8.66	32.35 ± 7.68	30.31 ± 7.27	34.01 ± 11.95	34.21 ± 8.61
Total eosinophils	2.70 ± 1.27	2.61 ± 1.40	2.50 ± 1.22	2.54 ± 1.46	2.37 ± 4.13
Total basophils	0.12 ± 0.20	0.07 ± 0.16	0.08 ± 0.10	0.09 ± 0.09	0.11 ± 0.14
Total myeloid cells	63.19 ± 9.10	35.03 ± 8.09	32.90 ± 7.85	36.64 ± 2.26	36.69 ± 8.91
Monocytes	0.88 ± 0.85	1.01 ± 0.89	0.91 ± 0.83	0.68 ± 0.56	0.75 ± 0.75
Miscellaneous					
Megakaryocytes	0.06 ± 0.15	0.05 ± 0.09	0.10 ± 0.13	0.06 ± 0.09	0.06 ± 0.06
Plasma cells	0.00 ± 0.02	0.02 ± 0.06	0.02 ± 0.05	0.00 ± 0.02	0.01 ± 0.03
Unknown blasts	0.31 ± 0.31	0.62 ± 0.50	0.58 ± 0.50	0.63 ± 0.60	0.56 ± 0.53
Unknown cells	0.22 ± 0.34	0.21 ± 0.25	0.16 ± 0.24	0.19 ± 0.21	0.23 ± 0.25
Damaged cells	5.79 ± 2.78	5.50 ± 2.46	5.09 ± 1.78	4.75 ± 2.30	4.80 ± 2.29
Total	6.38 ± 2.84	6.39 ± 2.63	5.94 ± 1.94	5.63 ± 2.36	5.66 ± 2.30

*Percentages of cell types (means ± standard deviation) in tibial bone marrow of infants from birth to 18 months of age. Data were obtained from normal American infants of black, white, and Asian racial origin. The changes in the marrow during the first 18 months of postnatal life are based on differential counts of 1000 cells classified on stained smears on each of 10 serial marrow samples aspirated from the same population of infants. Criteria for including bone marrow data in this study consisted of absence of any clinical evidence of disease, normal rate of growth, and normal serum proteins and transferrin saturations.

†n = number of infants studied at each stage.

‡Expressed in round figures for facilitating comparison. Means ± SD were calculated from values obtained in individual infants, and statistical comparisons were performed.

From Rosse C, Kraemer MJ, et al: Bone marrow cell populations of normal infants: the predominance of lymphocytes. J Lab Clin Med 1977; 89:1228.

Appendix 31. BONE MARROW CELL POPULATIONS OF NORMAL INFANTS* *(Continued)*

		Month			
5(n = 22)	*6(n = 22)*	*9(n = 16)*	*12(n = 18)*	*15(n = 12)*	*18(n = 19)*
47.19 ± 9.93	47.55 ± 7.88	48.76 ± 8.11	47.11 ± 11.32	42.77 ± 8.94	43.55 ± 8.56
1.83 ± 0.89	2.31 ± 1.16	1.92 ± 1.39	2.32 ± 1.90	1.70 ± 0.82	1.99 ± 1.00
0.07 ± 0.10	0.09 ± 0.12	0.07 ± 0.09	0.02 ± 0.04	0.07 ± 0.12	0.08 ± 0.13
0.47 ± 0.33	0.32 ± 0.24	0.31 ± 0.24	0.30 ± 0.25	0.38 ± 0.37	0.50 ± 0.34
0.55 ± 0.36	0.41 ± 0.30	0.39 ± 0.28	0.39 ± 0.27	0.46 ± 0.36	0.59 ± 0.34
7.55 ± 2.35	7.30 ± 3.60	7.73 ± 3.39	6.83 ± 3.75	6.04 ± 1.56	6.97 ± 3.56
0.46 ± 0.51	0.38 ± 0.56	0.39 ± 0.48	0.37 ± 0.51	0.50 ± 0.65	0.44 ± 0.49
0.14 ± 0.11	0.16 ± 0.22	0.22 ± 0.25	0.23 ± 0.25	0.17 ± 0.12	0.21 ± 0.19
8.16 ± 2.58	7.85 ± 4.11	8.34 ± 3.31	7.42 ± 4.11	6.72 ± 1.80	7.62 ± 3.63
1:15	1:17	1:19	1:17	1:15	1:10
8.70 ± 2.69	8.25 ± 4.31	8.72 ± 3.34	7.81 ± 4.26	7.18 ± 1.95	8.21 ± 37.1
1.38 ± 0.65	1.74 ± 0.80	1.67 ± 0.52	1.79 ± 0.79	2.10 ± 0.91	1.84 ± 0.46
0.87 ± 0.80	0.67 ± 0.66	0.41 ± 0.34	0.69 ± 0.71	0.67 ± 0.58	0.64 ± 0.59
2.73 ± 1.82	2.22 ± 1.25	2.07 ± 1.20	2.32 ± 1.14	2.48 ± 0.94	2.49 ± 1.39
3.60 ± 2.50	2.89 ± 1.71	2.48 ± 1.46	3.02 ± 1.52	3.16 ± 1.19	3.14 ± 1.75
11.89 ± 3.24	11.02 ± 3.12	11.80 ± 3.90	11.10 ± 3.82	12.48 ± 7.45	12.42 ± 4.15
14.07 ± 5.48	14.00 ± 4.58	14.08 ± 4.53	14.02 ± 4.88	15.17 ± 4.20	14.20 ± 5.23
3.77 ± 2.44	4.85 ± 2.69	3.97 ± 2.29	5.65 ± 3.92	6.94 ± 3.88	6.31 ± 3.91
29.73 ± 7.19	29.86 ± 6.74	29.86 ± 7.36	30.77 ± 8.69	34.60 ± 7.35	32.93 ± 7.01
1:8	1:10	1:12	1:10	1:10	1:10
33.12 ± 8.34	32.75 ± 7.03	32.33 ± 7.75	33.79 ± 8.76	37.76 ± 7.32	36.06 ± 7.40
1.98 ± 0.86	2.08 ± 1.16	1.74 ± 1.08	1.92 ± 1.09	3.39 ± 1.93	2.70 ± 2.16
0.09 ± 0.13	0.10 ± 0.13	0.11 ± 0.13	0.13 ± 0.15	0.27 ± 0.37	0.10 ± 0.12
35.40 ± 8.54	34.93 ± 7.52	34.18 ± 8.13	35.83 ± 8.84	41.42 ± 7.43	38.86 ± 7.92
1.29 ± 1.06	1.21 ± 1.01	1.17 ± 0.97	1.46 ± 1.52	1.68 ± 1.09	2.12 ± 1.59
0.08 ± 0.09	0.04 ± 0.07	0.09 ± 0.12	0.05 ± 0.08	0.00 ± 0.00	0.07 ± 0.12
0.05 ± 0.11	0.03 ± 0.07	0.01 ± 0.03	0.03 ± 0.07	0.07 ± 0.12	0.06 ± 0.08
0.50 ± 0.37	0.56 ± 0.48	0.42 ± 0.50	0.37 ± 0.33	0.46 ± 0.32	0.43 ± 0.45
0.17 ± 0.22	0.10 ± 0.15	0.14 ± 0.17	0.11 ± 0.14	0.13 ± 0.18	0.20 ± 0.23
4.86 ± 1.25	5.04 ± 1.08	4.89 ± 1.60	5.34 ± 2.19	4.99 ± 1.96	5.05 ± 2.15
5.66 ± 1.41	5.78 ± 1.16	5.55 ± 1.74	5.90 ± 2.03	5.65 ± 2.02	5.81 ± 2.16

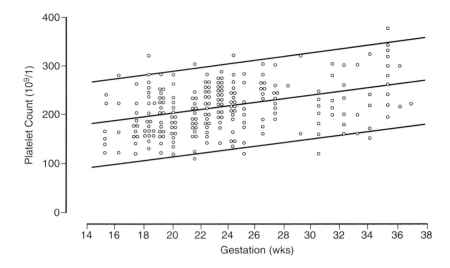

Appendix 32. Platelet counts as a function of gestational age.

Reference range (mean ± 2 SD) for fetal platelet counts as a function of gestational age in 229 pregnancies. (From Van den Hof MC, Nicolaides KH: Platelet count in normal, small and anemic fetuses. Am J Obstet Gynecol 1990; 162:735.)

Appendix 33. COMPARISON OF SELECTED COAGULATION FACTOR VALUES IN NEWBORNS

Age	Fibrinogen (mg/dL)	F II (U/mL)	F VIII (U/mL)	F IX (U/mL)	F XII (U/mL)	Antithrombin (U/mL)	Protein C (U/mL)
Term							
Hathaway and Bonnar (1987) and Manco-Johnson et al (1988)*	240 (150)	0.52 (0.25)	1.5 (0.55)	0.35 (0.15)	0.44 (0.16)	0.56 (0.32)	0.32 (0.16)
Andrews et al (1987, 1988)†	283 (177)	0.48 (0.26)	1.0 (0.50)	0.53 (0.25)	0.53 (0.20)	0.63 (0.25)	0.35 (0.17)
Corrigan (1992)‡	246 (150)	0.45 (0.22)	1.68 (0.50)	0.40 (0.20)	0.44 (0.16)	0.52 (0.20)	0.31 (0.17)
Preterm							
Hathaway and Bonnar (1987) and Manco-Johnson et al (1988)*	300 (120)	0.45 (0.26)	0.93 (0.54)	0.41 (0.20)	0.33 (0.23)	0.40 (0.25)	0.24 (0.18)
Andrews et al (1987, 1988)†	243 (150)	0.45 (0.20)	1.1 (0.50)	0.35 (0.19)	0.38 (0.10)	0.38 (0.14)	0.28 (0.12)
Corrigan (1992)‡	240 (150)	0.35 (0.21)	1.36 (0.21)	0.35 (0.10)	0.22 (0.09)	0.35 (0.10)	0.28 (0.12)

Data are expressed as mean and (lower limits of normal). Preterm, 30–36 wk gestational age.
From Hathaway W, Corrigan J: Report of scientific and standardization subcommittee on neonatal hemostasis. Thromb Haemost 1991; 65:323.
*Hathaway W, Bonnar J: Hemostatic Disorders of the Pregnant Woman and Newborn Infant. New York, Elsevier Science Publishing Co., 1987; Manco-Johnson M, Marlar R, et al: Severe protein C deficiency in newborn infants. J Pediatr 1988; 113:359.
†Andrews M, Paes B, et al: Development of the human coagulation system in the full-term infant. Blood 1987; 70:165; Andrew M, Paes B, et al: Development of the human coagulation system in the healthy premature infant. Blood 1988; 72:1651.
‡Corrigan JJ Jr: Normal hemostasis in fetus and newborn. Coagulation. In Polin RA, Fox WW (eds): Fetal and Neonatal Physiology. Philadelphia, WB Saunders, 1992, pp 1368–1371.

Appendix 34. CHANGES IN PROTHROMBIN TIME, ACTIVATED PARTIAL THROMBOPLASTIN TIME, AND THROMBIN TIME IN TERM AND PREMATURE INFANTS

	Prothrombin Time	Activated Partial Thromboplastin Time	Thrombin Time
Normal control	1	1	1
Term infants (ratio) (increase in sec)	1.15–1.3 (3–4 sec)	1.2–1.5	1.16–1.4
Small preterm (ratio) (increase in sec)	1.30 (4–5 sec)	1.4–2.4	1.31–1.50

Due to the variability of normal values for these tests, the results are expressed as a ratio of the newborn clotting times to the mean value for adult controls. Small preterm, less than 32 weeks of gestational age; From Hathaway W, Corrigan J: Report of scientific and standardization subcommittee on neonatal hemostasis. Thromb Haemost 1991; 65:323.

Appendix 35. REFERENCE VALUES FOR COAGULATION TESTS IN HEALTHY, FULL-TERM NEWBORNS COMPARED WITH NORMAL ADULTS

Test	Newborns	Adults	P <
PT (sec)	13.1±0.9	11.9±0.6	.0001
aPTT (sec)	35±4.5	28.8±2.7	.0001
Platelets (× 10⁹/L)	214±55	258±66	.0001
Fibrinogen (mg/dL)	251±51	262±44	NS
Factor II (%)	73±7	100±15	.0001
Factor V (%)	93±13	98±19	NS
Factor VII (%)	88±12	95±18	.005
Factor VIII (%)	113±38	92±21	.0001
Factor IX (%)	86±18	94±16	.003
Factor X (%)	72±10	97±15	.0001
Hematocrit (%)	59±3.0	44±2.5	.0001

Data were obtained in 71 newborns and 100 adults and expressed as mean±SD. Samples were collected with a constant anticoagulant-to-blood ratio, based on a previous determination of hematocrit.
From Cerneca F, de Vonderweid U, et al: The importance of hematocrit in the interpretation of coagulation tests in the full-term newborn infant. Haematologica 1994; 79:25.

Appendix 36. BLEEDING TIME IN CHILDREN

Age (y)	Number of Subjects	Bleeding Time (s)
0–2	33	180±30
2–4	33	240±60
4–9	75	300±60
9–18	66	300±70
0–18	201	270±60
Adults	90	320±90

Values are expressed as mean±SD, using a Disposable Simplate method.
From Aversa LA, Vázquez A, et al: Bleeding time in normal children. J Pediatr Hematol Oncol 1995; 17:25.

Appendix 37. REFERENCE VALUES FOR COAGULATION TESTS IN HEALTHY CHILDREN AGED 1 TO 16 YEARS COMPARED WITH ADULTS

Coagulation Tests	1 to 5 y Mean (Boundary)	6 to 10 y Mean (Boundary)	11 to 16 y Mean (Boundary)	Adult Mean (Boundary)
PT (s)	11 (10.6–11.4)	11.1 (10.1–12.1)	11.2 (10.2–12.0)	12 (11.0–14.0)
INR	1.0 (0.96–1.04)	1.01 (0.91–1.11)	1.02 (0.93–1.10)	1.10 (1.0–1.3)
APTT (s)	30 (24–36)	31 (26–36)	32 (26–37)	33 (27–40)
Fibrinogen (g/L)	2.76 (1.70–4.05)	2.79 (1.57–4.0)	3.0 (1.54–4.48)	2.78 (1.56–4.0)
Bleeding time (min)	6 (2.5–10)*	7 (2.5–13)*	5 (3–8)*	4 (1–7)
II (U/mL)	0.94 (0.71–1.16)*	0.88 (0.67–1.07)*	0.83 (0.61–1.04)*	1.08 (0.70–1.46)
V (U/mL)	1.03 (0.79–1.27)	0.90 (0.63–1.16)*	0.77 (0.55–0.99)*	1.06 (0.62–1.50)
VII (U/mL)	0.82 (0.55–1.16)*	0.85 (0.52–1.20)*	0.83 (0.58–1.15)*	1.05 (0.67–1.43)
VIII (U/mL)	0.90 (0.59–1.42)	0.95 (0.58–1.32)	0.92 (0.53–1.31)	0.99 (0.50–1.49)
vWF (U/mL)	0.82 (0.60–1.20)	0.95 (0.44–1.44)	1.00 (0.46–1.53)	0.92 (0.50–1.58)
IX (U/mL)	0.73 (0.47–1.04)*	0.75 (0.63–0.89)*	0.82 (0.59–1.22)*	1.09 (0.5–1.63)
X (U/mL)	0.88 (0.58–1.16)*	0.75 (0.55–1.01)*	0.79 (0.50–1.17)*	1.06 (0.70–1.52)
XI (U/mL)	0.97 (0.56–1.50)	0.86 (0.52–1.20)	0.74 (0.50–0.97)*	0.97 (0.67–1.27)
XII (U/mL)	0.93 (0.64–1.29)	0.92 (0.60–1.40)	0.81 (0.34–1.37)*	1.08 (0.52–1.64)
PK (U/mL)	0.95 (0.65–1.30)	0.99 (0.66–1.31)	0.99 (0.53–1.45)	1.12 (0.62–1.62)
HMWK (U/mL)	0.98 (0.64–1.32)	0.93 (0.60–1.30)	0.91 (0.63–1.19)	0.92 (0.50–1.36)
XIIIa (U/mL)	1.08 (0.72–1.43)*	1.09 (0.65–1.51)*	0.99 (0.57–1.40)	1.05 (0.55–1.55)
XIIIs (U/mL)	1.13 (0.69–1.56)*	1.16 (0.77–1.54)*	1.02 (0.60–1.43)	0.97 (0.57–1.37)

All factors except fibrinogen are expressed as units per milliliter, where pooled plasma contains 1.0 U/mL. All data are expressed as the mean, followed by the upper and lower boundary encompassing 95% of the population. Between 20 and 50 samples were assayed for each value for each age group. Some measurements were skewed due to a disproportionate number of high values. The lower limit, which excludes the lower 2.5% of the population, is given.
PT = prothrombin time; APTT = activated partial thromboplastin time; VIII = factor VIII procoagulant; vWF = von Willebrand factor; PK = prekallikrein; HMWK = high molecular weight kininogen.
*Values that are significantly different from adults.
From Andrew M, Vegh P, et al: Maturation of the hemostatic system during childhood. Blood 1992; 80:1998.

Appendix 38. REFERENCE VALUES FOR THE INHIBITORS OF COAGULATION IN HEALTHY CHILDREN AGED 1 TO 16 YEARS COMPARED WITH ADULTS

Coagulation Inhibitors	Age			
	1 to 5 y Mean (Boundary)	**6 to 10 y** Mean (Boundary)	**11 to 16 y** Mean (Boundary)	**Adult** Mean (Boundary)
ATIII (U/mL)	1.11 (0.82–1.39)	1.11 (0.90–1.31)	1.05 (0.77–1.32)	1.0 (0.74–1.26)
α_2M (U/mL)	1.69 (1.14–2.23)*	1.69 (1.28–2.09)*	1.56 (0.98–2.12)*	0.86 (0.52–1.20)
C_1-Inh (U/mL)	1.35 (0.85–1.83)*	1.14 (0.88–1.54)	1.03 (0.68–1.50)	1.0 (0.71–1.31)
α_1AT (U/mL)	0.93 (0.39–1.47)	1.00 (0.69–1.30)	1.01 (0.65–1.37)	0.93 (0.55–1.30)
HCII (U/mL)	0.88 (0.48–1.28)*	0.86 (0.40–1.32)*	0.91 (0.53–1.29)*	1.08 (0.66–1.26)
Protein C (U/mL)	0.66 (0.40–0.92)*	0.69 (0.45–0.93)*	0.83 (0.55–1.11)*	0.96 (0.64–1.28)
Protein S				
Total (U/mL)	0.86 (0.54–1.18)	0.78 (0.41–1.14)	0.72 (0.52–0.92)	0.81 (0.60–1.13)
Free (U/mL)	0.45 (0.21–0.69)	0.42 (0.22–0.62)	0.38 (0.26–0.55)	0.45 (0.27–0.61)

All values are expressed in units per milliliter, where for all factors pooled plasma contains 1.0 U/mL, with the exception of free protein S, which contains a mean of 0.4 U/mL. All values are given as a mean, followed by the lower and upper boundary encompassing 95% of the population. Between 20 and 30 samples were assayed for each value for each age group. Some measurements were skewed due to a disproportionate number of high values. The lower limits, which exclude the lower 2.5% of the population, are given.
*Values that are significantly different from adults.
From Andrew M, Vegh P, et al: Maturation of the hemostatic system during childhood. Blood 1992; 80:1998.

Appendix 39. REFERENCE VALUES FOR THE FIBRINOLYTIC SYSTEM IN HEALTHY CHILDREN AGED 1 TO 16 YEARS COMPARED WITH ADULTS

	Age			
	1 to 5 y Mean (Boundary)	**6 to 10 y** Mean (Boundary)	**11 to 16 y** Mean (Boundary)	**Adult** Mean (Boundary)
Plasminogen (U/mL)	0.98 (0.78–1.18)	0.92 (0.75–1.08)	0.86 (0.68–1.03)*	0.99 (0.77–1.22)
Tissue plasminogen activator (TPA) (ng/mL)	2.15 (1.0–4.5)*	2.42 (1.0–5.0)*	2.16 (1.0–4.0)*	4.90 (1.40–8.40)
Alpha$_2$-antiplasmin (α_2-AP) (U/mL)	1.05 (0.93–1.17)	0.99 (0.89–1.10)	0.98 (0.78–1.18)	1.02 (0.68–1.36)
Plasminogen activator inhibitor (PAI) (U/mL)	5.42 (1.0–10.0)	6.79 (2.0–12.0)*	6.07 (2.0–10.0)*	3.60 (0–11.0)

For α_2AP, values are expressed as units per milliliter, where pooled plasma contains 1.0 U/mL. Values for TPA are given as nanograms per milliliter. Values for PAI are given as U/mL, where 1 U of PAI activity is defined as the amount of PAI that inhibits 1 IU of human single-chain TPA. All values are given as the mean, followed by the lower and upper boundary encompassing 95% of the population (boundary).
*Values that are significantly different from adults.
From Andrew M, Vegh P, et al: Maturation of the hemostatic system during childhood. Blood 1992; 80:1998.

Appendix 40. ENDOGENOUS PLASMA CONCENTRATIONS OF THROMBIN–ANTITHROMBIN COMPLEXES (TATs) AND PROTHROMBIN FRAGMENT 1.2 (F1.2) IN CHILDREN AND ADULTS

	1–5 years	**6–10 years**	**11–16 years**	**20–45 years**
TAT (μg/L)	2.30 ± 0.08	2.38 ± 0.13	2.80 ± 0.18	2.15 ± 0.09
F1.2 (nm/L)	1.04 ± 0.06	0.87 ± 0.07	0.82 ± 0.06	0.83 ± 0.06

Data are expressed as mean ± SEM.
From Andrew M, Mitchell L, et al: Thrombin regulation in children differs from adults in the absence and presence of heparin. Thromb Haemost 1994; 72:836.

Appendix 41. COAGULATION SCREENING TESTS AND FACTOR LEVELS IN FETUSES AND FULL-TERM NEWBORNS

Parameter	Fetuses (weeks' gestation)			Newborns (n = 60)	Adults (n = 40)
	19–23 (n = 20)	24–29 (n = 22)	30–38 (n = 22)		
PT (s)	32.5 (19–45)	32.2 (19–44)†	22.6 (16–30)†	16.7 (12.0–23.5)*	13.5 (11.4–14.0)
PT (INR)	6.4 (1.7–11.1)	6.2 (2.1–10.6)†	3.0 (1.5–5.0)*	1.7 (0.9–2.7)*	1.1 (0.8–1.2)
APTT (s)	168.8 (83–250)	154.0 (87–210)†	104.8 (76–128)†	44.3 (35–52)*	33.0 (25–39)
TCT (s)	34.2 (24–44)*	26.2 (24–28)*	21.4 (17.0–23.3)	20.4 (15.2–25.0)†	14.0 (12–16)
Factor					
I (g/L Von Clauss)	0.85 (0.57–1.50)	1.12 (0.65–1.65)	1.35 (1.25–1.65)	1.68 (0.95–2.45)†	3.0 (1.78–4.50)
I Ag (g/L)	1.08 (0.75–1.50)	1.93 (1.56–2.40)	1.94 (1.30–2.40)	2.65 (1.68–3.60)†	3.5 (2.50–5.20)
IIc (%)	16.9 (10–24)	19.9 (11–30)*	27.9 (15–50)†	43.5 (27–64)†	98.7 (70–125)
VIIc (%)	27.4 (17–37)	33.8 (18–48)*	45.9 (31–62)	52.5 (28–78)†	101.3 (68–130)
IXc (%)	10.1 (6–14)	9.9 (5–15)	12.3 (5–24)†	31.8 (15–50)†	104.8 (70–142)
Xc (%)m	20.5 (14–29)	24.9 (16–35)	28.0 (16–36)†	39.6 (21–65)†	99.2 (75–125)
Vc (%)	32.1 (21–44)	36.8 (25–50)	48.9 (23–70)†	89.9 (50–140)	99.8 (65–140)
VIIIc (%)	34.5 (18–50)	35.5 (20–52)	50.1 (27–78)†	94.3 (38–150)	101.8 (55–170)
XIc (%)	13.2 (8–19)	12.1 (6–22)	14.8 (6–26)†	37.2 (13–62)†	100.2 (70–135)
XIIc (%)	14.9 (6–25)	22.7 (6–40)	25.8 (11–50)†	69.8 (25–105)†	101.4 (65–144)
PK (%)	12.8 (8–19)	15.4 (8–26)	18.1 (8–28)†	35.4 (21–53)†	99.8 (65–135)
HMWK (%)	15.4 (10–22)	19.3 (10–26)	23.6 (12–34)†	38.9 (28–53)†	98.8 (68–135)

Values are the mean, followed in parentheses by the lower and upper boundaries including 95% of the population.
Abbreviations: Ag, antigenic value; c, coagulant activity.
*P < .05.
†P < .01.
From Reverdiau-Moalic P, Delahousse B, et al: Evaluation of blood coagulation activators and inhibitors in the healthy human fetus. Blood 1996; 88:900.

Appendix 42. COAGULATION INHIBITORS IN FETUSES AND FULL-TERM NEWBORNS

Parameter	Fetuses (weeks' gestation)			Newborns (n = 60)	Adults (n = 40)
	19–23 (n = 20)	24–29 (n = 22)	30–38 (n = 22)		
ATIII (%)	20.2 (12–31)*	30.0 (20–39)	37.1 (24–55)†	59.4 (42–80)†	99.8 (65–130)
HCII (%)	10.3 (6–16)	12.9 (5.5–20)	21.1 (11–33)†	52.1 (19–99)†	101.4 (70–128)
TFPI (ng/mL)‡	21.0 (16.0–29.2)	20.6 (13.4–33.2)	20.7 (10.4–31.5)†	38.1 (22.7–55.8)†	73.0 (50.9–90.1)
PC Ag (%)	9.5 (6–14)	12.1 (8–16)	15.9 (8–30)†	32.5 (21–47)†	100.8 (68–125)
PC Act (%)	9.6 (7–13)	10.4 (8–13)	14.1 (8–18)*	28.2 (14–42)†	98.8 (68–129)
Total PS (%)	15.1 (11–21)	17.4 (14–25)	21.0 (15–30)†	38.5 (22–55)†	99.6 (72–118)
Free PS (%)	21.7 (13–32)	27.9 (19–40)	27.1 (18–40)†	49.3 (33–67)†	98.7 (72–128)
Ratio of free PS to total PS	0.82 (0.75–0.92)	0.83 (0.76–0.95)	0.79 (0.70–0.89)†	0.64 (0.59–0.98)†	0.41 (0.38–0.43)
C4b-BP (%)	1.8 (0.6)	6.1 (0–12.5)	9.3 (5–14)	18.6 (3–40)†	100.3 (70–124)

Values are the mean, followed in parentheses by the lower and upper boundaries including 95% of the population.
Abbreviations: Ag, antigen; Act, activity.
*P < .05.
†P < .01.
‡Twenty samples were assayed for each group, but only 10 for 19- to 23-week-old fetuses.
From Reverdiau-Moalic P, Delahousse B, et al: Evaluation of blood coagulation activators and inhibitors in the healthy human fetus. Blood 1996; 88:900.

Appendix 43. SERUM FERRITIN, IRON, TOTAL IRON-BINDING CAPACITY, AND TRANSFERRIN SATURATION

Age	Male Subjects		Female Subjects	
Ferritin	ng/mL	μg/L	ng/mL	μg/L
1–30 d†	6–400	6–400	6–515	6–515
1–6 mo†	6–410	6–410	6–340	6–340
7–12 m†	6–80	6–80	6–45	6–45
1–5 y*‡	6–24	6–24	6–24	6–24
6–9 y*‡	10–55	10–55	10–55	10–55
10–14 y‡	23–70	23–70	6–40	6–40
14–19 y‡	23–70	23–70	6–40	6–40
Iron	μg/dL	μmol/L	μg/dL	μmol/L
1–5 y*‡	22–136	4–25	22–136	4–25
6–9 y*‡	39–136	7–25	39–136	7–25
10–14 y‡	28–134	5–24	45–145	8–26
14–19 y‡	34–162	6–29	28–184	5–33
Iron-Binding Capacity				
1–5 y*‡	268–441	48–79	268–441	48–79
6–9 y*‡	240–508	43–91	240–508	43–91
10–14 y‡	302–508	54–91	318–575	57–103
14–19 y‡	290–570	52–102	302–564	52–101
Transferrin Saturation				
1–5 y*‡	0.07–0.44		0.07–0.44	
6–9 y*‡	0.17–0.42		0.17–0.42	
10–14 y‡	0.11–0.36		0.02–0.40	
14–19 y‡	0.06–0.33		0.06–0.33	
Transferrin	U/L (males and females)			
0–5 d§	1.43–4.46			
1–3 y§	2.18–3.47			
4–6 y§	2.08–3.78			
7–9 y§	2.25–3.61			
10–13 y§	2.24–4.42			
14–19 y§	2.33–4.44			

*No significant differences between males and females; range derived from combined data.
†Soldin SJ, Morales A, et al: Pediatric reference ranges on the Abbott IMx for FSH, LH, prolactin, TSH, T4, T3, free T3, T-Uptake, IgE, and ferritin. Clin Biochem 1995; 28:603. Study based on hospitalized patients; values represent 2.5 and 97.5th percentiles.
‡Lockitch G, Halstead AC, et al: Age- and sex-specific pediatric reference intervals for zinc, copper, selenium, iron, vitamins A and E and related proteins. Clin Chem 1988; 34:1625. Study based on healthy children; values represent the 0.025 and 0.975 fractiles. Transferrin saturation calculated from iron (μmol/L)/TIBC. Note that the lower reference limits for serum iron and transferrin saturation in this study are below the limits used to define acceptable levels for these two analytes (see O'Neal RM, Johnson OC, Schaefer AE: Guidelines for the classification and interpretation of group blood and urine data collected as part of the National Nutritional Survey. Pediatr Res 1970; 4:103).
§Lockitch G, Halstead AC, et al: Age- and sex-specific pediatric reference intervals: study design and methods illustrated by measurement of serum proteins with the Behring LN nephelometer. Clin Chem 1988; 34:1618. Results are 2.5–97.5 percentiles.

Appendix 44. PLASMA LEVELS OF FOLIC ACID AND VITAMIN B$_{12}$ IN CHILDREN

	Males	Females
Folic Acid	nmol/L	nmol/L
0–1 y	16.3–50.8	14.3–51.5
2–3 y	5.7–34.0	3.9–35.6
4–6 y	1.1–29.4	6.1–31.9
7–9 y	5.2–27.0	5.4–30.4
10–12 y	3.4–24.5	2.3–23.1
13–18 y	2.7–19.9	2.7–16.3
Vitamin B$_{12}$	pmol/L	pmol/L
0–1 y	216–891	168–1117
2–3 y	195–897	307–892
4–6 y	181–795	231–1038
7–9 y	200–863	182–866
10–12 y	135–803	145–752
13–18 y	158–638	134–605

Hicks JM, Cook J, et al: Vitamin B$_{12}$ and folate: pediatric reference ranges. Arch Pathol Lab Med 1993; 117:704. Data collected from hospitalized patients; 2.5–97.5th percentile values obtained with the Hoffman technique.

Appendix 45. PLASMA LEVELS OF VITAMIN E (α-TOCOPHEROL) IN CHILDREN

	Males and Females	
Age	μ**mol/L**	μ**g/mL**
Prematures*	1–8	0.5–3.5
Full term*	2–8	1.0–3.5
2–5 mo*	5–14	2.0–6.0
6–24 mo*	8–19	3.5–8.0
2–12 y*	13–21	5.5–9.0
1–6 y†	7–21	3.0–9.0
7–12 y†	10–21	4.0–9.0
13–19 y†	13–24	6.0–10.1

*Meites S (ed): Pediatric Clinical Chemistry. 3rd ed. Washington, DC, AACC Press, 1989, pp 295–296.
†Lockitch G, Halstead AC, et al: Age- and sex-specific pediatric reference intervals for zinc, copper, selenium, iron, vitamins A and E and related proteins. Clin Chem 1988; 34:1625. Study based on healthy children; values represent the 0.025 and 0.975 fractiles.

Appendix 46. SERUM ERYTHROPOIETIN LEVELS DURING THE FIRST YEAR OF LIFE

Days After Birth	Erythropoietin (mU/mL)	Hemoglobin (g/dL)	RBC (× 10⁶/μL)
0–6	33.0 ± 31.4 (11)	15.6 ± 2.2 (11)	4.51 ± 0.74 (11)
7–50	11.7 ± 3.6 (7)	12.8 ± 1.1 (5)	3.92 ± 0.35 (5)
51–100	21.1 ± 5.5 (13)	11.4 ± 1.0 (10)	4.09 ± 0.51 (10)
101–150	15.1 ± 3.9 (5)	11.2 ± 1.1 (3)	4.21 ± 0.31 (3)
151–200	17.8 ± 6.3 (6)	—	—
>201	23.1 ± 9.7 (10)	11.8 ± 0.8 (9)	4.57 ± 0.24 (9)

Values are expressed as mean ± SD; ( ), number of specimens.
From Yamashita H, Kukita J, et al: Serum erythropoietin levels in term and preterm infants during the first year of life. Am J Pediatr Hematol Oncol 1994; 16:213.

Appendix 47. PLASMA ERYTHROPOIETIN REFERENCE RANGES IN CHILDREN

Age (y)	Male Subjects 2.5%	Male Subjects 97.5%	Female Subjects 2.5%	Female Subjects 97.5%
1–3	1.7	17.9	2.1	15.9
4–6	3.5	21.9	2.9	8.5
7–9	1.0	13.5	2.1	8.2
10–12	1.0	14.0	1.1	9.1
13–15	2.2	14.4	3.8	20.5
16–18	1.5	15.2	2.0	14.2

Values expressed in mIU/mL. Data obtained from a total of 1122 hospitalized and outpatient children age 1–18 years.
Levels found in anemic patients cannot be compared with normal values. In fact, as long as the erythropoietin-generating apparatus in the kidney is efficient, serum levels increase exponentially as the hematocrit decreases. Serum erythropoietin must therefore be evaluated in relation to the degree of anemia, and every single laboratory should determine the exponential regression of serum erythropoietin versus hematocrit (or hemoglobin) in a home-made reference population of anemic subjects and define the 95% confidence limits. The patients gathered to calculate a reference regression equation should have an anemia with a single simple mechanism and no evidence of either renal failure or excessive cytokine production (i.e., normal values for C-reactive protein and α_2-globulins). Chronic iron deficiency anemia patients due to non-neoplastic and noninflammatory chronic blood loss have the advantages of being easily found, unequivocably defined, and homogeneous. They could become the universal reference population, although patients with hemolytic anemia or thalassemia intermedia also may be studied as reference subjects. Serum erythropoietin levels are also much higher for hemoglobin concentration in hypoplastic than in hyperplastic states. Thus, for the same hemoglobin concentration, serum erythropoietin levels are lower in thalassemia intermedia than in Diamond-Blackfan anemia.
From Krafte-Jacobs B, Williams J, Soldin SJ: Plasma erythropoietin reference ranges in children. J Pediatr 1995; 126:601.

Appendix 48. COMPLEMENT FRACTIONS C3 AND C4 IN MALES AND FEMALES

	Age	g/L
C3		
Zilow et al (1993)*	Healthy infants	0.30–0.98
Lockitch et al (1988)†	0–5 d	0.26–1.04
	1–19 y	0.51–0.95
	Adult	0.45–0.83
C4		
Lockitch et al (1988)†	0–5 d	0.06–0.37
	1–19 y	0.08–0.44
	Adult	0.11–0.41

*Zilow G, Zilow EP, et al: Complement activation in newborn infants with early onset infection. Pediatr Res 1993; 34:199. Results are 0–100th percentiles.
†Lockitch G, Halstead AC, et al: Age- and sex-specific pediatric reference intervals: study design and methods illustrated by measurement of serum proteins with the Behring LN nephelometer. Clin Chem 1988; 34:1618. Results are 0.025–0.975 fractiles.

Appendix 49. ACUTE PHASE PROTEINS AND COMPLEMENT ACTIVATION PRODUCTS IN HEALTHY NEWBORNS

	Median	Range
C3a-desArg (μg/L)	157	19–494
C3 (g/L)	0.67	0.30–0.98
C3bBbP (U/mL)	9.5	1.0–33.9
C1rsC1-inactivator (U/mL)	5.8	0.1–25.7
C-reactive protein (mg/L)	2	0–4

From Zilow G, Zilow EP, et al: Complement activation in newborn infants with early onset infection. Pediatr Res 1993; 34:199.

xxiv • Appendices

Appendix 50. PLASMA LEVELS OF IMMUNOGLOBULIN A
IN MALES AND FEMALES

Age	g/L	mg/dL
Lockitch et al (1988)*		
0–12 mo	0.00–1.00	0–100
1–3 y	0.24–1.21	24–121
4–6 y	0.33–2.35	33–235
7–9 y	0.41–3.68	41–368
10–11 y	0.64–2.46	64–246
12–13 y	0.70–4.32	70–432
14–15 y	0.57–3.00	57–300
16–19 y	0.74–4.19	74–419
Children's Hospital†		
Newborn	0.00–0.11	0–11
1–3 mo	0.06–0.05	6–50
4–6 mo	0.08–0.90	8–90
7–12 mo	0.16–1.00	16–100
1–3 y	0.20–2.30	20–230
3–6 y	0.50–1.50	50–150
Adult	0.50–2.00	50–200

*Lockitch G, Halstead AC, et al: Age- and sex-specific pediatric
reference intervals: study design and methods illustrated by
measurement of serum proteins with the Behring LN nephelometer.
Clin Chem 1988; 34:1618. Results are 0.025–0.975 percentiles.
†Children's Hospital, Boston, Massachusetts. Radial immunodiffusion
by Mancini.

Appendix 51. SERUM LEVELS OF IMMUNOGLOBULIN D
IN MALES AND FEMALES

Age	mg/L
Cord blood*	0.04–1.02
Adult†	2.0–173

*Ownby DR, Johnson CC, Peterson EL: Maternal smoking does not
influence cord serum IgE or IgD concentrations. J Allergy Clin
Immunol 1991; 88:555. Values constitute 95% of the measured
samples.
†Tozawa T, Nakata N, Adachi K: Serum IgD concentrations in normal
individuals 20–39 years of age. Rinsho Byori Jpn J Clin Pathol 1994;
42:656.

Appendix 52. SERUM LEVELS OF IMMUNOGLOBULIN E
IN MALES AND FEMALES

Age	IU/mL		
Cord blood*	0.02–2.08		
<1 y†	0–6.6		
1–2 y†	0–20.0		
2–3 y†	0.1–15.8		
3–4 y†	0–29.2		
4–5 y†	0.3–25.0		
5–6 y†	0.2–17.6		
6–7 y†	0.2–13.1		
7–8 y†	0.3–46.1		
8–9 y†	1.8–60.1		
9–10 y†	3.6–81.0		
10–11 y†	8.0–95.0		
11–12 y†	1.5–99.7		
12–13 y†	3.9–83.5		
13–16 y†	3.3–188.0		
<3 y‡	<30		
<10 y‡	<120		
10–14 y‡	<120		
Adult‡	<120		
	Females (KIU/L)	**Males (KIU/L)**	
0–12 mo§	0–20	2–24	
1–3 y§	2–55	2–149	
4–10 y§	8–279	4–249	
11–15 y§	5–295	7–280	
16–18 y§	7–698	5–268	

*Ownby DR, Johnson CC, Peterson EL: Maternal smoking does not
influence cord serum IgE or IgD concentrations. J Allergy Clin
Immunol 1991; 88:555. Values constitute 95% of the measured
samples.
†Lindenberg RE, Arroyave C: Levels of IgE in serum from normal
children and allergic children as measured by an enzyme
immunoassay. J Allergy Clin Immunol 1986; 78:614.
‡Children's Hospital, Boston, Massachusetts.
§Soldin SJ, Morales A, et al: Pediatric reference ranges on the Abbott
IMx for FSH, LH, prolactin, TSH, T4, T3, free T3, T-Uptake, IgE, and
ferritin. Clin Biochem 1995; 28:603. Study based on hospitalized
patients; values represent 2.5 and 97.5th percentiles.

Appendix 53. PLASMA LEVELS OF IMMUNOGLOBULIN M
IN MALES AND FEMALES

Age	g/L	mg/dL
Lockitch et al (1988)*		
0–12 mo	0.0–2.16	0–216
1–3 y	0.28–2.18	28–218
4–6 y	0.36–3.14	36–314
7–9 y	0.47–3.11	47–311
10–11 y	0.46–2.68	46–268
12–13 y	0.52–3.57	52–357
14–15 y	0.23–2.81	23–281
16–19 y	0.35–3.87	35–387
Children's Hospital†		
Newborn	0.05–0.30	5–30
1–3 mo	0.15–0.70	15–70
4–6 mo	0.10–0.80	10–80
7–12 mo	0.25–1.15	25–115
1–3 y	0.30–1.20	30–120
3–6 y	0.22–1.0	22–100
Adult	0.50–2.0	50–200

*Lockitch G, Halstead AC, et al: Age- and sex-specific pediatric
reference intervals: study design and methods illustrated by
measurement of serum proteins with the Behring LN nephelometer.
Clin Chem 1988; 34:1618. Results are 0.025–0.975 percentiles.
†Children's Hospital, Boston, Massachusetts.

Appendix 54. PLASMA LEVELS OF IMMUNOGLOBULIN G
IN MALES AND FEMALES

Age	g/L	mg/dL
Lockitch et al (1988)*		
0–12 mo	2.73–16.60	273–1660
1–3 y	5.33–10.78	533–1078
4–6 y	5.93–17.23	593–1723
7–9 y	6.73–17.34	673–1734
10–11 y	8.21–18.35	821–1835
12–13 y	8.93–18.23	893–1823
14–15 y	8.42–20.13	842–2013
16–19 y	6.46–18.64	646–1864
Children's Hospital†		
Newborn	7.0–1.30	700–1300
1–3 mo	2.80–7.50	280–750
4–6 mo	2.0–12.0	200–1200
7–12 mo	3.0–15.0	300–1500
1–3 y	4.0–13.0	400–1300
3–6 y	6.0–15.0	600–1500
Adult	6.0–15.0	600–1500

*Lockitch G, Halstead AC, et al: Age- and sex-specific pediatric
reference intervals: study design and methods illustrated by
measurement of serum proteins with the Behring LN nephelometer.
Clin Chem 1988; 34:1618. Results are 0.025–0.975 percentiles.
†Children's Hospital, Boston, Massachusetts.

Appendix 55. SERUM LEVELS OF IMMUNOGLOBULIN G SUBCLASSES (IgG_1, IgG_2, IgG_3, IgG_4)*

Age	IgG_1	IgG_2	IgG_3	IgG_4
Miles and Riches (1994)†				
Cord blood, preterm	3.4–9.7	0.7–1.7	0.2–0.5	0.2–0.7
Cord blood, term	5.8–13.7	0.6–5.2	0.2–1.2	0.2–1.0
5 y	5.6–12.7	0.4–4.4	0.3–1.0	0.1–0.8
6 y	6.2–11.3	0.5–4.0	0.3–0.8	0.2–0.9
7 y	5.4–10.5	0.9–3.5	0.3–1.1	0.2–1.1
8 y	5.6–10.5	0.7–4.5	0.2–1.1	0.1–0.8
9 y	3.9–11.4	0.7–4.7	0.4–1.2	0.2–1.0
10 y	4.4–10.8	0.6–4.0	0.3–1.2	0.1–0.9
11 y	6.4–10.9	0.9–4.3	0.3–0.9	0.2–1.0
12 y	6.0–11.5	0.9–4.8	0.4–1.0	0.2–0.9
13 y	6.1–11.5	0.9–7.9	0.2–1.1	0.1–0.8
Adults	4.8–9.5	1.1–6.9	0.3–0.8	0.2–1.1
Children's Hospital‡				
Cord	4.35–10.84	1.43–4.53	0.27–1.46	0.01–0.47
0–2 mo	2.18–4.96	0.40–1.67	0.04–0.23	0.01–0.33
3–5 mo	1.43–3.94	0.23–1.47	0.04–1.0	0.01–0.14
6–8 mo	1.90–3.88	0.37–0.60	0.12–0.62	<0.01
9 mo–2 y	2.86–6.80	0.30–3.27	0.13–0.82	0.01–0.65
3–4 y	3.81–8.84	0.70–4.43	0.17–0.90	0.01–1.16
5–6 y	2.92–8.16	0.83–5.13	0.08–1.11	0.01–1.21
7–8 y	4.22–8.02	1.13–4.80	0.15–1.33	0.01–0.84
9–10 y	4.56–9.38	1.63–5.13	0.26–1.13	0.01–1.21
11–12 y	4.56–9.52	1.47–4.93	0.12–1.79	0.01–1.68
13–14 y	3.47–9.93	1.40–4.40	0.23–1.17	0.01–0.83
Adults	4.22–12.92	1.17–7.47	0.41–1.29	0.01–2.91

*Values for males and females, expressed in g/L.
†Miles J, Riches P: The determination of IgG subclass concentrations in serum by enzyme linked immunosorbent assay: establishment of age-
related reference ranges for cord blood samples, children aged 5–13 years and adults. Ann Clin Biochem 1994; 31:245.
‡Children's Hospital, Boston, Massachusetts, by electron immunoassay.

Appendix 56. SERUM LEVELS OF IMMUNOGLOBULIN
LIGHT CHAINS IN MALES AND FEMALES

Age	(Kappa) g/L	(Lambda) g/L
Newborn	7.7–8.7	1.7–1.9
Premature	3.1–4.9	1.6–1.9
1 mo	3.6–4.8	1.6–2.0
2 mo	2.4–2.7	1.6–1.7
3 mo	1.7–2.5	1.0–1.3
4 mo	1.9–2.4	0.8–1.0
5 mo	2.0–3.2	1.0–1.1
1 y	3.0–5.3	0.9–1.2
2 y	3.6–6.4	1.3–1.5
3 y	4.1–5.4	1.1–1.4
4 y	4.8–8.3	1.2–1.7
5 y	5.4–7.1	1.3–1.7
6 y	6.0–8.5	1.6–1.7
7 y	4.6–7.5	1.4–1.8
8 y	7.3–9.1	1.4–1.7
9 y	7.1–9.6	1.5–1.8
10 y	8.2–9.6	1.3–1.9
11 y	6.0–8.3	1.4–1.8
12 y	8.2–9.6	1.7–2.0
13 y	8.2–10.5	1.4–1.7
14 y	8.0–10.8	1.9–2.2
15 y	7.2–11.0	1.7–2.3
16 y	7.0–11.2	1.5–2.2

From Herkner KR, Salzer H, et al: Pediatric and perinatal reference
intervals for immunoglobulin light chains kappa and lambda. Clin
Chem 1992; 38:548. Ranges are for 10th–90th percentiles.

Appendix 57. CONJUGATED BILIRUBIN IN
MALES AND FEMALES

	μmol/L	mg/dL
Neonates*	<10	<0.6
>Neonates*	<7	<0.4
Preterm infants†	<10	<0.6

*Children's Hospital, Boston, Massachusetts.
†Lockitch G, Halstead AC, et al: Age- and sex-specific pediatric
reference intervals for biochemistry analytes as measured with the
Ektachem 700 analyzer. Clin Chem 1988; 34:1622.

Appendix 58. TOTAL BILIRUBIN IN MALES AND FEMALES

	μmol/L	mg/dL
Birth–1 d*	<103	<6.0
1–3 d*	<137	<8.0
3–7 d*	<205	<12.0
7 d–1 mo	<120	<7.0
1 mo–adult*	<21	<1.2
Bottle-fed infants†	<212	<12.4
Breast-fed infants†	<253	<14.8

*Children's Hospital, Boston, Massachusetts.
†Maisels MJ, Gifford K: Normal serum bilirubin levels in the newborn
and the effect of breast feeding. Pediatrics 1986; 78:837.

Appendix 59. SELECTED BIOCHEMICAL PARAMETERS IN CORD BLOOD

	Cord Blood (Term)	Cord Blood (Preterm)	Adult or Maternal Blood
Erythrocytes			
Magnesium (mmol/L)*	1.76 ± 0.15 (44)	—	—
Copper (μmol/L)*	12.9 ± 3.0 (39)	—	—
Zinc (μmol/L)*	40.4 ± 13.6 (44)	—	—
Ferritin (ag/cell)†	265 (47)	92.7 (47)	
Serum/Plasma			
Ferritin (μg/L)†	56.8 (47)	17.7 (47)	—
Free riboflavin (nM)‡	20.2 (31)‖	25.0‖	4.7 (31)
Flavocoenzymes (nM)‡	55.8 (31)‖	71.8‖	90.7 (31)
Vitamin B_2 (nM)‡	77.2 (31)‖	92.6	94.9 (31)
Flavocoenzymes uptake (nmol/min per kg)‡	0.4	1.5¶	—
Free riboflavin release (nmol/min per kg)‡	0.2	0.4¶	—
Selenium (μmol/L)§	1.04 ± 0.21‖	0.89 ± 0.27‖	1.56 ± 0.27
Retinol (μmol/L)§	0.66 ± 0.22‖	0.52 ± 0.12‖	1.26 ± 0.45
Alpha-Tocopherol (μmol/L)§	7.10 ± 2.1‖	8.81 ± 2.8‖	32.4 ± 9.2
Glutathione peroxidase (U/L)§	456 ± 108‖	305 ± 89‖	873 ± 176

*Speich M, Murat A, et al: Magnesium, total calcium, phosphorus, copper and zinc in plasma and erythrocytes of venous cord blood from infants of diabetic mothers: comparison with a reference group by logist discriminant analysis. Clin Chem 1992; 38:2002. Values expressed as mean ± SD; ( ), n of samples.
†Carpani G, Marini F, et al: Red cell and plasma ferritin in a group of normal fetuses at different ages of gestation. Eur J Haematol 1992; 49:260. Values expressed as mean geometrical value; ( ), n of samples.
‡Zempleni J, Link G, Bitsch I: Intrauterine vitamin B_2 uptake of preterm and full-term infants. Pediatr Res 1995; 38:585. Concentrations measured in the umbilical vein are reported in this table; values for umbilical artery are reported in the chapter text as well.
§Dison PJ, Lockitch G, et al: Influence of maternal factors on cord and neonatal plasma micronutrient levels. Am J Perinatol 1993; 10:30. Data obtained in 107 term, 23 preterm (<32 wk), and 58 maternal samples.
‖$P < .05$ compared with full term.
¶$P < .05$ compared with adult/maternal.

Appendix 60. RELATIONSHIP OF SERUM PROTEIN LEVELS TO AGE

	Total Proteins (g/dL) Mean ± 1 SD and Range	Albumin (g/dL) Mean ± 1 SD and Range	Alpha-1 (g/dL) Mean ± 1 SD and Range	Alpha-2 (g/dL) Mean ± 1 SD and Range	Beta (g/dL) Mean ± 1 SD and Range	Gamma (g/dL) Mean ± 1 SD and Range
Cord blood	6.22 ± 1.21 (4.78–8.04)	3.23 ± 0.82 (2.17–4.04)	0.41 ± 0.10 (0.25–0.66)	0.68 ± 0.14 (0.44–0.94)	0.74 ± 0.30 (0.42–1.56)	1.28 ± 0.23 (0.81–1.16)
1–3 mo	5.64 ± 1.04 (3.64–7.38)	3.41 ± 0.72 (2.05–4.46)	0.24 ± 0.09 (0.08–0.43)	0.74 ± 0.24 (0.40–1.13)	0.59 ± 0.20 (0.39–1.14)	0.66 ± 0.24 (0.25–1.05)
4–6 mo	5.43 ± 0.84 (4.29–6.10)	3.46 ± 0.36 (3.17–3.88)	0.17 ± 0.04 (0.12–0.25)	0.67 ± 0.11 (0.52–0.84)	0.61 ± 0.14 (0.44–0.76)	0.61 ± 0.26 (0.24–0.90)
7–12 mo	6.54 ± 0.76 (5.10–7.31)	3.62 ± 0.60 (3.22–4.31)	0.35 ± 0.15 (0.15–0.55)	0.99 ± 0.30 (0.78–1.46)	0.79 ± 0.16 (0.63–0.91)	0.84 ± 0.36 (0.32–1.18)
13–24 mo	6.66 ± 0.93 (3.69–7.50)	3.63 ± 0.80 (1.89–5.03)	0.31 ± 0.15 (0.09–0.58)	0.88 ± 0.42 (0.41–1.36)	0.77 ± 0.31 (0.36–1.41)	1.09 ± 0.32 (0.36–1.62)
25–36 mo	6.98 ± 0.66 (6.38–8.06)	4.11 ± 0.78 (3.57–5.50)	0.23 ± 0.09 (0.19–0.26)	0.89 ± 0.14 (0.68–1.09)	0.67 ± 0.14 (0.47–0.91)	1.08 ± 0.28 (0.73–1.46)
3–5 y	6.65 ± 0.85 (4.88–8.06)	3.95 ± 0.57 (2.93–5.21)	0.21 ± 0.08 (0.08–0.40)	0.70 ± 0.15 (0.43–0.99)	0.67 ± 0.11 (0.47–1.01)	1.13 ± 0.31 (0.54–1.66)
6–8 y	6.95 ± 0.55 (5.97–7.94)	4.03 ± 0.45 (3.26–4.95)	0.22 ± 0.09 (0.09–0.45)	0.67 ± 0.10 (0.50–0.83)	0.72 ± 0.11 (0.45–0.93)	1.21 ± 0.32 (0.70–1.95)
9–11 y	7.43 ± 0.84 (6.32–9.00)	4.24 ± 0.79 (3.16–4.97)	0.30 ± 0.07 (0.12–0.38)	0.75 ± 0.27 (0.67–0.87)	0.84 ± 0.16 (0.63–1.02)	1.46 ± 0.41 (0.79–2.03)
12–16 y	7.25 ± 0.85 (6.25–8.75)	4.26 ± 0.64 (3.19–5.13)	0.19 ± 0.07 (0.09–0.32)	0.71 ± 0.15 (0.50–0.97)	0.68 ± 0.15 (0.48–0.88)	1.40 ± 0.31 (1.08–1.96)
Adult	7.41 ± 0.96 (6.44–8.32)	4.31 ± 0.59 (3.46–4.78)	0.23 ± 0.06 (0.16–0.30)	0.61 ± 0.14 (0.51–0.86)	0.81 ± 0.22 (0.59–1.06)	1.45 ± 0.46 (0.68–2.11)

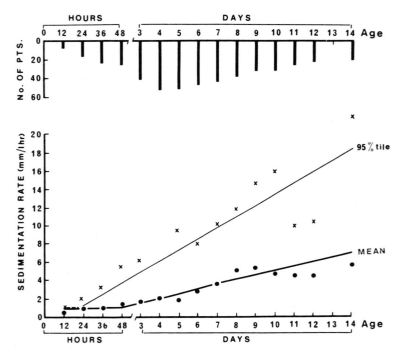

Appendix 61. Sedimentation rate in the newborn period.

The erythrocyte sedimentation rate was measured in capillary blood in healthy full-term and low-birth-weight newborns. Normal values ranged from 1 mm/h at 12 hours of age to 17 mm/h at 14 days of age. All values of neonates with hematocrit values less than 40% were corrected to 40%. (From Adler SM, Denton RL: The erythrocyte sedimentation rate in the newborn period. J Pediatr 1975; 86:942.)

Index

Note: Page numbers in *italics* refer to illustrations; page numbers followed by t refer to tables. Page numbers in roman numerals refer to the appendices.

Anemia *(Continued)*
  hemolytic, autoimmune, 499–516. See also
    Hemolytic anemia, autoimmune.
    Heinz body, 598, 745–748, *747*
    nonspherocytic, 665–693. See also *Hemo-*
      lytic anemia, nonspherocytic, congeni-
      tal.
    schistocytic, 528–537. See also *Hemolytic*
      anemia, schistocytic.
    spherocytic, 578–601. See also *Spherocyto-*
      sis, hereditary.
    stomatocytic, 616–619. See also *Stomato-*
      cytosis, hereditary.
    xerocytic, 619–621. See also *Xerocytosis,*
      hereditary.
  historical studies of, 4–8
  in acquired immunodeficiency syndrome,
    1877–1878
  in Addison's disease, 1851–1852
  in bacterial endocarditis, 1844
  in chronic disorders, 450–451, 1613, 1853–
    1855, 1854t
  in chronic inflammation, 450–451
  in chronic renal failure, 1613
  in copper deficiency, 436–437
  in cystic fibrosis, 1845
  in diabetes mellitus, 1867
  in Diamond-Blackfan syndrome, 42
  in DIDMOAD syndrome, 1852
  in dyskeratosis congenita, 1869
  in eczema, 1869
  in hookworm infection, 1904
  in hypothyroidism, 1850, *1851*
  in lead poisoning, 485–487
  in liver disease, 1846
  in myelodysplastic syndromes, 1311
  in Pearson's syndrome, 42, 278–280, *279,*
    1845–1846
  in polyarteritis nodosa, 1857
  in psoriasis, 1869
  in Rh hemolytic disease, 74
  in rheumatoid arthritis, 1855
  in sarcoidosis, 1853
  in Shwachman-Diamond syndrome, 277,
    1845
  in systemic lupus erythematosus, 1856
  in visceral leishmaniasis, 1902
  iron deficiency, 439–440. See also *Iron defi-*
    ciency; Iron deficiency anemia.
  macrocytic, 377t
  malarial, 1897–1901
    hemolysis in, 1897, 1898–1899
    splenic pathology in, 1897–1898
  megaloblastic, 385–415. See also *Folate;*
    Megaloblastic anemia; Vitamin B₁₂ (cobal-
    amin).
  microcytic, 377t
  neonatal, 34–42, 34t, 39t. See also specific
    disorders.
    blood sampling in, 37, *38*
    α chain hemoglobinopathy in, 39
    β chain hemoglobinopathy in, 39–40
    chain hemoglobinopathy in, 40, 40t
    diagnosis of, 42, *43*
    erythropoiesis failure in, 42
    fetal-to-fetal hemorrhage in, 36
    fetal-to-maternal hemorrhage in, 34–36,
      35t
    hemoglobin H disease in, 40
    hemoglobinopathies in, 39–41, 40t
    hemolytic processes in, 38–42, 39t, 40t
    hemorrhage in, 34–38, 35t, *38,* 38t
    hydrops fetalis in, 40–41
    iatrogenic, 37, *38*
    in developing countries, 33, 1894–1895,
      1894, 1894t, 1910

Anemia *(Continued)*
    in Diamond-Blackfan syndrome, 42
    in Pearson's syndrome, 42
    internal hemorrhage in, 36–37
    nuchal cord and, 31
    obstetric accidents in, 36
    placental malformations in, 36
    red cell enzyme deficiencies in, 42
    red cell membrane disorders in, 41
    α-thalassemia syndromes in, 40–41
    β-thalassemia syndromes in, 41
    γ-thalassemia syndromes in, 41
    umbilical cord malformations in, 36
  normocytic, 377t
  of prematurity, 42–46, *43,* 45t, 1792
  pernicious, 386, 393–395. See also *Perni-*
    cious anemia; Vitamin B₁₂ (cobalamin).
  physiologic, of prematurity, 42–46, *43,* 45t,
    1792
  recombinant erythropoietin in, 1774
  refractory, 1309–1312, 1310t
    granulocyte colony-stimulating factor
      in, 213–214
    granulocyte-macrophage colony-stimu-
      lating factor in, 213
    of Pearson's syndrome, 42, 278–280,
      279, 1845–1846
    with excess blasts, 1309–1312, 1310t
    with excess blasts in transformation,
      1309–1312, 1310t
    with ringed sideroblasts, 1309–1312,
      1310t
  sideroblastic, 448–450, 448t, *449*
    refractory (Pearson's syndrome), 42,
      278–280, *279,* 1845–1846
  spur cell, 628–630, *629*
  third-world, 33, 1894–1895, *1894,* 1894t
    treatment of, 1910
  with thrombocytopenia, 1588
Anemia of chronic disease, 450–451,
  1853–1855, 1854t
Anemia of prematurity, 42–46, *43,* 45t
  rHuEPO in, 1792
Anemia pseudoleucaemica infantum, 4
Anergy, clonal, of T lymphocytes, *1002,*
  1005, 1012
Anesthesia, epidural, in sickle cell disease,
  789
Anesthetics, methemoglobinemia with, 756
Aneurysm, in sickle cell disease, 779
Angioedema, eosinophilia in, 923
Angioid streaks, in hereditary spherocytosis,
  598
  in sickle cell disease, 785
Angioneurotic edema, hereditary, 1044
Anhidrotic ectodermal dysplasia,
  immunodeficiency in, 1035t
Aniline, methemoglobinemia with, 756
Anion exchanger–1 (band 3), 573t
  erythrocyte, *551,* 552t–553t, 557–559, *558*
    antibodies to, 524, 577, 772
    COOH-terminal domain of, 557–559,
      558
    defects of, 559
    fetal, 576
    glycophorin A association with, 555,
      559
    in hereditary spherocytosis, 582t, 585–
      586, 588, *589*
    in sickle cell disease, 772
    in Southeast Asian ovalocytosis, 615
    NH₂-terminal domain of, 557, *558*
    peripheral membrane protein interac-
      tions with, 557
    self-association of, 559
    synthesis of, 575–576

Anion exchanger–1 (band 3) *(Continued)*
    variants of, 559
    nonerythroid, 559
Aniridia, in Wilms' tumor, 1084
  sporadic, 1382t
Anisocytosis, in G6PD deficiency, 710
Anisoylated plasminogen streptokinase
  activator complex, 1561
Ankylosing spondylitis, radiation treatment
  in, aplastic anemia with, 243
Ankyrin, erythrocyte, *551,* 552t–553t,
  565–566
  death domain of, 566
  in hereditary spherocytosis, 581t, 583–
    585, *584,* 588
  isoforms of, 566
  phosphorylation of, 566, 572
  regulatory domain of, 566
  repeat domain of, 565, *565*
  spectrin-binding domain of, 565–566,
    565
  structure of, 565, *565*
  synthesis of, 575–576
  in spectrin membrane binding, 563–564
  nonerythroid, 566
Annexin II, 1564, 1564t
Anorexia nervosa, acanthocytosis in, 628
  hematologic manifestations of, 1868–1869
  neutropenia in, 919
Anthracyclines, as cancer risk factor, 1075
  biotransformation of, 1213–1214, *1213*
  cardiac toxicity of, 1218–1219
  CNS penetration of, 1223t
  distribution of, 1213
  elimination of, 1215–1216, 1215t
  extravasation of, 1216, 1217t
  in acute lymphoblastic leukemia, 1265–
    1266
  leukemia after, 1161, 1161t
  mechanisms of action of, 1208, 1208t
  resistance to, 1221t
  toxicity of, 1217t, 1218–1219
Anti-A antibodies, neonatal erythrocyte
  uptake of, 26
Anti–band 3 antibodies, 577, 772
  in red cell clearance, 524
Antibiotics, after exchange transfusion, 73
  antitumor, CNS penetration of, 1223t
    elimination of, 1215t
    mechanisms of action of, 1208, 1208t
    resistance to, 1221t
    toxicity of, 1217t
  aplastic anemia with, 241t, 242–243, 242t
  autoimmune hemolytic anemia with, 512
  in acquired aplastic anemia, 252
  in chronic granulomatous disease, 943–944
  in febrile neutropenic patient, 1746–1747
  in fever of unknown origin, 1747, *1748*
  postsplenectomy, in hereditary spherocyto-
    sis, 601
  prophylactic, in hyperimmunoglobulin E
    syndrome, 930
    in sickle cell disease, 1063–1064
Antibody(ies). See also *Autoantibody(ies);*
    Immunoglobulin(s); B Lymphocyte(s).
  anion exchanger–1 (band 3), 524, 577, 772
  anti-A, neonatal erythrocyte uptake of, 26
  anticoagulant-dependent, in *in vitro* plate-
    let agglutination, 1587
  bacterial, developmental changes in, 1063
  blood group, 1762, 1768t, 1770–1776,
    1771t, 1773t. See also *ABO hemolytic*
    disease; Rh hemolytic disease.
  cardiolipin, thrombotic disorders and,
    1583, 1697
  deficiency of, 932–933

England and Fraser function, in β-
thalassemia trait diagnosis, 850t
English springer spaniels,
phosphofructokinase deficiency in, 674
Enhancer region, of globin genes, 817
ENL gene, 1114t
in acute monoblastic leukemia, 1160
Enolase, 27
activity of, x, xi
deficiency of, 680–681
in hereditary spherocytosis, 586
Enteritis, regional, iron deficiency in, 1845
vitamin B$_{12}$ deficiency in, 1845
Enterobacter spp., infection with, 1740
Enterocolitis, 1742t
necrotizing, after exchange transfusion, 73
in acute lymphoblastic leukemia, 1255–
1256
thrombocytopenia with, 125
Enterocytes, in megaloblastic anemia, 388
vitamin B$_{12}$ transport defects of, 400–401
Enteropathy, milk-induced, iron deficiency
with, 438
Enuresis, in sickle cell disease, 784
Enzymes, lysosomal, 1463
assays for, 1469–1471, 1470t, 1473
disorders of, 1460–1499. See also specific lysosomal storage diseases.
genes for, 1464t, 1471
replacement of, 1472
Eosinopenia, 924, 1872
Eosinophil(s), 893–894, 894t
fetal, iii
functions of, 908–909, 908t
granules of, 893–894, 894t
hereditary hypersegmentation of, 1870
in acute lymphoblastic leukemia, 1257
in acute myelomonocytic leukemia, 1159
reference values for, xv
Eosinophilia, 921–923, 922t, 1872–1873, 1872t
embolic renal disease and, 1850
in developing countries, 1905–1906, 1905t,
1909
in parasitic infection, 1858
in polyarteritis nodosa, 1857
in pulmonary disease, 1853
tropical, 1905–1906, 1905t
Eosinophilic fasciitis, aplastic anemia with,
246
Eosinophilic gastroenteritis, 1845
Eosinophilic granuloma, 1372, 1372. See also
*Langerhans cell histiocytosis (histiocytosis
X).*
Ependymoma, 1435, 1435t
epidemiology of, 1082
treatment of, 1440t, 1441–1442
Epidermal growth factor receptor, in human
cancer, 1106–1107
Epimerase, activity of, x
Epinephrine, in blood transfusion reaction,
1796t
neutrophil effects of, 921, 928
Epipodophyllotoxin, as cancer risk factor,
1075
biotransformation of, 1213
CNS penetration of, 1223t
elimination of, 1216
in acute lymphoblastic leukemia, 1266
leukemia after, 1161, 1161t
mechanisms of action of, 1208, 1208t
resistance to, 1221t
Epistasis. See *Bleeding.*
Epithelial cells, hematopoietic growth factor
expression by, 191
EPO gene, 181–182, 181t
mutations in, 205–206

EPO gene *(Continued)*
regulation of, hypoxia in, 192
EPOR gene, 181t
Epsilon-aminocaproic acid, in acquired
aplastic anemia, 252
in Fanconi's anemia, 269
in sickle cell disease, 784
Epstein-Barr virus, antibody to, 1865, *1865*
congenital transmission of, 1861
infection with, 1741
African Burkitt's lymphoma and, 1076,
1081–1082, 1326
aplastic anemia with, 245–246
B-cell lymphoma and, 1195
CRAF1 interaction with, 980
hematologic manifestations of, 1739t
hemophagocytic lymphohistiocytoses
with, 1364–1366, *1364*, 1364t, *1365*
Hodgkin's disease and, 1340
in infectious mononucleosis, 1860. See
also *Infectious mononucleosis.*
in lymphomatoid granulomatosis, 1370–
1371
in sinus histiocytosis with massive
lymphadenopathy, 1370
in X-linked lymphoproliferative syndrome, 1366–1370, 1368t
lymphoreticular response to, 1361
malignancy and, 1865–1866
marrow toxicity of, *244*
non-Hodgkin's lymphoma and, 1325–
1326
prevention of, in X-linked lymphoproliferative syndrome, 1370
transfusion-associated, 1790, 1860–1861
vs. acute lymphoblastic leukemia, 1258
vs. juvenile chronic myelogenous leukemia, 1306
transmission of, 1361, 1790, 1860–1861
Er blood group, 1761t
c-*erb B*, in glioma, 1106
v-*erb B*, 1106
Erlenmeyer flask deformity, in Gaucher's
disease, 1476
Erythroblast(s), 169, 170, *170*
fetal, 21, 21t
in malaria, 1899, *1900*
in umbilical cord blood, iv
Erythroblastopenia, transient, *vs.* Diamond-
Blackfan anemia, 1777
Erythroblastosis fetalis, 54. See also *ABO
hemolytic disease; Rh hemolytic disease.*
blood sampling in, 29
Erythrocytapheresis, in cyanotic congenital
heart disease, 1843
in polycythemia, 1832
in sickle cell anemia, 1830–1832
in thalassemia, 1832
indications for, 1831t, 1832t
isovolemic, 1832
Erythrocyte(s), 19–29
at two weeks of life, vi
automated counting of, 376–379, 378t
basophilic stippling of, in lead poisoning,
485
crenated, 579t
diagnostic associations of, 381t
daily renewal of, 427
deformability of, 570–571. See also *Erythrocyte membrane.*
in glucose phosphate isomerase deficiency, 671–672
reduction of, 527, 527t
density of, *1828*
development of. See *Erythropoiesis.*
diameter of, reference values for, xiv

Erythrocyte(s) *(Continued)*
during first year, vii
fetal, iii
membrane of, 576
film examination of, 379, 381t, 382t
formation of, 19–23. See also *Erythropoiesis.*
glucose metabolism of, 27–29
G6PD in, 704, *705*
glycolysis of. See *Glycolysis, erythrocyte.*
historical studies on, 13
in acute lymphoblastic leukemia, 1257
in anorexia nervosa, 1868
in diabetes mellitus, 1866–1867
in hypothyroidism, 1850, *1851*
in liver disease, 1846
in megaloblastic anemia, 387–388, *388*
in muscular dystrophy, 1868
in myasthenia gravis, 1868
in myelodysplastic syndromes, 1311, *1311*
in psoriasis, 1869
in renal disease, 1848
in rheumatoid arthritis, 1855
inclusion in, in β-thalassemia, 851–852,
852
irradiation of, for blood transfusion, 1791,
1791t
life span of, 24, 24t, 88
hemolysis-related shortening of, 38–39,
39t
mass of, reference values for, xiv
membrane of, 24–27, *25, 26*, 544–632. See
also *Erythrocyte membrane.*
neonatal, 23, *25*
antigen expression of, 27
2,3-diphosphoglycerate metabolism of,
29
Embden-Meyerhof pathway of, 27
filtration rate of, 27
glucose consumption of, 27–29
intramembrane particles of, 26
life span of, 24, 24t, 88
lipids of, 27
membrane of, 24–27, *25, 26*. See also
Erythrocyte membrane.
metabolism of, 27–29, 28t
morphologic abnormalities of, 26
oxidant-induced injury response of, 29
pentose-phosphate pathway of, 29
phosphofructokinase deficiency in, 27,
28–29
pocks of, 25–26
protein binding sites of, 26–27
transport systems of, 27
vacuoles of, 26
volume of, 23, *23*
nucleotide metabolism of, defects of, 689–
692
adenosine deaminase overproduction
in, 691–692
adenylate kinase deficiency in, 691
pyrimidine–5'-nucleotidase deficiency
in, 689–691
of cord blood, iii, iv
of premature infant, 25–26
osmotic fragility of, 578
in hereditary spherocytosis, 594–595,
594
osmotic fragility test of, prosthetic cardiac
valves and, 1842
polyagglutination of, 1776
protoporphyrin accumulation in, iron deficiency–associated, 484–485
lead poisoning–associated, 483–484, *484*
reference values for, iii, iv, viii

Erythropoiesis (*Continued*)
negative regulation of, 206–207
normoblastic, 20
precursor cells in, 169–170, *170*
progenitor cells in, 168, *168*
steel factor in, 206
stress, 170, 205
transcription factors in, 205
transferrin receptor generation and, 436
transferrin receptors in, 432
Erythropoietin, 175t, 176
cellular expression of, 184
cost of, 217
during first year, xxii
gene for, 175t, 179–180, 181–182, 181t
mutations in, 205–206
regulation of, hypoxia in, 192
in acquired aplastic anemia, 249, 257
in acquired immunodeficiency syndrome, 215
in anemia of chronic disease, 217, 218, 451, 1854
in anemia of prematurity, 44–46, 45t, 217
in aplastic anemia, 214, 247
in blood transfusion, 1774
in cord blood, 43
in cystic fibrosis, 1853
in Diamond-Blackfan anemia, 215, 295, 298
in end-stage renal disease, 451, 452
in erythropoiesis, 22, 205–206
in fetal erythropoiesis, 22
in premature infant, 1792
in Rh hemolytic disease, 74–75
in sickle cell disease, 772
in transient erythroblastopenia of childhood, 300
iron interaction with, 451–452, *452*
receptor for, 196
fetal, 206
in cancer, 1108
in cell growth, 1097
reference values for, xxii
side effects of, 217
Erythrostasis, in hereditary spherocytosis, 590
Escherichia coli, infection with, hematologic manifestations of, 1739t
in hemolytic-uremic syndrome, 532–534, *533*
in sickle cell disease, 781t
E-selectin, in leukocyte migration, 899–900, *899*, *900*
in lymphocyte–endothelial cell adhesion, 1009–1010, *1010*
Esophagitis, 1742t
Candida causing, 1749–1750
Essential fatty acid deficiency, hematologic manifestations of, 1867–1868
Estrogen, hematologic effects of, 1852
in β-thalassemia–related delayed puberty, 859
interleukin–6 expression and, 191
Eta–1 (osteopontin), *1003*, 1010
Ethamsylate, in periventricular-intraventricular hemorrhage prevention, 134t, 135
Ethylene-diaminetetraacetic acid (EDTA)-dependent antibodies, in *in vitro* platelet agglutination, 1587
Etiocholanolone, in acquired aplastic anemia, 257–258
in Fanconi's anemia, 268
ETO gene, in acute myeloblastic leukemia, 1157
Etoposide, as cancer risk factor, 1075

Etoposide (*Continued*)
elimination of, 1215t, 1216
for stem cell transplantation, 340
mechanisms of action of, 1208
radiation therapy interaction with, 1237
toxicity of, 1217t
ETS genes, 186
Ets transcription factor, 185t, 186
in cell growth, 1098
ETV6 gene, in pre–B-cell acute lymphoblastic leukemia, 1165–1166
Evans' syndrome, 502, 512, 1594
Ewing's sarcoma, 1415–1420, 1415t. See also *Primitive neuroectodermal tumor.*
chromosomal translocations in, 1115t, 1123
clinical features of, 1416–1419
cytogenetics of, 1392t, 1415–1416
epidemiology of, 1083
extraosseous, 1419–1420
histopathology of, 1392t
metastatic, 1416, 1419
molecular biology of, 1392t
prognosis for, 1416
treatment of, 1416–1419
chemotherapy in, 1417–1419, 1418t
dose intensity of, 1206, *1207*
preoperative, 1417, 1418–1419
marrow ablative therapy in, 1419
radiation therapy in, 1417, 1418
surgical, 1416–1417
EWS gene, 1415
EWS-ATF1 fusion gene, 1115t
EWS-ERG fusion gene, 1115t, 1123
EWS-FLI1 fusion gene, 1112, 1115t, 1123
EWS-WT1 fusion gene, 1115t
Exchange transfusion, 1792. See also *Blood transfusion.*
antibiotics after, 73
breast feeding after, 73
complications of, 72–73, 72t
in acute myelogenous leukemia, 1297
in alloimmune thrombocytopenia, 1603
in autoimmune hemolytic anemia, 509t, 510
in G6PD deficiency, 720
in Rh hemolytic disease, 70–73, 72t
necrotizing enterocolitis after, 73
technique of, 71–72
thrombocytopenia with, 125
Exercise, hemoglobinuria with, 530–531, 622
neutrophilia with, 921
schistocytic hemolytic anemia with, 530
Extracorporeal membrane oxygenation, hemorrhage with, 1792–1793, 1793t
in respiratory insufficiency, 142
plasmapheresis with, 1835
Extremities, rhabdomyosarcoma of, 1407. See also *Rhabdomyosarcoma.*
Eye, disorders of, after stem cell transplantation, 351
in acute lymphoblastic leukemia, 1256, 1266
in G6PD deficiency, 722
in neuronal ceroid lipofuscinoses, 1497, 1498
in sickle cell disease, 785

F cells, in sickle cell disease, 768, 793–794
Fäber, E., 4
Fabry's disease, *1475*
clinical features of, 1474
kidney transplantation in, 1472
FACC gene, 1125t
in Fanconi's anemia, 267

Face, hypertrichosis of, in porphyria cutanea tarda, 472, *472*
Factor D, deficiency of, 1042
Factor H, deficiency of, 1044
Factor I. See also *Fibrinogen.*
deficiency of, 1044
in liver disease, 1846
in renal disease, 1849
Factor II, after cardiopulmonary bypass, 1685t
deficiency of, 128t, 129, 129t, 1665
fetal, 118t
in full-term infant, 119t
in liver disease, 1846–1847
in premature infant, 118t, 119t
in renal disease, 1849
reference values for, 118t, 119t, 1678t, xix, xviii
Factor V, 1534t
acquired antibodies to, 1681
activation of, 1538–1540, *1539*
after cardiopulmonary bypass, 1685t
antibody to, 1662
deficiency of, 128t, 129–130, 129t, 1662
clinical evaluation of, 1582, *1582*
fetal, 118t
gene organization of, 1537t
in full-term infant, 119t
in liver disease, 1847
in platelet alpha granules, 1609
in premature infant, 118t, 119t
in renal disease, 1849
reference values for, 118t, 119t, 1678t, xix
variant in, *1550*, 1551
Factor V Leiden, 1665–1666, 1666t
Factor Va, 1532, *1533*, 1534, 1538
activated protein C inhibition of, 1545–1546, *1545*, *1546*
Factor VII, 1533, 1534t, *1536*
after cardiopulmonary bypass, 1685t
assay for, 1533–1534
deficiency of, 128t, 129t, 130, 1532, 1662–1663, 1665
after stem cell transplantation, 352
classification of, 1663
fetal, 118t, 122, *123*
gene organization of, 1537t
in factor VII deficiency, 1663
in full-term infant, 119t
in liver disease, 1846–1847
in premature infant, 118t, 119t
in renal disease, 1849
reference values for, 118t, 119t, 1678t, xix
Factor VIIa, 1532, 1533, *1533*
assay for, 1533–1534
inhibition of, *1543*, 1544–1545
Factor VIII, 1534t, 1632, *1633*
activation of, 1538–1540, *1540*
after cardiopulmonary bypass, 1685t
antibodies to, 1638–1639, 1681
in hemophilia A patient, 1642–1644
continuous infusion of, in hemophilia A, 1643
cryoprecipitation-produced, in hemophilia A, 1641
deficiency of, 128t, 129t, 130, 1662. See also *Hemophilia A.*
fetal, 118t, 122
gene for, 1633–1634
immune tolerance to, in hemophilia A, 1643–1644
immunoassay for, 1638
in full-term infant, 119t
in hemophilia A, 1637t, 1639–1641, 1643–1644
in liver disease, 1847

Glucose-6-phosphate dehydrogenase (G6PD) deficiency *(Continued)*
  pathophysiology of, 718–719
  phenotypic expression of, 717–719, 718t
  polymorphic gene mutation in, 710, 717–719, 718t, *720*
  sickle cell disease and, 722, 764
  sickle cell trait and, 722
  sporadic gene mutation in, 710
  tests for, 716–717, 717t
  thalassemia and, 722
  treatment of, 719–722
    blood transfusion in, 720, 721
    exchange transfusion in, 720
    preventive, 719–720, *721*
Glucosylceramide lipidosis, 1465t, 1466t, 1470t, 1474, *1475,* 1476–1478. See also *Gaucher's disease (glucosylceramide lipidosis).*
β-Glucuronidase, deficiency of, 1466t, 1470t
  gene for, 1487
  in bilirubin metabolism, 87
Glutamate formiminotransferase, deficiency of, 412t, 413–414
Glutamic oxaloacetic transaminase, activity of, x
γ-Glutamyl-cysteine synthetase, activity of, x
Glutathione, in adult erythrocytes, x
  metabolism of, disorders of, 947–949, 947t
Glutathione cycle, 704–705, *705*
Glutathione peroxidase, activity of, x
  in cord blood, xi, xxvi
  in neonate, 29
  in phagocytosis, *905,* 907
Glutathione reductase, activity of, x
  deficiency of, 947–949, 947t
  in cord blood, xi
Glutathione synthetase, deficiency of, 947–949, 947t
Glutathione-S-transferase, activity of, x
Glyceraldehyde phosphate dehydrogenase, activity of, x
Glyceraldehyde-3-phosphate, reference values for, xi
Glyceraldehyde-3-phosphate dehydrogenase, *551,* 552t–553t
  activity of, xi
  deficiency of, 676–677
  of neonatal erythrocytes, 27
L-α-Glycerol-3-phosphate dehydrogenase, 29
Glycocalicin, in platelet function, 1514
Glycogen storage disease, immunodeficiency in, 1035t
  neutropenia in, 918
Glycolipids, erythrocyte-membrane, 546t, 549
  distribution of, 547
Glycolysis, erythrocyte, 27–29, 28t
  defects of, 665–693, *666,* 667t
    acquired, 692–693
    aldolase deficiency in, 675
    2,3-bisphosphoglycerate mutase deficiency in, 679–680
    enolase deficiency in, 680–681
    glucose phosphate isomerase deficiency in, 670–672, 671t
    glyceraldehyde-3-phosphate dehydrogenase deficiency in, 676–677
    hexokinase deficiency in, 667–670, 668t, *669*
    lactate dehydrogenase deficiency in, 689
    phosphofructokinase deficiency in, 673–675, 673t
    phosphoglycerate kinase deficiency in, 677–679, *678,* 678t, *679*

Glycolysis *(Continued)*
    pyruvate kinase deficiency in, 681–689, *682, 684, 685,* 687t
    triose phosphate isomerase deficiency in, 675–676
  in hereditary spherocytosis, 587
Glycophorin(s), 552–557, 552t–553t
  functions of, 555–556
  hybrid, 556
  in sickle erythrocytes, 770
  variants of, 556–557
Glycophorin A, 552–553, 552t–553t, *554,* 554t
  band 3 association with, 555
  P. falciparum receptors of, 556
  variants of, 556
Glycophorin B, 552t–553t, 553, *554,* 554t
  variants of, 556
Glycophorin C, 552t–553t, 553–555, *555*
  in hereditary elliptocytosis, 613
  variants of, 556–557
Glycophorin D, 552t–553t, *555*
  variants of, 556–557
Glycophorin E, 552t–553t, 553, 554t
  variants of, 556
Glycoproteins, platelet, antibodies to, 1592–1594, 1593t, *1594, 1595,* 1808–1809, 1808t
Glycoprotein Ia-IIa receptor complex, in platelet adhesion, 1513, 1513t
Glycoprotein Ib, absence of, in Bernard-Soulier syndrome, 1609
Glycoprotein Ibα, 1514
Glycoprotein Ib receptor, defect in (pseudo von Willebrand's disease), *1646,* 1654
Glycoprotein Ib-IX receptor complex, in platelet activation, 1516
  in platelet adhesion, 1513, 1513t
  structure of, 1514, *1514*
Glycoprotein IIb-IIIa receptor complex, absence of, in Glanzmann's thrombasthenia, 1609–1610, 1610t
  biosynthesis of, 1518
  fibrinogen binding to, 1518–1519, *1519*
  in platelet adhesion, 1513, 1513t
  in platelet aggregation, 1518–1519, *1518, 1519*
  monoclonal antibody inhibition of, 1524
  structure of, 1518, *1518*
Glycosylphosphatidylinositol anchor, of erythrocyte membrane, 571
Glycosylphosphatidyl-inositol–linked proteins, in paroxysmal nocturnal hemoglobinuria, 514–515, *514,* 515t
GM-CSF gene, 181t, 182
G_M1-Gangliosidosis, *1475,* 1481–1482
  laboratory diagnosis of, 1466t, 1470t
  peripheral blood smear in, *1467*
  type 1, 1464t, 1481
  type 2, 1465t, 1481
  type 3, 1481–1482
G_M2-Gangliosidosis, 1464t, 1466t, 1470t, 1482. See also *Sandhoff's disease; Tay-Sachs disease.*
Gold therapy, aplastic anemia with, 241t
  neutropenia with, 915
Gonads, disorders of, after acute lymphoblastic leukemia treatment, 1265
  after stem cell transplantation, 353
Gonadoblastoma, 1425
Gonadotropins, in severe β-thalassemia, 858
Gonadotropin-releasing hormone, in β-thalassemia–related delayed puberty, 859
Goodpasture's syndrome, hematologic manifestations of, 1853

Goodpasture's syndrome *(Continued)*
  iron deficiency in, 439
  microangiopathy, 537
  plasmapheresis in, 1835
Gout, in hereditary spherocytosis, 597
G6PD. See *Glucose-6-phosphate dehydrogenase (G6PD).*
gp91^phox, 905, 906t
  in chronic granulomatous disease, 940–941
Graft-versus-host disease, acute, after stem cell transplantation, 346–349, 347t, 349t
    prevention of, 348
    risk factors for, 348
    treatment of, 348–349
  blood transfusion–associated, 1791
    in preterm infant, 1792
  chronic, after stem cell transplantation, 349–351, 349t
    diagnosis of, 349–350, 350t
    risk factors for, 349
    treatment of, 350–351
  in allogeneic stem cell therapy, 1821
  platelet transfusion–related, 1813–1814
Granule(s), basophil, 894, 894t
  eosinophil, 893–894, 894t
  mast cell, 895
  neutrophil, 891, 891t, 892
    azurophil, 891, 891t, 892
      contents of, 904
      in Chédiak-Higashi syndrome, 934
    contents of, 904
    deficiency of, 936–938, 937t
    degranulation of, 903–904
    in Batten-Spielmeyer-Vogt disease, 1872
    in Chédiak-Higashi syndrome, 934, 1871–1872
    specific, 891t, 892
      deficiency of, 936–938, 937t
  platelet, alpha granules of, 1519–1520, 1520t, 1608–1609, 1611
    dense, 1519, 1608
Granulocyte(s), 891–895, 891t, 893t, 894t. See also *Basophil(s); Eosinophil(s); Neutrophil(s).*
  circulating pool of, 170, 172, *172*
  development of, 207–208
  fetal, 21t
  G6PD deficiency in, 722
  in systemic lupus erythematosus, 1856
  marginating pool of, 170, 172, *172*
  marrow release of, *165,* 172
  transfusion of, 1833
Granulocyte colony-stimulating factor, 175t, 176
  after chemotherapy, 211
  animal studies of, 211
  endothelial cell expression of, 191
  fibroblast expression of, 191
  gene for, 175t, 179–182, 181t
    mutations in, 208
  in acquired aplastic anemia, 249, 257
  in acute lymphoblastic leukemia, 1264
  in alloimmune neutropenia, 918
  in aplastic anemia, 214
  in bone marrow transplantation, 213
  in chronic idiopathic neutropenia, 216
  in cyclic neutropenia, 216, *912,* 913
  in dyskeratosis congenita, 276
  in human immunodeficiency virus infection, 214–215
  in Kostmann's disease, 215–216, 306, 1287, 1310
  in malignancy, 211–212
  in myelodysplasia, 213–214
  in neutropenia, 920

Hemophilia B *(Continued)*
  clinical evaluation of, 1574, *1575*
  clinical manifestations of, 1634–1636, *1635*
  demography of, 1632
  gastrointestinal bleeding in, 1636
  genetic testing for, 1639
  hematuria in, 1636
  hemorrhage in, 1634, 1636, 1637t
  inheritance of, 1634
  intracranial hemorrhage in, 1634, 1636
  laboratory evaluation of, 1581, 1638–1639
  musculoskeletal bleeding in, 1634–1636, *1635*
    complications of, 1636–1638
  oral bleeding in, 1636
  pathophysiology of, 1632
  screening tests in, *1575*
  surgery in, 1636
  treatment of, 1637t, 1642
    complications of, 1644
    factor IX concentrates in, 1642
    factor IX dose calculation in, 1642
    factor IX inhibitor antibodies and, 1644
    fresh frozen plasma in, 1642
    gene therapy in, 1644
    home therapy in, 1644
    immunoadsorbent columns in, 1836
    prothrombin complex concentrates in, 1642
    team approach to, 1644
Hemophilia C, 1663–1664
Hemorrhage. See also *Bleeding.*
  blood transfusion for, 1787
  CNS, in acute myelogenous leukemia, 1297
  fetal-to-fetal, neonatal anemia with, 36
  fetal-to-maternal, clinical features of, 35, 35t
    diagnosis of, 35–36
    neonatal anemia with, 34–36, 34t
  in acute lymphoblastic leukemia, 1264
  in extracorporeal membrane oxygenation, 1792–1793, 1793t
  in hemophilia, 1634–1636, 1637t
  in neonatal iron overload syndrome, 443
  in premature infant, 133–135, 134t
  in thrombocytosis, 1607
  intracranial, 133–135, 134t
    diagnosis of, 128
    extracorporeal membrane oxygenation and, 142
    heparin-induced, 145
    in hemophilia, 1634, 1636, 1637t
    in idiopathic thrombocytopenic purpura, 1597–1598
    in neonate, 37
    in premature infant, 133–135, 134t
    in sickle cell disease, 779
  iron deficiency with, 438–439
  neonatal, 34t
    clinical features of, 35t
    diagnosis of, 38, 38t
    internal, 36–37
    laboratory features of, 35t
    plasminogen activator inhibitor–1 deficiency and, 1568
  retinal, in acute lymphoblastic leukemia, 1256
  transplacental, in Rh hemolytic disease, 56–57, *56*, 57t
Hemorrhagic cystitis, after stem cell transplantation, 352
  chemotherapy-related, 1217–1218
Hemorrhagic disease of the newborn, 136–142. See also *Vitamin-K-deficiency bleeding.*

Hemorrhagic disease of the newborn *(Continued)*
  classical, 137, 138t
  clinical presentation of, 137, 138t
  early, 137, 138t
  historical studies of, 8–9
  laboratory diagnosis of, 137–138
  late, 137, 138t
  vitamin K prophylaxis in, 136–137
Hemorrhagic fever, 1907
Hemosiderin, 430–431
Hemosiderosis, pulmonary, hematologic manifestations of, 1852–1853
  iron deficiency in, 439
Hemostasis, 114–146, 1677–1706. See also *Coagulation; Coagulation factors; Platelet(s).*
  age-dependent features of, 1680–1681
  developmental, 1678–1681, 1678t, *1679,* 1679t, *1680,* 1680t
    coagulation system in, 118–123, 119t, 120t, *121*
    fibrinolytic system in, 120t, 123
    inhibitors of, 120t, 121
    physiology of, 122–123
    proteins of, 118, 119t, 121
    screening tests of, 118, 119t, 120t
    thrombin in, 121–122, *121*
  disorders of, 123–146, 1681–1706. See also specific disorders and coagulation factor deficiencies.
    hemorrhagic, 123–124, 1681–1687. See also specific disorders, e.g., *Disseminated intravascular coagulation.*
    thromboembolic, 142–146, 144t, 1688–1706. See also *Thrombotic disorders.*
  fibrinolytic system in, 120t, 123, 1680, 1680t
  in Osler-Weber-Rendu disease, 1845
  platelet adhesion in, 1513–1514, 1513t
  serotonin in, 1519
  thrombin in, 121–122, *121,* *1679,* 1679–1680
  vessel wall–platelet interactions in, 1680
Henoch-Schönlein purpura, 1576
Heparan sulfate, accumulation of, 1470t
  degradation of, *1483*
Heparan-*N*-sulfatase, deficiency of, 1465t, 1466t, 1470t, *1483,* 1483t, 1486
Heparin, adverse effects of, 1702–1703
  anticoagulant action of, 1543–1544, *1543*
  dose response to, 1702
  during cardiopulmonary bypass, 1685
  in apheresis, 1829
  in disseminated intravascular coagulation, 1683
  in ischemic stroke, 1698
  in newborn, 145
  in renal vein thrombosis, 1692
  in respiratory distress syndrome, 136, 136t
  in thrombotic disorders, 1523–1524, 1691, 1692, 1702–1703, 1702t
  in thrombotic thrombocytopenic purpura, 1701
  monitoring of, 1702, 1702t
  prophylactic, for catheter patency, 144, 144t
    for venous thromboembolism, 1691
  therapeutic range for, 1702
  thrombocytopenia with, 126, 1605
Heparin cofactor II, after cardiopulmonary bypass, 1685t
  fetal, 118t
  in infant, 120t, 121
  in premature infant, 120t
  reference values for, 1679t, xx
  thrombin inhibition by, 121, *122*

Hepatic nuclear factor 4, in *EPO* gene expression, 192
Hepatitis, aplastic anemia with, 244
  fibrinogen catabolism in, 1846
  hematologic manifestations of, 1739t
  pure red cell aplasia with, 287–288
Hepatitis A virus, blood transfusion–acquired, 1797
  platelet transfusion–acquired, 1812, 1812t
Hepatitis B virus, as cancer risk factor, 1077
  blood transfusion–acquired, 861, 1797
  in hepatic cancer, 1084, 1421–1422
  platelet transfusion–acquired, 1812, 1812t
Hepatitis C virus, blood transfusion–acquired, 861, 1797
  marrow toxicity of, *244*
  platelet transfusion–acquired, 1812, 1812t
Hepatitis D virus, blood transfusion–acquired, 1797
  platelet transfusion–acquired, 1812, 1812t
Hepatitis G virus, blood transfusion–acquired, 1797
Hepatoblastoma, 1421–1422
  epidemiology of, 1084–1085
  genetic disorders and, 1079t
  pathology of, 1420–1421
  polyposis coli and, 1421
  treatment of, 1422–1423
Hepatocellular carcinoma, 1421–1422
  epidemiology of, 1084–1085
  genetic disorders and, 1079t
  hepatitis B virus in, 1421–1422
  pathology of, 1421
  treatment of, 1422–1423
Hepatocyte, bilirubin uptake by, 84
  cholate injury to, 102
Hepatomegaly, in acute myelogenous leukemia, 1295
  in Rh hemolytic disease, 73–74
  in β-thalassemia, 851
Hereditary angioneurotic edema, 1044
Hereditary hemochromatosis, 442
  evolutionary advantage of, 442
  gene for, 442
  iron toxicity in, 857
Hereditary hemochromatosis trait, 442
Hereditary hemorrhagic telangiectasia (Osler-Weber-Rendu syndrome), 1614, 1615–1616
  bleeding in, 1578
  hematologic manifestations of, 1869
  hemostasis in, 1845
  iron deficiency with, 438
  pathophysiology of, 1615
  treatment of, 1615–1616
  von Willebrand's disease in, 1650
Hereditary nonpolyposis colorectal cancer, genetics of, 1129–1130
Hereditary persistence of fetal hemoglobin, 837–839
  deletion mutations in, 834t, 837–838
  globin gene mutation in, 833, 833t, 834t, 835t, 837–838
  β-globin synthesis in, 839
  haplotype analysis in, 838–839
  hemoglobin A₂ in, 839
  nondeletion mutations in, 794, 835t, 838–839
  pancellular, Hb S with, 793
  Swiss type, 838, 842–843
Hermansky-Pudlak syndrome, 1608t, 1611, 1872
Herpes simplex virus, infection with, 1740–1741, 1752
  after stem cell transplantation, 344
  hematologic manifestations of, 1739t

ISBN 0-7216-5952-7

90038